> Canadian drugs identified with a maple-leaf icon

> Pediatric, geriatric, and other special dosages included throughout

> Common and life-threatening adverse effects grouped by body system

calcium carbonate (Rx) (PO-OTC, Rx)

Alka-Mints, Amitone, Apo-Cal ✦, BioCal, Calcarb, Calci-Chew, Calciday, Calci-Mix, Calcite ✦, Caltrate, Chooz, Maalox Antacid, Os-Cal, Rolaids Extra Strength Soft-chew, Tums, Tums E-X
Func. class.: Antacid, calcium supplement
Chem. class.: Calcium product

calcium acetate (OTC)

(kal'see-um ass'e-tate)
Eliphos, PhosLo, Phoslyra
Pregnancy category C

Do not confuse: Os-Cal/Asacol

ACTION: Neutralizes gastric acidity

Therapeutic outcome: Neutralized gastric acidity; calcium at normal levels

USES: Antacid, calcium supplement; not suitable for chronic therapy, hyperphosphatemia, hypertension in pregnancy, osteoporosis, prevention/treatment of hypocalcemia, hypoparathyroidism

CONTRAINDICATIONS
Hypersensitivity, hypercalcemia

Precautions: Pregnancy **C**, breastfeeding, geriatric, fluid restriction, decreased GI motility, GI obstruction, dehydration, renal disease, hyperparathyroidism, bone tumors

DOSAGE AND ROUTES
Nutritional supplement including osteoporosis prophylaxis
Adult ≥51 yr: PO 1000-1500 mg/day elemental calcium (2500-3750 calcium carbonate)
Adult 19-50 yr: PO 1000 mg/day elemental calcium (2500 mg calcium carbonate)

Chronic hypocalcemia
Adult: PO 2-4 g/day elemental calcium (5-10 g calcium carbonate) in 3-4 divided doses
Child: PO 45-65 mg/kg/day elemental calcium (112.5-162.5 mg/kg calcium carbonate) in 4 divided doses
Neonate: PO 50-150 mg/kg/day elemental calcium (125-375 mg/kg/day in 4-6 divided doses, max 1 g/day)

Supplementation
Adolescent and child 9-18 yr: PO 1300 mg elemental calcium (3250 mg calcium carbonate)
Child 4-8 yr: PO 800 mg/day elemental calcium (2000 mg calcium carbonate)

✦ Canada only

---

calcium acetate **149**

Child 1-3 yr: PO 500 mg/day elemental calcium (1250 mg calcium carbonate)
Infant 6-12 mo: PO 270 mg/day elemental calcium based on total intake
Neonate and infant <6 mo: PO 210 mg/day elemental calcium based on total intake

Hyperphosphatemia
Adult: PO Individualized on response

Heartburn, dyspepsia, hyperacidity (OTC)
Adult: PO 1-2 tabs q2hr, max 9 tabs/24 hr (Alka-mints); chew 2-4 tab q1hr prn, max 16 tabs (Tums regular strength); chew 2-4 tab q1hr prn, max 10 tabs (Tums E-X); chew 2-3 tabs q1hr prn, max 10 tabs/24 hr (Tums Ultra); chew 2 tabs q2-3hr, max 19 tabs/24 hr (Titralac Extra Strength)

Available forms: Calcium carbonate: chewable tabs 350, 420, 450, 500, 750, 1000, 1250 mg; **tabs** 500, 600, 650, 667, 1000, 1250, 1500 mg; **gum** 300, 450 500 mg; **susp** 1250 mg/5 ml; **caps** 1250 mg; **powder** 6.5 g/packet; **calcium acetate: tabs** 667 mg (169 mg Ca), **caps** 500 mg (125 mg Ca); **gelcaps:** 667 mg (169 mg elemental Ca)

Implementation
PO route
• Administer as antacid 1 hr after meals and at bedtime
• Administer as supplement 1½ hr after meals and at bedtime
• Administer only with regular tablets or capsules; do not give with enteric-coated tablets
• Administer laxatives or stool softeners if constipation occurs

ADVERSE EFFECTS
GI: *Constipation*, anorexia, nausea, vomiting, flatulence, diarrhea, rebound hyperacidity, eructation
GU: Calculi, hypercalciuria

Pharmacokinetics

Absorption	⅓ absorbed by small intestines, must have adequate vit D for absorption
Distribution	Unknown
Metabolism	Unknown
Excretion	Feces, urine, crosses placenta
Half-life	Unknown

Pharmacodynamics

Peak	Unknown

evolve   ELSEVIER

YOU'VE JUST PURCHASED
MORE THAN
A TEXTBOOK!

Evolve Student Resources for *Skidmore-Roth:*
Mosby's Drug Guide for Nursing Students,
Twelfth Edition, **include the following:**

Canadian Resources

- High Alert Canadian Medications
- Canadian Controlled Substance Chart
- Vaccines Approved for Use in Canada
- Content Changes
- Drug Monographs—Additional Monographs
- Drug Monographs—Recently Approved

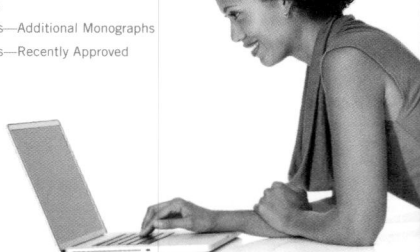

Activate the complete learning experience that comes with each
NEW textbook purchase by registering with your scratch-off access code at

http://evolve.elsevier.com/
nursingdrugupdates/Skidmore/NDG

REGISTER TODAY!

SKIDMORE

MOSBY'S
DRUG GUIDE
for NURSING
STUDENTS

TWE

ELSEVIER

9 8 7 6 5

Printed in the United States of America

...ght is the print number: 9 8 7 6 5

Project Manager: Sonya Seigafuse

...ment Manager: Billie Sharp

...ment Development: Lisa A. P. Bushey

...design Direction: Paula Catalano

Design Specialist: Jeff Patterson

...Number: 978-0-323-44807-9

ELSEVIER

3251 Riverport Lane
St. Louis, Missouri 63043

MOSBY'S DRUG GUIDE FOR NURSING STUDENTS,
TWELFTH EDITION

ISBN: 978-0-323-44807-9
ISSN: 2213-4409

Notices

International Standard Book N...

Executive Content Strat...
Content Developm...
Associate C...
Publi...

Consultants

Amanda Buckallew, PharmD
Pharmacist
Inpatient Pharmacy
Missouri Baptist Medical Center
St. Louis, Missouri

David S. Chun, PharmD, BCPS
Pharmacist in Charge
Omnicare of St. Louis
Florissant, Missouri

Joshua J. Neumiller, PharmD, CDE, CGP, FASCP
Associate Professor
Washington State University
Spokane, Washington

Travis E. Sonnett, PharmD, FASCP
Clinical Pharmacy Specialist/Inpatient Pharmacy
  Supervisor
Mann-Grandstaff VA Medical Center
Spokane, Washington
Adjunct Clinical Professor
Pharmacotherapy
Washington State University
Spokane, Washington

Patricia A. Talbert, AAS Nursing, AAS Horticulture, AA
Employee Health Nurse
Wellness
Baxter Regional Medical Center
Mountain Home, Arkansas
Aromatherapist
Gainesville, Missouri

Shamim Tejani, PharmD
Director of Quality and Medication Safety
Adelante Healthcare
Phoenix, Arizona

Preface

Mosby's Drug Guide for Nursing Students, twelfth edition, is the most in-depth handbook available for nursing students! Since its first publication in 1996, more than 100 U.S. and Canadian pharmacists and consultants have reviewed the book's content closely. Today, *Mosby's Drug Guide for Nursing Students* is more up-to-date than ever—with features that make it easy to find critical information fast!

NEW FEATURES
• Over 10 recent FDA-approved drugs for 2016 are located throughout the book and in Appendix A.

NEW FACTS
This edition features thousands of new drug facts, including:
• New drugs and new dosage information
• Newly researched adverse effects
• New Black Box Warnings
• The latest precautions, interactions, and contraindications
• IV therapy updates
• Revised nursing considerations
• Updated patient/family education guidelines
• Updates on key new drug research

ORGANIZATION
This handbook is organized into four main sections:
• Individual drug monographs (in alphabetical order by generic name)
• Drug Categories
• Appendixes
• Illustrated mechanisms and sites of action
The guiding principle behind this book is to provide fast, easy access to drug information and nursing considerations. Every detail—from the cover, binding, and paper to the typeface, four-color design, and appendixes—has been carefully chosen with the user in mind. Here's what you'll find in each section of the handbook:

Individual Drug Monographs
This book includes monographs for more than 4000 generic and trade medications—those most commonly administered by students. Common trade names are given for all drugs regularly used in the United States and Canada, with drugs available only in Canada identified by a maple leaf icon (🍁). Select monographs, important to learn and know for the NCLEX examination, have been identified by a ⭐. You'll see drug-specific information within monographs identified with a >>.

Each monograph provides the following information, whenever possible, for safe, effective administration of each drug:

High-alert status: Identifies drugs with the most potential to cause harm to patients if administered incorrectly.

"Tall Man" lettering: Uses the capitalization of distinguishing letters to avoid medication errors and is required by the FDA for drug manufacturers.

Pronunciation: Helps the nurse master complex generic names.

Rx, OTC: Identifies prescription or over-the-counter drugs.

Functional and chemical classifications: Helps the nurse recognize similarities and differences among drugs in the same functional but different chemical classes.

Pregnancy category: Notes FDA pregnancy categories A, B, C, D, and X at the beginning of each monograph, as well as under Precautions or Contraindications, depending on FDA category. Appendix D provides a detailed explanation of each category.

Do not confuse: Presents drug names that might easily be confused within each appropriate monograph.

Action: Describes pharmacologic properties concisely.

Therapeutic outcome: Details all possible results of medication use.

Uses: Lists the conditions the drug is used to treat.

Unlabeled uses: Describes drug uses that may be encountered in practice but are not yet FDA approved.

Dosages and routes: Lists all available and approved dosages and routes for adult, pediatric, and geriatric patients.

Available forms: Includes tablets, capsules, extended release, injectables (IV, IM,

SUBCUT), solutions, creams, ointments, lotions, gels, shampoos, elixirs, suspensions, suppositories, sprays, aerosols, and lozenges.

Adverse effects: Groups these reactions by alphabetical body system, with common side effects *italicized* and life-threatening reactions in **bold, red type** for emphasis.

Contraindications: Lists conditions under which the drug absolutely should not be given, including FDA pregnancy safety categories D and X.

Precautions: Lists conditions that require special consideration when the drug is prescribed, including FDA pregnancy safety categories A, B, and C.

Black Box Warnings: Identifies FDA warnings that highlight serious and life-threatening adverse effects.

Pharmacokinetics/pharmacodynamics: Features a quick-reference chart of concise facts of pharmacokinetics (absorption, distribution, metabolism, excretion, half-life) and pharmacodynamics (onset, peak, duration).

Interactions: Lists confirmed drug, food, herb, and lab test interactions.

Nursing considerations: Identifies key nursing considerations for each step of the nursing process: Assessment, Implementation, Patient/Family Education, and Evaluation, including positive therapeutic outcomes. Instructions for giving drugs by various routes (e.g., **IV**, PO, IM, SUBCUT, topically, rectally) appear under Implementation, with route subheadings in bold.

Compatibilities: Lists syringe, Y-site, and additive compatibilities and incompatibilities. If no compatibilities are listed for a drug, the necessary compatibility testing has not been done and that compatibility information is unknown. To ensure safety, assume that the drug may not be mixed with other drugs unless specifically stated.

Nursing Alert icon ⚠: Highlights situations in which the patient could potentially be at risk.

Treatment of overdose: Lists drugs and treatments for overdoses where appropriate.

Drug Categories

The Drug Categories section, following the individual drug monographs, provides general information about the various functional classes to promote learning about the similarities and differences among drugs in the same functional class. It summarizes action, uses, adverse effects, contraindications, precautions, pharmacokinetics, interactions, and nursing considerations for each functional class.

Appendixes

Selected new drugs: Includes comprehensive information on 11 key drugs approved by the FDA during the last 12 months.

Ophthalmic, nasal, topical, and otic products: Provides essential information for 140 ophthalmic, nasal, topical, and otic products commonly used today, grouped by chemical drug class.

Vaccines and toxoids: Features an easy-to-use table with generic and trade names, uses, dosages and routes, and contraindications for 39 key vaccines and toxoids.

Abbreviations and pregnancy categories: Lists abbreviations alphabetically with their meanings and explains the five FDA pregnancy categories.

Immunization schedule: Recommended childhood and adolescent immunization schedules.

Standard Precautions: Used in the care of all patients regardless of their diagnosis or disease.

Illustrated mechanisms and sites of action: These 13 detailed, full-color illustrations are added to help enhance the understanding of the mechanism or site of action for the following drugs and drug classes:

- Anticholinergic bronchodilators
- Antidepressants
- Antidiabetic agents
- Antifungal agents
- Antiinfective agents
- Antiretroviral agents
- Benzodiazepines
- Diuretics
- Laxatives
- Narcotic agonist-antagonist analgesics
- Narcotic analgesics
- Phenytoin
- Sympatholytics

Photo atlas of drug administration: This practical resource for students and practitioners lists standard precautions and provides more than 20 full-color illustrations depicting the physical landmarks and administration techniques used for IV, IM, SUBCUT, and ID drug delivery.

The following sources were consulted in the preparation of this edition:

Blumenthal M: *The Complete German Commission E Monographs: Therapeutic Guide to Herbal Medicines,* Austin, 1998, American Botanical Council.

Brunton L, Lazo J, Parker K: *Goodman and Gilman's The Pharmacological Basis of Therapeutics,* ed 11, New York, 2006, McGraw-Hill.

Clinical Pharmacology [database online], Tampa, 2014, Gold Standard, Inc. http://www.clinicalpharmacology.com. Updated March 2014.

Gahart BL, Nazareno AR: *Intravenous Medications,* ed 29, St. Louis, 2013, Mosby.

McKenry LM, Tessier E, Hogan MA: *Mosby's Pharmacology in Nursing,* ed 22, St. Louis, 2006, Mosby.

Acknowledgments

I am indebted to the nursing and pharmacology consultants who reviewed the manuscript and pages and thank them for their criticism and encouragement. I would also like to thank Billie Sharp and Sarah Vora, my editors, whose active encouragement and enthusiasm have made this book better than it might otherwise have been. I am likewise grateful to Lisa Bushey at Elsevier, and Suzanne Kastner and Evelyn Dayringer at Graphic World Inc., for the coordination of the production process and assistance with the development of the new edition, and to Craig Roth for his editorial assistance.

Linda Skidmore-Roth

Contents

INDIVIDUAL DRUG MONOGRAPHS, 1

DRUG CATEGORIES, 1080

APPENDIXES

INDEX, 1173

EVOLVE WEBSITE CONTENTS

A HIGH ALERT

abacavir (Rx)

(a-ba-ka′veer)

Ziagen

Func. class.: Antiretroviral

Chem. class.: Nucleoside reverse transcriptase inhibitor (NRTI)

Pregnancy category C

ACTION: Inhibitory action against HIV; inhibits replication of HIV by incorporating into cellular DNA by viral reverse transcriptase, thereby terminating the cellular DNA chain

Therapeutic outcome: Decreased symptoms of HIV

USES: In combination with other antiretroviral agents for HIV-1 infection

CONTRAINDICATIONS

BLACK BOX WARNING: Hypersensitivity, moderate to severe hepatic disease, lactic acidosis

Precautions: Pregnancy **C**, breastfeeding, child <3 mo, granulocyte count <1000/mm³ or Hgb <9.5 g/dl, severe renal disease, impaired hepatic function, HLA B5701 (Black, Caucasian, Asian patients), abrupt discontinuation; Guillain-Barré syndrome, immune reconstitution syndrome, MI, obesity, polymyositis

DOSAGE AND ROUTES

Adult/adolescent ≥16 hr: PO 300 mg bid or 600 mg daily with other antiretrovirals

Adolescent <16 yr/child ≥3 mo: PO 8 mg/kg bid or 16mg/kg q day, max 300 mg bid with other antiretrovirals

Hepatic dose

Adult: (Child-Pugh 5-6) PO oral/sol 200 mg bid; moderate to severe hepatic disease, do not use

Available forms: Tabs 300 mg; oral sol 20 mg/ml

Implementation

PO route

• May give without regard to food q12hr around the clock

• Give in combination with other antiretrovirals with or without food; do not use triple therapy as a beginning treatment, resistance may occur

• Store in cool environment; protect from light; do not freeze

ADVERSE EFFECTS

CNS: *Fever, headache, malaise, insomnia,* paresthesia

GI: *Nausea, vomiting, diarrhea, anorexia, cramps, abdominal pain, increased AST, ALT,* hepatotoxicity, hepatomegaly with steatosis

HEMA: Granulocytopenia, anemia, lymphopenia

INTEG: Rash, urticaria, hypersensitivity reactions

META: Lactic acidosis

MISC: Increased CPK, fatal hypersensitivity reactions, fat redistribution, immune reconstitution, decreased bone density

RESP: Dyspnea

Pharmacokinetics

Absorption	Rapid/extensive (PO)
Distribution	50% protein binding, extravascular space, then erythrocytes
Metabolism	To inactive metabolite
Excretion	Kidneys, feces
Half-life	1½-2 hr

Pharmacodynamics

Unknown

INTERACTIONS

Individual drugs

Do not coadminister with abacavir-containing products, ribavarin, interferon

Alcohol: increased abacavir levels; do not use with alcohol

Ribavirin: possible lactic acidosis

Methadone: decreased levels of methadone

Tipranavir: decreased abacavir levels

Drug/lab test

Increased: glucose, triglycerides, LFTs

NURSING CONSIDERATIONS

Assessment

• Assess for symptoms of HIV and possible infection, increased temp

BLACK BOX WARNING: **Assess for lactic acidosis** (elevated lactate levels, increased liver function tests) and severe hepatomegaly with steatosis; discontinue treatment and do not restart, women are at greater risk for lactic acidosis

BLACK BOX WARNING: **Assess for fatal hypersensitivity reactions:** fever, rash, nausea, vomiting, fatigue, cough, dyspnea, diarrhea, abdominal discomfort; treatment should be discontinued and not restarted, register at the Abacavir Hypersensitivity Registry (800-270-0425)

Adverse effects: *italics* = common; **bold** = life-threatening

BLACK BOX WARNING: ⚠ Assess for pancreatitis: abdominal pain, nausea, vomiting, elevated liver enzymes; product should be discontinued because condition can be fatal

• Monitor CBC, differential, platelet count qmo; withhold product if WBC is <4000/mm³ or platelet count is <75,000/mm³; notify prescriber of results; monitor viral load and CD4 counts during treatment, perform hepatitis B virus (HBr) screening to confirm correct treatment
• Monitor renal function studies; BUN, serum uric acid, urine CCr before, during therapy; these may be elevated throughout treatment
• Monitor temp q4hr; may indicate beginning of infection

BLACK BOX WARNING: Monitor liver function tests before, during therapy (bilirubin, AST, ALT, amylase, alkaline phosphatase, creatine phosphokinase, creatinine prn or qmo)

⚠ **Immune reconstitution syndrome:** may occur anytime during treatment; response to CMV, mycobacterium avium infection

Patient/family education
• Advise patient to report signs of infection: increased temp, sore throat, flulike symptoms; to avoid crowds and those with known infections, to carry emergency ID with condition, products taken, do not take other products that contain abacavir
• Instruct patient to report signs of anemia: fatigue, headache, faintness, shortness of breath, irritability
• Advise patient to report bleeding; avoid use of razors or commercial mouthwash
• Inform patient that product is not a cure but will control symptoms
• Inform patient that major toxicities may necessitate discontinuing product
• **Consider the use of contraception during treatment,** that body fat redistribution may occur, not to share product
• Caution patient to avoid OTC products or other medications without approval of prescriber
• Caution patient not to have any sexual contact without use of a condom; needles should not be shared; blood from infected individual should not come in contact with another's mucous membranes
• Give Medication Guide and Warning Card; discuss points on guide
• Advise patient to notify prescriber if skin rash, fever, cough, shortness of breath, GI symptoms occur; advise all health care providers that allergic reactions have occurred with this product
• To use exactly as prescribed

Evaluation
Positive therapeutic outcome
• Increased CD4 count
• Decreased viral load

abatacept (Rx)
(ab-a-ta′sept)
Orencia
Func. class.: Antirheumatic agent (disease modifying)
Chem class.: immunomodulator
Pregnancy category C

ACTION: A selective costimulation modulator, inhibits production of T lymphocytes, inhibits tumor necrosis factor (TNF-α), interferon-γ, interleukin-2, which are involved in immune and inflammatory reactions

Therapeutic outcome: Decreased pain, inflammation in joints

USES: Polyarticular juvenile rheumatoid arthritis; acute chronic rheumatoid arthritis that has not responded to other disease-modifying agents; may use in combination with DMARDs; do not use with TNF antagonists (adalimumab, etanercept, infliximab) or anakinra

CONTRAINDICATIONS
Hypersensitivity

Precautions: Pregnancy **C,** breastfeeding, children, geriatric, recurrent infections, COPD, immunosuppression, neoplastic disease, respiratory infection, TB, viral hepatitis

DOSAGE AND ROUTES
Rheumatoid arthritis
Adult: SUBCUT 125 mg within a day after single IV loading dose, then 125 mg weekly, weekly subcut may be initiated without IV loading dose for those unable to receive an infusion; give at 2, 4 wk after first infusion, then q4wk
Adult >100 kg (220 lb): IV INF 1 g over 30 min; give at 2, 4 wk after first infusion, then q4wk
Adult 60-100 kg (132-220 lb): IV INF 750 mg over 30 min; give at 2, 4 wk after first infusion, then q4wk
Adult <60 kg (132 lb): IV INF 500 mg over 30 min; give at 2, 4 wk after first infusion, then q4wk

Juvenile rheumatoid arthritis (JRA)/ juvenile idiopathic arthritis (JIA)
Child/adolescent ≥6 yr >100 kg: IV 1000 mg over 30 min q2wk × 2 doses, then 1 g over 30 min q4wk starting at wk 8
Child/adolescent >6 yr >75 kg: IV INF 750 mg over 30 min q2wk × 2 doses, then 750 mg over 30 min q4wk starting at wk 8

Child/adolescent ≥6 yr <75 kg: IV INF 10 mg/kg over 30 min q2wk × 2 doses, then 10 mg/kg q4wk starting at wk 8

Available forms: Lyophilized powder, single-use vials 250 mg, sol for subcut injection 125 mg/ml

Implementation
• Store in refrigerator; do not use expired vials, protect from light, do not freeze

Intermittent IV infusion route
• To **reconstitute,** use 10 ml of sterile water for injection; insert syringe needle into vial and direct stream of sterile water for inj on the wall of vial; rotate vial until mixed; vent with needle to rid foam after reconstitution 25 mg/ml; **further dilute** in 100 ml from a 100 ml NS infusion bag/bottle; withdraw the needed volume (2 vials remove 20 ml; 3 vials remove 30 ml, 4 vials remove 40 ml); slowly add the reconstituted sol from each vial into the infusion bag/bottle using the same disposable syringe supplied; mix gently, discard unused portions of vials; do not use if particulate is present or if discolored; **give** over 30 min; use non–protein binding filter (0.2-1.2 mcg)
• Do not admix with other sol or medications
• Store in refrigerator; do not use expired vials; protect from light

Subcut route
• Use prefilled syringe for subcut only, do not use for IV; allow syringe to warm to room temperature (30-60 min) do not speed up warming process; the amount of liquid should be between the two lines on the barrel, do not use the syringe if there is more or less liquid; use front of thigh, outer area of the upper arm, or abdomen except 2-inch area around the navel, do not inject into tender, bruised area
• Gently pinch skin and hold firmly, insert needle at 45-degree angle, inject full amount in 125 mg syringe, rotate injection sites

ADVERSE EFFECTS
CNS: Headache, asthenia, dizziness
CV: *Hypertension, hypotension*
GI: Abdominal pain, dyspepsia, nausea
INTEG: Rash, *inj site reaction,* flushing, urticaria, pruritus
RESP: *Pharyngitis, cough, URI,* non-URI, *rhinitis,* wheezing
SYST: Anaphylaxis, malignancies, angioedema, serious infections, antibody development

Pharmacokinetics

Absorption	Unknown
Distribution	Unknown; steady state 60 days
Metabolism	Increased clearance in obesity (subcut); clearance increases with increased body weight
Excretion	Unknown
Half-life	Terminal IV 13 days, subcut 14.3 days

Pharmacodynamics

Unknown

INTERACTIONS
Individual drugs
Anakinra: do not use
Atropine, scopolamine, halothane: avoid concurrent use

Drug classifications
Corticosteroids, immunosuppressives: avoid concurrent use, nitrous oxide
TNF antagonists (adalimumab, etanercept, inFLIXimab): do not use
Vaccines: do not give concurrently; immunizations should be brought up to date before treatment

NURSING CONSIDERATIONS
Assessment
• **RA:** Assess for pain, stiffness, ROM, swelling of joints during treatment
• Assess for latent/active TB before beginning treatment
• Assess for inj site pain, swelling
• Monitor patient's overall health on each visit; product should not be given with active infections; parenteral product contains maltose; glucose monitoring must be done with glucose-specific testing
• **Infection:** sinusitis, urinary tract infection, influenza, bronchitis, serious infections have occurred

Patient/family education
• Teach patient that product must be continued for prescribed time to be effective
• Advise patient to use caution when driving; dizziness may occur
• Advise patient not to have vaccinations while taking this product or use alcohol, TNF antagonists, other immunosuppressants
• Discuss with patient information included in packaging
• How to inject and rotate injection sites
• To report signs of infection

Evaluation
Positive therapeutic outcome
• Decreased inflammation, pain in joints; decreased erythrocyte sedimentation rate (ESR)

⚠ HIGH ALERT

abiraterone
Zytiga
(a-bir-a'ter-one)
Func Class.: Antineoplastic
Chem Class.: Androgen inhibitor
Pregnancy category X

ACTION: Converted to abiraterone, which inhibits CYP17, the enzyme required for androgen biosynthesis; androgen-sensitive prostate cancer responds to treatment that decreases androgens

Therapeutic outcome: Decreases spread of malignancy

USES: Metastatic castration-resistant prostate cancer in combination with prednisone in patients who have received prior chemotherapy containing docetaxel

CONTRAINDICATIONS
Pregnancy (X), women, children

Precautions
Adrenal insufficiency, cardiac disease, MI, heart failure, hepatic disease, hypertension, hypokalemia, infection, surgery, ventricular dysrhythmia

DOSAGE AND ROUTES
Adult Males: PO 1000 mg q day with predniSONE 5 mg bid

Hepatic dose
Adult Males: (Child-Pugh B, 7-9) PO 250 mg qday with predniSONE, permanently discontinue if AST/ALT >5 times of the upper normal limit (ULN) or total bilirubin >3 times (ULN); (Child-Pugh C, >10) do not use

Available forms: Tab 250 mg

Implementation
PO route
• Give whole, on empty stomach two hrs before or 1 hr after meals with full glass of water
⚠ Women who are pregnant or may become pregnant should not touch tabs without gloves
• Storage of tabs at room temperature

ADVERSE EFFECTS
CV: Angina, **dysrhythmia exacerbation, atrial flutter/fibrillation/tachycardia, AV block,** chest pain, edema, **heart failure, MI,** hypertension, **QT prolongation, sinus tachycardia, supraventricular tachycardia, ventricular tachycardia**
ENDO: Hot flashes
GI: Diarrhea, dyspepsia, **hepatotoxicity**
GU: Increased urinary frequency, nocturia, urinary tract infection
META: Adrenocortical insufficiency, hyperbilirubinemia, hypertriglyceridemia, hypokalemia, hypophosphatemia
MS: Arthralgia, myalgia
RESP: Cough, upper respiratory infection
SYST: Infection

Pharmacokinetics
Absorption	Food increases effect; give on empty stomach; increased effect in hepatic disease
Distribution	99% protein binding
Metabolism	Converted to abiraterone (active metabolite)
Excretion	88% (feces), 5% (urine)
Half-life	Mean terminal half-life 12 hr

Pharmacodynamics
Onset	Unknown
Peak	Unknown
Duration	Unknown

INTERACTIONS
Drug classifications
CYP3A4 inhibitors (Decrease: abiraterone effect-clarithromycin, atazanavir, nefazodone, saquinavir, telithromycin, ritonavir, indinavir, nelfinavir, voriconazole, ketoconazole, itraconazole); CYP3A4 inducers (carBAMazepine, phenytoin, rifampin, rifabutin, rifapentine, PHENobarbital)
CYP2D6 substrates (dextromethorphan, thioridazine): increased action, testosterone of these products; dose of these products should be reduced

Drug/Lab
Increase: ALT, AST, bilirubin, triglycerides
Decrease: Potassium, phosphate

NURSING CONSIDERATIONS
Assessment
• Monitor prostate-specific antigen (PSA), serum potassium, serum bilirubin
• Monitor liver function tests (AST/ALT) baseline and every 2 wk for 3 mo and monthly thereafter in those with no known hepatic disease; interrupt treatment in patients without known hepatic disease at baseline who develop ALT/AST >5 times ULN or total bilirubin >3 times ULN; in baseline moderate hepatic disease, measure ALT, AST, and bilirubin before the start of treatment, every week

---

for the first month, every 2 weeks for the following 2 months, and monthly thereafter; if elevations in ALT and/or AST >5 times ULN or total bilirubin >3 times ULN occur in patients with baseline moderate hepatic impairment, discontinue and do NOT restart. Measure serum total bilirubin, AST, and ALT if hepatotoxicity is suspected. Elevations of AST, ALT, bilirubin from baseline should prompt more frequent monitoring.

• Monitor musculoskeletal pain, joint swelling, discomfort: Arthritis, arthralgia, joint swelling, and joint stiffness, some severe. Muscle discomfort that included muscle spasms, musculoskeletal pain, myalgia, musculoskeletal discomfort, and musculoskeletal stiffness may be relieved with analgesics.

• Assess for signs and symptoms of adrenocorticoid insufficiency; monthly for hypertension, hypokalemia, and fluid retention

⚠ Monitor ECG for QT prolongation, ejection fraction in those with cardiac disease, small increases in the QTc interval such as <10 ms have occurred; monitor for arrhythmia exacerbation such as sinus tachycardia, atrial fibrillation, supraventricular tachycardia (SVT), atrial tachycardia, ventricular tachycardia, atrial flutter, bradycardia, AV block complete, conduction disorder, and bradyarrhythmia

Patient/family education
⚠ Teach patient that women must not come in contact with tabs, wear gloves if product needs to be handled, pregnancy (X)
• Instruct patient to report chest pain, swelling of joints, burning/pain when urinating

acarbose (Rx)
(a-kar'bose)
Glucobay ✦, Prandase, Precose
Func. class.: Oral antidiabetic
Chem. class.: α-Glucosidase inhibitor
Pregnancy category B

Do not confuse: Precose/PreCare

ACTION: Delays the digestion/absorption of ingested carbohydrates by inhibiting α-glucosidase, results in a smaller rise in blood glucose after meals; does not increase insulin production

Therapeutic outcome: Decreased blood glucose levels in diabetes mellitus

USES: Type 2 diabetes mellitus, alone or in combination with a sulfonylurea, metformin, insulin

CONTRAINDICATIONS
Hypersensitivity, breastfeeding, diabetic ketoacidosis, cirrhosis, inflammatory bowel disease,

ileus, colonic ulceration, partial intestinal obstruction, chronic intestinal disease, serum creatinine >2 mg/dl

Precautions: Pregnancy **B**, children, renal/hepatic disease

DOSAGE AND ROUTES
Initial dose
Adult >60 kg (>132 lb): PO 25 mg tid with first bite of meal

Maintenance dose
Adult: PO May be increased to 50-100 mg tid; dosage adjustment at 4-8 wk intervals, individualized
Adult <60 kg (<132 lb): PO Max 50 mg tid

Available forms: Tabs 25, 50, 100 mg

Implementation
• Give tid with first bite of each meal
• Provide storage in tight container in cool environment

ADVERSE EFFECTS
GI: *Abdominal pain, diarrhea, flatulence*

Pharmacokinetics
Absorption	Poor systemic
Distribution	Unknown
Metabolism	GI tract
Excretion	Kidneys as intact drug
Half-life	Elimination 2 hr

Pharmacodynamics
Onset	Unknown
Peak	1 hr
Duration	2-4 hr

INTERACTIONS
Individual drugs
Acetaminophen: increased toxicity combined with alcohol
Digoxin: decreased acarbose effect
Phenytoin: increased hypoglycemia
Baclofen, cycloSPORINE, tacrolimus, isoniazid: increased hyperglycemia

Drug classifications
Androgens, quinolones: increased or decreased glycemic control
Corticosteroids, diuretics, estrogens, oral contraceptives, phenothiazines, progestins, sympathomimetics: digestive enzymes, intestinal absorbents, thiazide diuretics, loop diuretics, corticosteroids, protease inhibitors, atypical antipsychotics, carbonic anhydrase inhibitors: increased hyperglycemia, decreased effect of acarbose

MAOIs, salicylates, fibric acid derivatives, bile acid sequestrants, ACE inhibitors, angiotensin II receptor antagonists, β-blockers, sulfonylureas, insulins: increased hypoglycemia

Drug/herb
Chromium, garlic, horse chestnut: increased hypoglycemia

Drug/lab test
Increased: ALT, AST, bilirubin
Decreased: calcium, vit B_6, Hgb , Hct
Interference: Urine glucose tests, 1,5-AG assay

NURSING CONSIDERATIONS
Assessment
• Assess for hypoglycemia (weakness, hunger, dizziness, tremors, anxiety, tachycardia, sweating), hyperglycemia; even though this product does not cause hypoglycemia, if on a sulfonylurea or insulin, hypoglycemia may be additive; if hypoglycemia occurs, treat with glucose or if severe, **IV** dextrose or IM glucagon
• Monitor 1 hr postprandial glucose for establishing effectiveness, then glycosylated Hgb q3mo, 1 hr PP throughout treatment
• Monitor AST, ALT q3mo × 1 yr, and periodically thereafter, if elevated dose, may need to be reduced or discontinued, usually increased with doses ≥ 300 mg/day; dose-related elevations may occur, and patients are usually asymptomatic; if symptomatic, dosage reduction or withdrawal is needed; obtain glycosylated Hgb periodically
• Assess for stress, surgery, or other trauma that may require change in dose

Patient/family education
• Teach patient the symptoms of hypoglycemia, hyperglycemia, and what to do about each
• Instruct that medication must be taken as prescribed; must be taken with food; explain consequences of discontinuing the medication abruptly; that insulin may need to be used during stress such as trauma, surgery, fever
• Tell patient to avoid OTC medications, herbal products unless approved by prescriber
• Teach patient that diabetes is a lifelong illness; product will not cure condition; that diet and exercise regimen must be followed
• Instruct patient to carry/wear emergency ID as diabetic
• Teach patient to avoid breastfeeding if using acarbose with other antidiabetics
• Inform that GI side effects may occur

Evaluation
Positive therapeutic outcome
• Improved signs, symptoms of diabetes mellitus (decreased polyuria, polydipsia, polyphagia; clear sensorium, absence of dizziness, stable gait)

acetaminophen (OTC) (Paracetamol)
(a-seat-a-mee′noe-fen)
222AF ✹, Abenol ✹, ACET ✹, Aceta, Acetab ✹, Aminofen, Apacet, APAP, Apra, Atasol ✹, Children's Feverall, Equaline Children's Pain Relief, Equaline Infant's Pain Relief, Exdol ✹, Fortolin ✹, Genapap, Good Sense Acetaminophen, Good Sense Children's Pain Relief, Infantaire, Leader Children's Pain Reliever, Mapap, Maranox, Meda, Neopap, Novo-Gesic ✹, Ofirmev, Oraphen-PD, Pediaphen ✹, Pediatrix ✹, Q-Pap, Q-Pap Children's, Rapid Action Relief ✹, Redutemp, Ridenol, Robigesic ✹, Rounox ✹, Silapap, Taminol ✹, Tapanol, Tempra ✹, T-Painol, Tylenol, Uni-Ace, Vick's Custom Care Body Aches ✹, Walgreen's Acetaminophen, Walgreen's Non-Aspirin, XS Pain Reliever
Func. class.: Nonopioid analgesic
Chem. class.: Nonsalicylate, paraaminophenol derivative
Pregnancy category B

ACTION: May block pain impulses peripherally that occur in response to inhibition of prostaglandin synthesis; does not possess antiinflammatory properties; antipyretic action results from inhibition of prostaglandins in the CNS (hypothalamic heat-regulating center)

Therapeutic outcome: Decreased pain, fever

USES: Mild to moderate pain or fever; arthralgia, dental pain, dysmenorrhea, headache, myalgia, osteoarthritis

CONTRAINDICATIONS
Hypersensitivity to this product or phenacetin

Precautions: Pregnancy **B; C (IV)** breastfeeding, geriatric, anemia, renal/hepatic disease, chronic alcoholism

DOSAGE AND ROUTES
Adult and child >12 yr: PO/RECT 325-650 mg q4-6hr prn, max 4 g/day; weight ≥50 kg IV 1000 mg q6hr or 650 mg q4hr prn, max single dose 1000 mg, minimum dosing interval 4 hr; weight <50 kg IV 15 mg/kg/dose q6hr or 12.5 mg/kg/dose q4hr, max single dose 15 mg/kg minimum dosing interval

4 hr, max 75 mg/kg/day from all sources, ext rel 650-1300 mg q8hr as needed, max 4 g/day

Child ≥2 yr and <50 kg: IV 15 mg/kg/dose q6hr or 12.5 mg/kg/dose q4hr, max single dose 15 mg/kg, minimum dosing interval 4 hr, max 75 mg/kg/day from all sources

Available forms: Rectal supp 120, 325, 650 mg; chewable tabs 80 mg; caps 500 mg; elix 120, 160, 325 mg/5 ml; tabs 160, 325, 500, 650 mg; sol for injection 1000 mg/100 ml; disintegrating tab 80, 160 mg; oral drops 80 mg/10.8 ml; liquid 500 mg/5 ml, 160 mg/5 ml, 1000 mg/30 ml, 80 mg/ml; ext rel tabs 650 mg

Implementation
PO route
⚠ **Do not confuse: 2 × 325 (650 mg), with 650 mg ER tab**
- Administer to patient crushed or whole; chewable tabs may be chewed; do not crush or chew EXT REL product
- Give with food or milk to decrease gastric symptoms; give 30 min before or 2 hr after meals; absorption may be slowed
- Shake susp well; check all product concentrations carefully; check elixir, liquid, suspension concentration carefully; susp and cups are bioequivalent

Intermittent IV infusion route
- No further dilution needed, do not add other medications to vial or infusion device
- For doses equal to single vial, a vented IV set may be used to deliver directly from vial; for doses less than a single vial, withdraw and place in an empty sterile syringe, plastic IV container, or glass bottle, infuse over 15 mins
- Discard unused portion, once seal is broken or vial penetrated or transferred to another container, give within 6 hr

> **BLACK BOX WARNING:** Check IV dose carefully to prevent dosing errors

Rectal route
- Store suppositories <80° F (27° C)

ADVERSE EFFECTS
GI: Nausea, vomiting, abdominal pain; **hepatotoxicity, hepatic seizure (overdose), GI bleeding**
GU: Renal failure (high, prolonged doses)
HEMA: Leukopenia, neutropenia, hemolytic anemia (long-term use), thrombocytopenia, pancytopenia
INTEG: Rash, urticaria, injection site pain
SYST: Stevens-Johnson syndrome, toxic epidermal necrolysis
TOXICITY: Cyanosis, anemia, neutropenia, jaundice, pancytopenia, CNS stimulation, delirium followed by vascular collapse, seizures, coma, death

Pharmacokinetics

Absorption	Well absorbed (PO), variable (RECT)
Distribution	Widely distributed; crosses placenta in low concentrations
Metabolism	Liver 85%-95%; metabolites are toxic at high levels
Excretion	Kidneys—metabolites, breast milk
Half-life	3-4 hr

Pharmacodynamics

	PO	RECT	IV
Onset	½-1 hr	½-1 hr	Unknown
Peak	1-3 hr	1-3 hr	30-120 min
Duration	3-4 hr	3-4 hr	3-4 hr

INTERACTIONS
Individual drugs
Alcohol, carBAMazepine, dasatinib mipomersen, diflunisal, imatinib, isoniazid, lamoTRIgine, rifabutin, rifampin, zidovudine: increased hepatotoxicity
Colestipol, cholestyramine: decreased absorption of acetaminophen
Decrease: zidovudine effect
Avoid use with salicylates
Warfarin: hypoprothrombinemia; long-term use, high doses of acetaminophen

Drug classifications
Barbiturates, hydantoins: decreased effect; increased hepatotoxicity
NSAIDs, salicylates: increased renal adverse reactions

Drug/herb
St. John's wort: increased hepatotoxicity due to acetaminophen metabolism

Drug/lab test
Interference: urinary 5-HIAA
Increased: LFTs, potassium, bilirubin, LDH, protime
Decreased: Hgb/Hct, WBC, RBC, platelets; albumin, magnesium, phosphate (pediatrics)

NURSING CONSIDERATIONS
Assessment
⚠ Monitor liver function studies: AST, ALT, bilirubin, creatinine before therapy if long-term therapy is anticipated; may cause hepatic toxicity at doses >4 g/day with chronic use

Adverse effects: *italics* = common; **bold** = life-threatening

- Monitor renal function studies: BUN, urine creatinine, occult blood; albumin indicates nephritis
- Monitor blood studies: CBC, PT if patient is on long-term therapy
- Check I&O ratio; decreasing output may indicate renal failure (long-term therapy)
- Assess for fever and pain: type of pain, location, intensity, duration, temp, diaphoresis
⚠ **Assess for chronic poisoning: rapid, weak pulse; dyspnea; cold, clammy extremities; report immediately to prescriber**

> **BLACK BOX WARNING: Assess hepatotoxicity:** dark urine, clay-colored stools, yellowing of skin and sclera; itching, abdominal pain, fever, diarrhea if patient is on long-term therapy; **doses > 4 gm/day**

- Stevens-Johnson syndrome, toxic epidermal necrolysis may occur when beginning treatment or any other dose

Patient/family education

> **BLACK BOX WARNING: ⚠ Teach patient not to exceed recommended dosage; the elixir, liquid, and suspension come in several concentrations, read label carefully; acute poisoning with liver damage may result; acute toxicity includes symptoms of nausea, vomiting, and abdominal pain; prescriber should be notified immediately**

- Inform patient that toxicity may occur when used with other combination products
- Advise patient not to use with alcohol, OTC products, or herbals without prescriber approval
- Teach patient to recognize signs of chronic overdose: bleeding, bruising, malaise, fever, sore throat
- Inform patient that urine may become dark brown as a result of phenacetin (metabolite of acetaminophen)
- Tell patient to notify prescriber for pain or fever lasting more than 3 days, not to be used in <2 yr unless approved by prescriber
- May be used when breastfeeding, short-term

Evaluation
Positive therapeutic outcome
- Decreased pain, use pain scoring
- Decreased fever

TREATMENT OF OVERDOSE:
Product level q4hr, gastric lavage, activated charcoal; administer oral acetylcysteine to prevent hepatic damage (*see acetylcysteine monograph*, p. 10)

acetaZOLAMIDE (Rx)
(a-set-a-zole′-a-mide)
Diamox ❖, Novo-zolamide ❖
Func. class.: Diuretic carbonic anhydrase inhibitor; antiglaucoma agent, antiepileptic
Chem. class.: Sulfonamide derivative
Pregnancy category C

Do not confuse: acetaZOLAMIDE/
acetoHEXAMIDE, **Diamox**/Dobutrex/
Trimox

ACTION: Decreases the aqueous humor in the eye, which lowers intraocular pressure by the inhibition of carbonic anhydrase; also inhibits carbonic anhydrase activity in proximal renal tubules to decrease reabsorption of water, sodium, potassium, bicarbonate; decreases carbonic anhydrase in CNS, increasing seizure threshold; prevents uric acid or cysteine buildup in the renal system by the decrease in pH, causing increased urine volume and alkaline urine

Therapeutic outcome: Decreased intraocular pressure; control of seizures; prevention and treatment of acute mountain sickness; prevention of uric acid/cysteine renal stones; decreased edema in lung tissue and peripherally; decreased B/P

USES: Open-angle glaucoma, angle closure glaucoma (preoperatively if surgery delayed), mixed, tonic-clonic, myclonic, refractory, epilepsy (petit mal, grand mal, absence), edema in CHF, product-induced edema, acute altitude sickness

CONTRAINDICATIONS
Hypersensitivity to sulfonamides, severe renal/hepatic disease, electrolyte imbalances (hyponatremia, hypokalemia), hyperchloremic acidosis, Addison's disease, long-term use in closed-angle glaucoma, adrenalcortical insufficiency, metabolic acidosis, acidemia, anuria

Precautions: Pregnancy **C**, breastfeeding, hypercalciuria, COPD, respiratory acidosis, pulmonary obstruction/emphysema

DOSAGE AND ROUTES
Angle closure glaucoma
Adult: PO/IV 250 mg q4hr or 250 mg bid, to be used for short-term therapy

Chronic open-angle glaucoma
Adult: PO/IV 250 mg/day in divided doses for amounts over 250 mg or 500 mg **EXT REL** bid, max 1 g/day

Child: PO 8-30 mg/kg/day in divided doses tid or qid, or 300-900 mg/m²/day, max 1 g/day; IV 5 to 10 mg/kg q6hr, max 1 g/day

Edema in CHF
Adult: PO/**IV** 250-375 mg/day or 5 mg/kg in AM, give for 2 days, then 1-2 days drug-free
Child: PO/**IV** 5 mg/kg/day or 150 mg/m² in AM

Seizures
Adult: PO/**IV** 8-30 mg/kg/day in 1-4 divided doses, usual range 375-1000 mg/day; EXT REL not recommended in seizures

Altitude sickness
Adult 125 mg bid/Child ≥ 12 yrs: PO (Ext Rel) 500-1000 mg q12hr, start therapy 24-48 hr prior to ascent and ≥48 hr after arrival at high altitude
Geriatric: PO 250 mg bid; use lowest effective dose

Renal dose
Adult: PO/IV CCr 50-80 ml/min, give dose ≥q6hr regular release of IV; CCr 10-50 ml/min, give dose q12hr; CCr <10 ml/min, avoid use

Available forms: Tabs 125, 250 mg; ext rel caps 500 mg; inj 500 mg

Implementation
• Give in AM to avoid interference with sleep
• Administer fluids 2-3 L/day to prevent renal calculi, unless contraindicated
• Potassium replacement if potassium level is <3.0 ml/dl

PO route
• Do not crush or chew ext rel caps; caps may be opened and sprinkled on food; store at room temperature
• Give with food; if nausea occurs, crush tabs and mix with sweet substance to counteract bitter taste

IV route
• Do not use solution that is yellow or has a precipitate or crystals
• **Reconstitute with** 500 mg of product/5 ml or more sterile water for inj: use within 24 hr, **give** at 100-500 mg/min

IV, direct route
• Give over 1 min or more
• Store in cool, dark area, use reconstituted solution within 24 hr

Additive compatibilities: Cimetidine, ranitidine

Additive incompatibilities: Multivitamins

ADVERSE EFFECTS
CNS: Drowsiness, paresthesia, anxiety, depression, headache, dizziness, confusion, stimulation, fatigue, *seizures*

EENT: Myopia, tinnitus
ENDO: Hyperglycemia, hypoglycemia
GI: Nausea, vomiting, anorexia, diarrhea, melena, weight loss, **hepatic insufficiency, cholestatic jaundice, fulminant hepatic necrosis**, taste alterations, **bleeding**
GU: Frequency, polyuria, **uremia**, glucosuria, hematuria, dysuria, crystalluria, renal calculi
HEMA: Aplastic anemia, hemolytic anemia, leukopenia, thrombocytopenia purpura, pancytopenia
INTEG: Rash, pruritus, urticaria, fever, **Stevens-Johnson syndrome,** photosensitivity, flushing, toxic epidermal necrolysis
META: *Hypokalemia, hyperchloremic acidosis,* hyponatremia, sulfonamide-like reactions, metabolic acidosis, growth inhibition in children, hyperuricemia, hypercalcemia

Pharmacokinetics

Absorption	GI tract—65% if fasting, 75% with food; **IV**—complete
Distribution	Crosses placenta; widely distributed
Metabolism	None
Excretion	Kidneys, unchanged (80% within 24 hr); breast milk
Half-life	2½-5½ hr

Pharmacodynamics

	PO	PO–ext rel	IV
Onset	1 hr	2 hr	2 min
Peak	8-12 hr	3-6 hr	15 min
Duration	8-12 hr	18-24 hr	4-5 hr

INTERACTIONS
Individual drugs
Amphotericin B, corticotropin, ACTH: increased hypokalemia
Arsenic trioxide, levomethadyl: increased cardiac toxicity if hypokalemia develops
CarBAMazepine, ethotoin: increased osteomalacia
CycloSPORINE: increased toxicity
Diflunisal: increased side effects
Lithium: increased excretion of lithium
Increase: acidosis (respiratory disorders) beta blockers
Methenamine: decreased acetaZOLAMIDE effect
Primidone: decreased primidone level
Topiramate: increased renal stone formation, heat stroke, avoid concurrent use

Drug classifications
Amphetamines: increased action
Anticholinergics, folic acid antagonists: increased action of each product

Adverse effects: *italics* = common; **bold** = life-threatening

Cardiac glycosides: increased cardiac toxicity if hypokalemia develops

Corticosteroids: increased hypokalemia

Flecainide, memantine, phenytoin, procainamide, quiNIDine, mecamylamine, mexiletine: increased effect of each product

Salicylates: increased toxicity

Drug/lab test

Increased: glucose, bilirubin, calcium, uric acid

Decreased: thyroid iodine uptake, sodium, Hct/Hgb

False positive: urinary protein, 17-hydroxysteroids

NURSING CONSIDERATIONS

Assessment

• Assess patient for tinnitus, hearing loss, ear pain; periodic testing of hearing is needed when high doses of this product are given by **IV** route

• **Assess for seizures: type, location, duration; provide seizure precautions**

• Assess fluid volume status: I&O ratio and record, count or weigh diapers as appropriate, distended neck veins, crackles in lung, color, quality, and specific gravity of urine, skin turgor, adequacy of pulses, moist mucous membranes, bilateral lung sounds, peripheral pitting edema; dehydration symptoms of decreasing output, thirst, hypotension, dry mouth, and mucous membranes should be reported

• Monitor electrolytes: potassium, sodium, calcium, magnesium; also include BUN, blood pH, ABGs, uric acid, CBC, blood glucose

• Assess B/P before and during therapy with patient lying, standing, and sitting as appropriate; orthostatic hypotension can occur rapidly

• Monitor blood, urine glucose in diabetic patients; glucose levels may be increased

• Assess for eye pain, change in vision when using product for intraocular pressure

• Assess neurologic status when using product for seizures

• **Assess for decreased symptoms of acute mountain sickness:** headache, nausea, vomiting, dizziness, fatigue, drowsiness, shortness of breath, insomnia

Patient/family education

• Teach patient to take the medication early in the day to prevent nocturia

• Instruct patient to take with food or milk if GI symptoms of nausea and anorexia occur

• Teach patient to maintain a record of weight on a weekly basis and notify prescriber of weight loss of >5 lb

• Caution patient that this product causes a loss of potassium, so food rich in potassium should be added to the diet; refer to a dietitian for assistance in planning

• Advise patient to wear protective clothing and sunscreen in the sun to prevent photosensitivity

• Teach patient not to use alcohol or any OTC medications without prescriber's approval; serious product reactions may occur

⚠ Emphasize the need to contact prescriber immediately if muscle cramps, weakness, nausea, dizziness, or numbness, rapid weight changes, change in stools, rash, sore throat, bleeding/bruising, Stevens-Johnson syndrome, toxic epidermal necrolysis (red rash that spreads, blistering) occur

• Avoid prolonged sun exposure

• Teach patient to take own B/P and pulse and record

• Teach patient to continue taking medication even if feeling better; this product controls symptoms but does not cure the condition

• Teach patient to see ophthalmologist periodically; glaucoma is a slow process

• Advise patient to increase fluids to 2-3 L/day if not contraindicated

Evaluation

Positive therapeutic outcome

• Decreased intraocular pressure (glaucoma)

• Decreased edema in feet, legs, sacral area daily (CHF)

• Decreased frequency of seizures

• Prevention of altitude sickness

TREATMENT OF OVERDOSE:

Lavage if taken orally, monitor electrolytes, administer dextrose in saline, monitor hydration, CV, renal status

acetylcholine ophthalmic

See Appendix B

acetylcysteine (Rx)

(a-se-teel-sis'tay-een)

Acetadote, Airbron ✦, Mucomyst ✦, Parvolex ✦

Func. class.: Mucolytic; antidote—acetaminophen

Chem. class.: Amino acid L-cysteine

Pregnancy category B

Do not confuse: acetylcysteine/ acetylcholine, **Mucomyst/Mucinex**

ACTION: Decreases viscosity of secretions in respiratory tract by breaking disulfide links of mucoproteins; serves as a substrate of glutathione, which is necessary to inactivate toxic metabolites in acetaminophen overdose

Therapeutic outcome: Decreased hepatotoxicity from acetaminophen overdose (PO); decreased viscosity of mucus in respiratory disorders (inh)

USES: Acetaminophen toxicity, bronchitis, cystic fibrosis, COPD, atelectasis, meconium ileus

CONTRAINDICATIONS
Hypersensitivity

Precautions: Pregnancy **B,** breastfeeding, hypothyroidism, Addison's disease, CNS depression, brain tumor, asthma, renal/hepatic disease, COPD, psychosis, alcoholism, seizure disorders, bronchospasms, asthma, anaphylactoid reactions, fluid restriction, weight <40 kg, increased intracranial pressure, status asthmaticus

DOSAGE AND ROUTES
Mucolytic
Adult and child: Instill 1-2 ml (10%-20% sol) q2-8hr prn, or 3-5 ml (20% sol) or 6-10 ml (10% sol) tid or qid; nebulization (face, mask, mouthpiece, tracheostomy) 1-10 ml of a 20% sol or 2-20 ml of a 10% sol q2-6hr; nebulization (tent, croupette) may require large dose, up to 300 ml/contrast-induced nephrotoxicity (unlabeled) Adult PO 600-1200 mg bid × 2 days (beginning the day before the procedure)

Acetaminophen toxicity
Adult and child >40 kg: PO 140 mg/kg, then 70 mg/kg q4hr × 17 doses to total 1330 mg/kg; **>40 kg IV** loading dose 150 mg/kg over 60 min (dilution 150 mg/kg in 200 ml of D_5W); then 1:50 mg/kg over 4 hr (dilution 50 mg/kg in 500 ml D_5); then 2:100 mg/kg over 16 hr (dilution 100 mg/kg in 1000 ml D_5W)
Child/Adolescents 21-40 kg: IV 150 mg/kg in 100 ml of diluent over 1 hr, then 50 mg/kg in 250 ml over 4 hr, then 100 mg/kg in 500 mg over 16 hr
Infants/Child 5-20 kg: IV 150 mg/kg in 3 ml/kg diluent over 1 hr, then 50 mg/kg in 7 ml/kg diluent over 4 hr, then 100 mg/kg in 14 ml/kg diluent over 16 hr.

Available forms: Oral sol 10%, 20%; inj 20% (200 mg/ml)

Implementation
• Give decreased dosage to geriatric patients; their metabolism may be slowed; give gum, hard candy, frequent rinsing of mouth for dryness of oral cavity
• Use only if suction machine is available
PO route (Antidotal use)
• Give within 24 hr; dilute 10% or 20% sol to a 5% sol with diet soda; may use water if giving via gastric tube; dilution of 10% sol 1:1, 20%

sol 1:3; use within 1 hr, store open undiluted solution refrigerated ≤96 hr
Direct intratracheal INSTILL
• Use ½-1 hr before meals for better absorption to decrease nausea; only after patient clears airway by deep breathing, coughing
• Give by syringe 2-3 doses of 1-2 ml of 10%-20% sol up to q1hr
• Store in refrigerator: use within 96 hr of opening
• Provide assistance with inhaled dose: bronchodilator if bronchospasm occurs; wash face and rinse mouth after use to remove sticky feeling
• Use decreased dose in geriatric, metabolism may be slowed
• Use mechanical suction if cough insufficient to remove excess bronchial secretions
• Store in refrigerator; use within 96 hr of opening

IV route
21-hr regimen:
• **Loading dose:** dilute 150 mg/kg in 200 ml D_5W; maintenance dose no. 1 **dilute** 50 mg/kg in 500 ml D_5W; maintenance dose no. 2 **dilute** 100 mg/kg in 1000 ml D_5W
• **Give** loading over 15 min; **give** maintenance dose no. 1 over 4 hr; **give** maintenance dose no. 2 over 16 hr; **give** sequentially without time between doses

Incompatibilities: Rubber, metals, stability with other products unknown

ADVERSE EFFECTS
CNS: Chills, *dizziness, drowsiness,* fever, headache
CV: Flushing, hypotension, tachycardia
EENT: *Rhinorrhea,* tooth damage
GI: Anorexia, constipation, diarrhea, **hepatotoxicity,** *nausea,* stomatitis, vomiting
INTEG: Clamminess, fever, pruritus, rash, urticaria
MISC: **Anaphylaxis, angioedema,** unpleasant odor
RESP: **Bronchospasm,** burning, chest tightness, cough, **hemoptysis,** dyspnea

Pharmacokinetics

Absorption	Extensive (PO), locally (inh)
Distribution	Protein binding 83%
	Peak ½-1 hr
Metabolism	Liver
Excretion	Kidneys
Half-life	5.6 hr (adult), 11 hr (newborn)

INTERACTIONS
Individual drugs
Activated charcoal, do not use with acetylcysteine

NURSING CONSIDERATIONS
Assessment
Mucolytic use
- **Assess cough:** type, frequency, character, including sputum; bronchospasm
- **Assess characteristics, rate, rhythm of respirations,** increased dyspnea, sputum; discontinue if bronchospasm occurs; ABGs for increased CO_2 retention in asthma patients
- Monitor VS, cardiac status including checking for dysrhythmias, increased rate, palpitations

Antidotal use
- Assess liver function tests, acetaminophen levels, PT, glucose, electrolytes, BUN, creatinine; inform prescriber if dose is vomited or vomiting is persistent; 150 mg/kg may be toxic, check acetaminophen level q4hr; provide adequate hydration; decrease dosage in hepatic encephalopathy
- Assess for nausea, vomiting, rash; notify prescriber if these occur

⚠ **Hypersensitivity: Anaphylaxis may occur with IV dose; if present, stop infusion, treat, restart**

Patient/family education
Mucolytic use
- Tell patient to avoid driving or other hazardous activities until patient is stabilized on this medication; avoid alcohol, other CNS depressants; will enhance sedating properties of this product
- Inform patient that foul odor and smell may be unpleasant
- Instruct patient to clear airway for inhalation; avoid smoking, smoke-filled rooms, perfume, dust, environmental pollutants, cleaners
- Teach patient to report vomiting, as dose may need to be repeated

Evaluation
Positive therapeutic outcome
- Absence of purulent secretions when coughing (mucolytic use)
- Clear lung sounds bilaterally (mucolytic use)
- Absence of hepatic damage (acetaminophen toxicity)
- Decreasing blood toxicology (acetaminophen toxicity)

---

acyclovir (Rx)
(ay-sye′kloe-veer)
Sitavig, Zovirax
Func. class.: Antiviral
Chem. class.: Acyclic purine nucleoside analog
Pregnancy category B

Do not confuse: Zovirax/Zyvox/Valtrex/Zostrix

ACTION: Interferes with DNA synthesis by conversion to acyclovir triphosphate, causing decreased viral replication

Therapeutic outcome: Decreased amount and time of healing of lesions

USES: Mucocutaneous herpes simplex virus, herpes genitalis (HSV-1, HSV-2), varicella infections, herpes zoster, herpes simplex encephalitis

CONTRAINDICATIONS
Hypersensitivity to this product or valacyclovir

Precautions: Pregnancy **B**, breastfeeding, renal/hepatic disease, electrolyte imbalance, dehydration, neurologic disease; hypersensitivity to famciclovir, ganciclovir, penciclovir, valganciclovir, obesity

DOSAGE AND ROUTES
Renal dose
Adult and child: PO/IV CCr >50 ml/min 100% dose q8hr; CCr 25-50 ml/min 100% dose q12hr; CCr 10-24 ml/min 100% dose q24hr; CCr 0-10 ml/min 50% of dose q24hr
Base dose in obese patients on ideal body weight, not actual body weight

Herpes simplex
Adult: PO 400 mg 3 ×/day for 5 days or 200 mg 5 ×/day × 5 days
Adult and child >12 yr (use ideal weight in obesity): IV INF 5 mg/kg over 1 hr q8hr × 5 days
Infant >3 mo/child <12 yr: IV INF 250 mg/m² or 30 mg/kg/day divided q8hr over 1 hr × 5 days

Genital herpes
Adult: PO 200 mg q4hr (5 times a day while awake) × 5 days to 12 mo depending on whether initial, recurrent, or chronic; **IV** 5 mg/kg q8hr × 5 days

Genital herpes, initial limited, mucocutaneous HSV in immunocompromised patients, non-life-threatening
Adult and child ≥12 yr: TOP cover lesions q3hr 6 times/day

Herpes simplex encephalitis
Adult: IV 10 mg/kg over 1 hr q8hr × 10 days
Child 3 mo-12 yr: IV 20 mg/kg q8hr × 10 days
Child birth-3 mo: IV 20 mg/kg q8hr × 21 days

Herpes labialis, recurrent
Adult and child ≥12 yr: TOP apply cream 5 times a day × 4 days, start as soon as symptoms appear

Herpes, labialis, recurrent in immunocompetent patients:
Adult: buccal 50 mg as a single dose in upper gum region within 1 hr after prodromal symptoms and before cold sore formation

Herpes zoster (shingles): immunocompromised patients
Adult and adolescent: PO 800 mg q4hr 5 times/day × 7-10 days; IV 10 mg/kg q8hr × 7 days
Child ≥12 yr: IV 10 mg/kg q8hr × 7 days
Infant and child <12 yr: IV 20 mg/kg q8hr × 7-10 days

Herpes zoster (shingles): immunocompetent patient
Adult: PO 800 mg q4hr 5 times/day × 7-10 days; start within 48-72 hr of rash onset

Varicella (chickenpox): immunocompetent patient
Adult, adolescent, and child: PO 800 mg 4 times/day × 5 days
Child ≥2 yr: PO 20 mg/kg (max 800 mg) PO 4 times per day × 5 days

Mucosal/cutaneous herpes simplex infections in immunosuppressed patients
Adult and child >12 yr: IV 5 mg/kg q8hr × 7 days
Infant >3 mo/child <12 yr: IV 10 mg/kg q8hr × 7 days

Recurrent ocular herpes, prevention (unlabeled)
Adult and child ≥12 yr: PO 600-800 mg/day × 8-12 mo

Available forms: Caps 200 mg; tabs 400, 800 mg; powder for inj 500, 1000 mg; sol for inj 50 mg/ml; oral susp 200 mg/5 ml; ointment/cream 5%; buccal tab 50 mg

Implementation
PO route
• Do not break, crush, or chew caps
• Give with food to lessen GI symptoms; may give without regard to meals with 8 oz of water
• Store at room temperature in dry place

• May be taken orally before infection occurs or when itching or pain occurs, usually before eruptions
• Must be taken at equal intervals around the clock
• Shake susp before use

IV route
• Provide increased fluids to 3 L/day to decrease crystalluria, most critical during first 2 hr after IV infusion
Intermittent IV infusion route
• Reconstitute with 10 ml sterile water for injection/500 mg of product (50 mg/ml); shake; **further dilute** in 50-125 ml compatible sol, use within 12 hr; **give** over at least 1 hr (constant rate) by infusion pump to prevent nephrotoxicity; do not reconstitute with sol containing benzyl alcohol or parabens; check infusion site for redness, pain, induration; rotate sites
• Lower dosage in acute or chronic renal failure
• Store at room temp for up to 12 hr after reconstitution; if refrigerated, sol may show a precipitate that clears at room temperature; yellow discoloration does not affect potency

Y-site compatibilities: Alemtuzumab, allopurinol, amikacin, aminophylline, amphotericin B cholesteryl, amphotericin B liposome, ampicillin, anidulafungin, argatroban, atracurium, bivalirudin, buprenorphine, busulfan, butorphanol, calcium chloride/gluconate, CARBOplatin, ceFAZolin, cefonicid, cefotaxime, cefOXitin, cefTAZidime, ceftizoxime, cefTRIAXone, cefuroxime, chloramphenicol, chlolesteryl sulfate complex, cimetidine, clindamycin, dexamethasone sodium phosphate, dimenhyDRINATE, DOXOrubicin, doxycycline, erythromycin, famotidine, filgrastim, fluconazole, gentamicin, granisetron, heparin, hydrocortisone sodium succinate, HYDROmorphone, imipenemcilastatin, LORazepam, magnesium sulfate, melphalan, methylPREDNISolone sodium succinate, metoclopramide, metroNIDAZOLE, multivitamin, nafcillin, oxacillin, PACLitaxel, penicillin G potassium, PENTobarbital, perphenazine, piperacillin, potassium chloride, propofol, ranitidine, remifentanil, sodium bicarbonate, teniposide, theophylline, thiotepa, ticarcillin, tobramycin, trimethoprimsulfamethoxazole, vancomycin, vasopressin, voriconazole, zidovudine

Y-site incompatibilities: DOBUTamine, DOPamine, ondansetron, verapamil
Topical route
• Use finger cot or glove to cover all lesions completely, do not get in eye, wash hands after use

Adverse effects: *italics* = common; **bold** = life-threatening

ADVERSE EFFECTS

CNS: Tremors, confusion, lethargy, hallucinations, **seizures,** *dizziness, headache,* encephalopathic changes

EENT: Gingival hyperplasia

GI: Nausea, vomiting, diarrhea, increased ALT, AST, abdominal pain, glossitis, colitis

GU: Oliguria, proteinuria, hematuria, vaginitis, moniliasis, glomerulonephritis, acute renal failure, changes in menses, polydipsia

HEMA: Thrombotic thrombocytopenia purpura, hemolytic uremic syndrome (immunocompromised patient)

INTEG: Rash, urticaria, pruritus, pain or phlebitis at **IV** site, unusual sweating, alopecia, Stevens-Johnson syndrome

MS: Joint pain, leg pain, muscle cramps

Pharmacokinetics

Absorption	Minimal (PO)
Distribution	Widely distributed, crosses placenta; CSF concentration 50% plasma; protein binding 9%-33%
Metabolism	Liver, minimal
Excretion	Kidneys, 95% unchanged
Half-life	2.0-3.5 hr, increased in renal disease

Pharmacodynamics

	PO	IV
Onset	Unknown	Rapid
Peak	2.5-3.3 hr	Infusion's end
Duration	Unknown	Unknown

INTERACTIONS

Individual drugs

Aminoglycosides: increased nephrotoxicity

Entecavir, PEMEtrexed, tenofovir: increased concentration of each product

Probenecid: increased neurotoxicity, nephrotoxicity

Valproic acid: decreased action of valproic acid

Zidovudine, IT methotrexate: increased CNS side effects

Drug classifications

Hydantoins: decreased actions of hydantoins

NURSING CONSIDERATIONS

Assessment

• **Monitor for signs of infection,** type of lesions, area of body covered, purulent drainage

• Check I&O ratio; report hematuria, oliguria, fatigue, weakness; may indicate nephrotoxicity; check for protein in urine during treatment

• **Toxicity:** monitor any patient with compromised renal system, since product is excreted slowly in poor renal system function; toxicity may occur rapidly

• Monitor liver studies: AST, ALT

⚠ Monitor renal studies: urinalysis, protein, BUN, creatinine, CCr; increased BUN, creatinine indicates renal failure and nephrotoxicity

• Monitor bowel pattern before, during treatment; if severe abdominal pain with bleeding occurs, product should be discontinued

• Assess allergies before treatment, reaction of each medication; place allergies on chart in bright red letters; allergic reaction: burning, stinging, swelling, redness, rash, vulvitis, pruritus

• Assess neurologic status in herpes encephalitis

Patient/family education

PO route

• Teach patient that product may be taken orally before infection occurs or when itching or pain occur, usually before eruptions; that partners need to be told that patient has herpes; they can become infected, so condoms must be worn to prevent reinfections

⚠ Tell patient to report sore throat, fever, fatigue; may indicate superinfection; that product must be taken at equal intervals around the clock to maintain blood levels for duration of therapy

• Tell patient to notify prescriber of side effects: bruising, bleeding, fatigue, malaise; may indicate blood dyscrasias

• Adequate intake of fluids (2 L) to prevent deposits in kidneys, more likely to occur with rapid administration or in dehydration

• Tell patient to seek dental care during treatment to prevent gingival hyperplasia

• Teach female patients with genital herpes to have regular Pap smears to prevent undetected cervical cancer

Evaluation

Positive therapeutic outcome

• Absence of itching, painful lesions

• Crusting and healed lesions

TREATMENT OF OVERDOSE:

Discontinue product, hemodialysis, resuscitate if needed

---

acyclovir topical
See Appendix B

adalimumab (Rx)
(add-a-lim'yu-mab)
Humira
Func. class.: Antirheumatic agent (disease modifying), immunomodulator, anti-TNF
Pregnancy category B

Do not confuse: Humira/Humalin/Humalog

ACTION: A form of human IgG1 monoclonal antibody specific for human tumor necrosis factor (TNFα); elevated levels of TNFα are found in patients with rheumatoid arthritis

Therapeutic outcome: Decreased pain, inflammation in joints, better ROM

USES: Reduction in signs and symptoms and inhibiting progression of structural damage in patients with moderate to severe active rheumatoid arthritis in patients ≥18 years of age who have not responded to other disease-modifying agents, JRA, psoriatic arthritis, Crohn's disease, moderate-severe plaque psoriasis, ankylosing spondylitis

CONTRAINDICATIONS
Hypersensitivity

Precautions: Pregnancy **B**, breastfeeding, children, geriatric, CNS demyelinating disease, lymphoma, latent TB, CHF, hepatitis B carriers, mannitol hypersensitivity, latex allergy, neoplastic disease

> **BLACK BOX WARNING:** Active infections, risk of lymphomas/leukemias, TB

DOSAGE AND ROUTES
Rheumatoid arthritis, ankylosing spondylitis, psoriatic arthritis
Adult: SUBCUT 40 mg every other wk or every week if not combined with methotrexate

Juvenile rheumatoid arthritis (JRA)
Child ≥2 yr/adolescent ≥30 kg: SUBCUT 40 mg every other wk
Child ≥2 yr/adolescent ≥15 kg to <30 kg: SUBCUT 20 mg every other wk
Child ≥2 yr/adolescent 10 kg to <15 kg: SUBCUT 10 mg every other wk

Crohn's disease
Adult: SUBCUT 160 mg given as 4 inj on day 1, or 2 inj on days 1 and 2, then 80 mg at wk 2 and 40 mg every other wk, starting at wk 4

Plaque psoriasis
Adult: SUBCUT 80 mg baseline as 2 inj, then 40 mg every other week starting 1 wk after initial dose × 16 wk

Available forms: Inj 40 mg/0.8 ml; 20 mg/0.4 ml (pediatric)

Implementation
SUBCUT route
• Do not admix with other sol or medications, do not use filter, protect from light

ADVERSE EFFECTS
CNS: Headache, **Guillain-Barré syndrome**
CV: Hypertension, CHF
EENT: Sinusitis
GI: Abdominal pain, nausea, hepatic damage, **GI bleeding**
HEMA: **Leukopenia, pancytopenia, aplastic anemia, agranulocytopenia, thrombocytopenia**
INTEG: Rash, *inj site reaction*
MISC: Flulike symptoms, UTI, hypertension, back pain, lupuslike syndrome, risk of cancer, antibody development to this drug, **risk of infection (TB, invasive fungal infections, other opportunistic infections); may be fatal, Stevens-Johnson syndrome,** anaphylaxis, hypercholesterolemia, hyperlipidemia
RESP: *URI, pulmonary fibrosis,* bronchitis

Pharmacokinetics

Absorption	Unknown
Distribution	Unknown
Metabolism	Unknown
Excretion	Unknown
Half-life	Terminal 2 wk

Pharmacodynamics
Unknown

INTERACTIONS
Individual drugs
Anakinra: do not use together, serious infections may occur
Rilonacept: increase serious infections

Drug classifications
Live-virus vaccines: do not give concurrently; immunization should be brought up to date before treatment

> **BLACK BOX WARNING:** Other TNF blockers: increased serious infections

Drug/lab test
Increased: ALT, cholesterol, lipids

NURSING CONSIDERATIONS
Assessment
• Rheumatoid arthritis: assess for pain, stiffness, ROM, swelling of joints during treatment
• Check for inj site pain, swelling, redness; usually occur after 2 inj (4-5 days) use cold compress to relieve pain/swelling

> **BLACK BOX WARNING:** Check for infections, fever, flulike symptoms, dyspnea, change in urination, redness/swelling around wounds, stop treatment if present, some serious infections, including sepsis, may occur; patients with active infections should not be started on this product

• **May reactivate hepatitis B in chronic carriers, may be fatal**

> **BLACK BOX WARNING:** Assess for latent TB prior to therapy; treat before starting this product

• **Assess for anaphylaxis, latex allergic; stop therapy if lupuslike syndrome develops**
• Assess for blood dyscrasias: CBC, differential periodically

> **BLACK BOX WARNING:** Assess for neoplastic disease (lymphomas/leukemia); in children, adolescents, hepatosplenic T-cell lymphoma is more likely in adolescent males with Crohn's disease or ulcerative colitis

Patient/family education
• Teach patient about self-administration if appropriate: inj should be made in thigh, abdomen, upper arm; rotate sites at least 1 inch from old site; do not inject in areas that are bruised, red, hard
• Advise patient that if medication is not taken when due, inject next dose as soon as remembered and inject next dose as scheduled
• Advise patient not to take any live-virus vaccines during treatment
⚠ **Instruct patient to report signs of infection, allergic reactions, lupuslike syndrome, immediately**

Evaluation
Positive therapeutic outcome
• Decreased inflammation, pain in joints, decreased joint destruction

---

adefovir (Rx)
(add-ee-foh′veer)
Hepsera
Func. class.: Antiviral Nucleoside
Pregnancy category C

ACTION: Inhibits hepatitis B virus DNA polymerase by competing with natural substrates and by causing DNA termination after its incorporation into viral DNA; causes viral DNA death

Therapeutic outcome: Improving liver function tests, lessening symptoms of chronic hepatitis B

USES: Chronic hepatitis B

CONTRAINDICATIONS
Hypersensitivity

Precautions: Pregnancy **C**, breastfeeding, children, geriatric, dialysis, females, labor, obesity, organ transplant

> **BLACK BOX WARNING:** Severe renal disease, impaired hepatic disease, lactic acidosis, HIV

DOSAGE AND ROUTES
Adult/adolescent: PO 10 mg daily, optimal duration unknown

Renal dose
Adult: PO CCr ≥50 ml/min 10 mg q24hr; CCr 30-49 ml/min 10 mg q48hr; CCr 10-29 ml/min 10 mg q72hr; hemodialysis 10 mg q7 days following dialysis

Available forms: Tabs 10 mg

Implementation
• Give by mouth without regard to food
• Store in cool environment; protect from light
• Take with full glass of water

ADVERSE EFFECTS
CNS: *Headache*
GI: *Dyspepsia*, abdominal pain, nausea, vomiting, diarrhea, hepatomegaly, flatulence, pancreatitis
GU: Hematuria, glycosuria, nephrotoxicity, Fanconi syndrome, renal failure
MISC: Fever, rash, weight loss, cough

Pharmacokinetics

Absorption	Rapidly from GI tract
Distribution	Unknown
Metabolism	Unknown
Excretion	Kidneys 45%
Half-life	7.48 hr

Pharmacodynamics

Onset	Unknown
Peak	1¾ hr
Duration	Unknown

INTERACTIONS
Individual drugs
AMILoride, cimetidine, cycloSPORINE, digoxin, dofetilide, efavirenz, emtricitabine, memantine, metformin, midodrine, morphine, PEMEtrexed, procainamide, quiNIDine, quinine, ranitidine, tacrolimus, tenofovir, triamterene, trospium, vancomycin: increased serum concentrations, nephrotoxicity

Do not use in combination with emtricitabine/tenofovir, emtricitabine/rilpivirine, emtricitabine/efavirenz/tenofovir

Drug classifications
Benzodiazepines, nucleoside analogs (experimental), NSAIDs, sulfonamides: increased serum concentrations, toxicity

> BLACK BOX WARNING: Lactic acidosis, severe hepatomegaly, NNRTIs, NRTIs, antiretroviral protease-inhibitors, aminoglycosides

Drug/lab test
Increased: ALT, AST, amylase, creatine kinase

NURSING CONSIDERATIONS
Assessment

> BLACK BOX WARNING: Assess **nephrotoxicity:** increasing CCr, BUN

> Pregnancy: Pregnant women should call the Antiretroviral Pregnancy Registry (800-258-4263) for monitoring fetal outcome

> BLACK BOX WARNING: Assess for HIV antibody testing before beginning treatment because HIV resistance may occur in chronic hepatitis B patients

> BLACK BOX WARNING: Assess **lactic acidosis,** severe hepatomegaly with stenosis, more common in females, obesity, and prolonged nucleoside use

• Assess geriatric patients more carefully; may develop renal, cardiac symptoms more rapidly

> BLACK BOX WARNING: Assess exacerbations of **hepatitis** after discontinuing treatment, monitor liver function tests, hepatitis B serology

Patient/family education
• Advise patient that optimal duration of treatment is unknown, that drug is not a cure; transmission may still occur
• Advise patient to avoid use with other medications unless approved by prescriber
• Advise patient to notify prescriber of decreased urinary output
• Teach patient not to stop abruptly unless directed, worsening of hepatitis may occur
• Teach patient to report immediately dyspnea, nausea, vomiting, abdominal pain, weakness, dizziness, cold extremities
• Teach patient to notify prescriber if pregnancy is planned or suspected, avoid breastfeeding

Evaluation
Positive therapeutic outcome
• Decreased symptoms of chronic hepatitis B, improving liver function tests

> **▲ HIGH ALERT**
>
> ## adenosine (Rx)
> (ah-den′oh-seen)
> **Adenocard**
> *Func. class.:* Antidysrhythmic—miscellaneous
> *Chem. class.:* Endogenous nucleoside
> **Pregnancy category C**

ACTION: Slows conduction through AV node, can interrupt reentry pathways through AV node, and can restore normal sinus rhythm in patients with paroxysmal supraventricular tachycardia (PSVT), decreases cardiac oxygen demand decreasing hypoxia

Therapeutic outcome: Normal sinus rhythm in patients diagnosed with SVT or diagnosis of perfusion defect

USES: PSVT, as a diagnostic aid to assess myocardial perfusion defects in CAD; Wolff-Parkinson-White (WPW) syndrome

CONTRAINDICATIONS
Hypersensitivity, 2nd- or 3rd-degree heart block, AV block, sick sinus syndrome, bradycardia

Precautions: Pregnancy C, breastfeeding, children, geriatric, asthma, atrial flutter, atrial fibrillation, ventricular tachycardia, bronchospastic lung disease, symptomatic bradycardia, bundle branch block, heart transplant, unstable angina, COPD, hypotension, hypovolemia, vascular heart disease, CV disease

---

DOSAGE AND ROUTES
Antidysrhythmic

Adult and child >50 kg: IV BOL 6 mg; if conversion to normal sinus rhythm does not occur within 1-2 min, give 12 mg by rapid IV BOL; may repeat 12 mg dose again in 1-2 min

Infant and child <50 kg: IV BOL 0.05 mg/kg; if not effective, increase dose by 0.05-0.1 mg/kg q2min to a max of 0.3 mg/kg/dose

Neonate: IV BOL: 0.05 mg/kg by rapid IV BOL, may increase by 0.05 mg/kg q2min, max 0.3 mg/kg/dose

Implementation

IV, direct (bolus) route
- Give **IV** BOL undiluted; give 6 mg or less by rapid inj; if using an **IV** line, use port near insertion site, flush with 0.9% NaCl (20 ml), then elevate arm
- Store at room temperature; sol should be clear; discard unused product

Solution compatibilities: D_5LR, D_5W, LR, 0.9% NaCl

ADVERSE EFFECTS

CNS: Light-headedness, dizziness, arm tingling, numbness, headache

CV: Chest pain/pressure, *atrial tachydysrhythmias,* sweating, palpitations, hypotension, *facial flushing,* AV block, cardiac arrest, ventricular dysrhythmias, atrial fibrillation

GI: *Nausea,* metallic taste

RESP: *Dyspnea, chest pressure,* hyperventilation, bronchospasm (asthmatics)

Pharmacokinetics

Absorption	Complete bioavailability
Distribution	Erythrocytes, cardiovascular endothelium
Metabolism	Liver, converted to inosine and adenosine monophosphate
Excretion	Kidneys
Half-life	10 sec

Pharmacodynamics

Onset	Rapid
Peak	Unknown
Duration	1-2 min

INTERACTIONS
Individual drugs

Caffeine, theophylline: decreased effects of adenosine

CarBAMazepine: increased heart block

Digoxin, verapamil: increased ventricular fibrillation

Dipyridamole: increased effects of adenosine

Smoking: increased tachycardia

Drug/herb

Ginger: increased effect

Green tea, guarana: decreased effect

NURSING CONSIDERATIONS
Assessment

- **Assess cardiopulmonary status:** pulse, respiration, ECG intervals (PR, QRS, QT); check for transient dysrhythmias (PVCs, PACs, sinus tachycardia, AV block)
- Assess respiratory status: rate, rhythm, lung fields for crackles, watch for respiratory depression; bilateral crackles may occur in CHF patient; if increased respiration, increased pulse occurs, product should be discontinued
- Assess CNS effects: dizziness, confusion, paresthesias; product should be discontinued

Patient/family education

- Tell patient to report facial flushing, dizziness, sweating, palpitations, chest pain

Evaluation
Positive therapeutic outcome

- Normal sinus rhythm
- Diagnosis of perfusion defect

⚠ HIGH ALERT

ado-trastuzumab
(a'doe-tras-tooz'ue-mab)
Kadcyla
Func. class.: Antineoplastic-biologic response modifier
Chem. class.: Signal transduction inhibitor (STI), humanized anti-HER2 antibody
Pregnancy category D

ACTION: Humanized anti-HER2 monoclonal antibody that is linked to DM1, a small molecule microtubular inhibitor. Once the antibody is bound to the HER2 receptor, the complex is internalized and the DM1 is released to bind with tubulin to lead to apoptosis

Therapeutic outcome: Decrease in size of tumors

USES: Breast cancer, metastatic with overexpression of HER2, in patients who previously received trastuzumab and a taxane separately or in combination

CONTRAINDICATIONS
Hypersensitivity to this product, Chinese hamster ovary cell protein, pregnancy **(D)**

Precautions: Breastfeeding, children, acute bronchospasm, anticoagulants, Asian patients,

---

asthma, cardiomyopathy/CHF, COPD, extravasation, fever, hepatitis, human anti-human antibody, hypotension, neuropathy, hepatotoxicity, interstitial lung disease/pneumonitis; pulmonary disease, thrombocytopenia

DOSAGE AND ROUTES

Adult: IV 3.6 mg/kg over 30-90 min q3wk; give first infusion over 90 min; if tolerated, give over 30 min

Dosage adjustments for toxicities

Hepatotoxicity
AST/ALT >5 to ≤20× ULN: withhold, resume at a reduced dose when AST/ALT is ≤5× ULN
• **First dose reduction: reduce the dose to 3 mg/kg**
• **Second dose reduction: reduce the dose to 2.4 mg/kg**
• **Requirement for further dose reduction: discontinue**
AST/ALT >20× ULN: discontinue
Total bilirubin >3 to ≤10× ULN: withhold; resume treatment at a reduced dose when total bilirubin recovers to ≤1.5
• **First dose reduction: reduce the dose to 3 mg/kg**
• **Second dose reduction: reduce the dose to 2.4 mg/kg**
• **Requirement for further dose reduction: discontinue treatment**
Total bilirubin >10× ULN: permanently discontinue
• **Permanently discontinue treatment in patients with AST/ALT > 3× ULN and total bilirubin > 2× ULN**
• **Permanently discontinue treatment in patients diagnosed with nodular regenerative hyperplasia (NRH)**
• **Left ventricular ejection fraction (LVEF) 40%-45% and decrease is <10% points from baseline: continue treatment; repeat LVEF assessment within 3 wk**
• **LVEF 40%-45% and decrease is ≥10% points from baseline: withhold; repeat LVEF assessment within 3 wk; if LVEF remains ≥10% points from baseline, discontinue**
• **LVEF < 40%: withhold; repeat LVEF assessment within 3 wk; if LVEF remains <40%, discontinue**
• **Symptomatic congestive heart failure (CHF): discontinue**
Thrombocytopenia
Platelet count 25,000/mm³ to <50,000/ mm³: withhold; resume treatment at same dose when platelet count recovers to ≥75,000/mm³

Platelet count <25,000/mm³: withhold; resume treatment at a reduced dose when platelet count recovers to ≥75,000/mm³
• **First dose reduction: reduce the dose to 3 mg/kg**
• **Second dose reduction: reduce the dose to 2.4 mg/kg**
• **Requirement for further dose reduction: discontinue**
Pulmonary toxicity
• **Permanently discontinue in patients diagnosed with interstitial lung disease or pneumonitis**
Peripheral neuropathy
• **Withhold in patients experiencing grade 3 or 4 peripheral neuropathy; resume treatment upon resolution to ≤ grade 2**

Available forms: Lyophilized powder 100, 160 mg

Implementation

IV route
• Visually inspect for particulate matter and discoloration prior to use
• Give as IV infusion with a 0.22-micron in-line filter; do not administer as an IV push or bolus
• Use cytotoxic handling procedures; do not mix with, or administer as an infusion with, other IV products
Reconstitution
• Slowly inject 5 ml of sterile water for injection into each 100 mg vial, or 8 ml of sterile water for injection into each 160 mg vial, to yield a single-use solution of 20 mg/ml
• Direct the stream of sterile water toward the wall of the vial and not directly at the cake or powder
• Gently swirl the vial to aid in dissolution; do not shake
• After reconstitution, withdraw desired amount from the vial and dilute immediately in 250 ml of 0.9% sodium chloride; do not use dextrose 5% solution; gently invert the bag to mix the solution in order to avoid foaming
• The reconstituted single-use product does not contain a preservative. Use the diluted solution immediately or store at 2-8 °C (36-46 °F) for up to 24 hr after reconstitution; discard any unused drug after 24 hr. Do not freeze.
IV infusion
• Closely monitor for possible subcutaneous infiltration during drug administration
• First infusion: Give over 90 min. The infusion rate should be slowed or interrupted if the patient develops an infusion-related reaction. Patients should be observed for at least 90 min following the initial dose for fever, chills, or

other infusion-related reactions. Permanently discontinue for life-threatening infusion-related reactions.
• Subsequent infusions: Administer over 30 min if prior infusions were well tolerated. The infusion rate should be slowed or interrupted if the patient develops an infusion-related reaction. Patients should be observed for at least 30 min after the infusion. Permanently discontinue for life-threatening infusion-related reactions

ADVERSE EFFECTS
CNS: Dizziness, insomnia, neuropathy, chills, fatigue, fever, flushing, headache
CV: Heart failure, tachycardia
EENT: Blurred vision, conjunctivitis, stomatitis
GI: Diarrhea, nausea, vomiting, abdominal pain, constipation, dyspepsia, hepatotoxicity
HEMA: Anemia, bleeding, thrombocytopenia
INTEG: Rash
MISC: Elevated LFTs, hand-foot syndrome
MS: Arthralgia
RESP: Cough, dyspnea, bronchospasm, pneumonitis, interstitial lung disease
SYST: Anaphylaxis

Pharmacokinetics
Absorption	Unknown
Distribution	93% Protein binding
Metabolism	Liver
Excretion	Unknown
Half-life	Unknown

Pharmacodynamics
Onset	Unknown
Peak	Unknown
Duration	Unknown

INTERACTIONS
Drug classifications
Anticoagulants, 5% dextrose, strong CYP3A4 inhibitors, platelets: avoid concurrent use
Do not give with other IV products

NURSING CONSIDERATIONS
Assessment
• Monitor liver function tests; pregnancy test;
• Monitor CBC, HER2 overexpression

> **BLACK BOX WARNING:** CHF, other cardiac symptoms: assess for dyspnea, coughing; gallop; obtain full cardiac workup including ECG, echo, MUGA

• Monitor for symptoms of infection; may be masked by product
• CNS reaction: monitor LOC, mental status, dizziness, confusion

> **BLACK BOX WARNING:** Monitor hypersensitive reactions, anaphylaxis

• Infusion reactions that may be fatal: monitor fever, chills, nausea, vomiting, pain, headache, dizziness, hypotension; discontinue product
• Pulmonary toxicity: monitor dyspnea, interstitial pneumonitis, pulmonary hypertension, ARDs: can occur after infusion reaction; those with lung disease may have more severe toxicity

> **BLACK BOX WARNING:** Hepatic disease: may be fatal

Patient/family education
• Teach patient to take acetaminophen for fever
• Teach patient to avoid hazardous tasks because confusion, dizziness may occur
• Teach patient to report signs of infection: sore throat, fever, diarrhea, vomiting, bleeding, decreased heart function/SOB with exertion, neuropathy, liver toxicity
• Teach patient that emotional lability is common: to notify prescriber if severe or incapacitating
• Teach patient to use contraception while taking this product; and for additional 6 months after discontinuing this drug; pregnancy (D); to avoid breastfeeding
• Teach patient to report pain at infusion site

Evaluation
Positive therapeutic outcome
• Decrease in size of tumors

> ⚠ **HIGH ALERT**
>
> ## afatinib
> (a-fat′i-nib)
> **Gilotrif**
> *Func. class.:* Antineoplastic biologic response modifiers
> *Chem. class.:* Signal transduction inhibitors (STIs), epidermal growth factor receptor tyrosine kinase inhibitor
> **Pregnancy category D**

Do not confuse: afatinib/afinitor/axitinib

ACTION: Selective inhibitor of EGFR (ErbB1), HER2 (ErbB2), and HER4 (ErbB4); irreversible, covalent binding of intracellular tyrosine kinase inhibiting (and causing regression in) tumor growth by decreasing EGFR signal transduction, cell cycle arrest, and inhibition of angiogenesis.

Therapeutic outcome: Decrease in progression of disease

USES: Treatment of non-small cell lung cancer whose tumors have epidermal growth factor receptor Exon 19 deletions or 21 substitution mutations

CONTRAINDICATIONS
Pregnancy **(D)**, hypersensitivity

Precautions: Contact lenses, dehydration, inflammation, keratitis, ocular disease, pneumonitis, pulmonary disease, renal disease, respiratory distress syndrome, serious rash, skin disease, diarrhea, hepatic disease, ocular disease

DOSAGE AND ROUTES
Adult: PO 40 mg/day

Dosage adjustments for toxicities
Hepatotoxicity
AST/ALT >5 to ≤20×ULN: withhold; resume at a reduced dose when AST/ALT is ≤5× ULN:
• First dose reduction: reduce the dose to 3 mg/kg
• Second dose reduction: reduce the dose to 2.4 mg/kg
• Requirement for further dose reduction: discontinue
AST/ALT >20× ULN: discontinue
Total bilirubin > 3 to ≤10× ULN: withhold; resume treatment at a reduced dose when total bilirubin recovers to ≤1.5:
• First dose reduction: reduce the dose to 3 mg/kg
• Second dose reduction: reduce the dose to 2.4 mg/kg
• Requirement for further dose reduction: discontinue treatment
Total bilirubin >10× ULN: permanently discontinue
• Permanently discontinue treatment in patients with AST/ALT >3× ULN and total bilirubin >2× ULN
• Permanently discontinue treatment in patients diagnosed with nodular regenerative hyperplasia (NRH)
Left ventricular ejection fraction *(LVEF)* 40%-45% and decrease is <10% points from baseline: continue treatment. Repeat LVEF assessment within 3 wk.
LVEF 40%-45% and decrease is ≥10% points from baseline: withhold; repeat LVEF assessment within 3 wk; if LVEF remains ≥10% points from baseline, discontinue
LVEF <40%: withhold; repeat LVEF assessment within 3 wk; if LVEF remains <40%, discontinue
Symptomatic congestive heart failure (CHF): discontinue

Thrombocytopenia
Platelet count 25,000/mm³ to <50,000/mm³: withhold; resume treatment at same dose when platelet count recovers to $75,000 /mm³
Platelet count <25,000/mm³: withhold; resume treatment at a reduced dose when platelet count recovers to ≥75,000/mm³.
• First dose reduction: reduce the dose to 3 mg/kg
• Second dose reduction: reduce the dose to 2.4 mg/kg
• Requirement for further dose reduction: discontinue
Pulmonary toxicity
• Permanently discontinue in patients diagnosed with interstitial lung disease or pneumonitis
Peripheral neuropathy
• Withhold in patients experiencing grade 3 or 4 peripheral neuropathy. Resume treatment upon resolution to ≤ grade 2

Available forms: Tabs 20, 30, 40 mg

Implementation
PO route
• Give on empty stomach 1 hr before, 2 hr after food
• Give at same time of day
• Do not take a missed dose if within 12 hr of next dose

ADVERSE EFFECTS
CNS: Fatigue, fever
CV: **Heart failure**
EENT: Blurred vision, conjunctivitis
GI: Diarrhea, nausea, vomiting, stomatitis, decreased appetite
HEMA: Anemia, **neutropenia, leukopenia,** epistaxis
INTEG: Rash, pruritus, acne vulgaris, photosensitivity, nail bed infections
MISC: Elevated LFTs, infection, **hand-foot syndrome,** dehydration, **renal failure,** cystitis, hypokalemia
MS: Arthralgia
RESP: Cough, dyspnea, **acute respiratory distress syndrome, interstitial lung disease, pneumonitis**

Pharmacokinetics	
Absorption	Unknown
Distribution	95% protein binding; time to steady state is approx. 8 days
Metabolism	Unknown
Excretion	Primarily excreted as unchanged drug in feces
Half-life	37 hr

Adverse effects: *italics* = common; **bold** = life-threatening

Pharmacodynamics

Onset	Unknown
Peak	2-5 hr
Duration	Unknown

INTERACTIONS
Drug classifications
P-gp inhibitors: increased afatinib effect

Drug/food
Grapefruit juice: increased afatinib effect; avoid use while taking product

Drug/herb
St. John's wort: increased afatinib concentrations

NURSING CONSIDERATIONS
Assessment

> **BLACK BOX WARNING:** Myelosuppression: anemia, neutropenia; obtain a CBC weekly × 1 mo, then monthly as needed; LFTs every mo × 3 mo, then as clinically indicated, hepatic failure may occur

Patient/family education
• Teach patient to report adverse reactions immediately, bleeding
• Teach patient about reason for treatment, expected results
• Teach patient to use effective contraception during treatment and up to 30 days after discontinuing treatment
• Teach patient to treat skin rash with topicals and oral antibiotics; use loperamide for diarrhea; if any side effect is severe or is persistent, contact prescriber
• Teach patient that complicated dosing changes may occur based on toxicity or drug-drug interaction
• Teach patient to take on empty stomach (at least 1 hr before or 2 hr after meal); do not take missed dose within 12 hr of next scheduled dose

Evaluation
Positive therapeutic outcome
• Decrease in progression of disease

> **albumin, human 5% (Rx)**
> (al-byoo'min)
> **Albumarc, Albuminar-5, Albutein 5%, Buminate 5%, Plasbumin-5**
> **albumin, human 25% (Rx)**
> Albuminar-25, Albutein 25%, Buminate 25%, Plasbumin-25
> *Func. class.:* Blood derivative—plasma volume expander
> **Pregnancy category C**

ACTION: Exerts colloidal oncotic pressure, which expands volume of circulating blood by pulling fluid from extravascular to intravascular spaces, and maintains cardiac output

Therapeutic outcome: Increased B/P, decreased edema, increased serum albumin levels, increased plasma protein

USES: Restores plasma volume in burns, hyperbilirubinemia, shock, hypoproteinemia, prevention of cerebral edema, cardiopulmonary bypass procedures, ARDS, hemorrhage; also replacement in nephrotic syndrome

CONTRAINDICATIONS
Hypersensitivity, CHF, severe anemia, renal insufficiency, pulmonary edema

Precautions: Pregnancy **C**, decreased salt intake, decreased cardiac reserve, lack of albumin deficiency, renal/hepatic disease, chronic anemia

DOSAGE AND ROUTES
Burns
Adult: **IV** dose to maintain plasma albumin at 3-4 mg/dl

Hypovolemic shock
Adult: **IV** Rapidly give 5% sol; when close to normal, infuse at ≤2-4 ml/min; 25% sol ≤1 ml/min
Child: 0.5-1 g/kg/dose, 5% sol, may repeat as needed; max 6 g/kg/day

Nephrotic syndrome
Adult: **IV** 100-200 mg of 25% and loop diuretic × 7-10 days

Hypoproteinemia
Adult: **IV** 25 g, may repeat in 15-30 min, or 50-75 g of 25% albumin infused at ≤2 ml/min
Child/infant: **IV** 0.5-1 g/kg/dose over 2-4 hr, may repeat q1-2days

Hyperbilirubinemia/erythroblastosis fetalis
Child: **IV** 1 g/kg 1-2 hr before transfusion

Available forms: Inj 50, 250 mg/ml (5%, 25%)

Implementation
IV route
• Check type of albumin; some are stored at room temperature, some need to be refrigerated; use only amber-colored sol without precipitate; solution should be clear, use within 4 hr of opening
• Give **IV** slowly to prevent fluid overload; 5% sol may be given undiluted; 25% sol may be given diluted (D₅W, 0.9% NaCl) or undiluted; give over 4 hr, use infusion pump
• Provide adequate hydration before, during administration; whole blood may need to be

given to prevent anemia; monitor hydration during treatment
• 5% sol may be used in hypovolemic/intravascular depletion
• 25% sol may be used in sodium/fluid restriction

Y-site compatibilities: Diltiazem

Solution compatibilities: LR, NaCl, Ringer's, D₅W, D₁₀W, D₂½W, dextrose/saline, dextran₆ D₅, dextran₆ NaCl 0.9%, dextrose/Ringer's, dextrose/LR

ADVERSE EFFECTS
CNS: Fever, chills, flushing, headache
CV: Fluid overload, hypotension, erratic pulse, tachycardia
GI: Nausea, vomiting, increased salivation
INTEG: Rash, urticaria
RESP: Altered respirations, **pulmonary edema**

Pharmacokinetics
Absorption	Complete bioavailability
Distribution	Intravascular spaces
Metabolism	Liver
Excretion	Unknown
Half-life	Terminal, 16-24 hr

Pharmacodynamics
Onset	15-30 min
Peak	Unknown
Duration	Unknown

INTERACTIONS
Drug/lab test
Increased: alkaline phosphatase

NURSING CONSIDERATIONS
Assessment
• Monitor blood studies: Hct, Hgb; if serum protein declines, dyspnea, hypoxemia can result; check for decreasing B/P, erratic pulse, respiration
• Adequate hydration before, during administration
• Check type of albumin; some stored at room temp, some need to be refrigerated, use within 4 hr of opening
⚠ Monitor CVP: **pulmonary wedge pressure will increase if overload occurs; I&O ratio: urinary output may decrease; CVP reading: distended neck veins indicate circulatory overload; shortness of breath, anxiety, insomnia, expiratory crackles, frothy blood-tinged sputum, cough, cyanosis indicate pulmonary overload**
• Assess for allergy: fever, rash, itching, chills, flushing, urticaria, nausea, vomiting, hypotension; requires discontinuation of infusion, use of new lot if therapy reinstituted; premedicate with diphenhydrAMINE

Patient/family education
• Explain use, reason for albumin; provide information on what to report to prescriber (hypersensitivity, fluid overload)

Evaluation
Positive therapeutic outcome
• Increased B/P, decreased edema (shock, burns)
• Increased serum albumin levels
• Increased plasma protein (hypoproteinemia)

---

albuterol (Rx)
(al-byoo′ter-ole)
AccuNeb, Salbutamol ✦, Airomir, ProAir HFA, ProAir RespiClick, Proventil, Proventil HFA, ReliOn, Ventolin HFA, Vospire ER
Func. class.: Bronchodilator
Chem. class.: Adrenergic β₂-agonist, sympathomimetic, bronchodilator
Pregnancy category C

Do not confuse: albuterol/atenolol/Albutein, **Proventil**/Prinivil, **Ventolin**/Vantin

ACTION: Causes bronchodilatation by action on β₂ (pulmonary) receptors by increasing levels of cyclic AMP, which relaxes smooth muscle; produces bronchodilatation; CNS, cardiac stimulation, increased diuresis, and increased gastric acid secretion; longer acting than isoproterenol

Therapeutic outcome: Increased ability to breathe because of bronchodilatation

USES: Prevention of exercise-induced asthma, acute bronchospasm, bronchitis, emphysema, bronchiectasis, reversible airway obstruction

Unlabeled uses: Hyperkalemia in dialysis patients, COPD, emphysema

CONTRAINDICATIONS
Hypersensitivity to sympathomimetics

Precautions: Pregnancy **C**, breastfeeding, exercise-induced bronchospasm (aerosol) in children <12 yr, cardiac/renal disease, hyperthyroidism, diabetes mellitus, hypertension, prostatic hypertrophy, closed-angle glaucoma, seizures, hypoglycemia, tachydysrhythmias, severe cardiac disease, heart block

DOSAGE AND ROUTES
Bronchospasm
Adult and child ≥4 yr: INH (metered dose inhaler) 2 puffs (180 mcg) q4-6hr prn;

Powdered inhaler (ProAir RespiClick) >12 yrs 180 mcg (2 INH) q4-6hr as needed

Other respiratory conditions
Adult and child ≥12 yr: INH (metered dose inhaler) 1 puff q4-6hr; PO 2-4 mg tid-qid, max 32 mg/day, depending on formulation; NEB/IPPB 2.5 mg tid-qid

Geriatric: PO 2 mg tid-qid, may increase gradually to 8 mg tid-qid

Child 2-12 yr: INH (metered dose inhaler) 0.1 mg/kg tid (max 2.5 mg tid-qid); NEB/IPPB 0.1-0.15 mg/kg/dose tid or 1.25 mg tid-qid for child 10-15 kg or 2.5 mg tid-qid >15 kg

Available forms: INH aerosol 108 mcg/actuation; tabs 2, 4 mg; oral syr 2 mg/5 ml; ext rel 4, 8 mg; inh sol 0.083, 0.5, 0.042%, 0.02%; powder inhaler 90 mcg/actuation

Implementation
PO route
• Do not break, crush, or chew ext rel tabs
• Give PO with meals to decrease gastric irritation; oral sol for children (no alcohol, sugar)
• In geriatric patients, a spacing device is advised

Aerosol route
• Give after shaking metered dose inhaler; have patient exhale and place mouthpiece in mouth, inhale slowly while depressing inhaler, hold breath, remove inhaler, exhale slowly; allow at least 1 min between inhalations; avoid using near flames or source of heat
• Track number of inhalations used and discard when labeled inhalations have been used
• Store in light-resistant container; do not expose to temperatures >86° F (30° C)

Albuterol Administration
ProAir RespiClick: Instruct patient on inhalation use; before using for the first time, check the dose counter window that the number 200 is in the window. The dose counter will count down each time the mouthpiece cap is opened and closed. The dose counter only displays even numbers; hold the inhaler upright while opening the cap fully; when the cap is opened, a dose will be activated for delivery; make sure a "click" is heard; do not open the cap unless ready to give dose; the patient should breathe out through the mouth and push as much air from the lungs as he or she can; be careful that the patient does not breathe out into the inhaler mouthpiece; put the mouthpiece in the mouth and have patient close lips around it; the patient should breathe in deeply through the mouth, until the lungs feel completely full of air; ensure that the vent above the mouthpiece is not blocked by the patient's lips or fingers; hold breath for about 10 sec; remove the inhaler; check dose counter on the back of the inhaler to make sure the dose was received; close the cap over the mouthpiece after each use of the inhaler; make sure the cap closes firmly into place; to inhale another dose, close the cap and then repeat inhaler steps; do not wash or put any part of the inhaler in water; if the mouthpiece needs cleaning, gently wipe with a dry cloth or tissue; when there are 20 doses left, the counter will change to red; refill

Nebulizer/IPPB route
• **Dilute** 5 mg/ml sol/2.5 ml 0.9% NaCl for inhalation; other solutions do not require dilution for nebulizer O_2 flow or compressed air 6-10 L/min

ADVERSE EFFECTS
CNS: *Tremors, anxiety,* insomnia, headache, dizziness, stimulation, *restlessness,* hallucinations, flushing, irritability
CV: *Palpitations, tachycardia, hypertension,* angina, hypotension, dysrhythmias
EENT: Dry nose, irritation of nose and throat
GI: *Heartburn, nausea, vomiting*
MISC: Flushing, sweating, anorexia, bad taste/smell changes, hypokalemia
MS: Muscle cramps
RESP: Cough, wheezing, dyspnea, **bronchospasm,** dry throat

Pharmacokinetics

Absorption	Well absorbed (PO)
Distribution	Unknown
Metabolism	Liver extensively, tissues
Excretion	Unknown, breast milk
Half-life	3-4 hr

Pharmacodynamics

	PO	PO–ext rel	INH
Onset	½ hr	½ hr	5-15 min
Peak	2½ hr	2-3 hr	1½-2hr
Duration	2 hr	12 hr	4-6 hr

INTERACTIONS
Individual drugs
Atomoxetine, selegiline: increased CV effects
Digoxin: increased digoxin level

Drug classifications
Adrenergics: increased action of albuterol; do not use together
β-Adrenergic blockers: block therapeutic effect
Bronchodilators (aerosol): increased action of bronchodilator
CNS stimulants: increased CNS stimulation
Diuretics (potassium-losing): increased ECG changes/hypokalemia

MAOIs, tricyclics: increased chance of hypertensive crisis; do not use together
Other drugs that increase QT prolongation: increased QTc prolongation
Oxytocics: severe hypotension; do not use together
Theophylline: toxicity

Drug/herb
Black tea, green tea, kola nut, guarana, yerba maté: increased stimulation

Drug/food
Caffeine products, chocolate: increased stimulation

Drug/lab test
Decreased: potassium

NURSING CONSIDERATIONS
Assessment
• Assess respiratory function: vital capacity, forced expiratory volume, ABGs, lung sounds; heart rate, rhythm; B/P, sputum (baseline and during therapy)
• Determine that patient has not received theophylline therapy before giving dose, to prevent additive effect; client's ability to self-medicate
• **Monitor for evidence of allergic reactions; paradoxic bronchospasm; withhold dose; notify prescriber if bronchospasm occurs**

Patient/family education
• Tell patient not to use OTC medications before consulting prescriber; excess stimulation may occur; instruct patient to use this medication before other medications and allow at least 5 min between each to prevent overstimulation; to limit caffeine products such as chocolate, coffee, tea, and cola
• Teach patient to use inhaler; review package insert with patient; to avoid getting aerosol in eyes or blurring may result; to wash inhaler in warm water and dry daily; to rinse mouth after using; to avoid smoking, smoke-filled rooms, persons with respiratory infections, about when to empty and when to renew
⚠ Teach patient that if paradoxic bronchospasm occurs to stop product immediately and notify prescriber
• Instruct patient on administration of dose, not to use more than prescribed; serious side effects may occur; if taking PO regularly and dose is missed, take when remembered; space other doses on new time schedule; do not double doses
• In geriatric patients, a spacing device is advised

Evaluation
Positive therapeutic outcome
• Absence of dyspnea and wheezing after 1 hr
• Improved airway exchange
• Improved ABGs

TREATMENT OF OVERDOSE:
Administer a β_1-adrenergic blocker, **IV** fluids

RARELY USED

alemtuzumab
(al'em-tooz'ue-mab)
Lemtrada
Func. class.: Biologic response modifier

USES: Reserved for those with multiple sclerosis with inadequate response to ≥ 2 drugs because of severe adverse reactions

CONTRAINDICATIONS: HIV

DOSAGE AND ROUTES
Adult: IV 12 mg/day for 5 consecutive days (total 60 mg) for a first treatment course; follow 12 mo later with 12 mg/day for 3 consecutive days (total 36 mg) for a second treatment course

---

alendronate (Rx)
(al-en'droe-nate)
Apo-Alendronate ✦, CO Alendronate, Fosamax, Fosamax plus D
Func. class.: Bone-resorption inhibitor
Chem. class.: Bisphosphonate
Pregnancy category C   ✳

Do not confuse: Fosamax/Flomax

ACTION: Decreases rate of bone resorption and may directly block dissolution of hydroxyapatite crystals of bone; inhibits osteoclast activity

Therapeutic outcome: Decreased symptoms of osteoporosis, Paget's disease

USES: Treatment and prevention of osteoporosis in postmenopausal women, treatment of osteoporosis in men, Paget's disease, treatment of corticosteroid-induced osteoporosis in postmenopausal women not receiving estrogen, or in men who are continuing corticosteroid treatment with low bone mass

CONTRAINDICATIONS
Hypersensitivity to bisphosphonates, delayed esophageal emptying, inability to sit or stand for 30 min, hypocalcemia

Precautions: Pregnancy **C,** breastfeeding, children, CCr <35 ml/min, esophageal disease, increased esophageal cancer risk, ulcers, gastritis, poor dental health

DOSAGE AND ROUTES
Osteoporosis in postmenopausal women
Adult and geriatric: PO 10 mg daily or 70 mg qwk

Paget's disease
Adult and geriatric: PO 40 mg daily × 6 mo, consider retreatment for relapse

Prevention of osteoporosis
Adult (postmenopausal females): PO 5 mg daily or 35 mg qwk

Renal dose
Adult: PO CCr ≤35 ml/min, not recommended

Available forms: Tabs 5, 10, 35, 40, 70 mg, tabs 70 mg with 2800 IU Vit D$_3$, 70 mg with 5600 IU Vit D$_3$; oral sol 70 mg/75 ml

Implementation
• Give PO for 6 mo to be effective in Paget's disease; take with 8 oz of water 30 min before 1st food, beverage, or medication of the day
• Patient to remain upright for 30 min after dose to prevent esophageal irritation
• Store in cool environment out of direct sunlight
Tablet:
• Do not lie down for ≥30 min after dose, do not take at bedtime
Liquid:
• Use oral syringe or calibrated device; give in AM with ≥2 oz of water ≥30 min before food, beverage, or medication

ADVERSE EFFECTS
CNS: Headache
GI: Abdominal pain, constipation, nausea, vomiting, esophageal ulceration, acid reflux, dyspepsia, **esophageal perforation**, diarrhea, **esophageal cancer**
META: Hypophosphatemia, hypocalcemia
MS: Bone pain, **osteonecrosis of the jaw, bone fractures**
SYST: Angioedema, Stevens-Johnson syndrome, toxic epidermal necrolysis

Pharmacokinetics

Distribution	Mainly to bones; protein binding 78%
Metabolism	Unknown
Excretion	Via kidneys after bound to bone
Half-life	>10 yrs

Pharmacodynamics
Unknown

INTERACTIONS
Drug classifications
Antacids, calcium supplements: decreased absorption
H$_2$ blockers, proton pump inhibitors (PPIs), gastric mucosal agents, NSAIDs, salicylates: adverse GI reactions

Drug/food
Caffeine, food, orange juice: decreased product absorption

Drug/lab test
Decreased: calcium, phosphate

NURSING CONSIDERATIONS
Assessment
⚠ **Assess for serious reactions: angioedema, Stevens-Johnson syndrome, toxic epidermal necrolysis, atrial fibrillation**
• Assess dental status, regular dental exams should be done; dental extractions (cover with antiinfectives) prior to procedure
• Hormonal status if a woman, prior to treatment
• Assess for **osteoporosis:** bone density testing
• For **Paget's disease:** increased skull size, bone pain, headache
• Monitor renal studies and electrolytes (calcium, potassium, magnesium, phosphorous) BUN/creatinine
• Assess for **hypercalcemia:** paresthesia, twitching, laryngospasm, Chvostek's, Trousseau's signs
• Monitor alkaline phosphatase; level of 2 × upper limit of normal is indicated for Paget's disease

Patient/family education
• Teach patient to remain upright for 30 min after dose to prevent esophageal irritation; if dose is missed, skip dose, do not double doses or take later in day
• Teach patient to take in AM, only before food, other meds, to take with 6-8 oz of water (not mineral water)
• Teach patient to take calcium, vit D if instructed by provider
• Teach patient to use weight-bearing exercise to increase bone density
• Teach patient to let provider know if pregnancy is planned or suspected or if nursing
• Advise to maintain good oral hygiene

Evaluation
Positive therapeutic outcome
• Increased bone mass, absence of fractures

alfuzosin (Rx)

(al-fyoo'zoe-sin)
Uroxatral, Xatral ✣
Func. class.: Urinary tract, antispasmodic,
α_1-agonist
Chem. class.: Quinazolone
Pregnancy category B

ACTION: Binds preferentially to α_{1A}-adrenoceptor subtype located mainly in the prostate, relaxing smooth muscles

Therapeutic outcome: Resolution of symptoms of benign prostatic hyperplasia

USES: Symptoms of benign prostatic hyperplasia

CONTRAINDICATIONS

Hypersensitivity, moderate to severe hepatic impairment, not indicated for use in women or children, breastfeeding (but not used in women)

Precautions: Pregnancy **B**, geriatric, coronary artery disease, coronary insufficiency, mild hepatic disease, mild/moderate/severe renal disease, history of QT prolongation or coadministration with medications known to prolong QT interval, torsades de pointes, syncope, surgery, prostate cancer, orthostatic hypotension, ocular surgery, CAD, dysrhythmias, angina

DOSAGE AND ROUTES
Adult: PO EXT REL 10 mg daily, taken after same meal each day

Available forms: EXT REL tabs 10 mg

Implementation
• Swallow tabs whole; do not break, crush, or chew tabs
• Store in tight container in cool environment

ADVERSE EFFECTS
CNS: *Dizziness, headache,* fatigue, flushing
CV: Postural hypotension (dizziness, light-headedness, fainting) within a few hours of administration, chest pain, tachycardia, angina
GI: Nausea, abdominal pain, dyspepsia, constipation, diarrhea, liver injury, jaundice
GU: Impotence, priapism
HEMA: **Thrombocytopenia**
INTEG: Rash, urticaria, **angioedema**, pruritus, **toxic epidermal necrolysis**
MISC: Body pain in general, xerostomia, rhinitis
RESP: Upper respiratory tract infection, pharyngitis, bronchitis, sinusitis

Absorption	Unknown
Distribution	Moderately protein bound (82%-90%)
Metabolism	Liver (by CYP3A4 enzyme)
Excretion	Urine
Half-life	10 hr

Unknown

INTERACTIONS
Individual drugs
Alcohol: possible increased effects of alfuzosin
Doxaconazole, itraconazole, ketoconazole, prazosin, ritonavir, terazosin: do not take concurrently

Drug classifications
b-Blockers, nitrates, antihypertensives, phosphodiesterase 5 inhibitors: increased hypotension
CYP3A4 inhibitors, cimetidine (ketoconazole, itraconazole, ritonavir): do not take concurrently, **toxic epidermal necrolysis**

NURSING CONSIDERATIONS
Assessment
• Assess for prostatic hyperplasia: change in urinary patterns, baseline and throughout treatment
• Monitor CBC with differential and liver function tests; B/P and heart rate; QT prolongation
• Monitor BUN, uric acid, urodynamic studies (urinary flow rates, residual volume)
• Monitor I&O ratios, weight daily, edema; report weight gain or edema

Patient/family education
• Advise not to drive or operate machinery for 4 hr after first dose or after dosage increase, meds, herbs

Evaluation
Positive therapeutic outcome
• Decreased symptoms of benign prostatic hyperplasia

aliskiren (Rx)

(a-lis'kir-en)
Tekturna, Rasilez ✣
Func. class.: Antihypertensive
Chem. class.: Direct renin inhibitor
Pregnancy category D

ACTION: Renin inhibitor that acts on the renin-angiotensin system (RAS)

Adverse effects: *italics* = common; **bold** = life-threatening

Therapeutic outcome: Decrease in B/P

USES: Hypertension, alone or in combination with other antihypertensives

CONTRAINDICATIONS
Hypersensitivity

BLACK BOX WARNING: Pregnancy **D**

Precautions: Breastfeeding, children, geriatric, angioedema, aortic/renal artery stenosis, cirrhosis, CAD, dialysis, hyper/hypokalemia, hyponatremia, hypotension, hypovolemia, renal/hepatic disease, surgery, diabetes

DOSAGE AND ROUTES
Adult: PO 150 mg/day, may increase to 300 mg/day if needed, max 300 mg/day

Available forms: Tabs 150, 300 mg

Implementation
- May use with other antihypertensives
- PO; do not use with a high-fat meal
- Give daily with a full glass of water, titrate up to achieve correct dose
- Do not discontinue abruptly; correct electrolyte/volume depletion prior to treatment
- Store in tight container at room temperature

ADVERSE EFFECTS
CNS: Headache, dizziness, seizures
CV: Orthostatic hypotension, hypotension
GI: *Diarrhea*
GU: Renal stones, increased uric acid
INTEG: Rash
META: Hyperkalemia
MISC: Angioedema, cough

Pharmacokinetics

Absorption	Poor, bioavailability 2.5%
Distribution	Steady state 7-8 days
Metabolism	Unknown
Excretion	91% unchanged in the feces
Half-life	Unknown

Pharmacodynamics

Onset	Unknown
Peak	1-3 hr
Duration	Unknown

INTERACTIONS
Individual drugs
Atorvastatin, cycloSPORINE, itraconazole, ketoconazole: increased aliskiren levels, concurrent use is not recommended
Warfarin: decreased levels of warfarin

Drug classifications
Do not use with ACE inhibitors, angiotensin II receptor antagonists, potassium-sparing diuretics, potassium supplements: increased potassium levels
Diuretics, other antihypertensives: increased hypotension
Do not use ACE inhibitors, angiotensin II receptor antagonists in diabetes mellitus

Drug/food
High-fat meal: aliskiren effect, grapefruit

Drug/lab test
Increased: uric acid, BUN, serum creatinine, potassium

NURSING CONSIDERATIONS
Assessment
- Monitor renal tests: uric acid, serum creatinine, BUN may be increased; hyperkalemia may occur
- Assess for allergic reactions: angioedema may occur
- Monitor daily dependent edema in feet, legs; weight, B/P, orthostatic hypotension
- Diabetes: Identify the use of ACE inhibitors, angiotensin II receptor antagonists, do not use with aliskiren

Patient/family education

BLACK BOX WARNING: Teach patient to notify prescriber if pregnancy is planned or suspected; if pregnant, product will need to be discontinued (pregnancy **D**)

- Teach patient the importance of complying with dosage schedule even if feeling better
- Instruct patient to notify if pregnancy is planned or suspected; if pregnant, product needs to be discontinued
- Teach patient how to take B/P and normal reading for age-group
- Advise patient that if dose is missed, take as soon as possible; if it is almost time for the next dose, take only that dose; do not double dose
- Instruct patient not to use OTC products, including herbs, supplements unless approved by prescriber
- Advise patient to report to prescriber immediately: dizziness, faintness, chest pain, palpitations, uneven or rapid heart beat, headache, severe diarrhea, swelling of tongue or lips, trouble breathing, difficulty swallowing, tightening of the throat
- Caution patient not to operate machinery or perform hazardous tasks if dizziness occurs
- Advise patient to rise slowly in order to avoid faintness

Evaluation
Positive therapeutic outcome
• Decrease in B/P

allopurinol (Rx)
(al-oh-pure′i-nole)
Alloprin ✚, Purinol 1, Aloprim, Zyloprim
Func. class.: Antigout drug, antihyperuricemic
Chem. class.: Xanthine enzyme inhibitor
Pregnancy category C

Do not confuse: Zyloprim/Zovirax/ZORprin/zolpidem

ACTION: Inhibits the enzyme xanthine oxidase, reducing uric acid synthesis

Therapeutic outcome: Decreasing serum uric acid levels, decreasing joint pain

USES: Chronic gout, hyperuricemia associated with malignancies, recurrent calcium oxalate calculi, uric acid calculi

CONTRAINDICATIONS
Hypersensitivity

Precautions: Pregnancy **C**, breastfeeding, children, renal/hepatic disease

DOSAGE AND ROUTES
Increased uric acid levels in malignancies
Adult: PO 600-800 mg/day in divided doses, for 2-3 days; start up to 1-2 days prior to chemotherapy; **IV** INF 200-400 mg/m²/day, max 600 mg/day 24-48 hr prior to chemotherapy, may be divided at 6-, 8-, 12-hr intervals
Child 6-10 yr: PO 300 mg/day, adjust dose after 48 hr
Child <6 yr: PO 150 mg/day, adjust dose after 48 hr
Child: **IV** INF 200 mg/m²/day, initially as a single dose or divided q6-12hr

Gout (mild)
Adult: PO 200-300 mg/day, increase qwk based on uric acid levels, max 800 mg/day

Gout (moderate-severe)
Adult: PO 400-600 mg/day in a single dose or divided bid-tid, max 800 mg/day, doses >300 mg should be given in divided doses, may start during an acute attack as long as antiinflammatories are being used

Recurrent calculi
Adult: PO 200-300 mg/day in a single dose or divided bid-tid

Uric acid nephropathy prevention
Adult and child >10 yr: PO 600-800 mg daily × 2-3 days

Renal dose
Adult: PO/IV CCr 81-100 ml/min 300 mg/day; CCr 61-80 ml/min 250 mg/day; CCr 41-60 ml/min 200 mg/day; CCr 21-40 ml/min 150 mg/day; CCr 10-20 ml/min 100-200 mg/day; CCr 3-9 ml/min 100 mg/day or 100 mg every other day; CCr <3 ml/min 100 mg q24hr or longer or 100 mg every third day

Available forms: Tabs, scored, 100, 300 mg; powder for inj 500 mg/vial

Implementation
PO route
• Give with meals to prevent GI symptoms; crush and mix with food or fluids for patients with swallowing difficulties
• Increase fluid intake to 2 L/day
• Begin 1-2 days before antineoplastic therapy if using for hyperuricemia associated with malignancy

Intermittent IV infusion route
• Reconstitute 30-ml vial with 25 ml of sterile water for inj; dilute to desired conc (≤6 mg/ml) with 0.9% NaCl for inj or D₅ for inj, begin inf within 10 hr

IV compatibilities: Acyclovir, aminophylline, amphotericin B lipid complex, anidulafungin, argatroban, atenolol, aztreonam, bivalirudin, bleomycin, bumetanide, buprenorphine, butorphanol, calcium gluconate, CARBOplatin, caspofungin, ceFAZolin, cefoTEtan, cefTAZidime, ceftizoxime, cefTRIAXone, cefuroxime, CISplatin, cyclophosphamide, DACTINomycin, DAUNOrubicin liposome, dexamethasone, dexmedetomidine, DOCEtaxel, DOXOrubicin liposomal, enalaprilat, etoposide, famotidine, fenoldopam, filgrastim, fluconazole, fludarabine, fluorouracil, furosemide, gallium, ganciclovir, gatifloxacin, gemcitabine, gemtuzumab, granisetron, heparin, hydrocortisone phosphate, hydrocortisone succinate, HYDROmorphone, ifosfamide, linezolid, LORazepam, mannitol, mesna, methotrexate, metroNIDAZOLE, milrinone, mitoXANtrone, morphine, nesiritide, octreotide, oxytocin, PACLitaxel, pamidronate, pantoprazole, PEMEtrexed, piperacillin, piperacillin-tazobactam, plicamycin, potassium chloride, ranitidine, sodium, sulfamethoxazole-trimethoprim, teniposide, thiotepa, ticarcillin, ticarcillin clavulanate, tigecycline, tirofiban, vancomycin, vasopressin, vinBLAStine, vinCRIStine, voriconazole, zidovudine, zoledronic acid

Adverse effects: *italics* = common; **bold** = life-threatening

ADVERSE EFFECTS
GI: *Nausea, vomiting, malaise,* cramps, diarrhea
INTEG: rash
MS: Acute gouty attack

Pharmacokinetics

Absorption	80%
Distribution	Widely distributed
Metabolism	Liver to oxypurinol
Excretion	Kidneys
Half-life	1-2 hr

Pharmacodynamics

	PO	IV
Onset	Unknown	Unknown
Peak	1½ hr	Up to 30 min
Duration	Unknown	Unknown

INTERACTIONS
Individual drugs
Ammonium chloride, potassium/sodium phosphate, vit C: increased kidney stone formation
Ampicillin, amoxicillin: increased risk of rash, avoid concurrent use
AzaTHIOprine: increased bone marrow depression
Mercaptopurine: increased bone marrow depression
Rasburicase: increased xanthine nephropathy, calculi
Theophylline: increased action of theophylline

Drug classifications
ACE inhibitors: increased hypersensitivity, toxicity
Anticoagulants (oral): increased action of oral anticoagulants
Antidiabetics (oral): increased action of antidiabetics
Antineoplastics: increased bone marrow suppression
Diuretics (thiazide): increased hypersensitivity

NURSING CONSIDERATIONS
Assessment
• Assess for **pain** including location, characteristics, onset/duration, frequency, quality, intensity or severity of pain, precipitating factors; **gout:** joint pain, swelling, may use with NSAIDs for acute gouty attacks
• Monitor uric acid levels q2wk; normal uric acid levels are 6 mg/dl or less; effect may take several wk; check I&O ratio, increase fluids to 2 L/day to prevent stone formation, toxicity
• Monitor CBC, AST, BUN, creatinine before starting treatment, monthly; check blood glucose in diabetic patients receiving oral antidiabetic agents

Patient/family education
• Tell patient to increase fluid intake to 2 L/day; to avoid taking large doses of vit C; kidney stone formation may occur; to maintain a diet enhancing urine alkalinity (e.g., milk, other dairy products); if taking for calcium oxalate stones, reduce dairy products, refined sugar, sodium, meat
• Tell patient to report skin rash, stomatitis, malaise, fever, aching; product should be discontinued
• Advise patient to avoid hazardous activities if drowsiness or dizziness occurs; response may take several days to determine
• Tell patient to avoid alcohol, caffeine; these substances increase uric acid levels and decrease allopurinol levels
• Teach patient to report side effects and adverse reactions to prescriber, including rash, itching, nausea, vomiting

Evaluation
Positive therapeutic outcome
• Decreased pain in joints
• Decreased stone formation in kidney
• Decreased uric acid level to 6 mg/dl

almotriptan (Rx)
(al-moh-trip′tan)
Axert
Func. class.: Antimigraine agent
Chem. class.: 5-HT₁ receptor agonist, triptan
Pregnancy category C

Do not confuse: Axert/Antivert

ACTION: Binds selectively to the vascular 5-HT$_{1B/1D/1F}$ receptor subtype, exerts antimigraine effect; causes vasoconstriction in cranial arteries

Therapeutic outcome: Absence of migraines

USES: Acute treatment of migraine with or without aura (Adults/adolescents/children ≥12 yr)

CONTRAINDICATIONS
Hypersensitivity, acute MI, angina, CV disease, CAD, stroke, vasospastic angina, ischemic heart disease or risk for, peripheral vascular syndrome; uncontrolled hypertension, basilar or hemiplegic migraine

Precautions: Pregnancy **C**, breastfeeding, children <18 yr, geriatric, postmenopausal women, men >40 yr, risk factors for coronary artery disease, MI, hypercholesterolemia, obesity, diabetes, impaired renal/hepatic function, sulfonamide hypersensitivity, cardiac dysrhythmias, Raynaud's disease, tobacco smoking, Wolff-Parkinson-White syndrome

DOSAGE AND ROUTES

Adult/adolescent/child ≥12 yr: PO 6.25-12.5 mg, may repeat dose after 2 hr; max 2 doses/24 hr, 25 mg/day, or 4 treatment cycles within any 30-day period

Renal/hepatic dose (CCr 10-30 ml/hr)
Adult: PO 6.25 mg initially, max 12.5 mg

Available forms: Tabs 6.25 or 12.5 mg

Implementation

• Swallow tabs whole; do not break, crush, or chew tabs, without regard to food 2 times/24 hr
• Provide quiet, calm environment with decreased stimulation from noise, bright light, excessive talking

ADVERSE EFFECTS

CNS: *Dizziness,* headache, **seizures,** paresthesias
CV: *Flushing,* palpitations, tachycardia, **coronary artery vasospasm, MI, ventricular fibrillation, ventricular tachycardia**
EENT: Throat, mouth, nasal discomfort; vision changes
GI: Nausea, xerostomia
INTEG: Sweating, rash
MS: *Weakness, neck stiffness,* myalgia
RESP: Chest tightness, pressure

Pharmacokinetics

Absorption	Well absorbed (~70%)
Distribution	35% protein bound
Metabolism	Liver (metabolite); metabolized by MAO-A, CYP2D6, CYP3A4
Excretion	Urine 40%, feces 13%
Half-life	3-4 hr

Pharmacodynamics

Onset	Unknown
Peak	1-3 hr
Duration	3-4 hr

INTERACTIONS
Individual drugs

Ergot: increased vasospastic effects, avoid concurrent use

Erythromycin, itraconazole, ketoconazole, ritonavir: increased plasma concentration of almotriptan, avoid concurrent use in renal/hepatic disease

Drug classifications

5-HT$_1$ agonists, ergot derivatives: increased vasospastic effects, avoid concurrent use

CYP2D6 inhibitors: increased almotriptan effect; do not use together

MAOIs: increased almotriptan effect; do not use together

SSRIs, SNRIs, serotonin-receptor agonists, sibutramine: increased serotonin syndrome

Drug/herb

Feverfew: avoid use
St. John's wort: increased serotonin syndrome

NURSING CONSIDERATIONS
Assessment

• Assess B/P, signs/symptoms of coronary vasospasms
• Assess for tingling, hot sensation, burning, feeling of pressure, numbness, flushing
• Assess for stress level, activity, recreation, coping mechanisms
• Assess neurologic status: LOC, blurring vision, nausea, vomiting, tingling in extremities preceding headache
• Assess for ingestion of **tyramine-containing foods** (pickled products, beer, wine, aged cheese), food additives, preservatives, colorings, artificial sweeteners, chocolate, caffeine, which may precipitate these types of headaches
• Assess for **migraine:** pain, location, aura, duration, intensity, nausea, vomiting
• **Assess for serotonin syndrome: occurs in those taking SSRIs, SNRIs; agitation, confusion, hallucinations, diaphoresis, hypertension, diarrhea, fever, tremor, usually occurs when dose is increased**

Patient/family education

• Instruct patient to use contraception while taking product, notify prescriber if pregnancy is planned or suspected, avoid breastfeeding
• Advise patient to have dark, quiet environment available
• Inform patient that product does not prevent or reduce number of migraine attacks, max 4 doses/30 days, do not take MAOIs for ≥ 24 hr
• Advise patient to report chest pain, drowsiness, dizziness, tingling, flushing

Evaluation

Positive therapeutic outcome
• Decrease in severity of migraine

Adverse effects: *italics* = common; **bold** = life-threatening

TREATMENT OF OVERDOSE:
Gastric lavage followed by activated charcoal; clinical and ECG monitoring for ≥20 hr after overdose

alogliptin
(al'oh glip'tin)
Nesina
Func. class.: Antidiabetic
Chem. class.: Dipeptidyl peptidase-4 (DPP-4) inhibitor
Pregnancy category B

ACTION: A dipeptidyl peptidase-4 (DPP-4) inhibitor for the treatment of type 2 diabetes mellitus (monotherapy or in combination with other antidiabetic agents), potentiates the effects of the incretin hormones by inhibiting their breakdown by DPP-4

Therapeutic outcome: Decrease in polyuria, polydipsia, polyphagia; clear sensorium, absence of dizziness; improvement in A1c, daily blood glucose monitoring

USES: Type 2 diabetes mellitus (T2DM)

CONTRAINDICATIONS
Hypersensitivity

Precautions: Pregnancy (B), breastfeeding, hepatic disease, burns, ketoacidosis, diarrhea, fever, GI obstruction, hyper/hypoglycemia, hyper/hypothyroidism, type 1 diabetes, hypercortisolism, children, ileus, malnutrition, pancreatitis, surgery, trauma, vomiting, kidney disease, adrenal insufficiency, angioedema

DOSAGE AND ROUTES
Adult: **PO** 25 mg/day; when used in combination, a lower dose of the other antidiabetic may be needed

Renal dose
Adult: PO CCr 30-59 ml/min: 12.5 mg/day; CCr 30 ml/min: 6.25 mg/day; intermittent hemodialysis: 6.25 mg/day; give without regard to the timing of hemodialysis

Available forms: Tab 6.25, 12.5, 25

Implementation
Give without regard to food

ADVERSE EFFECTS
CNS: Headache
GI: Pancreatitis
META: Hypoglycemia
RESP: Upper respiratory infection, nasopharyngitis
SYST: Rash, hypersensitivity, angioedema, Stevens–Johnson syndrome, anaphylaxis

Pharmacokinetics
Absorption	Unknown
Distribution	Unknown
Metabolism	Unknown
Excretion	Unchanged (urine)
Half-life	Unknown

Pharmacodynamics
Onset	Unknown
Peak	1-2 hr
Duration	Effect decreased (liver disease), increased (kidney disease), half-life 21 hr

INTERACTIONS
Increase: Hypoglycemia-insulin, sulfonylureas

Drug/lab test
Increased: LFTs
Decrease: Glucose

NURSING CONSIDERATIONS
Assessment
• Diabetes: monitor blood glucose, glycosylated hemoglobin (A1c), LFTs, serum creatinine/BUN
• **Assess for pancreatitis: can occur anytime during use**
• **Monitor for hypersensitivity reactions: angioedema**
• **Assess for Stevens-Johnson syndrome**

Patient/family education
• Inform patient that diabetes is a life-long condition; product does not cure disease
• Advise patient to consume all food on diet plan, to continue other medical and lifestyle regimens
• Teach patient to carry emergency ID with prescriber, medications, and condition listed
• Teach patient to test blood glucose using a blood glucose meter

Evaluation
Positive therapeutic outcome
• Decrease in polyuria, polydipsia, polyphagia, clear sensorium, absence of dizziness, improvement in A1c, daily blood glucose monitoring
• To report allergic reactions, nausea, vomiting, abdominal pain, dark urine

alosetron
(ah-loss'a-tron)
Lotronex
Func. class.: Antidiarrheal, anti-IBS agent; serotonin receptor antagonist
Pregnancy category B

Do not confuse: Lotronex/Lovenox

ACTION: A potent and selective antagonist at serotonin 5-HT3 receptors; 5-HT3 receptors are extensively distributed on enteric neurons in the GI tract; antagonism at these receptors in the GI tract modulate the regulation of visceral pain, colonic transit, and GI secretions

Therapeutic outcome: Decreased irritable bowel syndrome (IBS) symptoms

USES: Severe-diarrhea-predominant IBS

CONTRAINDICATIONS: Crohn's disease, severe hepatic disease, toxic megacolon, GI adhesions/strictures/obstruction, thrombophlebitis, ulcerative colitis

> **BLACK BOX WARNING:** Ischemic colitis, severe constipation

Precautions: Pregnancy B, breastfeeding, child <18 yr, mild to moderate hepatic disease

DOSAGE AND ROUTES
Adult (woman): **PO** 0.5 mg bid, may increase to 1 mg bid after 4 wk if well tolerated; discontinue if symptoms are not controlled after 4 wk

Available forms: Tab 0.5 mg

Implementation
• Give without regard to meals with full glass of water
• Store at room temperature, protect from light and moisture

> **BLACK BOX WARNING:** Use only after "Patient Acknowledgement Form" is signed

ADVERSE EFFECTS
GI: Constipation, abdominal pain, distention, reflux, nausea, **obstruction**, impaction, **ischemic colitis, ileus perforation, small-bowel mesenteric ischemia**

Pharmacokinetics

Absorption	Unknown
Distribution	Unknown
Metabolism	Extensively in the liver
Excretion	Unknown, mainly excreted in urine
Half-life	1½ hr

Pharmacodynamics

Onset	Unknown
Peak	1 hr
Duration	Unknown

INTERACTIONS
Drug classifications
CYP3A4 inhibitors, hydrALAZINE, procainamide: decreased alosetron metabolism
CYP3A4 inducers: increased alosetron metabolism

Drug/lab test
Increased: ALT

NURSING CONSIDERATIONS
Assessment

> **BLACK BOX WARNING:** Irritable bowel syndrome: Assess for constipation, diarrhea, abdominal pain, fecal incontinence; discontinue immediately if bloody diarrhea, severe constipation, rectal bleeding, or severe abdominal pain occur

> **BLACK BOX WARNING:** Only clinicians enrolled in the Lotronex prescribing program should use this product

• Geriatric women: assess for more severe side effects

Patient/family education

> **BLACK BOX WARNING:** Teach patient to report immediately, severe constipation, bloody diarrhea, rectal bleeding or worsening abdominal pain

• Instruct patient not to double doses; if a dose is missed, it should be skipped, do not take with other meds or herbs without prescriber approval
• Advise patient that product may be taken without regard to food
• Advise patient that product does not cure disorder, but only controls symptoms
• Provide medication guide and clarify if needed, improvement in symptoms can take 1-4 wk
• Teach patient that product is used only for women with IBS
• **Advise patient to report if pregnancy is planned or suspected; product should not be used during pregnancy—effects are unknown**

Evaluation
Positive therapeutic outcome
• Decreasing symptoms of IBS

ALPRAZolam (Rx)

(al-pray′zoe-lam)
**Apo-Alpraz ✹, Novo-Alprazol ✹,
Niravam, Nu-Alpraz ✹, Xanax,
Xanax XR**

Func. class.: Antianxiety/sedative/
hypnotic
Chem. class.: Benzodiazepine, short/
intermediate acting
Pregnancy category D
Controlled substance schedule IV

Do not confuse: ALPRAZolam/
LORazepam, **X**anax/Lanoxin/Tylox/
Zantac

ACTION: Depresses subcortical levels of
CNS, including limbic system, reticular formation

Therapeutic outcome: Decreased anxiety

USES: Anxiety, panic disorders with or without
agoraphobia, anxiety with depressive symptoms

Unlabeled uses: Premenstrual dysphoric
disorder, insomnia, PMS, alcohol withdrawal
syndrome

CONTRAINDICATIONS

Pregnancy **D**, breastfeeding, hypersensitivity to
benzodiazepines, closed-angle glaucoma, psychosis, addiction

Precautions: Geriatric, debilitated, hepatic
disease, obesity, severe pulmonary disease

DOSAGE AND ROUTES
Anxiety disorder
Adult: PO 0.25-0.5 mg tid, may increase q3-
4days if needed, max 4 mg/day in divided doses
Geriatric: PO 0.125-0.25 mg bid; increase by
0.125 mg prn

Panic disorder
Adult: PO 0.5 mg tid, may increase up to 1 mg/
day q3-4days, max 10 mg/day; EXT REL TABS
(Xanax XR) give daily in AM 0.5-1 mg initially,
maintenance 3-6 mg daily

Premenstrual dysphoric disorder (unlabeled)
Adult: PO 0.25 mg tid-qid, starting on day 16-
18 of menses cycle, taper over 2-3 days when
menses occurs, max 4 mg/day

Hepatic dose
Reduce dose

Available forms: Tabs 0.25, 0.5, 1, 2 mg;
ext rel tabs (Xanax XR) 0.5, 1, 2, 3 mg; orally
disintegrating tabs 0.25, 0.5, 1, 2 mg; oral sol,
1 mg/ml

Implementation
• Give with food or milk for GI symptoms;
high-fat meal decreases absorption; tab may be
crushed, if patient is unable to swallow medication whole, and mixed with foods or fluids; may
divide total daily dose into more times/day, if
anxiety occurs between doses
• Give sugarless gum, hard candy, frequent sips
of water for dry mouth
• Discontinue, decrease by 0.5 mg q3days
• Place orally disintegrating tabs on tongue to
dissolve and swallow, protect from moisture
• Give ext rel tab in AM

ADVERSE EFFECTS
CNS: *Dizziness, drowsiness,* confusion, headache, anxiety, tremors, stimulation, fatigue, depression, insomnia, hallucinations, memory impairment, poor coordination, suicide
CV: *Orthostatic hypotension,* ECG changes,
tachycardia, hypotension
EENT: *Blurred vision,* tinnitus, mydriasis
GI: Constipation, dry mouth, nausea, vomiting,
anorexia, diarrhea, weight gain/loss, increased
appetite, ileus perforation, ischemic colitis
GU: Decreased libido
INTEG: Rash, dermatitis, itching, angioedema

Pharmacokinetics

Absorption	Slow, complete
Distribution	Widely distributed; crosses placenta; crosses blood-brain barrier, protein binding 80%
Metabolism	Liver, to active metabolites
Excretion	Kidneys, breast milk
Half-life	12-15 hr

Pharmacodynamics

	PO	Oral Disintegrating
Onset	1 hr	
Peak	1-2 hr	1.5-2 hr
Duration	4-6 hr, therapeutic response 2-3 days	

INTERACTIONS
Individual drugs
Alcohol: increased CNS depression
Cigarette smoking: decreased drug level
Levodopa: decreased action of levodopa
Rifampin: decreased action of ALPRAZolam

Drug classifications
Anticonvulsants, antihistamines, opioids, seda-
tives/hypnotics: increased CNS depression

CYP3A4 inducers (barbiturates): decreased action of ALPRAZolam

CYP3A4 inhibitors (cimetidine, disulfiram, erythromycin, fluoxetine, isoniazid, itraconazole, ketoconazole, metoprolol, propranolol, valproic acid): increased action of ALPRAZolam

Xanthines: decreased sedation

Drug/herb
Chamomile, kava, melatonin, St. John's wort, valerian: increased CNS depression

Drug/food
Grapefruit juice: increased product level, avoid concurrent use

Drug/lab test
Increased: ALT, AST, alkaline phosphatase

NURSING CONSIDERATIONS
Assessment
⚠ **Assess mental status: mood, sensorium, anxiety, affect, sleeping pattern, drowsiness, dizziness, especially geriatric; physical dependency, withdrawal symptoms: anxiety, panic attacks, agitation, seizures, headache, nausea, vomiting, muscle pain, weakness; suicidal tendencies; withdrawal seizures may occur after rapid decrease in dose or abrupt discontinuation; short duration of action makes it the product of choice in the geriatric, suicidal thoughts, behaviors**
• Monitor B/P (with patient lying, standing), pulse; if systolic B/P drops 20 mm Hg, hold product, notify prescriber
• Monitor blood studies: CBC during long-term therapy; blood dyscrasias have occurred rarely; decreased hematocrit, neutropenia may occur
• Monitor hepatic studies: AST, ALT, bilirubin, creatinine LDH, alkaline phosphatase, if on long-term treatment
• Monitor I&O; indicate renal dysfunction if on long-term treatment
⚠ **Pregnancy: Assess if planned or suspected, pregnancy (D), to avoid breastfeeding**

Patient/family education
• Tell patient that product may be taken with food or fluids and tabs may be crushed or swallowed whole
• Tell patient not to use for everyday stress or longer than 4 mo unless directed by prescriber; not to take more than prescribed amount; may be habit forming; not to double doses or skip doses; memory impairment is a sign of long-term use
• Tell patient to avoid OTC preparations unless approved by prescriber; alcohol and CNS depressants increase CNS depression

• **Teach patient not to use during pregnancy (D), avoid breastfeeding**
• Tell patient to avoid driving, activities that require alertness, since drowsiness may occur; to avoid alcohol ingestion or other psychotropic medications; to rise slowly, or fainting may occur, especially geriatric; that drowsiness may worsen at beginning of treatment
• **Tell patient not to discontinue medication abruptly after long-term use; withdrawal symptoms include vomiting, cramping, tremors, seizures**

Evaluation
Positive therapeutic outcome
• Decreased anxiety, restlessness, sleeplessness (short-term treatment only)

TREATMENT OF OVERDOSE:
Lavage, VS, supportive care, flumazenil

⚠ **HIGH ALERT**

alteplase (Rx)
(al-ti-plaze')
Activase, Cathflo
Func. class.: Thrombolytic enzyme
Chem. class.: Tissue plasminogen activator (TPA)
Pregnancy category C

Do not confuse: alteplase/Altace, Activase/Cathflo Activase

ACTION: Produces fibrin conversion of plasminogen to plasmin; able to bind to fibrin, convert plasminogen in thrombus to plasmin, which leads to local fibrinolysis, limited systemic proteolysis

Therapeutic outcome: Lysis of thrombi in MI, pulmonary emboli (life threatening)

USES: Lysis of obstructing thrombi associated with acute MI; conditions requiring thrombolysis (e.g., PE, unclotting arteriovenous shunts, acute ischemic CVA); central venous catheter occlusion (Cathflo)

Unlabeled uses: Arterial thromboembolism, deep vein thrombosis (DVT), occlusion prophylaxis, percutaneous coronary intervention (PCI)

CONTRAINDICATIONS
Active internal bleeding, recent CVA, severe uncontrolled hypertension, intracranial/intraspinal surgery/trauma (within 3 mo), aneurysm, brain tumor, platelets <100,000 mm³, bleeding diathesis including INR >1.7 or PT >15 sec,

arteriovenous malformation, subarachnoid hemorrhage, intracranial hemorrhage, uncontrolled hypertension, seizure at onset of stroke

Precautions: Pregnancy **C,** breastfeeding, children, geriatric, neurologic deficits, mitral stenosis, recent GI/GU bleeding, diabetic retinopathy, subacute bacterial endocarditis, arrhythmias, diabetic hemorrhage retinopathy, CVA, recent major surgery, hypertension, acute pericarditis, hemostatic defects, significant hepatic disease, septic thrombophlebitis, occluded AV cannula at seriously infected site

DOSAGE AND ROUTES
Pulmonary embolism (Activase)
Adult: IV 100 mg over 2 hr, then heparin

Acute ischemic stroke (Activase)
Adult: IV 0.9 mg/kg, max 90 mg; give as INF over 1 hr, give 10% of dose IV BOL over 1st min

Myocardial infarction (standard infusion)
Adult >65 kg: IV a total of 100 mg, given over 3 hr; 6-10 mg given IV BOL over 1-2 min, then the remaining 50-54 mg over the remainder of the hr, during 2nd, 3rd hr 20 mg is given by cont IV INF (20 mg/hr)
Adult <65 kg: IV 1.25 mg/kg over 3 hr; 60% in first 1 hr (10% as a bolus), remaining 40% over next 2 hr

Myocardial infarction (accelerated infusion) (Activase)
Adult >67 kg: 100 mg total dose: give 15 mg IV BOL, then 50 mg over 30 min, then 35 mg over 60 min
Adult <67 kg: 15 mg IV BOL: then 0.75 mg/kg over 30 min (max 50 mg); 0.5 mg/kg over the next 60 min (max 35 mg)

Occlusion prophylaxis (unlabeled) (Cathflo, Activase)
Adult ≥30 kg: Max 2 mg in 2 ml; may use up to 2 doses (120 min apart)

Complicated pleural effusions (unlabeled): **Adult:** intrapleural 10 mg in 30 ml ns bid in well time of 1 hr X 3 days, then after 2 hr or more intrapleural dornase alfa

Available forms: Powder for inj 50 mg (29 million international units/vial), 100 mg (58 million international units/vial); Cathflo Activase: lyophilized powder for injection 2 mg

Implementation
Intermittent IV infusion route
• Give after reconstituting with provided diluent; add appropriate amount of sterile water for inj (no preservatives); 20-mg vial/20 ml or 50-mg

vial/50 ml (1 mg/ml); mix by slow inversion or dilute with 0.9% NaCl, D₅W to a concentration of 0.5 mg/ml further dilution; 1.5 to <0.5 mg/ml may result in precipitation of product; use 18-G needle; flush line with 0.9% NaCl after administration; use reconstituted **IV** sol within 8 hr or discard, within 6 hr of coronary occlusion for best results

⚠️ **Do not use 150 mg or more total dose; intracranial bleeding may occur**

• Give heparin therapy after thrombolytic therapy is discontinued and when thrombin time, ACT, and APTT <2 times control (about 3-4 hr), treatment can be initiated before coagulation study results, infusion should be discontinued if pretreatment is INR >1.7, PT >15 sec, or an elevated APPT is identified

• Avoid invasive procedures, inj, rect temp; apply pressure for 30 sec to minor bleeding sites; 30 min to sites of atrial puncture, followed by pressure dressing; inform prescriber if this does not attain hemostasis; apply pressure dressing

• **Cathflo Activase:** Use this product after other options used for declotting a line; reconstitute by using 2.2 ml of sterile water provided and injecting in vial, direct flow into powder (1 mg/ml), foam will disappear after standing, swirl, do not shake, sol will be pale yellow or clear, use sol within 8 hr, instill 2 ml of reconstituted sol into occluded catheter, try to aspirate after ½ hr, if unable to remove allow 2 hrs; a second dose may be used; aspirate 5 ml of blood to remove clot and product; irrigate with normal saline

• Store powder at room temperature or refrigerate; protect from excessive light

• Avoidance of invasive procedures, inj, rectal temp

• Pressure for 30 sec to minor bleeding sites; 30 min to sites of atrial puncture followed by pressure dressing; inform prescriber if this does not attain hemostasis; apply pressure dressing

Y-site compatibilities: Eptifibatide, lidocaine, metoprolol, propranolol

Y-site incompatibilities: DOBUTamine, DOPamine, heparin, nitroglycerin

ADVERSE EFFECTS
CV: Sinus bradycardia, ventricular tachycardia, accelerated idioventricular rhythm, bradycardia, recurrent ischemic stroke, cholesterol microembolization, hypotension
EENT: Orolingual angioedema
INTEG: Urticaria, rash
SYST: GI, GU, intracranial, retroperitoneal bleeding, *surface bleeding*, anaphylaxis, fever

Pharmacokinetics

Absorption	Complete
Distribution	Unknown
Metabolism	>80% liver
Excretion	Kidneys
Half-life	35 min

Pharmacodynamics

Onset	Immediate

INTERACTIONS
Individual drugs
Abciximab, clopidogrel, dipyridamole, eptifibatide, plicamycin, ticlopidine, tirofiban, valproic acid: increased bleeding

ACE inhibitors: increased orolingual angio-edema

Nitroglycerin: decreased effect

Drug classifications
Anticoagulants (oral), cephalosporins (some), NSAIDs, salicylates: increased bleeding

Drug/herb
Feverfew, garlic, ginger, ginkgo, ginseng, green tea: increased risk of bleeding

Drug/lab test
Increased: PT, APTT, TT

NURSING CONSIDERATIONS
Assessment
• Treatment is not recommended in patient with acute ischemic stroke >3 hr after symptom onset, with minor neurologic deficit, or with rapidly improving symptoms
• Monitor VS q15min, B/P, pulse, respirations (including peripheral), neurologic signs, temp at least q4hr; temp >104° F (40° C) indicates internal bleeding; monitor rhythm closely; ventricular dysrhythmias may occur with hyperfusion; monitor heart, breath sounds, neurologic status, and peripheral pulses, those with severe neurologic deficit (NIHSS >22) at presentation (increased risk of hemorrhage)
⚠ Assess for bleeding during first hr of treatment and 24 hr after procedure: hematuria, hematemesis, bleeding from mucous membranes, epistaxis, ecchymosis, puncture sites; guaiac all body fluids and stools; obtain blood studies (Hct, platelets, PTT, PT, TT, APTT) before starting therapy; PT or APTT must be <2 times control before starting therapy; TT or PT q3-4hr during treatment; obtain CPK-MB to identify product effectiveness; do not use in severe uncontrolled hypertension, aneurysm, head trauma, for MI, pulmonary embolism

• Assess hypersensitivity: fever, rash, facial swelling, dyspnea, itching, chills; mild reaction may be treated with antihistamines; report to prescriber
• Occlusion: have patient exhale then hold breath when connecting/disconnecting syringe to prevent air embolism
• Cholesterol embolism: assess for purple toe syndrome, acute renal failure, gangrenous digits, hypertension, livedo reticularis, pancreatitis, MI, cerebral infarction, spinal cord infarction, retinal artery occlusion, bowel infarction, rhabdomyolysis
• Myocardial infarction: monitor ECG; on monitor, watch for segment changes, changes in rhythm: sinus bradycardia, ventricular tachycardia, accelerated idioventricular rhythm may occur due to reperfusion, cardiac enzymes, radionuclide myocardial scanning/coronary angiography
• Pulmonary embolism: monitor pulse, B/P, ABGs, rate/rhythm of respirations; symptoms include dyspnea, tachypnea, chest pain, cough, hemoptysis

Patient/family education
• Teach patient reason for alteplase, signs and symptoms of bleeding, allergic reactions, when to notify prescriber

Evaluation
Positive therapeutic outcome
• Lysis of pulmonary thrombi
• Adequate hemodynamic state
• Absence of congestive heart failure

aluminum hydroxide (OTC)
Func. class.: Antacid, hypophosphatemic, antiulcer
Chem. class.: Aluminum product, phosphate binder
Pregnancy category C

ACTION: Neutralizes gastric acidity, binds phosphates in GI tract; these phosphates are excreted

Therapeutic outcome: Decreased acidity, healing of ulcers; decreased phosphate levels in chronic renal failure

USES: Antacid, adjunct in peptic, gastric, duodenal ulcers; hyperphosphatemia in chronic renal failure; reflux esophagitis, hyperacidity, heartburn, stress ulcer prevention in critically ill, GERD

Unlabeled uses: GI bleeding

CONTRAINDICATIONS

Hypersensitivity to this product or aluminum products

Precautions: Pregnancy **C,** breastfeeding, geriatric, fluid restriction, decreased GI motility, GI obstruction, dehydration, renal disease, sodium-restricted diets, GI bleeding, hypokalemia

DOSAGE AND ROUTES
Antacid
Adult: SUSP PO 500-1500 mg 3-6 times/day; max 6 times/day

Hyperphosphatemia
Adult: PO 300-600 mg tid
Child: PO 50-150 mg/kg/day in 4-6 divided doses

GI bleeding (unlabeled)
Infant: PO 2-5 ml/dose q1-2hr
Child: PO 5-15 ml/dose q1-2hr

Available forms: SUSP 320 mg/5 ml, 600 mg/5 ml

Implementation
• 2 tsp (10 ml) neutralizes 20 mEq of acid
PO route
• Give laxatives or stool softeners if constipation occurs, especially geriatric
• Give after shaking suspension; follow with water to facilitate passage
• Tab may be chewed if patient is unable to swallow, drink 8 oz of water after chewing; or by nasogastric tube if patient unable to swallow
• Give with 8 oz of water for hyperphosphatemia unless contraindicated
• Give 1 hr before or after other medications to prevent poor absorption
• Give 15 ml 30 min after meals and at bedtime (esophagitis)
NG tube route
• May be given as prescribed q1-2hr and given by gastric tube after diluting with water (peptic ulcer)

ADVERSE EFFECTS
GI: *Constipation,* anorexia, obstruction, fecal impaction
META: *Hypophosphatemia,* hypercalciuria, hypomagnesemia, aluminum toxicity

Absorption	Not usually absorbed
Distribution	Widely distributed if absorbed; crosses placenta
Metabolism	Unknown
Excretion	Feces, kidneys (small amounts), breast milk
Half-life	Unknown

Onset	20-40 min
Peak	½ hr
Duration	1-3 hr

INTERACTIONS
Individual drugs
Allopurinol, amprenavir, delavirdine, digoxin, gabapentin, gatifloxacin, isoniazid, ketoconazole, penicillamine, phenytoin, quiNIDine, ticlopidine: decreased effect of each of these drugs

Drug classifications
Anticholinergics, cephalosporins, corticosteroids, H₂ antagonists, iron salts, phenothiazines, quinolones, tetracyclines, thyroid hormones: decreased effect of each of these drug classifications

Drug/food
High-protein meal: decreased product effect

Drug/lab test
Decreased: Phosphate Interference: Tc-99m

NURSING CONSIDERATIONS
Assessment
• Assess pain symptoms: location, duration, intensity, alleviating/precipitating factors
• Monitor phosphate levels, since product is bound in GI system; urinary pH, calcium, electrolytes; hypophosphatemia: anorexia, weakness, fatigue, bone pain, hyperreflexia
• Monitor constipation; increase bulk in diet if needed, may use stool softeners or laxatives; record amount and consistency of stools
• Monitor aluminum toxicity: severe renal disease; may also be used for hyperphosphatemia

Patient/family education
• Instruct patient to avoid phosphate-containing foods (most dairy products, eggs, fruits, carbonated beverages) during product therapy; to add cheese, corn, pasta, plums, prunes, lentils after product (hypophosphatemia)
• Instruct patient not to use for prolonged periods if serum phosphate is low or if on a low-sodium diet, shake liquid well; CHF patients should check for sodium content and use sodium-reduced products

---

• Instruct patient that stools may appear white or speckled; constipation may result; to report black tarry stools, which indicate gastric bleeding

• Instruct patient to check with prescriber after 2 wk of self-prescribed antacid use; may be used for 4-6 wk after symptoms subside or as prescribed

• Instruct patient to separate other medications by 2 hr

• **Teach patient to notify prescriber of black tarry stools, which may indicate bleeding**

Evaluation
Positive therapeutic outcome
• Absence of pain, decreased acidity
• Increased pH of gastric secretions
• Decreased phosphate levels

alvimopan (Rx)
(al-vi′moe-pan)
Entereg
Func. class.: Functional GI disorder agent
Chem. class.: Peripheral μ-opioid receptor antagonist
Pregnancy category B

ACTION: Acts within the GI tract, antagonizes opioid-induced GI dysfunction

Therapeutic outcome: Resolution of ileus

USES: Ileus, postoperative

CONTRAINDICATIONS
Hypersensitivity

> **BLACK BOX WARNING:** No more than 15 doses, MI

Precautions: Pregnancy **B**, breastfeeding, renal/hepatic disease, children, GI obstruction, MI, complete GI obstruction surgery

DOSAGE AND ROUTES
Ileus, postoperative
Adult: PO 12 mg given ½-5 hr before surgery, then 12 mg bid beginning the day after surgery, max 7 days (15 doses)

Available forms: Caps 12 mg

Implementation
• Use in hospital only; therapeutic doses of opiates should not be used for >7 consecutive days
• Must register in EASE program
• Do not give >15 doses (short-term hospital only)
• Give without regard to food
• Store at room temperature

ADVERSE EFFECTS
CV: MI
GI: Dyspepsia, flatulence, constipation
GU: Urinary retention
MISC: Anemia, hypokalemia
MS: Back pain

Pharmacokinetics
Absorption	High-fat meal decreases absorption
Distribution	Protein binding 80%-94%
Metabolism	Unknown
Excretion	Kidneys (35%)
Half-life	Terminal 10-18 hr

Pharmacodynamics
Unknown

INTERACTIONS
Individual drugs
Amiodarone, bepridil, cycloSPORINE, diltiazem, itraconazole, quiNIDine, quinine, spironolactone, verapamil: increased alvimopan effect
Methylnaltrexone: duplicate therapy

Drug classifications

> **BLACK BOX WARNING:** Opiate agonists: increased GI adverse reactions; do not give if opiate agonists were taken for ≥7 days

Opiate antagonists: duplicate therapy

NURSING CONSIDERATIONS
Assessment
• Monitor Hgb, Hct, serum potassium

Patient/family education
• Instruct the patient in the reason for the product

Evaluation
Positive therapeutic outcome
• Resolution of ileus

amantadine (Rx)
(a-man′ta-deen)
Func. class.: Antiviral, antiparkinsonian agent
Chem. class.: Tricyclic amine
Pregnancy category C

Do not confuse: amantadine/ranitidine/rimantadine

ACTION: Prevents uncoating of nucleic acid in viral cell, preventing penetration of virus to host; causes release of dopamine from neurons

Adverse effects: *italics* = common; **bold** = life-threatening

Therapeutic outcome: Resolution of infection, lessening of parkinsonism symptoms

USES: Prophylaxis or treatment of influenza type A, extrapyramidal reactions, parkinsonism, Parkinson's disease

Unlabeled uses: Neuroleptic malignant syndrome, MS-associated fatigue

CONTRAINDICATIONS
Breastfeeding, child <1 yr, hypersensitivity, eczematic rash

Precautions: Pregnancy **C**, geriatric, epilepsy, CHF, orthostatic hypotension, psychiatric disorders, renal/hepatic disease, peripheral edema, CV disease

DOSAGE AND ROUTES
Influenza type A
Adult and child >9 yr: PO 200 mg/day in single dose or divided bid
Geriatric: PO no more than 100 mg/day
Child 9-12 yr: PO 100 mg bid
Child 1-8 yr: PO 4.4-8.8 mg/kg/day divided bid-tid, max 150 mg/day

Drug-induced EPS
Adult: PO 100 mg bid up to 300 mg/day in divided doses

Parkinsonism
Adult: PO 100 mg bid, up to 400 mg/day in EPS; in divided doses

Renal dose
Adult: PO CCr 30-50 ml/min 200 mg first day, then 100 mg/day; CCr 15-29 ml/min 100 mg first day, then 100 mg on alternate days; CCr 15 ml/min reduce dose and interval to 200 mg q7days

MS-associated fatigue (unlabeled)
Adult: PO 200 mg daily or 100 mg bid

Neuroleptic malignant syndrome (unlabeled)
Adult: PO 100 mg bid × 3 wk

Available forms: Caps 100 mg; oral sol 50 mg/5 ml, tab 100 mg

Implementation
• **Prophylaxis:** give before exposure to influenza; continue for 10 days after contact; **treatment:** initiate within 24-48 hr after onset of symptoms, continue for 24-48 hr after symptoms disappear
• Give at least 4 hr before bedtime to prevent insomnia
• Give after meals for better absorption, to decrease GI symptoms

• Give in divided doses to prevent CNS disturbances: headache, dizziness, fatigue, drowsiness
• Store in tight, dry container
• Caps may be opened and mixed with food

ADVERSE EFFECTS
CNS: *Headache, dizziness,* drowsiness, fatigue, *anxiety,* psychosis, *depression, hallucinations,* tremors, seizures, confusion, *insomnia*
CV: *Orthostatic hypotension,* CHF
EENT: Blurred vision
GI: *Nausea, vomiting,* constipation, dry mouth, anorexia
GU: *Frequency, retention*
HEMA: Leukopenia, agranulocytosis
INTEG: Photosensitivity, dermatitis, livedo reticularis

Pharmacokinetics
Absorption	Unknown
Distribution	Crosses placenta
Metabolism	Not metabolized
Excretion	Urine unchanged (90%), breast milk
Half-life	11-15 hr

Pharmacodynamics
Onset	48 hr
Peak	2-4 hr
Duration	Unknown

INTERACTIONS
Individual drugs
Atropine: increased anticholinergic response
H1N1 influenza A virus vaccine: decreased effect of vaccine; avoid use 2 wk before or 48 hr after amantadine
Metoclopramide: decreased amantadine effect
Triamterene, hydrochlorothiazide: decreased excretion of amantadine

Drug classifications
Anticholinergics (other): increased anticholinergic response
CNS stimulants: increased CNS stimulation
Phenothiazines: decreased amantadine effect

Drug/lab test
Increase: BUN, creatinine, alk phos, CK, LDH, bilirubin, AST, ALT, GGT

NURSING CONSIDERATIONS
Assessment
• Mental status: may cause increased psychiatric disorders, especially in the elderly
• Assess **CHF,** confusion, mottling of skin
• Assess bowel pattern before, during treatment

- Assess skin eruptions, photosensitivity after administration of product
- Serum creatinine, BUN in renal impairment
- Assess signs of infection
- Assess for **livedo reticularis:** mottling of the skin, usually red, edema, itching in lower extremities, usually in Parkinson's disease
- Assess for **Parkinson's disease:** gait, tremors, akinesia, rigidity, may be effective if anticholinergics have not been effective
- Assess for toxicity: confusion, behavioral changes, hypotension, seizures

Patient/family education
- Advise patient to change body position slowly to prevent orthostatic hypotension
- Teach about aspects of product therapy: need to report dyspnea, weight gain, dizziness, poor concentration, dysuria, complex sleep behaviors
- Advise patient to avoid hazardous activities if dizziness, blurred vision occurs
- Advise patient to take product exactly as prescribed; parkinsonian crisis may occur if product is discontinued abruptly; do not double dose; if a dose is missed, do not take within 4 hr of next dose
- Teach to avoid alcohol

Evaluation
Positive therapeutic outcome
- Absence of fever, malaise, cough, dyspnea in infection; tremors, shuffling gait in Parkinson's disease

TREATMENT OF OVERDOSE:
Withdraw product, maintain airway, administer EPINEPHrine, aminophylline, O₂, **IV** corticosteroids, physostigmine

ambrisentan (Rx)
(am-bri-sen'tan)
Letairis, Volibris ✤
Func. class.: Antihypertensive
Chem. class.: Vasodilator/endothelin receptor antagonist
Pregnancy category X

ACTION: Endothelin-1A receptor antagonist; endothelin-1A is vasoconstrictor

Therapeutic outcome: Decreased shortness of breath, dizziness

USES: Pulmonary arterial hypertension, alone or in combination with other antihypertensives in WHO class II (significant exertion), III (mild exertion)

CONTRAINDICATIONS
Breastfeeding, hypersensitivity

BLACK BOX WARNING: Pregnancy **X**

Precautions: Children, women, geriatric, hepatitis, anemia, heart failure, jaundice, peripheral edema, hepatic disease, pulmonary edema

DOSAGE AND ROUTES
Adult: PO 5 mg/day; may increase to 10 mg if needed

Hepatic dose
Adult: Discontinue if AST/ALT >5 or if elevations are accompanied by bilirubin >2 ULN or other signs of liver dysfunction

Available forms: Tabs 5, 10 mg

Implementation
- Do not break, crush, or chew tabs
- Give daily with a full glass of water without regard to food
- Do not discontinue abruptly
- Only those facilities enrolled in the LEAP program (866-664-5327) may administer this product
- Store in tight container at room temperature

ADVERSE EFFECTS
CNS: Headache, fever, flushing, fatigue
CV: Orthostatic hypotension, hypotension, peripheral edema, palpitations
EENT: Sinusitis, rhinitis
GI: Abdominal pain, constipation, anorexia, hepatotoxicity
GU: Decreased sperm counts
HEMA: Anemia
INTEG: Rash, angioedema
RESP: Pharyngitis, dyspnea, pulmonary edema, venoocclusive disease (VOD)

Pharmacokinetics

Absorption	Rapid
Distribution	Protein binding 99%
Metabolism	By CYP3A4, CYP2C19, UGTa
Excretion	Unknown
Half-life	Terminal 15 hr, effective half-life 9 hr

Pharmacodynamics

Onset	Unknown
Peak	2 hr
Duration	Unknown

INTERACTIONS
Individual drugs
Cimetidine, clopidogrel, efavirenz, felbamate, FLUoxetine, modafinil, OXcarbazepine, ticlopidine: possibly increased ambrisentan

Mefloquine, niCARdipine, propafenone, quiNI-Dine, ranolazine, tacrolimus, testosterone: decreased ambrisentan absorption

Drug classifications
Antihypertensives (other), diuretics, MAOIs: increased hypotension
Barbiturates: need for ambrisentan dosage change
CYP3A4 inhibitors (amprenavir, aprepitant, atazanavir, clarithromycin, conivaptan, cycloSPORINE, dalfopristin, danazol, darunavir, erythromycin, estradiol, imatinib, itraconazole, ketoconazole, nefazodone, nelfinavir, propoxyphene, quinupristin, ritonavir, RU-486, saquinavir, tamoxifen, telithromycin, troleandomycin, zafirlukast), CYP2C19/CYP3A4 (chloramphenicol, delavirdine, fluconazole, fluvoxaMINE, isoniazid, voriconazole): increased ambrisentan
CYP3A4 inducers (carBAMazepine, PHENobarbital, phenytoin, rifampin): decreased ambrisentan

Drug/herb
Ephedra (ma huang), St. John's wort: need for ambrisentan dosage change

Drug/food
Grapefruit products: avoid use

Drug/lab test
Decreased: Hct, Hgb
Increased: LFTs

NURSING CONSIDERATIONS
Assessment
• Assess pulmonary status: improvement in breathing, ability to exercise; pulmonary edema that may indicate venooclusive disease
• Monitor blood studies: CBC with differential; Hct, Hgb may be decreased
• Monitor liver function tests: AST, ALT, blirubin

> **BLACK BOX WARNING:** Assess pregnancy status before giving this product and monthly; pregnancy category **X**

⚠ **Hepatotoxicity: assess for nausea, vomiting, pain/cramping, jaundice, anorexia, itching**

Patient/family education
• Teach patient the importance of complying with dosage schedule even if feeling better
• Advise patient that if a dose is missed, take as soon as possible; if it is almost time for the next dose, take only that dose; do not double dose
• Instruct patient not to use OTC products, including herbs, supplements unless approved by prescriber
• **Advise patient to report to prescriber immediately: dizziness, faintness, chest pain,** palpitations, uneven or rapid heart rate, headache, edema, weight gain
• Caution patient not to operate machinery or perform hazardous tasks if dizziness occurs
• Advise patient to avoid faintness; do not get up or stand up rapidly

> **BLACK BOX WARNING:** To notify if pregnancy is planned or suspected; if pregnant, product will need to be discontinued, pregnancy test done monthly, to use two contraception methods while taking this product

• To report hepatic dysfunction: nausea/vomiting, anorexia, fatigue, jaundice, right upper quadrant abdominal pain, itching, fever, malaise
• Advise patient of importance of follow-up with labs

Evaluation
Positive therapeutic outcome
• Decrease in B/P
• Decreased shortness of breath

amikacin (Rx)
(am-i-kay'sin)
Func. class.: Antibiotic
Chem. class.: Aminoglycoside
Pregnancy category D

Do not confuse: Amikacin/Anakinra

ACTION: Interferes with protein synthesis in bacterial cell by binding to ribosomal subunit, which causes misreading of genetic code; inaccurate peptide sequence forms in protein chain, causing bacterial death

Therapeutic outcome: Bactericidal effects for the following organisms: *Pseudomonas aeruginosa, Escherichia coli, Enterobacter, Acinetobacter, Providencia, Citrobacter, Staphylococcus, Serratia, Proteus*

USES: Severe systemic infections of CNS, respiratory, GI, urinary tract, bone, skin, soft tissues caused by *Staphylococcus aureus (MSSA), Pseudomonas aeruginosa, Escherichia coli, Enterobacter, Acinetobacter, Providencia, Citrobacter, Serratia, Proteus, Klebsiella pneumoniae*

Unlabeled uses: *Mycobacterium avium* complex (intrathecal or intraventricular) in combination; actinomycotic mycetoma, cystic fibrosis

CONTRAINDICATIONS
Pregnancy **D**, hypersensitivity to aminoglycosides, sulfites

Precautions: Neonates, breastfeeding, geriatric, myasthenia gravis, Parkinson's disease, dehydration, mild to moderate infections

> **BLACK BOX WARNING:** Hearing impairment, renal/neuromuscular disease

DOSAGE AND ROUTES
Severe systemic infections
Adult and child: IV INF 10-15 mg/kg/day in 2-3 divided doses q8-12hr in 100-200 ml D₅W over 30-60 min, not to exceed 1.5 g/day; **pulse dosing** (once-daily dosing) may be used with some infections; IM 10-15 mg/kg/day in divided doses q8-12hr; or extended internal dosing as an alternative dosing regimen

Neonate: IM/IV 10 mg/kg initially, then 7.5 mg/kg q12hr

Severe urinary tract infections
Adult: IM 10-15 mg/kg/day divided q8-12hr

Hemodialysis
Adult: IM/IV 7.5 mg/kg followed by 5 mg/kg 3 ×/ wk after each dialysis session (for TIW dialysis)

Mycobacterium avian complex (unlabeled)
Adult and adolescent: IV 7.5-15 mg/kg divided q12-24hr as part of a multiple-drug regimen
Child: IV 15-30 mg/kg/day divided q12-24hr as part of a multiple-drug regimen, max 1.5 g/day

Renal dose (extended interval dosing)
Adult: IV/IM CCr 40-59 ml/min 15 mg/kg IV q36hr; CCr 20-39 ml/min 15 mg/kg IV q48hr; <20 ml/min adjust based on serum concentrations and MIC (use traditional dosing)

Traditional dosing
• Decrease dose and maintain interval or maintain dose and decrease interval

Available forms: Inj IM, IV 50, 250 mg/ml

Implementation
• Obtain C&S before administration, begin treatment before results

IM route
• Give deeply in large muscle mass, rotate inj sites
• Obtain peak 1 hr after IM, trough before next dose

Intermittent IV INF route
• **Dilute** 500 mg of product/100-200 ml of **IV** D₅W, 0.9% NaCl and **give** over ½-1 hr; dilute insufficient volume to allow inf over 1-2 hr (infants); **flush** after administration with D₅W or 0.9% NaCl; solution is clear or pale yellow; discard if precipitate or dark color develops
• In children, amount of fluid depends on ordered dose; in infants infuse over 1-2 hr
• Give in evenly spaced doses to maintain blood level

Y-site compatibilities: Acyclovir, alatrofloxacin, aldesleukin, alemtuzumab, alfentanil, amifostine, aminophylline, amiodarone, amsacrine, anidulafungin, argatroban, ascorbic acid, atracurium, atropine, aztreonam, benztropine, bivalirudin, bumetanide, buprenorphine, butorphanol, calcium chloride/gluconate, CARBOplatin, caspofungin, ceFAZolin, cefepime, cefonicid, cefotaxime, cefoTEtan, cefOXitin, cefTAZidime, ceftizoxime, cefTRIAXone, cefuroxime, chloramphenicol, chlorproMAZINE, cimetidine, cisatracurium, CISplatin, clindamycin, codeine, cyanocobalamin, cyclophosphamide, cycloSPORINE, cytarabine, DACTINomycin, DAPTOmycin, dexamethasone, dexmedetomidine, digoxin, diltiazem, diphenhydrAMINE, DOBUTamine, DOCEtaxel, DOPamine, doripenem, doxacurium, DOXOrubicin, doxycycline, enalaprilat, ePHEDrine, EPINEPHrine, epirubicin, epoetin alfa, eptifibatide, ertapenem, erythromycin, esmolol, etoposide, famotidine, fentaNYL, filgrastim, fluconazole, fludarabine, fluorouracil, foscarnet, furosemide, gemcitabine, gentamicin, glycopyrrolate, granisetron, hydrocortisone, HYDROmorphone, IDArubicin, ifosfamide, IL-2, imipenemcilastatin, isoproterenol, ketorolac, labetalol, levofloxacin, lidocaine, linezolid, LORazepam, magnesium sulfate, mannitol, mechlorethamine, melphalan, meperidine, metaraminol, methotrexate, methoxamine, methyldopate, methylPREDNISolone, metoclopramide, metoprolol, metroNIDAZOLE, midazolam, milrinone, mitoXANtrone, morphine, multivitamins, nafcillin, nalbuphine, naloxone, niCARdipine, nitroglycerin, nitroprusside, norepinephrine, octreotide, ondansetron, oxaliplatin, oxytocin, PACLitaxel, palonosetron, pantoprazole, papaverine, PEMEtrexed, penicillin G, pentazocine, perphenazine, PHENobarbital, phenylephrine, phytonadione, piperacillin-tazobactam, potassium chloride, procainamide, prochlorperazine, promethazine, propranolol, protamine, pyridoxime, quinupristindalfopristin, ranitidine, remifentanil, riTUXimab, rocuronium, sargramostim, sodium acetate, sodium bicarbonate, succinylcholine, SUFentanil, tacrolimus, teniposide, theophylline, thiamine, thiotepa, ticarcillin/clavulanate, tigecycline, tirofiban, tobramycin, tolazoline, trimetaphan, urokinase, vancomycin, vasopressin, vecuronium, verapamil, vinCRIStine, vinorelbine, voriconazole, warfarin, zidovudine, zoledronic acid

ADVERSE EFFECTS
CNS: Confusion, depression, numbness, tremors, *seizures,* muscle twitching, **neurotoxicity,** dizziness, vertigo, tinnitus, **neuromuscular blockade with respiratory paralysis**

Adverse effects: *italics* = common; **bold** = life-threatening

CV: Hypotension or hypertension
EENT: Ototoxicity, deafness
GI: *Nausea, vomiting, anorexia,* bilirubin
GU: **Oliguria, hematuria, renal damage, azotemia, renal failure, nephrotoxicity**
HEMA: **Eosinophilia, anemia**
INTEG: *Rash,* burning, urticaria, dermatitis, alopecia

Pharmacokinetics

Absorption	Well absorbed (IM), completely absorbed (**IV**)
Distribution	Widely distributed in extracellular fluids, poor in CSF; crosses placenta
Metabolism	Minimal; liver
Excretion	Mostly unchanged (79%) in kidneys, removed by hemodialysis
Half-life	2-3 hr, prolonged up to 7 hr in infants; increased in renal disease

Pharmacodynamics

	IM	IV
Onset	Rapid	Rapid
Peak	15-30 min	1-2 hr
Duration	Unknown	Unknown

INTERACTIONS
Individual drugs
Increased: masking
Acyclovir, amphotericin B, cidofovir, cycloSPO-RINE, vancomycin: nephrotoxicity
DimenhyDRINATE, ethacrynic acid: increased masking of ototoxicity

Drug classifications
Anesthetics, nondepolarizing neuromuscular blockers: increased neuromuscular blockade, respiratory depression

> **BLACK BOX WARNING:** Increased: Ototoxici-to-IV loop diuretics

> **BLACK BOX WARNING:** Cephalosporins: inactivation of amikacin, nephrotoxicity

NSAIDs: increased serum trough and peak

Drug/lab test
Increased: BUN, creatinine, urea levels (urine)

NURSING CONSIDERATIONS
Assessment
• Assess patient for previous sensitivity reaction
• Assess patient for signs and symptoms of infection, including characteristics of wounds,
sputum, urine, stool, WBC $>10,000/mm^3$, ear-ache, temp; obtain baseline information before and during treatment
• Assess for allergic reactions: rash, urticaria, pruritus

> **BLACK BOX WARNING:** Assess renal impair-ment; obtain urine for CCr, BUN, serum creati-nine; lower dosage should be given in renal impairment; nephrotoxicity may be reversible if product is stopped at first sign

• Notify prescriber of increased BUN and creati-nine, urine CCr <80 ml/min; urinalysis daily for protein, cells, casts
• Monitor blood studies: AST, ALT, CBC, Hct, bilirubin, LDH, alkaline phosphatase; Coombs' test monthly if patient is on long-term therapy
• Monitor electrolytes: potassium, sodium, chloride, magnesium monthly if patient is on long-term therapy
• Assess bowel pattern daily; if severe diarrhea occurs, product should be discontinued
• Monitor for bleeding: ecchymosis, bleeding gums, hematuria, stool guaiac daily if on long-term therapy
• Assess for **overgrowth of infection:** perineal itching, fever, malaise, redness, pain, swelling, drainage, rash, diarrhea, change in cough, sputum
• Obtain weight before treatment; calculation of dosage is usually based on ideal body weight but may be calculated on actual body weight, in those underweight and nonobese, use total body weight (TBW) instead of ideal body weight
• Monitor VS during infusion, watch for hypo-tension, change in pulse
• Assess **IV** site for thrombophlebitis including pain, redness, swelling q30min; change site if needed; apply warm compresses to discontinued site

> **BLACK BOX WARNING:** Deafness by audio-metric testing, ringing, roaring in ears, vertigo; assess hearing before, during, after treatment

• **Dehydration:** high specific gravity, decrease in skin turgor, dry mucous membranes, dark urine
• **Vestibular dysfunction:** nausea, vomiting, dizziness, headache; product should be discon-tinued if severe

Patient/family education
• Teach patient to report sore throat, bruising, bleeding, joint pain; may indicate blood dyscra-sias (rare)
• Advise patient to contact prescriber if vaginal itching, loose foul-smelling stools, furry tongue occur; may indicate superinfection

---

- Advise patient to report hypersensitivity: rash, itching, trouble breathing, facial edema and notify prescriber

Evaluation

Positive therapeutic outcome

- Absence of signs/symptoms of infection: WBC <10,000/mm³, temp WNL; absence of red draining wounds; absence of earache
- Reported improvement in symptoms of infection

TREATMENT OF OVERDOSE:

Withdraw product; administer EPINEPHrine, O₂, hemodialysis, exchange transfusion in the newborn; monitor serum levels of product; may give ticarcillin or carbenicillin

---

aMILoride (Rx)

(a-mill'oh-ride)

Apo-Amilzide ✦, Midamor, Moduretic ✦, Novamilor ✦, Nu-Amilzide

Func. class.: Potassium-sparing diuretic
Chem. class.: Pyrazine
Pregnancy category B

Do not confuse: aMILoride/amLODIPine/ amiodarone

ACTION: Inhibits sodium, potassium ATPase ion exchange in the distal tubule, cortical collecting duct resulting in inhibition of sodium reabsorption and decreasing potassium secretion

Therapeutic outcome: Diuretic and antihypertensive effect while retaining potassium

USES: Edema in CHF in combination with other diuretics; for hypertension, adjunct with other diuretics to maintain potassium

Unlabeled uses: Ascites

CONTRAINDICATIONS

Anuria, hypersensitivity, diabetic neuropathy, renal failure

> BLACK BOX WARNING: Hyperkalemia

Precautions: Pregnancy **B,** breastfeeding, children, geriatric, dehydration, diabetes, acidosis, respiratory hyponatremia, impaired renal function

DOSAGE AND ROUTES

Adult: PO 5-10 mg daily in 1-2 divided doses; may be increased to 10-20 mg daily if needed
Infant/child (6-20 kg): PO 0.625 mg/kg/day

Renal dose

Adult: PO CCr 10-50 ml/min reduce dose by 50%; however, avoid if possible, CCr <10 ml/min contraindicated

Ascites (unlabeled)

Adult: PO 10 mg/day, max 40 mg

Available forms: Tabs 5 mg

Implementation

- Give in AM to avoid interference with sleep
- With food; if nausea occurs, absorption may be increased

ADVERSE EFFECTS

CNS: *Headache,* dizziness, fatigue, weakness, paresthesias, tremor, depression, anxiety, **encephalopathy**
CV: Orthostatic hypotension, dysrhythmias, angina
EENT: Blurred vision, increased intraocular pressure
ELECT: **Hyperkalemia,** dehydration, hyponatremia, hypochloremia
GI: *Nausea, diarrhea,* dry mouth, *vomiting, anorexia,* cramps, constipation, abdominal pain, jaundice
GU: *Polyuria,* dysuria, frequency, impotence
HEMA: **Aplastic anemia, neutropenia**
INTEG: *Rash, pruritus,* alopecia, urticaria
MS: *Cramps*
RESP: *Cough, dyspnea,* shortness of breath

Pharmacokinetics

Absorption	Variable (10%-50%)
Distribution	Widely distributed
Metabolism	Unchanged in urine (50%), in feces (40%)
Excretion	Renal; breast milk
Half-life	6-9 hr

Pharmacodynamics

Onset	2 hr
Peak	6-10 hr
Duration	24 hr

INTERACTIONS

Individual drugs

> BLACK BOX WARNING: CycloSPORINE, tacrolimus: increased hyperkalemia

Lithium: increased lithium toxicity, monitor lithium levels

Drug classifications

> **BLACK BOX WARNING:** ACE inhibitors, diuretics (potassium-sparing), potassium products, salt substitutes: increased hyperkalemia. Avoid concurrent use; if using together, monitor K level

Antihypertensives: increased action
NSAIDs: decreased effectiveness of aMILoride, avoid concurrent use

Drug/herb
Hawthorn, horse chestnut: increased aMILoride effect

Drug/food
Potassium foods: increased hyperkalemia, potassium-based salt substitutes

Drug/lab test

> **BLACK BOX WARNING:** Interference: GTT

Increased: LFTs, BUN, potassium, sodium

NURSING CONSIDERATIONS
Assessment
• Monitor for **hyperkalemia:** *MS:* fatigue, muscle weakness; *CARDIAC:* dysrhythmias, hypotension; *NEURO:* paresthesias, confusion; *RESP:* dyspnea
• Monitor for **hypokalemia:** weakness, polyuria, polydipsia, fatigue, ECG U wave
• Assess fluid volume status: distended red veins, crackles in lung, color, quality, and specific gravity of urine, skin turgor, adequacy of pulses, moist mucous membranes, bilateral lung sounds, peripheral pitting edema; dehydration symptoms of decreasing output, thirst, hypotension, dry mouth and mucous membranes should be reported
• Monitor electrolytes: potassium, sodium, calcium, magnesium; also include BUN, ABGs, uric acid, CBC, blood glucose
• Assess B/P before, during therapy with patient lying, standing, and sitting as appropriate; orthostatic hypotension can occur rapidly

Patient/family education
• Teach patient to take medication early in the day to prevent nocturia, to avoid alcohol
• Instruct patient to take with food or milk if GI symptoms of nausea and anorexia occur
• Teach patient to maintain a weekly record of weight and notify prescriber of weight loss >5 lb
• Caution patient that this product causes an increase in potassium levels, so foods high in potassium and potassium supplements should be avoided; refer to dietitian for assistance, planning

• Caution patient not to exercise in hot weather or stand for prolonged periods since orthostatic hypotension is enhanced
• Teach patient not to use alcohol or any OTC medications without prescriber's approval; serious product reactions may occur
• Emphasize the need to contact prescriber immediately if muscle cramps, weakness, nausea, dizziness, or numbness occurs
• Teach patient to take own B/P and pulse and record
• Advise patient that dizziness and confusion may occur; avoid driving or other hazardous activities if alertness is decreased
• Teach patient to continue taking medication even if feeling better; this product controls symptoms but does not cure the condition
• Advise patient with hypertension to continue other medical treatment (exercise, weight loss, relaxation techniques, cessation of smoking)
• Teach patient to avoid hazardous activities if dizziness occurs

Evaluation
Positive therapeutic outcome
• Prevention of hypokalemia (diuretic use)
• Decreased edema
• Decreased B/P
• Increased diuresis

TREATMENT OF OVERDOSE:
Lavage if taken orally; monitor electrolytes; administer **IV** fluids; monitor hydration, CV, renal status

amino acid (Rx)
(a-mee'noe)
Injection: FreAmine, HepatAmine
Solution: Aminess, Aminosyn, Branch Amin, FreAmine III, NephrAmine, Novamine, ProcalAmine, Ren Amin, Travasol, TrophAmine
Func. class.: Caloric agent
Chem. class.: Nitrogen product
Pregnancy category C

ACTION: Needed for anabolism to maintain structure; decreases catabolism, promotes healing

Therapeutic outcome: Positive nitrogen balance, decreased catabolism

USES: Hepatic encephalopathy, cirrhosis, hepatitis, nutritional support in cancer, burn, or solid organ transplant patients; to prevent nitrogen loss when adequate nutrition by mouth, gastric, or duodenal tube cannot be

---

used; intestinal obstruction, short bowel syndrome, severe malabsorption

CONTRAINDICATIONS
Hypersensitivity, severe electrolyte imbalances, anuria, severe liver damage, maple syrup urine disease, PKU, azotemia, genetic disease of amino acid metabolism

Precautions: Pregnancy C, children, renal disease, diabetes mellitus, CHF, breastfeeding, sulfite sensitivity

DOSAGE AND ROUTES
Amino acid injection
Adult: IV 80-120 g/day; 500 ml of amino acids/500 ml D$_{50}$ given over 24 hr

Amino acid solution
Adult: IV 1-1.5 g/kg/day titrated to patient's needs
Child: IV 2-3 g/kg/day titrated to patient's needs

Available forms: Inj; many strengths, types

Implementation
Continuous IV route
• Give up to 40% protein and dextrose (up to 12.5%) via peripheral vein; stronger solutions require central IV administration; TPN only mixed with dextrose to promote protein synthesis
• Use immediately after mixing in pharmacy under strict aseptic technique using laminar flowhood; use infusion pump, in-line filter (0.22 μm) unless mixed with fat emulsion and dextrose (3 in 1)
⚠ Use careful monitoring technique; do not speed up infusion; pulmonary edema, glucose overload will result
• Storage depends on type of solution; consult manufacturer
• Change dressing and IV tubing to prevent infection q24-48hr or q5-7days if transparent dressing is used

ADVERSE EFFECTS
CNS: *Dizziness, headache,* confusion, loss of consciousness
CV: Hypertension, CHF, pulmonary edema
ENDO: *Hyperglycemia, rebound hypoglycemia, electrolyte imbalances, hyperosmolar syndrome, hyperosmolar hyperglycemic non-ketotic syndrome,* alkalosis, acidosis, hypophosphatemia, hyperammonemia, dehydration, hypocalcemia
GI: Nausea, vomiting, liver fat deposits, abdominal pain, jaundice, cholestasis
GU: Glycosuria, osmotic diuresis, diuresis

INTEG: Chills, flushing, warm feeling, rash, urticaria, extravasation necrosis, phlebitis at inj site

Pharmacokinetics
Absorption	Complete bioavailability
Distribution	Widely distributed
Metabolism	Anabolism
Excretion	Kidney to urea nitrogen
Half-life	Unknown

Pharmacodynamics
Unknown

INTERACTIONS
Drug classifications
Tetracycline: decreased protein-sparing effects (inj only)

NURSING CONSIDERATIONS
Assessment
• Monitor electrolytes (potassium, sodium, calcium, chloride, magnesium), blood glucose, ammonia, phosphate, ketones; renal, liver function studies: BUN, creatinine, ALT, AST, bilirubin; urine glucose q6hr using Chemstrips, which are not affected by infusion substances; if BUN increases over 15%, therapy may need to be discontinued
• Check inj site for extravasation: redness along vein, edema at site, necrosis, pain; for a hard, tender area
• Monitor respiratory function q4hr: auscultate lung fields bilaterally for crackles; monitor respirations for quality, rate, rhythm that indicates fluid overload
• Monitor temp q4hr for increased fever, indicating infection; if infection is suspected, infusion is discontinued and tubing, bottle, catheter tip cultured; blood catheter may be obtained
⚠ Monitor for impending hepatic coma: asterixis, confusion, fetor, lethargy
• **Hyperammonemia:** nausea, vomiting, malaise, tremors, anorexia, seizures; increased ammonia, ketone levels may occur

Patient/family education
• Teach reason for use of amino acids as part of nutrition (TPN), how to care for tubing/site
• Instruct patient to report at once to prescriber if chills, sweating are experienced, risk of infection is higher

Evaluation
Positive therapeutic outcome
• Weight gain
• Decreased jaundice in liver disorders
• Increased LOC

aminophylline (theophylline ethylenediamine) (Rx)
(am-in-off′i-lin)

Elixophyllin, Techtron, Teho-24

Func. class.: Bronchodilator, spasmolytic
Chem. class.: Xanthine, ethylenediamine

Pregnancy category C

ACTION: Exact mechanism unknown; relaxes smooth muscle of respiratory system by blocking phosphodiesterase, which increases cyclic AMP; increased cyclic AMP alters intracellular calcium ion movements; produces bronchodilatation, increased pulmonary blood flow, relaxation of respiratory tract

Therapeutic outcome: Increased ability to breathe

USES: Apnea in infancy for respiratory/myocardial stimulation, bronchial asthma, bronchospasm associated with chronic bronchitis, emphysema

Unlabeled uses: Methotrexate toxicity, sleep apnea, status asthmaticus

CONTRAINDICATIONS
Hypersensitivity to xanthines, tachydysrhythmias

Precautions: Pregnancy **C,** breastfeeding, children, geriatric, CHF, cor pulmonale, hepatic disease, diabetes mellitus, hyperthyroidism, hypertension, seizure disorder, irritation of the rectum or lower colon, alcoholism, active peptic ulcer disease

DOSAGE AND ROUTES
Adult: PO 6 mg/kg, then 3 mg/kg q6hr × 2 doses, then 3 mg/kg q8hr maintenance, max 900 mg/day or 13 mg/kg; PO in CHF 6 mg/kg, then 2 mg/kg q8hr × 2 doses, then 1-2 mg/kg q12hr maintenance; **IV** 4.7 mg/kg, then 0.55 mg/kg/hr × 12 hr, then 0.36 mg/kg/hr maintenance; **IV** in CHF 4.7 mg/kg, then 0.39 mg/kg/hr × 12 hr; then 0.08-0.16 mg/kg/hr maintenance
Geriatric and in cor pulmonale: PO 6 mg/kg, then 2 mg/kg q6hr × 2 doses, then 2 mg/kg q8hr maintenance; **IV** 4.7 mg/kg, then 0.47 mg/kg/hr × 12 hr, then 0.24 mg/kg/hr maintenance
Child 9-16 yr: PO 6 mg/kg, then 3 mg/kg q4hr × 3 doses, then 3 mg/kg q6hr maintenance, max 18 mg/kg/day 12-16 yr, or 20 mg/kg/day 9-12 yr; **IV** 4.7 mg/kg, then 0.79 mg/kg/hr × 12 hr, then 0.63 mg/kg/hr maintenance
Child 6 mo-9 yr: PO 4 mg/kg q4hr × 3 doses, then 4 mg/kg q6hr maintenance, max 24 mg/kg/day; **IV** 4.7 mg/kg, then 0.95 mg/kg/hr × 12 hr, then 0.79 mg/kg/hr maintenance
Infant 6-52 wk: Dose (0.2 × age in wk) ÷ 5 × kg = 24 hr dose in mg
Neonate up to 40 wk premature postconception age: PO/**IV** 1 mg/kg q12hr
Neonate at birth or 40 wk postconception age: PO/**IV** >8 wk postnatal 1-3 mg/kg q6hr; 4-8 wk postnatal 1-2 mg/kg q8hr; up to 4 wk postnatal 1-2 mg/kg q12hr

Hepatic disease
Adult: PO 6 mg/kg, then 2 mg/kg q8hr × 2 doses, then 1-2 mg/kg q12hr maintenance; IV 4.7 mg/kg, then 0.39 mg/kg/hr × 12 hr, then 0.08-0.16 mg/kg/hr maintenance

Available forms: Inj 250 mg/10 ml, 500 mg/20 ml, 100 mg/100 ml in 0.45% NaCl; 200 mg/100 ml in 0.45% NaCl; extended release tab or cap 100, 200, 300, 400 mg; oral solution 80 mg/15 ml

Implementation
• Give around the clock to maintain blood (theophylline) levels
• If switching from **IV** to PO, give controlled-release dose at time **IV** infusion is discontinued; if giving tab (immediate release), discontinue **IV** and wait >4 hr
• If GI upset occurs, take with 8 oz of water or food
• Increase fluids to 2 L/day
PO route
• Do not break, crush, or chew enteric-coated or extended release caps/tabs
• Avoid giving with food

Continuous IV infusion route
• May be diluted for **IV** inf in 100-200 ml in D_5W, $D_{10}W$, $D_{20}W$, 0.9% NaCl, 0.45% NaCl, LR
• Give loading dose over ½ hr, max rate of inf 25 mg/min, use infusion pump; after loading dose, give by cont inf
• Avoid IM inj; pain and tissue damage may occur
• Only clear sol; flush **IV** line before dose; store diluted sol for 24 hr if refrigerated

Syringe compatibilities: Heparin, metoclopramide, PENTobarbital, thiopental

Y-site compatibilities: Allopurinol, amifostine, amphotericin B sulfate complex, inamrinone, aztreonam, cefTAZidime, cimetidine, cladribine, DOXOrubicin liposome, enalaprilat, esmolol, famotidine, filgrastim, fluconazole, fludarabine, foscarnet, gallium, granisetron, heparin sodium with hydrocortisone sodium succinate, labetalol, melphalan, meropenem, netilmicin, PACLitaxel, pancuronium, piperacil-lin/tazobactam, potassium chloride, propofol, ranitidine, remifentanil, sargramostim, tacroli-mus, teniposide, thiotepa, tolazoline, vecuronium

Y-site incompatibilities: DOBUTamine, hydrALAZINE, ondansetron

ADVERSE EFFECTS

CNS: Anxiety, restlessness, insomnia, *dizzi-ness, seizures,* headache, light-headedness, muscle twitching, tremors
CV: *Palpitations, sinus tachycardia,* hypoten-sion, flushing, **dysrhythmias,** edema
GI: *Nausea, vomiting,* diarrhea, dyspepsia, anal irritation (suppositories), epigastric pain, reflux, anorexia
GU: Urinary frequency, SIADH
INTEG: Flushing, urticaria
MISC: Hyperglycemia
RESP: Tachypnea, increased respiratory rate

Pharmacokinetics

Absorption	Well absorbed (PO), slow (PO–EXT REL), erratic (RECT)
Distribution	Widely distributed; crosses placenta
Metabolism	Liver to caffeine
Excretion	Kidneys
Half-life	3-12 hr, increased in renal disease, CHF, geriatric patients, smokers, crosses into CSF (cerebrospinal fluid)

Pharmacodynamics

	PO	PO–EXT REL	IV
Onset	15-60 min	Unknown	Immediate
Peak	1-2 hr	4-7 hr	Infusion's end
Duration	6-8 hr	8-12 hr	6-8 hr

INTERACTIONS
Individual drugs

Allopurinol (high doses), cimetidine, clarithro-mycin, disulfiram, erythromycin, fluvoxamine, interferon, mexiletine: decreased metabolism, increased toxicity of aminophylline
CarBAMazepine, isoniazid: increased or de-creased aminophylline levels
Halothane: increased risk of dysrhythmias
Ketoconazole, phenytoin, rifampin: decreased aminophylline effect
Lithium: decreased effect of lithium
Smoking: increased metabolism, decreased effect

Drug classifications

Barbiturates, β-adrenergic blockers: decreased effect of aminophylline
Benzodiazepines, β-blockers (nonselective), corticosteroids, diuretics (loop), fluoroqui-nolones, influenza vaccines, oral contracep-tives: increased aminophylline levels
Corticosteroids, influenza vaccines: increased aminophylline toxicity
Diuretics (loop): may increase or decrease aminophylline levels
Dose-dependent reversal of neuromuscular blockade
Fluoroquinolones: decreased metabolism, in-creased toxicity
Sympathomimetics: increased CNS, CV adverse reactions
Tetracyclines: increased adverse reactions

Drug/herb

Cola tree, ginseng, guarana, horsetail, Siberian ginseng, tea (black, green), yerba maté: in-creased effects
St. John's wort: decreased effects

Drug/food

High-carbohydrate, low-protein diet: decreased elimination
Low-carbohydrate, high-protein diet, charcoal-broiled beef: increased elimination
Xanthines: increased effect

Drug/lab test

Increased: plasma free fatty acids

NURSING CONSIDERATIONS
Assessment

• **Monitor theophylline blood levels (thera-peutic level is 10-20 mcg/ml); toxicity may occur with small increase above 20 mcg/ml, especially geriatric; determine whether theophylline was given recently (24 hr); check for toxicity: nausea, vomiting, anxi-ety, restlessness, insomnia, tachycardia, dysrhythmias, seizures; notify prescriber immediately**
• Monitor I&O; diuresis will occur; dehydra-tion may result in geriatric or children in whom diuresis is great
• Monitor liver function tests: periodically, lower doses may be required in those with moderate to severe hepatic disease
• Monitor respiratory rate, rhythm, depth; auscultate lung fields bilaterally, pulmonary function tests; notify prescriber of abnormali-ties; check ECG for tachycardia, PVCs, PACs in patients with cardiac problems
• Monitor allergic reactions: rash, urticaria; if these occur, product should be discontinued, prescriber notified

Patient/family education
• Teach patient to take doses as prescribed, not to skip dose; to check OTC medications, current prescription medications for ephedrine, which will increase CNS stimulation; advise patient not to drink alcohol or caffeine products (tea, coffee, chocolate, colas), which will increase action
• Teach patient to avoid hazardous activities; dizziness may occur
• Teach patient if GI upset occurs, to take product with 8 oz of water or food; absorption may be decreased
• Instruct patient to avoid smoking because it increases metabolism; decreases blood levels and terminal half-life; dosage may need to be increased
• Teach patient to obtain blood levels of product every few months to prevent toxicity; not to change brands, since effect may not be the same
• Teach patient to increase fluids to 2 L/day to decrease viscosity of secretions
• Advise patient to report toxicity: nausea, vomiting, anxiety, insomnia, rapid pulse, seizures, flushing, headache, diarrhea

Evaluation
Positive therapeutic outcome
• Decreased dyspnea
• Respiratory stimulation in infants
• Clear lung fields bilaterally

⚠ HIGH ALERT

amiodarone (Rx)
(a-mee-oh′da-rone)
Cordarone, Nexterone, Pacerone
Func. class.: Antidysrhythmic (Class III)
Chem. class.: Iodinated benzofuran derivative
Pregnancy category D

Do not confuse: amiodarone/inamrinone, Cordarone/Inocor

ACTION: Prolongs action potential duration and effective refractory period, noncompetitive α- and β-adrenergic inhibition; increases PR and QT intervals, decreases sinus rate, decreases peripheral vascular resistance

Therapeutic outcome: Decreased amount and severity of ventricular dysrhythmias

USES: Hemodynamically unstable ventricular tachycardia, supraventricular tachycardia, ventricular fibrillation not controlled by 1st-line agents

CONTRAINDICATIONS
Pregnancy **D**, breastfeeding, neonates, infants, severe sinus node dysfunction, hypersensitivity to this product/iodine/benzyl alcohol, cardiogenic shock

> **BLACK BOX WARNING:** 2nd-3rd degree AV block, bradycardia

Precautions: Goiter, Hashimoto's thyroiditis, electrolyte imbalances, CHF, severe respiratory disease, children, torsades de pointes

> **BLACK BOX WARNING:** Cardiac arrhythmias, pneumonitis, pulmonary fibrosis, severe hepatic disease

DOSAGE AND ROUTES
Ventricular dysrhythmias
Adult: PO loading dose 800-1600 mg/day for 1-3 wk; then 600-800 mg/day × 1 mo; maintenance 400 mg/day; **IV** loading dose (first rapid) 150 mg over the first 10 min then slow 360 mg over the next 6 hr; maintenance 540 mg given over the remaining 18 hr, decrease rate of the slow infusion to 0.5 mg/min

Supraventricular tachycardia
Adult: PO 600-800 mg/day × 7 days or until desired response, then 400 mg/day × 21 days, then 200-400 mg/day maintenance
Child: PO 10 mg/kg/day (800 mg/1.72 m²/day) × 10 days or until desired response, then 5 mg/kg/day (400 mg/1.72 m²/day) × 21-28 days, then 2.5 mg/kg/day (200 mg/1.72 m²/day) (not recommended in children)

Available forms: Tabs 100, 200, 400 mg; inj 50 mg/ml

Implementation
Start with patient hospitalized and monitored
PO route
• Give reduced dosage slowly with ECG monitoring only
• Loading dose with food to decrease nausea

IV, direct route
• **Peripheral:** max 2 mg/ml for longer than 1 hr; preferred through central venous line with in-line filter; concentration >2 mg/ml should be given by central line
• **Cardiac arrest:** give 300 mg IV bol diluted to a total volume of 20 ml D₅W; may repeat 150 mg after 3-5 min
Intermittent IV INF route
• **Rapid loading:** add 3 ml (150 mg), 100 ml D₅W (1.5 mg/ml), give over 10 min
• **Slow loading:** add 18 ml (900 mg), 500 ml D₅W (1.8 mg/ml), give over next 6 hr

---

A

Continuous IV infusion route
• After 24 hr, dilute 50 ml to 1-6 mg/ml, give 1-6 mg/ml at 1 mg/ml for the first 6 hr, then 0.5 mg/min

Y-site compatibilities: Amikacin, bretylium, clindamycin, DOBUTamine, DOPamine, doxycycline, erythromycin, esmolol, gentamicin, insulin (regular), isoproterenol, labetalol, lidocaine, metaraminol, metroNIDAZOLE, midazolam, morphine, nitroglycerin, norepinephrine, penicillin G potassium, phentolamine, phenylephrine, potassium chloride, procainamide, tobramycin, vancomycin

Solution compatibilities: D₅W, 0.9% NaCl

ADVERSE EFFECTS

CNS: *Headache, dizziness,* involuntary movement, tremors, peripheral neuropathy, malaise, fatigue, ataxia, paresthesias, insomnia
CV: *Hypotension,* **bradycardia, sinus arrest, CHF, dysrhythmias, SA node dysfunction, AV block,** increased defibrillation energy requirement
EENT: Blurred vision, halos, photophobia, *corneal microdeposits,* dry eyes
ENDO: Hyper/hypothyroidism
GI: Nausea, vomiting, diarrhea, abdominal pain, anorexia, constipation, **hepatotoxicity**
GU: Epididymitis, ED
INTEG: Rash, photosensitivity, blue-gray skin discoloration, alopecia, spontaneous ecchymosis, **toxic epidermal necrolysis,** urticaria, **pancreatitis,** phlebitis (IV)
MISC: Flushing, abnormal taste or smell, edema, abnormal salivation, coagulation abnormalities
MS: Weakness, pain in extremities
RESP: **Pulmonary fibrosis/toxicity,** pulmonary inflammation, **ARDS, gasping syndrome in neonates**

Pharmacokinetics

Absorption	Slow, variable (PO) up to 65%
Distribution	Body tissues; crosses placenta
Metabolism	Liver, an inhibitor of CYP1A2, CYP3A4, CYP2C8, CYP2C9, CYP2C19, CYP2A6, CYP2B6, CYP2D6, P-glycoprotein, organic cation transporter
Excretion	Bile, kidney (minimal)
Half-life	15-100 days, increased in geriatrics

Pharmacodynamics

	PO
Onset	1-3 wk
Peak	3-7 hr
Duration	Up to several months

INTERACTIONS
Individual drugs
CycloSPORINE, dextromethorphan, digoxin, disopyramide, flecainide, methotrexate, phenytoin, procainamide, quiNIDine, theophylline: increased blood levels, increased toxicity
Warfarin: increased bleeding, dabigatran

Drug classifications
Azoles, fluoroquinolones, macrolides: increased QT prolongation
β-Adrenergic blockers, calcium channel blockers: increased bradycardia
Class I antidysrhythmics: increased levels
HMG-CoA reductase inhibitors: increased myopathy
Protease inhibitors: increased amiodarone concentrations, possible serious dysrhythmias, reduce dose

Drug/herb
St. John's wort: decreased amiodarone effect

Drug/food
Grapefruit juice: toxicity

Drug/lab test
Increased: T₄, ALT, AST, GGT, alk phos, cholesterol, lipids, PT, INR
Decrease: T₃

NURSING CONSIDERATIONS
Assessment
• Monitor electrolytes: potassium, sodium, chloride
• Monitor chest x-ray, thyroid function tests
• Monitor liver function studies: AST, ALT, bilirubin, alkaline phosphatase

> **BLACK BOX WARNING:** Monitor ECG continuously to determine product effectiveness; measure PR, QRS, QT intervals; check for PVCs, other dysrhythmias; monitor B/P continuously for hypo/hypertension; check for rebound hypertension after 1-2 hr

• Monitor for dehydration or hypovolemia, monitor PT, INR if using warfarin
• Assess for CNS symptoms: confusion, psychosis, numbness, depression, involuntary movements; if these occur, product should be discontinued

---

• Assess for hypothyroidism: lethargy, dizziness, constipation, enlarged thyroid gland, edema of extremities, cool, pale skin
• Monitor hyperthyroidism: restlessness, tachycardia, eyelid puffiness, weight loss, frequent urination, menstrual irregularities, dyspnea, warm, moist skin

> **BLACK BOX WARNING:** Assess for pulmonary toxicity including ARDS, pulmonary fibrosis: dyspnea, fatigue, cough, fever, chest pain; product should be discontinued if these occur, increased at higher doses, toxicity is common

• Monitor cardiac rate, respiration: rate, rhythm, character, chest pain, ventricular tachycardia, supraventricular tachycardia or fibrillation
• Assess sight and vision before treatment and throughout therapy; microdeposits on the cornea may cause blurred vision, halos, and photophobia, to prevent corneal deposits use methylcellulose

Patient/family education

• Instruct patient to report side effects immediately to prescriber; more common at high dose NO
• Instruct patient that skin discoloration is usually reversible, but skin may turn bluish on neck, face, arms when used for long periods
• Advise patient that dark glasses may be needed for photophobia
• Instruct patient to use sunscreen and protective clothing to prevent burning associated with photosensitivity
• Instruct patient to take medication as prescribed, not to double doses, do not discontinue abruptly, not to use other drugs, herbs without prescriber approval, many interactions
• Instruct patient to complete follow-up appointment with health care provider, including pulmonary function studies, chest x-ray, ophthalmic examinations

Evaluation

Positive therapeutic outcome
• Decreased ventricular tachycardia
• Decreased supraventricular tachycardia or fibrillation

TREATMENT OF OVERDOSE:
Administer O_2, artificial ventilation, ECG, DOPamine for circulatory depression, diazepam or thiopental for seizures, isoproterenol

---

amitriptyline (Rx)
(a-mee-trip′ti-leen)
Elavil ✱, **Levate** ✱, **Novo-Triptyn** ✱
Func. class.: Antidepressant—tricyclic
Chem. class.: Tertiary amine
Pregnancy category C

Do not confuse: amitriptyline/ nortriptyline/aminophylline

ACTION: Blocks reuptake of norepinephrine, serotonin into nerve endings that increase action of norepinephrine, serotonin in nerve cells

Therapeutic outcome: Decreased symptoms of depression after 2-3 wk

USES: Major depression

Unlabeled uses: Neuropathic pain, prevention of cluster/migraine headaches, fibromyalgia

CONTRAINDICATIONS
Hypersensitivity to tricyclics, recovery phase of MI

Precautions: Pregnancy C, breastfeeding, geriatric, seizure disorders, prostatic hypertrophy, schizophrenia, psychosis, severe depression, increased intraocular pressure, closed-angle glaucoma, urinary retention, cardiac disease, renal/ hepatic disease, hyperthyroidism, electroshock therapy, elective surgery

> **BLACK BOX WARNING:** Child <12 yr, suicidal patients

DOSAGE AND ROUTES
Depression
Adult/adolescent: PO 25-75 mg/day as a single dose at bedtime or in divided doses; may increase to 200 mg/day, max 300 mg/day (hospitalized)
Geriatric: PO 10-25 mg at bedtime; may be increased to 150 mg/day

Cluster/migraine headaches (unlabeled)
Adult: PO 25-200 mg/day, initiate at lowest dose, titrate

Pain (unlabeled)
Adult: PO 75-300 mg/day

Fibromyalgia/insomnia (unlabeled)
Adult: PO 10-50 mg nightly

Available forms: Tabs 10, 25, 50, 75, 100, 150 mg

Implementation
• Give with food or milk for GI symptoms
• Crush if patient is unable to swallow medication whole
• Give dose at bedtime if oversedation occurs during day; may take entire dose at bedtime; geriatric may not tolerate once/day dosing
• Store at room temperature; do not freeze

ADVERSE EFFECTS
CNS: *Dizziness, drowsiness,* confusion, headache, anxiety, tremors, stimulation, weakness, *insomnia,* nightmares, EPS (geriatric), increased psychiatric symptoms, **seizures, suicidal thoughts,** anxiety
CV: *Orthostatic hypotension,* **ECG changes, tachycardia, hypertension,** palpitations, dysrhythmias
EENT: *Blurred vision,* tinnitus, mydriasis, ophthalmoplegia, amblyopia
GI: *Constipation, dry mouth,* weight gain, nausea, vomiting, **paralytic ileus,** increased appetite, cramps, epigastric distress, jaundice, **hepatitis,** stomatitis
GU: *Urinary retention,* sexual dysfunction
HEMA: **Agranulocytosis, thrombocytopenia, eosinophilia, leukopenia, aplastic anemia**
INTEG: Rash, urticaria, sweating, pruritus, photosensitivity
RESP: Asthma exacerbation, rhinitis
SYST: **Neuroleptic malignant syndrome, serotonin syndrome**

Pharmacokinetics

Absorption	Well absorbed
Distribution	Widely distributed; crosses placenta
Metabolism	Liver, extensively
Excretion	Kidneys, breast milk
Half-life	10-46 hr

Pharmacodynamics

	PO
Onset	45 min
Peak	2-12 hr
Duration	Unknown

INTERACTIONS
Individual drugs
Alcohol: increased CNS depression
Amiodarone, procainamide, quiNIDine: increased QT prolongation
CarBAMazepine: increased amitriptyline levels, increased toxicity
Cimetidine, fluoxetine: increased levels, increased toxicity

CloNIDine: decreased effects
Guanethidine: decreased effects
Linezolid, methylene blue: increased serotonin syndrome, use cautiously

Drug classifications
Antidepressants, antidysrhythmics (class IC), phenothiazines: increased amitriptyline levels, toxicity
Antidysrhythmics (class IA, III), tricyclic antidepressants: increased QT prolongation
Antithyroid agents: increased risk of agranulocytosis
Barbiturates, benzodiazepines, CNS depressants, opioids, sedative/hypnotics, sympathomimetics (direct acting): increased CNS effects
MAOIs: hypertensive crisis, seizures, hyperpyretic crisis, do not use 14 days of MAOIs
Oral contraceptives: increased effects, toxicity
Sympathomimetics (indirect acting): decreased effects

Drug/herb
Chamomile, hops, kava, lavender, valerian: increased CNS depression
SAM-e, St. John's wort, yohimbe: serotonin syndrome

Drug/lab test
Increased: serum bilirubin, blood glucose, alkaline phosphatase, LFTs
Decreased: WBCs, platelets, granulocytes

NURSING CONSIDERATIONS
Assessment
• Monitor B/P (with patient lying, standing), pulse q4hr; if systolic B/P drops 20 mm Hg, hold product, notify prescriber; take VS q4hr in patients with cardiovascular disease
• Monitor blood studies: CBC, leukocytes, differential, cardiac enzymes if patient is receiving long-term therapy, thyroid function tests
• Monitor hepatic studies: AST, ALT, bilirubin
• Check weight weekly; appetite may increase with product
• Assess ECG for flattening of T wave, bundle branch block, AV block, prolongation of QTc interval, dysrhythmias in cardiac patients, avoid use immediately after MI
• Assess for EPS primarily in geriatric: rigidity, dystonia, akathisia
• Assess mental status: mood, sensorium, affect, suicidal tendencies; increase in psychiatric symptoms: depression, panic
⚠ Assess for serotonin syndrome: may occur with other serotonergic products (hyperthermia, hypertension, rigidity, delirium)
• Monitor urinary retention, constipation; constipation is more likely to occur in children or geriatric

• Assess for paralytic ileus, glaucoma exacerbation
• Assess for **withdrawal symptoms:** headache, nausea, vomiting, muscle pain, weakness; do not usually occur unless product was discontinued abruptly
• Identify alcohol consumption; if alcohol is consumed, hold dose until morning
• Assess for sexual dysfunction: erectile dysfunction, decreased libido; usually resolves after discontinuing product

Patient/family education
• Teach patient that therapeutic effects may take 2-3 wk
• Instruct patient to use caution in driving or other activities requiring alertness because of drowsiness, dizziness, blurred vision; to avoid rising quickly from sitting to standing, especially geriatric; management of anticholinergic effects
⚠ Teach patient the symptoms of serotonin syndrome
• Advise patient to avoid alcohol ingestion, other CNS depressants; overheating
• Teach patient not to discontinue medication quickly after long-term use; may cause nausea, headache, malaise
• Advise patient to wear sunscreen or large hat, since photosensitivity occurs; hyperthermia can occur
• Teach patient to increase fluids, bulk in diet if constipation, urinary retention occur, especially geriatric
• Teach patient to use gum, hard sugarless candy, or frequent sips of water for dry mouth
• Instruct patient to use contraception during treatment
⚠ Teach patient to watch for suicidal ideation

Evaluation
Positive therapeutic outcome
• Decreased depression
• Absence of suicidal thoughts

TREATMENT OF OVERDOSE:
ECG monitoring, lavage, administer anticonvulsant, sodium bicarbonate

---

amLODIPine (Rx)
(am-loe′di-peen)
Norvasc
Func. class.: Antianginal, calcium channel blocker, antihypertensive
Chem. class.: Dihydropyridine
Pregnancy category C

Do not confuse: amLODIPine/aMILoride

ACTION: Inhibits calcium ion influx across cell membrane during cardiac depolarization; produces relaxation of coronary vascular smooth muscle and peripheral vascular smooth muscle; dilates coronary vascular arteries; increases myocardial oxygen delivery in patients with vasospastic angina

Therapeutic outcome: Decreased angina pectoris, dysrhythmias, B/P

USES: Chronic stable angina pectoris, hypertension, variant angina (Prinzmetal's angina); may coadminister with other antihypertensives, antianginals

CONTRAINDICATIONS
Hypersensitivity to this product or dihydropyridine, severe aortic stenosis, severe obstructive CAD

Precautions: Pregnancy C, breastfeeding, children, geriatric, CHF, hypotension, hepatic injury, GERD

DOSAGE AND ROUTES
Coronary artery disease
Adult: PO 5-10 mg daily
Geriatric: PO 5 mg daily, may increase; max 10 mg/day

Hypertension
Adult: PO 5 mg daily initially, max 10 mg/day
Geriatric: PO 2.5 mg/day; may increase to 5 mg/day, max 10 mg/day

Hepatic dose
Adult: PO 2.5 mg/day, may increase to 10 mg/day (antihypertensive); 5 mg/day, may increase to 10 mg/day (antianginal)

Available forms: Tabs 2.5, 5, 10 mg

Implementation
• Give once a day, without regard to meals

ADVERSE EFFECTS
CNS: Headache, fatigue, dizziness, asthenia, anxiety, depression, insomnia, paresthesia, somnolence
CV: Peripheral edema, bradycardia, hypotension, palpitations, syncope, chest pain
GI: Nausea, vomiting, diarrhea, gastric upset, constipation, flatulence, anorexia, gingival hyperplasia, dyspepsia
GU: Nocturia, polyuria, sexual difficulties
INTEG: Rash, pruritus, urticaria, alopecia
MISC: Flushing, muscle cramps, cough, weight gain, tinnitus, epistaxis, pulmonary edema, dyspnea

---

Pharmacokinetics

Absorption	Well absorbed up to 90%
Distribution	Crosses placenta, protein binding 93%
Metabolism	Liver, extensively by CYP3A4
Excretion	Kidneys to metabolites (90%)
Half-life	30-50 hr; increased in geriatric, hepatic disease

Pharmacodynamics

Onset	Unknown
Peak	6-10 hr
Duration	24 hr

INTERACTIONS
Individual drugs
Diltiazem: increased amLODIPine level; Conivaptan; CYP3A4 inhibitors

Drug classifications
Antihypertensives, nitrates: increased hypotension
Increase: level of cyclosporine
Increase: myopathy simvastatin

NURSING CONSIDERATIONS
Assessment
• Assess fluid volume status: distended red veins, crackles in lung; color, quality, and specific gravity of urine, skin turgor, adequacy of pulses, moist mucous membranes, bilateral lung sounds, peripheral pitting edema; dehydration symptoms of decreasing output, thirst, hypotension, dry mouth and mucous membranes should be reported
• Assess for angina: intensity, location, duration of pain
• Monitor B/P and pulse; if B/P drops, call prescriber
• Monitor ALT, AST, bilirubin daily; if these are elevated, hepatotoxicity is suspected
• Monitor platelet count: if <150,000/mm³, product is usually discontinued and another product started
• Monitor cardiac status: B/P, pulse, respiration, ECG

Patient/family education
• Advise patient to avoid hazardous activities until stabilized on product, dizziness is no longer a problem
• Instruct patient to avoid alcohol and OTC products unless directed by prescriber
• Advise patient to comply in all areas of medical regimen: diet, exercise, stress reduction, smoking cessation, product therapy; to notify prescriber of irregular heartbeat, shortness of breath, swelling of feet, face, and hands, severe dizziness, constipation, nausea, hypotension; use nitroglycerin when angina is severe
• Teach patient to use as directed even if feeling better; may be taken with other cardiovascular products (nitrates, β-blockers)
• Advise to avoid large amounts of grapefruit juice or alcohol

Evaluation
Positive therapeutic outcome
• Decreased anginal pain
• Decreased B/P
• Increased exercise tolerance

TREATMENT OF OVERDOSE:
Defibrillation, β-agonists, **IV** calcium inotropic agents, diuretics, atropine for AV block, vasopressor for hypotension

amoxicillin (Rx)
(a-mox-i-sill'in)
Amoxil ✤, Apo-Amoxi ✤, Lin-Amox ✤, Moxatag, Novamoxin ✤, Nu-Amoxi ✤
Func. class.: Antiinfective, antiulcer
Chem. class.: Aminopenicillin
Pregnancy category B

Do not confuse: amoxicillin/amoxapine/Amoxil

ACTION: Interferes with cell wall replication of susceptible organisms by binding to the bacterial cell wall; the cell wall; bactericidal, lysis mediated by bacterial cell wall autolysis

Therapeutic outcome: Bactericidal effects for the following organisms: effective for gram-positive cocci *(Staphylococcus aureus, Streptococcus pyogenes, Streptococcus faecalis, Streptococcus pneumoniae)*, gram-negative cocci *(Neisseria gonorrhoeae, Neisseria meningitidis)*, gram-negative bacilli *(Haemophilus influenzae, Proteus mirabilis, Escherichia coli, Salmonella)*, in combination for *Helicobacter pylori*, gram-positive bacilli *(Corynebacterium diphtheriae, Listeria monocytogenes)*; gastric ulcer, β-lactamase-negative organisms

USES: Infections of respiratory tract, skin, GI tract, GU tract, otitis media, meningitis, septicemia, sinusitis

Unlabeled uses: Lyme disease, anthrax treatment and prophylaxis, and bacterial endocarditis prophylaxis in combination with other products used for treatment of *Helicobacter pylori*

CONTRAINDICATIONS
Hypersensitivity to penicillins

Precautions: Pregnancy **B,** breastfeeding, neonates, hypersensitivity to cephalosporins, carbapenems; severe renal disease, mononucleosis, phenylketonuria, diabetes, geriatrics, asthma, child, colitis, dialysis, eczema, pseudomembranous colitis, syphilis

DOSAGE AND ROUTES
Upper respiratory infections
Adult/adolescent and child ≥40 kg: *Mild to moderate infections:* PO 500 mg q12hr or 250 mg q8hr; *Severe infections:* 875 mg q12hr or 500 mg q8hr
Child <40 kg: *Mild to moderate infections:* 25-90 mg/kg/day in individual doses q12hr; *Severe infections:* 40 mg/kg/day divided q8hr or 45 mg/kg/day divided q12hr

Otitis media
Adult: PO 500 mg q12hr or 250 mg q8hr
Infant >3 months/child/adolescent PO: 80-90 mg/kg/day in divided doses q8-12hr, max 500 mg/dose if given q8hr or 875 mg/dose if given q12hr

Gonorrhea (not CDC approved)
Adult: PO 3 g given with 1 g probenecid as a single dose; followed by tetracycline or erythromycin

Chlamydia trachomatis
Adult: PO 500 mg/day × 1 wk

Bacterial endocarditis prophylaxis
Adult: PO 2 g 1 hr prior to procedure
Child: PO 50 mg/kg/hr 1 hr prior to procedure, max 2 g

Helicobacter pylori
Adult: PO 1000 mg bid given with lansoprazole 30 mg bid, clarithromycin 500 mg bid × 2 wk; or 1000 mg bid given with omeprazole 20 mg bid, clarithromycin 500 mg bid × 2 wk; or 1000 mg tid given with lansoprazole 30 mg tid × 2 wk

Renal disease
Adult: PO CCr 10-30 ml/min 250-500 mg q12hr; CCr <10 ml/min 250-500 mg q24hr; do not use 775, 875 mg strength if CCr <30 ml/min

Available forms: Caps 250, 500 mg; chewable tabs 125, 200, 250, 400 mg; tabs 250, 500, 875 mg; ext rel tab (Moxatag) 775 mg; susp 125, 200, 250, 400 mg/5 ml

Implementation
PO route
• Identify allergies before use
• Give in even doses around the clock without regard to food; if GI upset occurs, give with food; product must be given for 10-14 days to ensure organism death and prevent superinfection; store in tight container
• The caps may be opened and contents taken with fluids
• **Suspension:** shake well before each dose, may be used alone or mixed in drinks, use immediately; susp may be stored in refrigerator for 14 days
• **Extended release:** do not crush, chew, or break; take with food

ADVERSE EFFECTS
CNS: Headache, seizures, agitation, confusion, dizziness, insomnia
GI: *Nausea, vomiting, diarrhea,* increased AST, ALT, abdominal pain, glossitis, colitis, pseudomembranous colitis, jaundice, cholestasis
HEMA: Anemia, increased bleeding time, bone marrow depression, granulocytopenia, hemolytic anemia, eosinophilia, thrombocytopenia, agranulocytosis
INTEG: *Urticaria, rash*
SYST: Anaphylaxis, respiratory distress, serum sickness, Stevens-Johnson syndrome, toxic epidermal necrolysis, exfoliative dermatitis

Pharmacokinetics
Absorption	Well absorbed (90%)
Distribution	Readily in body tissues, fluids, CSF; crosses placenta
Metabolism	Liver (30%)
Excretion	Breast milk, kidney, unchanged (70%)
Half-life	1-1.3 hr, extended in renal disease

Pharmacodynamics
Onset	½ hr
Peak	1-2 hr
Duration	Unknown

INTERACTIONS
Individual drugs
Methotrexate: increased methotrexate levels
Decreased: Hgb, WBC, platelets
Probenecid: increased amoxicillin levels, decreased renal excretion
Warfarin: increased anticoagulant effects

Drug classifications
Contraceptives (oral): decreased contraceptive effectiveness

Drug/lab test
Decreased: Hgb, WBC, platelets
Increase: AST/ALT, alk phos, LDH, eosinophils

Interference: urine glucose test (Clinitest, Benedict's reagent, cupric SO_4)

NURSING CONSIDERATIONS
Assessment
• Assess patient for previous sensitivity reaction to penicillins or other cephalosporins; cross-sensitivity between penicillin products and cephalosporins is common
• Assess patient for signs and symptoms of **infection**, including characteristics of wounds, sputum, urine, stool, WBC $>10,000/mm^3$, earache, fever; obtain baseline information and monitor symptoms during treatment
• Obtain C&S before beginning product therapy to identify if correct treatment has been initiated
• **Assess for allergic reactions during treatment: rash, urticaria, pruritus, chills, fever, joint pain; angioedema may occur a few days after therapy begins; EPINEPHrine and resuscitation equipment should be available for anaphylactic reactions, rash is more common if allopurinol is taken concurrently**
• Identify urine output; if decreasing, notify prescriber (may indicate nephrotoxicity); also, increased BUN, creatinine, urinalysis, protein, blood
• Monitor blood studies: AST, ALT, CBC, Hct, bilirubin, LDH, alkaline phosphatase, Coombs' test monthly if patient is on long-term therapy
• Monitor electrolytes: potassium, sodium, chloride monthly if patient is on long-term therapy
• **Assess bowel pattern daily; diarrhea, cramping, blood in stools; if severe diarrhea occurs, notify prescriber; product should be discontinued; pseudomembranous colitis may occur**
• Monitor for bleeding: ecchymosis, bleeding gums, hematuria, stool guaiac daily if on long-term therapy
• Assess for overgrowth of infection: perineal itching, fever, malaise, redness, pain, swelling, drainage, rash, diarrhea, change in cough, sputum

Patient/family education
⚠ **Teach patient to report sore throat, bruising, bleeding, joint pain; may indicate blood dyscrasias (rare)**
• **Advise patient to contact prescriber if vaginal itching, loose foul-smelling stools, diarrhea, sore throat, fever, fatigue, furry tongue occur; may indicate superinfection or agranulocytopenia**
• Instruct patient to take all medication prescribed for the length of time ordered; not to double dose; chew form is available

• **Advise patient to notify prescriber of diarrhea with blood or pus, abdominal pain, which may indicate pseudomembranous colitis**

Evaluation
Positive therapeutic outcome
• Absence of signs/symptoms of infection (WBC $<10,000/mm^3$, temp WNL, absence of red draining wounds or earache)
• Prevention of endocarditis
• Resolution of ulcer symptoms

TREATMENT OF ANAPHYLAXIS:
Withdraw product, maintain airway, administer EPINEPHrine, aminophylline, O_2, **IV** corticosteroids

amoxicillin/clavulanate (Rx)
(a-mox-i-sill′in)
Apo-Amoxi Clav ✦, Augmentin, Augmentin XR, Clavulin ✦
Func. class.: Broad-spectrum antiinfective (extended spectrum)
Chem. class.: Aminopenicillin-β-lactamase inhibitor
Pregnancy category B

Do not confuse: Augmentin/amoxicillin

ACTION: Interferes with cell wall replication of susceptible organisms; lysis mediated by bacterial cell wall autolytic enzymes, combination increases spectrum of activity against β-lactamase resistance organisms

Therapeutic outcome: Bactericidal effects for *Actinomyces, Bacillus anthracis, Bacteroides, Bordetella pertussis, Borrelia burgdorferi, Brucella, Burkholderia pseudomallei, Clostridium perfringens, Clostridium tetani, Corynebacterium diphtheriae, Eikenella corrodens, Enterobacter, Enterococcus faecalis, Erysipelothrix rhusiopathiae, Escherichia coli, Eubacterium, Fusobacterium, Haemophilus ducreyi, Haemophilus parainfluenzae* (positive/negative beta-lactamase), *Helicobacter pylori, Klebsiella, Lactobacillus, Listeria monocytogenes, Moraxella catarrhalis, Neisseria gonorrhoeae, Neisseria meningitis, Nocardia brasiliensis, Peptococcus, Peptostreptococcus, Prevotella melaninogenica, Propionibacterium, Salmonella, Shigella, Staphylococcus aureus* (MSSA), *Staphylococcus epidermidis, Staphylococcus saprophyticus, Streptococcus agalactiae* (group B Streptococci), *Streptococcus dysgalactiae, Streptococcus pneumoniae,*

Adverse effects: *italics* = common; **bold** = life-threatening

Streptococcus pyogenes (group A Streptococci), *Treponema pallidum, Vibrio cholerae,* viridans streptococci

USES: Infections of lower respiratory tract, skin, GU tract; impetigo; otitis media, sinusitis, pneumonia, and endocarditis prophylaxis

CONTRAINDICATIONS
Hypersensitivity to penicillins, severe renal disease, dialysis, jaundice

Precautions: Pregnancy **B,** breastfeeding, neonates, children, hypersensitivity to cephalosporins, GI/renal disease, asthma, colitis, diabetes, eczema, leukemia, mononucleosis, viral infections, phenylketonuria

DOSAGE AND ROUTES
Adult: PO 250-500 mg q8hr or 500-875 mg q12hr depending on severity of infection
Child ≤40 kg: PO 20-90 mg/kg/day in divided doses q8-12hr

Community-aquired pneumonia or acute bacterial sinusitis
Adult: PO 2000 mg/125 mg (Augmentin XR) q12hr x 7-10 days (pneumonia), 10 days (sinusitis)

Renal dose
Adult: PO CCr 10-30 ml/min dose q12hr; CCr <10 ml/min dose q24hr; do not use 875 mg strength if CCr <30 ml/min; Augmentin XR is contraindicated in renal disease

Available forms: Tabs 250, 500, 875 mg/125 mg clavulanate; chewable tabs 200/28.5, 400/57 mg; powder for oral susp 125, 250/28.5, 200/28.5, 400/57, 600/42.9 mg/5 ml; (XR) ext rel tabs 1000 mg amoxicillin/62.5 mg clavulanate; (ES) powder for oral susp 600 mg amoxicillin; 42.9 mg clavulanate 5 ml

Implementation
PO route
• Give in even doses around the clock; if GI upset occurs, give with food; product must be taken for 10-14 days to ensure organism death and prevent superinfection; store in tight container; cap can be opened and mixed with food or liquid; chewable tabs should be chewed
• Administer only as directed; two 250-mg tabs not equivalent to one 500-mg tab due to strength of clavulanate
• Shake susp well before each dose; may be used alone or mixed in drinks, use immediately; susp may be stored in refrigerator for 10 days

ADVERSE EFFECTS
CNS: Headache, fever, seizures, agitation, insomnia

GI: *Nausea, diarrhea, vomiting,* increased AST, ALT, abdominal pain, glossitis, colitis, black tongue, **pseudomembranous colitis,** jaundice
GU: Oliguria, proteinuria, hematuria, *vaginitis, moniliasis,* **glomerulonephritis**
HEMA: Anemia, **bone marrow depression, granulocytopenia, leukopenia, eosinophilia,** thrombocytopenic purpura
INTEG: Rash, urticaria, dermatitis, **toxic epidermal necrolysis**
META: Hyperkalemia, hypokalemia, alkalosis, hypernatremia
SYST: Anaphylaxis, respiratory distress, serum sickness, superinfection, Stevens-Johnson syndrome , superinfection, candidiasis

Pharmacokinetics
Absorption	Well absorbed (90%)
Distribution	Readily in body tissues, fluids, CSF; crosses placenta
Metabolism	Liver (30%)
Excretion	Breast milk; kidney, unchanged (70%), removed by hemodialysis
Half-life	1-1.3 hr

Pharmacodynamics
Onset	½ hr
Peak	1-2.5 hr
Duration	Unknown

INTERACTIONS
Individual drugs
Allopurinol: increased skin rash
Probenecid: increased amoxicillin levels
Warfarin: increased anticoagulant effect, monitor closely: dose adjustment may be needed

Drug/food
High-fat meal: decreased absorption

Drug/lab test
Increased: AST/ALT, alk phos, LDH
Interference: urine glucose tests (Clinitest, Benedict's reagent, cupric SO_4)

NURSING CONSIDERATIONS
Assessment
• Assess patient for previous sensitivity reaction to penicillins or other cephalosporins; cross-sensitivity between penicillins and cephalosporins is common
• Assess patient for signs and symptoms of **infection,** including characteristics of wounds, sputum, urine, stool, WBC >10,000/mm³,

earache, fever; obtain baseline information and during treatment

• Complete C&S before beginning product therapy to identify if correct treatment has been initiated

• **Assess for anaphylaxis: rash, urticaria, pruritus, chills, dyspnea, laryngeal edema, fever, joint pain; angioedema may occur a few days after therapy begins; EPINEPHrine and resuscitation equipment should be available for anaphylactic reaction**

• **Identify urine output; if decreasing, notify prescriber (may indicate nephrotoxicity)**

• Monitor renal studies: urinalysis, protein, blood, BUN, creatinine

• Monitor blood studies: AST, ALT, CBC, Hct, bilirubin, LDH, alkaline phosphatase, Coombs' test monthly if patient is on long-term therapy

• Monitor electrolytes: potassium, sodium, chloride monthly if patient is on long-term therapy

• **Assess bowel pattern daily; diarrhea, cramping, blood in stools, report to prescriber; if severe diarrhea occurs, product should be discontinued; may indicate pseudomembranous colitis**

• Monitor for bleeding: ecchymosis, bleeding gums, hematuria, stool guaiac daily if on long-term therapy

• Assess for **overgrowth of infection:** perineal itching, fever, malaise, redness, pain, swelling, drainage, rash, diarrhea, change in cough, sputum

Patient/family education

⚠ **Teach patient to report sore throat, bruising, bleeding, joint pain; may indicate blood dyscrasias (rare)**

• **Advise patient to contact prescriber if vaginal itching, loose foul-smelling stools occur; may indicate superinfection**

• Instruct patient to take all medication prescribed for the length of time prescribed

• **Advise patient to notify prescriber of diarrhea with blood or pus, which may indicate pseudomembranous colitis**

Evaluation

Positive therapeutic outcome

• Absence of signs/symptoms of infection (WBC <10,000/mm³, temp WNL)

• Reported improvement in symptoms of infection

TREATMENT OF ANAPHYLAXIS:

Withdraw product, maintain airway, administer EPINEPHrine, aminophylline, O₂, **IV** corticosteroids

---

⚠ HIGH ALERT

amphotericin B lipid complex (ABLC)
(am-foe-ter'i-sin)

Abelcet

Func. class.: Antifungal

Chem. class.: Amphoteric polyene

Pregnancy category B

ACTION: Increases cell membrane permeability in susceptible fungi by binding sterols; alters cell membrane, thereby causing leakage of cell components, cell death

Therapeutic outcome: Decreased fever, malaise, rash; negative C&S for infecting organism

USES: Indicated for the treatment of invasive fungal infections in patients who cannot tolerate or have failed conventional amphotericin B therapy; broad-spectrum activity against many fungal, yeast and mold pathogen infections, including *Aspergillus, Zygomycetes, Fusarium, Cryptococcus,* and many hard-to-treat *Candida* species; *Aspergillus fumigatus, Aspergillus, Blastomyces dermatitidis, Candida albicans, Candida guilliermondii, Candida stellatoidea, Candida tropicalis, Coccidioides immitis, Cryptococcus, Histoplasma, sporotrichosis*

Precautions: Hypersensitivity, anemia, breastfeeding, cardiac disease, children, electrolyte imbalance, geriatric, hematological/hepatic/renal disease, hypotension pregnancy (B)

DOSAGE AND ROUTES

Adult: IV 3-5 mg/kg/day as a single inf given at 2.5 mg/kg/hr

Renal dose
Adult: IV CCr <10 ml/min; give 5 mg/kg q24-36hr

Available forms: Susp for inj 100 mg/20-ml vial

Implementation

• **Do not confuse four different types; these are not interchangeable: conventional amphotericin B, amphotericin B cholesteryl, amphotericin B lipid complex, amphotericin B liposome**

• May premedicate with acetaminophen, diphenhydrAMINE

• Use only after C&S confirms organism

IV route
- Give product only after C&S confirms organism, product needed to treat condition; make sure product is used for life-threatening infections
- Handle with aseptic technique because amphotericin B lipid complex (ABLC) has no preservatives; visually inspect parenteral products for particulate matter and discoloration before use

Filtration and dilution
- Prior to dilution, store at 36°-46° F (2°-8° C), protected from moisture and light; do not freeze; the diluted, ready-for-use admixture is stable for up to 48 hours at 36°-46° F (2°-8° C) and an additional 6 hr at room temperature; do not freeze
- Prepare the admixture for infusion by first shaking the vial until there is no evidence of yellow sediment on the bottom of the vial
- Transfer the appropriate amount of drug from the required number of vials into one or more sterile syringes using an 18-gauge needle
- Attach the provided 5-micron filter needle to the syringe; inject the syringe contents through the filter needle, into an IV bag containing the appropriate amount of D₅W injection; each filter needle may be used on the contents of no more than four 100-mg vials
- The suspension must be diluted with D₅W injection to a final concentration of 1 mg/ml; for pediatric patients and patients with cardiovascular disease, the final concentration may be 2 mg/ml; DO NOT USE SALINE SOLUTIONS OR MIX WITH OTHER DRUGS OR ELECTROLYTES
- The diluted ready-for-use admixture is stable for up to 48 hr at 36°-46° F (2°-8° C) and an additional 6 hr at room temperature; do not freeze

IV INF
- Flush IV line with D₅W injection before use or use a separate IV line; DO NOT USE AN IN-LINE FILTER
- Before infusion, shake the bag until the contents are thoroughly mixed; max rate 2.5 mg/kg/hr; if the infusion time exceeds 2 hr, mix the contents by shaking the infusion bag every 2 hr

Y-site compatibilities: Acyclovir, allopurinol, aminocaproic acid, aminophylline, amiodarone, anidulafungin, argatroban, arsenic trioxide, atracurium, azithromycin, aztreonam, bumetanide, buprenorphine, busulfan, butorphanol, CARBOplatin, carmustine, ceFAZolin, cefepime, cefotaxime, cefoTEtan, cefOXitin, cefTAZidime, ceftizoxime, cefTRIAXone, cefuroxime, chloramphenicol, chlorproMAZINE, cimetidine, cisatracurium, clindamycin, cyclophosphamide, cycloSPORINE, cytarabine, DACTINomycin dexamethasone, digoxin, diphenhydrAMINE, DOCEtaxel, doxacurium, DOXOrubicin liposomal, enalaprilat, EPINEPHrine, eptifibatide, ertapenem, etoposide, famotidine, fentaNYL, fludarabine, fluorouracil, fosphenytoin, furosemide, ganciclovir, granisetron, heparin, hydrocortisone, HYDROmorphone, ifosfamide, insulin, regular ketorolac, lepirudin, lidocaine, linezolid, LORazepam, mannitol, melphalan, meperidine, methotrexate, methylPREDNISolone, metoclopramide, mitoMYcin, mivacurium, nafcillin, nesiritide, nitroglycerin, nitroprusside, octreotide, oxaliplatin, PACLitaxel, pamidronate, pantoprazole, PEMEtrexed, pentazocine, PENTobarbital, PHENobarbital, phentolamine, piperacillin-tazobactam, procainamide, ranitidine, succinylcholine, SUFentanil, tacrolimus, telavancin, teniposide, theophylline, thiopental, thiotepa, ticarcillin, ticaracillin-clavulanate, trimethobenzamide, verapamil, vinBLAStine, vinCRIStine, zidovudine, zoledronic acid

ADVERSE EFFECTS

CNS: *Headache, fever, chills,* peripheral nerve pain, paresthesias, peripheral neuropathy, **seizures,** dizziness
CV: Bradycardia, hypotension, **cardiac arrest,** chest pain, hypertension
EENT: Tinnitus, deafness, diplopia, blurred vision
GI: *Nausea, vomiting, anorexia,* diarrhea, cramps, **hemorrhagic gastroenteritis, acute liver failure,** jaundice, bilirubinemia
GU: *Hypokalemia,* **azotemia, hyposthenuria, renal tubular acidosis, nephrocalcinosis, permanent renal impairment, anuria, oliguria**
HEMA: Normochromic, normocytic ane**mia, thrombocytopenia, agranulocytosis, leukopenia, eosinophilia**
INTEG: *Burning, irritation,* pain, **necrosis at inj site with extravasation,** flushing, dermatitis
META: Hyponatremia, hypomagnesemia, hypokalemia
MS: Arthralgia, myalgia, generalized pain, weakness, weight loss
RESP: **Bronchospasm, dyspnea**
SYST: **Toxic epidermal neurolysis, exfoliative dermatitis, anaphylaxis,** sepsis, infection, infusion reactions

Pharmacokinetics

Absorption	Complete bioavailability (IV)
Distribution	Body tissues
Metabolism	Liver
Excretion	Kidneys, detectable for several weeks
Half-life	Terminal lipid complex mean 7 days

Pharmacodynamics

Onset	Immediate
Peak	2 hr
Duration	Unknown

INTERACTIONS
Individual drugs
Cidofovir: do not use concurrently
Digoxin: increased hypokalemia
Pentamidine, tacrolimus, tenofovir: increased nephrotoxicity

Drug classifications
Other nephrotoxic antibiotics (aminoglycosides, CISplatin, vancomycin, cycloSPORINE, polymyxin B), antineoplastics, salicylates): increased nephrotoxicity
Azole antifungals: decreased amphotericin B lipid complex effect; antifungals may still be used concurrently in serious resistant infections
Corticosteroids, skeletal muscle relaxants, thiazides, loop diuretics: increased hypokalemia

Drug/lab test
Increased: AST/ALT, alk phos, BUN, creatinine, LDH, bilirubin
Decreased: magnesium, potassium, Hgb, WBC, platelets

NURSING CONSIDERATIONS
Assessment
• VS every 15-30 min during first inf; note changes in pulse, B/P
• I&O ratio; watch for decreasing urinary output, change in specific gravity; discontinue product to prevent permanent damage to renal tubules
• Blood studies: CBC, potassium, sodium, calcium, magnesium every 2 wk; BUN, creatinine 2-3 ×/wk
• Weight weekly; if weight increases by more than 2 lb/wk, edema is present; renal damage should be considered
⚠ For renal toxicity: increasing BUN, serum creatinine; if BUN is >40 mg/dl or if serum creatinine is >3 mg/dl, product may be discontinued, dosage reduced
⚠ For hepatotoxicity: increasing AST, ALT, alk phos, bilirubin
⚠ For allergic reaction: dermatitis, rash; product should be discontinued, antihistamines (mild reaction) or EPINEPHrine (severe reaction) should be administered
• For hypokalemia: anorexia, drowsiness, weakness, decreased reflexes, dizziness, increased urinary output, increased thirst, paresthesias

• Infusion reactions: fever, chills, pain, swelling at site
• For ototoxicity: tinnitus (ringing, roaring in ears), vertigo, loss of hearing (rare)

Patient/family education
• Teach patient that long-term therapy may be needed to clear infection (2 wk-3 mo, depending on type of infection)
⚠ Instruct patient to notify prescriber of bleeding, bruising, or soft-tissue swelling, neurologic, renal symptoms

Evaluation
Positive therapeutic outcome
• Decreased fever, malaise, rash; negative C&S for infecting organism

---

⚠ **HIGH ALERT**

amphotericin B liposomal (LAmB)
(am-foe-ter′i-sin)
AmBisome
Func. class.: Antifungal
Chem. class.: Amphoteric polyene
Pregnancy category B

ACTION: Increases cell membrane permeability in susceptible fungi by binding to membrane sterols; alters cell membrane, thereby causing leakage of cell components, cell death

Therapeutic outcome: Resolution of infection

USES: Empirical therapy for presumed fungal infection in febrile neutropenic patients; treatment of *Cryptococcal* Meningitis in HIV-infected patients; treatment of *Aspergillus, Candida,* and/or *Cryptococcus* infections refractory to amphotericin B deoxycholate, or in patients where renal impairment or unacceptable toxicity precludes the use of amphotericin B deoxycholate *(Aspergillus flavus, Aspergillus fumigatus, Blastomyces dermatitidis, Candida albicans, Candida krusei, Candida lusitaniae, Candida parapsilosis, Candida tropicalis, Cryptococcus neoformans)*; treatment of visceral leishmaniasis

Unlabeled uses: Coccidioidomycosis, histoplasmosis

CONTRAINDICATIONS
Hypersensitivity

Precautions: Anemia, breastfeeding, cardiac disease, children, electrolyte imbalance, geriatric, hematological/hepatic/renal disease, hypotension, pregnancy (B), severe bone marrow depression

Adverse effects: *italics* = common; **bold** = life-threatening

DOSAGE AND ROUTES
Visceral leishmaniasis
Adult and child ≥1 mo: IV 3 mg/kg every 24 hr days 1-5, and days 14, 21 (immunocompetent), 4 mg/kg every 24 hr days 1-5, and days 10, 17, 24, 31, 38 (immunocompromised)

Cryptococcal meningitis in HIV
Adult and child ≥1 mo: IV 6 mg/kg/ day

Fungal infection, empirical
Adult and child ≥1 mo: IV 3 mg/kg/day

Fungal infection, systemic
Adult and child ≥1 mo: IV 3-5 mg/kg/ day

Renal dose
Adult: IV CCr <10 ml/min; use 3 mg/kg q24hr

Available forms: Powder for inj 50-mg vial

Implementation
⚠ **Do not confuse four different types; these are not interchangeable: conventional amphotericin B, amphotericin B cholesteryl, amphotericin B lipid complex, amphotericin B liposome**
• May premedicate with acetaminophen, diphenhydrAMINE

IV route
• Make sure product is used for life-threatening infections
• Administer by IV infusion only; handle with aseptic technique as LAmB does not contain any preservatives
• Visually inspect products for particulate matter and discoloration
Reconstitution
• LAmB *must* be reconstituted using sterile water for injection (without a bacteriostatic agent); **do not reconstitute with saline or add saline to the reconstituted suspension, do not mix with other drugs;** doing so can cause a precipitate to form
• Reconstitute vials containing 50 mg of LAmB/12 ml of sterile water (4 mg/ml)
• Immediately after the addition of water, SHAKE THE VIAL VIGOROUSLY for 30 sec; the suspension should be yellow and translucent; visually inspect vial for particulate matter and continue shaking until product is completely dispersed
• Store suspension for up to 24 hours refrigerated if using sterile water for injection; do not freeze
Filtration and dilution
• Calculate the amount of reconstituted (4 mg/ml) suspension to be further diluted and withdraw this amount into a sterile syringe

• Attach the provided 5-micron filter to the syringe; inject the syringe contents through the filter, into the appropriate amount of D$_5$W injection; use only one filter per vial
• The suspension must be diluted with D$_5$W injection to a final concentration of 1-2 mg/ml before administration; for infants and small children, lower concentrations (0.2-0.5 mg/ml) may be appropriate to provide sufficient volume for infusion
• Use injection of LAmB within 6 hr of dilution with D$_5$W
IV INF
• Flush intravenous line with D$_5$W injection before infusion; if this cannot be done, then a separate IV line must be used
• An inline membrane filter may be used provided the mean pore diameter of the filter is not less than 1 micron
• Administer by IV infusion using a controlled infusion device over a period of approximately 120 min; infusion time may be reduced to approximately 60 min in patients who tolerate the infusion; if discomfort occurs during infusion, the duration of infusion may be increased
Acetaminophen and diphenhydrAMINE
• 30 min before inf to reduce fever, chills, headache
• Store protected from moisture and light; diluted solution is stable for 24 hr at room temp

Y-site compatibilities: Acyclovir, amifostine, aminophylline, anidulafungin, atropine, azithromycin, bivalirudin, bumetanide, buprenorphine, busulfan, butorphanol, CARBOplatin, carmustine, ceFAZolin, ceFOXitin, ceftizoxime, cefTRIAXone, cefuroxime, cimetidine, clindamycin, cyclophosphamide, cytarabine, DACTINomycin, DAPTOmycin, dexamethasone, dexmedetomidine, diphenhydrAMINE, doxacurium, enalaprilat, ePHEDrine, EPINEPHrine, eptifibatide, ertapenem, esmolol, etoposide, famotidine, fenoldopam, fentaNYL, fludarabine, fluorouracil, fosphenytoin, furosemide, granisetron, haloperidol, heparin, hydrocortisone, HYDROmorphone, ifosfamide, isoproterenol, ketorolac, levorphanol, lidocaine, linezolid, mesna, methotrexate, methylPREDNISolone, metoprolol, milrinone, mitoMYcin, nesiritide, nitroglycerin, nitroprusside, octreotide, oxaliplatin, oxytocin, palonosetron, pancuronium, pantoprazole, PEMEtrexed, PENTobarbital, PHENobarbital, phenylephrine, piperacillin/tazobactam, potassium chloride, procainamide, ranitidine, SUFentanil, tacrolimus, theophylline, thiopental, thiotepa, ticarcillin/clavulanate, tigecycline, trimethoprim-sulfamethoxazole, vasopressin, vinCRIStine, voriconazole, zidovudine

ADVERSE EFFECTS

CNS: *Headache, fever, chills,* peripheral nerve pain, paresthesias, peripheral neuropathy, seizures, dizziness, insomnia
CV: Bradycardia, hypotension, cardiac arrest
EENT: Tinnitus, deafness, diplopia, blurred vision
ENDO: Hyperglycemia
GI: *Nausea, vomiting, anorexia,* diarrhea, cramps, **hemorrhagic gastroenteritis, acute liver failure**
GU: *Hypokalemia,* **azotemia, hyposthenuria,** renal tubular acidosis, **nephrocalcinosis,** permanent renal impairment, anuria, oliguria
HEMA: Normochromic normocytic anemia, thrombocytopenia, agranulocytosis, leukopenia, eosinophilia, hyponatremia, hypomagnesemia
INTEG: *Burning, irritation,* pain, necrosis at inj site with extravasation, flushing, dermatitis, skin rash (topical route)
MS: Arthralgia, myalgia, generalized pain, weakness, weight loss
RESP: Dyspnea
SYST: Stevens–Johnson syndrome, toxic epidermal neurolysis, exfoliative dermatitis, anaphylaxis

Pharmacokinetics

Absorption	Complete bioavailability (IV)
Distribution	Body tissues
Metabolism	Liver
Excretion	Kidneys, detectable for several weeks
Half-life	Liposomal mean 4-6 days

Pharmacodynamics

Onset	Immediate
Duration	Unknown

INTERACTIONS
Individual drugs
Digoxin: increased hypokalemia

Drug classifications
Other nephrotoxic antibiotics (aminoglycosides, CISplatin, vancomycin, cycloSPORINE, polymyxin B): increased nephrotoxicity
Corticosteroids, skeletal muscle relaxants, thiazides: increased hypokalemia

NURSING CONSIDERATIONS
Assessment
• VS every 15-30 min during first inf; note changes in pulse, B/P
• I&O ratio; watch for decreasing urinary output, change in specific gravity; discontinue product to prevent permanent damage to renal tubules
• Blood studies: CBC, potassium, sodium, calcium, magnesium every 2 wk, BUN, creatinine 2-3 ×/wk
• Weight weekly; if weight increases by more than 2 lb/wk, edema is present; renal damage should be considered
⚠ **For renal toxicity: increasing BUN, serum creatinine; if BUN is >40 mg/dl or if serum creatinine is >3 mg/dl, product may be discontinued, dosage reduced**
⚠ **For hepatotoxicity: increasing AST, ALT, alk phos, bilirubin, monitor LFTs**
⚠ **For allergic reaction: dermatitis, rash; product should be discontinued, antihistamines (mild reaction) or EPINEPHrine (severe reaction) administered**
⚠ **For hypokalemia: anorexia, drowsiness, weakness, decreased reflexes, dizziness, increased urinary output, increased thirst, paresthesias**
⚠ **For ototoxicity: tinnitus (ringing, roaring in ears), vertigo, loss of hearing (rare)**
⚠ **Infusion reaction: chills, fever, pain, swelling at site**

Patient/family education
• Teach patient that long-term therapy may be needed to clear infection (2 wk-3 mo, depending on type of infection)
⚠ **Instruct patient to notify prescriber of bleeding, bruising, or soft-tissue swelling, renal, neurological side effects**

Evaluation
Positive therapeutic outcome
• Decreased fever, malaise, rash; negative C&S for infecting organism

ampicillin (Rx)
(am-pi-sill'in)
Ampicin ✤, Apo-Ampi ✤, Nu-Ampi ✤, Penbritin ✤
Func. class.: Broad-spectrum antiinfective
Chem. class.: Aminopenicillin
Pregnancy category B

ACTION: Interferes with cell wall replication of susceptible organisms; the cell wall, rendered osmotically unstable, swells and bursts from osmotic pressure, lysis mediated by cell wall autolysis

Therapeutic outcome: Bactericidal effects for the following organisms: effective for gram-positive cocci *(Streptococcus aureus,*

Streptococcus pyogenes, Streptococcus faecalis, Streptococcus pneumoniae), gram-negative cocci *(Neisseria meningitidis)*, gram-negative bacilli *(Haemophilus influenzae, Proteus mirabilis, Salmonella, Shigella, Listeria monocytogenes)*, gram-positive bacilli

USES: Infections of respiratory tract, skin, skin structures, GI/GU tract; otitis media, meningitis, septicemia, sinusitis, and endocarditis prophylaxis, bacterial endocarditis

CONTRAINDICATIONS
Hypersensitivity to penicillins, antimicrobial resistance, skin infection

Precautions: Pregnancy **B**, breastfeeding, neonates, hypersensitivity to cephalosporins, renal disease, mononucleosis

DOSAGE AND ROUTES
Renal dose
Adult and child: CCr 10-50 ml/min extend to q6-12hr; CCr <10 ml/min dose q12-16hr

Systemic infections
Adult and child ≥40 kg (88 lb): PO 250-500 mg q6hr; IV/IM 2-8 g daily in divided doses q4-6hr
Child <40 kg: PO 50-100 mg/kg/day in divided doses q6-8hr; IV/IM 50-500 mg/kg/day in divided doses q6-8hr

Bacterial meningitis
Adult/adolescent: IM/IV 150-200 mg/kg/day in divided doses, q3-4hr; IDSA IV 12 g divided q4hr
Infant/child: IM/IV 150-200 mg/kg/day in divided doses q3-4hr; IDSA dose IV 300 mg/kg/day divided q6hr
Neonate >7 days and >2000 g: IM/IV 200 mg/kg/day divided q6hr; IDSA dose IV 200 mg/kg/day divided q6-8hr

Prevention of bacterial endocarditis
Adult: IM/IV 2 g 30 min before procedure
Child: IM/IV 50 mg/kg 30 min before procedure, max 2 g

GI/GU infections other than caused by *N. gonorrhoeae*
Adult and child >40 kg: PO 250-500 mg q6hr, may use larger dose for more serious infections
Child <40 kg: PO 50 mg/kg/day in divided doses q6-8hr

Available forms: Powder for inj 125, 250, 500 mg, 1, 2, 10 g; IV inf 500 mg, 1, 2 g; caps 250, 500 mg; powder for oral susp 125, 250, 500 mg/5 mg

Implementation
PO route
• Give in even doses around the clock; product must be taken for 10-14 days to ensure organism death and prevent superinfection; store caps in tight container; store after reconstituting in refrigerator up to 2 wk, 1 wk room temperature
• Tabs may be crushed or caps opened and mixed with water
• Shake susp well before each dose; store for 2 wk in refrigerator or 1 wk at room temperature
IM route (painful)
• **Reconstitute** with 125 mg/0.9-1.2 ml; 250 mg/0.9-1.9 ml; 500 mg/1.2-1.8 ml; 1 g/2.4-7.4 ml; 2 g/6.8 ml
• **Give** deep in large muscle mass

IV route
• **Reconstitute** with 125 mg/0.9-1.2 ml; 250 mg/0.9-1.9 ml; 500 mg/1.2-1.8 ml; 1 g/2.4-7.4 ml; 2 g/6.8 ml
Direct IV route
• **Give** over 3-5 min in lower dosages (125-500 mg) or over 15 min in higher dosages (1-2 g)
Intermittent IV infusion route
• **Give** after diluting with 0.9% NaCl, LR, D₅W, D₅/0.45% NaCl; use 50 ml of sol and dilute to concentration of <30 mg/ml

Y-site compatibilities: Acyclovir, alemtuzumab, amifostine, allopurinol, argatroban, azithromycin, aztreonam, carmustine, cyclophosphamide, cytarabine, DAUNOrubicin, dexrazoxane, doxapram, DOXOrubicin liposome, enalaprilat, esmolol, etoposide phosphate, famotidine, filgrastim, fludarabine, foscarnet, gallium, gemtuzumab, granisetron, heparin, regular insulin, labetalol, lepirudin, leucovorin, liposome, magnesium sulfate, mannitol, melphalan, meperidine, milrinone, morphine, multivitamins, oflaxacin, penicillin G potassium, perphenazine, phytonadione, potassium acetate, potassium chloride, propofol, remifentanil, thiotepa, tolazoline, vecuronium, vinBLAStine, vit B with C, zoledronic acid

Y-site incompatibilities: Calcium gluconate, EPINEPHrine, fluconazole, hetastarch, HYDROmorphone, hydrALAZINE, ondansetron, sargramostim, verapamil, vinorelbine

ADVERSE EFFECTS
GI: *Nausea, vomiting, diarrhea,* pseudomembranous colitis, stomatitis, black hairy tongue
GU: Oliguria, proteinuria, hematuria, *vaginitis, moniliasis,* glomerulonephritis
HEMA: Anemia, increased bleeding time, bone marrow depression, granulocytopenia, leukopenia, eosinophilia, hemolysis

INTEG: *Rash*, urticaria, **toxic epidermal necrolysis**, erythema, multiforme
SYST: **Anaphylaxis**, **serum sickness**, **Stevens-Johnson syndrome**

Pharmacokinetics

Absorption	Moderate, in duodenum (35%-50%)
Distribution	Readily in body tissues, fluids, CSF; crosses placenta
Excretion	Breast milk; kidney unchanged (70%), removed by dialysis
Half-life	50-110 min

Pharmacodynamics

	PO	IM	IV
Onset	Rapid	Rapid	Rapid
Peak	2 hr	1 hr	Rapid
Duration	Unknown	Unknown	Unknown

INTERACTIONS
Individual drugs
Allopurinol: increased ampicillin-induced skin rash, monitor for rash
Probenecid: increased ampicillin levels, decreased renal excretion

Drug classifications
Contraceptives (oral): decreased contraceptive effectiveness; use reliable contraception, use alternative contraception
H2 antagonists, proton pump inhibitors: decreased ampicillin level
Oral anticoagulants: increased bleeding, monitor INR/PTT

Drug/lab test
Increased: eosinophil
Decreased: conjugated estrone in pregnancy, conjugated estriol, Hgb, WBC, platelets
False positive: urine glucose
Interfere: urine glucose (Clinitest, Benedict's reagent, cupric SO_4)

NURSING CONSIDERATIONS
Assessment
• Assess patient for previous sensitivity reaction to penicillins or other cephalosporins; cross-sensitivity between penicillins and cephalosporins is common
• Assess patient for signs and symptoms of **infection**, including characteristics of wounds, sputum, urine, stool, WBC >10,000/mm³, earache, fever; obtain baseline information and during treatment

• Obtain C&S before beginning product therapy to identify if correct treatment has been initiated
• **Assess for allergic reactions: rash, urticaria, pruritus, chills, fever, joint pain; angioedema may occur a few days after therapy begins; EPINEPHrine and resuscitation equipment should be on unit for anaphylactic reaction; also, check for ampicillin rash: pruritic, red, raised; identify allergies before using**
⚠ **Identify urine output, hematuria; if decreasing, notify prescriber (may indicate nephrotoxicity)**
• Monitor renal studies: urinalysis, protein, blood, BUN, creatinine
• Monitor blood studies: AST, ALT, CBC, Hct, bilirubin, LDH, alkaline phosphatase, Coombs' test monthly if patient is on long-term therapy
• Monitor electrolytes: potassium, sodium, chloride monthly if patient is on long-term therapy
• Assess bowel pattern daily; if severe diarrhea occurs, product should be discontinued; may indicate pseudomembranous colitis
• Assess for **overgrowth of infection:** perineal itching, fever, malaise, redness, pain, swelling, drainage, rash, diarrhea, change in cough, sputum

Patient/family education
⚠ **Teach patient to report sore throat, bruising, bleeding, joint pain; may indicate blood dyscrasias (rare)**
• **Advise patient to contact prescriber if vaginal itching, loose foul-smelling stools, furry tongue occur; may indicate superinfection**
• Instruct patient to take all medication prescribed for the length of time ordered
• **Advise patient to notify prescriber of diarrhea with blood or pus, which may indicate pseudomembranous colitis**
• Tab may be crushed; cap may be opened and mixed with water; to use alternative contraception

Evaluation
Positive therapeutic outcome
• Absence of signs/symptoms of infection (WBC <10,000, temp WNL)
• Reported improvement in symptoms of infection

TREATMENT OF ANAPHYLAXIS:
Withdraw product, maintain airway, administer EPINEPHrine, aminophylline, O_2, **IV** corticosteroids

---

Adverse effects: *italics* = common; **bold** = life-threatening

ampicillin/sulbactam (Rx)
(am-pi-sill'in/sul-bak'tam)
Unasyn
Func. class.: Broad-spectrum antiinfective
Chem. class.: Aminopenicillin
Pregnancy category B (ampicillin)

ACTION: Interferes with cell wall replication of susceptible organisms; the cell wall, rendered osmotically unstable, swells and bursts from osmotic pressure; lysis due to cell wall autolytic enzymes; this combination extends the spectrum of activity and inhibits β-lactamase that may inactivate ampicillin

Therapeutic outcome: Bactericidal against *Staphylococcus aureus, Klebsiella, Bacteroides fragilis, Enterobacter, Acinetobacter calcoaceticus, Pneumococcus, Enterococcus, Streptococcus, Escherichia coli, Proteus mirabilis, Neisseria meningitidis, Neisseria gonorrhoeae, Shigella, Salmonella,* and *Haemophilus influenzae* organisms; use only with β-lactamase–producing strain of infection

USES: Skin infections, intraabdominal infections, gynecological infections, asthma, cellulitis, diabetes mellitus, diabetic foot ulcer, dialysis, diarrhea, eczema, IBS, leukemia, meningitis, nosocomial pneumonia, ulcerative colitis; *Actinobacter, Actinomyces, Bacillus anthracis, Bacteroides, Bifidobacterium, Bordetella pertussis, Borrelia burgdorferi, Brucella, Clostridium, Corynebacterium diptheriae/xerosis, Eikenella corrodens, Enterococcus faecalis, Erysipelothrix rhusiopathiae, Escherichia coli, Eubacterium, Fusobacterium, Gardnerella vaginalis, Haemophilus influenzae* (beta-lactamase negative/positive), *Helicobacter pylori, Klebsiella, Lactobacillus, Leptospira, Listeria monocytogenes, Moraxella catarrhalis, Morganella morganii, Neisseria gonorrhoeae, Pasteurella multocida, Peptococcus, Peptostreptococcus, Porphyromonas, Prevotella, Propionibacterium, Proteus mirabilis, Proteus vulgaris, Providencia rettgeri, Providencia stuartii, Salmonella, Shigella, Staphylococcus aureus* (MSSA)/*epidermidis/saprophyticus, Streptococcus agalactiae/dysgalactiae/pneumoniae/pyrogenes, Treponema pallidum,* viridans streptococci

Unlabeled uses: Hospital/community-acquired pneumonia, infective endocarditis, pelvic inflammatory disease

CONTRAINDICATIONS
Hypersensitivity to ampicillin, or sulbactam

Precautions: Pregnancy **B**, breastfeeding, neonates, hypersensitivity to cephalosporins, renal disease, mononucleosis, viral infections, syphilis

DOSAGE AND ROUTES
Adult and child >40 kg: IM/IV 1 g ampicillin and 0.5 g sulbactam to 2 g ampicillin, and 1 g sulbactam q6hr, not to exceed 4 g/day sulbactam
Child <40 kg: IV 100-200 mg/kg/day (ampicillin component) divided q6hr, max 4 g/day

Renal dose
Adult ≥40 kg: IM/IV CCr 15-29 ml/min dose q12hr; CCr 5-14 ml/min dose q24hr

Community-aquired pneumonia (unlabeled)
Adult: IV 3 g q12hr in combination X ≥ 5 days

Endocarditis (unlabeled)
Adult: IV 12 g divided q8hr
Child: IV 300 mg/kg per day divided q8hr

Pelvic inflammatory disease (unlabeled)
Adult/adolescent: IV 3 g q6hr in combination

Available forms: Powder for inj 1.5 g (1 g ampicillin, 0.5 g sulbactam), 3 g (2 g ampicillin, 1 g sulbactam), 15 g (10 g ampicillin, 5 g sulbactam)

Implementation
• Scratch test to assess allergy after securing order from prescriber; usually done when penicillin is only product choice
IM route
• Reconstitute by adding 3.2 ml/1.5 g or 6.4 ml/3 g; use sterile water, 0.5% or 2% lidocaine; give within 1 hr of preparation; give deep in large muscle mass, aspirate
• Do not give IM in child
• Give after C&S completed; on empty stomach

IV direct route
• Give **IV** after diluting 1.5 g/3.2 ml sterile water for inj; or 3 g/6.4 ml (250 mg ampicillin/125 mg sulbactam); allow to stand until foaming stops; give directly over 10-15 min, inject slowly
Intermittent IV infusion route
• Dilute further in 50 ml or more of D₅W, D₅/10.45% NaCl, 10% invert sugar in water, LR, 6% sodium lactate, isotonic NaCl; administer within 1 hr after reconstitution; give as an intermittent inf over 15-30 min

Y-site compatibilities: Alemtuzumab, amifostine, aminocaproic acid, anidulafungin, argatroban, atenolol, bivalirudin, bleomycin, CARBOplatin, carmustine, cefepime, CISplatin, codeine, cyclophosphamide, cytarabine, DAPTOmycin, DAUNOrubicin liposome, dexmedetomidine, DOCEtaxel, doxacurium, DOXOrubicin liposomal, eptifibatide, etoposide, fenoldopam, filgrastim, fludarabine, fluorouracil, foscarnet, gallium, gatifloxacin, gemcitabine, granisetron, irinotecan, levofloxacin, linezolid, methotrexate, metroNIDAZOLE, octreotide, oxaliplatin, PACLitaxel, palonosetron, pamidronate, pancuronium, pantoprazole, PEMEtrexed, remifentanil, riTUXimab, rocuronium, tacrolimus, teniposide, thiotepa, tigecycline, tirofiban, TNA, TPN, trastuzumab, vecuronium, vinCRIStine, voriconazole, zoledronic acid

Y-site incompatibilities: IDArubicin, ondansetron, sargramostim

ADVERSE EFFECTS

CNS: Lethargy, hallucinations, anxiety, depression, twitching, **coma, seizures**

GI: *Nausea, vomiting, diarrhea,* increased AST, ALT, abdominal pain, glossitis, colitis, **pseudomembranous colitis, hepatic necrosis/ failure,** black hairy tongue

GU: Oliguria, proteinuria, hematuria, *vaginitis, moniliasis,* **glomerulonephritis,** dysuria

HEMA: Anemia, increased bleeding time, **bone marrow depression, granulocytopenia, leukopenia, eosinophilia, hemolysis**

INTEG: Injection site reactions, rash, edema, urticaria

SYST: **Anaphylaxis, serum sickness, toxic epidermal necrolysis, Stevens-Johnson syndrome,** hypoalbuminemia

Pharmacokinetics

Absorption	Well absorbed (IM)
Distribution	Readily in body tissues, fluids, CSF; crosses placenta
Metabolism	Liver (10%-50%)
Excretion	Breast milk; kidney unchanged (75%)
Half-life	50-110 min (ampicillin)

Pharmacodynamics

	IM	IV
Onset	Rapid	Immediate
Peak	1 hr	Infusion's end
Duration	Unknown	Unknown

INTERACTIONS
Individual drugs

Allopurinol: ampicillin-induced skin rash, check for rash

Methotrexate: increased methotrexate level

Probenecid: increased ampicillin levels, decreased renal excretion

Drug classifications

Oral anticoagulants: increased bleeding risk, check INR, PT

Drug/lab test

False positive: urine glucose, urine protein

NURSING CONSIDERATIONS
Assessment

• Assess patient for previous sensitivity reaction to penicillins or cephalosporins; cross-sensitivity between penicillins and cephalosporins is common

• Assess patient for signs and symptoms of **infection,** including characteristics of wounds, sputum, urine, stool, WBC >10,000/mm^3, earache, fever; obtain baseline information and during treatment; complete C&S before beginning product therapy to identify if correct treatment has been initiated

• **Assess for allergic reactions: rash, urticaria, pruritus, chills, fever, joint pain; angioedema may occur a few days after therapy begins; EPINEPHrine and resuscitation equipment should be on unit for anaphylactic reaction**

⚠ **Identify urine output; if decreasing, notify prescriber (may indicate nephrotoxicity)**

• Assess renal studies: urinalysis, protein, BUN, creatinine

• Monitor blood studies: AST, ALT, CBC, Hct, bilirubin, LDH, alkaline phosphatase, Coombs' test monthly if patient is on long-term therapy

• Monitor electrolytes: potassium, sodium, chloride monthly if patient is on long-term therapy

• **Assess bowel pattern daily; if severe diarrhea occurs, product should be discontinued; may indicate pseudomembranous colitis**

• Monitor for bleeding: ecchymosis, bleeding gums, hematuria, stool guaiac daily if on long-term therapy

• Assess for superinfection: perineal itching, fever, malaise, redness, pain, swelling, drainage, rash, diarrhea, change in cough, sputum

Patient/family education

• Teach patient to report sore throat, bruising, bleeding, joint pain, persistent diarrhea; may indicate blood dyscrasias (rare) or superinfection

• **Advise patient to contact prescriber if vaginal itching, loose foul-smelling stools, furry tongue occur; may indicate pseudomembraneous colitis**

• Instruct patient to use another form of contraception other than oral contraceptives

⚠ **Instruct patient to report immediately pseudomembranous colitis: fever, diarrhea**

Adverse effects: *italics* = common; **bold** = life-threatening

with pus, blood, or mucus; may occur up to 4 wk after treatment

• Instruct patient to wear or carry emergency ID if allergic to penicillin products

Evaluation
Positive therapeutic outcome
• Absence of signs/symptoms of infection (WBC <10,000/mm^3, temp WNL, absence of red draining wounds, earache)
• Reported improvement in symptoms of infection

TREATMENT OF OVERDOSE:
Withdraw product, maintain airway, administer EPINEPHrine, aminophylline, O$_2$, **IV** corticosteroids for anaphylaxis

anakinra (Rx)
(an-ah-kin′rah)
Kineret
Func. class.: Antirheumatic agent (disease modifying), immunomodulator
Chem. class.: Recombinant form of human interleukin-1 receptor antagonist (IL-1Ra)
Pregnancy category B

Do not confuse: anakinra/amikacin

ACTION: A form of human interleukin-1 receptor antagonist (IL-1Ra) produced by DNA technology; blocks activity of IL-1, resulting in decreased inflammation, cartilage degradation, bone resorption

Therapeutic outcome: Decreased pain, inflammation

USES: Reduction in signs and symptoms of moderate to severe active rheumatoid arthritis in patients 18 years of age or older who have not responded to other disease-modifying agents, neonatal-onset multisystem inflammatory disease

CONTRAINDICATIONS
Hypersensitivity to *Escherichia coli*–derived proteins or this product, sepsis, latex

Precautions: Pregnancy **B**, breastfeeding, children, geriatric, renal impairment, active infections, immunosuppression, neoplastic disease, asthma

DOSAGE AND ROUTES
Rheumatoid arthritis
Adult: SUBCUT 100 mg daily

Renal dose
Adult: CCr <30 ml/min; SUBCUT 100 mg every other day

Neonatal-onset multisystem inflammatory disease
Adult/child: SUBCUT 1-2 mg/kg/day; may increase by 0.5-1 mg to max 8 mg/kg/day (adult) or 7.6 mg/kg/day (child)

Available forms: Inj, 100 mg/0.67 ml prefilled glass syringe

Implementation
• Do not use if cloudy or discolored or if particulate is present; protect from light
• Do not admix with other sol or medications, do not use filter

ADVERSE EFFECTS
CNS: Headache
CV: Cardiac arrest
EENT: Sinusitis
GI: Abdominal pain, nausea, diarrhea
HEMA: Neutropenia
INTEG: Rash, *inj site reaction,* allergic reaction
MISC: Flulike symptoms, infection
MS: *Worsening of RA, arthralgia*
RESP: *URI*

Pharmacokinetics
Absorption	Well absorbed (SUBCUT)
Distribution	Unknown
Metabolism	Unknown
Excretion	Urine
Half-life	4-6 hr

Pharmacodynamics
Onset	Unknown
Peak	3-7 hr
Duration	Unknown

INTERACTIONS
Individual drugs
Rilonacept: do not use

Drug classifications
Antibody reactions: decreased
Etanercept, TNF-blocking agents: increased risk of severe infection, do not use together
Vaccines: Avoid concurrent use; immunizations should be brought up to date before treatment

NURSING CONSIDERATIONS
Assessment
• **Rheumatoid arthritis:** assess pain, stiffness, ROM, swelling of joints during treatment
• Assess for inj site pain, swelling; usually occur after 2 inj (4-5 days)
• Assess for **infections**, stop treatment if present, do not start if patient has active infection

---

Patient/family education
• Teach patient about self-administration if appropriate: inj should be made in thigh, abdomen, upper arm; rotate sites at least 1 in from old site, store in refrigerator, do not freeze
• Advise patient to notify prescriber if pregnancy is planned or suspected, avoid breastfeeding
• Advise patient not to receive vaccines while taking this product, update vaccines before treatment

Evaluation
Positive therapeutic outcome
• Decreased inflammation, pain in joints

⚠ HIGH ALERT

anastrozole (Rx)
(an-ass-stroh'zole)
Arimidex
Func. class.: Antineoplastic
Chem. class.: Aromatase inhibitor
Pregnancy category X

ACTION: Highly selective nonsteroidal aromatase inhibitor that lowers serum estradiol concentrations; many breast cancers have strong estrogen receptors

Therapeutic outcome: Prevention of rapidly growing malignant cells

USES: Advanced breast carcinoma in estrogen-receptor-positive patients (usually postmenopausal); patients with advanced disease on tamoxifen, adjunct therapy, endometriosis

CONTRAINDICATIONS
Pregnancy **X**, hypersensitivity, breastfeeding

Precautions: Children, geriatric, cardiac/hepatic disease, premenopausal females, osteoporosis

DOSAGE AND ROUTES
Adult: PO 1 mg daily; continue for 5 yr in ERT early breast cancer who have already received 2-3 yr of tamoxifen and are switched to anastrozole, max 5 yr; may also combine with tamoxifen for up to 10 yr

Available forms: Tabs 1 mg

Implementation
• Do not break, crush, or chew enteric products
• Give with food or fluids for GI upset; repeat dose may be needed if vomiting occurs
• Store in light-resistant container at room temperature

ADVERSE EFFECTS
CNS: Hot flashes, headache, light-headedness, depression, dizziness, confusion, insomnia, anxiety, fatigue, mood changes
CV: Chest pain, hypertension, **thrombophlebitis**, edema, **MI, CVA, cerebral infarction**, angina, *vasodilation*, **PE, DVT**
GI: Nausea, vomiting, altered taste leading to anorexia, diarrhea, constipation, abdominal pain, dry mouth, weight gain
GU: Vaginal bleeding, pruritus vulvae, vaginal dryness, pelvic pain, UTI
HEMA: Leukopenia, anemia
INTEG: Rash, **Stevens-Johnson syndrome**
MISC: Hypercholesterolemia
MS: Bone pain, myalgia, asthenia, bone loss, osteoporosis, arthralgia, fractures
RESP: Cough, sinusitis, dyspnea, **pulmonary embolism**

Pharmacokinetics
Absorption	Adequately absorbed
Distribution	Unknown
Metabolism	Liver
Excretion	Feces, urine
Half-life	50 hr

Pharmacodynamics
Onset	Unknown
Peak	4-7 hr
Duration	Unknown

INTERACTIONS
Drug/drug
• Do not use with oral contraceptives, estrogen, tamoxifen, androstenedione, DHEA

Drug/lab test
Increased: GGT, AST, ALT, alkaline phosphatase, cholesterol, LDL

NURSING CONSIDERATIONS
Assessment
• Monitor bone mineral density, cholesterol, lipid panel periodically
• Assess serious skin reactions: Stevens-Johnson syndrome
• Not effective in hormone receptor-negative disease, use only in postmenopausal women
• That tumor flare—increase in size of tumor, increased bone pain—may occur and will subside rapidly; may take analgesics for pain

---

Adverse effects: *italics* = common; **bold** = life-threatening

Patient/family education

- Instruct patient to report any complaints, side effects to health care prescriber; if dose is missed, do not double next dose
- Advise patient that vaginal bleeding, pruritus, hot flashes, can occur and are reversible after discontinuing treatment
- Teach patient to take adequate calcium, vitamin D; risk of bone loss/fractures
- Inform patient that rash or lesions are temporary and may become large during beginning therapy

Evaluation

Positive therapeutic outcome
- Decreased spread of malignant cells in breast cancer

---

anidulafungin (Rx)

(a-nid-yoo-luh-fun′jin)

Eraxis

Func. class.: Antifungal, systemic
Chem. class.: Echinocandin

Pregnancy category C

ACTION: Inhibits fungal enzyme synthesis; causes direct damage to fungal cell wall

Therapeutic outcome: Decreased symptoms of candida infection, negative culture

USES: Esophageal candidiasis, *Aspergillosis, Candida albicans, Candida glabrata, Candida parapsilosis, Candida tropicalis*

CONTRAINDICATIONS

Hypersensitivity to this product or other echinocandins

Precautions: Pregnancy **C**, breastfeeding, children, severe hepatic disease

DOSAGE AND ROUTES

Candidemia and other candidal infections; serious systemic infections (unlabeled)

Adult: IV loading dose 200 mg on day 1, then 100 mg/day until 14 days or more since last positive culture

Esophageal candidiasis

Adult: IV loading dose 100 mg on day 1, then 50 mg/day for at least 14 days and for at least 7 days after symptoms are resolved

Available forms: Powder for injection, lyophilized 50, 100 mg

Implementation

IV route

- Visually inspect prepared infusions for particulate matter and discoloration—do not use if present; give by IV infusion only, after dilution
- **Reconstitution:** Reconstitute each 50 mg or 100 mg vial/15 ml or 30 ml of sterile water for injection, respectively (3.33 mg/ml)
- **Storage:** Reconstituted solutions are stable for ≤24 hr at room temperature
- **Dilution:** Do not use any other diluents besides dextrose 5% in water (D_5W) or sodium chloride 0.9% (NS)
- *Preparation of the 200-mg loading dose infusion:* Withdraw the contents of either four 50-mg reconstituted vials OR two 100-mg reconstituted vials and add to an IV infusion bag or bottle containing 200 ml of D_5W or NS to give a total infusion volume of 260 ml
- *Preparation of the 100-mg daily infusion:* Withdraw the contents of one 100-mg reconstituted vial OR two 50-mg reconstituted vials and add to an IV infusion bag or bottle containing 100 ml of D_5W or NS to give a total infusion volume of 130 ml
- *Preparation of a 50-mg daily infusion:* Withdraw the contents of one 50-mg reconstituted vial and add to an IV infusion bag or bottle containing 50 ml of D_5W or NS to give a total infusion volume of 65 ml

Intermittent IV INF route

- Do not mix or co-infuse with other medications
- Administer as a slow IV infusion at a rate of 1.4 ml/min or 84 ml/hr; minimum duration of infusion is 180 min for the 200-mg dose, 90 min for the 100-mg dose, and 45 min for the 50-mg dose
- Store reconstituted vials at 59°-86° F (15°-30° C) for up to 24 hr; do not freeze (dehydrated alcohol); store reconstituted vials at 36°-46° F (2°-7° C) (sterile water) for up to 24 hr; do not freeze

IV compatibilities: Acyclovir, alemtuzumab, alfentanil, allopurinol, amifostine, amikacin, aminocaproic acid, aminophylline, amiodarone hydrochloride, amphotericin B lipid complex, amphotericin B liposome, ampicillin, ampicillin sulbactam, argatroban, arsenic trioxide, atenolol, atracurium, azithromycin, aztreonam, bivalirudin, bleomycin, bumetanide, buprenorphine, busulfan, butorphanol, calcium chloride/gluconate, CARBOplatin, carmustine, caspofungin, ceFAZolin, cefepime, cefotaxime, cefoTEtan, cefOXitin, cefTAZidime, ceftizoxime, cefTRIAXone, cefuroxime, chloramphenicol, chlorproMAZINE, cimetidine, ciprofloxacin, cisatracurium, CISplatin, clindamycin, cyclophosphamide, cycloSPORINE, cytarabine, dacarbazine, DACTINomycin, DAUNOrubicin, DAUNOrubicin liposome, dexamethasone, dexmedetomidine, dexrazoxane, diazepam, digoxin, diltiazem, diphenhydrAMINE, DOBUTamine, DOCEtaxel, dolasetron, DOPamine, doripenem, doxacurium, DOXOrubicin, DOXOrubicin liposomal, doxycycline, droperidol, enalaprilat, ePHEDrine, EPINEPHrine, epirubicin, eptifibatide, erythromycin, esmolol, etoposide, etoposide phosphate, famotidine, fenoldopam, fentaNYL, fluconazole, fludarabine, fluorouracil, foscarnet, fosphenytoin, furosemide, gallium, ganciclovir, gatifloxacin, gemcitabine, gentamicin, glycopyrrolate, granisetron, haloperidol, heparin, hydrALAZINE, hydrocortisone, HYDROmorphone, hydrOXYzine, IDArubicin, ifosfamide, imipenem-cilastatin, inamrinone, insulin (regular), irinotecan, isoproterenol, ketorolac, labetalol, leucovorin, levofloxacin, lidocaine, linezolid injection, LORazepam, mannitol, mechlorethamine, melphalan, meperidine, meropenem, mesna, metaraminol, methotrexate, methyldopate, methylPREDNISolone, metoclopramide, metoprolol, metroNIDAZOLE, midazolam, milrinone, mitoMYcin, mitoXANtrone, mivacurium, morphine, moxifloxacin, mycophenolate mofetil, nafcillin, naloxone, nesiritide, niCARdipine, nitroglycerin, nitroprusside, norepinephrine, octreotide, ondansetron, oxaliplatin, oxytocin, PACLitaxel, palonosetron, pamidronate, pancuronium, pantoprazole, pentamidine, pentazocine, PENTobarbital, PHENobarbital, phentolamine, phenylephrine, piperacillin-tazobactam, polymyxin B, potassium acetate/chloride, procainamide, prochlorperazine, promethazine, propranolol, quiNIDine, quinupristin-dalfopristin, ranitidine, remifentanil, rocuronium, sodium acetate, streptozocin, succinylcholine, SUFentanil citrate, sulfamethoxazole-trimethoprim, tacrolimus, teniposide, theophylline, thiopental, thiotepa, ticarcillin, ticarcillin-clavulanate, tirofiban, tobramycin, topotecan, trimethobenzamide, vancomycin, vasopressin, vecuronium, verapamil, vinBLAStine, vinCRIStine, vinorelbine, voriconazole, zidovudine, zoledronic acid

ADVERSE EFFECTS
Candidemia/other candida infections
CNS: *Seizures,* dizziness, *headache*
CV: Deep vein thrombosis, **atrial fibrillation, right bundle branch block,** hypotension, **QT prolongation, sinus arrhythmia, thrombophlebitis superficial, ventricular extrasystoles (rare)**
GI: *Nausea; anorexia; vomiting; diarrhea; increased AST, ALT*
META: Hypokalemia

Esophageal candidiasis
CNS: *Headache*
GI: *Nausea, anorexia, vomiting, diarrhea,* **hepatic necrosis**
HEMA: **Neutropenia, thrombocytopenia, leukopenia, coagulopathy**
INTEG: *Rash,* urticaria, itching, flushing
META: Hypocalcemia, hyperglycemia, hyperkalemia, hypernatremia, hypomagnesemia (rare)
MS: *Back pain, rigors*

Pharmacokinetics

Absorption	Unknown
Distribution	Steady state after loading dose, protein binding 84%
Metabolism	Unknown
Excretion	Unknown
Half-life	Distribution 0.5-1 hr, terminal 40-50 hr

Pharmacodynamics

Unknown

INTERACTIONS
Drug/lab test
Increased: amylase, bilirubin, CPK, creatinine, ECG, lipase, PT, alk phos
Decreased: platelets, magnesium, potassium, transferase, urea

NURSING CONSIDERATIONS
Assessment
• Assess for **infection,** clearing of cultures during treatment; obtain culture at baseline and throughout; product may be started as soon as culture is taken, those with HIV pharyngeal candidiasis may need antifungals
• **Blood dyscrasias (rare):** monitor CBC (RBC, Hct, Hgb), differential, platelet count periodically; notify prescriber of results
• Monitor hepatic studies before and during treatment: bilirubin, AST, ALT, alk phosphatase; uric acid, as needed
• Assess for **bleeding:** hematuria, heme-positive stools, bruising or petechiae, mucosa or orifices; blood dyscrasias can occur
• Assess for GI symptoms: frequency of stools, cramping, if severe diarrhea occurs, electrolytes may need to be given

Patient/family education
• Advise patient to notify prescriber if pregnancy is suspected or planned; use nonhormonal form of contraception while taking this product
• Instruct patient to avoid breastfeeding while taking this product

- Advise patient to inform prescriber of kidney or liver disease
- Advise patient to report bleeding
- Teach patient to report signs of infection: increased temp, sore throat, flulike symptoms
- **Teach patient to notify prescriber of nausea, vomiting, diarrhea, jaundice, anorexia, clay-colored stools, dark urine; heptatotoxicity may occur**

Evaluation
Positive therapeutic outcome
- Decreased symptoms of candidal infection, negative culture

apraclonidine ophthalmic
See Appendix B

apremilast
(a-pre'mi-last)
Otezla
Func. class.: Musculoskeletal agent: disease-modifying antirheumatic drug (DMARD)
Pregnancy category C

ACTION: A phosphodiesterase-4 (PDE4) inhibitor specific for cyclic adenosine monophosphate (cAMP). Inhibition of PDE4 results in an increase in intracellular concentration of cAMP, with a partial inhibition of proinflammatory mediators and an increase in the production of some antiinflammatory mediators

Therapeutic outcome: Resolution of symptoms of psoriatic arthritis or plaque psoriasis

USES: Treatment of active psoriatic arthritis; severe plaque psoriasis (in those not a candidate for phototherapy)

CONTRAINDICATIONS: Hypersensitivity

Precautions: Pregnancy **C**, breastfeeding, depression/suicidal, renal disease (CCr <30 ml/min)

DOSAGE AND ROUTES
Treatment of active psoriatic arthritis/severe plaque psoriasis
Adult: PO To reduce the risk for gastrointestinal symptoms, titrate to a final dose of 30 mg bid; day 1: 10 mg PO AM; day 2: 10 mg AM and PM; day 3: 10 mg AM and 20 mg PM; day 4: 20 mg AM and PM; day 5: 20 mg AM and 30 mg PM; day 6 and thereafter: 30 mg bid

Renal dose
Adult: PO CCr ≥30 ml/min: no change; CCr <30 ml/min: 30 mg every day. Initially, 10 mg AM days 1-3; 20 mg AM days 4 and 5; 30 mg every day for day 6 and thereafter

Available forms: Tab 30 mg; starter pack

Implementation
Give whole; do not crush, break, or chew; give without regard to meals

ADVERSE EFFECTS
CNS: *Headache,* depression, suicidal ideation, fatigue, insomnia
GI: Diarrhea, nausea, vomiting, abdominal pain, frequent bowel movements, dyspepsia, weight loss
MS: Back pain
RESP: URI, pharyngitis, bronchitis
SYST: Hypersensitivity reactions

Pharmacokinetics

Absorption	Unknown
Distribution	68% bound to plasma proteins
Metabolism	Liver, metabolized by CYP3A4
Excretion	Urine (58%), feces (39%)
Half-life	6-9 hr

Pharmacodynamics

Onset	Unknown
Peak	2.5 hr
Duration	Unknown

INTERACTIONS
Drug classifications
CYP3A4 inducers (rifampin, isoniazid, pyrazinamide, barbiturates, phenytoin, carbamazepine, enzalutamide), avoid concurrent use; decreased effect of apremilast

Drug/herb
CYP3A4 inducers (St. Johns' wort), avoid concurrent use: decreased effect of apremilast

NURSING CONSIDERATIONS
Assessment
- **Psoriatic arthritis/severe plaque psoriasis:** assess for hypersensitivity reactions
- **Pregnancy and breastfeeding: if used during pregnancy, call 877-311-8972; avoid use in breastfeeding**
- **Assess for depression and suicidal ideation, mood changes; for renal failure or severe renal impairment (CCr <30 ml/min), dosage reduction is required**

A

Patient/family education
• Teach patient to report rash, hypersensitivity reactions
• Teach patient to avoid use in pregnancy and breastfeeding; if used during pregnancy, call 877-311-8972
• **Advise patient to be alert for depression and suicidal ideation, mood changes; if these occur, notify prescriber immediately**

Evaluation
Positive therapeutic outcome
• Resolution of symptoms of psoriatic arthritis or plaque psoriasis

---

aprepitant (Rx)
(ap-re′pi-tant)
Emend
fosaprepitant
Emend
Func. class.: Antiemetic
Chem. class.: Miscellaneous
Pregnancy category B

Do not confuse: aprepitant/fosaprepitant

ACTION: Selective antagonist of human substance P/neurokinin 1 (NK$_1$) receptors, decreasing emetic reflex

Therapeutic outcome: Decreased nausea, vomiting during chemotherapy

USES: Prevention of nausea, vomiting associated with cancer chemotherapy (highly emetogenic/moderately emetogenic) including high-dose cisplatin; used in combination with other antiemetics; postop nausea, vomiting

CONTRAINDICATIONS
Hypersensitivity to this product, polysorbate 80

Precautions: Pregnancy **B**, breastfeeding, children, geriatric, hepatic disease

DOSAGE AND ROUTES
Prevention of nausea/vomiting after chemotherapy antineoplastics
Adult: PO day 1 (1 hr prior to chemotherapy) aprepitant 125 mg with 12 mg 1st dose of aprepitant on day 1 of regimen (fosaprepitant)

Prevention of postop nausea/vomiting
Adult: PO 40 mg within 3 hr of induction of anesthesia

Available forms: Caps 40, 80, 125 mg; powder for inj, 150 mg; combo pack cap 80-125 mg

Implementation
PO route
• Give PO on 3-day schedule, given with other antiemetics
• Take first dose 1 hr prior to chemotherapy
• Store at room temperature; keep in original bottles, blisters

IV route
• Only approved as a substitute for the 1st dose of aprepitant in 3-day regimen
• Reconstitution: use aseptic technique; inject 5 ml 0.9% NaCl into the vial, directing stream to wall of vial to prevent foam; swirl; do not shake
• Prepare inf bag with 145 ml/150 mg do not dilute or reconstitute with any divalent cations such as calcium, magnesium, including LR, Hartmann's sol
• Withdraw the entire volume from vial and transfer to inf bag; total volume 115 ml (1 mg/1 ml)
• Gently invert bag 2-3 times; reconstituted sol is stable for 24 hr at lower room temperature or <25° C
• Visually inspect for particulates and discoloration
• Infuse over 20-30 min, stable for 24 hr at room temperature

ADVERSE EFFECTS
CNS: *Headache, dizziness,* insomnia, anxiety, depression, confusion, peripheral neuropathy
CV: Bradycardia, tachycardia, **DVT,** hypertension, hypotension
GI: *Diarrhea; constipation;* abdominal pain; anorexia; gastritis; increased AST, ALT; *nausea;* vomiting; heartburn
GU: Increased BUN, serum creatine, proteinuria, dysuria
HEMA: Anemia, **thrombocytopenia, neutropenia**
INTEG: Pruritus, rash, urticaria, infection reaction
MISC: Asthenia, fatigue, dehydration, fever, hiccups, tinnitus, alopecia
SYST: **Anaphylaxis**

Pharmacokinetics
Absorption	Unknown
Distribution	95% protein bound
Metabolism	Liver (CYP3A4 enzymes to an active metabolite)
Excretion	Not in kidneys
Half-life	10-12 hr

Pharmacodynamics
Unknown

Adverse effects: *italics* = common; **bold** = life-threatening

INTERACTIONS
Individual drugs
Paroxetine: decreased action of both products

Drug classifications
CYP2C9 substrates (phenytoin, TOLBUTamide, warfarin), oral contraceptives: decreased action
CYP3A4 inhibitors (clarithromycin, diltiazem, itraconazole, ketoconazole, nefazodone, nelfinavir, ritonavir, troleandomycin): increased aprepitant action
CYP3A4 inducers (carBAMazepine, phenytoin, rifampin): decreased aprepitant action
CYP3A4 substrates (ALPRAZolam, cisapride, dexamethasone, DOCEtaxel, etoposide, ifosfamide, imatinib, irinotecan, methylPREDNISolone, midazolam, PACLitaxel, pimozide, triazolam, vinBLAStine, vinCRIStine, vinorelbine): increased action

Drug/food
Grapefruit juice: decreased effect

NURSING CONSIDERATIONS
Assessment
• Assess for hypersensitivity reactions: pruritus, rash, urticaria, anaphylaxis
• Assess for absence of nausea, vomiting during chemotherapy
• CBC, LFTs, creatinine baseline and periodically

Patient/family education
• Teach to report diarrhea, constipation
• Advise to take only as prescribed
• Advise to report all medication to prescriber prior to taking this medication
• Instruct to use nonhormonal form of contraception while taking this agent
• Advise those on warfarin to have clotting monitored closely during 2-wk period following administration of aprepitant
• Teach to avoid breastfeeding

Evaluation
Positive therapeutic outcome
• Absence of nausea, vomiting during cancer chemotherapy

---

arformoterol (Rx)
(ar-for-moe′ter-ole)
Brovana
Func. class.: Long-acting adrenergic β_2-agonist, sympathomimetic, bronchodilator
Pregnancy category C

Do not confuse: Brovana/Boniva

ACTION: Causes bronchodilation by action on β_2 (pulmonary) receptors by increasing levels of cyclic AMP, which relaxes smooth muscle; produces bronchodilation, CNS, and cardiac stimulation, and increased diuresis and gastric acid secretion; longer acting than isoproterenol

Therapeutic outcome: Absence of dyspnea, wheezing after 1 hr, improved airway exchange, improved ABGs

USES: Maintenance bronchospasm prevention in COPD, including chronic bronchitis, emphysema

CONTRAINDICATIONS
Hypersensitivity to sympathomimetics, this product, or racemic formoterol; tachydysrhythmias, severe cardiac disease, heart block, children, monotherapy in asthma

Precautions: Pregnancy **C**, breastfeeding, cardiac disorders, hyperthyroidism, diabetes mellitus, hypertension, prostatic hypertrophy, closed-angle glaucoma, seizures, hypoglycemia

> **BLACK BOX WARNING:** Asthma-related death

DOSAGE AND ROUTES
COPD
Adult: NEB 15 mcg, bid, AM, PM

Available forms: Inh sol 15 mcg/2 ml

Implementation
• Must be used by nebulization; give over 5-10 min
• Store in refrigerator; if stored at room temp, discard after 6 wk or if past expiration date, whichever is sooner

ADVERSE EFFECTS
CNS: *Tremors, anxiety,* insomnia, headache, dizziness, stimulation, *restlessness,* hallucinations, flushing, irritability
CV: Palpitations, tachycardia, hypo/hypertension, angina, dysrhythmias, AV block, heart failure, prolonged QT, supraventricular tachycardia
EENT: Dry nose, irritation of nose and throat
GI: Heartburn, nausea, vomiting
MISC: Flushing, sweating, anorexia, bad taste/smell changes, hypokalemia, anaphylaxis, *hypoglycemia*
MS: Muscle cramps, back pain
RESP: Cough, wheezing, dyspnea, bronchospasm, dry throat

Pharmacokinetics

Absorption	Unknown
Distribution	Crosses placenta, protein binding 52%-65%
Metabolism	Direct conjugation by CYP2D6, CYP2C19, extensively
Excretion	Urine 63%, feces 11%
Half-life	Terminal (COPD) 26 hr

Pharmacodynamics

Onset	Rapid
Peak	1-1½ hr
Duration	4-6 hr

INTERACTIONS
Individual drugs
Oxytoxics: increased severe hypotension
Theophylline: increased toxicity

Drug classifications
Adrenergics, MAOIs, tricyclics: increased action of arformoterol; do not use together

Class IA/III antidysrhythmics, MAOIs, tricyclics: increased QT prolongation

Nebulized bronchodilators: increased action of nebulized bronchodilators

Other β-blockers: decreased arformoterol action, asthma-related death

Potassium-losing diuretics: increased ECG changes/hypokalemia

Drug/herb
Caffeine (kola nut, green/black tea, guarana, yerba maté, coffee, chocolate): increased stimulation

NURSING CONSIDERATIONS
Assessment

> BLACK BOX WARNING: Assess respiratory function: vital capacity, forced expiratory volume, ABGs; lung sounds, heart rate and rhythm, B/P, sputum (baseline and peak); actively deteriorating COPD may occur; a rescue inhaler should be readily available

• Determine that patient has not received theophylline therapy or other bronchodilators before giving dose
• Assess patient's ability to self-medicate
• Assess for allergic reactions
• Assess **paradoxical bronchospasm;** hold medication, notify prescriber if bronchospasm occurs

Patient/family education

> BLACK BOX WARNING: Teach patient to use exactly as prescribed, that death has resulted from asthma with products similar to this one, to have a rescue inhaler always

• Advise patient not to use OTC medications; excess stimulation may occur
• An opened unit-dose vial should be used immediately
• To notify prescriber if there is more frequent use needed

Evaluation
Positive therapeutic outcome
• Absence of dyspnea, wheezing after 1 hr, improved airway exchange, improved ABGs

⚠ HIGH ALERT

argatroban (Rx)
(are-ga-troe′ban)
Argatroban
Func. class.: Anticoagulant
Chem. class.: Thrombin inhibitor
Pregnancy category B

Do not confuse: argatroban/Aggrastat

ACTION: Direct inhibitor of thrombin that is derived from L-arginine; it reversibly binds to the thrombin active site

Therapeutic outcome: Absence or decrease of thrombosis

USES: Thrombosis prophylaxis or treatment; anticoagulation prevention/treatment of thrombosis in heparin-induced thrombocytopenia (HIT); percutaneous coronary intervention (PCI) in those with a history of HIT, deep vein thrombosis, pulmonary embolism

CONTRAINDICATIONS
Hypersensitivity, overt major bleeding

Precautions: Pregnancy **C,** breastfeeding, children, intracranial bleeding, impaired renal function, hepatic disease, severe hypertension, after lumbar puncture, spinal anesthesia, major surgery/trauma, congenital or acquired bleeding, GI ulcers, abrupt discontinuation

DOSAGE AND ROUTES
DVT, pulmonary embolism
Adult: CONT **IV** inf 2 mcg/kg/min; adjust dose until steady-state aPPT is 1.5-3 × initial baseline, not to exceed 100 sec, max dose 10 mcg/kg/min

Percutaneous coronary intervention (PCI) in HIT

Adult: IV inf 25 mcg/kg/min and a bol of 350 mcg/kg given over 3-5 min, check ACT 5-10 min after bol is completed, **proceed if ACT >300 sec; if ACT <300 sec, give another 150 mcg/kg bol and increase infusion rate to 30 mcg/kg/min; recheck ACT in 5-10 min; if ACT >450 sec, decrease infusion rate to 15 mcg/kg/min; recheck ACT in 5-10 min; once ACT is therapeutic, continue for duration of procedure**

Hepatic dose

Adult: Cont inf 0.5 mcg/kg/min, adjust rate based on APTT

Available forms: Inj 100 mg/ml (2.5 ml) (must dilute 100-fold), 50 mg/50 ml, 125 mg/125 ml

Implementation

- Avoid all IM inj that may cause bleeding

IV, direct route
- **For PCI:** 350 mg/kg bol, and continuous inf of 25 mcg/kg/min, check ACT 5-10 min after bolus

Intermittent IV INF route
- **Dilute** in 0.9% NaCl, D₅W, LR to a final conc 1 mg/ml; **dilute** each 2.5-ml vial 100-fold by mixing with 250 ml of diluent, mix by repeated inversion of the diluent bag for 1 min; may be slightly hazy briefly
- Dosage adjustment may be made after review of aPTT, not to exceed 10 mcg/kg/min

ADVERSE EFFECTS

CNS: Fever, intracranial bleeding, headache
CV: Atrial fibrillation, ventricular tachycardia, coronary thrombosis, MI, myocardial ischemia, coronary occlusion, bradycardia, chest pain, hypotension
GI: Nausea, vomiting, abdominal pain, diarrhea, GI bleeding
GU: Hematuria, abnormal kidney function, UTI
HEMA: Hemorrhage
MISC: *Back pain*, infection
RESP: Dyspnea, coughing, hemoptysis, pulmonary edema
SYST: Sepsis

Pharmacokinetics

Absorption	Unknown
Distribution	To extracellular fluid, 54% plasma protein binding
Metabolism	Liver
Excretion	Feces
Half-life	39-51 min

Pharmacodynamics

Unknown

INTERACTIONS

Individual drugs

Clopidogrel, dipyridamole, heparin, ticlodipine, warfarin: increased bleeding risk

Drug classifications

Antiplatelets, glycoprotein IIb/IIIa antagonists (abciximab, eptifibatide, tirofiban), NSAIDs, other anticoagulants, salicylates, thrombolytics (alteplase, reteplase, tenecteplase, urokinase): increased risk of bleeding

Drug/herb

Garlic, ginger, ginkgo, horse chestnut: increased bleeding risk

Drug/lab

Decrease: Hgb/HcT

NURSING CONSIDERATIONS

Assessment

- Obtain baseline aPTT before treatment; do not start treatment if aPTT ratio ≥2.5, then aPTT 4 hr after initiation of treatment and at least daily thereafter; if aPTT above target, stop inf for 2 hr, then restart at 50%, take aPTT in 4 hr; if below target, increase inf rate by 20%, take aPTT in 4 hr, do not exceed inf rate of 0.21 mg/kg/hr without checking for coagulation abnormalities
- Monitor aPTT, which should be 1.5-3 × control, draw blood for ACT q20-30min during long PCI
- ⚠ Assess for bleeding gums, petechiae, ecchymosis, black tarry stools, hematuria/epistaxis, decreased B/P, HCT, vaginal bleeding, and possible hemorrhage
- Fever, skin rash, urticaria
- **Anaphylaxis:** assess for dyspnea, rash during treatment

Patient/family education

- Advise patient to use soft-bristle toothbrush to avoid bleeding gums, avoid contact sports, use electric razor, avoid IM inj
- Instruct patient to report any signs of bleeding: gums, under skin, urine, stools; trouble breathing, wheezing, skin rash

Evaluation

Positive therapeutic outcome
- Absence or decrease of thrombosis
- Not to use OTC meds, herbal products unless approved by prescriber

A

ARIPiprazole (Rx)

(a-rip-ip-pra'zol)

Abilify, Abilify Discmelt, Abilify Maintena

Func. class.: Antipsychotic/neuroleptic

Pregnancy category C

ACTION: Exact mechanism unknown; may be mediated through both dopamine type 2 (D_2) and serotonin type 2 (5-HT_2) antagonism, dopamine system stabilizer

Therapeutic outcome: Decreased excitement, hallucinations, delusions, paranoia, reorganization of patterns of thought, speech

USES: Schizophrenia and bipolar disorder (adults and adolescents), agitation, mania, major depressive disorder, short-term mania or mixed episodes of bipolar disorder, irritability in autism

CONTRAINDICATIONS

Hypersensitivity, breastfeeding, seizure disorders

Precautions: Pregnancy **C**, geriatric, renal/cardiac/hepatic disease, neutropenia

> **BLACK BOX WARNING:** Children with depression, dementia, suicidal ideation

DOSAGE AND ROUTES
Schizophrenia
Adult: PO 10-15 mg/day; if needed, dosage may be increased to 30 mg daily after 2 wk; maintenance 15 mg/day, periodically reassess; IM/EXT REL (monthly inj susp) 400 mg qmo

Adolescent 13-17 yr: 2 mg/day, may increase to 5 mg after 2 days, then 10 mg after 2 more days, max 30 mg/day

Major depressive disorder
Adult: PO 2-5 mg/day as an adjunct to other antidepressant treatment; adjust by 5 mg at ≥1 wk (range, 2-15 mg/day)

Agitation in bipolar disorder/ schizophrenia
Adult: IM 9.75 mg as a single dose; may start with a lower dose, max 30 mg/day

Bipolar disorder
Adult: 15 mg/day, may increase to 30 mg/day if needed (monotherapy): adjunctive to lithium or valproate PO 10-15 mg qd, may increase to 30 mg as needed

Child ≥10 yr/adolescent: PO 2 mg, titrate to 5 mg/day after 2 days to a target of 10 mg/day after another 2 days

Irritability associated with autism
Child ≥6 yr/adolescent: PO 2 mg/day, increase to 5 mg/day after 1 wk, may increase to 10-15 mg/day if needed, dose changes should not occur more frequently than q1wk

Potential CYP2D6 inhibitor, strong CYP3A4 inhibitors
Adult: PO reduce to 50% of usual dose, increase dose when CYP2D6, CYP3A4 inhibitor is withdrawn

Combination of strong CYP3A4/ CYP2D6 inhibitors
Adult: PO reduce to 25% of usual dose

Available forms: Tabs 2, 5, 10, 15, 20, 30 mg; inj 9.75 mg/1.3 ml; orally disintegrating tab 10, 15 mg; oral sol 1 mg/ml; susp for injection 441 mg/1.6 ml, 662 mg/2.4 ml, 882 mg/3.2 ml; susp EXT REL 300, 400 mg

Implementation
• Administer reduced dose in geriatric
• Decreased stimulus by dimming lights, avoiding loud noises
• Supervise ambulation until patient is stabilized on medication; do not involve in strenuous exercise program because fainting is possible; patient should not stand still for a long time
• Store in tight, light-resistant container
• Available as ready to use
• Oral sol can be substituted for tablet mg per mg up to 25-mg dose; patients receiving 30-mg tablets should receive 25 mg of sol
• IM route: EXT REL monthly (Abilify Maintena)
• Do not give IV or subcut

ADVERSE EFFECTS
CNS: *Drowsiness, insomnia, agitation, anxiety, headache,* seizures, **neuroleptic malignant syndrome,** *lightheadedness, akathisia, asthenia, tremor,* stroke, suicidal ideation, dystonia, cogwheel rigidity

CV: Orthostatic hypotension, tachycardia, chest pain, hypertension, peripheral edema

EENT: Blurred vision, rhinitis

GI: Constipation, *nausea,* vomiting, jaundice, weight gain

INTEG: *Rash*

META: Hyperglycemia, dyslipidemia

MS: Musculoskeletal pain/stiffness, myalgia

RESP: *Cough*

SYST: Death in geriatric patients with dementia

Pharmacokinetics

Absorption	Unknown
Distribution	Protein binding, 90%
Metabolism	Liver, extensively to major active metabolism
Excretion	Unknown
Half-life	Unknown

Pharmacodynamics

Unknown

INTERACTIONS
Individual drugs

Alcohol: increased sedation

CarBAMazepine: decreased effects of ARIPiprazole

Erythromycin, FLUoxetine, ketoconazole, quiNIDine, PARoxetine: increased effects of ARIPiprazole, reduce dose

Famotidine, valproate: decreased ARIPiprazole level

Lithium: increased EPS

Drug classifications

Antipsychotics: increased EPS

CNS depressants: increased sedation

CYP3A4/CYP2D6 inhibitors: increased effects of ARIPiprazole, reduce dose

CYPA34 inducers: decreased effects of ARIPiprazole; increase dose

Drug/herb

St. John's wort: decreased ARIPiprazole effect

Drug/Lab

False positive: amphetemine drug screen

NURSING CONSIDERATIONS
Assessment

> **BLACK BOX WARNING:** Assess mental status before initial administration, children/young adults may exhibit suicidal thoughts/behaviors, the smallest amount of product should be given; elderly patients with dementia-related psychosis are at increased risk of death

• Check for swallowing of PO medication; check for hoarding or giving of medication to other patients

• Monitor I&O ratio; palpate bladder if urinary output is low

• Monitor liver function tests qmo, AIMS assessment, neurologic function

• Assess affect, orientation, LOC, reflexes, gait, coordination, sleep pattern disturbances

• Monitor B/P standing and lying; also pulse, respirations; take q4hr during initial treatment; establish baseline before starting treatment; report drops of 30 mm Hg; watch for ECG changes

• Assess for dizziness, faintness, palpitations, tachycardia on rising

• Assess for EPS, including akathisia (inability to sit still, no pattern to movements), tardive dyskinesia (bizarre movements of the jaw, mouth, tongue, extremities), pseudoparkinsonism (rigidity, tremors, pill rolling, shuffling gait)

⚠ **Assess for neuroleptic malignant syndrome: hyperthermia, increased CPK, altered mental status, muscle rigidity**

• Monitor weight, lipid profile, fasting blood glucose

• Assess skin turgor daily

• Assess for constipation, urinary retention daily; if these occur, increase bulk and water in diet

Patient/family education

• Advise patient that orthostatic hypotension may occur and to rise from sitting or lying position gradually

• Advise patient to avoid hot tubs, hot showers, tub baths; hypotension may occur

• Instruct patient to avoid abrupt withdrawal of this product; EPS may result; product should be withdrawn slowly

• Teach patient to avoid OTC preparations (cough, hayfever, cold) unless approved by prescriber, because serious product interactions may occur; avoid use with alcohol, CNS depressants; increased drowsiness may occur

• Advise patient to avoid hazardous activities if drowsy or dizzy

• Explain importance of compliance with product regimen

• Advise patient, family to report impaired vision, tremors, muscle twitching, urinary retention

• Instruct patient to take extra precautions to stay cool in hot weather, that heat stroke may occur

> **BLACK BOX WARNING:** Teach patient to report suicidal thoughts/behaviors, dementia immediately

Evaluation
Positive therapeutic outcome

• Decreased emotional excitement, hallucinations, delusions, paranoia; reorganization of patterns of thought, speech

TREATMENT OF OVERDOSE:

Lavage if orally ingested; provide airway; *do not induce vomiting*

---

asenapine (Rx)

(a-sen'a-peen)

Saphris

Func. class.: Antipsychotic, atypical

Chem. class.: Dibenzazepine

Pregnancy category C

ACTION: Unknown; may be mediated through both dopamine type 2 (D_2) and serotonin type 2 (5-HT_{2A}) antagonism

Therapeutic outcome: Decrease in delusions, hallucinations

USES: Bipolar 1 disorder, schizophrenia

CONTRAINDICATIONS

Breastfeeding, hypersensitivity

Precautions: Pregnancy **C**, children, geriatric patients, cardiac/renal/hepatic disease, breast cancer, Parkinson's disease, dementia, seizure disorder, CNS depression, agranulocytosis, QT prolongation, torsades de pointes, suicidal ideation, substance abuse, diabetes mellitus

> **BLACK BOX WARNING:** Increased mortality in elderly patients with dementia-related psychosis

DOSAGE AND ROUTES

Schizophrenia

Adult: SL 5 mg bid, max 20 mg/day

Bipolar 1 disorder

Adult: SL 10 mg bid, may decrease to 5 mg bid as needed, max 20 mg/day

Available forms: SL tab 2.5, 10 mg

Implementation

PO route

• Give anticholinergic agent for EPS

• Avoid use with CNS depressants

• **SL tab:** remove tab, place tab under tongue; after it dissolves, swallow; advise not to chew, crush or swallow tabs, not to eat or drink for 10 min

• Supervise ambulation until patient is stabilized on medication; do not involve in strenuous exercise program because fainting is possible; patient should not stand still for a long time

• Increase fluids to prevent constipation

• Store in tight, light-resistant container

ADVERSE EFFECTS

CNS: *EPS, pseudoparkinsonism, akathisia, dystonia, tardive dyskinesia, drowsiness, insomnia, agitation, anxiety, headache,* seizures, neuroleptic malignant syndrome, dizziness, suicidal ideation, drowsiness, depression

CV: Orthostatic hypotension, sinus tachycardia, heart failure, QT prolongation, stroke, bundle branch block

ENDO: Hyperglycemia, hyperlipidemia

GI: *Nausea,* vomiting, *constipation,* weight gain, increased appetite; oral hypoesthesia/parasthesia (SL)

HEMA: Thrombocytopenia, agranulocytosis, anemia, leukopenia

INTEG: Serious allergic reaction (anaphylaxis, angioedema)

Pharmacokinetics

Absorption	Unknown
Distribution	Protein binding 95%
Metabolism	Liver
Excretion	Unknown
Half-life	Terminal 24 hr

Pharmacodynamics

Onset	Unknown
Peak	½-1½ hr
Duration	Unknown

INTERACTIONS

Individual drugs

Alcohol: increased sedation

Chloroquine, clarithromycin, droperidol, erythromycin, haloperidol, methadone, pentamidine: increased QT prolongation

CarBAMazepine: increased asenpine excretion

Drug classifications

Other CNS depressants: increased sedation

CYP2D6 inhibitors/substrates (SSRIs), other antipsychotics: increased EPS

Class IA/III antidysrhythmics, some phenothiazines, β-agonists, local anesthetics, tricyclics: increased QT prolongation

CYP2D6 inducers (carBAMazepine, barbiturates, phenytoin, rifampin): decreased asenapine action

SSRIs: increased serotonin syndrome

Drug/herb

Kava: increased CNS depression, increased EPS

Betel palm: increased EPS

Drug/lab test

Increased: cholesterol, glucose, LFTs, lipids, prolactin levels, triglycerides

Decreased: sodium

NURSING CONSIDERATIONS

Assessment

> **BLACK BOX WARNING:** ⚠ Assess mental status before initial administration; watch for suicidal thoughts and behaviors; dementia and death may occur in the elderly

• Assess for affect, orientation, LOC, reflexes, gait, coordination, sleep pattern disturbances
• Monitor B/P standing and lying, pulse, respirations; take these q4hr during initial treatment; establish baseline before starting treatment; report drops of 30 mm Hg; watch for ECG changes; QT prolongation may occur
• Monitor for dizziness, faintness, palpitations, tachycardia on rising
• Assess for **EPS,** including akathisia, tardive dyskinesia (bizarre movements of the jaw, mouth, tongue, extremities), pseudoparkinsonism (rigidity, tremors, pill rolling, shuffling gait)
⚠ **Assess for neuroleptic malignant syndrome: hyperthermia, increased CPK, altered mental status, muscle rigidity**
• Assess for constipation daily; increase bulk and water in diet if needed
• Assess for weight gain, hyperglycemia, metabolic changes in diabetes

Patient/family education
• Caution patient that orthostatic hypotension may occur and to rise from sitting or lying position gradually
• Teach patient to avoid hot tubs, hot showers, tub baths; hypotension may occur
• Advise patient to avoid abrupt withdrawal of this product; EPS may result; product should be withdrawn slowly
• Advise patient to avoid OTC preparations (cough, hay fever, cold) unless approved by prescriber, serious product interactions may occur; avoid use of alcohol, increased drowsiness may occur
• Advise patient to avoid hazardous activities if drowsy or dizzy
• Weight, thyroid function studies, serum prolactin, lipid profile, serum electrolytes, creatinine, pregnancy test, neurologic function, LFTs, glycosylated hemoglobulin A1C, CBC, blood glucose, AIMS assessment baseline and periodically
• Advise patient about compliance with product regimen
• Advise patient that heat stroke may occur in hot weather; take extra precautions to stay cool
• Advise patient to use contraception, inform prescriber if pregnancy is planned or suspected
• **Advise patient to report suicidal thoughts/behaviors immediately**

Evaluation
Positive therapeutic outcome
• Therapeutic response: decrease in emotional excitement, hallucinations, delusions, paranoia; reorganization of patterns of thought, speech

TREATMENT OF OVERDOSE:
Lavage if orally ingested; provide airway; *do not induce vomiting*

aspirin (OTC)
(as′pir-in)
APC-ASA Coated Aspirin 🍁, **Apo-Asa** 🍁, **A.S.A., Asaphen** 🍁, **Asatab** 🍁, **Ascriptin Enteric, Aspergum, Aspirin** 🍁, **Aspir-Low, Aspirtrin** 🍁, **Bayer Aspirin, Bayer Children's Aspirin, Bufferin, Ecotrin, Entrophen** 🍁, **Equaline, Good Sense Aspirin, Halfprin, Lowprin** 🍁, **Novasen** 🍁, **PMS-ASA** 🍁, **Rivasa** 🍁, **St. Joseph Children's, St. Joseph's Adult, Walgreens Aspirin Adult**
Func. class.: Nonopioid analgesic
Chem. class.: Salicylate
Pregnancy category D (3rd trimester)

Do not confuse: Aspirin/Ascendin/Afrin

ACTION: Blocks pain impulses by blocking COX-1 in CNS, reduces inflammation by inhibition of prostaglandin synthesis; antipyretic action results from vasodilatation of peripheral vessels; decreases platelet aggregation

Therapeutic outcome: Decreased pain, inflammation, fever; absence of MI, transient ischemic attacks, thrombosis

USES: Mild to moderate pain or fever including rheumatoid arthritis, osteoarthritis, thromboembolic disorders, transient ischemic attacks, rheumatic fever, post-MI, prophylaxis of MI, ischemic stroke, angina; acute MI

Unlabeled uses: Prevention of cataracts (long-term use), prevention of pregnancy loss in women with clotting disorders, polycythemia vera

CONTRAINDICATIONS
Pregnancy **D** (3rd trimester), breastfeeding, children <12 yr, children with flulike symptoms, hypersensitivity to salicylates, tartrazine (FDC yellow dye #5), GI bleeding, bleeding disorders, vit K deficiency, peptic ulcer, acute bronchospasm, agranulocytosis, increased intracranial pressure, intracranial bleeding, nasal polyps, urticaria

Precautions: Abrupt discontinuation, acetaminophen/NSAIDs hypersensitivity, acid/base imbalance, alcoholism, ascites, asthma, bone marrow suppression, geriatric patients, dehydration, G6PD deficiency, gout, heart failure, anemia, renal/hepatic disease, pre/postoperatively, gastritis, pregnancy **C** 1st trimester

DOSAGE AND ROUTES
Arthritis
Adult: PO 3 g/day in divided doses q4-6hr, target salicylate level 150-300 mcg/ml
Child: PO or RECT 90-130 mg/kg/day in divided doses, target salicylate level 150-300 mcg/ml

Kawasaki's disease (unlabeled)
Child: PO 80-100 mg/kg/day in 4 divided doses, maintenance 3-5 mg/kg/day

MI, stroke prophylaxis
Adult: PO 50-325 mg/day

Pain/fever
Adult: PO/RECT 325-1000 mg q4hr prn, max 4 g/day
Child 2-11 yr: PO 10-15 mg/kg/dose q4hr, max 4 g/day

Thromboembolic disorders
Adult: PO 325-650 mg/day or bid

Transient ischemic attacks (risk)
Adult: PO 50-325 mg/day (grade 1A)

Prevention of recurrent MI
Adult: PO 75-162 mg/day

CABG
Adult: PO 325 mg/day starting 6 hr post-procedure, continue for 1 yr

PTCA
Adult: PO 325 mg 2 hr presurgery, then 160-325 mg daily

Polycythemia vera (unlabeled)
Adult: PO 75-100 mg/day during pregnancy and 6 wk after birth

Evolving MI with ST segment elevation (STEMI)
Adult: PO 160-325 mg nonenteric, chewed and swallowed immediately, maintenance 75-162 mg qd

Available forms: Tabs 81, 325, 500, 650, 800 mg; chewable tabs 81 mg; supp 300, 600, mg; gum 227 mg; enteric coated tabs 81, 325, 500, 975 mg; ext rel 800 mg; del rel tabs 325, 500 mg; supp 300, 600 mg

Implementation
PO route
• Do not break, crush, or chew enteric product
• Administer to patient crushed or whole; chewable tab should be chewed

• Give with food or milk to decrease gastric symptoms; separate by 2 hr of enteric product; absorption may be slowed
• Give antacids 1-2 hr after enteric products
• Give with 8 oz of water and have patient sit upright for 30 min after dose; discard tabs if vinegar-like smell is present; avoid if allergic to tartrazine
• Give ½ hr before planned exercise
Rectal route
• Place suppository in refrigerator for at least 30 min before removing wrapper

ADVERSE EFFECTS
CNS: Stimulation, drowsiness, dizziness, confusion, seizures, headache, flushing, hallucinations, coma, intracranial hemorrhage
CV: Rapid pulse, pulmonary edema, dysrhythmias
EENT: Tinnitus, hearing loss
ENDO: Hypoglycemia, hyponatremia, hypokalemia
GI: *Nausea, vomiting,* GI bleeding, diarrhea, heartburn, anorexia, hepatitis, GI ulcer
HEMA: Thrombocytopenia, agranulocytosis, leukopenia, neutropenia, hemolytic anemia, increased PT, PTT, bleeding time
INTEG: *Rash,* urticaria, bruising
RESP: Wheezing, hyperpnea, bronchospasm
SYST: Reye's syndrome (children), anaphylaxis, laryngeal edema, angioedema

Pharmacokinetics

Absorption	Well absorbed, small intestine (PO); erratic (enteric); slow (RECT)
Distribution	Rapidly, widely distributed; crosses placenta, protein binding 90%
Metabolism	Liver, extensively
Excretion	Inactive metabolites, kidney; breast milk
Half-life	15-20 min (low doses); 9 hr (high doses)

Pharmacodynamics

	PO	RECT
Onset	15-30 min	Slow
Peak	1-2 hr	4-5 hr
Duration	4-6 hr	6-7 hr

PO: Enteric-coated: Onset 10-30 min, duration 2-4 hr,
Solution: Onset 10-30 min, peak 15-30 min, duration 2-4 hr

INTERACTIONS
Individual drugs
Alcohol, cefamandole, clopidogrel, eptifibatide, heparin, plicamycin, ticlopidine, tirofiban: increased risk of bleeding

Ammonium chloride, nizatidine: increased salicylate level

Insulin, methotrexate, phenytoin, valproic acid, increased effects of each specific product

Nitroglycerin: increased hypotension

Probenecid: decreased effects of probenecid

Spironolactone, sulfinpyrazone: decreased effects

Drug classifications
ACE inhibitors: decreased antihypertensive effect

Antacids (high doses), corticosteroids, urinary alkalizers: decreased effects of aspirin

Anticoagulants, thrombolytics: increased risk of bleeding

Diuretics (loop), sulfonylamides, NSAIDs, β-blockers: decreased effect of each specific product

NSAIDs, antiinflammatories, steroids: increased gastric ulcers

Penicillins, oral hypoglycemics, sulfonamides, thrombolytic agents: increased effects of each specific product

Salicylates: decreased blood glucose levels

Urinary acidifiers: increased salicylate levels

Drug/herb
Feverfew, garlic, ginger, ginkgo, ginseng *(Panax),* horse chestnut: increased risk of bleeding

Drug/food
Foods acidifying urine may increase aspirin levels

Fish oil (omega-3-fatty acids): increased risk of bleeding

Drug/lab test
Increased: coagulation studies, liver function studies, serum uric acid, amylase, CO_2, urinary protein

Decreased: serum potassium, cholesterol

Interference: VMA, 5-HIAA, xylose tolerance test, TSH, pregnancy test

NURSING CONSIDERATIONS
Assessment
• Assess for **pain:** character, location, intensity, ROM before and 1 hr after administration

• Monitor liver function studies: AST, ALT, bilirubin, creatinine if patient is on long-term therapy

• Monitor renal function studies: BUN, urine creatinine if patient is on long-term therapy

• Monitor blood studies: CBC, Hct, Hgb, PT if patient is on long-term therapy

• Check I&O ratio; decreasing output may indicate renal failure (long-term therapy)

⚠ **Assess hepatotoxicity: dark urine, clay-colored stools, yellowing of the skin and sclera, itching, abdominal pain, fever, diarrhea if patient is on long-term therapy**

• **Assess for allergic reactions: rash, urticaria; if these occur, product may have to be discontinued; in patients with asthma, nasal polyps, allergies, severe allergic reactions may occur**

• Assess for **ototoxicity:** tinnitus, ringing, roaring in ears; audiometric testing needed before, after long-term therapy

• Monitor **salicylate level:** therapeutic level 150-300 mcg/ml for chronic inflammation

• Check edema in feet, ankles, legs

• Identify prior product history; there are many product interactions

Patient/family education
• Teach patient to report any symptoms of renal/hepatic toxicity, visual changes, ototoxicity, allergic reactions, bleeding (long-term therapy)

• Instruct patient to take with 8 oz of water and sit upright for 30 min after dose to facilitate product passing into the stomach; to discard tabs if vinegar-like smell is present; to avoid if allergic to tartrazine

• **Instruct patient not to exceed recommended dosage; acute poisoning may result**

• Advise patient to read label on other OTC products; many contain aspirin

• Inform patient that the therapeutic response takes 2 wk (arthritis)

• Teach patient to report tinnitus, confusion, diarrhea, sweating, hyperventilation

• Advise patient to avoid alcohol ingestion; GI bleeding may occur

• Advise patient with allergies, nasal polyps, asthma, that allergic reactions may develop

• Instruct patient to read labels on other OTC products: may contain salicylates

• Teach patient not to give to children or teens with flulike symptoms or chicken pox; Reye's syndrome may develop

⚠ **Instruct patient not to use during 3rd trimester of pregnancy (D)**

• Teach patient to take with a full glass of water

Evaluation
Positive therapeutic outcome
• Decreased pain

• Decreased inflammation

• Decreased fever

• Absence of MI

• Absence of transient ischemic attacks, thrombosis

TREATMENT OF OVERDOSE:
Lavage, activated charcoal; monitor electrolytes, VS

atazanavir (Rx)
(at-a-za-na'veer)
Reyataz
Func. class.: Antiretroviral
Chem. class.: Protease inhibitor
Pregnancy category B

ACTION: Inhibits human immunodeficiency virus (HIV-1) protease, which prevents maturation of the infectious virus

Therapeutic outcome: Decreasing symptoms of HIV

USES: HIV-1 infection in combination with other antiretroviral agents

CONTRAINDICATIONS
Hypersensitivity, Child-Pugh Class C

Precautions: Pregnancy **B,** breastfeeding, children, geriatric, liver disease, alcoholism, antimicrobial resistance, AV block, diabetes, dialysis, elderly, women, hemophilia, hypercholesterolemia, immune reconstitution syndrome, lactic acidosis, pancreatitis, cholelithiasis, serious rash

DOSAGE AND ROUTES
Antiretroviral-naive patients
Adult: PO 400 mg daily
Child ≥6 yr/adolescent ≤40 kg: PO 300 mg with ritonavir 100 mg qd
Child ≥6 yr/adolescent 20 to <40 kg: PO 200 mg with ritonavir 100 mg qd
Child ≥6 yr/adolescent 15 to <20 kg: PO 150 mg with ritonavir 80 mg qd

Antiretroviral-experienced patients
Adult: PO 300 mg daily and ritonavir 100 mg daily
Pregnant adult/adolescent (2nd/3rd trimester) with H₂ blocker or tenofovir: PO 400 mg with ritonavir 100 mg qd
Child ≥6 yr/adolescent ≥40 kg: PO 300 mg with ritonavir 100 mg qd
Child ≥6 yr/adolescent 20 to <40 kg: PO 200 mg with ritonavir 100 mg qd
Infants ≥ 3 months and children 10 to <25 kg: Oral powder 15 to <25 kg 250 mg/dose q24hr with ritonavir 80 mg/dose q24hr; 10 to <15 kg 200 mg/dose q24hr with ritonavir 80 mg/dose q24hr

Hepatic dose
Adult: PO (Child-Pugh B) 300 mg daily; (Child-Pugh C) do not use

Available forms: Caps 100, 150, 200, 300 mg, oral powder 50 mg

Implementation
• Administer with food; take 2 hr before or 1 hr after antacid or didanosine; swallow cap whole, do not open

ADVERSE EFFECTS
CNS: Headache, depression, dizziness, insomnia, peripheral neuropathy
CV: Increased PR interval
EENT: Yellowing of sclera
GI: *Diarrhea, abdominal pain, nausea,* vomiting, **hepatotoxicity,** cholelithiasis
INTEG: *Rash,* **Stevens-Johnson syndrome,** *photosensitivity,* **DRESS**
MISC: Fatigue, fever, arthralgia, back pain, cough, lipodystrophy, pain, gynecomastia, nephrolithiasis, **lactic acidosis, hyperbilirubinemia** (pregnancy, females, obesity)

Pharmacokinetics

Absorption	Rapid, increased with food
Distribution	86% protein bound
Metabolism	Liver extensively by CYP3A4
Excretion	27% excreted unchanged in urine/feces (minimal)
Half-life	7 hr

Pharmacodynamics

Onset	Unknown
Peak	2 hr
Duration	Unknown

INTERACTIONS
Individual drugs
Chlorazepate, clarithromycin, cycloSPORINE, diazepam, irinotecan, midazolam, pimozide, sildenafil, sirolimus, tacrolimus, triazolam, warfarin: increased levels resulting in toxicity
Didanosine, efavirenz, rifampin: decreased atazanavir levels
Indinavir: increased hyperbilirubinemia
Ritonavir, teleprevir: decreased teleprevir levels when used with atazanavir and ritonavir

Drug classifications
Antacids, H₂-receptor antagonists, proton pump inhibitors, CYP3A4 inducers: decreased atazanavir levels
Antidepressants (tricyclics), antidysrhythmics, ergots, calcium channel blockers, HMG-CoA reductase inhibitors, immunosuppressants, other protease inhibitors: increased levels resulting in increased toxicity

Contraceptives (oral), estrogens: increased effects (unboosted), decreased (boosted with ritonavir)

CYP3A4 substrates, CYP3A4 inhibitors: increased atazanavir levels

Drug/herb
Red yeast rice: myopathy, rhabdomyolysis
St. John's wort: decreased atazanavir levels, avoid concurrent use

Drug/lab test
Increased: AST, ALT, total bilirubin, amylase, lipase, CK
Decreased: Hgb, neutrophils, platelets

Drug/food
Increased: drug bioavailability (to be taken with food)

NURSING CONSIDERATIONS
Assessment
⚠ **Immune reconstitution syndrome: when given with combination antiretroviral therapy**
⚠ **Assess for hepatic failure**
• Assess for signs of infection, anemia
• Monitor liver function studies: ALT, AST, bilirubin
• Monitor bowel pattern before, during treatment; if severe abdominal pain with bleeding occurs, product should be discontinued; monitor hydration
• **If pregnant, call Antiretroviral Pregnancy Registry 800-258-4263**
• PR interval in those taking calcium channel blockers, digoxin
• Monitor viral load, CD4 count throughout treatment
⚠ **Serious rash (Stevens-Johnson syndrome, DRESS): most rashes last 1-4 wk; if serious, discontinue product**
⚠ **Immune Reconstitution syndrome: time of onset is variable**

Patient/family education
• Advise to take as prescribed with other antiretrovirals as prescribed; if dose is missed, take as soon as remembered up to 1 hr before next dose; do not double dose; do not share with others
• Teach that product must be taken daily to maintain blood levels for duration of therapy
• To report yellowing of skin, sclera
• Instruct to notify prescriber if diarrhea, nausea, vomiting, rash occur; dizziness, lightheadedness; ECG may be altered
• Inform that product interacts with many products and St. John's wort; advise prescriber of all products, herbal products used

• Advise that redistribution of body fat may occur; the effect is not known
• Teach that product does not cure HIV-1 infection or prevent transmission to others, only controls symptoms
⚠ **Advise that if taking sildenafil with atazanavir, there may be an increased risk of phosphodiesterase type 5 inhibitor–associated adverse events, including hypotension and prolonged penile erection; notify physician promptly of these symptoms**

Evaluation
Positive therapeutic outcome
• Increasing CD4 counts; decreased viral load, resolution of symptoms of HIV-1 infection

---

atenolol (Rx)
(a-ten′oh-lole)
Tenormin
Func. class.: Antihypertensive
Chem. class.: β-Blocker; β₁-, β₂-blocker (high doses)
Pregnancy category D

Do not confuse: atenolol/albuterol/Altenol, Tenormin/thiamine/Imuran

ACTION: Competitively blocks stimulation of β-adrenergic receptor within vascular smooth muscle; produces negative chronotropic activity (decreases rate of SA node discharge, increases recovery time), slows conduction of AV node, decreases heart rate, negative inotropic activity, decreases O_2 consumption in myocardium; also decreases renin-aldosterone-angiotensin system at high doses, inhibits β₂-receptors in bronchial system at higher doses

Therapeutic outcome: Decreased B/P, heart rate, prevention of angina pectoris, MI

USES: Mild to moderate hypertension; prophylaxis of angina pectoris; suspected or known MI (**IV** use), MI prophylaxis, atrial fibrillation/flutter

CONTRAINDICATIONS
Pregnancy **D**, hypersensitivity to β-blockers, cardiogenic shock, 2nd- or 3rd-degree heart block, sinus bradycardia, cardiac failure

Precautions: Major surgery, breastfeeding, diabetes mellitus, renal disease, thyroid disease, CHF, COPD, asthma, well-compensated heart failure, dialysis, myasthenia gravis, Raynaud's disease, pulmonary edema

BLACK BOX WARNING: Abrupt discontinuation, **may precipitate angina, MI**

DOSAGE AND ROUTES

Adult: PO 25-50 mg daily, increasing q1-2wk to 100 mg daily; may increase to 200 mg daily for angina or up to 100 mg for hypertension
Child: PO 0.8-1 mg/kg/dose initially, range 0.8-1.5 mg/kg/day, max 2 mg/kg/day
Geriatric: PO 25 mg/day initially

Chronic stable angina
Adult: PO 50 mg q day, then 100 mg/day prn after 7 days, max 200 mg/day

Post MI, MI prophylaxis
Adult: PO 1000 mg/day, in 1-2 divided doses, may need for 1-3 yr post MI

Renal dose
Adult: PO CCr 15-35 ml/min, max 50 mg/day; CCr <15 ml/min max 25 mg/day; hemodialysis 25-50 mg after dialysis

Available forms: Tabs 25, 50, 100 mg

Implementation
PO route
• Given before meals, at bedtime; tablet may be crushed or swallowed whole; give with food, same time of day to prevent GI upset; reduced dosage in renal dysfunction; take at same time each day
• Store protected from light, moisture; place in cool environment

ADVERSE EFFECTS

CNS: *Insomnia, fatigue, dizziness, mental changes,* memory loss, hallucinations, depression, lethargy, drowsiness, strange dreams, catatonia
CV: **Profound hypotension, bradycardia, CHF,** *cold extremities, postural hypotension,* **2nd- or 3rd-degree heart block**
ENDO: Increased hypoglycemic response to insulin
GI: *Nausea, diarrhea,* vomiting, **mesenteric arterial thrombosis, ischemic colitis**
GU: Impotence, decreased libido
HEMA: **Agranulocytosis, thrombocytopenia, purpura**
INTEG: Rash, fever, alopecia
RESP: **Bronchospasm,** dyspnea, wheezing, pulmonary edema

Pharmacokinetics

Absorption	50%-60% (PO)
Distribution	Crosses placenta; protein binding (5%-15%)
Metabolism	Not metabolized
Excretion	Breast milk, kidneys (50%), feces (50%— unabsorbed product)
Half-life	7 hr

Pharmacodynamics

	PO
Onset	1 hr
Peak	2-4 hr
Duration	24 hr

INTERACTIONS

Individual drugs
Digoxin, diltiazem, hydrALAZINE, methyldopa, prazosin, reserpine, verapamil: increased hypotension, bradycardia
EPHEDrine, pseudoephedrine: increased hypertension
DOPamine, insulin, theophylline: decreased effect of each of these drugs

Drug classifications
Amphetamines: increased hypertension
Anticholinergics, antihypertensives: cardiac glycosides, increased hypotension, bradycardia
Antidiabetic agents (oral) MAOIs: decreased effect of each of these drugs
Sympathomimetics (cough, cold preparations): mutual inhibition

Drug/herb
Hawthorn: increased atenolol effect
Ephedra (ma huang): decreased atenolol effect

Drug/lab test
Increased: uric acid, potassium, triglyceride, blood, BUN, ANA titer, platelets, alkaline phosphatase, creatinine, LDH, AST/ALT
Decreased: glucose

NURSING CONSIDERATIONS

Assessment
• Monitor **hypertension,** B/P during beginning treatment, periodically thereafter; pulse q4hr; note rate, rhythm, quality: apical/radial pulse before administration; notify prescriber of any significant changes (pulse <50 bpm); ECG
• Hypotension: may be caused in hemodialysis
• Hypoglycemia: may be masked in diabetes mellitus
• Check for baselines in renal, liver function tests before therapy begins
• Assess for edema in feet, legs daily; monitor I&O, daily weight; check for jugular vein distention, crackles bilaterally, dyspnea (CHF)

Patient/family education

> **BLACK BOX WARNING:** Teach patient not to discontinue product abruptly; taper over 2 wk (angina) as directed, **may precipitate angina, MI,** if stopped abruptly; take at same time each day

- Teach patient not to use OTC products containing α-adrenergic stimulants (such as nasal decongestants, OTC cold preparations); to limit alcohol, smoking; to limit sodium intake as prescribed
- Teach patient how to take pulse and B/P at home; advise when to notify prescriber
- Instruct patient to comply with weight control, dietary adjustments, modified exercise program
- Advise patient to carry/wear emergency ID for products, allergies, conditions being treated; tell patient product controls symptoms but does not cure
- Caution patient to avoid hazardous activities if dizziness, drowsiness is present
- Teach patient to report symptoms of CHF: difficult breathing, especially on exertion or when lying down, night cough, swelling of extremities or bradycardia, dizziness, confusion, depression, fever
- Teach patient to take product as prescribed, not to double doses, skip doses; take any missed doses as remembered if at least 6 hr until next dose
- Advise to change position slowly
- Advise patient that product may mask symptoms of hypoglycemia in diabetic patients
⚠ **Advise patient to use contraception while taking this product, avoid breastfeeding**

Evaluation
Positive therapeutic outcome
- Decreased B/P in hypertension (after 1-2 wk)
- Absence of dysrhythmias
- Absence of MI
- Decreased angina/pain
- Increased activity tolerance

TREATMENT OF OVERDOSE:
Lavage, **IV** atropine for bradycardia, **IV** theophylline for bronchospasm, digoxin, O₂, diuretic for cardiac failure, hemodialysis, **IV** glucose for hyperglycemia, **IV** diazepam (or phenytoin) for seizures

atomoxetine (Rx)
(at-o-mox′eh-teen)
Strattera
Func. class.: Psychotherapeutic—miscellaneous
Pregnancy category C

ACTION: A selective norepinephrine reuptake inhibitor; may inhibit the presynaptic norepinephrine transporter; exact mechanism of action is unknown

Therapeutic outcome: Decreased hyperactivity, impulsivity, increased attention, organization, ability to complete tasks

USES: Attention deficit hyperactivity disorder

CONTRAINDICATIONS
Hypersensitivity, closed-angle glaucoma, MAOI therapy, history of pheochromocytoma

Precautions: Pregnancy **C**, breastfeeding, hypertension, hepatic disease, angioedema, bipolar disorder, dysrhythmias, CAD, hypo/hypertension, arteriosclerosis, cardiac disease, cardiomyopathy, heart failure, jaundice

> **BLACK BOX WARNING:** Children <6 yr, suicidal ideation

DOSAGE AND ROUTES
Child ≤70 kg, <6 yr: PO 0.5 mg/kg/day, increase after 3 days to a target daily dose of 1.2 mg/kg in AM or evenly divided doses AM, late afternoon; max 1.4 mg/kg/day or 100 mg daily, whichever is less
Adult and child >70 kg: PO 40 mg daily, increase after 3 days to a target daily dose of 80 mg in AM or evenly divided doses AM, late afternoon; max 100 mg daily

Maintenance
Adolescent ≤15 yr and child ≥6 yr: PO 1.2-1.8 mg/kg/day

Initial dosage titration with strong CYP2D6 inhibitors
Adult and child >6 yr weighing >70 kg: PO 40 mg/day each AM or 2 evenly divided doses, titrate to target of 80 mg/day if symptoms do not improve after 4 wk and dose is well tolerated

Hepatic dose
Child-Pugh B: reduce dose by 50%
Child-Pugh C: reduce dose by 75%

Available forms: Caps 10, 18, 25, 40, 60, 80, 100 mg

Implementation
- Swallow whole; do not break, crush, or chew
- Give without regard to food
- Provide gum, hard candy, frequent sips of water for dry mouth

ADVERSE EFFECTS
CNS: *Insomnia,* dizziness, headache, irritability, crying, mood swings, fatigue, hypoesthesia, lethargy, paresthesia
CV: *Palpitations,* hot flushes, tachycardia, increased B/P
ENDO: Growth retardation

GI: Dyspepsia, nausea, anorexia, dry mouth, weight loss, vomiting, diarrhea, constipation, hepatic injury
GU: Urinary hesitancy, retention, dysmenorrhea, erectile disturbance, ejaculation failure, impotence, prostatitis, abnormal orgasm, male pelvic pain
INTEG: Exfoliative dermatitis, sweating, rash
MISC: Cough, rhinorrhea, dermatitis, ear infection, rhabdomyolysis

Pharmacokinetics

Absorption	Unknown
Distribution	Protein binding, 98%
Metabolism	Liver
Excretion	Kidneys
Half-life	Unknown, half-life 5 hr

Pharmacodynamics

Unknown

INTERACTIONS
Individual drug
Albuterol: increased cardiovascular effects

Drug classifications
CYP2D6 inhibitors (amiodarone, cimetidine [weak], citalopram, clomiPRAMINE, delavirdine, escitalopram, FLUoxetine, gefitinib, imatinib, PARoxetine, propafenone, quiNIDine [potent], ritonavir, sertraline, thioridazine, venlafaxine): increased effects of atomoxetine
Increase: B/P pressor agents
⚠ MAOIs or within 14 days of MAOIs, vasopressors: hypertensive crisis
Increase: QT prolongation, torsade de pointes dofetilide, grepfloxacin, mesoridazine, pimozide, probucol, sperfloxacin, ziprasidone
Pressor agents: increased cardiovascular effects

NURSING CONSIDERATIONS
Assessment
• Monitor VS, B/P; check patients with cardiac disease more often for increased B/P
• Hepatic injury: may cause liver failure: monitor LFT; assess for jaundice, pruritus, flu-like symptoms, upper right quadrant pain

> BLACK BOX WARNING: Assess mental status: mood, sensorium, affect, stimulation, insomnia, aggressiveness, suicidal ideation in children/young adults

• Assess appetite, sleep, speech patterns
• Assess for attention span, decreased hyperactivity in ADHD persons, growth rate, weight; therapy may need to be discontinued

Patient/family education
• Advise patient to avoid OTC preparations, other medications, herbs, supplements unless approved by prescriber, no tapering needed when discontinuing product
• Advise patient to avoid alcohol ingestion
• Advise patient to avoid hazardous activities until stabilized on medication
• Advise patient to get needed rest; patients will feel more tired at end of day; do not take dose late in day, insomnia may occur

> BLACK BOX WARNING: Advise to report suicidal ideation

• Teach patient to notify prescriber immediately if erection >4 hr

Evaluation
Positive therapeutic outcome
• Decreased hyperactivity (ADHD)

atorvastatin (Rx)
(a-tore′va-stat-in)
Lipitor
Func. class.: Antilipidemic
Chem. class.: HMG-CoA reductase inhibitor
Pregnancy category X

ACTION: Inhibits HMG-CoA reductase enzyme, which reduces cholesterol synthesis, high doses lead to plaque regression

Therapeutic outcome: Decreased cholesterol levels and LDLs, increased HDLs

USES: As an adjunct in primary hypercholesterolemia (types Ia, Ib), dysbetalipoproteinemia, elevated triglyceride levels; prevention of cardiovascular disease by reduction of heart risk in those with mildly elevated cholesterol

CONTRAINDICATIONS
Pregnancy **X**, breastfeeding, hypersensitivity, active liver disease

Precautions: Past liver disease, alcoholism, severe acute infections, trauma, severe metabolic disorders, electrolyte imbalance

DOSAGE AND ROUTES
Adult: PO 10-20 mg daily, usual range 10-80 mg, dosage adjustments may be made in 2-4 wk intervals, max 80 mg/day; patients requiring >45% reduction in LDL may be started at 40 mg daily

Heterozygous familial hypercholesterolemia
Child 10-17 yr: PO 10 mg q day, adjust q4 wk, max 20 mg/day

Available forms: Tabs 10, 20, 40, 80 mg

Implementation
- Administer total daily dose at any time of day
- Store in cool environment in airtight, light-resistant container

ADVERSE EFFECTS
CNS: Headache, asthenia, insomnia
EENT: Lens opacities
GI: *Abdominal cramps, constipation, diarrhea, heartburn,* nausea, dyspepsia, *flatus, liver dysfunction, pancreatitis,* increased serum transaminase
GU: Impotence
INTEG: Rash, pruritus, alopecia, photosensitivity (rare)
MISC: Hypersensitivity; gynecomastia (child)
MS: Myalgia, **rhabdomyolysis**, arthralgia, myositis
RESP: Pharyngitis, sinusitis

Pharmacokinetics

Absorption	Unknown
Distribution	Unknown
Metabolism	Liver
Excretion	Bile, feces, kidneys
Half-life	14 hr

Pharmacodynamics

Unknown

INTERACTIONS
Individual drugs
Clofibrate, cycloSPORINE, gemfibrozil, niacin: increased risk of rhabdomyolysis
Colestipol: decreased action of atorvastatin, myopathy
Digoxin: increased action of digoxin CYP3A4 inhibitors
Erythromycin: increased levels of atorvastatin
Warfarin: increased action of warfarin

Drug classifications
Antifungals (azole): possible rhabdomyolysis
Contraceptives (oral): increased levels

Drug/herb
St. John's wort: decreased effect

Drug/food
Grapefruit juice: possible toxicity
Oat bran may reduce effectiveness

Drug/lab test
Increased: ALT, AST, CK
Interference: thyroid function tests

NURSING CONSIDERATIONS
Assessment
- **Hypercholesterolemia:** assess nutrition: fat, protein, carbohydrates; nutritional analysis should be completed by dietitian before treatment; assess for muscle pain, tenderness; obtain CPK if these occur, product may need to be discontinued; monitor triglycerides, cholesterol at baseline and throughout treatment; LDL and VLDL should be watched closely; if increased, product should be discontinued
- Monitor bowel pattern daily; diarrhea may be a problem
- Monitor liver function studies q1-2mo during the first 1½ yr of treatment; AST, ALT, liver function tests may be increased
- Monitor renal studies in patients with compromised renal system: BUN, I&O ratio, creatinine
- Assess eyes via ophthalmic exam 1 mo after treatment begins, annually

Patient/family education
- Inform patient that compliance is needed for positive results to occur, not to double doses
- Teach patient that risk factors should be decreased: high-fat diet, smoking, avoid alcohol consumption, absence of exercise
- Advise patient to notify prescriber if the GI symptoms of diarrhea, abdominal or epigastric pain, nausea, vomiting; chills, fever, sore throat; muscle pain, weakness occur
- Advise patient that treatment will take several years
- Advise patient that blood work and eye exam will be necessary during treatment
- **Advise not to take if pregnant (pregnancy X) or breastfeeding**
- Advise patient to stay out of the sun, use protective clothing, or use sunscreen to prevent photosensitivity (rare)

Evaluation
Positive therapeutic outcome
- Decreased cholesterol levels, serum triglyceride
- Improved HDL:LDL ratio

atovaquone (Rx)
(a-toe′va-kwon)
Mepron
Func. class.: Antiprotozoal
Chem. class.: Analog of ubiquinone
Pregnancy category C

ACTION: Interferes with DNA/RNA synthesis in protozoa

Therapeutic outcome: Antiprotozoal for *Pneumocystis jiroveci* only

USES: *P. jiroveci* infections in patients intolerant of trimethoprim/sulfamethoxazole (co-trimoxazole), prophylaxis, *Toxoplasma gondii*, toxoplasmosis

CONTRAINDICATIONS
Hypersensitivity or history of developing life-threatening allergic reactions to any component of the formulation, benzyl alcohol sensitivity

Precautions: Pregnancy **C**, breastfeeding, GI/hepatic disease, neonates, respiratory insufficiency

DOSAGE AND ROUTES
Acute, mild, moderate *Pneumocystis jiroveci* pneumonia (PCP)
Adult and adolescent 13-16 yr: PO 750 mg tid with food for 21 days

Pneumocystis jiroveci pneumonia prophylaxis
Adult and adolescent: PO 1500 mg daily with meal

Available forms: Susp 750 mg/5 ml

Implementation
• Give with food (preferably fatty); to increase absorption of the product and higher plasma concentrations; give tid × 3 wk
• Give oral suspension after shaken
• Take all contents of foil pouch

ADVERSE EFFECTS
CNS: *Dizziness, headache, anxiety,* insomnia, asthenia, fever
CV: Hypotension
GI: *Nausea, vomiting, diarrhea,* anorexia, increased AST and ALT, **acute pancreatitis,** constipation, abdominal pain
HEMA: Anemia, **neutropenia**
INTEG: Pruritus, urticaria, *rash*
META: Hypoglycemia, hyponatremia
OTHER: Cough, dyspnea

Pharmacokinetics
Absorption	Poor; increased when taken with fatty foods
Distribution	Unknown
Metabolism	Hepatic recycling
Excretion	Feces, unchanged (94%)
Half-life	2-3 days

Pharmacodynamics
Onset	Unknown
Peak	1-8 hr
Duration	Unknown

INTERACTIONS
Individual drugs
Rifampin, rifabutin, tetracycline: decreased effectiveness of atovaquone, avoid concurrent use
Zidovudine: increased level of zidovudine, monitor for toxicity

Drug/lab test
Increase: AST, ALT, alk phos
Decrease: glucose, neutrophils, Hgb, sodium

NURSING CONSIDERATIONS
Assessment
• Assess for *Pneumocystis jiroveci:* monitor WBC, bilateral lung sounds, sputum for C&S; these should be checked before, periodically during, after treatment; after collection of 1st sputum, therapy may begin
• Monitor for signs of **infection;** anemia; monitor bowel pattern before, during treatment
• Monitor respiratory status: rate, character, wheezing, dyspnea; ABGs, chest films
• Assess for dizziness, confusion, hallucination
• Assess for allergies before treatment, reaction of each medication; place allergies on chart; notify all people giving products

Patient/family education
• Instruct patient to take with food, preferably fatty foods, to increase plasma concentrations
• Advise patient to take product exactly as prescribed

Evaluation
Positive therapeutic outcome
• Decreased temperature
• Ability to breathe
• Three negative sputum cultures

⚠ HIGH ALERT

atropine (Rx)
(a'troe-peen)
Func. class.: Antidysrhythmic, anticholinergic parasympatholytic, antimuscarinic
Chem. class.: Belladonna alkaloid
Pregnancy category C

Do not confuse: atropine/Akarpine

ACTION: Blocks acetylcholine at parasympathetic neuroeffector sites; increases cardiac output, heart rate by blocking vagal stimulation in heart; dries secretions by blocking vagus

Therapeutic outcome: Drying of secretions, increased heart rate, cycloplegia, mydriasis

Adverse effects: *italics* = common; **bold** = life-threatening

USES: Bradycardia <40-50 bpm, bradydys-rhythmia, reversal of anticholinesterase agents, insecticide poisoning, blocking cardiac vagal reflexes, decreasing secretions before surgery, antispasmodic with GU and biliary surgery, bronchodilator, AV heart block, irinotecan-induced diarrhea, rapid-sequence intubation

CONTRAINDICATIONS

Hypersensitivity to belladonna alkaloids, closed-angle glaucoma, GI obstructions, myasthenia gravis, thyrotoxicosis, ulcerative colitis, prostatic hypertrophy, tachycardia/tachydysrhythmias, asthma, acute hemorrhage, severe hepatic disease, myocardial ischemia, paralytic ileus

Precautions: Pregnancy **C**, breastfeeding, child <6 yr, geriatric, renal disease, CHF, hyperthyroidism, COPD, hypertension, intraabdominal infections, Down syndrome, spastic paralysis, gastric ulcer

DOSAGE AND ROUTES
Bradycardia/bradydysrhythmias
Adult: IV bol 0.5-1 mg given q3-5min, not to exceed 2 mg
Child: IV 0.02 mg/kg, may repeat X1, min dose 0.1 mg to avoid paradoxical reaction, max single dose 0.5 mg, max total dose 1 mg

Organophosphate poisoning
Adult and child: IM (AtroPen)/IV 1-2 mg q 20-30 min until muscarinic symptoms disappear; may need 6 mg qhr
Adult and child ≥90 lb, usually >10 yr: 2 mg IM (AtroPen)
Child 40-90 lb, usually 4-10 yr: 1 mg IM (AtroPen)
Child 15-40 lb, 6 mo-4 yr: 0.5 mg IM (AtroPen)
Infant <15 lb: IM/IV 0.05 mg/kg q5-20min

Presurgery
Adult and child >20 kg: SUBCUT/IM/ IV 0.4-0.6 mg 30-60 min before anesthesia
Child <20 kg: IM/SUBCUT 0.01 mg/kg up to 0.4 mg ½-1 hr preop, max 0.6 mg/dose

Available forms: Inj 0.05, 0.1, 0.4, 0.5, 0.8, 1 mg/ml; inj prefilled autoinjectors (AtroPen) 0.5, 1, 2 mg

Implementation
PO route
• PO without regard to meals
IM route
• Expect atropine flush 15-20 min after inj; it may occur in children and is not harmful
AtroPen
• Use no more than 3 AtroPen injections unless under the supervision of trained provider

• Use as soon as symptoms appear (tearing, wheezing, muscle fasciculations, excessive oral secretions), may use through clothing

IV route
• Give IV undiluted or diluted with 10 ml sterile water; give at a rate of 0.6 mg/min; give through Y-tube or 3-way stopcock; do not add to IV sol; may cause paradoxical bradycardia lasting 2 min

Y-site compatibilities: Amrinone, etomidate, famotidine, heparin, hydrocortisone sodium succinate, meropenem, nafcillin, potassium chloride, SUFentanil, vit B/C

ADVERSE EFFECTS
CNS: Headache, dizziness, involuntary movement, confusion, psychosis, anxiety, **coma**, flushing, drowsiness, insomnia, weakness, delirium (geriatric)
CV: Hypo/hypertension, paradoxical bradycardia, angina, PVCs, **tachycardia**, ectopic ventricular beats, **bradycardia**, palpitations
EENT: Blurred vision, photophobia, glaucoma, eye pain, pupil dilatation, nasal congestion, increased intraoccular pressure
GI: Dry mouth, nausea, vomiting, abdominal pain, anorexia, constipation, **paralytic ileus**, abdominal distention, altered taste
GU: Retention, hesitancy, impotence, dysuria
INTEG: Rash, urticaria, contact dermatitis, dry skin, flushing
MISC: Suppression of breastfeeding, decreased sweating, **anaphylaxis**

Pharmacokinetics
Absorption	Well absorbed (PO, SUBCUT, IM)
Distribution	Crosses blood-brain barrier, placenta
Metabolism	Liver
Excretion	Kidneys, unchanged (70%-90%); breast milk
Half-life	13-40 hr

Pharmacodynamics
	IM/ SUBCUT	IV	Ophth
Onset	15 min	2-4 min	½ hr
Peak	30 min	2-4 min	30-60 min
Duration	4-6 hr	4-6 hr	1-2 wk

INTERACTIONS
Individual drugs
Amantadine: increased anticholinergic effects

Ketoconazole, levodopa: decreased absorption
Potassium chloride (oral): increased mucosal
lesions

Drug classifications

Antacids: decreased absorption of atropine
Antidepressants (tricyclic), antiparkinson
agents: increased anticholinergic effect

NURSING CONSIDERATIONS
Assessment

• Monitor I&O ratio; check for urinary retention and daily output in geriatric or postoperative patients
• Monitor ECG for ectopic ventricular beats,
PVC, tachycardia in cardiac patients
• Monitor for bowel sounds; check for constipation; abdominal distention and constipation
may occur
• Monitor respiratory status: rate, rhythm, cyanosis, wheezing, dyspnea, engorged neck veins
• Monitor cardiac rate: rhythm, character, B/P
continuously
• Monitor allergic reaction: rash, urticaria

Patient/family education

• Advise patient not to perform strenuous activity in high temperatures; heat stroke may result
• Instruct patient to take as prescribed; not to
skip doses
• Instruct patient to report change in vision;
blurring or loss of sight; trouble breathing;
sweating; flushing, chest pain, allergic reactions, constipation, urinary retention, to use
sunglasses to protect the eyes
• Caution patient not to operate machinery if
drowsiness occurs
• Advise patient not to take OTC products
without approval of physician
• Teach patient not to freeze or expose to light
(Astropen)

Evaluation
Positive therapeutic outcome

• Decreased dysrhythmias
• Increased heart rate
• Decreased secretions, GI, GU spasms
• Bronchodilatation

TREATMENT OF OVERDOSE:

O_2, artificial ventilation, ECG; administer DOPamine for circulatory depression; administer diazepam or thiopental for seizure; assess need for antidysrhythmics

atropine ophthalmic
See Appendix B

⚠ HIGH ALERT
axitinib
Inlyta
Func. class.: Antineoplastic, biologic
response modifier, signal transduction in-
hibitor (STI)
Chem. class.: Tyrosine kinase inhibitor
Pregnancy category D

ACTION: Inhibits receptor tyrosine kinases including vascular endothelial growth factor receptors (VEGFR)-1, VEGFR-2, and
VEGFR-3; inhibits tumor growth and phosphorylation of VEGFR-2 and VEGF-mediated endothelial cell proliferation

Therapeutic outcome: Decreased spread
of malignancy

USES: Treatment of advanced renal cell cancer after failure of one prior systemic therapy

CONTRAINDICATIONS
Pregnancy (D), breastfeeding

Precautions: Risk for or history of thromboembolic disease, recent bleeding, untreated
brain metastasis, recent GI bleeding, GI perforation, fistula, surgery, moderate hepatic disease,
uncontrolled hypertension, hyper/hypothyroid-
ism, proteinuria, infertility, end-stage renal disease (CrCl <15 ml/min); not intended for use in
adolescents, children, infants, neonates

DOSAGE AND ROUTES
Adult: PO 5 mg bid (at 12 hr intervals), may
increase to 7 mg bid and then to 10 mg bid in
those not receiving antihypertensives who tolerate the lower dosage for at least 2 consecutive wk
with no more than grade 2 adverse reactions.
Reduce to 3 mg bid if a dose reduction is
needed; if further reduction is necessary, reduce
to 2 mg bid
**Adult receiving a strong CYP 3A4/5 inhibi-
tor:** Reduce dose by 1/2, adjust as needed

Available forms: Tab 1, 5 mg

Implementation
• Give with or without food; swallow tablet
whole with a glass of water
• If patient vomits or misses a dose, an additional dose should not be taken; the next dose
should be taken at the usual time
• Store at room temperature

ADVERSE EFFECTS
CNS: Dizziness, headache, reversible posterior
leukoencephalopathy syndrome (RPLS), fatigue

CV: Hypertension, arterial thromboembolic events (ATE), venous thromboembolic events (VTE)

ENDO: Hypothyroidism, hyperthyroidism

GI: Lower GI bleeding/perforation/fistula. abdominal pain, constipation, diarrhea, dysgeusia, dyspepsia, dysphonia, hemorrhoids, nausea, mucosal inflammation, stomatitis, vomiting, increased ALT/AST

GU: Proteinuria

HEMA: Bleeding, intracranial bleeding, anemia, polycythemia, decreased/increased hemoglobin, lymphopenia, thrombocytopenia, neutropenia

INTEG: Palmar-plantar erythrodysesthesia (hand and foot syndrome), rash, dry skin, pruritus, alopecia, erythema

MISC: Weight loss dehydration metabolic and electrolyte laboratory abnormalities included

MS: Asthenia, arthralgia, musculoskeletal pain, myalgia

RESP: Cough, dyspnea

Pharmacokinetics

Absorption	Unknown
Distribution	Protein binding >99%
Metabolism	Liver
Excretion	Unknown
Half-life	2.5-6.1 hr

Pharmacodynamics

Onset	Unknown
Peak	Unknown
Duration	Unknown

INTERACTIONS
Individual drugs

CYP3A4/5 inhibitor, strong, moderate (ketoconazole, boceprevir, chloramphenicol, conivaptan, delavirdine, fosamprenavir, imatinib, indinavir, isoniazid, itraconazole, dalfopristin; quinupristin, posaconazole, ritonavir, telithromycin, tipranavir [boosted with ritonavir], darunavir [boosted with ritonavir], aldesleukin, IL-2, amiodarone, aprepitant, fosaprepitant atazanavir, bromocriptine, clarithromycin, crizotinib, danazol, diltiazem, dronedarone, erythromycin, fluvoxaMINE, lanreotide, lapatinib, miconazole, mifepristone, nefazodone, nelfinavir, niCARdipine, octreotide, pantoprazole, saquinavir, tamoxifen, verapamil, voriconazole, grapefruit juice): increased axitinib effect

CYP3A4/5 inducers, strong/moderate (rifampin, carBAMazepine, dexamethasone, phenytoin, PHENobarbital, rifabutin, rifapentine, St. John's wort, ethanol, bexarotene, bosentan, efavirenz, etravirine, griseofulvin, metyrapone, modafinil, nafcillin, nevirapine, OXcarbazepine, vemurafenib, pioglitazone, topiramate): decreased effect of axitinib

CYP3A4/5 inhibitor and inducers (quiNINE): increased or decreased axitinib effect

Drug/lab test

Increase: creatinine, lipase, amylase, potassium
Decrease: bicarbonate, calcium, albumin, glucose, phosphate, sodium
Increase or decrease: sodium, glucose

Drug/food

Increase drug effect: grapefruit or grapefruit juice

Drug/herb

St. John's wort: decreased effect of axitinib

NURSING CONSIDERATIONS
Assessment

• Bleeding: monitor for GI bleeding or perforation; temporarily discontinue therapy if a patient develops any bleeding that requires treatment

• Surgery: discontinue ≥24 hr before surgery, may be resumed after adequate wound healing

• Hepatic/renal disease: dosage should be reduced in patients with moderate (Child-Pugh Class B) hepatic disease, monitor liver function tests (ALT, AST, bilirubin) before and periodically during therapy; monitor CCr before and during treatment

• Hypertension: B/P should be well controlled before starting treatment; monitor patients for hypertension and administer antihypertensive therapy as needed before and during therapy; dose should be reduced for persistent hypertension; therapy should be discontinued if B/P remains elevated after a dosage reduction or if there is evidence of hypertensive crisis; after discontinuation monitor B/P for hypotension in those receiving antihypertensives

• Hyper/hypothyroidism: monitor thyroid function tests before and periodically during therapy; thyroid disease should be treated with thyroid medications

• Monitor for proteinuria before and periodically during therapy; product may need to be decreased or discontinued if moderate to severe proteinuria occurs

• Pregnancy/breastfeeding: pregnancy category D; determine if the patient is pregnant or breastfeeding before using this product; may also cause infertility

Patient/family education

• Instruct patient to use contraception during treatment (pregnancy category D)

---

or to avoid use of this product; to notify prescriber if pregnancy is planned or suspected, not to breastfeed
• Instruct patient to notify prescriber of bleeding that is severe or that requires treatment
• Teach patient that product will be discontinued ≥24 hr before surgery; may be resumed after adequate wound healing
• Teach patient that laboratory testing will be required before and periodically during product use
• Teach patient how to monitor B/P and that B/P products should be continued as directed by prescriber

Evaluation
Positive therapeutic outcome
• Decreased spread of malignancy

⚠ HIGH ALERT

azaCITIDine (Rx)
(a-za-sie-ti′deen)
Vidaza
Func. class.: Antineoplastic hormone
Chem. class.: Pyrimidine nucleoside analogue
Pregnancy category D

Do not confuse: azaCITIDine/ azaTHIOprine

ACTION: Cytotoxic by producing damage to double-strand DNA during DNA synthesis

Therapeutic outcome: Improved blood counts in refractor anemia

USES: Myelodysplastic syndrome (MDS)

CONTRAINDICATIONS
Pregnancy **D**, hypersensitivity to this product or mannitol, advanced malignant hepatic tumors

Precautions: Breastfeeding, children, geriatric, renal/hepatic disease; baseline albumin <30 g/L; a man should not father a child while taking this product

DOSAGE AND ROUTES
Adult: SUBCUT 75 mg/m^2 daily × 7 days, q4wk, premedicate with antiemetic; dose may be increased to 100 mg/m^2 if no response is seen after 2 treatment cycles; minimum treatment 4 cycles

Available forms: Powder for inj, 100 mg

Implementation
• Increase patient's fluid intake to 2-3 L/day to prevent dehydration, unless contraindicated
• Assist patient with rinsing of mouth tid-qid with water, club soda; brushing of teeth bid-tid with soft brush or cotton-tipped applicator for stomatitis; use unwaxed dental floss
• Provide a nutritious diet with iron, vitamin supplement, low fiber, few dairy products
• Use cytotoxic handling procedures
SUBCUT route
• **Reconstitute** with 4 ml sterile water for inj (25 mg/ml), **inject** diluents slowly into vial, **invert** vial 2-3 times and gently rotate; sol will be cloudy, use immediately; divide doses >4 ml into two syringes; invert the contents 2-3 times and gently roll syringe between the palms for 30 sec immediately before administration; rotate inj site

┃ IV intermittent INF route
• **Reconstitute** each vial with 4 ml sterile water for inj, **shake** well until all solids are dissolved, (10 mg/ml) withdraw sol and **inject** in 50-100 NS or LR, **infuse** over 10-40 min

ADVERSE EFFECTS
CNS: Anxiety, depression, dizziness, fatigue, headache, fever, insomnia
CV: Cardiac murmur, hypotension, tachycardia, peripheral edema, chest pain
GI: Diarrhea, nausea, vomiting, anorexia, constipation, abdominal pain, distention, tenderness, hemorrhoids, mouth hemorrhage, tongue ulceration, stomatitis, dyspepsia, **hepatotoxicity, hepatic coma**
GU: **Real failure, renal tubular acidosis,** dysuria, UTI
HEMA: **Leukopenia, anemia, thrombocytopenia, neutropenia,** ecchymosis, febrile neutropenia, petechiae
INTEG: Irritation at site, rash, sweating, pyrexia, pruritus
META: Hypokalemia
MS: Weakness, arthralgia, muscle cramps, myalgia, back pain
RESP: Cough, dyspnea, pharyngitis, **pleural effusion**

Pharmacokinetics

Absorption	Rapid
Distribution	Unknown
Metabolism	Liver
Excretion	Urine
Half-life	35-49 min

Pharmacodynamics

Onset	Unknown
Peak	½ hr
Duration	Unknown

INTERACTIONS
Drug classifications
Antineoplastics, other: increased bone marrow depression
Increase: bleeding, anticoagulants

Drug/lab
Increase: BUN/creatinine
Decrease: WBC, platelets, neutrophils, potassium

NURSING CONSIDERATIONS
Assessment
• Assess for CNS symptoms: fever, headache, chills, dizziness
• **Monitor bone marrow suppression with patients with baseline WBC 3 × 10⁹/L, absolute neutrophil count (ANC) = 1.5 × 10⁹/L, and platelets = 75 × 10⁹/L, adjust dose; ANC < 0.5 × 10⁹/L, platelets < 25 × 10⁹/L, give 50% dose next course; ANC 0.5-1.5 × 10⁹/L, platelets 25-50 × 10⁹/L, give 67% next course**
• Assess buccal cavity q8hr for dryness, sores, or ulceration, white patches, oral pain, bleeding, dysphagia
• Assess for bruising, bleeding, blood in stools, urine, sputum, emesis; myelodysplastic syndrome (MDS), splenomegaly

Patient/family education
• Instruct patient to avoid foods with citric acid or hot or rough texture if stomatitis is present; to drink adequate fluids
• Instruct patient to report stomatitis; any bleeding, white spots, ulcerations in mouth; tell patient to examine mouth daily, report symptoms
• Instruct patient to avoid crowds, persons with known infections; not to receive immunizations
• **Advise patient to use contraception during and for several months after therapy, pregnancy D not to breastfeed, not to father a child while receiving this product**

Evaluation
Positive therapeutic outcome
• Improvement in blood counts in refractory anemia, or refractory anemia with excess blasts

---

azaTHIOprine (Rx)
(ay-za-thye′oh-preen)
Azasan, Imuran
Func. class.: Immunosuppressant
Chem. class.: Purine antagonist
Pregnancy category D

Do not confuse: Imuran/Imferon/Elmiron/IMDUR/Enduron/Tenormin, azaTHIOprine/azaCITIDine

ACTION: Produces immunosuppression by inhibiting purine synthesis in cells

Therapeutic outcome: Absence of graft rejection, slowing of rheumatoid arthritis

USES: Renal transplants to prevent graft rejection, refractory rheumatoid arthritis

Unlabeled uses: Myasthenia gravis, chronic ulcerative colitis, Crohn's disease, Behçet's syndrome

CONTRAINDICATIONS
Pregnancy **D**, breastfeeding, hypersensitivity

Precautions: Severe renal/hepatic disease, geriatric, thiopurine methyltransferase deficiency, infection

> **BLACK BOX WARNING:** Bone marrow suppression, neoplastic disease; must be used by experienced clinician

DOSAGE AND ROUTES
Prevention of rejection
Adult and child: IV 3-5 mg/kg/day, then maintenance (PO) of at least 1-3 mg/kg/day,

Renal dose
Adult: PO; give lower dose in tubular necrosis in immediate postcadaveric transplant period, CCr 10-50 ml/min 75% of dose; CCr <10 ml/min 50% of dose

Refractory rheumatoid arthritis
Adult: PO 1 mg/kg/day; may increase dosage after 2 mo by 0.5 mg/kg/day and then q4wk; not to exceed 2.5 mg/kg/day

Idiopathic thrombocytopenia purpura (unlabeled)
Adult: PO 1-2 mg/kg/day X 3-6 mo max 150 mg/day

Available forms: Tabs 50, 75, 100 mg; inj **IV** 100 mg

Implementation
PO route
• Give with meals to reduce GI upset; nausea is common

IV route
• Prepare in biological cabinet using gown, gloves, mask
Direct, IV route
• **Dilute** to 10 mg/ml with 0.9% NaCl, 0.45% NaCl, D₅W, **give** over 5 min
Intermittent IV INF route
• **Reconstitute** 100 mg/10 ml of sterile water for inj; rotate to dissolve; **further dilute** with 50 ml or more saline or glucose in saline, **give** over ½-1 hr

---

Y-site compatibilities: Alfentanil, atracurium, atropine, benztropine, calcium gluconate, cycloSPORINE, enalaprilat, epoetin alfa, erythromycin, fentaNYL, fluconazole, folic acid, furosemide, glycopyrrolate, heparin, insulin, mannitol, mechlorethamine, metoprolol, naloxone, nitroglycerin, oxytocin, penicillin G, potassium chloride, propranolol, protamine, SUFentanil, trimetaphan, vasopression

Solution compatibilities: D$_5$W, NaCl 0.9%, NaCl 0.45%

ADVERSE EFFECTS

GI: Nausea, vomiting, stomatitis, esophagitis, **pancreatitis, hepatotoxicity, jaundice, hepatic veno-occlusive disease**
HEMA: Leukopenia, thrombocytopenia, anemia, pancytopenia, bleeding
INTEG: Rash, alopeia
MISC: Raynaud's symptoms, serum sickness, secondary malignancy, infection
MS: Arthralgia, muscle wasting

Pharmacokinetics

Absorption	Readily (PO)
Distribution	Crosses placenta
Metabolism	Liver to mercaptopurine
Excretion	Kidney, minimal
Half-life	3 hr

Pharmacodynamics

	PO	IV
Onset	Unknown	Unknown
Peak	4 hr	Unknown
Duration	Unknown	Unknown

INTERACTIONS
Individual drugs
Do not admix with other products
Allopurinol: increased action of azaTHIOprine
CycloSPORINE: increased myelosuppression
Sulfamethoxazole-trimethoprim: increased leukopenia
Warfarin: decreased action of warfarin

Drug classifications
ACE inhibitors: increased leukopenia
Antineoplastics: increased myelosuppression
Toxoids, vaccines: decreased immune response

Drug/lab test
Increased: liver function tests
Decreased: uric acid
Interference: CBC, diff count

NURSING CONSIDERATIONS
Assessment
• Assess symptoms of **rheumatoid arthritis:** pain in joints, stiffness, poor range of motion, mobility, inflammation before and during treatment
• Monitor **blood studies:** CBC, Hgb, WBC, platelets during treatment monthly; if leukocytes are <3000/mm^3 or platelets <100,000/mm^3, product should be discontinued or reduced; decreased Hgb level may indicate bone marrow suppression
• **Bone marrow suppression: severe leukopenia, pancytopenia, thrombocytopenia**
• **Monitor liver function studies: alkaline phosphatase, AST, ALT, amylase, bilirubin; and for hepatotoxicity: dark urine, jaundice, itching, light-colored stools; product should be discontinued**
• Monitor I&O, weight daily, report decreasing urine output, toxicity may occur
• Assess for **infection:** increased temp, WBC; sputum, urine

Patient/family education
• Teach patient to take as prescribed, do not miss doses; if dose is missed on daily regimen, skip dose; if on multiple dosing/day, take as soon as remembered
• Teach patient that therapeutic response may take 3-4 mo in rheumatoid arthritis, to continue with prescribed exercise, rest, other medications; that product is needed for life in renal transplant
• **Instruct patient to report fever, rash, severe diarrhea, chills, sore throat, fatigue, since serious infections may occur; or clay-colored stools and cramping (hepatotoxicity)**
• **Advise patient to use contraceptive measures during treatment for 16 wk after ending therapy; product is teratogenic (pregnancy D)**
• Advise patient to avoid vaccinations
• Tell patient to avoid crowds and persons with known infections to reduce risk of infection
• Teach patient to take with food to decrease GI intolerance
• Teach patient regarding multiple significant drug/drug interactions
• Instruct patient not to use OTC medications without approval of prescriber
• Advise patient to use soft-bristled toothbrush to prevent bleeding

Evaluation
Positive therapeutic outcome
• Absence of graft rejection
• Immunosuppression in autoimmune disorders
• Increased joint mobility without pain in rheumatoid arthritis

azelaic acid topical
See Appendix B

azelastine (Rx)
(ay′ze-lass-teen)
Optivar
Func. class.: Leukotriene synthesis inhibitor
Chem. class.: Phthalazinone derivative
Pregnancy category C

ACTION: Inhibits the synthesis and release of leukotrienes; antagonizes action of acetylcholine, histamine, serotonin

Therapeutic outcome: Decreased nasal stuffiness, itching, swollen eyes

USES: Seasonal allergic rhinitis

CONTRAINDICATIONS
Hypersensitivity

Precautions: Pregnancy **C**

DOSAGE AND ROUTES
Adult and child ≥12 yr: NASAL 2 sprays/nostril bid

Available forms: Spray 137 mcg/actuation

Implementation
• Remove cap/safety clip from spray pump
• Prime pump if using for first time, push 4 times quickly, away from face, blow your nose, then place tip of pump into one nostril, while holding other nostril closed, tilt head forward, and spray into nostril
• Put cover/safety clip back on

ADVERSE EFFECTS
CNS: Sedation (more common with increased dosages), drowsiness
MISC: Weight increase, myalgia

Pharmacokinetics

Absorption	Unknown
Distribution	Unknown
Metabolism	Liver, extensively
Excretion	Feces
Half-life	25-42 hr

Pharmacodynamics

Onset	Unknown
Peak	4-5 hr
Duration	Unknown

INTERACTIONS
Individual drugs
Alcohol: increased CNS depression

Drug classifications
CNS depressants, opioids, sedative/hypnotics: increased CNS depression

NURSING CONSIDERATIONS
Assessment
• Assess respiratory status: rate, rhythm, increase in bronchial secretions, wheezing, chest tightness; provide fluids to 2 L/day to decrease secretion thickness

Patient/family education
• Teach patient all aspects of product uses; to notify prescriber if confusion, sedation occur; to avoid driving and other hazardous activity if drowsiness occurs; to avoid alcohol and other CNS depressants that may potentiate effect
• Caution patient not to exceed recommended dosage; dysrhythmias may occur

Evaluation
Positive therapeutic outcome
• Absence of runny or congested nose

azelastine nasal agent
See Appendix B

azelastine ophthalmic
See Appendix B

azilsartan
(ay-zil-sar′tan)
Edarbi
(Pronunciation)
Func. class.: Antihypertensive
Chem class.: Angiotensin II receptor antagonist
Pregnancy category D

ACTION: Antagonizes angiotensin II at the AT_1 receptor in tissues like vascular smooth muscle and the adrenal gland. Two angiotensin II receptors, AT_1 and AT_2, have been identified; azilsartan exhibits more than a 10,000-fold greater affinity for the AT_1 receptor than the AT_2 receptor.

Therapeutic outcome: Decreased B/P

USES: Hypertension, alone or in combination with other antihypertensives

CONTRAINDICATIONS

BLACK BOX WARNING: Pregnancy **D** (2nd/3rd trimesters)

Precautions: Angioedema, African descent, renal disease, renal artery stenosis, children, geriatrics, heart failure, hypovolemia, breastfeeding, pregnancy C 1st trimester

DOSAGE AND ROUTES
Adult: PO 80 mg/day, may give an initial dose of 40 mg/day in patients receiving high-dose diuretic therapy

Available forms: Tabs 40, 80 mg

Implementation
• May administer without regard to food
• Use original package to protect from light, moisture, and heat

ADVERSE EFFECTS
CNS: Dizziness, fatigue, asthenia, syncope
CV: Hypotension, orthostatic hypotension
GI: Nausea, diarrhea
HEMA: Anemia
INTEG: Angioedema, rash, pruritus
MS: Muscle cramps
RESP: Cough

Pharmacokinetics

Absorption	Absolute bioavailability (60%) not affected by food; steady state within 5 days and no accumulation in plasma occurs with once-daily dosing; hydrolyzed to the active metabolite, azilsartan, in GI tract during absorption, rapidly absorbed
Distribution	Protein binding, >99%, to serum albumin
Metabolism	Metabolized by CYP2C9
Excretion	55% eliminated (feces), 42% (urine)
Half-life	Elimination half-life 11 hr

Pharmacodynamics

Onset	Unknown
Peak	1.5-3 hr
Duration	Unknown

INTERACTIONS
Individual drugs
CycloSPORINE: in those with poor renal function, increased renal failure risk: monitor closely
Lithium: increased lithium toxicity
Sodium phosphate monobasic monohydrate, sodium phosphate dibasic anhydrous: increased phosphate nephropathy

Drug classifications
Antidiabetics: increased hypoglycemia
NSAIDs in those with poor renal function: monitor closely: Increased renal failure risk
Other antihypertensives, other angiotensin receptor antagonists, MAOIs: increased hypotensive effect

Drug/herb
Ephedra: decreased antihypertensive effect
Hawthorn: increased antihypertensive effect

NURSING CONSIDERATIONS
Assessment
• **Angioedema: Assess for facial swelling, difficulty breathing**

> **BLACK BOX WARNING:** Pregnancy **D** (2nd/3rd trimester), can cause fetal death

• Response and adverse reactions especially in renal disease
• B/P, pulse during beginning therapy and periodically thereafter; note rhythm, rate, quality; obtain electrolytes before beginning therapy

Patient/family education
• Instruct patient to comply with dosage schedule even if feeling better
• **Instruct patient to notify prescriber of facial swelling; if pregnancy is planned or suspected (D 2nd/3rd trimester)**
• Advise patient that diarrhea, dehydration, excessive perspiration, vomiting, may lead to fall in B/P, to consult prescriber if these occur
• Instruct patient to rise slowly from lying or sitting to minimize orthostatic hypotension; that product may cause dizziness
• Instruct patient to avoid OTC medications unless approved by prescriber; to inform all health care providers of product use
• Instruct patient to use proper technique for obtaining B/P

Evaluation
Positive therapeutic outcome
• Decreased B/P

azithromycin (Rx)
(ay-zi-thro-my′sin)
AzaSite, Zithromax, Zmax
Func. class.: Antiinfective
Chem. class.: Macrolide (azalide)
Pregnancy category B

Do not confuse: azithromycin/erythromycin, Zithromax/Zinacef

ACTION: Binds to 50S ribosomal subunits of susceptible bacteria and suppresses protein synthesis; much greater spectrum of activity than erythromycin; more effective against gram-negative organisms

Therapeutic outcome: Bacteriostatic against the following susceptible organisms: PO, acute pharyngitis/tonsillitis (group A

Adverse effects: *italics* = common; **bold** = life-threatening

streptococcal); acute skin/soft tissue infections; community-acquired pneumonia

USES: Mild to moderate infections of the upper respiratory tract, in children: acute otitis media, lower respiratory tract; uncomplicated skin and skin structure infections, nongonococcal urethritis, or cervicitis; prophylaxis of disseminated *Mycobacterium avium* complex (MAC); *Bacillus anthracis, Bacteroides bivius, Bordetella pertussis, Borrelia burgdorferi, Campylobacter jejuni,* CDC coryneform group G, *Chlamydia trachomatis, Chlamydophila pneumoniae, Clostridium perfringens, Gardnerella vaginalis, Haemophilus ducreyi/influenzae* (beta-lactamase negative/positive), *Helicobacter pylori, Klebsiella granulomatis, Legionella pneumoniae/moraxella/catarrhalis, Mycobacterium avium/intracellulare, Mycoplasma genitalium/hominis/pneumoniae, Neisseria gonorrhoeae, Peptostreptococcus, Prevotella bivia, Rickettsia tsutsugamushi, Salmonella typhi, Staphylococcus aureus* (MSSA)/*epidermidis, Streptococcus, Toxoplasma gondii, Treponema pallidum, Ureaplasma urealyticum, Vibrio cholerae,* viridans streptococci; **opthalmic: bacterial conjunctivitis**

CONTRAINDICATIONS

Hypersensitivity to azithromycin, erythromycin, or any macrolide, hepatitis, jaundice

Precautions: Pregnancy **B,** breastfeeding, child <6 mo for otitis media, child <2 yr for pharyngitis, geriatric, renal/hepatic/cardiac disease, tonsillitis, QT prolongation, ulcerative colitis, torsades de pointes, sunlight exposure, sodium restriction, myasthenia gravis, pseudomembranous colitis, contact lenses, hypokalemia, hypomagnesemia

DOSAGE AND ROUTES
Most infections
Adult: PO 500 mg on day 1, then 250 mg daily on days 2-5 for a total dose of 1.5 g or 500 mg a day × 3 days
Child 2-15 yr: PO 10 mg/kg on day 1, then 5 mg/kg × 4 days

Pelvic inflammatory disease
Adult: PO/**IV** 500 mg **IV** q24hr × 2 doses, then 250 mg PO q24hr × 7-10 days

Cervicitis, chlamydia, chancroid, nongonococcal urethritis, syphilis
Adult: PO 1 g single dose

Gonorrhea
Adult: PO 2 g single dose

Endocarditis prophylaxis
Adult: PO 500 mg 1 hr prior to procedure
Child: PO 15 mg/kg 1 hr prior to procedure

Community-acquired pneumonia
Adult: PO 500 mg on day 1, then 250 mg PO once daily on days 2-5
Adolescent/child, infant ≥6 mo: Susp PO 10 mg/kg on day 1, then 5 mg/kg/day on days 2-5
Adult/adolescent, child ≥34 kg: Ext Rel Susp PO 2 g as a single dose (≥1 hr before or 2 hr after a meal)
Infant ≥6 mo and child weighing 5 to <34 kg and adolescent weighing <34 kg: Ext Rel Susp PO 60 mg/kg as a single dose (≥1 hr before or 2 hr after a meal)
Adult and adolescent ≥16 yr: Initially, 500 mg **IV** infusion as a single daily dose × 2 days or more then 500 mg PO/day to complete a 7-10 day course
Adolescent <16 yr, child, infant ≥3 mo: **IV** 10 mg/kg, max 500 mg qd × 2 days, then conversion to oral therapy as soon as possible to complete a 5-day course. After **IV** loading doses have been given, oral dosage is 5 mg/kg/day, max 250 mg/dose

Disseminated MAC infections
Adult: PO 600 mg/day in combination with ethambutol 15 mg/kg/day

MAC in HIV
Adult/adolescent: PO 1.2 g qwk, alone or with rifabutin

Lower respiratory tract infections
Adult: PO 500 mg day 1, then 250 mg × 4 days
Child: PO 5-12 mg/kg/day × 5 days

Acute otitis media
Child >6 mo: PO 30 mg/kg as a single dose or 10 mg/kg daily × 3 days or 10 mg/kg as a single dose on day 1, max 500 mg/day, then 5 mg/kg on days 2-5, max 250 mg/day

Prevention of acute otitis media
Child: PO 10 mg/kg qwk × 6 mo

Bacterial conjunctivitis
Adult/child ≥ 1 yr: opthalmic instill 1 drop in affected eye bid × 2 days then 1 drop in eye q day × 5 days

Available forms: Tabs 250, 500, 600 mg; powder for inj 500 mg; powder for oral susp 1 g/packet; susp 100, 200 mg/5 ml; ophthalmic drops 1% sol

Implementation
Opthalmic route
- Store in refrigerator
- Do not touch dropper to eye

PO route

- Provide adequate intake of fluids (2 L) during diarrhea episodes
- Give with a full glass of water; give susp 1 hr before or 2 hr after meals; tabs may be taken without regard to food; do not give with fruit juices
- Store at room temperature
- Reconstitute 1 g packet for susp with 60 ml water, mix, rinse glass with more water and have patient drink to consume all medication; packets not for pediatric use
- Do not take aluminum/magnesium-containing antacids or food simultaneously with this product

Intermittent IV infusion route

- **Reconstitute** 500 mg product/4.8 ml sterile water for inj (100 mg/ml), shake, **dilute** with ≥ 250 ml 0.9% NaCl, 0.45% NaCl, or LR to 1-2 mg/ml; diluted solution is stable for 24 hr or 7 days if refrigerated
- **Give** 1 mg/ml sol over 3 hr or 2 mg/ml sol over 1 hr, never give IM or as a bolus

Y-site compatibilities: Alemtuzumab, alfentanil, aminophylline, ampicillin, ampicillin-sulbactam, bumetanide, buprenorphine, butorphanol, calcium chloride/gluconate, carmustine, ceFAZolin, cefepime, cefoTEtan, cefOXitin, ceftaroline, cefTAZidime, ceftizoxime, cimetidine, cisatracurium, cyclophosphamide, cycloSPORINE, DAUNOrubicin liposome, dexamethasone, dexrazoxane, digoxin, diltiazem, DOBUTamine, DOXOrubicin liposomal, doxycycline, enalaprilat, EPINEPHrine, esmolol, etoposide, etoposide phosphate, fluconazole, foscarnet, fosphenytoin, gallium, ganciclovir, gatifloxacin, gemcitabine, granisetron, haloperidol, heparin, hydrocortisone phosphate/succinate, HYDROmorphone, hydrOXYzine, ifosfamide, inamrinone, isoproterenol, labetalol, lepirudin, magnesium sulfate, mannitol, meropenem, mesna, methohexital, methotrexate, methylPREDNISolone, metoclopramide, metroNIDAZOLE, milrinone, minocycline, mivacurium, nalbuphine, naloxone, nitroglycerin, nitroprusside, ofloxacin, oxytocin, PACLitaxel, PENTobarbital, phenylephrine, piperacillin, potassium acetate/phosphates, procainamide, prochlorperazine, promethazine, propranolol, ranitidine, remifentanil, succinylcholine, SUFentanil, sulfamethoxazole-trimethoprim, tacrolimus, telavancin, teniposide, thiotepa, ticarcillin, trimethobenzamide, vancomycin, vecuronium, verapamil, zidovudine, zoledronic acid

ADVERSE EFFECTS
CNS: Dizziness, headache, vertigo, somnolence, fatigue

CV: Palpitations, chest pain, QT prolongation, torsades de pointes (rare)
EENT: Hearing loss, tinnitus, loss of smell (anosmia)
GI: *Nausea, diarrhea,* hepatotoxicity, abdominal pain, stomatitis, heartburn, dyspepsia, flatulence, melena, cholestatic jaundice, pseudomembranous colitis, tongue discoloration
GU: Vaginitis, moniliasis, nephritis
HEMA: Anemia
INTEG: Rash, urticaria, pruritus, photosensitivity, pain at injection site
SYST: Angioedema, Stevens-Johnson syndrome, toxic epidermal necrolysis

Pharmacokinetics

Absorption	Rapid (PO) up to 50%
Distribution	Widely distributed
Metabolism	Unknown, minimal metabolism
Excretion	Unchanged (bile); kidneys, minimal
Half-life	11-70 hr

Pharmacodynamics

	PO	IV
Onset	Unknown	Unknown
Peak	2-4 hr	End of infusion
Duration	24 hr	24 hr

INTERACTIONS
Individual drugs
Bromocriptine, carBAMazepine, cycloSPORINE, digoxin, disopyramide, methylPREDNISolone, nelfinavir, phenytoin, tacrolimus, theophylline, triazolam: increased effects of specific products
Ergotamine: ergot toxicity
⚠ Amiodarone, droperidol, methadone, nilotinib, propafenone, quiNIDine: increased QT prolongation
⚠ Pimozide: increased dysrhythmias; fatal reaction; do not use concurrently
Triazolam: decreased clearance of triazolam

Drug classifications
Aluminum, magnesium antacids: decreased levels of azithromycin, separate by ≥2 hr
Anticoagulants (orals): increased effect of oral anticoagulants

Drug/food
Decreased: absorption—food (suspension)

Drug/lab test
Increased: bilirubin, alkaline phosphatase, CPK, BUN, creatinine, AST, ALT, potassium, blood glucose
Decreased: blood glucose, potassium, sodium

NURSING CONSIDERATIONS
Assessment
⚠ **QT prolongation, torsades de pointes: assess for patients with serious bradycardia, ongoing pro-arrhythmic conditions, or elderly; more common in these patients**
- Assess for signs and symptoms of **infection:** drainage, fever, increased WBC >10,000/mm^3, urine culture positive, sore throat, sputum culture positive
- Monitor respiratory status: rate, character, wheezing, tightness in chest; discontinue product if these occur
- Monitor allergies before treatment, reaction of each medication; place allergies on chart, notify all people giving products; skin eruptions, itching
- Monitor I&O ratio, renal studies; report hematuria, oliguria in renal disease; check urinalysis, protein, blood
- Monitor liver studies: AST, ALT, bilirubin, LDH, alkaline phosphatase; CBC with diff
- Monitor C&S before product therapy; product may be taken as soon as culture is taken; C&S may be repeated after treatment
- **Assess for serious skin reactions: Stevens-Johnson syndrome, toxic epidermal necrolysis, angioedema, discontinue if rash occurs**
- **Assess for pseudomembranous colitis: blood or pus in diarrhea stool, abdominal pain, fever, fatigue, anorexia; obtain CBC, serum albumin**
- Assess for **superinfection:** sore throat, mouth, tongue; fever, fatigue, diarrhea, anogenital pruritus

Patient/family education
- Instruct patient to report sore throat, black furry tongue, fever, loose foul-smelling stool, vaginal itching, discharge, fatigue; may indicate **superinfection**
- Caution patient not to take aluminum/magnesium-containing antacids or food simultaneously with this product; blood levels of azithromycin will be decreased
- **Instruct patient to notify prescriber of diarrhea stools, dark urine, pale stools, yellow discoloration of eyes or skin, severe abdominal pain; cholestatic jaundice is a severe adverse reaction**
- Teach patient to take Zmax 1 hr prior to or 2 hr after a meal; shake well before use
- Teach patient to complete dosage regimen; to notify prescriber if symptoms continue
- Teach patient to use protective clothing or stay out of the sun: photosensitivity may occur
- Teach patient to notify prescriber if pregnancy is suspected
⚠ **Cardiovascular death has occurred in those with serious bradycardia or ongoing hypokalemia, hypomagnesemia; avoid use**

Evaluation
Positive therapeutic outcome
- C&S negative for infection
- WBC within 5000-10,000/mm^3

azithromycin ophthalmic
See Appendix B

baclofen (Rx)

(bak'loe-fen)

Gablofen, Lioresal Intrathecal

Func. class.: Skeletal muscle relaxant, central acting

Chem. class.: GABA, chlorophenyl derivative

Pregnancy category C

Do not confuse: Lioresal/Lotensin, baclofen/Bactroban

ACTION: Inhibits synaptic responses in CNS by stimulating $GABA_B$ receptor subtype, which decreases neurotransmitter function, decreasing frequency, severity of muscle spasms

Therapeutic outcome: Decreased spasticity of muscles

USES: Spasticity in spinal cord injury, multiple sclerosis

CONTRAINDICATIONS

Hypersensitivity

Precautions: Pregnancy **C**, breastfeeding, geriatric, peptic ulcer, renal/hepatic disease, stroke, seizure disorder, diabetes mellitus, psychosis

> **BLACK BOX WARNING:** Abrupt discontinuation

DOSAGE AND ROUTES

Adult: PO 5 mg tid × 3 days, then 10 mg tid × 3 days, then 15 mg tid × 3 days, then 20 mg tid × 3 days, then titrated to response, max 80 mg/day; IT use implantable IT inf pump; use screening trial of 3 separate bol doses if needed 24 hr apart (50 mcg/ml, 75 mcg/1.5 ml, 100 mcg/2 ml); patients who do not respond to 100 mcg should not be considered for chronic IT therapy; spinal origin spasticity 12-2003 mcg/day; cerebral origin spasticity 22-1400 mcg/day

Child 2-7 yr: PO 10-15 mg/day divided q8hr; titrate every 3 days by 5-15 mg/day to max 40 mg/day

Child ≥8 yr: As above, max 60 mg/day

Child: IT initial test dose same as adult; for small children, initial dose of 25 mcg/dose may be used; 25-1200 mcg/day inf, titrated to response in screening phase

Available forms: Tabs 10, 20 mg; IT inj 10,000 mcg/20 ml, 20,000 mcg/20 ml, 40,000 mcg/20 ml; 50 mcg/ml, 0.05 mcg/ml, 10 mg/20 ml, 10 mg/5 ml, 50 mg/20 ml; pharmacy can prepare extemporaneous liquid preparations

Implementation

PO route

- Give with meals for GI symptoms; gum, frequent sips of water for dry mouth
- Store in airtight container at room temperature

IT route

- **For screening,** dilute to a concentration of 50 mcg/ml with NaCl for inj (preservative free); give test over 1 min; watch for decreasing muscle tone, frequency of spasm; if inadequate, use two more test doses q24hr; **maintenance inf** via implantable pump of 500-2000 mcg/ml dosage because individual titration is required
- Do not give IT dose by inj, **IV**, IM, SUBCUT, epidural

ADVERSE EFFECTS

CNS: *Dizziness, weakness, fatigue, drowsiness,* headache, disorientation, insomnia, paresthesias, tremors, seizures, coma; life-threatening CNS depression, impaired cognition, memory loss, insomnia, somnolence, CNS infection (IT)

CV: Hypotension, bradycardia, flushing, orthostatic hypotension, chest pain, palpitations, edema; cardiovascular collapse (IT)

EENT: Nasal congestion, blurred vision, mydriasis, tinnitus

GI: *Nausea,* constipation, vomiting, abdominal pain, dry mouth, anorexia, weight gain

GU: Urinary frequency, hematuria

INTEG: Rash, pruritus

RESP: Dyspnea, respiratory failure (IT)

Pharmacokinetics

Absorption	Good (PO)
Distribution	Widely, crosses placenta
Metabolism	Liver, partially
Excretion	Kidney, unchanged 70%-80%
Half-life	2½-4 hr

Pharmacodynamics

	PO/IT
Onset	0.5-1 hr
Peak	2-3 hr
Duration	>8 hr

INTERACTIONS

Individual drugs

Alcohol: CNS depression

Drug classifications

Antidepressants (tricyclics), barbiturates, MAOIs, opioids, sedative/hypnotics: increased CNS depression

Antihypertensives: increased hypotension

Drug/herb
Kava, valerian: increased CNS depression

Drug/lab test
Increased: AST, ALT, alkaline phosphatase, blood glucose, CK

NURSING CONSIDERATIONS
Assessment

> **BLACK BOX WARNING: Abrupt discontinu-ation** Serious adverse reactions may occur with intrathecal route

• **Multiple sclerosis:** spasms, spasticity, ataxia, mobility, improvement should occur
• Monitor B/P, weight, blood glucose, and hepatic function periodically
⚠ **Check for increased seizure activity in patients with epilepsy; this product de-creases seizure threshold, monitor ECG**
• Check I&O ratio; check for urinary retention, frequency, hesitancy
• Allergic reactions: rash, fever, respiratory dis-tress; severe weakness, numbness in extremities
• Assess CNS depression: dizziness, drowsiness, psychiatric symptoms
• Check dosage, as individual titration is required
• Assess for **withdrawal symptoms:** CNS depression, dizziness, drowsiness, psychiatric symptoms
• **Intrathecal: Have emergency equipment nearby; assess test dose and titration, if there is no response, check pump and catheter for proper functioning**

Patient/family education
⚠ **Advise patient not to discontinue medi-cation quickly; hallucinations, spasticity, tachycardia will occur; product should be tapered off over 1-2 wk**
• Advise patient not to take with alcohol, other CNS depressants
• Teach patient to avoid hazardous activities if drowsiness, dizziness occurs; to rise slowly to prevent orthostatic hypotension
• Teach patient to avoid using OTC medications: cough preparations, antihistamines, unless directed by prescriber
• Teach patient to notify prescriber if nausea, headache, tinnitus, insomnia, confusion, constipation, or inadequate, painful urination continues
• May require 1-2 mo for full response

Evaluation
Positive therapeutic outcome
• Decreased pain, spasticity

TREATMENT OF OVERDOSE: Induce emesis of conscious patient, activated charcoal, dialysis, physostigmine to reduce life-threatening CNS side effects

> **⚠ HIGH ALERT**
>
> ## basiliximab (Rx)
> (bas-ih-liks′ih-mab)
> **Simulect**
> *Func. class.:* Immunosuppressant
> *Chem. class.:* Murine/human monoclonal antibody (interleukin-2) receptor antagonist
> **Pregnancy category B**

ACTION: Binds to and blocks the IL-2 re-ceptor, which is selectively expressed on the surface of activated T lymphocytes; impairs the immune system to antigenic challenges

Therapeutic outcome: Prevention of graft rejection

USES: Acute allograft rejection in renal transplant patients when used with cycloSPO-RINE and corticosteroids

CONTRAINDICATIONS
Breastfeeding

Precautions: Pregnancy **B,** children, geriat-ric, human anti-murine antibody, hypersensitivity to mannitol/murine, exposure to viral infections

> **BLACK BOX WARNING:** Infections

DOSAGE AND ROUTES
Adult/child ≥35 kg: IV 20 mg × 2 doses; first dose within 2 hr before transplant surgery; sec-ond dose given 4 days after transplantation
Child <35 kg: IV 10 mg × 2 doses; first dose within 2 hr before transplant surgery; second dose given 4 days after transplantation

Available forms: Powder for inj 10, 20 mg

Implementation
Intermittent IV INF route
• **Reconstitute** 10 mg vial/2.5 ml or 20 mg vial in 5 ml sterile water for inj; shake gently to dis-solve, **dilute** reconstituted sol in 25 ml (10 mg vial) or 50 ml (20 mg vial) with 0.9% NaCl or D₅W, gently invert bag, do not shake, **give** over ½ hr, do not admix
• Storage of reconstituted sol refrigerated for up to 24 hr or at room temp for 4 hr

ADVERSE EFFECTS
CNS: *Pyrexia, chills, tremors, headache, in-somnia, weakness,* dizziness; psychiatric/behav-ioral changes (child)

CV: *Chest pain,* angina, **cardiac failure,** hypo/ hypertension, edema
GI: *Vomiting, nausea, diarrhea,* constipation, abdominal pain, GI bleeding, gingival hyperplasia, stomatitis
GU: Urinary retention/ frequency
INTEG: *Acne,* pruritus, impaired wound healing
META: Acidosis, hypercholesterolemia, hyperuricemia, hypo/hyperkalemia, hypocalcemia, hypophosphatemia
MISC: Infection, moniliasis, **anaphylaxis,** anemia, allergic reaction, dysuria, CMV infection, candidiasis, abnormal vision
MS: Arthralgia, myalgia
RESP: *Dyspnea, wheezing, cough,* **pulmonary edema**

Pharmacokinetics

Absorption	Unknown
Distribution	Unknown
Metabolism	Unknown
Excretion	Unknown
Half-life	7 days (adult) 9½ days (child)

Pharmacodynamics

Onset	Unknown
Peak	½ hr (adult)
Duration	Unknown

INTERACTIONS
Drug classifications
Immunosuppressants: increased immunosuppression

Drug/lab test
Increased: BUN, cholesterol, uric acid, creatinine, potassium, calcium, blood glucose, Hgb, Hct
Decreased: Hgb, Hct, platelets, magnesium, phosphate

NURSING CONSIDERATIONS
Assessment

> **BLACK BOX WARNING:** Assess for infection, increased temp, WBC, sputum, urine, may be fatal (bacterial, protozoal, fungal)

• Monitor blood studies: Hgb, WBC, platelets during treatment qmo; if leukocytes are <3000/ mm³, product should be discontinued
• Monitor liver function studies: alkaline phosphatase, AST, ALT, bilirubin
• **Assess hepatotoxicity: dark urine, jaundice, itching, light-colored stools; product should be discontinued**

⚠ Assess for anaphylaxis, hypersensitivity: dyspnea, wheezing, rash, pruritus, hypotension, tachycardia; if severe hypersensitivity reactions occur, product should not be used again

Patient/family education

> **BLACK BOX WARNING:** Instruct patient to report fever, chills, sore throat, fatigue, since serious infection may occur; avoid crowds, persons with known upper respiratory infections; use contraception during treatment

Evaluation
Positive therapeutic outcome
• Absence of graft rejection

beclomethasone (Rx)
(be-kloe-meth'a-sone)
QVAR
Func. class.: Synthetic glucocorticoid (long acting)
Chem. class.: Beclomethasone diester
Pregnancy category C

Do not confuse: beclomethasone/ betamethasone

ACTION: Prevents inflammation by suppression of migration of polymorphonuclear leukocytes, fibroblasts, reversal of increased capillary permeability and lysosomal stabilization; does not suppress hypothalamus and pituitary function

Therapeutic outcome: Decreased inflammation and normal immunity

USES: Seasonal, perennial allergic/vasomotor rhinitis, nasal polyps, chronic steroid-dependent asthma

CONTRAINDICATIONS
Hypersensitivity, status asthmaticus (primary treatment)

Precautions: Pregnancy **C,** breastfeeding, child <12, nasal disease/surgery, nonasthmatic bronchial disease, bacterial, fungal, viral infections of mouth, throat, lungs, HPA suppression, osteoporosis, Cushing's syndrome, diabetes mellitus, measles, cataracts, corticosteroid hypersensitivity, glaucoma, herpes infection

DOSAGE AND ROUTES
Adult and child >12 yr: inh 48-80 mcg bid (alone) or 40-160 mcg bid (with inhaled corticosteroids), max 320 bid

Child 5-12 yr: inh 40 mcg bid, max 80 mcg bid

Available forms: Oral inh 40, 80, 250 ♣ mcg /metered spray

Implementation
Oral route
• Give PO, using a spacer device for proper dose
• Shake oral inhaler well, use spacer
• Use after cleaning aerosol top daily with warm water; dry thoroughly
• Store in cool environment; do not puncture or incinerate container

Nasal route
• Shake inhaler, invert, tilt head backward, insert nozzle into nostril, away from septum; hold other nostril closed and depress activator, inhale through nose, exhale through mouth

ADVERSE EFFECTS
CNS: *Headache;* psychiatric/behavioral changes (child)
EENT: *Candidal infection of oral cavity, hoarseness,* sore throat, dysgeusia, loss of taste/smell, pharyngitis, rhinitis, sinusitis, cataracts, fungal infections, epistaxis
ENDO: Hypothalamic-pituitary (HPA) suppression
GI: Dry mouth, dyspepsia
MISC: Angioedema, adrenal insufficiency, facial edema, Churg-Strauss syndrome (rare)
RESP: Bronchospasm, wheezing, cough

Pharmacokinetics

Absorption	Locally only
Distribution	Not distributed
Metabolism	Lungs, liver (by CYP3A)
Excretion	Feces, urine
Half-life	2.8 hr

Pharmacodynamics

	Inh	Nasal
Onset	1-4 wk	10 min
Peak	Unknown	Unknown
Duration	Unknown	Unknown

NURSING CONSIDERATIONS
Assessment
• Assess adrenal suppression: 17-KS, plasma cortisol for decreased levels, adrenal function periodically for HPA axis suppression during prolonged therapy; monitor growth and development
• Assess blood studies, neutrophils, decreased platelets; WBC with diff at baseline and q3mo; if neutrophils are <1000/mm³, discontinue treatment

• Check nasal passages during long-term treatment for changes in mucus; check for burning, stinging; assess for glucocorticoid withdrawal: dizziness, hypotension, fatigue, muscle/joint pain; notify prescriber immediately
• Assess respiratory status: rest, rhythm, characteristics; auscultate lung bilaterally before and throughout treatment
• Assess for fungal infections in mucous membranes

Patient/family education
• Teach patient to gargle/rinse mouth after each use to prevent oral fungal infections
• Teach patient that in times of stress, systemic corticosteroids may be needed to prevent adrenal insufficiency; do not discontinue oral product abruptly, taper slowly
• Teach patient to continue using product even if mild nasal bleeding occurs; is usually transient
• Teach patient method of administration after providing written instructions from manufacturer
• Clean inhaler by wiping with dry cloth, need for spacer or face mask
• Teach patient the symptoms of **adrenal insufficiency:** nausea, anorexia, fatigue, dizziness, dyspnea, weakness, joint pain, depression

Evaluate
Positive therapeutic outcome
• Decrease in runny nose, improved symptoms of bronchial asthma

beclomethasone nasal agent
See Appendix B

belatacept (Rx)
(bel-a-ta′sept)
Nulojix
Func. class.: Biologic response modifier
Chem. class.: Fusion protein
Pregnancy category C

ACTION: Activated T lymphocytes are the mediators of immunologic rejection, and this product is a selective T-cell costimulation blocker; blocks the CD28 mediated costimulation of T lymphocytes by binding to CD80 and CD86 on antigen-presenting cells; inhibits T-lymphocyte proliferation and the production of the cytokines interleukin-2, interferon-gamma, interleukin-4, and TNF-alpha.

Therapeutic outcome: Absence of kidney transplant rejection

B

USES: Kidney transplant rejection prophylaxis given with basiliximab induction, mycophenolate mofetil, corticosteroids

CONTRAINDICATIONS
Hypersensitivity, EBV seronegative, EBV status unknown

> **BLACK BOX WARNING:** Infection, organ transplant, requires an experienced clinician, secondary malignancy, posttransplant lymphoproliferation disorder (PTLD)

Precautions: Breastfeeding, child/infant/neonate, pregnancy C, diabetes mellitus, progressive multifocal leukoencephalopathy, immunosuppression, sunlight exposure, TB

DOSAGE AND ROUTES
Adult: IV 10 mg/kg rounded to nearest 12.5 mg increment give over 30 min the day of transplantation (day 1) but before transplantation, on day 5 approximately 96 hours after the day 1 dose 1, at the end of wk 2, at the end of wk 4, at the end of wk 8, and at the end of wk 12; maintenance dosage is 5 mg/kg rounded to nearest 12.5 mg increment given over 30 min at the end of wk 16 and q4wk ± 3 days thereafter; doses should be calculated on actual body weight on the transplantation day unless the patient's weight varies by >10%

Available forms:
Powder for inj 250 mg

Implementation

> **BLACK BOX WARNING:** Only providers skilled in the use of immunosuppressant and management of transplant should use these products

IV route
• Visually inspect for particulate matter, discoloration, discard if present
• Calculate the number of drug vials required to provide total infusion dose
• Reconstitute each vial/10.5 ml of sterile water for injection, 0.9% sodium chloride, D₅W using the silicone-free disposable syringe provided with each vial and an 18G to 21G needle. If silicone-free disposable syringe is dropped or becomes contaminated, use a new silicone-free disposable syringe. If you need additional silicone-free disposable syringes, call 888-685-6549. If the powder is accidentally reconstituted using a different syringe than the one provided, the solution may develop a few translucent particles. Discard any solutions prepared using siliconized syringes.

• Using aseptic technique, inject the diluent into the vial and direct the stream of diluent to the glass wall of the vial. To minimize foaming, rotate the vial and invert with gentle swirling until the contents are dissolved. Do not shake when reconstituted (25 mg/ml), should be clear to slightly opalescent and colorless to pale yellow. Do not use if opaque particles, discoloration, or other foreign particles are present.
• Calculate the total volume of the reconstituted 25 mg/ml sol required to provide the prescribed dose. Further dilute this volume with a volume of inf fluid equal to the volume of the reconstituted drug sol required. Use either NS or D₅W if drug was reconstituted with SWFI; use NS if drug was reconstituted with NS; use D₅W if drug was reconstituted with D₅W. With the same silicone-free disposable syringe used for reconstitution, withdraw the required amount of belatacept sol from the vial, inject it into the inf container, gently rotate; final concentration in inf container should range (2-10 mg/ml). Volume of 100 ml will be appropriate for most doses, but total inf volumes ranging from 50-250 ml may be used. Discard any unused drug solution; after reconstitution, immediately transfer the reconstituted sol from the vial to the inf bag or bottle; complete within 24 hr.

IV INF route
• Give over 30 min, use an infusion set and a sterile, nonpyrogenic low-protein-binding filter (0.2-1.2 mm), use a separate line
• Storage: refrigerate, protect from light ≤24 hr; max 4 hr of the total 24 hr can be at room temp and room light

ADVERSE EFFECTS
CV: Hypo/hypertension
CNS: Guillain-Barré syndrome, anxiety, dizziness, fever, insomnia, tremor
EENT: Pharyngitis, stomatitis
GI: Abdominal pain, constipation, diarrhea, nausea, vomiting
GU: Renal tubular necrosis, renal failure, proteinuria, urinary incontinence, dysuria, UTI
HEMA: Anemia, neutropenia, leukopenia, leukoencephalopathy
INTEG: Acne, alopecia, infusion reaction
META: Hypercholesterolemia, hyperglycemia, hyper/hypokalemia, hypocalcemia, hypophosphatemia, hypomagnesemia
MS: Arthralgia
SYST: Secondary malignancy, posttransplant lymphoproliferative disorder (PTLD), wound dehiscence, BK-virus associated neuropathy

Absorption	Unknown
Distribution	Steady state by week 8 after transplantation and by month 6 during the maintenance phase
Metabolism	Unknown
Excretion	Unknown
Half-life	Half-life range 6.1-15.1 days during receipt of 10 mg/kg IV doses; 3.1-11.9 days during receipt of 5 mg/kg IV doses

Pharmacodynamics

Onset	Unknown
Peak	Unknown
Duration	Unknown

INTERACTIONS
Individual drugs
• Do not use 30 days before or with this product: Live virus vaccines
• Do not use with cyclophosphamide IV

Drug classifications
Corticosteroids: increased belatacept effect
Vaccines: avoid concurrent use
Immunosuppressives: avoid increased dose

NURSING CONSIDERATIONS
Assessment

> **BLACK BOX WARNING:** Transplant rejection: flulike symptoms, decreasing urinary output, malaise; some may experience pain in area (rare; monitor BUN/Creatinine)

> **BLACK BOX WARNING:** Infection: Monitor for fever, chills, increased WBC, wound dehiscences

> **BLACK BOX WARNING:** Posttransplant lymphoproliferative disorder (PTLD): May lead to secondary malignancy (lymphoma) or infectious mononucleosislike lesions; may be treated with antivirals or immunosuppressant may need to be discontinued

• Hyperlipidemia: Monitor cholesterol, triglycerides; an antilipidemic may be needed
• Store refrigerated, protected from light ≤24 hr; max 4 hr of the total 24 hr can be at room temperature and room light

Evaluation
Positive therapeutic outcome
• Absence of renal transplant rejection

Patient/family education
• Teach reason for product and expected result, use REMS guidelines
• Teach to avoid exposure to sunlight, tanning beds, risk of secondary malignancy
• Teach to avoid crowds, persons with known infections
• Advise that repeated lab test will be needed
• Advise to avoid with vaccines
• Advise that immunosuppressants will be needed for life to prevent rejection/infection; teach symptoms of rejection and to call provider immediately

belimumab (Rx)
(be-lim'ue-mab)
Benlysta
Func. class.: Monoclonal antibody
Chem. class.: Disease-modifying antirheumatic drugs (DMARDs)
Pregnancy category C

ACTION: Inhibits B-lymphocyte stimulator (BLyS), which is needed for B-cell survival; normally, soluble BLyS binds to its receptors on B cells and allows B-cell survival; binds BLyS and prevents binding to its receptors on B cells

Therapeutic outcome: Decreasing symptoms of SLE: decreased fever, malaise, joint pains, myalgias, fatigue

USES: Active, autoantibody-positive, systemic lupus erythematosus (SLE) in combination with standard therapy

CONTRAINDICATIONS
Hypersensitivity

Precautions: African descent patients, depression, children/infants, immunosuppression, infection, pregnancy C, breastfeeding, suicidal ideation, vaccination, geriatrics, secondary malignancy, cardiac disease, requires experienced clinician

DOSAGE AND ROUTES
Adult: 10 mg/kg IV over 1 hr q2wk for the first 3 doses, then q4wk

Available forms: Powder for injection 120, 400 mg

Implementation
• Only health care providers prepared to manage anaphylaxis should administer this product, may give premedication for prophylaxis against infusion and hypersensitivity reactions

Intermittent IV infusion route
• Visually inspect particulate matter and discoloration whenever solution and container permit

• Give as IV infusion only, do not give IV bolus or push, give over 1 hr and slow or stop if infusion reactions occur
• Do not give with any other agents in the same IV line
• Allow to stand at room temperature for 10-15 min before using
• Reconstitute with the appropriate amount of sterile water for injection (80 mg/ml); add 1.5 ml of sterile water (120 mg/vial) or 4.8 ml of sterile water (400 mg/vial)
• Direct the stream of sterile water toward the side of the vial to minimize foaming; gently swirl for 60 sec and allow to sit during reconstitution, gently swirling for 60 secs q5min until the powder is dissolved; do not shake; reconstitution is complete in 10 to 30 min
• If a mechanical reconstitution device (swirler) is used, max 500 rpm swirled for ≤30 min
• The solution should be opalescent, and colorless to pale yellow, and without particles; small air bubbles are expected; protect from sunlight
• Dilution: Only dilute in NS for injection; dilute reconstituted solution with enough normal saline to 250 ml. From a 250-ml infusion bag or bottle of normal saline, withdraw and discard a volume equal to the volume of the reconstituted solution required for dose; add the required volume of the reconstituted solution the infusion bag/bottle; gently invert to mix
• Discard any unused solution
• Storage in refrigerator or at room temp; total time from reconstitution to completion of inf max 8 hr

ADVERSE EFFECTS
CNS: Anxiety, depression, dizziness, fever, headache, insomnia, migraine, suicidal ideation
CV: Bradycardia, hypotension
GU: UTI
GI: Diarrhea, nausea
MISC: Bronchitis, cystitis, dyspnea, leukopenia, myalgia, nasopharyngitis, pharyngitis, rash
SYST: Anaphylaxis, angioedema, antibody formation, infection, influenza, infusion reactions, secondary malignancy

Pharmacokinetics
Absorption	Unknown
Distribution	Unknown
Metabolism	Unknown
Excretion	Unknown
Half-life	Terminal half-life 19.4 days; distribution half-life 1.75 days

Pharmacodynamics
Onset	Unknown
Peak	Unknown
Duration	Unknown

INTERACTIONS
Individual drugs
IV cyclophosphamide, biologic therapies (riTUXimab, ofatumumab): avoid concurrent use

Drug classifications
Vaccines: avoid concurrent use

NURSING CONSIDERATIONS
Assessment
• **SLE:** Monitor for decreasing fever, malaise, fatigue, joint pain, myalgias
• **Suicidal ideation:** More common in those with preexisting depression
• **Infection:** Determine if a chronic or acute infection is present, may be fatal when used with this product; do not begin therapy if any products are being used for a chronic infection; leukopenia may occur with this product and susceptibility to infections increased
• **Anaphylaxis, infusion site reactions:** If these occur, stop infusion
• **African descent patients:** Use cautiously in these patients, may not respond to this product
• Cardiac disease: Monitor closely for cardiovascular side effects, bradycardia, hypotension
⚠ **Pregnancy:** Determine if pregnant or if pregnancy is planned or suspected, if pregnant call 877-681-6269 to enroll in registry

Patient/family education
⚠ Teach patient to notify prescriber if pregnancy is planned or suspected, use reliable contraception during and for 4 mo after final treatment, to avoid breastfeeding
⚠ Advise patient to seek treatment immediately for serious hypersensitive reactions
• Advise patient not to receive live vaccinations during treatment

Evaluation
• Decreasing symptoms of SLE: decreasing fatigue, fever, malaise

> **⚠ HIGH ALERT**

belinostat

(beh-lih′noh-stat′)

Beleodaq

Func. class.: Antineoplastic-biologic response modifier

Chem. class.: Histone deacetylase inhibitors

Pregnancy category D

ACTION: A class I and II inhibitor of the histone deacetylase (HDAC) enzymes. Overexpression of HDACs is present in some cancer cells. HDAC inhibitors have been shown to activate differentiation, inhibit the cell cycle, and induce apoptosis

Therapeutic outcome: Prevention of spread of disease

USES: For the treatment of relapsed or refractory peripheral T-cell lymphoma (PTCL)

CONTRAINDICATIONS: Hypersensitivity, pregnancy **D**

Precautions: Hematologic toxicity (thrombocytopenia, leukopenia, neutropenia, lymphopenia, anemia), serious infections (pneumonia, sepsis), fatal hepatic toxicity, tumor lysis syndrome (TLS), breastfeeding

DOSAGE AND ROUTES

Adult: IV 1000 mg/m² over 30 min on days 1-5 q21d. Reduce the dose to 750 mg/m² in those who are homozygous for the UGT1A1*28 allele. Cycles should be repeated until disease progression or unacceptable toxicity.

Available forms: Powder for injection 500 mg

Implementation

Intermittent IV route

• Reconstitution: Add 9 ml of sterile water for injection/500 mg, swirl until there are no visible particles in the solution (50 mg/ml); stable at room temperature for up to 12 hr

• Withdraw the appropriate amount from the reconstituted vial and further dilute in 250 ml 0.9% sodium chloride for injection; the final solution is stable at room temperature for up to 36 hr, including infusion time; use a 0.22-micron in-line filter; give over 30 min; if pain occurs at infusion site, run over 45 min

Dose adjustments due to treatment-related toxicity

Hematologic toxicities:

• Do not begin the next cycle of treatment until the absolute neutrophil count (ANC) is ≥1000/mm³ and platelet count ≥50,000/mm³

• ANC nadir ≥500/mm³ and platelet count nadir ≥25,000/mm³: no dose adjustment

• ANC nadir <500/mm³ (any platelet count): begin next cycle of treatment at a reduced dose of 750 mg/m². For the second occurrence of an ANC nadir <500/mm³, reduce the dose of the next cycle to 500 mg/m², if the ANC nadir is <500/mm³ after 2 dose reductions, discontinue therapy

• Platelet nadir <25,000/mm³ (any ANC): begin next cycle of treatment at a reduced dose of 750 mg/m². For the second occurrence of a platelet nadir <25,000/mm³, reduce the dose of the next cycle to 500 mg/m². If the platelet nadir is <25,000/mm³ after 2 dose reductions, discontinue therapy.

Nonhematologic toxicities:

• Grade 3 or 4 nausea, vomiting, or diarrhea for >7 days with supportive management; or other grade 3 or 4 toxicity of any duration: hold treatment. When toxicity resolves to grade ≤2, restart the next cycle at a reduced dose of 750 mg/m². For the second occurrence of grade 3 or 4 toxicity (for a duration >7 days with supportive management for GI toxicities), resume therapy at 500 mg/m² upon resolution to grade ≤2. If the grade 3 or 4 toxicity recurs after 2 dose reductions, discontinue therapy.

ADVERSE EFFECTS

CNS: Fatigue headache dizziness, fever, chills

CV: Hypotension, QT prolongation

GI: *Constipation, anorexia, abdominal pain, nausea, vomiting, diarrhea,* hepatotoxicity

HEMA: Anemia, thrombocytopenia, neutropenia

INTEG: Injection-site reactions, rash, phlebitis

MISC: Hypokalemia

RESP: Dyspnea, cough

SYST: Multiorgan failure, TLS, serious infections

Pharmacokinetics

Absorption	Unknown
Distribution	92.9%-95.8% protein bound
Metabolism	80%-90% metabolized by hepatic UGT1A1; liver
Excretion	40% excreted renally, primarily as metabolites
Half-life	1.1 hr

Pharmacodynamics

Onset	Unknown
Peak	Unknown
Duration	Unknown

INTERACTIONS
Drug classifications
Strong UGT1A1 inhibitors: increased belinostat

NURSING CONSIDERATIONS
Assessment
• **Hematologic toxicity (thrombocytopenia, leukopenia, neutropenia, lymphopenia, anemia): Monitor CBC before starting therapy and then every week. Dose modifications may be necessary in patients with bone marrow suppression and should be determined by the ANC and platelet count nadirs of the previous cycle of therapy. Platelet counts should be ≥50,000/mm³ and ANC >1000/mm³ before starting each cycle.**
• **Serious infections (pneumonia, sepsis): May be fatal. Do not use in those with an active infection. Use caution in patients with a history of extensive or intensive chemotherapy, as they may be at higher risk for life-threatening infections.**
• **Fatal hepatic toxicity: Monitor LFTs before the start of each cycle. Those with signs of hepatic disease may require dose modification or discontinuation.**
• **TLS: Those with high tumor burden or advanced-stage disease are at greater risk for development of TLS; consider tumor lysis prophylaxis with antihyperuricemic agents and hydration beginning 12-24 hr before treatment; for TLS treatment, administer aggressive IV hydration, antihyperuricemic agents, correct electrolyte abnormalities, and monitor renal function**
• **Pregnancy (D) and breastfeeding: Consider discontinuing breastfeeding, identify whether the patient is pregnant before using**
• **Renal studies:** Monitor BUN/creatinine periodically

Patient/family education
• **Teach patient to avoid use in breastfeeding, and not to use in pregnancy (D)**
• Advise patient to report infusion-site reactions, rash, severe constipation or diarrhea, abdominal pain

Evaluation
Positive therapeutic outcome
• Prevention of spread of disease

benazepril (Rx)
(ben-a′za-pril)
Lotensin
Func. class.: Antihypertensive
Chem. class.: ACE inhibitor
Pregnancy category D

Do not confuse: benazepril/Benadryl

ACTION: Selectively suppresses renin-angiotensin-aldosterone system; inhibits ACE, preventing conversion of angiotensin I to angiotensin II

Therapeutic outcome: Decreased B/P in hypertension

USES: Hypertension, alone or in combination with thiazide diuretics

Unlabeled uses: CHF

CONTRAINDICATIONS
Breastfeeding, children, hypersensitivity to ACE inhibitors, angioedema

> BLACK BOX WARNING: Pregnancy **D**

Precautions: Impaired renal/liver function, dialysis patients, hypovolemia, blood dyscrasias, CHF, COPD, asthma, geriatric, bilateral renal artery stenosis

DOSAGE AND ROUTES
Adult: PO 10 mg daily initially, then 20-40 mg/day divided bid or daily (without a diuretic); 5 mg PO daily (with a diuretic); max 80 mg daily
Geriatric: PO based on clinical response

Renal dose
Adult: PO 5 mg daily with CCr <30 ml/min; increase as needed to max of 40 mg/day

Available forms: Tabs 5, 10, 20, 40 mg

Implementation
• Store in airtight container at 86° F (30° C) or less
• Severe hypotension may occur after 1st dose of this medication; decreased hypotension may be prevented by reducing or discontinuing diuretic therapy 3 days before beginning benazepril therapy
• Storage in tight container at 86° F (30° C) or less

ADVERSE EFFECTS
CNS: Anxiety, hypertonia, insomnia, paresthesia, headache, dizziness, fatigue
CV: Hypotension, postural hypotension, syncope, palpitations, angina
GI: Nausea, constipation, vomiting, gastritis, diarrhea, melena, *hepatotoxicity, pancreatitis*
GU: Increased BUN, creatinine, decreased libido, impotence, urinary tract infection, renal insufficiency
HEMA: *Agranulocytosis, neutropenia*
INTEG: Rash, flushing, sweating, alopecia
META: Hyperkalemia, hyponatremia
MISC: *Angioedema, Stevens-Johnson syndrome,* hypersensitivity
MS: Arthralgia, arthritis, myalgia

Adverse effects: *italics* = common; **bold** = life-threatening

RESP: Cough, asthma, bronchitis, dyspnea, sinusitis

Pharmacokinetics

Absorption	<40%
Distribution	Unknown; crosses placenta
Metabolism	Liver metabolites; protein binding 97%
Excretion	Kidney, breast milk (minimal)
Half-life	10-11 hr (metabolite); increased in renal disease

Pharmacodynamics

Onset	Unknown
Peak	½-1 hr
Duration	Unknown

INTERACTIONS

Individual drugs

Alcohol: increased hypotension (large amounts)
Azathioprine: increased myelosuppression
Digoxin, lithium: increased serum levels

Drug classifications

Antihypertensives, diuretics, nitrates, phenothiazines: increased hypotension
Diuretics (potassium-sparing), potassium supplements: increased hyperkalemia
NSAIDs: decreased hypotensive effects

Drug/herb

Ephedra (Ma huang): decreased antihypertensive effect
Hawthorn: increased antihypertensive effect

Drug/lab test

Increased: AST, ALT, alkaline phosphatase, bilirubin, uric acid, blood glucose, potassium
False positive: ANA titer
Positive: ANA titer

NURSING CONSIDERATIONS

Assessment

• **Hypertension:** B/P, pulse baseline and periodically; monitor, check for orthostatic hypotension, syncope; if changes occur, dosage change may be required; notify prescriber of changes; monitor compliance

• **Monitor blood dyscrasias: neutrophils, decreased platelets; WBC with differential at baseline, q3mo; if neutrophils <1000/ mm³, discontinue treatment**

• Monitor renal studies: protein, BUN, creatinine; watch for increased levels that may indicate nephrotic syndrome and renal failure; monitor urine for protein; monitor renal symptoms: polyuria, oliguria, frequency, dysuria

• Establish baselines in renal, liver function tests before therapy begins

• Check potassium levels throughout treatment, although hyperkalemia rarely occurs; diuretic should be discontinued 3 days prior to initiation with benazepril; if hypertension is not controlled, a diuretic can be added; measure B/P at peak 2-4 hr and trough (before next dose); this product is less effective in African-American descendants

• **Assess for allergic reactions: rash, fever, pruritus, urticaria; product should be discontinued if antihistamines fail to help; angioedema is more common in African-American descendants, Stevens-Johnson syndrome**

Patient/family education

• Instruct patient not to discontinue product abruptly; advise patient to tell all persons associated with care

• Teach patient not to use OTC products (cough, cold, allergy) unless directed by prescriber; serious side effects can occur; xanthines such as coffee, tea, chocolate, cola can prevent action of product

• Emphasize the importance of complying with dosage schedule, even if feeling better; to continue with medical regimen to decrease B/P: exercise, cessation of smoking, decreasing stress, diet modifications

• Emphasize the need to rise slowly to sitting or standing position to minimize orthostatic hypotension, not to exercise in hot weather because increased hypotension can occur

⚠ **Teach patient to notify prescriber of mouth sores, sore throat, fever, swelling of hands or feet, irregular heartbeat, chest pain, coughing, shortness of breath, bruising, bleeding, swelling of face, tongue, lips, difficulty breathing**

• Caution patient to report excessive perspiration, dehydration, vomiting, diarrhea; may lead to fall in B/P

• Instruct patient to use caution in hot weather

• Caution patient that product may cause dizziness, fainting, light-headedness; may occur during first few days of therapy; to avoid activities that may be hazardous

• Teach patient how to take B/P; teach normal readings for age group; ensure patient takes own B/P

• Instruct patient to avoid potassium-containing products (salt substitutes)

> **BLACK BOX WARNING:** Advise patient to notify prescriber of pregnancy (**D**), product will need to be discontinued

Evaluation
Positive therapeutic outcome
• Decreased B/P in hypertension

TREATMENT OF OVERDOSE:
0.9% NaCl **IV** inf, hemodialysis

RARELY USED

bendamustine (Rx)
(ben-da-muss'teen)
Treanda
Func. class.: Antineoplastic alkylating agent
Chem. class.: Nitrogen mustard
Pregnancy category D

Therapeutic outcome: Improvement in blood counts and morphology

USES: Chronic lymphocytic leukemia, non-Hodgkin's lymphoma

CONTRAINDICATIONS
Pregnancy **D**, fetal harm may occur; hypersensitivity to this product or mannitol, children, hepatic disease, renal impairment, breastfeeding

DOSAGE AND ROUTES
Chronic lymphocytic leukemia
Adult: **IV** inf 100 mg/m^2 over 30 min on days 1, 2, q28days up to 6 cycles

Non-Hodgkin's lymphoma
Adult: **IV** inf 120 mg/m^2 over 60 min on days 1, 2, q21days up to 8 cycles

Renal/hepatic dose
Adult: **IV** inf CCr <40 ml/min, do not use; AST or ALT 2.5-10 × upper limit normal (ULN) or bilirubin 1.5-3 × ULN, do not use

Available forms: Powder for inj 25, 100 mg; solution for injection 180 mg/2 ml, 45 mg/0.5 ml

Implementation
⚠ Give allopurinol for 1-2 wk to those at high risk for tumor lysis syndrome; usually develops in first treatment cycle
• Give blood transfusions; or RBC colony-stimulating factors to counter anemia unless cure is the intent
• Give antiemetic 30-60 min before giving product to prevent vomiting
• Give all medications PO, if possible avoid IM inj if platelets are <100,000/mm^3

benzocaine topical
See Appendix B

---

benztropine (Rx)
(benz'troe-peen)
Cogentin
Func. class.: Cholinergic blocker, antiparkinson agent
Chem. class.: Tertiary amine
Pregnancy category C

ACTION: Blockade of central acetylcholine receptors in the CNS; neurotransmitters are balanced, balances cholinergic activity

Therapeutic outcome: Decreased involuntary movements

USES: Parkinsonian symptoms, EPS associated with neuroleptic products, acute dystonia

Unlabeled Uses: Hypersalivation

CONTRAINDICATIONS
Hypersensitivity, closed-angle glaucoma, dementia, tardive dyskinesia

Precautions: Pregnancy **C**, breastfeeding, children, geriatric, tachycardia, renal/hepatic disease, product abuse history, dysrhythmias, hypo/hypertension, psychosis; myasthenia gravis, GI/GU obstruction, child ≤3 yr, peptic ulcer, megacolon, prostate hypertrophy

DOSAGE AND ROUTES
Drug-induced extrapyramidal symptoms
Adult: IM/IV 1-4 mg daily/bid; give PO dose as soon as possible; PO 1-2 mg bid/tid; increase by 0.5 mg q5-6days
Child >3 yr: IM/IV 0.02-0.05 mg/kg/dose 1-2 ×/day
Geriatric: PO 0.5 mg daily-bid, increase by 0.5 mg q5-6days; max 4 mg/day

Parkinsonian symptoms
Adult: PO 1-2 mg daily, in 1-2 divided doses; increased 0.5 mg q5-6days titrated to patient response; max 6 mg daily

Acute dystonic reactions
Adult: IM/IV 1-2 mg, may increase to 1-2 mg bid (PO)

Available forms: Tabs 0.5, 1, 2 mg; inj 1 mg/ml

Implementation
PO route
• Give with or after meals to prevent GI upset; may give with fluids other than water; hard candy, frequent drinks, gum to relieve dry mouth

---

Adverse effects: *italics* = common; **bold** = life-threatening

- Give at bedtime to avoid daytime drowsiness in patient with parkinsonism
- May be crushed and mixed with food
- Store at room temperature

IM route
- Inject deeply in muscle; use filtered needle to remove solution from ampule
- Give in large muscle mass for dystonic symptoms

IV direct route
- Use in emergencies

Syringe compatibilities: ChlorproMAZINE, fluphenazine, metoclopramide, perphenazine, thiothixene

Y-site compatibilities: Alfentanil, amikacin, aminophylline, ascorbic acid injection, atracurium, atropine, azaTHIOprine, aztreonam, bumetanide, buprenorphine, butorphanol, calcium chloride, gluconate, ceFAZolin, cefotaxime, cefoTEtan, cefOXitin, cefTAZidime, ceftizoxime, cefTRIAXone, cefuroxime, chlorproMAZINE, cimetidine, clindamycin, cyanocobalamin, cycloSPORINE, dexamethasone, digoxin, diphenhydrAMINE, DOBUTamine, DOPamine, Doxycycline, enalaprilat, ePHEDrine, EPINEPHrine, epoetin alfa, erythromycin lactobionate, esmolol, famotidine, fentaNYL, fluconazole, folic acid (as sodium salt), gentamicin, glycopyrrolate, heparin, hydrocortisone sodium succinate, hydrOXYzine, imipenem-cilastatin, inamrinone, insulin, regular, isoproterenol, ketorolac, labetalol, lactated Ringer's, lidocaine, magnesium sulfate, mannitol, meperidine, metaraminol, methyldopate, methylPREDNISolone, metoclopramide, metoprolol, midazolam, minocycline, morphine, multiple vitamins injection, nafcillin, nalbuphine, naloxone, netilmicin, nitroglycerin, nitroprusside, norepinephrine, ondansetron, oxacillin, oxytocin, papaverine, penicillin G potassium, sodium, pentamidine, pentazocine, phenobarbital, phentolamine, phenylephrine, phytonadione, piperacillin, polymyxin B, potassium chloride, procainamide, prochlorperazine, promethazine, propranolol, protamine, pyridoxine, quiNIDine, ranitidine, Ringer's injection, sodium bicarbonate, succinylcholine, SUFentanil, tacrolimus

ADVERSE EFFECTS
CNS: Confusion; anxiety, restlessness, irritability, delusions, hallucinations, headache, sedation, depression, incoherence, dizziness, memory loss; delirium (geriatric)
CV: Palpitations, tachycardia, hypotension, bradycardia
EENT: Blurred vision, photophobia, dilated pupils, difficulty swallowing

GI: *Dryness of mouth, constipation,* nausea, vomiting, abdominal distress, **paralytic ileus**
GU: Hesitancy, retention, dysuria
INTEG: Rash, urticaria, dermatoses
MISC: Increased temperature, flushing, decreased sweating, **hyperthermia, heat stroke,** numbness of fingers

Pharmacokinetics

Absorption	Good (PO, IM), complete (IV)
Distribution	Unknown
Metabolism	Unknown
Excretion	Unknown
Half-life	Unknown

Pharmacodynamics

	IM/IV	PO
Onset	15 min	1 hr
Peak	Unknown	Unknown
Duration	6-10 hr	6-10 hr

INTERACTIONS
Individual drugs
Bethanechol: decreased cholinergic effects
Disopyramide, quiNIDine: increased anticholinergic 5 effects, reduce dose

Drug classifications
Antidepressants (tricyclic), antihistamines, phenothiazines: increased anticholinergic amantadine effects
Antidiarrheals, antacids: decreased absorption

NURSING CONSIDERATIONS
Assessment
- Assess for **parkinsonism**, EPS: shuffling gait, muscle rigidity, involuntary movements, loss of balance, pill rolling, muscle spasms, drooling before and during treatment
- **Paralytic ileus:** assess for abdominal pain, intermittent constipation/diarrhea
- Monitor I&O ratio; retention commonly causes decreased urinary output, distention, frequency, incontinence
- Monitor for urinary hesitancy, retention; palpate bladder if retention occurs
- Monitor for constipation, cramping, pain in abdomen, abdominal distention; increase fluids, bulk, exercise if this occurs
- Assess for tolerance over long-term therapy; dosage may have to be increased or changed
- Assess for mental status: affect, mood, CNS depression, worsening of mental symptoms during early therapy
- Assess for benztropine "buzz" or "high," patients may imitate EPS

Patient/family education

• Teach patient to report urinary hesitancy/retention, dysuria
• Teach patient to use caution in hot weather; product may increase susceptibility to stroke since perspiration is decreased; patient should remain indoors
• Advise patient not to discontinue this product abruptly; to taper off over 1 wk to prevent withdrawal symptoms (insomnia, involuntary movements, anxiety, tachycardias), to take as directed, not to double doses
• Advise patient that tabs may be crushed, mixed with food; may take whole dose at bedtime if approved by prescriber
• Caution patient to avoid driving or other hazardous activities; drowsiness, dizziness may occur
• Teach patient to avoid OTC medication: cough, cold preparations with alcohol, antihistamines, antacids, or antidiarrheals within 2 hr unless directed by prescriber; increased CNS depression may occur
• Advise patient to rise from sitting or recumbent position slowly to minimize orthostatic hypotension
• Teach patient to use good oral hygiene; to use sugarless gum, hard candy, frequent sips of water to decrease dry mouth; if dry mouth continues, saliva substitutes may be prescribed
• Instruct patient that doses should not be doubled, but missed dose may be taken up to 2 hr before next dose

Evaluation
Positive therapeutic outcome
• Absence of involuntary movements (pill rolling, tremors, muscle spasms) after 2 days of treatment

betamethasone topical
See Appendix B

betamethasone (augmented) topical
See Appendix B

betaxolol ophthalmic
See Appendix B

⚠ HIGH ALERT

bevacizumab (Rx)
(beh-va-kiz′you-mab)
Avastin
Func. class.: Antineoplastic—miscellaneous
Chem. class.: Monoclonal antibody
Pregnancy category C

Do not confuse: Avastin/Astelin

ACTION: Monoclonal antibody selectively binds to and inhibits activity of human vascular endothelial growth factor to reduce microvascular growth and inhibition of metastatic disease progression

Therapeutic outcome: Decreased tumor size

USES: Metastatic carcinoma of the colon or rectum in combination, renal cell carcinoma, glioblastoma, non–small cell lung cancer

Unlabeled uses: Adjunctive in breast, renal/ovarian cancer, (wet) macular degeneration

CONTRAINDICATIONS
Hypersensitivity, serious bleeding, hypertensive crisis, recent surgery

Precautions: Pregnancy **C**, breastfeeding, children, geriatric, CHF, blood dyscrasias, CV disease, hypertension, surgery, thromboembolic disease, hamster protein/murine hypersensitivity

> **BLACK BOX WARNING:** GI perforation, wound dehiscence, bleeding

DOSAGE AND ROUTES
Metastatic colorectal cancer
Adult: IV INF in combination with 5-fluorouracil 5 mg/kg q14 days given over 90 min; if well tolerated, the next infusion may be given over 60 min; if 60 min infusions are well tolerated, subsequent infusions may be given over 30 min; (second-line) 5 mg/kg q2wk or 7.5 mg/kg q3wk with fluoropyrimidine and irinotecan or fluoropyramide and oxaliplatin-based agent

Non–small cell lung cancer
Adult: IV 15 mg/kg over 60-90 min with CARBOplatin and paclitaxel

Metastatic cervical cancer
Adult: IV 15 mg/kg q3wk with paclitaxel and cisplatin or paclitaxel and topotecan

---

Metastatic renal cell carcinoma
Adult: IV 15 mg/kg q2wk with interferon alfa 9 million units SUBCUT 3 × per wk, up to 52 wk

Available forms: Inj 25 mg/ml

Implementation

IV intermittent infusion route
- Do not give by **IV** bolus or **IV** push
- Give as **IV** inf over 90 min for first dose and 60 min thereafter, if well tolerated

> **BLACK BOX WARNING: Wound dehiscence:** do not give for ≥28 days after surgery, make sure wounds are healed prior to use

ADVERSE EFFECTS

CNS: *Asthenia, dizziness,* **intracranial hemorrhage (malignant glioma)**, headache, fatigue, confusion, weakness
CV: **Deep vein thrombosis**, arterial thrombosis, hypo/hypertension, **hypertensive crisis, heart failure**
GI: Nausea, vomiting, anorexia, diarrhea, constipation, abdominal pain, colitis, taste change, dyspepsia, stomatitis, **GI hemorrhage/perforation**
GU: Proteinuria, urinary frequency/urgency, **nephrotic syndrome**, ovarian failure
HEMA: **Leukopenia, neutropenia, thrombocytopenia, microangiopathic hemolytic anemia, thromboembolism, bleeding**
META: Bilirubinemia, hypokalemia, hyponatremia
MISC: **Exfoliative dermatitis, hemorrhage,** non-GI fistula formation, *alopecia, impaired wound healing*, **osteonecrosis of the jaw,** antibody formation, back pain myalgia
RESP: Dyspnea, upper respiratory infection
INTEG: Skin discoloration, infusion reactions

Pharmacokinetics

Absorption	Unknown
Distribution	Steady state 100 days
Metabolism	Unknown
Excretion	Unknown
Half-life	20 days

Pharmacodynamics

Onset	Unknown
Peak	Unknown
Duration	Steady state 100 days

INTERACTIONS
Individual drugs
SUNItinib: avoid concurrent use; microangiopathic hemolytic anemia may occur

NURSING CONSIDERATIONS
Assessment
- Monitor B/P q3-4wk
- Assess for symptoms of infection; may be masked by product
- Monitor **CNS reaction:** dizziness, confusion
- Assess for **CHF:** crackles, jugular vein distention, dyspnea during treatment
- Assess **GU status** (proteinuria); nephrotic syndrome may occur; monitor urinalysis for increasing protein level; products should be held if protein ≥2 g/24 hr

> **BLACK BOX WARNING: Wound dehiscence:** hold for ≥28 days until incision is healed

> **BLACK BOX WARNING: Bleeding:** if severe discontinue product, occurs primarily in small cell lung cancer

⚠ Assess for GI perforation, serious bleeding, nephrotic syndrome, hypertensive crisis; product should be discontinued permanently; for surgery, product should be discontinued temporarily
⚠ Reversible posterior leukoencephalopathy syndrome (RPLS): discontinue if this disorder develops
Pregnancy/Breastfeeding: Drug may lead to fetal harm, avoid pregnancy, do not breastfeed

Patient/family education
- Instruct patient to avoid hazardous tasks, since confusion, dizziness may occur
- Instruct patient to report signs of infection: sore throat, fever, diarrhea, vomiting
- Advise patient not to become pregnant while taking this product, or for several months after discontinuing treatment
- Advise patient to notify prescriber if pregnant or planning a pregnancy
- Need to discontinue a month before surgery and not restart until wound is healed

Evaluation
Positive therapeutic outcome
- Decrease in size of tumors

bimatoprost ophthalmic
See Appendix B

bisacodyl (Rx, OTC)
(bis-a-koe′dill)
**Carter's Little Pills ♣, Codulax ♣,
Dacodyl, Doxiden, Dulcolax,
Ex-Lax Ultra Tab, Femilax,
Soflax-Ex ♣**
Func. class.: Laxative, stimulant
Chem. class.: Diphenylmethane
Pregnancy category C

ACTION: Acts directly on intestine by increasing motor activity; thought to irritate colonic intramural plexus; increases water in the colon

Therapeutic outcome: Decreased constipation

USES: Short-term treatment of constipation, bowel or rectal preparation for surgery, examination

CONTRAINDICATIONS
Hypersensitivity, abdominal pain, nausea, vomiting, appendicitis, acute surgical abdomen, ulcerated hemorrhoids, acute hepatitis, fecal impaction, intestinal/biliary tract obstruction

Precautions: Pregnancy **C**, breastfeeding, rectal fissures, severe CV disease

DOSAGE AND ROUTES
Adult ≥12 yr: PO 5-15 mg in PM or AM; may use up to 30 mg for bowel or rectal preparation; RECT 10 mg (single dose), 30 ml enema
Child 6-11 yr: PO 5 mg as a single dose; RECT 5 mg as a single dose

Available forms: Tabs del rel 5, 10 mg; enteric-coated tabs 5 mg; supp 5, 10 mg; enema 10 mg/30 ml

Implementation
Oral route
• Swallow tabs whole; do not break, crush, or chew
• Give alone with water only for better absorption; do not take within 1 hr of antacids, milk
• Administer in AM or PM (oral dose)
Rectal route
• Lubricate before insertion, patient should retain for ½ hr
• Insert high in rectum

ADVERSE EFFECTS
CNS: Muscle weakness
GI: *Nausea, vomiting, anorexia, cramps,* diarrhea, rectal burning (supp)

META: Protein-losing enteropathy, alkalosis, hypokalemia, **tetany,** electrolyte and fluid imbalances

Pharmacokinetics

Absorption	Poor
Distribution	Unknown
Metabolism	Liver, minimally
Excretion	Kidneys
Half-life	Unknown

Pharmacodynamics

	PO	Rect
Onset	6-10 hr	15-60 min
Peak	Unknown	Unknown
Duration	Unknown	Unknown

INTERACTIONS
Drug classifications
Antacids, gastric acid pump inhibitors, H$_2$-blockers: increased gastric irritation

Drug/food
Increased irritation—dairy products: separate by 2 hr

Drug/lab test
Increased: sodium phosphate
Decreased: calcium, magnesium

Drug/herb
Flax, lily of the valley, pheasant's eye, senna, squill: increased laxative action

NURSING CONSIDERATIONS
Assessment
• Monitor blood, urine electrolytes if used often by patient; check I&O ratio to identify fluid loss
• Assess **GI symptoms:** cramping, rectal bleeding, nausea, vomiting; if these symptoms occur, product should be discontinued; identify cause of constipation; identify whether fluids, bulk, or exercise are missing from lifestyle
• Multiple products/routes may be used for bowel prep

Patient/family education
• Discuss with the patient that adequate fluid and bulk consumption is necessary
• Advise patient that normal bowel movements do not always occur daily
• Teach patient not to use in presence of abdominal pain, nausea, vomiting; tell patient to notify prescriber if constipation is unrelieved or if symptoms of electrolyte imbalance occur: muscle cramps, pain, weakness, dizziness, excessive thirst
• Teach patient to take with a full glass of water; do not take with dairy products, separate by 1 hr

• Teach patient to identify bulk, water, constipating products, exercise in patient's life
• Instruct patient not to use laxatives for long-term therapy because bowel tone will be lost; 1 wk use is usually sufficient

Evaluation
Positive therapeutic outcome
• Decreased constipation within 3 days

bismuth subsalicylate (OTC)

(bis'meth sub-sa-li'si-late)

Bismatrol, Bismed ✦, Bismylate ✦, Kaopectate, Kao-Tin, Maalox Total Stomach Relief, Peptic Relief, Pepto-Bismol, Pink Bismuth, StomaK-care ✦

Func. class.: Antidiarrheal/weak antacid
Chem. class.: Salicylate
Pregnancy category C

ACTION: Inhibits prostaglandin synthesis responsible for GI hypermotility, intestinal inflammation; stimulates absorption of fluid and electrolytes; binds toxins produced by *Escherichia coli*

Therapeutic outcome: Absence of loose, watery stools

USES: Diarrhea (cause undetermined); prevention of diarrhea when traveling; may be included to treat *Helicobacter pylori,* heartburn, indigestion, nausea

Unlabeled uses: Chronic infantile diarrhea, traveler's diarrhea, gastric/duodenal ulcer, *H. pylori* eradication

CONTRAINDICATIONS
Child <3 yr; flulike symptoms; history of GI bleeding; varicella, hypersensitivity to this product or salicylates, PUD

Precautions: Pregnancy **C**, breastfeeding, geriatric, gout, diabetes mellitus, bleeding disorders, previous hypersensitivity to NSAIDs, *Clostridium difficile*–associated diarrhea when used with antiinfectives for *H. pylori*

DOSAGE AND ROUTES
Antidiarrheal
Adult: PO 2 tab or 30 ml/15 ml extra/max strength q30min or 2 tabs q6min, max 4.2 g/24 hr

Antiulcer
Adult: PO 524 mg q30-60min or 1048 mg q1hr, max 4.2 g/24 hr; given with metronidazole or tetracycline

Traveler's diarrhea (Unlabeled)
Adult: PO 30 ml q30min (8 times/day regular strength) (4 times/day max strength)

Available forms: Tabs 262 mg; chewable tabs 262 mg/15 ml, liquid 262 mg/15 ml, 525 mg/ml

Implementation
• **Suspension:** Shake susp before use; chewable tabs should not be swallowed whole, use measuring cup/syringe

ADVERSE EFFECTS
CNS: Confusion, twitching, neurotoxicity (high dose)
EENT: Hearing loss, tinnitus, metallic taste, blue gums, black tongue (chew tabs)
GI: Increased fecal impaction (high doses), dark stools, constipation, diarrhea, nausea
HEMA: Increased bleeding time

Pharmacokinetics	
Absorption	Salicylate >90%
Distribution	None
Metabolism	None
Excretion	Feces (unchanged)
Half-life	Unknown

Pharmacodynamics	
Onset	1 hr
Peak	2 hr
Duration	4 hr

INTERACTIONS
Individual drugs
Methotrexate: increased toxicity
Tetracycline: decreased absorption, phenytoin, separate by ≥2 hr
Increase: effect of anticoagulants (PO), antidiabetics (PO)

Drug classifications
Anticoagulants (oral): increased effect of anticoagulants
Quinolones: decreased absorption of quinolones
Salicylates: increased risk of salicylate toxicity

Drug/lab test
Interference: radiographic studies of GI system

NURSING CONSIDERATIONS
Assessment
• **Diarrhea:** Assess bowel pattern (frequency, consistency, shape, volume, color) before product therapy, after treatment; check weight, bowel sounds; identify factors contributing to diarrhea (bacteria, diet, medications, tube feedings)
• Monitor skin turgor; dehydration may occur in severe diarrhea; monitor electrolytes (potassium, sodium, chloride) if diarrhea is severe or continues long term

Patient/family education
• Teach patient to stop use if symptoms do not improve within 2 days or become worse, or if diarrhea is accompanied by high fever
• Teach patient to increase fluids for rehydration
• Tell patient to chew or dissolve chewable tabs in mouth; do not swallow whole; shake susp before using, maintain hydration
• Tell patient to avoid other salicylates unless directed by prescriber; not to give to children because of possibility of Reye's syndrome
• Tell patient that stools may turn gray; tongue may darken; impaction may occur in debilitated patients
• Separate quinolones, phenytoin, tetracycline by ≥ 2 hrs

Evaluation
Positive therapeutic outcome
• Decreased diarrhea or absence of diarrhea when traveling; resolution of ulcers

---

bisoprolol (Rx)
(bis-oh′pro-lole)
Zebeta
Func. class.: Antihypertensive
Chem. class.: β₁-Blocker (selective)

Pregnancy category C

Do not confuse: Zebeta/Diabeta/Zetia

ACTION: Preferentially and competitively blocks stimulation of β₁-adrenergic receptor within cardiac muscle (decreases rate of SA node discharge, increases recovery time), slows conduction of AV node, decreases heart rate, which decreases O₂ consumption in myocardium; decreases renin-aldosterone-angiotensin system; inhibits β₂-receptors in bronchial and vascular smooth muscle at high doses

Therapeutic outcome: Decreased B/P, heart rate

USES: Mild to moderate hypertension

Unlabeled uses: Stable angina, stable CHF

CONTRAINDICATIONS
Hypersensitivity to β-blockers, cardiogenic shock, heart block (2nd or 3rd degree), sinus bradycardia, acute cardiac failure

Precautions: Pregnancy **C,** breastfeeding, children, major surgery, diabetes mellitus, CHF, renal/hepatic/thyroid/peripheral vascular/aortic/mitral valve disease, COPD, asthma, well-compensated heart failure, myasthenia gravis

BLACK BOX WARNING: Abrupt discontinuation

DOSAGE AND ROUTES
Renal/hepatic dose
Adult: PO CCr <40 ml/min 2.5 mg, titrate upward

Hypertension
Adult: PO 2.5-5 mg/day, may increase if necessary to 20 mg once daily, max 20 mg/day; reduce to 2.5 mg in bronchospastic disease

Angina (unlabeled)
Adult: PO 5-20 mg/day

Heart failure (unlabeled)
Adult: PO 1.25 mg/day × 48 hr, then 2.5 mg/day for 1st mo, then 5 mg/day, max 10 mg/day

Available forms: Tabs 5, 10 mg

Implementation
• Give daily; give with food to prevent GI upset; may be crushed
• Store protected from light, moisture; place in cool environment

ADVERSE EFFECTS
CNS: Vertigo, headache, insomnia, fatigue, dizziness, mental changes, memory loss, hallucinations, depression, lethargy, drowsiness, strange dreams, catatonia, peripheral neuropathy
CV: Ventricular dysrhythmias, profound hypotension, bradycardia, CHF, cold extremities, postural hypotension, 2nd- or 3rd-degree heart block, peripheral edema
EENT: Sore throat, dry burning eyes
ENDO: Increased hypoglycemic response to insulin
GI: Nausea, diarrhea, vomiting, mesenteric arterial thrombosis, ischemic colitis, flatulence, gastritis, gastric pain
GU: Impotence, decreased libido
HEMA: Agranulocytosis, thrombocytopenia, purpura, eosinophilia
INTEG: Rash, flushing, alopecia, pruritus, sweating
MISC: Facial swelling, weight gain, decreased exercise tolerance
MS: Joint pain, arthralgia
RESP: Bronchospasm, dyspnea, wheezing, cough, nasal stuffiness, upper respiratory infection

Pharmacokinetics

Absorption	Well absorbed
Distribution	Unknown; protein binding (30%)
Metabolism	Liver, inactive metabolites
Excretion	Urine, unchanged (50%)
Half-life	9-12 hr

Adverse effects: *italics* = common; **bold** = life-threatening

Pharmacodynamics

Onset	Unknown
Peak	2-4 hr
Duration	24 hr

INTERACTIONS
Individual drugs
Amiodarone, digoxin: increased bradycardia
Guanethidine, reserpine: increased hypotension

Drug classifications
ACE inhibitors, α-blockers, calcium channel blockers, diuretics: increased antihypertensive effect
Antidiabetics: increased antidiabetic effect
Calcium channel blockers: increased myocardial depression
Ergots: increased peripheral ischemia
NSAIDs, salicylates: decreased antihypertensive effects, may mask hypoglycemic symptoms

Drug/herb
Hawthorn: increased β-blocking effect
Ephedra: decreased β-blocking effect

Drug/lab test
Increased: AST, ALT, blood glucose, BUN, uric acid, potassium, lipoprotein, ANA titer
Interference: glucose/insulin tolerance tests

NURSING CONSIDERATIONS
Assessment
• **Hypertension:** Monitor B/P during beginning treatment, periodically thereafter; pulse: note rate, rhythm, quality; apical/radial pulse before administration; notify prescriber of any significant changes (pulse <50 bpm)
• Check for baselines in renal, liver function tests before therapy begins
• **CHF:** assess for edema in feet, legs daily, monitor I&O, daily weight; check for jugular vein distention, crackles, bilaterally, dyspnea (CHF)
• Monitor skin turgor, dryness of mucous membranes for hydration status, especially geriatric

Patient/family education

> **BLACK BOX WARNING:** Teach patient not to discontinue product abruptly; may cause precipitate angina if stopped abruptly; evaluate noncompliance

• Teach patient not to use OTC products containing α-adrenergic stimulants (such as nasal decongestants, cold preparations); to avoid alcohol, smoking; to limit sodium intake as prescribed
• Teach patient how to take pulse and B/P at home; advise when to notify prescriber

• Instruct patient to comply with weight control, dietary adjustments, modified exercise program
• Tell patient to carry/wear emergency ID to identify product being taken, allergies; tell patient product controls symptoms but does not cure
• Caution patient to avoid hazardous activities if dizziness, drowsiness present
• Teach patient to take product as prescribed, not to double doses, skip doses; take any missed doses as soon as remembered if at least 8 hr until next dose
• Advise patient to report bradycardia, dizziness, confusion, depression, fever, cold extremities
• Teach diabetic patient drug may mask signs of hypoglycemia or alter blood glucose levels

Evaluation
Positive therapeutic outcome
• Decreased B/P in hypertension (after 1-2 wk)

TREATMENT OF OVERDOSE:
Lavage, **IV** atropine for bradycardia, **IV** theophylline for bronchospasm, digoxin, O$_2$, diuretic for cardiac failure, hemodialysis, **IV** glucose for hypoglycemia, **IV** diazepam (or phenytoin) for seizures

---

⚠ HIGH ALERT

bivalirudin (Rx)
(bye-val-i-rue′din)
Angiomax
Func. class.: Anticoagulant
Chem. class.: Thrombin inhibitor
Pregnancy category B

ACTION: Direct inhibitor of thrombin that is highly specific; able to inhibit free and clot-bound thrombin

Therapeutic outcome: Anticoagulation in percutaneous transluminal coronary angioplasty (PTCA), used with aspirin; heparin-induced thrombocytopenia with thrombosis syndrome

USES: Unstable angina in patients undergoing PTCA, used with aspirin; heparin-induced thrombocytopenia; heparin-induced thrombocytopenia with thrombosis syndrome, PCI with IIb/IIIa

CONTRAINDICATIONS
Hypersensitivity, active bleeding, cerebral aneurysm, intracranial hemorrhage, recent surgery, CVA

Precautions: Pregnancy **B**, breastfeeding, children, geriatric, renal function impairment, hepatic disease, asthma, blood dyscrasias, thrombocytopenia, GI ulcers, hypertension, inflammatory bowel disease, vitamin K deficiency

DOSAGE AND ROUTES
PCI/PTCA
Adult: IV bol 0.75 mg/kg, then IV inf 1.75 mg/kg/hr for 4 hr; another IV inf may be used at 0.2 mg/kg/hr for ≤20 hr; this product is intended to be used with aspirin (325 mg daily) adjusted to body weight

HIT/HITTS
Adult: IV bol 0.75 mg/kg, then cont INF 1.75 mg/kg/hr for duration of procedure

Renal dose
Adult: IV GFR 30-59 ml/min, give 1.75 mg/kg/hr; GFR 10-29 ml/min, give 1 mg/kg/hr; dialysis-dependent patients, give 0.25 mg/kg/hr

Available forms: Inj, lyophilized 250 mg vial

Implementation
• Prior to PTCA, give with aspirin, 325 mg IV direct 1 mg/kg as a bolus; then intermittent infusion

Intermittent IV infusion route
• To each 250-mg vial add 5 ml of sterile water for inj, swirl until dissolved, further dilute reconstituted vial with 50 ml of D₅W or 0.9% NaCl (5 mg/ml); the dose is adjusted to body weight, run at 2.5 mg/hr, do not admix before or during administration
• Give reduced dose in renal impairment

Y-site compatibilities: Abciximab, acyclovir, alfentanil, allopurinol, amifostine, amikacin, aminocaproic acid, aminophylline, amphotericin B liposome, ampicillin, ampicillin-sulbactam, anidulafungin, argatroban, arsenic trioxide, atenolol, atracurium, atropine, azithromycin, aztreonam, bleomycin, bumetanide, buprenorphine, busulfan, butorphanol, calcium chloride/gluconate, capreomycin, CARBOplatin, carmustine, ceFAZolin, cefepime, cefotaxime, cefoTEtan, cefOXitin, cefTAZidime, ceftizoxime, cefTRIAXone, cefuroxime, chloramphenicol, cimetidine hydrochloride, ciprofloxacin, cisatracurium, CISplatin, clindamycin, cyclophosphamide, cycloSPORINE, cytarabine, dacarbazine, DACTINomycin, DAPTOmycin, DAUNOrubicin, DAUNOrubicin liposome, dexamethasone, dexmedetomidine, dexrazoxane, digoxin, diltiazem, diphenhydrAMINE, DOCEtaxel, dolasetron, DOPamine, DOXOrubicin, DOXOrubicin liposomal, doxycycline, droperidol, enalaprilat, ePHEDrine, EPINEPHrine, epirubicin, epoprostenol, eptifibatide, ertapenem, erythromycin, esmolol, etoposide, etoposide phosphate, famotidine, fenoldopam, fentaNYL, fluconazole, fludarabine, fluorouracil, foscarnet, fosphenytoin, furosemide, gallium, ganciclovir, gatifloxacin, gemcitabine, gentamicin, glycopyrrolate, granisetron, haloperidol, heparin, hydrALAZINE, hydrocortisone, HYDROmorphone, hydrOXYzine, IDArubicin, ifosfamide, imipenem-cilastatin, inamrinone, insulin, irinotecan, isoproterenol, ketorolac, labetalol, leucovorin, levofloxacin, lidocaine, linezolid, LORazepam, magnesium, mannitol, mechlorethamine, methohexital, methotrexate, methyldopate, methylPREDNISolone, metoclopramide, metoprolol, metroNIDAZOLE, midazolam, milrinone, mitoMYcin, mitoXANtrone, mivacurium, morphine, moxifloxacin, mycophenolate, nafcillin, nalbuphine, naloxone, nesiritide, niCARdipine, nitroglycerin, nitroprusside, norepinephrine, octreotide, ofloxacin, ondansetron, oxaliplatin, oxytocin, PACLitaxel, palonosetron, pamidronate, pancuronium, PEMEtrexed, PENTobarbital, PHENobarbital, phenylephrine, piperacillin, piperacillin-tazobactam, polymyxin B, potassium acetate/chloride/phosphates, procainamide, promethazine, propranolol, ranitidine, remifentanil, rocuronium, sodium acetate/bicarbonate/phosphates, streptozocin, succinylcholine, SUFentanil, sulfamethoxazole-trimethoprim, tacrolimus, teniposide, theophylline, thiopental, thiotepa, ticarcillin, ticarcillin-clavulanate, tigecycline, tirofiban, tobramycin, topotecan, vasopressin, vecuronium, verapamil, vinBLAStine, vinCRIStine, vinorelbine, voriconazole, warfarin, zidovudine, zoledronic acid

ADVERSE EFFECTS
CNS: *Headache, insomnia, anxiety, nervousness*
CV: *Hypo/hypertension, bradycardia,* ventricular fibrillation
GI: *Nausea, vomiting, abdominal pain, dyspepsia*
HEMA: Hemorrhage, **thrombocytopenia**
MISC: Pain at inj site, pelvic pain, urinary retention, fever, **anaphylaxis,** infection
MS: *Back pain*
GU: Urinary retention, **renal failure, oliguria**

Pharmacokinetics

Absorption	Unknown
Distribution	No protein binding
Metabolism	Unknown
Excretion	Kidneys
Half-life	25 min

Pharmacodynamics

Onset	Unknown
Peak	Unknown
Duration	1 hr

INTERACTIONS
Individual drugs
Aspirin, treprostinil: increased risk of bleeding, GPIIb/IIIa inhibitors

Drug classifications
Anticoagulants, thrombolytics: increased risk of bleeding, NSAIDs, salicylates, cephalosporins, antineoplastics, sulfinpyrazone

Drug/herb
Angelica, chamomile, devil's claw, dong quai, garlic, ginger, ginkgo, ginseng, horse chestnut, saw palmetto

NURSING CONSIDERATIONS
Assessment
⚠ Assess for fall in B/P or Hct that may indicate hemorrhage, hematoma, hemorrhage at puncture site are more common in the elderly
• Assess for fever, skin rash, urticaria
• Assess **bleeding:** check arterial and venous sites, IM inj sites, catheters; all punctures should be minimized
• PCI use: assess for possible thrombosis, stenosis, unplanned stent, prolonged ischemia, decreased reflow

Patient/family education
• Explain reason for product and expected results
• Teach patient not to use other OTC products unless approved by prescriber
• Teach patient not to use hard-bristle toothbrush, regular razor to avoid any injury: hemorrhage may result

Evaluation
Positive therapeutic outcome
• Anticoagulation in PTCA

⚠ HIGH ALERT

bleomycin (Rx)
(blee-oh-mye′sin)
Blenoxane ✤
Func. class.: Antineoplastic, antibiotic
Chem. class.: Glycopeptide
Pregnancy category D

ACTION: Inhibits synthesis of DNA, RNA, protein; derived from *Streptomyces verticillus;* phase specific in the G_2 and M phases; a nonvesicant, sclerosing agent

Therapeutic outcome: Prevention of rapidly growing malignant cells

USES: Cancer of head, neck, penis, cervix, vulva of squamous cell origin, Hodgkin's/non-Hodgkin's disease, testicular carcinoma, as a sclerosing agent for malignant pleural effusion

CONTRAINDICATIONS
Pregnancy **D**, breastfeeding, hypersensitivity, prior idiosyncratic reaction

Precautions: Renal/hepatic/respiratory disease, patients >70 yr old

> **BLACK BOX WARNING:** Idiosyncratic reaction, pulmonary fibrosis, fever, requires specialized care setting, experienced clinician

Hodgkin's lymphoma
Adult/adolescent/child: IV, IM, SUBCUT 5-20 units/m2 may give in combination

DOSAGE AND ROUTES
Adult and child: IM/SUBCUT/IV 0.25-0.5 units/kg q1-2wk or 10-20 units/m²; then 1 unit/day or 5 units/wk; may also be given by cont INF; max total dose, 400 units in lifetime

Hodgkin's disease (test dose)
Adult and child (unlabeled): IM/IV/SUBCUT <2 units for first 2 doses followed by 24 hr observation

Malignant pleural effusion
Adult: 60 units diluted in 100 ml of 0.9% NaCl intrapleural inj given through a thoracotomy tube following drainage of excess pleural fluid and complete lung expansion, remove after 4 hr

Testicular cancer
Adult: IV 10-20 units/m2 q1-2 × 1wk, may be given in combination

Renal Dose
Adult/child: CCr 40-50 ml/min reduce dose by 30%; CCr 30-39 ml/min reduce dose by 40%; CCr 20-29 ml/min reduce dose by 45%; CCr 10-19 ml/min reduce dose by 55%; CCr 5-10 ml/min reduce dose by 60%

Available forms: Powder for inj 15, 30 units/vial

Implementation
• Avoid contact with skin; very irritating; wash completely to remove

- Give fluids **IV** or PO before chemotherapy to hydrate patient
- Give antacid before oral agent; give antiemetic 30-60 min before giving product and prn to prevent vomiting; give antibiotics for prophylaxis of infection
- Provide liquid diet: carbonated beverages, gelatin may be added if patient is not nauseated or vomiting
- Rinse mouth tid-qid with water, club soda; brush teeth bid-qid with soft brush or cotton-tipped applicators for stomatitis; use unwaxed dental floss

IM/SUBCUT route
- IM test dose in lymphoma
- Reconstitute with 1-5 ml sterile water for inj; max conc 5 units/ml, D₅W, 0.9% NaCl, rotate inj sites

IV route
- Product should be prepared by experienced personnel using proper precautions
- Two test doses 2-5 units before initial dose in lymphoma; monitor for anaphylaxis
- Give by direct **IV** after reconstituting 15 units or less/5 ml or more of 0.9% NaCl; give 15 units or less/10 min through Y-tube or 3-way stopcock initial dose; monitor for anaphylaxis

Intermittent IV infusion route
- Administer after diluting 50-100 ml 0.9% NaCl, D₅W and giving at prescribed rate

Y-site compatibilities: Acyclovir, alfentanil, allopurinol, amifostine, amikacin, aminocaproic acid, aminophylline, amiodarone, ampicillin, ampicillin-sulbactam, anidulafungin, atenolol, atracurium, azithromycin, aztreonam, bivalirudin, bumetanide, buprenorphine, busulfan, butorphanol, calcium chloride/gluconate, CARBOplatin, carmustine, caspofungin, ceFAZolin, cefepime, cefotaxime, cefoTEtan, cefOXitin, cefTAZidime, ceftizoxime, cefTRIAXone, cefuroxime, chloramphenicol, chlorproMAZINE, cimetidine, ciprofloxacin, cisatracurium, CISplatin, clindamycin, codeine, cyclophosphamide, cycloSPORINE, cytarabine, dacarbazine, DACTINomycin, DAPTOmycin, DAUNOrubicin, dexamethasone, dexmedetomidine, dexrazoxane, digoxin, diltiazem, diphenhydrAMINE, DOBUTamine, DOCEtaxel, DOPamine, doxacurium, DOXOrubicin, DOXOrubicin liposomal, doxycycline, droperidol, enalaprilat, ePHEDrine, EPINEPHrine, epirubicin, ertapenem, erythromycin, esmolol, etoposide, famotidine, fenoldopam, fentaNYL, filgrastim, fluconazole, fludarabine, fluorouracil, foscarnet, fosphenytoin, furosemide, ganciclovir, gatifloxacin, gemcitabine, gentamicin, glycopyrrolate, granisetron, haloperidol, heparin, hydrALAZINE, hydrocortisone sodium succinate, HYDROmorphone, hydrOXYzine, IDArubicin, ifosfamide, imipenem-cilastatin, inamrinone, insulin (regular), irinotecan, isoproterenol, ketorolac, labetalol, leucovorin, levofloxacin, levorphanol, lidocaine, linezolid, LORazepam, magnesium sulfate, mannitol, mechlorethamine, melphalan, meperidine, meropenem, mesna, metaraminol, methohexital, methotrexate, methyldopate, methylPREDNISolone, metoclopramide, metoprolol, metroNIDAZOLE, midazolam, milrinone, minocycline, mitoMYcin, mitoXANtrone, mivacurium, morphine, nafcillin, nalbuphine, naloxone, nesiritide, niCARdipine, nitroglycerin, nitroprusside, norepinephrine, octreotide, ondansetron, oxaliplatin, palonosetron, pamidronate, pancuronium, pantoprazole, PEMEtrexed, pentamidine, pentazocine, PENTobarbital, PHENobarbital, phenylephrine, piperacillin, piperacillin-tazobactam, polymyxin B, potassium chloride, potassium phosphates, procainamide, prochlorperazine, promethazine, propranolol, quiNIDine, ranitidine, remifentanil, riTUXimab, rocuronium, sargramostim, sodium acetate, sodium bicarbonate, sodium phosphates, succinylcholine, SUFentanil, sulfamethoxazole-trimethoprim, tacrolimus, teniposide, theophylline, thiopental, thiotepa, ticarcillin, ticarcillin-clavulanate, tirofiban, tobramycin, tolazoline, trastuzumab, trimethobenzamide, vancomycin, vasopressin, vecuronium, verapamil, vinBLAStine, vinCRIStine, vinorelbine, voriconazole, zidovudine

ADVERSE EFFECTS
CNS: Pain at tumor site, headache, confusion, fever, chills, malaise
CV: MI, stroke
GI: *Nausea, vomiting, anorexia, stomatitis, weight loss,* ulceration of mouth, lips
GU: Hemolytic-uremic syndrome
IDIOSYNCRATIC REACTION: Hypotension, confusion, fever, chills, wheezing
INTEG: *Rash, hyperkeratosis, nail changes, alopecia,* pruritus, acne, striae, peeling, hyperpigmentation, phlebitis
RESP: Fibrosis, pneumonitis, wheezing, pulmonary toxicity
SYST: Anaphylaxis, radiation recall, Raynaud's phenomenon

Pharmacokinetics

Absorption	Well absorbed (IM, SUBCUT, intrapleural, intraperitoneal)
Distribution	Widely distributed
Metabolism	Liver, 30%
Excretion	Kidneys, unchanged (50%)
Half-life	2-4 hr; increased in renal disease

Pharmacodynamics

Unknown

INTERACTIONS
Individual drugs
Filgrastim, sargramostim: increased toxicity

Fosphenytoin, phenytoin: decreased phenytoin levels

Radiation: increased toxicity, bone marrow suppression

Drug classifications
Anesthetics (general), antineoplastics: increased toxicity

Live virus vaccines: avoid concurrent use

Drug/lab test
Increased: uric acid

Decrease: Pulmonary function tests

NURSING CONSIDERATIONS
Assessment
• Assess buccal cavity q8hr for dryness, sores or ulceration, white patches, oral pain, bleeding, dysphagia; obtain prescription for viscous lidocaine (Xylocaine)

⚠ **Assess symptoms indicating anaphylaxis: rash, pruritus, urticaria, purpuric skin lesions, itching, flushing, wheezing, hypotension; have emergency equipment available**

> **BLACK BOX WARNING: Pulmonary toxicity/ fibrosis:** Assess pulmonary function tests; chest x-ray before, during therapy; monitor q2wk during treatment; pulmonary diffusion capacity for carbon monoxide (DL_{CO}) monthly; if <40% of pretreatment value, stop treatment; assess for dyspnea, crackles, unproductive cough, chest pain, tachypnea, fatigue, increased pulse, pallor, lethargy, more common in the elderly, radiation therapy, pulmonary disease; **usually occurs with cumulative doses >400 units**

• Monitor CBC, differential, platelet count weekly; withhold product for WBC <4000/ mm³ or platelet count <100,000/mm³; notify prescriber of results for WBC <20,000/mm³, platelets <150,000/mm³

> **BLACK BOX WARNING: Idiosyncratic reaction:** assess hypotension, mental confusion, fever, chills, wheezing in lymphoma

• Monitor temp (may indicate beginning of infection)

• Monitor liver function tests before, during therapy (bilirubin, AST, ALT, LDH) as needed or monthly

• Assess for bleeding: hematuria, stool guaiac, bruising or petechiae, mucosa or orifices q8hr; inflammation of mucosa, breaks in skin

• Treat pulmonary infection prior to treatment; identify dyspnea, crackles, unproductive cough, chest pain, tachypnea

• Identify effects of alopecia on body image; discuss feelings about body changes; if edema in feet, joint pain, stomach pain, shaking present, prescriber should be notified; identify inflammation of mucosa, breaks in skin

Patient/family education
• Teach patient to avoid use of products containing aspirin or ibuprofen, razors, commercial mouthwash; bleeding may occur; to report symptoms of bleeding (hematuria, tarry stools); decreased urination

• Instruct patient to report signs of anemia (fatigue, headache, irritability, faintness, shortness of breath)

• Instruct patient to report any changes in breathing or coughing even several months after treatment; to avoid crowds and persons with respiratory tract or other infections

• Inform patient that hair may be lost during treatment; a wig or hairpiece may make patient feel better; new hair may be different in color, texture

• Caution patient not to have any vaccinations without the advice of the prescriber; serious reactions can occur

• **Advise patient contraception is needed during treatment and for several months after completion of therapy, pregnancy D**

Evaluation
Positive therapeutic outcome
• Prevention of rapid division of malignant cells

> ## boceprevir
> (boe-se′pro-vir)
> **Victrelis**
> *Func. class.:* Antiviral, antihepatitis agents
> **Pregnancy category X**

ACTION: Prevents hepatitis C viral (HCV) replication by blocking the activity of HCV NS3/4A serine protease. Hepatitis C virus NS3/4A serine protease is an enzyme responsible for the conversion of HCV encoded polyproteins to mature/functioning viral proteins.

Theurapeutic outcome: Resolution of hepatitis C infection

USES: Hepatitis C infection in combination with peginterferon alfa and ribavirin with compensated liver function

---

CONTRAINDICATIONS
Pregnancy (**X**), male partners of women who are pregnant

Precautions: Breastfeeding, anemia, neutropenia, thrombocytopenia, HIV, hepatitis B, decompensated hepatic disease, in liver or other organ transplants, neonates, infants, children, adolescents <18 years of age, hypersensitivity

DOSAGE AND ROUTES
Chronic hepatitis C infection (genotype 1) compensated liver disease (without cirrhosis, previously untreated with interferon and ribavirin therapy, null responders/partial responders/relapsers)
Adult: PO Before starting therapy, give peginterferon alfa and ribavirin 4 wk, then add boceprevir 800 mg (four 200-mg capsules) PO tid (7-9 hr). Treatment length is determined by HCV RNA concentrations at treatment wk 4, 8, 12, and 24. If the patient has undetectable HCV RNA concentrations at wk 8 and 24, discontinue all three medications at wk 28 (previously untreated); wk 36 (partial responders/relapsers). If HCV RNA is detectable at wk 8 but undetectable at wk 24, the three-drug regimen through wk 36, then give only peginterferon alfa and ribavirin through treatment wk 48. If the patient has a poor response to peginterferon alfa and ribavirin during the initial 4 wk, continue treatment with all three medications for a total of 48 wks. Discontinue the three-drug regimen if the HCV RNA concentration >100 IU/ml at treatment wk 12 or a detectable HCA RNA concentration at treatment wk 24.

Chronic hepatitis C infection (genotype 1) compensated liver disease with cirrhosis
Adult: PO Before starting therapy with boceprevir, peginterferon alfa and ribavirin must be given 4 wk; then add boceprevir 800 mg (four 200-mg capsules) PO tid (q7-9hr) to peginterferon alfa and ribavirin for an additional 44 wk (48 wk total)

Available forms: Cap 200 mg

Implementation
• Only use in combination with peginterferon alfa and ribavirin; never give as monotherapy
• Discontinue in hepatitis C virus (HCV) RNA concentrations ≥100 IU/ml at wk 12 or a confirmed detectable HCV RNA concentrations at wk 24
• Any contraindication to peginterferon alfa or ribavirin also applies to boceprevir
• Give with food

ADVERSE EFFECTS
When used in combination with peginterferon/ribavarin
CNS: *Asthenia, chills,* dizziness, *fatigue,* insomnia, irritability
GI: Diarrhea, decreased appetite, dysgeusia, nausea, vomiting, xerostomia
HEMA: Anemia (Hgb <10 g/dl), neutropenia, thrombocytopenia
INTEG: *Alopecia, rash,* xerosis
MISC: *Arthralgia, exertional dyspnea,* **drug rash with eosinophilia and systemic symptoms (DRESS) syndrome, exfoliative dermatitis, Stevens-Johnson syndrome, toxic epidermal necrolysis**

Pharmacokinetics
Absorption	Unknown
Distribution	75% protein binding
Metabolism	By the enzyme aldoketoreductase (AKR) to a ketone-reduced metabolite; undergoes oxidative metabolism by the hepatic isoenzyme CYP3A4/5 and is a substrate for the drug efflux transporter, P-glycoprotein (PGP)
Excretion	Feces (79%),urine (9%)
Half-life	3.4 hrs

Pharmacodynamics
Onset	Unknown
Peak	2 hrs
Duration	Unknown

INTERACTIONS
Individual drugs
Alfuzosin, cisapride, ezetimibe, lovastatin, niacin with simvastatin and boceprevir, oral midazolam, pimozide, sildenafil, simvastatin, tadalafil (pulmonary arterial hypertension), triazolam: Increased, life-threatening reactions of each product: do not use concurrently

Acetaminophen, alfentanil, aliskiren, almotriptan, alosetron, ALPRAZolam, aminophylline, amiodarone, amitriptyline, amLODIPine, ARIPiprazole, astemizole, atorvastatin, bepridil, boceprevir, bosentan, budesonide, bupivacaine, buprenorphine, busPIRone, carvedilol, cevimeline, chloroquine, cilostazol, cinacalcet, citalopram, clarithromycin, clomiPRAMINE, clonazePAM, clopidogrel, cloZAPine, colchicine, cyclobenzaprine, cycloSPORINE, dapsone, DAUNOrubicin, desipramine, desloratadine, dexamethasone, dexlansoprazole, dextromethorphan, diazepam, diclofenac, digoxin, diltiazem, disopyramide, disulfiram, DOCEtaxel, dolasetron, donepezil, DOXOrubicin, droperidol, dutasteride, ebastine, eletriptan, eplerenone, erlotinib, erythromycin, estazolam, eszopiclone, ethosuximide, etoposide, exemestane, felodipine, fentaNYL, fexofenadine, finasteride, flecainide, flunitrazepam, flurazepam, galantamine, gefitinib, glyburide, granisetron, halofantrine, haloperidol, HYDROcodone, ifosfamide, imipramine, indiplon, irinotecan, isradipine, itraconazole, ivermectin, ixabepilone, ketoconazole, lansoprazole, lidocaine, loperamide, loratadine, losartan, maraviroc, mefloquine, meloxicam, mirtazapine, mitoMYcin, montelukast, morphine, nateglinide, niCARdipine, NIFEdipine, nisoldipine, nortriptyline, omeprazole, ondansetron, oxybutynin, oxyCODONE, PACLitaxel, palonosetron, paricalcitol, plicamycin, posaconazole, prasugrel, praziquantel, propafenone, quazepam, QUEtiapine, quinacrine, quiNIDine, ramelteon, repaglinide, rifabutin, risperiDONE, ropivacaine, salmeterol, selegiline, sertraline, sibutramine, silodosin, sirolimus, sitaxsentan, solifenacin, SUFentanil, SUNItinib, systemic corticosteroids, tacrolimus, telithromycin, teniposide, terfenadine, testosterone, theophylline, tiaGABine, tinidazole, tolterodine, tolvaptan, traMADol, traZODone, vardenafil, venlafaxine, verapamil, vinBLAStine, vinCRIStine, voriconazole, warfarin, and others: increased effect, adverse reactions of each product; use cautiously; may need to reduce dose

Drosperinone: increased hyperkalemia

Ethinyl estradiol: decreased estrogen levels

Methadone: decreased effect of this product

Efavirenz, ritonavir, atazanavir, lopinavir with ritonavir: possible treatment failure

Drug classifications

Ergots (dihydroergotamine, ergotamine, ergonovine, methylergonovine): do not use concurrently

Phosphodiesterase type 5 (PDE5) inhibitors (for erectile dysfunction): increased effect, adverse reactions of each product

CYP3A4 inhibitors (phenytoin, carBAMazepine, PHENobarbital, rifampin): decreased boceprevir effect

Drug/herb
Do not use with St. John's wort

Drug/lab test
Decreased: Hgb, platelets

NURSING CONSIDERATIONS
Assessment
⚠ **Pregnancy: Obtain a pregnancy test prior to, monthly during, and for 6 months after treatment is completed; those who are not willing to practice strict contraception should not receive treatment; report any cases of prenatal ribavirin exposure to the Ribavirin Pregnancy registry at (800) 593-2214**

• **Anemia:** Monitor Hgb, CBC with differential prior to, at treatment wks 2, 4, 8, and 12, and as needed. If Hgb is less than 10 g/dl, decrease ribavirin dosage; if Hgb is less than 8.5 g/dl, discontinuation of therapy is recommended; dosage should not be altered based on adverse reactions; anemia may be managed through ribavirin dose modifications; never alter the dose of boceprevir. If anemia persists despite a reduction in ribavirin dose, consider discontinuing boceprevir. If management of anemia requires permanent discontinuation of ribavirin, treatment with boceprevir MUST also be permanently discontinued. Once boceprevir has been discontinued, it must not be restarted; monitor CBC with differential at treatment wks 4, 8, 12, and at other treatment points as needed

⚠ **Serious skin disorders (DRESS, Stevens-Johnson syndrome, toxic epidermal necrolysis, exfoliative dermatitis): These reactions may be due to combination use with peginterferon alfa, ribavirin; if serious skin reactions occur, discontinue all three products**

Patient/family education
⚠ **Instruct patient to use 2 forms of effective contraception (intrauterine devices and barrier methods)**

• Instruct patient to take with food to increase absorption, do not start new meds/herbs without prescriber's approval

• Instruct patient to use precautions to prevent transmission of hepatitis C

• Instruct patient to inform prescriber of all medications, herbs, supplements used

Evaluation
Positive therapeutic outcome
• Resolution of hepatitis C infection

B

⚠ HIGH ALERT

bortezomib (Rx)

(bor-tez'oh-mib)

Velcade

Func. class.: Antineoplastic—miscellaneous

Chem. class.: Proteasome inhibitor

Pregnancy category D

ACTION: Reversible inhibitor of chymotrypsin-like activity in mammalian cells; causes a delay in tumor growth by disrupting normal homeostatic mechanisms 26S proteasome

Therapeutic outcome: Decreased growth and spread of malignant cells

USES: Multiple myeloma previously untreated or when at least two other treatments have failed; mantle cell lymphoma

CONTRAINDICATIONS

Pregnancy **D**, breastfeeding, hypersensitivity to this product, boron, or mannitol

Precautions: Peripheral neuropathy, children, geriatric, cardiac/hepatic disease, hypotension, tumor lysis syndrome, thrombocytopenia, infection, diabetes mellitus, bone marrow suppression, intracranial bleeding, injection-site irritation

DOSAGE AND ROUTES
Multiple myeloma (previously untreated)

Adult: IV bol/subcut Give for 9 6-wk cycles; cycle 1-4, 1.3 mg/m²/dose given on days 1, 4, 8, 11, then a 10-day rest period (days 12-21) and again on days 22, 25, 29, 32, then a 10-day rest period (days 33-42) given with melphalan (9 mg/m²/day on days 1-4) and predniSONE (60 mg/m²/day on days 1-4); this 6-wk cycle is considered one course; in cycles 5-9, give bortezomib 1.3 mg/m²/dose on days 1, 8, 22, 29 with melphalan (9 mg/m²/day on days 1-4) and predniSONE (60 mg/m²/day on days 1-4); this 6-wk cycle is considered one course; at least 72 hr should elapse between consecutive doses

Mantle cell lymphoma in combination

Adult: IV bol/subcut 1.3 mg/m²/dose (days 1, 4, 8, 11) followed by 10-day rest period (days 12 to 21); × 6 (3wk) cycles with rituximab 375 mg/m2, cyclophosphamide 750 mg/m2, doxorubicin 50mg/m2 all on day 1, and prednisone 100mg/m2 q day on day 1-5, give bortezomib before rituximab

Neuropathic pain

Grade 1 with pain or grade 2, reduce to 1 mg/m²; grade 2 with pain or grade 3, hold product until toxicity resolves, then start at 0.7 mg/m² qwk; grade 4 hematologic toxicities, withhold use

Relapsed mantle cell lymphoma

who have received ≥ 1 prior therapy

Adult: IV BOL/SUBCUT 1.3 mg/m2/dose on days 1, 4, 8, 11 followed by a 10-day rest period

Hepatic dose

Adult: IV bilirubin >1.5 × ULN reduce to 0.7 mg/m² in cycle 1, consider dose escalation to 1 mg/m² or further reduction to 0.5 mg/m² in next cycles based on tolerability

Available forms: Lyophilized powder for inj 3.5 mg

Implementation
Subcut Route

• Use 2.5 mg/ml, rotate injection sites
• If injection reaction occurs, use 1 mg/ml

IV direct

• **Reconstitute** each vial with 3.5 ml 0.9% NaCl (1 mg/ml), sol should be clear/colorless; **inject** bol over 3-5 sec
• Store unopened product at room temperature, protect from light
• Use protective clothing during handling, preparation; avoid contact with skin
• Monitor for extravasation at inj site

SC route

• Reconstitute with 1.4 ml NS (2.5 mg/ml) or 3.5 ml NS (1 mg/ml); the 1 mg/ml may be used for local inj site reaction with the 2.5 mg/ml solution; if injection-site reaction occurs, use 1 mg/ml; the final product should be a clear, colorless solution; if any discoloration or particulate matter is observed, do not use
• Store reconstituted at room temperature, give within 8 hr of reconstitution, store ≤8 hr in a syringe; total storage time must be ≤8 hr when exposed to normal light
• Determine the volume of reconstituted bortezomib to be administered by multiplying the desired dose in mg/m² by the patient's BSA and dividing the result by the concentration (1 mg/ml or 2.5 mg/ml); discard unused drug, as no preservative is present
• Place a sticker that indicates subcut use on the syringe

SC inj

• Inject subcutaneously in the thigh or abdomen; do not inject into a site that is tender, bruised, erythematous, or indurated; rotate injection sites; new sites should be at least 1 inch from an old site

• Use of gloves and protective clothing are recommended to prevent skin contact

ADVERSE EFFECTS

CNS: Anxiety, insomnia, dizziness, headache, peripheral neuropathy, rigors, paresthesia, fever, headache

CV: Hypotension, edema, CHF

GI: Abdominal pain, constipation, diarrhea, dyspepsia, *nausea,* vomiting, anorexia

HEMA: Anemia, neutropenia, thrombocytopenia

MISC: Dehydration, weight loss, herpes zoster, *rash,* pruritus, blurred vision

MS: Fatigue, malaise, weakness, arthralgia, bone pain, muscle cramps, myalgia, back pain, tumor lysis syndrome

RESP: Cough, pneumonia, dyspnea, URI, ARDs, pneumonitis, interstitial pneumonia, lung infiltration

Pharmacokinetics

Absorption	Unknown
Distribution	Protein binding 83%
Metabolism	P450 enzymes (3A4, 2D6, 2C19, 2C9, 1A2)
Excretion	Unknown
Half-life	9-15 hr

Pharmacodynamics

Unknown

INTERACTIONS

Individual drugs

Amiodarone, amprenavir, chloramphenicol, CISplatin, colchicine, cycloSPORINE, dapsone, didanosine, disulfiram, gold salts, INH, iodoquinal, isoniazid, lamiVUDine, metroNIDAZOLE, nitrofurantoin, oxaliplatin, PACLitaxel, penicillamine, phenytoin, ritonavir, stavudine, sulfaSALAzine, thalidomide, vinBLAStine, vinCRIStine, zacatabine, zidovudine, and others: increased peripheral neuropathy

Drug classifications

Anticoagulants, NSAIDs, platelet inhibitors, salicylates, thrombolytics: increased bleeding risk

Antihypertensives: increased hypotension

Antivirals, statins, HMG-CoA reductase inhibitors: increased peripheral neuropathy

Hematopoietic pregenitor cells (sargramostim, filgrastim): do not use within 24 hr of chemotherapy

Oral hypoglycemics: increased hypo/hyperglycemia

Products that induce or inhibit CYP3A4: increased toxicity or decreased efficacy

Decreased: effect of norethindrone, estradiol, combination oral contraceptives, another nonhormonal contraceptive should be used

Fatal pulmonary toxicity: assess for risk factors, or new worsening pulmonary symptoms

Tumor lysis syndrome: usually with those with a high tumor burden

Drug/herb

St. John's wort: toxicity or decreased efficacy

NURSING CONSIDERATIONS

Assessment

• Assess hematologic status: platelets, CBC throughout treatment

Patient/family education

⚠ Teach to use contraception while on this product, avoid breastfeeding

• Advise diabetic to monitor blood glucose levels

• Instruct to contact prescriber if new or worsening peripheral neuropathy, severe vomiting, diarrhea

• Advise to avoid driving, operating machinery until effect is known

• Advise to avoid using other medications unless approved by prescriber

• To report peripheral neuropathy (burning, discomfort)

• Bleeding risk (report bruising, bleeding)

Evaluation

Positive therapeutic outcome

• Improvement of multiple myeloma symptoms

bosentan (Rx)

(boh-sen-tan)

Tracleer

Func. class.: Vasodilator

Chem. class.: Endothelin receptor antagonist

Pregnancy category X

ACTION: Peripheral vasodilation occurs via antagonism of the effect of endothelin on endothelium and vascular smooth muscle

Therapeutic outcome: Decreased pulmonary arterial hypertension

USES: Pulmonary arterial hypertension with WHO class III, IV symptoms

Unlabeled uses: Septic shock to improve microcirculatory blood flow

CONTRAINDICATIONS

Hypersensitivity, CVA, CAD

⚠ Nurse Alert　　★ Key NCLEX® Drug　　≫ Drug Specifics

Precautions: Breastfeeding, children, geriatric, mitral stenosis, impaired hepatic function, anemia, edema, jaundice, hypovolemia, hypotension

> **BLACK BOX WARNING:** Pregnancy **X,** hepatic disease

DOSAGE AND ROUTES
Adult ≥40 kg and child >12 yr: PO 62.5 mg bid × 4 wk, then 125 mg bid
Adult <40 kg and child >12 yr: PO 62.5 mg bid

Adults taking a protease inhibitor for ≥10 days
Adult: PO 62.5 mg qday or every other day based on tolerance, max 125 mg/day

Hepatic dose
Adult: PO
- **Baseline AST/ALT <3× ULN: no dosage change, monitor LFTs qmo, reduce or interrupt if elevated**
- **AST/ALT >3 and ≤5× ULN: repeat test; if confirmed, reduce to 62.5 mg bid or interrupt; monitor LFTs q2wk, if interrupted, restart when LFTs <3× ULN, check LFTs within 3 days**
- **Increase in AST/ALT >5 and ≤5× ULN: during treatment, repeat test to confirm, discontinue, monitor LFTs q2wk until LFTs <3× ULN, restart at starting dose**
- **AST/ALT >8× ULN: discontinue permanently**

Available forms: Tabs 62.5, 125 mg

Implementation
- Store at room temperature
- Only available through the TAP program 866-228-3546

ADVERSE EFFECTS
CNS: Headache, flushing, fatigue, fever
CV: *Hypotension, chest pain,* palpitations, edema of lower limbs, fluid retention
GI: Abnormal liver function, dyspepsia, **hepatotoxicity,** diarrhea
HEMA: **Anemia, leukopenia, neutropenia, lymphopenia, thrombocytopenia**
INTEG: Pruritus, **Stevens-Johnson syndrome, toxic epidermal necrolysis,** rash
MISC: **Anaphylaxis,** oligospermia, **tumor lysis syndrome,** respiratory infection, arthralgia
SYST: **Secondary malignancy**

Pharmacokinetics

Absorption	50% absorbed
Distribution	Protein binding >98%
Metabolism	Liver (metabolites); metabolized CYP2C9, CYP3A4, and possibly CYP2C19; steady state 3-5 days
Excretion	Biliary
Half-life	5 hr

Pharmacodynamics

Unknown

INTERACTIONS
Individual drugs
CycloSPORINE, glyBURIDE: do not coadminister
CycloSPORINE, ketoconazole: increased bosentan level
CycloSPORINE: decreased cycloSPORINE level
GlyBURIDE: glyBURIDE level decreased significantly, bosentan also decreased, increased liver function tests
Ketoconazole: increased bosentan level
Simvastatin: decreased effects
Warfarin: decreased anticoagulation

Drug classifications
Contraceptives (hormonal), statins: decreased effects
CYP2C9, CYP3A4 inhibitors: increased bosentan effects

Drug/lab test

> **BLACK BOX WARNING:** Increased: ALT, AST

Decreased: Hgb, Hct

NURSING CONSIDERATIONS
Assessment
⚠ **Serious skin toxicities: angioedema occurring 8-21 days after initiating therapy**
- Assess B/P, pulse during treatment until stable
- **Assess hepatic toxicity: AST, ALT, bilirubin; liver enzymes may increase; if ALT/AST >3 and ≤5 × ULN, decrease dose or interrupt treatment and monitor AST/ALT q2wk; if >2 × ULN, and bilirubin >2 × ULN or signs of hepatitis, hepatic disease, stop treatment; vomiting, jaundice; product should be discontinued**
- Assess blood studies: Hct, Hgb after 1 mo, 3 mo, then q3mo may be decreased
- **Pulmonary hypertension/CHF:** fluid retention, weight gain, increased leg edema; may occur within wks

Patient/family education
• Instruct patient to report jaundice, dark urine, joint pain, fatigue, malaise, bruising, easy bleeding, fluid retention

> **BLACK BOX WARNING:** Pregnancy (**X**), monitor pregnancy test monthly; patient must use nonhormonal contraception during and ≥ 1 month after conclusion of treatment

• Instruct patient to take without regard to food, do not take new meds/herbs without prescriber approval

Evaluation
Positive therapeutic outcome
• Decrease in pulmonary hypertension

RARELY USED

bosutinib
(boe-sue′ti-nib)
Bosulif
Func. class.: Antineoplastic biologic response modifiers
Chem. class.: Signal transduction inhibitors (STIs), tyrosine kinase inhibitor
Pregnancy category D

USES: Treatment of CML; (chronic accelerator phase) Philadelphia-chromosome–positive patients in blast-cell crisis

CONTRAINDICATIONS
Pregnancy (**D**), hypersensitivity

Precautions: Breastfeeding, children, diarrhea, geriatric patients, hepatic disease, bone marrow suppression, infection, thrombocytopenia, neutropenia, immunosuppression, fluid retention

DOSAGE AND ROUTES
Adult: **PO** 500 mg daily with food, may increase to 600 mg/day in those who have not developed grade 3 toxicity or in patients who do not reach complete hematological response by wk 8 or complete cytogenic response (CCyR) by wk 12

Hepatic dosage
Adult: PO Any baseline hepatic impairment: Start at 200 mg/day; liver transaminase >5 × ULN hold dose until levels ≤2.5 × ULN, then resume at 400 mg/day; liver transaminase level ≥3 × ULN and bilirubin >2 × ULN and alk phos <2 × ULN, discontinue

Dosage adjustments for treatment related toxicity
Hematologic toxicity: ANC <1000 × 10^6/L or platelet count <50,000 × 10^6/L: hold dose until ANC ≥1000 × 10^6/L and platelets ≥50,000 × 10^6/L; if recovery within 2 wks, resume therapy at the same dose; if blood counts remain low after 2 wks, upon recovery, resume at 100 mg/day less than the previous dose
Diarrhea: Grade 3 or 4 diarrhea (≥7 stools/day compared with baseline): hold therapy until recovery to grade 1 toxicity or lower; resume therapy at 400 mg/day
Other nonhematologic toxicity: Significant or moderate or severe toxicity: hold therapy until toxicity resolves; resume therapy at 400 mg/day

Available forms: Tabs 100, 500 mg

ADVERSE EFFECTS
CNS: Headache, dizziness, fever, fatigue, weakness
GI: Nausea, vomiting, anorexia, abdominal pain, diarrhea
HEMA: Neutropenia, thrombocytopenia, bleeding
INTEG: Rash, pruritus
MS: Arthralgia, myalgia
RESP: Cough, dyspnea, pleural effusion, edema
OTHER: Elevated LFTs

Pharmacokinetics

Absorption	Unknown
Distribution	Protein binding 96%
Metabolism	CYP3A4
Half-life	22.5 hr

Pharmacodynamics

Onset	Unknown
Peak	Unknown
Duration	Unknown

INTERACTIONS
Individual drugs
Simvastatin: Increased plasma concentrations

Drug classifications
CYP3A4 inhibitors (ketoconazole, itraconazole, erythromycin, clarithromycin), P-gb inhibitors: increased bosutinib concentrations
Simvastatin, calcium channel blockers, ergots: increased plasma concentrations
CYP3A4 inducers (dexamethasone, phenytoin, carBAMazepine, rifampin, PHENobarbital), antacids, proton-pump inhibitors: decrease bosutinib concentrations

Drug/food
Grapefruit juice: increased bosutinib effect; avoid use while taking product

---

Drug/herb
St. John's wort: decreased bosutinib
concentration

Drug/Lab
Increase: LFTs, magnesium
Decrease: Bicarbonates, magnesium

NURSING CONSIDERATIONS
Assessment
• **Myelosuppression:** Assess for anemia,
thrombocytopenia, neutropenia; obtain a CBC
weekly × 1 mo, then monthly as needed
• Monitor LFTs every mo × 3 mo, then as clinically indicated

Patient/family education
• **Teach patient to immediately report adverse reactions, bleeding; report diarrhea,
hepatic, hematologic symptoms/toxicity**
• Teach patient about reason for treatment,
expected results
• **Advise patient to use effective contraception during treatment and up to 30 days after
discontinuing treatment**

Evaluation
Positive therapeutic outcome
• Decrease in leukemic cells or size of tumor

⚠ HIGH ALERT

brentuximab (Rx)
(bren-tak'see-mab)
Adcetris
Func. class.: antineoplastic
Chem. class.: monoclonal antibody
Pregnancy category D

ACTION: The anticancer activity is due to
the binding of the ADC to CD30-expressing cells,
followed by the internalization and transportation of the ADC-CD30 complex to lysosomes, and
the release of MMAE via selective proteolytic
cleavage. MMAE binds to tubulin and disrupts the
microtubule network within the cell, inducing
cell cycle arrest and apoptotic death of the cells

Therapeutic outcome: Decreasing symptoms of Hodgkin's disease (increased lymph
nodes, night sweats, weight loss, splenomegaly,
hepatomegaly)

USES: For the treatment of Hodgkin's disease
after failure of autologous stem cell transplant
(ASCT) or after failure of at least 2 prior multia-
gent chemotherapy regimens in patients who are
not ASCT candidates; For the treatment of non-
Hodgkin's lymphoma (NHL): For the treatment
of systemic anaplastic large cell lymphoma

(sALCL) after failure of at least one prior multia-
gent chemotherapy regimen

CONTRAINDICATIONS
Hypersensitivity, pregnancy **D**

> **BLACK BOX WARNING:** Progressive multifo-
> cal leukoencephalopathy (PML)

Precautions: Breastfeeding, children, infants,
neonates, neutropenia, peripheral neuropathy,
tumor lysis syndrome (TLS)

DOSAGE AND ROUTES
Adult: IV 1.8 mg/kg IV over 30 minutes every
3 weeks until disease progression or unacceptable toxicity. For patients >100 kg, max weight
used for dosage calculation should be 100 kg,
which translates to no more than 180 mg/dose

Dose adjustments for toxicity due to peripheral neuropathy:
For Grade <3: No dosage adjustments are
recommended; For new or worsening grade
2/3: Interrupt treatment until toxicity resolves to grade ≤1; when resuming treatment, reduce dosage to 1.2 mg/kg IV q3wk;
For Grade 4: Discontinue treatment

Dose adjustments for toxicity due to neutropenia:
For neutropenia Grade <3: No dosage adjustments; For Grade 3/4 neutropenia: Interrupt treatment until toxicity resolves to baseline or grade ≤2; consider the use of growth
factors (CSFs) for subsequent cycles of therapy; For Grade 4 neutropenia despite the use
of growth factors: Discontinue treatment or
reduce the dose to 1.2 mg/kg IV q3wk

Available forms: Powder for injection 50 mg

Implementation:

Intermittent IV infusion route
• Visually inspect for particulate matter and
discoloration whenever solution and container
permit
• Give only as an IV infusion, do not give as an
IV push or bolus
• Use cytoxic handling procedures
• Do not mix with, or administer as an infusion
with, other IV products
• Calculate the dose (mg) and the number of
vials required. For patients weighing >100 kg,
use 100 kg to calculate the dose; reconstitute
each 50 mg vial/10.5 ml of sterile water for
injection (5 mg/ml)
• Direct the stream of sterile water toward the
wall of the vial and not directly at the cake or
powder; gently swirl the vial to aid in dissolution, do not shake

---

Adverse effects: *italics* = common; **bold** = life-threatening

- Discard any unused portion left in the vial
- After reconstitution, dilute immediately with ≥100 ml of 0.9% sodium chloride, 5% dextrose, or lactated ringers solution to a final concentration (0.4 mg/ml-1.8 mg/ml)
- Use the diluted solution immediately or store in refrigerator for ≤24 hrs after reconstitution; do not freeze
- Infuse over 30 min

ADVERSE EFFECTS

CNS: Headache, dizziness, *fever,* peripheral neuropathy, anxiety, chills, confusion, *fatigue,* paresthesias, insomnia, night sweats, **progressive multifocal leukoencephalopathy (PML)**
CV: Peripheral edema, supraventricular arrhythmia
GI: *Abdominal pain, nausea, vomiting,* constipation, *diarrhea,* weight loss
HEMA: **Anemia, neutropenia, thrombocytopenia,** lymphadenopathy
INTEG: *Rash,* pruritus, alopecia, xerosis
RESP: **Pneumothorax, pneumonitis, pulmonary embolism,** dyspnea, *cough*
SYST: **Anaphylaxis, tumor lysis syndrome, antibody formation, Stevens-Johnson syndrome,** infusion reactions

Pharmacokinetics

Absorption	Unknown
Distribution	Protein binding, 68%-82%
Metabolism	Small amount, potent inhibitors or inducers of CYP3A4, may alter action
Excretion	Unknown
Half-life	Terminal 4-6 days; three components are released: MMAE (monomethyl auristatin E), ADC, and the total antibody; the half-life of MMAE a component is 3.43-3.6 days

Pharmacodynamics

Onset	Unknown
Peak	ADC: End of infusion MME: 1-3 days
Duration	Unknown

INTERACTIONS
Individual drugs

Boceprevir, dalfopristin; delavirdine, isoniazid, indinavir, itraconazole, ketoconazole, quinupristin, rifampin, ritonavir; telithromycin, tipranavir: increased brentuximab component action:
Bleomycin: increased noninfectious pulmonary toxicity; do not use together

Drug/herb
St. John's wort: increased brentuximab CYP3A4 inducers P-gb inhibitors action
Decrease: brentuximab action-CYP3A4 inducers

NURSING CONSIDERATIONS
Assessment

⚠ Tumor lysis syndrome (TLS): Assess for **hyperkalemia, hyperphosphatemia, hypocalcemia; may develop renal failure may use allopurinol or rasburicase to prevent TLS; monitor serum BUN/Creatinine**
⚠ Pregnancy: determine if pregnancy is planned or suspected, pregnancy D
⚠ Progressive multifocal leukoencephalopathy (PML): Assess for weakness, or paralysis, vision loss, impaired speech, and cognitive deterioration; often fatal
- Monitor CBC and differential, LFTs, serum bilirubin (direct and indirect), electrolytes, uric acid, neurologic function

Patient/family education

⚠ Teach patient to report immediately weakness, change in vision, impaired speech; peripheral neuropathy, neutropenia if severe
⚠ Advise patient to use reliable contraception, pregnancy D; avoid breastfeeding
- Use the diluted sol immediately or store in refrigerator for ≤24 hr after reconstitution; do not freeze

Evaluation
Positive therapeutic outcome
- Decreasing symptoms of Hodgkin's disease (increased lymph nodes, night sweats, weight loss, splenomegaly, hepatomegaly)

brimonidine ophthalmic
See Appendix B

brinzolamide ophthalmic
See Appendix B

bromfenac ophthalmic
See Appendix B

bromocriptine (Rx)
(broe-moe-krip′teen)
Cycloset, Parlodel
Func. class.: Antiparkinsonian agent; DOPamine receptor agonist
Pregnancy category B

Do not confuse: bromocriptine/benztropine/brimonidine, **Parlodel**/pindolol/Provera

ACTION: Inhibits prolactin release by activating postsynaptic dopamine receptors; activation of striatal dopamine receptors may be reason for improvement in Parkinson's disease

Therapeutic outcome: Decreased involuntary movements in Parkinson's disease; decreased breastfeeding; decreased hormone levels in acromegaly; absence of amenorrhea in hyperprolactinemia

USES: Parkinson's disease, amenorrhea/galactorrhea caused by hyperprolactinemia, infertility, acromegaly, pituitary adenomas, adjunct in type 2 diabetes

Unlabeled uses: Neuroleptic malignant syndrome, alcoholism, premenstrual syndrome, mastalgia, cocaine withdrawal, premenstrual breast syndromes

CONTRAINDICATIONS
Hypersensitivity to ergot, bromocriptine; severe ischemic disease, severe peripheral vascular disease, uncontrolled hypertension, preeclampsia, migraine

Precautions: Pregnancy **B,** breastfeeding, children, hepatic/renal disease, pituitary tumors, peptic ulcer disease, sulfite hypersensitivity, pulmonary fibrosis, dementia, GI bleeding, bipolar disorder

DOSAGE AND ROUTES
Parkinson's disease
Adult: PO 1.25 mg bid with meals; may increase q2-4wk by 2.5 mg/day; not to exceed 100 mg/day, levodopa should be continued while bromocriptine is being instituted

Hyperprolactinemia
Adult: PO 1.25-2.5 mg with meals; may increase by 2.5 mg q3-7days; usual dosage 2.5-15 mg/day

Acromegaly
Adult: PO 1.25-2.5 mg/day × 3 days at bedtime; may increase by 1.25-2.5 mg q3-7days; usual range 20-30 mg/day; max 100 mg/day

Type 2 diabetes (Cycloset only)
Adult: PO (initially) 0.8 mg qd in AM within 2hr of waking, titrate by 0.8 mg/day no more than qwk to max 1.6-4.8 mg/day

Pituitary adenoma
Adult: PO 1.25 mg bid-tid, may increase over several weeks to 10-20 mg/day

Traumatic brain injury (unlabeled)
Adult: PO 2.5 mg daily, continue if response occurs

Available forms: Caps 5 mg; tabs 2.5 mg; (Perodel), 0.8mg (cycloset)

Implementation
• Give with meals or milk to prevent GI symptoms; crush tab if patient has swallowing difficulty
• Give at bedtime so dizziness, orthostatic hypotension do not occur
• Store at room temperature in airtight container

ADVERSE EFFECTS
CNS: *Headache,* depression, restlessness, anxiety, nervousness, confusion, **seizures,** hallucinations, *dizziness,* fatigue, drowsiness, abnormal involuntary movements, psychosis, weakness

CV: *Orthostatic hypotension,* decreased B/P, palpitations, extrasystole, **shock,** dysrhythmias, bradycardia, **MI**

EENT: Blurred vision, diplopia, burning eyes, nasal congestion

GI: *Nausea, vomiting, anorexia,* cramps, constipation, diarrhea, dry mouth, GI hemorrhage

GU: Frequency, retention, incontinence, diuresis

INTEG: *Rash on face, arms,* alopecia, coolness, pallor of fingers, toes, peripheral edema

META: Hypoglycemia

Pharmacokinetics
Absorption	Poorly absorbed
Distribution	Unknown
Metabolism	Liver, completely
Excretion	85%-98% feces
Half-life	4 hr (initial); 50 hr (terminal)

Pharmacodynamics
Onset	½-1½ hr
Peak	1-3 hr
Duration	8-12 hr

INTERACTIONS
Individual drugs
Alcohol: increased disulfiramlike reaction

Chloramphenicol, levodopa, probenecid: increased neurologic effects

Haloperidol, loxapine, methyldopa, metoclopramide, reserpine: decreased levels of bromocriptine

Levodopa: increased neurologic effects

Metoclopramide: decreased effect of bromocriptine

Drug classifications
Antihypertensives: increased hypotension

Butyrophenones, CYP3A4 inhibitors, phenothiazines, thioxanthenes: decreased bromocriptine effect

Contraceptives (oral), estrogens, MAOIs, phenothiazines, progestins: decreased levels of bromocriptine

CYP3A4 inducers: increased bromocriptine effect

Salicylates, sulfonamides: increased neurologic effects

Drug/herb
Horehound: increased serotonin effect

Drug/lab test
Increased: growth hormone, AST, ALT, BUN, CK, uric acid, alkaline phosphatase

NURSING CONSIDERATIONS
Assessment
• Assess symptoms of **Parkinson's disease** (EPS): shuffling gait, muscle rigidity, involuntary movements, pill rolling, muscle spasms, drooling before, during treatment
• **Assess for resolution of symptoms of neuroleptic malignant syndrome: decreased temp, seizures, sweating, pulse**
• Monitor for change in size of soft-tissue volume in acromegaly
• **Pregnancy: may cause postpartum conception, use pregnancy testing q4wk or if menstruation does not occur**
• Monitor B/P; establish baseline, compare with other readings; this product decreases B/P and causes orthostatic hypotension; patient should remain recumbent for 2-4 hr after first dose; supervise ambulation

Patient/family education
• Advise patient to change position slowly to prevent orthostatic hypotension
• Tabs may be crushed and mixed with food; bromocriptine to be taken within 2 hr of rising
• **Caution patient to use contraceptives during treatment with this product; pregnancy may occur; to use methods other than oral contraceptives/subdermal implants**
• Teach patient that therapeutic effect for Parkinson's disease may take 2 mo, titrate slowly: galactorrhea, amenorrhea
• Caution patient to avoid hazardous activity if dizziness, drowsiness occurs during treatment start-up
• Advise patient to avoid alcohol and OTC medication unless approved by prescriber
• **Teach patients with acromegaly to notify prescriber immediately if severe headache, nausea, vomiting, blurred vision occur; indicates change in or enlargement of tumor**

• **Advise patient to report symptoms of MI immediately**
• Teach patient to take with food, avoid alcohol

Evaluation
Positive therapeutic outcome
• Parkinson's disease: decreased slow movements, decreased drooling
• Decreased breast engorgement with accompanied pain, tenderness
• Acromegly: decreased growth hormone levels

budesonide (Rx)
(byoo-des´oh-nide)
Eceris, Entocort EC, Pulmicort, Pulmicort Flexhaler, Pulmicort Respules, Pulmicort Turbohaler, Rhinocort Aqua, Uceris
Func. class.: Glucocorticoid
Pregnancy category C

ACTION: Prevents inflammation by depression of migration of polymorphonuclear leukocytes, fibroblasts, reversal of increased capillary permeability and lysosomal stabilization; does not suppress hypothalamus and pituitary function

USES: Rhinitis; prophylaxis for asthma; Crohn's disease, ulcerative colitis

CONTRAINDICATIONS
Hypersensitivity, status asthmaticus, acute bronchospasm

Precautions: Pregnancy **C**; inhaled form pregnancy **B**; breastfeeding, children, TB, fungal, bacterial, systemic viral infections, ocular herpes simplex, nasal septal ulcers; hepatic disease, diabetes, GI disease, increased intraocular pressure

DOSAGE AND ROUTES
Rhinitis
Adult and child >6 yr: Spray/inh 2 sprays in each nostril AM, PM, or 4 sprays in each nostril AM

Asthma
Adult and child >6 yr: INH 400-1200 mcg/day
Child 1-8 yrs previously taking bronchodilator alone: (Re spules) 0.5 mg q day or 0.25 mg bid susp via jet nebulizer, max 0.5 mg q day; previously using inhaled corticosteroid 0.5 mg q day or 0.25 mg bid susp via jet nebulizer, max 0.5 mg bid

Crohn's disease, ulcerative colitis (Uceris)
Adult: PO 9 mg daily AM × 8 wk

Laryngotracheobronchitis (croup) (unlabeled)

Infant ≥3 months-child ≤5 yr: (Pulmicort Respules INH susp) 2 mg inhaled as a single dose

Available forms: Dry powder for INH 90, 180, 32 mcg/actuation (Rhinocort Aqua) nasal spray; susp for inh 0.5 mg/2 ml, 0.25 mg/2 ml; ext rel tab (Uceris) 9 mg; cap 3 mg, rectal foam 2 mg/actuation

Implementation
PO route (Crohn's disease)
• Swallow caps whole; do not break, crush, or chew, take in AM
• May repeat 8-wk course if needed; may taper to 6 mg/day for 2 wk before cessation
Oral inh route (dry powder for inh) (Pulmicort Turbuhaler)
• A new Turbuhaler should be primed before use, per the priming instructions that come with the device; while priming the Turbuhaler and loading the dose, hold in upright position; to load the dose on a primed inhaler, twist the brown grip fully to the right as far as it will go, then twist it back fully to the left; there will be the sound of a "click"
• When inhaling, the Turbuhaler may be held upright or horizontally; turn head away from the inhaler and breathe out; place the mouthpiece between the lips and inhale deeply and forcefully; remove the inhaler from the mouth and exhale normally; do not blow or exhale into the mouthpiece; do not chew or bite on the mouthpiece; if more than one dose is required, repeat the steps
• After the last dose, rinse the mouth with water; do not swallow the water; keep inhaler clean and dry
Inh susp route for nebulization (Pulmicort Respules)
• Use via jet nebulizer connected to an air compressor with adequate airflow and equipped with a mouthpiece or suitable face mask; do not use ultrasonic nebulizers
• See manufacturer's direction on use of nebulizer and preparation of the solution
• Gently shake the ampule in a circular motion before opening it and placing the suspension in the nebulizer reservoir; using the "blow by" technique (i.e., holding the face mask or open tube near the patient's nose and mouth) is not recommended; use inh susp separately in the nebulizer
• Store inhal susp upright at controlled room temperature and protected from light; after opening the envelope, the shelf life of the unused respules is 2 wk; return unused respules to the aluminum foil envelope to protect from light; opened respule should be used promptly

Intranasal inhalation route
• Instruct patient on proper nasal inhalation priming and use; shake inhaler well; prior to initial use, the Rhinocort Aqua container must be shaken gently and the pump must be primed by actuating 8 times; if used daily, the pump does not need to be reprimed; if not used for 2 consecutive days, reprime with 1 spray or until a fine spray appears; if not used for more than 14 days, rinse the applicator and reprime with 2 sprays or until a fine spray appears; blow nose gently, without squeezing; with head upright, spray into each nostril; sniff while squeezing the bottle quickly and firmly; after use, rinse the tip of the bottle with hot water, taking care not to suck water into the bottle, and dry with a clean tissue; replace the cap
• To avoid the spread of infection, do not use the container for more than one person
• Store at 59°-86° F (15°-30° C); keep away from heat, open flame
Rectal Foam Route
• Product is flammable, may use prior to bedtime, applicators are single use only

ADVERSE EFFECTS
CNS: *Headache,* insomnia, hypertonia, syncope, dizziness, drowsiness
CV: Chest pain, hypertension, sinus tachycardia, palpitation
EENT: *Sinusitis, pharyngitis,* rhinitis, oral candidiasis
ENDO: Adrenal insufficiency, growth suppression in children
GI: Dry mouth, dyspepsia, nausea, vomiting, abdominal pain
MISC: Ecchymosis, fever, *hypersensitivity,* flu-like symptoms, epistaxis, dysuria
MS: Back pain, myalgias, fractures
RESP: Nasal irritation, cough, nasal bleeding, *respiratory infections,* **bronchospasm**

Pharmacokinetics

Absorption	39%
Distribution	In airways, protein binding 85%-90%
Metabolism	Liver
Excretion	In urine (60%), small amounts in feces, enters breast milk
Half-life	2-3.6 hr

Pharmacodynamics

Onset	Respules 2-8 days, Rhinocort Aqua 10 hr
Peak	Respules 4-6 wk, Rhinocort Aqua 2 wk
Duration	Unknown

INTERACTIONS
Individual drugs
Varicella live vaccine: avoid concurrent use in pediatric patients

Drug classifications
CYP3A inhibitors: increased budesonide effect; dose adjustment may be required

NURSING CONSIDERATIONS
Assessment
• Assess respiratory status: rate, rhythm, increase in bronchial secretions, wheezing, chest tightness; provide fluids to 2 L/day to decrease thickness of secretions; check for oral candidiasis
• **For bronchospasm, stop treatment and give bronchodilator**
• With viral infections, corticosteroid use can mask infections
• For increased intraocular pressure, discontinue use if increase occurs

Patient/family education
• Teach patient to notify prescriber of pharyngitis, nasal bleeding, oral candidiasis
• Instruct patient not to exceed recommended dosage; adrenal suppression may occur
• Teach patient to carry/wear emergency ID identifying steroid use
• Instruct patient to read and follow package directions
• Instruct patient to prevent exposure to infections, especially viral
• Advise to use good oral hygiene if using by nebulizer or inhaler
• Teach patient to avoid breastfeeding
• Teach patient that product is not a bronchodilator and is not to be used for asthma; to use regularly
• Teach how to use as described in "administer"
• Advise to notify prescriber if symptoms persist after 3 wk, that results usually take 2 wk
• Advise to notify prescriber if exposure to measles, chickenpox occurs

Evaluation
Positive therapeutic outcome
• Absence of asthma, rhinitis

budesonide nasal agent
See Appendix B

bumetanide (Rx)
(byoo-met′a-nide)
Bumex, Burinex ❧
Func. class.: Loop diuretic, antihypertensive
Chem. class.: Sulfonamide derivative
Pregnancy category C

ACTION: Acts on the ascending loop of Henle in the kidney to inhibit the reabsorption of the electrolytes sodium and chloride

Therapeutic outcome: Decreased edema in lung tissue and peripherally; decreased B/P

USES: Edema in congestive heart failure, ascites, heart failure

CONTRAINDICATIONS
Hypersensitivity to sulfonamides, anuria, hepatic coma

> **BLACK BOX WARNING:** Electrolyte imbalance

Precautions: Pregnancy **C**, breastfeeding, neonates, severe renal disease, ascites, hepatic cirrhosis, blood dyscrasias, ototoxicity, hyperuricemia, hypokalemia, hyperglycemia, oliguria, hypomagnesemia, hypovolemia

> **BLACK BOX WARNING:** Dehydration

DOSAGE AND ROUTES
Adult/adolescent: PO 0.5-2 mg daily may give 2nd or 3rd dose at 4-5 hr intervals; max 10 mg/day; may be given on alternate days or intermittently; **IM/IV** 0.5-1 mg; may give 2nd or 3rd dose at 2-3 hr intervals; max 10 mg/day
Child (unlabeled): PO/IM/IV 0.015-0.1 mg/kg/day or every other day, max 10 mg/day

Available forms: Tabs 0.5, 1, 2, 5 mg ❧; inj 0.25 mg/ml

Implementation
• Give in AM to avoid interference with sleep
• Potassium replacement if potassium level is <3.0 mg/dl whole, or use oral solutions; product may be crushed if patient is unable to swallow
PO route
• Use in AM to prevent nocturia
• The safest dosage schedule is on alternate days, without regard to food

IV route
- Do not use solution that is yellow or has a precipitate or crystals

IV, direct route
- Give undiluted through Y-tube or 3-way stopcock; give 20 mg or less/min

Intermittent IV infusion route
- May be added to 0.9% NaCl, D_5W, $D_{10}W$, $D_{20}W$, invert sugar 10% in electrolyte #1, LR, sodium lactate $\frac{1}{6}$ mol/L; use within 24 hr to ensure compatibility; give through Y-tube or 3-way stopcock; give at 4 mg/min or less; use infusion pump

Syringe compatibility: Doxapram

Y-site compatibilities: Acyclovir, alfentanil, allopurinol, amifostine, amikacin, aminocaproic acid, aminophylline, amiodarone, amoxicillin, amphotericin B lipid complex (Abelcet), amphotericin B liposome (AmBisome), anidulafungin, ascorbic acid injection, atenolol, atracurium, atropine, aztreonam, benztropine, bivalirudin, bleomycin, buprenorphine, butorphanol, calcium chloride/gluconate, CARBOplatin, caspofungin, cefamandole, ceFAZolin, cefepime, cefmetazole, cefonicid, cefotaxime, cefoTEtan, cefOXitin, cefTAZidime, ceftizoxime, ceftobiprole, cefTRIAXone, cefuroxime, cephapirin, chloramphenicol, cimetidine, cisatracurium, CISplatin, cladribine, clarithromycin, clindamycin, codeine, cyanocobalamin, cyclophosphamide, cycloSPORINE, cytarabine, DACTINomycin, DAPTOmycin, dexamethasone, dexmedetomidine, digoxin, diltiazem, diphenhydrAMINE, DOBUTamine, DOCEtaxel, DOPamine, doripenem, doxacurium, DOXOrubicin, doxycycline, enalaprilat, ePHEDrine, EPINEPHrine, epirubicin, epoetin alfa, eptifibatide, ertapenem, erythromycin, esmolol, etoposide, famotidine, fentaNYL, filgrastim, fluconazole, fludarabine, fluorouracil, folic acid, furosemide, gatifloxacin, gemcitabine, gentamicin, glycopyrrolate, granisetron, heparin, hydrocortisone sodium succinate, HYDROmorphone, hydrOXYzine, IDArubicin, ifosfamide, imipenem-cilastatin, indomethacin, insulin (regular), irinotecan, isoproterenol, ketorolac, labetalol, levofloxacin, lidocaine, linezolid, LORazepam, magnesium sulfate, mannitol, mechlorethamine, melphalan, meperidine, metaraminol, methotrexate, methoxamine, methyldopa, methylPREDNISolone, metoclopramide, metoprolol, metroNIDAZOLE, mezlocillin, micafungin, miconazole, milrinone, mitoXANtrone, morphine, moxalactam, multiple vitamins injection, mycophenolate, nafcillin, nalbuphine, naloxone, netilmicin, nitroglycerin, nitroprusside, norepinephrine, octreotide, ondansetron, oxacillin, oxaliplatin, oxytocin, palonosetron, pamidronate, pancuronium, pantoprazole, PEMEtrexed, penicillin G potassium/sodium, pentazocine, PENTobarbital, PHENobarbital, phenylephrine, phytonadione, piperacillin, piperacillin-tazobactam, polymyxin B, potassium chloride, procainamide, promethazine, propofol, propranolol, protamine, pyridoxine, quiNIDine, ranitidine, remifentanil, rifampin, ritodrine, riTUXimab, rocuronium, sodium acetate, sodium bicarbonate, succinylcholine, SUFentanil, tacrolimus, teniposide, theophylline, thiamine, thiotepa, ticarcillin, ticarcillin-clavulanate, tigecycline, tirofiban, TNA, tobramycin, tolazoline, TPN, traMADol, trastuzumab, trimetaphan, urokinase, vancomycin, vasopressin, vecuronium, verapamil, vinCRIStine, vinorelbine, voriconazole

ADVERSE EFFECTS
CNS: Headache, fatigue, weakness, vertigo, encephalopathy
CV: *Hypotension,* chest pain, ECG changes, **circulatory collapse,** dehydration
EENT: Loss of hearing
ELECT: *Hypokalemia, hypochloremic alkalosis, hypomagnesemia, hyperuricemia, hypocalcemia, hyponatremia*
ENDO: *Hyperglycemia*
GI: *Nausea,* diarrhea, dry mouth, vomiting, anorexia, cramps, upset stomach, abdominal pain
GU: *Polyuria,* **renal failure,** *glycosuria,* premature ejaculation, hypercholesterolemia
HEMA: **Thrombocytopenia, leukopenia, granulocytopenia, hemoconcentration**
INTEG: *Rash, pruritus, purpura,* **Stevens-Johnson syndrome,** sweating, photosensitivity
MS: Muscular cramps, stiffness, arthritis

Pharmacokinetics

	PO/IM
Absorption	Rapidly, completely absorbed
	PO/IM/IV
Distribution	Crosses placenta, protein binding >91%
Metabolism	Liver (30%-40%)
Excretion	Breast milk, urine (50% unchanged), feces (20%)
Half-life	1-1½ hr

Pharmacodynamics

	PO	IM	IV
Onset	½-1 hr	40 min	5 min
Peak	1-2 hr	1-2 hr	½ hr
Duration	3-6 hr	4-6 hr	3-6 hr

INTERACTIONS
Individual drugs
Digoxin: increased toxicity

Indomethacin: decreased diuretic and antihypertensive effects of bumetanide

Lithium: decreased renal clearance causing increased toxicity

Metolazone: increased diuresis, electrolyte loss

Probenecid: decreased diuretic effect, other diuretics

Drug classifications
Aminoglycosides: increased ototoxicity, cisplatin

Antidiabetics: decreased antidiabetic effects

NSAIDs: decreased diuretic effect

Potassium-wasting products: increased hypokalemia

Drug/herb
Hawthorn, horse chestnut: increased diuretic effect

Drug/Lab
Increase: Glucose

Decrease: Chloride, potassium, sodium, calcium, phosphorus

NURSING CONSIDERATIONS
Assessment
• Assess patient for tinnitus, hearing loss, ear pain; periodic testing of hearing is needed when high doses of this product are given by **IV** route

• Assess fluid volume status: I&O ratio and record, distended red veins, crackles in lung, color, quality and specific gravity of urine, skin turgor, adequacy of pulses, moist mucous membranes, bilateral lung sounds, peripheral pitting edema; dehydration symptoms of decreasing output, thirst, hypotension, dry mouth and mucous membranes should be reported; if urinary output decreases or azotemia occurs, product should be discontinued

• Monitor for electrolyte imbalances: potassium, sodium, calcium, magnesium; also include BUN, blood pH, ABGs, uric acid, CBC, blood glucose; severe electrolyte imbalances should be corrected before starting treatment

• Assess B/P before and during therapy with patient lying, standing, and sitting as appropriate; orthostatic hypotension can occur rapidly

• **Monitor for digoxin toxicity (anorexia, nausea, vomiting, confusion, paresthesia, muscle cramps) in patients taking digoxin; lithium toxicity in those taking lithium**

Patient/family education
• Teach patient to take the medication early in the day to prevent nocturia

• Instruct the patient to take with food or milk if GI symptoms of nausea and anorexia occur

• Teach patient to maintain weekly record of weight and notify prescriber of weight loss of >5 lb

• Caution the patient that this product causes a loss of potassium, so food rich in potassium should be added to the diet; refer to a dietitian for assistance in planning

• Caution the patient not to exercise in hot weather or stand for prolonged periods since orthostatic hypotension will be enhanced

• Teach patient not to use alcohol or any OTC medications without prescriber's approval; serious product reactions may occur

• Emphasize the need to contact prescriber immediately if muscle cramps, weakness, nausea, dizziness, or numbness occur

• Teach patient to take own B/P and pulse and record

• Caution the patient that orthostatic hypotension may occur; patient should rise slowly from sitting or reclining positions and lie down if dizziness occurs

• Teach patient to continue taking medication even if feeling better; this product controls symptoms but does not cure the condition

• Advise the patient with hypertension to continue other medical treatment (exercise, weight loss, relaxation techniques, cessation of smoking), edema, weight gain

Evaluation
Positive therapeutic outcome
• Decreased edema
• Decreased B/P
• Increased diuresis

⚠ HIGH ALERT

buprenorphine (Rx)
(byoo-pre-nor′feen)

Belbuca, Buprenex, Butrans, Subutex

Func. class.: Opioid analgesic, partial agonist

Chem. class.: Thebaine derivative

Pregnancy category C

Controlled substance schedule V (parenteral); schedule III (tablet)

Do not confuse: Buprenex/Bumex

ACTION: Depresses pain impulse transmission at the spinal cord level by interacting with opioid receptors, partial agonist at MU-opiod receptor

Therapeutic outcome: Relief of pain

USES: Moderate to severe pain, opiate agonist withdrawal/dependence

Unlabeled uses: Cocaine

CONTRAINDICATIONS

Hypersensitivity, ileus, status asthmaticus

> **BLACK BOX WARNING:** Respiratory depression

Precautions: Pregnancy **C**, breastfeeding, substance abuse/alcoholism, increased intracranial pressure, MI (acute), severe heart disease, respiratory depression, renal/hepatic/pulmonary disease, hypothyroidism, Addison's disease

> **BLACK BOX WARNING:** QT prolongation, use of heating pad, accidental exposure, potential for overdose/poisoning, substance abuse

DOSAGE AND ROUTES

Adult: IM/IV 0.3 mg q6-8hr prn; may repeat; reduce dosage in geriatric, may repeat after 30-60 min; EPIDURAL (unlabeled) 4 mcg/kg or 2 mcg/kg (epidural injection), remove over 48 hr; TD: each patch is worn for 7 days (moderate-severe pain); **opioid-naive patients** (those taking <30 mg oral morphine or equivalent prior to beginning treatment with TD buprenorphine), 5 mcg/hr q7days, overestimating dose can be fatal; **conversion from other opiate agonist therapy,** titrate from other opioids for up to 7 days to no more than 30 mg oral morphine or equivalent prior to beginning TD therapy, begin with 5 mcg/hr q7days; for those with daily dose of 30-80 mg oral morphine or equivalent, start with 10 mcg/hr q7days; for those >80 mg oral morphine or equivalent start with 20 mcg/hr q7days; Transmucosal: 75 mcg qd or q12hrs

Child 2-12 yr: IM/IV 2-6 mcg/kg q4-8hr

Opiate dependence

Adult/adolescent ≥16 yr: SL 8 mg day 1, 16 mg day 2, then maintenance 16 mg daily

Available forms: Inj 0.3 mg/ml (1-ml vials); SL tab 2, 8 mg as base, TD system 5, 7.5, 10, 15, 20 mcg/hr (weekly); oral dissolving film 75, 300, 450, 600, 750, 900 mcg

Implementation

• Give by inj (IM, **IV**), only with resuscitative equipment available; give slowly to prevent rigidity

SL route

• Do not chew, dissolve under tongue or take 2 or more at same time

Transdermal route

• Apply to clean, dry, intact skin, each patch should be worn for 7 days, may use first aid tape if edge of patch is not adhering

> **BLACK BOX WARNING:** Do not apply direct heat source to patch

• Apply to upper outer arm, upper chest/back, or side of chest

IM route

• **Give** deep in large muscle mass; rotate sites of inj

IV route

• **Give IV** direct undiluted over ≥3-5 min (0.3 mg/2 min); give slowly

• With antiemetic if nausea, vomiting occur

• When pain is beginning to return; determine dosage interval by patient response; rapid injection will increase side effects

Y-site compatibilities: Acyclovir, alfentanil, allopurinol, amifostine, amikacin, aminocaproic acid, amphotericin B liposome (AmBisone), anidulafungin, ascorbic acid injection, atenolol, atracurium, atropine, aztreonam, benztropine, bivalirudin, bleomycin, bumetanide, butorphanol, calcium chloride/gluconate, CARBOplatin, cefamandole, ceFAZolin, cefepime, cefotaxime, cefoTEtan, cefOXitin, cefTAZidime, ceftizoxime, cefTRIAXone, cefuroxime, chloramphenicol, chlorproMAZINE, cimetidine, cisatracurium, CISplatin, cladribine, clindamycin, cyanocobalamin, cyclophosphamide, cycloSPORINE, cytarabine, D₅W-dextrose 5%, DACTINomycin, DAPTOmycin, dexamethasone, dexmedetomidine, digoxin, diltiazem, diphenhydrAMINE, DOBUTamine, DOCEtaxel, DOPamine, doxacurium, DOXOrubicin HCl, doxycycline, enalaprilat, ePHEDrine, EPINEPHrine, epirubicin, epoetin alfa, eptifibatide, ertapenem, erythromycin, esmolol, etoposide, famotidine, fenoldopam, fentaNYL, filgrastim, fluconazole, fludarabine, gatifloxacin, gemcitabine, gentamicin, glycopyrrolate, granisetron, heparin, hydrocortisone, hydrOXYzine, IDArubicin, ifosfamide, imipenem-cilastatin, inamrinone, insulin (regular), irinotecan, isoproterenol, ketorolac, labetalol, lactated Ringer's injection, levofloxacin, lidocaine, linezolid, LORazepam, magnesium sulfate, mannitol, mechlorethamine, melphalan, meperidine, metaraminol, methicillin, methotrexate, methoxamine, methyldopate, methylPREDNISolone, metoclopramide, metoprolol, metroNIDAZOLE, mezlocillin, miconazole, midazolam, milrinone, minocycline, mitoXANtrone, morphine, moxalactam, multiple vitamins injection, mycophenolate mofetil, nafcillin, nalbuphine, naloxone, nesiritide, netilmicin, nitroglycerin, nitroprusside, norepinephrine, octreotide, ondansetron, oxacillin, oxaliplatin, oxytocin, palonosetron, pamidronate, pancuronium, papaverine, PEMEtrexed, penicillin G potassium/sodium, pentamidine, pentazocine, phenylephrine, phytonadione, piperacillin, piperacillin-tazobactam, polymyxin B, potassium chloride, procainamide, prochlorperazine promethazine, propofol, propranolol, protamine, pyridoxine, quiNIDine, ranitidine, remifentanil, Ringer's injection, riTUXimab, rocuronium, sodium acetate, succinylcholine, SUFentanil, tacrolimus, teniposide, theophylline, thiamine, thiotepa, ticarcillin, ticarcillin-clavulanate, tigecycline, tirofiban, TNA (3-in-1), tobramycin, tolazoline, TPN, trastuzumab, trimetaphan, urokinase, vancomycin, vasopressin, vecuronium, verapamil, vinCRIStine, vinorelbine, voriconazole

Additive incompatibilities: Diazepam, floxacillin, furosemide, LORazepam

ADVERSE EFFECTS

CNS: *Drowsiness, dizziness, confusion, headache, sedation, euphoria,* increased intracranial pressure, amnesia, weakness, CNS depression
CV: Palpitations, bradycardia, change in B/P, tachycardia, QT prolongation, hypo/hypertension
EENT: Tinnitus, blurred vision, *miosis,* diplopia
GI: *Nausea,* vomiting, anorexia, constipation, cramps, dry mouth, abdominal pain, hepatotoxicity
GU: Dysuria, urinary retention
INTEG: *Rash,* urticaria, bruising, flushing, diaphoresis, pruritus
RESP: Respiratory depression, dyspnea, hypo/hyperventilation

Pharmacokinetics

Absorption	Well absorbed (IM)
Distribution	Crosses placenta
Metabolism	Liver, extensively by CYP3A4
Excretion	Kidneys, feces, breast milk
Half-life	2.2 hr (**IV**); 26 hr (transdermal); 37 hr (SL)

Pharmacodynamics

	IM	IV
Onset	15 min	Immediate
Peak	1 hr	5 min
Duration	6-10 hr (Epidural route: duration is dose-dependent)	6 hr

INTERACTIONS
Individual drugs
Alcohol: increased respiratory depression, hypotension, sedation

Drug classifications

> **BLACK BOX WARNING:** Antidysrhythmics (class IA, III): increased QT prolongation

Antihistamines, antipsychotics, CNS depressants, MAOIs, sedatives/hypnotics, skeletal muscle relaxants: increased respiratory depression, hypotension
CYP3A4 inducers (carBAMazepine, PHENobarbital, phenytoin, rifampin): decreased buprenorphine effect
CYP3A4 inhibitors (erythromycin, indinavir, ketoconazole, ritonavir, saquinavir): increased buprenorphine effect
Opioids: increased CNS depression

Drug/herb
St. John's wort: increased CNS depression

NURSING CONSIDERATIONS
Assessment
• Assess **pain characteristics:** location, intensity, type, severity before medication administration and after treatment

> **BLACK BOX WARNING:** Potential for overdose may occur from chewing, swallowing, snorting, or injecting extracted product from TD formulation

> **BLACK BOX WARNING: QT prolongation:** Assess often in those taking class Ia, III antidysrhythmics; patients with hypokalemia or cardiac instability (TD), max TD 20 mcg/hr q7 days

• Monitor VS after parenteral route; note muscle rigidity, product history, liver, kidney function tests, respiratory dysfunction: respiratory depression, character, rate, rhythm; notify prescriber if respirations are <10/min
• Monitor CNS changes: dizziness, drowsiness, hallucinations, euphoria, LOC, pupil reaction; withdrawal in opioid-dependent persons; if dependence occurs within 2 wk of discontinuing product, **withdrawal symptoms** will occur
• Monitor allergic reactions: rash, urticaria
• Monitor bowel pattern; severe constipation can occur

Patient/family education
• Instruct patient to report any symptoms of CNS changes, allergic reactions
• Caution patients to avoid CNS depressants: alcohol, sedative/hypnotics for at least 24 hr after taking this product

BLACK BOX WARNING: Advise that psychologic dependence leading to substance abuse may result when used for extended periods; long-term use is not recommended

• Advise to avoid driving, other hazardous activities until reaction is known
• Discuss with patient that dizziness, drowsiness, and confusion are common; to avoid getting up without assistance; to avoid hazardous activities
• Discuss in detail all aspects of the product
• Do not start new meds/herbs without prescriber approval
• Start stool softner/ laxatives to lessen constipation

Evaluation
Positive therapeutic outcome
• Relief of pain

TREATMENT OF OVERDOSE:
Naloxone 0.4 mg ampule diluted in 10 ml 0.9% NaCl, give by direct **IV** push 0.02 mg q2min (adult)

buPROPion (Rx)
(byoo-proe′pee-on)
Aplenzin, Buproban, Forfivo XL, Wellbutrin, Wellbutrin SR, Wellbutrin XL, Zyban
Func. class.: Antidepressant—miscellaneous, smoking deterrent
Chem. class.: Aminoketone
Pregnancy category C

Do not confuse: buPROPion/busPIRone, **Zyban**/Diovan/Zagam

ACTION: Inhibits reuptake of DOPamine, norepinephrine, serotonin

Therapeutic outcome: Decreased symptoms of depression after 2-3 wk

USES: Depression (Wellbutrin), smoking cessation (Zyban); seasonal affective disorder, substance abuse, glaucoma, smoking, cardiac disease, heart failure

Unlabeled uses: Neuropathic pain, enhancement of weight loss, attention-deficit/hyperactivity disorder (ADHD)

CONTRAINDICATIONS
Hypersensitivity, head trauma, stroke, intracranial mass, eating disorders, seizure disorder

Precautions: Pregnancy **C,** breastfeeding, geriatric, renal/hepatic disease, recent MI, cranial trauma, seizure disorders, substance abuse, glaucoma, smoking, cardiac disease, heart failure

BLACK BOX WARNING: Children <18 yr, suicidal thinking/behavior (young adults)

DOSAGE AND ROUTES
Depression
Adult: PO 100 mg bid initially, then increase after 3 days to 100 mg tid if needed, max 150 mg single dose; ER/SR, initially 150 mg AM, increase to 300 mg/day if initial dose is tolerated, after no less than 4 days; after several wk, titrate to 200 mg bid; Aplenzin 174 mg qAM; may increase to 348 mg qAM on day 4; may increase to 522 mg after several weeks if needed; Forfivo XL (not for initial treatment) 450 mg q day after titration with another product (300mg/day × ≥ 2 wks)
Geriatric: PO 50-100 mg/day, may increase by 50-100 mg q3-4days

Smoking cessation (Zyban)
Adult: SR 150 mg q day × 3 days, then 150 mg bid for remainder of treatment, initiate 1-2 wk before targeted "quit day," continue for 7-12 wk; in combination with nicotine TD, 150 mg q day × 3 days, then 150 mg bid for remainder of treatment, give ≥8 hr apart, max 300 mg/day, initiate 1-2 wk before targeted "quit day," continue for 7-12 wk, may be continued for 8-20 wk

Seasonal affective disorder
Adult: PO (Wellbutrin XL) 150 mg as a single dose in the AM, after 1 wk may be increased to 300 mg/day; (Aplenzin) 174 mg/day in AM, after 7 days may increase to 348 mg/day

Available forms: Tabs 75, 100 mg; sus rel tabs (**SR**), 100, 150, 200 mg; ext rel tab (XL) 100, 150, 300, 450 mg (SR-12 hr, XL-24 hr); ext rel tab (Aplenzin) 174, 348, 522 mg

Implementation
• Give with food or milk for GI symptoms
• Give sugarless gum, hard candy, or frequent sips of water for dry mouth
• **When switching to Aplenzin from Wellbutrin, Wellbutrin SR, or XL use these equivalents: 174 buPROPion HBr = 150 mg buPROPion HCl; 348 mg buPROPion HBr = 300 mg buPROPion HCl; 522 mg buPROPion HBr = 450 mg buPROPion HCl**
• **Wellbutrin immediate rel,** separate by ≥6 hr, give in 3 divided doses; **Wellbutrin SR,** if multiple doses are used, separate by ≥8 hr; **Wellbutrin XL,** give q day in AM; Zyban SR, give in 2 divided doses ≥8 hr apart; **Aplenzin ER,** give q day in AM, a larger dose of Aplenzin is needed because these products are not equivalent

Adverse effects: *italics* = common; **bold** = life-threatening

• Store at room temperature; do not freeze

ADVERSE EFFECTS

CNS: *Headache, agitation, confusion, seizures,* delusions, *insomnia, sedation, tremors,* dizziness, akinesia, bradykinesia, suicidal ideation, mania, hot flashes, myoclonia, chest pain, flushing

CV: Dysrhythmias, *hypertension,* palpitations, *tachycardia,* hypotension, complete AV block, QRS prolongation (overdose)

EENT: *Blurred vision, auditory disturbance,* tinnitus

GI: *Nausea, vomiting, dry mouth,* anorexia, diarrhea, increased appetite, *constipation,* altered taste

GU: Impotence, frequency, retention, *menstrual irregularities,* nocturia, altered libido

INTEG: *Rash,* pruritus, *sweating,* Stevens-Johnson syndrome

MISC: *Weight loss or gain*

Pharmacokinetics

Absorption	Well absorbed; bioavailability poor
Distribution	Unknown
Metabolism	Liver extensively
Excretion	Kidneys
Half-life	14 hr, steady state (immediate release) 1½-5 wk

Pharmacodynamics

Onset	Up to 4 wk
Peak	Unknown
Duration	Unknown

INTERACTIONS

Individual drugs

Alcohol, levodopa, theophylline: increased risk of seizures

CarBAMazepine, cimetidine, PHENobarbital, phenytoin: decreased buPROPion effect

Cimetidine: increased buPROPion levels

Ritonavir: increased buPROPion toxicity

Tamoxifen: decreased effect of tamoxifen

Do not use within 14 days of MAOIs

Drug classifications

Antidepressants, benzodiazepines, MAOIs, phenothiazines, steroids (systemic): increased risk of seizures

CYP2D6/CYP2B6 inhibitors: increased buPROPion effect

CYP450, CYP2D6 products: decreased buPROPion effects

CYP2D6, CYP2B6 inducers: decreased buPROPion effect

MAOIs: acute toxicity

Drug/herb

Kava, valerian: increased CNS depression

Drug/lab test

Positive urine drug screen for amphetamine possible

NURSING CONSIDERATIONS

Assessment

• Monitor B/P (with patient lying, standing), pulse q4hr; if systolic B/P drops 20 mm Hg hold product, notify prescriber; take vital signs q4hr in patients with CV disease

• Assess smoking cessation progress after 7-12 wk, if progress has not been made, product should be discontinued

⚠ Assess for increased risk of seizures; if patient has used CNS depressant or CNS stimulants, dosage of buPROPion should not be exceeded

• Monitor blood studies: CBC, leukocytes, differential, cardiac enzymes if patient is receiving long-term therapy

• Monitor hepatic studies: AST, ALT, bilirubin if on long-term treatment

• Check weight weekly; appetite may increase with product

• Assess ECG for flattening of T wave, bundle branch block, AV block, dysrhythmias in cardiac patients

• Assess for EPS primarily in geriatric: rigidity, dystonia, akathisia

> **BLACK BOX WARNING:** Assess mental status: mood, sensorium, affect, suicidal tendencies; increase in psychiatric symptoms: depression, panic

• Monitor urinary retention, constipation; constipation is more likely to occur in children or geriatric

• Identify alcohol consumption; if alcohol was consumed, hold dose

Patient/family education

• Teach patient that therapeutic effects may take 2-3 wk; not to increase dose without prescriber's approval; that treatment for smoking cessation lasts 7-12 wk

• Teach patient to use caution in driving or other activities requiring alertness because of drowsiness, dizziness, blurred vision; to avoid rising quickly from sitting to standing, especially geriatric

• Teach patient to avoid alcohol ingestion; alcohol may increase risk of seizures, obtain approval for other products

• Teach patient to increase fluids, bulk in diet if constipation, urinary retention occur, especially

geriatric; notify prescriber immediately if urinary retention occurs
• Teach patient to take gum, hard sugarless candy, or frequent sips of water for dry mouth
• Advise patient not to use with nicotine patches unless directed by prescriber, may increase B/P

> **BLACK BOX WARNING:** Teach patient that risk of seizures increases when dose is exceeded or if patient has seizure disorder; suicidal ideas, behavior, hostility, depression may occur in children or young adults

• Teach patient to notify prescriber if pregnancy is suspected or planned
• Report hearing, visual, CNS changes
• May need to use stool softener/laxative

Evaluation
Positive therapeutic outcome
• Decrease in depression
• Absence of suicidal thoughts
• Smoking cessation

TREATMENT OF OVERDOSE:
ECG monitoring, induce emesis, lavage, activated charcoal, administer anticonvulsant

busPIRone (Rx)
(byoo-spye′rone)
BuSpar, BuSpar Dividose, Buspirex ✦, Bustab ✦, PMS-Buspirone ✦
Func. class.: Antianxiety, sedative
Chem. class.: Azaspirodecanedione
Pregnancy category B

Do not confuse: busPIRone/buPROPion

ACTION: Acts by inhibiting the action of serotonin (5-HT) by binding to serotonin and dopamine receptors; also increases norepinephrine metabolism; has shown little potential for abuse, a good choice in substance abuse

Therapeutic outcome: Decreased anxiety

USES: Management and short-term relief of generalized anxiety disorders

CONTRAINDICATIONS
Hypersensitivity, child <18 yr

Precautions: Pregnancy **B**, breastfeeding, geriatric, impaired renal/hepatic function

DOSAGE AND ROUTES
Adult: PO 7.5 mg bid; may increase by 5 mg/day q2-3days; max 60 mg/day

Renal/hepatic dose
Adult: PO reduce by 25%-50% in mild to moderate hepatic disease, do not use in severe hepatic disease, CCr 11-70 ml/min reduce dose by 25%-50%, CCr <10 ml/min do not use

Available forms: Tabs 5, 7.5, 10, 15, 30 mg

Implementation
• Give with food or milk for GI symptoms (avoid grapefruit juice); sugarless gum, hard candy, frequent sips of water for dry mouth
• May be crushed

ADVERSE EFFECTS
CNS: *Dizziness, headache, depression, stimulation, insomnia, nervousness, light-headedness, numbness, paresthesia, incoordination, tremors,* excitement, involuntary movements, confusion, akathisia, nightmares, hostility
CV: *Tachycardia, palpitations,* hypo/hypertension, **CVA, CHF, MI,** chest pain
EENT: *Sore throat, tinnitus, blurred vision, nasal congestion,* red, itching eyes, change in taste, smell
GI: *Nausea, dry mouth, diarrhea, constipation,* flatulence, increased appetite, rectal bleeding
GU: Frequency, hesitancy, menstrual irregularity, change in libido
INTEG: *Rash,* edema, pruritus, alopecia, dry skin
MISC: *Sweating,* fatigue, weight gain, fever, **serotonin syndrome**
MS: *Pain, weakness,* muscle cramps, spasms, myalgia
RESP: Hyperventilation, chest congestion, shortness of breath

Pharmacokinetics

Absorption	Rapid
Distribution	Protein binding 86%
Metabolism	Liver, extensively
Excretion	Feces
Terminal half-life	2-4 hr

Pharmacodynamics

Onset	Unknown
Peak	40-90 min
Duration	Unknown

INTERACTIONS
Individual drugs
Alcohol: increased CNS depression; avoid use

Drug classifications

Products metabolized by CYP3A4 (erythromycin, itraconazole, nefazodone, ketoconazole, ritonavir, verapamil, diltiazem, several other protease inhibitors): increased busPIRone levels

MAOIs, procarbazine: increased B/P, do not use together

Products induced by CYP3A4 (rifampin, phenytoin, PHENobarbital, carBAMazepine, dexamethasone): decreased busPIRone action

Psychotropics: increased CNS depression, avoid use

Selective serotonin reuptake inhibitors (SNRIs, serotonin receptor agonists): increase serotonin syndrome

Drug/food

Grapefruit juice: increased peak concentration of busPIRone

NURSING CONSIDERATIONS
Assessment

• Assess anxiety reaction: inability to sleep, apprehension, dread, foreboding, or uneasiness related to unidentified source of danger
• Assess for previous product dependence or tolerance; if patient is product dependent or tolerant, amount of medication should be restricted
• Monitor B/P (lying, standing), pulse; if systolic B/P drops 20 mm Hg, hold product, notify prescriber; check I&O; may indicate renal dysfunction
• Monitor mental status: mood, sensorium, affect, sleeping patterns, drowsiness, dizziness, suicidal tendencies; withdrawal symptoms when dose is reduced or product discontinued
• Assess for CNS reaction, some reactions may be unpredictable

Patient/family education

• Teach patient that product may be taken consistently with or without food; if dose is missed take as soon as remembered; do not double doses
• Caution patient to avoid OTC preparations unless approved by the prescriber; to avoid alcohol ingestion and other psychotropic medications unless prescribed; that 2 wk of therapy may be required before therapeutic effects occur; to avoid large amounts of grapefruit juice, max effect 3-6 wk
• Caution patient to avoid driving and activities requiring alertness since drowsiness may occur; until medication response is known, tell patient that drowsiness may worsen at beginning of treatment
• Instruct patient not to discontinue medication abruptly after long-term use; if dose is missed, do not double

• Advise patient to rise slowly or fainting may occur, especially in geriatric

⚠ Serotonin syndrome: Teach patient to report immediately (fever, tremor, sweating, diarrhea, delirium)

Evaluation
Positive therapeutic outcome

• Increased well-being
• Decreased anxiety, restlessness, sleeplessness, dread

RARELY USED

busulfan (Rx)
(byoo-sul'fan)
Busulfex, Myleran
Func. class.: Antineoplastic alkylating agent
Chem. class.: Bifunctional alkylating agent
Pregnancy category D

USES: Chronic myelocytic leukemia, bone marrow ablation, stem cell transplant preparation in CML

CONTRAINDICATIONS

Pregnancy **D** (3rd trimester), breastfeeding, radiation, chemotherapy, blastic phase of chronic myelocytic leukemia, hypersensitivity

DOSAGE AND ROUTES
Chronic myelocytic leukemia

Adult: PO 4-8 mg/day or 1.8-4 mg/m²/day initially; reduce dosage if WBC levels reach 30,000-40,000/mm³; stop if WBC ≤20,000/mm³; maintenance 1-3 mg/day

Child: PO 0.06-0.12 mg/kg/day or 1.8-4.6 mg/m²/day, reduce if WBC is 30,000-40,000/mm³; discontinue if WBC ≤20,000/mm³

Allogenic hemopoietic stem cell transplantation in chronic myelogenous leukemia

Adult: IV 0.8 mg/kg over 2 hr, q6hr × 4 days (total 16 doses); give cyclophosphamide **IV** 60 mg/kg over 1 hr/day for 2 days, starting after 16th dose of busulfan

Available forms: Tabs 2 mg; sol for inj 6 mg/ml

ADVERSE EFFECTS

CV: *Hypotension,* thrombosis, *chest pain,* tachycardia, atrial fibrillation, heart block, pericardial effusion, cardiac tamponade (high dose with cyclophosphamide)

GI: Anorexia, constipation, dry mouth, nausea, vomiting, *diarrhea*
RESP: Alveolar hemorrhage, atelectasis, cough, hemoptysis, hypoxia, pleural effusion, pneumonia, sinusitis, pulmonary fibrosis
CNS: *Depression, dizziness, insomnia, headache*
EENT: *Blurred vision*
GU: Impotence, sterility, amenorrhea, gynecomastia, renal toxicity, hyperuremia, adrenal insufficiency–like syndrome
HEMA: Thrombocytopenia, leukopenia, pancytopenia, severe bone marrow depression
INTEG: Dermatitis, hyperpigmentation, alopecia
MISC: Chromosomal aberrations
RESP: Irreversible pulmonary fibrosis, pneumonitis

⚠ Advise patient that contraception is needed during treatment and for ≥3 months after the completion of therapy (pregnancy D); avoid breastfeeding; may cause infertility; discuss family planning before initiating therapy

Evaluation
Positive therapeutic outcome
• Decreased leukocytes to normal limits
• Absence of sweating at night
• Increased appetite, increased weight

butoconazole vaginal antifungal
See Appendix B

⚠ **HIGH ALERT**
butorphanol (Rx)
(byoo-tor′fa-nole)
Stadol ♣
Func. class.: Mixed opiate analgesic
Chem. class.: Opioid antagonist, partial agonist
Pregnancy category C
Controlled substance schedule IV

ACTION: Depresses pain impulse transmission at the spinal cord level by interacting with opioid receptors

Therapeutic outcome: Relief of pain

USES: Moderate to severe pain, general anesthesia induction/maintenance, headache, migraine, preanesthesia

CONTRAINDICATIONS
Hypersensitivity to this product or preservative, addiction (opioid)

Precautions: Pregnancy **C,** breastfeeding, child <18 yr, addictive personality, increased ICP, respiratory depression, renal/hepatic disease, ileus, COPD

DOSAGE AND ROUTES
Moderate to severe pain
Adult: IM 1-4 mg q3-4hr prn; **IV** 0.5-2 mg q3-4hr prn; **nasal** spray in 1 nostril; may give another dose 1-1½ hr later; may repeat if needed in q3-4hr after last dose
Geriatric: **IV** ½ adult dose at 2× the interval; **intranasal** if no relief in 90-120 min, may repeat with 1 spray

Severe pain
Adult: INTRANASAL 1 spray in each nostril q3-4hr

Renal/hepatic dose
Adult: INTRANASAL max 1 mg, followed by 1 mg in 90-120 min; IM/IV give 50% of dose (0.5 mg IV, 1 mg IM); do not repeat within 6 hr

Available forms: Inj 1, 2 mg/ml; INTRANASAL 10 mg/ml

Implementation
• Store in light-resistant container at room temperature
Nasal route
• Prime before first use, point sprayer away from face, pump activator 7 times until a fine, wide spray occurs; if not used for 48 hr, reprime by pumping 1-2 times
• If more than 1 spray is needed, use other nostril
• Do not share with others
• Nasal congestion/irritation may occur
IM route
• Give deeply in large muscle mass; rotate inj sites
Intranasal route
• Give 1 spray in nostril
• Remove clip and cover, prime before using until spray appears; pump must be reprimed q48hr; close nostril with finger and spray once quickly; have patient sniff
IV direct route
• Give **IV** undiluted at a rate of ≤2 mg/>3-5 min; titrate to patient response

Syringe incompatibilities: Dimenhy-DRINATE, PENTobarbital

Y-site compatibilities: Acyclovir, alfentanil, allopurinol, amifostine, amikacin, aminocaproic acid, aminophylline, amphotericin B liposome (AmBisome), anidulafungin, ascorbic acid injection, atenolol, atracurium, atropine, aztreonam, benztropine, bivalirudin, bleomycin, bumetanide, buprenorphine, calcium chloride/gluconate, CARBOplatin, caspofungin, cefamandole, ceFAZolin, cefepime, cefotaxime, cefoTEtan, cefOXitin, cefTAZidime, ceftizoxime, cefTRIAXone, cefuroxime, cephalothin, chlorproMAZINE, cimetidine, cisatracurium, CISplatin, cladribine, clindamycin, cyanocobalamin, cyclophosphamide, cycloSPORINE, cytarabine, DACTINomycin, DAPTOmycin, dexamethasone phosphate, dexmedetomidine, digoxin, diltiazem, diphenhydrAMINE, DOBUTamine, DOCEtaxel, DOPamine, doxacurium, DOXOrubicin, DOXOrubicin liposomal, doxycycline, enalaprilat, ePHEDrine, EPINEPHrine, epirubicin, epoetin alfa, eptifibatide, ertapenem, erythromycin, esmolol, etoposide, famotidine, fenoldopam, fentaNYL, filgrastim, fluconazole, fludarabine, fluorouracil, gatifloxacin, gemcitabine, gentamicin, glycopyrrolate, granisetron, heparin, hydrocortisone, hydrOXYzine, IDArubicin, ifosfamide, imipenem-cilastatin, irinotecan, isoproterenol, ketorolac, labetalol, lactated Ringer's injection, levofloxacin, lidocaine, linezolid injection, LORazepam, magnesium, mannitol, mechlorethamine, melphalan, meperidine, metaraminol, methicillin, methotrexate, methoxamine, methyldopa, methylPREDNISolone, metoclopramide, metoprolol, metroNIDAZOLE, mezlocillin, milrinone, minocycline, mitoXANtrone, morphine, multiple vitamins injection, mycophenolate mofetil, nafcillin, nalbuphine, naloxone, nesiritide, netilmicin, niCARdipine, nitroglycerin, nitroprusside, norepinephrine, octreotide, ondansetron, oxacillin, oxaliplatin, oxytocin, palonosetron, pamidronate, pancuronium, papaverine, PEMEtrexed, penicillin G potassium/sodium, pentazocine, PHENobarbital, phenylephrine, phytonadione, piperacillin, piperacillin-tazobactam, polymyxin B, potassium chloride, procainamide, prochlorperazine, promethazine, propofol, propranolol, protamine, pyridoxine, quiNIDine, ranitidine, remifentanil, Ringer's injection, riTUXimab, rocuronium, sargramostim, sodium acetate, succinylcholine, SUFentanil, tacrolimus, teniposide, theophylline, thiamine, thiotepa, ticarcillin, ticarcillin-clavulanate, tigecycline, tirofiban, TNA, tobramycin, tolazoline, TPN, trastuzumab, urokinase, vancomycin, vasopressin, vecuronium, verapamil, vinCRIStine, vinorelbine, voriconazole

ADVERSE EFFECTS

CNS: *Drowsiness, dizziness, confusion, headache, sedation, euphoria, weakness, hallucinations,* insomnia (nasal)

CV: Palpitations, bradycardia, hypotension
EENT: Tinnitus, blurred vision, miosis, diplopia, nasal congestion, unpleasant taste
GI: *Nausea, vomiting, anorexia, constipation, cramps*
GU: Urinary retention
INTEG: Rash, urticaria, bruising, flushing, diaphoresis, pruritus
RESP: Respiratory depression

Pharmacokinetics

Absorption	Well absorbed (IM, nasal); complete (**IV**)
Distribution	Crosses placenta, protein binding 80%
Metabolism	Liver, extensively
Excretion	Feces (10%-15%); kidneys, unchanged (small amounts)
Half-life	2-9 hr

Pharmacodynamics

	IM	IV	Nasal
Onset	5-15 min	1 min	15 min
Peak	30-60 min	4-5 min	1-2 hr
Duration	3-4 hr	2-4 hr	4-5 hr

INTERACTIONS
Individual drugs
Alcohol: increased respiratory depression, hypotension, sedation

Drug classifications
Antipsychotics, CNS depressants, opioids, MAOIs, sedative/hypnotics, skeletal muscle relaxants: increased respiratory depression, hypotension

MAOIs: do not use 2 wk before butorphanol, fatal reaction

NURSING CONSIDERATIONS
Assessment
• Monitor VS after parenteral administration; note muscle rigidity, product history, liver, kidney function tests, respiratory dysfunction: respiratory depression, character, rate, rhythm; notify prescriber if respirations are <10/min
• Monitor CNS changes: dizziness, drowsiness, hallucinations, euphoria, LOC, pupil reaction
• Monitor allergic reactions: rash, urticaria
• Assess for withdrawal symptoms in opioid-dependent patient; pulmonary embolism, vascular occlusion, abscesses, ulcerations

Patient/family education
• Instruct patient to report any symptoms of CNS changes, allergic reactions; to avoid CNS depressants: alcohol, sedative/hypnotics for at least 24 hr after taking this product

• Discuss with patient that dizziness, drowsiness, and confusion are common; to avoid getting up without assistance, hazardous activities
• Discuss in detail all aspects of the product
Nasal route
• Teach patient to blow nose to clear both nostrils before using
• Patient should replace clip and cover after use; caution patient not to shake medication

• Teach patient how to use nasal product
• Teach patient to avoid hazardous activities

Evaluation
Positive therapeutic outcome
• Pain relief

TREATMENT OF OVERDOSE:
Narcan 0.4-2 mg **IV**, O$_2$, **IV** fluids, vasopressors

Adverse effects: *italics* = common; **bold** = life-threatening

RARELY USED

cabozantinib
(ka′boe-zan′ti-nib)
Cometriq
Func. class.: Antineoplastic biologic response modifiers
Chem. class.: Signal transduction inhibitor (STI)
Pregnancy category D

USES: Treatment of progressive metastatic medullary thyroid cancer

CONTRAINDICATIONS
Pregnancy (D), hypersensitivity

DOSAGE AND ROUTES
Adult: PO 140 mg/day until disease progression or unacceptable toxicity
• Avoid the concomitant use of strong 3A4 inhibitors or inducers if possible; temporary interruption of therapy and a dosage reduction may be necessary in patients who develop toxicity or intolerable side effects

calcitonin (salmon) (Rx)
Fortical, Miacalcin
Func. class.: Parathyroid agents (calcium regulator)
Chem. class.: Polypeptide hormone
Pregnancy category C

ACTION: Decreases bone resorption, blood calcium levels; increases deposits of calcium in bones; opposes parathyroid hormone

Therapeutic outcome: Lowered calcium level, decreasing symptoms of Paget's disease

USES: Paget's disease, postmenopausal osteoporosis, hypercalcemia

CONTRAINDICATIONS
Hypersensitivity to this product or fish

Precautions: Pregnancy **C**, breastfeeding, children, hypotension

DOSAGE AND ROUTES
Postmenopausal osteoporosis
Adult: SUBCUT/IM 100 units/day; nasal 200 units (1 spray) alternating nostrils daily, activate pump before 1st dose

Paget's disease
Adult: SUBCUT/IM 100 units daily, maintenance 50-100 units daily or every other day, or 3 × per wk

Hypercalcemia
Adult: SUBCUT/IM 4 units/kg q12hr, increase to 8 units/kg q12hr if response is unsatisfactory, no more than 4-7 days

Available forms: Inj 200 units/ml; nasal spray 200 units/actuation

Implementation
• Store at <77° F (25° C); protect from light
SUBCUT route
• Rotate inj sites
IM route (salmon)
• Give after test dose of 10 international units/ml, 0.1 ml intradermally; watch 15 min; **give** only with EPINEPHrine and emergency meds available
• IM inj in deep muscle mass slowly; rotate sites; preferred route if volume is >2 ml
Nasal route
• Use alternating nostrils for nasal spray; allow to warm to room temperature, prime to get full spray

ADVERSE EFFECTS
CNS: Headache, **tetany,** chills, weakness, dizziness, fever, tremors
CV: Chest pressure, hypertension
EENT: Nasal congestion, eye pain
GI: Nausea, diarrhea, vomiting, anorexia, abdominal pain, salty taste, epigastric pain
GU: Diuresis, nocturia, urine sediment, frequency, cystitis
INTEG: Rash, flushing, pruritus of earlobes, edema of feet, inj site reaction
MS: Swelling, tingling of hands, backache, myalgia
RESP: Dyspnea, flulike symptoms
SYST: Anaphylaxis

Pharmacokinetics

Absorption	Completely absorbed
Distribution	Unknown
Metabolism	Rapid; kidneys, tissue, blood
Excretion	Kidneys, inactive metabolite
Half-life	1 hr

Pharmacodynamics

	SUBCUT
Onset	15 min
Peak	4 hr
Duration	8-24 hr

INTERACTIONS
Individual drugs
Lithium: decreased lithium effect

Drug classifications
Bisphosphonates (Paget's disease): decreased effect of nasal spray

NURSING CONSIDERATIONS
Assessment
• **Anaphylaxis, hypersensitivity: inability to breathe, rash, fever; have emergency equipment nearby**
• Assess for GI symptoms, polyuria, flushing, head swelling, tingling, headache; may indicate hypercalcemia; nervousness, irritability, twitching, seizures, spasm, paresthesia indicate hypocalcemia during beginning of treatment
• Identify nutritional status; check diet for sources of vit D (milk, some seafood), calcium (dairy products, dark green vegetables), phosphates
• Monitor BUN, creatinine, uric acid, chloride, electrolytes, urine pH, urinary calcium, magnesium, phosphate, urinalysis; vit D 50-135 international units/dl), alkaline phosphatase baseline and q3-6mo; check urine sediment for casts throughout treatment; monitor urine hydroxyproline in Paget's disease, biochemical markers of bone formation/absorption, radiologic evidence of fracture; bone density (osteoporosis)
• **Toxicity (can occur rapidly): Assess for increased product level, since toxic reactions occur rapidly; have parenteral calcium or gluconate on hand if calcium level drops too low; check for tetany (irritability, paresthesia, nervousness, muscle twitching, seizure, tetanic spasm)**

Patient/family education
• Teach method of inj if patient will be responsible for self-medication
• Instruct patient to notify prescriber for hypercalcemic relapse: renal calculi, nausea, vomiting, thirst, lethargy, deep bone or flank pain
• Teach patient that warmth and flushing occur and last 1 hr
• Provide a low-calcium diet as prescribed (Paget's disease, hypercalcemia)

• Advise patients with osteoporosis to increase calcium and vit D in diet and to continue with moderate exercise to prevent continued bone loss
• **Advise patients to report difficulty swallowing or change in side effects to prescriber immediately**

Evaluation
Positive therapeutic outcome
• Calcium levels 9-10 mg/dl
• Decreasing symptoms of Paget's disease, including pain
• Decreased bone loss in osteoporosis

calcitriol (Rx)
(kal-si-tree′ole)
Calcijex, Rocaltrol, Vectical
Func. class.: Parathyroid agent (calcium regulator)
Chem. class.: Vitamin D hormone
Pregnancy category C

Do not confuse: calcitriol/Calciferol

ACTION: Increases intestinal absorption, renal reabsorption of calcium, provides calcium for bones, increases renal tubular resorption of phosphate

Therapeutic outcome: Calcium at normal level

USES: Hypocalcemia in chronic renal disease, hyperparathyroidism, pseudohypoparathyroidism, psoriasis, renal osteodystrophy

CONTRAINDICATIONS
Hypersensitivity, hyperphosphatemia, hypercalcemia, vit D toxicity

Precautions: Pregnancy **C**, breastfeeding, renal calculi, CV disease

DOSAGE AND ROUTES
Hypocalcemia (stage 5 chronic kidney disease, on dialysis)
Adult and child ≥6 yr: **PO** 0.25 mcg/day
IV 1-2 mcg three times/wk, initially; may increase by 0.5-1 mcg q4-8wk
Child 1-5 yr: **PO** 0.25-2 mcg/day

Renal osteodystrophy
Adult and child ≥3 yr: **PO** 0.25 mcg/day, may increase to 0.5 mcg/day
Child <3 yr: **PO** 0.01-0.015 mcg/kg/day

Hypoparathyroidism
Adult and child ≥6 yr: **PO** 0.25 mcg/day, may increase q2-4wk, maintenance 0.5-2 mcg/day

Adverse effects: *italics* = common; **bold** = life-threatening

Child 1-5 yr: PO 0.25-0.75 mcg daily
Child <1 yr: PO 0.04-0.08 mcg/kg/day

Available forms: Caps 0.25, 0.5 mcg; inj 1 mcg/ml, 2 mcg/ml; oral sol 1 mcg/ml; top 3 mcg/g

Implementation
PO route
- Do not break, crush, or chew caps
- Give with meals for GI symptoms
- Store protected from light, heat, moisture

IV route
- Give by direct **IV** over 1 min

ADVERSE EFFECTS
CNS: Drowsiness, headache, vertigo, fever, lethargy, hallucinations
CV: Palpitations, hypertension
ENDO: Hypercalcemia
EENT: Blurred vision, photophobia
GI: Nausea, diarrhea, vomiting, jaundice, anorexia, dry mouth, constipation, cramps, metallic taste
GU: Polyuria, hypercalciuria, hyperphosphatemia, hematuria, thirst
MS: Myalgia, arthralgia, decreased bone development, weakness
SYST: Anaphylaxis
INTEG: Pain at injection site, rash, pruritus

Pharmacokinetics

Absorption	Well absorbed
Distribution	To liver, crosses placenta
Metabolism	Liver
Excretion	Bile
Half-life	3-6 hr, undergoes hepatic recycling, excreted in bile

Pharmacodynamics

Onset	2-6 hr
Peak	10-12 hr
Duration	Up to 5 days

INTERACTIONS
Individual drugs
Cholestyramine, mineral oil: decreased absorption of calcitriol
Phenytoin: increased vit D metabolism
Verapamil: increased dysrhythmias

Drug classifications
Antacids (magnesium): increased hypermagnesemia
Calcium supplements, diuretics (thiazide): increased hypercalcemia
Cardiac glycosides: increased dysrhythmias
Vitamin D products: increased toxicity

Vitamins (fat-soluble): decreased calcitriol absorption

Drug/food
Large amounts of high-calcium foods may cause hypercalcemia

Drug/lab test
Increase: AST/ALT
False: increased cholesterol
Interference: alkaline phosphatase, electrolytes

NURSING CONSIDERATIONS
Assessment
- Assess GI symptoms, polyuria, flushing, head swelling, tingling, headache; may indicate hypercalcemia
- **Hypercalcemia:** dry mouth, metallic taste, polyuria, bone pain, muscle weakness, headache, fatigue, change in LOC, dysrhythmias, increased respirations, anorexia, nausea, vomiting, cramps, diarrhea, constipation, confusion, paresthesia, twitching, Chvostek's/Trousseau's sign, **hypocalcemia**
- Identify nutritional status; check diet for sources of vit D (milk, some seafood), calcium (dairy products, dark green vegetables), phosphates
- Monitor BUN, creatinine, uric acid, chloride, electrolytes, urine pH, urinary calcium, magnesium, phosphate, urinalysis (calcium should be kept at 9-10 mg/dl; vit D 50-135 international units/dl), alkaline phosphatase baseline and q3-6mo

Patient/family education
- Teach patient the symptoms of hypercalcemia (renal stones, nausea, vomiting, anorexia, lethargy, thirst, bone or flank pain) and about foods rich in calcium
- Advise patient to avoid products with sodium: cured meats, dairy products, cold cuts, olives, beets, pickles, soups, meat tenderizers in chronic renal failure
- Advise patient to avoid products with potassium: oranges, bananas, dried fruit, peas, dark green leafy vegetables, milk, melons, beans in chronic renal failure
- Advise patient to avoid OTC products containing calcium, potassium, or sodium in chronic renal failure
- Instruct patient to avoid all preparations containing vit D
- Instruct patient to monitor weight weekly; maintain fluid intake

Evaluation
Positive therapeutic outcome
- Calcium levels 9-10 mg/dl

C

calcium carbonate (Rx) (PO-OTC, Rx)
Alka-Mints, Amitone, Apo-Cal ✦, BioCal, Calcarb, Calci-Chew, Calciday, Calci-Mix, Calcite ✦, Caltrate, Chooz, Maalox Antacid, Os-Cal, Rolaids Extra Strength Soft-chew, Tums, Tums E-X
Func. class.: Antacid, calcium supplement
Chem. class.: Calcium product

calcium acetate (OTC)
(kal'see-um ass'e-tate)
Eliphos, PhosLo, Phoslyra
Pregnancy category C

Do not confuse: Os-Cal/Asacol

ACTION: Neutralizes gastric acidity

Therapeutic outcome: Neutralized gastric acidity; calcium at normal levels

USES: Antacid, calcium supplement; not suitable for chronic therapy, hyperphosphatemia, hypertension in pregnancy, osteoporosis, prevention/treatment of hypocalcemia, hypoparathyroidism

CONTRAINDICATIONS
Hypersensitivity, hypercalcemia

Precautions: Pregnancy **C**, breastfeeding, geriatric, fluid restriction, decreased GI motility, GI obstruction, dehydration, renal disease, hyperparathyroidism, bone tumors

DOSAGE AND ROUTES
Nutritional supplement including osteoporosis prophylaxis
Adult ≥51 yr: PO 1000-1500 mg/day elemental calcium (2500-3750 calcium carbonate)
Adult 19-50 yr: PO 1000 mg/day elemental calcium (2500 mg calcium carbonate)

Chronic hypocalcemia
Adult: PO 2-4 g/day elemental calcium (5-10 g calcium carbonate) in 3-4 divided doses
Child: PO 45-65 mg/kg/day elemental calcium (112.5-162.5 mg/kg calcium carbonate) in 4 divided doses
Neonate: PO 50-150 mg/kg/day elemental calcium (125-375 mg/kg/day in 4-6 divided doses, max 1 g/day)

Supplementation
Adolescent and child 9-18 yr: PO 1300 mg elemental calcium (3250 mg calcium carbonate)
Child 4-8 yr: PO 800 mg/day elemental calcium (2000 mg calcium carbonate)

Child 1-3 yr: PO 500 mg/day elemental calcium (1250 mg calcium carbonate)
Infant 6-12 mo: PO 270 mg/day elemental calcium based on total intake
Neonate and infant <6 mo: PO 210 mg/day elemental calcium based on total intake

Hyperphosphatemia
Adult: PO Individualized on response

Heartburn, dyspepsia, hyperacidity (OTC)
Adult: PO 1-2 tabs q2hr, max 9 tabs/24 hr (Alka-mints); chew 2-4 tab q1hr prn, max 16 tabs (Tums regular strength); chew 2-4 tab q1hr prn, max 10 tabs (Tums E-X); chew 2-3 tabs q1hr prn, max 10 tabs/24 hr (Tums Ultra); chew 2 tabs q2-3hr, max 19 tabs/24 hr (Titralac Extra Strength)

Available forms: Calcium carbonate: **chewable tabs** 350, 420, 450, 500, 750, 1000, 1250 mg; **tabs** 500, 600, 650, 667, 1000, 1250, 1500 mg; **gum** 300, 450 500 mg; **susp** 1250 mg/5 ml; **caps** 1250 mg; **powder** 6.5 g/packet; calcium acetate: **tabs** 667 mg (169 mg Ca), **caps** 500 mg (125 mg Ca); **gelcaps:** 667 mg (169 mg elemental Ca)

Implementation
PO route
• Administer as antacid 1 hr after meals and at bedtime
• Administer as supplement 1½ hr after meals and at bedtime
• Administer only with regular tablets or capsules; do not give with enteric-coated tablets
• Administer laxatives or stool softeners if constipation occurs

ADVERSE EFFECTS
GI: *Constipation,* anorexia, nausea, vomiting, flatulence, diarrhea, rebound hyperacidity, eructation
GU: Calculi, hypercalciuria

Pharmacokinetics
Absorption	⅓ absorbed by small intestines, must have adequate vit D for absorption
Distribution	Unknown
Metabolism	Unknown
Excretion	Feces, urine, crosses placenta
Half-life	Unknown

Pharmacodynamics
Peak	Unknown

INTERACTIONS
Individual drugs
Atenolol, etidronate, phenytoin, risedronate, ketoconazole: decreased levels of each drug
Digoxin: increased toxicity from hypercalcemia
QuiNIDine: increased quiNIDine levels

Drug classifications
Amphetamines: increased levels of amphetamines
Calcium channel blockers, calcium supplements, fluoroquinolones, iron products, salicylates, tetracyclines: PO decreased levels of each specific product
Thiazide diuretics: increased hypercalcemia

Drug/lab test
Decrease: phosphates
False increase: chloride
False decrease: magnesium, oxalate, lipase
False positive: benzodiazepines

NURSING CONSIDERATIONS
Assessment
• Monitor Ca^+ (serum, urine); Ca^+ should be 8.5-10.5 mg/dl, urine Ca^+ should be 150 mg/day, monitor weekly
⚠ Assess for milk-alkali syndrome: nausea, vomiting, disorientation, headache
• Assess for constipation; increase bulk in the diet if needed
• Assess for **hypercalcemia**: headache, nausea, vomiting, confusion; hypocalcemia: paresthesia, twitching, colic, dysrhythmias, Chvostek's/Trousseau's sign
• Assess those taking digoxin for toxicity
• Assess those taking for abdominal pain, heartburn, indigestion before, after administration

Patient/family education
• Advise patient to increase fluids to 2 L unless contraindicated, to add bulk to diet for constipation; notify prescriber of constipation
• Advise patient not to switch antacids unless directed by prescriber, not to use as antacid for >2 wk without approval by prescriber
• Teach patient that therapeutic dose recommendations are figured as elemental calcium
• Advise to avoid excessive use of alcohol, caffeine, tobacco
• Teach to avoid spinach, cereals, dairy products in large amounts

Evaluation
Positive therapeutic outcome
• Absence of pain, decreased acidity
• Decreased hyperphosphatemia in renal failure (Acetate)

CALCIUM SALTS

calcium chloride (Rx)
calcium gluceptate (Rx)
calcium gluconate (Rx)
calcium lactate (PO-OTC, IV-Rx)

Func. class.: Electrolyte replacement—calcium product
Pregnancy category C

ACTION: Calcium needed for maintenance of nervous, muscular, skeletal systems, enzyme reactions, normal cardiac contractility, coagulation of blood; affects secretory activity of endocrine, exocrine glands

Therapeutic outcome: Calcium at normal level, absence of increased magnesium, potassium

USES: Prevention and treatment of hypocalcemia, hypermagnesemia, hypoparathyroidism, neonatal tetany, cardiac toxicity caused by hyperkalemia, lead colic, hyperphosphatemia, vit D deficiency, osteoporosis prophylaxis, calcium antagonist toxicity (calcium channel blocker toxicity)

CONTRAINDICATIONS
Hypercalcemia, digoxin toxicity, ventricular fibrillation, renal calculi

Precautions: Pregnancy **C**, breastfeeding, children, renal disease, respiratory disease, cor pulmonale, digitalized patient, respiratory failure, diarrhea, dehydration

DOSAGE AND ROUTES
>> **Acute hypocalcemia (calcium chloride 10%):**
Adults: IV 0.5-1 g; **for tetany**, give over 5-10 min. Repeat q4-6 hrs, as needed by calcium concentrations or IV INF 15 mg/kg of elemental calcium (37.5 mg/kg calcium chloride) over 4-6 hr.
Child/infant: IV range from 2.7-5 mg/kg/dose (0.027-0.05 ml/kg/dose of 10%). **For tetany**, slow IV 10 mg/kg/dose over 5-10 min, may repeat initial dosage in 4-6 hr. The initial dose can be followed by a **CONT INF** max 200 mg/kg/day.

>> **(Calcium gluconate):**
Adults: IV 2-3 g slowly, max 5 ml/min (47.5 mg/min of calcium ion). **For tetany**, give over 5-10 min, repeat q6hr, as needed, as determined by serum calcium concentrations, max 15 g/day or IV INF 15 mg/kg of elemental calcium (167 mg/kg) over 4-6 hr may be administered if symptoms recur after initial IV calcium replacement
Child/infant: IV 200-500 mg/kg/day **CONT INF** or given in 4 divided doses, at max rate 5 ml/min (47.5 mg/min of calcium ion); **for tetany**,

IV 100-200 mg/kg over 5-10 min, may repeat after 6 hr or followed by 500 mg/kg/day IV as a **CONT INF** or in 3-4 divided doses.
Neonate: IV 200-800 mg/kg/day as a **CONT INF** or given in 3-4 divided doses. **For tetany,** 100-200 mg/kg IV is recommended, followed by 500 mg/kg/day **CONT INF** or given in 3-4 divided doses.

>> (Calcium lactate):
Adults: IM 10 ml 1-2/wk for 4-5 wk, may repeat if needed.

>> PO (calcium citrate):
Adults: PO 9.5-19 g/day in divided doses 2-4 times a day after meals

>> PO (calcium gluconate):
Adults: PO 22.5-45 g/day in 3-4 divided doses
Child/infant: PO 500-725 mg/kg/day in 4 divided doses
Neonate: PO 500-1500 mg/kg/day in 4-6 divided doses

>> PO (calcium lactate):
Adults: PO 15.4-30.8 g/day divided q8hr
Child: PO 345-500 mg/kg/day in divided doses q6-8 hrs, max 9 g/day
Infant: PO 400-500 mg/kg/day in divided doses q4-6 hr
CPR/cardiac arrest associated with hyperkalemia, hypermagnesemia, or ionized hypocalcemia (unlabeled)

>> IV (calcium chloride 10%):
Adult: IV 5-10 ml of a 10% solution (500-1000 mg) or 8-16 mg/kg given by slow IV inj; may repeat

>> IV (calcium gluconate):
Adult: IV 500-800 mg of 10% solution (5-8 ml) max 3 g
Infant/child: IV 60-100 mg/kg or intraosseous (0.6-1 ml/kg) max 3 g

>> For nutritional supplementation:
PO (any oral calcium salt; dosage expressed as elemental calcium):
Adults ≥ 51 yrs: PO 1200 mg per day (range 1000-1500 mg/day)
Adults 19-50 yrs: PO 1000 mg per day
Children/adolescents 9-18 years of age: PO 1300 mg per day
Children 4-8 years of age: PO 800 mg per day
Children 1-3 years of age: PO 500 mg per day
Infants 6-12 months of age: PO 270 mg per day based on total intake (consumption from breast milk/infant formula and solid food)
Neonate/infant <6 months of age: PO 210 mg per day based on total intake (content in human milk/infant formula). Source of calcium intake should come from food/breast milk only in order to prevent high levels of intake.

Therapeutic Drug Monitoring:
Ionized calcium concentrations are the preferred measure to determine true hypocalcemia. If total serum calcium concentrations are obtained, calcium concentrations should be adjusted if hypoalbuminemia or hyperalbuminemia is present. The corrected calcium concentration may be estimated from the following formula:

Corrected calcium (mg/dl) =

serum calcium (mg/dl) +

0.8 [4 − serum albumin (g/dl)]

Available forms: Many; check product listings

Implementation
PO route
• Give PO with or following meals to enhance absorption
• Store at room temperature
IM route
• Do not give chloride, gluconate IM

IV route
• Administer **IV** undiluted or diluted with equal amounts of 0.9% NaCl for inj to a 5% sol; give 0.5-1 ml/min
• Give through small-bore needle into large vein; if extravasation occurs, necrosis will result **(IV)**; IM inj may cause severe burning, necrosis, and tissue sloughing; warm sol to body temp before administering (only gluconate/glucceptate)
• Provide seizure precautions: padded side rails, decreased stimuli (noise, light); place airway suction equipment, padded mouth gag if calcium levels are low
• Patient should remain recumbent 30 min after IV dose

>> Calcium chloride

Y-site compatibility: Acyclovir, alemtuzumab, alfentanil, amikacin, aminocaproic acid, aminophylline, amiodarone, anidulafungin, argatroban, arsenic trioxide, ascorbic acid injection, asparaginase, atenolol, atracurium, atropine, azithromycin, aztreonam, benztropine, bivalirudin, bleomycin, bumetanide, buprenorphine, butorphanol, calcium gluconate, CARBOplatin, carmustine, caspofungin acetate, cefotaxime, cefoTEtan, cefOXitin, ceftaroline, ceftizoxime, chloramphenicol, chlorothiazide, chlorpheniramine, chlorproMAZINE, cimetidine, CISplatin, clindamycin, cloxacillin, colistimethate, cyanocobalamin, cyclophosphamide, cycloSPORINE, cytarabine, DACTINomycin, DAPTOmycin, DAUNOrubicin, dexmedetomidine, dexrazoxane, digoxin, diltiazem, diphenhydrAMINE, DOBUTamine, DOCEtaxel, dolasetron, DOPamine, doxacurium, doxapram, DOXOrubicin, doxycycline, edetate calcium disodium, enalaprilat, ePHEDrine, EPINEPHrine, epirubicin, epoetin alfa, eptifibatide, ergonovine, ertapenem, erythromycin, esmolol, etoposide, etoposide phosphate, famotidine, fenoldopam, fentaNYL, fluconazole, fludarabine, furosemide, gallamine, gallium, ganciclovir, gatifloxacin, gemcitabine, gentamicin, glycopyrrolate, granisetron, heparin sodium, HYDROmorphone, hydrOXYzine, IDArubicin, ifosfamide, inamrinone, insulin, regular, irinotecan, isoproterenol, kanamycin, labetalol, lactated Ringer's, lepirudin, leucovorin, lidocaine, lincomycin, linezolid, LORazepam, mannitol, mechlorethamine, meperidine, mephentermine, mesna, metaraminol, methohexital, methotrexate, methyldopate, metoclopramide, metoprolol, metroNIDAZOLE, micafungin, midazolam, milrinone, minocycline, mitoMYcin, mitoXANtrone, mivacurium, morphine, moxifloxacin, multiple vitamins injection, mycophenolate mofetil, nafcillin, nalbuphine, nalorphine, naloxone, nesiritide, niCARdipine, nitroglycerin, nitroprusside, norepinephrine, octreotide, ondansetron, oxytocin, PACLitaxel (solvent/surfactant), pancuronium, papaverine, penicillin G potassium/sodium, pentazocine, PENTobarbital, PHENobarbital, phentolamine, phenylephrine, phytonadione, piperacillin, piperacillin-tazobactam, polymyxin B, potassium, potassium chloride, procainamide, prochlorperazine, promazine, promethazine, propranolol, protamine, pyridoxine, quinupristin-dalfopristin, ranitidine, Ringer's injection, rocuronium, streptomycin, succinylcholine, SUFentanil, tacrolimus, teniposide, theophylline, thiamine, thiotepa, ticarcillin-clavulanate, tigecycline, tirofiban, TNA (3-in-1), tobramycin, tolazoline, topotecan, trimetaphan, tubocurarine, urokinase, vancomycin, vasopressin, vecuronium, verapamil, vinBLAStine, vinCRIStine, vinorelbine, voriconazole

Calcium gluconate Y-site compatibilities: Acyclovir, aldesleukin, alemtuzumab, alfentanil, allopurinol, amifostine, amikacin, aminocaproic acid, aminophylline, amiodarone, anidulafungin, argatroban, arsenic trioxide, ascorbic acid injection, asparaginase, atenolol, atracurium, atropine, azaTHIOprine, azithromycin, aztreonam, benztropine, bivalirudin, bleomycin, bumetanide, buprenorphine, butorphanol,

calcium chloride, CARBOplatin, carmustine, caspofungin, cefamandole, ceFAZolin, cefepime, cefoperazone, cefotaxime, cefoTEtan, cefOXitin, ceftaroline, cefTAZidime, ceftizoxime, cefuroxime, chloramphenicol sodium succinate, chlorothiazide, chlorpheniramine, chlorproMAZINE, cimetidine, ciprofloxacin, cisatracurium, CISplatin, cladribine, clindamycin, cloxacillin, codeine, colistimethate, cyanocobalamin, cyclophosphamide, cycloSPORINE, cytarabine, DACTINomycin, DAPTOmycin, DAUNOrubicin, DAUNOrubicin liposome, dexmedetomidine, dexrazoxane, digoxin, diltiazem, dimenhyDRINATE, diphenhydrAMINE, DOBUTamine, DOCEtaxel, dolasetron, DOPamine, doripenem, doxacurium, doxapram, DOXOrubicin, DOXOrubicin liposomal, doxycycline, edetate calcium disodium, enalaprilat, ePHEDrine, EPINEPHrine, epirubicin, epoetin alfa, eptifibatide, ergonovine, ertapenem, erythromycin, esmolol, etoposide, etoposide phosphate, famotidine, fenoldopam, fentaNYL, filgrastim, fludarabine, fluorouracil, folic acid (as sodium salt), furosemide, gallamine, gallium, ganciclovir, gatifloxacin, gemcitabine, gentamicin, glycopyrrolate, granisetron, heparin sodium, HYDROmorphone, hydrOXYzine, IDArubicin, ifosfamide, insulin, regular, irinotecan, isoproterenol, kanamycin, ketamine, labetalol, lactated Ringer's injection, lepirudin, leucovorin, levofloxacin, lidocaine, lincomycin, linezolid, LORazepam, magnesium sulfate, mannitol, mechlorethamine, melphalan, meperidine, mephentermine, mesna, metaraminol, methohexital, methotrexate, methyldopate, metoclopramide, metoprolol, metroNIDAZOLE, micafungin, midazolam, milrinone, mitoMYcin, mitoXANtrone, mivacurium, morphine, moxifloxacin, multiple vitamins injection, nafcillin, nalbuphine, nalorphine, naloxone, nesiritide, netilmicin, niCARdipine, nitroglycerin, nitroprusside, norepinephrine, octreotide, ondansetron, oritavancin, oxaliplatin, oxytocin, PACLitaxel (solvent/surfactant), palonosetron, pancuronium, papaverine, penicillin G potassium/sodium, pentamidine, pentazocine, PENTobarbital, PHENobarbital, phentolamine, phenylephrine, phytonadione, piperacillin, polymyxin B, potassium acetate/chloride, procainamide, prochlorperazine, promazine, promethazine, propofol, propranolol, protamine, pyridoxine, quiNIDine, ranitidine, remifentanil, Ringer's, riTUXimab, rocuronium, sargramostim, sodium acetate, streptomycin, succinylcholine, SUFentanil, tacrolimus, telavancin, teniposide, theophylline, thiamine, thiotepa, ticarcillin, ticarcillin-clavulanate, tigecycline, tirofiban, TNA (3-in-1), tobramycin, tolazoline, TPN (2-in-1), trastuzumab, trimethaphan, tubocurarine, urokinase, vancomycin, vasopressin, vecuronium, verapamil, vinBLAStine, vinCRIStine, vinorelbine, vitamin B complex with C, voriconazole

ADVERSE EFFECTS

CV: Shortened QT interval, heart block, hypotension, bradycardia, dysrhythmias; **cardiac arrest (IV)**
GI: Vomiting, nausea, constipation
HYPERCALCEMIA: Drowsiness, lethargy, muscle weakness, headache, constipation, coma, anorexia, nausea, vomiting, polyuria, thirst
INTEG: Pain, burning at **IV** site, severe venous thrombosis, necrosis, extravasation

Pharmacokinetics

Absorption	Complete bioavailability (**IV**)
Distribution	Readily extracellular; crosses placenta, protein binding 40%-50%
Metabolism	Liver
Excretion	Feces (80%), kidney (20%), breast milk
Half-life	Unknown

Pharmacodynamics

	PO	IV
Onset	Unknown	Immediate
Peak	Unknown	Rapid
Duration	Unknown	½-1½ hr

INTERACTIONS
Individual drugs
Atenolol: decreased effect
Phenytoin, tetracyclines, thyroid: decreased absorption when calcium is taken PO
Diltiazem, verapamil: decreased effects, increased toxicity

Drug classifications
Antacids: milk-alkali syndrome (renal disease)
Digoxin glycosides: increased dysrhythmias
Diuretics (thiazide): increased hypercalcemia
Fluoroquinolones: decreased absorption of fluoroquinolones when calcium is taken PO
Iron salts: decreased absorption of iron when calcium is taken PO

Drug/herb
Lily of the valley, pheasant's eye, shark cartilage, squill: increased side effects, action

Drug/lab test
Increased: calcium

NURSING CONSIDERATIONS
Assessment
• Monitor ECG for decreased QT interval and T-wave inversion: in hypercalcemia, product should be reduced or discontinued
• Monitor calcium levels during treatment (9-10 mg/dl is normal level), urine calcium if hypercalciuria occurs
• Assess cardiac status: rate, rhythm, CVP (PWP, PAWP if being monitored directly)
• Assess digitalized patients closely, an increase in calcium increases digoxin toxicity risk
• **Hypocalcemia:** muscle twitching, paresthesia, dysrhythmias, laryngospasm

Patient/family education
• Caution patient to add food high in vit D content; to add calcium-rich foods to diet: dairy products, shellfish, dark green leafy vegetables; decrease oxalate-rich and zinc-rich foods: nuts, legumes, chocolate, spinach, soy
• Advise patient to prevent injuries, avoid immobilization

Evaluation
Positive therapeutic outcome
• Decreased twitching, paresthesias, muscle spasms
• Absence of tremors, seizures, dysrhythmias, dyspnea, laryngospasm, negative Chvostek's sign, negative Trousseau's sign

canagliflozin
(kan′a-gli-floe′zin)
Invokana
Func. class.: Oral antidiabetic
Chem. class.: SGLT-2 inhibitor
Pregnancy category B

ACTION: Blocks reabsorption by the kidney, increases glucose excretion, lowers blood glucose concentrations

Therapeutic outcome: Improved signs/symptoms of diabetes mellitus (decreased polyuria, polydipsia, polyphagia; clear sensorium; absence of dizziness; stable gait

USES: Type 2 diabetes mellitus, with diet and exercise

CONTRAINDICATIONS

Dialysis, renal failure, hypersensitivity, breast-feeding, diabetic ketoacidosis

Precautions: Pregnancy (B), children, renal/hepatic disease, hypothyroidism, hyperglycemia, hypotension, pituitary insufficiency, type 1 diabetes mellitus, malnutrition, fever, dehydration, adrenal insufficiency, geriatrics

DOSAGE AND ROUTES

Renal dose
Adult: PO eGFR 45-59 ml/min/1.73 m², max 100 mg/day; <45 ml/min/1.73 m², do not use

Available forms: Tabs 100, 300 mg

Implementation
PO route
- Once daily with first meal of the day

ADVERSE EFFECTS

CNS: Dizziness, fatigue
GI: Abdominal pain, pancreatitis, constipation, nausea
GU: Candidiasis, urinary frequency, polydipsia, polyuria
INTEG: Photosensitivity, rash, pruritus
META: Hypercholesterolemia, lipidemia, hypoglycemia, hyperkalemia, hypermagnesemia, hyperphosphatemia
MISC: Bone fractures

Pharmacokinetics

Absorption	Unknown
Distribution	99% protein binding
Metabolism	By UGT1A9, UGT2B4
Excretion	33% in urine
Half-life	Unknown

Pharmacodynamics

Onset	Unknown
Peak	Unknown
Duration	Unknown

INTERACTIONS
Individual drugs

Baclofen, cycloSPORINE, estrogen, isoniazid, tacrolimus: decreased effect, hyperglycemia
Gatifloxacin: do not use concurrently
Lithium: increased or decreased glycemic control

Drug classifications

ACE inhibitors, angiotensin II receptor antagonists, β-blockers, bile acid sequestrants, fibric acid derivatives, insulin, MAOIs, salicylates, sulfonylureas: increased hypoglycemia

Atypical antipsychotics, carbonic anhydrase inhibitors, corticosteroids, digestive enzymes, intestinal absorbents, loop diuretics, oral contraceptives, phenothiazines, progestins, protease inhibitors, sympathomimetics, thiazide diuretics: decreased effect, hyperglycemia

NURSING CONSIDERATIONS
Assessment
- Assess for hypoglycemia (weakness, hunger, dizziness, tremors, anxiety, tachycardia, sweating), hyperglycemia; even though product does not cause hypoglycemia, if patient is on sulfonylureas or insulin, hypoglycemia may be additive; if hypoglycemia occurs, treat with dextrose, or, if severe, with IV glucagon
- Monitor for stress, surgery, or other trauma that may require a change in dose
- A1c q3mo, monitor serum glucose; 1 hr PP throughout treatment; serum cholesterol, serum creatinine/BUN, serum electrolytes

Patient/family education
- Teach patient the symptoms of hypoglycemia/hyperglycemia, what to do about each
- Instruct patient that medication must be taken as prescribed; explain consequences of discontinuing medication abruptly; that insulin may need to be used for stress, including trauma, fever, surgery
- Instruct patient to avoid OTC medications and herbal supplements unless approved by health care provider
- Instruct patient that diabetes is a lifelong illness; that the diet and exercise regimen must be followed; that this product is not a cure
- Instruct patient to carry emergency ID and glucose source; to avoid sugar, because sugar is blocked by acarbose
- Teach patient that blood glucose monitoring is required to assess product effect
- Teach patient that GI side effects may occur

Evaluation: Therapeutic response: improved signs/symptoms of diabetes mellitus (decreased polyuria, polydipsia, polyphagia; clear sensorium, absence of dizziness, stable gait

---

candesartan (Rx)
(can-deh-sar′tan)
Atacand
Func. class.: Antihypertensive
Chem. class.: Angiotensin II receptor (type AT₁)
Pregnancy category
C (1st trimester),
D (2nd/3rd trimesters)

ACTION: Blocks the vasoconstrictor and aldosterone-secreting effects of angiotensin II;

---

selectively blocks the binding of angiotensin II to the AT_1 receptor found in tissues

Therapeutic outcome: Decreased B/P

USES: Hypertension, alone or in combination; CHF NYHA Class II-IV and ejection fraction ≤40%

CONTRAINDICATIONS

Hypersensitivity

> **BLACK BOX WARNING:** Pregnancy **D** (2nd/ 3rd trimesters)

Precautions: Pregnancy **C** (1st trimester), breastfeeding, children, geriatric, hypersensitivity to ACE inhibitors, volume depletion, renal/hepatic impairment, renal artery stenosis, hypotension, electrolyte abnormalities

DOSAGE AND ROUTES

Adult: PO (single agent) 16 mg daily initially in patients who are not volume depleted, range 8-32 mg/day; with diuretic or volume depletion, 8-32 mg/day as a single dose or divided bid

Adult and child ≥6 yr and weight >50 kg: PO 8-16 mg/day or divided bid, adjust to B/P, usual range 4-32 mg/day max 32 mg/day

Child ≥6 yr and weight <50 kg: PO 4-8 mg/day or divided bid, adjust to B/P

Child ≥1 yr and <6 yr: PO 0.2 mg/kg/day in 1 dose or divided in 2 doses/day, adjust B/P, max 0.4 mg/kg/day, max 16 mg/day

Heart failure

Adult: PO 4 mg/day, may be doubled ≥2 wk, target dose 32 mg/day

Renal/hepatic dose

Adult: PO ≤8 mg/day in severe renal disease/moderate hepatic disease, adjust dose as needed

Available forms: Tabs 4, 8, 16, 32 mg

Implementation

• Administer without regard to meals
• Oral liquid (compounded) shake well, do not freeze

ADVERSE EFFECTS

CNS: *Dizziness,* fatigue, headache, syncope
CV: Chest pain, peripheral edema, hypotension, palpitations
EENT: Sinusitis, rhinitis, pharyngitis
GI: *Diarrhea,* nausea, abdominal pain, vomiting
GU: Renal failure
MS: Arthralgia, pain
RESP: *Cough, upper respiratory infection*
SYST: Angioedema

Pharmacokinetics

Absorption	Well absorbed
Distribution	Bound to plasma proteins
Metabolism	Extensive
Excretion	Feces, urine, breast milk
Half-life	9 hr

Pharmacodynamics

Onset	Unknown
Peak	2 hr
Duration	24 hr

INTERACTIONS

Individual drugs

Lithium: increased lithium level
Potassium: increased hyperkalemia

Drug classifications

α-Blockers, ACE inhibitors, β-blockers, calcium channel blockers, MAOIs: increased hypotension
Diuretics (potassium sparing): increased hypokalemia
NSAIDs, salicylates: decreased effect

Drug/herb

Astragalus, cola tree: increased or decreased antihypertensive effect
Ephedra: decreased antihypertensive effect
Hawthorn: increased antihypertensive effect

Drug/Lab

Increase: albumin, ALT/AST, potassium

NURSING CONSIDERATIONS

Assessment

• **Serious hypersensitivity reactions: Assess for angioedema, anaphylaxis; facial swelling, difficulty breathing (rare)**
• **Heart failure: Assess for jugular vein distention, weight, edema, dyspnea, crackles**
• Assess B/P, pulse q4hr; note rate, rhythm, quality
• Monitor electrolytes: potassium, sodium, chloride; total CO_2
• Obtain baselines in renal, liver function tests before therapy begins
• Assess blood studies: BUN, creatinine, liver function tests before treatment
• Monitor for edema in feet, legs daily
• Assess for skin turgor, dryness of mucous membranes for hydration status; for angioedema: facial swelling, dyspnea

> **BLACK BOX WARNING:** Assess for pregnancy; this product can cause fetal death when given in pregnancy (**D**), 2nd/3rd trimester

---

- Assess for adverse reactions, especially in renal disease

Patient/family education
- **Teach patient not to take the product if breastfeeding or pregnant, or having had an allergic reaction to this product**
- If a dose is missed, instruct patient to take as soon as possible, unless it is within 1 hour before next dose
- Advise patient to comply with dosage schedule, even if feeling better
- Teach patient to notify prescriber of fever, swelling of hands or feet, irregular heartbeat, chest pain
- Advise patient that excessive perspiration, dehydration, diarrhea may lead to fall in blood pressure—consult prescriber if these occur
- Inform patient that product may cause dizziness, fainting; light-headedness may occur
- Advise patient to avoid all OTC medications unless approved by prescriber; to inform all health care providers of medication use, full effect 4 wk, onset 2 wk
- Caution patient to rise slowly to sitting or standing position to minimize orthostatic hypotension
- Teach proper technique for obtaining B/P and acceptable parameters

> **BLACK BOX WARNING:** Teach patient to notify prescriber immediately if pregnant **(D)** 2nd/3rd trimester, **(C)** 1st trimester, not to use if breastfeeding

Evaluation
Positive therapeutic outcome
- Decreased B/P

> **⚠ HIGH ALERT**
>
> ## capecitabine (Rx)
> (cap-eh-sit′ah-bean)
> **Xeloda**
> *Func. class.:* Antineoplastic, antimetabolite
> *Chem. class.:* Fluoropyrimidine carbamate
> **Pregnancy category D**

Do not confuse: Xeloda/Xenical

ACTION: Competes with physiologic substrate of DNA synthesis, thus interfering with cell replication in the S phase of cell cycle (before mitosis); also interferes with RNA and protein synthesis; product is converted to 5-fluorouracil (5-FU)

Therapeutic outcome: Decreasing symptoms of breast cancer

USES: Paclitaxel and anthracycline metastatic breast, colorectal cancer when 5-FU monotherapy is preferred; treatment of patients with colorectal cancer who have undergone complete resection of their primary tumor

CONTRAINDICATIONS
Pregnancy **D**, infants, hypersensitivity to 5-FU, severe renal impairment (CCr <30 ml/min), DPD deficiency

Precautions: Renal/hepatic/cardiac disease, breastfeeding, children, geriatric infections, radiation therapy, anticoagulation

DOSAGE AND ROUTES
Metastatic breast cancer resistant to both PAClitaxel and anthracycline or resistant to PAClitaxel and when further anthracycline therapy is not indicated
Adult: PO 2500 mg/m²/day divided q12hr after meal ×2 wk, repeat q3wk

Breast cancer (locally advanced/metastatic) with DOCEtaxel, previously treated with anthracycline
Adult: PO 2500 mg/m²/day divided q12hr after a meal on days 1-14, with DOCEtaxel 75 mg/m² IV on day 1

Advanced/metastatic breast cancer (HER2 positive), who have received anthracycline, taxane, and trastuzumab
Adult: PO 2000 mg/m²/day divided q12hr after a meal on days 1-14 with lapatinib 1250 mg/day on days 1-21, repeat q21days

Metastatic/locally advanced breast cancer, resistant to anthracycline, and a taxane or taxane resistant and when further anthracycline is contraindicated
Adult: PO 2000 mg/m²/day divided q12hr on days 1-14 with ixabepilone 40 mg/m² IV over 3 hr, repeat q3wk

As an adjuvant in Dukes C colorectal cancer with a complete resection when fluoropyrimidine alone is preferred
Adult: PO 2500 mg/m²/day divided q12hr within 30 min of a meal ×2 wk, repeat q3wk for 8 cycles

First-line in metastatic colorectal cancer when fluoropyrimidine alone is preferred
Adult: PO 2500 mg/m²/day divided q12hr after a meal ×2 wk repeat q3wk

Renal dose
Adult: PO CCr 30-50 ml/min; decrease initial dose to 75% of usual dose; CCr < 30 ml/min contraindicated

Available forms: Tabs 150, 500 mg

Implementation

• **Dosage adjustments of capecitabine monotherapy based on the most severe toxicity OR when used in combination with ixabepilone based on nonhematologic toxicity:** Grade 1 toxicity: Maintain current dosage; Grade 2 toxicity (1st appearance): interrupt therapy until toxicity is resolved to grade 0–1; do not replace missed doses, begin the next cycle with 100% of the starting dose; Grade 2 toxicity (2nd appearance): interrupt therapy until toxicity is resolved to grade 0–1; do not replace missed doses, begin the next cycle with 75% of the starting dose; Grade 2 toxicity (3rd appearance): interrupt therapy until toxicity is resolved to grade 0–1; do not replace missed doses, begin the next cycle with 50% of the starting dose; Grade 2 toxicity (4th appearance): discontinue treatment permanently; Grade 3 toxicity (1st appearance): interrupt therapy until toxicity is resolved to grade 0-1

• Help patient to rinse mouth tid-qid with water or club soda, brush teeth bid-qid with soft brush or cotton-tipped applicators for stomatitis, use unwaxed dental floss

ADVERSE EFFECTS

CNS: Dizziness, headache, *paresthesia, fatigue,* insomnia

CV: **Venous thrombosis**

GI: *Nausea, vomiting, anorexia, diarrhea, stomatitis, abdominal pain, constipation, dyspepsia,* intestinal obstruction, necrotizing enterocolitis, hyperbilirubinemia, **hepatic failure,** GI bleeding

HEMA: **Neutropenia, lymphopenia, thrombocytopenia,** anemia

INTEG: *Hand and foot syndrome,* dermatitis, nail disorder, alopecia, rash

MISC: Eye irritation, edema, myalgia, limb pain, *pyrexia,* dehydration, renal impairment

RESP: *Cough, dyspnea,* **pulmonary embolism**

Pharmacokinetics

Absorption	Readily absorbed, decreased with food
Distribution	Unknown
Metabolism	Liver, extensively
Excretion	Kidneys
Half-life	45 min

Pharmacodynamics

Onset	Unknown
Peak	1½ hr
Duration	Unknown

INTERACTIONS

Individual drugs

Leucovorin: increased toxicity
Phenytoin: increased phenytoin level

Drug classifications

Antacids (aluminum, magnesium): increased capecitabine

> **BLACK BOX WARNING:** Anticoagulants: increased risk of bleeding, NSAIDs, salicylates, platelet inhibitors, thrombolytics

Food/drug

Increased absorption; give within 30 min of a meal

Drug/lab test

Increased: bilirubin
Decreased: Hgb/Hct/RBC, neutrophils, platelets, WBC

NURSING CONSIDERATIONS

Assessment

• **Bone marrow suppression: Monitor CBC, differential, platelet count weekly; withhold product if WBC <1000/mm³ or platelet count is <50,000/mm³ or RBC, Hct, Hgb is low; notify prescriber of results; frequently monitor INR in those receiving warfarin**

• Assess buccal cavity q8hr for dryness, sores or ulceration, white patches, pain, bleeding, dysphagia; obtain prescription for viscous lidocaine (Xylocaine)

• Assess symptoms indicating severe allergic reaction: rash, pruritus, urticaria, purpuric skin lesions, itching, flushing; product should be discontinued

• Monitor temp q4hr (may indicate beginning of infection)

• **Assess for hand/foot syndrome: paresthesia, tingling, painful/painless swelling, blistering, erythema with severe pain of hands/feet**

• **Assess for toxicity: severe diarrhea (multiple times/day or at night), nausea, vomiting, stomatitis**

• Assess **GI symptoms:** frequency of stools, cramping; if severe diarrhea occurs, fluids/electrolytes may need to be given

• Monitor liver function tests before and during therapy (bilirubin, AST, ALT, LDH) as needed or monthly; note jaundice of skin or sclera, dark urine, clay-colored stools, itchy skin, abdominal pain, fever, diarrhea

---

BLACK BOX WARNING: Assess for bleeding: hematuria, stool guaiac, bruising or petechiae, mucosa or orifices q8hr; inflammation of mucosa, breaks in skin, monitor INR and PT in those taking anticoagulants

---

Patient/family education
• Advise patient to avoid use of products containing aspirin or ibuprofen, razors, commercial mouthwash, since bleeding may occur; to report symptoms of bleeding (hematuria, tarry stools)
• Instruct patient to report signs of **anemia** (fatigue, headache, irritability, faintness, shortness of breath); **infection:** increased temp, sore throat, flulike symptoms
⚠ **Advise patient not to become pregnant while taking this product; not to use while breastfeeding**
• Advise patient not to double dose, if dose is missed
• Advise patient to report immediately severe diarrhea, vomiting, stomatitis, fever ≥100° F, hand/foot syndrome, anorexia

Evaluation
Positive therapeutic outcome
• Prevention of rapid division of malignant cells

---

captopril (Rx)
(kap′toe-pril)
Apo-Capto ✦, Capoten
Func. class.: Antihypertensive
Chem. class.: Angiotensin-converting enzyme (ACE) inhibitor
Pregnancy category D (2nd/3rd trimesters)

Do not confuse: captopril/Capitrol/carvedilol

ACTION: Selectively suppresses renin-angiotensin-aldosterone system; inhibits ACE; prevents conversion of angiotensin I to angiotensin II

Therapeutic outcome: Decreased B/P in hypertension; decreased preload, afterload in CHF

USES: Hypertension, CHF, left ventricular dysfunction (LVD) after MI, diabetic nephropathy, proteinuria

CONTRAINDICATIONS
Breastfeeding, children, hypersensitivity, heart block, potassium-sparing diuretics, bilateral renal artery stenosis, angioedema

---

BLACK BOX WARNING: Pregnancy **D** (2nd/3rd trimester)

Precautions: Dialysis patients, hypovolemia, leukemia, scleroderma, LE, blood dyscrasias, CHF, diabetes mellitus, renal/hepatic disease, thyroid disease, African descent, pregnancy (C) 1st trimester, collagen-vascular disease, hyperkalemia, hyponatremia

DOSAGE AND ROUTES
Hypertension
Adult: Initial dose: PO 12.5-25 mg bid-tid; may increase to 50 mg bid-tid at 1-2 wk intervals; usual range 25-150 mg bid-tid; max 450 mg/day
Child: PO 0.3-0.5 mg/kg/dose, may titrate up to 6 mg/kg/day in 2-4 divided doses

Neonate: PO 0.05-0.1 mg/kg bid-tid, may increase as needed

CHF
Adult: PO 25 mg tid; may increase to 50 mg bid-tid; after 14 days may increase to 150 mg tid if needed

Diabetic nephropathy
Adult: PO 25 mg tid

Renal dose
Adult: PO CCr >50 ml/min, no change; CCr 10-50 ml/min, decrease dose by 25%; CCr <10 ml/min, decrease dose by 50%

Available forms: Tabs 12.5, 25, 50, 100 mg

Implementation
• Store in air-tight container at 86° F (30° C) or less
• Severe hypotension may occur after first dose of this medication; decreasing hypotension may be prevented by reducing or discontinuing diuretic therapy 3 days before beginning captopril therapy
• Administer 1 hr before or 2 hr after meals
• **Oral sol:** May crush tab and dissolve in water, give within ½ hr, make sure tab is completely dissolved

ADVERSE EFFECTS
CNS: Fever, chills
CV: *Hypotension,* postural hypotension, *tachycardia,* angina
GI: Loss of taste, increased liver function tests
GU: Impotence, dysuria, nocturia, proteinuria, **nephrotic syndrome, acute reversible renal failure,** polyuria, oliguria, frequency
HEMA: Neutropenia, agranulocytosis, pancytopenia, thrombocytopenia, anemia
INTEG: Rash, pruritus
MISC: Angioedema, hyperkalemia
RESP: Bronchospasm, *dyspnea, cough*

Pharmacokinetics

Absorption	Well absorbed
Distribution	Widely distributed; crosses placenta, excreted in breast milk (small amounts)
Metabolism	Liver (50%)
Excretion	Kidneys, unchanged (50%)
Half-life	2 hr increase in renal disease

Pharmacodynamics

Onset	¼-1 hr
Peak	1 hr
Duration	6-12 hr

INTERACTIONS

Individual drugs

Alcohol (acute ingestion): increased hypotension (large amounts)

Digoxin, lithium: increased serum levels, toxicity

Insulin: increased hypoglycemia

Drug classifications

Antacids, NSAIDs, salicylates: decreased captopril effect

Antidiabetics (oral): increased hypoglycemia

Antihypertensives, diuretics, nitrates, phenothiazines: increased hypotension

Diuretics (potassium-sparing), potassium supplements: increased toxicity, do not use

Sympathomimetics: do not use

Drug/herb

Ephedra: decreased antihypertensive effect

Hawthorn: increased antihypertensive effect

Drug/food

Food: decreased absorption of captopril

Drug/lab test

Increased: AST, ALT, alkaline phosphatase, bilirubin, uric acid, potassium

Decreased: platelets, WBC, RBC, Hgb/Hct

False positive: urine acetone, ANA titer

NURSING CONSIDERATIONS

Assessment

⚠ **Blood dyscrasias:** Monitor blood studies: decreased platelets; WBC with diff baseline, periodically q3mo; if neutrophils are <1000/mm³, discontinue treatment

• **Hypertension:** Monitor B/P, check for orthostatic hypotension, syncope; if changes occur, dosage change may be required

• Monitor renal studies: protein, BUN, creatinine; watch for increased levels that may indicate nephrotic syndrome and renal failure; monitor renal symptoms: polyuria, oliguria, frequency, dysuria, potassium

• Establish baselines in renal, liver function tests before therapy begins and check periodically; monitor for increased liver function studies; watch for increased uric acid, glucose

• Check potassium levels throughout treatment, although hyperkalemia rarely occurs

• **CHF:** Assess for edema, dyspnea, wet crackles, increased B/P, weight gain

• **Assess for allergic reactions:** rash, fever, pruritus, urticaria; product should be discontinued if antihistamines fail to help

Patient/family education

• Caution patient not to discontinue product abruptly; advise patient to tell all persons associated with care

• Teach patient not to use OTC products (cough, cold, allergy) unless directed by prescriber; serious side effects can occur; xanthines such as coffee, tea, chocolate, cola can prevent action of product

• Teach patient importance of complying with dosage schedule, even if feeling better; to continue with medical regimen to decrease B/P: exercise, smoking cessation, decreasing stress, diet modifications

• Emphasize the need to rise slowly to sitting or standing position to minimize orthostatic hypotension; not to exercise in hot weather or increased hypotension can occur

• Teach patient to notify prescriber of mouth sores, sore throat, fever, swelling of hands or feet, irregular heartbeat, chest pain, coughing, shortness of breath

• Caution patient to report excessive perspiration, dehydration, vomiting, diarrhea; may lead to fall in B/P

• Caution patient that product may cause dizziness, fainting, light-headedness; may occur during first few days of therapy; to avoid activities that may be hazardous, avoid activities that require concentration

• Teach patient how to take B/P, and teach normal readings for age-group; ensure patient takes regularly

> **BLACK BOX WARNING:** Advise patient to tell prescriber if pregnancy is suspected or planned, pregnancy **(D)**

Evaluation

Positive therapeutic outcome

• Decreased B/P in hypertension

TREATMENT OF OVERDOSE:
0.9% NaCl **IV** infusion, hemodialysis

carbachol ophthalmic
See Appendix B

carBAMazepine (Rx)
(kar-ba-maz′e-peen)
Carbatrol, Equetro, Mazepine, Novo-Carbamaz, TEGretol, TEGretol-XR
Func. class.: Anticonvulsant
Chem. class.: Iminostilbene derivative
Pregnancy category D

Do not confuse: TEGretol/Toradol

ACTION: Exact mechanism unknown; appears to decrease polysynaptic responses and block posttetanic potentiation

Therapeutic outcome: Absence of seizures; decreased trigeminal neuralgia pain

USES: Tonic-clonic, complex-partial, mixed seizures; trigeminal neuralgia; bipolar disorder; diabetic neuropathy

Unlabeled uses: Neurogenic pain, psychotic behavior with dementia, agitation, hiccups

CONTRAINDICATIONS
Pregnancy **D**, hypersensitivity to carBAMazepine or tricyclics

> **BLACK BOX WARNING:** Bone marrow suppression

Precautions: Glaucoma, renal/hepatic/cardiac disease, psychosis, breastfeeding, child <6 yr, alcoholism, hepatic porphyria, AV or bundle branch block

> **BLACK BOX WARNING:** Hematologic disease, agranulocytosis, leukopenia, neutropenia, thrombocytopenia, Asian patients

DOSAGE AND ROUTES
Seizures
Adult and child >12 yr: PO 200 mg bid; may be increased by 200 mg/day in weekly intervals, give in divided doses q6-8hr; maintenance 800-1200 mg/day; max 1600 mg/day (adult); max child 12-15 yr 1000 mg/day; max child >15 yr 1200 mg/day; adjustment is needed to minimum dose to control seizures; EXT REL give bid; RECT administration of oral SUSP 200 mg/10 ml or 6 mg/kg as a single dose
Child 6-12 yr: PO tabs 100 mg bid or SUSP 50 mg qid; may increase by <100 mg qwk, max

1000 mg/day, usual dose 15-30 mg/kg/day; EXT REL tabs daily-bid
Child <6 yr: PO 10-20 mg/kg/day in 2-3 divided doses or 4 divided doses (susp), may increase qwk, don't use ext rel

Trigeminal neuralgia
Adult: PO 100 mg/bid; may increase 100 mg q12hr until pain subsides; max 1200 mg/day; maintenance is 200-400 mg bid

Bipolar disorder
Adult: PO (Equetro only) (regular release) 200 mg bid, may adjust dose 3-4 days to achieve carBAMazepine level to 8-12 mcg/ml micro response; max 1600 mg/day

Agitation due to dementia (unlabeled)
Adult: PO 100 mg bid, may increase to 250-300 mg/day

Hiccups (unlabeled)
Adult: PO 200 mg tid

Available forms: Chewable tabs 100, 200 mg; oral susp 100 mg/5 ml; ext rel tabs 100, 200, 400 mg; ext rel caps (Carbatrol) 200, 300 mg

Implementation
• Do not break, crush, or chew ext rel tabs and caps: ext rel caps may be opened and beads mixed with food; chewable tabs should be chewed, not swallowed whole
• Give with food for GI symptoms
• Shake oral susp before use
• **Suspension:** Turn off N/G, internal feeding 15 min before and hold for 15 min after; mix an equal amount of water, D₅W, 0.9% NaCl when giving by NG tube, flush tube with 15-30 ml of above sol
• Store at room temperature

ADVERSE EFFECTS
CNS: *Drowsiness*, dizziness, confusion, fatigue, paralysis, headache, hallucinations, worsening of seizures, unsteadiness, speech disturbances, suicidal ideation, neuroleptic malignant syndrome (when used with psychotropics), tremor
CV: Hypertension, CHF, hypotension, aggravation of CAD, dysrhythmias, AV block
EENT: Tinnitus, dry mouth, blurred vision, diplopia, nystagmus, conjunctivitis
ENDO: Syndrome of inappropriate antidiuretic hormone (SIADH) (geriatric)
GI: *Nausea, constipation, diarrhea,* anorexia, vomiting, abdominal pain, stomatitis, glossitis, increased liver enzymes, hepatitis, hepatic porphyria, hypercholesterolemia, pancreatitis

---

GU: Frequency, retention, albuminuria, glycosuria, impotence, increased BUN, renal failure
HEMA: Thrombocytopenia, leukopenia, agranulocytosis, leukocytosis, aplastic anemia, eosinophilia, increased pro-time, lymphadenopathy
INTEG: *Rash*, Stevens-Johnson syndrome, urticaria, photosensitivity, toxic epidermal necrolysis, DRESS, alopecia, pruritus
MS: Osteoporosis
RESP: Pulmonary hypersensitivity (fever, dyspnea, pneumonitis)

Pharmacokinetics

Absorption	Slow; completely absorbed
Distribution	Widely distributed; protein binding 76%
Metabolism	Extensively, liver, metabolized by CYP3A4
Excretion	Urine, feces, breast milk
Half-life	18-65 hr, then 8-29 hr after first month

Pharmacodynamics

Onset	Slow
Peak	4-5 hr (PO), 1.5 hr (susp)
Duration	Unknown

INTERACTIONS
Individual drugs

Benzodiazepines, darunavir, delavirdine, doxycycline, felbamate, haloperidol, nefazodone, OXcarbazepine, PHENobarbital, phenytoin, primidone: decreased effect of these products
Cimetidine, clarithromycin, danzol, diltiazem, erythromycin, FLUoxetine, fluvoxaMINE, isoniazid, propoxyphene, valproic acid, verapamil, voriconazole: increased carBAMazepine levels
CISplatin, darunavir, delavirdine, DOXOrubicin, felbamate, nefazodone, OXcarbazepine, PHENobarbital, phenytoin, primidone, rifampin, theophylline: decreased carBAMazepine levels
Contraceptives (oral): decreased effect of oral contraceptives
Desmopressin, lithium, hypressin, vasopressin: increased effects of each specific product
Doxycycline: decreased effect of doxycycline
Lithium: increased CNS toxicity
Phenytoin: increased and decreased plasma levels; decreased carBAMazepine plasma levels
Thyroid hormones: decreased effect of thyroid hormones
Warfarin: decreased effect of warfarin

Drug classifications

CYP3A4 inducers: decreased carBAMazepine levels
CYP3A4 inhibitors: increased carBAMazepine levels
⚠ **MAOIs: fatal reaction; do not use together**
⚠ **Do not use with: NNRTIs (non-nucleoside reverse-transcriptase inhibitors), nefazodone**

Drug/herb

Echinacea: decreased carBAMazepine metabolism, increased levels
St. John's wort: decreased anticonvulsant action

Drug/food

Grapefruit juice: increased peak concentration of carBAMazepine

Drug/lab test

Decreased: serum calcium, sodium
Increased: cholesterol

NURSING CONSIDERATIONS
Assessment

> **BLACK BOX WARNING:** Serious skin reactions: Asian patient, obtain genetic test prior to administration

• Assess for seizures: character, location, duration, intensity, frequency, presence of aura
• Assess for **trigeminal neuralgia:** facial pain including location, duration, intensity, character, activity that stimulates pain
• Monitor liver function tests (AST, ALT) and urine function tests, BUN, urine protein periodically during treatments; serum calcium may be decreased and lead to osteoporosis; cholesterol periodically
• Bone marrow supression: Assess blood studies: RBC, Hct, Hgb, reticulocyte counts qwk for 4 wk then q3-6mo if on long-term therapy; if myelosuppression occurs, product should be discontinued
⚠ Serious skin, multiorgan hypersensitivity (Stevens-Johnson syndrome, toxic epidermal necrolysis, DRESS): May be increased in HLA-A 3101 gene and may be fatal
• Check blood levels during treatment or when changing dose; therapeutic level 4-12 mcg/ml
• Assess for **blood dyscrasias:** fever, sore throat, bruising, rash, jaundice, epistaxis (long-term treatment only)
⚠ Assess mental status: mood, sensorium, affect, behavioral changes, suicidal thoughts/behaviors
• Toxicity: Assess for bone marrow suppression, nausea, vomiting, ataxia, diplopia, CV collapse, Stevens-Johnson syndrome

---

Patient/family education
• Teach patient to carry/wear emergency ID stating patient's name, products taken, condition, prescriber's name, phone number
• Caution patient to avoid driving, other activities that require alertness until stabilized on medication
• Teach patient not to discontinue medication quickly after long-term use
• Teach patient to use a nonhormonal type of contraception to prevent harm to the fetus
• Advise patient to use sunscreen to prevent burns
• Teach patient to take exactly as prescribed; do not double or omit doses
• **Teach patient to report immediately chills, rash, light-colored stools, dark urine, yellowing of skin/eyes, abdominal pain, sore throat, mouth ulcers, bruising, blurred vision, dizziness, skin rash, fever**
• **Teach patient to notify if pregnancy is planned or suspected, pregnancy (D), avoid breastfeeding**

Evaluation
Positive therapeutic outcome
• Decreased seizure activity

TREATMENT OF OVERDOSE:
Lavage, VS

⚠ HIGH ALERT

CARBOplatin (Rx)
(kar'boe'pla-tin)
Func. class.: Antineoplastic alkylating agent
Chem. class.: Platinum coordination compound
Pregnancy category D

Do not confuse: CARBOplatin/CISplatin

ACTION: Produces interstrand DNA crosslinks and to a lesser extent DNA-protein crosslinks; activity is not cell cycle phase specific

Therapeutic outcome: Prevention of rapidly growing malignant cells

USES: Initial treatment of advanced ovarian cancer in combination with other agents; palliative treatment of recurrent ovarian carcinoma after treatment with other antineoplastic agents

CONTRAINDICATIONS
Pregnancy **D,** hypersensitivity to this product, breastfeeding, significant bleeding, aluminum products used to prepare or administer CARBOplatin

---

BLACK BOX WARNING: Severe bone marrow depression, platinum compound hypersensitivity

Precautions: Geriatric patients, radiation therapy within 1 mo, other cancer, chemotherapy within 1 mo, renal disease, liver disease, hearing impairment

BLACK BOX WARNING: Anemia, infection

DOSAGE AND ROUTES
Dosing with the Calvert equation GFR capped at max 12.5 ml/min
Adult: The total CARBOplatin dose (in mg) for adults may be calculated using the Calvert equation: *total dose (mg/m²) = target AUC × (GFR + 25)*
Child: Calculate CARBOplatin dose (mg/m²) in children as follows: *total dose (mg/m²) = target AUC × [(0.93 × GFR) + 15]*

Advanced ovarian cancer
Adult (single agent): IV INF initially 300 mg/m² on day 1 with cyclophosphamide, 600 mg/m² IV on day 1, repeat q4wk × 6 cycles; refractory tumors 360 mg/m² single dose, may repeat q4wk as needed; do not repeat until neutrophils are >2000 mm³ and platelets are >100,000/mm³

Renal dose
Adult: IV INF CCr 41-59 ml/min 250 mg/m², CCr 16-40 ml/min 200 mg/m²; do not use in CCr <15 ml/min

Available forms: Lyophilized powder for inj 50, 150, 450 mg vials; aqueous sol for inj 50 mg/5 ml vial, 150 mg/15 ml vial, 450 mg/45 mg vial, 600 mg/60 ml vial

Implementation
• Antiemetic 30-60 min before giving product to prevent vomiting, and prn

IV route
• Do not use needles or IV administration sets containing aluminum; may cause precipitate or loss of potency
• Use cytotoxic handling procedures
• **Reconstitute** CARBOplatin 50, 150, or 450 mg with 5, 15, or 45 ml, respectively, of sterile water for inj, D₅W, or NaCl (10 mg/ml); then further **dilute** with the same sol to 0.5-4 mg/ml; **give** over 15 min - 1hr (**intermittent INF**)
• **Continuous IV INF** over 24 hr; max dose based on (GFR = 125 mg/ml)
• Store protected from light at room temperature; reconstituted sol is stable for 8 hr at room temperature

---

Y-site compatibilities: Acyclovir, alfentanil, allopurinol, amifostine, amikacin, aminocaproic acid, aminophylline, amiodarone, amphotericin B lipid complex, amphotericin B liposome, ampicillin, ampicillin sulbactam, anidulafungin, atenolol, atracurium, azithromycin, aztreonam, bivalirudin, bleomycin, bumetanide, buprenorphine, butorphanol, calcium chloride/gluconate, caspofungin, ceFAZolin, cefepime, cefoperazone, cefotaxime, cefoTEtan, cefOXitin, cefTAZidime, ceftizoxime, cefTRIAXone, cefuroxime, cimetidine, ciprofloxacin, cisatracurium, CISplatin, cladribine, clindamycin, codeine, cyclophosphamide, cycloSPORINE, cytarabine, DAPTOmycin, DAUNOrubicin, dexamethasone, dexmedetomidine, dexrazoxane, digoxin, diltiazem, diphenhydrAMINE, DOBUTamine, DOCEtaxel, DOPamine, doripenem, doxacurium, DOXOrubicin, DOXOrubicin liposomal, doxycycline, droperidol, enalaprilat, ePHEDrine, EPINEPHrine, epirubicin, ertapenem, erythromycin, esmolol, etoposide, famotidine, fenoldopam, fentaNYL, filgrastim, fluconazole, fludarabine, fluorouracil, foscarnet, fosphenytoin, furosemide, ganciclovir, gatifloxacin, gemcitabine, gentamicin, granisetron, haloperidol, heparin, hydrocortisone, HYDROmorphone, hydrOXYzine, IDArubicin, ifosfamide, imipenem-cilastatin, inamrinone, insulin (regular), irinotecan, isoproterenol, ketorolac, labetalol, levofloxacin, levorphanol, lidocaine, linezolid injection, LORazepam, magnesium sulfate, mannitol, melphalan, meperidine, meropenem, mesna, methohexital, methotrexate, methylPREDNISolone, metoclopramide, metoprolol, metroNIDAZOLE, micafungin, midazolam, milrinone, minocycline, mitoXANtrone, mivacurium, morphine, nafcillin, nalbuphine, naloxone, nesiritide, niCARdipine, nitroglycerin, nitroprusside, norepinephrine, octreotide, ofloxacin, ondansetron, oxaliplatin, PACLitaxel, palonosetron, pamidronate, pancuronium, pantoprazole, PEMEtrexed, pentamidine, PENTobarbital, PHENobarbital, phentolamine, piperacillin, piperacillin-tazobactam, potassium chloride, potassium phosphates, prochlorperazine, promethazine, propofol, propranolol, ranitidine, remifentanil, riTUXimab, rocuronium, sargramostim, sodium acetate, sodium bicarbonate, sodium phosphates, succinylcholine, SUFentanil, sulfamethoxazole-trimethoprim, tacrolimus, teniposide, theophylline, thiotepa, ticarcillin, ticarcillin-clavulanate, tigecycline, tirofiban, TNA, tobramycin, topotecan, TPN, trastuzumab, trimethobenzamide, vancomycin, vasopressin, vecuronium, verapamil, vinBLAStine, vinCRIStine, vinorelbine, voriconazole, zidovudine

Solution compatibilities: D$_5$/0.2% NaCl, D$_5$/0.45% NaCl, D$_5$/0.9% NaCl, 0.9% NaCl, D$_5$W, sterile water for inj

Solution incompatibilities: Sodium bicarbonate

ADVERSE EFFECTS

CNS: *Seizures, central neurotoxicity,* peripheral neuropathy, dizziness, confusion
CV: Cardiac abnormalities **(fatal CV events), stroke**
EENT: Tinnitus, hearing loss, vestibular toxicity, visual changes
GI: Severe nausea, vomiting, diarrhea, weight loss, mucositis, anorexia, constipation, taste change
HEMA: **Thrombocytopenia, leukopenia, pancytopenia, neutropenia, anemia,** bleeding
INTEG: Alopecia, dermatitis, rash, erythema, pruritus, urticaria
META: Hypomagnesemia, hypocalcemia, hypokalemia, hyponatremia, hyperuremia
SYST: **Anaphylaxis**

Pharmacokinetics

Absorption	Complete
Distribution	Unknown
Metabolism	Liver
Excretion	Kidneys
Half-life	Initial 1-2 hr; postdistribution 2½-6 hr; increased in renal disease

Pharmacodynamics

Onset	½ hr
Peak	Unknown
Duration	4-6 hr

INTERACTIONS
Individual drugs
Amphotericin B: increased nephrotoxicity or ototoxicity
Aspirin, anticoagulants, platelet inhibitors: increased risk of bleeding
Phenytoin: decreased levels, monitor levels
Radiation: increased toxicity, bone marrow suppression

Drug classifications
Aminoglycosides: ototoxicity, increased nephrotoxicity
Antineoplastics, bone marrow–suppressing products: increased bone marrow suppression
Myelosuppressives: increased myelosuppression
NSAIDs: increased risk of bleeding
Thrombolytic agents: increased risk of bleeding

Drug/lab test
Increased: AST, BUN, alkaline phosphatase, bilirubin, creatinine

Decreased: platelets, neutrophils, WBC, RBC, Hgb/Hct, calcium, potassium, magnesium, phosphate

NURSING CONSIDERATIONS
Assessment

> **BLACK BOX WARNING:** To be used only by person experienced in the use of chemotherapeutic products, in a specialized care setting

> **BLACK BOX WARNING: Bone marrow depression:** Monitor CBC, differential, platelet count weekly; withhold product if neutrophil count is <2000/mm³ or platelet count is <100,000/mm³; notify prescriber of results, calcium, magnesium, phosphate, potassium, sodium, uric acid, CCR, bilirubin; creatinine clearance < 60 ml/min may be responsible for increased bone marrow suppression; assess frequently for infection

• **Assess for anaphylaxis: pruritus, wheezing, tachycardia; may occur within a few minutes of use; notify physician after discontinuing products; resuscitation equipment should be available**
• **Peripheral neuropathy:** may be increased in geriatrics
• Delay dental work until blood counts have returned to normal; regular toothbrushes, dental floss and toothpicks should not be used, use soft bristle toothbrush
• Monitor renal function studies: BUN, creatinine, serum uric acid, urine CCr before, during therapy; I&O ratio; report fall in urine output to <30 ml/hr
• Monitor temp q4hr (may indicate beginning of infection)
⚠ **Monitor liver function tests before, during therapy (bilirubin, AST, ALT, LDH) as needed or monthly; note jaundice of skin or sclera, dark urine, clay-colored stools, itchy skin, abdominal pain, fever, diarrhea**
• Assess for **bleeding:** hematuria, stool guaiac, bruising or petechiae, mucosa or orifices; inflammation of mucosa, breaks in skin; avoid all IM injections if platelets <50,000/mm³
• Identify effects of alopecia on body image; discuss feelings about body changes

Patient/family education
• Advise patient to report ringing/roaring in the ears, numbness, tingling in face, extremities, weight gain

• Teach patient to avoid use of products containing aspirin or ibuprofen, NSAIDs, alcohol, razors, commercial mouthwash, since bleeding may occur; to report symptoms of bleeding (hematuria, tarry stools)
• Instruct patient to report signs of **anemia** (fatigue, headache, irritability, faintness, shortness of breath); sore throat, bleeding, bruising, chills, back pain, blood in stools, dyspnea
• Instruct patient to report any changes in breathing or coughing even several months after treatment; to avoid crowds and persons with respiratory tract or other infections
• Advise patient that hair may be lost during treatment; a wig or hairpiece may make patient feel better; new hair may be different in color, texture
• Caution patient not to have any vaccinations without the advice of the prescriber; serious reactions can occur
⚠ **Teach patient that impotence or amenorrhea can occur; that this is reversible after treatment is discontinued; to notify prescriber if pregnancy is planned or suspected; pregnancy (D), that contraception should be used if patient is fertile**
⚠ **Teach patient not to breastfeed**
• Teach patient to notify prescriber immediately of fever, fatigue, sore throat, bleeding, bruising, chills, back pain, blood in stools, dyspnea

Evaluation
Positive therapeutic outcome
• Prevention of rapid division of malignant cells

carboprost (Rx)
(kar′boe-prost)
Hemabate
Func. class.: Oxytocic, abortifacient
Chem. class.: Prostaglandin
Pregnancy category C

ACTION: Stimulates uterine contractions, causing complete abortion in approximately 16 hr

Therapeutic outcome: Loss of fetus; decreased postpartum bleeding

USES: Abortion between 13 and 20 wk gestation; postpartum hemorrhage caused by uterine atony not controlled by other methods

CONTRAINDICATIONS
Hypersensitivity to this product or benzyl alcohol, severe renal/hepatic/cardiac/respiratory disease, PID

Precautions: Pregnancy **C**, asthma, anemia, jaundice, diabetes mellitus, seizure disorders, past uterine surgery

DOSAGE AND ROUTES
To induce abortion
Adult: IM 100 mcg (0.4 ml) test dose, then IM 250 mcg, then 250 mcg q1½-3½hr, may increase to 500 mcg if no response, max 12 mg total dose

Postpartum hemorrhage
Adult: IM 250 mcg, repeat at 15-90 min intervals, max total dosage 2 mg

Available forms: Inj 250 mcg/ml

Implementation
• Give only by trained personnel in a hospital that can provide emergency services
• Incomplete abortion may occur in 20% of patients
• Give antiemetics to prevent nausea/vomiting
• Give IM inj in deep muscle mass; rotate inj sites if additional doses are given
• Have crash cart available on unit
• Store in refrigerator

ADVERSE EFFECTS
CNS: *Fever, chills,* headache
GI: *Nausea, vomiting, diarrhea*
CV: Hypertension

Pharmacokinetics

Absorption	Well absorbed (nasal)
Distribution	Widely distributed (extracellular fluid)
Metabolism	Liver, rapidly
Excretion	Kidneys
Half-life	3-9 min

Pharmacodynamics

Onset	Unknown
Peak	16 hr
Duration	Unknown

INTERACTIONS
Drug classifications
Oxytocics: increased effects

NURSING CONSIDERATIONS
Assessment
• Monitor B/P, pulse; watch for change that may indicate hemorrhage
⚠ For length, duration of contraction; notify physician if contractions lasting >1 min or absence of contractions
⚠ Assess for incomplete abortion; pregnancy must be terminated by another method; product is teratogenic

Patient/family education
• Advise patient to report increased blood loss, abdominal cramps, increased temp, or foul-smelling lochia

Evaluation
Positive therapeutic outcome
• Loss of fetus
• Control of bleeding

carfilzomib
(car-fil′zoe-mib)
Kyprolis
Func. class.: Antineoplastic biologic response modifiers
Chem. class.: Signal transduction inhibitors (STIs)
Pregnancy category D

ACTION: Antiproliferative and proapoptotic activity

USES: Multiple myeloma in those who have received 2 therapies (including bortezomib and immunomodulatory agents)

CONTRAINDICATIONS
Pregnancy (**D**), hypersensitivity

Precautions: Breastfeeding, children, cardiac disease, cardiac arrest, dysrhythmias, MI, infusion-related reactions, pulmonary/hepatic disease, edema, thrombocytopenia, neutropenia, tumor lysis syndrome

DOSAGE AND ROUTES
Adult: IV 20 mg/m^2 over 2-10 min on days 1, 2, 8, 9, 15, 16, then 12 days' rest (days 17-28), then may increase to 27 mg/m^2 on days 1, 2, 8, 9, 15, 16, repeated every 28 days; refer to package insert for dosage adjustments for treatment-related toxicity

Available forms: Powder for injection 60 mg

Implementation
• Premedicate with dexamethasone 4 mg PO/IV before all carfilzomib 20-mg/m^2 doses during cycle 1 and before all carfilzomib 27-mg/m^2 doses in cycle 2; dexamethasone may be given in subsequent cycles if infusion-related reactions occur
• Hydration with 250-500 ml of NS or other IV fluids before each dose in cycle 1; additional hydration with 250-500 ml may be given after the carfilzomib infusion in cycle 1, continue hydration as needed
• Do not mix with other products
• Flush IV line with NS or D$_5$ for injection, before and after use

Adverse effects: *italics* = common; **bold** = life-threatening

Reconstitution:
- Add 29 ml of sterile water for injection to the inside wall of the vial to minimize foaming (2 mg/mL); to mix, gently swirl and/or invert the vial slowly for about 1 min or until the cake or powder completely dissolves; do not shake; if foaming occurs, allow the solution to rest for 2-5 min or until foaming subsides; visually inspect for particulate and discoloration before use

IV injection route
- Give over 2-10 min; do not give as an IV bolus; the reconstituted sol may be stored in the vial/syringe at room temperature × 4 hr or ≤24 hr refrigerated
IV infusion route
- May further dilute in D₅W; measure and inject the correct dose from the reconstituted vial into 50 ml D₅W
- Administer IV over 2-10 min
- The diluted solution may be stored at room temperature × 4 hr or ≤24 hr refrigerated

ADVERSE EFFECTS
CNS: Headache, dizziness, insomnia
CV: Heart failure, hypertension
GI: Nausea, vomiting, dyspepsia, anorexia, diarrhea, hepatic failure, constipation
HEMA: Neutropenia, thrombocytopenia
META: Hyperglycemia, hypercalcemia, hypomagnesemia, hyponatremia, hypophosphatemia
MISC: Fatigue, infusion-related reactions
MS: Arthralgia, myalgia

Pharmacokinetics

Absorption	Protein binding 97%

NURSING CONSIDERATIONS
Assessment
- **Tumor lysis syndrome (TLS): hydrate well;** assess for hyperuricemia, hyperkalemia, hyperphosphatemia, hypocalcemia, uremia
- **Hematologic toxicity grade 3 and 4, neutropenia, and thrombocytopenia:** platelet nadirs occur day 8 of each 28-day cycle; counts return to baseline before the start of the next cycle; monitor blood and platelet counts frequently; hold dose for grade 3 or 4 neutropenia or grade 4 thrombocytopenia, can require dosage reduction
- **Serious liver toxicity:** AST/ALT and bilirubin elevations and rare cases of fatal hepatic failure have occurred; monitor hepatic enzymes frequently; withhold doses until resolution or return to baseline in grade 3 or 4 AST/ALT or bilirubin elevations

- **Serious cardiac toxicity:** fatal cardiac arrest, CHF with decreased left ventricular function/ejection fraction, myocardial ischemia, and pulmonary edema; those with NYHA class III/IV CHF, MI within 6 mo, cardiac arrhythmias (conduction abnormalities) may be at increased risk; monitor for cardiac complications; withhold doses until resolution or return to baseline for grade 3 or 4 cardiac toxicity
- Infusion-related reactions: can occur 24 hr after dose; premedication with dexamethasone is recommended; assess for fever, chills, arthralgia, myalgia, facial flushing, facial edema, vomiting, weakness, shortness of breath, hypotension, syncope, chest tightness, angina, report renal/liver symptoms, avoid infections

Patient/family education
⚠ Teach patient/family to promptly report infusion-related symptoms (fever, chills, arthralgia, myalgia, facial flushing, facial edema, vomiting, weakness, shortness of breath, hypotension, syncope, chest tightness, angina)

Evaluation
Positive therapeutic outcome
- Decreased spread of multiple myeloma

carisoprodol (Rx)
(kar-i-soe-proe′dole)
Soma
Func. class.: Skeletal muscle relaxant, central acting
Chem. class.: Meprobamate congener
Pregnancy category C
Controlled substance schedule IV

Do not confuse: Soma/Soma compound

ACTION: Depresses CNS by blocking interneuronal activity in descending reticular formation of spinal cord, producing sedation

Therapeutic outcome: Relaxation of skeletal muscles

USES: Relieving pain, stiffness in musculoskeletal disorders

CONTRAINDICATIONS
Hypersensitivity to these products or carbamates, intermittent porphyria

Precautions: Pregnancy **C**, breastfeeding, geriatric, renal/hepatic disease, substance abuse, seizure disorder, CNS depression, abrupt discontinuation, Asian patients

---

DOSAGE AND ROUTES

Adult and child ≥16 yr: PO 250-350 mg tid and at bedtime, max 3 wk of use

Available forms: Tabs 250, 350 mg

Implementation

- Give with meals for GI symptoms
- Have patient use gum, frequent sips of water for dry mouth
- Store in tight container at room temperature
- Use for short term (2-3 wk), potential for habituation

ADVERSE EFFECTS

CNS: *Dizziness, weakness, drowsiness,* headache, tremor, depression, insomnia, ataxia, irritability, **seizures**, confusion, flushing
CV: Postural hypotension, tachycardia
EENT: Diplopia, temporary loss of vision
GI: Nausea, vomiting, hiccups, epigastric discomfort
HEMA: Eosinophilia, pancytopenia
INTEG: Rash, pruritus, fever, facial flushing, **erythema multiforme**
RESP: Asthmatic attack
SYST: **Angioedema, anaphylaxis**

Pharmacokinetics

Absorption	Well absorbed
Distribution	Crosses placenta
Metabolism	Liver, extensively, substrate of CYP2C19
Excretion	Kidney, unchanged; breast milk
Half-life	8 hr

Pharmacodynamics

Onset	½ hr
Peak	4 hr
Duration	4-6 hr

INTERACTIONS

Individual drugs

Alcohol: increased CNS depression
Meprobamate: do not use together

Drug classifications

Antidepressants (tricyclic), barbiturates, opioids, sedative/hypnotics: increased CNS depression
CYP2C19 inhibitors (FLUoxetine, fluvoxaMINE, isoniazid, modafinil): increased carisoprodol effect
CYP2C19 inducers (rifampin): decreased carisoprodol effect

Drug/herb

Kava, valerian: increased CNS depression
St. John's wort: increased metabolism of carisoprodol

Drug/lab test

Increased: eosinophils
Decreased: RBC, WBC, platelets

NURSING CONSIDERATIONS

Assessment

- Pain: Monitor ROM, atrophy, stiffness, and pain in muscles; assess throughout treatment
- Monitor ECG in seizure patients; poor seizure control has occurred with patients taking this product
- Assess for idiosyncratic reaction within a few min or 1 hr of administration (disorientation, restlessness, weakness, euphoria, blurred vision); patient should be reassured that reaction is temporary, withhold and notify prescriber
- Check for allergic reactions: rash, fever
- CNS depression: Assess for dizziness, drowsiness, psychiatric symptoms, abuse potential
- Abrupt discontinuation: withdrawal reactions do occur but may be mild; dependence may occur

Patient/family education

- Caution patient not to take with alcohol, other CNS depressants
- Advise patient to avoid altering activities while taking this product, to avoid rapid position changes, postural hypotension occurs, not to use for >2-3 wk
- Caution patient to avoid hazardous activities if drowsiness or dizziness occurs
- Caution patient to avoid using OTC medication such as cough preparations, antihistamines, unless directed by prescriber
- Teach patient to report allergic reactions immediately: rash, swelling of tongue/lips, hives, dyspnea
- Advise patient to take with food for GI symptoms

Evaluation

Positive therapeutic outcome
- Decreased pain, spasticity

TREATMENT OF OVERDOSE:

Activated charcoal, lavage, dialysis

> **⚠ HIGH ALERT**

carmustine (Rx)

(kar-mus'teen)

BiCNU, Gliadel

Func. class.: Antineoplastic alkylating agent
Chem. class.: Nitrosourea

Pregnancy category D

ACTION: Alkylates DNA, RNA; inhibits enzymes that allow synthesis of amino acids in proteins; also responsible for cross-linking DNA strands; activity is not cell cycle phase specific

Therapeutic outcome: Prevention of rapidly growing malignant cells

USES: Brain tumors such as glioblastoma, medulloblastoma, astrocytoma, ependymoma, brain stem glioma, metastic brain tumors; multiple myeloma (with prednisone), non-Hodgkin's, Hodgkin's disease, other lymphomas; GI, breast, bronchogenic, and renal carcinomas; wafer, as adjunct to surgery/radiation in newly diagnosed high-grade malignant glioma patients

Unlabeled uses: Malignant melanoma

CONTRAINDICATIONS

Pregnancy **D**, breastfeeding, hypersensitivity, leukopenia, thrombocytopenia

Precautions: Dental disease, extravasation, females, infection, secondary malignancy, thrombocytopenia, renal disease

> **BLACK BOX WARNING:** Bone marrow suppression, pulmonary fibrosis, bleeding, infection

DOSAGE AND ROUTES

Brain tumors, Hodgkin's disease, malignant lymphoma, multiple myeloma

Adult: IV 75-100 mg/m² over 1-2 hr × 2 days or 150-200 mg/m² × 1 dose q6-8wk or 40 mg/m²/day × 5 days q6wk

Child (unlabeled): IV 200-250 mg/m² as a single dose q4-6wk

Adult: Intracavitary up to 8 wafers inserted into resection cavity

Available forms: Powder for inj 100 mg; wafer 7.7 mg intracavitary

Implementation

• RBC colony-stimulating factors to counter anemia may be required

• Give fluids **IV** or PO before chemotherapy to hydrate patient

• Provide antiemetic, serotonin antagonists, dexamethasone prn; antibiotics for prophylaxis of infection

• Give all medications PO, if possible; avoid IM inj if platelets are <100,000/mm³

> **BLACK BOX WARNING:** Carmustine should not be given until platelets >100,000/mm³ and WBC >4000/mm²

Wafer route

• Use cytotoxic handling procedures

• Foil pouches may be kept at room temperature for 6 hr, if unopened

• If wafers are broken into several pieces, do not use

Intermittent IV infusion route

• **Do not use with PVC IV tubing, do not admix**

• Administer after **diluting** 100 mg/3 ml ethyl alcohol (provided); then **further dilute** 27 ml sterile water for inj; **then dilute** with 100-500 ml 0.9% NaCl or D₅W; **give** over 1 hr or more; use only glass containers; reduce rate if discomfort is felt

• Flush **IV** line after carmustine with 10 ml 0.9% NaCl to prevent irritation at site

• Store reconstituted sol in refrigerator for 24 hr or room temperature for 8 hr

Y-site compatibilities: Amifostine, amphotericin B lipid complex, amphotericin B liposome, anidulafungin, aztreonam, bivalirudin, bleomycin, caspofungin, cefepime, codeine, DAPTOmycin, dexmedetomidine, DOCEtaxel, ertapenem, etoposide, fenoldopam, filgrastim, fludarabine, gemcitabine, granisetron, levofloxacin, melphalan, meperidine, mitoXANtrone, nesiritide, octreotide, ondansetron, PACLitaxel, palonosetron, pamidronate, pantoprazole, PEMEtrexed, piperacillintazobactam, riTUXimab, sargramostim, sodium acetate, tacrolimus, teniposide, thiotepa, tigecycline, tirofiban, trastuzumab, vinCRIStine, vinorelbine, voriconazole

ADVERSE EFFECTS

GI: *Nausea, vomiting, anorexia, stomatitis,* **hepatotoxicity**

GU: *Azotemia,* **renal failure**

HEMA: **Thrombocytopenia, leukopenia, myelosuppression, anemia**

INTEG: Pain, burning, hyperpigmentation at inj site, alopecia

RESP: **Fibrosis, pulmonary infiltrate**

SYST: **Secondary malignant neoplastic disease**

Pharmacokinetics

Absorption	Completely absorbed
Distribution	Readily penetrates CSF
Metabolism	Liver, rapid
Excretion	Kidneys, breast milk
Half-life	Unknown

Pharmacodynamics

Unknown

INTERACTIONS
Individual drugs
Aspirin: increased risk of bleeding
Cimetidine, radiation: increased toxicity
Digoxin: decreased effects of digoxin
Phenytoin: decreased effects of phenytoin

Drug classifications
Anticoagulants: increased risk of bleeding
Antineoplastics: increased toxicity
Live vaccines: increased adverse reactions; decreased antibody reaction
Myelosuppressive agents: increased myelosuppression

Drug/lab test
Increased: bilirubin, prolactin, uric acid, LFTs
Decreased: platelets, WBC, neutrophils, Hct

NURSING CONSIDERATIONS
Assessment
• Assess buccal cavity q8hr for dryness, sores or ulceration, white patches, pain, bleeding, dysphagia; obtain prescription for viscous lidocaine (Xylocaine)
• **Assess symptoms indicating severe allergic reaction: rash, pruritus, urticaria, purpuric skin lesions, itching, flushing; product should be discontinued**

> **BLACK BOX WARNING: Bone marrow depression:** Monitor CBC, differential, platelet count weekly; withhold product if WBC <4000/mm³ or platelet count is <100,000/mm³; notify prescriber of results

• Monitor renal function studies: BUN, creatinine, urine CCr before and during therapy; I&O ratio; report fall in urine output to <30 ml/hr, may use allopurinol for hyperuricemia with increased fluids
• Monitor temp q4hr (may indicate beginning of infection)
• Monitor liver function tests before, during therapy (bilirubin, AST, ALT, LDH), monitor regularly, hepatotoxicity occurs rarely; note yellowing of skin or sclera, dark urine, clay-colored stools, itchy skin, abdominal pain, fever, diarrhea; hepatotoxicity can be serious and fatal
• Assess for **bleeding:** hematuria, stool guaiac, bruising or petechiae, mucosa or orifices q8hr; inflammation of mucosa, breaks in skin

> **BLACK BOX WARNING:** Only to be used by an experienced clinician in use of cancer, immune suppression

> **BLACK BOX WARNING: Pulmonary fibrosis/ infiltrate:** Monitor pulmonary function tests, chest x-ray films before, during therapy; chest film should be obtained q2wk during treatment; monitor for dyspnea, cough, pulmonary fibrosis; infiltrate occurs after high doses or several low-dose courses (>1400 mg/m² cumulative dose), may occur months or years after treatment

• Identify effects of alopecia on body image; discuss feelings about body changes

Patient/family education
• Teach patient to avoid use of products containing aspirin or ibuprofen, razors, commercial mouthwash, since bleeding may occur; to report symptoms of bleeding (hematuria, tarry stools)
• Advise patient to avoid foods with citric acid, hot flavor, or rough texture if stomatitis is present

> **BLACK BOX WARNING:** Instruct patient to report signs of anemia (fatigue, headache, irritability, faintness, shortness of breath); avoid smoking

• Advise patient that hair may be lost during treatment; a wig or hairpiece may make patient feel better; new hair may be different in color, texture
• Caution patient not to have any vaccinations without the advice of the prescriber; serious reactions can occur
⚠ Advise patient that contraception is needed during treatment and for several months after completion of therapy; product has teratogenic properties
• Teach patient infusion can be painful to veins and product contains ethanol, report chest pain

Evaluation
Positive therapeutic outcome
• Prevention of rapid division of malignant cells

carteolol ophthalmic
See Appendix B

Adverse effects: *italics* = common; **bold** = life-threatening

carvedilol (Rx)

(kar-veh′dee-lol)

Coreg, Coreg CR

Func. class.: Antihypertensive α/β-blocker

Pregnancy category C

Do not confuse: carvedilol/Captopril/ Carteolol

ACTION: A mixture of nonselective β-blocking and α-blocking activity; decreases cardiac output, exercise-induced tachycardia, reflex orthostatic tachycardia; causes reduction in peripheral vascular resistance and vasodilatation

Therapeutic outcome: Decreased B/P in hypertension

USES: Essential hypertension alone or in combination with other antihypertensives, CHF, LV dysfunction following MI, cardiomyopathy

CONTRAINDICATIONS

Hypersensitivity, asthma, class IV decompensated cardiac failure, 2nd- and 3rd-degree heart block, cardiogenic shock, severe bradycardia, pulmonary edema, severe hepatic disease

Precautions: Pregnancy **C**, breastfeeding, children, geriatric, cardiac failure, hepatic injury, peripheral vascular disease, anesthesia, major surgery, diabetes mellitus, thyrotoxicosis, emphysema, chronic bronchitis, renal disease

> **BLACK BOX WARNING:** Abrupt discontinuation

DOSAGE AND ROUTES
Essential hypertension

Adult: PO 6.25 mg bid × 7-14 days if tolerated well, then increase to 12.5 mg bid × 7-14 days if tolerated well, may be increased if needed to 25 mg bid, max 50 mg daily; ext rel cap 20 mg/ day, may increase after 7-14 days to 40 mg/day, max 80 mg/day

Congestive heart failure

Adult: PO 3.125 mg bid × 2 wk; if well tolerated, give 6.25 mg bid × 2 wk, then double q2wk to max dose 25 mg bid <85 kg or 50 mg bid >85 kg; ext rel cap (Coreg CR) 10 mg/day × 2 wk, increase to 20, 40, 80 mg/day over successive intervals of 2 wk

Postmyocardial infarction

Adult: PO 6.25 mg bid with food ×3-10 days, a lower starting dose may be used if indicated, titrate upward as tolerated, may increase to 12.5 mg bid, then titrate to 25 mg bid; PO ext rel 20 mg/day with food, a lower starting dose of 10 mg/day may be used and titrate upwards after 3-10 days, increase to 40 mg/day as required

Available forms: Tabs 3.125, 6.25, 12.5, 25 mg; ext rel cap 10, 20, 40, 80 mg

Implementation

• Give with food in morning; tablets may be crushed or swallowed whole, give with food to decrease orthostatic hypotension; do not break, crush, or chew ext rel cap; decreased anginal pain

• Administer reduced dosage in renal dysfunction

> **BLACK BOX WARNING:** Do not discontinue prior to surgery

ADVERSE EFFECTS

CNS: *Dizziness,* somnolence, insomnia, ataxia, hyperesthesia, paresthesia, vertigo, depression, *fatigue,* weakness, headache

CV: *Bradycardia, postural hypotension,* dependent edema, *peripheral edema,* **AV block, extrasystoles,** hypo/hypertension, palpitations, peripheral ischemia, **CHF, pulmonary edema**

GI: *Diarrhea,* abdominal pain, increased alkaline phosphatase, increased ALT/AST, nausea, vomiting

GU: Decreased libido, *impotence,* UTI

INTEG: Rash, Stevens-Johnson syndrome

MISC: Injury, back pain, viral infection, hypertriglyceridemia, **thrombocytopenia,** *hyperglycemia,* abnormal weight gain, aplastic anemia

RESP: Rhinitis, pharyngitis, dyspnea, **bronchospasm,** cough, **lung edema**

Pharmacokinetics

Absorption	Readily and extensively absorbed
Distribution	>98% protein binding
Metabolism	Extensively liver
Excretion	Via bile into feces
Half-life	Terminal half-life 7-10 hr, increased in the geriatric, hepatic disease

Pharmacodynamics

Unknown

INTERACTIONS
Individual drugs

Alcohol (acute ingestion), cimetidine: increased toxicity

Clonidine: decreased heart rate, B/P

Digoxin: increased concentrations of digoxin

Reserpine, levodopa: increased hypotension, bradycardia

Rifampin: decreased levels of carvedilol

Drug classifications

Antihypertensives, nitrates: increased toxicity

Antidiabetic agents: increased hypoglycemia

Calcium channel blockers: increased conduction disturbance

CYP2D6 inhibitors (FLUoxetine, quiNIDine): increased digoxin

MAOIs: increased bradycardia, hypotension

NSAIDs, thyroid hormones: decreased levels of carvedilol

Drug/herb
Ephedra: decreased antihypertensive effect
Hawthorn: increased antihypertensive effect

Drug/lab test
Increased: blood glucose, potassium, triglycerides, uric acid, bilirubin, cholesterol, creatinine
Decreased: sodium, HDL

NURSING CONSIDERATIONS
Assessment
• Monitor I&O, weight daily
• **Hypertension:** Monitor B/P during beginning treatment and periodically thereafter; pulse q4hr, note rate, rhythm, quality
• Monitor apical/radial pulse before administration; notify prescriber of significant changes, pulse <50 bpm hold product, notify prescriber
• **CHF: Assess for edema in feet and legs daily, fluid overload: dyspnea, weight gain, jugular vein distention, fatigue, crackles**

Patient/family education
• Teach patient not to break, crush, or chew ext rel cap
• Instruct patient to comply with dosage schedule even if feeling better, that improvement may take several weeks
• Teach patient to rise slowly to sitting or standing position to minimize orthostatic hypotension
• Encourage patient to report bradycardia, dizziness, confusion, depression, fever, weight gain, shortness of breath, cold extremities, rash, sore throat, bleeding, bruising
• Teach patient to take pulse at home; advise when to notify prescriber

> BLACK BOX WARNING: Encourage patient not to discontinue product abruptly, taper over 1-2 wk, life-threatening dysrhythmias may occur

• Advise patient to avoid hazardous activities until stabilized on medication; dizziness may occur
• Teach patient that product may mask hypoglycemia
• Advise patient to avoid all OTC medications unless approved by prescriber
• Advise patient to carry/wear emergency ID with product name, prescriber at all times
• Advise patient to inform all health care providers of products, supplements taken

• Teach patient to report if pregnancy is planned or suspected, pregnancy (C), avoid breastfeeding

Evaluation
Positive therapeutic outcome
• Decreased B/P
• Decreased symptoms of CHF or angina

cefaclor
See cephalosporins—2nd generation

cefadroxil
ceFAZolin
See cephalosporins—1st generation

cefdinir
cefditoren pivoxil
cefepime
cefotaxime
See cephalosporins—3rd generation

cefoTEtan
cefOXitin
See cephalosporins—2nd generation

cefpodoxime
See cephalosporins—3rd generation

cefprozil
See cephalosporins—2nd generation

ceftaroline (Rx)
(sef-tar'oh-leen)
Teflaro
Func. class.: Cephalosporin
Pregnancy category B

ACTION: Inhibits cell wall synthesis through binding to essential penicillin-binding protein (PBP)

Therapeutic outcome: Negative C&S, resolution of symptoms of infection

USES: Acute bacterial skin/skin structure infections (ABSSI), bacterial community acquired pneumonia

CONTRAINDICATIONS
Cephalosporin hypersensitivity

Precautions: Antimicrobial resistance, breastfeeding, carbapenem/penicillin hypersensitivity, child/infant/neonate, coagulopathy, colitis, dialysis, diarrhea, geriatrics, GI disease, hypoprothrombinemia, IBS, pregnancy **B**, pseudomembranous colitis, renal disease, ulcerative colitis, viral infection, vitamin K deficiency

DOSAGE AND ROUTES

Adult: IV 600 mg q12hr × 5-14 days (skin/skin structure infections), × 5-7 days (bacterial community acquired pneumonia)

Renal dose
Adult: IV CCr >30-≤50 ml/min 400 mg q12hr; CCr ≥15-≤30 ml/min 300 mg q12hr, CCr <15 ml/min 200 mg q12hr

Available forms: Powder for injection 400 mg, 600 mg

Implementation

- Obtain C&S before use
- Visually inspect for particulate matter or discoloration if solution or container permit
- **Reconstitute:** add 20 mg of sterile water to 400 or 600 mg vial (20 ml/ml for 400 mg), (30 mg/ml for 600 mg), mix gently until dissolved: **Dilute:** in 250 ml of 0.9% NaCl, 0.45% NaCl, LR, D5, D2.5, give over 1 hr, do not admix, use within 6 hrs at room temperature or 24 hr refrigerated
- Store reconstituted solution in the refrigerator

ADVERSE EFFECTS

CNS: Dizziness, seizures
CV: Bradycardia, palpitations, phlebitis
ENDO: Hyperkalemia, hypokalemia
GI: Diarrhea, nausea, vomiting, constipation, abdominal pain, pseudomembranous colitis (rare), elevated hepatic enzymes
HEMA: Thrombocytopenia, neutropenia, anemia, eosinophilia
INTEG: Rash, anaphylaxis

Pharmacokinetics	
Absorption	Unknown
Distribution	Unknown
Metabolism	Not hepatically metabolized
Excretion	In urine 88%, feces 6%
Half-life	1.6 hr

Pharmacodynamics
Unknown

INTERACTIONS

Drug classifications
Anticoagulants: increased prothrombin time risk

Drug/lab test
Increased: LFTs
Decreased: potassium, eosinophils, platelets

NURSING CONSIDERATIONS

Assessment
- Assess for infection: vital signs, sputum, WBC prior to and during therapy
- Assess for hypersensitivity: prior to use, obtain a history of hypersensitivity reactions to cephalosporins, carbapenems, penicillins; cross sensitivity may occur
- Assess for anaphylaxis (rare): rash, pruritus, laryngeal edema, dyspnea, wheezing; discontinue and notify health care provider immediately, keep emergency equipment nearby
- Monitor for pseudomembranous colitis: diarrhea, abdominal pain, fever, bloody stools; report immediately if these occur, may occur several weeks after terminating therapy

Patient/family education
- Explain reason for treatment and expected result
⚠ Instruct patient to report immediately rash, itching, difficulty breathing, bloody diarrhea, fever, abdominal pain

Evaluation
Positive therapeutic outcome
- Negative C&S, resolution of symptoms of infection

cefTAZidime
ceftibuten
ceftizoxime
cefTRIAXone
See cephalosporins—3rd generation

cefuroxime
See cephalosporins—2nd generation

⚠ HIGH ALERT

celecoxib (Rx)
(cel-eh-cox'ib)
CeleBREX
Func. class.: Nonsteroidal antiinflammatory, antirheumatic
Chem. class.: COX-2 inhibitor
Pregnancy category C (<30 wks), D (>30 wks)

Do not confuse: CeleBREX/CeleXA/Cerebra/Cerebyx

ACTION: Inhibits prostaglandin synthesis by selectively inhibiting cyclooxygenase 2 (COX-2), an enzyme needed for biosynthesis

Therapeutic outcome: Decreased pain, inflammation

USES: Acute, chronic rheumatoid arthritis, osteoarthritis, acute pain, primary dysmenorrhea, ankylosing spondylitis, juvenile rheumatoid arthritis (JRA)

Unlabeled uses: Colorectal adenoma prophylaxis

CONTRAINDICATIONS
Pregnancy **D** (3rd trimester), hypersensitivity to salicylates, iodides, other NSAIDs, sulfonamides, severe hepatic impairment

> BLACK BOX WARNING: CABG

Precautions: Pregnancy **C** (1st/2nd trimester), breastfeeding, children <18 yr, geriatric, renal/hepatic disease, hypertension, severe dehydration, bleeding, GI, cardiac disorders, PVD, asthma

> BLACK BOX WARNING: GI bleeding/perforation, peptic ulcer disease, MI, stroke

DOSAGE AND ROUTES
Do not exceed recommended dose, deaths have occurred

Acute pain/primary dysmenorrhea
Adult: PO 400 mg initially, then 200 mg if needed on first day, then 200 mg bid prn on subsequent days, if needed; start with ½ dose in poor CYP2C9 metabolizers
Geriatric: PO use lowest possible dose

Osteoarthritis
Adult: PO 200 mg/day as a single dose or 100 mg bid; start with ½ dose in poor CYP2C9 metabolizers

Rheumatoid arthritis
Adult: PO 100-200 mg bid; start with ½ dose in poor CYP2C9 metabolizers

Ankylosing spondylitis
Adult: PO 200 mg daily or in divided dose (bid); start with ½ dose in poor CYP2C9 metabolizers

Juvenile rheumatoid arthritis (JRA)
Adolescent and child ≥2 yr (>25 kg): PO 100 mg bid; start with ½ dose in poor CYP2C9 metabolizers
Child ≥2 yr (10-25 kg): PO 50 mg bid; start with ½ dose in poor CYP2C9 metabolizers

Colorectal adenoma prophylaxis (unlabeled)
Adult: PO 200-400 mg bid for up to 3 yr

Hepatic dose
(Child-Pugh class II)
Adult: PO reduce dose by 50%; (Child-Pugh C) do not use

Available forms: Caps 50, 100, 200, 400 mg

Implementation
• Do not break, crush, chew, or dissolve caps; caps may be opened and mixed with applesauce, ingest immediately with water
• Administer with food or milk to decrease gastric symptoms
• Do not increase dose

ADVERSE EFFECTS
CNS: *Fatigue, anxiety, depression, nervousness, paresthesia,* dizziness, insomnia, headache
CV: Stroke, MI, tachycardia, CHF, angina, palpitations, dysrhythmias, hypertension, fluid retention
EENT: Tinnitus, hearing loss, blurred vision, glaucoma, cataract, conjunctivitis, eye pain
GI: *Nausea, anorexia, vomiting, constipation, dry mouth,* diverticulitis, gastritis, gastroenteritis, hemorrhoids, hiatal hernia, stomatitis, GI bleeding/ulceration
GU: Nephrotoxicity: dysuria, hematuria, azotemia, cystitis, UTI, renal papillary necrosis
HEMA: Blood dyscrasias, epistaxis, anemia
INTEG: Purpura, rash, pruritus, sweating, erythema, petechiae, photosensitivity, alopecia, bruising, hot flashes, serious sometimes fatal Stevens-Johnson syndrome, toxic epidermal necrolysis
RESP: Pharyngitis, shortness of breath, pneumonia, coughing

Pharmacokinetics

Absorption	Well absorbed (PO)
Distribution	Crosses placenta, protein binding ~97%
Metabolism	Liver by CYP2C9
Excretion	Feces/kidneys, small amount
Half-life	11 hr

Pharmacodynamics

Onset	Unknown
Peak	3 hr
Duration	Unknown

INTERACTIONS
Individual drugs
Aspirin: decreased effectiveness; increased adverse reactions
Fluconazole: increased celecoxib level
Furosemide, cidofovir: decreased effect of each drug
Lithium: increased toxicity
Warfarin: increased anticoagulant effects

Drug classifications
ACE inhibitors: may decrease effects of ACE inhibitors

Anticoagulants, antiplatelets, SSRIs, salicylates, thrombolytics: increased risk of bleeding

Antineoplastics: increased risk of hematologic toxicity

Bisphosphonates: increased toxicity

Glucocorticoids, NSAIDs: increased adverse reactions

Thiazide diuretics: decreased effectiveness of diuretics

Drug/herb
Feverfew: decreased effect of feverfew

Garlic, ginger, ginkgo: increased bleeding risk

Drug/lab test
Increased: ALT, AST, BUN, cholesterol, glucose, potassium, sodium

Decreased: glucose, sodium, WBC, platelets

NURSING CONSIDERATIONS
Assessment
• Assess for **pain** of rheumatoid arthritis, osteoarthritis; check ROM, inflammation of joints, characteristics of pain

> **BLACK BOX WARNING:** Assess for cardiac disease that may be worse after taking this product; MI, stroke, do not use in coronary artery bypass graft (CABG)

• Monitor CBC during therapy; watch for decreasing platelets; if low, therapy may need to be discontinued, restarted after hematologic recovery; LFTs, serum creatinine BUN, stool guaiac

> **BLACK BOX WARNING:** Assess for blood dyscrasias (thrombocytopenia): bruising, fatigue, bleeding, poor healing

• **Assess for GI toxicity: black, tarry stools; abdominal pain**

⚠ **Assess for serious skin disorders: Stevens-Johnson syndrome, toxic epidermal necrolysis; may be fatal**

Patient/family education

> **BLACK BOX WARNING:** Do not exceed recommended dose; notify prescriber, immediately of chest pain, skin eruptions, stop product

• Teach patient that product must be continued for prescribed time to be effective; to avoid other NSAIDs, sulfonamides

> **BLACK BOX WARNING:** Caution patient to report bleeding, bruising, fatigue, malaise, since blood abnormalities do occur; to report GI symptoms: black tarry stools, cramping

• Teach patient to take with a full glass of water to enhance absorption

• Teach patient to check with prescriber to determine when product should be discontinued before surgery; advise patient to notify prescriber if pregnancy is planned or suspected

• Advise patient to report possible respiratory infection: fever, shortness of breath, coughing, painful swallowing

⚠ **Teach patient to report if pregnancy is planned or suspected, pregnancy (C) prior to 30 wk, (D) after 30 wk**

Evaluation
Positive therapeutic outcome
• Decreased pain in arthritic conditions
• Decreased inflammation in arthritic conditions
• Decreased number of polyps (FAP)

cephalexin
See cephalosporins—1st generation

CEPHALOSPORINS— 1ST GENERATION

cefadroxil (Rx)
(sef-a-drox'ill)
Apo-Cefadroxil ✦
ceFAZolin (Rx)
(sef-a'zoe-lin)
cephalexin (Rx)
(sef-a-lex'in)
Keflex, Panixine
Pregnancy category B

Do not confuse: cephalexin/cefaclor

ACTION: Inhibits bacterial cell wall synthesis, rendering cell wall osmotically unstable, leading to cell death by binding to cell wall membrane, lysis mediated by cell wall autolytic enzymes

≫ cefadroxil
Therapeutic outcome: Bactericidal effects for the following: gram-negative bacilli *Escherichia coli, Proteus mirabilis, Klebsiella pneumoniae* (UTI only); gram-positive organisms *Streptococcus pneumoniae, Streptococcus pyogenes, Staphylococcus aureus/epidermidis*

USES: Upper, lower respiratory tract, urinary tract, skin infections; otitis media; tonsillitis, UTI

≫ ceFAZolin
Therapeutic outcome: Bactericidal effects for the following: gram-negative organisms *Haemophilus influenzae, Escherichia coli, Proteus mirabilis, Klebsiella;* gram-positive organisms *Staphylococcus aureus*

USES: Upper, lower respiratory tract, urinary tract, skin infections; bone, joint, biliary, genital infections; endocarditis, surgical prophylaxis, septicemia; *Streptococcus*

>> cephalexin
Therapeutic outcome: Bactericidal effects for the following: gram-negative organisms *Haemophilus influenzae, Escherichia coli, Proteus mirabilis, Klebsiella pneumoniae;* gram-positive organisms *Streptococcus pneumoniae, Streptococcus pyogenes, Streptococcus agalactiae, Staphylococcus aureus*

USES: Upper, lower respiratory tract, urinary tract, skin, bone infections; otitis media

CONTRAINDICATIONS
Hypersensitivity to cephalosporins, infants <1 mo

Precautions: Pregnancy **B**, breastfeeding, hypersensitivity to penicillins, renal disease

DOSAGE AND ROUTES
>> cefadroxil
Adult: PO 1-2 g daily or divided q12hr, give a loading dose of 1 g initially
Child: PO 30 mg/kg/day in divided doses bid, max 2 g/day

Renal dose
Adult: PO CCr 25-50 ml/min, 1 g, then 500 mg q12hr; CCr 10-24 ml/min, 1 g, then 500 mg q24hr; CCr < 10 ml/min, 1 g, then 500 mg q36hr

Available forms: Caps 500 mg; tabs 1 g; oral susp 250, 500 mg/5 ml

>> ceFAZolin
Life-threatening infections
Adult: IM/IV 1-2 g q6-8hr, max 12 g/day
Child >1 mo: IM/IV 75-100 mg/kg/day in 3-4 divided doses, max 6 g/day

Mild/moderate infections
Adult: IM/IV 250 mg-1 g q8hr, max 12 g/day
Child >1 mo: IM/IV 25-50 mg/kg in 3-4 equal doses, max 6 g/day or 2 g as a single dose

Renal dose
Adult: IM/IV following loading dose CCr 35-54 ml/min dose q8hr; CCr 10-34 ml/min 50% of dose q12hr; CCr <10 ml/min 50% of dose q18-24hr
Child: IM/IV CCr >70 ml/min, no dosage adjustment; CCr 40-70 ml/min following loading dose, reduce dose to 7.5-30 mg/kg q12hr; CCr 20-39 ml/min, give 3.125-12.5 mg/kg after loading dose q12hr; CCr 5-19 ml/min, 2.5-10 mg/kg after loading dose q24hr

Available forms: Inj 500 mg, 1, 10, 20 g; infusion 500 mg, 1 g/50 ml, 50 mg/500 ml vial

>> cephalexin
Moderate infections
Adult: PO 250-500 mg q6hr, max 4 g/day
Child: PO 25-100 mg/kg/day in 4 equal doses, max 4 g/day

Moderate skin infections
Adult: PO 500 mg q12hr

Endocarditis prophylaxis
2 g 1 hr before procedure

Severe infections
Adult: PO 500 mg-1 g q6hr, max 4 g
Child: PO 50-100 mg/kg/day in 4 equal doses, max 4 g/day

Renal dose
Adult: PO CCr 30-59 ml/min max 1000 mg/day; CCr 15-29 ml/min 250 mg q 8-12 hr; CCr 5-14 ml/min 250 mg q 24 hr; CCr 1-4 ml/min 250 mg q 48-60 hrs

Available forms: Caps 250, 500, 750 mg; tabs 250, 500 mg, 1 g; oral susp 125, 250 mg/5 ml

>> cefadroxil
Implementation
• Give in even doses around the clock; if GI upset occurs, give with food; product must be given for prescribed time to ensure organism death and prevent superinfection
• Shake susp, refrigerate, discard after 2 wk

>> ceFAZolin
Implementation
IM route
• Reconstitute 250-500 mg of product with 2 ml sterile or bacteriostatic water for inj, or 0.9% NaCl; reconstitute 1 g of product with 2.5 ml; give deep in large muscle mass, massage

IV route
• Check for irritation, extravasation, phlebitis daily, change site q72hr
• For direct **IV** dilute in 2 ml/500 mg or 2.5 ml/1 g of sterile water for inj; give over 5 min
• For intermittent inf dilute reconstituted sol (500 mg or 1 g) in 50-100 ml D_5W, $D_{10}W$, D_5/0.25% NaCl, D_5/0.45% NaCl, D_5/0.9% NaCl, D_5/LR, or LR, 0.9% NaCl; give over 30-60 min; may be refrigerated up to 96 hr or stored 24 hr at room temperature

Syringe compatibilities: Heparin, Salbutamol, vit B complex

Syringe incompatibilities: Ascorbic acid inj, cimetidine, lidocaine, vit B/C

Adverse effects: *italics* = common; **bold** = life-threatening

Y-site compatibilities: Acyclovir, alfentanil, allopurinol, alprostadil, amifostine, amikacin, aminocaproic acid, aminophylline, amphotericin B liposome, anidulafungin, ascorbic acid injection, atenolol, atracurium, atropine, aztreonam, benztropine, bivalirudin, bleomycin, bumetanide, buprenorphine, butorphanol, calcium gluconate, CARBOplatin, cefamandole, cefmetazole, cefonicid, cefoperazone, cefoTEtan, cefOXitin, cefpirome, cefTAZidime, ceftizoxime, cefTRIAXone, cefuroxime, cephalothin, cephapirin, chloramphenicol, cimetidine, CISplatin, clindamycin, codeine, cyanocobalamin, cyclophosphamide, cycloSPORINE, cytarabine, DACTINomycin, DAPTOmycin, dexamethasone, dexmedetomidine, digoxin, diltiazem, DOCEtaxel, doxacurium, doxapram, DOXOrubicin liposomal, enalaprilat, ePHEDrine, EPINEPHrine, epirubicin, epoetin alfa, eptifibatide, esmolol, etoposide, fenoldopam, fentaNYL, filgrastim, fluconazole, fludarabine, fluorouracil, folic acid (as sodium salt), foscarnet, furosemide, gallium, gatifloxacin, gemcitabine, gentamicin, glycopyrrolate, granisetron, heparin, hydrocortisone, hydrOXYzine, IDArubicin, ifosfamide, imipenem-cilastatin, indomethacin, insulin (regular), irinotecan, isoproterenol, ketorolac, lidocaine, linezolid, LORazepam, LR's injection, mannitol, mechlorethamine, melphalan, meperidine, metaraminol, methicillin, methotrexate, methoxamine, methyldopate, methylPREDNISolone, metoclopramide, metoprolol, metroNIDAZOLE, mezlocillin, miconazole, midazolam, milrinone, morphine, moxalactam, multiple vitamins injection, nafcillin, nalbuphine, naloxone, nesiritide, niCARdipine, nitroglycerin, nitroprusside, norepinephrine, octreotide, ondansetron, oxacillin, oxaliplatin, oxytocin, PACLitaxel, palonosetron, pamidronate, pancuronium, pantoprazole, penicillin G potassium/sodium, peritoneal dialysis solution, perphenazine, PHENobarbital, phenylephrine, phytonadione, piperacillin, Plasma-Lyte M in dextrose 5%, polymyxin B, potassium chloride, procainamide, propofol, propranolol, ranitidine, remifentanil, Ringer's injection, ritodrine, riTUXimab, sargramostim, sodium acetate, sodium bicarbonate, succinylcholine, SUFentanil, tacrolimus, teniposide, tenoxicam, theophylline, thiamine, thiotepa, ticarcillin, ticarcillin-clavulanate, tigecycline, tirofiban, TNA, tolazoline, trastuzumab, trimetaphan, urokinase, vasopressin, vecuronium, verapamil, vinCRIStine, vitamin B complex with C, voriconazole, warfarin, zoledronic acid

Y-site incompatibilities: Amiodarone, hetastarch, HYDROmorphone, IDArubicin, vinorelbine tartrate

>> cephalexin
Implementation
• Do not break, crush, or chew caps
• Give in even doses around the clock; if GI upset occurs, give with food; product must be taken for 10-14 days to ensure organism death and prevent superinfection
• Shake susp, refrigerate, discard after 2 wk, use calibrated oral syringe, spoon or measuring cup

ADVERSE EFFECTS
CNS: Headache, dizziness, weakness, paresthesia, fever, chills, seizures (high doses)
GI: Nausea, vomiting, *diarrhea, anorexia*, pain, glossitis, bleeding; increased AST, ALT, bilirubin, LDH, alkaline phosphatase; abdominal pain, pseudomembranous colitis
GU: Proteinuria, vaginitis, pruritus, candidiasis, increased BUN, nephrotoxicity, renal failure
HEMA: Leukopenia, thrombocytopenia, agranulocytosis, anemia, neutropenia, lymphocytosis, eosinophilia, pancytopenia, hemolytic anemia
INTEG: Rash, urticaria, dermatitis
MS: Arthralgia, arthritis
RESP: Dyspnea
SYST: Anaphylaxis, serum sickness, superinfection, Stevens-Johnson syndrome

>> cefadroxil
Pharmacokinetics

Absorption	Well absorbed
Distribution	Widely distributed; crosses placenta
Metabolism	Not metabolized
Excretion	Unchanged by kidneys; enters breast milk
Half-life	1½-2 hr

Pharmacodynamics

	PO
Onset	Rapid
Peak	1½-2 hr
Duration	12-24 hr

>> ceFAZolin
Pharmacokinetics

Absorption	Well absorbed
Distribution	Widely distributed; crosses placenta
Metabolism	Not metabolized
Excretion	Unchanged by kidneys; enters breast milk
Half-life	1½-2½ hr

Pharmacodynamics

	IM	IV
Onset	Rapid	10 min
Peak	1-2 hr	Infusion's end
Duration	6-12 hr	Unknown

>> cephalexin
Pharmacokinetics

Absorption	Well absorbed
Distribution	Widely distributed; crosses placenta
Metabolism	Not metabolized
Excretion	Kidneys, unchanged; enters breast milk
Half-life	½-1 hr; increased in renal disease

Pharmacodynamics

Onset	15-30 min
Peak	1 hr
Duration	6-12 hr

INTERACTIONS
Individual drugs
Probenecid: increased toxicity

Drug classifications
Aminoglycosides, diuretics (loop): increased toxicity
Anticoagulants: increased protime; use cautiously
Oral contraceptives: decreased effectiveness possible; use another form of contraception

Drug/lab test
Increased: AST, ALT, alkaline phosphatase, LDH, BUN, creatinine, bilirubin
False positive: urinary protein, direct Coombs' test, urine glucose
Interference: cross-matching

NURSING CONSIDERATIONS
Assessment
• **Assess patient for previous sensitivity reaction to penicillins or other cephalosporins; cross-sensitivity between penicillins and cephalosporins is common**
• Assess patient for signs and symptoms of **infection** including characteristics of wounds, sputum, urine, stool, WBC >10,000/mm³, earache, fever; obtain baseline information and during treatment
• Obtain C&S before beginning product therapy to identify if correct treatment has been initiated

• **Assess for anaphylaxis: rash, urticaria, pruritus, chills, fever, joint pain; angioedema may occur a few days after therapy begins; EPINEPHrine and resuscitation equipment should be available for anaphylactic reaction**
• **Identify urine output; if decreasing, notify prescriber (may indicate nephrotoxicity); also check for increased BUN, creatinine**
• Monitor blood studies: AST, ALT, CBC, Hct, bilirubin, LDH, alkaline phosphatase, Coombs' test monthly if patient is on long-term therapy
• Monitor electrolytes: potassium, sodium, chloride monthly if patient is on long-term therapy
• **Assess bowel pattern daily; if severe diarrhea occurs, product should be discontinued; may indicate pseudomembranous colitis**
• Monitor for bleeding: ecchymosis, bleeding gums, hematuria, stool guaiac daily if on long-term therapy
• **Assess for superinfection: perineal itching, fever, malaise, redness, pain, swelling, drainage, rash, diarrhea, change in cough, sputum**

Patient/family education
• **Teach patient to report sore throat, bruising, bleeding, joint pain; may indicate blood dyscrasias (rare)**
• **Advise patient to contact prescriber if vaginal itching, loose foul-smelling stools, furry tongue occur; may indicate superinfection**
• Instruct patient to take all medication prescribed for the length of time ordered
• **Advise patient to notify prescriber of diarrhea with blood, pus, mucus, which may indicate pseudomembranous colitis**

Evaluation
Positive therapeutic outcome
• Absence of signs/symptoms of infection (WBC <10,000/mm³, temp WNL, absence of red draining wounds, earache)
• Reported improvement in symptoms of infection
• Negative C&S

TREATMENT OF ANAPHYLAXIS: EPINEPHrine, antihistamines, resuscitate if needed

CEPHALOSPORINS—2ND GENERATION

cefaclor (Rx)
(sef′a-klor)
Ceclor, Raniclor
cefoTEtan (Rx)
(sef′oh-tee-tan)
Cefotan
cefOXitin (Rx)
(se-fox′i-tin)
Mefoxin
cefprozil (Rx)
(sef-proe′zill)
Cefzil
cefuroxime (Rx)
(sef-yoor-ox′eem)
Ceftin, Cefuroxime, Zinacef
Func. class.: Antiinfective
Chem. class.: Cephalosporin (2nd generation)
Pregnancy category B

Do not confuse: cefaclor/cephalexin, Cefotan/Ceftin, cefprozil/ceFAZolin/cefuroxime, Cefzil/Ceftin

ACTION: Inhibits bacterial cell wall synthesis, rendering cell wall osmotically unstable, leading to cell death by binding to cell wall membrane

>> cefaclor
Therapeutic outcome: Bactericidal effects for the following: gram-negative bacilli *Haemophilus influenzae, Escherichia coli, Proteus mirabilis, Klebsiella;* gram-positive organisms *Streptococcus pneumoniae, Streptococcus pyogenes, Staphylococcus aureus*

USES: Lower respiratory tract, urinary tract, skin infections; otitis media; infections

>> cefoTEtan
Therapeutic outcome: Bactericidal effects for the following: gram-negative organisms *Citrobacter, Haemophilus influenzae, Escherichia coli, Enterobacter aerogenes, Proteus mirabilis, Klebsiella, Salmonella, Shigella, Acinetobacter, Bacteroides fragilis, Neisseria, Serratia;* gram-positive organisms *Streptococcus pneumoniae, Streptococcus pyogenes, Staphylococcus aureus*

USES: Serious upper or lower respiratory tract, urinary tract, gynecologic, skin, bone, joint, gonococcal, intraabdominal infections

>> cefOXitin
Therapeutic outcome: Bactericidal effects for the following: gram-negative bacilli *Bacteroides fragilis, Haemophilus influenzae, Escherichia coli, Proteus, Klebsiella, Neisseria gonorrhoeae;* gram-positive organisms *Streptococcus pneumoniae, Streptococcus pyogenes, Staphylococcus aureus;* anaerobes including *Clostridium*

USES: Lower respiratory tract, urinary tract, skin, bone, gynecologic, gonococcal infections; septicemia, peritonitis

>> cefprozil
Therapeutic outcome: Bactericidal effects for the following: gram-negative bacilli *Haemophilus influenzae, Escherichia coli;* gram-positive organisms *Streptococcus pneumoniae, Streptococcus pyogenes, Staphylococcus aureus*

USES: Pharyngitis/tonsillitis, otitis media, secondary bacterial infection of acute bronchitis, and acute bacterial exacerbation of chronic bronchitis and uncomplicated skin and skin structure infections; acute sinusitis

>> cefuroxime
Therapeutic outcome: Bactericidal effects for the following: gram-negative bacilli *Haemophilus influenzae, Escherichia coli, Neisseria, Proteus mirabilis, Klebsiella;* gram-positive organisms: *Streptococcus pneumoniae, Streptococcus pyogenes, Staphylococcus aureus*

USES: Serious lower respiratory tract, urinary tract, skin, bone, joint, gonococcal infections; septicemia, meningitis, surgery prophylaxis

CONTRAINDICATIONS
Hypersensitivity to cephalosporins or related antibiotics, seizures

Precautions: Pregnancy **B,** breastfeeding, children, renal/GI disease, diabetes mellitus, coagulopathy, pseudomembranous colitis

DOSAGE AND ROUTES
>> cefaclor
Adult: PO 250-500 mg q8hr; EXT REL 500 mg q12hr; max 1.5 g/day (cap, oral susp); 1 g/day (EXT REL)
Child >1 mo: PO 20-40 mg/kg daily in divided doses q8hr, or total daily dose may be divided and given q12hr, max 1 g/day

Available forms: Caps 250, 500 mg; oral susp 125, 187, 250, 375 mg/5 ml; EXT REL tab 500 mg

C

>> cefoTEtan
Adult: IV/IM 1-3 g q12hr × 5-10 days

Perioperative prophylaxis
Adult: IV 1-2 g ½-1 hr before surgery

Renal dose
Adult: IM/IV CCr 30-50 ml/min 1-2 g, then 1-2 g q8-12hr; CCr 10-29 ml/min 1-2 g, then 1-2 g q12-24hr; CCr 5-9 ml/min 1-2 g, then 0.5-1 g q12-24hr; CCr <5 ml/min 1-2 g, then 0.5-1 g q24-48hr

Available forms: Inj 1, 2, 10 g

>> cefOXitin
Adult: IM/IV 1-2 g q6-8hr

Uncomplicated gonorrhea (outpatient)
Adult/adolescent/child ≥45 kg: IM 2 g as single dose with 1 g PO probenecid at same time

Severe infections
Adult: IM/IV 2 g q4hr
Child ≥3 mo: IM/IV 80-160 mg/kg/day divided q4-6hr; max 12 g/day

Available forms: Powder for inj 1, 2, 10 g

>> cefprozil
Renal dose
CCr <30 ml/min 50% of dose

Upper respiratory infections
Adult: PO 500 mg q24hr × 10 days

Otitis media
Child 6 mo-12 yr: PO 15 mg/kg q12hr × 10 days

Lower respiratory infections
Adult: PO 500 mg q12hr × 10 days

Skin/skin structure infections
Adult: PO 250-500 mg q12hr × 10 days

Available forms: Tabs 250, 500 mg; susp 125, 250 mg/5 ml

>> cefuroxime
Oral tablets and suspension are not bioequivalent

Lower respiratory tract infections (mild-moderate)/uncomplicated skin/skin structure infections
Adult/adolescent: PO 250-500 mg q12hr × 5-10 days; IV/IM 750 mg q8hr
Child (unlabeled): PO 125 mg q12hr; 750 mg IV or IM q8hr
Adolescent/child/infant ≥3 mo: IV/IM 50-100 mg/kg/day divided q6-8hr (not to exceed adult dose)

Serious lower respiratory tract infections/serious skin/skin structure infections
Adult: IV/IM 0.75-1.5 g q8hr; life-threatening infections or infections caused by less-susceptible organisms, IV 1.5 g q6hr
Adolescent/child/infant ≥3 mo: IV/IM 50-150 mg/kg/day divided q6-8hr; max 6 g/day

Impetigo
Child: PO (tab unlabeled) 250 mg PO q12hr
Child/infant ≥3 mo: (PO-Susp) 30 mg/kg/day divided into two doses; max 1000 mg/day

Urinary tract infection (UTI)
Adult/adolescent: PO 250 mg q12hr × 7-10 days; IV/IM 0.75-1.5 g q8hr (general) or 0.75 g q8hr (uncomplicated)
Adolescent/child/infant ≥3 mo: IV/IM 50-100 mg/kg/day in divided doses q6-8hr (max adult dose)

Bone and joint infections
Adult: IV/IM 1.5 g q8hr; for life-threatening infections or infections caused by less-susceptible organisms, 1.5 g IV q6hr
Adolescent/child/infant ≥3 mo: IV/IM 150 mg/kg/day in divided doses q8hr; max 6 g/day

Upper respiratory tract infections (e.g., pharyngitis, tonsillitis)
Adult/adolescent: PO (tabs) 250 mg q12hr × 10 days
Child/infant ≥3 mo: PO (susp) 20 mg/kg/day divided into 2 doses × 10 days, max 500 mg/day

Acute bacterial maxillary sinusitis
Adult/adolescent: PO (tabs) 250 mg bid × 10 days
Child (who can swallow tablets whole): PO (tabs) 250 mg bid × 10 days
Child/infant ≥3 mo: PO (susp) 15 mg/kg bid × 10 days, max 1000 mg/day

Early Lyme disease
Adult/adolescent: PO (tabs) 500 mg q12hr × 20 days
Child (unlabeled): PO (susp) 30 mg/kg/day in 2 divided doses (max 1000 mg/day) or 1000 mg/day × 14-21 days

Acute otitis media
Child (who can swallow whole tablets): PO (tabs) 250 mg bid × 10 days
Child/infant ≥3 mo: PO (susp) 30 mg/kg/day divided into 2 doses × 10 day, max 1000 mg/day

Septicemia
Adult: IV/IM 1.5-3 g q8hr, max 9 g/day

Adolescent/child/infant ≥3 mo: IV/IM 200-240 mg/kg/day divided doses q6-8hr, max 9 g/day

Renal dose
Adult: CCr 10-20 ml/min: IV/IM 0.75-1.5 g, then 750 mg q12hr; **CrCl <10 ml/min:** IV/IM 0.75-1.5 g, then 750 mg q24hr
Child: The frequency of dosing should be modified consistent with the recommendations for adults

Available forms: Tabs 125, 250, 500 mg; inj 150, 750 mg, 1.5, 7.5 g; inj 750 mg; 1.5 g powder, susp 125, 250 mg/5 ml

Implementation

>> cefaclor
- Do not break, crush, chew, or cut EXT REL tabs
- Give in even doses around the clock; if GI upset occurs, give with food; product must be given for 10-14 days to ensure organism death and prevent superinfection
- Shake susp, refrigerate, discard after 2 wk
- Swallow EXT REL whole

>> cefoTEtan
IM route
- Reconstitute 1 g/2 ml or 2 g/3 ml of sterile or bacteriostatic water for inj; may be diluted with 0.5% of 1% lidocaine to prevent pain; give deep in large muscle mass, massage

IV route
- May be stored 96 hr refrigerated or 24 hr at room temperature
- Check for irritation, extravasation, phlebitis daily; change site q72hr
- For direct **IV** dilute in 1 g/10 ml or more and give over 5 min
- For intermittent inf further dilute in 50-100 ml of 0.9% NaCl or D$_5$W; give over 3-5 min; discontinue primary line while running intermittent inf

Y-site compatibilities: Allopurinol, amifostine, aztreonam, diltiazem, famotidine, filgrastim, fluconazole, fludarabine, heparin, regular insulin, melphalan, meperidine, morphine, PACLitaxel, sargramostim, tacrolimus, teniposide, theophylline, thiotepa

>> cefOXitin
IM route
- Reconstitute 1 g/2 ml of sterile water for inj; may be diluted with 0.5% or 1% lidocaine to prevent pain; give deep in large muscle mass, massage

IV route
- Check for irritation, extravasation, phlebitis daily; change site q72hr
- For direct **IV**, dilute 1 g/10 ml or 2 g/20 ml of sterile water for inj; shake, let stand until clear; give over 3-5 min
- For intermittent inf further dilute with 50-100 ml of D$_5$W, D$_{10}$W, D$_5$/0.25% NaCl, D$_5$/0.45% NaCl, D$_5$/0.9% NaCl, 0.9% NaCl D$_5$/LR, D$_5$/0.02%, sodium bicarbonate, Ringer's, or LR; give over 15-30 min; may store 96 hr refrigerated or 24 hr room temperature
- For cont inf dilute in 500-1000 ml; give over prescribed rate

Syringe compatibilities: Heparin, insulin

Y-site compatibilities: Acyclovir, amifostine, aztreonam, cyclophosphamide, diltiazem, famotidine, fluconazole, foscarnet, HYDROmorphone, magnesium sulfate, meperidine, morphine, ondansetron, perphenazine, temiposide, thiotepa

Y-site incompatibilities: Hetastarch

>> cefprozil
IM route
- Reconstitute with 1 g/2 ml or 2 g/3 ml of sterile or bacteriostatic water for inj; may be diluted with 0.5% or 1% lidocaine to prevent pain; give deep in large muscle mass, massage

IV route
- Check for irritation, extravasation, phlebitis daily; change site q72hr
- For direct **IV**, dilute 1 g/10 ml or more and give over 5 min
- For intermittent inf further dilute with 50-100 ml of 0.9% NaCl or D$_5$W; give over 3-5 min; discontinue primary line while running intermittent inf

Syringe incompatibilities: Doxapram

Y-site compatibilities: Famotidine, fluconazole, fludarabine, regular insulin, meperidine, morphine, sargramostim

Additive incompatibilities: Aminoglycosides, tetracyclines, heparin

>> cefuroxime
- Give for 10-14 days to ensure organism death, prevent superinfection, discard after 14 days
- Give with food if needed for GI symptoms
- Five after C&S obtained

ADVERSE EFFECTS
CNS: Dizziness, headache, fatigue, paresthesia, fever, chills, confusion

GI: *Diarrhea,* nausea, vomiting, anorexia, dysgeusia, glossitis, bleeding; increased AST, ALT, bilirubin, LDH, alkaline phosphatase; abdominal pain, loose stools, flatulence, heartburn, stomach cramps, colitis, jaundice, **pseudomembranous colitis**

GU: Vaginitis, pruritus, candidiasis, increased BUN, **nephrotoxicity, renal failure,** pyuria, dysuria, reversible interstitial nephritis

HEMA: **Leukopenia, thrombocytopenia, agranulocytosis,** anemia, neutropenia, lymphocytosis, eosinophilia, pancytopenia, hemolytic anemia, leukocytosis, granulocytopenia

INTEG: Rash, urticaria, dermatitis, **Stevens-Johnson syndrome**

RESP: Dyspnea

SYST: **Anaphylaxis, serum sickness,** superinfection

>> cefaclor
Pharmacokinetics

Absorption	Well absorbed
Distribution	Widely distributed; crosses placenta
Metabolism	Not metabolized
Excretion	Unchanged by kidneys (60%-80%); enters breast milk
Half-life	36-54 min; increased in renal disease

Pharmacodynamics

Onset	15 min
Peak	½-1 hr
Duration	Unknown

>> cefoTEtan
Pharmacokinetics

Absorption	Well absorbed (IM)
Distribution	Widely distributed; crosses placenta
Metabolism	Not metabolized
Excretion	Kidneys, unchanged; enters breast milk
Half-life	5 hr; increased in renal disease

Pharmacodynamics

	IM	IV
Onset	Rapid	Immediate
Peak	1-3 hr	Infusion's end
Duration	Unknown	Unknown

>> cefOXitin
Pharmacokinetics

Absorption	Well absorbed (IM)
Distribution	Widely distributed; crosses placenta
Metabolism	Not metabolized
Excretion	Kidneys, unchanged; enters breast milk
Half-life	½-1 hr; increased in renal disease

Pharmacodynamics

	IM	IV
Onset	Rapid	Immediate
Peak	½ hr	Infusion's end
Duration	Unknown	Unknown

>> cefprozil
Pharmacokinetics

Absorption	Well absorbed
Distribution	Widely distributed; crosses placenta
Metabolism	Not metabolized
Excretion	Kidneys (60%), unchanged; enters breast milk
Half-life	1.3 hr (normal renal function); 2 hr (hepatic disease); 5¼-6 hr (end-stage renal disease)

Pharmacodynamics
Unknown

INTERACTIONS
Individual drugs
Antacids: decreased absorption of cephalosporins
Furosemide: increased effect/toxicity
Plicamycin, valproic acid: increased bleeding
Probenecid: decreased excretion of product and increased blood levels/toxicity

Drug classifications
Aminoglycosides: increased effect/toxicity
Anticoagulants, antiplatelets, NSAIDs, thrombolytics: increased bleeding (cefotetan)
H$_2$-blockers: decreased effects of cephalosporins
Oral contraceptives: decreased effectiveness possible; use additional form of contraception

Drug/lab test
False: increased creatinine (serum urine), urinary 17-KS

Adverse effects: *italics* = common; **bold** = life-threatening

False positive: urinary protein, direct Coombs' test, urine glucose (Clinitest)
Interference: cross-matching

NURSING CONSIDERATIONS
Assessment
• Assess patient for previous sensitivity reaction to penicillins or other cephalosporins; cross-sensitivity between penicillins and cephalosporins is common
• Assess patient for signs and symptoms of **infection** including characteristics of wounds, sputum, urine, stool, WBC $>10,000/mm^3$, earache, fever; obtain baseline information and during treatment
• Obtain C&S before beginning product therapy to identify if correct treatment has been initiated
• **Assess for anaphylaxis: rash, urticaria, pruritus, dyspnea, chills, fever, joint pain; angioedema may occur a few days after therapy begins; EPINEPHrine and resuscitation** equipment should be available for anaphylactic reaction
• **Identify urine output; if decreasing, notify prescriber (may indicate nephrotoxicity); also check for increased BUN, creatinine**
• Monitor blood studies: AST, ALT, CBC, Hct, bilirubin, LDH, alkaline phosphatase, Coombs' test monthly if patient is on long-term therapy
• Monitor electrolytes: potassium, sodium, chloride monthly if patient is on long-term therapy
• **Assess bowel pattern daily; if severe diarrhea occurs, product should be discontinued; may indicate pseudomembranous colitis**
• Monitor for bleeding: ecchymosis, bleeding gums, hematuria, stool guaiac daily if on long-term therapy
• Assess for **overgrowth of infection:** perineal itching, fever, malaise, redness, pain, swelling, drainage, rash, diarrhea, change in cough, sputum

Patient/family education
• Teach patient to report sore throat, bruising, bleeding, joint pain; may indicate **blood dyscrasias** (rare); symptoms of hypersensitivity
• Advise patient to contact prescriber if vaginal itching, loose foul-smelling stools, furry tongue occur; may indicate **superinfection**
• Instruct patient to take all medication prescribed for the length of time ordered; to use yogurt or buttermilk to maintain intestinal flora, decrease diarrhea
• **Advise patient to notify prescriber of diarrhea with blood or pus, which may indicate pseudomembranous colitis**

Evaluation
Positive therapeutic outcome
• Absence of signs/symptoms of infection (WBC $<10,000/mm^3$, temp WNL, absence of red draining wounds, earache)
• Reported improvement in symptoms of infection
• Negative C&S

TREATMENT OF ANAPHYLAXIS: EPINEPHrine, antihistamines, resuscitate if needed

CEPHALOSPORINS—3RD/4TH GENERATION

cefdinir (Rx)
(sef'dih-ner)
Omnicef
cefditoren pivoxil (Rx)
(sef-dit'oh-ren pih-vox'il)
Spectracef
(4th generation) cefepime (Rx)
(sef'e-peem)
Maxipime
cefixime (Rx)
(sef-iks'ime)
Cefixime, Suprax
cefotaxime (Rx)
(sef-oh-taks'eem)
Claforan
cefpodoxime (Rx)
(sef-poe-docks'eem)
Vantin
cefTAZidime (Rx)
(sef'tay-zi-deem)
Ceptaz, Fortaz, Tazicef, Tazidime
ceftibuten (Rx)
(sef-ti-byoo'tin)
Cedax
ceftizoxime (Rx)
(sef-ti-zox'eem)
Cefizox
cefTRIAXone (Rx)
(sef-try-ax'one)
Rocephin
Func. class.: Broad-spectrum antibiotic
Chem. class.: Cephalosporin (3rd generation)
Pregnancy category B

Do not confuse: cefTAZidime/ceftizoxime, Vantin/Ventolin

ACTION: Inhibits bacterial cell wall synthesis, rendering cell wall osmotically unstable, leading to cell death

>> **cefdinir**
Therapeutic outcome: Bactericidal effects for the following: *Citrobacter diversus, Escherichia coli, Haemophilus influenzae, Haemophilus parainfluenzae, Klebsiella pneumoniae, Moraxella catarrhalis, Proteus mirabilis, Staphylococcus aureus, Staphylococcus epidermidis, Streptococcus agalactiae* (group B), *Streptococcus pneumoniae, Streptococcus pyogenes,* viridans streptococci alpha

USES: Uncomplicated skin and skin structure infections, community-acquired pneumonia, acute exacerbations of chronic bronchitis, acute maxillary sinusitis, pharyngitis, tonsillitis, otitis media

>> **cefditoren pivoxil**
Therapeutic outcome: Bactericidal effects for the following organisms: *Haemophilus influenzae, Haemophilus parainfluenzae, Streptococcus pneumoniae, Moraxella catarrhalis, Streptococcus pyogenes, Staphylococcus aureus*

USES: Acute bacterial exacerbation of chronic bronchitis, pharyngitis/tonsillitis; uncomplicated skin, skin structure infections, community-acquired pneumonia, viridans streptococci

>> **cefepime**
Therapeutic outcome: Bactericidal effects for the following: *Acinetobacter calcoaceticus, Acinetobacter lwoffii, Aeromonas hydrophila, Citrobacter diversus, Citrobacter freundii, Enterobacter, Escherichia coli, Gardnerella vaginalis, Hafnia alvei, Klebsiella, Moraxella catarrhalis, Morganella morganii, Neisseria gonorrhoeae, Neisseria meningitidis, Proteus, Providencia rettgeri, Providencia stuartii, Pseudomonas aeruginosa, Salmonella, Serratia liquefaciens, Serratia marcescens, Shigella, Staphylococcus epidermidis, Staphylococcus saprophyticus, Streptococcus agalactiae, Streptococcus bovis, viridans streptococci, Yersinia enterocolitica*

USES: Lower respiratory tract, urinary tract, skin, bone, febrile neutropenia, intraabdominal infection

>> **cefixime**
Therapeutic outcome: Bactericidal effects for the following organisms: *Escherichia coli, Proteus mirabilis, Streptococcus pyogenes, Haemophilus influenzae, Moraxella catarrhalis, Streptococcus pneumoniae*

USES: Uncomplicated UTI, pharyngitis/tonsillitis, otitis media, acute bronchitis, exacerbations of chronic bronchitis, uncomplicated gonorrhea

>> **cefotaxime**
Therapeutic outcome: Bactericidal effects for the following: *Haemophilus influenzae, Haemophilus parainfluenzae, Escherichia coli, Enterococcus faecalis, Neisseria gonorrhoeae, Neisseria meningitidis, Proteus mirabilis, Klebsiella, Citrobacter, Serratia, Salmonella, Shigella Pseudomonas;* gram-positive organisms *Streptococcus pneumoniae, Streptococcus pyogenes, Staphylococcus aureus*

USES: Lower serious respiratory tract, urinary tract, skin, bone, gonococcal infections; bacteremia, septicemia, meningitis, skin, skin structure infections, CNS infections, perioperative prophylaxis, intraabdominal infections, PID, UTI, ventriculitis

>> **cefpodoxime**
Therapeutic outcome: Bactericidal effects for the following: *Neisseria gonorrhoeae, Haemophilus influenzae, Escherichia coli, Proteus mirabilis, Klebsiella;* gram-positive organisms *Streptococcus pneumoniae, Streptococcus pyogenes, Staphylococcus aureus*

USES: Upper and lower respiratory tract, urinary tract, skin infections; otitis media, STDs

>> **cefTAZidime**
Therapeutic outcome: Bactericidal effects for the following: *Haemophilus influenzae, Escherichia coli, Enterobacter aerogenes, Proteus mirabilis, Klebsiella, Citrobacter, Enterobacter, Salmonella, Serratia, Pseudomonas aeruginosa, Shigella, Acinetobacter, Bacteroides fragilis, Neisseria; Streptococcus pneumoniae, Streptococcus pyogenes, Staphylococcus aureus*

USES: Serious upper or lower respiratory tract, urinary tract, skin, gynecologic, bone, joint, intraabdominal infections; septicemia, meningitis, febrile neutropenia

>> **ceftibuten**
Therapeutic outcome: Bactericidal effects for the following: *Haemophilus influenzae, Escherichia coli; Streptococcus pneumoniae, Streptococcus pyogenes, Staphylococcus aureus*

USES: Pharyngitis, tonsillitis, otitis media, secondary bacterial infection of acute bronchitis

>> ceftizoxime
Therapeutic outcome: Bactericidal effects for the following: *Bacteroides, Haemophilus influenzae, Escherichia coli, Enterobacter aerogenes, Proteus mirabilis, Klebsiella, Enterobacter; Streptococcus pneumoniae, Streptococcus pyogenes, Staphylococcus aureus, Neisseria gonorrhoeae*

USES: Serious lower respiratory tract, urinary tract, skin, intraabdominal infections; septicemia, meningitis; bone, joint infections, PID

>> cefTRIAXone
Therapeutic outcome: Bactericidal effects on the following: gram-negative organisms *Haemophilus influenzae, Escherichia coli, Enterobacter aerogenes, Proteus mirabilis, Klebsiella, Citrobacter, Enterobacter, Salmonella, Shigella, Acinetobacter, Bacteroides fragilis, Neisseria, Serratia;* gram-positive organisms *Streptococcus pneumoniae, Streptococcus pyogenes, Staphylococcus aureus*

USES: Serious lower respiratory tract, urinary tract, skin, gonococcal, intraabdominal infections; septicemia, meningitis; bone, joint infections, otitis media, PID

CONTRAINDICATIONS
Hypersensitivity to cephalosporins, infants <1 mo

Precautions: Pregnancy **B**, breastfeeding, children, hypersensitivity to penicillins, renal/GI disease, geriatrics, pseudomembranous colitis, viral infection, vit K deficiencies, diabetes

DOSAGE AND ROUTES

>> cefdinir
Uncomplicated skin and skin structure infections/community-acquired pneumonia
Adult and child ≥13 yr: PO 300 mg q12hr × 10 days
Child 6 mo-12 yr: PO 7 mg/kg q12hr or 14 mg/kg q24hr × 10 days

Acute exacerbations of chronic bronchitis/acute maxillary sinusitis
Adult and child ≥13 yr: PO 300 mg q12hr or 600 mg q24hr × 10 days

Pharyngitis/tonsillitis
Adult and child ≥13 yr: PO 300 mg q12hr or 600 mg q24hr × 5-10 days
Child 6 mo-12 yr: PO 7 mg/kg q12hr × 5-10 days or 14 mg/kg q24hr × 5-10 days

Renal dose
(CCr <30 ml/min)
Adult: 300 mg/day
Child: 7 mg/kg/day

Available forms: Caps 300 mg, oral susp 125 mg/5 ml, 250 mg/5 ml

>> cefditoren pivoxil
Adult: PO 200-400 mg bid × 10-14 days

Renal dose
Adult: PO CCr 30-49 ml/min, max 200 mg bid; CCr <30 ml/min, max 200, 400 mg daily

Available forms: Tabs 200 mg

>> cefepime
Febrile neutropenia
Adult/adolescent >16 yr/child ≥40 kg: IV 2 g q8hr × 7 days or until neutropenia resolves
Infant ≥2 mo/child/adolescent ≤16 yr and weighing up to 40 kg: IV 50 mg/kg/dose q8hr × 7-10 days or until resolution

Urinary tract infections (mild to moderate)
Adult: IV/IM 0.5-1 g q12hr × 7-10 days

Urinary tract infections (severe)
Adult/adolescent >16 yr/child ≥40 kg: IV 2 g q12hr × 10 days

Pneumonia (moderate to severe)
Adult: IV 1-2 g q12hr × 10 days

Available forms: Powder for inj 500 mg, 1, 2 g; 1 g/50 ml, 2 g/100 ml

>> cefixime
Mild to moderate pharyngitis, tonsillitis, bronchitis
Adult/adolescent/child >45 kg: PO 400 mg/day q12-24hr
Child ≤45 kg and infant ≥6 mo: PO 8 mg/kg/day divided q12-24hr

Uncomplicated urinary tract infection (UTI)
Adult/adolescent/child >45 kg: PO 400 mg/day divided q12-24hr
Child ≤45 kg and infant ≥6 mo: PO 8 mg/kg/day divided q12-24hr max: 400 mg/day × 7-14 days is recommended by the American Academy of Pediatrics (AAP) for the treatment of initial UTI in febrile infants and young children 2-24 mo
Infant 2-5 mo (unlabeled): PO 8 mg/kg/day × 7-14 days is recommended by the American Academy of Pediatrics (AAP) for the treatment of initial UTI in febrile infants and young children

Mild to moderate otitis media
Adult/adolescent/child >45 kg: PO 400 mg/day divided q12-24hr

Child ≤45 kg: PO 8 mg/kg/day divided q12-24hr, max: 400 mg/day

Infant ≥6 mo: PO 8 mg/kg/day divided q12-24hr

Gonorrhea of uncomplicated cervicitis, or urethritis due to *N. gonorrhoeae*
Adult/adolescent: PO As alternative therapy, 400 mg as a single dose with a regimen effective against uncomplicated genital *C. trachomatis* infection (e.g., azithromycin as a single dose or doxycycline for 7 days) if chlamydial infection is not ruled out. The CDC states that cefixime is only acceptable if IM cefTRIAXone is not an option due to rising cefixime MICs for gonorrhea. If cefixime is used, test-of-cure should be done at the infected site 1 wk after treatment. Cefixime is not recommended for infections of the pharynx.

Child ≥45 kg: PO 400 mg as a single dose with a regimen effective against uncomplicated genital *C. trachomatis* infection (e.g., azithromycin as a single dose or doxycycline for 7 days) if chlamydial infection is not ruled out. Cefixime is not recommended for infections of the pharynx. Cefixime is an alternative to cefTRIAXone per the American Academy of Pediatrics (AAP).

Renal dose
CCr 21-59 ml/min give 65% of dose; CCr <20 ml/min give 50% of dose

Available forms: Tabs 400 mg; powder for oral susp 100 mg/5 ml; cap 400 mg

>> cefotaxime
Adult/adolescent/child ≥50 kg: IV/IM (uncomplicated infections) 1 g q12hr, (moderate-severe infections) 1-2 g q8hr, (severe infections) 2 g q6-8hr, (life-threatening infections) 2 g q4hr, max 12 g/day

Adolescent/child <50 kg and infant: IV/IM 50-180 mg/kg/day divided q6-8hr, max 2 g/dose, (severe infections) 200-225 mg/kg/day divided q4-6hr max 12 g)

Neonate >7 days: IV/IM 50 mg/kg/dose q8-12hr

Renal dose
Adult: IM CCr <20 ml/min 50% dose reduction

Available forms: Powder for inj 500 mg, 1, 2, 10 g; 1, 2 g premixed frozen

>> cefpodoxime
Pneumonia
Adult >13 yr: PO 200 mg q12hr for 14 days

Skin and skin structure
Adult >13 yr: PO 400 mg q12hr for 7-14 days

Pharyngitis and tonsillitis
Adult >13 yr: PO 100 mg q12hr for 5-10 days

Child 5 mo-12 yr: PO 5 mg/kg q12hr (max 100 mg/dose or 200 mg/day) × 5-10 days

Uncomplicated UTI
Adult >13 yr: PO 100 mg q12hr for 7 days; dosing interval increased in presence of severe renal impairment

Acute otitis media
Child 5 mo-12 yr: PO 5 mg/kg q12hr for 5 days

Available forms: Tabs 100, 200 mg; granules for susp 50, 100 mg/5 ml

>> cefTAZidime
Adult: IV/IM 1-2 g q8-12hr × 5-10 days

Child: IV 30-50 mg/kg q8hr, max 6 g/day

Neonate: IV 30-50 mg/kg q8-12hr

Renal dose
Adult: IV CCr 31-50 ml/min 1 g q12hr; CCr 16-30 ml/min 1 g q24hr; CCr 6-15 ml/min 1 g loading dose, then 0.5 g q24hr; CCr <5 ml/min 1 g loading dose, then 0.5 g q48hr

Available forms: Inj 250, 500 mg, 1, 2, 6 g

>> ceftibuten
Adult: PO 400 mg daily × 10 days

Child 6 mo-12 yr: PO 9 mg/kg daily × 10 days

Renal dose
Adult: PO CCr 30-49 ml/min 200 mg q24hr; CCr 5-29 ml/min 100 mg q24hr

Available forms: Caps 400 mg; susp 90, 180 mg/5 ml

>> ceftizoxime
Adult: IM/IV 1-2 g q8-12hr, may give up to 4 g q8hr in life-threatening infections

Child >6 mo: IM/IV 50 mg/kg q6-8hr

Renal dose
Adult: IM/IV CCr 50-79 ml/min; give loading dose 0.5-1 g, then 0.5 g q8h; CCr 5-49 ml/min give loading dose then 250-500, mg q12hr; CCr <5 ml/min give loading dose then 250-500 mg q24hr

PID
Adult: IV 2 g q8hr, may increase to 4 g q8hr in severe infections

Available forms: Premixed 1 g, 2 g/50 ml

>> cefTRIAXone
Adult: IM/IV 1-2 g daily, max 4 g q24hr

Child: IM/IV 50-75 mg/kg/day in equal doses q12-24hr

Uncomplicated gonorrhea
Adult: 250 mg IM as single dose
Reduce dosage in severe renal impairment (CCr <10 ml/min)

Available forms: Inj 250, 500 mg, 1, 2, 10 g

Implementation

>> cefdinir
PO route
• Give oral susp after adding 39 ml water to the 60 ml bottle; 65 ml water to the 12.0 ml bottle; discard unused portion after 10 days, give without regard to food, do not give within 2 hr of antacids, iron supplements

>> cefditoren pivoxil
• Give for 10 days to ensure organism death, prevent superinfection
• Give with food if needed, do not give with antacids
• Give after C&S is completed

>> cefepime
IV route
• Check for irritation, extravasation, phlebitis daily; change site q72hr
• For **intermittent inf** dilute with 50-100 ml of D5W, give over 30 min

Solution compatibilities: 0.9% NaCl, D5, 0.5, 1.0% lidocaine, bacteriostatic water for inj with parabens/benzyl alcohol

>> cefixime
• Give for 10-14 days to ensure organism death, prevent superinfection

>> cefotaxime
IV route
• **Dilute** 1 g/10 ml D5W, NS, sterile water for inj and **give** over 3-5 min by Y-tube or 3-way stopcock; may be **diluted further** with 50-100 ml of 0.9% NaCl or D5W; **run** over ½-1 hr; discontinue primary inf during administration; or may be diluted in larger volume of sol and given as a cont inf
• Give for 10-14 days to ensure organism death, prevent superinfection
• Thaw frozen container at room temperature or refrigeration, do not force thaw by immersion or microwave; visually inspect container for leaks

Syringe compatibilities: Heparin, ofloxacin

Y-site compatibilities: Acyclovir, alfentanil, alprostadil, amifostine, amikacin, aminocaproic acid, aminophylline, anidulafungin, ascorbic acid injection, atenolol, atracurium, atropine, aztreonam, benztropine, bivalirudin, bleomycin, bumetanide, buprenorphine, butorphanol, caffeine, calcium chloride/gluconate, CARBOplatin, cefamandole, cefmetazole, cefonicid, cefoperazone, cefoTEtan, cefOXitin, cefTAZidime (L-arginine), cefTRIAXone sodium, cefuroxime, cimetidine, CISplatin, clindamycin, codeine, cyanocobalamin, cyclophosphamide, cycloSPORINE, cytarabine, DACTINomycin, DAPTOmycin, dexamethasone, dexmedetomidine, digoxin, diltiazem, DOCEtaxel, DOPamine, doxacurium, doxycycline, enalaprilat, ePHEDrine, EPINEPHrine, epirubicin, epoetin alfa, eptifibatide, erythromycin, esmolol, etoposide, famotidine, fenoldopam, fentaNYL, fludarabine, fluorouracil, folic acid, furosemide, gatifloxacin, gentamicin, glycopyrrolate, granisetron, heparin, hydrocortisone, HYDROmorphone, ifosfamide, imipenem-cilastatin, insulin (regular), isoproterenol, ketorolac, lidocaine, linezolid, LORazepam, LR, magnesium sulfate, mannitol, mechlorethamine, melphalan, meperidine, metaraminol, methicillin, methotrexate, methoxamine, methyldopate, metoclopramide, metoprolol, metroNIDAZOLE, mezlocillin, miconazole, midazolam, milrinone, minocycline, mitoXANtrone, morphine, moxalactam, multiple vitamins, mycophenolate, nafcillin, nalbuphine, naloxone, nesiritide, netilmicin, nitroglycerin, nitroprusside, norepinephrine, normal saline, octreotide, ofloxacin, ondansetron, ornidazole, oxacillin, oxaliplatin, oxytocin, PACLitaxel, palonosetron, pamidronate, pancuronium, pantoprazole, papaverine, pefloxacin, PEMEtrexed, penicillin G potassium/sodium, pentamidine, pentazocine, PENTobarbital, peritoneal dialysis solution, perphenazine, PHENobarbital, phenylephrine, phenytoin, phytonadione, piperacillin, polymyxin B, potassium chloride, procainamide, prochlorperazine, promethazine, propofol, propranolol, protamine, quiNIDine, quinupristin, ranitidine, remifentanil, Ringer's injection, ritodrine, riTUXimab, rocuronium, sargramostim, sodium acetate/bicarbonate, sodium fusidate, sodium lactate, succinylcholine, SUFentanil, sulfamethoxazole-trimethoprim, tacrolimus, teniposide, theophylline, thiamine, thiotepa, ticarcillin, ticarcillin-clavulanate, tigecycline, tirofiban, TNA, tobramycin, tolazoline, TPN, trastuzumab, trimetaphan, urokinase, vancomycin, vasopressin, vecuronium, verapamil, vinorelbine, voriconazole

>> cefpodoxime
PO route
• Do not break, crush, or chew tabs due to taste
• Give for 10-14 days to ensure organism death, prevent superinfection

---

- With food for better absorption, do not give within 2 hr of antacids, H_2 receptor antagonists
- Shake susp well, refrigerate, discard after 2 wk

>> cefTAZidime

IM route

- **Fortaz, Tazidime vials:** Reconstitute 500 mg or 1 g with 1.5 or 3 ml, respectively, of sterile or bacteriostatic water for injection, or 0.5%-1% lidocaine (approx. 280 mg/ml)
- **Tazicef vials:** Reconstitute 1 g/3 ml sterile water for injection (approx. 280 mg/ml)
- **Ceptaz vials:** Reconstitute 1 g/3 ml sterile or bacteriostatic water for injection or 0.5%-1% lidocaine (approx. 250 mg/ml)
- Withdraw the dose, making sure the needle remains in the vial; ensure that no CO_2 bubbles are present; inject deeply in large muscle mass; aspirate prior to injection

IV route

- If possible, visually inspect for particulate matter and discoloration
- **Fortaz, Tazicef, Tazidime packs:** Reconstitute 1 or 2 g/100 ml sterile water for injection or other compatible **IV** sol (10 or 20 mg/ml, respectively). Reconstitution is done in two stages. First, inject 10 ml of the diluents into the pack and shake well to dissolve and become clear; CO_2 pressure inside the container will occur; insert a vent needle to release the pressure; add remaining diluents and remove vent needle
- **Fortaz, Tazicef, Tazidime vials:** Reconstitute 500 mg, 1 g, 2 g with 5, 10, 10 ml, respectively, of sterile water for injection or other compatible **IV** sol (100, 95-100, or 170-180 mg/ml, respectively; shake well to dissolve
- **Fortaz, Tazidime-ADD-Vantage vials** (for **IV** only): Reconstitute 1 or 2 g with NS, ½ NS, D_5W in either 50 or 100 ml flexible diluents container; to release CO_2 pressure, insert a vent needle after dissolving; remove vent before using
- **Ceptaz packs:** Reconstitute 1 or 2 g/100 ml sterile water for injection or compatible **IV** sol (10 or 20 mg/ml, respectively). Reconstitution is done in two stages. First, inject 10 ml of the diluent into the pack and shake well to dissolve; add the remaining diluents; insert as vent needle before giving
- **Ceptaz vials:** Reconstitute 1 or 2 g/10 ml of sterile water for injection or compatible **IV** sol (90-95, or 170-180 mg/ml, respectively)

- **Ceptaz ADD-Vantage vials** (for **IV** infusion only): Reconstitute 1 or 2 g with NS, ½ NS, or D_5W in either 50 or 100 ml diluent container as appropriate

Direct intermittent IV infusion route

- **Vials:** Withdraw the correct dose, making sure the needle opening remains in the solution; make sure there are no CO_2 bubbles in the syringe before injection; inject directly over 3-5 min or slowly into the tubing of a free-flowing compatible **IV** solution

Intermittent IV infusion route

- **Vials:** Withdraw the correct dose, making sure the needle opening remains in the solution; make sure there are no CO_2 bubbles in the syringe before injection; infusion packs and ADD-Vantage systems are ready for infusion after reconstitution; infuse over 15-30 min

>> ceftibuten

- Administer for 10 days to ensure organism death, prevent superinfection
- Administer after C&S
- Administer on empty stomach

>> ceftizoxime

IM route

- Reconstitute 250 mg/0.9 ml, 500 mg/1.8 ml, 1 g/3.6 ml, 2 g/7.2 ml; may be diluted with 0.5% or 1% lidocaine to prevent pain; give deep in large muscle mass, massage

IV route

- Check for irritation, extravasation, phlebitis daily; change site q72hr
- For intermittent inf reconstitute 250 mg/2.4 ml, 500 mg/4.8 ml, 1 g/9.6 mg/2 g/19.2 ml sterile water for inj, D_5W, or 0.9% NaCl; do not use sol with benzyl alcohol for neonates; may be further diluted in 50-100 ml of D_5W, $D_{10}W$, 0.9% NaCl, or LR; give over 15-30 min
- May store 96 hr refrigerated, 24 hr room temperature

Y-site compatibilities: Acetaminophen, acyclovir, allopurinol, amifostine, argatroban, aztreonam, enalaprilat, esmolol, famotidine, fludarabine, foscarnet, HYDROmorphone, labetalol, melphalan, meperidine, morphine, ondansetron, sargramostim, teniposide, thiotepa, vinorelbine

Additive compatibilities: Clindamycin, metroNIDAZOLE

Additive incompatibilities: Aminoglycosides

>> cefTRIAXone
- Give IM inj deep in large muscle mass
- Give for 10-14 days to ensure organism death, prevent superinfection

IV route
- Give **IV** after diluting 250 mg/2.4 ml of 500 mg/4.8 ml, 1 g/9.6 ml, 2 g/19.2 ml D$_5$W, water for inj, 0.9% NaCl; may be further diluted with 50-100 ml of 0.9% NaCl, D$_5$W, D$_{10}$W, shake; run over ½-1 hr
- Do not mix with calcium salts

Y-site compatibilities: Acyclovir, allopurinol, aztreonam, cisatracurium, diltiazem, DOXOrubicin liposome, fludarabine, foscarnet, heparin, melphalan, meperidine, methotrexate, morphine, PACLitaxel, remifentanil, sargramostim, tacrolimus, teniposide, theophylline, vinorelbine, warfarin, zidovudine

Additive compatibilities: Amino acids or sodium bicarbonate, metroNIDAZOLE

ADVERSE EFFECTS
CNS: Headache, dizziness, weakness, paresthesia, fever, chills, seizures, dyskinesia (cefdinir)
CV: Heart failure, syncope (cefdinir)
EENT: *Oral candidiasis*
GI: *Nausea, vomiting, diarrhea, anorexia, pain,* glossitis, bleeding; increased AST, ALT, bilirubin, LDH, alkaline phosphatase; abdominal pain, pseudomembranous colitis, cholestasis (cefotaxime)
GU: Proteinuria, vaginitis, pruritus, *candidiasis,* increased BUN, nephrotoxicity, renal failure
HEMA: Leukopenia, thrombocytopenia, agranulocytosis, anemia, neutropenia, lymphocytosis, eosinophilia, pancytopenia, hemolytic anemia
INTEG: Rash, urticaria, dermatitis
MS: Arthralgia (cefditoren)
RESP: Dyspnea
SYST: Anaphylaxis, serum sickness, Stevens-Johnson syndrome, toxic epidermal necrolysis

>> cefdinir
Pharmacokinetics

Absorption	Well absorbed
Distribution	Widely distributed; crosses placenta
Metabolism	Not metabolized
Excretion	Kidneys, unchanged; enters breast milk
Half-life	1.7 hr

Pharmacodynamics

Unknown

>> cefditoren pivoxil
Pharmacokinetics

Absorption	Well absorbed after it is broken down (prodrug)
Distribution	Widely
Metabolism	Unknown
Excretion	Unknown
Half-life	100 mins

Pharmacodynamics

Onset	Rapid
Peak	1.5-3 hr
Duration	12 hrs

>> cefepime
Pharmacokinetics

Absorption	Well absorbed (IM)
Distribution	Widely distributed; crosses placenta
Metabolism	Not metabolized
Excretion	Kidneys, unchanged; enters breast milk
Half-life	2 hr; increased in renal disease

Pharmacodynamics

	IM	IV
Onset	Rapid	Immediate
Peak	79 min	Infusion's end
Duration	Unknown	Unknown

>> cefixime
Pharmacokinetics

Absorption	Unknown
Distribution	Protein binding 65%-70%
Metabolism	Unknown
Excretion	Urine, bile
Half-life	3-4 hr

Pharmacodynamics

Onset	Unknown
Peak	2-6 hr
Duration	Unknown

>> cefotaxime
Pharmacokinetics

Absorption	Widely distributed
Distribution	Breast milk, small amounts
Metabolism	Liver, active metabolites
Excretion	40%-65% unchanged, kidney
Half-life	1 hr

Pharmacodynamics

	IV	IM
Onset	5 min	30 min
Peak	Unknown	Unknown
Duration	Unknown	Unknown

>> cefpodoxime
Pharmacokinetics

Absorption	Well absorbed
Distribution	Widely distributed; crosses placenta, protein binding 13%-38%
Metabolism	Not metabolized
Excretion	Kidneys, unchanged; enters breast milk
Half-life	1-1.5 hr, increased in renal disease

Pharmacodynamics
Unknown

>> cefTAZidime
Pharmacokinetics

Absorption	Well absorbed (IM)
Distribution	Widely distributed; crosses placenta
Metabolism	Not metabolized
Excretion	Kidneys, unchanged; enters breast milk
Half-life	1-2 hr; increased in renal disease

Pharmacodynamics

	IM	IV
Onset	Rapid	Immediate
Peak	1.5-2 hr	Infusion's end

>> ceftibuten
Pharmacokinetics

Absorption	Well absorbed
Distribution	Widely distributed; crosses placenta
Metabolism	Not metabolized
Excretion	Kidneys, unchanged; enters breast milk
Half-life	1-1½ hr; increased in renal disease

Pharmacodynamics
Unknown

>> ceftizoxime
Pharmacokinetics

Absorption	Well absorbed (IM)
Distribution	Widely distributed; crosses placenta, protein binding 30%
Metabolism	Not metabolized
Excretion	Kidneys, unchanged; enters breast milk
Half-life	1½-2 hr; increased in renal disease

Pharmacodynamics

	IM	IV
Onset	Rapid	Immediate
Peak	1 hr	Infusion's end

>> cefTRIAXone
Pharmacokinetics

Absorption	Well absorbed
Distribution	Widely distributed; crosses placenta; enters CSF, protein binding 58%-96%
Metabolism	Liver
Excretion	Kidneys, partly
Half-life	6-9 hr

Pharmacodynamics

	IM	IV
Onset	Rapid	Immediate
Peak	1.5-4 hr	30 min

INTERACTIONS
Individual drugs
Many products should not be used with calcium salts (mixed or administered) or H$_2$ blockers antacids (PO)

CycloSPORINE: increased cycloSPORINE levels
Furosemide, probenecid: increased toxicity
Iron: decreased absorption of cefdinir
Plicamycin, valproic acid: increased bleeding

Drug classifications
Aminoglycosides: increased toxicity
Anticoagulants, NSAIDs, thrombolytics: increased bleeding

Drug/food
Iron-rich cereal, infants' formula: decreased absorption

Drug/lab test
Increased: ALT, AST, alkaline phosphatase, LDH, bilirubin, BUN, creatinine
False increase: creatinine (serum urine), urinary 17-KS
False positive: urinary protein, direct Coombs' test, urine glucose
Interference: cross-matching

NURSING CONSIDERATIONS
Assessment
• Assess patient for previous sensitivity reaction to penicillins or other cephalosporins; cross-sensitivity between penicillins and cephalosporins is common
• Assess patient for signs and symptoms of **infection** including characteristics of wounds, sputum, urine, stool, WBC >10,000/mm³, fever; obtain baseline information and during treatment
• Obtain C&S before beginning product therapy to identify if correct treatment has been initiated
• **Assess for anaphylaxis: rash, urticaria, pruritus, chills, fever, joint pain; angioedema may occur a few days after therapy begins; EPINEPHrine and resuscitation equipment should be available for anaphylactic reaction**
• **Identify urine output; if decreasing, notify prescriber (may indicate nephrotoxicity); also check for increased BUN, creatinine**
• Monitor blood studies: AST, ALT, CBC, Hct, bilirubin, LDH, alkaline phosphatase, Coombs' test monthly if patient is on long-term therapy
• Monitor electrolytes: potassium, sodium, chloride monthly if patient is on long-term therapy
• **Assess bowel pattern daily; if severe diarrhea occurs, product should be discontinued; may indicate pseudomembranous colitis**
• Monitor for **bleeding:** ecchymosis, bleeding gums, hematuria, stool guaiac daily if on long-term therapy
• Assess for **overgrowth of infection:** perineal itching, fever, malaise, redness, pain,

swelling, drainage, rash, diarrhea, change in cough, sputum
• Monitor heart rate during direct IV infusion (cefotaxime)

Patient/family education
• Teach patient to report sore throat, bruising, bleeding, joint pain; may indicate blood dyscrasias (rare)
• Advise patient to contact prescriber if vaginal itching, loose foul-smelling stools, furry tongue occur; may indicate superinfection
• **Advise patient to notify prescriber of diarrhea with blood or pus, may indicate pseudomembranous colitis**

Evaluation
Positive therapeutic outcome
• Absence of signs/symptoms of infection (WBC <10,000/mm³, temp WNL, absence of red draining wounds, earache)
• Reported improvement in symptoms of infection
• Negative C&S

TREATMENT OF ANAPHYLAXIS: EPINEPHrine, antihistamines, resuscitate if needed

cephradine
See cephalosporins—1st generation

certolizumab pegol (Rx)
(ser'tue-liz'oo-mab) (pegh'ol)
Cimzia
Func. class.: Biologic response modifier
Chem. class.: Anti-TNF (tissue necrosis factor) agent
Pregnancy category B

ACTION: Monoclonal antibody that neutralizes the activity of tumor necrosis factor-α (TNF-α) found in Crohn's disease; decreased infiltration of inflammatory cells

Therapeutic outcome: Absence of fever, mucus in stools

USES: Crohn's disease (moderate-severe) that has not responded to conventional therapy, rheumatoid arthritis (moderate-severe), psoriatic arthritis, ankylosing spondylitis

CONTRAINDICATIONS
Influenza, **IV** administration, sepsis, hypersensitivity

Precautions: Pregnancy **B**, breastfeeding, children, geriatric patients, AIDS, coagulopathy, diabetes, fungal infection, heart failure, hepatitis, human anti-chimertic antibody, immunosuppression, leukopenia, MS, cancer, neurologic disease, surgery, thrombocytopenia, TB, vaccinations, renal disease

> **BLACK BOX WARNING:** Infection, neoplastic disease

DOSAGE AND ROUTES
Crohn's disease (moderate-severe)
Adult: SUBCUT 400 mg given as 2 inj at wk 0, 2, 4; if clinical response occurs, give 400 mg q4wk

Rheumatoid arthritis (moderate-severe)
Adult: SUBCUT 400 mg q2wk × 3 doses, then 200 mg q2wk; given with methotrexate

Available forms: Powder for inj 200, 400 mg kit

Implementation
• Store in refrigerator; do not freeze
SUBCUT route
• Give by SUBCUT only
• Allow reconstitution to warm to room temp; add 1 ml sterile water for inj to each vial; two vials will be needed for Crohn's disease
• Gently swirl; do not shake; full reconstitution may take up to 30 min; reconstituted product may remain at room temp for up to 2 hr or refrigerated up to 24 hr
• Warm to room temperature if reconstituted product has been refrigerated
• Use 2 syringes and 2 20-G needles
• Withdraw reconstituted sol from each vial into separate syringes; each will contain 200 mg; switch 20-G to 23-G needle; inject into 2 separate sites in abdomen or thigh

ADVERSE EFFECTS
CNS: *Dizziness*, syncope, peripheral neuropathy, fever, **seizures, demyelinating disease of CNS**
CV: **Heart failure, MI, cardiac dysrhythmia**
EENT: Optic neuritis, retinal hemorrhage, uveitis
GI: Increased LFTs, **hepatitis, bowel obstruction**
GU: UTI, renal disease
HEMA: **Anemia, aplastic anemia, pancytopenia, thrombocytopenia**
INTEG: *Rash, urticaria,* **angioedema**
RESP: Dyspnea, URI

SYST: **Anaphylaxis, malignancies, serum sickness,** bleeding, antibody formation, infection, lupus-like symptoms, lymphadenopathy, arthralgia, **suicidal ideation**

Pharmacokinetics

Absorption	Unknown
Distribution	Unknown
Metabolism	Unknown
Excretion	Unknown
Half-life	Terminal 14 days

Pharmacodynamics

Onset	Unknown
Peak	54-171 hr
Duration	Unknown

INTERACTIONS
Individual drugs
Abatacept, adalimumab, anakinra, etanercept, infliximab, do not use concurrently, rilonacept: increased possible infections
Adalimumab, etanercept, infliximab: increased possible malignancies

Drug classifications
Immunosuppressive agents: increased possible infections, do not use concurrently
Live vaccines, toxoids: do not administer concurrently

NURSING CONSIDERATIONS
Assessment
• Monitor antibody test (ANA), hepatitis B serology, CBC
• Assess for rheumatoid arthritis, ROM, pain
• Assess GI symptoms: nausea, vomiting, abdominal pain, hepatitis, increased LFTs
• Monitor periodic blood counts (CBC)
• Assess CV status: B/P, pulse, chest pain
⚠ Assess for allergic reaction, anaphylaxis: **rash, dermatitis, urticaria, dyspnea, hypotension, fever, chills; discontinue if severe, administer EPINEPHrine, corticosteroids, antihistamines; assess for allergies to murine proteins before starting therapy**

> **BLACK BOX WARNING:** Assess **infections:** discontinue if infection occurs; do not administer to patients with active infections

> **BLACK BOX WARNING:** Identify TB, risk for HBV before beginning treatment; a TB test should be obtained; if present, TB should be treated prior to receiving inFLIXimab

Patient/family education
• Instruct patient not to breastfeed while taking this product

> **BLACK BOX WARNING:** Advise patient to notify prescriber of GI symptoms, hypersensitivity reactions, infections, fluid retention, redness, pain, swelling at injection site

> **BLACK BOX WARNING:** Caution patient not to operate machinery, drive if dizziness, vertigo occur

Evaluation
Positive therapeutic outcome
• Absence of fever, mucus in stools

cetirizine (Rx)
(se-tear'i-zeen)
All Day Allergy, All Day Allergy Children's, Reactine ✦, ZyrTEC, ZyrTEC Children's
Func. class.: Antihistamine, peripherally selective (2nd generation)
Chem. class.: Piperazine, H_1 histamine antagonist
Pregnancy category B   ⭐

Do not confuse: ZyrTEC/Xanax/Zantac

ACTION: Acts on blood vessels, GI, respiratory system by competing with histamine for H_1-receptor site; decreases allergic response by blocking pharmacologic effects of histamine; minimal anticholinergic/sedative action

Therapeutic outcome: Absence of allergy symptoms, rhinitis, and chronic idiopathic urticaria

USES: Rhinitis, allergy symptoms, and chronic idiopathic urticaria

CONTRAINDICATIONS
Hypersensitivity to this product or hydrOXYzine, breastfeeding, newborn or premature infants, severe hepatic disease

Precautions: Pregnancy **B**, children, geriatric, respiratory disease, closed-angle glaucoma, prostatic hypertrophy, bladder neck obstruction, asthma

DOSAGE AND ROUTES
Perennial/seasonal allergic rhinitis or idiopathic urticaria
Adult and child ≥6 yr: PO 5-10 mg daily

Child 2-5 yr: PO 2.5 mg daily, may increase to 5 mg daily or 2.5 mg bid
Child 1-2 yr: PO 2.5 mg daily, may increase to 2.5 mg q12hr
Child 6-11 mo: PO 2.5 mg daily
Geriatric: PO 5 mg daily, may increase to 10 mg/day

Self-treatment of hay fever/other respiratory allergies
Adult/adolescent/child ≥6 yr: PO 10 mg/day, oral SOL 5-10 mg/day

Renal dose
Adult: PO CCr 11-31 ml/min 5 mg daily

Hemodialysis
Adult: PO 5 mg/day

Hepatic dose
Adult: PO 5 mg daily

Available forms: Tabs 5, 10 mg; syr 5 mg/5 ml; prefilled spoons 1 mg/ml; oral sol 5 mg/5 ml; liquid filled cap 10 mg; chew tab 5, 10 mg; orally disintegrating tab 10 mg

Implementation
• Give without regard to meals
• Store in tight, light-resistant container
• **Caps:** swallow whole, do not break, cut, chew, crush
• **Chew tabs:** chew before swallowing, may use without or with water
• **Oral liquid:** use calibrated measuring device

ADVERSE EFFECTS
CNS: *Headache*, stimulation, *drowsiness*, sedation, *fatigue*, confusion, blurred vision, tinnitus, restlessness, tremors, paradoxical excitation in children or geriatric
GI: *Dry mouth*, increased liver function tests, constipation
INTEG: Rash, eczema, photosensitivity, urticaria
RESP: *Thickening of bronchial secretions;* dry nose, throat

Pharmacokinetics
Absorption	Well absorbed, rapid
Distribution	Protein binding 93%
Metabolism	Liver
Excretion	Kidneys
Half-life	8.3 hr, decreased in children, increased in renal/hepatic disease

Pharmacodynamics
Onset	½ hr
Peak	1-2 hr
Duration	24 hr

INTERACTIONS
Individual drugs
Alcohol: increased CNS depression
Ritonavir: increased cetirizine effect

Drug classifications
CNS depressants, opioids, sedative/hypnotics: increased CNS depression
MAOIs: increased anticholinergic effect

Drug/food
Prolongs absorption by 1.7 hr

Drug/lab test
False negative: skin allergy tests (discontinue antihistamine 3 days before testing)

NURSING CONSIDERATIONS
Assessment
• Assess respiratory status: rate, rhythm; increase in bronchial secretions, wheezing, chest tightness; provide fluids to 2 L/day to decrease secretion thickness
• Assess for **allergy symptoms:** pruritus, urticaria, watering eyes, baseline, during treatment

Patient/family education
• Teach all aspects of product uses; to notify prescriber if confusion, sedation, hypotension occur; to avoid driving or other hazardous activity if drowsiness occurs; to avoid alcohol or other CNS depressants that may potentiate effect
• Instruct patient to take without regard to meals
• Instruct patient not to exceed recommended dose; dysrhythmias may occur
• Advise patient to avoid using if breastfeeding
• Advise patient to avoid exposure to sunlight; burns may occur
• Advise patient to use sugarless gum, candy, frequent sips of water to minimize dry mouth
• Advise patient to avoid alcohol, OTC antihistamines, other CNS depressants

Evaluation
Positive therapeutic outcome
• Absence of runny or congested nose, rashes

TREATMENT OF OVERDOSE:
Lavage, diazepam, vasopressors, phenytoin IV

▲ HIGH ALERT

cetrorelix (Rx)
(set-roe-ree′lix)
Cetrotide
Func. class.: Gonadotropin-releasing
Chem. class.: Synthetic decapeptide
Pregnancy category X

ACTION: Inhibitor of pituitary gonadotropin secretion; initially increases LH and FSH, induces a rapid suppression of gonadotropin secretion

Therapeutic outcome: Pregnancy

USES: For inhibition of premature LH surges in women undergoing controlled ovarian hyperstimulation

CONTRAINDICATIONS
Pregnancy **X,** breastfeeding, hypersensitivity, latex allergy, renal disease, KRA5 mutation

Precautions: Geriatric, bronchospasm

DOSAGE AND ROUTES
Single-dose regimen
Adult: SUBCUT 3 mg when serum estradiol level is at appropriate stimulation response, usually on stimulation day 7; if hCG has not been given within 4 days after inj of 3 mg cetrorelix, give 0.25 mg daily until day of hCG administration

Multiple-dose regimen
Adult: SUBCUT 0.25 mg is given on stimulation day 5 (either morning or evening) or 6 (morning) and continued daily until day hCG is given

Available forms: Inj 0.25 mg

Implementation
SUBCUT route
• Give SUBCUT using abdomen, 1 inch away from navel, or upper thigh; swab inj area with disinfectant, clean a 2-in circle and allow to dry, pinch up area between thumb and finger, insert needle at 45-90 degrees to surface; if blood is drawn into the syringe, reposition needle without removing it; rotate inj sites
• Do not administer if patient is pregnant
• Protect from light

ADVERSE EFFECTS
CNS: Headache, hot flashes
CV: Edema
ENDO: Ovarian hyperstimulation syndrome, abdominal pain (gyn)
GI: Nausea, vomiting, diarrhea

INTEG: Pain on inj; local site reactions, bruising, pruritus
OTHER: Rapid weight gain
RESP: Shortness of breath
SYST: Fetal death, anaphylaxis

Pharmacokinetics

Absorption	Unknown
Distribution	Protein binding 86%
Metabolism	Liver to metabolites
Excretion	Feces/urine
Half-life	Depends on dosage

Pharmacodynamics
Unknown

NURSING CONSIDERATIONS
Assessment
• **Assess for suspected pregnancy; product should not be used, pregnancy X**
• Assess for **latex allergy**; product should not be used
• Monitor ALT, AST, GGT, alkaline phosphatase, serum progesterone, LH; ovarian ultrasound days 7-14
• **Assess for anaphylaxis during first infusion**

Patient/family education
• Instruct to report abdominal pain, vaginal bleeding, nausea, vomiting, diarrhea, shortness of breath, peripheral edema
• Teach self-administration technique if needed

Evaluation
Positive therapeutic outcome
• Pregnancy

cetuximab (Rx)
(se-tux′i-mab)
Erbitux
Func. class.: Antineoplastic—miscellaneous, monoclonal antibody
Chem. class.: Epidermal growth factor receptor inhibitor
Pregnancy category C

ACTION: Not fully understood; binds to epidermal growth factor receptors (EGFRs); inhibits phosphorylation and activation of receptor-associated kinase resulting in inhibition of cell growth

Therapeutic outcome: Decrease in tumor size

USES: Alone or in combination with irinotecan for EGFR expressing metastatic colorectal carcinoma, head/neck cancer

CONTRAINDICATIONS
Hypersensitivity to this product or murine proteins

Precautions: Pregnancy **C**, breastfeeding, child, geriatric, CV/renal/hepatic disease, ocular, pulmonary disorders

> **BLACK BOX WARNING:** Arrhythmias, CAD, platinum-based therapy infusion-related reactions, radiation, cardiac, respiratory arrest

DOSAGE AND ROUTES
Adult: IV INF 400 mg/m² loading dose given over 120 min, max INF rate 5 ml/min, weekly maintenance dose (all other infusions) is 250 mg/m² given over 60 min, max INF rate 5 ml/min (10 mg/min); premedicate with an H₁ antagonist (diphenhydrAMINE 50 mg **IV**); dosage adjustments are made for INF reactions or dermatologic toxicity; other protocols are used

Available forms: Sol for inj 100 mg/50 ml, 200 mg/100 ml

Implementation
Intermittent infusion route
• Administer by **IV** infusion only, do not give by **IV** push or bolus
• Do not shake or dilute
• Do not dilute with other products
• **Infusion pump:** draw up volume of a vial using appropriate syringe/needle (a vented spike or other appropriate transfer device); fill Erbitux into sterile evacuated container/bag, repeat until calculated volume has been put into the container. Use a new needle for each vial; give through in-line filter (low protein binding 0.22-micrometer); affix inf line and prime before starting inf, max rate 5 ml/min; flush line at end of inf with 0.9% NaCl
• **Syringe pump:** Draw up volume of a vial using appropriate syringe/needle (a vented spike); place syringe into syringe driver of a syringe pump and set rate; use an in-line filter 0.22 micrometer (low protein binding); connect inf line and start inf after priming; repeat until calculated volume has been given
• Use a new needle and filter for each vial, max 5 ml/min rate; use 0.9% NaCl to flush line after inf
• Do not piggyback to patient inf line
• Observe patient for adverse reactions for 1hr after inf

BLACK BOX WARNING: Inf reactions: if mild (grade 1 or 2) reduce all doses by 50%; if severe (grade 3 or 4) permanently discontinue

• Store refrigerated 36°-46° F, discard unused portions

ADVERSE EFFECTS

CNS: *Headache, insomnia, depression,* aseptic meningitis

CV: Cardiac arrest

GI: *Nausea, diarrhea, vomiting, anorexia, mouth ulceration, dehydration, constipation, abdominal pain*

HEMA: Leukepenia, anemia, neutropenia

INTEG: Rash, pruritus, acne, dry skin, toxic epidermal necrolysis, angioedema, *blepharitis, cheilitis, cellulitis, cysts, alopecia, skin/ nail disorder,* acute infusion reactions, other skin toxicities

MISC: *Conjunctivitis, asthma, malaise, fever,* renal failure, hypomagnesemia

MS: *Back pain*

RESP: Interstitial lung disease, *cough, dyspnea,* pulmonary embolus, *peripheral edema,* respiratory arrest

SYST: Anaphylaxis, sepsis, infection, Stevens-Johnson syndrome, toxic epidermal necrolysis

Pharmacokinetics

Absorption	Unknown
Distribution	Unknown
Metabolism	Unknown
Excretion	Unknown
Half-life	114 hrs

Pharmacodynamics

Onset	Unknown
Peak	168-235 g/ml
Duration	Steady state by 3rd weekly infusion

INTERACTIONS
Drug/lab test
Increase: LFTs

NURSING CONSIDERATIONS
Assessment

BLACK BOX WARNING: Monitor pulmonary changes: lung sounds, cough, dyspnea; interstitial lung disease may occur, may be fatal; discontinue therapy if confirmed

• **Cardiac arrest: monitor electrolytes; in those undergoing radiation therapy, electrolytes may be decreased**

⚠ **Assess for toxic epidermal necrosis, angioedema, anaphylaxis, Stevens-Johnson syndrome**
• Assess GI symptoms: frequency of stools, dehydration, abdominal pain, stomatitis
• Obtain **K-RAS mutation** in metastatic colorectal carcinoma; if K-RAS mutation in codon 12 or 13 is detected, then patient should not receive anti-EGFR antibody therapy

Patient/family education

BLACK BOX WARNING: Instruct patient to report adverse reactions immediately: SOB, severe abdominal pain, skin eruptions

• Explain reason for treatment, expected results

BLACK BOX WARNING: Instruct patient to use contraception during treatment

• Advise patient to wear sunscreen and hat to limit sun exposure; sun exposure can exacerbate any skin reactions

Evaluation
Positive therapeutic outcome
• Decrease growth, spread of EGFR expressing metastatic colorectal carcinoma

chlordiazePOXIDE (Rx)
(klor-dye-az-e-pox′ide)
Librium
Func. class.: Antianxiety
Chem. class.: Benzodiazepine, long-acting
Pregnancy category D
Controlled substance schedule IV

Do not confuse: Librium/Librax

ACTION: Potentiates the actions of GABA, an inhibitory neurotransmitter, especially in the limbic system, reticular formation, which depresses the CNS

Therapeutic outcome: Decreased anxiety, successful alcohol withdrawal, relaxation

USES: Short-term management of anxiety, acute alcohol withdrawal, preoperative relaxation

CONTRAINDICATIONS
Pregnancy **D**, breastfeeding, child <6 yr, hypersensitivity to benzodiazepines, closed-angle glaucoma, psychosis

Precautions: Geriatric, debilitated, renal/ hepatic disease, suicidal ideation, abrupt discontinuation, respiratory depression, Parkinson's disease, myasthenia gravis

DOSAGE AND ROUTES
Mild anxiety
Adult: PO 5-10 mg tid-qid
Geriatric: PO 5 mg bid initially, increase as needed
Child >6 yr: PO 5 mg bid-qid, max 10 mg bid-tid

Severe anxiety
Adult: PO 20-25 mg tid-qid

Preoperatively
Adult: PO 5-10 mg tid-qid on day before surgery

Alcohol withdrawal
Adult: PO 50-100 mg q4-6hr prn, max 300 mg/day

Renal disease
Adult: PO CCr <10 ml/min give 50% dose

Available forms: Caps 5, 25 mg

Implementation
PO route
• Give with food or milk for GI symptoms; do not open capsules; provide sugarless gum, hard candy, frequent sips of water for dry mouth

ADVERSE EFFECTS
CNS: *Dizziness, drowsiness,* confusion, headache, anxiety, tremors, stimulation, fatigue, depression, insomnia, hallucinations
CV: *Orthostatic hypotension,* ECG changes, tachycardia, hypotension, edema
EENT: *Blurred vision,* tinnitus, mydriasis
GI: Constipation, dry mouth, nausea, vomiting, anorexia, diarrhea
GU: Irregular periods, decreased libido
HEMA: Agranulocytosis
INTEG: Rash, dermatitis, itching

Pharmacokinetics
Absorption	Well absorbed (PO); slow, erratic (IM)
Distribution	Widely distributed; crosses placenta, blood-brain barrier
Metabolism	Liver extensively
Excretion	Kidneys, breast milk
Half-life	5-30 hr (increased in geriatric)

Pharmacodynamics
	PO	IM	IV
Onset	30 min	15-30 min	1-5 min
Peak	Within 2 hr	Unknown	Unknown
Duration	4-6 hr	Unknown	Up to 1 hr

INTERACTIONS
Individual drugs
Alcohol: increased CNS depression
Cimetidine, disulfiram, FLUoxetine, isoniazid, ketoconazole, metoprolol, propranolol, valproic acid: increased action of chlordiazePOXIDE
Levodopa: decreased action of levodopa

Drug classifications
CNS depressants: increased CNS depression
Contraceptives (oral): increased effect of chlordiazePOXIDE
CYP3A4 inhibitors (barbiturates, protease inhibitors, rifamycins): decreased effect of chlordiazePOXIDE

Drug/lab test
Increased: LFTs
False increase: 17-OHCS
False positive: pregnancy test (some methods)

NURSING CONSIDERATIONS
Assessment
• Assess **anxiety reaction:** inability to sleep, apprehension, dread, foreboding, or uneasiness related to unidentified source of danger
• Assess for previous **product dependence** or tolerance; if product dependent or tolerant, amount of medication should be restricted
• Monitor B/P (with patient lying, standing), pulse; if systolic B/P drops 20 mm Hg, hold product, notify prescriber
• Monitor blood studies: CBC during long-term therapy; **blood dyscrasias** have occurred rarely
• Monitor hepatic studies: AST, ALT, bilirubin, creatinine, LDH, alkaline phosphatase during long-term therapy
⚠ Monitor mental status: mood, sensorium, affect, sleeping patterns, drowsiness, dizziness, suicidal tendencies, paradoxical reactions such as excitement, stimulation, acute rage
⚠ Assess for pregnancy, product should not be used during pregnancy D

Patient/family education
• Instruct patient that product may be taken with food; if dose is missed take as soon as remembered; do not double doses
• Tell patient to avoid OTC preparations unless approved by prescriber; to avoid alcohol ingestion or other psychotropic medications unless directed by a prescriber, tolerance occurs
• Caution patient to avoid driving and activities requiring alertness, since drowsiness may occur; until medication response is known, tell patient that drowsiness may worsen at beginning of treatment

⚠ Instruct patient not to discontinue medication abruptly after long-term use; product should be tapered over 1 wk

• Caution patient to rise slowly or fainting may occur, especially in geriatric

⚠ Advise patient that product should be avoided during pregnancy

⚠ Advise patient to report immediately suicidal thoughts/behaviors

Evaluation
Positive therapeutic outcome
• Increased well being
• Decreased anxiety, restlessness, sleeplessness, dread
• Successful alcohol withdrawal

TREATMENT OF OVERDOSE:
Lavage, VS, supportive care

---

chloroquine (Rx)
(klor'oh-kwin)
Aralen
Func. class.: Antimalarial
Chem. class.: Synthetic 4-aminoquinoline derivative
Pregnancy category C

ACTION: Inhibits parasite replications, transcription of DNA to RNA by forming complexes with DNA of parasite

Therapeutic outcome: Decreased symptoms of malaria, amebiasis

USES: Malaria caused by *Plasmodium vivax, Plasmodium malariae, Plasmodium ovale, Plasmodium falciparum* (some strains), amebiasis

CONTRAINDICATIONS
Hypersensitivity, retinal field changes

Precautions: Pregnancy **C**, breastfeeding, children, blood dyscrasias, severe GI, neurologic disease, alcoholism, cardiac/hepatic disease, G6PD deficiency, psoriasis, eczema, seizures, preexisting auditory damage, infection, torsades de pointes

---

BLACK BOX WARNING: Infection

DOSAGE AND ROUTES
Acute malaria attacks
Adult: **PO** 1000 mg (600 mg base), then 500 mg (300 mg base) in 6-8 hr, then 500 mg (300 mg base) q day × 2 days for a total of 2.5 g (1.5 g base) in 3 days
Adult/adolescent of low body weight, child/infant: **PO** 16.5 mg (10 mg base)/kg, max 600 mg base, then 8.3 mg (5 mg base)/kg max 300 mg

base, 6 hr after 1st dose, then 8.3 mg (5 mg base)/kg, max 300 mg base 24 hr after 1st dose, then 8.3 mg (5 mg base)/kg max 300 mg base 36 hr after 1st dose

Malaria prophylaxis (in areas with chloroquine-sensitive *P. falciparum*)
Adult: **PO** 500 mg (300 mg base) q wk on same day of each wk, starting 2 wk before travel and 8 wk after leaving

Extraintestinal amebiais
Adult: **PO** 1 g (600 mg base) q day × 2 days, then 500 mg (300 mg base) for ≥2-3 wk
Child (unlabeled): **PO** 16.6 mg (10 mg base)/kg (max 300 mg base) q day × 2-3wk

Available forms: Tabs 250 mg (150 mg base), 500 mg (300 mg base) phosphate

Implementation
PO route
• Give with meals to decrease GI symptoms; better to take on empty stomach 1 hr before or 2 hr after meals
• Give antiemetic if vomiting occurs
• Give after C&S is completed; monthly to detect resistance
IM route
• Give IM after aspirating to prevent inj into bloodstream
• Store in tight, light-resistant container at room temp; keep inj in cool environment

Additive compatibility: Promethazine

ADVERSE EFFECTS
CNS: Headache, stimulation, fatigue, *seizure,* psychosis, hallucinations, insomnia
CV: Hypotension, **heart block, asystole with syncope,** ECG changes, cardiomyopathy
EENT: *Blurred vision, corneal changes, retinal changes, difficulty focusing,* tinnitus, vertigo, deafness, photophobia, corneal edema
GI: *Nausea, vomiting, anorexia,* diarrhea, cramps
HEMA: **Thrombocytopenia, agranulocytosis, hemolytic anemia, leukopenia**
INTEG: Pruritus, pigmentary changes, skin eruptions, lichen planus–like eruptions, eczema, **exfoliative dermatitis**

Pharmacokinetics

Absorption	Well absorbed
Distribution	Widely
Metabolism	Liver
Excretion	Kidneys, feces
Half-life	3-5 days

Pharmacodynamics

	PO	IM
Onset	Rapid	Rapid
Peak	1-3 hr	30 min
Duration	6-8 hr	Unknown

INTERACTIONS
Individual drugs
Ampicillin, rabies vaccine (ID): decreased effects
Cimetidine: decreased oral clearance, metabolism
Kaolin: decreased absorption
Magnesium: decreased action of chloroquine

Drug classifications
CYP2D6 inhibitors (amiodarone, chlorphenira-mine, FLUoxetine, haloperidol, ritonavir, PARoxetine, terbinafine, ticlopidine), CYP3A4 inhibitors (clarithromycin, diltiazem, doxycy-cline, erythromycin, itraconazole, ketocon-azole, verapamil): increased effects
Antacids (aluminum): decreased absorption
Class IA, III antidysrhythmics: increased QT prolongation, torsades de pointes

Drug/lab test
Decreased: Hgb, platelets, WBC

NURSING CONSIDERATIONS
Assessment

> **BLACK BOX WARNING:** Assess for **infection:** resistance is common, not to be used for *P. falciparum* acquired in areas of resistance or where prophylaxis has failed

• Monitor **ECG,** baseline and periodically during therapy; watch for depression of T waves, widening of QRS complex
• **Assess for allergic reactions: pruritus, rash, urticaria**
• Assess for **ototoxicity:** tinnitus, vertigo, change in hearing; audiometric testing should be done before, after treatment
• Assess for **blood dyscrasias:** malaise, fever, bruising, bleeding (rare)
• Assess mental status often: affect, mood, behavioral changes; psychosis may occur
• **Assess for toxicity: blurring vision, difficulty focusing, headache, dizziness, decreased knee and ankle reflexes, product should be discontinued immediately**

Patient/family education
• Advise patient that compliance with dosage schedule, duration is necessary
• Instruct patient that scheduled appointments must be kept or relapse may occur
• Caution patient to avoid alcohol while taking product

• Instruct diabetic to use blood glucose monitor to obtain correct result
• Teach patient to report weakness, fatigue, loss of appetite, nausea, vomiting, yellowing of skin or eyes, tingling/numbness of hands/feet
• Advise patient that urine may turn rust brown color
• Instruct patient to use sunglasses in bright sunlight to prevent photophobia
⚠ **Keep away from pets, children; overdose is fatal**

Evaluation
Positive therapeutic outcome
• Decreased symptoms of malaria

TREATMENT OF OVERDOSE:
Induce vomiting, gastric lavage, administer bar-biturate (ultrashort-acting), vasopressor; trache-ostomy may be necessary

---

chlorpheniramine (OTC, Rx)
(klor-fen-ir′a-meen)
AHIST, Aller-Chlor, Allergy, Chlor-Pheniton, Chlor-Trimeton, Diabetic Tussin Allergy Relief, ED-Chlor-Tann, Equaline Allergy, Equate Chlortabs Allergy, Novopheniram ✦, P-Tann, Tana Hist-PD, Teldrin, Tripolon ✦
Func. class.: Antihistamine (1st generation, nonselective)
Chem. class.: Alkylamine, H_1-receptor antagonist
Pregnancy category B

Do not confuse: Teldrin/Tedral

ACTION: Acts on blood vessels, GI, respira-tory system by competing with histamine for H_1-receptor site; decreases allergic response by blocking histamine

Therapeutic outcome: Absence of allergy symptoms and rhinitis

USES: Allergy symptoms, rhinitis, conjuncti-vitis (allergic)

CONTRAINDICATIONS
Newborns/neonates

Precautions: Pregnancy **B,** breastfeeding, geriatric, increased intraocular pressure, renal/cardiac disease, hypertension, bronchial asthma, seizure disorder, hyperthyroidism, prostatic hy-pertrophy, GI obstruction, peptic ulcer disease, emphysema, hypersensitivity to H_1-receptor an-tagonists, lower respiratory tract disease, ste-nosed peptic ulcers, bladder neck obstruction, closed-angle glaucoma, children

---

DOSAGE AND ROUTES

Adult/child ≥12 yr: PO 4 mg tid-qid, max 24 mg/day; EXT REL 8-12 mg bid-tid, max 24 mg/day

Child 6-12 yr: PO 2 mg q4-6hr, max 12 mg/day; EXT REL 8 mg at bedtime or daily; EXT REL not recommended for child <6 yr

Available forms: Chewable tabs 2 mg; tabs 4, 8, 12 mg; ext rel tabs 8, 12 mg; ext rel caps 8, 12 mg; syr 1, 2, 2.5 mg/5 ml; drops 2 mg/ml

Implementation

PO route

- Swallow time rel tabs and caps whole
- Do not break, crush, chew, or open time rel tabs
- Chewable tabs should be chewed and not swallowed whole
- Avoid use in children ≤6 yr
- May give without regard to meals
- Store in tight container at room temp

IM/SUBCUT route

- Use only 20 and 100 mg/ml strengths; does not need to be reconstituted or diluted

Syrup

- Use dosing utensil to measure correct dose

IV route

Give undiluted by direct **IV** (10 mg/ml strength only); administer 10 mg over 1 min or more

Additive incompatibilities: Calcium chloride, kanamycin, norepinephrine, pentobarbital

ADVERSE EFFECTS

CNS: *Dizziness, drowsiness,* poor coordination, fatigue, anxiety, euphoria, confusion, paresthesia, neuritis

EENT: Blurred vision, dilated pupils, tinnitus, nasal stuffiness, dry nose, throat, mouth

GI: Nausea, anorexia, diarrhea

GU: *Retention,* dysuria, frequency

HEMA: **Thrombocytopenia, agranulocytosis, hemolytic anemia**

INTEG: Photosensitivity

RESP: Increased thick secretions, wheezing, chest tightness

Pharmacokinetics

Absorption	Well absorbed (PO, SUBCUT, IM, **IV**)
Distribution	Widely distributed; crosses blood-brain barrier
Metabolism	Liver, mostly
Excretion	Kidneys, metabolite; breast milk (minimal)
Half-life	12-15 hr

Pharmacodynamics

	PO	PO-ER	SUB-CUT	IM	IV
Onset	15-30 min	Unknown	Unknown	Unknown	Unknown
Peak	1-2 hr	Unknown	Unknown	Unknown	Unknown
Duration	4-12 hr	8-24 hr	4-12 hr	4-12 hr	4-12 hr

INTERACTIONS

Individual drugs

Alcohol: increased CNS depression

Atropine, haloperidol, quiNIDine: increased anticholinergic reactions

Drug classifications

Barbiturates, CNS depressants, opiates, sedative/hypnotics, tricyclics: increased CNS depression

MAOIs: increased effect of chlorpheniramine

Phenothiazines: increased anticholinergic reactions

Drug/lab test

False negative: skin allergy tests (discontinue antihistamines 3 days before testing)

NURSING CONSIDERATIONS

Assessment

- Assess respiratory status: rate, rhythm, increase in bronchial secretions, wheezing, chest tightness; provide fluids to 2 L/day to decrease secretion thickness
- Monitor I&O ratio: be alert for urinary retention, frequency, dysuria, especially geriatric; product should be discontinued if these occur
- **IV** administration may result in rapid drop in B/P, sweating, dizziness, especially in geriatric

Patient/family education

- Teach all aspects of product use; to notify prescriber if confusion, sedation, hypotension, or difficulty voiding occurs; to avoid driving and other hazardous activity if drowsiness occurs; to avoid alcohol and other CNS depressants that may potentiate effect
- Teach patient not to exceed recommended dosage; dysrhythmias may occur
- Advise patient hard candy, gum, frequent rinsing of mouth may be used for dryness

Evaluation

Positive therapeutic outcome

- Absence of running or congested nose, rashes, conjunctivitis

TREATMENT OF OVERDOSE:
Administer lavage, diazepam, vasopressors, phenytoin IV

---

chlorproMAZINE (Rx)
(klor-proe′ma-zeen)
Func. class.: Antipsychotic/neuroleptic/antiemetic
Chem. class.: Phenothiazine, aliphatic
Pregnancy category C

Do not confuse: chlorproMAZINE/chlorothiazide/ chlorproPAMIDE/chlorthalidone/ prochlorperazine

ACTION: Depresses cerebral cortex, hypothalamus, limbic system, which control activity, aggression; blocks neurotransmission produced by dopamine at synapse; exhibits a strong α-adrenergic, anticholinergic blocking action; mechanism for antipsychotic effects is unclear

Therapeutic outcome: Decreased signs and symptoms of psychosis; control of nausea, vomiting, intractable hiccups, decreased anxiety preoperatively

USES: Psychotic disorders, Tourette's syndrome, mania, schizophrenia, anxiety, intractable hiccups (adults), nausea, vomiting, preoperative relaxation, acute intermittent porphyria, behavioral problems in children, nonpsychotic patients with dementia

Unlabeled uses: Vascular headache

CONTRAINDICATIONS
Hypersensitivity, circulatory collapse, liver damage, cerebral arteriosclerosis, coronary disease, coma, child <6 mo

Precautions: Pregnancy **C**, breastfeeding, geriatric, seizure disorders, hypertension, hepatic/cardiac disease, prostate enlargement, pulmonary/Parkinson's disease, severe hypo/hypertension, blood dyscrasias, brain damage, bone marrow depression, alcohol and barbiturate withdrawal, closed-angle glaucoma

> **BLACK BOX WARNING:** Dementia; increased mortality in elderly patients with dementia-related psychosis

DOSAGE AND ROUTES
Psychosis
Adult: PO 10-50 mg q1-4hr initially, then increase up to 2 g/day if necessary; IM 10-50 mg q1-4hr, usual dose 300-800 mg/day

Geriatric: PO 10-25 mg daily-bid, increased by 10-25 mg/day q4-7day, max 800 mg/day
Child >6 mo: PO 0.55 mg/kg q4-6hr; IM 0.5 mg/kg q6-8hr

Nausea and vomiting
Adult: PO 10-25 mg q4-6hr prn; IM 25-50 mg q3hr prn; max 400 mg/day; **IV** 25-50 mg daily-qid
Child ≥6 mo: PO 0.55 mg/kg q4-6hr; IM q6-8hr; IM ≤5 yr or ≤22.7 kg 40 mg; max IM 5-10 yr or 22.7-45.5 kg 75 mg

Intractable hiccups/acute intermittent porphyria
Adult: PO 25-50 mg tid-qid; IM 25-50 mg (used only if PO dose does not work); **IV** 25-50 mg in 500-1000 ml saline (only for severe hiccups)

Available forms: Tabs 10, 25, 50, 100; inj 25 mg/ml

Implementation
PO route
• Periodically attempt dosage reduction in patients with behavioral problems
• Give with full glass of water, milk; or give with food to decrease GI upset
• Store in tight, light-resistant container, oral sol in amber bottle
Syrup: Use calibrated measuring device, do not spill on skin or clothes
IM route
• Store in tight, light-resistant container
• Use gloves to prepare product; if product touches skin, wash with soap and water to prevent contact dermatitis
• Inject in deep muscle mass; do not give SUBCUT; may be diluted with 0.9% NaCl, 2%, patient procaine as prescribed; do not administer sol with a precipitate
• Remain lying down after IM inj for at least 30 min
Rectal route
• Give after placing in refrigerator for 30 min if too soft to insert; this route is used for nausea, vomiting, hiccups
• Avoid skin contact with injection solution; may cause contact dermatitis

Direct IV
• Give by direct **IV** by diluting with 0.9% NaCl to a concentration of 1 mg/1 ml; administer at a rate of 1 mg/2 min, never give undiluted
• Give by intermittent IV infusion diluting 50 mg/500-1000 ml of D_5W, $D_{10}W$, 0.9% NaCl, 0.45% NaCl, LR, Ringer's over ½ hr or combinations (used for intractable hiccups)

Y-site compatibilities: Alfentanil, amikacin, amphotericin B lipid complex, amsacrine, anidulafungin, ascorbic acid injection, atenolol, atracurium, atropine, benztropine, bleomycin

---

sulfate, buprenorphine, butorphanol, calcium chloride/gluconate, caspofungin, cimetidine, cisatracurium, CISplatin, cladribine, codeine, cyanocobalamin, cyclophosphamide, cycloSPORINE, cytarabine, DACTINomycin, DAPTOmycin, dexmedetomidine, digoxin, diltiazem, diphenhydrAMINE, DOBUTamine, DOCEtaxel, DOPamine, doxacurium, DOXOrubicin, DOXOrubicin liposomal, doxycycline, enalaprilat, ePHEDrine, EPINEPHrine, epirubicin, erythromycin, esmolol, etoposide, famotidine, fenoldopam, fentaNYL, filgrastim, fluconazole, gatifloxacin, gemcitabine, gentamicin, glycopyrrolate, granisetron, hydrocortisone, HYDROmorphone, hydrOXYzine, IDArubicin, ifosfamide, isoproterenol, labetalol, levofloxacin, lidocaine, LORazepam, LR, magnesium sulfate, mannitol, mechlorethamine, meperidine, methicillin, methoxamine, methyldopate, methylPREDNISolone, metoclopramide, metoprolol, metroNIDAZOLE, miconazole, midazolam, milrinone, minocycline, mitoXANtrone, morphine, multiple vitamins injection, mycophenolate mofetil, nafcillin, nalbuphine, naloxone, netilmicin, nitroglycerin, norepinephrine, octreotide, ondansetron, oxacillin, oxaliplatin, palonosetron, pamidronate, pancuronium, papaverine, penicillin G potassium, pentamidine, pentazocine, phytonadione, polymyxin B, potassium chloride, procainamide, prochlorperazine, promethazine, propofol, propranolol, protamine sulfate, pyridoxine, quiNIDine, quinupristin-dalfopristin, ranitidine, Ringer's injection, ritodrine, riTUXimab, rocuronium, sodium acetate, succinylcholine, SUFentanil, tacrolimus, teniposide, theophylline, thiamine, thiotepa, tirofiban, TNA, tolazoline, TPN, trimetaphan, vancomycin, vasopressin, vecuronium, verapamil, vinCRIStine, vinorelbine, vitamin B complex with C, voriconazole, zoledronic acid

ADVERSE EFFECTS
CNS: Neuroleptic malignant syndrome, dizziness, *extrapyramidal symptoms: pseudoparkinsonism, akathisia, dystonia, tardive dyskinesia*, seizures, *headache*
CV: *Orthostatic hypotension,* hypertension, cardiac arrest, ECG changes, tachycardia
EENT: Blurred vision, glaucoma, dry eyes
ENDO: SIADH
GI: *Dry mouth, nausea, vomiting, anorexia, constipation,* diarrhea, cholestatic jaundice, weight gain
GU: Urinary retention, enuresis, impotence, amenorrhea, gynecomastia, breast engorgement
HEMA: Anemia, leukopenia, leukocytosis, agranulocytosis
INTEG: *Rash,* photosensitivity, dermatitis
RESP: Laryngospasm, dyspnea, respiratory depression

SYST: Death in geriatric patients with dementia

Pharmacokinetics
Absorption	Variable (PO); well absorbed (IM)
Distribution	Widely distributed; crosses placenta
Metabolism	Liver, GI mucosa extensively
Excretion	Kidneys
Half-life	23-37 hr

Pharmacodynamics
	PO	RECT	IM	IV
Onset	½-1 hr	12 hr	Unknown	Rapid
Peak	Unknown	Unknown	Unknown	Unknown
Duration	4-6 hr*	3-4 hr	4-8 hr	Unknown

*Duration PO ext rel is 10-12 hr.

INTERACTIONS
Individual drugs
Alcohol: increased effects of both products, oversedation
Aluminum hydroxide, magnesium hydroxide, cimetidine: decreased absorption
Bromocriptine, levodopa: decreased antiparkinsonian activity
EPINEPHrine: increased toxicity
Lithium: decreased chlorproMAZINE levels
Valproic acid: increased valproic acid level
Warfarin: decreased anticoagulant effect

Drug classifications
Antacids: decreased absorption
Anticholinergic, antidepressants, antiparkinsonian agents: increased anticholinergic effects
Anticonvulsants: decreased seizure threshold
Antidepressants, antihistamines, barbiturate anesthetics, opioids, sedative/hypnotics, MAOIs: increased CNS depression
Antithyroid agents: increased agranulocytosis
Barbiturates: decreased serum chlorproMAZINE
β-Adrenergic blockers: increased effect of both products

Drug/lab test
Increased: liver function tests
Decreased: WBC, platelets, Hgb/Hct
False positive: pregnancy tests, PKU
False negative: urinary steroids, 17-OHCS

NURSING CONSIDERATIONS
Assessment
• Assess mental status: orientation, mood, behavior, presence of hallucinations, and type

before initial administration and monthly; this product should significantly reduce psychotic behavior

• Assess any potentially reversible cause of behavior problems in geriatric before, during therapy

• Check for swallowing of PO medication; check for hoarding or giving of medication to other patients

• Monitor I&O ratio; palpate bladder if low urinary output occurs, especially in geriatric; urinalysis recommended before, during prolonged therapy

• Monitor bilirubin, CBC, liver function studies, ocular exam; agranulocytosis, glaucoma, cholestatic jaundice may occur

• **Assess respirations q4hr during initial treatment; establish baseline before starting treatment; report drops of 30 mm Hg; obtain baseline ECG, Q-wave, and T-wave changes**

• Check for dizziness, faintness, palpitations, tachycardia on rising; severe orthostatic hypotension is common

⚠ **Identify for neuroleptic malignant syndrome: hyperpyrexia, muscle rigidity, increased CPK, altered mental status; product should be discontinued**

• Assess for **EPS** including akathisia (inability to sit still, no pattern to movements), tardive dyskinesia (bizarre movements of the jaw, mouth, tongue, extremities), pseudoparkinsonism (rigidity, tremors, pill rolling, shuffling gate); an antiparkinsonian product should be prescribed

• Assess for constipation, urinary retention daily; if these occur, increase bulk, water in diet

Patient/family education

• Teach patient to use good oral hygiene; frequent rinsing of mouth, sugarless gum, candy, or ice chips for dry mouth

• Caution patient to avoid hazardous activities until product response is determined; dizziness, blurred vision may occur

• Inform patient that orthostatic hypotension occurs often and to rise from sitting or lying position gradually, to remain lying down after IM inj for at least 30 min; tell patient to avoid hot tubs, hot showers, tub baths, since hypotension may occur; tell patient that in hot weather heat stroke may occur; take extra precautions to stay cool

• Advise patient to avoid abrupt withdrawal of this product, or extrapyramidal symptoms may result; product should be withdrawn slowly

• Teach patient to avoid OTC preparations (cough, hay fever, cold) unless approved by prescriber, since serious product interactions may occur; avoid use with alcohol, CNS depressants, since increased drowsiness may occur

• Caution patient to use sunscreen and sunglasses to prevent burns

• Teach patient about extrapyramidal symptoms and necessity of meticulous oral hygiene, since oral candidiasis may occur

• Instruct patient to take antacids 2 hr before or after taking this product

• Instruct patient to report sore throat, malaise, fever, bleeding, mouth sores; if these occur, CBC should be drawn and product discontinued

• Teach that urine may turn pink or reddish-brown

• **Teach patient to use contraceptive measures**

Evaluation
Positive therapeutic outcome

• Decrease in emotional excitement, hallucinations, delusions, paranoia

• Reorganization of patterns of thought, speech

• Increase in target behaviors

TREATMENT OF OVERDOSE:
Lavage if orally ingested; provide airway, *do not induce vomiting or use EPINEPHrine*

cholecalciferol
See vitamin D

cholestyramine (Rx)
(koe-less-tear′a-meen)
Prevalite, Questran, Questran Light
Func. class.: Antilipemic
Chem. class.: Bile acid sequestrant
Pregnancy category C

Do not confuse: Questran/Quarzan

ACTION: Adsorbs, combines with bile acids to form an insoluble complex that is excreted through feces; loss of bile acids lowers LDL, cholesterol levels

Therapeutic outcome: Decreasing cholesterol levels and low-density lipoproteins, decreased pruritus

USES: Primary hypercholesterolemia (especially type IIa/IIb hyperlipoproteinemia), pruritus associated with biliary obstruction

Unlabeled uses: Diarrhea caused by excess bile acid

CONTRAINDICATIONS

Hypersensitivity; complete biliary obstruction; hyperlipidemia III, IV, V

Precautions: Pregnancy **C**, breastfeeding, children, PKU, renal disease, coagulopathy

DOSAGE AND ROUTES

Adult: PO 4 g daily-bid, max 24 g/day
Child: PO 240 mg/kg/day in 3 divided doses; administer with food or drink, max 8 g/day, titrated up over several weeks to decrease GI effects

Available forms: Powder for susp 4 g/cholestyramine/packet or scoop

Implementation

• Give product daily-bid, at bedtime; give all other medications 1 hr before cholestyramine or 4-6 hr after cholestyramine to avoid poor absorption; do not take dry; mix product with applesauce or stir into beverage (2-6 oz); let stand for 2 min; do not mix with carbonated beverages; avoid inhaling powder, avoid GI tube administration, take with food
• Provide supplemental doses of vit A, D, E, K if levels are low
• Doses are expressed in anhydrous cholestyramine resin; amount of resin varies with each product

ADVERSE EFFECTS

CNS: Headache, dizziness, drowsiness, vertigo, tinnitus, anxiety
GI: *Constipation, abdominal pain, nausea,* fecal impaction, hemorrhoids, flatulence, vomiting, steatorrhea, peptic ulcer
HEMA: **Bleeding,** increased pro-time
INTEG: Rash, irritation of perianal area, tongue, skin
META: Decreased vit A, D, K, red cell folate content, **hyperchloremic acidosis**
MS: Muscle, joint pain

Pharmacokinetics

Absorption	Not absorbed
Distribution	Not distributed
Metabolism	Not metabolized; LDL lowered in 4-7 days, serum cholesterol lowered in 1 mo
Excretion	Binds with bile acids, feces
Half-life	Unknown

Pharmacodynamics

Onset	24-48 hr
Peak	1-3 wk
Duration	2-4 wk

INTERACTIONS

Individual drugs

Acetaminophen, amiodarone, clofibrate, gemfibrozil, glipiZIDE, iron, oral vancomycin, penicillin G, propranolol, thyroid hormones, warfarin: decreased absorption of each specific product

Drug classifications

Cardiac glycosides, corticosteroids, tetracyclines, thiazides, vit A, D, E, K: decreased absorption

Drug/lab test

Increased: AST, ALT, alkaline phosphatase
Decreased: Na, K

NURSING CONSIDERATIONS

Assessment

• Assess nutrition: fat, protein, carbohydrates, nutritional analysis should be completed by dietitian
• Assess skin integrity after patient has been receiving product; itching, pruritus often occur from bile deposits on skin
• Monitor cardiac glycoside level if both products are being administered; cardiac glycoside levels will be decreased, may need to adjust dose of cardiac glycoside, if this product is increased or decreased
• **Hypercholesterolemia:** Monitor for signs of vit A, D, E, K deficiency; fasting LDL, HDL, total cholesterol, triglyceride levels, electrolytes if on extended therapy, diet history
• Monitor bowel pattern daily; increase bulk, water in diet if constipation develops
• **Pruritus:** Assess for itching

Patient/family education

⚠ **Teach patient symptoms of hypoprothrombinemia: bleeding mucous membranes, dark tarry stools, hematuria, petechiae; report immediately**
• Teach patient to take with food, never use dry
• Teach patient importance of compliance
• Teach patient that risk factors should be decreased: high-fat diet, smoking, alcohol consumption, absence of exercise
• Have patient mix product with 6 oz of milk, water, fruit juice; do not mix with carbonated beverages; rinse glass to make sure all medication is taken or may mix product in applesauce; allow to stand for 2 min before mixing

Evaluation
Positive therapeutic outcome
• Decreased cholesterol level (hyperlipidemia)
• Decreased diarrhea, pruritus (excess bile acids)

cidofovir (Rx)

(si-doh-foh′veer)
Vistide
Func. class.: Antiviral
Chem. class.: Nucleotide analog
Pregnancy category C

ACTION: Suppresses cytomegalovirus (CMV) replication by selective inhibition of viral DNA synthesis

Therapeutic outcome: Decreased symptoms of CMV

USES: CMV retinitis in patients with HIV, used with probenecid

CONTRAINDICATIONS

Hypersensitivity to this product or probenecid; sulfa products, direct intraocular injection

> **BLACK BOX WARNING:** Proteinuria, renal disease/failure

Precautions: Pregnancy **C**, breastfeeding, children <6 mo, geriatric, preexisting cytopenias, renal function impairment, platelet count <25,000/mm³, dehydration

> **BLACK BOX WARNING:** Neutropenia, infertility, secondary malignancy

DOSAGE AND ROUTES

Adult: **IV** 5 mg/kg qwk × 2 wk; then 3 mg/kg q2wk, give with probenecid

Renal dose
Adult: IV CCr ≤55 ml/min, do not use; SCr increase of 0.3-0.4 mg/dl above baseline, decrease dose to 3 mg/kg; SCr increase of ≥0.5 mg/dl above baseline or ≥2+ proteinuria, discontinue

Available forms: Inj 75 mg/ml

Implementation

• Allow to warm to room temperature
• If product comes in contact with skin, wash with soap and water immediately
• If zidovudine is used, reduce dose to 50% in cidofovir treatment days

Intermittent IV infusion route

• **Dilute** in 100 ml 0.9% NaCl sol before administration; probenecid must be given PO 2 g 3 hr before the cidofovir INF and 1 g at 2 and 8 hr after ending the cidofovir INF; **give** 1 L of 0.9% NaCl sol **IV** with each INF of cidofovir, **give** saline INF over 1-2 hr period immediately before cidofovir; patient should be given a second L if the patient can tolerate the fluid load (second L

given at time of cidofovir or immediately afterward and should be given over a 1-3 hr period)

> **BLACK BOX WARNING:** Use cytotoxic handling procedures

• **Administer** after diluting in 100 ml of 0.9% NaCl
• **Give** slowly; do not give by BOL **IV, IV,** SUBCUT inj
• **Use** diluted sol within 24 hr, do not refrigerate or freeze; do not use sol with particulate matter or discoloration
• Do not admix

ADVERSE EFFECTS

CNS: *Fever, chills,* coma, confusion, abnormal thought, *dizziness,* bizarre dreams, *headache,* psychosis, tremors, somnolence, paresthesia, *amnesia, anxiety, insomnia,* seizures
CV: Dysrhythmias, hypo/hypertension
EENT: Retinal detachment in CMV retinitis
GI: Abnormal liver function tests, *nausea, vomiting, anorexia, diarrhea,* abdominal pain, hemorrhage
GU: Hematuria, increased creatinine, BUN, nephrotoxicity
HEMA: Granulocytopenia, thrombocytopenia, irreversible neutropenia, anemia, eosinophilia
INTEG: *Rash, alopecia, pruritus, acne,* urticaria, pain at inj site, phlebitis
RESP: Dyspnea

Pharmacokinetics	
Absorption	Unknown
Distribution	Unknown
Metabolism	Unknown
Excretion	Unknown
Half-life	Terminal 2.6 hr

Pharmacodynamics
Unknown

INTERACTIONS
Individual drugs

> **BLACK BOX WARNING:** Amphotericin B, foscarnet, pentamidine **IV:** increased nephrotoxicity; wait 7 days after use to begin cidofovir

Drug classifications
Aminoglycosides, NSAIDs, salicylates: increased nephrotoxicity; wait 7 days after use to begin cidofovir

NURSING CONSIDERATIONS
Assessment

• Obtain culture before treatment is initiated; cultures of blood, urine, and throat may all be taken; CMV is not confirmed by this method; the diagnosis is made by an ophthalmic exam

• Assess for GI symptoms: severe nausea, vomiting, diarrhea; severe symptoms may necessitate discontinuing product
• Assess electrolytes and minerals: calcium, phosphorous, magnesium, sodium, potassium; watch closely for tetany during first administration
• **Assess for symptoms of blood dyscrasias (anemia, granulocytopenia); bruising, fatigue, bleeding, poor healing; assess for leukopenia, neutropenia, thrombocytopenia: WBCs, platelets q2day during 2 × / day dosing and qwk thereafter; check for leukopenias, with daily WBC count in patients with prior leukopenia, with other nucleoside analogs, or for whom leukopenia counts are <1000 cells/mm³ at start of treatment**
• Assess allergic reactions: flushing, rash, urticaria, pruritus
• Monitor serum creatinine or CCr at least q2wk; give only to those with creatinine levels ≤1.5 mg/dl, CCr >55 ml/min, urine protein <100 mg/dl

Patient/family education

• Advise to report perioral tingling, numbness in extremities, and paresthesias; report rash immediately, mental/vision changes, urinary problems, abnormal bleeding
⚠ **Teach that serious product interactions may occur if OTC products are ingested; check first with prescriber**
• Teach that product is not a cure, but will control symptoms
• Advise that regular ophthalmic exams, renal studies must be continued
• Advise that major toxicities may necessitate discontinuing product
⚠ **Advise to use contraception during treatment and that infertility may occur;**

men should use barrier contraception for 90 days after treatment

Evaluation
Positive therapeutic outcome
• Decreased symptoms of CMV

TREATMENT OF OVERDOSE:
Discontinue product; use hemodialysis, and increase hydration

cilastatin
See imipenem/cilastatin

cilostazol (Rx)
(sih-los′tah-zol)
Pletal
Func. class.: Platelet aggregation inhibitor
Chem. class.: Quinolinone derivative
Pregnancy category C

Do not confuse: Pletal/Plendil

ACTION: Multifactorial effects (antithrombotic, antiplatelet vasodilation)

Therapeutic outcome: Increased walking distance

USES: Intermittent claudication associated with PVD

CONTRAINDICATIONS
Hypersensitivity, acute MI, active bleeding conditions, hemostatic conditions

Precautions: Pregnancy **C,** breastfeeding, children, geriatric, past liver disease, renal/cardiac disease, increased bleeding risk, low platelet count, platelet dysfunction, smoking

DOSAGE AND ROUTES
Adult: PO 100 mg bid taken ≥30 min before or 2 hr after breakfast and dinner or 50 mg bid, if using products that inhibit CYP3A4 and CYP2C19; 12 wk of treatment may be needed for beneficial effect

Available forms: Tabs 50, 100 mg

Implementation
• Give bid ≥1 hr before or 2 hr after meals with a full glass of water; do not give with grapefruit juice

ADVERSE EFFECTS
CNS: *Dizziness, headache*
CV: *Palpitations, tachycardia,* **nodal dysrhythmia,** postural hypotension, chest pain

EENT: Blindness, diplopia, ear pain, tinnitus, retinal hemorrhage

GI: *Nausea, vomiting, diarrhea, GI discomfort,* colitis, cholelithiasis, ulcer, esophagitis, gastritis, anorexia, *flatulence, dyspepsia*

GU: Cystitis, frequency, vaginitis, vaginal hemorrhage, hematuria

HEMA: Bleeding (epistaxis, hematuria, retinal hemorrhage, GI bleeding), thrombocytopenia, anemia, polycythemia; aplastic anemia

INTEG: *Rash,* urticaria, dry skin, Stevens-Johnson syndrome

MISC: *Back pain,* headache, *infection, myalgia, peripheral edema,* chills, fever, malaise, diabetes mellitus

RESP: *Cough, pharyngitis, rhinitis,* asthma, pneumonia

Pharmacokinetics

Absorption	Unknown
Distribution	95%-98% protein binding
Metabolism	Hepatic extensively by CYP450 enzymes (active metabolite)
Excretion	Urine (74%), feces (20%)
Half-life	11-13 hr

Pharmacodynamics

Unknown

INTERACTIONS
Individual drugs
Abciximab, eptifibatide, ticlopidine, tirofiban: increased bleeding tendencies

Clarithromycin, diltiazem, erythromycin, omeprazole, verapamil: increased cilostazol levels

Fluconazole, FLUoxetine, fluvoxaMINE, gemfibrozil, isoniazid, itraconazole, ketoconazole, omeprazole, voriconazole: may increase cilostazol levels; exercise caution when coadministering and reduce dose to 50 mg bid

Drug classifications
Anticoagulants, NSAIDs, thrombolytics: may increase bleeding tendencies

CYP3A4 inducers: decreased cilostazol

Protease inhibitors, CYP3A4 inhibitors, CYP2C19 inhibitors: increased cilostazol levels

Drug/food
Grapefruit juice: do not use; toxicity may occur

High-fat meals: increased cilostazol action; avoid giving with food

Drug/herb
Feverfew, garlic, ginger, ginkgo biloba: decreased cilostazol action

NURSING CONSIDERATIONS
Assessment

> **BLACK BOX WARNING:** Assess for underlying CV disease since CV risk is great; for severe headache, signs of toxicity

- Assess for CV lesions with repeated oral administration
- Assess for CHF
- Monitor blood studies: CBC, Hct, Hgb, pro-time if patient is on long-term therapy; thrombocytopenia, neutropenia may occur

Patient/family education
- Teach patient to avoid hazardous activities until effect is known
- Advise patient to report any unusual bleeding to prescriber
- Caution patient to report side effects such as diarrhea, skin rashes, subcutaneous bleeding
- Teach patient that effects may take 2-4 wk, treatment of up to 12 wk may be required for necessary effect
- Teach patients with CHF about potential risks
- Advise patient to take ≥1 hr before or 2 hr after meals
- Advise patient that reading patient package insert is necessary
- Advise patient to discontinue tobacco use, not to drink grapefruit juice
- Advise that there are many drug and herb interactions; obtain approval by prescriber before use

Evaluation
Positive therapeutic outcome
- Increased walking distance and duration
- Decreased pain

cimetidine (OTC, Rx)
(sye-met'i-deen)

Acid Reducer, Equaline Acid Reducer, Nu-Cimet ✦, Tagamet, Tagamet HB

Func. class.: H₂-receptor antagonist
Chem. class.: Imidazole derivative

Pregnancy category B

ACTION: Inhibits histamine at H₂-receptor site in the gastric parietal cells, which inhibits gastric acid secretion

Therapeutic outcome: Healing of duodenal or gastric ulcers; prevention of duodenal ulcers; decreases symptoms of gastroesophageal reflux disease (GERD) and Zollinger-Ellison syndrome

USES: Short-term treatment of duodenal and gastric ulcers and maintenance; management of GERD, Zollinger-Ellison syndrome; prevention of upper GI bleeding; prevent, relieve heartburn, acid indigestion, upper GI bleeding

Unlabeled uses: Prevention of aspiration pneumonitis, stress ulcers

CONTRAINDICATIONS
Hypersensitivity to this product, H$_2$ blockers, benzyl alcohol

Precautions: Pregnancy **B**, breastfeeding, child <16 yr, geriatric, organic brain syndrome, renal/hepatic disease

DOSAGE AND ROUTES
Treatment of active ulcers
Adult/adolescent ≥16 yr: PO 300 mg qid with meals, at bedtime × 8-12 wk or 400 mg bid, 800 mg at bedtime; after 8 wk give at bedtime dose only; **IV BOL** 300 mg/20 ml 0.9% NaCl over 1-2 min q6hr; **IV INF** 300 mg/50 ml D$_5$W over 15-20 min; IM 300 mg q6hr, max 2400 mg
Child: PO 20-40 mg/kg/day, divided q6hr IM/IV 5-10 mg/kg q6-8hr

Prophylaxis of duodenal ulcer
Adult and child >16 yr: 400 mg at bedtime or 300 mg bid

GERD
Adult: PO 800-1600 mg/day in divided doses × ≤12 wk

Hypersecretory conditions (Zollinger-Ellison syndrome)
Adult: PO/IM/IV 300-600 mg q6hr; may increase to 12 g/day if needed; OTC use up to 200 mg daily or bid, max 2 ×/wk

Upper GI bleeding prophylaxis
Adult: IV 50 mg/hr; lowered in renal disease

Heartburn
Adult/child ≥12 yr: PO 200 mg Tagamet HB up to bid, may use prior to eating, max 400 mg/day, max daily use up to 2 wk

Renal dose
Adult: PO/IV CCr <30 ml/min 300 mg q12hr

Available forms: Tabs 200, 300, 400, 800 mg; liquid 300 mg/5 ml; inj 300 mg/2 ml, 300 mg/50 ml 0.9% NaCl

Implementation
PO route
• Give with meals for lengthened product effect; antacids 1 hr before or 1 hr after cimetidine
IM route
• May give undiluted
• Give at end of dialysis
• Inject deeply into large muscle mass, aspirate

IV route
• Give by **direct IV** after diluting 300 mg/20 ml of 0.9% NaCl for inj; give over ≥5 min
• Give **intermittent IV** by diluting 300 mg/50 ml of D$_5$W; run over ≥30 min
• Give by **cont inf** after using total daily dose (900 mg) diluted in 100-1000 ml D$_5$W given over 24 hr
• Store diluted sol at room temperature up to 48 hr

Y-site incompatibilities: Amsacrine

Y-site compatibilities: Acetaminophen, acyclovir, alfentanil, amifostine, amikacin, aminocaproic acid, aminophylline, amphotericin B lipid complex/liposome, anakinra, anidulafungin, ascorbic acid injection, atenolol, atracurium, atropine, aztreonam, benztropine, bivalirudin, bleomycin, bumetanide, buprenorphine, butorphanol, calcium chloride/gluconate, CARBOplatin, caspofungin, cefamandole, ceFAZolin, cefmetazole, cefonicid, cefotaxime, cefoTEtan, cefOXitin, cefTAZidime, ceftizoxime, cefTRIAXone, cefuroxime, cephalothin, cephapirin, chlorproMAZINE, cisatracurium, CISplatin, cladribine, clarithromycin, clindamycin, codeine, cyanocobalamin, cyclophosphamide, cycloSPORINE, cytarabine, DACTINomycin, DAPTOmycin, dexamethasone, dexmedetomidine, digoxin, diltiazem, diphenhydrAMINE, DOBUTamine, DOCEtaxel, DOPamine, doripenem, doxacurium, doxapram, DOXOrubicin, DOXOrubicin liposome, enalaprilat, ePHEDrine, EPINEPHrine, epirubicin, epoetin alfa, eptifibatide, ertapenem, erythromycin, esmolol, etoposide, famotidine, fenoldopam, fentaNYL, filgrastim, fluconazole, fludarabine, fluorouracil, folic acid, foscarnet, gallium, gatifloxacin, gemcitabine, gentamicin, glycopyrrolate, granisetron, heparin, hydrocortisone, HYDROmorphone, hydrOXYzine, IDArubicin, ifosfamide, imipenem-cilastatin, irinotecan, isoproterenol, ketorolac, labetalol, levofloxacin, lidocaine, linezolid, LORazepam, LR, magnesium sulfate, mannitol, mechlorethamine, melphalan, meperidine, metaraminol, meropenem, methicillin, methotrexate, methoxamine, methyldopate, methylPREDNISolone, metoclopramide, metoprolol, metroNIDAZOLE, mezlocillin, miconazole, midazolam, milrinone, minocycline, mitoXANtrone, morphine, moxalactam, multiple vitamins injection, mycophenolate, nafcillin, nalbuphine, naloxone, nesiritide, netilmicin, niCARdipine, nitroglycerin, nitroprusside, norepinephrine, octreotide, ondansetron, oxacillin, oxaliplatin, oxytocin, PACLitaxel, palonosetron, pamidronate, pancuronium, pantoprazole, papaverine, PEMEtrexed, penicillin G sodium/potassium, pentamidine, pentazocine, phenylephrine, phytonadione, piperacillin, piperacillin/tazobactam, polymyxin B, potassium chloride, procainamide, prochlorperazine, promethazine, propofol, propranolol, protamine, pyridoxine, quiNIDine, quinupristin-dalfopristin, ranitidine, remifentanil, Ringer's ritodrine, riTUXimab, rocuronium, sargramostim, sodium acetate/bicarbonate, succinylcholine, SUFentanil, tacrolimus, teniposide, theophylline, thiamine, thiotepa, ticarcillin, ticarcillin-clavulanate, tigecycline, tirofiban, TNA, tobramycin, tolazoline, topotecan, TPN, trastuzumab, trimetaphan, urokinase, vancomycin, vasopressin, vecuronium, verapamil, vinCRIStine, vinorelbine, voriconazole, zidovudine, zoledronic acid

ADVERSE EFFECTS

CNS: *Confusion, headache,* depression, dizziness, anxiety, weakness, psychosis, tremors, **seizures**

CV: Bradycardia, tachycardia, **dysrhythmias**

GI: *Diarrhea,* abdominal cramps, **paralytic ileus,** *jaundice*

GU: Gynecomastia, galactorrhea, impotence, increase in BUN, creatinine

HEMA: Agranulocytosis, thrombocytopenia, neutropenia, aplastic anemia, increase in pro-time

INTEG: Urticaria, rash, alopecia, sweating, flushing, **exfoliative dermatitis**

RESP: Pneumonia

Pharmacokinetics

Absorption	Well absorbed (PO, IM); completely absorbed (**IV**)
Distribution	Widely distributed; crosses placenta
Metabolism	Liver (30%)
Excretion	Kidneys, unchanged (70%); breast milk
Half-life	1½-2 hr; increased in renal disease

Pharmacodynamics

	PO	IM/IV
Onset	½ hr	10 min
Peak	45-90 min	½ hr
Duration	4-5 hr	4-5 hr

INTERACTIONS

Individual drugs

CarBAMazepine, chloroquine, lidocaine, metronidazole, moricizine, phenytoin, quiNIDine, quiNINE, valproic acid, warfarin: increased toxicity (CYP450 pathway)

Carmustine: increased bone marrow suppression

Itraconazole: decreased absorption of itraconazole

Ketoconazole: decreased absorption of ketoconazole

Sucralfate: decreased cimetidine absorption

Drug classifications

Antacids: decreased absorption of cimetidine

Antidepressants (tricyclic), benzodiazepines, β-adrenergic blockers, calcium channel blockers, phenytoins, sulfonylureas, theophyllines: increased toxicity (CYP450 pathway)

Drug/lab test

Increased: alkaline phosphatase, AST, creatinine, prolactin

False positive: Hemoccult, Gastroccult tests

False negative: TB skin tests

NURSING CONSIDERATIONS

Assessment

• **Ulcer symptoms:** Assess patient with ulcers or suspected ulcers: epigastric or abdominal pain, hematemesis, occult blood in stools, blood in gastric aspirate before and/or throughout treatment

Patient/family education

• Advise patient that any gynecomastia or impotence that develops is reversible after treatment is discontinued

• Caution patient to avoid driving, other hazardous activities until stabilized on this medication; drowsiness or dizziness may occur

• Advise patient to avoid black pepper, caffeine, alcohol, harsh spices, extremes in temperature of food; tell patient to avoid OTC preparations: aspirin, cough, cold preparations; condition may worsen, OTC therapy is used for short term (2 wk)

• Advise patient that smoking decreases the effectiveness of the product; smoking cessation should be considered

• Teach patient that product must be continued for prescribed time to be effective and taken exactly as prescribed; doses are not to be doubled; to take missed dose when remembered up to 1 hr before next dose

• Instruct patient to report bruising, fatigue, malaise; blood dyscrasias may occur

⚠ Have patient report to prescriber immediately any diarrhea, black tarry stools, sore throat, dizziness, confusion, or delirium

Evaluation

Positive therapeutic outcome

• Decreased pain in abdomen
• Healing of ulcers
• Absence of gastroesophageal reflux
• Gastric pH of ≥5

cinacalcet (Rx)

(sin-a-kal′set)

Sensipar

Func. class.: Calcium receptor agonist

Chem. class.: Polypeptide hormone

Pregnancy category C

ACTION: Directly lowers PTH levels by increasing sensitivity of calcium sensing receptors to extracellular calcium

Therapeutic outcome: Decreased symptoms of hypercalcemia

USES: Hypercalcemia in parathyroid carcinoma, secondary hyperparathyroidism in chronic kidney disease on dialysis, primary hyperparathyroidism

CONTRAINDICATIONS

Hypersensitivity, hypocalcemia

Precautions: Pregnancy **C**, breastfeeding, children, seizure disorders, hepatic disease

DOSAGE AND ROUTES
Parathyroid carcinoma

Adult: PO 30 mg bid, titrate q2-4wk, with sequential doses of 30 mg bid, 60 mg bid, 90 mg bid, 90 mg tid-qid to normalize calcium levels

Secondary hyperparathyroidism

Adult: PO 30 mg daily, titrate no more frequently than 2-4 wks with sequential doses of 30, 60, 90, 120, 180 mg daily

Available forms: Tabs 30, 60, 90 mg

Implementation

• Swallow tabs whole; do not break, crush, chew, or divide tabs

• Can be used alone or in combination with vit D sterols and/or phosphate binders

• Take with food or shortly after meal

Secondary hyperthyroidism

• Titrate q2-4wk to target iPTH consistent with National Kidney Foundation—Kidney Disease Outcomes Quality Initiative (NKF-K/DOQI) for chronic kidney disease patient on dialysis of 150-300 pg/ml; if iPTH drops below 150-300 pg/ml, reduce dose of cinacalcet and/or vit D sterols or discontinue treatment

• Store at <77° F (25° C)

ADVERSE EFFECTS

CNS: Dizziness, asthenia, *seizures,* tetany, hallucinations, depression, headache

CV: Hypertension, dysrhythmia exacerbation

GI: Nausea, diarrhea, vomiting, anorexia

MISC: Access infection, noncardiac chest pain, hypocalcemia

MS: Myalgia, bone fractures

Pharmacokinetics

Absorption	93%-97% bound to plasma
Distribution	Unknown
Metabolism	Proteins metabolized by CYP3A4, 2D6, 1A2
Excretion	Renal (80% renal, 15% feces)
Half-life	30-40 hr

Pharmacodynamics

Unknown

INTERACTIONS
Individual drugs

Flecainide, thioridazine, vinBLAStine: increased levels of CYP2D6 inhibitors; adjustments may be necessary

Drug classifications

Products metabolized by CYP3A4 inhibitors (erythromycin, itraconazole, ketoconazole): increased cinacalcet levels

Tricyclics: increased levels of CYP2D6 inhibitors)

Drug/food

High-fat meal: increased action

NURSING CONSIDERATIONS
Assessment

• Assess for **hypocalcemia:** cramping, seizures, tetany, myalgia, paresthesia

• Monitor calcium, phosphorous within 1 wk and iPTH 1-4 wk after initiation or dosage adjustment when maintenance is established; measure calcium, phosphorus monthly; iPTH q1-3mo, target range 150-300 pg/ml for iPTH level; biochemical markers of bone formation/resorption, radiologic evidence of fracture; if calcium <8.4 mg/dl, do not start therapy

• **Renal disease (without dialysis): These patients should not receive treatment with this product, high risk of hypocalcemia**

Patient/family education

• Instruct patient to take with food or shortly after a meal, to take tabs whole, not to take any other meds, supplements without prescriber approval

• **Instruct patient to immediately report cramping, seizures, muscle pain, tingling, tetany**

Evaluation
Positive therapeutic outcome

• Calcium levels 9-10 mg/dl, decreasing symptoms of hypercalcemia

ciprofloxacin (Rx)

(sip-ro-floks′a-sin)
Cipro, Cipro XR
Func. class.: Antiinfectives, broad-spectrum
Chem. class.: Fluoroquinolone
Pregnancy category C

Do not confuse: ciprofloxacin/cephalexin

ACTION: Interferes with conversion of intermediate DNA fragments into high-molecular-weight DNA in bacteria; DNA gyrase inhibitor

Therapeutic outcome: Bactericidal action against the following: gram-positive organisms *Staphylococcus epidermidis,* methicillin-resistant strains of *Staphylococcus aureus;* gram-negative organisms *Escherichia coli, Klebsiella* species, *Enterobacter, Salmonella, Proteus vulgaris, Pseudomonas aeruginosa, Serratia, Campylobacter jejuni*

USES: Adult urinary tract infections (including complicated); chronic bacterial prostatitis; acute sinusitis; infectious diarrhea; typhoid fever; complicated intraabdominal infections; nosocomial pneumonia; exposure to inhalation anthrax

CONTRAINDICATIONS

Hypersensitivity to quinolones

Precautions: Pregnancy **C,** breastfeeding, children, geriatric, renal disease, seizure disorder, stroke, CV disease, hepatic disease, QT prolongation, hypokalemia, colitis

> **BLACK BOX WARNING:** Tendon pain/rupture, tendonitis, myasthenia gravis

DOSAGE AND ROUTES
Uncomplicated urinary tract infections
Adult: PO 250 mg q12hr × 3 days or XL 500 mg q24hr × 3 days

Complicated/severe urinary tract infections
Adult: PO 500 mg q12hr or XL 1000 mg q24hr × 7-14 days; **IV** 400 mg q12hr

Respiratory, bone, skin, joint infections (mild-moderate)
Adult: PO 500-750 mg q12hr × 7-14 days; **IV** 400 mg q12hr

Nosocomial pneumonia
Adult: **IV** 400 mg q8hr × 10-14 days

Intraabdominal infections, complicated
Adult: PO 500 mg q12hr × 7-14 days, **IV** 400 mg q12hr × 7-14 days, usually given with metroNIDAZOLE

Acute sinusitis, mild/moderate
Adult: PO 500 mg q12hr × 10 days; **IV** 400 mg q12hr × 10 days

Inhalational anthrax (postexposure)
Adult: PO 500 mg q12hr × 60 days; **IV** 400 mg q12hr × 60 days
Child: PO 15 mg/kg/dose q12hr × 60 days, max 500 mg/dose; **IV,** 10 mg/kg q12hr, max 400 mg/dose

Infectious diarrhea
Adult: PO 500-750 mg q12hr × 5-7 days

Chronic bacterial prostatitis
Adult: PO 500 mg q12hr × 28 days; **IV** 400 mg q12hr × 28 days

Renal dose
Adult: PO CCr 30-50 ml/min PO 250-500 mg q12hr; CCr 5-29 ml/min PO 250-500 mg q18hr; IV 200-400 mg q18-24hr

Available forms: Tabs 100, 250, 500, 750 mg; ext rel tabs (XR) 500, 1000 mg; powder for oral susp 5%, 10%; inj 200 mg/20 ml, 400 mg/40 ml, 200 mg/100 ml D_5, 400 mg/200 ml D_5; oral susp 250, 500 mg/5 ml

Implementation
PO route
- Obtain C&S before use
- Give around the clock to maintain proper blood levels
- Administer 6 hr before or 2 hr after antacids, zinc, iron, calcium; use adequate fluids to prevent crystalluria
- Do not give oral sup by GI tube
- Limit intake of alkaline soda, products with milk, dairy products, alkaline antacids, sodium bicarbonate
- Ext rel and regular release are not interchangeable
- Do not add or stop products without prescriber's approval
- Use calibrated measuring device for suspension

IV route
- Check for irritation, extravasation, phlebitis daily
- For **intermittent inf,** dilute to 1-2 mg/ml of D_5W, 0.9% NaCl; give over 60 min; it will remain stable under refrigeration for 2 wk, diluted vials can be stored for 14 days at room temperature or in refrigerator, do not freeze

Y-site incompatibilities: Argatroban, arsenic, heparin, mezlocillin

ADVERSE EFFECTS
CNS: *Headache,* dizziness, fatigue, insomnia, depression, *restlessness,* **seizures,** confusion, hallucinations
GI: *Nausea,* increased ALT, AST, flatulence, heartburn, *vomiting, diarrhea,* oral candidiasis, dysphagia, **pseudomembranous colitis,** dry mouth, **abdominal pain, pancreatitis**
GU: Crystalluria, interstitial neuritis
HEMA: **Bone marrow depression,** agranulocytosis, eosinophilia
INTEG: *Rash,* pruritus, urticaria, photosensitivity, flushing, fever, chills, **toxic epidermal necrolysis,** injection site reactions
MISC: **Anaphylaxis, Stevens-Johnson syndrome,** visual impairment, **QT prolongation, pseudotumor cerebri**
MS: Tremor, arthralgia, tendon rupture

Pharmacokinetics
Absorption	Well absorbed (75%) (PO)
Distribution	Widely distributed
Metabolism	Liver (15%)
Excretion	Kidneys (40%-50%)
Half-life	4 hr; increased in renal disease

Pharmacodynamics
	PO	IV
Onset	Rapid	Immediate
Peak	4 hr	Infusion's end

INTERACTIONS
Individual drugs
Alfuzosin, arsenic trioxide, astemizole, chloroquine, cloZAPine, cyclobenzaprine, dasatinib, dolasetron, droperidol, flecainide, haloperidol, lapatinib, levomethadyl, methadone, octreotide, ondansetron, paliperidone, palonosetron, pentamidine, probucol, propafenone, ranolazine, risperiDONE, sertindole, SUNItinib, tacrolimus, terfenadine, vardenafil, vorinostat, ziprasidone: increased QT prolongation; less likely than other quinolones
CYP1A2 inhibitors: increased levels of CYP1A2 inhibitors
Calcium, enteral feeding, iron, sucralfate, sevelamer, zinc sulfate: decreased ciprofloxacin absorption
CycloSPORINE: increased nephrotoxicity

Probenecid: increased blood levels of ciprofloxacin, increased toxicity
Theophylline: increased theophylline levels, monitor blood levels, reduce dose
Warfarin: increased warfarin effect, monitor blood levels

Drug classifications
Antacids (containing magnesium, aluminum), iron salts: decreased absorption of ciprofloxacin
β-agonists, class IA/III antidysrhythmics, halogenated anesthetics, local anesthetics, macrolides, phenothiazines, tetracyclines, tricyclics: increased QT prolongation

> **BLACK BOX WARNING:** Corticosteroids: increased tendonitis, tendon rupture

Drug/food
Dairy products, food: decreased absorption

Drug/lab test
Increased: AST, ALT, bilirubin, BUN, creatinine, alkaline phosphatase, LDH, glucose, proteinuria, albuminuria
Decreased: WBC, glucose

NURSING CONSIDERATIONS
Assessment
• Assess patient for previous sensitivity reaction
• Assess patient for signs and symptoms of **infection** including characteristics of wounds, sputum, urine, stool, WBC >10,000/mm³, fever; obtain baseline information before, during treatment
• Obtain C&S before beginning product therapy to identify if correct treatment has been initiated
• **Assess for anaphylaxis: rash, urticaria, dyspnea, pruritus, chills, fever, joint pain; may occur a few days after therapy begins; EPINEPHrine and resuscitation equipment should be available for anaphylactic reaction**
• Identify urine output; if decreasing, notify prescriber (may indicate nephrotoxicity); also check for increased BUN, creatinine
• Monitor blood studies: AST, ALT, CBC, Hct, bilirubin, LDH, alkaline phosphatase, Coombs' test monthly if patient is on long-term therapy
• Monitor electrolytes: potassium, sodium, chloride monthly if patient is on long-term therapy

> **BLACK BOX WARNING:** Myasthenia gravis: avoid use in these patients, increases muscle weakness

> ⚠ **QT prolongation:** monitor for changes in QTc if taking other products that increase QT

• Assess for **CNS symptoms:** headache, dizziness, fatigue, insomnia, depression, seizures

• Monitor for bleeding: ecchymosis, bleeding gums, hematuria, stool guaiac daily if on long-term therapy

• Assess for **overgrowth of infection:** perineal itching, fever, malaise, redness, pain, swelling, drainage, rash, diarrhea, change in cough, sputum

> **BLACK BOX WARNING:** Assess for tendon pain, especially in children

> **BLACK BOX WARNING:** Tendonitis, tendon rupture: discontinue at first sign of tendon pain, inflammation; increased in those >60 yr, those taking corticosteroids, organ transplant recipients

⚠ **Pseudomotor cerebri:** may occur at excessive doses

Patient/family education

• Teach patient to report sore throat, bruising, bleeding, joint pain; may indicate blood dyscrasias (rare)

• Teach patient to contact prescriber if adverse reaction occurs or if inflammation or pain in tendon occurs before, 6 hr after

• Instruct patient to take all medication prescribed for the length of time ordered; product must be taken around the clock to maintain blood levels; do not give medication to others

> **BLACK BOX WARNING:** Teach patient to report tendon pain, chest pain, palpitations

• Advise patient to rinse mouth frequently, use sugarless candy or gum for dry mouth, to drink fluids to prevent crystals in urine

⚠ **Teach patient to notify prescriber if rash occurs, discontinue product**

• Teach patient to notify prescriber if pregnancy is planned or suspected, **(C)** do not breastfeed

• Teach patient to contact prescriber if taking theophylline, warfarin

Evaluation
Positive therapeutic outcome

• Absence of signs/symptoms of infection (WBC <10,000/mm^3, temp WNL, absence of red draining wounds)

• Reported improvement in symptoms of infection

ciprofloxacin ophthalmic
See Appendix B

> ⚠ **HIGH ALERT**

cisatracurium (Rx)
(sis-a-tra-cyoor'ee-um)
Nimbex
Func. class.: Neuromuscular blocker (nondepolarizing)
Pregnancy category B

ACTION: Inhibits transmission of nerve impulses by binding with cholinergic receptor sites, antagonizing action of acetylcholine

Therapeutic outcome: Paralysis of body for administration of anesthesia

USES: Facilitation of endotracheal intubation, skeletal muscle relaxation during mechanical ventilation surgery, or general anesthesia

CONTRAINDICATIONS
Hypersensitivity

Precautions: Pregnancy **B**, breastfeeding, children <2 yr, electrolyte imbalances, dehydration, cardiac/neuromuscular/respiratory disease, metabolic alkalosis, respiratory acidosis, myopathy, myasthenia gravis

DOSAGE AND ROUTES
Adult: IV 0.15 and 0.2 mg/kg depending on desired time to intubate and length of surgery: use peripheral nerve stimulation to evaluate dosage

Child 2-12 yr: IV 0.1 mg/kg over 5-10 sec with halothane or opioid anesthesia

Available forms: Inj 2, 10 mg/ml

Implementation

IV route

• Use nerve stimulator by anesthesiologist to determine neuromuscular blockade

• Give anticholinesterase to reverse neuromuscular blockade

• Give by slow **IV** only by qualified person; do not administer IM

• Store in light-resistant area

• Reassure if communication is difficult during recovery from neuromuscular blockage

ADVERSE EFFECTS
CV: Bradycardia, tachycardia; increased, decreased B/P
EENT: Increased secretions
INTEG: Rash, flushing, pruritus, urticaria
RESP: Prolonged apnea, bronchospasm, cyanosis, respiratory depression

---

Pharmacokinetics
Unknown

Pharmacodynamics

Onset	1-3 min
Peak	2-5 min
Duration	30-40 min

INTERACTIONS
Individual drugs
CarBAMazepine, phenytoin: decreased duration of neuromuscular blockade

Isoflurane, lithium: increased neuromuscular blockade

Succinylcholine: decreased neuromuscular blockade

Drug classifications
Aminoglycosides, antibiotics (polymix), β-adrenergic blockers, opioids: increased neuromuscular blockade

NURSING CONSIDERATIONS
Assessment
• This product is not an analgesic, treat pain with other agents

• Assess for electrolyte imbalances (K, Mg), may lead to increased action of this product

• Assess vital signs (B/P, pulse, respirations, airway) until fully recovered; rate, depth, pattern of respirations; strength of handgrip

• Assess I&O ratio: check for urinary retention, frequency, hesitancy

• Assess recovery: decreased paralysis of face, diaphragm, legs, arms, rest of body

• Assess allergic reactions: rash, fever, respiratory distress, pruritus; product should be discontinued

Evaluation
Positive therapeutic outcome
• Paralysis of jaw, eyelid, head, neck, rest of body

TREATMENT OF OVERDOSE:
Edrophonium or neostigmine, atropine, monitor VS; mechanical ventilation

---

⚠ HIGH ALERT

CISplatin (Rx)
(sis′pla-tin)
Platinol ✤
Func. class.: Antineoplastic alkylating agent
Chem. class.: Inorganic heavy metal
Pregnancy category D

Do not confuse: CISplatin/CARBOplatin

ACTION: Alkylates DNA, RNA; inhibits enzymes that allow synthesis of amino acids in proteins; activity is not cell cycle phase specific

Therapeutic outcome: Prevention of rapidly growing malignant cells

USES: Advanced bladder cancer; adjunctive in metastatic testicular cancer and metastatic ovarian cancer

CONTRAINDICATIONS
Pregnancy **D,** breastfeeding

> **BLACK BOX WARNING:** Bone marrow suppression, platinum compound hypersensitivity, renal disease/failure, preexisting hearing impairment

Precautions: Geriatric patients, vaccination, infections, extravasation, peripheral neuropathy, radiation therapy

DOSAGE AND ROUTES
Dosage protocols may vary

Metastatic testicular cancer
Adult: IV 20 mg/m^2 daily × 5 days, repeat q3wk for 2 cycles or more, depending on response

Advanced bladder cancer
Adult: IV 50-70 mg/m^2 q3-4wk

Metastatic ovarian cancer
Adult: IV 100 mg/m^2 q4wk or 75-100 mg/m^2 q3wk with cyclophosphamide therapy

Available forms: Inj 0.5 mg/ml ✤, 1 mg/ml

Implementation
• Hydrate patient with 0.9% NaCl over 8-12 hr before treatment

• Give all medications PO, if possible; avoid IM inj when platelets <100,000/mm^3

• Give EPINEPHrine, antihistamines, corticosteroids for hypersensitivity reaction; antiemetic 30-60 min before giving product to prevent vomiting, and prn; allopurinol or sodium bicarbonate to maintain uric acid level, alkalinization of urine; antibiotics for prophylaxis of infection; diuretic (furosemide 40 mg **IV**) or mannitol after infusion

• Prepare in biological cabinet using gown, gloves, mask; do not allow product to come in contact with skin; use soap and water if contact occurs

Intermittent IV infusion route
• Give after **diluting** 10 mg/10 ml or 50 mg/50 ml sterile water for inj; **withdraw** prescribed dose, **dilute** ½ dose with 1000 ml D$_5$ 0.2 NaCl or D$_5$ 0.45 NaCl with 37.5 g mannitol; **IV** inf is **given** over 3-4 hr; use a 0.45 μm filter; total dose 2000 ml over 6-8 hr; check site for irritation, phlebitis; do not use equipment containing aluminum

Continuous IV infusion route
• Give over 24 hr × 5 days

Adverse effects: *italics* = common; **bold** = life-threatening

Syringe compatibilities: Bleomycin, cyclophosphamide, doxapram, droperidol, fluorouracil, furosemide, heparin, leucovorin, methotrexate, metoclopramide, vinBLAStine, vinCRIStine

Y-site compatibilities: Acyclovir, alfentanil, allopurinol, amikacin, aminophylline, amiodarone, ampicillin, ampicillin-sulbactam, anidulafungin, atenolol, atracurium, azithromycin, aztreonam, bivalirudin, bleomycin, bumetanide, buprenorphine, butorphanol, calcium chloride/gluconate, carmustine, caspofungin, ceFAZolin, cefoperazone, cefotaxime, cefoTEtan, cefOXitin, cefTAZidime, ceftizoxime, cefTRIAXone, cefuroxime, chlorproMAZINE, cimetidine, ciprofloxacin, cisatracurium, cladribine, clindamycin, codeine, cyclophosphamide, cycloSPORINE, cytarabine, DACTINomycin, DAPTOmycin, DAUNOrubicin, dexamethasone, dexmedetomidine, dexrazoxane, digoxin, diltiazem, diphenhydrAMINE, DOBUTamine, DOCEtaxel, DOPamine, doripenem, doxacurium, DOXOrubicin, DOXOrubicin liposomal, doxycycline, droperidol, enalaprilat, ePHEDrine, EPINEPHrine, epirubicin, ertapenem, erythromycin, esmolol, etoposide, famotidine, fenoldopam, fentaNYL, filgrastim, fluconazole, fludarabine, fluorouracil, foscarnet, fosphenytoin, furosemide, ganciclovir, gatifloxacin, gemcitabine, gentamicin, glycopyrrolate, granisetron, haloperidol, heparin, hydrocortisone, HYDROmorphone, IDArubicin, ifosfamide, imipenem-cilastatin, inamrinone, indomethacin, irinotecan, isoproterenol, ketorolac, labetalol, leucovorin, levofloxacin, levorphanol, lidocaine, linezolid, LORazepam, magnesium sulfate, mannitol, melphalan, meperidine, meropenem, methohexital, methotrexate, methylPREDNISolone, metoclopramide, metoprolol, metroNIDAZOLE, midazolam, milrinone, minocycline, mitoMYcin, mitoXANtrone, mivacurium, nafcillin, naloxone, nesiritide, niCARdipine, nitroglycerin, nitroprusside, norepinephrine, octreotide, ofloxacin, ondansetron, oxaliplatin, PACLitaxel, palonosetron, pamidronate, pancuronium, PEMEtrexed, pentamidine, pentazocine, PENTobarbital, PHENobarbital, phenylephrine, phenytoin, piperacillin, polymyxin B, potassium chloride/phosphates, procainamide, prochlorperazine, promethazine, propofol, propranolol, quiNIDine, quinupristin-dalfopristin, ranitidine, remifentanil, riTUXimab, sargramostim, sodium acetate/bicarbonate/phosphates, succinylcholine, SUFentanil, sulfamethoxazole-trimethoprim, tacrolimus, teniposide, theophylline, thiopental, ticarcillin, ticarcillin-clavulanate, tigecycline, tirofiban, TNA, tobramycin, topotecan, trastuzumab, vancomycin, vasopressin, vecuronium, verapamil, vinBLAStine, vinCRIStine, vinorelbine, voriconazole, zidovudine, zoledronic acid

Solution compatibilities: D₅/0.225% NaCl, D₅/0.45% NaCl, D₅/0.9% NaCl, D₅/0.45% NaCl with mannitol 1.875%, D₅/0.33% NaCl with mannitol 1.875%, D₅/0.33% NaCl with KCl 20 mEq and mannitol 1.875%, 0.9% NaCl, 0.45% NaCl, 0.3% NaCl, 0.225% NaCl, water

Solution incompatibilities: Sodium bicarbonate 5%, 0.1% NaCl, water

ADVERSE EFFECTS

CNS: Seizures, *peripheral neuropathy*
CV: Cardiac abnormalities
EENT: *Tinnitus, hearing loss, vestibular toxicity*, blurred vision, altered color perception
GI: *Severe nausea, vomiting, diarrhea, weight loss*
GU: Renal tubular damage, *renal insufficiency*, impotence, sterility, amenorrhea, gynecomastia, hyperuremia
HEMA: Thrombocytopenia, leukopenia, pancytopenia
INTEG: *Alopecia,* dermatitis
META: *Hypomagnesemia,* hypocalcemia, hypokalemia, hypophosphatemia
RESP: Fibrosis
SYST: Anaphylaxis

Pharmacokinetics

Absorption	Complete
Distribution	Widely distributed, accumulates in body tissues for several months
Metabolism	Liver
Excretion	Kidneys
Half-life	30-100 hr

Pharmacodynamics

Unknown

INTERACTIONS
Individual drugs
Alcohol, aspirin: increased risk of bleeding
Bumetanide, ethacrynic acid, furosemide: ototoxicity
Phenytoin: decreased phenytoin effect

Drug classifications
Aminoglycosides, diuretics (loop), salicylates: increased nephrotoxicity
Myelosuppressive agents, radiation: increased myelosuppression
NSAIDs: increased risk of bleeding
Vaccines, live virus: decreased antibody response

⚠ Nurse Alert   ✳ Key NCLEX® Drug   >> Drug Specifics

Drug/lab test
Increased: uric acid, BUN, creatinine
Decreased: CCr, calcium, phosphate, potassium, magnesium
Positive: Coombs' test

NURSING CONSIDERATIONS
Assessment

> **BLACK BOX WARNING:** Monitor for **bone marrow depression:** CBC, differential, platelet count weekly; withhold product if WBC count is <4000/mm³ or platelet count is <100,000/mm³; notify prescriber of results if WBC <20,000/mm³, platelets <150,000/mm³

> **BLACK BOX WARNING:** Monitor **renal toxicity:** BUN, creatinine, serum uric acid, urine CCr before, during therapy; I&O ratio; report fall in urine output to <30 ml/hr; dose should not be given if BUN <25 mg/dl; creatinine <1.5 mg/dl

• Assess for anaphylaxis: wheezing, tachycardia, facial swelling, fainting; discontinue product and report to prescriber; resuscitation equipment should be nearby, may occur within minutes; often EPINEPHrine, corticosteroids, antihistamines may alleviate symptoms
• Monitor temp q4hr (may indicate beginning of infection)
• Monitor liver function tests before, during therapy (bilirubin, AST, ALT, LDH) as needed or monthly; note yellowing of skin or sclera, dark urine, clay-colored stools, itchy skin, abdominal pain, fever, diarrhea
• Assess for increased uric acid levels, swelling, joint pain primarily in extremities; patient should be well hydrated to prevent urate deposits
• Assess for **bleeding:** hematuria, stool guaiac, bruising or petechiae, mucosa or orifices q8hr; note inflammation of mucosa, breaks in skin
• Identify dyspnea, crackles, nonproductive cough, chest pain, tachypnea

> **BLACK BOX WARNING: Ototoxicity:** more common in genetic variants TPMT 3B and 3C in children; use audiometric testing baseline and before each dose

• Identify effects of alopecia on body image; discuss feelings about body changes
• Identify edema in feet, joint pain, stomach pain, shaking; prescriber should be notified

Patient/family education
⚠ Teach patient to avoid use of products containing aspirin or ibuprofen, NSAIDs, alcohol (may cause GI bleeding), razors, commercial mouthwash; to report symptoms of bleeding (hematuria, tarry stools, bruising, petechiae)
• Advise patient to report numbness, tingling in face or extremities, poor hearing or joint pain, swelling
⚠ Instruct patient to report signs of anemia (fatigue, headache, irritability, faintness, shortness of breath)
• Instruct patient to report any changes in breathing or coughing even several months after treatment; to avoid crowds and persons with respiratory tract or other infections
• Advise patient that hair may be lost during treatment; a wig or hairpiece may make patient feel better; new hair may be different in color, texture
• Tell patient not to have any vaccinations without the advice of the prescriber; serious reactions can occur
⚠ Caution patient contraception is needed during treatment and for 4 months after the completion of therapy, pregnancy D

> **BLACK BOX WARNING: Ototoxicity:** teach patient to report loss of hearing, ringing or roaring in the ears

Evaluation
Positive therapeutic outcome
• Prevention of rapid division of malignant cells

citalopram (Rx)
(sigh-tal'oh-pram)
CeleXA
Func. class.: Antidepressant
Chem. class.: Selective serotonin reuptake inhibitor (SSRI)
Pregnancy category C

Do not confuse: CeleXA/CelebREX/Cerebyx/Cerebra/Zyprexa

ACTION: Inhibits CNS neuron uptake of serotonin but not of norepinephrine; weak inhibitor of CYP450 enzyme system, making it more appealing than other products

Therapeutic outcome: Decreased symptoms of depression after 2-3 wk

USES: Major depressive disorder

Unlabeled uses: Premenstrual disorders, panic disorder, social phobia, obsessive-compulsive disorder in adolescents, anxiety, hot flashes, menopause, adjunct in schizophrenia, PTSD

CONTRAINDICATIONS
Hypersensitivity

Precautions: Pregnancy **C**, breastfeeding, geriatric, renal/hepatic disease, seizure disorder, hypersensitivity to escitalopram, bradycardia, recent MI, abrupt discontinuation, QT prolongation

> **BLACK BOX WARNING:** Children, suicidal ideation

DOSAGE AND ROUTES
Depression
Adult: PO 20 mg daily AM or PM, may increase if needed to 40 mg/day after 1 wk; maintenance: after 6-8 wk of initial treatment, continue for 24 wk (32 wk total)

Hepatic dose/geriatric
Adult: PO 20 mg/day, may increase to 40 mg/ day if no response

Panic disorder (unlabeled)
Adult: PO 20-40 mg/day

Premenstrual dysphoria, social phobia (unlabeled)
Adult: PO 10-30 mg/day used intermittently in premenstrual dysphoria

Available forms: Tabs 10, 20, 40 mg; oral SOL 10 mg/5 ml

Implementation
- Give with food or milk for GI symptoms
- Give dosage at bedtime if oversedation occurs during day
- Leave orally disintegrating tabs on tongue and allow to dissolve before swallowing
- Store at room temperature; do not freeze
- **⚠ Do not give within 14 days of MAOIs**

ADVERSE EFFECTS
CNS: *Headache, nervousness, insomnia, drowsiness, anxiety, tremor, dizziness, fatigue, sedation, poor concentration, abnormal dreams, agitation,* **seizures,** apathy, euphoria, hallucinations, delusions, psychosis, **suicidal attempts, malignant neuroleptic-like syndrome reactions**

CV: *Hot flashes, palpitations,* angina pectoris, **hemorrhage,** hypertension, tachycardia, 1st-degree AV block, bradycardia, **MI, thrombophlebitis, QT prolongation,** orthostatic hypotension, **torsades de pointes**

EENT: Vision changes, ear/eye pain, photophobia, tinnitus

GI: *Nausea, diarrhea, dry mouth, anorexia, dyspepsia, constipation, cramps, vomiting, taste changes, flatulence, decreased appetite*

GU: *Dysmenorrhea, decreased libido, urinary frequency, urinary tract infection,* amenorrhea, cystitis, impotence, urine retention

INTEG: *Sweating, rash, pruritus,* acne, alopecia, urticaria, photosensitivity

MS: *Pain,* arthritis, twitching

RESP: *Infection, pharyngitis, nasal congestion, sinus headache, sinusitis, cough, dyspnea, bronchitis,* asthma, hyperventilation, pneumonia

SYST: *Asthenia, viral infection, fever, allergy, chills,* hyponatremia (geriatric patients), **serotonin syndrome,** neonatal abstinence syndrome

Pharmacokinetics

Absorption	Well absorbed
Distribution	Unknown
Metabolism	Liver, by CYP1A2, CYP2D6
Excretion	Kidneys, steady state 28-35 days
Half-life	Unknown

Pharmacodynamics
Unknown

INTERACTIONS
Individual drugs
Alcohol: increased CNS depression

CarBAMazepine, cloNIDine: decreased citalopram levels

Lithium, tramadol, traZODone: increased serotonin syndrome

Pimoside, ziprasidone: increased QTc interval; do not use together

Drug classifications
Anticoagulants, antiplatelets, NSAIDs, salicylates, thrombolytics: increased risk of bleeding

Antidepressants (tricyclics): increased effect, use cautiously

Antifungals (azole), macrolides: increased citalopram levels

β-Adrenergic blockers: increased plasma levels of β-blockers

Barbiturates, benzodiazepines, CNS depressants, sedatives/hypnotics: increased CNS depression

MAOIs: hypertensive crisis, seizures, fatal reactions; do not use together

Quinolones: increased QTc interval; do not use together

Serotonin receptor agonists, SNRIs, SSRIs: increased serotonin syndrome

Drug/herb
SAM-e, St. John's wort: serotonin syndrome; do not use with citalopram; fatal reaction may occur
Yohimbe: increased CNS stimulation

Drug/lab test
Increased: serum bilirubin, blood glucose, alkaline phosphatase
Decreased: VMA, 5-HIAA
False increase: increased urinary catecholamines

NURSING CONSIDERATIONS
Assessment
• Monitor B/P (lying, standing), pulse q4hr; if systolic B/P drops 20 mm Hg, hold product and notify prescriber; take vital signs q4hr in patients with cardiovascular disease
• Monitor blood studies: CBC, leukocytes, differential, cardiac enzymes if patient is receiving long-term therapy; check platelets; bleeding can occur
• Monitor hepatic studies: AST, ALT, bilirubin
• Check weight qwk; appetite may increase with product
⚠ Assess ECG for flattening of T wave, bundle branch block, AV block, dysrhythmias in cardiac patients, torsades de pointes, QT prolongation (effect is dose dependent)
• Assess EPS primarily in geriatric: rigidity, dystonia, akathisia

> BLACK BOX WARNING: Assess mental status: mood, sensorium, affect, suicidal tendencies; increase in psychiatric symptoms: depression, panic

• Monitor urinary retention, constipation; constipation is more likely to occur in children or geriatric
• Assess for serotonin syndrome: increased heart rate, sweating, dilated pupils, tremors, twitching, hyperthermia, agitation
• Identify patient's alcohol consumption; if alcohol is consumed, hold dose until AM

Patient/family education
• Teach patient that therapeutic effects may take 4-6 wk, not to discontinue abruptly
• Instruct patient to use caution in driving or other activities requiring alertness because of drowsiness, dizziness, blurred vision; to avoid rising quickly from sitting to standing, especially geriatric patients

> BLACK BOX WARNING: Advise that suicidal ideas, behavior may occur in children or young adults

• Caution patient to avoid alcohol ingestion, other CNS depressants
• Instruct patient to increase fluids, bulk in diet if constipation, urinary retention occur, especially geriatric
• Advise patient to take gum, hard sugarless candy, or frequent sips of water for dry mouth
• Teach patient how to use orally disintegrating tabs
• Teach patient to report serotonin syndrome: sweating, dilated pupils, tremors, twitching, extreme heat, agitation

Evaluation
Positive therapeutic outcome
• Decrease in depression
• Absence of suicidal thoughts

clarithromycin (Rx)
(clare-i-thro-mye′sin)
Biaxin, Biaxin XL
Func. class.: Antiinfective
Chem. class.: Macrolide
Pregnancy category C

ACTION: Binds to 50S ribosomal subunits of susceptible bacteria and suppresses protein synthesis

Therapeutic outcome: Bactericidal action against the following: *Streptococcus pneumoniae, Streptococcus pyogenes, Mycoplasma pneumoniae, Corynebacterium diphtheriae, Bordetella pertussis, Listeria monocytogenes, Haemophilus influenzae, Staphylococcus aureus, Mycobacterium avium (MAC), Legionella pneumophila, Moxarella catarrhalis, Neisseria gonorrhoeae,* complex infections in AIDS patients, *Helicobacter pylori* in combination with omeprazole, *Helicobacter parainfluenzae*

USES: Mild to moderate infections of the upper respiratory tract, lower respiratory tract; uncomplicated skin and skin structure infections

CONTRAINDICATIONS
Hypersensitivity to this product or other macrolides, torsades de pointes, QT prolongation

Precautions: Pregnancy **C**, breastfeeding, geriatric, renal/hepatic disease, QT prolongation

DOSAGE AND ROUTES
Acute exacerbation of chronic bronchitis
Adult: PO 250-500 mg q12hr × 7-14 days or 1000 mg/day × 7 days (XL)

Pharyngitis/tonsillitis
Adult: PO 250 mg q12hr × 10 days

Community-acquired pneumonia
Adult: PO 250 mg q12hr × 7-14 days or 1000 mg/day × 7 days (XL)

Endocarditis prophylaxis
Adult: PO 500 mg 1 hr before procedure

MAC prophylaxis/treatment
Adult: PO 500 mg bid, will require an additional antiinfective for active infection

H. pylori infection
Adult: PO 500 mg with 30 mg lansoprazole and 1 g amoxicillin together q12hr × 10-14 days or 500 mg with omeprazole 20 mg and 1 g amoxicillin together q12hr × 10 days or 500 mg q8hr and omeprazole 40 mg q d × 14 days, continue omeprazole for 14 more days

Acute maxillary sinusitis
Adult: PO 500 mg q12hr × 14 days

Most infections
Child: PO 7.5 mg/kg q12hr × 10 days, max 500 mg/dose for MAC

Renal dose
Adult: PO CCr 30-60 ml/min; decrease dose by 50% if using with ritonavir; CCr < 30 ml/min reduce dose by 50%

Available forms: Tabs 250, 500 mg; oral susp 125, 250 mg/5 ml; ext rel tab (XL) 500 mg

Implementation
• Do not break, crush, or chew ext rel tab
• Ensure adequate fluid intake (2 L) during diarrhea episodes
• Give q12hr to maintain serum level
• Store at room temperature
• **Susp:** Shake well, store at room temperature, discard after 2 wk
• **Ext Rel:** Give with food

ADVERSE EFFECTS
CV: Ventricular dysrhythmias, QT prolongation
GI: Nausea, vomiting, diarrhea, hepatotoxicity, abdominal pain, stomatitis, heartburn, anorexia, abnormal taste, pseudomembranous colitis, tooth/tongue discoloration, pancreatitis
GU: Vaginitis, moniliasis, interstitial nephritis, azotemia
HEMA: Leukopenia, thrombocytopenia, increased INR
INTEG: Rash, urticaria, pruritus, Stevens-Johnson syndrome, toxic epidermal necrolysis
MISC: Headache, hearing loss

Pharmacokinetics
Absorption	50%
Distribution	Widely distributed
Metabolism	Liver
Excretion	Kidneys, unchanged (20%-30%)
Half-life	5-7 hr

Pharmacodynamics
Onset	Unknown
Peak	2 hr; Ext release: 5-7 hr;
Duration	Unknown

INTERACTIONS
Individual drugs
ALPRAZolam, busPIRone, carBAMazepine, cycloSPORINE, digoxin, disopyramide, felodipine, fluconazole, omeprazole, tacrolimus, theophylline: increased levels, increased toxicity
CarBAMazepine: increased toxicity, from increased levels of carBAMazepine
Cisapride, pimozide: increased effect, increased dysrhythmias
Midazolam, tacrolimus: increased effects
Rifabutin, rifampin, nevirapine, etravirine, benzodiazepine: decreased levels
Theophylline: increased toxicity from increased levels of theophylline, increased oral anticoagulant effect
Zidovudine: increased or decreased action

Drug classifications
All products metabolized by CYP3A enzyme system: increased action, risk of toxicity
Antidiabetics: increased toxicity
Digoxin: increased blood levels of digoxin, increased digoxin effects
Calcium channel blockers, benzodiazepines: increased effects
Class IA, III antidysrhythmics or other products that prolong QT: increased QT prolongation
Ergots: increased levels, increased toxicity
HMG-CoA reductase inhibitors: increased levels
Oral anticoagulants: increased effects of oral anticoagulants

Drug/food
Do not use with grapefruit juice

Drug/lab test
Increased: 17-OHCS/17-KS, AST, ALT, BUN, creatinine, LDH, total bilirubin
Decreased: folate assay, WBC

NURSING CONSIDERATIONS
Assessment
• Assess patient for signs and symptoms of **infection** including characteristics of wounds, sputum, urine, stool, WBC >10,000/mm³, earache, fever; obtain baseline information before, during treatment; obtain C&S before beginning product therapy to identify if correct treatment has been initiated, product may be given as soon as culture is taken, repeat after treatment
• Bleeding: check INR if anticoagulants are taken
• Monitor blood studies: AST, ALT, CBC, Hct, bilirubin, LDH, alkaline phosphatase, Coombs' test monthly if patient is on long-term therapy
• Assess bowel pattern daily; if severe diarrhea occurs, product should be discontinued and prescriber should be notified of all products used
• Assess for overgrowth of infection: perineal itching, fever, malaise, redness, pain, swelling, drainage, rash, diarrhea, change in cough, sputum
⚠ Assess for QT prolongation, ventricular dysrhythmias: monitor ECG, cardiac status in those with cardiac abnormalities
⚠ Assess for serious skin reaction: Stevens-Johnson syndrome, toxic epidermal necrolysis, product should be discontinued immediately

Patient/family education
• Advise patient to contact physician if vaginal itching, loose foul-smelling stools, furry tongue occur; may indicate superinfection
• Instruct patient to take all medication prescribed for the length of time ordered, ext rel with food
• Advise prescriber if pregnancy is planned or suspected
• Teach patient to notify prescriber of diarrhea, dark urine, pale stools, yellowing of eyes/skin, severe abdominal pain

Evaluation
Positive therapeutic outcome
• Absence of signs/symptoms of infection: WBC <10,000/mm³, temp WNL, absence of red draining wounds
• Reported improvement in symptoms of infection

clavulanate
See amoxicillin/clavulanate, ticarcillin/ clavulanate

clevidipine (Rx)
(klev-id′i-peen)
Cleviprex
Func. class.: Calcium channel blocker (L-type)
Chem. class.: Dihydropyridine
Pregnancy category C

ACTION: L-type calcium channels mediate the influx of calcium during depolarization in arterial smooth muscle; reduces mean arterial B/P by decreasing systemic vascular resistance

Therapeutic outcome: Decreased B/P

USES: Treatment of hypertension when oral therapy is not feasible

CONTRAINDICATIONS
Hypersensitivity to this product, eggs, or soya lecithin; defective lipid metabolism; severe aortic stenosis; pancreatitis

Precautions: Pregnancy **C**, breastfeeding, children <18 yr, heart failure, hyperlipidemia, hypertension, labor, pheochromocytoma

DOSAGE AND ROUTES
Adult: CONT **IV** 1-2 mg/hr; dose may be doubled q90sec initially; as B/P reaches goal, adjust dose less frequently (5-10 min) with smaller increases in dose; most patients require 4-6 mg/hr, max 32 mg/hr; no more than 1000 ml should be infused per 24 hr period due to lipid load restrictions

Available forms: Single dose vial 50, 100 ml (0.5 mg/ml)

Implementation
Intermittent IV infusion route
• Do not give through same line as other medications, do not dilute, do not filter
• Gently invert several times before use; do not use if discolored or if particulate matter is present
• Give through central or peripheral line at 1-2 mg/hr, use infusion device
• Store vials in refrigerator, do not freeze; leave vials in carton until use; product is photosensitive but protection from light during administration is not required

ADVERSE EFFECTS

CNS: Headache

CV: Hypotension, MI, sinus tachycardia, syncope, reflex tachycardia, atrial fibrillation

GI: Nausea, vomiting

GU: Renal failure

Pharmacokinetics

Absorption	Unknown
Distribution	Protein binding >99%
Metabolism	By esterases in blood, extravascular tissues
Excretion	Urine 63%-74%, feces 7%-22%
Half-life	Initially 1 min; terminal 15 min; increased in hepatic disease

Pharmacodynamics

Onset	2-4 min
Peak	6-12 hr
Duration	Unknown

NURSING CONSIDERATIONS

Assessment

• Assess cardiac status: B/P, pulse, respiration, ECG; some patients have developed severe angina, acute MI after calcium channel blockers if obstructive CAD is severe; if not transitioned to other antihypertensive therapies following clevidipine infusion, patients should be monitored ≥8 hr for rebound hypertension; monitor for rebound hypertension following drug stoppage

• **Renal failure: Monitor I&O ratio, weight daily; peripheral edema, dyspnea, jugular vein distention, crackles (perioperative hypertensive patients)**

Patient/family education

⚠ **Instruct patient to notify prescriber immediately if neurological symptoms, visual changes, or symptoms of CHF occur**

• Instruct patient to continue follow-up for hypertension

• Teach patient to notify prescriber if pregnancy is planned or suspected or if breastfeeding

Evaluation

Positive therapeutic outcome

• Decreased B/P

---

clindamycin HCl (Rx)

(klin-dah-my'sin)

Cleocin HCl

clindamycin palmitate (Rx)

Cleocin Pediatric

clindamycin phosphate (Rx)

Cleocin Phosphate

Func. class.: Antiinfective—miscellaneous

Chem. class.: Lincomycin derivative

Pregnancy category B

ACTION: Binds to 50S subunit of bacterial ribosomes; suppresses protein synthesis

Therapeutic outcome: Absence of infection

USES: Infections caused by staphylococci, streptococci, *Rickettsia, Fusobacterium, Actinomyces, Peptococcus, Bacteroides, Pneumocystis jiroveci*

CONTRAINDICATIONS

Hypersensitivity to this product or lincomycin, tartrazine dye, ulcerative colitis/enteritis

> **BLACK BOX WARNING:** Pseudomembranous colitis

Precautions: Pregnancy **B**, breastfeeding, geriatric, renal/liver/GI disease, asthma, allergy

> **BLACK BOX WARNING:** Diarrhea

DOSAGE AND ROUTES

Adult: PO 150-450 mg q6hr, max 2.7 g/day; IM/IV 1.2-2.7 g/day in 2-4 divided doses q6-12hr, max 4.8 g/day

Child >1 mo: PO 8-25 mg/kg/day in divided doses q6-8hr; IM/IV 20-40 mg/kg/day in divided doses q6-8hr in 3-4 equal doses

Neonate: 15-20 mg/kg/day divided q6-8hr

PID

Adult: IV 900 mg q8hr plus gentamicin

Bacterial endocarditis prophylaxis

Adult: 600 mg 1 hr before procedure

P. jiroveci pneumonia (unlabeled)

Adult: PO 1200-1800 mg/day in divided doses with 15-30 mg primaquine/day × 21 days

---

Available forms: Phosphate: inj 150, 300, 600 mg base/4 ml; 900 mg base/6 ml; inj inf in D₅ 300, 600, 900 mg; **HCl:** caps 75, 150, 300 mg; **palmitate:** oral sol 75 mg/5 ml

Implementation
• Obtain C&S before use

PO route
• Do not break, crush, or chew caps
• Give with 8 oz of water; give with meals for GI symptoms
• Shake liquids well
• Do not refrigerate oral preparations; stable at room temperature for 2 wk

Oral sol
• Do not refrigerate reconstituted product, store at room temperature ≤2 wk
• Reconstitute granules with most of 75 ml of water, shake well, add remaining water, shake well (75 mg/5 ml)

IM route
• If more than 600 mg must be given, divide into 2 inj
• Give deeply in large muscle mass; rotate sites

IV route
• Visually inspect parenteral products for particulate matter and discoloration prior to use
• **Vials:** Dilute 300 and 600 mg doses with 50 ml of a compatible diluent. Dilute 900 mg doses with 50-100 ml of a compatible diluent. Dilute 1200 mg doses with 100 ml of a compatible diluent, final concentration max 18 mg/ml
• **ADD-Vantage vials:** Dilute 300 and 600 mg ADD-Vantage containers with 50 or 100 mg, respectively, of NS or D₅W
• **Storage:** When diluted in D₅W, NS, or LR, solutions with concentrations of 6, 9, or 12 mg/ml are stable for 16 days at room temperature or 32 days under refrigeration when stored in glass bottles or minibags. When diluted in D₅W, solutions with a concentration of 18 mg/ml are stable for 16 days at room temperature

Intermittent IV infusion
• Infuse over at least 10-60 min, infusion rates max 30 mg/min and ≤1.2 g should be infused in a 1 hr period
• Infuse 300 mg doses over 10 min; 600 mg doses over 20 min, 900 mg doses over 30 min, and 1200 mg doses over 40 min

Continuous IV infusion
• Give first dose rapidly, and then follow with continuous infusion; rate is based on desired serum clindamycin levels

• To maintain serum concentrations above 4 mcg/ml, use a rapid infusion rate of 10 mg/min for 30 min and a maintenance rate of 0.75 mg/min; to maintain serum concentrations above 5 mcg/ml, use a rapid infusion rate of 15 mg/min for 30 min and a maintenance rate of 1 mg/min; to maintain serum concentrations above 5 mcg/ml, use a rapid infusion rate of 20 mg/min for 30 min and a maintenance rate of 1.25 mg/min

Syringe incompatibilities: Tobramycin

Y-site compatibilities: Acyclovir, alfentanil, amifostine, amikacin, aminocaproic acid, aminophylline, amiodarone, amphotericin B cholesteryl, amphotericin B lipid complex, amsacrine, anakinra, anidulafungin, ascorbic acid injection, atenolol, atracurium, atropine, aztreonam, benztropine, bivalirudin, bleomycin, bumetanide, buprenorphine, butorphanol, calcium chloride/gluconate, CARBOplatin, cefamandole, ceFAZolin, cefmetazole, cefonicid, cefoperazone, cefotaxime, cefoTEtan, cefOXitin, cefpirome, cefTAZidime, ceftizoxime, ceftobiprole, cefuroxime, cephalothin, cephapirin, chloramphenicol, cimetidine, cisatracurium, CISplatin, codeine, cyanocobalamin, cyclophosphamide, cycloSPORINE, cytarabine, DACTINomycin, DAPTOmycin, dexamethasone, dexmedetomidine, digoxin, diltiazem, diphenhydrAMINE, DOCEtaxel, DOPamine, doxacurium, DOXOrubicin, DOXOrubicin liposomal, doxycycline, enalaprilat, ePHEDrine, EPINEPHrine, epirubicin, epoetin alfa, eptifibatide, esmolol, etoposide, famotidine, fenoldopam, fentaNYL, fludarabine, fluorouracil, folic acid, foscarnet, furosemide, gatifloxacin, gemcitabine, gemtuzumab, gentamicin, glycopyrrolate, granisetron, heparin, hydrocortisone, HYDROmorphone, ifosfamide, imipenem-cilastatin, indomethacin, insulin (regular), irinotecan, isoproterenol, ketorolac, levofloxacin, lidocaine, linezolid, LORazepam, LR, magnesium sulfate, mannitol, mechlorethamine, melphalan, meperidine, metaraminol, methicillin, methotrexate, methoxamine, methyldopate, methylPREDNISolone, metoclopramide, metoprolol, metroNIDAZOLE, mezlocillin, miconazole, milrinone, morphine, moxalactam, multiple vitamins injection, nafcillin, nalbuphine, naloxone, nesiritide, netilmicin, niCARdipine, nitroglycerin, nitroprusside, norepinephrine, octreotide, ondansetron, oxacillin, oxaliplatin, oxytocin, PACLitaxel, palonosetron, pamidronate, pancuronium, pantoprazole, PEMEtrexed, penicillin G potassium/sodium, pentazocine, perphenazine, PHENobarbital, phenylephrine, phytonadione, piperacillin, piperacillin-tazobactam, potassium chloride, procainamide, propofol, propranolol, protamine, pyridoxine, ranitidine, remifentanil, Ringer's, ritodrine, riTUXimab, rocuronium, sargramostim, sodium acetate/bicarbonate, succinylcholine, SUFentanil, tacrolimus, teniposide, theophylline, thiamine, thiotepa, ticarcillin, ticarcillin-clavulanate, tigecycline, tirofiban, TNA, tobramycin, tolazoline, TPN, trimetaphan, urokinase, vancomycin, vasopressin, vecuronium, verapamil, vinCRIStine, vinorelbine, vitamin B complex/C, voriconazole, zidovudine, zoledronic acid

Y-site incompatibilities: IDArubicin

ADVERSE EFFECTS

GI: *Nausea, vomiting, abdominal pain, diarrhea,* **pseudomembranous colitis,** *anorexia, weight loss,* increased AST, ALT, bilirubin, alkaline phosphatase, jaundice
GU: *Vaginitis,* urinary frequency
INTEG: Rash, urticaria, pruritus, erythema, pain, abscess at inj site
SYST: Stevens-Johnson syndrome, exfoliative dermatitis

Pharmacokinetics

Absorption	Well absorbed (PO, IM), minimal (TOP)
Distribution	Widely distributed; crosses placenta
Metabolism	Liver, extensively
Excretion	Kidneys, breast milk
Half-life	2½ hr

Pharmacodynamics

	PO	IM	IV
Onset	Rapid	Rapid	Rapid
Peak	6-8 hr	1½ hr	Infusion's end

INTERACTIONS
Individual drugs
Erythromycin, chloramphenicol: decreased action of clindamycin
Kaolin: decreased absorption

Drug/lab test
Increased: alkaline phosphatase, bilirubin, CPK, AST, ALT

NURSING CONSIDERATIONS
Assessment
• Assess any patient with compromised renal system; product is excreted slowly in poor renal system function; toxicity may occur rapidly
• Assess patient for signs and symptoms of

infection including characteristics of wounds, sputum, urine, stool, WBC >10,000/mm³, fever; obtain baseline information before, during treatment; complete C&S testing before beginning product therapy; this will identify if correct treatment has been initiated, give product as soon as culture is taken
• Assess for allergic reactions: rash, urticaria, pruritus, chills, fever, joint pain; may occur a few days after therapy begins; EPINEPHrine and resuscitation equipment should be available in case of an anaphylactic reaction
• **Identify urine output; if decreasing, notify prescriber (may indicate nephrotoxicity); also look for increased BUN and creatinine levels**
• Monitor blood studies: AST, ALT, CBC, Hct, bilirubin, LDH, alkaline phosphatase, Coombs' test monthly if patient is on long-term therapy
• Monitor electrolytes: potassium, sodium, chloride monthly if patient is on long-term therapy

> **BLACK BOX WARNING:** Assess bowel pattern daily; if severe diarrhea occurs, product should be discontinued; may indicate **pseudomembranous colitis**

• Monitor for bleeding: ecchymosis, bleeding gums, hematuria, stool guaiac daily if on long-term therapy, may occur several weeks after therapy is terminated
• Assess for overgrowth of infection: perineal itching, fever, malaise, redness, pain, swelling, drainage, rash, diarrhea, change in cough, sputum
⚠ Assess for serious skin infections: Stevens-Johnson syndrome, exfoliative dermatitis

Patient/family education
• Tell patient to take oral product with full glass of water; may take with food if GI symptoms occur; antiperistaltic products may worsen diarrhea
• Teach patient aspects of product therapy: need to complete entire course of medication to ensure organism death (10-14 days); culture may be taken after medication course has been completed
• **Advise patient to report sore throat, fever, fatigue; may indicate superinfection**
• Advise patient that product must be taken at equal intervals around clock to maintain blood levels

> **BLACK BOX WARNING:** Teach patient to report diarrhea with pus, mucus

---

Evaluation
Positive therapeutic outcome
• Decreased temp, negative C&S

TREATMENT OF HYPERSEN-SITIVITY: Withdraw product; maintain airway; administer EPINEPHrine, aminophylline, O_2, **IV** corticosteroids

clindamycin topical
See Appendix B

clobetasol topical
See Appendix B

clomiPHENE (Rx)
(kloe'mi-feen)
Clomid, Serophene
Func. class.: Ovulation stimulant
Chem. class.: SERM (selective estrogen receptor modulator)
Pregnancy category X

Do not confuse: clomiPHENE/clomiPRAMINE, Serophene/Sarafem

ACTION: Increases LH, FSH release from the pituitary, which increases maturation of ovarian follicle, ovulation, development of corpus luteum

Therapeutic outcome: Pregnancy

USES: Female infertility (ovulatory failure)

CONTRAINDICATIONS
Pregnancy **X**, hypersensitivity, hepatic disease, undiagnosed uterine bleeding, uncontrolled thyroid or adrenal dysfunction, intracranial lesion, ovarian cysts, endometrial carcinoma

Precautions: Hypertension, depression, seizures, diabetes mellitus, abnormal ovarian enlargement, ovarian hyperstimulation

DOSAGE AND ROUTES
Adult: PO 50-100 mg daily × 5 days or 50 mg daily beginning on day 5 of the menstrual cycle, may increase to 100 mg/day × 5 days with next cycle; may be repeated until conception occurs or 3 (max 6) cycles of therapy have been completed

Available forms: Tabs 50 mg

Implementation
• Give after discontinuing estrogen therapy
• Give at same time daily to maintain product level; begin on 5th day of menstrual cycle

• Avoid heat, moisture, light, store at room temperature
• Give without regard to food

ADVERSE EFFECTS
CNS: *Headache, depression,* restlessness, anxiety, nervousness, fatigue, insomnia, dizziness, flushing
CV: Vasomotor flushing, phlebitis, **deep vein thrombosis**
EENT: Blurred vision, diplopia, photophobia
GI: *Nausea, vomiting, constipation,* abdominal pain, bloating
GU: Polyuria, frequency of urination, **birth defects, spontaneous abortions,** multiple ovulation, breast pain, oliguria, abnormal uterine bleeding, ovarian cyst, hypertrophy of ovary, hot flashes
INTEG: *Rash, dermatitis,* urticaria, alopecia

Pharmacokinetics	
Absorption	Well distributed
Distribution	Unknown
Metabolism	Liver, extensively
Excretion	Feces
Half-life	5 days

Pharmacodynamics

Unknown

NURSING CONSIDERATIONS
Assessment
• Verify infertility workup, pelvic exam
• Determine liver function tests before therapy: AST, ALT, alkaline phosphatase
• Monitor serum progesterone, urinary excretion of pregnanediol to identify occurrence of ovulation
• Pelvic exam should be done to determine ovary size, condition of cervix
• Endometrial biopsy may be done in women over 35 to rule out endometrial carcinoma

Patient/family education
• Advise patient that multiple births are common after product is taken
• Instruct patient to notify prescriber immediately if low abdominal pain occurs; may indicate ovarian cyst, cyst rupture
⚠ **Advise patient to notify prescriber of photophobia, blurred vision, diplopia, abnormal bleeding**
• Teach patient if dose is missed, double at next time; if more than one dose is missed, call prescriber

• Instruct patient that response usually occurs 4-10 days after last day of treatment
• Teach patient method for taking, recording basal body temp to determine whether ovulation has occurred; if ovulation can be determined (there is a slight decrease in temp, then a sharp increase for ovulation), to attempt coitus 3 days before and every other day until after ovulation
⚠ Teach patient if pregnancy (X) is suspected, to notify prescriber immediately

Evaluation
Positive therapeutic outcome
• Fertility

---

clomiPRAMINE (Rx)
(klom-ip′ra-meen)
Anafranil
Func. class.: Tricyclic antidepressant
Chem. class.: Tertiary amine
Pregnancy category C

Do not confuse: clomiPRAMINE/ clomiPHENE/desipramine/Norpramin

ACTION: Potentiates serotonin and norepinephrine uptake; moderate anticholinergic effect

Therapeutic outcome: Decreased signs and symptoms of obsessive-compulsive disorder, decreased depression

USES: Obsessive-compulsive disorder

Unlabeled uses: Dysphoria, anxiety, agoraphobia and other phobias

CONTRAINDICATIONS
Hypersensitivity to this product, carBAMazepine, tricyclics, immediately after MI, MAOI therapy

Precautions: Pregnancy **C,** breastfeeding, geriatric, seizures, cardiac disease, glaucoma, prostatic hypertrophy, urinary retention

> **BLACK BOX WARNING:** Suicidal ideation, children

DOSAGE AND ROUTES
Obsessive-compulsive disorder
Adult: PO 25 mg at bedtime; increase gradually over 4 wk to a dosage of 75-250 mg/day in divided doses
Child 10-18 yr: PO 25 mg/day gradually increased max over 2 wk 3 mg/kg/day or 200 mg/ day, whichever is smaller

Available forms: Caps 25, 50, 75 mg

Implementation
• Do not break, crush, or chew caps

• Give without regard to food; during initial dosing and titration, give with meals
• Store in tight container, at room temperature; do not freeze

ADVERSE EFFECTS
CNS: *Dizziness, tremors, mania,* seizures, aggressiveness, drowsiness, headache, EPS, neuroleptic malignant syndrome, insomnia, agitation, anxiety, impaired memory
CV: Hypotension, tachycardia, cardiac arrest, hypertension, palpitations
EENT: Blurred vision, altered taste, tinnitus, increased intraocular pressure
ENDO: Galactorrhea, hyperprolactinemia
GI: *Constipation, dry mouth, nausea, dyspepsia,* weight gain, hepatic toxicity
GU: *Delayed ejaculation, anorgasmia,* retention, decreased libido
HEMA: Agranulocytosis, neutropenia, pancytopenia
INTEG: Diaphoresis, photosensitivity, abnormal skin odor, flushing, rash, pruritus
META: Hyponatremia
RESP: Pharyngitis, rhinitis, bronchospasm
SYST: Suicide in children/adolescents

Pharmacokinetics

Absorption	Well absorbed
Distribution	Widely distributed
Metabolism	Liver, extensively
Excretion	Kidneys, breast milk
Half-life	20-32 hr; steady state 1-2 wk

Pharmacodynamics

Onset	≥2 wk
Peak	2-6 hr
Duration	Unknown

INTERACTIONS
Individual drugs
Alcohol: increased CNS depression
CarBAMazepine: decreased clomiPRAMINE action
Cimetidine, FLUoxetine, fluvoxaMINE, sertraline: increased clomiPRAMINE level; do not use together
CloNIDine, EPINEPHrine, norepinephrine: severe hypertension; avoid use
CloNIDine, haloperidol, levodopa: decreased effect of droperidol, mefloquine, mesoridazine, moxifloxacin, pentamide, pimozide, tacrolimus, ziprasidone: Increased QT prolongation these products
Phenytoin: decreased clomiPRAMINE action

Drug classifications
Barbiturates: decreased clomiPRAMINE levels
CNS depressants, general anesthetics: increased effects; do not use together
CYP1A2, CYP2D6: increased clomiPRAMINE level
MAOIs: hypertensive crisis, seizures; do not use together
SSRIs, SNRIs: increased serotonin syndrome
Antidysrhythmics, other tricyclics, phenothiazines, quinolones: QT prolongation
Skeletal muscle relaxants, opiates: decreased action of these products

Drug/herb
SAM-e, St. John's wort: serotonin syndrome, do not use together

Drug/lab test
Increased: prolactin, TBG, AST, ALT, blood glucose
Decreased: serum thyroid hormone (T_3, T_4)

NURSING CONSIDERATIONS
Assessment
• Monitor B/P (with patient lying, standing), pulse q4hr; if systolic B/P drops 20 mm Hg hold product, notify prescriber; take VS q4hr in patients with cardiovascular disease
• Monitor blood studies: CBC, leukocytes, differential, cardiac enzymes if patient is receiving long-term therapy and signs of blood dyscrasias
⚠ Serotonin syndrome: hyperpyrexia, rigidity, irregular pulse, diaphoresis
⚠ Monitor hepatic studies: AST, ALT, bilirubin
⚠ Check weight weekly; appetite may increase with product
⚠ Assess ECG for flattening of T wave, QTc prolongation bundle branch block, AV block, dysrhythmias in cardiac patients, may lead to cardiac collapse
• Assess for EPS primarily in geriatric: rigidity, dystonia, akathisia

BLACK BOX WARNING: Assess mental status: mood, sensorium, affect, suicidal tendencies; increase in psychiatric symptoms: depression, panic, frequency of obsessive-compulsive behaviors

• Monitor urinary retention, constipation; constipation is more likely to occur in children or geriatric
• Assess for **withdrawal symptoms:** headache, nausea, vomiting, muscle pain, weakness; do not usually occur unless product was discontinued abruptly

• Identify alcohol consumption; if alcohol is consumed, hold dose until morning

Patient/family education
• Teach patient that therapeutic effects may take 4-6 wk
• Teach patient to use caution in driving or other activities requiring alertness because of drowsiness, dizziness, blurred vision; to avoid rising quickly from sitting to standing, especially geriatric
• Teach patient to avoid alcohol ingestion, other CNS depressants
• Teach patient not to discontinue medication quickly after long-term use: may cause nausea, headache, malaise
• Teach patient to wear sunscreen or large hat, since photosensitivity occurs
• Teach patient to increase fluids, bulk in diet if constipation, urinary retention occur, especially geriatric
⚠ Serotonin syndrome: teach patient to report immediately sweating, diarrhea, twitching
⚠ Abrupt discontinuation: do not stop abruptly
• Teach patient to take gum, hard sugarless candy, or frequent sips of water for dry mouth
• Advise patient to notify prescriber if pregnancy is planned or suspected

BLACK BOX WARNING: Teach patient that suicidal ideas, behavior may occur in children/young adults, report immediately

Evaluation
Positive therapeutic outcome
• Decrease in depression
• Absence of suicidal thoughts

TREATMENT OF OVERDOSE:
ECG monitoring, induce emesis, lavage, activated charcoal, administer anticonvulsant

⚠ HIGH ALERT
clonazePAM (Rx)
(kloe-na′zi-pam)
KlonoPIN, Rivotril ♦
Func. class.: Anticonvulsant
Chem. class.: Benzodiazepine derivative
Pregnancy category D
Controlled substance schedule IV

Do not confuse: clonazePAM/LORazepam/clorazepate/cloNIDine, KlonoPIN/cloNIDine

ACTION: Inhibits spike, wave formation in absence seizures (petit mal), decreases amplitude, frequency, duration, spread of discharge in minor motor seizures

Therapeutic outcome: Decreased frequency, severity of seizures

USES: Absence, atypical absence, akinetic, myoclonic seizures, Lennox-Gastaut syndrome, panic disorder

CONTRAINDICATIONS
Pregnancy **D**, hypersensitivity to benzodiazepines, acute closed-angle glaucoma, psychosis, severe liver disease

Precautions: Open-angle glaucoma, chronic respiratory disease, renal/hepatic disease, breastfeeding, geriatric

DOSAGE AND ROUTES
Lennox-Gastaut syndrome/atypical absence seizures/akinetic and myoclonic seizures
Adult: PO 1.5 mg/day in 3 divided doses; may be increased 0.5-1 mg q3day until desired response; max 20 mg/day
Child <10 yr or <30 kg: PO 0.01-0.03 mg/kg/day in divided doses q8hr, max 0.05 mg/kg/day; may be increased 0.25-0.5 mg q3day until desired response; max 0.1-0.2 mg/kg/day
Geriatric: PO 0.25 daily-bid initially, increase by 0.25 daily q7-14day as needed

Panic disorder
Adult: PO 0.25 mg bid, increase to 1 mg/day after 3 days, max 4 mg/day

Available forms: Tabs 0.5, 1, 2 mg; **orally disintegrating tabs** 0.125, 0.25, 0.5, 1, 2 mg

Implementation
PO route
• Give on empty stomach for best absorption
Rectal route
• IV sol may be used rectally, 1 ml syringe inserted 3 cm into rectum
• Oral susp may be used rectally (1 mg/ml of product with 1 ml of water), use plastic tube (volume 2.2-3.3 ml)
• Store at room temperature

ADVERSE EFFECTS
CNS: *Drowsiness,* dizziness, confusion, behavioral changes, tremors, insomnia, headache, suicidal tendencies, slurred speech, anterograde amnesia, fatigue, poor coordination
CV: Palpitations, bradycardia, tachycardia
EENT: *Increased salivation, nystagmus, diplopia,* abnormal eye movements

GI: *Nausea, constipation,* polyphagia, anorexia, xerostomia, diarrhea, gastritis, sore gums, blurred vision
GU: Dysuria, enuresis, nocturia, retention, libido changes
HEMA: Thrombocytopenia, leukocytosis, eosinophilia
INTEG: Rash, alopecia, hirsutism
RESP: Respiratory depression, dyspnea, congestion
MS: Myalgia, muscle weakness

Pharmacokinetics
Absorption	Well absorbed
Distribution	Crosses blood-brain barrier, placenta
Metabolism	Liver, protein binding 85%
Excretion	Kidneys
Half-life	18-50 hr

Pharmacodynamics
Onset	½-1 hr
Peak	1-2 hr
Duration	6-12 hr

INTERACTIONS
Individual drugs
Alcohol: increased CNS depression
CarBAMazepine: decreased clonazePAM effect
Cimetidine, clarithromycin, diltiazem, erythromycin, FLUoxetine: increased clonazePAM effect
PHENobarbitol: decreased clonazePAM effect
Phenytoin: decreased clonazePAM levels

Drug classifications
Anticonvulsants, antidepressants, barbiturates, general anesthetics, opiates, sedative/hypnotics: increased CNS depression
Azoles, oral contraceptives: increased clonazePAM effect
CYP3A4 inducers: decreased clonazePAM effect

Drug/herb
Ginkgo, melatonin: increased clonazePAM effect
Ginseng, St. John's wort: decreased clonazePAM effect
Kava, chamomile, valerian: increased sedative effect

Drug/lab test
Increased: AST, alkaline phosphatase
Decreased: platelets, WBC

NURSING CONSIDERATIONS
Assessment
• Assess for **blood dyscrasias:** fever, sore throat, bruising, rash, jaundice, epistaxis (long-term treatment only)
• Assess **seizures:** duration, type, intensity, with or without aura

---

⚠ Nurse Alert   ★ Key NCLEX® Drug   ≫ Drug Specifics

⚠ Assess mental status: mood, sensorium, affect, memory (long, short), especially geriatric; behavioral changes, suicidal thoughts/behaviors
• Assess seizure activity including type, location, duration, and character; provide seizure precaution
• Assess renal studies: urinalysis, BUN, urine creatinine
• Monitor blood studies: RBCs, Hct, Hgb, reticulocyte counts weekly for 4 wk, then monthly
• Monitor hepatic studies: ALT, AST, bilirubin, creatinine
⚠ Abrupt discontinuation: do not discontinue abruptly, seizures may increase
• Assess for signs of physical withdrawal if medication suddenly discontinued
• Assess eye problems: need for ophthalmic examinations before, during, after treatment (slit lamp, fundoscopy, tonometry)
• Assess allergic reaction: red raised rash; if this occurs, product should be discontinued
• Monitor for toxicity: bone marrow depression, nausea, vomiting, ataxia, diplopia, cardiovascular collapse; monitor drug levels during initial treatment (therapeutic 20-80 ng/ml)

Patient/family education
• Teach patient to carry/wear emergency ID card stating patient's name, products taken, condition, physician's name, phone number, discuss tolerance, withdrawal
• Caution patient to avoid driving, other activities that require alertness
• Caution patient to avoid alcohol ingestion or CNS depressants; increased sedation may occur
⚠ Teach patient not to discontinue medication quickly after long-term use; taper off over several weeks
⚠ Teach patient to notify prescriber of yellowing skin/eyes, pale stools, bleeding, fever, extreme fatigue, sore throat, suicidal thoughts/behaviors
⚠ Teach patient to notify prescriber immediately if suicidal thoughts, behaviors occur

Evaluation
Positive therapeutic outcome
• Decreased seizure activity

TREATMENT OF OVERDOSE:
Lavage, activated charcoal, VS, flumazenil, monitor electrolytes

cloNIDine (Rx)
(klon'i-deen)
Catapres, Catapres-TTS, Diyaril ✦, Duraclon, Kapvay
Func. class.: Antihypertensive, centrally acting analgesic
Chem. class.: Centrally acting α-adrenergic agonist
Pregnancy category C

Do not confuse: cloNIDine/KlonoPIN/clonazePAM, Catapres/Cataflam/catarase

ACTION: Inhibits sympathetic vasomotor center in CNS, which reduces impulses in sympathetic nervous system; B/P, pulse rate, cardiac output decreased; prevents pain signal transmission in CNS by α-adrenergic receptor stimulation of the spinal cord

Therapeutic outcome: Decreased B/P in hypertension

USES: Mild to moderate hypertension, used alone or in combination; severe pain in cancer patients (epidural), attention-deficit/hyperactivity disorder (ADHD)

Unlabeled uses: Opioid withdrawal, prevention of vascular headaches, treatment of menopausal symptoms, dysmenorrhea, attention-deficit/hyperactivity disorder (ADHD), autism, cycloSPORINE nephrotoxicity prophylaxis, diabetic neuropathy, ethanol/nicotine/opiate agonist withdrawal, Tourette's syndrome, hypertensive emergency, neonatal abstinence syndrome, scleroderma renal crisis

CONTRAINDICATIONS
Hypersensitivity; (epidural) bleeding disorders, anticoagulants

Precautions: Pregnancy **C**, breastfeeding, child <12 yr (transdermal), geriatric, MI (recent), diabetes mellitus, chronic renal failure, Raynaud's disease, thyroid disease, depression, COPD, asthma, noncompliant patients

> **BLACK BOX WARNING:** Labor (transdermal)

DOSAGE AND ROUTES
Hypertension
Adult: PO 0.1 mg bid, then increase by 0.1-0.2 mg/day at weekly intervals, until desired response; range 0.2-0.6 mg/day in divided doses or transdermal **q7 days,** start 0.1 mg and adjust q1-2wk
Geriatric: PO 0.1 mg at bedtime, may increase gradually

Adverse effects: *italics* = common; **bold** = life-threatening

Child: PO 5-10 mcg/kg/day in divided doses q8-12hr, max 0.9 mg/day

Opioid withdrawal (unlabeled)
Adult: PO 0.3-1.2 mg/day; may decrease by 50% × 3 days, then decrease by 0.1-0.2 mg/day or discontinue

Severe pain
Adult: CONT EPIDURAL INF 30 mcg/hr
Child: CONT EPIDURAL INF 0.5 mcg/kg/hr, then titrate to response

Menopausal symptoms (unlabeled)
Adult: TD 0.1 mg patch q1wk; PO 0.05-0.4 mg daily

ADHD/TIC disorders in children/ autism (unlabeled)
Adolescent/child ≥6 yr: PO 0.05 mg/kg/day in 3-4 divided doses; may increase by 0.1 mg/day qwk up to 0.4 mg/day; EXT REL (Kapvay): 0.1 mg at bedtime, increase dose by 0.1 mg/day up to 0.4 mg/day

Tourette's syndrome (unlabeled)
Adult: PO 0.15-0.2 mg/day

Available forms: Tabs 0.025 ♣, 0.1, 0.2, 0.3 mg; transdermal sys 2.5, 5, 7.5 mg delivering 0.1, 0.2, 0.3 mg/24 hr, respectively; inj 100, 500 mcg/ml, ext rel tab 0.1 mg (Kapvay), 0.17 mg (Nexiclon)

Implementation
PO route
• Give last dose at bedtime
• Do not crush, cut, chew, or break ER tabs; Kapvay is not interchangeable with other products

Transdermal route
• Apply patch weekly; remove old patch and wash off residue; apply to site without hair; best absorption over chest or upper arm; rotate sites with each application; clean site before application; apply firmly, especially around edges, may secure with adhesive tape if loose; fold sticky sides together and discard
• Should be removed before MRI
• Store patches in cool environment, tabs in tight container

> **BLACK BOX WARNING:** Do not use for labor

ADVERSE EFFECTS
CNS: *Drowsiness, sedation, headache, fatigue,* nightmares, insomnia, mental changes, anxiety, depression, hallucinations, delirium, syncope, dizziness
CV: *Orthostatic hypotension, palpitations,* **CHF,** ECG abnormalities, sinus tachycardia

EENT: Taste change, parotid pain
ENDO: Hyperglycemia
GI: *Nausea, vomiting, malaise,* constipation, *dry mouth*
GU: Impotence, dysuria, *nocturia,* gynecomastia
INTEG: *Rash,* alopecia, facial pallor, pruritus, hives, edema, burning papules, excoriation (TD patches)
MISC: *Withdrawal symptoms*
MS: Muscle, joint pain, leg cramps

Pharmacokinetics

Absorption	Well absorbed (PO, TD)
Distribution	Widely distributed; crosses blood-brain barrier
Metabolism	Liver, extensively
Excretion	Kidneys, unchanged (45%)
Half-life	12-21 hr

Pharmacodynamics

	PO	TD
Onset	½-1 hr	3 days
Peak	2-4 hr	Unknown
Duration	8-12 hr	8 hr (after removal)

INTERACTIONS
Individual drugs
Alcohol: increased CNS depression
Levodopa: decreased levodopa effect
Prazosin: decreased hypotensive effects
Verapamil, diltiazem: AV block

Drug classifications
Amphetamines, appetite suppressants, MAOIs, tricyclics: decreased hypotensive effects
Anesthetics, opiates, sedatives/hypnotics: increased CNS depression
Antidepressants (tricyclic), β-adrenergic blockers: life-threatening increase in B/P
Diuretics, nitrates: increased hypotensive effects

Drug/herb
Aconite: increased toxicity, death
Ephedra, ginseng: decreased antihypertensive effect
Hawthorn: increased antihypertensive effect

Drug/lab test
Increased: blood glucose
Decreased: VMA, urinary catecholamines, aldosterone

NURSING CONSIDERATIONS
Assessment
• Assess **cancer pain:** location, intensity, character, alleviating, aggravation factors, baseline and frequency

---

- Perform blood studies: neutrophils, decreased platelets
- **Perform renal studies: protein, BUN, creatinine; watch for increased levels that may indicate nephrotic syndrome: polyuria, oliguria, frequency**
- Monitor baselines for renal/liver function tests before therapy begins; check potassium levels, although hyperkalemia rarely occurs
- Monitor B/P, pulse if the product is being used for **hypertension;** notify prescriber of changes
- Assess for **opiate withdrawal** (unlabeled) in patients receiving the product for opioid withdrawal, including fever, diarrhea, nausea, vomiting, cramps, insomnia, shivering, dilated pupils, weakness
- Check for edema in feet, legs daily; monitor I&O; check for decreasing output
- Assess **allergic reaction:** rash, fever, pruritus, urticaria; product should be discontinued if antihistamines fail to help
- ADHD: monitor B/P, pulse, palpitations, syncope
- Assess for symptoms of **CHF:** edema; dyspnea, wet crackles, B/P, weight gain, report significant changes, more common in the elderly

Patient/family education
⚠ **Instruct patient not to discontinue product abruptly, or withdrawal symptoms may occur: anxiety, increased B/P, headache, insomnia, increased pulse, tremors, nausea, sweating**
- Caution patient not to use OTC (cough, cold, or allergy), alcohol or CNS depressant products unless directed by prescriber
- Teach patient to comply with dosage schedule even if feeling better; product controls symptoms, does not cure
- Caution patient to change position slowly, to rise slowly to sitting or standing position to minimize orthostatic hypotension, especially geriatric
- **Instruct patient to notify physician of mouth sores, sore throat, fever, swelling of hands or feet, irregular heartbeat, chest pain, signs of angioedema, increased weight**
- Teach patient about excessive perspiration, dehydration, vomiting; diarrhea may lead to fall in B/P; consult prescriber if these occur
- Tell patient that product may cause dizziness, fainting; light-headedness may occur during first few days of therapy; use hard candy, saliva product, or frequent rinsing of mouth for dry mouth
- **Transdermal:** teach patient how to use patch; that patch comes in two parts: product

patch and overlay to keep patch in place; not to trim or cut patch; remove for MRI; can use during bathing, swimming
- Advise patient that compliance is necessary; not to skip or stop product unless directed by prescriber
- Teach patient that product may cause skin rash or impaired perspiration
- Teach patient that response may take 2-3 days if product is given TD; instruct on administration of patch; return demonstration
- Teach patient to avoid hazardous activities, since product may cause drowsiness, dizziness
- Teach patient to administer 1 hr before meals

Evaluation
Positive therapeutic outcome
- Decrease in B/P in hypertension
- Decrease in withdrawal symptoms
- Decrease in pain
- Decrease in vascular headaches
- Decrease in dysmenorrhea
- Decrease in menopausal symptoms

TREATMENT OF OVERDOSE:
Supportive treatment; administer tolazoline, atropine, DOPamine prn

clopidogrel (Rx)
(klo-pid'oh-grel)
Plavix
Func. class.: Platelet aggregation inhibitor
Chem. class.: Thienopyridine derivative
Pregnancy category B

Do not confuse: Plavix/Paxil/Elavil

ACTION: Inhibits first and second phases of ADP-induced effects in platelet aggregation

Therapeutic outcome: Decreased possibility of stroke, MI by decreasing platelet aggregation

USES: Reducing the risk of stroke, MI, vascular death, peripheral arterial disease in high-risk patients, acute coronary syndrome, transient ischemic attack (TIA), unstable angina

CONTRAINDICATIONS
Hypersensitivity, active bleeding

Precautions: Pregnancy **B,** breastfeeding, children, past liver disease, increased bleeding risk, neutropenia, agranulocytosis, renal disease, Asian/Black/Caucasian patients

> **BLACK BOX WARNING:** CYP2C19 allele (poor metabolizers)

Adverse effects: *italics* = common; **bold** = life-threatening

DOSAGE AND ROUTES
Recent MI, stroke, peripheral arterial disease, TIA
Adult: PO 75 mg daily with aspirin

Acute coronary syndrome
Adult: PO loading dose 300 mg then 75 mg daily with aspirin

Available forms: Tabs 75, 300 mg

Implementation
• Give with food to decrease gastric symptoms
• Product should be discontinued 5 days before elective surgery if an antiplatelet action is not desired

ADVERSE EFFECTS
CNS: Headache, dizziness, depression, syncope, hyperesthesia, neuralgia, confusion, hallucinations
CV: Edema, hypertension, chest pain
GI: Nausea, vomiting, diarrhea, GI discomfort, GI bleeding, pancreatitis, hepatic failure
GU: Glomerulonephritis
HEMA: *Epistaxis,* purpura, bleeding (major/minor from any site), neutropenia, aplastic anemia, agranulocytosis, thrombotic thrombocytopenic purpura
INTEG: Rash, pruritus
MISC: UTI, hypercholesterolemia, chest pain, fatigue, intracranial hemorrhage, toxic epidermal necrolysis, Stevens-Johnson syndrome, flu-like syndrome, anaphylaxis
MS: Arthralgia, back pain
RESP: Upper respiratory tract infection, dyspnea, rhinitis, bronchitis, cough, bronchospasm

Pharmacokinetics

Absorption	Rapidly absorbed
Distribution	Unknown
Metabolism	Liver, extensively, protein binding 95%, CYP2B6, CYP1A2, CYP2C8
Excretion	Kidneys, unchanged product
Half-life	6 hr

Pharmacodynamics

Onset	Unknown
Duration	Unknown

INTERACTIONS
Individual drugs
Abciximab, aspirin, eptifibatide, rifampin, ticlopidine, tirofiban, treprostinil: increased bleeding tendencies

Fluvastatin, phenytoin, tamoxifen, TOLBUTamide, torsemide, warfarin: increased action of each specific product

Drug classifications
Anticoagulants, NSAIDs, SSRIs, thrombolytics: increased bleeding tendencies
CYP3A4 inhibitors/substrates (atorvastatin, cerivistatin, esomeprazole, omeprazole, simvastatin): decreased effects

> **BLACK BOX WARNING:** CYP2C19 inhibitors: avoid use

NSAIDs: increased action of some NSAIDs
Proton pump inhibitors (PPIs): decreased clopidogrel effect

Drug/herb
Bilberry, saw palmetto: decreased clopidogrel effect
Feverfew, fish oil, garlic, ginger, ginkgo biloba, green tea, horse chestnut, omega-3 fatty acids: increased clopidogrel effect

Drug/lab test
Increased: AST, ALT, bilirubin, uric acid, total cholesterol, nonprotein nitrogen (NPN)

NURSING CONSIDERATIONS
Assessment

> **BLACK BOX WARNING:** CYP2C19 allele (poor metabolizers): Consider using another antiplatelet product, higher CV reaction occurs after acute coronary syndrome or PCI, tests are available to determine CYP2C19 allele

• Assess for symptoms of stroke, MI during treatment
• Assess for thrombotic/thrombocytic purpura; fever, thrombocytopenia, neurolytic anemia
• Monitor liver function tests: AST, ALT, bilirubin, creatinine if patient is on long-term therapy (4 mo or more)
• Monitor blood studies: CBC, Hct, Hgb, protime, cholesterol if patient is on long-term therapy; thrombocytopenia, neutropenia may occur

Patient/family education
• Advise patient that blood work will be necessary during treatment
• Advise patient to report any unusual bleeding to prescriber, that it may take longer to stop bleeding
• Teach patient to take without regard to food
• Caution patient to report diarrhea, skin rashes, subcutaneous bleeding, chills, fever, sore throat

---

- Teach patient to tell all health care providers that clopidogrel is being used; may be held for 5 days before surgery

Evaluation
Positive therapeutic outcome
- Absence of stroke

clotrimazole topical
See Appendix B

clotrimazole vaginal antifungal
See Appendix B

cloZAPine (Rx)
(kloz′a-peen)
Clozaril, Fazaclo, Versacloz
Func. class.: Antipsychotic
Chem. class.: Tricyclic dibenzodiazepine derivative
Pregnancy category B

Do not confuse: Clozaril/Colazal/cloZAPine/clonidine/clofazimine/clonazepam/Klonopin

ACTION: Interferes with dopamine receptor binding with lack of EPS and tardive dyskinesia; also acts as an adrenergic, cholinergic, histaminergic, serotoninergic antagonist

Therapeutic outcome: Decreased psychotic behavior

USES: Management of psychotic symptoms in schizophrenic patients for whom other antipsychotics have failed, recurrent suicidal behavior; orally disintegrating tabs are not used for recurrent suicidal behavior

Unlabeled uses: Agitation, bipolar disorder, dementia, psychosis in Parkinson's disease

CONTRAINDICATIONS
Hypersensitivity, severe granulocytopenia (WBC $<3500/mm^3$ before therapy), coma

> **BLACK BOX WARNING:** Myeloproliferative disorders, severe CNS depression, agranulocytosis, leukopenia, neutropenia, seizure disorders

Precautions: Pregnancy **B**, breastfeeding, children <16 yr, geriatric, renal/hepatic/cardiac/CV/pulmonary disease, seizures, prostatic enlargement, closed-angle glaucoma, stroke

> **BLACK BOX WARNING:** Bone marrow suppression, hypotension, myocarditis, orthostatic hypotension, elderly patients with dementia-related psychosis

DOSAGE AND ROUTES
Schizophrenia
Adult: PO 12.5 mg daily or bid; may increase by 25-50 mg/day; normal range 300-450 mg/day 1-2 ×/wk; do not increase dosage more than 2 times/wk; dose > 500 mg requires 3 divided doses; max 900 mg/day; use lowest dosage to control symptoms; if dose is to be discontinued, taper over 1-2 wk
Adolescent, child ≥9 yr (unlabeled): PO 6.25-12.5 mg initially slowly titrate

Dementia with multiple behavioral disturbances (unlabeled)
Geriatric: PO 12.5 mg qd at bedtime, may increase by 12.5 mg every other day; max 50 mg/day

Available forms: Tabs 12.5, 25, 50, 100, 200 mg; orally disintegrating tabs 12.5, 25, 100 150, 200 mg; oral suspension 50 mg/ml

Implementation
- Decrease dosage in geriatric since metabolism is slowed
- Give with full glass of water, milk; or give with food to decrease GI upset
- Store in tight, light-resistant container; oral sol in amber bottle
- **Patient-specific registration is required before administration; if WBC <3500 cells/mm³ or ANC <2000 cells/mm², therapy should not be started, pharmacist may only dispense the 7, 14, 28 day supply upon receipt of lab report that is appropriate**
- **Orally disintegrating tab:** do not push through foil, leave in foil blister until ready to take, peel back foil, place tab in mouth, allow to dissolve, swallow; water is not needed
- **Oral suspension:** Shake before using, use oral syringe and syringe adapter

ADVERSE EFFECTS
CNS: *Sedation, salivation, dizziness, headache, tremors, sleep problems, akinesia, fever,* seizures, *sweating, akathisia, confusion, fatigue, insomnia, depression, slurred speech,* anxiety, **neuroleptic malignant syndrome,** *agitation, dystonia, obsessive-compulsive symptoms*
CV: *Tachycardia, hypo/hypertension,* chest pain, ECG changes, orthostatic hypotension
EENT: Blurred vision

GI: *Drooling or excessive salivation, constipation, nausea, abdominal discomfort, vomiting, diarrhea,* anorexia, weight gain, dry mouth, heartburn, dyspepsia, gastroesophageal reflux
GU: *Urinary abnormalities,* incontinence, ejaculation dysfunction, frequency, urgency, retention, dysuria
HEMA: Leukopenia, neutropenia, agranulocytosis, eosinophilia
MS: Weakness; pain in back, neck, legs; spasm; rigidity
RESP: Dyspnea, nasal congestion, lower respiratory tract infection
OTHER: Diaphoresis
SYST: Death in geriatric patients with dementia, aggravation of diabetes mellitus

Pharmacokinetics

Absorption	Well absorbed
Distribution	Widely distributed; crosses blood-brain barrier, placenta; 95% protein binding
Metabolism	Liver, CYP1A2, 2D6, 3A4
Excretion	Kidneys (50%), feces (30%) (metabolites)
Half-life	8-12 hr

Pharmacodynamics

Onset	Unknown
Peak	Unknown
Duration	8-12 hr

INTERACTIONS
Individual drugs
Alcohol: increased CNS depression
Caffeine, citalopram, erythromycin, FLUoxetine, fluvoxaMINE, ketoconazole, risperiDONE, ritonavir, sertraline: increased cloZAPine levels
CarBAMazepine, omeprazole, PHENobarbital, rifampin: decreased cloZAPine level
Digoxin: increased plasma concentration of digoxin
Warfarin: increased plasma concentrations

Drug classifications
Benzodiazepines: increased hypotension, respiratory, cardiac arrest, collapse
β-blockers, class IA/III antidysrhythmics, and other drugs that increase QT: increased QT prolongation
CNS depressants, psychoactives: increased CNS depression
CYPIA2 inducers: decreased cloZAPine levels
CYP1A2 inhibitors, CYP3A4 inhibitors: increased cloZAPine level

Highly protein-bound products: increased plasma concentrations
Drug/food
Caffeine: increased cloZAPine levels
Drug/lab test
Increased: liver function tests, cardiac enzymes, cholesterol, blood glucose, bilirubin, PBI, cholinesterase, ^{131}I, Hct/Hgb, erythrocyte sedimentation rate
Decreased: WBC
False positive: pregnancy tests, PKU
False negative: urinary steroids, 17-OHCS

NURSING CONSIDERATIONS
Assessment
• Assess for **myocarditis** if suspected, discontinue; myocarditis usually occurs during first month of treatment
• AIMS assessment, blood glucose, CBC differential, glycosylated hemoglobin A1C, LFTs, neurologic function, pregnancy test, serum creatinine, electrolytes, lipid profile, prolactin, thyroid function tests, weight

> **BLACK BOX WARNING:** Assess for **seizures;** usually occurs with higher doses (>600 mg/day) or dosage change >100 mg/day; do not use in uncontrolled seizure disorder; use cautiously in those with a predisposition to seizures

• Assess mental status: orientation, mood, behavior, presence of hallucinations, and type before initial administration and monthly; this product should significantly reduce psychotic behavior
• Check for swallowing of PO medication; check for hoarding or giving of medication to other patients

> **BLACK BOX WARNING: Bone marrow depression:** Monitor bilirubin, CBC, liver function test monthly; discontinue treatment if WBC <3000-3500/mm³ or if ANC <1500/mm³; test qwk; may resume when normal; if WBC <2000/mm³ or ANC <1000/mm³, discontinue; **if agranulocytosis develops, never restart product**

• Assess affect, orientation, LOC, reflexes, gait, coordination, sleep pattern disturbances

> **BLACK BOX WARNING: Hypotension:** Monitor B/P with patient sitting, standing, and lying; take pulse and respirations q4hr during initial treatment; establish baseline before starting treatment; report drops of 30 mm Hg

---

• Check for dizziness, faintness, palpitations, tachycardia on rising
• **Assess for neuroleptic malignant syndrome: hyperpyrexia, muscle rigidity, increased CPK, altered mental status; product should be discontinued**
• Assess for **EPS** including akathisia (inability to sit still, no pattern to movements), tardive dyskinesia (bizarre movements of the jaw, mouth, tongue, extremities), pseudoparkinsonism (rigidity, tremors, pill rolling, shuffling gate)
• Assess for constipation, urinary retention daily; if these occur, increase bulk, water in diet

Patient/family education
• Teach patient to use good oral hygiene; frequent rinsing of mouth, sugarless gum for dry mouth
• Caution patient to avoid hazardous activities until product response is determined
• Inform patient that orthostatic hypotension occurs often and to rise from sitting or lying position gradually
• Caution patient to avoid hot tubs, hot showers, tub baths, since hypotension may occur
• Teach patient to avoid OTC preparations (cough, hay fever, cold) unless approved by prescriber, since serious product interactions may occur; avoid use with alcohol, CNS depressants; increased drowsiness may occur
• Teach patient about EPS and necessity of meticulous oral hygiene, since oral candidiasis may occur
• Teach patient to report sore throat, malaise, fever, bleeding, mouth sores; if these occur, CBC should be performed and product discontinued
• Advise patient that in hot weather, heat stroke may occur; take extra precautions to stay cool

> **BLACK BOX WARNING:** Teach patient symptoms of agranulocytosis and need for blood test qwk for 6 mo, then q2wk; report flulike symptoms

Evaluation
Positive therapeutic outcome
• Decrease in emotional excitement, hallucinations, delusions, paranoia
• Reorganization of patterns of thought, speech

TREATMENT OF ANAPHYLAXIS: Withdraw product, maintain airway; if diabetic, check blood glucose levels

codeine (Rx)
(koe′deen)
Func. class.: Opiate, phenanthrene derivative
Pregnancy category C
Controlled substance schedule II, III, IV, V (depends on content)

Do not confuse: codeine/Lodine/Iodine/Cardene

ACTION: Depresses pain impulse transmission at the spinal cord level by interacting with opioid receptors; decreases cough reflex, GI motility

Therapeutic outcome: Pain relief, decreased cough, decreased diarrhea depending on route

USES: Mild to moderate to severe pain

Unlabeled uses: Diarrhea, nonproductive cough

CONTRAINDICATIONS
Hypersensitivity to opiates, respiratory depression, increased intracranial pressure, seizure disorders, severe respiratory disorders, breastfeeding

> **BLACK BOX WARNING:** Children (tonsillectomy/adenoidectomy)

Precautions: Pregnancy **C**, geriatric, cardiac dysrhythmias,prostatic hypertrophy, bowel impaction

DOSAGE AND ROUTES
Pain
Adult: PO IM/IV/SUBCUT 15-60 mg q4hr prn; use phosphate product for IM/IV
Child: PO 6-17 yr 3 mg/kg/day in divided doses q4hr prn
Renal dose
Adult: PO CCr 10-50 ml/min 75% of dose; CCr <10 ml/min 50% of dose

Cough (unlabeled)
Adult: PO 10-20 mg q4-6hr, max 120 mg/day

Diarrhea (unlabeled)
Adult: PO 30 mg; may repeat qid prn

Available forms: Tabs 15, 30 mg; oral sol 30, 60 mg/5 ml; inj 15, 30 mg/ml; syrup 5 mg/ml ✤

Implementation
• Give with antiemetic if nausea, vomiting occur
• Administer when pain is beginning to return, determine dosage interval by patient response; continuous dosing of medication is more effective given prn; explain analgesic effect
• Medication should be slowly withdrawn after long-term use to prevent withdrawal symptoms, use stool softener, laxative for constipation
• Store in light-resistant container at room temp

PO route
• May be given with food or milk to lessen GI upset

IM/SUBCUT route
• Do not give if cloudy, or a precipitate has formed

ADVERSE EFFECTS
CNS: *Drowsiness, sedation,* dizziness, agitation, dependency, lethargy, restlessness, euphoria, seizures, hallucinations, headache, confusion
CV: Bradycardia, palpitations, orthostatic hypotension, tachycardia, circulatory collapse
GI: *Nausea, vomiting, anorexia, constipation,* dry mouth
GU: Urinary retention
INTEG: Flushing, rash, urticaria, pruritus
RESP: Respiratory depression, respiratory paralysis, dyspnea
SYST: Anaphylaxis

Pharmacokinetics

Absorption	Bioavailability 60%-90%
Distribution	Widely distributed; crosses placenta, protein binding 7%
Metabolism	Liver, extensively by CYP3A4 to morphine; altered in ethnic groups
Excretion	Kidneys (up to 15%), breast milk
Half-life	3-4 hr

Pharmacodynamics

	PO	IM	SUBCUT
Onset	30-60 min	30-60 min	15-30 min
Peak	1-2 hr	30-60 min	Unknown
Duration	4 hr	4 hr	4 hr

INTERACTIONS
Individual drugs
Alcohol: increased CNS depression

Drug classifications
Antipsychotics, CYP2D6, sedative, hypnotics, opiates, skeletal muscle relaxants: increased CNS depression
MAOIs: increased toxicity; use cautiously

Drug/lab test
Increased: amylase, lipase

NURSING CONSIDERATIONS
Assessment
• Assess **pain:** intensity, type, alleviating factors, type, location, need for pain medication, tolerance, use pain scoring
• Assess GI function: nausea, vomiting, constipation
• Assess **cough:** type, duration, ability to raise secretion for productive cough; do not use to suppress a productive cough
• Monitor VS after parenteral route; note muscle rigidity, product history, renal/hepatic function tests, respiratory dysfunction: respiratory depression, character, rate, rhythm; notify prescriber if respirations are <10/min
• Monitor CNS changes: dizziness, drowsiness, hallucinations, euphoria, LOC, pupil reaction

> **BLACK BOX WARNING:** Child (tonsillectomy/ adenoidectomy): deaths have occurred, use is contraindicated

• Monitor allergic reactions: rash, urticaria
• Respiratory dysfunction: respiratory depression, character, rate, rhythm; notify prescriber if respirations are <10/min, shallow

Patient/family education
• Teach patient to report any symptoms of CNS changes, allergic reactions; to avoid CNS depressants: alcohol, sedative/hypnotics for at least 24 hr after taking this product
• Discuss with patient that dizziness, drowsiness, and confusion are common
• Advise patient to avoid getting up without assistance
• Discuss in detail with patient all aspects of the product
• Advise patient not to breastfeed
• Teach patient that physical dependency may result after extended periods
• Advise patient to use sugarless gum, rinse mouth after, for dry mouth

Evaluation
Positive therapeutic outcome
• Decreased pain
• Decreased cough
• Decreased diarrhea

TREATMENT OF OVERDOSE:
Naloxone 0.4 ample diluted in 10 ml 0.9% NaCl and given by direct **IV** push 0.02 mg q2min (adult)

colchicine (Rx)

(kol'chih-seen)

Colcrys

Func. class.: Antigout agent

Chem. class.: *Colchicum autumnale* alkaloid

Pregnancy category C

ACTION: Inhibits microtubule formation of lactic acid in leukocytes, which decreases phagocytosis and inflammation in joints

Therapeutic outcome: Decreased pain, inflammation of joints

USES: Gout, gouty arthritis (prevention, treatment); to arrest progression of neurologic disability in multiple sclerosis

Unlabeled uses: Hepatic cirrhosis, familial Mediterranean fever, pericarditis, amyloidosis, Behçet's syndrome, biliary cirrhosis, dermatitis herpetiformis, idiopathic thrombocytopenic purpura, Paget's disease, pseudogout, pulmonary fibrosis

CONTRAINDICATIONS

Hypersensitivity; serious GI disorders, severe renal/hepatic/cardiac disorders

Precautions: Pregnancy **C**, breastfeeding, children, geriatric, blood dyscrasias, hepatic disease

DOSAGE AND ROUTES
Gout prevention
Adult: PO 0.6-1.8 mg in 1-2 divided doses daily depending on severity

Gout treatment
Adult: PO 1.2 mg initially, then 0.6 mg 1 hr later (1.8 mg); those on strong CYP3A4 inhibitor (past 14 days) 0.6 mg initially, then 0.3 mg 1 hr later

Renal dose
Adult: PO CCr <30 ml/min for acute gout, do not repeat course for 2 wk; familial Mediterranean fever 0.3 mg daily, increase cautiously

Pericarditis (unlabeled)
Adult: PO 0.5 mg bid

Mediterranean fever (unlabeled)
Adult: PO (on no interacting products): 1.2-2.4 mg/day in 1-2 divided doses; strong CYP3A4 inhibitor/increase cautiously; P-glycoprotein inhibitors within 14 days: max 0.6 mg/day in 1-2 divided doses; moderate CYP3A4 inhibitors with 14 day max 1.2 mg/day in 1-2 divided doses

Adolescent: PO 1.2-2.4 mg/day in 1-2 divided doses, titrate by 0.3 mg/day

Child 6-12 yr: PO 0.9-1.8 mg/day in 1-2 divided doses

Child 4-6 yr: PO 0.3-1.8 mg/day in 1-2 divided doses

Available forms: Tabs 0.6 mg; caps 0.6 mg

Implementation
PO route
• Give without regard to food
• Cumulative doses ≤4 mg, renal patients ≤2 mg, when reached, administer only for 3 wks

ADVERSE EFFECTS

GI: *Nausea, vomiting, anorexia, malaise,* metallic taste, cramps, peptic ulcer, diarrhea

GU: Hematuria, *oliguria, renal damage*

HEMA: **Agranulocytosis, thrombocytopenia, aplastic anemia, pancytopenia**

INTEG: Chills, dermatitis, pruritus, purpura, erythema

MISC: Myopathy, alopecia, reversible azoospermia, peripheral neuritis

Pharmacokinetics

Absorption	Well absorbed
Distribution	WBCs
Metabolism	Deacetylates in liver
Excretion	Feces (metabolites/active product)
Half-life	4.4 hr

Pharmacodynamics

	PO
Onset	Unknown
Peak	½-2 hr
Duration	Unknown

INTERACTIONS
Individual drugs
CycloSPORINE, radiation: increased bone marrow depression

Ethanol: increased GI effects

Vitamin B_{12}: decreased action of vit B_{12}; may cause reversible malabsorption

Drug classifications
Bone marrow depressants: increased bone marrow depression

Moderate/strong CYP3A4 inhibitors, reduce dose: increased colchicine level/toxicity

NSAIDs: increased GI effects

Drug/food
Grapefruit juice: increased colchicine level

Drug/lab test
Increased: alkaline phosphatase, AST
Decreased: platelets, WBC, granulocytes
False positive: urine Hgb
Interference: urinary 17-hydroxycorticosteroids

NURSING CONSIDERATIONS
Assessment
• Assess pain and mobility of joints, uric acid levels returning to normal
• Monitor I&O ratio; observe for decrease in urinary output; CBC, platelets, reticulocytes before, during therapy (q3mo); may cause aplastic anemia, agranulocytosis, decreased platelets
• **Assess for toxicity: weakness, abdominal pain, nausea, vomiting, diarrhea, product should be discontinued, report symptoms immediately**

Patient/family education
• Caution patient to avoid alcohol, OTC preparations that contain alcohol
• Instruct patient to report any pain, redness, or hard area, usually in legs; rash, sore throat, fever, bleeding, bruising, weakness, numbness, tingling, nausea, vomiting, abdominal pain
• Teach patient importance of complying with medical regimen (diet, weight loss, product therapy); bone marrow depression may occur
• Advise patient to tell all providers of product use, surgery may increase possibility of acute gout symptoms

Evaluation
Positive therapeutic outcome
• Decreased stone formation on x-ray
• Decreased pain in kidney region
• Absence of hematuria
• Decreased pain in joints

TREATMENT OF OVERDOSE:
Discontinue medication, may need opioids to treat diarrhea

---

colesevelam (Rx)
(coal-see-vel′am)
Welchol
Func. class.: Antilipemic
Chem. class.: Bile acid sequestrant
Pregnancy category B

ACTION: Adsorbs, combines with bile acids to form insoluble complex that is excreted through feces; loss of bile acids lowers cholesterol levels

Therapeutic outcome: Decreasing LDL cholesterol

USES: Elevated LDL cholesterol, alone or in combination with HMG-CoA reductase inhibitor; type 2 diabetes (adjunct)

CONTRAINDICATIONS
Hypersensitivity, bowel disease, primary biliary cirrhosis, triglycerides >300 mg/dl, bowel obstruction, pancreatitis, biliary obstruction; dysphagia, fat-soluble vitamin deficiency

Precautions: Pregnancy **B,** breastfeeding, children

DOSAGE AND ROUTES
Monotherapy
Adult: PO 3 625 mg tabs bid with meals or 6 tabs daily with a meal; may increase to 7 tabs if needed

Combination therapy
Adult: PO 3 tabs bid with meals or 6 tabs daily with a meal given with an HMG-CoA reductase inhibitor

Type 2 diabetes, adjunct (to improve glycemic control)
Adult and geriatric: PO approx 3.8 g (6 tabs)/day or approx 1.9 g (3 tabs) bid

Heterozygous familial hypercholesterolemia
Females (postmenarchal and >10 yr) and males ≥10 yr: PO 1.875 g packet bid or 3.75 g packet q day dissolved in 4-8 oz of water with a meal

Available forms: Tabs 625 mg, powder for oral susp 3.75 g/packet

Implementation
• Give product daily, bid with meals; give all other medications 4 hr before colesevelam to avoid poor absorption; take with liquid
• Give supplemental doses of vit A, D, K if levels are low

Powder for oral susp
• Empty contents of packet into a cup/glass; add ½-1 cup (4-8 oz) of water, fruit juice, or diet soda; stir well before drinking

ADVERSE EFFECTS
GI: *Constipation, abdominal pain, nausea,* fecal impaction, hemorrhoids, flatulence, vomiting, GI obstruction
MISC: Hypertriglycerides, hypoglycemia
MS: Muscle, joint pain

⚠ Nurse Alert   ✸ Key NCLEX® Drug   ≫ Drug Specifics

C

Pharmacokinetics

Absorption	Unknown
Distribution	Unknown
Metabolism	Unknown
Excretion	Feces
Half-life	Unknown

Pharmacodynamics

LDL decreased in 4-7 days

INTERACTIONS
Individual drugs

Digoxin, diltiazem, gemfibrozil, glyBURide, fluoroquinolones, iron, mycophenolate, penicillin G, phenytoin, propanolol, warfarin: decreased absorption of each specific product

Thyroid hormones: decreased absorption of thyroid

Drug classifications

Corticosteroids: decreased corticosteroid action

Oral contraceptives: decreased action of oral contraceptives

Tetracyclines: decreased absorption of tetracyclines

Thiazides: decreased absorption of thiazides

Vitamins (fat-soluble): decreased absorption of fat-soluble vitamins

Drug/lab test

Increased: liver function tests

NURSING CONSIDERATIONS
Assessment

• Assess cardiac glycoside level if both products are being administered
• Assess for signs of vit A, D, K deficiency
• Monitor fasting LDL, HDL, total cholesterol, triglyceride levels, electrolytes if on extended therapy
• Monitor bowel pattern daily; increase bulk, H_2O in diet for constipation

Patient/family education

• Teach the importance of compliance; toxicity may result if doses missed, timing of dose 4 hr after other meds
• Teach that risk factors should be decreased: high-fat diet, smoking, alcohol consumption, absence of exercise

Evaluation
Positive therapeutic outcome

• Decreased cholesterol level (hyperlipidemia); diarrhea, pruritus (excess bile acids), collagenase *Clostridium histolyticum*

conivaptan (Rx)

(kon-ih-vap'tan)
Vaprisol
Func. class.: Vasopressin receptor antagonist
Pregnancy category C

ACTION: Dual arginine vasopressin (AVP) antagonist with affinity for V_{1A}, V_2 receptors; level of AVP in circulating blood is critical for regulation of water, electrolyte balance and is usually elevated in euvolemic/hypervolemic hyponatremia

Therapeutic outcome: Correct serum sodium levels

USES: Euvolemia hyponatremia in those hospitalized, not indicated for CHF, hypervolemia, hyponatremia

CONTRAINDICATIONS

Hypersensitivity, hypovolemia

Precautions: Pregnancy **C,** breastfeeding, orthostatic/renal disease, heart failure, rapid correction of serum sodium

DOSAGE AND ROUTES

Adult: **IV** INF loading dose 20 mg given over 30 min, then CONT **IV** over 24 hr; after 1 day, give for an additional 1-3 days as a CONT INF of 20 mg/day total, can be titrated up to 40 mg/day if serum sodium is not rising at the desired rate; max time 4 days

Hepatic/renal dose
Adult: IV Child-Pugh A-C or CCr 30-60 ml/ min: Give IV loading dose over 10 min, then cont IV INF 10 mg over 24 hr × 2-4 days

Available forms: Injection (premixed) 0.2 mg/ml in 100 ml D_5W

Implementation

IV route

• Withdraw 4 ml (20 mg) of conivaptan, add to 100 ml D_5W, gently invert several times to mix, give over 30 min; in large vein, change site q24hr to minimize vascular irritation

Continuous IV infusion route

• Withdraw 4 ml (20 mg) of conivaptan, add to 250 ml D_5W, gently invert several times to mix, give over 24 hr; or 40 mg in 250 ml D_5W, gently invert several times to mix, give over 24 hr

ADVERSE EFFECTS

CNS: Headache, confusion, insomnia
CV: *Atrial fibrillation,* hypo/hypertension, orthostatic hypotension, phlebitis

---

GI: Nausea, vomiting, constipation, dry mouth
GU: Hematuria, polyuria, UTI, pollakiuria
HEMA: Anemia
INTEG: Erythemia, inj site reaction
META: Dehydration, hypo/hyperglycemia, hypokalemia, hypomagnesia, hyponatremia
MISC: Oral candidiasis, pain, peripheral edema, pneumonia

Pharmacokinetics

Absorption	Unknown
Distribution	Protein binding 99%
Metabolism	By CYP3A4
Excretion	Unknown
Half-life	Terminal 5 hr

Pharmacodynamics

Unknown

INTERACTIONS
Drug classifications
CYP3A4 substrates (alfuzosin, ARIPiprazole, bexarolene, bortezomib, bosentan, bupivacaine, buprenorphine, carBAMazepine, cevimeline, cilostazol, cinacalcet, clopidogrel, colchicine, cyclobenzaprine, dapsone, darifenacin, disopyramide, DOCEtaxel, donepezil, DOXOrubicin, dutasteride, eletriptan, eplerenone, ergots, erlotinib, eszopiclone, ethinyl estradiol, ethosuximide, etoposide, fentaNYL, galantamine, gefitinib, halofantrine, ifosfamide, irinotecan, levobupivacaine, levomethadyl, lidocaine, loperamide, loratadine, mefloquine, methadone, modafinil, PACLitaxel, pimozide, praziquantel, quiNIDine, quiNINE, ramelteon, reboxetine, repaglinide, rifabutin, sibutramine, sildenafil, sirolimus, SUFentanil, SUNItinib, tacrolimus, tamoxifen, teniposide, testosterone, tiaGABine, tinidazole, trimetrexate, vardenafil, vinca alkaloids, ziprasidone, zolpidem, zonisamide): increased effects, do not use concurrently

NURSING CONSIDERATIONS
Assessment
⚠ Monitor renal/hepatic function
⚠ Assess frequent sodium volume status; overly rapid correction of sodium concentration (>12 mEq/L per 24 hr) may result in osmotic demyelination syndrome
• Assess neurologic status: confusion, headache
• Assess CV status: atrial fibrillation, hyper/hypotension, orthostatic hypotension; monitor B/P, pulse
• Monitor other electrolytes (magnesium and potassium)

Patient/family education
• Advise patient to report neurologic changes: headache, insomnia, confusion
• Teach patient administration procedure and expected result
• Advise patient to report inj site pain, redness, swelling

Evaluation
Positive therapeutic outcome
• Correction of serum sodium levels

CONTRACEPTIVES, HORMONAL

MONOPHASIC, ORAL
ethinyl estradiol/ desogestrel (Rx)
Apri, Cesia, Desogen, Kariva, Mircette, Ortho-Cept, Reclipsen, Solia, Velivet
ethinyl estradiol/ drospirenone (Rx)
Ocella, Yasmin, Yaz 28
ethinyl estradiol/ ethynodiol (Rx)
Kelnor 1/35, Zovia 1/35, Zovia 1/50
ethinyl estradiol/ levonorgestrel (Rx)
Alesse, Aviane-28, Enpresse, Jolessa, Lessina, Levlen, Levlite, Levora, Lutera, Nordette, Portia, Quasense, Seasonique, Sronyx

C

**ethinyl estradiol/
norethindrone (Rx)**
Brevicon, Genora 0.5/35, Genora
1/35, Junel 21 1/20, Junel 21 1.5/20,
Loestrin 21 1.5/30, Loestrin 21 1/20,
Microgestin, Modicon, Necon 0.5/35,
N.E.E 1/35, Nelova 0.5/35E, Nelova
1/35E, Norcept-E 1/35, Norethin
1/35E, Norinyl 1+35, Norlestrin 1/50,
Norlestrin 2.5/50, Nortrel 1/35, Nortrel
7/7/7
**ethinyl estradiol/
norgestimate (Rx)**
MonoNessa, Ortho-Cyclen, Previfem,
Sprintec, Tri-Sprintec
**ethinyl estradiol/norgestrel
(Rx)**
Cryselle, Lo/Ovral, Low-Ogestrel,
Ogestrel, Ovral
**mestranol/norethindrone
(Rx)**
Genora 1/50, Nelova 1/50m, Norethin
1/50m, Norinyl 1+50, Ortho-Novum 1/50

BIPHASIC, ORAL
**ethinyl estradiol/
norethindrone (Rx)**
Nelova 10/11, Ortho-Novum 10/11

TRIPHASIC, ORAL
**ethinyl estradiol/
desogestrel (Rx)**
Cyclessa
**ethinyl estradiol/
norethindrone (Rx)**
Necor 7/7/7, Nortrel 7/7/7, Ortho-
Novum 7/7/7, Tri-Norinyl
**ethinyl estradiol/
norgestimate (Rx)**
Ortho Tri-Cyclen, Ortho Tri-Cyclen Lo
**ethinyl estradiol/
levonorgestrel (Rx)**
Enpresse, Tri-Levlen, Triphasil

EXTENDED CYCLE, ORAL
**ethinyl estradiol/
levonorgestrel (Rx)**
Seasonale

PROGESTIN, ORAL
norethindrone (Rx)
Errin, Ortho Micronor, Camila,
Jolivette, Nor-Q D

PROGRESSIVE ESTROGEN, ORAL
**ethinyl estradiol/
norethindrone acetate (Rx)**
Estrostep, Estrostep Fe

EMERGENCY
**levonorgestrel/ethinyl
estradiol (Rx)**
Preven
levonorgestrel (Rx)
Plan B
**medroxyPROGESTERone
(Rx)**
Depo-Provera

INTRAUTERINE
levonorgestrel (Rx)
Mirena

IMPLANT
etonogestrel (Rx)
Implanon

VAGINAL RING
**ethinyl estradiol/
etonogestrel (Rx)**
Nuva Ring

TRANSDERMAL
**ethinyl estradiol/
norelgestromin (Rx)**
Ortho Evra

ACTION: Prevents ovulation by contraceptives suppressing FSH, LH; *monophasic:* estrogen/progestin (fixed dose) used during a 21-day cycle; ovulation is inhibited by suppression of FSH and LH; thickness of cervical mucus and endometrial lining prevents pregnancy; *biphasic:* ovulation is inhibited by suppression of FSH and LH; alteration of cervical mucus, endometrial lining prevents pregnancy; *triphasic:* ovulation is inhibited by suppression of FSH and LH; change of cervical mucus, endometrial lining prevents pregnancy; variable doses of estrogen/progestin combinations may be similar to natural hormonal fluctuations; *extended cycle:* estrogen/progestin continuous for 84 days, off for 7 days, result 4 menstrual periods/yr; *progressive estrogen:* constant progestin with 3 progressive doses of estrogen; *progestin-only pill, implant, intrauterine:* change of cervical mucus and endometrial lining prevents pregnancy; ovulation may be suppressed

Therapeutic outcome: Prevention of pregnancy, decreased severity of endometriosis, hypermenorrhea

USES: To prevent pregnancy, regulation of menstrual cycle, treatment of acne in women >14 yr that other treatment has failed, emergency contraception; *injection:* inhibits gonadotropin secretion, ovulation, follicular maturation; *emergency:* inhibits ovulation and fertilization, decreases transport of sperm and egg from fallopian tube to uterus; *vaginal ring, transdermal:* inhibits ovulation, prevents sperm entry into uterus; *antiacne:* may decrease sex hormone binding globulin, results in decreased testosterone

CONTRAINDICATIONS
Pregnancy **X,** breastfeeding, women 40 yr and over, reproductive cancer, thrombophlebitis, MI, hepatic tumors, hepatic disease, CAD, CVA, breast cancer, jaundice, stroke, vaginal bleeding

Precautions: Depression, hypertension, renal disease, seizure disorders, lupus erythematosus, rheumatic disease, migraine headache, amenorrhea, irregular menses, gallbladder disease, diabetes mellitus, heavy smoking, acute mononucleosis, sickle cell disease

> **BLACK BOX WARNING:** Tobacco smoking

DOSAGE AND ROUTES
Monophasic
Adult: PO take first tab on Sunday after start of menses × 21 days; skip 7 days; then repeat cycle; start on 1st day of menses × 21 days; skip 7 days, then repeat cycle; may contain 7 placebo tabs, where 1 tab is taken daily

Biphasic
Adult: PO Take 10 days of small progestin, then large progestin; estrogen is the same during cycle; skip 7 days, then repeat cycle; may contain 7 placebo tabs, where 1 tab is taken daily

Triphasic
Adult: PO estrogen dose remains constant, progestin changes throughout 21 day cycle, some products contain 28 tabs per month

Extended cycle
Adult: PO start taking on first day of menses; continue for 84 days of active tab, then 7 days of placebo; repeat cycle

Progestin
Adult: PO start on 1st day of menses, then daily and continuously

Progressive estrogen
Adult: PO progestin dose remains constant, estrogen increases q7days throughout 21-day cycle, may include 7 placebo tabs for 28-day cycle

Emergency
Adult and adolescent: Give within 72 hr of intercourse, repeat 12 hr later; Plan B 1 tab, then 1 tab 12 hr later; Preven 2 tab, then 2 tab 12 hr later; Ovral (unlabeled) 2 white tabs; Lo/Ovral (unlabeled) 4 white tabs; Levlen (unlabeled), Nordette (unlabeled) 4 orange tabs; Triphasil (unlabeled), Tri-Levlen (unlabeled) 4 yellow tabs

Injectable
Adult: IM (Depo-Provera) 150 mg within 5 days of start of menses, or within 5 days postpartum (must not be breastfeeding); if breastfeeding, give 6 wk postpartum, repeat q3mo

Intrauterine
Adult: To be inserted using the levonorgestrel-releasing intrauterine system (LRIS) by those trained in procedure; inserted into uterine cavity within 7 days of the onset of menstruation; use should not exceed 5 years per implant

Vaginal ring
Adult: VAG insert 1 ring on or prior to day 5 of cycle, leave in place 3 wk; remove for 1 wk, then repeat

Transdermal
Adult: Transdermal apply patch within 7 days of menses, change weekly × 3 wk; no patch wk 4, repeat cycle

Implant
Adult: Subdermal in inner side of upper arm on days 1-5 of menses, replace q3yr

Acne
Adult: PO (Ortho Tri-Cyclen) take daily × 21 days, off 7 days

Implementation
PO route
• If GI symptoms occur, medication may be taken with food; take at same time each day
Implant route
• Inject 6 cap subdermally
• Implant is effective for 5 yr, should be removed after that
IM route
• Administer inj deep in large muscle mass after shaking susp well; ensure pregnancy has not occurred if inj are 2 wk or more apart

ADVERSE EFFECTS
CNS: Depression, fatigue, dizziness, nervousness, anxiety, headache

CV: Increased B/P, **cerebral hemorrhage, thrombosis, pulmonary embolism,** fluid retention, edema, MI
EENT: Optic neuritis, retinal thrombosis, cataracts
ENDO: Decreased glucose tolerance, increased TBG, PBI, T_4, T_3, temporary infertility
GI: *Nausea,* vomiting, cramps, diarrhea, bloating, constipation, change in appetite, **cholestatic jaundice,** weight change
GU: Breakthrough bleeding, amenorrhea, spotting, dysmenorrhea, galactorrhea, endocervical hyperplasia, vaginitis, cystitis-like syndrome, breast change
HEMA: Increased fibrinogen, clotting factor
INTEG: *Chloasma, melasma,* acne, rash, urticaria, erythema, pruritus, hirsutism, alopecia, photosensitivity

Pharmacokinetics

Absorption	Unknown
Distribution	Unknown
Metabolism	Unknown
Excretion	Breast milk
Half-life	Unknown

Pharmacodynamics

Unknown

INTERACTIONS
Individual drugs
Griseofulvin, rifampin: decreased effectiveness of oral contraceptive

Drug classifications
Analgesics, antibiotics, anticonvulsants, antihistamines: decreased action of oral contraceptives
Anticoagulants (oral): decreased action of oral anticoagulants

Drug/herb
Black cohosh: altered action
Saw palmetto, St. John's wort: decreased oral contraceptive effect

Drug/food
Grapefruit juice: increased peak level

Drug/lab test
Increased: pro-time; clotting factors VII, VIII, IX, X; TBG, PBI, T_4, platelet aggregation, BSP, triglycerides, bilirubin, AST, ALT
Decreased: T_3, antithrombin III, folate, metyrapone test, GTT, 17-OHCS

NURSING CONSIDERATIONS
Assessment
• Assess for reproductive changes: change in breasts, tumors, positive Pap smear; product should be discontinued if changes occur

• Monitor glucose, thyroid function, liver function tests, B/P

Patient/family education
• Teach patient about detection of clots using Homans' sign; teach monitoring technique for heat, redness, pain, swelling
• Teach patient to use sunscreen or to avoid sunlight; photosensitivity can occur
• Teach patient to take at same time each day to ensure equal product level; to take another tab as soon as possible if one is missed
• Teach patient that after product is discontinued, pregnancy may not occur for several mo
• Instruct patient to report GI symptoms that occur after 4 mo
⚠ Advise patient to use another birth control method during first 3 wk of oral contraceptive use
⚠ Teach patient to report abdominal pain, change in vision, shortness of breath, change in menstrual flow, spotting, breakthrough bleeding, breast lumps, swelling, headache, severe leg pain, mental changes; that continuing medical care is needed: Pap smear and gynecologic exam q6mo

> **BLACK BOX WARNING:** Teach patient not to smoke, increased risk of CV side effects

• Teach patient to notify physicians and dentist of oral contraceptive use

Evaluation
Positive therapeutic outcome
• Absence of pregnancy
• Decreased severity of endometriosis
• Decreased severity of hypermenorrhea

cotrimoxazole
See trimethoprim/sulfamethoxazole

⚠ HIGH ALERT

crizotinib
(kriz-oh'ti-nib)
XALKORI
Func. class.: Antineoplastic; biologic response modifiers
Pregnancy category D

ACTION: An inhibitor of receptor tyrosine kinases (anaplastic lymphoma kinase (ALK), hepatocyte growth factor receptor (HGFR, c-Met), recepteur d'origine nantais (RON).

Therapeutic outcome: Decreased spread of malignancy

Adverse effects: *italics* = common; **bold** = life-threatening

USES: Locally advanced or metastatic non–small-cell lung cancer (NSCLC) that is anaplastic lymphoma kinase (ALK)-positive as detected by an FDA-approved test

CONTRAINDICATIONS
Pregnancy D, breastfeeding, hypersensitivity

Precautions: Pneumonitis, severe hepatic disease, congenital long QT syndrome, neonates, infants, children, adolescents, severe renal impairment, end-stage renal disease, vision disorders

DOSAGE AND ROUTES
Adult: **PO** 250 mg bid; continue as long as is beneficial

Dose adjustments for hematologic toxicities
For Grade 1-2: No dosage adjustment needed

For Grade 3: Interrupt treatment until toxicity resolves to grade ≤2, then, continue with the same dosage schedule. In case of recurrence after a grade 4 event with dose reduction, interrupt treatment until toxicity resolves to grade ≤2; when resuming treatment, reduce dosage to 250 mg PO daily

For Grade 4: Interrupt treatment until toxicity resolves to grade ≤2; when resuming treatment, reduce dosage to 200 mg PO bid. In case of grade 4 recurrence, permanently discontinue treatment

Dose adjustment for hepatic laboratory abnormalities
For Grade 1: No dosage adjustment necessary:

For Grade 2 ALT/AST elevations with grade ≤1 total bilirubin elevations: No dosage adjustment necessary

For Grade 3-4 ALT/AST elevations with grade ≤1 total bilirubin elevations: Interrupt treatment until toxicity resolves to grade ≤1 or baseline; when resuming treatment, reduce dosage to 200 mg PO bid; in case of recurrence, interrupt treatment until toxicity resolves to ≤1, and when resuming treatment, reduce dosage to 250 mg PO daily; permanently discontinue treatment in case of further recurrence

For Grade 2-4 ALT/AST elevations with concurrent Grade 2-4 total bilirubin elevations (in the absence of cholestasis or hemolysis): Permanently discontinue treatment

Dose adjustment for pneumonitis not attributable to NSCLC progression, other pulmonary disease, infection, or radiation effect
For any grade pneumonitis: Permanently discontinue

Dose adjustment for QTc prolongation
For Grade 1–2 QTc prolongation: No dosage adjustment necessary

For Grade 3 QTc prolongation: Interrupt treatment until toxicity resolves to grade ≤1; when resuming treatment, reduce dosage to 200 mg PO bid; in case of recurrence, interrupt treatment until toxicity resolves to grade ≤1 and when resuming treatment, reduce dosage to 250 mg PO daily; permanently discontinue in case of further recurrence

For Grade 4 QTc prolongation: Permanently discontinue

Available forms: Caps 200, 250 mg

Implementation
- May be taken orally with or without food
- Have the patient swallow capsule whole; do not crush or chew
- If a dose is missed, it can be taken up to 6 hr before the next dose is due to maintain the twice daily regimen. Do not take both doses at the same time
- Store capsules at room temperature

ADVERSE EFFECTS
CNS: Dizziness, balance disorder, presyncope, neuropathy (motor and sensory), burning sensation, dysesthesia, hyperesthesia, hypoesthesia, neuralgia, paresthesias, peripheral neuropathy (motor and sensory), headache, insomnia

CV: QT prolongation, disseminated intravascular coagulation (DIC), septic shock, bradycardia

EENT: *Diplopia, photopsia,* photophobia, *blurred vision,* visual field defect, *vitreous floaters,* visual brightness, *reduced visual acuity,* esophageal disorders, dyspepsia

GI: *Nausea, diarrhea, vomiting, constipation,* decreased appetite, dysgeusia, abdominal pain, abdominal discomfort/pain, stomatitis, oral ulceration, elevated hepatic enzymes, hyperbilirubinemia, glossodynia, glossitis, cheilitis, mucosal inflammation, oropharyngeal pain/discomfort, oral pain, esophageal disorder, dysphagia, epigastric discomfort/pain, burning, esophagitis, **esophageal obstruction/pain/spasm, esophageal ulceration,** gastroesophageal reflux, odynophagia, and reflux esophagitis

HEMA: Grade 3/4 neutropenia, thrombocytopenia, lymphopenia

MISC: Fatigue, fever, *edema,* localized/peripheral edema, chest pain (unspecified), chest discomfort, musculoskeletal chest pain, arthralgia, back pain, rash

RESP: Severe, life-threatening pneumonitis, pneumonia, hypoxia, acute respiratory

---

distress syndrome (ARDS), dyspnea, empyema, **pulmonary hemorrhage, pulmonary embolism,** upper respiratory tract infection (nasopharyngitis, pharyngitis, rhinitis), cough

Pharmacokinetics

Absorption	43%
Distribution	Steady state 15 days, protein binding 91%, distribution tissue, plasma
Metabolism	By 3YPA4/5, oxidation to metabolites
Excretion	63% feces, unchanged 53%; 22% urine, unchanged 2, 3%
Half-life	Terminal 42 hr

Pharmacodynamics

Onset	Unknown
Peak	4-6 hr
Duration	Unknown

INTERACTIONS
Drug classifications

CYP2B6 substrates (prasugrel, selegiline, cyclophosphamide): increased action of these products

β-agonists, Class IA antiarrhythmics (disopyramide, procainamide, quiNIDine), Class III antiarrhythmics (amiodarone, dofetilide, ibutilide, sotalol), halogenated anesthetics, local anesthetics, tricyclic antidepressants: increased QT prolongation, torsades de pointes

CYP3A4 inhibitors (ketoconazole, atazanavir, indinavir, itraconazole, nefazodone, nelfinavir, ritonavir, voriconazole, boceprevir, delavirdine, isoniazid, dalfopristin-quinupristin, tipranavir): increased crizotinib

CYP3A4 inducers (rifampin, carBAMazepine, PHENobarbital, phenytoin, rifabutin); antacids, H2-blockers, proton pump inhibitors (PPIs): decreased crizotinib

CYP3A4 substrates (alfentanil, cycloSPORINE, ergotamine, dihydroergotamine fentaNYL, sirolimus, colchicine): avoid concurrent use

Individual drugs

Abarelix, alfuzosin, amoxapine, apomorphine, arsenic trioxide, asenapine, chloroquine, ciprofloxacin, citalopram, clarithromycin, cloZAPine, cyclobenzaprine, dasatinib, dolasetron, dronedarone, droperidol, eribulin, erythromycin, ezogabine, flecainide, fluconazole, gatifloxacin, gemifloxacin, grepafloxacin, halofantrine, haloperidol, iloperidone, indacaterol, lapatinib, levofloxacin, levomethadyl, lopinavir/ritonavir, magnesium sulfate, maprotiline, mefloquine, methadone, moxifloxacin, nilotinib, norfloxacin, octreotide, ofloxacin, OLANZapine, ondansetron, paliperidone, palonosetron, pentamidine, certain phenothiazines (chlorpromazine, mesoridazine, thioridazine, fluPHENAZine, perphenazine, prochlorperazine, trifluoperazine), pimozide, posaconazole, potassium sulfate, probucol, propafenone, QUEtiapine, quiNIDine, ranolazine, rilpivirine, risperidone, saquinavir, sodium, sparfloxacin, SUNItinib, tacrolimus, telavancin, telithromycin, tetrabenazine, troleandomycin, vardenafil, vemurafenib, venlafaxine, vorinostat, ziprasidone: increased QT prolongation, torsades de pointes
Midazolam: increased midazolam action

Drug/herb
Do not use with St. John's wort

Drug/food
Do not use with grapefruit juice

NURSING CONSIDERATIONS
Assessment

⚠ **Severe, life-threatening, or fatal treatment-related pneumonitis:** All cases occurred within 2 months of treatment initiation; monitor for pulmonary symptoms that may indicate pneumonitis and other causes of pneumonitis should be excluded; permanently discontinue in patients with treatment-related pneumonitis

⚠ **Hepatic disease:** Liver function test (LFT) abnormalities, altered bilirubin levels, may occur during treatment; monitor LFTs and bilirubin levels prior to treatment, then monthly; more frequent testing is needed in those presenting with grade 2 or greater toxicities; Laboratory alterations should be managed with dose reduction, treatment interruption, or discontinuation

⚠ **QT prolongation:** has been reported with the use of crizotinib; crizotinib should be avoided in these patients. Monitor ECG and electrolytes in those with CHF, bradycardia, electrolyte imbalance (hypokalemia, hypomagnesemia), or in those who are taking concomitant medications known to prolong the QT interval; treatment interruption, dosage adjustment, or treatment discontinuation may be needed in those who develop QT prolongation

• **Vision disorders:** Generally started within 2 weeks of the start of therapy; ophthalmologic evaluation should be considered, particularly if patients experience photopsia or new/ increased

Adverse effects: *italics* = common; **bold** = life-threatening

vitreous floaters; caution should be used when driving or operating machinery by patients who experience vision disorders

• **Pregnancy/breastfeeding: Identify if pregnancy is planned or suspected; pregnancy category D, avoid breastfeeding**

• CBC with differential; BUN/creatinine

Patient/family education

• Missed doses can be taken up to 6 hr before the next dose is due to maintain the twice daily regimen

• **Teach patient to use reliable contraception; both women and men of childbearing age should use adequate contraceptive methods during therapy and for at least 90 days after completing treatment; pregnancy D**

• **Teach patient to report immediately shortness of breath, cough, fatigue, visual changes**

• Teach patient not to take with grapefruit juice

• Teach patient to avoid activities requiring mental alertness until effects are known

• **Teach patient to report signs of QT prolongation (abnormal heartbeats, dizziness, syncope)**

• Teach patient to swallow caps whole and avoid contact with broken cap

Evaluation
Positive therapeutic outcome
• Decreased spread of malignancy

---

crofelemer
(kroe-fel´e-mer)
Fulyzaq
Func. class.: Antidiarrheal
Chem. class.: Red sap of *Croton lechleri* plant
Pregnancy category C

ACTION: Blocks chloride channel and high volume water loss in diarrhea

Therapeutic outcome: Decreasing diarrhea

USES: Noninfectious diarrhea in those with HIV/AIDS using antiretrovirals

CONTRAINDICATIONS
Hypersensitivity

Precautions: Pregnancy (C), breastfeeding, Black patients, children/ adolescents, GI disease, infection, malabsorption syndrome, pancreatitis

DOSAGE AND ROUTES
Adult: PO 125 mg bid

Available forms: Del rel tabs 125 mg

Implementation
PO route
• Do not break, crush, or chew
• Give without regard to meals

ADVERSE EFFECTS
CNS: Dizziness, depression
GI: Nausea, constipation, abdominal pain, anorexia, flatulence, hyperbilirubinemia
INTEG: Acne vulgaris, contact dermatitis
MISC: Arthralgia, cough, increased urinary frequency

Pharmacokinetics

Absorption	Unknown
Distribution	Unknown
Metabolism	Unknown
Excretion	Unknown
Half-life	Unknown

Pharmacodynamics

Onset	Unknown
Peak	Unknown
Duration	Unknown

INTERACTIONS
Individual drugs
Alosetron: increased serious constipation, bowel obstruction

Drug classifications
Antimuscarinics, opiate agonists: increased constipation

NURSING CONSIDERATIONS
Assessment
• Stools: volume, color, characteristic frequency; bowel pattern before protein rebound constipation
• Electrolytes (K, Na, Cl), hydration status
• Monitor effect in Black patients; may be less effective

Patient/family education
• Instruct patient to avoid OTC products unless directed by prescriber
• Instruct patient not to operate machinery if drowsiness occurs

Evaluation
Positive therapeutic outcome:
• Decreased diarrhea

---

cyclobenzaprine (Rx)

(sye-kloe-ben′za-preen)

Amrix, Fexmid, Flexeril

Func. class.: Skeletal muscle relaxant, central acting

Chem. class.: Tricyclic amine salt

Pregnancy category B

Do not confuse: cyclobenzaprine/cyproheptadine

ACTION: Reduction of tonic muscle activity at the brain stem; may be related to antidepressant effects

Therapeutic outcome: Relaxation of skeletal muscle

USES: Adjunct for relief of muscle spasm and pain in musculoskeletal conditions

Unlabeled uses: Fibromyalgia

CONTRAINDICATIONS

Acute recovery phase of MI, dysrhythmias, heart block, CHF, hypersensitivity, child <12 yr, intermittent porphyria, thyroid disease

Precautions: Pregnancy **B**, breastfeeding, geriatric, renal/hepatic disease, addictive personality

DOSAGE AND ROUTES
Musculoskeletal disorders

Adult/adolescent ≥15 yr: PO 5 mg tid × 1 wk, max 30 mg/day × 3 wk

Adult: EXT REL 15 mg q day, max 30 mg q day × 3 wk

Geriatric: PO 5 mg tid

Hepatic dose

Adult (mild hepatic disease): PO 5 mg, titrate slowly

Fibromyalgia (unlabeled)

Adult: PO 10 mg at bedtime, titrated up

Available forms: Tabs 5, 7.5, 10 mg; ext rel tab 15, 30 mg

Implementation

• Give without regard to meals, give with food for GI symptoms

• Store in airtight container at room temperature

ADVERSE EFFECTS

CNS: *Dizziness, weakness, drowsiness,* headache, tremor, depression, insomnia, confusion, paresthesia, nervousness

CV: Postural hypotension, tachycardia, **dysrhythmias**

EENT: Diplopia, temporary loss of vision, blurred vision

GI: *Nausea,* vomiting, hiccups, dry mouth, constipation, hepatitis

GU: Urinary retention, frequency, change in libido

INTEG: Rash, pruritus, fever, facial flushing, sweating

Pharmacokinetics

Distribution	Well
Metabolism	Liver, partially
Excretion	Kidney (unchanged)
Half-life	1-3 days, 32 hr ext rel

Pharmacodynamics

Onset	1 hr
Peak	3-8 hr
Duration	12-24 hr

INTERACTIONS
Individual drugs

Alcohol: increased CNS depression

TraMADol: do not use within 14 days

Drug classifications

Antidepressants (tricyclic), barbiturates, opiates, sedative/hypnotics: increased CNS depression

MAOIs: do not use within 14 days

Serotonin syndrome—SSRIs, SNRIs: increased action of these products

Drug/herb

Kava: increased CNS depression

NURSING CONSIDERATIONS
Assessment

⚠ **Serotonin syndrome: if using with SSRIs, SNRIs, monitor closely; if syndrome occurs, discontinue both products immediately**

• Assess pain periodically: location, duration, mobility, stiffness, baseline

• Monitor ECG in epileptic patients; poor seizure control has occurred in patients taking this product

• Check for allergic reactions: rash, fever, respiratory distress

• Check for severe weakness, numbness, in extremities

• Assess for CNS depression: dizziness, drowsiness, psychiatric symptoms

Patient/family education

⚠ **Teach patient not to discontinue medication quickly; insomnia, nausea, headache, spasticity, tachycardia will occur; product should be tapered off over 1-2 wk**

Adverse effects: *italics* = common; **bold** = life-threatening

- Caution patient not to take with alcohol, other CNS depressants
- Advise to avoid altering activities while taking this product
- Caution patient to avoid hazardous activities if drowsiness/dizziness occurs
- Caution patient to avoid using OTC medication: cough preparations, antihistamines, unless directed by prescriber
- Teach patient to use gum, frequent sips of water for dry mouth

Evaluation
Positive therapeutic outcome
- Decreased pain, spasticity; muscle spasms of acute, painful musculoskeletal conditions are generally short term; long-term therapy is seldom warranted

TREATMENT OF OVERDOSE:
Empty stomach with emesis, gastric lavage, then administer activated charcoal; use anticonvulsants if indicated; monitor cardiac function

---

cyclopentolate ophthalmic
See Appendix B

⚠ HIGH ALERT

cyclophosphamide (Rx)
(sye-kloe-foss'fa-mide)
Cytoxan, Procytox ✤
Func. class.: Antineoplastic alkylating agent
Chem. class.: Nitrogen mustard
Pregnancy category D

Do not confuse: cyclophosphamide/
cycloSPORINE,
Cytoxan/Cytosar/Cytotec/Cytarabine

ACTION: Alkylates DNA; responsible for cross-linking DNA strands; activity is not cell cycle phase specific

Therapeutic outcome: Prevention of rapidly growing malignant cells

USES: Hodgkin's disease, lymphomas, leukemia, multiple myeloma, neuroblastoma, retinoblastoma, Ewing's sarcoma, cancer of female reproductive tract, breast, nephrotic syndrome

CONTRAINDICATIONS
Pregnancy **D**, hypersensitivity, prostatic hypertrophy, bladder neck obstruction

Precautions: Radiation therapy, cardiac disease, anemia, dysrhythmias, child, dental disease/work, dialysis, geriatrics, heart failure, hematuria, infections, leukopenia QT prolongation, secondary malignancy surgery, tumor lysis syndrome, vaccinations, breastfeeding, severely depressed bone marrow function

DOSAGE AND ROUTES
Acute lymphocytic leukemia (ALL) (induction therapy)
Adult/adolescent/child: IV 300-1500 mg/m² have been used with induction, intensification, and consolidation regimens that may include prediSONE, vinCRIStine and others; PO 1-5 mg/kg/day adjusted to response

Neuroblastoma
Adult/child: IV For induction, 40-50 mg/kg in divided doses over 2-5 days or 10-15 mg/kg q7-10 days, 3-5 mg/kg 2 times/wk or 1-5 mg/kg daily

Child and infant: PO 150 mg/m²/day, days 1-7 with DOXOrubicin (**IV** 35 mg/m² on day 5) q21days × 5 cycles

Child: IV 70 mg/kg/day with hydration on days 1 and 2 with DOXOrubicin and vinCRIStine q21days for courses 1, 2, 4, 6, alternating with CISplatin and etoposide q21days for courses 3, 5, 7

Breast cancer
Adult: PO 100-200 mg/m²/day or 2 mg/kg/day × 4-14 days; IV 500-1000 mg/m² on day 1 in combination with fluorouracil and methotrexate or DOXOrubicin, or DOXOrubicin alone; also cyclophosphamide 600 mg/m², may be given dose-dense on day 1 of q14day with DOXOrubicin (60 mg/m²) with growth factor support

Operable node-positive breast cancer
IV (TAC regimen) Adult: 500 mg/m² with DOXOrubicin (50 mg/m² **IV**) then docetaxel (75 mg/m²) **IV** given 1 hr later × 6 cycles q3wk

Nephrotic syndrome
Child: PO 2.5-3 mg/kg q day × 60-90 days

Available forms: Inj IV 200 ✤, 500 mg, 1, 2 g; vials 25, 50 mg

Implementation
- Give fluids **IV** or PO before chemotherapy to hydrate patient
- Give antacid before oral agent, after PM meals, before bedtime; antiemetic 30-60 min before giving product to prevent vomiting and prn; antibiotics for prophylaxis of infection
- Give top or syst analgesics for pain; give in AM so product can be eliminated before bedtime
- Use cytotoxic handling procedures

PO route
- To be taken on empty stomach; do not crush, break, chew tab, wash hands immediately if in contact with tab
- May be taken as a single dose or divided doses
- Take in AM or afternoon, avoid evening

Direct IV
- Reconstitute with NS only
- Store in tight container at room temperature

Intermittent IV infusion route
- Use cytotoxic handling procedures
- Give **IV** after diluting 100 mg/5 ml of sterile or bacteriostatic water; shake; let stand until clear; may be further diluted in up to 250 ml D₅ 0.9% NaCl, 0.45% NaCl, LR, D₅NS; SWI, 0.45% NaCl Ringer's; give 100 mg or less/min through 3-way stopcock of glucose or saline inf
- Use 21-, 23-, or 25-G needle; check site for irritation, phlebitis

Syringe compatibilities: Bleomycin, CISplatin, doxapram, DOXOrubicin, droperidol, fluorouracil, furosemide, heparin, leucovorin, methotrexate, metoclopramide, mitoMYcin, mitoXANtrone, vinBLAStine, vinCRIStine

Y-site compatibilities: Amifostine, amikacin, ampicillin, azlocillin, aztreonam, bleomycin, cefamandole, ceFAZolin, cefepime, cefoperazone, cefotaxime, cefOXitin, cefuroxime, cephalothin, cephapirin, chloramphenicol, chlorproMAZINE, cimetidine, CISplatin, cladribine, clindamycin, dexamethasone, diphenhydrAMINE, DOXOrubicin, doxycycline, droperidol, erythromycin, famotidine, filgrastim, fludarabine, fluorouracil, furosemide, gallium, ganciclovir, gentamicin, granisetron, heparin, HYDROmorphone, IDArubicin, kanamycin, leucovorin, LORazepam, melphalan, methotrexate, methylPREDNISolone, metoclopramide, metroNIDAZOLE, mezlocillin, minocycline, mitoMYcin, moxalactam, nafcillin, ondansetron, oxacillin, PAClitaxel, penicillin G potassium, piperacillin, piperacillin/tazobactam, prochlorperazine, promethazine, propofol, ranitidine, sargramostim, sodium bicarbonate, teniposide, tetracycline, thiotepa, ticarcillin, ticarcillin-clavulanate, tobramycin, trimethoprim-sulfamethoxazole, vancomycin, vinBLAStine, vinCRIStine, vinorelbine

Solution compatibilities: Amino acids 4.25%/D₂₅, D₅/0.9% NaCl, D₅W, 0.9% NaCl

ADVERSE EFFECTS
CNS: Headache, dizziness
CV: *Cardiotoxicity (high doses), myocardial fibrosis, congestive heart failure, pericarditis*

ENDO: Syndrome of inappropriate antidiuretic hormone (SIADH), gonadal suppression
GI: *Nausea, vomiting, diarrhea, weight loss,* colitis, **hepatotoxicity**
GU: **Hemorrhagic cystitis,** hematuria, neoplasms, amenorrhea, azoospermia, sterility, ovarian fibrosis, **renal tubular fibrosis**
HEMA: **Thrombocytopenia, leukopenia, pancytopenia, myelosuppression**
INTEG: *Alopecia,* dermatitis
META: Hyperuricemia
MISC: Secondary neoplasms, **anaphylaxis**
RESP: **Pulmonary fibrosis, interstitial pneumonia**

Pharmacokinetics

Absorption	Well absorbed (PO)
Distribution	Widely distributed; crosses placenta, blood-brain barrier (50%)
Metabolism	Liver to active product
Excretion	Kidneys, unchanged (30%)
Half-life	4-6½ hr

Pharmacodynamics

Unknown

INTERACTIONS
Individual drugs
Allopurinol: increased bone marrow suppression
Chloramphenicol: decreased cyclophosphamide effect
Digoxin: decreased digoxin levels
Insulin: increased hypoglycemia
Succinylcholine: increased neuromuscular blockade
Warfarin: increased warfarin action

Drug classifications
Diuretics (thiazides): increased bone marrow suppression
Barbiturates: increased toxicity of cyclophosphamide
Corticosteroids: decreased cyclophosphamide effect
Live virus vaccines: decreased antibody reaction

Drug/herb
St. John's wort: increased toxicity

Drug/lab test
Increased: uric acid
Decreased: pseudocholinesterase
False positive: Pap smear
False negative: PPD, mumps trichophytin, *Candida, Trichophyton,* Pap smear

NURSING CONSIDERATIONS
Assessment
⚠ Assess symptoms indicating severe allergic reaction: rash, pruritus, urticaria, purpuric skin lesions, itching, flushing
• Assess for tachypnea, ECG changes, dyspnea, edema, fatigue
⚠ Bone marrow suppression: Monitor CBC, differential, platelet count weekly; withhold product if WBC count is <2500/mm³ or platelet count is <75,000/mm³; notify prescriber of results
⚠ Assess for hemorrhagic cystitis: renal function studies including BUN, creatinine, serum uric acid, urine CCr before, during therapy; I&O ratio; report fall in urine output to <30 ml/hr
⚠ Monitor temp q4hr (elevated temp may indicate beginning of infection)
⚠ Hepatotoxicity: Monitor liver function tests before, during therapy (bilirubin, AST, ALT, LDH) as needed or monthly; note jaundice of skin or sclera, dark urine, clay-colored stools, itchy skin, abdominal pain, fever, diarrhea
⚠ Assess for bleeding: hematuria, stool guaiac, bruising or petechiae, mucosa or orifices q8hr
• Identify dyspnea, crackles, unproductive cough, chest pain, tachypnea
• Identify effects of alopecia on body image; discuss feelings about body changes

Patient/family education
• Teach patient to avoid use of products containing aspirin or ibuprofen, razors, commercial mouthwash, since bleeding may occur; to report symptoms of bleeding (hematuria, tarry stools, bruising)
• Instruct patient to report signs of anemia (fatigue, headache, irritability, faintness, shortness of breath)
• Teach patient to report any changes in breathing or coughing even several months after treatment
• Advise patient that hair may be lost during treatment; a wig or hairpiece may make patient feel better; new hair may be different in color, texture
• Advise patient on proper handling and disposal of chemotherapy drugs
• Teach patient not to have any vaccinations without the advice of the prescriber; serious reactions can occur
⚠ Advise patient contraception is needed during treatment and for several months after the completion of therapy
⚠ Teach patient to take adequate fluids to eliminate product

Evaluation
Positive therapeutic outcome
• Prevention of rapid division of malignant cells
• Increased appetite, increased weight

cycloSPORINE (Rx)
(sye-kloe-spor′een)
SandIMMUNE
cycloSPORINE, modified
Gengraf, Neoral
Func. class.: Immunosuppressant
Chem. class.: Fungus-derived peptide
Pregnancy category C

Do not confuse: cycloSPORINE/Cyclo-SERINE/cyclophosphamide, SandIMMUNE/SandoSTATIN

ACTION: Produces immunosuppression by inhibiting T lymphocytes

Therapeutic outcome: Absence of transplant rejection

USES: Organ transplants (liver, kidney, heart, GVHD) to prevent rejection, rheumatoid arthritis, psoriasis

Unlabeled uses: Recalcitrant ulcerative colitis, aplastic anemia, Crohn's disease, thrombocytopenia purpura, lupus, nephritis, myasthenia gravis, psoriatic arthritis

CONTRAINDICATIONS
Hypersensitivity to polyoxyethylated castor oil (inj only), psoriasis or rheumatoid arthritis in renal disease (Neoral/Gengraf), Gengraf/Neoral used with PUVA/UVB; methotrexate, coal tar, breastfeeding, ocular infections

> **BLACK BOX WARNING:** Neoplastic disease, sunlight (UV) exposure, renal disease/failure, uncontrolled, malignant hypertension; radiation in psoriasis

Precautions: Pregnancy **C**, geriatric, severe renal/hepatic disease

DOSAGE AND ROUTES
Prevention of transplant rejection (unmodified)
Adult and child: PO 15 mg/kg several hr before surgery, daily for 2 wk, reduce dosage by 2.5 mg/kg/wk to 5-10 mg/kg/day; IV 5-6 mg/kg several hr before surgery, daily, switch to PO form as soon as possible

Prevention of transplant rejection (modified)
Adult and child: PO 4-12 mg/kg/day divided q12hr, depends on organ transplanted

Rheumatoid arthritis (Neoral/Gengraf)
Adult: PO 2.5 mg/kg/day divided bid, may increase 0.5-0.75 mg/kg/day after 8-12 wk, max 4 mg/kg/day

Psoriasis (Neoral/Gengraf)
Adult: PO 2.5 mg/kg/day divided bid × 4 wk, then increase by 0.5 mg/kg/day q2wk, max 4 mg/kg/day

Idiopathic thrombocytopenia purpura (unlabeled)
Adult: PO 1.25-2.5 mg/kg bid

Severe aplastic anemia (unlabeled)
Adult and child: PO 12 mg/kg/day or 15 mg/kg/day (child) with antithymocyte globulin (ATG)

Available forms: Oral sol (Neoral) 100 mg/ml; soft gel cap 25, 50, 100 mg; inj 50 mg/ml

Implementation
PO route
• Some brands are not interchangeable
• Do not break, crush, or chew caps
• Use pipette provided to draw up oral sol; may mix with milk or juice, wipe pipette, do not wash (Neoral)
• Give for several days before transplant surgery with corticosteroids
• Microemulsion products (Neoral) and other products are not interchangeable
• Give with meals for GI upset or place product in chocolate milk (SandIMMUNE)

Intermittent IV infusion route
• Give **IV** after diluting each 50 mg/20-100 ml of 0.9% NaCl or D₅W; run over 2-6 hr; use an inf pump, glass inf bottles only
Continuous IV infusion route
• May run over 24 hr
• **For Sandimmune parenteral:** give 1/3 of PO dose, initial dose 4-12 hr prior to transplantation as a single **IV** dose 5-6 mg/kg/day, continue the single daily dose until PO can be used

Additive compatibilities: Ciprofloxacin

Y-site compatibilities: Abciximab, alatrofloxacin, alfentanil, amikacin, aminocaproic acid, aminophylline, amphotericin B lipid complex, anidulafungin, argatroban, ascorbic acid injection, atenolol, atracurium, atropine, azaTHIOprine, aztreonam, benztropine, bivalirudin, bleomycin, bretylium, bumetanide, buprenorphine, butorphanol, calcium chloride/gluconate, CARBOplatin, carmustine, caspofungin, ceFAZolin, cefmetazole, cefonicid, cefotaxime, cefoTEtan, cefOXitin, cefTAZidime, ceftizoxime, cefTRIAXone, cefuroxime, chloramphenicol, chlorproMAZINE, cimetidine, ciprofloxacin, CISplatin, clindamycin, codeine, cyanocobalamin, cyclophosphamide, cytarabine, DACTINomycin, DAPTOmycin, DAUNOrubicin, dexamethasone, dexmedetomidine, digoxin, diltiazem, diphenhydrAMINE, DOBUTamine, DOCEtaxel, DOPamine, doripenem, doxacurium, DOXOrubicin, doxycycline, enalaprilat, ePHEDrine, EPINEPHrine, epirubicin, epoetin alfa, eptifibatide, ertapenem, erythromycin, esmolol, etoposide, famotidine, fenoldopam, fentaNYL, fluconazole, fludarabine, fluorouracil, folic acid, furosemide, gallium, ganciclovir, gatifloxacin, gemcitabine, gentamicin, glycopyrrolate, granisetron, heparin, hydrocortisone, HYDROmorphone, hydrOXYzine, ifosfamide, imipenem-cilastatin, indomethacin, irinotecan, isoproterenol, ketorolac, labetalol, lansoprazole, levofloxacin, lidocaine, linezolid, LORazepam, mannitol, mechlorethamine, meperidine, meropenem, methotrexate, methyldopate, methylPREDNISolone, metoclopramide, metoprolol, metroNIDAZOLE, micafungin, miconazole, midazolam, milrinone, minocycline, mitoXANtrone, morphine, multiple vitamins injection, nafcillin, naloxone, nesiritide, netilmicin, nitroglycerin, nitroprusside, norepinephrine, octreotide, ondansetron, oxacillin, oxaliplatin, oxytocin, paclitaxel, palonosetron, pamidronate, pancuronium, pantoprazole, papaverine, PEMEtrexed, penicillin G potassium/sodium, pentamidine, pentazocine, phentolamine, phenylephrine, phytonadione, piperacillin, piperacillin-tazobactam, polymyxin B, potassium acetate/chloride, procainamide, prochlorperazine, promethazine, propofol, propranolol, protamine, pyridoxine, quiNIDine, quinupristin-dalfopristin, ranitidine, ritodrine, sargramostim, sodium acetate/bicarbonate, succinylcholine, SUFentanil, tacrolimus, teniposide, theophylline, thiamine, thiotepa, ticarcillin, ticarcillin-clavulanate, tigecycline, tirofiban, tobramycin, trimetaphan, urokinase, vancomycin, vasopressin, vecuronium, verapamil, vinCRIStine, vinorelbine, zoledronic acid

Solution compatibilities: D₅W, NaCl 0.9%

ADVERSE EFFECTS
CNS: *Tremors, headache,* seizures, confusion, **encephalopathy**
GI: Nausea, vomiting, diarrhea, *oral candida, gum hyperplasia,* **hepatotoxicity,** pancreatitis
GU: Albuminuria, hematuria, proteinuria, renal failure, hemolytic uremic syndrome, nephrotoxicity
INTEG: Rash, acne, *hirsutism,* pruritus

META: Hyperkalemia, hypomagnesemia, hyperlipidemia, hyperuricemia
MISC: *Infection, hypertension*

Pharmacokinetics

Absorption	Poorly absorbed (PO)
Distribution	Crosses placenta
Metabolism	Liver to mercaptopurine
Excretion	Kidney, minimal
Half-life	Biphasic 1.2 hr, 25 hr

Pharmacodynamics

	PO
Onset	Unknown
Peak	4 hr
Duration	Unknown

INTERACTIONS
Individual drugs

Allopurinol, amiodarone, amphotericin B, bromocriptine, carvedilol, cimetidine, colchicine, foscarnet, imipenem-cilastatin, melphalan, metoclopramide: increased action, cycloSPORINE toxicity

Digoxin: increased digoxin level
Etoposide: increased etoposide level
Methotrexate: increased methotrexate level
Nafcillin, orlistat, PHENobarbital, phenytoin, terbinafine, ticlodipine, trimethoprim/sulfamethoxazole: decreased cycloSPORINE action
Sirolimus: increased sirolimus level
Tacrolimus: increased tacrolimus level

Drug classifications:

Androgens, antifungals (azole), β-blockers, calcium channel blockers, contraceptives (oral), corticosteroids, fluoroquinolones, macrolides, NSAIDs, selective serotonin reuptake inhibitors: increased cycloSPORINE levels, toxicity
Anticonvulsants, rifamycins: decreased cycloSPORINE levels
HMG-CoA reductase inhibitors, diuretics (potassium-sparing): increased effects of each product
Live virus vaccines: decreased antibody reaction

Drug/food

Grapefruit juice, food: increased slowed metabolism of product

NURSING CONSIDERATIONS
Assessment

• **Encephalopathy: Assess for impaired cognition, seizures, vision changes including blindness, loss of motor function, movement disorders, psychiatric changes; dosage reduction or discontinuation may be needed in severe cases**

• Monitor renal studies: BUN, creatinine at least monthly during treatment, 3 mo after treatment
• Monitor liver function studies: alkaline phosphatase, AST, ALT, bilirubin
• Monitor product blood levels during treatment (Therapeutic range: 100-400 mg/ml)
• **Assess for hepatotoxicity: dark urine, jaundice, itching, light-colored stools; product should be discontinued**
• **Assess for nephrotoxicity: 6 wk postop, CyA trough level >200 ng/ml, intracapsular pressure <40 mm Hg, rise in creatinine 0.15 mg/dl/day**

Patient/family education

• Advise patient to report fever, rash, severe diarrhea, chills, sore throat, fatigue, since serious infections may occur; also to report clay-colored stools, cramping (may indicate hepatotoxicity); tremors, bleeding gums, increased B/P

> **BLACK BOX WARNING:** Advise patient to limit UV exposure

• **Caution patient to use contraceptive measures during treatment and for 12 wk after ending therapy; product is teratogenic, to notify prescriber if pregnancy is planned or suspected**
• Caution patient to avoid crowds and persons with known infections to reduce risk of infection
• Teach patient to take at the same time of day, every day; do not skip or double a missed dose; not to use with grapefruit juice or receive vaccines; there are many drug interactions, do not add or discontinue products without prescriber approval
• Teach patient that treatment is lifelong to prevent rejection; to identify signs of rejection
• Advise patient to report severe diarrhea as drug loss may result
• **Nephrotoxicity: Teach patient to notify prescriber of increased B/P, tremors of the hands, change in gums, increased hair on body/face**
• Advise patient to continue with lab work and follow-up appointment
• Teach patient types of products are not interchangeable
• Teach patient not to wash syringe/container with water; a variation in dose may result

Evaluation
Positive therapeutic outcome
• Absence of graft rejection

> **⚠ HIGH ALERT**
>
> ## cytarabine (Rx)
> (sye-tare´a-been)
> **Ara-C, Cytosar ✤, Cytosar-U**
> ## cytarabine liposomal (Rx)
> **Depo Cyt**
> *Func. class.:* Antineoplastic, antimetabolite
> *Chem. class.:* Pyrimidine nucleoside
> **Pregnancy category D**

Do not confuse: Cytosar ✤/Cytovene/
Cytoxan

ACTION: Competes with physiologic substrate of DNA synthesis, thus interfering with cell replication in the S phase of the cell cycle (before mitosis)

Therapeutic outcome: Prevention of rapidly growing malignant cells

USES: Acute myelocytic leukemia, acute lymphocytic leukemia, chronic myelocytic leukemia, lymphomatous meningitis (IT/intraventricular)

Unlabeled uses: Hodgkin's/non-Hodgkin's lymphoma

CONTRAINDICATIONS
Pregnancy **D**, hypersensitivity

Precautions: Renal/hepatic disease, breastfeeding, children, tumor lysis syndrome, infection, hyperkalemia, hyperphosphatemia, hyperuricemia, hypocalcemia

> **BLACK BOX WARNING:** Bone marrow suppression

DOSAGE AND ROUTES
Acute myelogenous leukemia (AML)
Adult: cont **IV** infusion 100 mg/m^2/day × 7 days q2wk as a single agent or 2-3 divided doses × 5-10 days until remission used in combination; maintenance 70-200 mg/m^2/day × 2-5 days qmo; **SUBCUT** maintenance 100 mg/m^2/day × 5 days q28days
Adult/child: **IV** For induction, 40-50 mg/kg in divided doses over 2-5 days or 10-15 mg/kg q7-10 days, 3-5 mg/kg 2 times/wk or 1-5 mg/kg daily

Meningeal leukemia
Adult and child: Intrathecal For induction 50 mg (liposomal) q14 days × 2 doses (wk 1, 3); consolidation 50 mg (liposomal) q14 days × 3 doses (wk 5, 7, 9) then another dose at wk 13; maintenance 50 mg (liposomal) q28 days (wks 17, 21, 25, 29)

Carcinomatous meningitis (liposoma)
Adult: Intrathecal 50 mg over 1-5 min q14days, during induction and consolidation wk 1, 3, 5, 7, 9, give another 50 mg wk 13; maintenance 50 mg q28days on wk 17, 21, 25, 29 use with dexamethasone 4 mg PO/IV × 5 days on each day of cytarabine

Renal dose
Adult CCr ≤60 ml/min, serum creatinine 1.5-1.9 mg/dl or increase of 0.5-1.2 mg/dl from baseline: during treatment reduce to 1 g/m^2/dose; serum creatinine ≥2 mg/dl or change from baseline serum creatinine was 1.2 mg/dl reduce to 100 mg/m^2/day

Available forms: Powder for inj 100 ✤, 500 mg, 1, 2 g vials; sus rel (Depo Cyt) liposomal for intrathecal use 10 mg/ml

Implementation
• Avoid contact with skin; very irritating; wash completely to remove
• Give fluids **IV** or PO before chemotherapy to hydrate patient
• Give antiemetic 30-60 min before giving product to prevent vomiting, and prn; antibiotics for prophylaxis of infection
• Increase fluids to 3 L/day
• Give in AM so product can be eliminated before bedtime
• Use cytotoxic handling precautions
IM/SUBCUT route
• **Reconstitute** 100 mg/5 ml or 500 mg/10 ml with bacteriostatic water for inj with benzyl alcohol 0.9%; do not use sol with precipitate; stable for 48 hr
Intrathecal route
• **Liposomal: withdraw** product immediately before use; **use** within 4 hr, do not save unused portions or use in-line filter; **give** directly into CSF by intraventricular reservoir or by direct inj into lumbar site
• **Give** slowly over 1-5 min; follow with lumbar puncture; instruct patient to lie flat; **give** dexamethasone 4 mg bid PO or **IV** × 5 days beginning on day of liposomal inj

> **Direct IV route**
> • **Dilute** 100 mg/5 ml of sterile water for inj, **give** over 1-3 min through a free-flowing IV
> **Intermittent IV infusion route**
> • May be further diluted in 50-100 ml NS or D$_5$W and **give** over 30 min-24 hr, depending on dose
> **Continuous IV infusion route**
> • May be given as continuous IV infusion

Adverse effects: *italics* = common; **bold** = life-threatening

Y-site compatibilities: Acyclovir, alfentanil, amifostine, amikacin, aminocaproic acid, aminophylline, amphotericin B lipid complex, amphotericin B liposome, ampicillin, ampicillin-sulbactam, amsacrine, anidulafungin, atenolol, atracurium, azithromycin, aztreonam, bivalirudin, bleomycin, bumetanide, buprenorphine, butorphanol, calcium chloride/gluconate, CARBOplatin, ceFAZolin, cefepime, cefotaxime, cefoTEtan, cefOXitin, cefTAZidime, ceftizoxime, cefTRIAXone, cefuroxime, chlorproMAZINE, cimetidine, ciprofloxacin, cisatracurium, CISplatin, cladribine, clindamycin, codeine, cyclophosphamide, cycloSPORINE, DAUNOrubicin, dexamethasone, dexmedetomidine, dexrazoxane, digoxin, diltiazem, diphenhydrAMINE, DOBUTamine, DOCEtaxel, dolasetron, DOPamine, doxacurium, DOXOrubicin, DOXOrubicin liposomal, doxycycline, droperidol, enalaprilat, ePHEDrine, EPINEPHrine, ertapenem, erythromycin, esmolol, etoposide, famotidine, fenoldopam, fentaNYL, filgrastim, fluconazole, fludarabine, foscarnet, fosphenytoin, furosemide, gatifloxacin, gemcitabine, gemtuzumab, gentamicin, granisetron, haloperidol, heparin, hydrocortisone, HYDROmorphone, hydrOXYzine, IDArubicin, ifosfamide, imipenem-cilastatin, inamrinone, insulin (regular), irinotecan, isoproterenol, ketorolac, labetalol, leucovorin, levofloxacin, levorphanol, lidocaine, linezolid, LORazepam, magnesium sulfate, mannitol, melphalan, meperidine, meropenem, mesna, methohexital, methotrexate, methylPREDNISolone, metoclopramide, metoprolol, metroNIDAZOLE, midazolam, milrinone, minocycline, mitoXANtrone, mivacurium, morphine, nalbuphine, naloxone, nesiritide, niCARdipine, nitroglycerin, nitroprusside, norepinephrine, octreotide, ofloxacin, ondansetron, oxaliplatin, PACLitaxel, palonosetron, pamidronate, pancuronium, pantoprazole, PEMEtrexed, pentamidine, PENTobarbital, PHENobarbital, phenylephrine, piperacillin, piperacillin-tazobactam, potassium chloride/phosphates, procainamide, prochlorperazine, promethazine, propofol, propranolol, quinupristin-dalfopristin, ranitidine, rapacuronium, remifentanil, riTUXimab, rocuronium, sargramostim, sodium acetate/bicarbonate/phosphates, succinylcholine, SUFentanil, sulfamethoxazole-trimethoprim, tacrolimus, teniposide, theophylline, thiopental, thiotepa, ticarcillin, ticarcillin-clavulanate, tigecycline, tirofiban, TNA, tobramycin, trastuzumab, trimethobenzamide, vancomycin, vasopressin, vecuronium, verapamil, vinCRIStine, vinorelbine, voriconazole, zidovudine, zoledronic acid

Additive incompatibilities: Carbenicillin, fluorouracil, heparin, regular insulin, nafcillin, oxacillin, penicillin G sodium

Solution compatibilities: Amino acids, 4.25%/D_{25}, D_5/LR, D_5/0.2% NaCl, D_5/0.9% NaCl, D_{10}/0.9% NaCl, D_5W, invert glucose 10% in electrolyte #1, Ringer's LR, 0.9% NaCl, sodium lactate 1/6 mol/L, TPN #57

ADVERSE EFFECTS

CNS: Neuritis, dizziness, headache, cerebellar syndrome, personality changes, ataxia, mechanical dysphasia, **coma; chemical arachnoiditis** (IT)
CV: Chest pain, **cardiopathy**
EENT: Sore throat, conjunctivitis
GI: *Nausea, vomiting, anorexia, diarrhea, stomatitis,* **hepatotoxicity,** abdominal pain, hematemesis, **GI hemorrhage**
GU: Urinary retention, **renal failure, hyperuricemia**
HEMA: **Thrombophlebitis, bleeding, thrombocytopenia, leukopenia, myelosuppression, anemia**
INTEG: *Rash, fever,* freckling, cellulitis
META: Hyperuricemia
MISC: Cytarabine syndrome—fever, myalgia, bone pain, chest pain, rash, conjunctivitis, malaise (6-12 hr after administration)
RESP: **Pneumonia,** dyspnea, **pulmonary edema** (high doses)
SYST: **Anaphylaxis, tumor lysis syndrome**

Pharmacokinetics

Absorption	Complete
Distribution	Widely distributed; crosses blood-brain barrier, placenta
Metabolism	Liver, extensively
Excretion	Kidneys
Half-life	Distribution 10 min; elimination 1-3 hr; IT 100-236 hr

Pharmacodynamics

Unknown

INTERACTIONS
Individual drugs

Digoxin oral: decreased digoxin effects
Filgrastim, G-CSF, GM-CSF, sargramostim: do not use within 24 hr
Flucytosine, methotrexate: increased toxicity, immunosuppression
Gentamicin: decreased effects
Radiation: increased toxicity, bone marrow suppression

Drug classifications

Anticoagulants, NSAIDs, platelet inhibitors, salicylates, thrombolytics: increased bleeding risk

Immunosuppressants, antineoplastics: increased toxicity, bone marrow suppression

Live virus vaccines: do not use together

NURSING CONSIDERATIONS
Assessment

• Assess buccal cavity q8hr for dryness, sores or ulceration, white patches, pain, bleeding, dysphagia; obtain prescription for viscous lidocaine (Xylocaine)

• **Assess symptoms indicating anaphylaxis: rash, pruritus, urticaria, purpuric skin lesions, itching, flushing; resuscitation equipment should be nearby**

⚠ **Assess for chemical arachnoiditis (IT): headache, nausea, vomiting, fever; neck rigidity/pain, meningism, CSF pleocytosis; may be decreased by dexamethasone**

• Assess tachypnea, dyspnea, edema, fatigue; identify dyspnea, crackles, unproductive cough, chest pain, tachypnea; pulmonary edema may be fatal (rare)

⚠ **Assess for cytarabine syndrome 6-12 hr after infusion: fever, myalgia, bone pain, chest pain, rash, conjunctivitis, malaise; corticosteroid may be ordered**

• **Bone marrow suppression:** Monitor CBC, differential, platelet count weekly; withhold product if WBC count is <1000/mm³ or platelet count is <50,000/mm³

• Assess for increased uric acid levels, swelling, joint pain primarily in extremities; patient should be well hydrated to prevent urate deposits

• Monitor renal function studies: BUN, creatinine, serum uric acid, urine CCr before and during therapy; I&O ratio; report fall in urine output to <30 ml/hr

• Monitor temp q4hr (may indicate beginning of infection)

⚠ **Hepatotoxicity: Monitor liver function tests before and during therapy (bilirubin, AST, ALT, LDH) as needed or monthly; note yellowing of skin or sclera, dark urine, clay-colored stools, pruritus, abdominal pain, fever, diarrhea; an antispasmodic may be used for GI symptoms**

• Assess for bleeding: hematuria, stool guaiac, bruising or petechiae, mucosa or orifices q8hr; identify inflammation of mucosa, breaks in skin

Patient/family education

• **Advise patient that contraceptive measures are recommended during and 4 mo after therapy**

• Teach patient to avoid use of products containing aspirin or ibuprofen, NSAIDs, razors, commercial mouthwash, since bleeding may occur; to report symptoms of bleeding (hematuria, tarry stools)

• Advise that fever, headache, nausea, vomiting are likely to occur but to continue using dexamethasone with IT administration

• Provide liquid diet: carbonated beverages; gelatin may be added if patient is not nauseated or vomiting

• Provide rinsing of mouth tid-qid with water, club soda; brushing of teeth bid-qid with soft brush or cotton-tipped applicators for stomatitis; use unwaxed dental floss

• Advise patient to report signs of anemia (fatigue, headache, irritability, faintness, shortness of breath)

• Advise patient to avoid foods with citric acid, hot flavor, or rough texture if stomatitis is present, to use sponge brush and rinse with water after each meal; to report stomatitis: any bleeding, white spots, ulcerations in mouth; tell patient to examine mouth daily, report any symptoms

• Instruct patient to report any changes in breathing or coughing even several months after treatment; to avoid crowds and persons with respiratory tract or other infections; neurotoxicity

• Caution patient not to have any vaccinations without the advice of the prescriber; serious reactions can occur

• Advise patient to take 3 L/day fluids to prevent renal damage

Evaluation
Positive therapeutic outcome

• Prevention of rapid division of malignant cells

dabigatran (Rx)

(da-bye-gat'ran)

Pradaxa

Func. class.: Anticoagulant
Chem. Class.: Thrombin inhibitor

Pregnancy category C

ACTION: Direct thrombin inhibitor that inhibits both free and clot-bound thrombin, prevents thrombin-induced platelet aggregation and thrombus formation by preventing conversion of fibrinogen to fibrin

Therapeutic outcome: Decreased thrombus formation/extension, absence of emboli, postthrombotic effects

USES: Stroke/systemic embolism prophylaxis with nonvalvular atrial fibrillation, DVT, pulmonary embolism in hip replacement

CONTRAINDICATIONS

Hypersensitivity, bleeding

Precautions: Abrupt discontinuation, anticoagulant therapy, breastfeeding, pregnancy **C**, children, geriatrics, labor, obstetric delivery, renal disease, surgery

> BLACK BOX WARNING: Abrupt discontinuation

DOSAGE AND ROUTES

Stroke prophylaxis

Adult: PO 150 mg bid

For conversion from an alternative anticoagulant to dabigatran

• When converting from warfarin to dabigatran, discontinue warfarin and initiate dabigatran therapy when the INR is <2.0. When converting from a parenteral anticoagulant to dabigatran, initiate dabigatran 0-2 hr before the time of the next scheduled anticoagulant dose or at the time of discontinuation of a continuously administered anticoagulant (e.g., intravenous unfractionated heparin)

For conversion from dabigatran to warfarin

Adult: CCr >50 ml/min start warfarin 3 days before discontinuing dabigatran; CCr 31-50 ml/min start warfarin 2 days before discontinuing dabigatran; CCr 15-30 ml/min start warfarin 1 day before discontinuing dabigatran

For conversion from dabigatran to parenteral anticoagulants

Adult: PO discontinue dabigatran, start parenteral anticoagulant 12 hr (CCR ≥30 ml/min), 24 hr (CCR <30 ml/min) after the last dabigatran dose

DVT/PE/treated with a parenteral anticoagulant × 5-10 days

Adult: PO 150 mg bid

Deep vein thrombus (DVT)/pulmonary embolism prophylaxis

Adult: PO 220 mg or 150 mg/day 28-35 days, starting with ½ dose 1-4 hr after surgery (knee replacement); 110 on first day 1-4 hr after surgery, hemostasis achieved, then 220 mg qd × 28-35 days; those previously treated 150 mg bid (hip replacement)

Renal dose

Adult: PO CCr 15-30 ml/min 75 mg bid

Available forms: Cap 75, 150 mg

Implementation

• Do not crush, break, chew, or empty contents of capsule
• Take without regard to food
• Store in original package until time of use at room temperature, discard after 30 days, protect from moisture

ADVERSE EFFECTS

CV: Myocardial infarction
CNS: Intracranial bleeding
GI: Abdominal pain, dyspepsia, peptic ulcer, esophagitis, GERD, gastritis, GI bleeding
HEMA: Bleeding (any site)
INTEG: Rash, pruritus
SYST: Anaphylaxis (rare)

Pharmacokinetics

Absorption	Protein binding 35%
Distribution	Unknown
Metabolism	Unknown
Excretion	Unknown
Half-life	12-17 hr (extended in renal disease)

Pharmacodynamics

Onset	Unknown
Peak	1 hr; high-fat meal delays peak
Duration	Unknown

INTERACTIONS

Individual drugs

Amiodarone, clopidogrel, ketoconazole, quiNIDine, verapamil: increased bleeding risk
Rifampin: decreased dabigatran effect

Drug classifications

Anticoagulants, thrombolytics: increased bleeding risk

Drug/herb

St. John's wort: decreased dabigatran effect

NURSING CONSIDERATIONS
Assessment
• **Assess for bleeding:** blood in urine or emesis, dark tarry stools, lower back pain. Caution with arterial/venous punctures, catheters, NG tubes. Monitor vital signs frequently. The elderly are more prone to serious bleeding
• **Assess for thrombosis/MI/emboli: swelling, pain, redness, difficulty breathing, chest pain, tachypnea, cough, coughing up blood, cyanosis**
• **Assess for postthrombotic syndrome:** pain, heaviness, itching/tingling, swelling, varicose veins, brownish/reddish skin discoloration, ulcers; ambulation, compression stockings and adequate anticoagulation can prevent this syndrome
• Monitor serum creatinine

Patient/family education
• Explain the purpose and expected results of this product, store in original container
• If dose is missed take as soon as remembered if on the same day, do not administer if <6 hr before next dose
• Instruct patient to report if bleeding or bruising is present, check with prescriber about when to discontinue
• Advise patient not to use any other OTC products, herbs without prescriber approval
• Inform patient that lab tests will be required during treatment
• Advise patient to keep dry, do not use other containers

Evaluation
Positive therapeutic outcome
• Decreased thrombus formation/extension, absence of emboli, postthrombotic effects

---

dabrafenib
(da-braf′e-nib)
Tafinlar
Func. class.: Antineoplastic
Chem. class.: Signal transduction inhibitor, kinase inhibitor
Pregnancy category D

ACTION: Inhibits kinase, inhibitor against mutated forms of BRAF kinases in melanoma cells

Therapeutic outcome: Decrease in melanoma progression

USES: Unresectable or metastatic BRAD V600E-mutated malignant melanoma

CONTRAINDICATIONS
Pregnancy **D**, hypersensitivity

Precautions: Breastfeeding, children, infection, dehydration, diabetes mellitus, fever, G6PD deficiency, hemolytic anemia, hyperglycemia, hypotension, infertility, iritis, renal failure, secondary malignancy

DOSAGE AND ROUTES
Adult: PO 150 mg q12hr until disease progression, avoid strong CYP3A4/CYP2C8 inhibitors or inducers

Available forms: Caps 50, 75 mg

Implementation
PO route
• Swallow whole
• If dose is missed, take within 6 hr of missed dose, if >6 hr have passed, skip dose
• Space doses q12hr
• Take at least 1 hr before or 2 hr after a meal

ADVERSE EFFECTS
CNS: Headache, fever
GI: *Pancreatitis*
INTEG: Rash, alopecia
MISC: Arthralgia, back pain, hand-foot syndrome, hyperglycemia, hypophosphatemia, hyponatremia, myalgia, **secondary malignancy**

Pharmacokinetics
Absorption	Unknown
Distribution	Protein binding 99.7%
Metabolism	Unknown
Excretion	71% (feces), 23% (urine)
Half-life	8 hr (dabrafenib), 10 hr, 21-22 hr metabolites

Pharmacodynamics
Onset	Unknown
Peak	Unknown
Duration	Unknown

INTERACTIONS
Drug classifications
Antacids, CYP3A4 inducers (dexamethasome, phenytoin, carBAMazepine, rifampin, PHENobarbital), proton-pump inhibitors: decreased dabrafenib concentrations
CYP3A4 inhibitors (ketoconazole, itraconazole, erythromycin, clarithromycin): altered dabrafenib concentrations

Drug/food
Grapefruit juice: increased dabrafenib effect; avoid use while taking product

---

Adverse effects: *italics* = common; **bold** = life-threatening

Drug/herb
St. John's wort: decreased dabrafenib concentrations

NURSING CONSIDERATIONS
Assessment
• Toxicity: Assess for fever, grade 2, 3

Patient/family education
• Instruct patient to report adverse reactions immediately
• Teach patient about reason for treatment, expected results
• Instruct patient to use effective contraception during treatment and for 30 days after discontinuing treatment, pregnancy D

Evaluation

Positive therapeutic outcome
• Decrease in melanoma progression

⚠ HIGH ALERT

dacarbazine (Rx)
(da-kar′ba-zeen)
dacarbazine, DTIC ✤, DTIC-Dome
Func. class.: Antineoplastic—miscellaneous agent
Chem. class.: Imidazole
Pregnancy category C

ACTION: Alkylates DNA, RNA; inhibits RNA, DNA synthesis; also responsible for breakage, cross-linking DNA strands; activity is not cell cycle phase specific

Therapeutic outcome: Prevention of rapidly growing malignant cells

USES: Hodgkin's disease, malignant melanoma

Unlabeled uses: Malignant pheochromocytoma in combination with cyclophosphamide and vinCRIStine, metastatic soft tissue sarcoma in combination with other agents, carcinoma meningitis, neuroblastoma

CONTRAINDICATIONS
Hypersensitivity, breastfeeding

Precautions: Renal disease, infection

> BLACK BOX WARNING: Pregnancy C (1st trimester), radiation therapy, hepatic disease, bone marrow suppression, secondary malignancy

DOSAGE AND ROUTES
Metastatic malignant melanoma
Adult: IV 2-4.5 mg/kg daily × 10 days or 100-250 mg/m^2 daily × 5 days; repeat q3wk depending on response

Hodgkin's disease
Adult: IV 150 mg/m^2 daily × 5 days with other agents, repeat q4wk or 375 mg/m^2 on days 1 and 15 when given in combination, repeat q28day

Osteogenic sarcoma (unlabeled)
Adult and child: IV 250 mg/m^2/day as a cont INF × 4 days in combination with other agents q28day

Soft tissue sarcoma (unlabeled)
Adult and child: IV 250-300 mg/m^2/day as a cont INF × 3 days q21-28day

Available forms: Powder for inj 10, 100, 200 mg

Implementation
• Give fluids IV or PO before chemotherapy to hydrate patient
• Nausea/vomiting may be severe and last several hours
• Give antiemetic 30-60 min before giving product to prevent vomiting, and prn; antibiotics for prophylaxis of infection
• Provide liquid diet: carbonated beverages; gelatin may be added if patient is not nauseated or vomiting

Direct IV route
• After diluting 100 mg/9.9 ml or 200 mg/19.7 ml of sterile water for inj (10 mg/ml), give by direct IV over 2-3 min through Y-tube or 3-way stopcock

Intermittent IV infusion route
• May be further diluted in 50-250 ml of D$_5$W or normal saline for inj and given over 30 min
• Watch for extravasation; stop infusion, apply ice to area
• Store in light-resistant container in a dry area

Y-site compatibilities: Amifostine, aztreonam, filgrastim, fludarabine, granisetron, melphalan, ondansetron, PACLitaxel, sargramostim, teniposide, thiotepa, vinorelbine

ADVERSE EFFECTS
CNS: Facial paresthesia, flushing, fever, malaise, confusion, headache, seizures, cerebral hemorrhage, blurred vision (high doses)
GI: *Nausea, anorexia, vomiting,* hepatotoxicity (rare)
HEMA: Thrombocytopenia, leukopenia, anemia
INTEG: *Alopecia,* dermatitis, pain at inj site, photosensitivity, severe sun reactions (high doses)
MISC: Flulike symptoms, malaise, fever, myalgia, hypotension
SYST: Anaphylaxis

Pharmacokinetics

Absorption	Complete bioavailability (**IV**)
Distribution	Widely distributed; concentrates in liver
Metabolism	Liver (50%, 5% protein bound)
Excretion	Kidneys, unchanged (50%)
Half-life	Terminal 19 min; 5 hr

Pharmacodynamics

Unknown

INTERACTIONS
Individual drugs
PHENobarbital, phenytoin: increased metabolism; decreased dacarbazine effect

Radiation: bone marrow suppression, toxicity

Drug classifications
Aminoglycosides: increased nephrotoxicity

Anticoagulants, NSAIDs, salicylates: increased risk of bleeding

Antineoplastics, bone marrow–suppressing products: increased toxicity, bone marrow suppression

Diuretics, loop: increased ototoxicity

Live virus vaccines: increased adverse reactions; decreased antibody reaction

NURSING CONSIDERATIONS
Assessment
• **Assess symptoms indicating severe allergic reaction: rash, pruritus, urticaria, purpuric skin lesions, itching, flushing; product should be discontinued**

> **BLACK BOX WARNING: Assess for bone marrow suppression:** Monitor CBC, differential, platelet count weekly; withhold product if WBC is <4000/mm³ or platelet count is <75,000/mm³

• Monitor renal function tests: BUN, creatinine, urine CCr before, during therapy; I&O ratio; report fall in urine output to <30 ml/hr

• Monitor temp q4hr (may indicate beginning of infection), I&O, for nausea, appetite

> **BLACK BOX WARNING: Assess for hepatic disease:** Monitor liver function tests before, during therapy (bilirubin, AST, ALT, LDH) as needed or monthly; note jaundice of skin or sclera, dark urine, clay-colored stools, itchy skin, abdominal pain, fever, diarrhea; hepatotoxicity can be serious and fatal

• Assess for bleeding: hematuria, stool guaiac, bruising or petechiae, mucosa or orifices q8hr; check for inflammation of mucosa, breaks in skin

• Assess IV site for irritation, redness, pain; if infiltration occurs use hot packs at site

• Identify effects of alopecia on body image; discuss feelings about body changes

> **BLACK BOX WARNING: Secondary malignancy:** Assess for secondary malignancy that may occur with this product

Patient/family education
• Teach patient to avoid use of products containing aspirin or ibuprofen, razors, commercial mouthwash, since bleeding may occur; to report symptoms of bleeding (hematuria, tarry stools)

⚠ **Instruct patient to report signs of anemia (fatigue, headache, irritability, faintness, shortness of breath)**

• Advise patient that hair may be lost during treatment; a wig or hairpiece may make patient feel better; new hair may be different in color, texture

⚠ **Pregnancy: Teach patient to notify prescriber if pregnancy is planned or suspected pregnancy (D)**

• Caution patient not to have any vaccinations without the advice of prescriber; serious reactions can occur

> **BLACK BOX WARNING:** Advise patient contraception is needed during treatment and for several months after the completion of therapy; product has teratogenic properties

⚠ **Teach patient to report signs of infection: fever, sore throat, flulike symptoms**

Evaluation
Positive therapeutic outcome
• Prevention of rapid division of malignant cells

dalbavancin
(dal-ba-van′sin)
Dalvance
Func. class.: Antiinfective-glycopeptide
Pregnancy category C

ACTION: Binds to the bacterial cell walls, inhibiting their synthesis

Therapeutic outcome: Decreased symptoms of infection, negative C&S

USES: Treatment of acute bacterial skin and skin structure infections caused by gram-positive organisms (cellulitis, major abscess, wound infections)

CONTRAINDICATIONS: Hypersensitivity

Precautions: Antimicrobial resistance, breastfeeding, colitis, diarrhea, GI disease, inflammatory bowel disease, infusion-related reactions, pregnancy, pseudomembranous colitis, ulcerative colitis, vancomycin hypersensitivity, viral infection

DOSAGE AND ROUTES
Adult: **IV** 1000 mg once, then 500 mg **IV** 1 wk later

Available forms: Powder for injection 500 mg

Implementation
IV infusion route
- Visually inspect parenteral products for particulate matter and discoloration
- **Reconstitution:** Reconstitute each 500 mg/25 ml sterile water for injection; to avoid foaming, alternate between gentle swirling and inversion until completely dissolved, do not shake; further dilution is required
- **Storage:** Refrigerate or store at room temperature. Do not freeze. Total time from reconstitution to dilution to use should not exceed 48 hr
- **Dilution:** Transfer the dose of reconstituted solution from the vial(s) to an IV bag or bottle containing D₅W (1-5 mg/ml)

Intermittent IV INF
- Give over 30 min, do not infuse with other medications or electrolytes
- Saline-based infusion solutions may cause precipitation and should not be used
- If a common IV line is being used to administer other drugs, the line should be flushed before and after each dose

ADVERSE EFFECTS
CNS: Dizziness, headache, flushing
GI: Nausea, vomiting, pseudomembranous colitis, GI bleeding, abdominal pain, diarrhea
HEMA: Thrombocytopenia, neutropenia, leukopenia, anemia
INTEG: Rash, urticaria, infusion-related reactions, pruritus
SYST: Red man syndrome, hypersensitivity reactions

Pharmacokinetics

Absorption	Unknown
Distribution	Protein binding 93%, primarily to albumin
Metabolism	Decreased in renal disease
Excretion	Feces and urine
Half-life	Unknown

Pharmacodynamics

Onset	Unknown
Peak	Unknown
Duration	Unknown

INTERACTIONS
Drug classifications
Oral contraceptives: decreased with prolonged use

Drug/lab test
Increased: LFTs

NURSING CONSIDERATIONS
Assessment
- Assess: BUN/creatinine, lower dose may be required in severe renal disease
- Pseudomembranous colitis: bowel pattern daily, if severe diarrhea occurs, product should be discontinued
- IV site for INF-site reactions
- Anaphylaxis: rash, urticaria, pruritus, wheezing, may occur a few days after administration
- Red man syndrome: flushing, rash over upper torso and neck, may occur after a few minutes of infusion, may be treated with antihistamines and a slower infusion

Patient/family education
- Teach patient to report sore throat, bruising, bleeding, joint pain (blood dyscrasias), diarrhea with mucus, blood (pseudomembranous colitis)
- Advise patient to use nonhormonal contraceptive if on long-term therapy (controversial)

Evaluation
Positive therapeutic outcome
- Decreased symptoms of infection, negative C&S

---

dalfampridine (Rx)
(dal-fam′pri-deen)
Ampyra, Fampyra ✤
Func. class.: Neurological agent—MS
Chem. class.: Broad-spectrum potassium channel blocker
Pregnancy category C

ACTION: Mechanism of action is not fully understood, a broad-spectrum potassium channel blocker inhibits potassium channels and increased action potential conduction in demyelinated axons

Therapeutic outcome: Ability to walk at improved speed in MS

USES: For improved walking in patients with multiple sclerosis

CONTRAINDICATIONS
Renal failure (CCr <50 ml/min), seizures

Precautions: Pregnancy **C**, breastfeeding, renal disease, elderly

DOSAGE AND ROUTES
Adult: PO 10 mg q12hr

Renal dose
Adult: PO CCr 51-80 ml/min no dosage adjustment needed, but seizure risk is unknown; CCr ≤50 ml/min, do not use

Available forms: Ext rel tab 10 mg

Implementation
• Do not break, crush, or chew; give without regard to meals
• Do not give closer together than q12hr, seizures may occur
• Do not double doses, if a dose is missed, skip it

ADVERSE EFFECTS
CNS: Seizures, paresthesias, headache, dizziness, asthenia, insomnia
GI: Nausea, constipation, dyspepsia
GU: Urinary tract infection
MS: Back pain

Pharmacokinetics

Absorption	Bioavailability 96%
Distribution	Largely unbound to plasma proteins
Metabolism	Unknown
Excretion	96% is recovered in the urine
Half-life	Unknown

Pharmacodynamics

Onset	Unknown
Peak	3-4 hr (fasting), longer if taken with food
Duration	Unknown

INTERACTIONS
Individual drugs
Fampridine: do not use together

Drug classifications
4-aminopyridine (4-AP)-containing products: do not use together

NURSING CONSIDERATIONS
Assessment
• **Multiple sclerosis:** assess walking, including speed
• **Assess for seizures:** more common in those with previous seizure disorder

Patient/family education
• Advise patient to notify prescriber if pregnancy is planned or suspected, do not breastfeed

• Teach patient about expected results, side effects including seizures

Evaluation

Positive therapeutic outcome
• Ability to walk at improved speed in MS

▲ HIGH ALERT

D

dalteparin (Rx)
(dahl'ta-pear-in)
Fragmin
Func. class.: Anticoagulant
Chem. class.: Low-molecular-weight heparin
Pregnancy category B

ACTION: Inhibits factor Xa/IIa (thrombin), resulting in anticoagulation

Therapeutic outcome: Absence of deep vein thrombosis

USES: Unstable angina/non-Q-wave MI; prevention/treatment of deep vein thrombosis in abdominal surgery, hip replacement patients or those with restricted mobility during acute illness; pulmonary embolism

Unlabeled uses: Antiphospholipid antibody, arterial thromboembolism (after heart valve surgery), cerebral thromboembolism, acute MI

CONTRAINDICATIONS
Hypersensitivity to this product, heparin, pork products; active major bleeding, hemophilia, leukemia with bleeding, thrombocytopenic purpura, cerebrovascular hemorrhage, cerebral aneurysm, those undergoing regional anesthesia for unstable angina, non–Q-wave MI, dalteparin-induced thrombocytopenia

Precautions: Hypersensitivity to benzyl alcohol, pregnancy **B**, recent childbirth, breastfeeding, child, geriatric, hepatic disease, severe renal/cardiac disease, blood dyscrasias, bacterial endocarditis, acute nephritis, peptic ulcer disease, pericarditis, pericardial effusion, recent lumbar puncture, vasculitis, other diseases where bleeding is possible, uncontrolled hypertension; recent brain, spine, eye surgery; congenital or acquired disorders, hemorrhagic stroke, history of HIT

BLACK BOX WARNING: Epidural anesthesia, lumbar puncture

DOSAGE AND ROUTES
Deep vein thrombosis/pulmonary embolism
Adult: SUBCUT 200 international units/kg/day during 1st month (max single dose 18,000 international units), then 150 IU/kg/day in month 2-6 (max single dose 18,000 international units), use prefilled syringe that is closest to calculated dose; if platelets are 50,000-100,000/mm³ reduce dose by 2500 international units until platelets ≥100,000/mm³; if platelets <50,000/mm³ discontinue until >50,000/mm³

Hip replacement surgery/DVT prophylaxis
Adult: SUBCUT 2500 international units 2 hr before surgery and 2nd dose in the evening the day of surgery (4-8 hr postop), then 5000 international units SUBCUT 1st postop day and daily 5-10 days

Unstable angina/non-Q-wave MI
Adult: SUBCUT 120 international units/kg q12hr × 5-8 days; max 10,000 international units q12hr × 5-8 days with concurrent aspirin, continue until stable

Deep vein thrombosis, prophylaxis for abdominal surgery
Adult: SUBCUT 2500 international units 1-2 hr prior to abdominal surgery and repeat daily × 5-10 days; in high-risk patients >3400 international units should be used

Renal dose
Adult: SUBCUT cancer patient with CCr <30 ml/min, monitor and adjust based on antifactor Xa

Available forms: Prefilled syringes, 2500, 5000 international units/0.2 ml; 7500 international units/0.3 ml, 10,000, 12,500, 15,000, 18,000 international units/ml

Implementation
SUBCUT route
• Cannot be used interchangeably unit for unit with unfractionated heparin or other LMWHs
• Do not give IM or **IV** product route; approved in SUBCUT only; do not mix with other inj or sol
• Give by SUBCUT only; have patient sit or lie down; SUBCUT inj may be 2 in from umbilicus in a U-shape, upper outer side of thigh, around navel, or upper outer quadrangle of the buttocks; rotate inj sites
• Change inj site daily, use at same time of day

ADVERSE EFFECTS
CNS: Intracranial bleeding
HEMA: Thrombocytopenia
INTEG: Alopecia, pruritus, superficial wound infection, skin necrosis, injection site reaction

SYST: Hypersensitivity, hemorrhage, anaphylaxis possible, hematoma

Pharmacokinetics

Absorption	87%
Distribution	Unknown
Metabolism	Liver
Excretion	Kidney
Half-life	3-5 hr elimination

Pharmacodynamics

Onset	Unknown
Peak	2-4 hr
Duration	Unknown

INTERACTIONS
Individual drugs
Aspirin: increased bleeding risk

Drug classifications
Anticoagulants, NSAIDs, platelet inhibitors, some cephalosporins, salicylates, thrombolytics: increased risk of bleeding

Drug/herb
Feverfew, garlic, ginger, ginkgo, horse chestnut: increased bleeding risk

NURSING CONSIDERATIONS
Assessment
• Assess for bleeding (Hct, occult blood in stools) during treatment since bleeding can occur
⚠ Assess for bleeding gums, petechiae, ecchymosis, black tarry stools, hematuria, epistaxis, decrease in Hct, B/P; may indicate bleeding, possible hemorrhage; notify prescriber immediately; product should be discontinued
• Assess for hypersensitivity: fever, skin rash, urticaria; notify prescriber immediately
• Assess for needed dosage change q1-2wk; dosage may need to be decreased if bleeding occurs

> **BLACK BOX WARNING:** Epidural anesthesia: Assess for neurologic impairment frequently when neuraxial anesthesia has been used, spinal/epidural hematomas can occur, with paralysis

Patient/family education
• Advise patient to avoid OTC preparations that contain aspirin, other anticoagulants; serious product interaction may occur
• Advise patient to use soft-bristle toothbrush to avoid bleeding gums, avoid contact sports, use electric razor, avoid IM inj

D

- Instruct patient to report any signs of bleeding: gums, under skin, urine, stools; unusual bruising

Evaluation

Positive therapeutic outcome
- Absence of deep vein thrombosis

TREATMENT OF OVERDOSE:
Protamine sulfate 1% given **IV**; 1 mg protamine/100 anti-Xa international units of dalteparin given

dantrolene (Rx)
(dan′troe-leen)
Dantrium, Revonto
Func. class.: Skeletal muscle relaxant, direct acting
Chem. class.: Hydantoin
Pregnancy category C

Do not confuse: Dantrium/danazol

ACTION: Interferes with intracellular release from the sarcoplasmic reticulum of calcium necessary to initiate contraction; slows catabolism in malignant hyperthermia

Therapeutic outcome: Decreased muscle spasticity; absence of malignant hyperthermia

USES: Spasticity in multiple sclerosis, stroke, spinal cord injury, cerebral palsy, prevention and treatment of malignant hyperthermia

Unlabeled uses: Neuroleptic malignant syndrome

CONTRAINDICATIONS
Hypersensitivity, compromised pulmonary function, active hepatic disease, impaired myocardial function

BLACK BOX WARNING: Active hepatic disease

Precautions: Pregnancy **C,** breastfeeding, geriatric, peptic ulcer disease, renal/cardiac/hepatic, stroke, seizure disorder, diabetes mellitus, ALS, COPD, MS, mannitol/gelatin hypersensitivity, labor, lactase deficiency, extravasation

BLACK BOX WARNING: Females >35 yr, with MS or taking estrogens

DOSAGE AND ROUTES
Spasticity
Adult: PO 25 mg/day; may increase to 25-100 mg bid-qid, max 400 mg/day, may be increased q7days as needed
Child: PO 0.5 mg/kg/day given in divided doses bid; may be increased q7days as needed; max 400 mg daily

Malignant hyperthermia
Adult and child: **IV** 1 mg/kg; may repeat to total dose of 10 mg/kg; PO 4-8 mg/kg/day in 4 divided doses × 1-3 days to prevent further hyperthermia; postcrisis follow-up 4-8 mg/kg/day for 1-3 days

Prevention of malignant hyperthermia
Adult and child: PO 4-8 mg/kg/day in 3-4 divided doses × 1-2 days before procedures; give last dose 4 hr preoperatively; **IV** 2.5 mg/kg prior to anesthesia

Neuroleptic malignant syndrome (unlabeled)
Adult: PO 100-300 mg/day in divided doses, **IV** 1.25-1.5 mg/kg

Available forms: Caps 25, 50, 100 mg; powder for inj 20 mg/vial

Implementation
PO route
- Do not crush or chew caps; caps may be opened and mixed with juice and swallowed; drink immediately after mixing
- Give with meals for GI symptoms
- Store in airtight container at room temperature

IV route
- Administer **IV** after diluting 20 mg/60 ml sterile water for inj without bacteriostatic agent (333 mcg/ml); shake until clear; give by rapid **IV** push through Y-tube or 3-way stopcock; follow by prescribed doses immediately; may also give by intermittent inf over 1 hr before anesthesia; assess site for extravasation, phlebitis
- Protect diluted sol from light; use reconstituted sol within 6 hr
- Considered incompatible in sol or syringe, compatibility unknown

ADVERSE EFFECTS
CNS: *Dizziness, weakness, fatigue, drowsiness,* headache, disorientation, insomnia, paresthesias, tremors, seizures
CV: Hypotension, chest pain, palpitations, tachycardia
EENT: Nasal congestion, blurred vision, mydriasis, excessive lacrimation
GI: Hepatic injury, *nausea,* constipation, vomiting, increased AST and alkaline phosphatase, abdominal pain, dry mouth, anorexia, hepatitis, dyspepsia
GU: Urinary frequency, nocturia, impotence, crystalluria, hepatitis
HEMA: Eosinophilia, aplastic anemia, leukopenia, thrombocytopenia/lymphoma
INTEG: Rash, pruritus, photosensitivity, extravasation (tissue necrosis), phlebitis
RESP: Pleural effusion, pulmonary edema

Pharmacokinetics

Absorption	PO (30%-35%), poor
Distribution	Unknown
Metabolism	Liver, extensively
Excretion	Kidney
Half-life	9 hr

Pharmacodynamics

	PO	IV
Onset	Unknown	Immediate
Peak	5 hr	5 hr
Duration	Dose related	Dose related

INTERACTIONS
• Considered incompatible in sol or syringe; compatibility unknown

Individual drugs
Alcohol: increased CNS depression
Verapamil: increased dysrhythmias

Drug classifications
Antidepressants (tricyclic), antihistamines, barbiturates, opiates, sedative/hypnotics: increased CNS depression, tramadol
Estrogens, hepatotoxic agents: increased hepatotoxicity

NURSING CONSIDERATIONS
Assessment
• Monitor I&O ratio; check for urinary retention, frequency, hesitancy, especially geriatric
• **Seizures:** Monitor ECG in epileptic patients; poor seizure control has occurred with patients taking this product; assess for increased seizure activity in epilepsy patient

> **BLACK BOX WARNING: Active hepatic disease:** Monitor hepatic function by frequent determination of AST, ALT, bilirubin, alkaline phosphatase, GGTP; renal function studies; CBC; use lowest dose possible; check for jaundice, dark urine, diarrhea, weakness; product should be discontinued

• Assess for allergic reactions: rash, fever, respiratory distress
• Monitor for severe weakness, numbness in extremities
• Assess for CNS depression: dizziness, drowsiness, psychiatric symptoms

> **BLACK BOX WARNING: Assess for signs of hepatotoxicity:** Jaundice, yellow sclera, pain in abdomen, nausea, fever; product should be discontinued if these signs and symptoms occur

Patient/family education
• Caution patient not to discontinue product quickly, hallucinations, spasticity, tachycardia will occur; product should be tapered over 1-2 wk; notify prescriber of abdominal pain, jaundiced sclera, clay-colored stools, change in color of urine, rash, itching
• Caution patient not to take with alcohol, other CNS depressants; severe CNS depression can occur; avoid using OTC medication (cough preparations, antihistamines, alcohol, other CNS depressants), unless directed by prescriber, to take with meals
• Tell patient that if improvement does not occur within 6 wk, prescriber may discontinue
• Caution patient to avoid hazardous activities if drowsiness, dizziness, blurred vision occurs; wait several days to identify patient response to medication
• Advise patient to report severe weakness, seizures, signs of liver insufficiency
• Teach patient to use sunscreen, protective clothing for photosensitivity
• Instruct patient to take medication as prescribed; do not double doses; take missed dose within 1 hr of scheduled time
• **Malignant hyperthermia:** These patients should use a medical ID stating condition, products used

Evaluation
Positive therapeutic outcome
• Decreased pain, spasticity
• Absence or decreased symptoms of malignant hyperthermia

TREATMENT OF OVERDOSE:
Activated charcoal, supportive care

dapagliflozin
(dap'a-gli-floe'zin)
Farxiga
Func. class.: Oral antidiabetic
Chem. class.: SGLT-2 inhibitor
Pregnancy category C

ACTION: Blocks reabsorption of glucose by the kidneys, increases glucose excretion, lowers blood glucose concentrations

Therapeutic outcome: Improved signs/symptoms of diabetes mellitus (decreased polyuria, polydipsia, polyphagia; clear sensorium, absence of dizziness, stable gait); HbA1c WNL

USES: Type 2 diabetes mellitus, with diet and exercise

CONTRAINDICATIONS
Dialysis, renal failure, hypersensitivity, breast-feeding, diabetic ketoacidosis

Precautions: Pregnancy C, children, renal/hepatic disease, hypothyroidism, hyperglycemia, hypotension, bladder cancer, hypercholesterolemia, pituitary insufficiency, type 1 diabetes mellitus, malnutrition, fever, dehydration, adrenal insufficiency, geriatrics, genital fungal infections, hypoglycemia

DOSAGE AND ROUTES
Adult: PO 5 mg in AM; may increase to 10 mg/day if needed

Renal dose
Adult: PO eGFR ≥60 ml/min/1.73m², no change; eGFR<60 ml/min, do not use

Available forms: Tabs 5, 10 mg

Implementation
PO route
• Give once/day in AM without regard to food

ADVERSE EFFECTS
CNS: Dizziness, fatigue
GI: Abdominal pain, pancreatitis, constipation, nausea
GU: Cystitis, candidiasis, urinary frequency, polydipsia, polyuria, increased serum creatinine, renal impairment/failure, infections
META: Hypercholesterolemia, lipidemia, hypoglycemia, hyperkalemia, hypomagnesemia, hypophosphatemia/hyperphosphatemia
MISC: Bone fractures, hypotension, dehydration, orthostatic hypotension, hypersensitivity, new bladder cancer; increased hematocrit

Pharmacokinetics

Absorption	Unknown
Distribution	91% protein binding
Metabolism	Primarily metabolized by O-glucuronidation by UGT1A9; minor CYP3A4
Excretion	Urine
Half-life	12.9 hr

Pharmacodynamics

Onset	Unknown
Peak	Less than 2 hr
Duration	Unknown

INTERACTIONS
Individual drugs:
Baclofen, cycloSPORINE, isoniazid, tacrolimus: decreased effect, hyperglycemia

Bortezomib, lithium: increased or decreased glycemic control
Gatifloxacin: do not use concurrently

Drug classifications
Androgens, quinolones: increased or decreased glycemic control
ACE inhibitors, angiotensin II receptor antagonists, bile acid sequestrates, β-blockers, fibric acid derivatives, insulins, MAOIs, salicylates, sulfonylureas: increased hypoglycemia
Atypical antipsychotics, carbonic anhydrase inhibitors, corticosteroids, digestive enzymes, estrogen, intestinal absorbents, loop diuretics, oral contraceptives, phenothiazines, progestins, protease inhibitors, sympathomimetics, thiazide diuretics: decrease effect, hyperglycemia

NURSING CONSIDERATIONS
Assessment
• Hypoglycemia (assess hunger, dizziness, tremors, anxiety, tachycardia, sweating, weakness), hyperglycemia; even though product does not cause hyperglycemia, if patient is on sulfonylureas or insulin, hypoglycemia may be additive; if hypoglycemia occurs, treat with dextrose, or, if severe, with IV glucagon; HbA1c; lipid panel; renal function tests; volume status; blood pressure

Patient/family education
• Teach patient the symptoms of hypoglycemia and hyperglycemia, what to do about each
• Instruct patient that medication must be taken as prescribed; explain consequences of discontinuing medication abruptly; that insulin may need to be used for stress, including trauma, fever, surgery
• Instruct patient to avoid OTC medications and herbal supplements unless approved by health care provider
• Instruct patient that diabetes is a lifelong illness; that the diet and exercise regimen must be followed; that this product is not a cure
• Instruct patient to carry emergency ID and glucose source
• Instruct patient that blood glucose monitoring is required to assess product effect
• Instruct patient that GI side effects may occur
• Instruct patient that there is a risk of renal impairment, dehydration, and new bladder cancer

Evaluation
Positive therapeutic outcome
• Improved signs/symptoms of diabetes mellitus (decreased polyuria, polydipsia, polyphagia); clear sensorium, absence of dizziness, stable gait; HbA1c WNL

DAPTOmycin (Rx)

(dap'toe-mye-sin)

Cubicin

Func. class.: Antiinfective—miscellaneous
Chem. class.: Lipopeptides
Pregnancy category B

ACTION: New class of antiinfective; binds to the bacterial membrane and results in a rapid depolarization of the membrane potential, leading to inhibition of DNA, RNA, and protein synthesis

Therapeutic outcome: Absence of infections

USES: Complicated skin, skin structure infections caused by *Staphylococcus aureus,* (MRSA, MSSA) including methicillin-resistant strains, *Streptococcus pyogenes, S. agalactiae, S. dysgalactiae* (vancomycin-susceptible strains only), *Streptococcus pyogenes* (group A beta hemolytic), *Staphylococcus aureus, Staphylococcus epidermidis,* bone, joint infection, infectious arthritis, orthopedic device-related infection, osteomyelitis

CONTRAINDICATIONS

Hypersensitivity

Precautions: Pregnancy **B,** breastfeeding, children, geriatrics, GI/renal disease, myopathy, ulcerative/pseudomembranous colitis, rhabdomyolysis, eosinophilic pneumonia

DOSAGE AND ROUTES

Adult: IV INF 4-6 mg/kg over ½ hr diluted in 0.9% NaCl, give q24hr × 7-14 days
Adolescent/child/infant ≥5 mo (unlabeled): IV 4-6 mg/kg/day

Staphylococcus aureus bacteremia, including right-sided infective endocarditis

Adult: IV INF 6 mg/kg/day × 2-6 wk, up to 8-10 mg/kg/day, treatment failures should use another agent

Renal dose

Adult: IV CCr <30 ml/min; hemodialysis, CAPD 4 mg/kg q48hr, 6 mg/kg q48hr (bacteremia)

Available forms: Lyophilized powder for inj 500 mg

Implementation

Intermittent IV infusion route

• Give after reconstitution with 10 ml 0.9% NaCl (500 mg/10 ml), further dilution is needed with 0.9% NaCl; infuse over ½ hr

Direct IV route

• Give reconstituted sol (50 mg/ml) by direct IV inj over 2 min
• Refrigerate vials, for single use only, discard unused portion; prepared solutions are stable for 12 hr at room temperature or 48 hr refrigerated

Y-site compatibilities: Alfentanil, amifostine, amikacin, aminocaproic acid, aminophylline, amiodarone, amphotericin B liposome, ampicillin, ampicillin-sulbactam, argatroban, arsenic trioxide, atenolol, atracurium, azithromycin, aztreonam, bivalirudin, bleomycin, bumetanide, buprenorphine, busulfan, butorphanol, calcium chloride/gluconate, CARBOplatin, carmustine, caspofungin, ceFAZolin, cefepime, cefotaxime, cefoTEtan, cefOXitin, cefTAZidime, ceftizoxime, cefTRIAXone, cefuroxime, chloramphenicol, chlorproMAZINE, cimetidine, ciprofloxacin, cisatracurium, CISplatin, clindamycin, cyclophosphamide, cycloSPORINE, dacarbazine, DACTINomycin, DAUNOrubicin, dexamethasone, dexmedetomidine, dexrazoxane, diazepam, digoxin, diltiazem, diphenhydrAMINE, DOBUTamine, DOCEtaxel, DOPamine, doripenem, doxacurium, DOXOrubicin, DOXOrubicin liposomal, doxycycline, droperidol, enalaprilat, ePHEDrine, EPINEPHrine, epirubicin, eptifibatide, ertapenem, erythromycin, esmolol, etoposide, famotidine, fenoldopam, fentaNYL, fluconazole, fludarabine, fluorouracil, foscarnet, fosphenytoin, furosemide, ganciclovir, gentamicin, glycopyrrolate, granisetron, haloperidol, heparin, hydrALAZINE, hydrocortisone, HYDROmorphone, hydrOXYzine, IDArubicin, ifosfamide, inamrinone, insulin (regular), irinotecan, isoproterenol, ketorolac, labetalol, lepuridin, leucovorin, levofloxacin, lidocaine, linezolid, LORazepam, magnesium sulfate, mannitol, mechlorethamine, melphalan, meperidine, meropenem, mesna, metaraminol, methyldopate, methylPREDNISolone, metoclopramide, metoprolol, midazolam, milrinone, mitoXANtrone, mivacurium, morphine, moxifloxacin, mycophenolate mofetil, nafcillin, nalbuphine, naloxone, niCARdipine, nitroprusside, norepinephrine, octreotide, ondansetron, oxaliplatin, oxytocin, PACLitaxel, palonosetron, pamidronate, pancuronium, PEMEtrexed, pentamidine, PHENobarbital, phenylephrine, piperacillin-tazobactam, polymyxin B, potassium acetate/chloride/phosphates, procainamide, prochlorperazine, promethazine, propranolol, quinupristin-dalfopristin, ranitidine, rocuronium, sodium acetate/bicarbonate/citrate/phosphates, succinylcholine, sulfamethoxazole-trimethoprim, tacrolimus, teniposide, theophylline, thiotepa, ticarcillin, ticarcillin-clavulanate, tigecycline, tirofiban, tobramycin, topotecan, trimethobenzamide, vasopressin, vecuronium, verapamil, vinBLAStine, vinCRIStine, vinorelbine, voriconazole, zidovudine, zoledronic acid

Solution compatibilities: 0.9% NaCl, LR

ADVERSE EFFECTS
CNS: Headache, insomnia, dizziness, confusion, anxiety, fatigue, fever
CV: Hypo/hypertension, heart failure, chest pain
GI: Nausea, constipation, diarrhea, vomiting, dyspepsia, pseudomembranous colitis, abdominal pain, stomatitis, xerostomia, anorexia
GU: Nephrotoxicity: increased BUN
HEMA: Leukocytosis, anemia, thrombocytopenia
INTEG: Rash, pruritus
META: Electrolyte imbalances
MISC: Fungal infections, UTI, anemia, hypoglycemia
MS: Muscle pain or weakness, arthralgia, pain, rhabdomyolysis, myopathy
RESP: Cough, eosinophilic pneumonia, dyspnea
SYST: Anaphylaxis, DRESS, Stevens-Johnson syndrome

Pharmacokinetics
Absorption	Unknown
Distribution	Protein binding 92%
Metabolism	Unknown
Excretion	Breast milk
Half-life	Unknown

Pharmacodynamics
Unknown

INTERACTIONS
Drug classifications
Increase: daptomycin action-tobramycin
Increase: tobramycin levels
HMG-CoA reductase inhibitors: myopathy

Drug/lab test
Increased: CPK, AST, ALT, BUN, creatinine, albumin, LDH
Increased/decreased: glucose
Decreased: alk phos, magnesium, phosphate, bicarbonate

NURSING CONSIDERATIONS
Assessment
• Assess signs of infection, C&S, product may be given as soon as culture is taken
⚠ Rhabdomyolysis: check for myopathy CPK >1000 U/L (5×ULN), discontinue product, muscle pain, weakness
⚠ Nephrotoxicity: Monitor any patient with compromised renal system: BUN, creatinine; toxicity may occur

• Bowel function: Assess for diarrhea, fever, abdominal pain; report to prescriber; Pseudomembranous colitis may occur
⚠ Monitor I&O ratio: report hematuria, oliguria; nephrotoxicity may occur
• Eosinophilic pneumonia: Assess for dyspnea, fever, cough, shortness of breath, if left untreated can lead to respiratory failure and death
• Monitor blood tests: CBC
• Monitor C&S, product may be given as soon as culture is taken
• Monitor B/P during administration; hypo/hypertension may occur
• Identify allergies before treatment, reaction of each medication

Patient/family education
• Teach all aspects of product therapy
• Advise patient to report sore throat, fever, fatigue; could indicate **superinfection; shortness of breath;** diarrhea; muscle weakness, pain
• Instruct patient to avoid breastfeeding

Evaluation

Positive therapeutic outcome
• Negative culture

⚠ HIGH ALERT

darbepoetin (Rx)
(dar'bee-poh'-eh-tin)
Aranesp
Func. class.: Hematopoietic agent
Chem. class.: Recombinant human erythropoietin
Pregnancy category C

ACTION: Stimulates erythropoiesis by the same mechanism as endogenous erythropoietin; in response to hypoxia, erythropoietin is produced in the kidney and released into the bloodstream, where it interacts with progenitor stem cells to increase red cell production

Therapeutic outcome: Decreased anemia with increased RBCs

USES: Anemia associated with chronic renal failure in patients on and not on dialysis and anemic in nonmyeloid malignancies receiving coadministered chemotherapy

CONTRAINDICATIONS
Hypersensitivity to hamster proteins, human albumin, polysorbate 80; uncontrolled hypertension, red cell aplasia

Precautions: Pregnancy **C,** breastfeeding, children, seizure disorder, porphyria, hypertension, sickle cell disease, vit B$_{12}$, folate deficiency, chronic renal failure, dialysis, latex hypersensitivity, CABG, angina, anemia

> **BLACK BOX WARNING:** Hgb >11 g/dl, neoplastic disease

DOSAGE AND ROUTES
Correction of anemia in chronic renal failure
Adult: SUBCUT/**IV** 0.45 mcg/kg as a single inj, titrate max target Hgb of 11 g/dl

Chemotherapy treatment
Adult: SUBCUT 2.5 mcg/kg/wk or 500 mcg q3wk

Epoetin alfa to darbepoetin conversion
Adult: SUBCUT/**IV** (epoetin alfa <2500 units/wk) 6.25 mcg/wk; (epoetin alfa 2500-4999 units/wk) 12.5 mcg/wk; (epoetin alfa 5000-10,999 units/wk) 25 mcg/wk; (epoetin alfa 11,000-17,999 units/wk) 40 mcg/wk; (epoetin alfa 18,000-33,999 units/wk) 60 mcg/wk; (epoetin alfa 34,000-89,999 units/wk) 100 mcg/wk; (epoetin alfa >90,000 units/wk) 200 mcg/wk

Available forms: Sol for inj 25, 40, 60, 100, 150, 200, 300, 500 mcg/ml

Implementation
• Transfusions may still be required for anemia, use iron supplements with this product

IV/SUBCUT route
• Do not shake, do not dilute, do not mix with other products or solutions
• Check for discoloration, particulate matter; do not use if present; discard unused portion; do not pool unused portion
• Store refrigerated, do not freeze, protect from light

ADVERSE EFFECTS
CNS: *Seizures*, sweating, headache, dizziness, stroke
CV: *Hypo/hypertension*, cardiac arrest, *angina pectoris*, thrombosis, CHF, acute MI, dysrhythmias, chest pain, transient ischemic attacks, edema
GI: *Diarrhea, vomiting, nausea, abdominal pain, constipation*
HEMA: Red cell aplasia
MISC: *Infection, fatigue, fever,* death, *fluid overload*, vascular access hemorrhage, dehydration, sepsis
MS: *Bone pain, myalgia, limb pain, back pain*
RESP: *Upper respiratory infection, dyspnea, cough, bronchitis,* pulmonary embolism
SYST: Allergic reactions, anaphylaxis

Pharmacokinetics

Absorption	Slow, rate-limiting (SUBCUT)
Distribution	Vascular space
Metabolism	Metabolized in body (**IV**), extent unknown
Excretion	Unknown
Half-life	49 hr

Pharmacodynamics

Onset	Onset of increased reticulocyte count 1-6 wk
Peak	34 hr
Duration	Unknown

INTERACTIONS
Individual drugs
⚠ Do not use epoetin alfa with this product

Drug classifications
Androgens: increased darbepoetin alfa effect

Drug/lab test
Increased: WBC, platelets, Hgb
Decreased: bleeding time

NURSING CONSIDERATIONS
Assessment
• **Assess for serious allergic reactions:** rash, urticaria; if anaphylaxis occurs, stop product, administer emergency treatment (rare)

> **BLACK BOX WARNING:** Assess blood studies: ferritin, transferrin monthly; transferrin sat ≥20%, ferritin ≥100 ng/ml; Hgb 2 ×/wk until stabilized in target range (30%-33%), then at regular intervals; those with endogenous erythropoietin levels of <500 units/L respond to this agent, if there is lack of response, obtain folic acid, iron, B$_{12}$ levels

> **BLACK BOX WARNING:** Assess renal studies: urinalysis, protein, blood, BUN, creatinine, those with renal dysfunction may be at greater risk of death

• Assess B/P, Hct; check for rising B/P as Hct rises; antihypertensives may be needed
⚠ Assess CV status: hypertension may occur rapidly, leading to hypertensive encephalopathy; Hgb >11 g/dl may lead to death
• Assess I&O ratio; report drop in output to <50 ml/hr
• Assess for **seizures** if Hgb is increased within 2 wk by 4 points
• **Assess CNS symptoms: cold sensation, sweating, pain in long bones**

BLACK BOX WARNING: Assess **dialysis patients** for thrill, bruit of shunts; monitor for circulation impairment

BLACK BOX WARNING: Neoplastic disease: breast, non-small cell lung, head and neck, lymphoid or cervical cancers, increased tumor progression, use lowest dose to avoid RBC transfusion

Patient/family education
• Caution patient to avoid driving or hazardous activity during beginning of treatment
• Advise patient to monitor B/P, max Hgb 11 g/dl
• Advise patient to take iron supplements, vit B₁₂, folic acid as directed

BLACK BOX WARNING: Advise patient to report chest pain, shortness of breath, swelling/pain in legs, confusion, inability to speak to prescriber, to comply with treatment regimen

• Teach patient that menses may return, use contraception
• Teach home administration and review information for patients and caregivers if home administration is deemed appropriate

BLACK BOX WARNING: Seizures: discuss injury prevention in those that are prone to seizures

BLACK BOX WARNING: Facility must be enrolled in the ESA APPRISE oncology program (866-284-8089) to use this product in cancer treatment

Evaluation
Positive therapeutic outcome
• Increased reticulocyte count, Hgb/Hct
• Increased appetite
• Enhanced sense of well-being

TREATMENT OF OVERDOSE: If polycythemia occurs, discontinue product temporarily; perform phlebotomy if clinically indicated

darifenacin
(da-ree-fen′ah-sin)
Enablex
Func. class.: Antispasmodic/GU anticholinergic
Pregnancy category C

ACTION: Bladder smooth muscle relaxation by decreasing the action of muscarinic receptors, thereby relieving overactive bladder

Therapeutic outcome: Decreasing urgency, frequency of urination

USES: Urge incontinence, frequency, urgency in overactive bladder

CONTRAINDICATIONS
Hypersensitivity, urinary retention, narrow-angle glaucoma (uncontrolled)
    Concurrent use of solid dosage forms of potassium chloride (the passage of potassium chloride tablets through the GI tract may be delayed); potassium chloride liquid is suitable alternative

Precautions: Severe hepatic disease (Child-Pugh C), GI/GU obstruction, controlled narrow-angle glaucoma, ulcerative colitis, myasthenia gravis, moderate hepatic disease (Child-Pugh B), elderly patients

DOSAGE AND ROUTES
Adult: PO 7.5 mg/day, initially, may increase to 15 mg/day after 14 days if needed

With **taking a potent CYP3A4 inhibitor**
Adult: PO Max 7.5 mg/day

Hepatic dose
Adult: PO (Child-Pugh B) max 7.5 mg

Available forms: Tabs, EXT REL 7.5, 15 mg

Implementation
PO route
• Give without regard to meals
• Do not crush, break, chew EXT REL tabs
• Store at room temperature

ADVERSE EFFECTS
CNS: Dizziness, headache
EENT: Blurred vision, drying eyes, sinusitis, rhinitis
GI: Constipation, dry mouth, abdominal pain, nausea, vomiting, dyspepsia
GU: UTI, urine retention, vaginitis
INTEG: Rash, pruritus, skin drying
MISC: Bronchitis, flulike symptoms
MS: Back pain

Pharmacokinetics

Absorption	Unknown
Distribution	Unknown
Excretion	Unknown
Metabolism	Extensively in the liver
Half-life	12-19 hr

Pharmacodynamics

Onset	Unknown
Peak	7 hr
Duration	Unknown

INTERACTIONS
Drug classifications
Anticholinergics: increased anticholinergic effect
CYP3A4 and CYP2D6 inhibitors: increased darifenacin levels
Drugs metabolized by CYP2D6: increased levels of these products

NURSING CONSIDERATIONS
Assessment
• Urinary function: Assess for urgency, frequency, retention in bladder outflow obstruction

Patient/family education
• Instruct patient to advise prescriber if pregnancy (**C**) is planned or suspected; avoid breastfeeding
• Teach patient about anticholinergic symptoms (dry mouth, constipation, dry eyes, heat prostration), not to become overheated, not to use other products unless approved by prescriber
• Teach patient to avoid hazardous activities until reaction is known, dizziness, blurred vision may occur

Evaluation

Positive therapeutic outcome
• Decreasing urgency, frequency of urination

darunavir (Rx)
(dar-ue'na-vir)
Prezista
Func. class.: Antiretroviral
Chem. class.: Protease inhibitor
Pregnancy category B

ACTION: Inhibits human immunodeficiency virus (HIV-1) protease; this prevents maturation of virus

Therapeutic outcome: Decreased viral load, increase in CD4 counts

USES: HIV-1 in combination with ritonavir and other antiretrovirals

CONTRAINDICATIONS
Hypersensitivity

Precautions: Pregnancy **B,** breastfeeding, children, renal/hepatic disease, history of renal stones, diabetes, hypercholesterolemia, sulfonamide hypersensitivity, antimicrobial resistance, bleeding, elderly, immune reconstitution syndrome, pancreatitis

DOSAGE AND ROUTES
Treatment-naive patients
Adult: PO 800 mg with ritonavir 100 mg qd
Child/adolescent ≥40 kg and ≥12 yr: PO 800 mg with ritonavir 100 mg qday, avoid once daily darunavir dosing in those <12 yr

Child/adolescent 30 to 39 kg and ≥12 yr: PO 675 mg with ritonavir 100 mg qday, avoid once daily darunavir dosing in those <12 yr
Child ≥3 yr, 15 to 29 kg: PO 600 mg with ritonavir 100 mg qday, avoid once daily darunavir dosing in those <12 yr
Child ≥3 yr, 14 kg: PO 490 mg with ritonavir 96 mg qd; 13 kg: 455 mg with ritonavir 80 mg qday; 12 kg: 420 mg with ritonavir 80 mg qday; 11 kg: 385 mg with ritonavir 64 mg qday; 10 kg: 350 mg with ritonavir 64 mg qday, avoid once daily dosing in those <12 yr

Treatment-experienced patients with at least one darunavir resistance-associated substitution
Adult/adolescent/child ≥40 kg: PO 600 bid with ritonavir 100 mg bid
Child ≥3 yr/adolescent ≥30 kg, <40 kg: PO 450 mg bid with ritonavir 60 mg bid
Child ≥3 yr/adolescent ≥15 kg, <30 kg: PO 375 mg bid with ritonavir 50 mg bid
Child ≥ 3 yr (14 kg): PO 280 mg (with ritonavir 48 mg) bid with food
Child ≥ 3 yr (13 kg): PO 260 mg (with ritonavir 40 mg) bid with food
Child ≥ 3 yr (12 kg): PO 240 mg (with ritonavir 40 mg) bid with food
Child ≥ 3 yr (11 kg): PO 220 mg (with ritonavir 32 mg) bid with food
Child ≥ 3 yr (10 kg): PO 200 mg (with ritonavir 32 mg) bid with food

Available forms: Tabs 75, 150, 600, 800 mg; oral susp 100 mg/ml

Implementation
• Give with food and ritonavir
• Tab should be swallowed whole

ADVERSE EFFECTS
CNS: *Headache, insomnia,* dizziness, somnolence
GI: *Diarrhea, abdominal pain, nausea, vomiting,* anorexia, dry mouth, hepatitis, hepatotoxicity, pancreatitis
GU: Nephrolithiasis
INTEG: Rash, angioedema, Stevens-Johnson syndrome, toxic epidermal necrolysis, exanthematous pustulosis
MS: Pain
OTHER: Asthenia, insulin-resistant hyperglycemia, hyperlipidemia, ketoacidosis, lipodystrophy

Pharmacokinetics

Absorption	Unknown
Distribution	Protein binding 95%
Metabolism	By CYP3A4
Excretion	Feces 79.5%, urine 13.9%
Half-life	Terminal 15 hr

Pharmacodynamics

Onset	Unknown
Peak	2.5-4 hr
Duration	Unknown

INTERACTIONS
Individual drugs
Artemether/lumefantrine: increased side effects (CYP3A4 substrate)

Atorvastatin, lovastatin, simvastatin: increased myopathy

CarBAMazepine, efavirenz, fluconazole, fosphenytoin, nevirapine, PHENobarbital, phenytoin: decreased darunavir levels

Clarithromycin, zidovudine: increased levels of both products

Delavirdine, itraconazole, ketoconazole: increased darunavir levels

Telaprevir, rilpivirine: increased levels of these products; monitor for adverse reactions

Isoniazid: increased levels of isoniazid

⚠ Midazolam, pimozide, rifampin, triazolam: life-threatening dysrhythmias

Tenofovir: avoid concurrent use; decreased levels of both products

Drug classifications
⚠ Ergots: life-threatening dysrhythmias; do not use concurrently

Oral contraceptives: increased levels of oral contraceptives

Rifamycins: decreased darunavir levels

Drug/herb
Red yeast rice: increased myopathy, rhabdomyolysis

St. John's wort: decreased darunavir levels; avoid concurrent use

Drug/food
Darunavir: increased absorption

Drug/lab test
Increased: LFTs, bilirubin, uric acid, amylase, lipase

Decreased: WBC, neutrophils, platelets

NURSING CONSIDERATIONS
Assessment
• Assess for complaints of lower back, flank pain; indicates kidney stones

• Assess for signs of infection, anemia, the presence of other STDs

• **Serious skin reaction: angioedema, Stevens-Johnson syndrome, toxic epidermal necrolysis; discontinue immediately, notify prescriber**

• **Hepatotoxicity: Monitor liver function tests: ALT, AST, bilirubin, amylase; all may be elevated in those with underlying liver disease, product should be discontinued in those with increased LFTs**

• Monitor viral load, CD4 during treatment; viral load should be decreasing, CD4 increasing

• Assess bowel pattern before, during treatment; if severe abdominal pain with bleeding occurs, product should be discontinued; monitor hydration

• **Hyperlipidemia:** Cholesterol, triglycerides, LDL may be elevated, monitor serum cholesterol, lipid panel throughout treatment

Patient/family education
• Teach patient to use nonhormonal birth control, do not breastfeed

• Instruct patient to take as prescribed; if dose is missed, take as soon as remembered up to 1 hr before next dose; do not double dose

• Advise patient that product must be taken at same time of day to maintain blood levels for duration of therapy

⚠ Advise patient that hyperglycemia may occur; watch for increased thirst, weight loss, hunger; dry, itchy skin; notify prescriber

• Teach patient to increase fluids to prevent kidney stones; if stone formation occurs, treatment may need to be interrupted

• Teach patient that product does not cure AIDS, only controls symptoms; do not donate blood, do not share, notify all health care providers of use, do not use with any other products without prescriber's approval

Evaluation
Positive therapeutic outcome
• Decreased viral load, increased CD4 counts

---

dasatinib (Rx)
(da-si'ti-nib)
Sprycel
Func. class.: Miscellaneous antineoplastic
Chem. class.: Protein-tyrosine kinase inhibitor
Pregnancy category D

ACTION: Inhibits a tyrosine kinase enzyme, thereby reducing cell growth in leukemia, inhibitor of BCR-ABL and imatinib-resistant mutations of BCR-ABL

Therapeutic outcome: Decrease in number of leukemic cells or size of tumor

USES: Treatment of accelerated, chronic blast phase CML or acute lymphoblastic leukemia (ALL); chronic phase CML with resistance or intolerance to prior therapy; Philadelphia chromosome–positive CML in chronic phase

---

CONTRAINDICATIONS

Pregnancy **D**, hypersensitivity

Precautions: Breastfeeding, children, geriatric, QT prolongation, infection, thrombocytopenia, accidental exposure, edema, infertility, lactase deficiency, neutropenia, anemia, autoimmune disease with immune reconstitution syndrome

DOSAGE AND ROUTES

Accelerated or myeloid/lymphoid blast phase CML with resistance/intolerance to prior therapy
Adult: PO 140 mg daily, titrated up to 180 mg bid in those resistant to therapy

Chronic phase CML with resistance/intolerance to prior therapy
Adult: PO 100 mg daily either AM or PM

Dosage reduction for those taking a strong CYP3A4 inhibitor
Adult: 20 mg daily

Available forms: Tabs 20, 50, 70, 80, 100, 140 mg

Implementation
- Do not break, crush, or chew tab
- Give after meal and with large glass of water
- Give nutritious diet with iron, vitamin supplement
- Store at 25° C (77° F)
- Separate from antacids by 2 hr before and 2 hr after; do not use with H₂ blockers and PPIs

ADVERSE EFFECTS

CNS: CNS hemorrhage, headache, dizziness, insomnia, neuropathy, asthenia
CV: Dysrhythmias, chest pain, CHF, pericardial effusion, congestive cardiomyopathy; decreased injection fraction, QT prolongation
GI: *Nausea, vomiting, anorexia, abdominal pain*, constipation, diarrhea, GI bleeding, mucositis, stomatitis, hepatotoxicity
HEMA: Neutropenia, thrombocytopenia, bleeding
INTEG: *Rash, pruritus,* alopecia
META: Fluid retention, edema, hypocalcemia, hypophosphatemia
MISC: Increased/decreased weight, infection, fatigue
MS: Pain, arthralgia, myalgia
RESP: Cough, dyspnea, pulmonary edema/hypertension, pneumonia, URI, pleural effusion

Pharmacokinetics

Absorption	Unknown
Distribution	Protein binding 96%
Metabolism	By CYP3A4
Excretion	Feces 85%, urine 4%
Half-life	Terminal 3-5 hr

Pharmacodynamics

Onset	0.5-6 hr
Peak	Unknown
Duration	Unknown

INTERACTIONS

Individual drugs

Clarithromycin, erythromycin, itraconazole, ketoconazole, nefazodone, telithromycin: increased dasatinib concentrations
Simvastatin: increased concentrations of this product

Drug classifications

Class IA/III antidysrhythmics and other products that increase QT prolongation: increased QT prolongation
CYP3A4 inducers (dexamethasone, phenytoin, carBAMazepine, rifampin, PHENobarbital), H₂ blockers (famotidine), proton pump inhibitors (omeprazole): decreased dasatinib concentrations
HMG-CoA reductase inhibitors (rare): increased myopathy, rhabdomyolysis
CYP3A4 substrates (alfentanil, cycloSPORINE, ergots, fentaNYL, pimozide, quiNIDine, sirolimus, tacrolimus): altered action
Protease inhibitors: increased dasatinib concentrations

Drug/herb

St. John's wort: decreased dasatinib concentration

Drug/food

Grapefruit: do not use

NURSING CONSIDERATIONS

Assessment

- **Myelosuppression:** Monitor ANC and platelets; in chronic phase if ANC is <1 × 10⁹/L and/or platelets <50 ×10⁹/L, stop until ANC >1.5 × 10⁹/L and platelets >75 × 10⁹/L; in accelerated phase/blast crisis if ANC <0.5 × 10⁹/L and/or platelets <10 × 10⁹/L, determine whether cytopenia is related to biopsy/aspirate, if not, reduce dose by 200 mg; if cytopenia continues, reduce dose by another 100 mg; if cytopenia continues for 4 wk, stop product until ANC ≥1 × 10⁹/L, monitor CBC qwk × 8 wk, then qmo
- **Assess for hepatotoxicity:** monitor liver function tests before treatment and qmo; if liver transaminases >5 × IULN, withhold until transaminase levels return to <2.5 × IULN
- **Monitor for signs of fluid retention, edema:** weigh, monitor lung sounds, assess for edema, some fluid retention is dose dependent, may result in CHF, congestive cardiomyopathy, decreased injection fraction

⚠ QT prolongation: more common in those with hypokalemia, hypomagnesemia, congenital long QT syndrome, those taking products that prolong QT, correct electrolyte imbalances before use

Patient/family education
• Instruct patient to report adverse reactions immediately: SOB, swelling of extremities, bleeding, bruising
• Teach patient reason for treatment, expected result
• Teach patient to use contraception, pregnancy D, avoid breastfeeding; men should use condoms
• Teach patient to take at same time of day, not to crush or chew, not to use grapefruit juice

Evaluation

Positive therapeutic outcome
• Decrease in number of leukemic cells

⚠ HIGH ALERT

DAUNOrubicin (Rx)
(daw-noe-roo′bi-sin)
Cerubidine

DAUNOrubicin citrate liposome (Rx)
DaunoXome
Func. class.: Antineoplastic, antibiotic
Chem. class.: Anthracycline glycoside
Pregnancy category D

Do not confuse: DAUNOrubicin/
DOXOrubicin

ACTION: Inhibits DNA synthesis, primarily; derived from *Streptomyces coeruleorubidus;* replication is decreased by binding to DNA, binds DNA causing confirmational changes; a vesicant

Therapeutic outcome: Prevention of rapidly growing malignant cells; immunosuppression

USES: Acute lymphocytic leukemia (ALL), acute myelogenous leukemia (AML); liposomal Kaposi's sarcoma

CONTRAINDICATIONS
Pregnancy **D,** breastfeeding, hypersensitivity, systemic infections, cardiac disease, bone marrow depression

BLACK BOX WARNING: IM/Subcut use

Precautions: Renal/hepatic disease, gout, tumor lysis syndrome, MI, infection, thrombocytopenia

BLACK BOX WARNING: Bone marrow suppression, cardiac disease, extravasation, renal failure, hepatic disease, requires a specialized care setting and an experienced clinician

DOSAGE AND ROUTES
Use decreased dose for those >60 yr

≫ DAUNOrubicin
In combination
Adult: IV 45-60 mg/m^2/day × 3 days, then 2 days of subsequent courses in combination, max 400-600 mg/m^2 total cumulative dose
Child: IV 25-60 mg/m^2 depending on cycle (AML); ≤2 yr or <0.5 m^2: 1 mg/kg on day 1 weekly in combination with vinCRIStine and predniSONE, base dose on body weight, not surface area (ALL); >2 yr or 0.5 m^2: 25 mg/m^2 day 1 q wk in combination with vinCRIStine and predniSONE (ALL)

≫ DAUNOrubicin citrate liposome
Adult: IV 40 mg/m^2 q2wk (Kaposi's sarcoma); IV 100-140 mg/m^2 q3wk (non-Hodgkin's lymphoma, unlabeled); IV escalating doses of 75, 100, 125, 135, 150 mg/m^2/day × 3 days (AML, unlabeled)

Renal dose
Adult: IV serum Cr >3 mg/dl reduce dose by 50%

Hepatic dose
Adult: IV serum bilirubin 1.2-3 mg/dl reduce dose by 50%; bilirubin >3 mg/dl reduce dose by 75%; bilirubin >5 mg/dl omit dose

Available forms: Inj 20 mg powder/vial, sol for inj 5 mg/ml (DaunoXome); liposome: dispersion for inj 2 mg/ml

Implementation
• Avoid contact with skin; very irritating; wash completely to remove
• Give fluids **IV** or PO before chemotherapy to hydrate patient; give antiemetic 30-60 min before giving product to prevent vomiting, and prn; antibiotics for prophylaxis of infection
• Provide liquid diet: carbonated beverages; gelatin may be added if patient is not nauseated or vomiting

BLACK BOX WARNING: To be used in a care setting with emergency equipment available

BLACK BOX WARNING: To be used by a clinician knowledgeable in cytotoxic therapy

• Help patient rinse mouth tid-qid with water, club soda, brush teeth bid-qid with soft brush or cotton-tipped applicators for stomatitis, use unwaxed dental floss

---

- Product should be prepared by experienced personnel using proper precautions
- Do not give by IM/SUBCUT inj

>> Cerubidine

IV route
- Give after diluting 20 mg/4 ml sterile water for inj (5 mg/ml); rotate; further dilute in 10-15 ml 0.9% NaCl; give over 3-5 min by direct **IV** through Y-tube or 3-way stopcock of inf of D₅W or 0.9% NaCl, may use premix vial 5 mg/ml

Intermittent IV infusion route
- Dilute further in 50-100 ml 0.9% NaCl, LR, D₅W; give over 15 min (50 ml), 30 min (100 ml) for extravasation

Y-site compatibilities: Amifostine, anidulafungin, atenolol, bivalirudin, bleomycin, CARBOplatin, caspofungin, CISplatin, codeine, cyclophosphamide, cytarabine, DACTINomycin, DAPTOmycin, dexmedetomidine, etoposide, fenoldopam, filgrastim, gemcitabine, gemtuzumab, granisetron, melphalan, meperidine, methotrexate, nesiritide, octreotide, ondansetron, oxaliplatin, PACLitaxel, palonosetron, quinupristin-dalfopristin, riTUXimab, sodium acetate/bicarbonate, teniposide, thiotepa, tigecycline, trastuzumab, vinCRIStine, vinorelbine, voriconazole, zoledronic acid

Y-site incompatibilities: Fludarabine

Solution compatibilities: D₃.₃/0.3% NaCl, D₅W, Normosol-R, Ringer's, 0.9% NaCl

>> DaunoXome

IV route
- Dilute with D₅W (1 mg/ml), give over 60 min, do not use in-line filter, reconstituted sol may be stored ≤6 hr refrigerated; do not admix

ADVERSE EFFECTS

>> DAUNOrubicin
CNS: Fever, chills
CV: CHF, pericarditis, myocarditis, peripheral edema, fatal myocarditis, left ventricular failure, QT prolongation, ST-T wave changes, QRS voltage changes, tachycardia, SVT, PVCs
GI: *Nausea, vomiting, anorexia, mucositis, hepatotoxicity*
GU: Impotence, sterility, amenorrhea, gynecomastia
HEMA: Thrombocytopenia, leukopenia, anemia
INTEG: *Rash, extravasation,* dermatitis, reversible alopecia, cellulitis, thrombophlebitis at inj site
MISC: Anaphylaxis, tumor lysis syndrome, secondary malignancies

>> DAUNOrubicin citrate liposome
CNS: Fatigue, headache, depression, insomnia, dizziness, malaise, neuropathy
CV: Chest pain, edema
GI: Abdominal pain, nausea, vomiting, *diarrhea,* constipation, stomatitis
INTEG: *Alopecia,* sweating, *pruritus*
MISC: *Allergic reactions, chest pain, fever,* edema, flulike symptoms
MS: *Rigors,* arthralgia, back pain
RESP: *Cough, dyspnea, rhinitis, sinusitis*

Pharmacokinetics

Absorption	Complete
Distribution	Widely distributed; crosses placenta
Metabolism	Liver, extensively
Excretion	Biliary (40%-50%)
Half-life	18½ hr, liposome 55½ hr

Pharmacodynamics
Unknown

INTERACTIONS
Arsenic trioxide, chloroquine, clarithromycin, dasatinib, dolasetron, droperidol, erythromycin, flecainide, halofantrine, haloperidol, levomethadyl, methadone, ondansetron, palonosetron, pentamide, propafenone, risperiDONE, sparfloxacin, vorinstat, ziprasidone: increase QT prolongation, torsades de pointes

Individual drugs
Cyclophosphamide, radiation: increased toxicity

Drug classifications
Antineoplastics: increased toxicity
Class IA/III antidysrhythmics, some phenothiazines, tricyclic antidepressants (high doses): increased QT prolongation, torsades de pointes
Live virus vaccines: decreased antibody reaction
NSAIDs, salicylates: increased risk of bleeding, anticoagulants, platelet inhibitors, thrombolytics
Hematopoietic progenitor cells: given within 24 hr: decreased DAUNOrubicin given within 24 hr

Drug/lab test
Increased: uric acid

NURSING CONSIDERATIONS
Assessment
- Assess buccal cavity q8hr for dryness, sores or ulceration, white patches, pain, bleeding, dysphagia; obtain prescription for viscous lidocaine (Xylocaine)
- **Assess symptoms indicating severe allergic reaction: rash, pruritus, urticaria,**

purpuric skin lesions, itching, flushing; product should be discontinued

> **BLACK BOX WARNING: Cardiac toxicity:** assess chest x-ray, echocardiography, radionuclide angiography, MUGA, ECG; watch for ST-T wave changes, low QRS and T, QT prolongation possible, dysrhythmias (sinus tachycardia, heart block, PVCs); watch for CHF (jugular vein distention, weight gain, edema, crackles), may occur after 2-6 mo of treatment, cumulative dose (400-550 mg/m²), 450 mg/m² if used in combination with radiation, cyclophosphamide

> **BLACK BOX WARNING: Monitor CBC, bone marrow suppression,** differential, platelet count weekly, leukocyte nadir within 2 wk after administration, recovery within 3 wk; do not administer if absolute granulocyte count is <750/mm³ (liposome)

• Assess for increased uric acid levels, swelling, joint pain primarily in extremities; patient should be well hydrated to prevent urate deposits
• **Acute renal failure, uric acid nephropathy: Monitor renal function tests: BUN, creatinine, serum uric acid, urine CCr baseline and before each dose; I&O ratio; report fall in urine output to <30 ml/hr, provide aggressive alkalinization of the urine as use of allopurinol can prevent urate nephropathy**
• **Monitor temp q4hr (may indicate beginning of infection)**
• **Hepatotoxicity: Monitor liver function tests baseline and before each dose (bilirubin, AST, ALT, LDH) as needed or monthly; note jaundice of skin or sclera, dark urine, clay-colored stools, itchy skin, abdominal pain, fever, diarrhea; hepatotoxicity can be severe**
• Assess for bleeding: hematuria, stool guaiac, bruising or petechiae, mucosa or orifices q8hr; check for inflammation of mucosa, breaks in skin
• Identify effects of alopecia on body image; discuss feelings about body changes
⚠ Tumor lysis syndrome: hyperkalemia, hyperphosphatemia, hyperuricemia, hypocalcemia

> **BLACK BOX WARNING: Extravasation:** swelling, pain, decreased blood return, if extravasation occurs stop infusion, remove tubing, attempt to aspirate the drug prior to removing the needle, elevate area, treat with ice

Patient/family education
• Teach patient to avoid use of products containing aspirin or ibuprofen, razors, commercial mouthwash, since bleeding may occur; to report symptoms of bleeding (hematuria, tarry stools)
• Instruct patient to report signs of **anemia** (fatigue, headache, irritability, faintness, shortness of breath); signs of **infection;** bleeding, bruising, shortness of breath, swelling, change in heart rate; to avoid crowds, those with known infections
• Advise patient that hair may be lost during treatment; a wig or hairpiece may make patient feel better; new hair may be different in color, texture
• Caution patient not to have any vaccinations without the advice of the prescriber; serious reactions can occur
⚠ Advise patient that contraception is needed during treatment and for 4 mo after the completion of therapy, pregnancy D
• Advise patient to avoid alcohol, aspirin, NSAIDs
• Inform patient that urine and other body fluids may be red-orange for 48 hr
• Teach patient to avoid crowds, those with known infections

Evaluation
Positive therapeutic outcome
• Prevention of rapid division of malignant cells

delavirdine (Rx)
(de-la-veer'deen)
Rescriptor
Func. class.: Antiretroviral
Chem. class.: Nonnucleoside reverse transcriptase inhibitor (NNRTI)
Pregnancy category C

ACTION: Binds directly to reverse transcriptase and blocks RNA, DNA-dependent polymerase activities causing a disruption of the enzyme's site

Therapeutic outcome: Improvement of HIV-1 infection

USES: HIV-1 in combination with at least 2 other antiretrovirals

CONTRAINDICATIONS
Hypersensitivity

Precautions: Pregnancy **C,** breastfeeding, children, hepatic disease, exfoliative dermatitis, hepatitis, immune reconstitution syndrome, achlorhydria, antimicrobial resistance

DOSAGE AND ROUTES
Adult and child ≥16 yr: PO 400 mg tid; max 1200 mg/day

Available forms: Tabs 100, 200 mg

Implementation
• Add 4 tabs/3-4 oz of water, let stand, stir, swallow, rinse glass, swallow; use only 100 mg tabs for dispersion
• Do not give within 1 hr of antacids or didanosine
• Take in equal intervals around the clock
• Always use as combination therapy; this product is not recommended for initial treatment; due to inferior, virologic effect, it is no longer listed as part of any preferred regimens

ADVERSE EFFECTS
CNS: Headache, fatigue, anxiety, insomnia, fever
GI: Diarrhea, anorexia, abdominal pain, nausea, vomiting, dyspepsia, hepatotoxicity
GU: Nephrotoxicity
HEMA: Neutropenia, leukopenia, thrombocytopenia, anemia, granulocytopenia
INTEG: Rash, pruritis
MISC: Cough
MS: Pain, myalgia, rhabdomyolysis
SYST: Stevens-Johnson syndrome, immune reconstitution syndrome (combination therapy)

Pharmacokinetics

Absorption	Well
Distribution	98% protein bound
Metabolism	Liver, extensively by CYP3A4
Excretion	Kidneys, feces
Half-life	2-11 hr

Pharmacodynamics

Onset	Unknown
Peak	1 hr
Duration	8 hr

INTERACTIONS
Individual drugs
ALPRAZolam, amprenavir, atorvastatin, clarithromycin, dapsone, felodipine, indinavir, lovastatin, midazolam, NIFEdipine, saquinavir, simvastatin: increased level of each specific product
ALPRAZolam, astemizole, cisapride, midazolam, pimozide, sildenafil, terfenadine, triazolam: life-threatening reactions; do not combine
Clarithromycin, quiNIDine, warfarin: increased level of both products
Didanosine: decreased delavirdine levels, decreased action of didanosine, H₂ blockers, PPIs
FLUoxetine, ketoconazole: increased level of delavirdine

Drug classifications
Amphetamines, antidysrhythmics, benzodiazepines, calcium channel blockers, ergots,

sedative/hypnotics, opiates: increased serious life-threatening adverse reaction
Antacids, anticonvulsants, protease inhibitors, rifamycins: decreased delavirdine levels
Contraceptives (oral): decreased action of oral contraceptives
CYP3A4, 2D6 inhibitors: increased levels
Ergots: increased levels of ergots

Drug/herb
St. John's wort: decreased delavirdine level

NURSING CONSIDERATIONS
Assessment
• Assess CBC, blood chemistry, plasma HIV RNA, absolute CD4⁺/CD8⁺/cell counts/%, serum β₂ microglobulin, serum ICD+24 antigen levels
• Assess signs of infection, anemia
• Assess liver function tests: ALT, AST; renal studies
• Assess C&S before product therapy; product may be taken as soon as culture is taken; repeat C&S after treatment; determine the presence of other STDs
• Assess bowel pattern before, during treatment; if severe abdominal pain with bleeding occurs, product should be discontinued; monitor hydration
• Assess allergies before treatment, reaction to each medication; place allergies on chart
• Assess plasma delavirdine concentrations (trough 10 mcm)
• HIV: Obtain hepatitis B virus (HBV) screening to ensure proper treatment, if co-infected, a fully suppressive antiretroviral regimen with productions against both
• Serious skin reactions: Stevens-Johnson syndrome; any rash may occur within 1-3 wk of beginning treatment; if rash is not severe, manage with diphenhydrAMINE, hydrOXYzine, topical corticosteroids
• Immune reconstitution syndrome: When treated with combination therapy; development of opportunistic infections (Mycobacterium avium complex [MAC]), cytomegalovirus (CMV), Pneumocystis jiroveci pneumonia (PCP), or TB
• Delavirdine toxicity: severe nausea, vomiting, maculopapular rash

Patient/family education
• Advise patient to take as prescribed; if dose is missed, take as soon as remembered up to 1 hr before next dose; do not double dose, separate by 1 hr, do not take antacids concurrently
• Advise patient that product must be taken in equal intervals around the clock to maintain blood levels for duration of therapy

- Advise patient that tabs may be dissolved; drink right away (100 mg only), rinse cup with water, and drink that to get all medication
- Instruct patient to make sure health care provider knows of all the medications being taken
- Advise patient that if severe rash, mouth sores, swelling, aching muscles/joints, or eye redness occur, stop taking and notify health care provider
- Advise patient not to breastfeed if taking this product
- Teach patient that this product is not a cure, only controls symptoms

Evaluation

Positive therapeutic outcome
- Increased CD4$^+$ cell count
- Decreased viral load
- Improvement in symptoms of HIV

denosumab (Rx)

(den-oh′sue-mab)
Prolia, Xgeva
Func. class.: Bone resorption inhibitor
Chem. class.: Monoclonal antibody, bone resorption

Pregnancy category C

ACTION: Neutralizes activity of receptor activator nuclear factor kappa-B ligand (RANKL) by binding to it and blocking its interaction with cell surface receptors, use of a RANKL inhibitor may reduce bone turnover and decrease tumor burden

Therapeutic outcome: Increased/maintained bone density

USES: Osteoporosis in postmenopausal women or men at high risk for fractures, who are receiving androgen deprivation therapy for prostate cancer, and women receiving aromastase inhibitor therapy for breast cancer; prevention of skeletal-related events in bone metastases from solid tumors; giant cell tumor of bone (Xgeva); increase bone mass

CONTRAINDICATIONS

Hypersensitivity, hypocalcemia, pregnancy (Xgeva) **D**; (Prolia) **X**

Precautions: Anemia, breastfeeding, child/infant/neonate, coagulopathy, diabetes mellitus, dialysis, eczema, hypoparathyroidism, immunosuppression, latex hypersensitivity, malabsorption syndrome, neonates, neoplastic disease, pancreatitis, parathyroid disease, pregnancy **C**, dental/renal/thyroid disease, TB, vitamin D deficiency

DOSAGE AND ROUTES

Postmenopausal osteoporosis (Prolia)
Adult female: SUBCUT 60 mg q6mo with 1000 mg calcium and 400 international units vitamin D, max 60 mg q6mo

Bone metastases from solid tumors
Adult: SUBCUT 120 mg q4wk, max 120 mg q4wk; administer with calcium and vitamin D as necessary to prevent hypocalcemia

Giant cell tumor of bone (Xgeva)
Adult: SUBCUT 120 mg on days 1, 8, 15, then 120 mg q4wk; use calcium, vitamin D as needed

Available forms: Solution for injection 60 mg/ml (Prolia); 120 mg/1.7 ml (Xgeva)

Implementation
SUBCUT route
- Give acetaminophen before and for 72 hr after to decrease pain
- Do not use if particulate matter or discoloration is present; solution is clear and colorless to slightly yellow with small white/opalescent particles, remove from refrigerator and allow to warm to room temperature (15-30 min)
- **Use of prefilled syringe with needle safety guard:** Leave green guard in original position until after administration, remove and discard needle cap immediately before injection, give by SUBCUT injection in upper arm, thigh, or abdomen; after injection, point needle away from people and slide green guard over needle
- **Use of single-use vials:** Use 27G needle, give in upper arm/thigh, or abdomen, do not re-insert needle in vial, discard supplies as appropriate
- Avoid direct sunlight/heat, do not freeze, use within 14 days after removal from refrigerator, store unopened containers in refrigerator

ADVERSE EFFECTS

CNS: Chills, fever, flushing, headache, vertigo, neuropathic pain
CV: Angina, **atrial fibrillation**
GI: Abdominal pain, constipation, *diarrhea,* flatulence, GERD, *vomiting, nausea*
GU: Cystitis, lactation suppression
HEMA: Anemia, neutropenia
INTEG: Atopic dermatitis, pruritus
META: Hypercholesterolemia, hypocalcemia, hypophosphatemia
MS: Back/bone pain, MS pain, myalgia, **osteonecrosis of the jaw**
RESP: Cough, *dyspnea*
SYST: Infection, secondary malignancy

Pharmacokinetics

Absorption	Bioavailability 62%
Distribution	Unknown
Metabolism	Unknown
Excretion	Unknown
Half-life	25.4 days

Pharmacodynamics

Onset	Unknown
Peak	Maximum serum concentration 3-21 days
Duration	Steady state 6 months

INTERACTIONS
Drug classifications

Immunosuppressives, corticosteroids: possible increased infection

Antineoplastics, corticosteroids: possible increased osteonecrosis of the jaw

NURSING CONSIDERATIONS
Assessment

• **Assess for acute acute-phase reaction: fever, myalgia, headache, flulike symptoms, for 72 hr after injection, usually resolves after 72 hr**

• Monitor blood tests: serum calcium/creatinine/BUN/magnesium/phosphate

⚠ **Assess for hypocalcemia (may be fatal): paresthesia, twitching, laryngospasm, Chvostek's/Trousseau's signs; preexisting hypocalcemia prior to treatment; patient with vitamin D deficiency may require higher doses of vitamin D**

• **Assess for hypercalcemia:** nausea, vomiting, anorexia, weakness, thirst, constipation, dysrhythmias

• **Monitor dental status:** correct dental complications prior to product use, good oral hygiene should be maintained; if dental work is to be performed, antiinfectives should be given to prevent osteonecrosis of the jaw

• **Assess for infection:** Do not start treatment in those with active infections, infections should be resolved first

Patient/family education

• Advise patient to report hypercalcemic relapse: nausea, vomiting, bone pain, thirst

• Teach patient to continue with dietary recommendations including additional calcium 1000 mg/day and vitamin D ≥ 400 units (Prolia product labeling)

• Advise patient to avoid use in pregnancy and breastfeeding, notify prescriber if pregnancy is planned or suspected

• Instruct patient to use acetaminophen prior to and for 72 hrs after injection to lessen bone pain

• Explain the purpose of this product and expected results

• Advise patient to avoid OTC, Rx, or herbs and supplements unless approved by prescriber

• Teach patient to use regular exercise, stop smoking, and avoid alcohol to maintain bone health

• Advise patient to inform all health care providers of product use, avoid dental procedures/surgery if possible, practice good oral hygiene

• Teach patient that lab tests and follow-up exams will be required

Evaluation
Positive therapeutic outcome
• Increased/maintained bone density

desipramine (Rx)
(dess-ip'ra-meen)

Norpramin

Func. class.: Antidepressant, tricyclic

Chem. class.: Dibenzazepine, secondary amine

Pregnancy category C

ACTION: Blocks reuptake of norepinephrine, serotonin into nerve endings, increasing action of norepinephrine, serotonin in nerve cells

Therapeutic outcome: Decreased depression

USES: Depression

Unlabeled uses: Chronic pain, ADHD, bulimia, diabetic neuropathy, panic disorder, social phobia

CONTRAINDICATIONS

Hypersensitivity to tricyclics, carBAMazepine; closed-angle glaucoma, acute MI, MAOIs

Precautions: Pregnancy C, breastfeeding, geriatric, severe depression, increased intraocular pressure, seizure disorder, CV disease, urinary retention, cardiac dysrhythmias, cardiac conduction disturbances, family history of sudden death, prostatic hypertrophy, thyroid disease

> **BLACK BOX WARNING:** Suicidal patients, children <18 yr

DOSAGE AND ROUTES
Major depression

Adult: PO 50-75 mg/day in 1-4 divided doses; titrate by 25-50 mg qwk up to 300 mg/day in single or divided doses (inpatient), 200 mg/day (outpatient)

⚠ Nurse Alert　　　✴ Key NCLEX® Drug　　　>> Drug Specifics

Geriatric: PO 25 mg/day at bedtime, titrate qwk; may increase to 150 mg/day

Child >12 yr: PO 25-50 mg/day in divided doses, max 150 mg/day

Child 6-12 yr: PO 1-3 mg/kg/day in divided doses, give >3 mg/kg/day with close medical monitoring; max 5 mg/kg/day

Available forms: Tabs 10, 25, 50, 75, 100, 150 mg

Implementation

• Increase fluids, bulk in diet for constipation, especially in geriatric
• Take with food or milk for GI symptoms
• Crush if patient is unable to swallow medication whole
• Give dosage at bedtime if oversedation occurs during day; may take entire dose at bedtime; geriatric may not tolerate once a day dosing
• Store at room temperature
• Provide assistance with ambulation during beginning of therapy for drowsiness/dizziness
• Provide safety measures, primarily in the geriatric
• Check to see that PO medication is swallowed

ADVERSE EFFECTS

CNS: *Dizziness, drowsiness,* confusion, headache, anxiety, tremors, stimulation, weakness, insomnia, nightmares, EPS (geriatric), increased psychiatric symptoms, paresthesia, suicidal ideation, impaired memory, **seizures, serotonin syndrome**
CV: *Orthostatic hypo/hypertension,* ECG *changes, tachycardia, palpitations*
EENT: *Blurred vision,* tinnitus, mydriasis, ophthalmoplegia
ENDO: SIADH
GI: *Diarrhea, dry mouth,* nausea, vomiting, **paralytic ileus,** increased appetite, cramps, epigastric distress, jaundice, **hepatitis,** stomatitis, constipation, weight gain
GU: *Retention,* **acute renal failure**
HEMA: **Agranulocytosis, thrombocytopenia, eosinophilia, leukopenia**
INTEG: Rash, urticaria, sweating, pruritus, photosensitivity

Pharmacokinetics

Absorption	Well
Distribution	Widely, protein binding 92%
Metabolism	Extensively, liver
Excretion	Unknown
Half-life	12-24 hr

Pharmacodynamics

Unknown

INTERACTIONS
Individual drugs
Alcohol: increased CNS depression
Cimetidine, diltiazem, fluvoxaMINE, FLUoxetine, PARoxetine, sertraline, verapamil: increased desipramine level
CloNIDine: increased life-threatening B/P elevations, do not use concurrently
EPINEPHrine, norepinephrine: increased hypertension
Gatifloxacin, levofloxacin, moxifloxacin, sparfloxacin, SUNItinib, vorinostat, ziprasidone: increased serotonin syndrome, neuroleptic malignant syndrome

Drug classifications
Barbiturates, opioids, CNS depressants: increased CNS depression, skeletal muscle relaxants
MAOIs: increased hyperpyrexia, seizures, excitation; do not use within 14 days of MAOIs
SSRIs, SNRIs, serotonin-receptor agonists, other tricyclic antidepressants: increased serotonin syndrome, neuroloptic malignant syndrome
Class IA/III dysrhythmics, tricyclic antidepressants: increased QT interval

Drug/herb
Kava, valerian: increased CNS depression
St. John's wort: may increase serotonin syndrome; avoid concurrent use

Drug/lab test
Increase: serum bilirubin, blood glucose, alkaline phosphatase
Decreased: sodium

NURSING CONSIDERATIONS
Assessment
• Monitor B/P (lying, standing), pulse q4hr; if systolic B/P drops 20 mm Hg, hold product, notify prescriber; take vital signs q4hr in patients with CV disease
• Monitor blood studies: CBC, leukocytes, differential, cardiac enzymes if patient is receiving long-term therapy
• Monitor hepatic studies: AST, ALT, bilirubin
• Check weight qwk; appetite may increase with this product
• **Monitor ECG for flattening T wave, bundle branch block, AV block, dysrhythmias in cardiac patients**
• Assess for **EPS** primarily in geriatric: rigidity, dystonia, akathisia
• Assess for **seizure activity** in those with a history of seizures

---

Adverse effects: *italics* = common; **bold** = life-threatening

BLACK BOX WARNING: Assess mental status: mood, sensorium, affect, **suicidal tendencies,** increase in psychiatric symptoms: depression, panic; this product is not indicated for children, monitor mental status baseline and during first few months of treatment

• Assess for urinary retention, constipation; constipation most likely in children
• Assess for **withdrawal symptoms:** headache, nausea, vomiting, muscle pain, weakness; not usual unless product is discontinued abruptly
• Assess for alcohol consumption; if consumed, hold dose until morning

Patient/family education
• Advise patient that therapeutic effects may take 2-3 wk

BLACK BOX WARNING: Teach patient that suicidal thoughts and behavior may occur, notify prescriber immediately

• Advise patient to use caution in driving, other activities requiring alertness because of drowsiness, dizziness, blurred vision
• Teach patient to avoid alcohol ingestion, other CNS depressants
• Teach patient not to discontinue medication quickly after long-term use; may cause nausea, headache, malaise
• Teach patient to wear sunscreen or large hat, since photosensitivity occurs

Evaluation

Positive therapeutic outcome
• Decreased depression

TREATMENT OF OVERDOSE:
ECG monitoring; induce emesis; lavage, activated charcoal; administer anticonvulsant

RARELY USED

desirudin
(deh-sihr′uh-din)
Iprivask
Func. class.: Anticoagulant; thrombin inhibitor
Pregnancy category C

ACTION: Selectively inhibits free and clot-bound thrombin, prevents activation of clotting factors

Therapeutic outcome: Decreased occurrence of deep vein thrombosis (DVT) in hip-replacement surgery

USES: Prevents DVT in hip-replacement surgery

CONTRAINDICATIONS
Hypersensitivity to this product, mannitol (diluent), hirudins, active bleeding, coagulation disorders

Precautions: Renal disease (CCr <60 ml/min), hepatic disease, GI/respiratory bleeding ≤3 mo, severe uncontrolled hypertension, spinal/epidural anesthesia, bacterial endocarditis

DOSAGE AND ROUTES
Adult: SUBCUT 15 mg q12hr × 9-12 days; give first dose 5-15 min prior to surgery if a regional block is used

Renal dose
Adult: SUBCUT CCr 31-60 ml/min 5 mg q12hr; CCr <31 ml/min 1.7 mg q12hr

Available forms: Inj 15 mg and 0.6 mannitol diluent

Implementation
• Visually inspect particulate matter and discoloration prior to use, do not use solutions that are cloudy or contain particles
• Do not use IM
Subcut route
• Do not mix with other injections, solvents, or parenteral fluids
Reconstitution for subcut use
• Reconstitute each vial with 0.5 ml of provided diluent, shake gently until the drug is fully reconstituted; the injection should be clear, colorless; once reconstituted, each 0.5 ml contains 15.75 mg desirudin; use immediately; however, it remains stable ≤ 24 hrs at room temperature and protected from light. Discard any unused solution
Subcut inj
• Have patient sit or lie down; using a syringe with a 26 or 27 G needle which is approximately 0.5-inch in length, withdraw the entire reconstituted solution into the syringe; inject total volume subcut; alternate between the left and right anterolateral and left and right posterolateral thigh or abdominal wall; insert whole length of the needle in a skin fold held between the thumb and forefinger; the skin fold should be held throughout the injection; to minimize bruising, do not rub the site, rotate sites

ADVERSE EFFECTS
CV: Thrombosis, thrombophlebitis, hypotension
CNS: Dizziness, fever
EENT: Nosebleeding, occular bleeding
GI: Hematemesis, nausea, vomiting
HEMA: Hemorrhage, anemia
GU: Hematuria
MISC: Anaphylaxis, impaired healing edema, injection-site reaction

---

Pharmacokinetics

Absorption	Unknown
Distribution	Unknown
Metabolism	Unknown
Excretion	Unknown
Half-life	2 hr

Pharmacodynamics

Onset	½ hr
Peak	1-1½ hr
Duration	Unknown

INTERACTIONS
Drug classifications
Other anticoagulants, glycoprotein IIb/IIIa antagonists, NSAIDs, salicylates, thrombolytics, corticosteroids: increased bleeding risk

Drug/lab test
Decreased: Hct/Hgb

NURSING CONSIDERATIONS
Assessment
Bleeding:
• Assess for bleeding gums, black tarry stools, hematuria, epistaxis, decreased Hct/Hgb, guaiac-positive stools, bleeding from hip replacement site, notify prescriber if any of these occurs
• Observe for thrombosis, ecchymosis
• Monitor aPTT q day in those with bleeding risk, aPTT should not be > 2 times control

> **BLACK BOX WARNING:** Assess epidural/spinal anesthesia sites for hematomas, may result in irreversible paralysis

Patient/family education
• Teach patient to report any signs of bleeding
• Teach patient to use a soft-bristle toothbrush to avoid bleeding gums, to use an electric razor

Evaluation
Positive therapeutic outcome
• Decreased occurrence of DVT in hip replacement surgery

---

desloratadine (Rx)
(des-lor-at′ah-deen)
Clarinex, Clarinex RediTabs
Func. class.: Antihistamine, 2nd generation
Chem. class.: Selective histamine (H_1) receptor antagonist
Pregnancy category C

ACTION: Binds to peripheral histamine receptors, providing antihistamine action without sedation

Therapeutic outcome: Decreased nasal stuffiness, itching, swollen eyes

USES: Seasonal/perennial allergic rhinitis, chronic idiopathic urticaria

CONTRAINDICATIONS
Hypersensitivity, infants/neonates

Precautions: Pregnancy **C**, bronchial asthma, renal/hepatic impairment, child, breastfeeding, phenylketonuria

DOSAGE AND ROUTES
Adult and child ≥12 yr: PO 5 mg daily
Child 6-11 yr: PO 2.5 mg daily
Child 1-5 yr: PO 1.25 mg daily
Child 6-11 mo: PO 1 mg daily (urticaria only)

Renal/hepatic dose
Adult: PO 5 mg every other day

Available forms: Tabs 5 mg; orally disintegrating (Reditabs) 2.5, 5 mg; syr 0.5 mg/ml

Implementation
• May administer without regard to meals
• Store in airtight container at room temperature
• Use calibrated device for syrup

ADVERSE EFFECTS
CNS: Sedation (more common with increased dosages), headache, psychomotor hyperactivity, *seizures*, fatigue, dizziness
GI: *Hepatitis*, nausea, dry mouth
MISC: Flulike symptoms, pharyngitis, myalgias

Pharmacokinetics

Absorption	Unknown
Distribution	Bound to plasma proteins (82%-87%)
Metabolism	Liver (active metabolites)
Excretion	Urine, feces (metabolites)
Half-life	8½-28 hr

Pharmacodynamics

Peak	1½ hr
Duration	24 hr

INTERACTIONS
Drug/drug
Alcohol: increased CNS depression (rare)
Etravirine, nilotinib: increased desloratadine effect

Drug classification
Anxiolytics, antipsychotics, H_1 blockers, opiates, sedative/hypnotics, tricyclics, antidepressants: increased CNS depression (rare)

Adverse effects: *italics* = common; **bold** = life-threatening

NURSING CONSIDERATIONS
Assessment
• Assess for **allergy:** hives, rash, rhinitis; monitor respiratory status; stop product 4 days before antigen skin test

Patient/family education
• Advise patient to avoid driving, other hazardous activities if drowsiness occurs; to observe caution until product's effects are known
• Advise patient that product may cause photosensitivity; use sunscreen or stay out of the sun to prevent burns
• Instruct patient not to exceed max dose, take without regard to meals
• Caution patient to avoid use of other CNS depressants
• Teach not to remove Reditabs from blister until ready to use; to place Reditab directly on tongue; may take with or without water
• Advise patient to use Redi-Tab by removing from pack and allow to dissolve on tongue, without regard to water

Evaluation
Positive therapeutic outcome
• Absence of running or congested nose, other allergy symptoms

---

desmopressin (Rx)
(des-moe-press'in)
DDAVP, Minirin, Octostim ✳, Stimate
Func. class.: Pituitary hormone
Chem. class.: Synthetic antidiuretic hormone
Pregnancy category B

ACTION: Promotes reabsorption of water by action on renal tubular epithelium in the kidney; causes smooth muscle constriction and increase in plasma factor VIII levels, which increases platelet aggregation resulting in vasopressor effect; similar to vasopressin

Therapeutic outcome: Prevention of nocturnal enuresis, decreased bleeding in hemophilia A, von Willebrand's disease type 1, control and stabilization of water in diabetes insipidus

USES: Hemophilia A, von Willebrand's disease type 1, nonnephrogenic diabetes insipidus, symptoms of polyuria/polydipsia caused by pituitary dysfunction, nocturnal enuresis

CONTRAINDICATIONS
Hypersensitivity, nephrogenic diabetes insipidus, severe renal disease, hyponatremia

Precautions: Pregnancy **B,** breastfeeding, CAD, hypertension, cystic fibrosis, thrombus, electrolyte imbalances, male infertility

DOSAGE AND ROUTES
Primary nocturnal enuresis (unlabeled)
Adult and child ≥6 yr: INTRANASAL 20 mcg (half in each nostril) at bedtime, may increase to 40 mcg; PO 0.2 mg at bedtime, may be increased to max 0.6 mg at bedtime

Diabetes insipidus
Adult: INTRANASAL 10-40 mcg in divided doses (1-4 sprays with pump); SUBCUT/**IV** 2-4 mcg/day or SUBCUT in 2 divided daily in divided doses
Child 3 mo-12 yr: INTRANASAL 5-30 mcg 2-4 mcg/day or SUBCUT in 2 divided daily in divided doses

Hemophilia/von Willebrand's disease
Adult and child >3 mo: IV 0.3 mcg/kg in NaCl over 15-30 min; may repeat if needed

Antihemorrhagic
Adult and child >3 mo: IV 0.3 mcg/kg
Adult and child <50 kg: INTRANASAL 1 spray in one nostril
Adult and child >50 kg: 1 spray each nostril
Adult: SUBCUT/**IV** 0.2-0.4 mcg/kg dose

Available forms: Inj 4, 15 mcg/ml, Rhinal Tube delivery 2.5 mg/vial (0.1 mg/ml); tabs 0.1, 0.2 mg; nasal spray pump (DDAVP) 10 mcg/spray (0.1 mg/ml); nasal spray (Stimate) 1.5 mg/ml (150 mcg/dose)

Implementation
PO route
• Store at room temperature
• Draw medication into tube, insert tube into nostril to instill product and blow on other end to deliver sol into nasal cavity; rinse after use
• Store in refrigerator or cool environment
Nasal route
• DDAVP and Stimate are not interchangeable
• Prime prior to first dose (press down 4 times), pump stays primed for 1 wk; to reprime, press down 1 time

IV, direct route
• Give undiluted over 1 min in diabetes insipidus

Intermittent IV infusion route
• Give single dose diluted in 50 ml of 0.9% NaCl (adult and child >10 kg); a single dose/10 ml as an **IV** inf over 15-30 min in von Willebrand's disease or hemophilia A
• Store in refrigerator

ADVERSE EFFECTS
CNS: Drowsiness, headache, lethargy, flushing, seizures

CV: Increased B/P, palpitations, tachycardia
EENT: Nasal irritation, congestion, rhinitis
GI: Nausea, heartburn, cramps
GU: *Vulval pain*
META: Hyponatremia, hyponatremia-induced seizures
SYST: Anaphylaxis (IV)

Pharmacokinetics

Absorption	Nasal (up to 20%)
Distribution	Unknown
Metabolism	Unknown
Excretion	Unknown; breast milk

Pharmacodynamics

	PO	Intra-nasal	SUBCUT/IV
Onset	1 hr	1 hr	Rapid
Peak	4-7 hr	1-4 hr	15-30 min
Duration	Unknown	8-20 hr	3 hr

INTERACTIONS
Individual drugs
Alcohol, demeclocycline, EPHINEPHrine (large doses), heparin, lithium: decreased antidiuretic action
CarBAMazepine, chlorpropamide, clofibrate: increased antidiuretic action, SSRIs, lamotrigine

Drug classifications
Pressor products: increased pressor effect

NURSING CONSIDERATIONS
Assessment
• Monitor I&O ratio, urine osmolality, specific gravity, weight daily; check for edema in extremities; if water retention is severe, diuretic may be prescribed; check pulse, B/P when giving product **IV** or SUBCUT
• **Assess for water intoxication:** lethargy, behavioral changes, disorientation, neuromuscular excitability, dehydration, poor skin turgor, severe thirst, dry skin, tachycardia
• Assess intranasal use: nausea, congestion, cramps, headache; usually decreased with decreased dosage
• Monitor for enuresis during treatment (**nocturnal enuresis**)
• Assess for allergic reaction, including anaphylaxis (**IV route**), notify prescriber, discontinue use
• Assess for nasal mucosa changes: congestion, edema, discharge, scarring (nasal route)
• Monitor urine volume osmolality and plasma osmolality (diabetes insipidus)
• Nocturia enuresis: Identify how often enuresis is occurring, avoid use in those prone to water intoxication or sodium depletion

• Monitor factor VIII coagulant activity before using for hemostasis

Patient/family education
• Use demonstration, return demonstration to teach technique for nasal instillation, clear nasal passage before use
• Teach patient to notify prescriber of dyspnea, vomiting, cramping, drowsiness, headache, nasal congestion
• Caution patient to avoid OTC products (cough, hay fever), since these preparations may contain EPINEPHrine and decrease product response; do not use with alcohol
• Advise patient to carry/wear emergency ID or other identification specifying disease and medication used
• Advise patient if dose is missed, take when remembered, up to 1 hr before next dose; do not double doses; avoid fluids from 1 hr to up to 8 hr after PO dose
• Teach patient to report upper respiratory infection, nasal congestion
• How to use subcut, rotate sites

Evaluation
Positive therapeutic outcome
• Absence of severe thirst
• Decreased urine output, osmolality
• Absence of bleeding (hemophilia)

desonide topical
See Appendix B

desoximetasone topical
See Appendix B

desoxyribonuclease
See fibrinolysin/desoxyribonuclease

desvenlafaxine (Rx)
Khedezla, Pristiq
Func. class.: Antidepressant, serotonin-receptor norepinephrine reuptake inhibitor (SNRI)
Pregnancy category C

ACTION: May work by blocking the central presynaptic reuptake of 5-HT and NE, resulting in an increased sustained level of these neurotransmitters.

Therapeutic outcome: Decreased depression, increased sense of well-being and renewed interest in activities

USES: Major depressive disorder

Unlabeled uses: Vasomotor symptoms (hot flashes) associated with menopause

CONTRAINDICATIONS
Hypersensitivity to this product or venlafaxine, MAOI therapy

Precautions: CNS depression, abrupt discontinuation, hypertension, hepatic/renal disease, hyponatremia, geriatric patients, pregnancy C, labor and delivery, breastfeeding, angina, bleeding, cardiac dysrhythmias, MI, stroke, mania, hypovolemia, dehydration, increased intraocular pressure

> **BLACK BOX WARNING:** Children, suicidal ideation

DOSAGE AND ROUTES
Adult: PO Initially, 50 mg daily; max 400 mg/day with adjustments as needed

Available forms: Ext rel tabs 50, 100 mg

ADVERSE EFFECTS
CNS: *Dizziness,* drowsiness, *headache,* tremor, paresthesias, asthenia, suicidal thoughts and behaviors, seizures, chills, yawning, hot flashes, flushing, *irritability , insomnia, anxiety, abnormal dreams, fatigue*

CV: Palpitations, sinus tachycardia, increased blood pressure, orthostatic hypotension

EENT: Blurred vision, mydriasis, tinnitus, bruxism

GI: *Nausea,* xerostomia, *diarrhea,* constipation, vomiting, anorexia, weight loss, dysgeusia, hypercholesterolemia, hypertriglyceridemia

GU: Urinary retention/hesitancy, orgasm dysfunction, decreased libido, impotence, proteinuria

HEMA: Impaired platelet aggregation

INTEG: Photosensitivity, hyperhidrosis, diaphoresis

SYST: Serotonin syndrome, neuroleptic malignant syndrome-like symptoms, toxic epidermal necrolysis, rash, Stevens-Johnson syndrome, erythema multiforme, angioedema; neonatal abstinence syndrome (fetal exposure)

Pharmacokinetics

Absorption	Unknown
Distribution	Protein binding 30%; enters breast milk
Metabolism	Liver, 55%
Excretion	Urine, unchanged, 45%
Half-life	Elimination 11 hr, increased in hepatic/renal disease

Pharmacodynamics

Onset	Unknown
Peak	7.5 hr
Duration	24 hr

INTERACTIONS
Individual drugs
Dexfenfluramine, dexmethylphenidate, dextromethorphan, fenfluramine, linezolid, lithium, nefazodone, meperidine, methylphenidate, mirtazapine, pentazocine, phentermine, promethazine, sibutramine, SUMAtriptan, traZODone, tryptophan: do not administer concurrently; increased serotonin syndrome, neuroleptic malignant syndrome-like reactions

Zolpidem: increased hallucinations, delusions, disorientation

Drug classifications
Anticoagulants, NSAIDs, platelet inhibitors, salicylates, thrombolytics: increased bleeding risk

Alcohol, antihistamines, opioids, sedatives/hypnotics: increased CNS depression

Ergots, MAOIs, serotonin receptor agonists (almotriptan, eletriptan, frovatriptan, methylene blue IV, naratriptan, rizatriptan, SUMAtriptan, ZOLMitriptan), SSRIs, other SNRIs, TCAs, tricyclics: do not administer concurrently; increased serotonin syndrome, neuroleptic malignant syndrome-like reactions

Drug/herb
Kava, valerian: increased desvenlafaxine action

Drug/lab test
Increased: sodium, cholesterol, triglycerides
False positive: amphetamine, phencyclidine

NURSING CONSIDERATIONS
Assessment

> **BLACK BOX WARNING: Suicidal thoughts/behaviors:** Assess mental status and mood, identify suicidal ideation

- Serotonin syndrome, neuroleptic malignant syndrome-like symptoms: Assess for nausea/vomiting, sedation, dizziness, diaphoresis (sweating), facial flush, hallucinations, mental status changes, myoclonia, restlessness, shivering, elevated blood pressure, hyperthermia, muscle rigidity, autonomic instability, and mental status changes; if serotonin syndrome occurs discontinue desvenlafaxine, and any other serotonergic agents
- Monitor B/P baseline and periodically during treatment, lipid levels, signs of glaucoma
- Assess appetite and nutritional intake, weight loss is common, change diet as need to support weight

Patient/family education
- Teach patient to take as directed, not to double or skip doses; if a dose is missed, take as soon as remembered unless close to next dose, do not discontinue abruptly, decreased gradually

> **BLACK BOX WARNING:** Advise patient to report immediately suicidal thoughts or behaviors, have family members look for symptoms of suicidal ideation

- Inform patient not to operate machinery or engage in hazardous activities until reaction ins known, may cause dizziness, drowsiness
- Teach patient to avoid all others products unless approval by prescriber
- Teach patient to report if pregnancy is planned or suspected, pregnancy C, or if breastfeeding
- ⚠ Teach patient to report immediately allergic reactions including, rash, hives, difficulty breathing, or swelling of face, lips
- Advise patient that continuing follow-up exams will be needed

Evaluation

Positive therapeutic outcome
- Decreased depression, increased sense of well-being and renewed interest in activities

dexamethasone (Rx)
(dex-ah-meth′ah-sone)
Dexasone ✚, Zena-Pak

dexamethasone sodium phosphate (Rx)
Func. class.: Corticosteroid, synthetic
Chem. class.: Glucocorticoid, long-acting
Pregnancy category C

Do not confuse: Decadron/Percodan

ACTION: Decreases inflammation by suppressing migration of polymorphonuclear leukocytes, fibroblasts, reversing increased capillary permeability and lysosomal stabilization, suppresses normal immune response, no mineralocorticoid effects

USES: Inflammation, allergies, neoplasms, cerebral edema, septic shock, collagen disorders, dexamethasone suppression test for Cushing syndrome, adrenocortical insufficiency, TB, meningitis, acute exacerbations of MS

CONTRAINDICATIONS
Psychosis, hypersensitivity to corticosteroids, sulfites, or benzyl alcohol, idiopathic thrombocytopenia, acute glomerulonephritis, amebiasis, fungal infections, nonasthmatic bronchial disease, child <2 yr, AIDS, TB, glaucoma, ocular infection

Precautions: Pregnancy **C**, breastfeeding, diabetes mellitus, osteoporosis, seizure disorders, ulcerative colitis, CHF, myasthenia gravis, renal disease, peptic ulcer, esophagitis, recent MI, hypertension, TB, active hepatitis, psychosis, sulfite hypersensitivity, thromboembolic disorders, abrupt discontinuation, coagulopathy, ulcerative colitis, seizure disorders

DOSAGE AND ROUTES
Inflammation
Adult: PO 0.75-9 mg/day, in divided doses q6-12hr; or phosphate IM 0.5-9 mg/day divided q6-12hr
Child: PO 0.024-0.34 mg/kg/day in divided doses q6-12hr

Shock
Adult: IV (phosphate) single dose 1-6 mg/kg or IV 40 mg q2-6hr as needed up to 72 hr

Cerebral edema
Adult: IV (phosphate) 10 mg, then 4-6 mg IM q6hr × 2-4 days, then taper over 1 wk
Child: PO/IM/IV loading dose 1-2 mg/kg, then 1-1.5 mg/kg/day, max 16 mg/day divided q4-6hr for 2-4 days, then taper down qwk

Adrenocortical insufficiency
Adult: PO 0.75-9 mg/day in divided doses
Child: PO 0.03-0.3 mg/kg/day divided in 2-4 doses

Suppression test
Adult: PO 1 mg at 11 PM or 0.5 mg q6hr × 48 hr

Available forms: Dexamethasone: tabs 0.5, 0.75, 1, 1.5, 2, 4, 6 mg; elix 0.5 mg/5 ml; oral sol 0.5 mg/5 ml, 1 mg/ml; **sodium phosphate** 4, 10 mg/ml; ophth implant 0.7 mg; ophth susp drops/sol 0.1%

Implementation
PO route
- Give with food or milk to decrease GI symptoms
- Provide assistance with ambulation in patient with bone tissue disease to prevent fractures, give once a day in AM for less toxicity, less adverse reactions

IM route
- IM inj deep in large muscle mass; rotate sites; avoid deltoid; use 21-G needle
- In one dose in AM to prevent adrenal suppression; avoid SUBCUT administration, may damage tissue

Direct IV route (sodium phosphate)
- **IV** undiluted direct over 1 min or less
- Titrated dose; use lowest effective dose

Intermittent IV infusion route
- Diluted with 0.9% NaCl or D₅W and give as an **IV** inf at prescribed rate

Dexamethasone sodium phosphate

Syringe compatibilities: Acetaminophen, caffeine, dimenhydrAMINE, furosemide, granisetron, hyaluronidase, ketamine, metoclopramide, octreotide, oxyCODONE, palonosetron, ranitidine, salbutamol, SUFentanil, traMADol

Y-site compatibilities: Acetaminophen, acyclovir, alfentanil, allopurinol, amifostine, amikacin, aminocaproic acid, aminophylline, amphotericin B cholesteryl, amphotericin B lipid complex, amphotericin B liposome, amsacrine, anidulafungin, argatroban, ascorbic acid injection, atenolol, atracurium, atropine, aztreonam, benztropine, bivalirudin, bleomycin, bumetanide, buprenorphine, butorphanol, CARBOplatin, carmustine, ceFAZolin, cefepime, cefonicid, cefoTEtan, cefOXitin, cefpirome, ceftaroline, cefTAZidime, ceftizoxime, cefTRIAXone, chloramphenicol, cimetidine, cisatracurium, CISplatin, cladribine, clindamycin, codeine, cyanocobalamin, cyclophosphamide, cycloSPORINE, cytarabine, DACTINomycin, DAPTOmycin, DAUNOrubicin liposome, dexmedetomidine, digoxin, diltiazem, DOCEtaxel, DOPamine, doripenem, doxacurium, DOXOrubicin, DOXOrubicin liposomal, enalaprilat, ePHEDrine, EPINEPHrine, epoetin alfa, eptifibatide, ertapenem, etoposide, etoposide phosphate, famotidine, fentaNYL, filgrastim, fluconazole, fludarabine, fluorouracil, folic acid, fosaprepitant, foscarnet, furosemide, ganciclovir, gatifloxacin, gemcitabine, glycopyrrolate, granisetron, heparin, hydrocortisone, HYDROmorphone, ifosfamide, imipenem-cilastatin, indomethacin, insulin (regular), irinotecan, isoproterenol, ketorolac, lansoprazole, leucovorin, levofloxacin, lidocaine, linezolid, liposome, LORazepam, LR, mannitol, mechlorethamine, melphalan, meropenem, metaraminol, methadone, methyldopate, methylPREDNISolone, metoclopramide, metoprolol, metroNIDAZOLE, mezlocillin, milrinone, morphine, multiple vitamins injection, nafcillin, nalbuphine, naloxone, nitroglycerin, nitroprusside, norepinephrine, octreotide, ondansetron, oxacillin, oxaliplatin, oxyCODONE, oxytocin, PACLitaxel, palonosetron, pamidronate, pancuronium, PEMEtrexed, penicillin G potassium/sodium, PENTobarbital, PHENobarbital, phenylephrine, phytonadione, piperacillin, piperacillin-tazobactam, potassium chloride, procainamide, propofol, propranolol, pyridoxine, ranitidine, remifentanil, Ringer's, ritodrine, riTUXimab, sargramostim, sodium acetate/bicarbonate, succinylcholine, SUFentanil, tacrolimus, telavancin, teniposide, theophylline, thiamine, thiotepa, ticarcillin, ticarcillin-clavulanate, tigecycline, tirofiban, TNA, tolazoline, topotecan, trastuzumab, urokinase, vancomycin, vasopressin, vecuronium, verapamil, vinCRIStine, vinorelbine, vitamin B complex/C, voriconazole, zidovudine, zoledronic acid

ADVERSE EFFECTS
CNS: *Depression, flushing, sweating,* headache, mood changes, euphoria, psychosis, seizures, insomnia, **pseudotumor cerebri**
CV: *Hypertension,* circulatory collapse, thromboembolism, heart failure, dysrhythmias, tachycardia, edema, cardiomyopathy
EENT: Fungal infections, increased intraocular pressure, blurred vision, cataracts, glaucoma
ENDO: Hypothalmic-pituitary-adrenal axis suppression, hyperglycemia, sodium, fluid retention
GI: *Diarrhea, nausea, abdominal distention,* **GI hemorrhage,** *increased appetite,* **pancreatitis**
HEMA: Thrombocytopenia, transient leukocytosis, thromboembolism
INTEG: Acne, poor wound healing, ecchymosis, petechiae, hirsutism, **angioedema**
META: Hypokalemia
MS: Fractures, osteoporosis, weakness, arthralgia, myopathy

Pharmacokinetics

Absorption	Unknown
Distribution	Unknown
Metabolism	Liver
Excretion	Kidneys
Half-life	1-2 days

Pharmacodynamics

	PO	IM
Onset	1 hr	Unknown
Peak	1-2 hr	8 hr
Duration	2½ days	6 days-3 wk

INTERACTIONS
Individual drugs
Alcohol, amphotericin B, cycloSPORINE, digoxin, indomethacin: increased side effects

Ambemonium, isoniazid, neostigmine, sometrem: decreased effects of each specific product

Bosentan, carBAMazepine, cholestyramine, colestipol, ePHEDrine, ethotoin, phenytoin, rifampin, theophylline: decreased action of dexamethasone

CycloSPORINE, tacrolimus: increased effect of each drug

Ketoconazole, NSAIDs: increased action of dexamethasone

Drug classifications
Antacids, barbiturates: decreased action of dexamethasone

Antibiotics (macrolide), contraceptives (hormonal), estrogens, salicylates: increased action of dexamethasone

Anticholinesterases, anticoagulants, anticonvulsants, antidiabetics, salicylates, toxoids/vaccines: decreased effects of each specific product

Antidiabetics: increased effect of these products

Diuretics, NSAIDs, salicylates: increased side effects

Quinolones: increased risk of tendinitis, tendon rupture

Thiazide diuretics: decreased potassium levels/ loop, amphotericin B

Drug/lab test
Increased: cholesterol, Na, blood glucose, uric acid, Ca, urine glucose

Decreased: Ca, potassium, T_4, T_3, thyroid ^{131}I uptake test, urine 17-OHCS, 17-KS, PBI

False negative: skin allergy tests

NURSING CONSIDERATIONS
Assessment
• Monitor K, blood, urine glucose while on long-term therapy; hypokalemia and hyperglycemia
• Monitor weight daily; notify prescriber of weekly gain >5 lb
• Monitor B/P, pulse; notify prescriber of chest pain
• Monitor I&O ratio; be alert for decreasing urinary output, increasing edema
• **Epidural injections (unlabeled): may cause rare events (vision loss, paralysis, stroke, death)**
• Monitor plasma cortisol levels during long-term therapy (normal: 138-635 nmol/L when assessed at 8 AM), prolonged use can cause **cushingoid symptoms** (buffalo hump, moon face, increased B/P)
• **Assess infection:** fever, WBC even after withdrawal of medication; product masks infection

• **Assess potassium depletion:** paresthesias, fatigue, nausea, vomiting, depression, polyuria, dysrhythmias, weakness
• Assess edema, hypertension, cardiac symptoms
• Assess mental status: affect, mood, behavioral changes, aggression
⚠ **Abrupt withdrawal: acute adrenal insufficiency and death may occur following abrupt discontinuation of systemic therapy; withdraw gradually**

Patient/family education
• Advise that emergency ID as corticosteroid user should be carried or worn
• Teach to notify prescriber if therapeutic response decreases; dosage adjustment may be needed
• **Teach not to discontinue abruptly or adrenal crisis can result**
• Teach to avoid OTC products: salicylates, alcohol in cough products, cold preparations unless directed by prescriber
• Instruct patient to contact prescriber if surgery, trauma, stress occurs, dosage may need to be adjusted
• Teach patient all aspects of product use, including cushingoid symptoms
• Instruct patient to notify prescriber of infection
• Teach patient to take with food or milk
• Teach patient that bruising may occur easily
• Teach patient that if on long-term therapy, a high-protein diet may be needed
• Teach symptoms of adrenal insufficiency: nausea, anorexia, fatigue, dizziness, dyspnea, weakness, joint pain
• Advise patient to avoid exposure to chickenpox or measles, persons with infections

Evaluation
Positive therapeutic outcome
Decreased inflammation

dexamethasone ophthalmic
See Appendix B

dexlansoprazole (Rx)
(dex-lan-so-prey′zole)
Dexilant
Func. class.: Anti-ulcer—proton pump inhibitor
Chem. class.: Benzimidazole
Pregnancy category B

ACTION: Suppresses gastric secretion by inhibiting hydrogen/potassium ATPase enzyme system in gastric parietal cell; characterized as gastric acid pump inhibitor, since it blocks final step of acid production

Therapeutic outcome: Reduction in gastric pain, swelling, fullness

USES: Gastroesophageal reflux disease (GERD), severe erosive esophagitis, heartburn

CONTRAINDICATIONS
Hypersensitivity

Precautions: Pregnancy **B,** breastfeeding, children, proton-pump hypersensitivity, gastric cancer, hepatic disease, vit B_{12} deficiency, colitis

DOSAGE AND ROUTES
Erosive esophagitis
Adult: PO 60 mg qd for up to 8 wk; maintenance: PO 30 mg qd for up to 6 mo

GERD
Adult: PO: 30 mg qd × 4 wk

Hepatic disease
Adult: PO (Child-Pugh B): max 30 mg/day

Available forms: Del rel caps 30, 60 mg

Implementation
• Swallow del rel cap whole; do not break, crush, chew; caps may be opened and contents sprinkled on food, use immediately; do not chew contents of caps, give without regard to food

ADVERSE EFFECTS
CNS: Headache, dizziness, confusion, agitation, amnesia, depression, anxiety, seizures, insomnia
CV: Chest pain, angina, bradycardia, palpitations, CVA, hypertension, MI
EENT: Tinnitus
GI: Diarrhea, abdominal pain, vomiting, nausea, constipation, flatulence, colitis, dysgeusia, pseudomembranous colitis
HEMA: Anemia, neutropenia, thrombocytopenia, pernicious anemia, thrombosis
INTEG: Rash, urticaria, pruritus
META: Gout
MS: Arthralgia, myalgia
RESP: Upper respiratory infections, cough, epistaxis, dyspnea
SYST: Anaphylaxis, Stevens-Johnson syndrome, toxic epidermal necrolysis, exfoliative dermatitis, pneumonia

Pharmacokinetics
Absorption	57%-64%
Distribution	Protein binding 97%
Metabolism	Liver extensively
Excretion	Urine, feces; clearance decreased in geriatric, renal/hepatic disease
Half-life	Plasma 1-2 hr, 4-5 hr

Pharmacodynamics
Unknown

INTERACTIONS
Individual drugs
Ampicillin, calcium carbonate, delavirdine, iron, itraconazole, ketoconazole: decreased absorption of each specific product

Drug classifications
CYP2C19, CYP3A4 (fluvoxamine, voriconazole): increased dexlansoprazole effect
Sucralfate: delayed absorption of dexlansoprazole

Drug/lab test
Increased: LFTs, bilirubin, creatinine, glucose, lipids
Decreased: platelets, magnesium

NURSING CONSIDERATIONS
Assessment
• **Pseudomembranous colitis:** diarrhea, abdominal cramps, fever, report to prescriber promptly
⚠ Anaphylaxis, serious skin disorders requiring emergency intervention (rare)
⚠ Hepatotoxicity: Hepatitis, jaundice, monitor liver enzymes (AST, ALT, alkaline phosphatase) during treatment if hepatic adverse reactions occur (rare)
• **Hypomagnesemia:** Usually 3 months to 1 yr after beginning therapy; monitor magnesium level, assess for irregular heart beats, muscle spasms; in children fatigue, upset stomach, dizziness; magnesium supplement may be used

Patient/family education
• **Pseudomembranous colitis:** report to prescriber at once abdominal cramps, bloody diarrhea, fever
• Inform diabetic patient that hypoglycemia may occur
• Encourage patient to avoid hazardous activities; dizziness may occur
• Tell patient to avoid alcohol, salicylates, ibuprofen; may cause GI irritation

• Teach patient to report allergic reactions, symptoms of low magnesium levels

⚠ Teach patient to notify prescriber if pregnancy is planned or suspected, not to breastfeed

• Advise patient to swallow cap whole, not to chew, crush, to report all products being used to prescriber

Evaluation

Positive therapeutic outcome

• Absence of gastric pain, swelling, fullness; healing of erosive esophagitis

---

dexmethylphenidate (Rx)

(dex′meth-ul-fen′ih-dayt)

Focalin, Focalin XR

Func. class.: Central nervous system (CNS) stimulant, psychostimulant

Pregnancy category C

Controlled substance schedule II

Do not confuse: dexmethylphenidate/methylphenidate

ACTION: Increases release of norepinephrine and dopamine into the extraneuronal space, also blocks reuptake of norepinephrine and dopamine into the presynaptic neuron; mode of action in treating attention-deficit-hyperactivity disorder (ADHD) is unknown

Therapeutic outcome: Increased alertness, decreased fatigue, ability to stay awake (narcolepsy), increased attention span, decreased hyperactivity (ADHD)

USE: ADHD

CONTRAINDICATIONS

Hypersensitivity to methylphenidate, anxiety, history of Tourette's syndrome; glaucoma, concurrent treatment with MAOIs or within 14 days of discontinuing treatment with MAOIs, tics, psychosis

Precautions: Pregnancy C, hypertension, depression, seizures, CV disorders, breastfeeding, Child <6 yr, geriatrics, psychosis, thyrotoxicosis

> **BLACK BOX WARNING:** Substance abuse, alcoholism

DOSAGE AND ROUTES

Adult: PO EXT REL 10 mg/day, may adjust to 20 mg/day in 10 mg increments

Child >6 yr: PO 2.5 mg bid with doses at least 4 hr apart, gradually increase to a max of 20 mg/day (10 mg bid); for those taking methylphenidate, use ½ of methylphenidate dose initially, then increase as needed to max 20 mg/day; EXT REL 5 mg/day, may adjust to 20 mg/day in 5 mg increments

Available forms: Tabs 2.5, 5, 10 mg; ext rel caps 5, 10, 15, 20, 25, 30, 35, 40 mg

Implementation

• Do not break, crush, or chew ext rel caps
• Twice daily at least 4 hr apart; ext rel once a day
• Without regard to meals
• Med guide should be provided by dispenser

ADVERSE EFFECTS

CNS: Dizziness, headache, drowsiness, nervousness, insomnia, toxic psychosis, neuroleptic malignant syndrome (rare), Tourette's syndrome

CV: Palpitations, B/P changes, angina, dysrhythmias, tachycardia, **MI, stroke**

GI: *Nausea, anorexia*, abnormal liver function, hepatic coma, *abdominal pain*

HEMA: Leukopenia, anemia, thrombocytopenic purpura

INTEG: Exfoliative dermatitis, urticaria, rash, erythema multiforme

MISC: *Fever*, arthralgia, scalp hair loss, rhabdomyolysis

Pharmacokinetics

Absorption	Readily absorbed
Distribution	Unknown
Metabolism	Liver
Excretion	Kidneys
Half-life	2.2 hr

Pharmacodynamics

	PO	EXT REL
Onset	½-1 hr	Unknown
Peak	1-1½ hr	4 hr

INTERACTIONS

Drug classifications

Anticoagulants (coumarin), anticonvulsants, selective serotonin reuptake inhibitors, tricyclics: increased effects

Antihypertensives: decreased effects

Decongestants, vasoconstrictors: increased sympathomimetic effect

MAOIs: hypertensive crisis if coadministered or given within 14 days

Vasopressors: hypertensive crisis

Drug/herb

Melatonin: increased synergistic effect

NURSING CONSIDERATIONS

Assessment

> **BLACK BOX WARNING:** Assess for previous or current substance abuse; psychotic episodes may occur, especially with parental abuse

• Toxicity/ rhabdomyolysis: Assess for headache, flushing, vomiting, agitation, tachycardia, tremor, euphoria, hallucinations, hyperreflexia
• Assess VS, B/P; may reverse antihypertensives; check patients with cardiac disease more often for increased B/P
• Assess CBC, differential, platelet counts during long-term therapy, urinalysis; in diabetes: blood/urine glucose; insulin changes may have to be made, since eating will decrease
• Assess height, growth rate q3mo in children; growth rate may be decreased
• Assess mental status: mood, sensorium, affect, stimulation, insomnia, aggressiveness
⚠ Assess withdrawal symptoms: headache, nausea, vomiting, muscle pain, weakness
• Assess appetite, sleep, speech patterns
• Assess for attention span, decreased hyperactivity in persons with ADHD

Patient/family education
• Advise patient to decrease caffeine consumption (coffee, tea, cola, chocolate); may increase irritability, stimulation
• Advise patient to avoid OTC preparations unless approved by prescriber
• Caution patient to taper off product over several wk to avoid depression, increased sleeping, lethargy
• Caution patient to avoid alcohol ingestion
• Caution patient to avoid hazardous activities until stabilized on medication
• Advise patient to get needed rest; patients will feel more tired at end of day
• Notify all health providers including school nurse of medication and schedule
• Discuss information instructions provided in patient information section
• Teach patient to notify prescriber if pregnancy is planned or suspected, avoid breastfeeding
• Teach patient to report toxicity immediately: vomiting, agitation, tremor, hyperreflexia, euphoria, confusion, hallucinations, flushing, headache, tachycardia, rhabdomyolysis

Evaluation

Positive therapeutic outcome
• Decreased hyperactivity or ability to stay awake

TREATMENT OF OVERDOSE:
Administer fluids; hemodialysis or peritoneal dialysis; antihypertensive for increased B/P; administer short-acting barbiturate before lavage

dextroamphetamine (Rx)
(dex-troe-am-fet'a-meen)
Dexedrine, ProCentra
Func. class.: Cerebral stimulant
Chem. class.: Amphetamine
Pregnancy category C
Controlled substance schedule II

ACTION: Increases release of norepinephrine, dopamine in cerebral cortex to reticular activating system

Therapeutic outcome: Increased alertness, decreased fatigue, ability to stay awake (narcolepsy); increased attention span, decreased hyperactivity (ADHD)

USES: Narcolepsy, attention-deficit disorder with hyperactivity

Unlabeled use: Obesity

CONTRAINDICATIONS
Hypersensitivity to sympathomimetic amines, hyperthyroidism, hypertension, glaucoma, severe arteriosclerosis, drug abuse

> **BLACK BOX WARNING:** Symptomatic CV disease, substance abuse

Precautions: Pregnancy **C**, breastfeeding, child <3 yr, Gilles de la Tourette's disorder, depression, cardiomyopathy, bipolar disorder, abrupt discontinuation, acute MI; benzyl alcohol, salicylate hypersensitivity; hypercortisolism, obesity, psychosis, seizure disorder, anxiety, anorexia nervosa, tartrazine dye hypersensitivity

DOSAGE AND ROUTES
Narcolepsy
Adult: PO 5 mg bid, titrate daily dose by no more than 10 mg/wk, max 60 mg/day
Child 6-12 yr: PO 5 mg daily increasing by no more than 5 mg/day at weekly intervals

ADHD
Adult: PO 5-60 mg/day q day or divided bid
Child 6-12 yr: PO 5 mg daily-bid increasing by 5 mg/day at weekly intervals
Child 3-5 yr: PO 2.5 mg daily increasing by 2.5 mg/day at weekly intervals (max 40 mg/day)

Available forms: Tabs 5, 10 mg; oral sol 5 mg/5 ml; caps ext rel 5, 10, 15 mg

Implementation
• Give at least 6 hr before bedtime to avoid sleeplessness; titrate to patient's response; lowest dosage should be used to control symptoms

• Give gum, hard candy, frequent sips of water for dry mouth at beginning of treatment; these symptoms tend to lessen with time
• Store all forms at room temperature

ADVERSE EFFECTS

CNS: *Hyperactivity, insomnia, restlessness, talkativeness,* dizziness, headache, chills, stimulation, dysphoria, irritability, aggressiveness, tremor, dependence, addiction
CV: *Palpitations,* tachycardia, hypertension, decrease in heart rate, dysrhythmias
GI: *Anorexia,* dry mouth, diarrhea, constipation, weight loss, metallic taste
GU: Impotence, change in libido
INTEG: Urticaria
MISC: Rhabdomyolysis

Pharmacokinetics

Absorption	Well absorbed
Distribution	Widely distributed; crosses placenta
Metabolism	Liver
Excretion	Kidneys, pH dependent: increased pH, increased reabsorption
Half-life	10-30 hr; increased when urine is alkaline

Pharmacodynamics

Onset	½ hr; ext rel 1 hr
Peak	1-3 hr; ext rel 2 hr
Duration	4-10 hr; ext rel 8 hr

INTERACTIONS
Individual drugs
AcetaZOLAMIDE, sodium bicarbonate: increased effect of dextroamphetamine
Ammonium chloride, ascorbic acid, guanethidine: decreased effect of dextroamphetamine
Haloperidol: increased CNS effect
Phenytoin: decreased absorption of phenytoin

Drug classifications
Adrenergic blockers: decreased adrenergic blocking effect
Antacids: increased effect of dextroamphetamine
Antidepressants (tricyclic), phenothiazines: increased CNS effect
Antidiabetics: decreased antidiabetic effect
Antihistamines: decreased antihistamine effect
Antihypertensives: decreased antihypertensive effect
Barbiturates: decreased absorption of barbiturate
MAOIs: hypertensive crisis if used within 14 days
SSRIs, SNRIs, serotonin-receptor agonists: do not use concurrently: increased serotonin syndrome, neuroleptic malignant syndrome

Drug/herb
Eucalyptus: decreased stimulant effect
St. John's wort: increased serotonin syndrome

Drug/food
Caffeine (cola, coffee, tea [green/black]): increased amine effect

Drug/lab test
Increase: plasma corticosteroids, urinary steroids

NURSING CONSIDERATIONS
Assessment

> **BLACK BOX WARNING: Cardiac disease:** monitor VS, B/P, since this product may reverse antihypertensives; check patients with cardiac disease more often for increased B/P

• Monitor CBC, urinalysis; for diabetic patients monitor blood, urine glucose; insulin changes may be required, since eating will decrease
• Monitor height and weight q3mo since growth rate in children may be decreased; appetite is suppressed so weight loss is common during the first few months of treatment
• Toxicity: Symptoms may vary in children; anxiety, headache, flushing, vomiting, rhabdomyolysis, tremor, hyperreflexia, confusion, euphoria, tachycardia
• Monitor mental status: mood, sensorium, affect, stimulation, insomnia; aggressiveness may occur; depression with crying spells may occur after product has worn off
• Assess for **physical dependency;** should not be used for extended time except in ADHD; dosage should be decreased gradually to prevent withdrawal symptoms
• Assess for narcoleptic symptoms before medication and after; ability to stay awake should increase significantly
• In children or adults with ADHD, monitor for improved organizational skills, attention span, attending to tasks, impulse control, socialization, and ability to get along better with others
• Assess for withdrawal symptoms: headache, nausea, vomiting, muscle pain, weakness; product tolerance develops after long-term use; dosage should not be increased if tolerance develops; this medication has a high abuse potential

Patient/family education
• Advise patient to decrease caffeine consumption (coffee, tea, cola, chocolate), which may increase irritability and stimulation; to avoid OTC preparations unless approved by prescriber; to

avoid alcohol ingestion; these may cause serious drug interactions

- Advise patient to take before meals (obesity)
- Caution patient to taper off product over several weeks, or depression, increased sleeping, lethargy may occur
- Caution patient to avoid hazardous activities until patient is stabilized on medication
- Instruct patient not to double doses if medication is missed; prescriber may suggest product holidays (ADHD) during the school year to assess progress and determine continued need for product
- Instruct patient/family to notify prescriber if significant side effects occur: tremors, insomnia, palpitations, restlessness, product changes may be needed
- Inform patient that if dry mouth occurs, to use frequent sips of water, sugarless gum, hard candy during beginning therapy; dry mouth lessens with continued treatment
- Advise patient to get needed rest; patients will feel more tired at end of day; to give last dose at least 6 hr before bedtime to avoid insomnia

Evaluation
Positive therapeutic outcome

- Decreased activity in ADHD
- Absence of sleeping during day in narcolepsy

TREATMENT OF OVERDOSE:
Administer fluids, hemodialysis, peritoneal dialysis, antihypertensives for increased B/P; ammonium chloride for increased excretion

dextromethorphan (OTC)
(dex-troe-meth-or′fan)

Balminil ✦, Buckley's DM, Buckley's Mixture, Delsym 12-Hour, ElixSure Cough, Koffex, Robafen Cough Gels, Robitussin, Robitussin Cough with Honey, Robitussin Long-Acting Cough, Scot-Tussin Diabetes CF, Triaminic Long-Acting Cough, Vicks Formula 44 Cough Relief, Wal-Tussin

Func. class.: Antitussive, nonopioid
Chem. class.: Levorphanol derivative

Pregnancy category C

ACTION: Depresses cough center in medulla by direct effect related to levorphanol

Therapeutic outcome: Absence of cough

USES: Nonproductive cough carried by minor respiratory tract infections or irritants that might be inhaled

CONTRAINDICATIONS
Hypersensitivity

Precautions: Pregnancy **C**, fever, hepatic disease, asthma/emphysema, chronic cough

DOSAGE AND ROUTES
Adult and child ≥12 yr: PO 10-20 mg q4hr, or 30 mg q6-8hr, max 120 mg/day; SUS REL LIQUID 60 mg q12hr, max 120 mg/day
Child 6-11 yr: PO 5-10 mg q4hr; SUS REL LIQUID 30 mg bid, max 60 mg/day; LOZENGE 5-10 mg q1-4hr, max 60 mg/day

Available forms: Liquid 7.5, 15 mg/5 ml; syr 15 mg/15 ml, 10 mg/5 ml; 15 mg/5 ml, 30 mg/15 ml; caps 15 mg; gel caps 15 mg; EXT REL SUSP 30 mg/5 ml

Implementation
- Give **chew tabs:** chew well; **syrup:** use calibrated measuring device; **ext rel susp:** shake well, use calibrated measuring device
- Administer decreased dosage to geriatric patients; their metabolism may be slowed; do not provide water within 30 min of administration because it dilutes product
- Shake susp before administration

ADVERSE EFFECTS
CNS: *Dizziness,* sedation, confusion, ataxia, fatigue
GI: *Nausea*

Pharmacokinetics

Absorption	Rapid (PO); slow (SUS REL)
Distribution	Unknown
Metabolism	Liver
Excretion	Kidneys
Half-life	Terminal 11 hr

Pharmacodynamics

	PO	PO-sus
Onset	15-30 min	Unknown
Peak	Unknown	Unknown
Duration	3-6 hr	12 hr

INTERACTIONS
Individual drugs
Alcohol: increased CNS depression
Amiodarone, quiNIDine, sibutramine: increased adverse reactions
Furazolidone, linezolid, procarbazine: increased hypotension, hyperpyrexia; do not give within 2 wk (MAOI activity)

Drug classifications
Antihistamines, antidepressants, opiates, sedative-hypnotics: increased CNS depression
MAOIs: increased hypotension, hyperpyrexia, do not give within 2 wk of MAOIs

Serotonin receptor agonists, SSRIs: increased serotonin syndrome

NURSING CONSIDERATIONS
Assessment
• Assess **cough**: type, frequency, character including sputum; provide adequate hydration to 2 L/day to decrease viscosity of secretions

Patient/family education
• Caution patient to avoid driving or other hazardous activities until stabilized on this medication; may cause drowsiness, dizziness in some individuals
• Advise patient to avoid smoking, smoke-filled rooms, perfumes, dust, environmental pollutants, cleaners, which increase cough; may use gum, hard candy to prevent dry mouth
• Advise patient to avoid alcohol or other CNS depressants while taking this medication; drowsiness will be increased
• Caution patient that any cough lasting over a few days should be assessed by prescriber

Evaluation
Positive therapeutic outcome
• Absence of dry, irritating cough

RARELY USED
dextrose (D-glucose) (Rx)
Func. class.: Caloric agent

Therapeutic outcome: Provides calories, prevents severe hypoglycemia

USES: Increases intake of calories; increases fluids in patients unable to take adequate fluids, calories orally; acute hypoglycemia

CONTRAINDICATIONS
Hyperglycemia, delirium tremens, hemorrhage (cranial/spinal), CHF, anuria, allergy to corn products, concentrated products

DOSAGE AND ROUTES
Hypoglycemia
Adult: PO/IV 10-25 mg per mg/dose (20-50 ml of a 50% sol), may need subsequent continuous IV infusion of 10% dextrose

Acute symptomatic hypoglycemia (infants/neonates)
Neonate/infant: IV 250-500 mg/kg/dose (25% sol)

---

diazepam (Rx)
(dye-az'e-pam)
Diastat, Diazemuls ♣, Valium
Func. class.: Antianxiety, anticonvulsant, skeletal muscle relaxant, central acting
Chem. class.: Benzodiazepine, long-acting
Pregnancy category D
Controlled substance schedule IV

Do not confuse: diazepam/Ditropan/ LORazepam

ACTION: Potentiates the actions of GABA, especially in limbic system, reticular formation; enhances presympathetic inhibition, inhibits spinal polysynaptic afferent paths

Therapeutic outcome: Decreased anxiety, restlessness, insomnia

USES: Anxiety, acute alcohol withdrawal, adjunct in seizure disorders; preoperative skeletal muscle relaxation; rectally for acute repetitive seizures

CONTRAINDICATIONS
Pregnancy **D**, hypersensitivity to benzodiazepines, closed angle glaucoma, coma, myasthenia gravis, ethanol intoxication, hepatic disease, sleep apnea

Precautions: Breastfeeding, geriatric, debilitated, addiction, child <6 mo, asthma, renal disease, bipolar disorder, COPD, CNS depression, labor, Parkinson's disease, neutropenia, psychosis, seizures, substance abuse, smoking

DOSAGE AND ROUTES
Anxiety/convulsive disorders
Adult: PO 2-10 mg bid-qid; IM/IV 2-10 mg q3-4hr
Geriatric: PO 2-2.5 mg daily-bid, increase slowly as needed
Child >6 mo: IM/IV 0.04-0.3 mg/kg/dose q2-4hr, max 0.6 mg/kg in an 8-hr period

Precardioversion
Adult: IV 5-15 mg 5-10 min precardioversion

Preendoscopy
Adult: IV 2.5-20 mg, IM 5-10 mg ½ hr preendoscopy

Muscle relaxation
Adult: PO 2-10 mg tid-qid or EXT REL 15-30 mg daily; IM/IV 5-10 mg repeat in 2-4 hr

Tetanic muscle spasms
Child >5 yr: IM/IV 5-10 mg q3-4hr prn
Infant >30 days: IM/IV 1-2 mg q3-4hr prn

Status epilepticus
Adult: IM/IV 5-10 mg, 2 mg/min, may repeat q10-15min; max 30 mg; may repeat in 2-4 hr if seizures reappear
Child >5 yr: IV 1 mg slowly; IM 1 mg q2-5min
Child 1 mo-5 yr: IV 0.2-0.5 mg slowly; IM 0.2-0.5 mg slowly q2-5min up to 5 mg; may repeat in 2-4 hr prn

Seizures other than status epilepticus
Adult: RECT 0.2 mg/kg, may repeat 4-12 hr later
Child 6-11 yr: RECT 0.3 mg/kg, may repeat 4-12 hr later
Child 2-5 yr: RECT 0.5 mg/kg, may repeat 4-12 hr later

Alcohol withdrawal
Adult: IV 10 mg initially, then 5-10 mg q3-4hr prn

Available forms: Tabs 2, 5, 10 mg; inj 5 mg/ml; oral sol 5 mg/5 ml; rectal 2.5 (pediatric), 10, 20 mg, twin packs; ext rel cap 15 mg; rectal gel

Implementation
PO route
- Give with food or milk for GI symptoms
- Crush tab if patient is unable to swallow medication whole
- Reduce opioid dosage by one third if given concomitantly with diazepam
- Check to see if PO medication has been swallowed
- **Concentrate:** use calibrated dropper only; mix with water, juice, pudding, applesauce; consume immediately

Rectal route
- Do not use more than 5 ×/mo or for an episode q5day (Diastat)

Direct IV route
- Administer **IV** into large vein; do not dilute or mix with any other product; give **IV** 5 mg or less/min or total dose over 3 min or more (children, infants); cont inf is not recommended; inject closest vein insertion as possible; do not dilute or mix with other products
- Check **IV** site for thrombosis or phlebitis, which may occur rapidly

Sterile emulsion for injection route
- Use **IV** only, within 6 hr, flush line after use and after 6 hr

ADVERSE EFFECTS
CNS: *Dizziness, drowsiness,* confusion, headache, anxiety, tremors, stimulation, fatigue, depression, insomnia, hallucinations, ataxia, fatigue

CV: *Orthostatic hypotension, ECG changes, tachycardia,* hypotension
EENT: *Blurred vision,* tinnitus, mydriasis, nystagmus
GI: Constipation, dry mouth, nausea, vomiting, anorexia, diarrhea
HEMA: Neutropenia
INTEG: Rash, dermatitis, itching
RESP: Respiratory depression

Pharmacokinetics

Absorption	Rapid (PO); erratic (IM)
Distribution	Widely distributed; crosses blood-brain barrier, placenta; protein binding 99%
Metabolism	Liver, extensively, CYP2C19, CYP3A4
Excretion	Kidneys, breast milk
Half-life	1-12 days

Pharmacodynamics

	PO	IM	IV
Onset	½ hr	15 min	Immediate
Peak	Peak 2 hr	½-1½ hr	15 min
Duration	Up to 24 hr	1-1½ hr	15 min-1 hr

INTERACTIONS
Individual drugs
Alcohol: increased CNS depression
Amiodarone, cimetidine, clarithromycin, dalfopristin, delavirdine, diltiazem, disulfiram, efavirenz, erythromycin, fluconazole, fluvoxaMINE, imatinib, itraconazole, ketoconazole, IV miconazole, nefazodone, niCARdipine, quinupristin, ranolazine, troleandomycin, valproic acid, verapamil, voriconazole, zafirlukast, zileuton: increased diazepam effect
Cimetidine, valproic acid: increased toxicity
CYP3A4 inducers (carBAMazepine, ethetoin, fosphenytoin, phenytoins, rifampin), smoking: decreased diazepam effect
Disulfiram, isoniazid, propranolol, valproic acid: decreased metabolism of diazepam

Drug classifications
Barbiturates, CNS depressants, CYP3A4 inhibitors, SSRIs: increased toxicity
CNS depressants: increased CNS depression
CYP3A4 inducers (barbiturates): decreased diazepam effect
Oral contraceptives: decreased metabolism of diazepam

Drug/lab test
Increased: AST/ALT, serum bilirubin, alk phos

NURSING CONSIDERATIONS
Assessment
• **Assess degree of anxiety;** what precipitates anxiety and whether product controls symptoms; other signs of anxiety: dilated pupils, inability to sleep, restlessness, inability to focus
• **Assess for alcohol withdrawal symptoms,** including hallucinations (visual, auditory), delirium, irritability, agitation, fine to coarse tremors
• Monitor B/P (with patient lying, standing), pulse, respiratory rate; if systolic B/P drops 20 mm Hg, hold product, notify prescriber; monitor respirations q5-15min if given **IV**
• Monitor blood studies: CBC during long-term therapy; blood dyscrasias have occurred (rarely); hepatic studies: ALT, AST
• Monitor for seizure control: type, duration, and intensity of seizures; what precipitates seizures
• Monitor hepatic studies: AST, ALT, bilirubin, creatinine, LDH, alkaline phosphatase
• Assess mental status: mood, sensorium, affect, sleeping pattern, drowsiness, dizziness, suicidal tendencies, and ability of product to control these symptoms; check for tolerance, withdrawal symptoms: headache, nausea, vomiting, muscle pain, weakness after long-term use
• Assess for muscle spasms, pain relief

Patient/family education
• Advise patient that product may be taken with food; that product is not to be used for everyday stress or used longer than 4 mo unless directed by prescriber; take no more than prescribed amount; may be habit forming
• Caution patient to avoid OTC preparations unless approved by a prescriber; to avoid alcohol, other psychotropic medications unless prescribed; that smoking may decrease diazepam effect by increasing diazepam metabolism; not to discontinue medication abruptly after long-term use, gradually taper
• Inform patient to avoid driving, activities that require alertness; drowsiness may occur; to rise slowly or fainting may occur, especially in geriatric
• Advise patient not to become pregnant while using this product
• Inform patient that drowsiness may worsen at beginning of treatment
⚠ Teach patient to notify prescriber if pregnancy is planned or suspected (D), avoid breastfeeding

Evaluation

Positive therapeutic outcome
• Decreased anxiety, restlessness, insomnia

TREATMENT OF OVERDOSE:
Lavage, VS, supportive care, flumazenil

dibucaine topical
See Appendix B

diclofenac ophthalmic
See Appendix B

D

diclofenac epolamine (Rx)
(dye-kloe'fen-ak)
Flector
diclofenac potassium (Rx)
Cambia, Cataflam, Voltaren Rapide ✦, Zipsor
diclofenac sodium (Rx)
Apo-Diclo ✦, Novo-Difenac ✦, Nu-Diclo ✦, Pennsaid, Sandoz Diclofenac ✦, Solaraze Topical Gel, Voltram Topical Gel, Voltaren, Voltaren XR
Func. class.: Nonsteroidal antiinflammatory drug (NSAID), nonopioid analgesic
Chem. class.: Phenylacetic acid
Pregnancy category C

Do not confuse: Cataflam/Catapres

ACTION: Inhibits COX-1, COX-2 by blocking arachidonate, resulting in analgesic, antiinflammatory, antipyretic effects

Therapeutic outcome: Decreased pain, inflammation

USES: Acute, chronic rheumatoid arthritis, osteoarthritis, ankylosing spondylitis, analgesia, primary dysmenorrhea; patch: mild to moderate pain

CONTRAINDICATIONS
Hypersensitivity to aspirin, iodides, other NSAIDs, bovine protein; asthma, serious CV disease; eczema, exfoliative dermatitis, skin abrasions (gel patch)

> **BLACK BOX WARNING:** Treatment of perioperative pain in CABG surgery

Precautions: Breastfeeding, children, bleeding disorders, GI/cardiac disorders, hypersensitivity to other antiinflammatory agents, CCr <30 ml/min, accidental exposure, acute bronchospasm, hypersensitivity to benzyl alcohol; pregnancy (**C**) (tabs, del rel tab, ext rel tab, top gel); pregnancy (**B**) (top gel) (Solaraze); top patch, top sol, cap, powder for oral solution (pregnancy C <30 wk, D >30 wk)

> **BLACK BOX WARNING:** GI bleeding, MI, stroke

DOSAGE AND ROUTES
Osteoarthritis
Adult: PO (Cataflam) 50 mg bid-tid, max 150 mg/day; DEL REL (Voltaren) 50 mg bid-tid or 75 mg bid, max 150 mg/day; EXT REL (Voltaren-XR) 100 mg daily, max 150 mg/day; TOP gel 1% (Voltaren gel) 4 g for each lower extremity qid, max 16 g/day; 2 g for each upper extremity qid, max 8 g/day; TOP SOL (Pennsaid) apply 40 drops to each affected knee qid, apply 10 drops at a time, spread over entire knee

Rheumatoid arthritis
Adult: PO (Cataflam) 50 mg tid-qid, max 200 mg/day; DEL REL (Voltaren) 50 mg tid-qid or 75 mg bid, max 200 mg/day; EXT REL (Voltaren-XR) 100 mg qd, may increase to 200 mg/day, max 200 mg/day

Ankylosing spondylitis
Adult: PO DEL REL (Voltaren) 25 mg qid and 25 mg at bedtime, max 125 mg/day

Acute migraine with/without aura
Adult: PO (powder for oral SOL) (Cambia) 50 mg as a single dose; mix contents of packet in 1-2 oz water

Mild to moderate pain
Adult: PO (Zipsor) 25 mg qid

Dysmenorrhea or nonrheumatic inflammatory conditions
Adult: PO (Cataflam) 50 mg tid or 100 mg initially, then 50 mg tid, max 200 mg 1st day, then 150 mg/day, immediate release only

Pain of strains/sprains
Adult: TOP patch (Flector) apply patch to area bid

Actinic keratosis
Adult: TOP gel (Solaraze) apply to area bid

Renal dose
Avoid use of top gel, patch, sol, potassium oral tab in advanced renal disease

Available forms: Epolamine: topical patch 1.3%; **potassium:** tabs 50 mg tabs, liquid filled 25 mg; **sodium:** del rel tabs (enteric-coated) 25, 50, 75, 100 mg; oral powder for sol 50 mg; topical gel 1%, 3%

Implementation
PO route
• Do not break, crush, chew, or dissolve enteric-coated or ext rel tabs
• Administer with food or milk to decrease gastric symptoms
• Remain upright for ½ hr
• Store at room temperature

Topical route (patch) (Flector)
• Wash hands before handling patch
• Remove and release liner before administering
• Use only on normal, intact skin
• Remove before bath, shower, swimming, do not use heat or occlusive dressings
• Discard removed patch in trash away from children, pets
• Store at room temperature

Topical route (gel)
• Apply to intact skin, do not use heat or occlusive dressings
• Use only for osteoarthritis: mild-moderate pain
• Store at room temperature, avoid heat, do not freeze

Ophthalmic route
• Administer with patient recumbent or tilting head back; pull down on lower lid; when conjunctival sac is exposed, instill 1 drop; wait a few minutes before instilling other drops

ADVERSE EFFECTS
CNS: *Dizziness, headache,* drowsiness, fatigue, tremors, confusion, insomnia, anxiety, depression, nervousness, paresthesia, muscle weakness
CV: CHF, tachycardia, peripheral edema, palpitations, dysrhythmias, hypo/hypertension, fluid retention, MI, stroke
EENT: Tinnitus, hearing loss, blurred vision, laryngeal edema
GI: Nausea, anorexia, vomiting, diarrhea, jaundice, cholestatic hepatitis, constipation, flatulence, cramps, dry mouth, peptic ulcer, GI bleeding, hepatotoxicity, hematemesis
GU: Nephrotoxicity: dysuria, hematuria, oliguria, azotemia, cystitis, UTI
HEMA: Blood dyscrasias, epistaxis, anemia
INTEG: Purpura, rash, pruritus, sweating, erythema, petechiae, photosensitivity, alopecia
META: Hyperglycemia, hypoglycemia
RESP: Dyspnea, bronchospasm
SYST: Anaphylaxis, Stevens-Johnson syndrome

Pharmacokinetics

Absorption	Well absorbed (PO, ophth)
Distribution	Crosses placenta; 99% bound to plasma proteins
Metabolism	Liver (50%)
Excretion	Breast milk
Half-life	1-2 hr, patch 12 hr

Pharmacodynamics

	PO	Ophth	TOP (Patch)
Onset	Unknown	Unknown	Unknown
Peak	2-3 hr	Unknown	12 hr
Duration	Unknown	Unknown	Unknown

INTERACTIONS
Individual drugs
Aspirin: increased GI side effects

Cidofovir, cycloSPORINE, digoxin, lithium, methotrexate, phenytoin: increased toxicity

Drug classifications
ACE inhibitors, β-blockers, diuretics: decreased antihypertensive effect

Anticoagulants, NSAIDs, platelet inhibitors, salicylates, SSRIs, thrombolytics: increased risk of bleeding

Antidiabetic agents: increased need for dosage adjustment

Diuretics: decreased effect of these products

Diuretics (potassium-sparing): hyperkalemia

NSAIDs, bisphosphonates, corticosteroids: increased GI side effects

Drug/herb
Garlic, ginger, ginkgo: monitor for bleeding; increased bleeding risk

NURSING CONSIDERATIONS
Assessment

> **BLACK BOX WARNING: CABG:** do not use oral, top, gel, patch in perioperative pain in CABG surgery for 10-14 days

> **BLACK BOX WARNING: Stroke/MI:** may increase CHF and hypertension, increased CV thrombotic events that may be fatal; those with CV disease may be at greater risk

• **Assess for pain of rheumatoid arthritis, osteoarthritis, ankylosing spondylitis;** check ROM, inflammation of joints, characteristics of pain

• Assess ophthalmic patients for pain, inflammation, redness, swelling

• Assess for asthma, aspirin hypersensitivity, nasal polyps; may develop hypersensitivity

• Monitor liver function tests (may be elevated) and uric acid (may be decreased in serum, increased in urine) periodically; also BUN, creatinine, electrolytes (may be elevated)

⚠ Monitor for blood dyscrasias (thrombocytopenia): bruising, fatigue, bleeding, poor healing; monitor blood counts during therapy; watch for decreasing platelets; if low, therapy may need to be discontinued, restarted after hematologic recovery; stool guaiac

Patient/family education
• Teach patient that product must be continued for prescribed time to be effective; to avoid aspirin, NSAIDs, acetaminophen, or other OTC medications unless approved by prescriber, alcoholic beverages; to contact prescriber before surgery regarding when to discontinue this product

• Caution patient to report bleeding, bruising, fatigue, malaise, since blood dyscrasias do occur

• Advise patient to report hepatotoxicity: flulike symptoms, nausea, vomiting, jaundice, pruritus, lethargy

• Instruct patient to use sunscreen to prevent photosensitivity

• Instruct patient to use caution when driving; drowsiness, dizziness may occur

• Teach patient to take with a full glass of water to enhance absorption; remain upright for ½ hr; if dose is missed, take as soon as remembered within 2 hr if taking 1-2 ×/day; do not double doses

• Advise to notify all providers that product is being used

⚠ Teach patient to notify prescriber if pregnancy is planned or suspected (C, tabs) (C <30 wk, D >30 wk caps, topical patch/solution, powder for oral solution)

Evaluation

Positive therapeutic outcome
• Decreased pain in arthritic conditions
• Decreased inflammation in arthritic conditions
• Decreased ocular irritation

RARELY USED

dicyclomine
(dye-sye′kloe-meen)
Bentyl, Bentylol ✤**, Formulex** ✤**, Lomine** ✤
Func. class.: Gastrointestinal anticholinergic

USES: IBS

CONTRAINDICATIONS
Hypersensitivity to anticholinergics, closed-angle glaucoma, GI obstructions, myasthenia gravis, paralytic ileus, GI atony, toxic megacolon, dementia

DOSAGE AND ROUTES
Adult: PO 10-20 mg tid-qid; **IM** 20 mg q4-6hr, max 160/day
Child >2 yr: PO 10 mg tid-qid
Child 6 mo-2 yr: PO 5 mg tid-qid

didanosine (Rx)
(dye-dan'oh-seen)
ddI, Pediatric Videx, Videx EC
Func. class.: Antiretroviral
Chem. class.: Synthetic purine nucleoside reverse transcriptase inhibitor (NRTI)
Pregnancy category B

ACTION: Nucleoside analog incorporating into cellular DNA by viral reverse transcriptase, thereby terminating the cellular DNA chain and preventing viral replication

Therapeutic outcome: Antiviral against the retroviruses, primarily HIV-1

USES: HIV-1 infection in combination with at least 2 other antiretrovirals

CONTRAINDICATIONS
Hypersensitivity, lactic acidosis, pancreatitis, phenylketonuria

Precautions: Pregnancy **B,** breastfeeding, children, renal disease, sodium-restricted diets, elevated amylase, preexistent peripheral neuropathy, hyperuricemia, gout, CHF, noncirrhotic portal hypertension

> **BLACK BOX WARNING:** Hepatic disease, lactic acidosis, pancreatitis

DOSAGE AND ROUTES
Ext rel cap
Adult/adolescent/child ≥6 yr and ≥60 kg: PO ext rel cap 400 mg daily; if used with tenofovir, reduce to 250 mg daily
Adult/adolescent/child ≥6 yr and 25 kg to <60 kg: PO ext rel cap 250 mg daily; if used with tenofovir, reduce to 200 mg daily
Adolescent 20 kg to <25 kg: PO ext rel cap 200 mg daily

Oral dosage (powder for oral solution)
Adult ≥60 kg: PO 200 mg bid or 400 mg daily; if used with tenofovir, reduce to 250 mg daily

Adult <60 kg: PO 125 mg bid or 250 mg daily; if used with tenofovir, reduce to 200 mg daily
Adolescent/child/infant >8 mo: PO 120 mg/m^2 q12hr, max adult dosing
Infant ≤8 mo/neonate ≥2 wk: PO 100 mg/m^2 q12hr for up to 3 months

Renal dose
Adult: PO CrCl ≥60 ml/min: no change
Adult/adolescent ≥60 kg: PO CCr 30-59 ml/min: reduce oral solution to 100 mg q12hr or 200 mg q24hr, reduce ext rel capsules to 200 mg daily; CCr 10-29 ml/min: reduce oral solution to 150 mg q24hr, reduce ext rel capsules to 125 mg q24hr; CCr <10 ml/min: reduce oral solution to 100 mg q24hr, reduce ext rel capsules to 125 mg q24hr
Adult/adolescent <60 kg: PO CCr 30-59 ml/min: reduce oral solution to 75 mg q12hr or to 150 mg q24hr, reduce ext rel capsules to 125 mg daily; CCr 10-29 ml/min: reduce oral solution to 100 mg q24hr, reduce ext rel capsules to 125 mg daily; CCr <10 ml/min: reduce oral solution to 75 mg q24hr, ext rel capsules are not recommended

Intermittent hemodialysis/continuous ambulatory peritoneal dialysis
≥60 kg, give 100 mg oral solution or 125 mg ext rel capsules q24hr; <60 kg, give 75 mg oral solution q24hr, ext rel capsules are not recommended

Available forms: Powder for oral sol 10 mg/ml; del rel caps 125, 200, 250, 400 mg

Implementation
• Give on empty stomach 1 hr before or 2 hr after meals q12hr; food decreases effectiveness of product; adjust dose in renal impairment
• Pediatric powder for oral sol should be prepared in the pharmacy; shake before using
• Packets for oral sol must be mixed with ½ glass of water, not fruit juice; stir until dissolved; drink immediately
• Store caps, tabs in tightly closed bottle at room temperature; store oral sol after dissolving at room temperature ≤4 hr
• Do not take dapsone at same time as ddI

ADVERSE EFFECTS
CNS: Peripheral neuropathy, seizures, confusion, *anxiety,* hypertonia, abnormal thinking, asthenia, *insomnia, CNS depression,* pain, dizziness, chills, fever
CV: Hypertension, vasodilatation, dysrhythmia, syncope, CHF, palpitations
EENT: Ear pain, otitis, photophobia, visual impairment, retinal depigmentation, optic neuritis

GI: Pancreatitis, *diarrhea, nausea,* vomiting, *abdominal pain,* constipation, stomatitis, dyspepsia, liver abnormalities, flatulence, taste perversion, dry mouth, oral thrush, melena, increased ALT, AST, alkaline phosphatase, amylase, **hepatic failure,** noncirrhotic portal hypertension
GU: Increased bilirubin, uric acid
HEMA: **Leukopenia, granulocytopenia, thrombocytopenia, anemia**
INTEG: *Rash, pruritus,* alopecia, ecchymosis, hemorrhage, petechiae, sweating
MS: Myalgia, arthritis, myopathy, muscular atrophy
RESP: Cough, pneumonia, dyspnea, asthma, epistaxis, hypoventilation, sinusitis
SYST: **Lactic acidosis, anaphylaxis**

Pharmacokinetics

Absorption	Rapidly absorbed (up to 40%)
Distribution	Unknown
Metabolism	Not metabolized
Excretion	Kidneys (55%), feces
Half-life	48 min, shorter in children

Pharmacodynamics

Onset	Unknown
Peak	Up to 1 hr, del rel 2 hr
Duration	Unknown

INTERACTIONS
Individual drugs
Allopurinol, tenofovir

> **BLACK BOX WARNING:** Increase: fatal lactic acidosis: stavudine, tenofovir, other retrovirals

Dapsone, ketoconazole: decreased absorption of each specific product
Gatifloxacin, gemifloxacin, grepafloxacin, levofloxacin, lomefloxacin, moxifloxacin, norfloxacin, sparfloxacin, trovafloxacin: Do not use didanosine with these products (PO)
Itraconazole: decreased concentrations
Methadone: decreased didanosine level
Stavudine: increased pancreatitis risk

Drug classifications
Aluminum, antacids, magnesium: increased side effects
Antiretrovirals, other: decreased concentration
Fluoroquinolones, tetracyclines: decreased concentrations of each specific product

Drug/food
Do not use with acidic juices
Decreased: absorption 50%, do not use with food

NURSING CONSIDERATIONS
Assessment

> **BLACK BOX WARNING: Pancreatitis:** do not use in those with symptoms of pancreatitis (may be dose-related) or advanced HIV, alcoholism, history of pancreatitis

• **Assess for peripheral neuropathy:** tingling or pain in hands and feet, distal numbness; onset usually occurs 2-6 mo after beginning treatment; if these occur during therapy, product may be decreased or discontinued
• **Assess for pancreatitis: abdominal pain, nausea, vomiting, elevated liver enzymes; product should be discontinued since condition can be fatal**
• Assess children by dilated retinal examination q6mo to rule out retinal depigmentation
• Monitor CBC, differential, platelet count monthly, viral load, CD4$^+$ count; notify prescriber of results
• Monitor renal function studies: BUN, serum uric acid, urine CCr before, during therapy; these may be elevated throughout treatment

> **BLACK BOX WARNING:** Lactic acidosis, severe hepatomegaly, pancreatitis: assess for abdominal pain, nausea, vomiting, elevated hepatic enzymes; product should be discontinued because condition can be fatal

• Monitor temp; may indicate beginning of infection
• Monitor liver function tests before, during therapy (bilirubin, AST, ALT, amylase, alkaline phosphatase) as needed or monthly

Patient/family education
• Advise patient to take on empty stomach; not to mix powder with fruit juice; to drink powder immediately after mixing; to use exactly as prescribed
• Instruct patient to report signs of **infection:** increased temp, sore throat, flulike symptoms; to avoid crowds and those with known infections
• Instruct patient to report signs of **anemia:** fatigue, headache, faintness, shortness of breath, irritability
• Advise patient to report numbness/tingling in extremities
• Instruct patient to report **bleeding;** avoid use of razors and commercial mouthwash
• Advise patient that hair may be lost during therapy; a wig or hairpiece may make patient feel better
• Caution patient to avoid OTC products and other medications without approval of prescriber; to avoid alcohol

D

• Teach patient not to have any sexual contact without use of a condom; needles should not be shared; blood from infected individual should not come in contact with another's mucous membranes

Evaluation

Positive therapeutic outcome
• Absence of opportunistic infection, symptoms of HIV

difenoxin with atropine
See diphenoxylate with atropine

⚠ HIGH ALERT

digoxin (Rx)
(di-jox'in)
Apo-Digoxin ♣, Lanoxin
Func. class.: Inotropic antidysrhythmic, cardiac glycoside
Chem. class.: Digitalis preparation
Pregnancy category C

Do not confuse: Lanoxin/Lasix/Lonox/Lomotil/Xanax/Levoxine

ACTION: Inhibits sodium-potassium ATPase, which makes more calcium available for contractile proteins, resulting in increased cardiac output; increases force of contraction (positive inotropic effect); decreases heart rate (negative chronotropic effect); decreases AV conduction speed

Therapeutic outcome: Decreased edema, pulse, respiration, crackles

USES: Atrial fibrillation

CONTRAINDICATIONS
Hypersensitivity to digoxin, ventricular fibrillation, ventricular tachycardia, carotid sinus syndrome, 2nd- or 3rd-degree heart block

Precautions: Pregnancy **C**, breastfeeding, geriatric, renal disease, acute MI, AV block, severe respiratory disease, hypothyroidism, sinus nodal disease, hypokalemia, electrolyte disturbances, hypertension, cor pulmonale, Wolff-Parkinson-White syndrome

DOSAGE AND ROUTES
Loading dose: IV
Adult: IV 400-600 mcg as a single dose, effect in 5-30 min, max effect 1-4 hr, give subsequent doses of 100-300 mcg q6-8hr
Adolescent/child >10 yr: IV 8-12 mcg/kg, divided into 3 or more doses, with the first dose equaling approximately half of the total, give subsequent doses q4-8hr

Child 5-10 yr: IV 15-30 mcg/kg divided into 3 or more doses, with the first dose equaling approximately half of the total, give subsequent doses q4-8hr
Child 2-4 yr: IV 25-35 mcg/kg, divided into 3 or more doses, with the first dose equaling approximately half of the total, give subsequent doses q4-8hr
Child <2 yr/infant: IV 30-50 mcg/kg, divided into 3 or more doses, with the first dose equaling approximately half of the total, give subsequent doses q4-8hr
Full-term neonate: IV 20-30 mcg/kg, divided into 3 or more doses, with the first dose equaling approximately half of the total, give subsequent doses q4-8hr
Premature neonate: IV 15-25 mcg/kg, divided into 3 or more doses, with the first dose equaling approximately half of the total, give subsequent doses q4-8hr

Loading dose: oral dosage (tablets)
Tablets are 60%-80% bioavailable; oral elixir should be used to obtain the appropriate dose in infants, young pediatric patients, or patients with very low body weight
Adult/adolescent/child >10 yr: PO Total dose of 10-15 mcg/kg, in 3 divided doses, give half of the total loading dose initially, then one-fourth the loading dose q4-8hr × 2 doses
Child 5-10 yr: PO Total dose of 20-45 mcg/kg, in 3 divided doses, give half of the total loading dose initially, then one fourth of the loading dose q4-8hr × 2 doses

Loading dose: oral dosage (elixir)
Elixir is approximately 70%-85% bioavailable
Adult/adolescent/child >10 yr: PO Total dose of 10-15 mcg/kg, give half of the total loading dose initially, then additional fractions of the planned total dose at 4-8 hr
Child 5-10 yr: PO Total dose of 20-35 mcg/kg, give half of the total loading dose initially, then additional fractions of the planned total dose at 4-8 hr
Child 2-4 yr: PO Total dose of 30-45 mcg/kg, give half of the total loading dose initially, then additional fractions of the planned total dose at 4-8 hr
Infant/child <2 yr: PO Total dose of 35-60 mcg/kg, give half of the total loading dose initially then additional fractions of the planned total dose at 4-8 hr
Full-term neonate: PO Total dose of 25-35 mcg/kg, give half of the total loading dose initially, then additional fractions of the planned total dose at 4-8 hr

Premature neonate: PO Total dose of 20-30 mcg/kg, give half of the total loading dose initially, then additional fractions of the planned total dose at 4-8 hr

Maintenance dose: IV
Adult: IV 125-350 mcg/day, depending on CrCl, daily; usual daily maintenance dose for the CHF in adult based on corrected CrCl (ml/min per 70 kg) and lean body weight (LBW) are listed below
- LBW 50-59 kg
  CrCl ≥100 ml/min: 175 mcg IV daily
  CrCl 70-99 ml/min: 150 mcg IV daily
  CrCl 60-69 ml/min: 125 mcg IV daily
- LBW 60-69 kg
  CrCl ≥90 ml/min: 200 mcg IV daily
  CrCl 70-89 ml/min: 175 mcg IV daily
  CrCl 60-69 ml/min: 150 mcg IV daily
- LBW 70-79 kg
  CrCl ≥100 ml/min: 250 mcg IV daily
  CrCl 90-99 ml/min: 225 mcg IV daily
  CrCl 70-89 ml/min: 200 mcg IV daily
  CrCl 60-69 ml/min: 175 mcg IV daily
- LBW 80-89 kg
  CrCl ≥100 ml/min: 275 mcg IV daily
  CrCl 80-99 ml/min: 250 mcg IV daily
  CrCl 70-79 ml/min: 225 mcg IV daily
  CrCl 60-69 ml/min: 200 mcg IV daily
- LBW 90-99 kg
  CrCl ≥90 ml/min: 300 mcg IV daily
  CrCl 80-89 ml/min: 275 mcg IV daily
  CrCl 70-79 ml/min: 250 mcg IV daily
  CrCl 60-69 ml/min: 225 mcg IV daily
- LBW ≥100 kg
  CrCl ≥100 ml/min: 350 mcg IV daily
  CrCl 90-99 ml/min: 325 mcg IV daily
  CrCl 80-89 ml/min: 300 mcg IV daily
  CrCl 70-79 ml/min: 275 mcg IV daily
  CrCl 60-69 ml/min: 250 mcg IV daily

Full-term neonate to child >10 yr: 25%-35% of the IV digitalizing dose IV daily
Preterm neonate: 20%-30% of the IV digitalizing dose in 2 daily doses

Maintenance dose: oral dosage (tablets)
Adult/adolescent/child >10 yr: PO 3.4-5.1 mcg/kg/day
- LBW 40-49 kg
  CrCl ≥70 ml/min: 187.5 mcg PO daily
  CrCl ≥60-69 ml/min: 125 mcg PO daily
- LBW 50-59 kg
  CrCl ≥90 ml/min: 250 mcg PO daily
  CrCl 60-89 ml/min: 187.5 mcg PO daily
- LBW 60-69 kg
  CrCl ≥100 ml/min: 312.5 mcg PO daily
  CrCl 60-99 ml/min: 250 mcg PO daily
- LBW 70-79 kg
  CrCl ≥80 ml/min: 312.5 mcg PO daily
  CrCl 60-79 ml/min: 250 mcg PO daily
- LBW 80-89 kg
  CrCl ≥90 ml/min: 375 mcg PO daily
  CrCl 60-89 ml/min: 312.5 mcg PO daily
- LBW 90-99 kg
  CrCl ≥90 ml/min: 437.5 mcg PO daily
  CrCl 70-89 ml/min: 375 mcg PO daily
  CrCl 60-69 ml/min: 312.5 mcg PO daily
- LBW ≥100 kg
  CrCl ≥100 ml/min: 500 mcg PO daily
  CrCl 80-99 ml/min: 437.5 mcg PO daily
  CrCl 60-79 ml/min: 375 mcg PO daily

Child 5-10 yr: PO 6.4-12.9 mcg/kg/day PO in 2 divided doses is the recommended starting maintenance dose

Maintenance dose: oral dosage (elixir)
Adult/adolescent/child >10 yr: PO 3-4.5 mcg/kg/day daily
- LBW 40-49 kg
  CrCl ≥100 ml/min: 170 mcg PO daily
  CrCl 90-99 ml/min: 160 mcg PO daily
  CrCl 80-89 ml/min: 150 mcg PO daily
  CrCl 70-79 ml/min: 140 mcg PO daily
  CrCl 60-69 ml/min: 130 mcg PO daily
- LBW 50-59 kg
  CrCl ≥100 ml/min: 213 mcg PO daily
  CrCl 90-99 ml/min: 200 mcg PO daily
  CrCl 80-89 ml/min: 188 mcg PO daily
  CrCl 70-79 ml/min: 175 mcg PO daily
  CrCl 60-69 ml/min: 163 mcg PO daily
- LBW 60-69 kg
  CrCl ≥100 ml/min: 255 mcg PO daily
  CrCl 90-99 ml/min: 240 mcg PO daily
  CrCl 80-89 ml/min: 225 mcg PO daily
  CrCl 70-79 ml/min: 210 mcg PO daily
  CrCl 60-69 ml/min: 195 mcg PO daily
- LBW 70-79 kg
  CrCl ≥100 ml/min: 298 mcg PO daily
  CrCl 90-99 ml/min: 280 mcg PO daily
  CrCl 80-89 ml/min: 263 mcg PO daily
  CrCl 70-79 ml/min: 245 mcg PO daily
  CrCl 60-69 ml/min: 228 mcg PO daily
- LBW 80-89 kg
  CrCl ≥100 ml/min: 340 mcg PO daily
  CrCl 90-99 ml/min: 320 mcg PO daily
  CrCl 80-89 ml/min: 300 mcg PO daily
  CrCl 70-79 ml/min: 280 mcg PO daily
  CrCl 60-69 ml/min: 260 mcg PO daily
- LBW 90-99 kg
  CrCl ≥100 ml/min: 383 mcg PO daily
  CrCl 90-99 ml/min: 360 mcg PO daily
  CrCl 80-89 ml/min: 338 mcg PO daily
  CrCl 70-79 ml/min: 315 mcg PO daily
  CrCl 60-69 ml/min: 293 mcg PO daily

- LBW ≥100 kg
  CrCl ≥100 ml/min: 425 mcg PO daily
  CrCl 90-99 ml/min: 400 mcg PO daily
  CrCl 80-89 ml/min: 375 mcg PO daily
  CrCl 70-79 ml/min: 350 mcg PO daily
  CrCl 60-69 ml/min: 325 mcg PO daily

Child 5-10 yr: PO 5.6-11.3 mcg/kg/day in 2 divided doses

Child 2-4 yr: PO 9.4-13.1 mcg/kg/day in 2 divided doses

Child <2 yr/infant: PO 11.3-18.8 mcg/kg/day in 2 divided doses

Full-term neonate: PO 7.5-11.3 mcg/kg/day in 2 divided doses

Preterm neonate: PO 4.7-7.8 mcg/kg/day in 2 divided doses

Renal dose
IV route

- CrCl 50-59 ml/min
  LBW 50-59 kg: 125 mcg IV once daily
  LBW 60-69 kg: 150 mcg IV once daily
  LBW 70-79 kg: 175 mcg IV once daily
  LBW 80-89 kg: 200 mcg IV once daily
  LBW 90-99 kg: 225 mcg IV once daily
  LBW ≥100 kg: 250 mcg IV once daily
- CrCl 40-49 ml/min
  LBW 50-59 kg: 100 mcg IV once daily
  LBW 60-69 kg: 125 mcg IV once daily
  LBW 70-79 kg: 150 mcg IV once daily
  LBW 80-89 kg: 175 mcg IV once daily
  LBW 90-99 kg: 200 mcg IV once daily
  LBW ≥100 kg: 225 mcg IV once daily
- CrCl 30-39 ml/min
  LBW 50-59 kg: 100 mcg IV once daily
  LBW 60-69 kg: 125 mcg IV once daily
  LBW 70-89 kg: 150 mcg IV once daily
  LBW 90-99 kg: 175 mcg IV once daily
  LBW ≥100 kg: 200 mcg IV once daily
- CrCl 20-29 ml/min
  LBW 50-69 kg: 100 mcg IV once daily
  LBW 70-79 kg: 125 mcg IV once daily
  LBW 80-99 kg: 150 mcg IV once daily
  LBW ≥100 kg: 175 mcg IV once daily
- CrCl 10-19 ml/min
  LBW 50-59 kg: 75 mcg IV once daily
  LBW 60-79 kg: 100 mcg IV once daily
  LBW 80-89 kg: 125 mcg IV once daily
  LBW ≥90 kg: 150 mcg IV once daily
- CrCl <10 ml/min
  LBW 50-69 kg: 75 mcg IV once daily
  LBW 70-89 kg: 100 mcg IV once daily
  LBW 90-99 kg: 125 mcg IV once daily
  LBW ≥100 kg: 150 mcg IV once daily

Oral dosage (tablets)

- CrCl 40-59 ml/min
  LBW 50-69 kg: 187.5 mcg PO once daily

- CrCl 50-59 ml/min
  LBW 70-89 kg: 250 mcg PO once daily
  LBW ≥90 kg: 312.5 mcg PO once daily
- CrCl 30-39 ml/min
  LBW 50-59 kg: 125 mcg PO once daily
  LBW 60-79 kg: 187.5 mcg PO once daily
  LBW 80-99 kg: 250 mcg PO once daily
  LBW ≥100 kg: 312.5 mcg PO once daily
- CrCl 20-29 ml/min
  LBW 50-69 kg: 125 mcg PO once daily
  LBW 70-89 kg: 187.5 mcg PO once daily
  LBW ≥90 kg: 250 mcg PO once daily
- CrCl <20 ml/min
  LBW 50-69 kg: 125 mcg PO once daily
  LBW 70-99 kg: 187.5 mcg PO once daily
  LBW ≥100 kg: 250 mcg PO once daily

Oral dosage (elixir)

- CrCl 50-59 ml/min
  LBW 50-59 kg: 150 mcg PO once daily
  LBW 60-69 kg: 180 mcg PO once daily
  LBW 70-79 kg: 210 mcg PO once daily
  LBW 80-89 kg: 240 mcg PO once daily
  LBW 90-99 kg: 270 mcg PO once daily
  LBW ≥100 kg: 300 mcg PO once daily
- CrCl 40-49 ml/min
  LBW 50-59 kg: 138 mcg PO once daily
  LBW 60-69 kg: 165 mcg PO once daily
  LBW 70-79 kg: 193 mcg PO once daily
  LBW 80-89 kg: 220 mcg PO once daily
  LBW 90-99 kg: 248 mcg PO once daily
  LBW ≥100 kg: 275 mcg PO once daily
- CrCl 30-39 ml/min
  LBW 50-59 kg: 125 mcg PO once daily
  LBW 60-69 kg: 150 mcg PO once daily
  LBW 70-79 kg: 175 mcg PO once daily
  LBW 80-89 kg: 200 mcg PO once daily
  LBW 90-99 kg: 225 mcg PO once daily
  LBW ≥100 kg: 250 mcg PO once daily
- CrCl 20-29 ml/min
  LBW 50-59 kg: 113 mcg PO once daily
  LBW 60-69 kg: 135 mcg PO once daily
  LBW 70-79 kg: 158 mcg PO once daily
  LBW 80-89 kg: 180 mcg PO once daily
  LBW 90-99 kg: 203 mcg PO once daily
  LBW ≥100 kg: 225 mcg PO once daily
- CrCl <20 ml/min
  LBW 50-59 kg: 100 mcg PO once daily
  LBW 60-69 kg: 120 mcg PO once daily
  LBW 70-79 kg: 140 mcg PO once daily
  LBW 80-89 kg: 160 mcg PO once daily
  LBW 90-99 kg: 180 mcg PO once daily
  LBW ≥100 kg: 200 mcg PO once daily

The daily maintenance dose can also be estimated using the patient's CrCl and loading dose (LD) according to the method of Jelliffe and Brooker daily % loss = 14 + CrCl/5

Available forms: Caps 0.05, 0.1, 0.2 mg; elix 0.05 mg/ml; tabs 0.125, 0.25, 0.5, 0.0625, 0.1875 mg; inj 0.5 ♣, 0.25 mg/ml; pediatric inj 0.1 mg/ml

Implementation
• Do not give at same time as antacids or other products that decrease absorption
PO route
• **Bioavailability varies between different oral dosage forms of digoxin and between different brands of the same dosage form. Changing from one preparation to another may require dosage adjustments.**
• All dosage forms may be administered without regard to meals.
• Tab may be crushed and administered with food or fluids
• Pediatric elixir should be administered using a calibrated measuring device
Injectable routes
• When changing from PO to IM/IV use 20%-25% less
• IV is preferred over IM, as it is less painful
• PO should replace parenteral therapy as soon as possible
• Visually inspect parenteral products for particulate matter and discoloration prior to use

IV route
• May be given undiluted or each 1 ml may be diluted in 4 ml of sterile water for injection, NS, D₅W, or LR; diluent volumes less than 4 ml will cause precipitation; use diluted solutions immediately
• Inject over at least 5 min via Y-site or 3-way stopcock; in patients with pulmonary edema, administer over 10-15 min to avoid inadvertent overdosage, do not flush the syringe following administration

IM route
• Do not administer more than 2 ml at any one IM injection site
• Inject deeply into gluteal muscle, then massage area

Syringe compatibilities: Heparin, milrinone

Syringe incompatibility: Doxapram

Y-site compatibilities: Amrinone, ciprofloxacin, cisatracurium, diltiazem, famotidine, meperidine, meropenem, midazolam, milrinone, morphine, potassium chloride, propofol, remifentanil, tacrolimus, vit B/C

Y-site incompatibilities: Fluconazole, foscarnet

Additive compatibilities: Bretylium, cimetidine, furosemide, lidocaine, ranitidine, verapamil

Additive incompatibility: DOBUTamine

ADVERSE EFFECTS
CNS: *Headache,* drowsiness, apathy, confusion, disorientation, fatigue, depression, hallucinations
CV: *Dysrhythmias,* hypotension, bradycardia, **AV block**
EENT: Blurred vision, yellow-green halos, photophobia, diplopia
GI: Nausea, vomiting, anorexia, abdominal pain, diarrhea

Pharmacokinetics
Absorption	Unknown
Distribution	Widely distributed; 20%-25% protein bound
Metabolism	Liver, small amount; also intestinal bacteria
Excretion	Urine
Half-life	30-40 hr

Pharmacodynamics
	PO	IV
Onset	½-1½ hr	5-30 min
Peak	2-6 hr	1-4 hr
Duration	After steady state	2-6 days

INTERACTIONS
Individual drugs
AMILoride, cholestyramine, colestipol, metoclopramide, thyroid hormones: decreased digoxin levels
Amiodarone, diltiazem, indomethacin, NIFEdipine, propantheline, quiNIDine, verapamil: increased digoxin levels
Amphotericin B, carbenicillin, ticarcillin: increased hypokalemia, increased toxicity
Azole antifungals, macrolides, tetracyclines: increased toxicity
Calcium IV: increased hypercalcemia, hypomagnesemia, digoxin toxicity
Kaolin/pectin: decreased absorption

Drug classifications
Antacids: decreased digoxin absorption
Anticholinergics: increased digoxin blood levels
Antidysrhythmics, β-adrenergic blockers: increased bradycardia
Diuretics (thiazide) corticosteroids: increased hypokalemia, hypercalcemia, hypomagnesemia, digoxin toxicity
Sympathomimetics: increased cardiac dysrhythmia risk

Drug/herb
St. John's wort: decreased product effect

Drug/food
Flaxseed, psyllium: decreased digoxin absorption

Drug/lab test
Increased: CPK

NURSING CONSIDERATIONS
Assessment
• Assess and document apical pulse for 1 min before giving product; if pulse <60 in adult or <90 in an infant or is significantly different, take again in 1 hr; if <60 in adult, call prescriber; note rate, rhythm, character
• Monitor electrolytes: potassium, sodium, chloride, magnesium, calcium; renal function studies: BUN, creatinine; other blood studies: ALT, AST, bilirubin, Hct, Hgb, product levels (therapeutic level 0.5-2 ng/ml) before initiating treatment and periodically thereafter, draw ≥ 6-8 hr after last dose, optimally 12-24 hr after a dose
• Monitor resolution of atrial dysrhythmias by ECG; if tachydysrhythmia develops, hold product; delay cardioversion while product levels are determined
• Monitor ECG continuously during parenteral loading doses and for patients with suspected toxicity; provide hemodynamic monitoring for patients with heart failure or administer multiple cardiac products

Patient/family education
• Advise patient not to stop abruptly; teach all aspects of product
• Caution patient to avoid OTC medications including cough, cold, allergy preparations, antacids, since many adverse product interactions may occur; do not take antacid at same time
• Instruct patient to notify prescriber of any loss of appetite, lower stomach pain, diarrhea, weakness, drowsiness, headache, blurred or yellow-green vision, rash, depression; teach toxic symptoms of this product and when to notify prescriber
• Advise patient to maintain a sodium-restricted diet as ordered; to take potassium supplements as ordered to prevent toxicity
• Instruct patient to report shortness of breath, difficulty breathing, weight gain, edema, persistent cough
• Teach patient purpose of product is to regulate the heart's functioning
• Teach patient as outpatient to check and record pulse for 1 min before taking dose; if there is a change of >15 bpm from usual pulse, prescriber should be notified
• Teach patient to take medication at the same time each day, take missed doses within 12 hr; do not double doses; notify prescriber if doses are missed for 2 days or more; how to monitor heart rate
• Teach patient toxic symptoms and when to notify prescriber
• Advise patient to carry/wear emergency ID describing dosage and reason for digoxin
• Advise patient to use one brand consistently

Evaluation
Positive therapeutic outcome
• Decreased weight, edema, pulse, respiration, crackles
• Increased urine output
• Serum digoxin level 0.5-2 ng/ml

TREATMENT OF OVERDOSE:
Discontinue product, administer potassium, monitor ECG, administer an adrenergic blocking agent, digoxin immune FAB

RARELY USED

digoxin immune FAB (ovine) (Rx)
(di-jox′in)
DigiFab
Func. class.: Antidote, digoxin specific
Pregnancy category C

Therapeutic outcome: Correction of digoxin toxicity

USES: Reversal of life-threatening digoxin or digitoxin toxicity, including severe bradycardia, ventricular tachycardia/fibrillation, severe hypertension

CONTRAINDICATIONS
Mild digoxin toxicity, hypersensitivity to this product, papain, or ovine protein

DOSAGE AND ROUTES
1 (40 mg) DigiFab binds 0.5 mg digoxin

Digoxin toxicity (known amount) (tabs, oral sol, IM)
Adult and child: IV dose (mg) = dose ingested (mg) × 0.8/1000 × 38 or 40 mg vial

Toxicity (known amount) (cap, IV)
Adult and child: IV dose = dose ingested (mg)/0.5 × 38 or 40 mg vial

Toxicity (known amount) by serum digoxin concentrations (SDCs)
Adult and child: IV SDC (nanograms/ml) × kg of weight/100 × 38 or 40 mg vial

Digoxin toxicity (unknown amount)
Adult and child >20 kg: IV 228 mg (6 vials)

Infant and child <20 kg: **IV** 38 mg (1 vial)

Acute ingestion
Adult: **IV** 10 vials (380 mg)

Life-threatening ingestion
Adult: **IV** 20 vials (760 mg)

Skin test
Adult: ID 0.1 ml of 1:100 dilution check after 20 min

dihydroergotamine
See ergotamine

dihydrotachysterol (Rx)
(dye-hye-droh-tak-iss′ter-ole)
DHT Intensol ✷, Hytakerol
Func. class.: Parathyroid agent (calcium regulator)
Chem. class.: Vitamin D analog
Pregnancy category C

ACTION: Increases intestinal absorption of calcium, increases renal tubular absorption of phosphorus; is able to regulate calcium levels by regulation of calcitonin, parathyroid hormone

Therapeutic outcome: Prevention of continued calcium loss in bones

USES: Hypoparathyroidism, pseudohypoparathyroidism, postoperative tetany

CONTRAINDICATIONS
Hypersensitivity, renal disease, hyperphosphatemia, hypercalcemia, hypervitaminosis D

Precautions: Pregnancy **C**, breastfeeding, renal calculi, CV disease

DOSAGE AND ROUTES
Hypoparathyroidism/pseudohypoparathyroidism
Adult: PO 0.75-2.5 mg daily × 4 days, maintenance 0.2-1 mg daily regulated by serum calcium levels

Neonate: PO 0.05-0.1 mg/day
Child/infant: PO 1-5 mg qd × 4 days then 0.5-1.5 mg qd

Rickets (vit D resistant)
Child: PO 0.25-1 mg/day

Available forms: Tabs 0.125, 0.2, 0.4 mg; caps 0.125 mg; oral sol 0.2, 0.25 mg/5 ml, 0.2 mg/ml ✷ (Intensol)

Implementation
• Do not break, crush, or chew caps
• May be increased q4wk depending on blood level; give with meals for GI symptoms

• Store in tight, light-resistant containers at room temperature
• Restrict sodium, potassium if required
• Restriction of fluids may be required for chronic renal failure

ADVERSE EFFECTS
CNS: Drowsiness, headache, vertigo, fever, lethargy, depression
CV: *Dysrhythmias,* hypertension
EENT: Tinnitus
GI: Nausea, diarrhea, vomiting, jaundice, anorexia, dry mouth, constipation, cramps, metallic taste, thirst
GU: *Polyuria,* hypercalciuria, hyperphosphatemia, *hematuria,* nocturia, renal calculi
MS: Myalgia, arthralgia, decreased bone development, weakness, ataxia

Pharmacokinetics
Absorption	Well absorbed from small intestine
Distribution	Liver, fat
Metabolism	Liver
Excretion	Feces (inactive, active metabolites)
Half-life	Unknown

Pharmacodynamics
Onset	2 wk
Peak	2 wk
Duration	2-9 wk

INTERACTIONS
Individual drugs
Cholestyramine, colestipol, mineral oil: decreased absorption of dihydrotachysterol
Phenytoin: decreased effect of dihydrotachysterol
Verapamil: increased dysrhythmias

Drug classifications
Barbiturates, corticosteroids: decreased effect of dihydrotachysterol
Calcium supplements, diuretics (thiazide): increased hypercalcemia
Cardiac glycosides: increased dysrhythmias

Drug/lab test
False increase: cholesterol

NURSING CONSIDERATIONS
Assessment
• Monitor BUN, urinary calcium, AST, ALT, cholesterol, alkaline phosphatase, creatinine, uric acid, chloride, magnesium, electrolytes, urine pH, phosphate; may increase calcium; should be kept at 9-10 mg/dl; keep vit D at 50-135 international units/dl, phosphate at 70 mg/dl; these tests should be checked before and throughout treatment

- Monitor for increased blood level, since toxic reaction may occur rapidly
- Monitor for dry mouth, metallic taste, polyuria, bone pain, muscle weakness, headache, fatigue, tinnitus, change in LOC, irregular pulse, dysrhythmias, increased respirations, anorexia, nausea, vomiting, cramps, diarrhea, constipation; may indicate hypercalcemia; if these occur, discontinue product, give laxatives, low-calcium diet
- Monitor renal status: decreased urinary output (oliguria, anuria), edema in extremities, weight gain >5 lb, periorbital edema
- Assess nutritional status; check diet for sources of vit D (milk, some seafood), calcium (dairy products, dark green vegetables); phosphates (dairy products) must be avoided

Patient/family education
- Teach symptoms of hypercalcemia and when to report symptoms to prescriber
- Teach patient about foods rich in calcium, vit D; provide list of calcium-rich foods; renal failure patients are given a renal diet
- Caution patient not to double doses, take exactly as prescribed

Evaluation
Positive therapeutic outcome
- Prevention of bone deficiencies
- Calcium, phosphorus at normal levels

⚠ HIGH ALERT

diltiazem (Rx)
(dil-tye′a-zem)
Apo-Diltiaz ✤, Cardizem, Cardizem CD, Cardizem LA, Cartia XT, Dilacor-XR, Dilt-CD, Diltia XR, Diltia XT, Diltzac, Taztia XT, Tiamate, Tiazac
Func. class.: Calcium channel blocker, antianginal, antiarrhythmic class IV, antihypertensive
Chem. class.: Benzothiazepine
Pregnancy category C

Do not confuse: Cardizem/Cardene

ACTION: Inhibits calcium ion influx across cell membrane during cardiac depolarization, produces relaxation of coronary vascular smooth muscle, dilates coronary arteries, slows SA/AV node conduction times, dilates peripheral arteries

Therapeutic outcome: Decreased angina pectoris, dysrhythmias, B/P

USES

Oral: Angina pectoris due to hypertension, coronary artery spasm

Parenteral: Atrial fibrillation, flutter; paroxysmal supraventricular tachycardia

CONTRAINDICATIONS
Sick sinus syndrome, 2nd- or 3rd-degree heart block, hypotension less than 90 mm Hg systolic, acute MI, pulmonary congestion, cardiogenic shock

Precautions: Pregnancy **C**, breastfeeding, children, CHF, aortic stenosis, bradycardia, GERD, hepatic disease, hiatal hernia, ventricular dysfunction, elderly

DOSAGE AND ROUTES
Hypertension
Adult: PO 30 mg TID, increase to max 480 mg/day; EXT REL 120-240 mg qday, max 540 mg/day; SUS REL 60 mg bid, max 360 mg/day

Prinzmetal's or variant angina, chronic stable angina
Adult: PO 30 mg qid, increasing dose gradually to 180-360 mg/day in divided doses or EXT REL (LA, CD, XT, XR products) 180-360 mg, max 480-540 mg/day, depending on brand

Atrial fibrillation, flutter, paroxysmal supraventricular tachycardia
Adult: IV 0.25 mg/kg as BOL over 2 min initially, then 0.35 mg/kg may be given after 15 min; if no response, may give CONT INF 5-15 mg/hr for up to 24 hr

Available forms: Tabs 30, 60, 90, 120 mg; ext rel tab 120, 180, 240, 300, 360, 420 mg; ext rel caps 60, 90, 120, 180, 240, 300, 360, 420 mg; inj 5 mg/ml (5, 10 ml); powder for inj 100 mg

Implementation
PO route
- Not all products are interchangeable
- Store at room temperature
- **Cardizem LA ext rel tab 24 hr:** give daily, either AM or PM, without regard to meals
- **Dilacor XR/Diltia XT ext rel cap 24 hr** give daily, take on empty stomach, swallow whole, do not cut, crush, chew, open
- **Tiazac, Tiztia XT:** give daily without regard to meals
- **Conventional regular-rel tab:** give before meals and at bedtime
- **Cardizem CD or equivalent (Cartia XT) generic ext rel cap 24 hr:** give daily, without regard to meals
- Give with meals for GI symptoms; may crush and sprinkle (reg tab) on applesauce

---

Direct IV route
• Give direct **IV** undiluted over 2 min
Continuous IV infusion route
• **Dilute** 125 mg/100 ml (1.25 mg/ml) or 250 mg/250 ml (1 mg/ml) or 250 mg/500 ml (0.5 mg/ml) of D₅W, 0.9% NaCl, D₅/0.45% NaCl; give 10 mg/hr; may increase by 5 mg/hr to 15 mg/hr; may continue inf up to 24 hr

Y-site compatibilities: Albumin, amikacin, amphotericin B, aztreonam, bretylium, bumetanide, ceFAZolin, cefotaxime, cefoTEtan, cefOXitin, cefTAZidime, cefTRIAXone, cefuroxime, cimetidine, ciprofloxacin, clindamycin, digoxin, DOBUTamine, DOPamine, doxycycline, EPINEPHrine, erythromycin, esmolol, fentaNYL, fluconazole, gentamicin, hetastarch, HYDROmorphone, imipenem-cilastatin, labetalol, lidocaine, LORazepam, meperidine, metoclopramide, metroNIDAZOLE, midazolam, milrinone, morphine, multivitamins, niCARdipine, nitroglycerin, norepinephrine, oxacillin, penicillin G potassium, pentamidine, piperacillin, potassium chloride, potassium phosphates, ranitidine, sodium nitroprusside, theophylline, ticarcillin, ticarcillin/clavulanate, tobramycin, trimethoprim-sulfamethoxazole, vancomycin, vecuronium

ADVERSE EFFECTS
CNS: *Headache, fatigue, drowsiness,* dizziness, depression, weakness, insomnia, tremor, paresthesia
CV: *Dysrhythmia, edema, CHF,* bradycardia, hypotension, palpitations, **heart block**
GI: *Nausea,* vomiting, diarrhea, gastric upset, *constipation,* increased LFTs
GU: Nocturia, polyuria, **acute renal failure**
INTEG: *Rash,* pruritus at inj site, flushing, photosensitivity, burning
RESP: Rhinitis, dyspnea, pharyngitis

Pharmacokinetics
Absorption	Well absorbed
Distribution	Not known
Metabolism	Liver, extensively
Excretion	Metabolites (96%)
Half-life	3½-9 hr

Pharmacodynamics
	PO	PO–sus rel	IV
Onset	½ hr	Unknown	Unknown
Peak	2-3 hr	Unknown	Unknown
Duration	6-8 hr	11-18 hr	Unknown

INTERACTIONS
Individual drugs
CarBAMazepine, lithium, lovastatin, methylPREDNISolone: increased effects of each specific product

Cimetidine: increased effects of diltiazem
CycloSPORINE: increased cycloSPORINE effect
Digoxin: increased digoxin effect
Theophylline: increased effect, toxicity
Drug classifications
Anesthetics: increased effects of anesthetics
β-Adrenergic blockers: increased bradycardia, CHF, increased β-blocker effect
Benzodiazepines: increased effect of benzodiazepines
HMG-CoA reductase inhibitors: increased effects

NURSING CONSIDERATIONS
Assessment
• **CHF:** monitor for dyspnea, weight gain, edema, jugular vein distention, rales; monitor I&O ratios daily, weight
• **Angina:** location, duration, alleviating factors, activity when pain starts
• **Dysrhythmias: monitor B/P and pulse, respiration, ECG and intervals (PR, QRS, QT); PCWP, CVP often during infusion; if B/P drops 30 mm Hg, stop infusion and call prescriber**

Patient/family education
• Caution patient to avoid hazardous activities until stabilized on product and dizziness is no longer a problem
• Instruct patient to limit caffeine consumption; to avoid grapefruit juice; to avoid alcohol and OTC products unless directed by prescriber
⚠ Tell patient to comply in all areas of medical regimen; diet, exercise, stress reduction, product therapy; to notify prescriber of irregular heartbeat, shortness of breath, swelling of feet and hands, pronounced dizziness, constipation, nausea, hypotension
• Teach patient to use as directed even if feeling better; may be taken with other cardiovascular products (nitrates, β-blockers); how to take pulse, B/P before taking product; to change position slowly
• Teach patient not to discontinue abruptly

Evaluation
Positive therapeutic outcome
• Decreased anginal pain
• Decreased B/P
• Absence of dysrhythmias

TREATMENT OF OVERDOSE:
Atropine for AV block, vasopressor for hypotension

Adverse effects: *italics* = common; **bold** = life-threatening

dimenhyDRINATE (OTC, Rx)
(dye-men-hye′dri-nate)
Apo-DimenhyDRINATE ✦,
Dramamine, Driminate, Travol Motion
Sickness, TripTone, Wal-Dram
Func. class.: Antiemetic, antihistamine,
anticholinergic
Chem. class.: H1-receptor antagonist,
ethanolamine derivative

Do not confuse: dimenhyDRINATE/
diphenhydrAMINE

ACTION: Competes with histamine for H1
receptors in GI tract, blood vessels, respiratory
tract; central anticholinergic activity, which results in decreased vestibular stimulation and
blockade of chemoreceptor trigger zone

Therapeutic outcome: Absence of nausea, vomiting, or vertigo

USES: Motion sickness, nausea, vomiting,
vertigo

Unlabeled uses: Hyperemesis gravidarum,
Ménière's syndrome

CONTRAINDICATIONS
Hypersensitivity, infants, neonates, tartrazine dye
hypersensitivity

Precautions: Pregnancy (**B**), breastfeeding, children, geriatric patients, cardiac dysrhythmias, asthma, prostatic hypertrophy,
bladder-neck obstruction, closed-angle glaucoma, stenosing peptic ulcer, pyloroduodenal
obstruction

DOSAGE AND ROUTES
Adult: PO 50-100 mg q4hr; IM/IV 50 mg q4hr
as needed (Canada only)
Child 6-12 yr: PO 25-50 mg q6-8hr prn, max
150 mg/day
Child 2-5 yr: PO 12.5-25 mg q6-8hr, max
75 mg/day

Available forms: Tabs 50 mg; inj 50 mg/ml;
elixir 15 mg/5 ml; chew tabs 50 mg

Implementation
• Give IM inj in large muscle mass; aspirate to
avoid IV administration (Canada only)
• Tablets may be swallowed whole, chewed, or
allowed to dissolve

IV route (Canada only)
• After diluting 50 mg/10 ml of NaCl inj, give
50 mg over 2 min

ADVERSE EFFECTS
CNS: Drowsiness, restlessness, headache,
dizziness, insomnia, confusion, nervousness,
tingling, vertigo
CV: Hypertension, hypotension, palpitation
EENT: Dry mouth, blurred vision, diplopia,
nasal congestion, photosensitivity, xerostomia
GI: Nausea, anorexia, vomiting, constipation
INTEG: Rash, urticaria, fever, chills, flushing
MISC: Anaphylaxis

Pharmacokinetics
Absorption	Unknown
Distribution	May cross placenta, enter breast milk
Metabolism	Liver
Excretion	Kidneys
Half-life	Unknown

Pharmacodynamics
Onset	PO 15-30 min
Peak	PO 2 hr
Duration	PO 4-6 hr

INTERACTIONS
Individual drugs
Alcohol: increased effects

Drug classifications
Anticholinergics, tricyclics, MAOIs, opiates,
sedative/hypnotics, other CNS depressants:
increased effects

Drug/lab test
False negative: allergy skin testing

NURSING CONSIDERATIONS
Assessment
• Monitor VS, B/P; check patients with cardiac
disease more often
• Assess for signs of toxicity of other products
or masking of symptoms of disease: brain
tumor, intestinal obstruction
• Observe for drowsiness, dizziness

Patient/family education
• Advise patient to avoid hazardous activities,
activities requiring alertness because dizziness may occur; to request assistance with
ambulation
• Advise to avoid alcohol, other CNS depressants

Evaluation

Positive therapeutic outcome
• Absence of nausea, vomiting, or vertigo

dinoprostone (Rx)

(dye-noe-prost′one)

Cervidil, Prepidil, Prostin E-Z

Func. class.: Oxytocic, abortifacient

Chem. class.: Prostaglandin E_2

Pregnancy category C

Do not confuse: Prepidil/bepridil

ACTION: Stimulates uterine contractions similar to labor by myometrium stimulation, causing abortion; acts within 30 hr for complete abortion

Therapeutic outcome: Beginning of labor, fetal expulsion

USES: Abortion during 2nd trimester, benign hydatidiform mole, expulsion of uterine contents in fetal deaths to 28 wk, missed abortion, cervical effacement and dilatation in term pregnancy when they have not occurred spontaneously

CONTRAINDICATIONS

Hypersensitivity, C-section, surgery, fetal distress, multiparity, vaginal bleeding, cephalopelvic disproportion

Precautions: Pregnancy **C**, renal/hepatic/cardiac disease, asthma, anemia, jaundice, diabetes mellitus, seizure disorders, hypertension, glaucoma, uterine fibrosis, cervical stenosis, pelvic surgery, PID, respiratory disease

> BLACK BOX WARNING: Requires a specialized setting and an experienced clinician

DOSAGE AND ROUTES

Abortifacient/2nd trimester/missed abortion/benign hydatidiform mole/intrauterine fetal death

Adult: VAG SUPP 20 mg; repeat q3-5hr until abortion occurs; max dose 240 mg

Cervical ripening

Adult: GEL 0.5 mg vag gel placed in cervical canal, may repeat after 6 hr, max 1.5 mg/24 hr; vag insert 10 mg high in vagina, remove at onset of active labor or within 12 hr

Available forms: Vag supp 20 mg; gel 0.5 mg/3 g (prefilled syringe); vag insert 10 mg

Implementation

Suppository route

• Warm supp by running warm water over package; insert high in vagina, wear gloves to prevent absorption; have patient recumbent for at least 10 min

Gel route

• Do not allow to come in contact with skin; use soap and water to wash after use

• Gel should be at room temperature

• Place patient in dorsal or lithotomy position to insert gel into cervical canal; remove catheter; discard all items after use; keep supine 15-30 min

ADVERSE EFFECTS

CNS: *Headache,* dizziness, chills, fever, flushing

CV: Hypotension, **dysrhythmias,** DIC

EENT: Blurred vision

GI: *Nausea, vomiting, diarrhea*

GU: Vaginitis, vaginal pain, vulvitis, vaginismus

INTEG: Rash, skin color changes

MS: *Leg cramps, joint swelling,* weakness

SYST: **Anaphylactoid syndrome of pregnancy**

Insert: Uterine hyperstimulation, fever, nausea, vomiting, diarrhea, abdominal pain

Gel: Uterine contractile abnormality, GI side effects, back pain, fever

Fetal: Bradycardia (i.e., deceleration)

Suppository: **Uterine rupture, anaphylaxis**

Pharmacokinetics

Absorption	Rapidly absorbed
Distribution	Unknown
Metabolism	Enzymes
Excretion	Kidneys
Half-life	Unknown

Pharmacodynamics

	Gel	Supp
Onset	Rapid	10 min
Peak	30-45 min	Unknown
Duration	Unknown	2-3 hr

INTERACTIONS

Individual drugs

Alcohol: decreased oxytoxic effect

Drug classifications

Other oxytocics: increased effect

NURSING CONSIDERATIONS

Assessment

> BLACK BOX WARNING: Specialized setting, specialized clinician: use only with emergency equipment nearby, by a clinician experienced with use in pregnancy termination; complete abortion should result within 17 hr (insert)

• **Cervical ripening:** assess dilatation and effacement of the cervix, uterine contractions, fetal heart tones; watch for contractions lasting over 1 min, hypertonus, fetal distress; product should be slowed or discontinued

• Assess for fever that occurs approximately 30 min after supp insertion (abortion)

• Monitor for nausea, vomiting, diarrhea; these may require medication

• **Assess for hypersensitivity reaction:** dyspnea, rash, chest discomfort

• Assess respiratory rate, rhythm, depth; notify prescriber of abnormalities in pulse, B/P
• **Check vaginal discharge;** itching, irritation indicates vaginal infection

Patient/family education
• Teach patient all aspects of treatment including purpose of medication and expected results
• Tell patient that gel may produce warmth in her vagina
• Caution patient that if contractions are longer than 1 min to notify nurse or prescriber
• Advise patient to notify prescriber of cramping, pain, increased bleeding, chills, increased temp, or foul-smelling discharge; these symptoms may indicate uterine infection
• Advise patient to remain supine 10-15 min after insertion of suppository, 2 hr after insert, 15-30 min after gel

Evaluation

Positive therapeutic outcome
• Progression of labor
• Abortion

diphenhydrAMINE (OTC, Rx)

(dye-fen-hye′dra-meen)

Allerdryl ✿, AllerMax ✿, Altaryl, Banophen, Benadryl, Benadryl Allergy, Benadryl Allergy Dye Free, Benadryl Children's Allergy, Buckley's Bedtime, Diphedryl, Diphenhist, Dytan, ElixSure Allergy, Equaline Allergy, Equaline Children's Allergy, Equate Allergy, Equate Children's Allergy, Genahist, Good Sense Children's Allergy Relief, Good Sense Diphedryl, Leader Complete Allergy, Nytol, PediaCare Children's Allergy, PediaCare Nighttime Cough, Q-Dryl Allergy, Select Brand Allergy, Siladryl, Silphen, Simply Sleep, Sleepinal, Sleep Tabs, Sominex, Unisom ✿, Valu-Dryl, Wal-dryl Allergy, Wal-dryl Allergy Dye Free, Wal-dryl Children's Allergy, ZzzQuil

Func. class.: Antihistamine (1st generation, nonselective), antitussive
Chem. class.: Ethanolamine derivative, H_1-receptor antagonist
Pregnancy category B

Do not confuse: diphenhydrAMINE/dicyclomine/dimenhyDRINATE

ACTION: Acts on blood vessels, GI, respiratory system by competing with histamine for H_1-receptor site; decreases allergic response by blocking histamine

Therapeutic outcome: Absence of allergy symptoms and rhinitis, decreased dystonic symptoms, absence of motion sickness, absence of cough, ability to sleep

USES: Allergy symptoms, rhinitis, motion sickness, antiparkinsonism, nighttime sedation, infant colic, nonproductive cough, insomnia in children

CONTRAINDICATIONS
Hypersensitivity to H_1-receptor antagonist, neonates

Precautions: Pregnancy **B**, breastfeeding, children <2 yr, increased intraocular pressure, renal/cardiac disease, hypertension, bronchial asthma, seizure disorder, stenosed peptic ulcers, hyperthyroidism, prostatic hypertrophy, bladder neck obstruction

DOSAGE AND ROUTES
Adult and child >12 yr: PO 25-50 mg q4-6hr, max 300 mg/day; IM/IV 10-50 mg, max 300 mg/day
Child 6-12 yr: PO/IM/IV 5 mg/kg/day in 4 divided doses, max 300 mg/day

Nighttime sleep aid
Adult and child ≥12 yr: PO 25-50 mg at bedtime

Antitussive (syrup only)
Adult and child ≥12 yr: 25 mg q4hr, max 150 mg/24 hr
Child 6-12 yr: 12.5 mg q4hr, max 75 mg/24 hr

Available forms: Caps 25, 50 mg; tabs 25, 50 mg; chew tabs 12.5, 25 mg; elix 12.5 mg/5 ml; syr 12.5 mg/5 ml; inj 50 mg/ml; orally disintegrating tabs 12.5 mg; orally disintegrating strips 12.5, 25 mg

Implementation
• Avoid use in children <2 yr, death has occurred; overdose has occurred in topical gel taken orally (adult/child)
• Give 20 min before bedtime if using for sleep aid
PO route
• Give with meals if GI symptoms occur; absorption rate may be slightly decreased; cap may be opened and product mixed with food/fluids for patients with swallowing difficulties
IM route
• Give IM inj in large muscle mass; aspirate to avoid **IV** administration; rotate sites

Direct IV route
- Give **IV** undiluted ≤25 mg/min

Intermittent IV infusion route
May be diluted with 0.9% NaCl, D₅W, D₁₀W, 0.45% NaCl, D₅/0.9% NaCl, D₅/0.45% NaCl, D₅/0.25% NaCl, LR, Ringer's; give 25 mg/min or less

Syringe incompatibilities: PENTobarbital, phenytoin, thiopental

Y-site compatibilities: Acetaminophen, aldesleukin, alfentanil hydrochloride, amifostine, amikacin sulfate, aminocaproic acid, amphotericin B lipid complex (Abelcet), amphotericin B liposome (AmBisome), amsacrine, anidulafungin, argatroban, ascorbic acid injection, atenolol, atracurium besylate, atropine sulfate, azithromycin, benztropine mesylate, bivalirudin, bleomycin, bumetanide, buprenorphine, butorphanol, calcium chloride/gluconate, CARBOplatin, caspofungin, cefTAZidime, ceftizoxime, chlorproMAZINE, cimetidine, ciprofloxacin, cisatracurium, CISplatin, cladribine, clindamycin, codeine, cyanocobalamin, cyclophosphamide, cycloSPORINE, cytarabine, DACTINomycin, DAPTOmycin, digoxin, diltiazem, DOBUTamine, DOCEtaxel, DOPamine, doripenem, doxacurium, DOXOrubicin, DOXOrubicin liposomal, doxycycline, enalaprilat, ePHEDrine, EPINEPHrine, epirubicin, epoetin alfa, eptifibatide, ertapenem, erythromycin, esmolol, etoposide, famotidine, fenoldopam, fentaNYL, filgrastim, fluconazole, fludarabine, folic acid, gallium, gatifloxacin, gemcitabine, gemtuzumab, gentamicin, glycopyrrolate, granisetron, HYDROmorphone, hydrOXYzine, IDArubicin, ifosfamide, imipenem-cilastatin, irinotecan, isoproterenol, labetalol, levofloxacin, lidocaine, linezolid, LORazepam, LR, magnesium sulfate, mannitol, mechlorethamine, melphalan, meperidine, meropenem, metaraminol, methadone, methicillin, methotrexate, methoxamine, methyldopa, metoclopramide, metoprolol, metroNIDAZOLE, miconazole, midazolam, minocycline, mitoXANtrone, morphine, multiple vitamins injection, mycophenolate, nalbuphine, naloxone, nesiritide, netilmicin, nitroglycerin, norepinephrine, octreotide, ondansetron, oxaliplatin, oxytocin, PACLitaxel, palonosetron, pamidronate, pancuronium, papaverine, PEMEtrexed, penicillin G potassium/sodium, pentamidine, pentazocine, phenylephrine, phytonadione, piperacillin, piperacillin-tazobactam, polymyxin B, potassium chloride, procainamide, prochlorperazine, promethazine, propofol, propranolol, protamine, pyridoxine, quiNIDine, quinupristin-dalfopristin, ranitidine, remifentanil, Ringer's, ritodrine, riTUXimab, rocuronium, sargramostim, sodium acetate, succinylcholine, SUFentanil, tacrolimus, teniposide, theophylline, thiamine, thiotepa, ticarcillin, ticarcillin-clavulanate, tigecycline, tirofiban, TNA, tobramycin, tolazoline, TPN, trastuzumab, trimetaphan, urokinase, vancomycin, vasopressin, vecuronium, verapamil, vinCRIStine, vinorelbine, vitamin B complex/C, voriconazole, zoledronic acid

Y-site incompatibilities: Foscarnet

ADVERSE EFFECTS
CNS: *Dizziness, drowsiness,* poor coordination, fatigue, anxiety, euphoria, confusion, paresthesia, neuritis, **seizures**
CV: Hypotension, palpitations
EENT: Blurred vision, dilated pupils, tinnitus, nasal stuffiness, dry nose, throat, mouth
GI: Nausea, anorexia, diarrhea
GU: *Retention,* dysuria, frequency
HEMA: **Thrombocytopenia, agranulocytosis, hemolytic anemia**
INTEG: Photosensitivity
MISC: **Anaphylaxis**
RESP: Increased thick secretions, wheezing, chest tightness

Pharmacokinetics

Absorption	Well absorbed (PO, IM); completely absorbed (**IV**)
Distribution	Widely distributed; crosses placenta
Metabolism	Liver (95%)
Excretion	Kidneys, breast milk
Half-life	2½-7 hr

Pharmacodynamics

	PO	IM	IV
Onset	15-60 min	30 min	Immediate
Peak	2-4 hr	2-4 hr	Unknown
Duration	4-8 hr	4-8 hr	4-8 hr

INTERACTIONS
Individual drugs
Alcohol: increased CNS depression

Drug classifications
Antidepressants (tricyclic), barbiturates, CNS depressants, opiates, sedative/hypnotics: increased CNS depression
MAOIs: increased effect of diphenhydrAMINE

Drug/lab test
False negative: skin allergy tests (discontinue antihistamines 3 days before testing)

NURSING CONSIDERATIONS
Assessment
• Assess respiratory status: rate, rhythm, increase in bronchial secretions, wheezing, chest tightness; provide fluids to 2 L/day to decrease secretion thickness
• Monitor I&O ratio: be alert for urinary retention, frequency, dysuria, especially geriatric; product should be discontinued if these occur
• Monitor CBC during long-term therapy; blood dyscrasias may occur but are rare
• If giving for dystonic reactions, assess type of involuntary movements and evaluate response to this medication
• Assess cough characteristics including type, frequency, thickness of secretions; evaluate response to this medication if using for cough
• Product should be discontinued 4 days prior to skin allergy tests

Patient/family education
• Tell patient that a false-negative result may occur with skin testing; these procedures should not be scheduled until 3 days after discontinuing use
• Caution patient to avoid hazardous activities and activities requiring alertness, since dizziness may occur; instruct patient to request assistance with ambulation
• Teach patient to use sunscreen to prevent photosensitivity
• Advise patient to avoid alcohol, other depressants; may potentiate effect; CNS depression may occur
• Teach all aspects of product uses; to notify prescriber if confusion, sedation, hypotension occur; to avoid driving and other hazardous activity if drowsiness occurs; to avoid alcohol or other CNS depressants that may potentiate effect
• Advise patient to avoid breastfeeding; **not to breastfeed (injectable)**

Evaluation

Positive therapeutic outcome
• Absence of motion sickness
• Absence of nausea, vomiting
• Ability to sleep
• Absence of cough
• Decrease in involuntary movements

TREATMENT OF OVERDOSE:
• Administer lavage, diazepam, vasopressors, phenytoin **IV**

diphenoxylate with atropine (Rx)
(dye-fen-ox'i-late)
Lomotil, Lonox

difenoxin/atropine (Rx)
(dye-fen-ox'in/a'troe-peen)
Motofen
Func. class.: Antidiarrheal
Chem. class.: Phenylpiperidine derivative, opiate agonist
Pregnancy category C
Controlled substance schedule V (diphenoxylate/atropine); IV (difenoxin/atropine (US))

Do not confuse: Lomotil/Lamictal/Lamasil/Lanoxin/Lasix/Ludomil

ACTION: Inhibits gastric motility by acting on mucosal receptors responsible for peristalsis

Therapeutic outcome: Decreased loose stools

USES: Acute nonspecific and acute exacerbations of chronic functional diarrhea

CONTRAINDICATIONS
Hypersensitivity, pseudomembranous colitis, child <2 yr, severe electrolyte imbalances, diarrhea associated with organisms that penetrate intestinal mucosa

Precautions: Pregnancy C, breastfeeding, hepatic disease, ulcerative colitis, severe hepatic disease, substance abuse, dehydration

DOSAGE AND ROUTES
diphenoxylate/atropine
Adult: PO 5 mg qid, titrated to patient response, max 8 tabs/24 hr
Child 2-12 yr: PO (liquid only) 0.3-0.4 mg/kg/day in 4 divided doses

difenoxin/atropine
Adult: PO initially 2 tabs, then 1 tab after each loose stool or q3-4hr prn, max 8 tabs/day

Available forms: diphenoxylate/atropine: tab 2.5 mg diphenoxylate/0.025 mg atropine; liq 2.5 mg diphenoxylate/0.025 mg atropine/5 ml; **difenoxin/atropine:** tabs 1 mg difenoxin/0.025 atropine

Implementation
• Give for 48 hr only; tabs may be given with food, crushed and mixed with fluids; liquid should be measured accurately

ADVERSE EFFECTS

CNS: *Dizziness, drowsiness, light-headedness, headache,* fatigue, nervousness, insomnia, confusion
EENT: Blurred vision, burning eyes
GI: *Nausea, vomiting, dry mouth, epigastric distress,* constipation, **paralytic ileus, toxic megacolon**
MISC: **Anaphylaxis, angioedema**
RESP: Respiratory depression

Pharmacokinetics

Absorption	Well absorbed
Distribution	Unknown
Metabolism	Liver, active metabolite
Excretion	Kidneys
Half-life	2½ hr

Pharmacodynamics

Onset	45-60 min
Peak	3 hr
Duration	3-4 hr

INTERACTIONS

Individual drugs

Alcohol: increased action of alcohol
Amantadine, amoxapine, diphenhydrAMINE, clemastine, cloZAPine, cyclobenzaprine, disopyramide, loperamide, maprotiline, olanzapine: decreased GI motility, possible toxic megacolon

Drug classifications

Anticholinergics: increased anticholinergic effect
Antimuscarinics, phenothiazines, tricyclics: decreased GI motility, possible toxic megacolon
Barbiturates: increased action of barbiturates
CNS depressants: increased action of CNS depressants
MAOIs: hypertensive crisis; do not use together
Opiates: increased action of opioids

NURSING CONSIDERATIONS

Assessment

• Monitor electrolytes (potassium, sodium, chloride) if on long-term therapy; fluid status, skin turgor
• Assess bowel pattern before, during treatment; check for rebound constipation after termination of medication; check bowel sounds
• Check response after 48 hr; if no response, product should be discontinued and other treatment initiated
• Assess for abdominal distention and toxic megacolon, which may occur in ulcerative colitis
• Assess hepatic function if on long-term therapy

Patient/family education

• Advise patient to avoid alcohol and OTC products unless directed by prescriber; may cause increased CNS depression

• Caution patient not to exceed recommended dosage; that product may be habit forming
• Advise patient that product may cause drowsiness; to avoid hazardous activities until response to product is determined
• Teach patient that dry mouth can be decreased by frequent sips of water, hard candy, sugarless gum

Evaluation

Positive therapeutic outcome
• Decreased diarrhea

dipyridamole (Rx)

(dye-peer-id′a-mole)
Persantine
Func. class.: Coronary vasodilator, antiplatelet agent
Chem. class.: Nonnitrate
Pregnancy category B

ACTION: Inhibits adenosine uptake, which produces coronary vasodilatation; increases oxygen saturation in coronary tissues, coronary blood flow; acts on small vessels with little effect on vascular resistance; may increase development of collateral circulation; decreased platelet aggregation by the inhibition of phosphodiesterases (enzymes)

Therapeutic outcome: Inhibition of platelet aggregation; absence of ischemic attacks, reinfarction

USES: Prevention of transient ischemic attacks, inhibition of platelet adhesion to prevent myocardial reinfarction, thromboembolism, with warfarin in prosthetic heart valves, prevention of coronary bypass graft occlusion with aspirin; **IV** form used to evaluate coronary artery disease; used as alternative to exercise in thallium myocardial perfusion imaging to evaluate coronary artery disease

CONTRAINDICATIONS
Hypersensitivity

Precautions: Pregnancy **B**, breastfeeding, hypotension, unstable angina, asthma, hepatic disease, labor

DOSAGE AND ROUTES

Inhibition of platelet adhesion
Adult: PO 75-100 mg qid in combination with warfarin, 75 mg qid with aspirin

Thallium myocardial perfusion imaging

Adult: IV 570 mcg/kg, max 60 mg/day

Transient ischemic attacks with aspirin (unlabeled)

Adult: PO 225-400 mg/day, max 400 mg daily

Available forms: Tabs 25, 50, 75 mg; inj 10 mg/2 ml

Implementation

PO route

• Give with 8 oz of water; to improve absorption give on an empty stomach; if GI symptoms occur may give with meals
• Tabs may be crushed, mixed with food or fluids for swallowing difficulty, or swallowed whole
• Store at room temperature

Intermittent IV infusion route

• Give by IV after diluting to at least 1:2 ratio using D₅W, 0.45% NaCl, or 0.9% NaCl; 20-50 ml should be given; give over 4 min; do not give undiluted
• Inject thallium 201 within 5 min after product infusion
• Do not admix

ADVERSE EFFECTS

CNS: *Headache, dizziness, weakness, fainting, syncope;* **IV:** *transient cerebral ischemia, weakness*
CV: *Postural hypotension;* **IV:** MI
GI: *Nausea, vomiting,* anorexia, diarrhea
INTEG: *Rash,* flushing

Pharmacokinetics

Absorption	30%-50% (PO)
Distribution	Widely distributed; crosses placenta
Metabolism	Liver
Excretion	Bile, undergoes enterohepatic recirculation; enters breast milk
Half-life	10 hr

Pharmacodynamics

	PO	IV
Onset	Unknown	Unknown
Peak	1-3 hr	Unknown
Duration	Unknown	Unknown

INTERACTIONS

Individual drugs

Aspirin, cefoTEtan, sulfinpyrazone, valproic acid: increased risk of bleeding

Digoxin: increased digoxin effect
Theophylline: prevention of coronary vasodilation

Drug classifications

Anticoagulants, NSAIDs, salicylates, thrombolytics: increased risk of bleeding

NURSING CONSIDERATIONS

Assessment

• Monitor B/P, pulse baseline and during treatment until stable; take B/P with patient lying, standing; orthostatic hypotension is common
• Assess cardiac status: chest pain, what aggravates or ameliorates condition
• If using by IV route, monitor VS before, during, and after infusion; monitor for chest pain, bronchospasm; use ECG for identifying dysrhythmias; use aminophylline up to 250 mg IV for bronchospasm and chest pain; if chest pain is unrelieved with the 250 mg dose of aminophylline, give SL dose of nitroglycerin

Patient/family education

• Teach patient that this medication is not a cure; that product may have to be taken continuously in evenly spaced doses only as directed; if a dose is missed, take one when remembered up to 4 hr; do not double doses
• Advise patient to rise slowly from sitting or lying down to prevent orthostatic hypotension
• Caution patient not to use alcohol or OTC medication unless approved by prescriber
• Caution patient to avoid hazardous activities until stabilized on medication; dizziness may occur

Evaluation

Positive therapeutic outcome

• Absence of reinfarction, ischemic attacks

TREATMENT OF OVERDOSE:
Administer IV phenylephrine

> ### divalproex sodium
> *See valproate*

> **⚠ HIGH ALERT**
> ### DOBUTamine (Rx)
> (doe-byoo′ta-meen)
> *Func. class.:* Adrenergic direct-acting β₁-agonist, inotropic agent, cardiac stimulant
> *Chem. class.:* Catecholamine
> **Pregnancy category B**

Do not confuse: DOBUTamine/DOPamine

ACTION: Causes increased contractility, increased cardiac output without marked increase in heart rate by acting on β_1-receptors in heart; minor α/β_2 effects

Therapeutic outcome: Cardiac output increased with decreased fatigue and dyspnea

USES: Cardiac decompensation due to organic heart disease or cardiac surgery

Unlabeled uses: Cardiogenic shock in children, congenital heart disease in children undergoing cardiac catherization

CONTRAINDICATIONS
Hypersensitivity, idiopathic hypertrophic subaortic stenosis

Precautions: Pregnancy **B**, breastfeeding, children, hypertension, CAD, MI, hypovolemia, dysrhythmias, sulfite hypersensitivity, renal failure, geriatrics

DOSAGE AND ROUTES
Adult and child: IV INF 0.5-1 mcg/kg/min; titrate to 2-20 mcg/kg/min; may increase to 40 mcg/kg/min if needed

Available forms: Inj 12.5 mg/ml, 250 mg/20 ml

Implementation
Injectable administration
• Visually inspect parenteral products for particulate matter and discoloration prior to administration whenever solution and container permit

IV administration
NOTE: Infusions up to 72 hours have been given without development of tolerance. However, β-receptor desensitization may occur with prolonged infusions of any β-adrenergic agonist, including DOBUTamine, or as a consequence of sympathetic compensatory mechanisms associated with advanced congestive heart failure, resulting in alterations in DOBUTamine pharmacodynamics. Experience with intravenous DOBUTamine in controlled trials does not extend beyond 48 hours of repeated boluses and/or continuous infusions
• Must be diluted before administration
• Infuse into a large vein

Dilution
• Concentrate for injection must be diluted with at least 50 ml of a compatible IV solution (strongly alkaline [i.e., sodium bicarbonate] solutions are incompatible). A common dilution is 500 mg (40 ml) in 210 ml D_5W or NS (withdraw 40 ml from a 250 ml bag) to produce a final concentration of 2000 mcg/ml; or 1000 mg (80 ml) in 170 ml D_5W or NS (withdraw 80 ml from a 250 ml bag) to produce a final

concentration of 4000 mcg/ml. Maximum concentration should not exceed 5000 mcg/ml and should be adjusted according to the fluid requirements of the patient
Infusion
• Administer diluted solution by IV infusion using a controlled infusion device
• Premixed bags of DOBUTamine in D_5W solutions may exhibit a pink color that, if present, will increase with time; this color change is due to slight oxidation of the drug, but there is no significant loss of potency.
• Do not administer DOBUTamine simultaneously with solutions containing sodium bicarbonate or strong alkaline solutions (incompatible)
• Infusion of DOBUTamine should be started at a low rate and titrated frequently to reach the optimal dosage (see Dosage); dosage titration is guided by the patient's response, including systemic blood pressure, urine flow, frequency of ectopic activity, heart rate, and (whenever possible) measurements of cardiac output, central venous pressure, and/or pulmonary capillary wedge pressure

Syringe compatibilities: Heparin, ranitidine

Syringe incompatibility: Doxapram

Y-site compatibilities: Alfentanil, alprostadil, amifostine, amikacin, aminocaproic acid, amiodarone, anidulafungin, argatroban, ascorbic acid injection, atenolol, atracurium, atropine, aztreonam, benztropine, bleomycin, bumetanide, buprenorphine, butorphanol, calcium chloride/gluconate, CARBOplatin, caspofungin, chlorproMAZINE, cimetidine, ciprofloxacin, cisatracurium, CISplatin, cladribine, clarithromycin, cloNIDine, codeine, cyanocobalamin, cyclophosphamide, cycloSPORINE, cytarabine, DACTINomycin, DAPTOmycin, dexmedetomidine, digoxin, diltiazem, diphenhydrAMINE, DOCEtaxel, DOPamine, doripenem, doxacurium, DOXOrubicin, DOXOrubicin liposomal, doxycycline, enalaprilat, ePHEDrine, EPINEPHrine, epirubicin, epoetin alfa, eptifibatide, erythromycin, esmolol, etoposide, famotidine, fenoldopam, fentaNYL, fluconazole, fludarabine, gatifloxacin, gemcitabine, gentamicin, glycopyrrolate, granisetron, HYDROmorphone, hydrOXYzine, IDArubicin, ifosfamide, irinotecan, isoproterenol, labetalol, levofloxacin, lidocaine, linezolid, LORazepam, LR, magnesium sulfate, mannitol, mechlorethamine, meperidine, meropenem, metaraminol, methoxamine, methyldopa, methylPREDNISolone, metoclopramide, metoprolol, metroNIDAZOLE, miconazole, milrinone, minocycline, mitoXANtrone, morphine, multiple vitamins injection, mycophenolate mofetil, nafcillin, nalbuphine, naloxone, netilmicin, niCARdipine, nitroglycerin,

D

norepinephrine, octreotide, ondansetron, oxaliplatin, oxytocin, PACLitaxel, palonosetron, pamidronate, pancuronium, papaverine, pentamidine, pentazocine, phenylephrine, polymyxin B, potassium chloride, procainamide, prochlorperazine, promethazine, propofol, propranolol, protamine, pyridoxine, quiNIDine, ranitidine, remifentanil, Ringer's, ritodrine, riTUXimab, rocuronium, sodium acetate, succinylcholine, SUFentanil, tacrolimus, temocillin, teniposide, theophylline, thiamine, thiotepa, tigecycline, tirofiban, TNA, tobramycin, tolazoline, TPN, trastuzumab, trimetaphan, urokinase, vancomycin, vasopressin, vecuronium, verapamil, vinCRIStine, vinorelbine, voriconazole, zidovudine, zoledronic acid

Y-site incompatibilities: Acyclovir, alteplase, aminophylline, foscarnet, phytonadione

ADVERSE EFFECTS

CNS: *Anxiety,* headache, dizziness, fatigue
CV: Palpitations, tachycardia, hypo/hypertension, PVCs, angina
ENDO: Hypokalemia
GI: Heartburn, nausea, vomiting
MS: Muscle cramps (leg)
RESP: Dyspnea

Pharmacokinetics

Absorption	Complete
Distribution	Unknown
Metabolism	Liver
Excretion	Kidneys
Half-life	2 min

Pharmacodynamics

Onset	1-5 min
Peak	10 min
Duration	<10 min

INTERACTIONS
Individual drugs
Atomoxetine: increased pressor effect, dysrhythmias
Bretylium, oxytocin: increased dysrhythmias
Guanethidine: increased severe hypertension
Oxytocin: increased pressor effects

Drug classifications
Anesthetics (general): increased dysrhythmias
Antidepressants (tricyclic), COMT inhibitors, MAOIs, oxytocics: increased pressor response, dysrhythmias
β-Blockers: decreased action of DOBUTamine

NURSING CONSIDERATIONS
Assessment
• **Assess for hypovolemia;** if present, correct before beginning treatment with DOBUTamine;

avoid use in patients with atrial fibrillation before digitalization

• **Monitor ECG for dysrhythmias, ischemia** during treatment; some patients may not need continuous ECG monitoring; also monitor PCWP, CVP, CO_2, urinary output; notify prescriber if <30 ml/hr

• **Assess for heart failure:** bibasilar crackles, S_3 gallop, dyspnea, neck vein distention in patients with cardiomyopathy or CHF

• Assess for oxygenation or perfusion deficit: decreased B/P, chest pain, dizziness, loss of consciousness

• Monitor B/P and pulse q5min during infusion; if B/P drops 30 mm Hg, stop infusion and call prescriber

• Monitor ALT, AST, bilirubin daily

• **Monitor for sulfite sensitivity, which may be life threatening**

Patient/family education
• Teach patient reason for medication and expected results, reason for all monitoring and procedures
• Advise patient to report dyspnea, headache, IV site discomfort, chest pain, numbness of extremities

Evaluation
Positive therapeutic outcome
• Increased cardiac output
• Decreased PCWP, adequate CVP
• Decreased dyspnea, fatigue, edema, ECG
• Increased urine output

TREATMENT OF OVERDOSE:
Discontinue product, support circulation

⚠ HIGH ALERT

DOCEtaxel (Rx)
(doe-se-tax'el)
Docefrez, Taxotere
Func. class.: Antineoplastic, miscellaneous
Pregnancy category D

Do not confuse: Taxotere/Taxol

ACTION: Inhibits the reorganization of the microtubule network needed for interphase and mitotic cellular functions; also causes abnormal bundles of microtubules during cell cycle and multiple esters of microtubules during mitosis

Therapeutic outcome: Prevention of rapidly growing malignant cells

USES: Locally advanced or metastatic breast cancer, non–small cell lung cancer, androgen-independent metastatic prostate cancer, postsurgery operable node-positive breast cancer, induction treatment of locally advanced squamous cell cancer of the head/neck, adjuvant treatment of breast cancer with CARBOplatin and trastuzumab, gastric adenocarcinoma

CONTRAINDICATIONS

Pregnancy **D,** breastfeeding, hypersensitivity to this product, bilirubin exceeding upper normal limit

> **BLACK BOX WARNING:** Hypersensitivity to other products with polysorbate 80, neutropenia (neutrophils <1500/mm³)

Precautions: Children, CV disease, pulmonary disorders, bone marrow depression, herpes zoster, pleural effusion

> **BLACK BOX WARNING:** Edema, hepatic disease, lung cancer, taxane hypersensitivity

DOSAGE AND ROUTES

• Other regimens are used

Locally advanced or metastatic breast cancer after failure of other chemotherapy

Adult: IV 60-100 mg/m² given over 1 hr q3wk; if neutrophil count is <500/mm³ for >1 wk, reduce dose by 25%

Operable node-positive breast cancer; adjuvant postsurgery treatment of operable node-positive breast cancer

Adult: IV (TAC regimen) 75 mg/m² 1 hr after DOXOrubicin 50 mg/m² and cyclophosphamide 500 mg/m² q3wk for 6 cycles

Adjuvant treatment of operable stage I-III invasive breast cancer in combination with cyclophosphamide

Adult: IV (TAC) regimen DOCEtaxel 75 mg/m² with cyclophosphamide 600 mg/m² q21day × 4 cycles

Locally advanced or metastatic non–small cell lung cancer after failure of CISplatin chemotherapy

Adult: IV 75 mg/m² over 1 hr q3wk; if neutrophil count is <500/mm³ for >1 wk, reduce dose to 55 mg/m²; if patient develops grade 3 peripheral neuropathy, stop product

Unresectable, locally advanced or metastatic non–small cell lung cancer previously treated with chemotherapy

Adult: IV 75 mg/m² over 1 hr, then CISplatin 75 mg/m² IV given over 30-60 min q3wk; reduce dose to 65 mg/m² in those with hematologic or nonhematologic toxicities

Androgen-independent metastatic prostate cancer

Adult: IV 75 mg/m² given over 1 hr q3wk, with 5 mg predniSONE PO bid continuously; give dexamethasone 8 mg PO at 12 hr, 3 hr, and 1 hr prior to DOCEtaxel; if neutrophil count is <500 cells/mm³ for more than 1 wk or other toxicities occur, reduce dose to 60 mg/m²

Squamous cell cancer of head/neck

Adult: IV 75 mg/m² over 1 hr, then CISplatin 100 mg/m² over 1 hr on day 1, then 5-FU 1000 mg/m²/day CONT INF × 5 days, repeat cycle q3wk

Gastric adenocarcinoma

Adult: IV 75 mg/m² q3wk, given with CISplatin, fluorouracil

Available forms: Inj 10 mg/ml, 20 mg/0.5 ml, 20 mg/ml, 80 mg/2 ml, 80 mg/4 ml; 20, 80 mg powder for injection

Implementation

• Give top or systemic analgesics for pain to lessen effects of stomatitis
• Give liquid diet: carbonated beverages; gelatin may be added if patient is not nauseated or vomiting
⚠ Confirm that dexamethasone was given 12 hr and 6 hr before inf begins
• Store prepared sol up to 27 hr in refrigerator

Intermittent IV infusion route

• Use gloves and cytotoxic handling precautions
• Use non-PVC bag and use non-DEHP tubing
• Allow vials to warm to room temperature, withdraw all diluent and inject in vial of docetaxel, rotate gently to mix, allow to stand to decrease foaming, then withdraw the required amount (10 mg/ml) and inject in 250 ml of 0.9% NaCl or D₅W, mix gently, give over 1 hr

Y-site compatibilities: Acyclovir, alfentanil, allopurinol, amifostine, amikacin, aminocaproic acid, aminophylline, amiodarone, amphotericin B lipid complex, ampicillin, ampicillin-sulbactam, anidulafungin, atenolol, atracurium, azithromycin, aztreonam, bivalirudin, bleomycin, bumetanide, buprenorphine, busulfan, butorphanol, calcium chloride/gluconate, CARBOplatin, carmustine, caspofungin,

---

Adverse effects: *italics* = common; **bold** = life-threatening

ceFAZolin, cefepime, cefonicid, cefotaxime, cefoTEtan, cefOXitin, cefTAZidime, ceftizoxime, cefTRIAXone, cefuroxime, chloramphenicol, chlorproMAZINE, cimetidine, ciprofloxacin, cisatracurium, CISplatin, clindamycin, codeine, cyclophosphamide, cycloSPORINE, cytarabine, dacarbazine, DACTINomycin, DAPTOmycin, dexamethasone, dexmedetomidine, dexrazoxane, diazepam, digoxin, diltiazem, diphenhydrAMINE, DOBUTamine, DOPamine, doripenem, doxacurium, DOXOrubicin HCl, doxycycline, droperidol, enalaprilat, ePHEDrine, EPINEPHrine, epirubicin, ertapenem, erythromycin, esmolol, etoposide, famotidine, fenoldopam, fentaNYL, fluconazole, fludarabine, fluorouracil, foscarnet, fosphenytoin, furosemide, ganciclovir, gatifloxacin, gemcitabine, gentamicin, glycopyrrolate, granisetron, haloperidol, heparin, hydrALAZINE, hydrocortisone, HYDROmorphone, hydrOXYzine, ifosfamide, imipenem-cilastatin, inamrinone, insulin (regular), irinotecan, isoproterenol, ketorolac, labetalol, leucovorin, levofloxacin, levorphanol, lidocaine, linezolid, LORazepam, LR, magnesium sulfate, mannitol, meperidine, meropenem, mesna, methotrexate, methyldopa, metoclopramide, metoprolol, metroNIDAZOLE, midazolam, milrinone, minocycline, mitoXANtrone, mivacurium, morphine, nafcillin, naloxone, nesiritide, netilmicin, niCARdipine, nitroglycerin, nitroprusside, norepinephrine, octreotide, ofloxacin, ondansetron, oxaliplatin, palonosetron, pamidronate, pancuronium, pantoprazole, PEMEtrexed, pentamidine, pentazocine, PENTobarbital, PHENobarbital, phenylephrine, piperacillin, piperacillin-tazobactam, polymyxin B, potassium chloride/phosphates, procainamide, prochlorperazine, promethazine, propranolol, quiNIDine, quinupristin-dalfopristin, ranitidine, remifentanil, riTUXimab, rocuronium, sodium acetate/bicarbonate/phosphates, succinylcholine, SUFentanil, sulfamethoxazole-trimethoprim, tacrolimus, teniposide, theophylline, thiopental, thiotepa, ticarcillin, ticarcillin-clavulanate, tigecycline, tirofiban, tobramycin, tolazoline, trastuzumab, trimethobenzamide, vancomycin, vasopressin, vecuronium, verapamil, vinCRIStine, vinorelbine, voriconazole, zidovudine, zoledronic acid

ADVERSE EFFECTS
CNS: Seizures
CV: *Hypotension, fluid retention, peripheral edema,* flushing, MI, sinus tachycardia
GI: *Nausea, vomiting, diarrhea,* hepatotoxicity, stomatitis, colitis
HEMA: Neutropenia, leukopenia, thrombocytopenia, anemia, bleeding, infections, myelosuppression

INTEG: *Alopecia,* nail pain, rash, skin eruptions
MISC: Amenorrhea, fever of unknown origin, secondary malignancy, Stevens-Johnson syndrome, epiphora
MS: *Arthralgia, myalgia,* back pain, weakness
NEURO: *Peripheral neuropathy*
RESP: Dyspnea, pulmonary edema, fibrosis, embolism
SYST: Hypersensitivity reactions, AML, death

Pharmacokinetics

Absorption	Completely absorbed
Distribution	Unknown
Metabolism	Liver, extensively
Excretion	Fecal
Half-life	11.1 hr

Pharmacodynamics

Onset	Rapid
Peak	Unknown
Duration	Unknown

INTERACTIONS
Individual drugs
Anastrozole (high doses), aprepitant, clarithromycin, conivaptan, delavirdine, efavirenz (induces or inhibits), erythromycin, fluconazole, FLUoxetine, fluvoxaMINE, fosaprepitant, imatinib, itraconazole, ketoconazole, nefazodone, voriconazole, and others: increased CYP3A inhibition

Bosentan, carBAMazepine, nevirapine, phenytoin, fosphenytoin, rifabutin, rifampin, rifapentine: increased CYP3A induction

CycloSPORINE, erythromycin, ketoconazole, troleandomycin: altered metabolism of DOCEtaxel

Drug classifications
Antineoplastics, radiation: increased myelosuppression

Barbiturates: increased CYP3A induction

Live virus vaccines: decreased immune response

NURSING CONSIDERATIONS
Assessment
• **Assess CNS changes:** confusion, paresthesias, peripheral neuropathy, dysesthesia, pain, weakness: if severe, product should be discontinued
• Check buccal cavity q8hr for dryness, sores or ulceration, white patches, oral pain, bleeding, dysphagia; obtain prescription for viscous lidocaine (Xylocaine) to use in mouth

BLACK BOX WARNING: **Taxane: assess symptoms indicating severe allergic reaction, anaphylaxis:** rash, pruritus, urticaria, purpuric skin lesions, itching, flushing

BLACK BOX WARNING: Monitor CBC, differential, platelet count weekly; withhold product if WBC is <1500/mm³ or platelet count is <100,000/mm³, notify prescriber of results

BLACK BOX WARNING: Use of DOCEtaxel, polysorbate 80 are contraindicated

BLACK BOX WARNING: **Edema:** oral corticosteroids should be given as premedication; assess for fluid retention

BLACK BOX WARNING: **Lung cancer:** increased mortality in those with increased LFTs and a history of platinum-based products

• Monitor renal function tests: BUN, creatinine, serum uric acid, urine CCr before, during therapy; check I&O ratio; report fall in urine output to <30 ml/hr
• Monitor temp (may indicate beginning of infection)

BLACK BOX WARNING: **Hepatic disease:** Monitor liver function tests before, during therapy (bilirubin, AST, ALT, LDH) as needed or monthly; check for jaundice of skin and sclera, dark urine, clay-colored stools, itchy skin, abdominal pain, fever, diarrhea

BLACK BOX WARNING: **Assess for bone marrow depression/bleeding:** hematuria, stool guaiac, bruising or petechiae, mucosa or orifices q8hr; check for inflammation of mucosa, breaks in skin

• Assess effects of alopecia on body image; discuss feelings about body changes

Patient/family education
⚠ Inform patient that nonhormonal contraceptive measures are recommended during therapy and >4 mo after; teratogenic effects are possible, pregnancy D
• Teach patient to avoid use of products containing aspirin or ibuprofen, razors, commercial mouthwash, since bleeding may occur; to report symptoms of bleeding (hematuria, tarry stools)
• Instruct patient to report signs of **anemia** (fatigue, headache, irritability, faintness, shortness of breath) and CNS reactions (confusion, psychosis, nightmares, seizures, severe headaches)

• Instruct patient to report signs of **infection:** fever, sore throat, flulike symptoms
• Inform patient that hair may be lost during treatment; a wig or hairpiece may make patient feel better; new hair may be different in color and texture
• Inform patient that receiving vaccinations during therapy may cause serious reactions
• Instruct patient to rinse mouth tid-qid with water, club soda; brush teeth bid-qid with soft brush or cotton-tipped applicators for stomatitis; use unwaxed dental floss

Evaluation
Positive therapeutic outcome
• Prevention of rapid division of malignant cells

docosanol topical
See Appendix B

docusate calcium (OTC)
(dok'yoo-sate cal'see-um)
Kao-Tin, Kaopectate Stool Softener
docusate sodium (OTC)
Colace, Correctol, Diocto, Docu DOK, Doculace, Enemeez, Fleet Pedialax, Fleet Sof-Lax, Phillips Liquid-Gels, Selex ✦, Silace, Soflax ✦
Func. class.: Laxative, emollient
Chem. class.: Anionic surfactant
Pregnancy category C

ACTION: Increases water, fat penetration in intestine; allows for easier passage of stool

Therapeutic outcome: Passage of softened stool, absence of constipation

USES: Prevent hard, dry stools, prevent constipation, soften fecal impaction (rectal route)

CONTRAINDICATIONS
Hypersensitivity, obstruction, fecal impaction, nausea/vomiting

Precautions: Pregnancy **C**, breastfeeding

DOSAGE AND ROUTES
Adult: PO 50-300 mg/day (docusate sodium) or 240 mg (docusate calcium); enema 4 ml (docusate sodium)
Child >12 yr: Enema 2 ml (docusate sodium)
Child 6-12 yr: PO 40-150 mg/day (docusate sodium) in divided doses
Child 3-6 yr: PO 20-60 mg/day (docusate sodium) in divided doses
Child <3 yr: PO 10-40 mg/day (docusate sodium) in divided doses

---

Available forms: Docusate calcium: caps 240 mg; **docusate sodium:** caps 50, 100, 250 mg; tabs 100 mg; liquid syr 20 mg/5 ml, 50 mg/5 ml, enema 283 mg

Implementation
PO route
• Dilute oral sol in juice or other fluid to disguise taste
• Give tabs or caps with 8 oz of liquid; give on empty stomach for increased absorption, results
• Store in cool environment; do not freeze

ADVERSE EFFECTS
EENT: Bitter taste, throat irritation
GI: Nausea, anorexia, cramps, diarrhea
INTEG: Rash

Pharmacokinetics
Absorption	Minimal (PO)
Distribution	Unknown
Metabolism	Not metabolized
Excretion	Bile
Half-life	Unknown

Pharmacodynamics
	PO	RECT
Onset	24-72 hr	4-6 hr
Peak	Unknown	Unknown
Duration	Unknown	Unknown

INTERACTIONS
Individual drugs
Mineral oil: toxicity

Drug/herb
Flax, senna: increased laxative action

NURSING CONSIDERATIONS
Assessment
• Assess cramping, rectal bleeding, nausea, vomiting; if these symptoms occur, product should be discontinued; identify cause of constipation; identify fluids, bulk, or exercise is missing from lifestyle

Patient/family education
• Discuss with patient that adequate fluid consumption is as necessary as bulk, exercise for adequate bowel function
• Teach patient that normal bowel movements do not always occur daily
• Advise patient not to use in presence of abdominal pain, nausea, vomiting; tell patient to notify prescriber if unrelieved constipation or if symptoms of electrolyte imbalance occur: muscle cramps, pain, weakness, dizziness, excessive thirst

• Advise patient that product may take up to 3 days to soften stools
• Instruct patient to take oral preparation with a full glass of water and increase fluid intake unless on fluid restrictions
• Caution patients with heart disease to avoid using the Valsalva maneuver to expedite evacuation

Evaluation
Positive therapeutic outcome
• Decreased constipation within 3 days

> **⚠ HIGH ALERT**
> ## dofetilide
> (doff-ee-till′-lide)
> **Tikosyn**
> *Func. class.:* Antidysrhythmic (Class III)
> **Pregnancy category C**

ACTION: Blocks cardiac ion channel carrying the rapid component of delayed potassium current, no effect on sodium channels

Therapeutic outcome: Absence of atrial fibrillation

USES: Atrial fibrillation, flutter, maintenance of normal sinus rhythm

CONTRAINDICATIONS
Hypersensitivity, digoxin toxicity, aortic stenosis, pulmonary hypertension, children, severe renal disease

> **BLACK BOX WARNING:** QT prolongation, torsades de pointes, renal failure

Precautions: Pregnancy **C**, breastfeeding, AV block, bradycardia, electrolyte imbalance

> **BLACK BOX WARNING:** Renal disease, arrhythmias, ventricular arrhythmias/tachycardia

DOSAGE AND ROUTES
Conversion of atrial fibrillation/atrial flutter to normal sinus rhythm; or, maintenance therapy with highly symptomatic atrial fibrillation/atrial flutter of ≥1 wk duration
Adult: PO Individualize dosage based on renal function and QTc in a monitored facility. Refer to the step-by-step procedure for determining the initial dose of dofetilide

Maintenance therapy of atrial fibrillation/atrial flutter after hospital discharge

Adult: PO continue dosage at discharge as from initial dosage titration. Individualize dosage based on renal function and QTc, which should be re-evaluated q3mo or as medically warranted; if the QTc >500 milliseconds (550 msec in patients with ventricular conduction abnormalities) at any time, discontinue; carefully monitor until QTc returns to baseline; if renal function deteriorates, adjust the dose as described in the dosage guidelines for patients with renal impairment

Discontinuation of dofetilide before use of interacting drugs

Adult: PO discontinue dofetilide for ≥2 days before starting a potentially interacting drug

Renal dose
Adult: PO initial dose for CCr >60 mg/ml 500 mcg bid; CCr 40-60 mg/min 250 mcg bid; CCr 20-39 mg/min 125 mcg bid; CCr <20 mg/min do not use

Available forms: Caps 125, 250, 500 mcg

Implementation

• Physician and pharmacy must be registered to use product

Step 1: Assess cardiac conduction: Before first dose, the QTc interval must be determined using an average of 5-10 beats; if the QTc interval is >440 msec (or >500 msec in ventricular conduction abnormalities), do not use. If baseline heart rate is <60 bpm, then the QT interval should be used

Step 2: Assess renal function: Before first dose, determine renal function using the Cockroft-Gault equation, use actual body weight to calculate creatinine clearance

Step 3: Adjust starting dose according to renal function: Refer to the Renal dose section (above) to determine the appropriate initial dose

Step 4: ECG monitoring: Begin continuous ECG monitoring starting with the first dose

Step 5: Dose adjustments: Approximately 2-3 hr after the first dose, determine the QTc interval. If the QTc interval has increased by >15% (compared with baseline), or, if the QTc interval is >500 msec (>550 msec in patients with ventricular conduction abnormalities), the initial dosage should be reduced by half as follows:

• Decrease an initial dose of 500 mcg bid to 250 mcg bid
• Decrease an initial dose of 250 mcg bid to 125 mcg bid
• Decrease an initial dose of 125 mcg bid to 125 mcg daily

Step 6: Reassess QTc interval: Reassess the QTc interval 2-3 hr after each subsequent dose; if, the QTc interval lengthens to >500 msec (or >550 msec in patients with ventricular conduction abnormalities), **discontinue**

Step 7: ECG Monitoring: Monitor continuous ECG for a minimum of 3 days or for 12 hr after conversion to normal sinus rhythm, whichever is greater

ADVERSE EFFECTS

CNS: *Syncope, dizziness,* headache, **stroke**
CV: *Hypotension, postural hypotension, bradycardia,* angina, PVCs, substantial pressure, precipitation of angina, transient hypertension, **QT prolongation, torsades de pointes, ventricular dysrhythmias,** chest pain
GI: *Nausea, vomiting,* severe diarrhea, anorexia
MISC: Angioedema
RESP: Dyspnea, respiratory infections

Pharmacokinetics

Absorption	>90%
Distribution	Steady state 2-3 days
Metabolism	Not metabolized
Excretion	Kidneys 80%
Half-life	10 hr

Pharmacodynamics

Unknown

INTERACTIONS
Individual drugs

AMILoride, entecavir, lamiVUDine, memantine, metFORMIN, procainamide, triamterene, trospium: increased toxicity

Arsenic trioxide, chloroquine, ciprofloxacin, clarithromycin, droperidol, erythromycin, halofantrine, haloperidol, levomethadyl, methadone, pentamidine, ziprasidone: increased QT prolongation, torsades de pointes

Cimetidine, hydrochlorothiazide, ketoconazole, megestrol, metFORMIN, prochlorperazine, triamterene, trimethoprim/sulfamethoxazole, verapamil: do not use together

Drug classifications

Antiretroviral protease inhibitors: increased dofetilide levels

Class IA/III antidysrhythmics, some phenothiazines: increased QT prolongation, torsades de pointes

Diuretics, potassium depletion: increased hypokalemia

Drug/food
• Do not use with grapefruit juice

NURSING CONSIDERATIONS
Assessment

> **BLACK BOX WARNING: Severe renal impairment:** CCr <20 ml/min: do not use for mild to moderate renal disease, monitor BUN/creatinine; adjust dose based on creatinine clearance

⚠ **AF patients should receive anticoagulation prior to cardioversion**

Patient/family education
• Instruct patient to notify prescriber if fast heartbeats with fainting or dizziness occur
• Instruct patient to notify all prescribers of all medications and supplements taken
• Teach patient that if a dose is missed, do not double, take next dose at usual time

Evaluation

Positive therapeutic outcome
• Increased control in atrial fibrillation

dolasetron (Rx)
(do-la′se-tron)
Anzemet
Func. class.: Antiemetic
Chem. class.: 5-HT receptor antagonist
Pregnancy category B

ACTION: Prevents nausea, vomiting by blocking serotonin peripherally, centrally, and in the small intestine

Therapeutic outcome: Control of nausea, vomiting

USES: Prevention of postoperative nausea, vomiting

Unlabeled uses: Radiotherapy-induced nausea/vomiting

CONTRAINDICATIONS
Hypersensitivity

Precautions: Pregnancy **B**, breastfeeding, children, geriatric, hypokalemia, electrolyte imbalances, granisetron, ondansetron, palonosetron hypersensitivity, QT prolongation

DOSAGE AND ROUTES
Prevention of postoperative nausea/vomiting
Adult: IV 12.5 mg as a single dose 15 min before cessation of anesthesia; PO 100 mg 2 hr before surgery (prevention only)

Child 2-16 yr: IV 0.35 mg/kg as a single dose 15 min before cessation of anesthesia; PO 1.2 mg/kg within 2 hr before surgery (prevention only)

Available forms: Tabs 50, 100 mg; inj 20 mg/ml, 12.5 mg/0.625 ml

Implementation
PO route
• Do not mix product for oral administration in juice until immediately before administration; apple or apple-grape diluted can be kept for 2 hr at room temperature
• Store at room temp 48 hr after dilution

Intermittent IV infusion route
• Administer by inj 100 mg/30 sec or less or diluted in 50 ml of compatible sol; give over 15 sec
• Store at room temperature for 24 hr after dilution
• Do not admix

ADVERSE EFFECTS
CNS: *Headache,* dizziness, fatigue, drowsiness
CV: Dysrhythmias, ECG changes, hypo/hypertension, tachycardia, bradycardia, QT prolongation, torsades de pointes, ventricular tachycardia/fibrillation, cardiac arrest (IV)
GI: *Diarrhea,* constipation, increased AST, ALT, abdominal pain, anorexia
GU: Urinary retention, oliguria
MISC: Rash, bronchospasm

Pharmacokinetics
Absorption	Completely absorbed
Distribution	Unknown
Metabolism	Liver, extensively
Excretion	Kidneys
Half-life	Unknown

Pharmacodynamics
Unknown

INTERACTIONS
Individual drugs
Arsenic trioxide, chloroquine, clarithromycin, droperidol, erythromycin, halofantrine, haloperidol, levomethadyl, methadone, pentamidine, ziprasidone: increased QT prolongation; occurs at higher dose of dolasetron
Cimetidine: increased dolasetron levels
Rifampin: decreased dolasetron levels

Drug classifications
Antidysrhythmics: increased dysrhythmias
Class IA/III antidysrhythmics, some phenothiazines, loop diuretics, thiazide: increased QT prolongation

NURSING CONSIDERATIONS
Assessment
• QT prolongation and QRS, PR prolongation: do not use in those with congenital long QT syndrome, hypokalemia, hypomagnesemia, complete heart block (unless a pacemaker is in place); correct electrolytes before use; monitor ECG in the elderly, renal cardiac disease
• Assess for hypersensitivity reaction: rash, bronchospasm
• Assess for cardiac conduction conditions; electrolyte imbalances or dysrhythmias

Patient/family education
• Instruct patient to report diarrhea, constipation, rash, or changes in respirations; may cause headache; use analgesic
• Teach patient reason for medication and expected results

Evaluation

Positive therapeutic outcome
• Absence of nausea, vomiting during cancer chemotherapy

dolutegravir
(dole-oo-teg′ra-vir)
Tivicay
Func. class.: Antiretroviral
Chem. class.: HIV integrase strand transfer inhibitor (ISTIs)
Pregnancy category C

ACTION: Inhibits catalytic activity of HIV integrase, which is an HIV-encoded enzyme needed for replication

Therapeutic outcome: Improvement in cell counts, T-cell counts

USES: HIV in combination with other retrovirals

CONTRAINDICATIONS
Breastfeeding, hypersensitivity

Precautions: Pregnancy C, children, geriatric patients, hepatic disease, immune reconstitution syndrome, hepatitis, antimicrobial resistance, lactase deficiency

DOSAGE AND ROUTES
Adult and child >12 yr and ≥40 kg (treatment-naïve or treatment-experienced but integrase strand transfer inhibitor–naïve): PO 50 mg/day; if given with efavirenz, fosamprenavir/ritonavir, tipranavir/ritonavir or rifampin give 50 mg bid

Available forms: Tabs 50 mg

Implementation
• May give without regard to meals, with 8 oz of water
• Store at room temperature
• Give 2 hr before or 6 hr after cation-containing antacids or laxatives, sucralfate, oral iron, oral calcium, or buffered products

ADVERSE EFFECTS
CNS: Fatigue, fever, dizziness, headache, asthenia, suicidal ideation
CV: MI
GI: Nausea, vomiting, diarrhea, abdominal pain, asthenia, gastritis, hepatitis
INTEG: Rash, pruritis, urticaria
META: Hyperglycemia
SYST: Immune reconstitution syndrome

Pharmacokinetics

Absorption	Unknown
Distribution	Steady state 5 days, 98% protein binding
Metabolism	Liver
Excretion	Feces 53%, urine 31%
Half-life	Terminal 14 hr

Pharmacodynamics

Onset	Unknown
Peak	Peak 2-3 hr
Duration	Unknown

INTERACTIONS
Individual drugs
Efavirenz, rifampin tenofovir, tipranavir/ritonavir: decreased levels of each product

Drug classifications
Antacids, buffered products, laxatives/sucralfate, oral iron products, oral calcium products, buffered products: decreased effect of dolutegravir

Drug/herb
St. John's wort: avoid concurrent use

NURSING CONSIDERATIONS
Assessment
• HIV infection: monitor CD4, T-cell count, plasma HIV RNA, viral load; resistance testing before treatment, at treatment failure

- Perform drug resistance testing prior to use in treatment-naïve patients
- **Immune reconstitution syndrome, usually during initial phase of treatment, may be antiinfective before starting**
- Monitor total/HDL/LDL cholesterol baseline and periodically, all may be elected

Patient/family education
- Teach patient to take as prescribed; if dose missed to take as soon as remembered up to 1 hr before next dose; not to double dose; not to share with others
- Teach patient that sexual partners need to be told that patient has HIV; that product does not cure infection, just controls symptoms, does not prevent infecting others
- Teach patient to report sore throat, fever, fatigue (may indicate superinfection)
- Teach patient to notify prescriber if pregnancy is planned or suspected; to avoid breastfeeding and to continue follow-up exams and work

Evaluation

Positive therapeutic outcome
- Improvement in cell counts, T-cell counts

---

donepezil (Rx)
(don-ep-ee′zill)
Aricept, Aricept ODT
Func. class.: Anti-Alzheimer's agent
Chem. class.: Reversible cholinesterase inhibitor
Pregnancy category C

ACTION: Elevates acetylcholine concentrations (cerebral cortex) by slowing degradation of acetylcholine released in cholinergic neurons; does not alter underlying dementia

Therapeutic outcome: Decreased symptoms of Alzheimer's disease

USES: Treatment of mild to severe dementia in Alzheimer's disease

Unlabeled uses: Subcortical vascular dementia, dementia with Lewy bodies

CONTRAINDICATIONS
Hypersensitivity to this product or piperidine derivatives

Precautions: Pregnancy C, breastfeeding, children, sick sinus syndrome, history of ulcers, GI bleeding, hepatic disease, bladder obstruction, asthma, seizures, COPD, abrupt disconinuation, AV block, GI obstruction, Parkinson's disease, surgery

DOSAGE AND ROUTES
Adult: PO 5 mg/day at bedtime; may increase to 10 mg/day after 4-6 wk, may increase to 23 mg/day after 3 mo of 10 mg/day (moderate to severe)

Available forms: Tabs 5, 10, 23 mg; oral sol 1 mg/ml; orally disintegrating tabs 5, 10 mg (Aricept ODT)

Implementation
PO route
- Give between meals; may be given with meals for GI symptoms
- Administer dosage adjusted to response no more than q4-6wk, oral dosage forms are interchangeable
- Provide assistance with ambulation during beginning therapy; dizziness, ataxia may occur
- Oral sol: measure with calibrated oral syringe or other calibrated device
- Orally disintegrating tabs: allow to dissolve on tongue before swallowing

ADVERSE EFFECTS
CNS: Dizziness, insomnia, somnolence, headache, fatigue, abnormal dreams, syncope, seizures, drowsiness, agitation, depression, confusion, fever, hallucinations
CV: Atrial fibrillation, hypo/hypertension, sinus bradycardia, AV block
GI: *Nausea, vomiting,* anorexia, *diarrhea,* abdominal pain, weight loss, GI bleeding
GU: Frequency, UTI, incontinence
INTEG: Rash, flushing, diaphoresis, bruising
META: Hyperlipidemia
MS: Cramps, arthritis, arthralgia, back pain
RESP: Rhinitis, URI, cough, pharyngitis

Pharmacokinetics
Absorption	Well
Distribution	Unknown
Metabolism	Liver to metabolites
Excretion	Unknown
Half-life	10 hr (single dose)

Pharmacodynamics
Unknown

INTERACTIONS
Individual drugs
CarBAMazepine, dexamethasone, PHENobarbital, phenytoin, rifampin: decreased donepezil effect
Succinylcholine: synergistic effects

Drug classification
Anticholinergics: decreased activity
Cholinergic agonists, cholinesterase inhibitors: synergistic effects

---

Increase: QT prolongation: astemizole, cisapride, dofetilide, dronedarone, grepafloxacin, mesoridazine, pimozide, probucol, sparfloxacin, terfenadine, ziprasidone, do not use concurrently

NSAIDs: increased GI intolerance

CYP2D6, CYP3A4 inducers: decreased donepezil effects

CYP2D6, CYP3A4 inhibitors: increased donepezil effects

Drug/herb
St. John's wort: decreased donepezil effect

NURSING CONSIDERATIONS
Assessment
- Monitor B/P, heart rate: hypo/hypertension
- Assess mental status: affect, mood, behavioral changes, depression, complete suicide assessment
- Assess GI status: nausea, vomiting, anorexia, diarrhea
- Assess GU status: urinary frequency, incontinence

Patient/family education
- Advise patient to report side effects: twitching, nausea, vomiting, sweating, dizziness; indicates overdose
- Advise patient to use product exactly as prescribed, not to use with other products, unless approved by prescriber
- Advise patient to notify prescriber of nausea, vomiting, diarrhea (dose increase or beginning treatment), or rash
- Advise patient not to increase or abruptly decrease dosage, serious consequences may result
- Instruct patient that product is not a cure

Evaluation
Positive therapeutic outcome
- Decrease in confusion; improved mood

▲ HIGH ALERT

DOPamine (Rx)
(doe′pa-meen)
Func. class.: Agonist, vasopressor, inotropic agent
Chem. class.: Catecholamine
Pregnancy category C

Do not confuse: DOPamine/DOBUTamine

ACTION: Causes increased cardiac output; acts on β_1- and α-receptors, causing vasoconstriction in blood vessels; when low doses are administered, causes renal and mesenteric vasodilatation; β_1 stimulation produces inotropic effects with increased cardiac output

Therapeutic outcome: Increased B/P, cardiac output

USES: Shock; to increase perfusion; hypotension, cardiogenic/septic shock

CONTRAINDICATIONS
Hypersensitivity, ventricular fibrillation, tachydysrhythmias, pheochromocytoma, hypovolemia

Precautions: Pregnancy **C**, breastfeeding, geriatric, arterial embolism, peripheral vascular disease, sulfite hypersensitivity, acute MI

BLACK BOX WARNING: Extravasation

DOSAGE AND ROUTES
Adult: IV INF 2-5 mcg/kg/min, titrate upward 5-10 mcg/kg/min, max 50 mcg/kg/min; titrate to patient's response
Child: IV 1-5 mcg/kg/min initially; usual dosage range 2-20 mcg/kg/min

CHF
Adult: IV 3-10 mcg/kg/min

Available forms: Inj 40, 80, 160 mg/ml; conc for **IV** inf 0.8, 1.6, 3.2 mg/ml in 250, 500 ml D$_5$W

Implementation
- Store reconstituted sol for up to 24 hr if refrigerated
- Do not use discolored sol; protect from light

Continuous infusion route
- Dilute 200-400 mg/250-500 ml of D$_5$W, 0.9% NaCl, D$_5$/LR, D$_5$/0.45% NaCl, D$_5$/0.9% NaCl, LR; do not use discolored sol; sol is stable for 24 hr; give 0.5-5 mcg/kg/min; may increase by 1-4 mcg/kg/min q15-30min until desired patient response; use infusion pump

BLACK BOX WARNING: **Extravasation:** if extravasation occurs, stop infusion, may inject area with phentolamine 10 mg/15 ml NS

Y-site compatibilities: Alfentanil, alprostadil, amifostine, amikacin, aminocaproic acid, aminophylline, amiodarone, anidulafungin, argatroban, ascorbic acid injection, atenolol, atracurium, atropine, aztreonam, benztropine, bivalirudin, bleomycin, bumetanide, buprenorphine, butorphanol, calcium chloride/gluconate, CARBOplatin, caspofungin, cefmetazole, cefonicid, cefotaxime, cefoTEtan, cefOXitin, cefTAZidime, ceftizoxime, cefTRIAXone, cefuroxime, chlorproMAZINE, cimetidine, ciprofloxacin, cisatracurium, CISplatin, cladribine, clarithromycin, clindamycin, cloNIDine, codeine, cyanocobalamin, cyclophosphamide, cycloSPORINE,

---

Adverse effects: *italics* = common; **bold** = life-threatening

cytarabine, DACTINomycin, DAPTOmycin, dexamethasone, dexmedetomidine, digoxin, diltiazem, diphenhydrAMINE, DOBUTamine, DOCEtaxel, doripenem, doxacurium, DOXOrubicin, DOXOrubicin liposomal, doxycycline, droperidol, enalaprilat, ePHEDrine, EPINEPHrine, epirubicin, epoetin alfa, eptifibatide, ertapenem, erythromycin, esmolol, etoposide, famotidine, fenoldopam, fentaNYL, fluconazole, fludarabine, fluorouracil, folic acid, foscarnet, gatifloxacin, gemcitabine, gemtuzumab, gentamicin, glycopyrrolate, granisetron, heparin, hydrocortisone, HYDROmorphone, hydrOXYzine, IDArubicin, ifosfamide, imipenem-cilastatin, irinotecan, isoproterenol, ketorolac, labetalol, levofloxacin, lidocaine, linezolid, LORazepam, LR, magnesium sulfate, mannitol, mechlorethamine, meperidine, methicillin, methyldopa, methylPREDNISolone, metoclopramide, metoprolol, metroNIDAZOLE, micafungin, miconazole, midazolam, milrinone, minocycline, mitoXANtrone, morphine, multiple vitamins injection, mycophenolate, nafcillin, nalbuphine, naloxone, netilmicin, niCARdipine, nitroglycerin, nitroprusside, norepinephrine, octreotide, ondansetron, oxacillin, oxaliplatin, oxytocin, PACLitaxel, palonosetron, pancuronium, pantoprazole, papaverine, PEMEtrexed, penicillin G potassium/sodium, pentamidine, pentazocine, PENTobarbital, PHENobarbital, phenylephrine, phytonadione, piperacillin, piperacillin-tazobactam, polymyxin B, potassium chloride, procainamide, prochlorperazine, promethazine, propofol, propranolol, protamine, pyridoxine, quiNIDine, ranitidine, remifentanil, Ringer's, ritodrine, riTUXimab, rocuronium, sargramostim, sodium acetate, succinylcholine, SUFentanil, tacrolimus, temocillin, teniposide, theophylline, thiamine, thiotepa, ticarcillin, ticarcillin-clavulanate, tigecycline, tirofiban, TNA, tobramycin, tolazoline, TPN, trastuzumab, trimetaphan, urokinase, vancomycin, vasopressin, vecuronium, verapamil, vinCRIStine, vinorelbine, vitamin B complex/C, voriconazole, warfarin, zidovudine, zoledronic acid

ADVERSE EFFECTS

CNS: *Headache,* anxiety
CV: *Palpitations,* tachycardia, *hypertension, ectopic beats, angina,* wide QRS complex, peripheral vasoconstriction, hypotension
GI: *Nausea, vomiting, diarrhea*
INTEG: Necrosis, tissue sloughing with extravasation, gangrene
RESP: Dyspnea

Pharmacokinetics

Absorption	Complete
Distribution	Widely
Metabolism	Liver
Excretion	Kidney, plasma
Half-life	2 min

Pharmacodynamics

Onset	2-5 min
Peak	Unknown
Duration	<10 min

INTERACTIONS
Individual drugs
Phenytoin: bradycardia, hypotension

Drug classifications
α-Adrenergic blockers, β-adrenergic blockers: decreased action of DOPamine
Anesthetics (general): increased dysrhythmias
Antidepressants (tricyclic): increased pressor response
Ergots: severe hypertension
MAOIs: increased hypertension (severe), do not use within 2 wk; increased pressor effect; hypertensive crisis may result
Oxytocics: increased B/P

Drug/lab test
Increased: urinary catecholamine, serum glucose

NURSING CONSIDERATIONS
Assessment
• Monitor ECG for dysrhythmias, ischemia during treatment; some patients may not need continuous ECG monitoring; also monitor PCWP, CVP, CO_2, urinary output; notify prescriber if <30 ml/hr
• Assess for heart failure: bibasilar crackles, S_3 gallop, dyspnea, neck vein distention in patients with cardiomyopathy or CHF
• Assess for oxygenation or perfusion deficit: decreased B/P, chest pain, dizziness, loss of consciousness
• Monitor B/P and pulse q5min during inf; if B/P drops 30 mm Hg, stop inf and call prescriber
• Check for extravasation: if this occurs, administer phentolamine mixed with 0.9% NaCl

Patient/family education
• Teach patient reason for medication, expected results, reason for all monitoring and procedures
• Advise patient to report all side effects

Evaluation

Positive therapeutic outcome
• Increased cardiac output

TREATMENT OF OVERDOSE:
Discontinue product, support circulation; give a short-acting α-blocker

doripenem (Rx)
(dore-i-pen'em)
Doribax
Func. class.: Antiinfective, miscellaneous
Chem. class.: Carbapenem
Pregnancy category B

ACTION: Bactericidal, interferes with cell wall replication of susceptible organisms; osmotically unstable cell wall swells, bursts from osmotic pressure

Therapeutic outcome: Negative C&S; decreasing symptoms and signs of infection

USES: Serious infections caused by *Acinetobacter baumannii, Bacteroides caccae, Bacteroides fragilis, Bacteroides thetaiotaomicron, Bacteroides uniformis, Bacteroides vulgatus, Citrobacter freundii, Escherichia coli, Klebsiella pneumoniae, Peptostreptococcus micros, Proteus mirabilis, Pseudomonas aeruginosa, Serratia marcescens, Staphylococcus aureus, Streptococcus contellatus, Streptococcus intermedius;* complicated UTIs, pyelonephritis, complicated intraabdominal infections

CONTRAINDICATIONS
Hypersensitivity to carbapenems (meropenem, doripenem, imipenem), penicillin, β-lactam; viral infection

Precautions: Pregnancy **B**, breastfeeding, geriatric, renal disease, seizure disorder, pseudomembranous colitis, nebulizer or inhalation use, hypersensitivity to cephalosporins, children/adolescents

DOSAGE AND ROUTES
Adult: IV 500 mg every 8 hr × 5-14 days; if improvement occurs after 3 days, switch to an appropriate oral product

Renal dose
Adult: IV CCr 30-50 ml/min 250 mg over 1 hr q8hr; CCr >10 to <30 ml/min 250 mg over 1 hr q12hr; CCr ≤10 ml/min no data

Available forms: Powder for inj 500 mg

Implementation

IV route
• Visually inspect parenteral products for particulate matter and discoloration before use, diluted range in color from clear, colorless solutions to solutions that are clear and slightly yellow
• **Reconstitution:** No bacteriostatic preservative is present; observe aseptic technique while preparing the infusion
• **500-mg dose using the 500 mg vial:** Reconstitute the vial with 10 ml of sterile water for injection or sodium chloride 0.9% (normal saline). Gently shake (50 mg/ml); THE RECONSTITUTED SUSPENSION IS NOT FOR DIRECT INJECTION; FURTHER DILUTION IS REQUIRED. Using a syringe with a 21-G needle, withdraw the suspension and add it to an infusion bag containing 100 ml of NS or D₅W; gently shake until clear; final (4.5 mg/ml)
• **250-mg dose using the 500 mg vial:** Reconstitute the vial with 10 ml of sterile water for injection or sodium chloride 0.9% (normal saline). Gently shake (50 mg/ml); THE RECONSTITUTED SUSPENSION IS NOT FOR DIRECT INJECTION; FURTHER DILUTION IS REQUIRED. Using a syringe with a 21-G needle, withdraw the 5 ml (250 mg) and add it to an infusion bag containing 100 ml of normal saline or D₅W; gently shake until clear; remove 55 ml of this solution and discard. The remaining infusion solution contains 250 mg (4.5 mg/ml)
• **250-mg dose using the 250 mg vial:** Reconstitute the vial with 10 ml of sterile water for injection or sodium chloride 0.9% (normal saline). Gently shake (25 mg/ml); THE RECONSTITUTED SUSPENSION IS NOT FOR DIRECT INJECTION; FURTHER DILUTION IS REQUIRED. Using a syringe with a 21-G needle, withdraw the contents of the vial and add it to an infusion bag containing 50 or 100 ml of normal saline or D₅W; gently shake until clear; final concentration 4.2 mg/ml (50 ml infusion bag) or 2.3 mg/ml (100 ml infusion bag)
• **Storage:** Reconstituted suspensions may be held in vial for up to 1 hr prior to transfer and dilution in the infusion bag. Including storage and infusion time, diluted infusion solutions are stable for up to 12 hr (NS) or 4 hr (D₅W) at controlled room temperature; diluted infusion solutions are stable for up to 72 hr (NS) or 24 hr (D₅W) refrigerated, do not freeze reconstituted solutions.
• If Baxter Minibag Plus infusion bags are to be used, consult the instructions provided by the infusion bag manufacturer

Intermittent IV infusion route
• Do not mix with or physically add to solutions containing other drugs, infuse over 1 hr

---

Adverse effects: *italics* = common; **bold** = life-threatening

Solution compatibilities: D₅W, 0.9% NaCl, sterile water for inj

Y-site compatibilities: Acyclovir, amikacin, aminophylline, amiodarone, anidulafungin, atropine, azithromycin, bumetanide, calcium gluconate, CARBOplatin, caspofungin, ceftaroline, ceftobiprole, cimetidine, ciprofloxacin, CISplatin, cyclophosphamide, cycloSPORINE, DAPTOmycin, dexamethasone, digoxin, diltiazem, diphenhydrAMINE, DOBUTamine, DOCEtaxel, DOPamine, DOXOrubicin, enalaprilat, esmolol, esomeprazole, etoposide, famotidine, fentaNYL, fluconazole, fluorouracil, foscarnet, furosemide, gemcitabine, gentamicin, granisetron, heparin, hydrocortisone, HYDROmorphone, ifosfamide, insulin (regular), labetalol, levofloxacin, linezolid, LORazepam, magnesium sulfate, mannitol, meperidine, methotrexate, methylPREDNISolone, metoclopramide, metroNIDAZOLE, micafungin, midazolam, milrinone, morphine, moxifloxacin, norepinephrine, ondansetron, PACLitaxel, pantoprazole, PHENobarbital, phenylephrine, potassium chloride, ranitidine, sodium bicarbonate/phosphates, tacrolimus, telavancin, tigecycline, tobramycin, vancomycin, voriconazole, zidovudine

ADVERSE EFFECTS
CNS: Seizures, headache
GI: *Diarrhea, nausea,* vomiting, pseudomembranous colitis, hepatitis
GU: Renal impairments/failure
HEMA: Neutropenia, leukopenia, anemia
INTEG: *Rash,* urticaria, phlebitis, erythema at inj site, Stevens-Johnson syndrome, toxic epidermal necrolysis, pruritus
RESP: Pneumonitis (inhalation)
SYST: Anaphylaxis, Stevens-Johnson syndrome, toxic epidermal necrolysis

Pharmacokinetics

Absorption	Unknown
Distribution	To most body fluids/tissue
Metabolism	Unknown
Excretion	Mainly unchanged in urine, 70% recovered in 48 hr
Half-life	1 hr, extended in renal disease

Pharmacodynamics
Unknown

INTERACTIONS
Individual drugs
Probenecid: increased doripenem plasma levels
Divalproex sodium, valproic acid: decreased effects

Drug/lab test
Increased: AST, ALT, LDH, BUN, alkaline phosphatase, bilirubin, creatinine
False positive: direct Coombs' test

NURSING CONSIDERATIONS
Assessment
• **Assess sensitivity to carbapenem antibiotics, penicillins, cephalosporins, other beta lactams**
• Monitor renal disease: lower dose may be required
• **Monitor bowel pattern daily; if severe diarrhea occurs, product should be discontinued; may indicate pseudomembranous colitis**
• **Monitor for infection:** temp, sputum, characteristics of wound, before, during, and after treatment
⚠ **Monitor for allergic reactions, anaphylaxis: rash, urticaria, pruritus; may occur few days after therapy begins**
• **Monitor overgrowth of infection:** perineal itching, fever, malaise, redness, pain, swelling, drainage, rash, diarrhea, change in cough, sputum

Patient/family education
• **Instruct patient to report severe diarrhea; may indicate pseudomembranous colitis**
• Instruct patient to report sore throat, bruising, bleeding, joint pain; may indicate blood dyscrasias (rare)
• Instruct patient to report overgrowth of infection: black, furry tongue; vaginal itching; foul-smelling stools
• Advise patient to avoid breastfeeding; product is excreted in breast milk

Evaluation
Positive therapeutic outcome
• Negative C&S
• Absence of symptoms and signs of infection

TREATMENT OF HYPERSENSITIVITY: EPINEPHrine, antihistamines; resuscitate if needed (anaphylaxis)

dorzolamide ophthalmic
See Appendix B

doxazosin (Rx)
(dox-ay′zoe-sin)
Cardura, Cardura XL
Func. class.: Peripheral α-adrenergic blocker, antihypertensive
Chem. class.: Quinazoline
Pregnancy category C

Do not confuse: Cardura/Coumadin/Cardene/Ridaura

⚠ Nurse Alert   ✳ Key NCLEX® Drug   >> Drug Specifics

ACTION: Peripheral blood vessels are dilated, peripheral resistance lowered; reduction in B/P results from peripheral α-adrenergic receptors being blocked

Therapeutic outcome: Decreased B/P, decreased symptoms of benign prostatic hypertrophy (BPH)

USES: Hypertension, urinary outflow obstruction, symptoms of benign prostatic hyperplasia

CONTRAINDICATIONS
Hypersensitivity to quinazolines

Precautions: Pregnancy **C**, breastfeeding, children, hepatic disease, geriatrics

DOSAGE AND ROUTES
BPH
Adult: PO 1 mg/day at bedtime, increase in stepwise manner to 2, 4, 8 mg/day as needed at 1-2 wk intervals, max 8 mg; ext rel tab (Cardura XL) 4 mg/day with breakfast, adjust dose q3-4wk up to 8 mg/day

Hypertension
Adult: PO 1 mg/day at bedtime, increasing up to 16 mg daily if required; usual range 4-16 mg/day
Geriatric: PO 0.5 mg nightly, gradually increase

Available forms: Tabs 1, 2, 4, 8 mg; ext rel tabs 4, 8 mg

Implementation
PO route
• **Tabs** broken, crushed, or chewed; chewed tabs taste bitter; do not break, crush, chew **XL tabs**
• **Immediate release tab:** give without regard to meals; **EXT REL tabs:** give with breakfast; when switching from immediate release to EXT REL, the final evening dose of immediate release should be taken
• Store in tight container at room temperature (86° F [30° C] or less)
• May be used in combination with other antihypertensives
• May be given with food to prevent GI symptoms

ADVERSE EFFECTS
CNS: *Dizziness,* headache, drowsiness, anxiety, depression, vertigo, weakness, fatigue, asthenia, syncope
CV: Palpitations, *orthostatic hypotension,* tachycardia, *edema,* **dysrhythmias,** chest pain

EENT: Epistaxis, tinnitus, dry mouth, red sclera, pharyngitis, rhinitis
GI: *Nausea,* vomiting, diarrhea, constipation, abdominal pain, hepatitis
GU: Incontinence, polyuria, priapism, impotence

Pharmacokinetics

Absorption	Well absorbed
Distribution	Not known; 98% plasma protein bound
Metabolism	Liver, extensively ($<63\%$)
Excretion	Kidneys
Half-life	22 hr

Pharmacodynamics

Onset	2 hr
Peak	2-3 hr
Duration	up to 24 hr

INTERACTIONS
Individual drugs
Alcohol: increased hypotensive effects
CloNIDine: decreased antihypertensive effect

Drug classifications
Other antihypertensives, nitrates, PDE-5 inhibitors: increased hypotensive effects

NURSING CONSIDERATIONS
Assessment
• **Hypertension:** monitor B/P (lying, standing) and pulse, syncope; check for edema in feet, legs daily; I&O; monitor for weight daily; notify prescriber of changes
• **BPH:** urinary pattern changes (hesitancy, dribbling, incomplete bladder emptying, dysuria, urgency, nocturia, urgency incontinence, intermittency before and during treatment)
• Assess for orthostatic hypotension; tell patient to rise slowly from sitting or lying position; assess pulse, jugular venous distention q4hr, crackles, dyspnea, orthopnea with B/P

Patient/family education
• Teach patient not to discontinue product abruptly; emphasize the importance of complying with dosage schedule, even if feeling better; if dose is missed take as soon as remembered; take at same time each day
• Teach patient not to use OTC products (cough, cold, allergy) unless directed by prescriber; also to avoid large amounts of caffeine
• Emphasize the need to rise slowly to sitting or standing position to minimize orthostatic hypotension

- Teach patient to notify prescriber of mouth sores, sore throat, fever, swelling of hands or feet, irregular heartbeat, chest pain
- Caution patient to report excessive perspiration, dehydration, vomiting, diarrhea; may lead to fall in B/P
- Caution patient that product may cause dizziness, fainting, light-headedness; may occur during 1st few days of therapy; to avoid hazardous activities
- Teach patient how to take B/P, and normal readings for age-group; to take B/P q7days
- Inform patient that fainting occasionally occurs after 1st dose; do not drive or operate machinery for 4 hr after 1st dose or after dosage increase or take 1st dose at bedtime; may take 1-2 wk in BPH

Evaluation

Positive therapeutic outcome
- Decreased B/P in hypertension
- Decreased symptoms of BPH

TREATMENT OF OVERDOSE:
Administer volume expanders or vasopressors; discontinue product; place in supine position

---

doxepin (Rx)
(dox′e-pin)
Prudoxin Cream, Silenor ✤, Zonolon Topical Cream
Func. class.: Antidepressant, tricyclic; antianxiety
Chem. class.: Dibenzoxepin, tertiary amine
Pregnancy category
B (Topical)
C (PO)

ACTION: Blocks reuptake of norepinephrine, serotonin into nerve endings, increasing action of norepinephrine, serotonin in nerve cells; has anticholinergic effects

Therapeutic outcome: Decreased symptoms of depression after 2-3 wk

USES: Major depression, anxiety, topical: lichen simplex, atopic dermatitis, eczema, insomnia

Unlabeled uses: Migraine prophylaxis; topical: pruritus

CONTRAINDICATIONS
Hypersensitivity to tricyclics, urinary retention, closed-angle glaucoma, prostatic hypertrophy, acute recovery from MI

Precautions: Pregnancy **C** (PO), **B** (topical), breastfeeding, geriatric, seizures

---

> **BLACK BOX WARNING:** Suicidal patients, children

DOSAGE AND ROUTES
Depression/anxiety
Adult: PO 50-75 mg/day, may increase to 300 mg/day for severely ill, give in divided doses if >150 mg/day
Geriatric: PO 25-50 mg at bedtime, increase qwk by 25-50 mg to desired dose, max 150 mg/day

Pruritus
Adult: PO 10 mg at bedtime, may increase to 25 mg at bedtime; TOP apply a thin film qid ≥3 hr apart

Available forms: Caps 10, 25, 50, 75, 100, 150 mg; oral conc 10 mg/ml; cream 5%; tabs (Silenor) 3, 6 mg

Implementation
- **Oral conc** should be diluted with 120 ml of water, milk, or orange, grapefruit, tomato, prune, pineapple juice; do not mix with grape juice
- Give with food or milk for GI symptoms; do not give with carbonated beverages
- Give dose at bedtime if oversedation occurs during day; may take entire dose at bedtime; geriatric may not tolerate once/day dosing
- Store at room temperature; do not freeze
- Provide safety measures, primarily for geriatric
- Store in tight container protected from direct sunlight
- **Topical:** apply to affected area; rub slightly, do not use occlusive dressing

ADVERSE EFFECTS
CNS: *Dizziness, drowsiness,* confusion, headache, anxiety, tremors, stimulation, weakness, insomnia, nightmares, EPS (geriatric), increased psychiatric symptoms, paresthesia, suicidal ideation
CV: *Orthostatic hypotension, ECG changes,* tachycardia, hypertension, palpitations, dysrhythmias
EENT: *Blurred vision,* tinnitus, mydriasis, ophthalmoplegia, glossitis
GI: *Diarrhea, dry mouth,* nausea, vomiting, paralytic ileus, increased appetite, cramps, epigastric distress, jaundice, hepatitis, stomatitis, constipation
GU: *Retention, acute renal failure*
HEMA: Agranulocytosis, thrombocytopenia, eosinophilia, leukopenia, pancytopenia, purpuric disorder

---

INTEG: Rash, urticaria, sweating, pruritus, photosensitivity

Pharmacokinetics

Absorption	Well absorbed
Distribution	Widely distributed; crosses placenta
Metabolism	Liver, extensively
Excretion	Kidneys, breast milk
Half-life	8-24 hr

Pharmacodynamics

PO: Peak 2 hr

INTERACTIONS
Individual drugs

Alcohol: increased CNS depression

Cimetidine, FLUoxetine, fluvoxaMINE, PARoxetine, sertraline: increased doxepin effect

CloNIDine: increased hypertensive crisis; do not use together

EPINEPHrine, norepinephrine: increased hypertensive action

Drug classifications

Antiarrhythmics, 1C (propafenone, flecainide), class III, quinolones: increased QT interval

Anticholinergics: increased anticholinergic effect

Barbiturates, benzodiazepines, CNS depressants, sedative/hypnotics: increased CNS depression

MAOIs: hypertensive crisis, seizures, hyperpyretic crisis

SSRIs, SNRIs, serotonin receptor agonists: increased toxicity

Drug/herb

St. John's wort: increased serotonin syndrome

Drug/lab test

Increased: serum bilirubin, blood glucose, alkaline phosphatase, LFTs

NURSING CONSIDERATIONS
Assessment

• **Assess chronic pain:** location, severity, type, alleviating/aggravating factors before and during treatment

• Monitor B/P (with patient lying, standing), pulse q4hr; if systolic B/P drops 20 mm Hg, hold product, notify prescriber; take VS q4hr in patients with CV disease

• Monitor blood studies: CBC, leukocytes, differential, cardiac enzymes if patient is receiving long-term therapy

• Monitor liver function tests: AST, ALT, bilirubin

• Check weight weekly; appetite may increase with product

• **Assess ECG for flattening of T wave, bundle branch block, AV block, dysrhythmias in** cardiac patients; product should be discontinued gradually several days before surgery

• Assess for EPS primarily in geriatric: rigidity, dystonia, akathisia

• **Assess depression: mood, sensorium, affect, suicidal tendencies; increase in psychiatric symptoms**

• Monitor urinary retention, constipation; constipation is more likely to occur in children or geriatric

• **Assess for withdrawal symptoms:** headache, nausea, vomiting, muscle pain, weakness; do not usually occur unless product was discontinued abruptly

• Identify alcohol consumption; if alcohol is consumed, hold dose until AM

Patient/family education

• Tell patient that therapeutic effects of decreased depression may take 2-3 wk, antianxiety effects sooner; to use caution in driving and other activities requiring alertness because of drowsiness, dizziness, blurred vision

• Advise patient to avoid rising quickly from sitting to standing, especially geriatric

• Teach patient to avoid alcohol ingestion, other CNS depressants: may potentiate effects; not to discontinue medication quickly after long-term use: may cause nausea, headache, malaise

• Teach patient to wear sunscreen or large hat, since photosensitivity occurs

• **Teach patient that clinical worsening and suicidal ideation may occur**

• Teach patient to increase fluids, bulk in diet if constipation occurs, especially geriatric; to take gum, hard sugarless candy, or frequent sips of water for dry mouth

• Teach patient to report urinary retention immediately

Evaluation
Positive therapeutic outcome

• Decrease in depression
• Absence of suicidal thoughts

TREATMENT OF OVERDOSE:
ECG monitoring, induce emesis, lavage, activated charcoal, administer anticonvulsant

> **⚠ HIGH ALERT**

DOXOrubicin
(dox-oh-roo′bi-sin)
Adriamycin
Func. class.: Antineoplastic, antibiotic
Chem. class.: Anthracycline glycoside
Pregnancy category D

Do not confuse: DOXOrubicin/DOXOrubicin liposomal/DAUNOrubicin

ACTION: Inhibits DNA synthesis primarily; replication is decreased by binding to DNA, which causes strand splitting; active throughout entire cell cycle; a vesicant

USES: Wilms' tumor; bladder, breast, lung, ovarian, stomach, thyroid cancer; Hodgkin's/non-Hodgkin's disease; acute lymphoblastic leukemia; myeloblastic leukemia; neuroblastomas; soft tissue/bone sarcomas

CONTRAINDICATIONS: Pregnancy (D) 1st trimester, breastfeeding, hypersensitivity, systemic infections, cardiac disorders, severe myelosuppression, lifetime dose of 550 mg/m^2

> **BLACK BOX WARNING:** Hepatic disease

Precautions: Accidental exposure, cardiac disease, dental work, electrolyte imbalance, infection, hyperuricemia

> **BLACK BOX WARNING:** Bone marrow suppression, extravasation, heart failure, secondary malignancy; requires an experienced clinician

DOSAGE AND ROUTES

Adult: IV 60-75 mg/m^2 q3wk, or may be used in combination with other antineoplastics with 40-75 mg/m^2 q21-28d, max cumulative dose 550 mg/m^2 or 450 mg/m^2 if prior DAUNOrubicin, cyclophosphamide, mediastinal XRT

Hepatic dose
Adult: IV Bilirubin 1.2-3 mg/dl, give 50% of dose; bilirubin 3.1-5 mg/dl, give 25% of dose

Renal dose
Adult: IV CCr <10 ml/min give 75% of dose

Available forms: Powder for inj 10, 20, 50 mg; inj 2 mg/ml

Implementation

IV route
• Give antiemetic 30-60 min before product to prevent vomiting
• Give allopurinol or sodium bicarbonate to maintain uric acid levels, alkalization of urine
⚠ **Use cytotoxic handling procedures: inspect for particulate and discoloration before use**

> **BLACK BOX WARNING:** Do not give IM, subcut

> **BLACK BOX WARNING:** If extravasation occurs, stop inf and complete via another vein, preferably in another limb, use dexrazoxane topically

• Aluminum needles may be used during administration; avoid aluminum during storage
• Rapid injection can cause facial flushing or erythema along the vein
Reconstitution:
• To avoid risks with reconstitution, the commercially available injection may be used; there are still risks involved in handling the injection
• Do not use diluents containing preservatives to reconstitute powder for injection
• Reconstitute 10, 20, 50, 100 mg of DOXOrubicin with 5, 10, 25, 50 ml, respectively, of nonbacteriostatic NS injection (2 mg/ml), shake until completely dissolved; use reconstituted solution within 24 hr; do not expose to sunlight
• **IV injection:** Inject reconstituted solution over 0.3-5 min via Y-site or 3-way stopcock into a free-flowing IV inf of NS or D$_5$W; a butterfly needle inserted into a large vein is preferred

> **BLACK BOX WARNING:** Care should be taken to avoid extravasation because the drug is extremely irritating to extravascular tissue

• Increased fluid intake to 2-3 L/day to prevent urate, calculi formation
• Store at room temperature for 24 hr after reconstituting

Y-site compatibilities: Alemtuzumab, alfentanil, amifostine, amikacin, anidulafungin, argatroban, aztreonam, bivalirudin, bleomycin, bumetanide, buprenorphine, butorphanol, calcium chloride/gluconate, CARBOplatin, carmustine, caspofungin, ceftizoxime, chlorproMAZINE, cimetidine, ciprofloxacin, CISplatin, cladribine, clindamycin, cyclophosphamide, cycloSPORINE, cytarabine, DACTINomycin, DAPTOmycin, dexamethasone, diltiazem, diphenhydrAMINE, DOBUTamine, DOCEtaxel, dolasetron, DOPamine, doripenem, doxycycline, droperidol, enalaprilat, ePHEDrine, EPINEPHrine, erythromycin, esmolol, etoposide, etoposide phosphate, famotidine, fenoldopam, fentaNYL, filgrastim, fluconazole, fludarabine, gemcitabine, gentamicin, granisetron, haloperidol, hydrocortisone, HYDROmorphone, ifosfamide, imipenem cilastatin, inamrinone, isoproterenol, ketorolac, labetalol, leucovorin, levorphanol, lidocaine, linezolid, LORazepam, mannitol, mechlorethamine, melphalan, meperidine, mesna, methotrexate, metoclopramide, metoprolol, metroNIDAZOLE, midazolam, milrinone, mitoMYcin, morphine, nalbuphine, naloxone, nesiritide, niCARdipine, nitroglycerin, nitroprusside, octreotide, ofloxacin, ondansetron, oxaliplatin, PACLitaxel, palonosetron, pancuronium, phenylephrine, potassium chloride, procainamide, prochlorperazine, promethazine, propranolol, quinupristin-dalfopristin, ranitidine, sargramostim, sodium acetate, tacrolimus, teniposide, theophylline, thiotepa, ticarcillin/clavulanate, tigecycline, tirofiban, tobramycin, topotecan, trastuzumab, trimethobenzamide, vancomycin, vasopressin, vecuronium, verapamil, vinBLAStine, vinCRIStine, vinorelbine, zidovudine, zoledronic acid

ADVERSE EFFECTS

CV: Increased B/P, sinus tachycardia, PVCs, chest pain, bradycardia, extrasystoles, **irreversible cardiomyopathy, acute left ventricular failure**

GI: *Nausea, vomiting,* anorexia, *mucositis,* **hepatotoxicity**

GU: Impotence, sterility, amenorrhea, gynecomastia, hyperuricemia, urine discoloration

HEMA: **Thrombocytopenia, leukopenia, anemia**

INTEG: *Rash,* **necrosis at inj site,** radiation recall, dermatitis, reversible *alopecia,* cellulitis, thrombophlebitis at inj site

SYST: **Anaphylaxis, secondary malignancy**

Pharmacokinetics

Absorption	Complete
Distribution	Crosses placenta
Metabolism	Liver
Excretion	Urine, bile, breast milk
Half-life	30 min, terminal 16.5 hr

Pharmacodynamics

Onset	Unknown
Peak	Unknown
Duration	Unknown

INTERACTIONS
Individual drugs
CycloSPORINE, mercaptopurine: increased toxicity

Fluconazole, posaconazole: increased life-threatening dysrhythmias: do not use together

Fosphenytoin, phenytoin: increased effect of these drugs

Hematopoietic progenitor cell: decreased antineoplastic effect; do not use 24 hr before or after treatment

PACLitaxel: decreased clearance of DOXOrubicin

PHENobarbital: decreased DOXOrubicin effect

Progesterone: increased neutropenia, thrombocytopenia

Streptozocin: increased DOXOrubicin effect

Drug classifications
Antineoplastics, radiation: increased toxicity

Calcium channel blockers: increased cardiomyopathy

Drugs that increase QT prolongation: increased effect

Live virus vaccine: decreased antibody response

Drug/lab test
Increased: uric acid

NURSING CONSIDERATIONS
Assessment:

> **BLACK BOX WARNING: Bone marrow depression:** CBC, differential, platelet count weekly; withhold or reduce dose of product if WBC is <1500/mm³ or platelet count is <50,000/mm³; notify prescriber of these results

• Renal studies: BUN, serum uric acid, urine CCr, electrolytes before, during therapy
• I&O ratio: Report fall in urine output to <30 ml/hr
• Monitor temperature: Fever might indicate beginning infection

> **BLACK BOX WARNING: Hepatotoxicity:** hepatic studies before, during therapy: bilirubin, AST, ALT, alk phos as needed or monthly; check for jaundice of skin and sclera, dark urine, clay-colored stools, itchy skin, abdominal pain, fever, diarrhea

> **BLACK BOX WARNING: Dysrhythmias:** ECG; watch for ST-T wave changes, low QRS and T, possible dysrhythmias (sinus tachycardia, heart block, PVCs), ejection fraction before treatment, signs of irreversible cardiomyopathy, can occur up to 6 mo after treatment begins

• Bleeding: hematuria, guaiac, bruising, petechiae of mucosa or orifices every 8 hr
• Effects of alopecia on body image; discuss feelings about body changes; almost total alopecia is expected

- Buccal cavity every 8 hr for dryness, sores, ulceration, white patches, oral pain, bleeding, dysphagia
- Alkalosis if severe vomiting is present

> **BLACK BOX WARNING: Extravasation:** local irritation, pain, burning at inj site; a vesicant; if extravasation occurs, stop drug, restart at another site, apply ice, elevate extremity to reduce swelling; if resolution does not occur, surgical debridement may be required

- GI symptoms: frequency of stools, cramping
- Rinsing of mouth tid-qid with water, club soda; brushing of teeth bid-tid with soft brush or cotton-tipped applicators for stomatitis; use unwaxed dental floss

Patient/family education
- Instruct patient to add 2-3 L of fluids unless contraindicated before and for 24-48 hr after to decrease possible hemorrhagic cystitis
- Instruct patient to report any complaints, side effects to nurse or prescriber
- Advise patient that hair may be lost during treatment; that wig or hairpiece might make patient feel better; that new hair might be different in color, texture
- Instruct patient to avoid foods with citric acid, hot or rough texture
- Instruct patient to report any bleeding, white spots, ulcerations in mouth to prescriber; to examine mouth daily
- Advise patient that urine, other body fluids may be red-orange for 48 hr
- Instruct patient to avoid crowds and persons with infections when granulocyte count is low
- ⚠ Advise patient that barrier contraceptive measures are recommended during therapy and for 4 mo after (pregnancy [D]); to avoid breastfeeding
- Instruct patient to avoid vaccinations

Evaluation

Positive therapeutic outcome
- Decreased tumor size, decreased spread of malignancy

> **⚠ HIGH ALERT**
>
> ## DOXOrubicin liposomal
> (dox-oh-roo'bi-sin)
> **Doxil, Lipodex**
> *Func. class.:* Antineoplastic, antibiotic
> *Chem. class.:* Anthracycline glycoside
> **Pregnancy category D**

Do not confuse: DOXOrubicin liposomal/ DOXOrubicin/DAUNOrubicin

ACTION: Inhibits DNA synthesis primarily; replication is decreased by binding to DNA, which causes strand splitting; active throughout entire cell cycle; a vesicant

USES: AIDS-related Kaposi's sarcoma, multiple myeloma, metastatic ovarian carcinoma

CONTRAINDICATIONS:
Pregnancy (**D**), breastfeeding, hypersensitivity, systemic infections, cardiac disorders

> **BLACK BOX WARNING:** Cardiotoxicity, inf reactions, myelosuppression, hepatic disease

Precautions: Children, infection, leukopenia, stomatitis, thrombocytopenia

DOSAGE AND ROUTES
Max lifetime cumulative dose 550 mg/m²; 400 mg/m² for those who have received other cardiotoxics or mediastinal radiation

Kaposi's sarcoma
Adult: IV 20 mg/m² q3wk

Multiple myeloma
Adult: IV 30 mg/m² IV inf on day 4 every 3 wk plus bortezomib 1.3 mg/m²/dose IV bolus on days 1, 4, 8, 11 of each cycle; give DOXOrubicin liposomal after bortezomib receipt on day 4; administer up to 8 treatment cycles or until disease progression or unacceptable toxicity occurs

Breast cancer, metastatic (unlabeled)
Adult: IV 50 mg/m² day 1, q4wk

Available forms: Liposomal dispersion for inj: 2 mg/ml

Implementation
- Prepared liposomal DOXOrubicin is a translucent, red liposomal dispersion; visually inspect for particulate matter and discoloration before use
- Pegylated liposomal DOXOrubicin (Doxil) is for IV INF use only and should not be given IM/subcut, give under the supervision of a physician who is experienced in cancer chemotherapy

> **BLACK BOX WARNING:** Care should be taken to avoid extravasation because the drug is irritating to extravascular tissue

- Premedication with antiemetics is recommended

IV route
• **Reconstitution (Doxil):** dilute the appropriate dose, not to exceed 90 mg/250 ml D₅W; do not mix with any other diluent, drugs, or bacteriostatic agent, use aseptic technique; product contains no preservative or bacteriostatic agent; diluted solution must be refrigerated and used within 24 hr

• **IV INF (Doxil):** do not administer as a bolus injection or an undiluted solution; rapid injection can increase the risk of an inf-related reaction
• An acute inf reaction can occur during the first inf and is usually resolved by slowing the rate of inf; most patients can tolerate subsequent inf
• **Rate:** infuse at an initial rate of 1 mg/min; if no inf-related action, the rate can be increased to complete the inf over 1 hr; do not filter
• For hematologic toxicity in patients with ovarian cancer or HIV-related Kaposi's sarcoma: Grade 1 (ANC of 1500-1900/mm³, platelets ≥75,000/mm³): No dose reduction; Grade 2 (ANC of 1000-1499/mm³, platelets ≥50,000/ mm³ and <75,000/mm³: Wait until ANC ≥1500 cells/mm³ and platelets ≥75,000 cells/mm³; redose with no dose reduction; Grade 3 (ANC of 500-999/mm³, platelets ≥25,000/ mm³ and <50,000/mm³): Wait until ANC ≥1500 cells/ mm³ and platelets ≥75,000 cells/mm³; redose with no dose reduction; Grade 4 (ANC <500/ mm³, platelets <25,000/mm³): Wait until ANC ≥1500 cells/mm³ and platelets ≥75,000 cells/ mm³; reduce dose by 25% or continue with full dose with colony-stimulating factor
• Give antiemetic 30-60 min before product to prevent vomiting
• Use allopurinol or sodium bicarbonate to maintain uric acid levels, alkalinization of urine
• Avoid mixing with other products
• Increase fluid intake to 2-3 L/day to prevent urate, calculi formation
• Store refrigerated for 24 hr after reconstituting

ADVERSE EFFECTS
CNS: Paresthesias, headache, depression, insomnia, fatigue, fever
CV: Chest pain, decreased B/P, **cardiomyopathy, heart failure, dysrhythmias, tachycardia**
EENT: Optic neuritis, rhinitis, pharyngitis, stomatitis
GI: *Nausea, vomiting,* anorexia, *mucositis,* **hepatotoxicity,** constipation, **oral candidiasis,** abdominal pain
HEMA: **Thrombocytopenia, leukopenia, anemia, neutropenia**
INTEG: *Rash,* **necrosis at inj site,** dermatitis, reversible *alopecia,* **exfoliative dermatitis,** palmar-plantar erythrodysesthesia, thrombophlebitis at inj site
RESP: Dyspnea, cough, respiratory infections

Pharmacokinetics

Absorption	Complete
Distribution	Crosses placenta
Metabolism	Liver
Excretion	Urine, bile, breast milk
Half-life	55 hr

Pharmacodynamics

Onset	Unknown
Peak	Unknown
Duration	Unknown

INTERACTIONS
Individual drugs
CycloSPORINE, mercaptopurine: increased toxicity
Fluconazole, posaconazole: increased life-threatening dysrhythmias: do not use together
Fosphenytoin, phenytoin: increased effect of these drugs
Hematopoietic progenitor cell: decreased antineoplastic effect; do not use 24 hr before or after treatment
PACLitaxel: decreased clearance of DOXOrubicin
PHENobarbital: decreased DOXOrubicin effect
Progesterone: increased neutropenia, thrombocytopenia
Streptozocin: increased DOXOrubicin effect

Drug classifications
Antineoplastics, radiation: increased toxicity
Calcium channel blockers: increased cardiomyopathy
Drugs that increase QT prolongation: increased effect
Live virus vaccine: decreased antibody response

Drug/lab test
Increased: uric acid

NURSING CONSIDERATIONS
Assessment

> **BLACK BOX WARNING: Bone marrow depression:** CBC, differential, platelet count weekly; withhold or reduce dose of product if WBC is <1500/mm³ or platelet count is <50,000/mm³; notify prescriber of these results

• Renal studies: BUN, serum uric acid, urine CCr, electrolytes before, during therapy

- I&O ratio: Report fall in urine output to <30 ml/hr
- Monitor temperature: Fever might indicate beginning infection

> **BLACK BOX WARNING: Hepatotoxicity:** hepatic studies before, during therapy: bilirubin, AST, ALT, alk phos as needed or monthly; check for jaundice of skin and sclera, dark urine, clay-colored stools, itchy skin, abdominal pain, fever, diarrhea

> **BLACK BOX WARNING: Dysrhythmias:** ECG; watch for ST-T wave changes, low QRS and T, possible dysrhythmias (sinus tachycardia, heart block, PVCs), ejection fraction before treatment, watch for irreversible cardiomyopathy, can occur up to 6 mo after treatment begins

- Bleeding: hematuria, guaiac, bruising, petechiae of mucosa or orifices every 8 hr
- Effects of alopecia on body image; discuss feelings about body changes; almost total alopecia is expected
- Inflammation of mucosa, breaks in skin
- Buccal cavity every 8 hr for dryness, sores, ulceration, white patches, oral pain, bleeding, dysphagia
- Alkalosis if severe vomiting is present

> **BLACK BOX WARNING: Extravasation:** local irritation, pain, burning at inj site; a vesicant; if extravasation occurs, stop drug, restart at another site, apply ice, elevate extremity to reduce swelling; if resolution does not occur, surgical debridement may be required

- GI symptoms: frequency of stools, cramping
- Rinsing of mouth tid-qid with water, club soda; brushing of teeth bid-tid with soft brush or cotton-tipped applicators for stomatitis; use unwaxed dental floss

Patient/family education
- Instruct patient to add 2-3 L of fluids unless contraindicated before and for 24-48 hr after to decrease possible hemorrhagic cystitis
- Instruct patient to report any complaints, side effects to nurse or prescriber
- Advise patient that hair may be lost during treatment; that wig or hairpiece might make patient feel better; that new hair might be different in color, texture
- Instruct patient to avoid foods with citric acid, hot or rough texture
- Instruct patient to report any bleeding, white spots, ulcerations in mouth to prescriber; to examine mouth daily

- Advise patient that urine, other body fluids may be red-orange for 48 hr
- Instruct patient to avoid crowds and persons with infections when granulocyte count is low
- **⚠ Advise patient that barrier contraceptive measures are recommended during therapy and for 4 mo after (pregnancy [D]); to avoid breastfeeding**
- Instruct patient to avoid vaccinations because reactions can occur; to avoid alcohol

Evaluation
Positive therapeutic outcome
- Decreased tumor size, decreased spread of malignancy

---

doxycycline (Rx)
(dox-i-sye′kleen)
Adoxa, Apo-Doxy ✦, Doryx, Doxy, Doxycaps, Doxycin ✦, doxycycline calcium, doxycycline hyclate, doxycycline monohydrate, Monodox, Oracea, Periostat, Vibramycin, Vibra-Tabs
Func. class.: Antiinfective
Chem. class.: Tetracycline
Pregnancy category D

Do not confuse: doxycycline/doxepin/dicyclomine

ACTION: Inhibits protein synthesis, phosphorylation in microorganisms by binding to 30S ribosomal subunits, reversibly binding to 30S ribosomal subunits; bacteriostatic

Therapeutic outcome: Bactericidal action against the following: gram-positive pathogens: *Bacillus anthracis, Clostridium perfringens, Clostridium tetani, Listeria monocytogenes, Nocardia, Propionibacterium acnes, Actinomyces israelii;* gram-negative pathogens *Haemophilus influenzae, Legionella pneumophila, Yersinia enterocolitica, Yersinia pestis, Neisseria gonorrhoeae, Neisseria meningitidis, Mycoplasma, Chlamydia*

USES: Syphilis, gonorrhea, lymphogranuloma venereum, uncommon gram-negative or gram-positive organisms, malaria prophylaxis, *Acinetobacter, Actinomyces israelii, Bacillus anthracis, Bacteroides, Balantidium coli, Bartonella bacilliformis, Borrelia recurrentis, Brucella, Campylobacter fetus, Chlamydia psittaci, Chlamydia trachomatis, Clostridium, Entamoeba histolytica, Enterobacter aerogenes, Enterococcus, Escherichia coli, Francisella tularensis, Fusobacterium fusiforme,*

Haemophilus ducreyi, Haemophilus influenzae (beta-lactamase negative), *Haemophilus influenzae* (beta-lactamase positive), *Klebsiella granulomatis, Klebsiella, Leptospira, Listeria monocytogenes, Mycoplasma pneumoniae, Neisseria gonorrhoeae, Neisseria meningitidis, Orientia tsutsugamushi, Plasmodium falciparum, Propionibacterium acnes, Rickettsia akari, Rickettsia prowazekii, Rickettsia rickettsii, Shigella, Staphylococcus aureus* (MSSA), *Streptococcus pneumoniae, Streptococcus pyogenes* (group A beta-hemolytic streptococci), *Treponema pallidum, Treponema pertenue, Ureaplasma urealyticum, Vibrio cholerae,* viridans streptococci, *Yersinia pestis*

Unlabeled uses: Enterocolitis, biliary tract, intraabdominal infections; epididymitis *(Chlamydia trachomatis);* chronic prostatitis *(Ureaplasma urealyticum);* traveler's diarrhea (enterotoxigenic *Escherichia coli);* Legionnaire's disease *(Legionella pneumophila);* Lyme disease *(Borrelia burgdorferi),* Lyme disease (erythema migrans); Lyme arthritis; Lyme carditis; pleural effusion; malaria (chloroquine-resistant *Plasmodium falciparum);* pelvic inflammatory disease (PID), tubo-ovarian abscess in combination; acute dental infection, dentoalveolar infection, endodontic infection; aggressive juvenile periodontitis, plague prophylaxis *(Yersinia pestis);* tularemia prophylaxis *(Francisella tularensis);* Bancroft's filariasis (elephantiasis) *(Wuchereria bancrofti);* melioidosis due to *Burkholderia pseudomallei;* leptospirosis *(Leptospira);* infection prophylaxis for gynecologic procedures/surgical infection prophylaxis for hysterosalpingogram or chromotubation/induced abortion/dilation and evacuation; methicillin-resistant *Staphylococcus aureus* (MRSA)-associated bone and joint infections

CONTRAINDICATIONS

Pregnancy **D,** children <8 yr, esophageal ulceration, hypersensitivity to tetracyclines

Precautions: Hepatic disease, breastfeeding, pseudomembranous colitis, ulcerative colitis, sulfite hypersensitivity, excessive sunlight

DOSAGE AND ROUTES
Most infections
Adult: PO/**IV** 100 mg q12hr on day 1, then 100 mg/day; **IV** 200 mg in 1-2 INF on day 1, then 100-200 mg/day

Child >8 yr (≥45 kg): PO/**IV** 100 mg q12hr on day 1, then 100 mg/day; severe infections

100 mg q12hr; **IV** 200 mg on day 1, then 100-200 mg/day, give 200 mg dose as 1 or 2 infusions

Child ≥8 yr, <45 kg: PO 2.2 mg/kg q12hr on day 1, then 2.2 mg/kg/day, severe infections 2.2 mg/kg q12hr; **IV** 4.4 mg/kg divided on day 1, then 2.2-4.4 mg/kg/day in 1-2 divided doses

Gonorrhea (uncomplicated) (patients allergic to penicillin)
Adult: PO 100 mg q12hr × 7 days, or 300 mg followed 1 hr later by another 300 mg

Malaria prophylaxis
Adult: 100 mg/day 1-2 days before travel, daily during travel, and 4 wk after return

Adolescent/child ≥8 yr <45 kg: PO 2 mg/kg/day (up to 100 mg/day) begin 1-2 days before travel, continue for 4 wk after return

Chlamydia trachomatis
Adult: PO 100 mg bid × 7 days

Syphilis
Adult: PO 100 mg bid × 14 days

Anthrax
Adult and child >8 yr and ≥45 kg: **IV** 100 mg q12hr, change to PO when able × 60 days

Adolescent/child ≥8 yr and <45 kg: PO 2.2 mg/kg q12hr × 60 days; **IV** 100 mg q12hr, change to PO when able × 60 days

Lyme disease
Adult: PO 100 mg bid × 14-21 days

Periodontitis
Adult: 20 mg bid after sealing and root planing for ≤9 mo; give close to meal AM or PM

Available forms: Doxycycline: cap 40 mg; **doxycycline calcium:** susp 50 mg/5 ml; **doxycycline hyclate:** cap 20, 50, 100 mg; del rel tab 75, 100, 150 mg; del rel cap 75, 100 mg; inj 100 mg; tabs 20, 100, mg; **doxycycline monohydrate:** caps 50, 100, 150 mg; tabs 50, 75, 100 mg; oral susp 25 mg/5 ml

Implementation
PO route
• Do not break, crush, or chew caps
• Give around the clock to maintain proper blood levels; give with food to increase absorption of product; do not give within 3 hr of other agents; product reactions may occur
• Give with 8 oz of water 1 hr before bedtime to prevent ulceration
• Shake liquid preparation well before giving; use calibrated device for proper dosing

- Do not give with iron, calcium, magnesium products or antacids, which decrease absorption and form insoluble chelate
- **Del rel cap:** swallow whole or open and sprinkle on applesauce
- **Susp:** shake well, use calibrated device, may give with food/milk for GI irritation, store at room temperature, discard after 14 days

Intermittent IV infusion route
- Check for irritation, extravasation, phlebitis daily
- Dilute each 100 mg/10 ml or 200 mg/20 ml of 0.9% NaCl, sterile water for inj; each 100 mg must be further dilute in at least 100 ml of 0.9% NaCl, D₅W, Ringer's, LR, D₅W/LR; give over 1-4 hr
- Avoid rapid use, extravasation
- Store in tight, light-resistant container at room temperature; **IV** sol stable for 12 hr at room temperature, 72 hr if refrigerated; discard if precipitate forms

Y-site compatibilities: Acyclovir, alemtuzumab, alfentanil, amifostine, amikacin, aminophylline, amiodarone, anidulafungin, ascorbic acid, atracurium, atropine, aztreonam, bivalirudin, bumetanide, buprenorphine, butorphanol, calcium chloride, calcium gluconate, CARBOplatin, caspofungin, cefonicid, cefotaxime, cefTRIAXone, chlorproMAZINE, cimetidine, cisatracurium, CISplatin, clindamycin, codeine, cyanocobalamin, cyclophosphamide, cycloSPORINE, cytarabine, DACTINomycin, DAPTOmycin, dexmedetomidine, digoxin, diltiazem, diphenhydrAMINE, DOBUTamine, DOCEtaxel, DOPamine, doxacurium, DOXOrubicin, enalapril, ePHEDrine, EPINEPHrine, epirubicin, epoetin alfa, eftifibitide, ertapenem, esmolol, etoposide, etoposide phosphate, famotidine, fenoldopam, fentaNYL, filgrastim, fluconazole, fludarabine, gemcitabine, gentamicin, glycopyrrolate, granisetron, HYDROmorphone, IDArubicin, ifosfamide, imipenem/cilastatin, insulin, isoproterenol, labetalol, levofloxacin, lidocaine, linezolid, LORazepam, magnesium sulfate, mannitol, mechlorethamine, melphalan, meperidine, methyldopate, metoclopramide, metoprolol, metroNIDAZOLE, miconazole, midazolam, milrinone, mitoXANtrone, morphine, multivitamins, nalbuphine, naloxone, nesiritide, netilmicin, nitroglycerin, nitroprusside, norepinephrine, octreotide, ondansetron, oxaliplatin, oxytocin, PACLitaxel, pancuronium, pantoprazole, papaverine, pentamidine, pentazocine, perphenazine, phentolamine, phenylephrine, phytonadione, potassium chloride, procainamide, prochlorperazine, promethazine, propofol, propranolol, protamine, pyridoxime, quinupristin/dalfopristin, ranitidine, remifentanil, ritodrine, riTUXimab, rocuronium, sargramostim, sodium acetate, streptokinase, succinylcholine, SUFentanil, tacrolimus, telavancin, teniposide, theophylline, thiamine, thiotepa, tirofiban, tobramycin, tolazoline, TPN (2 in 1), trastuzumab, trimetaphan, urokinase, vancomycin, vasopressin, vecuronium, verapamil, vinCRIStine, vinorelbine, voriconazole, zoledronic acid

Y-site incompatibilities: Allopurinol, amphotericin B colloidal, amphotericin B liposome, ampicillin, ampicillin/sulbactam, azaTHIOprine, ceFAZolin, cefoperazone, cefoTEtan, cefOXitin, ceftizoxime, cefuroxime, chloramphenicol, dantrolene, dexamethasone, diazepam, diazoxide, erythromycin, fluorouracil, folic acid, furosemide, ganciclovir, heparin, hydrocortisone, inamrinone, indomethacin, ketorolac, methotrexate, methylPREDNISolone, mezlocillin, moxalactam, nafcillin, oxacillin, palonosetron, PEMEtrexed, penicillin G, PENTobarbital, PHENobarbital, phenytoin, piperacillin/tazobactam, potassium acetate, sodium bicarbonate, trimethoprim/sulfamethoxazole

ADVERSE EFFECTS
CNS: Fever, headache
CV: Pericarditis
EENT: Dysphagia, glossitis, decreased calcification of deciduous teeth, oral candidiasis, tooth discoloration
GI: *Nausea, abdominal pain, vomiting, diarrhea,* anorexia, enterocolitis, hepatotoxicity, flatulence, abdominal cramps, gastric burning, stomatitis
GU: *Increased BUN*
HEMA: Eosinophilia, neutropenia, thrombocytopenia, hemolytic anemia
INTEG: Rash, urticaria, photosensitivity, increased pigmentation, exfoliative dermatitis, pruritus, phlebitis, injection site reaction
MS: Bone growth retardation (child <8 yr), muscle, joint pain
RESP: Cough
SYST: Stevens-Johnson syndrome, angioedema, toxic epidermal necrolysis

Pharmacokinetics

Absorption	Well absorbed
Distribution	Widely distributed, crosses placenta
Metabolism	Some hepatic recycling, 90% protein binding
Excretion	Bile, feces; kidneys unchanged (20%-40%), enters breast milk
Half-life	1 day; increased in severe renal disease

⚠ Nurse Alert   ★ Key NCLEX® Drug   >> Drug Specifics

Pharmacodynamics

	PO	IV
Onset	1½-4 hr	Immediate
Peak	1½-4 hr	Infusion's end

INTERACTIONS
Individual drugs
Bismuth, calcium, carBAMazepine, cimetidine, cholestyramine, colestipol, kaolin/pectin, magnesium, NaHCO$_3$, phenytoin, rifampin, sucralfate, zinc: decreased effect of doxycycline

Digoxin: increased or decreased effect of digoxin, sevelamer

Iron: forms chelates, decreased absorption

Penicillins: decreased effects of penicillins

Warfarin: increased effect of warfarin

Drug classifications
Alkali products, antacids, barbiturates: decreased effect of doxycycline

Anticoagulants (oral): increased effect of anticoagulants, methotrexate

Drug/food
Decreased: absorption with dairy products

Drug/lab test
Increased: BUN, alkaline phosphatase, bilirubin, amylase, ALT, AST, eosinophils, WBC

False increase: urinary catecholamines

NURSING CONSIDERATIONS
Assessment
• Assess patient for previous sensitivity reaction

• **Assess patient for signs and symptoms of infection** including characteristics of wounds, sputum, urine, stool, WBC >10,000/mm^3, fever; obtain baseline information before, during treatment

• Obtain C&S before beginning product therapy to identify if correct treatment has been initiated

• **Assess for allergic reactions: rash, urticaria, pruritus, chills, fever, joint pain; angioedema may occur a few days after therapy begins**

• Assess bowel pattern daily; if severe diarrhea occurs, product should be discontinued

• Monitor for bleeding: ecchymosis, bleeding gums, hematuria, stool guaiac daily if on long-term therapy; blood dyscrasias may occur

• **Assess for overgrowth of infection:** perineal itching, fever, malaise, redness, pain, swelling, drainage, rash, diarrhea, change in cough, sputum

Patient/family education
• Teach patient to report sore throat, bruising, bleeding, joint pain; may indicate blood dyscrasias (rare)

• Advise patient to contact prescriber if vaginal itching, loose foul-smelling stools, furry tongue occur; may indicate superinfection; report itching, rash, pruritus, urticaria

• Instruct patient to take all medication prescribed for the length of time ordered; product must be taken around the clock to maintain blood levels; do not give medication to others

• Advise patient to notify prescriber of diarrhea with blood or pus

• Teach patient not to use with antacids, iron products, H$_2$ blockers, sevelamer

• Advise patient to take with full glass of water, if nausea occurs take with food

Evaluation
Positive therapeutic outcome
• Absence of signs/symptoms of infection (WBC <10,000/mm^3, temp WNL, absence of red draining wounds)

• Reported improvement in symptoms of infection

⚠ HIGH ALERT

dronedarone (Rx)
(drone-da-rone)
Multaq
Func. class.: Antidysrhythmic (Class III)
Chem. class.: Iodinated benzofuran derivative
Pregnancy category X

ACTION: Prolongs action potential duration and effective refractory period, noncompetitive α- and β-adrenergic inhibition; increases PR and QT intervals, decreases sinus rate, decreases peripheral vascular resistance

Therapeutic outcome: Decreased amount and severity of ventricular dysrhythmias

USES: Atrial fibrillation, atrial flutter

CONTRAINDICATIONS:
Pregnancy **X,** breastfeeding, severe sinus node dysfunction, 2nd- or 3rd-degree AV block; bradycardia, hypersensitivity, heart failure, hepatic disease, QT prolongation

BLACK BOX WARNING: NYHA class IV heart failure or class II-III with recent decompensation requiring hospitalization, permanent atrial fibrillation (cannot restore sinus rhythm)

Precautions: Children, electrolyte imbalances, elderly, Asian patients, females, atrial fibrillation/flutter

DOSAGE AND ROUTES
Adult: **PO** 400 mg bid; discontinue class I, III antidysrhythmias or strong CYP3A4 inhibitors prior to beginning treatment; max 800 mg/day
Available forms: Tabs 400 mg

Implementation
• Start with patient hospitalized and monitored
PO route
• Give reduced dosage slowly with ECG monitoring only
• Give loading dose with food to decrease nausea

ADVERSE EFFECTS
CNS: Weakness
CV: *Bradycardia, heart failure, QT prolongation, torsades de pointes,* atrial flutter
ENDO: Hypo/hyperthyroidism
GI: Nausea, vomiting, diarrhea, abdominal pain, severe hepatic injury, hepatic failure
INTEG: Rash, photosensitivity, angioedema
RESP: Interstitial pneumonitis, pulmonary fibrosis

Pharmacokinetics

Absorption	Slow, variable (PO) up to 65%
Distribution	Body tissues; crosses placenta
Metabolism	Liver
Excretion	Bile, kidney (minimal)
Half-life	15-100 day

Pharmacodynamics

	PO
Onset	1-3 wk
Peak	Unknown
Duration	Up to months

INTERACTIONS
Individual drugs
CycloSPORINE, dextromethorphan, digoxin, disopyramide, flecainide, methotrexate, phenytoin, procainamide, quiNIDine, theophylline: increased blood levels, increased toxicity
Dabigatran, warfarin: increased anticoagulant effect

Drug classifications
β-Adrenergic blockers, calcium channel blockers: increased bradycardia
CYP3A4 inhibitors, CYP2D6 inhibitors: increased dronedarone levels
CYP3A, CYP2D6 inducers: decreased dronedarone levels

Drug/herb
St. John's wort: decreased effect
Yohimbine: increased anticoagulant effect

Drug/food
Grapefruit juice: increased dronedarone effect, avoid use

Drug/lab test
Increased: T4, LFTs, bilirubin, creatinine
Decreased: potassium, magnesium

NURSING CONSIDERATIONS
Assessment
• Monitor I&O ratio; monitor electrolytes: potassium, creatinine, magnesium
• Monitor liver function studies: AST, ALT, bilirubin, alkaline phosphatase

> **BLACK BOX WARNING:** NYHA Class IV heart failure or symptomatic heart failure with recent decomposition requiring hospitalization doubles risk of death

• Monitor **ECG** to determine product effectiveness; measure PR, QRS, QT intervals; check for PVCs, other dysrhythmias; monitor B/P continuously for hypo/hypertension; check for rebound hypertension after 1-2 hr
• Monitor serum creatine, potassium, magnesium
• Monitor for dehydration or hypovolemia
• **Assess for hypothyroidism:** lethargy, dizziness, constipation, enlarged thyroid gland, edema of extremities, cool, pale skin
• **Monitor hyperthyroidism:** restlessness, tachycardia, eyelid puffiness, weight loss, frequent urination, menstrual irregularities, dyspnea, warm, moist skin
• Monitor cardiac rate, respiration: rate, rhythm, character, chest pain, ventricular tachycardia, supraventricular tachycardia or fibrillation
• Assess sight and vision before treatment and throughout therapy; microdeposits on the cornea may cause blurred vision, halos, and photophobia

Patient/family education
• Instruct patient to report weight gain, edema, difficulty breathing immediately to prescriber
• Instruct patient to use sunscreen and protective clothing to prevent burning associated with photosensitivity
• Instruct patient to take medication as prescribed, not to double doses, avoid use with all other products without approval of prescriber, do not use grapefruit juice
• Instruct patient to complete follow-up appointment with health care provider, including pulmonary function studies, chest x-ray

- Teach patient to use effective contraception during treatment, pregnancy **X**, do not breastfeed

Evaluation

Positive therapeutic outcome
- Decreased dysrhythmias

TREATMENT OF OVERDOSE:
Administer O_2, artificial ventilation, ECG, DOPamine for circulatory depression, diazepam or thiopental for seizures, isoproterenol

---

RARELY USED

droperidol (Rx)
(droe-per'i-dole)
Func. class.: Sedative-hypnotic
Chem. class.: Butyrophenone derivative
Pregnancy category C

Therapeutic outcome: Maintenance of anesthesia

USES: Premedication for surgery; induction, maintenance in general anesthesia; postoperatively for nausea and vomiting

CONTRAINDICATIONS
Hypersensitivity, breastfeeding, child <2 yr

> **BLACK BOX WARNING:** QT prolongation, torsades de pointes

DOSAGE AND ROUTES
Induction, adjunct
Adult: IV/IM 1.25-2.5 mg, may give additional 1.25 mg with caution
Child 2-12 yr: IV 0.1 mg/kg titrate to response

Premedication
Adult: IM 2.5 mg ½-1 hr before surgery, may give 1.25-2.5 mg additionally
Child 2-12 yr: IM 0.1 mg/kg

Available forms: Inj 2.5 mg/ml

droxidopa
(drox'-i-doe'-pa)
Northera
Func. class.: Cardiovascular agent-vasopressor
Pregnancy category C

ACTION: A synthetic amino acid precursor of norepinephrine. It is used to increase blood pressure with symptomatic neurogenic orthostatic hypotension (NOH) caused by primary autonomic failure (e.g., Parkinson's disease, multiple system atrophy, and pure autonomic failure), dopamine β-hydroxylase deficiency, or nondiabetic autonomic neuropathy

Therapeutic outcome: Decreased B/P

USES: Increased B/P

CONTRAINDICATIONS
Hypersensitivity

Precautions: Angina, breastfeeding, cardiac arrhythmias, cardiac disease, children, coronary artery disease, heart disease, hyperthermia, infants, mental status changes, myocardial infarction, neonates, pregnancy, salicylate/tartrazine dye hypersensitivity

> **BLACK BOX WARNING:** Hypertension

DOSAGE AND ROUTES
Adult: **PO** 100 mg tid: upon arising in the morning, at midday, and in the late afternoon at least 3 hr before bedtime; titrate to response, by 100 mg tid q24-48hr up to a dose of 600 mg PO tid, max 1800 mg/day

Available forms: Caps 100, 200, 300 mg

Implementation
- Give tid at the following times: upon arising in the morning, at midday, and in the late afternoon at least 3 hr before bedtime (to reduce the potential for supine hypertension during sleep)
- Use without regard to food, but should be taken consistently in regard to food to ensure consistent absorption
- Swallow capsules whole

ADVERSE EFFECTS
CNS: Headache, dizziness, fatigue
CV: Supine hypertension, arrhythmia exacerbation, chest pain
MISC: Urinary tract infection, **neuroleptic malignant syndrome**

Pharmacokinetics

Absorption	Unknown
Distribution	Unknown
Metabolism	Unknown
Excretion	Unknown
Half-life	Unknown

Pharmacodynamics

Onset	Unknown
Peak	Unknown
Duration	Unknown

INTERACTIONS
Drug classifications
Serotonin receptor agonists, sympathomimetics, carbidopa: Increased droxidopa effects

MAOIs: Increased hypertensive crisis

NURSING CONSIDERATIONS
Assessment
• Monitor supine B/P before and at every dosage increase, assess response periodically. Advise to elevate the head of the bed when resting or sleeping to lessen the risk for supine hypertension. B/P should be monitored in supine position and the recommended head-elevated sleeping position. Reduce or discontinue if supine hypertension persists.

• Neuroleptic malignant syndrome: hyperthermia, severe extrapyramidal dysfunction, alterations in consciousness, mental status changes, and autonomic instability (tachycardia, blood pressure fluctuations, diaphoresis). In those with Parkinson's disease, this condition may occur with abrupt reduction of products with dopaminergic properties.

• Arrhythmia exacerbation: exacerbation of existing ischemic cardiac disease (coronary artery disease, angina, myocardial infarction, CHF); consider the potential risk before initiating therapy; if chest pain occurs during use, assess cardiac status

Patient/family education
• Instruct patients to rest and sleep in an upper-body-elevated position and to monitor B/P (to reduce the potential for supine hypertension)

Evaluation
Positive therapeutic outcome
• Increased B/P

DULoxetine (Rx)
(du-lox′uh-teen)
Cymbalta
Func. class.: Antidepressant, miscellaneous
Chem. class.: Serotonin, norepinephrine reuptake inhibitor (SNRI)
Pregnancy category C

ACTION: Unknown, may potentiate serotoninergic, noradrenergic activity in the CNS. In studies duloxetine is a potent inhibitor of neuronal serotonin and norepinephrine reuptake

Therapeutic outcome: Decreased depression, decreased neuropathic pain

USES: Major depressive disorder (MDD), neuropathic pain associated with diabetic neuropathy, generalized anxiety disorder, fibromyalgia, chronic low back pain, osteoarthritis pain

CONTRAINDICATIONS:
Hypersensitivity, closed-angle glaucoma, alcohol intoxication, alcoholism, hepatic disease, hepatitis, jaundice

Precautions: Pregnancy **C**, breastfeeding, geriatric, mania, hypertension, cardiac/renal/hepatic disease, seizures, increased intraocular pressure, anorexia nervosa, bleeding, dehydration, diabetes, hyponatremia, hypotension, hypovolemia, orthostatic hypotension, abrupt drug withdrawal

> **BLACK BOX WARNING:** Children, suicidal ideation

DOSAGE AND ROUTES
Depression
Adult: PO 40-60 mg/day as a single dose or 2 divided doses

Diabetic neuropathy
Adult: PO 60 mg qday

Generalized anxiety disorder
Adult: PO 60 mg/day, may start with 30 mg/day × 1 wk, then increase to 60 mg/day, maintenance 60-120 mg/day

Fibromyalgia
Adult: PO 30 mg/day × 1 wk, then 60 mg/day

Musculoskeletal pain
Adult: PO 60 mg/day or 30 mg/day × 1 wk, then 60 mg/day

Renal dose
Adult: PO Start with 20 mg, gradually increase; avoid use in severe renal disease

Available forms: Caps 20, 30, 60 mg

Implementation
• Swallow caps whole; do not break, crush, or chew; do not sprinkle on food or mix with liquid
• Give without regard to food
• Store in tight container at room temperature; do not freeze
• Provide assistance with ambulation during beginning therapy, since drowsiness, dizziness occur
• Check to see if PO medication was swallowed

ADVERSE EFFECTS

CNS: Insomnia, anxiety, dizziness, tremor, somnolence, fatigue, decreased appetite, decreased weight, agitation, diaphoresis, hallucinations, **neuroleptic malignant syndrome–like reaction,** aggression, **seizures,** headache, abnormal dreams, flushing, hot flashes, chills

CV: **Thrombophlebitis,** peripheral edema, palpitations, hypertension, **supraventricular dysrhythmia,** orthostatic hypotension

EENT: *Abnormal vision*

ENDO: Hypoglycemia, SIADH

GI: Constipation, diarrhea, dysphagia, *nausea,* vomiting, anorexia, dry mouth, colitis, gastritis, abdominal pain, **hepatic failure**

GU: Abnormal ejaculation, urinary hesitation, ejaculation delayed, erectile dysfunction, urinary frequency/retention, gyn bleeding

INTEG: Photosensitivity, bruising, sweating, **Stevens-Johnson syndrome**

MS: Gait disturbances, muscle spasm, restless legs syndrome, myalgia

SYST: **Anaphylaxis, angioedema, serotonin syndrome, Stevens-Johnson syndrome**

Pharmacokinetics

Absorption	Well absorbed
Distribution	90% protein binding
Metabolism	Extensively metabolized (CYP2D6, CYP1A2) in the liver to an active metabolite
Excretion	70% of product recovered in urine, 20% in feces
Half-life	12 hr

Pharmacodynamics

Unknown

INTERACTIONS

Individual drugs

Alcohol: increased ALT, bilirubin

Drug classifications

⚠ **MAOIs: coadministration (or within 14 days of MAOIs use) is contraindicated: hyperthermia, rigidity, rapid fluctuations of VS, mental status changes, neuroleptic malignant syndrome**

Anticoagulants, antiplatelets, salicylates, NSAIDs: increased bleeding risk

Opioids, antihistamines, sedative/hypnotics: increased CNS depression

CYP1A2 inhibitors (fluvoxaMINE, quinolone anti-infectives); CYP2D6 inhibitors (FLUoxetine, quiNIDine, PARoxetine): increased action of DULoxetine

CYP2D6 extensively metabolized products (flecainide, phenothiazines, propafenone, tricyclics, thioridazine): narrow therapeutic index

SSRIs serotonin receptor agonists: increased serotonin syndrome, neuroleptic malignant syndrome

Drug/herb

Kava: increased CNS depression

St. John's wort: serotonin syndrome

Drug/lab test

Increased: blood glucose

NURSING CONSIDERATIONS
Assessment

> **BLACK BOX WARNING: Depression:** Assess mental status: mood, sensorium, affect, **suicidal tendencies,** increase in psychiatric symptoms; depression, panic

- Assess B/P lying, standing; pulse q4hr; if systolic B/P drops 20 mm Hg, hold product, notify prescriber; take VS q4hr in patients with CV disease
- Monitor hepatic studies: AST, ALT, bilirubin
- Monitor weight qwk; weight loss or gain; appetite may increase; peripheral edema may occur
- Offer sugarless gum, hard candy, frequent sips of water for dry mouth
- Assess for withdrawal symptoms: headache, nausea, vomiting, muscle pain, weakness; not usual unless product is discontinued abruptly

⚠ Assess for neuroleptic malignant syndrome–like reaction

- **Serotonin syndrome:** assess for nausea, vomiting, dizziness, facial flushing, shivering, sweating
- **Sexual dysfunction:** ejaculation dysfunction, erectile dysfunction, decreased libido, orgasm dysfunction

Patient/family education

- Advise that product is dispensed in small amounts because of suicide potential, especially in the beginning of therapy
- Teach patient/family to use caution when driving or other activities requiring alertness because of drowsiness, dizziness, blurred vision
- Advise patient to avoid alcohol ingestion, other CNS depressants, MAOIs

---

• **Abrupt discontinuation:** Advise patient not to discontinue medication quickly after long-term use; may cause nausea, headache, malaise
• Advise patient to wear sunscreen or large hat, since photosensitivity may occur
• Advise patient to notify prescriber if pregnancy is planned or suspected or if breastfeeding
• Tell patient that improvement may occur in 4-8 wk; up to 12 wk (geriatric patients)

> **BLACK BOX WARNING:** Advise that clinical worsening and suicide risk may occur

Evaluation
Positive therapeutic outcome
• Decreased depression

---

dutasteride (Rx)
(doo-tass´ter-ide)
Avodart
Func. class.: Sex hormone, 5α-reductase inhibitor
Chem. class.: Synthetic 4-azasteroid compound
Pregnancy category X

ACTION: Inhibits both types 1 and 2 forms of a steroid enzyme that converts testosterone to 5 μ-dihydrotestosterone (DHT), which is responsible for the initial growth of prostatic tissue

Therapeutic outcome: Decreased symptoms of benign prostatic hyperplasia (BPH)

USES: Treatment of symptomatic BPH in men with an enlarged prostate gland, or may be used in combination with tamsulosis

Unlabeled uses: Alopecia

CONTRAINDICATIONS
Pregnancy **X,** breastfeeding, children, women, hypersensitivity

Precautions: Hepatic disease

DOSAGE AND ROUTES
Benign prostatic hyperplasia (BPH)
Adult: PO 0.5 mg/day

Alopecia (unlabeled)
Adult: PO 0.5-2.5 mg/day

Available forms: Caps 0.5 mg

Implementation
• Swallow caps whole: do not break, crush, chew, or open
• May be given without regard to meals

ADVERSE EFFECTS
GU: Decreased libido, impotence, gynecomastia, ejaculation disorders (rare), mastalgia, teratogenesis
INTEG: Serious skin infections

Pharmacokinetics

Absorption	Absolute bioavailability ~60%
Distribution	Protein binding 99%
Metabolism	Liver (CYP3A4)
Excretion	Feces
Half-life	5 wk at steady state

Pharmacodynamics

Onset	Rapid
Peak	2-3 hr
Duration	Levels detectable 4-6 mo post-treatment

INTERACTIONS
Individual drugs
Cimetidine, ciprofloxacin, diltiazem, ketoconazole, ritonavir, verapamil: increased dutasteride concentrations

Drug classifications
Antiretroviral protease inhibitors or other CYP3A4-metabolized products: increased dutasteride concentrations

Drug/lab test
Decreased: PSA

NURSING CONSIDERATIONS
Assessment
• **Assess for decreasing symptoms in BPH:** decreasing urinary retention, frequency, urgency, nocturia
• Assess PSA levels, digital rectal exam, urinary obstruction; determine the absence of urinary cancer before starting treatment
• Assess liver function tests: ALT, AST, bilirubin; blood studies: CBC with differential, serum creatitine, serum electrolytes

Patient/family education
• Advise patient to notify prescriber if therapeutic response decreases, if edema occurs
• Caution patient not to discontinue product abruptly
• Inform patient about changes in sex characteristics
• Caution patient not to donate blood for at least 6 mo after last dose to prevent possible blood administration to pregnant woman
• Advise patient and family that caps should not be handled by pregnant women or those who may become pregnant since

---

this product can be absorbed through the skin

• Inform patient that ejaculate volume may decrease during treatment, that product rarely interferes with sexual function

• Advise patient to read patient information leaflet before starting therapy and reread it upon prescription renewal

• Teach patient product should not be used or handled by breastfeeding women

• Advise patient to swallow whole; do not crush, chew, or open

• Teach patient that drug may increase risk for developing high-grade prostate cancer

Evaluation
Positive therapeutic outcome

• Decreased levels of DHT (5 α-dihydrotestosterone)

• Decreased urinary frequency

• Decreased urinary retention

• Decreased urinary urgency

• Decreased nocturia

Adverse effects: *italics* = common; **bold** = life-threatening

econazole topical
See Appendix B

efavirenz (Rx)
(ef-ah-veer'enz)
Sustiva
Func. class.: Antiretroviral
Chem. class.: Nonnucleoside reverse
transcriptase inhibitor (NNRTI)
Pregnancy category D

ACTION: Binds directly to reverse transcriptase and blocks RNA polymerase and DNA polymerase, causing a disruption of the enzyme's site

Therapeutic outcome: Improvement of HIV-1 infection

USES: HIV-1 in combination with other antiretrovirals

CONTRAINDICATIONS
Pregnancy **D**, hypersensitivity, moderate/severe hepatic disease

Precautions: Liver disease, breastfeeding, children <3 yr, renal disease, myelosuppression, depression, seizures

DOSAGE AND ROUTES
Given in combination with protease inhibitor or nucleoside analog reverse transcriptase inhibitors (NRTIs)
Adult and child >40 kg: PO 600 mg/day at bedtime
Child ≥3 mo:
7-14.9 kg: PO 200 mg/day at bedtime
15-19.9 kg: PO 250 mg/day at bedtime
20-24.9 kg: PO 300 mg/day at bedtime
25-32.4 kg: PO 350 mg/day at bedtime
32.5-39.9 kg: PO 400 mg/day at bedtime
Child ≥3 mo, 5-<7.5 kg: PO 150 mg/day at bedtime
Child 3.5 ≤5 kg: PO 100 mg/day at bedtime

Available forms: Caps 50, 100, 200 mg; tabs 600 mg

Implementation
• Give at bedtime to decrease CNS side effects, give on empty stomach, or sprinkled on food, do not cut/break caps

ADVERSE EFFECTS
CNS: Headache, dizziness, fatigue, impaired cognition, insomnia, abnormal dreams, depression, anxiety, drowsiness, odd feeling, depersonalization

GI: *Diarrhea*, abdominal pain, *nausea*, hyperlipidemia, constipation, increased liver function tests, vomiting, **hepatotoxicity**
GU: Hematuria, kidney stones
INTEG: *Rash*, erythema multiforme, Stevens-Johnson syndrome, toxic epidermal necrolysis, exfoliative dermatitis

Pharmacokinetics

Absorption	Well absorbed, concentrations higher in females, Africans, Asians, Hispanics
Distribution	Highly protein bound (99%)
Metabolism	Liver
Excretion	Kidneys, feces
Half-life	Terminal 40-76 hr

Pharmacodynamics

Onset	Unknown
Peak	3-5 hr
Duration	Unknown

INTERACTIONS
Individual drugs
Alcohol: increased CNS depression
Amprenavir, indinavir, itraconazole, ketoconazole, lopinavir, posaconazole, saquinavir, voriconazole, cycloSPORINE, tacrolimus, sirolimus, buPROPion, sertraline: decreased level of each specific product
CarBAMazepine: decreased efavirenz levels
Cisapride, midazolam, triazolam, pimozide: do not give together
Ritonavir: increased levels of both products

Drug classifications
Anticonvulsants, ergots, statins (except pravastatin, fluvastatin): increased levels of each specific product
Antidepressants, antihistamines, opioids: increased CNS depression
Benzodiazepines, ergots: do not give together
CYP3A4 inhibitors (conivaptan, ambrisentan, sorafenib): decreased efavirenz metabolism
CYP3A4 inducers (carBAMazepine, rifamycins): decreased efavirenz effect
Estrogens: increased level of both products
Oral contraceptives: decreased level of these products
Rifamycins: decreased efavirenz action

Drug/herb
St. John's wort: decreased efavirenz level; do not use together

Drug/food
Increased: absorption of high-fat foods

Drug/lab test
Increased: ALT
False positive: cannabinoids

NURSING CONSIDERATIONS
Assessment
⚠ Pregnancy: Rule out pregnancy (D) before starting treatment; a type of contraception is needed, oral/non-oral contraceptives are decreased, use barrier methods also
• **HIV:** Assess CBC, blood chemistry, plasma HIV RNA, absolute $CD4^+/CD8^+$ cell counts/%, serum β_2 microglobulin, serum ICD + 24 antigen levels, cholesterol, hepatic enzymes
• Serious skin reactions: Stevens-Johnson syndrome, toxic epidermal necrolysis, usually occurs during first 2 wk, mild rash may resolve within 30 days; severe skin reactions including blistering, fever, product should be discontinued immediately and corticosteroids started
• Assess bowel pattern before, during treatment; if severe abdominal pain with bleeding occurs, product should be discontinued; monitor hydration
• Assess for signs of toxicity: severe nausea/vomiting, maculopapular rash
• Hepatotoxicity: Monitor LFTs in those with liver disease, hold if LFTs are moderately elevated; if severe or if LFTs increase after product is restarted, discontinue permanently

Patient/family education
• Advise patient to take as prescribed; if dose is missed, take as soon as remembered; do not double dose; take on empty stomach with water/juice
• Instruct patient to make sure health care provider knows of all the medications being taken, supplements, herbs, OTC products
• Advise patient that if severe rash occurs, stop taking and notify health care provider
⚠ Advise patient not to breastfeed or become pregnant (pregnancy D) if taking this product, use barrier method for ≥ 3 months after last dose
• Advise patient that adverse reactions (rash, dizziness, abnormal dreams, insomnia) lessen after a month
• Teach patient to avoid hazardous activities if dizziness, drowsiness occurs
• Teach patient that product does not cure disease but controls symptoms; HIV can be transmitted to others even while taking this product
• Advise patient to continue safer-sex practices

Evaluation
Positive therapeutic outcome
• Increased CD4, cell counts
• Decreased viral load
• Improvement in symptoms and progression of HIV-1 infection

efinaconazole topical
See Appendix B

eletriptan (Rx)
(el-ee-trip′tan)
Relpax
Func. class.: Antimigraine agent
Pregnancy category C

ACTION: Binds selectively to the vascular $5\text{-}HT_1$-receptor subtype, exerts antimigraine effect; causes vasoconstriction in cranial arteries

Therapeutic outcome: Decreased severity of migraine

USES: Acute treatment of migraine with or without aura

CONTRAINDICATIONS
Uncontrolled hypertension, hypersensitivity, basilar or hemiplegic migraine, ischemic bowel disease, severe renal/hepatic disease, coronary artery vasospasm, peripheral vascular disease, heart disease, acute MI, stroke, angina, postmenopausal women, men >40 yr, risk factors of CAD, MI, or other cardiac disease, hypercholesterolemia, obesity, diabetes

Precautions: Pregnancy **C**, breastfeeding, children, geriatric, impaired renal/hepatic function

DOSAGE AND ROUTES
Adult: PO 20 or 40 mg, may increase if needed, max 40 mg (single dose); may repeat in 2 hr if headache improves but returns, max 80 mg/24 hr

Available forms: Tabs 20, 40 mg

Implementation
• Swallow tabs whole; do not break, crush, or chew, take with 8 oz of water
• Provide quiet, calm environment with decreased stimulation from noise, bright light, excessive talking

ADVERSE EFFECTS
CNS: *Dizziness,* headache, anxiety, paresthesia, asthenia, somnolence, flushing, fatigue, hot/cold sensation, chills, vertigo, hypertonia, **seizures, serotonin syndrome**
CV: Chest pain, palpitations, hypertension, **MI, sinus tachycardia, stroke, ventricular fibrillation/tachycardia, atrial fibrillation, AV block, bradycardia, chest pressure syndrome, coronary vasospasm**

GI: Nausea, dry mouth, vomiting
MS: *Weakness,* back pain
RESP: Chest tightness, pressure

Pharmacokinetics

Absorption	Unknown
Distribution	Unknown
Metabolism	Liver
Excretion	Urine, feces
Half-life	4 hr

Pharmacodynamics

Onset	Of pain relief 1/2, peak 1 1/2-2 hr
Peak	Unknown
Duration	Unknown

INTERACTIONS
Individual drugs
Clarithromycin, erythromycin, itraconazole, ketoconazole, nelfinavir, propanolol, ritonavir: increased plasma concentration of eletriptan

Drug classifications
CYP3A4 inhibitors: increased concentration of ergots, eletriptan, avoid use within 72 hr of these products
SSRIs, SNRIs, serotonin-receptor agonists: increased serotonin syndrome
Ergots, ergot similar products: Increase: vasospastic reactions, avoid use within 24 hr of these products

NURSING CONSIDERATIONS
Assessment
• **Migraine:** pain location, character, intensity, nausea, vomiting, aura
• Monitor B/P; signs/symptoms of coronary vasospasms; geriatrics may be at higher risk
• Assess for tingling, hot sensation, burning, feeling of pressure, numbness, flushing
• Assess stress level, activity, recreation, coping mechanisms
• Assess neurologic status: LOC, blurring vision, nausea, vomiting, tingling in extremities preceding headache
• Identify ingestion of tyramine foods (pickled products, beer, wine, aged cheese), food additives, preservatives, colorings, artificial sweeteners, chocolate, caffeine, which may precipitate these types of headaches
• Determine if CYP3A4 inhibitors or other ergot type products have been given

Patient/family education
• Have patient report any side effects to prescriber
• Teach patient to use contraception while taking product

• Teach patient to have dark, quiet environment
• Teach patient that product does not prevent or reduce number of migraine attacks

Evaluation
Positive therapeutic outcome
• Decreased severity of migraine

eltrombopag
Promacta
See Appendix A, Selected New Drugs

emedastine ophthalmic
See Appendix B

empagliflozin
(em-pa-gli-floe′zin)
Jardiance
Func. class.: Antidiabetic
Chem. class.: Sodium-glucose cotransporter 2 (SGLT2) inhibitors
Pregnancy category C

ACTION: An inhibitor of sodium-glucose cotransporter 2 (SGLT2), the transporter responsible for reabsorbing the majority of glucose filtered by the tubular lumen in the kidney

Therapeutic outcome: Decreased blood glucose, A1c

USES: Type 2 diabetes mellitus with diet and exercise

CONTRAINDICATIONS: Hypersensitivity, dialysis, renal failure

Precautions: Adrenal insufficiency, breastfeeding, children, dehydration, diabetic ketoacidosis, fever, geriatric patients, hypercholesterolemia, hypercortisolism, hyperglycemia, hyperthyroidism, hypoglycemia, hypotension, hypothyroidism, hypovolemia, malnutrition, pituitary insufficiency, pregnancy **C**, renal impairment, type 1 diabetes mellitus, vaginitis

DOSAGE AND ROUTES
Adult: PO 10 mg daily, may increase to 25 mg daily

Available forms: Tabs 10, 25 mg

Implementation
• Give every day without regard to food in the AM

ADVERSE EFFECTS
CNS: Syncope
CV: Hypotension, orthostatic hypotension
ENDO: Hypercholesterolemia, hyperlipidemia, hypoglycemia

GU: Increased urinary frequency, nocturia, polyuria, cystitis, dehydration, diuresis
GI: Nausea
MISC: Infection
MS: Arthralgia

Pharmacokinetics

Absorption	Unknown
Distribution	Protein binding 82.6%
Metabolism	Unknown
Excretion	Unknown
Half-life	Terminal elimination half-life 12.4 hr

Pharmacodynamics

Onset	Unknown
Peak	1.5 hr
Duration	Unknown

INTERACTIONS
Individual drugs
Alcohol, bortezomib, cloNIDine, lithium: increased/decreased hypoglycemic effect

Baclofen, cycloSPORINE, dexfenfluramine, dextrothyroxine, ethotoin, fenfluramine, fosphenytoin, glucagon, phenytoin, tacrolimus, tobacco: decreased hypoglycemic effect

FLUoxetine, octreotide, OLANZapine: increased hypoglycemic effect

Gatifloxacin: do not use concurrently

Drug classifications
Androgens, sulfonamides: increase/decreased hypoglycemic effect

Angiotensin II receptor antagonists, angiotensin-converting enzyme (ACE) inhibitors, β-blockers, fibric acid derivatives, loop diuretics, MAOIs type A, thiazide diuretics: increased hypoglycemic effect

Atypical antipsychotics, carbonic anhydrase inhibitors, corticosteroids, estrogens, oral contraceptives, phenothiazines, progestins, salicylates: decreased hypoglycemic effect

Thyroid hormones: do not use concurrently

Drug/herb
Chromium, horse chestnut: increased hypoglycemia

Green tea: decreased hypoglycemia

Niacin: increased/decreased hypoglycemia

NURSING CONSIDERATIONS
Assessment
• Diabetes: Monitor blood glucose, glycosylated hemoglobin A1c (HbA1c), serum cholesterol profile, serum creatinine/BUN, assess for polydipsia, other products taken by patient

Patient/family education
• Teach patient how to check blood glucose, to continue with diet and exercise changes, to avoid smoking, alcohol
• Instruct patient to avoid other products unless approved by prescriber

Evaluation
Positive therapeutic outcome
• Decreased blood glucose, A1c

emtricitabine (Rx)
(em-tri-sit′uh-bean)
Emtriva
Func. class.: Antiretroviral
Chem. class.: Nucleoside reverse transcriptase inhibitor (NRTI)
Pregnancy category B

ACTION: Synthetic nucleoside analog of cytosine; inhibits replication of HIV virus by competing with the natural substrate and then becoming incorporated into cellular DNA by viral reverse transcriptase, thereby terminating cellular DNA chain

Therapeutic outcome: Decreasing symptoms of HIV

USES: HIV-1 infection with other antiretrovirals

Unlabeled uses: HBV (hepatitis B virus) infection

CONTRAINDICATIONS
Hypersensitivity

> **BLACK BOX WARNING:** Lactic acidosis

Precautions: Pregnancy **B,** breastfeeding, children, geriatric, renal disease

> **BLACK BOX WARNING:** Hepatic insufficiency, chronic hepatitis B virus (HBV) infection, **more common in females or those that are overweight; monitor lactic acid levels, LFTs**

DOSAGE AND ROUTES
Oral cap and sol are not interchangeable

Adult: PO (caps) 200 mg/day; oral SOL 240 mg (24 ml) daily

Adolescent/child >33 kg: PO (caps) 200 mg/day

Child 3 mo-17 yr: oral SOL 6 mg/kg/day, max 240 mg (24 ml)

Infant <3 mo: PO oral SOL 3 mg/kg daily, do not use caps

Renal dose

Adult: PO CCr 30-49 ml/min 200 mg q48hr, SOL 120 mg q24hr; caps CCr 15-29 ml/min 200 mg q72hr, SOL 80 mg q24hr; caps CCr ,15 ml/min 200 mg q96hr, SOL 60 mg q24hr

Available forms: Caps 200 mg; oral sol 10 mg/ml; oral cap and sol are not interchangeable

Implementation

- Give without regard to meals
- Store at 25° C (77° F)
- Take at same time every day
- **Oral cap and sol are not interchangeable**

ADVERSE EFFECTS

CNS: Headache, abnormal dreams, depression, dizziness, insomnia, neuropathy, paresthesia, *asthenia*

GI: *Nausea, vomiting, diarrhea, anorexia, abdominal pain, dyspepsia,* **hepatomegaly with stenosis (may be fatal)**

INTEG: Rash, skin discoloration

MS: Arthralgia, myalgia

RESP: Cough

SYST: Change in body fat distribution, **lactic acidosis**

Pharmacokinetics

Absorption	Rapidly, extensively absorbed
Distribution	Protein binding <4%
Metabolism	Unknown
Excretion	Excreted unchanged in urine (86%), feces (14%)
Half-life	10 hr

Pharmacodynamics

Onset	Unknown
Peak	1-2 hr
Duration	Unknown

INTERACTIONS

Efavirenz, lamiVUDine, tenofovir: Do not use together, treatment duplication

Ribavirin: Complex interactions

Drug classifications

Interferons: Decreased emtricitabine level

Drug/Lab

Increase: AST/ALT, glucose, amylase, bilirubin, CK, lipase

Decrease: neutrophils

NURSING CONSIDERATIONS

Assessment

- Monitor liver, renal function tests: AST, ALT, bilirubin, amylase, lipase, triglycerides periodically during treatment

BLACK BOX WARNING: Assess for lactic acidosis, severe hepatomegaly with steatosis; if lab reports confirm these conditions, discontinue treatment; more common in females, obese; monitor serum lactate levels, liver function tests

BLACK BOX WARNING: Confirm that patient is free of HBV (hepatitis B virus) before starting treatment

BLACK BOX WARNING: Hepatotoxicity: Do not use in those with risk factors such as alcoholism; discontinue if hepatotoxicity occurs

BLACK BOX WARNING: Hepatitis B and HIV coinfection (unlabeled): Perform HBV screening in any patient who has HIV to ensure appropriate treatment; avoid single-drug treatments in HBV

Patient/family education

- Teach that GI complaints resolve after 3-4 wk of treatment
- **Advise patient to report planned or suspected pregnancy, not to breastfeed while taking this product**
- Instruct that product must be taken at same time of day to maintain blood level, **solution and cap are not interchangeable**
- Advise that product will control symptoms, but is not a cure for HIV; patient is still infectious, may pass HIV virus on to others
- Instruct that other products may be necessary to prevent other infections
- Advise that changes in body fat distribution may occur

BLACK BOX WARNING: Lactic acidosis: Teach patient to notify prescriber immediately of fatigue, muscle aches/pains, abdominal pain, difficulty breathing, nausea, vomiting, change in heart rate

BLACK BOX WARNING: Hepatotoxicity: Teach patient to notify prescriber of dark urine, yellowing of skin/eyes, clay-colored stools, anorexia, nausea, vomiting

⚠ Instruct patient to avoid breastfeeeding to reduce postnatal HIV transmission

Evaluation

Positive therapeutic outcome

- Decrease in signs/symptoms of HIV
- Decrease viral load, increase CD4 counts

enalapril/enalaprilat (Rx)
(e-nal′a-pril/e-nal′a-pril-at)
Vasotec
Func. class.: Antihypertensive
Chem. class.: Angiotensin-converting enzyme (ACE) inhibitor
Pregnancy category D

Do not confuse: enalapril/Eldepryl/ramipril/Anafranil

ACTION: Selectively suppresses renin-angiotensin-aldosterone system; inhibits ACE; prevents conversion of angiotensin I to angiotensin II, resulting in dilatation of arterial and venous vessels

Therapeutic outcome: Decreased B/P in hypertension; decreased preload, afterload in CHF

USES: Hypertension, CHF, left ventricular dysfunction

CONTRAINDICATIONS
Hypersensitivity, history of angioedema

> BLACK BOX WARNING: Pregnancy **D**

Precautions: Breastfeeding, renal disease, hyperkalemia, hepatic failure, dehydration, bilateral renal artery/aortic stenosis

DOSAGE AND ROUTES
Hypertension
Adult: PO 2.5-5 mg/day, may increase or decrease to desired response, range 10-40 mg/day; **IV** 0.625-1.25 mg q6hr over 5 min
Child: PO 0.08 mg/kg/day in 1-2 divided doses, max 0.58 mg/kg/day in 1-2 divided doses; **IV** 5-10 mcg/kg/dose q8-24hr

CHF
Adult: PO 2.5-20 mg/day in 2 divided doses, max 40 mg/day in divided doses

Renal dose
Adult: PO CCr <30 ml/min 2.5 mg/day, increase gradually; IV CCr >30 ml/min 1.25 mg q6hr; CCr <30 ml/min 0.625 mg as one-time dose, increase as per B/P

Available forms: Enalapril: tabs 2.5, 5, 10, 20 mg; enalaprilat: inj 1.25 mg/ml

Implementation
PO route
• Store in airtight container at 86° F (30° C) or less
• Severe hypotension may occur after 1st dose of this medication; hypotension may be prevented by reducing or discontinuing diuretic therapy 3 days before beginning benazepril therapy

• Give by **IV** inf of 0.9% NaCl (as ordered) to expand fluid volume if severe hypotension occurs

Direct IV route/ intermittent IV infusion
• Give undiluted over ≥5 min; use diluent provided or 50 ml D₅W, 0.9% NaCl, 0.9% NaCl in D₅W, or LR, give over ≥5 min, sol is stable for 24 hr

Y-site compatibilities: Acyclovir, alemtuzumab, alfentanil, allopurinol, amifostine, amikacin, aminophylline, amphotericin B liposome, anidulafungin, ascorbic acid, atracurium, atropine, azaTHIOprine, aztreonam, benztropine, bivalirudin, bretylium, bumetanide, buprenorphine, butorphanol, calcium chloride/gluconate, CARBOplatin, ceFAZolin, cefonicid, cefotaxime, cefoTEtan, cefOXitin, cefTAZidime, ceftizoxime, cefTRIAXone, cefuroxime, chloramphenicol, cimetidine, cisatracurium, cladribine, clindamycin, cyanocobalamin, cyclophosphamide, cycloSPORINE, cytarabine, DACTINomycin, DAPTOmycin, dexamethasone, dexmedetomidine, dextran 40, digoxin, diltiazem, diphenhydrAMINE, DOBUTamine, DOCEtaxel, DOPamine, doripenem, doxacurium, DOXOrubicin, DOXOrubicin liposome, doxycycline, ePHEDrine, EPINEPHrine, epirubicin, epoetin, ertapenem, erythromycin, esmolol, etoposide, etoposide phosphate, famotidine, fenoldopam, fentaNYL, filgrastim, fluconazole, fludarabine, fluorouracil, folic acid, furosemide, ganciclovir, gemcitabine, gentamicin, granisetron, heparin, hydrocortisone, HYDROmorphone, ifosfamide, imipenem/cilastatin, indomethacin, insulin, isoproterenol, ketorolac, labetalol, levofloxacin, lidocaine, linezolid, LORazepam, magnesium sulfate, mannitol, mechlorethamine, melphalan, meperidine, meropenem, metaraminol, methicillin, methotrexate, methoxamine, methyldopate, methylPREDNISolone, metoclopramide, metoprolol, metroNIDAZOLE, mezlocillin, miconazole, midazolam, milrinone, minocycline, mitoXANtrone, morphine, moxalactam, multiple vitamin infusion, nafcillin, nalbuphine, naloxone, netilmicin, niCARdipine, nitroglycerin, nitroprusside, norepinephrine, octreotide, ondansetron, oxacillin, oxaliplatin, oxytocin, PACLitaxel, palonosetron, papaverine, PEMEtrexed, penicillin G potassium, pentamidine, pentazocine, PENTobarbital, PHENobarbital, phentolamine, phenylephrine, phytonadione, piperacillin/tazobactam, potassium chloride/phosphate, procainamide, prochlorperazine, promethazine, propofol, propranolol, protamine, pyridoxime, quinupristin/dalfopristin, ranitidine, remifentanil, ritodrine, riTUXimab, rocuronium, sodium acetate, sodium bicarbonate, succinylcholine, SUFentanil, tacrolimus, teniposide, tetracycline, theophylline, thiamine, thiotepa, ticarcillin/clavulanate, tigecycline, tirofiban, tobramycin, tolazoline, trastuzumab, trimetaphan, urokinase, vancomycin, vasopressin, vecuronium, verapamil, vinCRIStine, vinorelbine, voriconazole

Y-site incompatibilities: Amphotericin B cholesteryl sulfate, caspofungin, cefepime, dantrolene, diazepam, diazoxide, gemtuzumab, lansoprazole, phenytoin

ADVERSE EFFECTS

CNS: *Insomnia, dizziness,* paresthesias, headache, fatigue, anxiety

CV: *Hypotension,* chest pain, tachycardia, **dysrhythmias,** syncope, angina, **MI,** orthostatic hypotension

EENT: *Tinnitus,* visual changes, sore throat, double vision, dry burning eyes

GI: Nausea, vomiting, colitis, cramps, diarrhea, constipation, flatulence, dry mouth, loss of taste, hepatotoxicity

GU: Proteinuria, renal failure, increased frequency of polyuria or oliguria

HEMA: Agranulocytosis, neutropenia

INTEG: Rash, purpura, alopecia, hyperhidrosis, photosensitivity

META: Hyperkalemia

RESP: Dyspnea, dry cough, crackles

SYST: Toxic epidermal necrolysis, Stevens-Johnson syndrome, angioedema

Pharmacokinetics

Absorption	Well absorbed (PO), complete (**IV**)
Distribution	Unknown
Metabolism	Liver (active metabolite—enalaprilat)
Excretion	Kidneys (60%—enalaprilat, 20%—enalapril)
Half-life	Enalaprilat 35 hr, increased in renal disease

Pharmacodynamics

	PO	IV
Onset	1 hr	5-15 min
Peak	4-6 hr	1-4 hr
Duration	24 hr	4-6 hr

INTERACTIONS
Individual drugs

Alcohol: increased hypotension (large amounts)

Allopurinol: increased hypersensitivity

CycloSPORINE, NSAIDs: increased potassium levels

Digoxin, lithium: increased serum levels

Rifampin: decreased effects of enalapril

Drug classifications

Antacids: decreased effects of enalapril

Diuretics, general anesthesia, nitrates, other antihypertensives, phenothiazines: increased hypotension

Diuretics (potassium-sparing), potassium supplements, salt substitutes: increased potassium levels

Drug/lab test

Increased: ALT, AST, bilirubin, alkaline phosphatase, glucose, uric acid, BUN, creatinine

False positive: ANA titer

NURSING CONSIDERATIONS
Assessment

• **Bone marrow depression (rare): monitor blood studies: neutrophils, decreased platelets with differential baseline and q3mo; if neutrophils <1000/mm³, discontinue treatment**

• **Hypertension:** monitor B/P, orthostatic hypotension, syncope; if changes occur, dosage change may be required; obtain peak/trough levels, maintain adequate hydration

• **CHF: monitor for increased weight, rales, jugular vein distention, edema, difficulty breathing**

• Monitor electrolytes: K, Na, Cl during 1st 2 wk of therapy

• **Monitor renal studies: protein, BUN, creatinine; increased levels may indicate nephrotic syndrome and renal failure**

• Monitor renal symptoms: polyuria, oliguria, frequency, dysuria

• Establish baselines in renal, liver function tests before therapy begins and 1 wk into therapy, avoid activities requiring coordination

• Check potassium levels throughout treatment, although hyperkalemia rarely occurs

• Check for edema in feet, legs daily

• Assess for allergic reactions: rash, fever, pruritus, urticaria; product should be discontinued if antihistamines fail to help

Patient/family education

• Advise patient not to discontinue product abruptly; advise patient to tell all persons associated with health care that product is being taken

• Teach patient not to use OTC products (cough, cold, allergy medications) unless directed by physician, to avoid potassium, salt substitutes; serious side effects can occur; xanthines, such as coffee, tea, chocolate, cola, can prevent action of product

• Instruct patient on the importance of complying with dosage schedule, even if feeling better; to continue with medical regimen to decrease B/P: exercise, cessation of smoking, decreasing stress, diet modifications

• Emphasize the need to rise slowly to sitting or standing position to minimize orthostatic hypotension; not to exercise in hot weather, which can cause increased hypotension
• **Advise patient to notify prescriber of mouth sores, sore throat, fever, swelling of hands or feet, irregular heartbeat, chest pain, coughing, shortness of breath**
• Caution patient to report excessive perspiration, dehydration, vomiting, diarrhea; may lead to fall in B/P
• **Caution patient that product may cause skin rash or impaired perspiration; that angioedema may occur and to discontinue if it occurs**
• Caution patient that product may cause dizziness, fainting, light-headedness; may occur during 1st few days of therapy; to avoid activities that may be hazardous
• Teach patient how to take B/P, normal readings for age-group

> **BLACK BOX WARNING:** Teach patient to use contraception during treatment, pregnancy **D**, to notify prescriber if pregnancy is planned or suspected

Evaluation
Positive therapeutic outcome
• Decreased B/P in hypertension

TREATMENT OF OVERDOSE:
Lavage, **IV** atropine for bradycardia; **IV** theophylline for bronchospasm, digoxin, O_2; diuretic for cardiac failure, hemodialysis

---

enfuvirtide (Rx)
(en-fyoo´vir-tide)
Fuzeon
Func. class.: Antiretroviral
Chem. class.: Fusion inhibitor
Pregnancy category B

ACTION: Inhibitor of the fusion of HIV-1 with CD4+ cells

Therapeutic outcome: Decreasing symptoms of HIV

USES: Treatment of HIV-1 infection in combination with other antiretrovirals

CONTRAINDICATIONS
Breastfeeding, hypersensitivity

Precautions: Pregnancy **B,** (must be enrolled in the Antiretroviral Pregnancy Registry: 800-258-4263), children <6 yr, liver disease, myelosuppression, infections

DOSAGE AND ROUTES
Adult: SUBCUT 90 mg (1 ml) bid
Child 6-16 yr and <42.6 kg: SUBCUT 2 mg/kg bid, max 90 mg bid; 11-15.5 kg 27 mg/0.3 ml bid; 15.6-20 kg 36 ml/0.4 ml bid; 20.1-24.5 kg 45 mg/0.5 ml bid; 24.6-29 kg 54 mg/0.6 ml bid; 29.1-33.5 kg 63 mg/0.7 ml bid; 33.6-38 kg 72 mg/0.8 ml bid; 38.1-42.5 kg 81 mg/0.9 ml bid

Available forms: Powder for inj, lyophilized 108 mg (90 mg/ml when reconstituted)

Implementation
• Give SUBCUT, bid; rotate sites; preferred sites are upper arm, anterior thigh, abdomen

ADVERSE EFFECTS
CNS: Anxiety, peripheral neuropathy, taste disturbance, **Guillain-Barré syndrome,** insomnia, depression
GI: Nausea, abdominal pain, anorexia, constipation, **pancreatitis**
GU: Glomerulonephritis, renal failure
HEMA: Thrombocytopenia, neutropenia
INTEG: *Inj site reactions*
MISC: Influenza, cough, conjunctivitis, lymphadenopathy, myalgias, hyperglycemia, hypersensitivity, **pneumonia,** rhinitis, fatigue

Pharmacokinetics

Absorption	Well absorbed
Distribution	92% protein binding
Metabolism	Undergoes catabolism
Excretion	Unknown
Half-life	Terminal 3.8 hr

Pharmacodynamics

Onset	Unknown
Peak	8 hrs
Duration	Unknown

INTERACTIONS
Drug/lab
Increased: LFTs, lipase
Decreased: Hgb

NURSING CONSIDERATIONS
Assessment
• **Assess for signs of infection, inj site reactions, use analgesics; bacterial pneumonia may occur if blood counts are low or viral load is high**
• **Monitor renal studies: BUN, creatinine, renal failure may occur**
• Monitor bowel pattern before, during treatment; if severe abdominal pain or constipation occurs, notify prescriber; monitor hydration
• Assess skin eruptions, rash, urticaria, itching

- Identify allergies before treatment, reaction to each medication
- CBC, blood chemistry, plasma HIV RNA, absolute CD4/CD8 cell counts/%, serum β_2 microglobulin, serum ICD+24 antigen levels, cholesterol
- **Immune reconstitution syndrome: Occurs with combination therapy**

Patient/family education
- **Instruct to notify prescriber if pregnancy is suspected or if breastfeeding**
- **⚠ Advise that pneumonia may occur, to contact prescriber if cough, fever occur**
- Teach that hypersensitive reactions may occur: rash, pruritus; stop product, contact prescriber
- Teach that this product is not a cure for HIV-1 infection but controls symptoms; HIV-1 can still be transmitted to others
- Teach that this product is to be used in combination only with other antiretrovirals
- Teach patient how to prepare and give using subcut injection, watch for site reactions, rotate sites
- **Teach patient that pneumonia may occur; to contact prescriber if cough, fever occur**

Evaluation
Positive therapeutic outcome
- Increased CD4 cell counts; decreased viral load; slowing progression of HIV-1 infection

---

⚠ HIGH ALERT

enoxaparin (Rx)
(ee-nox′a-par-in)
Lovenox
Func. class.: Anticoagulant, antithrombotic
Chem. class.: Unfractionated porcine heparin (low-molecular-weight heparin)
Pregnancy category B

Do not confuse: enoxaparin/enoxacin, Lovenox/Lotronex

ACTION: Binds to antithrombin III inactivating factors Xa/IIa resulting in higher ratio of anti-factor Xa to anti-factor IIa

Therapeutic outcome: Prevention of deep vein thrombosis

USES: Prevention of DVT (inpatient or outpatient), pulmonary emboli (inpatient) in hip and knee replacement, abdominal surgery at risk for thrombosis; unstable angina/non–Q-wave MI, acute MI, coronary artery thrombosis

CONTRAINDICATIONS
Hypersensitivity to this product, heparin, or pork; hemophilia; leukemia with bleeding;

thrombocytopenic purpura, heparin-induced thrombocytopenia, active major bleeding

Precautions: Pregnancy **B**, breastfeeding, children, geriatric, severe renal/hepatic disease, blood dyscrasias, severe hypertension, subacute bacterial endocarditis, acute nephritis, recent burn, spinal surgery, indwelling catheters, low weight (men <57 kg, women <45 kg), hypersensitivity to benzyl alcohol

> **BLACK BOX WARNING:** Lumbar puncture, epidural/spinal anesthesia, aneurysm, coagulopathy

DOSAGE AND ROUTES
DVT/PE prophylaxis
Adult (moderate risk—general surgery, non-surgery 40-60 yr, major surgery <40 yr with no risk factors): SUBCUT 20 mg/day
Adult (higher risk—abdominal surgery, elderly-general surgery, major surgery <40 yr with no risk factors): SUBCUT 30 mg q12hr or 40 mg/day

DVT prevention before hip/knee surgery
Adult: SUBCUT 30 mg bid given 12-24 hr post-operatively for 7-10 days until DVT risk is diminished

DVT prevention before hip replacement
Adult: SUBCUT 40 mg/day started 9-15 hr preop or 30 mg q12hr started 12-24 hr postop, continued until DVT risk is diminished or patient is adequately on anticoagulant

DVT prophylaxis before abdominal surgery
Adult: SUBCUT 40 mg/day × 7-10 days to prevent thromboembolic complications, start 24 hr before surgery

Treatment of DVT/PE
Adult: SUBCUT (outpatient without PE) 1 mg/kg q12hr or 1.5 mg/kg/day (outpatient/inpatient); warfarin should be started within 72 hr and continued ≥5 days until INR is 2-3 (at least 3)

Prevention of ischemic complications in unstable angina/non–Q-wave/non-ST MI with aspirin
Adult: SUBCUT/**IV** 1 mg/kg q12hr until stable with aspirin 100-325 mg/day × ≥2 days

Renal dose
Adult: SUBCUT CCr <30 ml/min: 30 mg q day (thrombosis prophylaxis in abdominal surgery, hip or knee replacement surgery, during acute illness); 1 mg/kg q day (concurrently with aspirin to treat unstable angina

---

or non-Q-wave myocardial infarction); 1 mg/kg q day (STEMI in those ≥75 yrs, 30 mg IV bolus plus 1 mg/kg SC then 1 mg/kg q day (STEMI in those <75 yrs, or 1 mg/kg q day (concurrently with warfarin for inpatient or outpatient treatment of acute deep vein thrombosis (with or without pulmonary embolism)

Available forms: Prefilled syringes/inj 30 mg/0.3 ml, 40 mg/0.4 ml, 60 mg/0.6 ml, 80 mg/0.8 ml, 100 mg/1 ml, 120 mg/0.8 ml, 150 mg/ml; multidose vials 100 mg/ml (3 ml)

Implementation
• Give at same time each day to maintain steady blood levels
SUBCUT route
• Administer SUBCUT deeply; do not give IM, begin 1 hr before surgery, do not aspirate, do not expel bubble from syringe before administration; sol is clear to yellow; do not use sol with precipitate; apply gentle pressure for 1 min, do not use products with benzyl alcohol in pregnant women
• Give to recumbent patient, rotate sites (left/right anterolateral, left/right posterolateral abdominal wall)
• Leave vascular access sheath in place for 6 hr after dose, then give next dose 6 hr after sheath removed

Direct IV route
• Use multidose vial for IV administration; use TB syringe or other graduated syringe to measure dose; give **IV** BOL through **IV** line; flush after
• If withdrawing from multidose vial, use TB syringe for proper measurement
• Prefilled syringes (30, 40 mg) are not graduated; do not use for partial doses
• Do not mix with other products or infusion fluids
⚠ Give only this product when ordered; not interchangeable with heparin or LMWHs

ADVERSE EFFECTS
CNS: Fever, confusion
GI: Nausea
HEMA: **Hemorrhage from any site, hypochromic anemia, thrombocytopenia,** bleeding
INTEG: Ecchymosis, inj site hematoma
META: Hyperkalemia in renal failure
MS: Osteoporosis
SYST: Edema, peripheral edema

Pharmacokinetics
Absorption	Well absorbed (90%)
Distribution	Unknown
Metabolism	Unknown
Excretion	Kidneys
Half-life	4½ hr

Pharmacodynamics
Onset	Unknown
Peak	3-5 hr
Duration	Unknown

INTERACTIONS
Drug classifications
Anticoagulants, antiplatelets, NSAIDs, RU-486, salicylates, thrombolytics: increased bleeding

Drug/herb
Feverfew, garlic, ginger, ginkgo, horse chestnut: increased bleeding risk

Drug/lab test
Increased: AST/ALT
Decreased: platelets

NURSING CONSIDERATIONS
Assessment
• **Monitor antifactor Xa activity in chronic therapy (renal disease)**
• Monitor blood studies (Hct, CBC, coagulation studies, occult blood in stools), anti-Xa levels q3mo; platelet count q2-3day; thrombocytopenia may occur
• **Assess patient for bleeding gums, petechiae, ecchymosis, black tarry stools, hematuria, epistaxis, decrease in B/P; indicate bleeding and possible hemorrhage; notify prescriber immediately**

> **BLACK BOX WARNING:** Assess for neuro-symptoms in patients who have received spinal anesthesia, may develop spinal hematoma, those who have had trauma, spinal surgery are at greater risk

• **Hypersensitivity: Assess for rash, fever, chills, report to prescriber**
• **Neurologic status:** those with epidural catheters are at greater chance for impairments Injection site reactions: Assess for inflammation, redness, hematomas

Patient/family education
• Warn patient to avoid OTC preparations unless directed by prescriber because they could cause serious product interactions
• Instruct patient to use soft-bristled toothbrush to avoid bleeding gums; to avoid contact sports; to use electric razor; to avoid IM inj

---

• Advise patient to report any signs of bleeding, bruising: gums, under skin, urine, stools, dizziness, rash, breathing changes, do not rub injection site

Evaluation
Positive therapeutic outcome
• Absence of DVT/PE

entacapone (Rx)
(en-ta′ka-pone)
Comtan
Func. class.: Antiparkinsonian agent
Chem. class.: COMT
Pregnancy category C

ACTION: Inhibits COMT (catechol *O*-methyltransferase) and alters the plasma pharmacokinetics of levodopa; given with levodopa/carbidopa

Therapeutic outcome: Decreased symptoms of Parkinson's disease (involuntary movements)

USES: Parkinsonism in those experiencing end of dose, decreased effect as an adjunct to levodopa/carbidopa

CONTRAINDICATIONS
Hypersensitivity

Precautions: Pregnancy **C,** breastfeeding, children, renal/hepatic disease, affective disorders, psychosis

DOSAGE AND ROUTES
Adult: PO 200 mg given with carbidopa/levodopa, max 1600 mg/day; may allow 25% dosage reduction in levodopa therapy

Available forms: Tabs 200 mg film coated

Implementation
• Adjust dosage to patient response
• Give with meals to decrease GI upset; limit protein taken with product
• Give only after MAOIs have been discontinued for 2 wk

ADVERSE EFFECTS
CNS: *Involuntary choreiform movements, dyskinesia, hypokinesia, hyperkinesia, hand tremors, fatigue, headache, anxiety, twitching, numbness, weakness, confusion, agitation, nightmares,* psychosis, hallucinations, hypomania, severe depression, dizziness, neuroleptic malignant syndrome
CV: *Orthostatic hypotension*
GI: *Nausea, vomiting, anorexia, abdominal distress, dry mouth, flatulence,* gastritis, GI disorder, *diarrhea, constipation,* bitter taste

INTEG: Rash, sweating, alopecia
MISC: Dark urine and other body fluids, back pain, dyspnea, purpura, fatigue, asthenia, infection-bacterial, rhabdomyolysis

Pharmacokinetics

Absorption	Well absorbed
Distribution	Protein binding 98%
Metabolism	Liver extensively
Excretion	Kidneys, feces; breast milk
Half-life	0.5 hr initial, 2.5 hr second

Pharmacodynamics

Onset	Unknown
Peak	Unknown
Duration	≤8 hr

INTERACTIONS
Individual drugs
Ampicillin, chloramphenicol, erythromycin, probenecid, rifampin: decreased excretion of entacapone
Bitolterol, DOBUTamine, DOPamine, EPHINEPHrine, isoetharine, methyldopa, norepinephrine: increased CV reactions; avoid use

Drug classifications
MAOIs: prevent catecholamine metabolism; do not use together

Drug/herb
Kava: decreased effect
Ma huang: increased B/P

NURSING CONSIDERATIONS
Assessment
• Assess for neuroleptic malignant syndrome: high temp, increased CPK, rigidity, change in consciousness, usually during rapid withdrawal
• Monitor B/P, respiration during initial treatment; hypotension should be reported
• Assess mental status: affect, mood, behavioral changes, depression; complete suicide assessment
• Monitor liver function enzymes: AST, ALT, alkaline phosphatase; also check LDH, bilirubin, CBC
• Assess for involuntary movements in parkinsonism: akinesia, tremors, staggering gait, muscle rigidity, drooling; these symptoms should improve with therapy when given with levodopa/carbidopa
• Rhabdomyolysis: Assess for muscle pain, tenderness, weakness, swelling of affected muscles, may lead to decreased B/P, shock

Patient/family education
• Advise patient that hallucinations, mental changes, nausea, dyskinesia can occur
• Caution patient to change positions slowly to prevent orthostatic hypotension; not to drive

or operate machinery until stabilized on medication and mental performance is not affected
• Instruct patient to use product exactly as prescribed; if dose is missed, take as soon as remembered, up to 2 hr before next dose, not to discontinue abruptly, withdraw gradually
• Inform patient that urine, sweat may darken
• Instruct patient to notify prescriber if pregnancy is suspected; if breastfeeding, product is excreted in breast milk

Evaluation
Positive therapeutic outcome
• Decreased akathisia, other involuntary movements when used with levodopa/carbidopa
• Increased mood when used with levodopa/carbidopa

---

entecavir (Rx)
(en-te′ka-veer)
Baraclude
Func. class.: Antiretroviral nucleoside reverse transcriptase inhibitors (NRTIs)
Chem. class.: Guanosine nucleoside analog
Pregnancy category C

ACTION: Inhibits hepatitis B virus DNA polymerase by competing with natural substrates and by causing DNA termination after its incorporation into viral DNA; causes viral DNA death

Therapeutic outcome: Improved liver function tests in chronic hepatitis B (HBV)

USES: Chronic hepatitis B (HBV)

CONTRAINDICATIONS
Hypersensitivity

Precautions: Pregnancy **C**, breastfeeding, child, geriatric, severe renal disease, liver transplant

> BLACK BOX WARNING: Hepatic disease, hepatitis, lactic acidosis, HIV

DOSAGE AND ROUTES
Chronic hepatitis B (nucleoside treatment–naive)
Adult and adolescent ≥16 yr: PO tab 0.5 mg/day
Adult: PO (solution) 0.5 mg qday
Child/adolescent ≥2 yr, >30 kg: 0.5 mg (10 mL) qday
Child ≥2 yr, 27 to 30 kg: 0.45 mg (9 mL) qday
Child ≥2 yr, 24 to 26 kg: 0.4 mg (8 mL) qday
Child ≥2 yr, 21 to 23 kg: 0.35 mg (7 mL) qday
Child ≥2 yr, 18 to 20 kg: 0.3 mg (6 mL) qday
Child ≥2 yr, 15 to 17 kg: 0.25 mg (5 mL) qday
Child ≥2 yr, 12 to 14 kg: 0.2 mg (4 mL) qday
Child ≥2 yr: 0.15 mg (3 mL) qday

Chronic hepatitis B with compensated liver disease and history of hepatitis B viremia, while receiving lamiVUDine/telbivudine or known lamiVUDine resistance mutations
Adult and adolescent ≥16 yr: PO tab 1 mg/day
Adult: PO (solution) 1 mg qday
Child/adolescent ≥2 yr, >30 kg: 1 mg (20 mL) qday
Child ≥2 yr, 27 to 30 kg: 0.9 mg (18 mL) qday
Child ≥2 yr, 24 to 26 kg: 0.8 mg (16 mL) qday
Child ≥2 yr, 21 to 23 kg: 0.7 mg (14 mL)
Child ≥2 yr, 18 to 20 kg: 0.6 mg (12 mL) qday
Child ≥2 yr, 15 to 17 kg: 0.5 mg (10 mL) qday
Child ≥2 yr, 12 to 14 kg: 0.4 mg (8 mL) qday
Child ≥2 yr, 10 to 11 kg: 0.3 mg (6 mL) qday

Renal dose
Adult: PO CCr ≥50 ml/min 0.5 mg/day; CCr 30-49 ml/min 0.25 mg daily, 0.5 mg/day or 1 mg q48hr for lamiVUDine refractory patient; CCr 10-29 ml/min 0.15/day, 0.3 for lamiVUDine refractory patient; CCr <10 ml/min 0.05 mg PO/day, 0.1 mg/day or 1 mg q7days for lamiVUDine refractory patient

Available forms: Tabs, film coated 0.5, 1 mg; oral sol 0.05 mg/ml

Implementation
• After hemodialysis give by mouth on empty stomach 2 hr before or after food
• Tabs: Store at room temperature
• Oral liquid: Use calibrated oral dosing spoon provided, may be used interchangeably with tabs, do not dilute
• Store in cool environment; protect from light

ADVERSE EFFECTS
CNS: *Headache*, fatigue, dizziness, insomnia
ENDO: Hyperglycemia
GI: *Dyspepsia*, nausea, vomiting, diarrhea, elevated liver function enzymes, **hepatotoxicity with steatosis**
INTEG: Alopecia, rash
SYST: Lactic acidosis

Pharmacokinetics

Absorption	100%
Distribution	Extensively to tissues, protein binding 13%
Metabolism	Unknown
Excretion	Unchanged 62%-73% via kidneys
Half-life	Terminal 128-149 hr

Pharmacodynamics

Onset	Unknown
Peak	0.5-1.5 hr
Duration	Unknown

Adverse effects: *italics* = common; **bold** = life-threatening

INTERACTIONS
Drug/food
High-fat meal: decreased absorption

Drug/lab test
Increased: ALT, AST, total bilirubin, amylase, lipase, creatinine, blood glucose, urine glucose
Decreased: platelets, albumin

NURSING CONSIDERATIONS
Assessment

> **BLACK BOX WARNING:** Assess for HIV before beginning treatment because HIV resistance may occur in patients with chronic hepatitis B infection; monitor HIV RNA

> **BLACK BOX WARNING:** Assess for lactic acidosis and severe hepatomegaly with stenosis: increased serum lactate, increased hepatic enzymes, palpate liver; discontinue product if these occur

• Monitor geriatric patients more carefully; may develop renal, cardiac symptoms more rapidly

> **BLACK BOX WARNING:** Assess for exacerbations of hepatitis (jaundice, pruritus, fatigue, anorexia) after discontinuing treatment; and for several months monitor liver function tests

Patient/family education
• Teach patient not to take with food
• Teach patient to take exactly as prescribed, read the "Patient Information," take missed dose when remembered unless close to time of next dose, that compliance with dosage schedule is required, do not share product
• Advise patient not to stop medication without approval of prescriber
• Advise that optimal duration of treatment is unknown
• Teach patient to avoid use with other medications, supplements unless approved by prescriber
• Teach patient to notify prescriber of decreased urinary output, blood in urine

> **BLACK BOX WARNING: Teach patient symptoms of lactic acidosis:** muscle pain, severe tiredness, weakness, trouble breathing, stomach pain with nausea/vomiting, coldness in arms/legs, fast/irregular heartbeat, dizziness

> **BLACK BOX WARNING: Teach patient symptoms of hepatotoxicity:** eyes/skin turns yellow, dark urine, light bowel movements, no appetite for days, nausea, stomach pain

• Advise patient that product does not cure, but lowers the amount of HBV in body
• Teach patient that product does not stop the spreading of HBV to others by sex, sharing needles, or being exposed to blood
• Teach patient to notify prescriber if pregnancy is planned or suspected, not to breastfeed
• Teach patient not to operate machinery until effect is known, dizziness may occur
• Inform patient that regular follow-up and lab tests will be needed

Evaluation
Positive therapeutic outcome
• Decreased symptoms of chronic hepatitis B, improving liver function tests

RARELY USED

enzalutamide
(en-zal-u′ta-mide)
Xtandi
Func. class.: Antineoplastic hormone
Chem. class.: Nonsteroidal antiandrogen
Pregnancy category X

Therapeutic outcome: Decreased tumor size, decreased spread of malignancy

USES: Metastatic castration-resistant prostate cancer in those who have received DOCETaxel

CONTRAINDICATIONS
Pregnancy (**X**), women, hypersensitivity

DOSAGE AND ROUTES
Adult: PO 160 mg (4 × 40-mg caps) daily
If a patient experiences a grade 3 or higher toxicity or an intolerable adverse effect, withhold dosing for 1 wk or until symptoms improve to grade 2 or less, then resume at the same or a reduced dosage (120 or 80 mg), if warranted
The concomitant use of strong cytochrome P450 (CYP-450) 2C8 inhibitors should be avoided if possible; if a strong CYP2C8 inhibitor must be coadministered, reduce the enzalutamide dosage to 80 mg once daily

Available forms: Tabs 40 mg

epinastine ophthalmic
See Appendix B

A HIGH ALERT

EPINEPHrine (Rx, OTC)
(ep-i-nef´rin)
**Adrenaclick, Primatene Mist,
Twinject, Walgreens Bronchial Mist**
EPINEPHrine HCI
Adrenalin, EpiPen, EpiPen Jr.
Func. class.: Bronchodilator, nonselective
adrenergic agonist, cardiac stimulant,
vasopressor
Chem. class.: Catecholamine
Pregnancy category C

Do not confuse: EPINEPHrine/ePHEDrine

ACTION: β_1- and β_2-agonist causing increased levels of cyclic AMP producing bronchodilatation, cardiac and CNS stimulation; large doses cause vasoconstriction via α-receptors; small doses can cause vasodilation via β_2-vascular receptors

Therapeutic outcome: Vasoconstrictor, cardiac stimulator, bronchodilator, decreased aqueous humor

USES: Acute asthmatic attacks, hemostasis, bronchospasm, anaphylaxis, allergic reactions, cardiac arrest, adjunct in anesthesia, shock

CONTRAINDICATIONS
Hypersensitivity to sympathomimetics, sulfites, closed-angle glaucoma, nonanaphylactic shock during general anesthesia

Precautions: Pregnancy **C**, breastfeeding, cardiac disorders, hyperthyroidism, diabetes mellitus, prostatic hypertrophy, hypertension, organic brain syndrome, local anesthesia of certain areas, labor, cardiac dilatation, coronary insufficiency, cerebral arteriosclerosis, organic heart disease

DOSAGE AND ROUTES
Anaphylaxis/severe asthma exacerbation
Adult: IM/SUBCUT 0.3-0.5 mg, may repeat q10-15min (anaphylaxis) or q20min-4 hr (asthma)

Severe allergic reactions type 1
Adult/child ≥30 kg: IM 0.3 mg (EpiPen/EpiPen 2-Pak, 1:1000)

Child <30 kg: IM 0.15 mg (EpiPen Jr/EpiPen Jr 2-Pak 1:2000)

Adult/child ≥66 lb: IM/SUBCUT 0.3 mg (0.3 ml) initially (Twinject 1.1 ml 1:1000, 1 mg/ml, containing 2 doses of 0.3 mg)

Adult/child 33-66 lb: IM/SUBCUT 0.15 mg (0.15 ml) initially, may give another 0.15 mg after 10 min (Twinject 1.1 ml 1:1000 [1 mg/ml] containing 2 doses of 0.15 mg)

Status asthmaticus
Adult/adolescent: SUBCUT 0.3-0.5 mg (0.3-0.5 ml of the 1:1000 injection) q20min ×3 doses

Child/infant: SUBCUT 0.01 mg/kg-0.5 mg q20min ×3 doses

Available forms: Nasal spray (sol) 1 mg/ml; sol for inj 1 mg/ml; 1:10,000, 1:1000; inh vapor (sol) 0.22 mg/actuation; pressurized inh (sol) 0.22 mg/actuation; sol for inj 0.15 mg/0.15 ml autoinjector, 0.3 mg/0.3 ml autoinjector, 0.15 mg/0.3 ml

Implementation
• Give subcut, IM, intraosseously, IV; suspensions are for subcut use only; do not give IV
• Visually inspect parenteral products for particulate matter and discoloration prior to use; do not use solutions that are pinkish to brownish in color or contain a precipitate
• **Avoid extravasation during parenteral administration; if extravasation occurs, infiltrate the affected area with phentolamine diluted in NS**
• **Death has occurred from drug errors; make sure the right concentration is used**
• Store reconstituted sol refrigerated 24 hr

Direct IV injection route
• Inject EPINEPHrine directly into a vein over 5-10 min for adults or 1-3 min for children; may be given IV push in cardiac arrest
• In neonates, may administer via the umbilical vein
• During adult cardiopulmonary resuscitation (CPR): resuscitation drugs may be given IV by bolus injection into a peripheral vein, followed by an injection of 20 ml IV fluid; elevate the extremity for 10-20 sec to facilitate drug delivery to the central circulation
Continuous IV infusion route
• Dilute 1 mg EPINEPHrine in 250 or 500 ml of a compatible IV infusion solution to provide a concentration of 4 or 2 mcg/ml, respectively; give into a large vein, if possible
• More concentrated solutions (16-32 mcg/ml) may be used in fluid-restricted patients when administered through a central line

IM route
• EPINEPHrine injection should preferably be into the deltoid or anterior thigh (vastus lateralis); do not administer into the gluteal muscle
• Twinject is light-sensitive and should be stored in the carrying case provided; do not refrigerate; protect from freezing; replace if solution is discolored or contains a precipitate
Subcut route
• Inject taking care not to inject intradermally
• Massage injection site well after use to

enhance absorption and to decrease local vaso-constriction; injection can cause tissue irritation

Intraosseous infusion route (unlabeled)
• During CPR, the same EPINEPHrine dosage may be given via the intraosseous route when IV access is not available

Intracardiac route
• Should be reserved for extreme emergencies. Intracardiac injection should only be performed by properly trained medical personnel

Inhalation route
• Use 2.25% sol diluted in nebulizer/respirator
• Rinse mouth after inh
• 10 drops of a 1% sol should be placed in nebulizer
• Dilute racepinephrine 2.25% sol

Endotracheal route
• Per the ACLS or PALS guidelines, the EPI-NEPHrine parenteral product is administered via this route
• Endotracheal (ET) administration should only be used if access to IV or intraosseous routes is not possible
• **Adult:** Dilute dose in 5-10 ml NS or sterile distilled water; administer via ET tube; endo-tracheal absorption of EPINEPHrine may be improved by diluting with water instead of NS
• **Child:** After dose administration, flush the ET tube with a minimum of 5 ml NS

Y-site compatibilities: Alfentanil, amikacin, amiodarone, amphotericin B liposome, anidulafun-gin, ascorbic acid, atracurium, aztreonam, benztro-pine, bivalirudin, bleomycin, bumetanide, bu-prenorphine, butorphanol, calcium chloride/gluconate, CARBOplatin, caspofungin, ceFAZolin, cefotaxime, cefoTEtan, cefOXitin, cefTAZidime, ceftizoxime, cefTRIAXone, cefuroxime, chloram-phenicol, chlorproMAZINE, cimetidine, cisatracu-rium, CISplatin, clindamycin, cyanocobalamin, cy-clophosphamide, cycloSPORINE, cytarabine, DACTINomycin, DAPTOmycin, dexamethasone, dexmedetomidine, digoxin, diltiazem, diphenhydr-AMINE, DOBUTamine, DOCEtaxel, DOPamine, DOXOrubicin, doxycycline, enalaprilat, epirubicin, epoetin alfa, ertapenem, erythromycin, esmolol, et-oposide, etoposide phosphate, famotidine, fenoldo-pam, fentaNYL, fluconazole, fludarabine, folic acid, furosemide, gemcitabine, gentamicin, glycopyrro-late, granisetron, heparin, hydrocortisone, HYDRO-morphone, ifosfamide, imipenem/cilastatin, isopro-terenol, ketorolac, labetalol, levofloxacin, lidocaine, linezolid, LORazepam, magnesium sulfate, manni-tol, mechlorethamine, meperidine, metaraminol, methicillin, methotrexate, methoxamine, methyl-dopa, methylPREDNISolone, metoclopramide, metoprolol, metroNIDAZOLE, midazolam, milri-none, minocycline, mitoXANtrone, morphine, multiple vitamins, nafcillin, nalbuphine, naloxone, niCARDipine, nitroglycerin, nitroprusside, norepi-nephrine, octreotide, ondansetron, oxacillin, oxali-platin, oxytocin, PACLitaxel, palonosetron, pan-curonium, pantoprazole, PEMEtrexed, penicillin G potassium, pentamidine, pentazocine, phentol-amine, phenylephrine, phytonadione, piperacillin-tazobactam, potassium chloride, procainamide, prochlorperazine, promethazine, propofol, pro-pranolol, protamine, pyridoxime, quinupristin/dal-fopristin, ranitidine, remifentanil, ritodrine, ro-curonium, sodium acetate, streptomycin, succinylcholine, SUFentanil, tacrolimus, teniposide, theophylline, thiamine, thiotepa, ticarcillin/clavula-nate, tigecycline, tirofiban, tobramycin, tolazoline, trimethaphan, urokinase, vancomycin, vasopressin, vecuronium, verapamil, vinCRIStine, vinorelbine, vitamin B complex with C, voriconazole, warfarin, zoledronic acid

Y-site incompatibilities: Acyclovir, ami-nophylline, azaTHIOprine, carmustine, cephapi-rin, dantrolene, diazepam, diazoxide, fluoroura-cil, ganciclovir, gemtuzumab, indomethacin, micafungin, PENTobarbital, PHENobarbital, phe-nytoin, sodium bicarbonate, thiopental, sulfa-methoxazole/trimethoprim

ADVERSE EFFECTS
CNS: *Tremors, anxiety,* insomnia, headache, dizziness, weakness, drowsiness, confusion, hal-lucinations, cerebral hemorrhage
CV: *Palpitations, tachycardia,* hypertension, *dysrhythmias,* increased T wave
GI: *Anorexia, nausea, vomiting*
MISC: Sweating, dry eyes
RESP: *Dyspnea,* paradoxical broncho-spasm (inhalation)
META: Hypoglycemia

Pharmacokinetics

Absorption	Well absorbed (PO), com-plete (**IV**)
Distribution	Unknown, crosses placenta
Metabolism	Liver
Excretion	Breast milk
Half-life	Unknown

Pharmacodynamics

	SUB-CUT	IM	IV	INH
Onset	3-5 min	Variable	Imme-diate	1 min
Peak	Un-known	Un-known	Un-known	Un-known
Duration	1-4 hr	1-4 hr	Un-known	1-4 hr

INTERACTIONS
Drug classifications

β-Adrenergic blockers: decreased hypertensive effects, stop β blocker 3 days before starting product

Antidepressants (tricyclics): increased chance of hypertensive crisis; do not use together

MAOIs: increased chance of hypertensive crisis, do not use together

Other sympathomimetics: toxicity

α blockers: Increase: hypotension-antihistamines, thyroid replacement hormones: Increased: cardiac effects

Cardiac glycosides: Increase: dysrhythmias

NURSING CONSIDERATIONS
Assessment

• **Asthma:** Monitor respiratory function: vital capacity, forced expiratory volume, ABGs, lung sounds, heart rate, rhythm (baseline); amount, color of sputum

• **Vasopressor: Monitor ECG during administration continuously; if B/P increases, product should be decreased; check B/P, pulse q5min after parenteral route; CVP, PCWP, SVR; inadvertent high arterial B/P can result in angina, aortic rupture, cerebral hemorrhage**

• Check inj site for tissue sloughing; if this occurs, administer phentolamine mixed with 0.9% NaCl

• **Monitor for evidence of allergic reactions, paradoxical bronchospasm: (swelling of face/lips/eyelids, rash, difficulty breathing) withhold dose, notify prescriber; sulfite sensitivity, which may be life threatening**

Patient/family education

• Tell patient not to use OTC medications; extra stimulation may occur; to use this medication before other medications and allow at least 5 min between each, to prevent overstimulation

• Teach patient that paradoxical bronchospasm may occur and to stop product immediately and notify prescriber; to limit caffeine products such as chocolate, coffee, tea, and colas

• Patient should rinse mouth after inh

• Patient should report blurred vision, irritation with ophth preparations

Evaluation
Positive therapeutic outcome

• Absence of dyspnea, wheezing

• Improved airway exchange, improved ABGs

• Decreased aqueous humor

• Stabilization of heart rate and cardiac output

TREATMENT OF OVERDOSE:

Administer a β₂-adrenergic blocker, vasodilators, α-blocker

EPINEPHrine nasal agent
See Appendix B

⚠ HIGH ALERT

epirubicin (Rx)
(ep-i-roo′bi-sin)

Ellence, Pharmorubicin ✣

Func. class.: Antineoplastic, antibiotic

Chem. class.: Anthracycline

Pregnancy category D

Do not confuse: epirubicin/DOXOrubicin/DAUNOrubicin/eribulin/IDArubicin

ACTION: Inhibits DNA synthesis primarily; replication is decreased by binding to DNA, which causes strand splitting; maximum cytotoxic effects at S and G_2 phases; a vesicant

Therapeutic outcome: Prevention of rapidly growing malignant cells

USES: Breast cancer as an adjuvant therapy, with axillary node involvement, after resection

Unlabeled uses: Used in combination for treatment of advanced forms of cancer

CONTRAINDICATIONS

Pregnancy **D**, breastfeeding, hypersensitivity to this product, anthracyclines, anthracenediones, baseline neutrophil count <1500 cell/mm³, severe myocardial insufficiency, recent MI, heart failure, cardiomyopathy

> **BLACK BOX WARNING:** Severe hepatic disease, IM/subcut

Precautions: Children, geriatric, renal/hepatic/cardiac disease, previous anthracycline use, accidental exposure, angina, dental disease, herpes, hyperkalemia, hyperphosphatemia, hypertension, hyperuricemia, hypocalcemia, infection, infertility, tumor lysis syndrome, ventricular dysfunction

> **BLACK BOX WARNING:** Bone marrow suppression (severe), heart failure, extravasation, secondary malignancy, requires an experienced clinician

DOSAGE AND ROUTES
Breast cancer with axillary node involvement following resection of the primary tumor in combination with cyclophosphamide and fluorouracil

Adult: IV 100 mg/m² on day 1 with fluorouracil and cyclophosphamide (FEC regimen) q21 days × 6 cycles or 60 mg/m² on days 1 and 8 with oral cyclophosphamide and fluorouracil q28 days × 6 cycles

---

Breast cancer in combination with cyclophosphamide

Adult: IV 60 mg/m^2 day 1 with cyclophosphamide (500 mg/m^2 IV day 1), repeated q21 days × 8 cycles, or a higher-dose regimen of epirubicin 100 mg/m^2 IV day 1 with cyclophosphamide (830 mg/m^2 IV day 1), q21 days × 8 cycles

Dosage adjustments based upon hematologic and non-hematologic toxicities:
Nadir platelet counts <50,000/mm^3, absolute neutrophil counts (ANC) <250/mm^3, neutropenic fever, or Grades 3/4 non-hematologic toxicities: Day 1 dose in subsequent cycles should be reduced by 25% of the previous dose

For patients receiving divided-dose epirubicin (i.e., day 1 and 8): Day 8 dose should be reduced by 25% of the day 1 dose if the platelet counts are 75,000-100,000/mm^3 and the ANC is 1000-1499/mm^3; if day 8 platelet counts are <75,000/mm^3, ANC <1000/mm^3, or Grade 3/4 nonhematologic toxicity has occurred, omit the day 8 dose

Hepatic dose

Adult: IV Bilirubin 1.2-3 mg/dl or AST 2-4 × normal upper limit, 50% of starting dose; bilirubin >3 mg/dl or AST >4 × normal upper limit, 25% of starting dose

Available forms: Inj (2 mg/ml) 10 mg/5 ml, 50 mg/25 ml, 150 mg/75 ml, 200 mg/100 ml

Implementation

• Avoid contact with skin; very irritating; wash completely to remove; give fluids **IV** or PO before chemotherapy to hydrate patient
• Give antiemetic 30-60 min before giving product to prevent vomiting and prn
• Administer prophylactic antibiotic with a fluoroquinolone or trimethoprim/sulfamethoxazole if dose of epirubicin is 120 mg/m^2
• Provide liquid diet: carbonated beverages; gelatin may be added if patient is not nauseated or vomiting; monitor electrolytes

> **BLACK BOX WARNING:** To be used by a clinician experienced in giving cytotoxic products

> **BLACK BOX WARNING:** Do not use IM/subcut due to severe tissue necrosis

> **BLACK BOX WARNING:** Give IV, only; subcut; a vesicant: if extravasation occurs, stop and complete via another vein, preferably in another limb; avoid infusion into veins over joints or in extremities with compromised venous or lymphatic drainage

• Rapid injection may cause facial flushing or erythema along the vein; avoid administration time of less than 3 min
• **Product should be given to those with neutrophils ≥1500/mm^3, platelet count ≥100,000/mm^3, and non-hematologic toxicities recovered to ≤Grade 1**
• When refrigerated, the preservative-free, ready-to-use solution may form a gelled product; and will return to solution after 2-4 hr at room temperature
• Visually inspect for particulate matter and discoloration prior to use

IV route

• Product should be prepared by experienced personnel using proper precautions; pregnant women must not handle product
• Reconstitute 50 mg and 200 mg powder for injection vials with 25 ml and 100 ml, respectively, of sterile water for injection (2 mg/ml), shake vigorously for up to 4 min; reconstituted solutions are stable for 24 hr when stored refrigerated and protected from light or at room temperature in normal light
• Solution can be further diluted with sterile water for injection

IV injection route

• Give doses of 100-120 mg/m^2 into tubing of a freely flowing 0.9% sodium chloride (NS) or D$_5$W IV infusion over 15-20 min; the infusion time may be decreased, proportionally, in those who require lower doses; infusion times <3 min are not recommended
• Direct injection into the vein is not recommended due to the risk of extravasation; avoid use with any solution of alkaline pH as hydrolysis will occur

IV infusion route

• Dilute dose in 0.9% sodium chloride (NS) or D$_5$W; infuse over 30-60 min
• Avoid use with any solution of alkaline pH as hydrolysis will occur

Y-site compatibilities: Alemtuzumab, alfentanil, amifostine, amikacin, aminocaproic acid, anidulafungin, argatroban, atracurium, aztreonam, bivalirudin, bleomycin, bumetanide, buprenorphine, butorphanol, calcium chloride/gluconate, CARBOplatin, caspofungin, ceFAZolin, cefotaxime, ceftizoxime, chlorproMAZINE, cimetidine, ciprofloxacin, cisatracurium, CISplatin, clindamycin, cyclophosphamide, cycloSPORINE, DAPTOmycin, dexrazoxane, digoxin, diltiazem, diphenhydrAMINE, DOBUTamine, DOCEtaxel, dolasetron, DOPamine, doxacurium, doxycycline, droperidol, enalaprilat, ePHEDrine, EPINEPHrine, ertapenem, erythromycin, etoposide, famotidine, fenoldopam, fentaNYL, fluconazole, gatifloxacin, gemcitabine, gentamicin, granisetron, haloperidol, hydrocortisone, HYDROmorphone, hydrOXYzine, ifosfamide, imipenem-cilastatin, inamrinone, insulin (regular), isoproterenol, labetalol, levofloxacin, levorphanol, lidocaine, linezolid, LORazepam, mannitol, meperidine, mesna, methotrexate, metoclopramide, metoprolol, metroNIDAZOLE, midazolam, milrinone, minocycline, mitoMYcin, mivacurium, morphine, moxifloxacin, nalbuphine, naloxone, nesiritide, niCARdipine, nitroglycerin, nitroprusside, norepinephrine, octreotide, ofloxacin, ondansetron, oxaliplatin, PACLitaxel, palonosetron, pamidronate, pancuronium, pentamidine, pentazocine, phenylephrine, potassium chloride, procainamide, prochlorperazine, promethazine, propranolol, quinupristin-dalfopristin, ranitidine, remifentanil, rocuronium, sodium acetate, succinylcholine, SUFentanil, tacrolimus, teniposide, theophylline, thiotepa, tigecycline, tirofiban, tobramycin, trimethobenzamide, vancomycin, vasopressin, vecuronium, verapamil, vinBLAStine, vinCRIStine, vinorelbine, voriconazole, zidovudine, zoledronic acid

Y-site incompatibilities: Acyclovir, allopurinol, aminophylline, amphotericin B colloidal, amphotericin B lipid complex, amphotericin B liposome, ampicillin, ampicillin/sulbactam, azithromycin, cefepime, cefoperazone, cefoTEtan, cefOXitin, cefTAZidime, cefTRIAXone, cefuroxime, dexamethasone, diazepam, ertapenem, fluorouracil, foscarnet, fosphenytoin, furosemide, ganciclovir, gemtuzumab, heparin, hydrocortisone, ketorolac, leucovorin, magnesium sulfate, meropenem, methohexital, methylPREDNISolone, nafcillin, pantoprazole, PEMEtrexed, PENTobarbital, PHENobarbital, phenytoin, piperacillin/tazobactam, potassium phosphates, sodium bicarbonate, sodium phosphates, thiopental, ticarcillin/clavulanate, tigecycline, sulfamethoxazole/trimethoprim

ADVERSE EFFECTS
CV: Increased B/P, **sinus tachycardia, PVCs,** chest pain, **bradycardia, extrasystole,** cardiomyopathy
GI: Nausea, vomiting, diarrhea, anorexia, mucositis
GU: *Hot flashes, amenorrhea, hyperuricemia,* red urine
HEMA: **Thrombocytopenia, leukopenia, anemia, neutropenia, secondary AML**
INTEG: *Rash, necrosis, pain at inj site, reversible alopecia*
MISC: Infection, febrile neutropenia, lethargy, fever, conjunctivitis, tumor lysis syndrome

Pharmacokinetics

Absorption	Complete bioavailability
Distribution	Widely distributed, crosses placenta
Metabolism	Liver, extensively
Excretion	Bile (60%)
Half-life	3 min; 1hr; 30 hr

Pharmacodynamics
Unknown

INTERACTIONS
Individual drugs
Cimetidine, radiation: increased toxicity
PACLitaxel: give epirubicin before PACLitaxel if given concurrently
Trastuzumab: increased ventricular dysfunction, CHF

Drug classifications
Antineoplastics: increased toxicity
Calcium channel blockers: increased heart failure
Live virus vaccines: decreased antibody response

NURSING CONSIDERATIONS
Assessment

> **BLACK BOX WARNING: Heart failure:** monitor left ventricular ejection fraction, multigated acquisition scan or echocardiogram, ECG; watch for ST-T wave changes, low QRS and T; possible dysrhythmias (sinus tachycardia, heart block, PVCs) may occur; assess tachypnea, ECG changes, dyspnea, edema, fatigue; cardiac status: B/P, pulse, character, rhythm, rate, ABGs; identify cumulative amount of anthracycline received (lifetime)

• **Assess symptoms indicating severe allergic reaction: rash, pruritus, urticaria, purpuric skin lesions, itching, flushing; product should be discontinued**

> **BLACK BOX WARNING: Bone marrow depression (severe):** monitor CBC, differential, platelet count weekly; withhold product if baseline neutrophil count is <1500/mm³; notify prescriber of results if WBC <20,000/mm³, platelets <150,000/mm³; leukocyte nadir occurs 10-14 days after administration; recovery by 21st day

• Infection: treat before receiving this product in regimens >120 mg/m²; prophylactic antibiotics should be given (trimethoprim-sulfamethoxazole or a quinolone)

• Assess for increased uric acid levels, swelling, joint pain, primarily extremities; patient should be well hydrated to prevent urate deposits
• Monitor renal function studies: BUN, creatinine, serum uric acid, urine CCr before, during therapy; I&O ratio; report fall in urine output to <30 ml/hr; dosage adjustment is needed for serum creatinine >5 mg/dl

> **BLACK BOX WARNING: Severe hepatic disease:** monitor liver function tests before, during therapy (bilirubin, AST, ALT, LDH) as needed or monthly; note jaundice of skin or sclera, dark urine, clay-colored stools, itchy skin, abdominal pain, fever, diarrhea

• Assess for bleeding: hematuria, stool guaiac, bruising or petechiae, mucosa or orifices q8hr; inflammation of mucosa, breaks in skin
• Identify effects of alopecia on body image; discuss feelings about body changes

> **BLACK BOX WARNING: Extravasation (vesicant):** Assess for local irritation, pain, burning, necrosis at injection site; discontinue and start at another site

Patient/family education
• Advise patient to avoid use of products containing aspirin or NSAIDs, razors, commercial mouthwash, since bleeding may occur; to report symptoms of bleeding (hematuria, tarry stools)
• Instruct patient to report signs of anemia (fatigue, headache, irritability, faintness, shortness of breath)
• Inform patient that hair may be lost during treatment; a wig or hairpiece may make patient feel better; new hair may be different in color, texture, new hair growth occurs in ≤3 mo after treatment
• Caution patient not to have any vaccinations without the advice of the prescriber; serious reactions can occur

> **BLACK BOX WARNING:** Teach patient that irreversible myocardial damage, leukopenia, menopause may occur

⚠ Advise patient to use contraception during treatment and 4 mo afterward; pregnancy D
• Advise patient that urine may be red for 2 days
• Instruct patient to avoid crowds, persons with known infection
• Caution patient to avoid OTC medications, supplements unless approved by prescriber

• Teach patient to report rapid heartbeat, trouble breathing, fever, nausea, vomiting, oral sores
• To report pain at site immediately

Evaluation
Positive therapeutic outcome
• Prevention of rapid division of malignant cells

eplerenone (Rx)
(ep-ler-ee′known)
Inspra
Func. class.: Antihypertensive
Pregnancy category B

Do not confuse: Inspra/Spiriva

ACTION: Binds to mineralocorticoid receptor and blocks the binding of aldosterone, a component of the renin-angiotensin-aldosterone system (RAAS)

Therapeutic outcome: Absence of hypertension

USES: Hypertension, alone or in combination with thiazide diuretics, CHF, post-MI

CONTRAINDICATIONS
Hypersensitivity, increased serum creatinine >2 mg/dl (male) or >1.8 mg/dl (female), potassium >5.5 mEq/L, type 2 diabetes with microalbuminuria, hepatic disease, CCr <30 ml/min, CCr <50 ml/min in hypertension

Precautions: Pregnancy **B**, breastfeeding, children, geriatric, impaired renal/hepatic function, hyperkalemia

DOSAGE AND ROUTES
Hypertension
Adult: PO 50 mg/day initially, may increase to 50 mg bid after 4 wk; start dose at 25 mg/day if patient is taking CYP3A4 inhibitors

CHF/post-MI
Adult: PO 25 mg/day initially, may increase to 50 mg/day max

Available forms: Tabs 25, 50 mg

Implementation
• Store in tight container at 86° F (30° C) or less

ADVERSE EFFECTS
CNS: Headache, *dizziness, fatigue*
CV: Angina, **MI**
GI: Increased GGT *diarrhea,* abdominal pain, increased ALT
GU: Gynecomastia, mastodynia (males), abnormal vaginal bleeding

---

META: *Hyperkalemia,* hyponatremia, hypercholesteremia, hypertriglyceridemia, increased uric acid
RESP: *Cough*

Pharmacokinetics

Absorption	Unknown
Distribution	Protein binding 50%
Metabolism	Liver (CYP3A4)
Excretion	Urine, feces
Half-life	4-6 hr

Pharmacodynamics

Onset	Unknown
Peak	1½ hr
Duration	Unknown

INTERACTIONS
Individual drugs
Clarithromycin, imatinib, nelfinavir, nefazodone, ritonavir, troleandomycin: do not use concurrently
Erythromycin, fluconazole, verapamil: reduce dose of eplerenone; increased eplerenone levels
Itraconazole, ketoconazole, saquinavir, verapamil: increased levels of eplerenone; reduce dose of eplerenone
Lithium: increased serum lithium levels

Drug classifications
ACE inhibitors, angiotensin II antagonists, diuretics (potassium-sparing), NSAIDs, potassium supplements: increased hyperkalemia
CYP3A4 inhibitors: increased levels of eplerenone; reduce dose of eplerenone
NSAIDs: decreased antihypertensive effect

Drug/herb
Decreased antihypertensive effect: ephedra

Drug/food
Grapefruit, grapefruit juice: increased product level by 25%
• Do not use salt substitutes with potassium

Drug/lab test
Increased: BUN, creatinine, potassium, cholesterol, lipids, uric acid
Decreased: sodium

NURSING CONSIDERATIONS
Assessment
• **Hypertension:** monitor B/P at peak/trough level of product, orthostatic hypotension, syncope when used with diuretic
• Monitor renal studies: protein, BUN, creatinine; increased liver function tests; uric acid may be increased

• Monitor potassium levels, hyperkalemia may occur

Patient/family education
• Advise patient not to discontinue product abruptly
• Advise patient not to use OTC products (cough, cold, allergy) unless directed by prescriber; do not use salt substitutes containing potassium without consulting prescriber
• Teach patient the importance of complying with dosage schedule, even if feeling better
• Teach patient that product may cause dizziness, fainting, light-headedness; may occur during first few days of therapy
• Teach patient how to take B/P, normal readings for age group
• Teach patient to avoid activities that require coordination

Evaluation
Positive therapeutic outcome
• Decrease in B/P

⚠ HIGH ALERT

epoetin alfa (Rx)
(ee-poe′e-tin)
Epogen, Eprex ✦, Procrit
Func. class.: Antianemic, biologic modifier, hormone
Chem. class.: Amino acid polypeptide
Pregnancy category C

ACTION: Erythropoietin is a factor controlling rate of red cell production; product is developed by recombinant DNA technology

Therapeutic outcome: Decreased anemia with increased RBCs

USES: Anemia caused by reduced endogenous erythropoietin production, primarily end-stage renal disease; to correct hemostatic defect in uremia; anemia caused by AZT (zidovudine) treatment in HIV-positive patients; anemia caused by chemotherapy; reduction of allogeneic blood transfusion in surgery patients

Unlabeled uses: Anemia in premature preterm infants

CONTRAINDICATIONS
Hypersensitivity to mammalian cell–derived products or human albumin; uncontrolled hypertension

Precautions: Pregnancy **C**, breastfeeding, children <1 mo, seizure disorder, porphyria, CV disease, hemodialysis, latex allergy, hypertension, history of CABG; multidose preserved formulation

Adverse effects: italics = common; bold = life-threatening

contains benzyl alcohol and should not be used in premature infants

> **BLACK BOX WARNING:** Hgb >11 g/dl, surgery, neoplastic disease

DOSAGE AND ROUTES

Anemia due to chronic kidney disease including dialysis-dependent and dialysis-independent patients to decrease the need for red blood cell transfusion

Adult/adolescent ≥17 yr: SUBCUT/IV, initially, 50-100 units/kg 3×/wk; for patients on dialysis, administer IV and initiate treatment when hemoglobin (Hgb) is <10 g/dl. If Hgb approaches or exceeds 11 g/dl, reduce or interrupt the dose. For patients not on dialysis, consider initiating treatment only when Hgb is <10 g/dl and the rate of Hgb decline indicates the likelihood of requiring a RBC transfusion and reducing the risk of alloimmunization and/or other RBC transfusion-related risks is a goal. If Hgb is >10 g/dl, reduce or interrupt the dose, and use the lowest dose sufficient to reduce the need for RBC transfusions. If the Hgb rises >1 g/dl in any 2-wk period, reduce dose by 25% or more as needed to reduce rapid responses. In contrast, if Hgb has not increased >1 g/dl after 4 wk of therapy, increase the dose by 25%. For patients who do not respond adequately over a 12-wk escalation period, increasing the dose further is unlikely to improve response and may increase risks. Use the lowest dose that will maintain a Hgb concentration sufficient to reduce the need for RBC transfusions. Evaluate other causes of anemia, and discontinue if responsiveness does not improve

Adolescent ≤16 yr/child/infant: SUBCUT/IV 50 units/kg 3×/wk initially; for dosage adjustments, see adult dosage

Zidovudine-induced anemia in HIV-infected patients with circulating endogenous erythropoietin concentrations ≤500 mUnits/ml who are receiving a dose of zidovudine ≤4200 mg/wk

Adult: SUBCUT/IV initially, 100 units/kg 3×/wk. If Hgb does not increase after 8 wk, increase by 50-100 units/kg at 4 to 8 wk intervals until Hgb is at a concentration to avoid RBC transfusions or a dose of 300 units/kg is reached. If the Hgb >12 g/dl, withhold, once Hgb <11 g/dl resume at a dose 25% below the previous dose

Anemia in patients with nonmyeloid malignancies where the anemia is due to the effect of concomitantly administered chemotherapy and at least 2 additional months of chemotherapy is planned

Adult: SUBCUT 150 units/kg three times weekly or 40,000 units once weekly only when the hemoglobin is <10 g/dl and only until the chemotherapy course is completed. Adjust the dose to maintain the lowest Hgb concentration sufficient to avoid RBC transfusions. If no rise in Hgb ≥1 g/dl after 4 wk of therapy and Hgb is <10 g/dl, the dosage may be increased to 300 units/kg 3 times weekly or 60,000 units once wkly. Discontinue if after 8 wk of therapy there is no response as measured by Hgb rise of <1-2 g/dl concentrations or if transfusions are still required. Reduce the dose by approximately 25% if Hgb increases by more than 1 g/dl in any 2-week period or if Hgb reaches a concentration needed to avoid RBC infusion. If Hgb is increasing and exceeds a concentration necessary to avoid blood transfusions, hold therapy and reinstitute at a dose that is 25% lower when the Hgb reaches a concentration where transfusions may be needed

Adolescent/child ≥5 yr: IV 600 units/kg qwk only when the hemoglobin is <10 g/dl and only until the chemotherapy course is completed. Adjust the dose to maintain the lowest Hgb concentration sufficient to avoid RBC transfusions. If no rise in Hgb ≤1 g/dl after 4 wk of therapy and Hgb is <10 g/dl, the dosage may be increased to 900 units/kg (up to 60,000 units) IV weekly. Discontinue if after 8 wk there is no response as measured by Hgb concentrations or if transfusions are still required. Reduce the dose by approximately 25% if Hgb increases by more than 1 g/dl in any 2-wk period or if Hgb reaches a concentration needed to avoid RBC infusion. If the Hgb is increasing and exceeds a concentration necessary to avoid blood transfusions, hold therapy and reinstitute at a dose that is 25% lower when the Hgb reaches a concentration where transfusions may be needed

To reduce the need for allogenic blood transfusions in anemic patients (hemoglobin >10 and ≤13 g/dl) scheduled to undergo elective, noncardiac, nonvascular surgery

Adult: Subcut 300 units/kg/day × 10 days before surgery, on the day of surgery, and for 4 days after surgery (15 days total) or 600 units/kg once weekly, 21, 14, and 7 days before surgery plus one dose on the day of surgery

Available forms: Inj 2000, 3000, 4000, 10,000, 20,000, 40,000 units/ml

---

⚠ Nurse Alert　　✦ Key NCLEX® Drug　　>> Drug Specifics

Implementation
• Do not use if discolored or particulates are present
SUBCUT route
• Before injecting, preservative-free, single-dose formulation may be admixed by using 0.9% NaCl, USP, with benzyl alcohol 0.9% at a 1:1 ratio to reduce injection site discomfort, store solution in refrigerator, protect from light

Direct IV route
• Administer by direct route at end of dialysis by venous line, do not shake vial
• If Hgb increases by 1 g/dl in 2 wk, decrease dose by 25%; increase dose if Hgb does not increase by 5-6 points after 8 wk of therapy; suggested target Hgb range 30%-36%
• Give additional heparin to lower chance of clots

Solution compatibilities: Do not dilute or administer with other solutions

ADVERSE EFFECTS
CNS: Seizures, coldness, sweating, headache, fatigue, dizziness
CV: *Hypertension,* hypertensive encephalopathy, CHF, edema, DVT
INTEG: Pruritus, rash, inj site reaction
MISC: Iron deficiency
MS: Bone pain, arthralgia, myalgia
RESP: Cough

Pharmacokinetics

Absorption	Well absorbed (SUBCUT), completely absorbed (**IV**)
Distribution	Increased RBC count 2-6 wk
Metabolism	Unknown
Excretion	Unknown
Half-life	5-14 hr

Pharmacodynamics

	SUBCUT/IV
Onset	Unknown
Peak	Immediate; SUBCUT: Peak 5-24 hr
Duration	Unknown

INTERACTIONS
Drug classifications
Anticoagulants: need for increased heparin during hemodialysis

NURSING CONSIDERATIONS
Assessment
• Monitor renal studies: urinalysis, protein, blood, BUN, creatinine; I&O; report drop in output to <50 ml/hr

BLACK BOX WARNING: Monitor blood studies: ferritin, transferrin monthly, transferrin sat ≥20%; ferritin ≥100 ng/ml; Hct 2 ×/wk until stabilized in target range (30%-36%), then at regular intervals; those with endogenous erythropoietin levels of <500 units/L respond to this agent; check for symptoms of anemia: fatigue, pallor, dyspnea; monitor Hct 2 ×/wk in chronic renal failure; cancer patients and those being treated with zidovudine should be monitored weekly, then periodically after stabilization; death may occur in Hgb >12 g/dl

• Assess for CNS symptoms: coldness, sweating, pain in long bones
• Assess CV status: B/P before, during treatment; hypertension may occur rapidly, leading to hypertension encephalopathy; antihypertensives may be needed
• Assess patient during hemodialysis for bruits, thrills, or shunts; product prevents severe anemia in chronic renal failure; clotting may need to be treated with increased anticoagulant
• Seizures: place on seizure precautions; assess for seizures if Hct is increased within 2 wk by 4 points, increased B/P, more common in chronic renal failure in the first 90 days of treatment
• Monitor serum iron, ferritin, transferrin levels; iron therapy may be needed to prevent recurring anemia
• Monitor B/P, check for rising B/P as Hct rises
• Monitor blood studies: BUN, creatinine, uric acid, platelets, WBC, phosphorus, potassium, bleeding time; Hct, Hgb, RBCs, reticulocytes should be checked in chronic renal failure
• For hypersensitivity reactions: Skin rashes, urticaria (rare), antibody development does not occur
⚠ For pure cell aplasia (PRCA) in absence of other causes, evaluate by testing serum for recombinant erythropoietin antibodies; any loss of response to epoetin should be evaluated

Patient/family education
• Teach patient how to take B/P
• Advise patients to take iron supplements, vit B_{12}, folic acid as directed
• Teach patient to avoid driving or hazardous activity during treatment
• Teach patients with renal disease to include high-iron and low-potassium foods in their diets (meat, dark green leafy vegetables, eggs, enriched breads)
• Teach patient the reason for treatment, expected results
• Advise patient to use contraception

Evaluation
Positive therapeutic outcome
- Increased appetite
- Enhanced sense of well-being
- Increase in reticulocyte count in 2-6 wk, Hgb, Hct

eprosartan (Rx)
(ep-roh-sar'tan)
Teveten
Func. class.: Antihypertensive
Chem. class.: Angiotensin II receptor antagonist (Subtype AT$_1$)
Pregnancy category C (1st trimester), D (2nd/3rd trimesters)

ACTION: Blocks the vasoconstrictor and aldosterone-secreting effects of angiotensin II; selectively blocks the binding of angiotensin II to the AT$_1$ receptor found in tissues

Therapeutic outcome: Decreased B/P

USES: Hypertension, alone or in combination with other antihypertensives

CONTRAINDICATIONS
Hypersensitivity

> **BLACK BOX WARNING:** Pregnancy **D**

Precautions: Breastfeeding, children, geriatric, hypersensitivity to ACE inhibitors, renal/hepatic disease, angioedema, hyperkalemia

DOSAGE AND ROUTES
Adult: PO 600 mg/day; dose may be divided and given bid, with total daily doses ranging from 400-800 mg, max 900 mg/day

Renal dose
Adult: PO CCr ≤30 ml/min, max 600 mg/day

Available forms: Tabs 400, 600 mg

Implementation
- May be given without regard to meals

ADVERSE EFFECTS
CNS: *Dizziness*, depression, *fatigue*, headache
CV: Chest pain, palpitations
EENT: Sinusitis
GI: *Diarrhea, dyspepsia, abdominal pain*
GU: UTI
HEMA: Neutropenia
INTEG: Pruritus, angioedema
META: Hypertriglyceridemia
MS: *Myalgia*, arthralgia, rhabdomyolysis
RESP: *Cough, upper respiratory infection*, rhinitis, pharyngitis, viral infection
SYST: Anaphylaxis

Pharmacokinetics

Absorption	Absolute bioavailability ~13%; food delays absorption
Distribution	Protein binding 98%
Metabolism	Moderate renal impairment increases product levels by 30%, hepatic impairment increases levels by 40%
Excretion	Urine, feces
Half-life	5-9 hr

Pharmacodynamics

Onset	Unknown
Peak	1-2 hr
Duration	Unknown

INTERACTIONS
Drug classifications
Antidiabetics: Increase: hyperglycemia
ACE inhibitors, angiotensin II receptor antagonists, potassium sparing diuretics, potassium supplements: increased hyperkalemia
NSAIDs, salicylates: decreased antihypertensive effect
Other antihypertensives: increased antihypertensive effect

Drug/lab test
Increased: ALT, AST, alkaline phosphatase, potassium
Decreased: Hgb

NURSING CONSIDERATIONS
Assessment
- Assess B/P with position changes, pulse q4hr; note rate, rhythm, quality
- Assess electrolytes: K, Na, Cl
- Assess baselines in renal, liver function tests before therapy begins
- Assess for edema in feet, legs daily, weight
- Assess skin turgor, dryness of mucous membranes for hydration status

Patient/family education
- Advise patient to comply with dosage schedule, even if feeling better
- Advise patient to notify prescriber of fever, swelling of hands or feet, chest pain
- Inform patient that excessive perspiration, dehydration, diarrhea may lead to fall in blood pressure; consult prescriber if these occur, maintain adequate hydration
- Inform patient that product may cause dizziness; advise to avoid hazardous activities until effect is known, to rise slowly from sitting position

BLACK BOX WARNING: Advise patient not to take this medication if pregnant or breastfeeding, or if allergic reaction to this product has occurred

• Advise patient to take missed dose as soon as possible, unless within 1 hr of next dose

Evaluation
Positive therapeutic outcome
• Decreased B/P

⚠ HIGH ALERT

eptifibatide (Rx)
(ep-tih-fib′ah-tide)
Integrilin
Func. class.: Antiplatelet agent
Chem. class.: Glycoprotein IIb/IIIa inhibitor
Pregnancy category B

ACTION: Platelet glycoprotein antagonist; reversibly prevents fibrinogen, von Willebrand factor from binding to the glycoprotein IIb/IIIa receptor, inhibiting platelet aggregation

Therapeutic outcome: Decreased platelets

USES: Acute coronary syndrome, including those undergoing percutaneous coronary intervention (PCI)

CONTRAINDICATIONS
Hypersensitivity, active internal bleeding, recent history of bleeding, stroke within 30 days or any hemorrhagic stroke, major surgery with severe trauma, severe hypertension, history of intracranial bleeding, current or planned use of another parenteral GPIIb/IIIa inhibitor, dependence on renal dialysis, coagulopathy, AV malformation, aneurysm

Precautions: Pregnancy **B**, breastfeeding, children, geriatric, bleeding, renal function impairment

DOSAGE AND ROUTES
Acute coronary syndrome
Adult: IV BOL 180 mcg/kg as soon as diagnosed, max 22.6 mg; then **IV** CONT INF 2 mcg/kg/min × 72 hr or coronary artery bypass graft (CABG) discontinue ≥ 2-4 hr before procedure

PCI in patients without acute coronary syndrome
Adult: IV BOL 180 mcg/kg given immediately before PCI; then 2 mcg/kg/min × 18 hr by CONT IV INF and a 2nd 180 mcg/kg BOL, 10 min after 1st BOL; continue INF for up to 18-24 hr at a rate of 1 mcg/kg/min

Renal dose
Adult: IV BOL CCr <50 ml/min 2-4 mg/dl same loading dose, then ½ usual INF dose; CCr <10 ml/min contraindicated

Available forms: Sol for inj 2 mg/ml (10 ml), 0.75 mg/ml (100 ml)

Implementation
• Aspirin may be given with this product; check for bleeding
• Discontinue heparin before removing femoral artery sheath after PCI
• Do not give discolored solutions, those with particulates; discard unused amount, protect from light
• Discontinue product prior to CABG

Direct IV route
• After withdrawing the BOL dose from 10-ml vial, give **IV** push over 1-2 min
• Do not use discolored sol or sol with particulate
Continuous IV infusion route
• Follow BOL dose with cont inf using infusion pump, give product undiluted directly from the 100-ml vial, spike the 100-ml vial with a vented infusion set; use caution when centering the spike on the circle of the stopper top, refrigerate vials, store vials ≤2 months at room temperature

Y-site compatibilities: Alfentanil, alteplase, amikacin, aminophylline, amphotericin B lipid complex, amphotericin B liposome, ampicillin, ampicillin-sulbactam, anidulafungin, argatroban, atenolol, atracurium, atropine, azithromycin, aztreonam, bivalirudin, bumetanide, buprenorphine, butorphanol, calcium chloride/gluconate, ceFAZolin, cefepime, cefotaxime, cefoTEtan, cefOXitin, cefTAZidime, ceftizoxime, cefTRIAXone, cefuroxime, cimetidine, ciprofloxacin, cisatracurium, clindamycin, cycloSPORINE, DAPTOmycin, dexamethasone, D₅/NaCl 0.9%, diazepam, diltiazem, diphenhydrAMINE, DOBUTamine, dolasetron, DOPamine, doxycycline, droperidol, enalaprilat, ePHEDrine, EPINEPHrine, ertapenem, erythromycin, esmolol, famotidine, fentaNYL, fluconazole, fosphenytoin, ganciclovir, gatifloxacin, gentamicin, granisetron, haloperidol, heparin, hydrocortisone, HYDROmorphone, hydrOXYzine, imipenem-cilastatin, inamrinone, isoproterenol, ketorolac, labetalol, leucovorin, levofloxacin, levorphanol, lidocaine, linezolid, LORazepam, magnesium sulfate, mannitol, meperidine, meropenem, methylPREDNISolone, metoclopramide, metoprolol, metroNIDAZOLE, micafungin, midazolam, milrinone, minocycline, mivacurium, morphine, nalbuphine, naloxone, niCARdipine, nitroglycerin, nitroprusside, NS, octreotide, ofloxacin, ondansetron, oxytocin, palonosetron, pancuronium, PEMEtrexed, PENTobarbital, PHENobarbital, phenylephrine, piperacillin, piperacillin-tazobactam, potassium chloride/phosphates, procainamide, prochlorperazine, promethazine, propranolol, ranitidine, remifentanil, rocuronium, sodium bicarbonate/phosphates, succinylcholine, SUFentanil, sulfamethoxazole-trimethoprim, teniposide, theophylline, ticarcillin, ticarcillin-clavulanate, tigecycline, tirofiban, tobramycin, trimethobenzamide, vancomycin, vecuronium, verapamil, zidovudine, zoledronic acid

Solution compatibilities: 0.9% NaCl, D_5/0.9% NaCl

• Discontinue product before CABG
• Give all medications PO if possible, avoid IM inj and catheters

ADVERSE EFFECTS

CV: Stroke, hypotension
GU: Hematuria
HEMA: Thrombocytopenia, platelet dysfunction
SYST: Major/minor bleeding from any site, anaphylaxis

Pharmacokinetics

Absorption	Unknown
Distribution	Protein binding 25%
Metabolism	Limited
Excretion	Kidneys
Half-life	1.5-2 hr

Pharmacodynamics

Onset	Within 1 hr

INTERACTIONS
Individual drugs
Abciximab, aspirin, clopidogrel, dipyridamole, heparin, ticlopidine, valproate: increased bleeding

Drug classifications
Anticoagulants, NSAIDs, SSRIs, SNRIs, thrombolytics: increased bleeding
Platelet receptor inhibitors IIb, IIIa: do not give together

Drug/herb
Feverfew, garlic, ginger, ginkgo, ginseng

NURSING CONSIDERATIONS
Assessment
• **Thrombocytopenia: Monitor platelets, Hgb, Hct, creatinine, APTT baseline, INR, within 6 hr of loading dose and daily**

thereafter; patients undergoing PCI should have ACT monitored; maintain APTT 50-70 sec unless PCI is to be performed; during PCI, ACT should be 200-300 sec; if platelets drop <100,000/mm³, obtain additional platelet counts; if thrombocytopenia is confirmed, discontinue product; also draw Hct, Hgb, serum creatinine
• Assess for bleeding: gums, bruising, ecchymosis, petechiae; from GI, GU tract, cardiac catheter sites, IM inj sites

Patient/family education
• Teach patient to report bruising, bleeding, chest pain immediately
• Inform patient of reason for medication and expected results

Evaluation
Positive therapeutic outcome
• Decreased platelets

---

ergocalciferol
See vitamin D

---

eribulin (Rx)
(er'i-bue'lin)
Halaven
Func. class.: Antineoplastics, nontaxane
Pregnancy category D

Do not confuse: eribulin/epirubicin/erlotinib

ACTION: Potent antimitotic agent, different from taxes, vinca alkaloids, epothilones; blocks cell progression in G_2-M phase, inhibits the growth phase of microtubules and sequesters tubules, leading to disruption of mitotic spindles and apoptotic cell death

Therapeutic outcome: Decreased spread and size of tumor

USES: Metastatic breast cancer patients who have received at least 2 chemotherapy regimens

CONTRAINDICATIONS
Hypersensitivity, pregnancy **D**

Precautions: Bradycardia, breastfeeding, children, electrolyte imbalances, heart failure, hepatic disease, hypokalemia, hypomagnesemia, infants, infertility, neonates, neutropenia, peripheral neuropathy, QT prolongation, renal disease

DOSAGE AND ROUTES
Adult: IV 1.4 mg/m² over 2-5 min on days 1 and 8, repeat q21days

Recommendations for dose delay
• *For ANC< 1000/mm³, platelets< 75,000/ mm³ , or grade 3 or 4 nonhematologic toxicities:* Do not administer; the day 8 dose may be delayed a maximum of 1 wk
• *For the day 8 dose, if toxicities do not resolve to ≤grade 2 by day 15:* Omit the dose
• *For the day 8 dose, if toxicities resolve or improve to ≤grade 2 by day 15:* Administer eribulin at a reduced dose (see below) and initiate the next cycle no sooner than 2 wk later

Dosage adjustments for hematologic toxicity
• *ANC <500/mm³ for >7 days or ANC <1000/mm³ with fever or infection:* Permanently reduce dosage to 1.1 mg/m²
• *Platelets <25,000/mm³ or <50,000/mm³ requiring transfusion:* Permanently reduce dosage to 1.1 mg/m²
• *If day 8 of previous cycle omitted or delayed:* Permanently reduce dosage to 1.1 mg/m²
• *While receiving 1.1 mg/m², if recurrence of hematologic event occurs, or if day 8 of previous cycle omitted or delayed:* Permanently reduce dosage to 0.7 mg/m²
• *While receiving 0.7 mg/m², if recurrence of hematologic event occurs, or if day 8 of previous cycle omitted or delayed:* Discontinue

Dose adjustments of eribulin for nonhematologic toxicity during treatment
• *Any grade 3 or 4 nonhematologic toxicity:* Permanently reduce dosage to 1.1 mg/m²
• *If day 8 of previous cycle omitted or delayed:* Permanently reduce dosage to 1.1 mg/m²
• *While receiving 1.1 mg/m², if recurrence of grade 3 or 4 nonhematologic toxicity occurs, or if day 8 of previous cycle omitted or delayed:* Permanently reduce dosage to 0.7 mg/m²
• *While receiving 0.7 mg/m², if recurrence of grade 3 or 4 nonhematologic toxicity occurs, or if day 8 of previous cycle omitted or delayed:* Discontinue

Available forms: Solution for injection 1 mg/2 ml

Implementation

IV direct, intermittent route
• Visually inspect for particulate matter or discoloration as solution and container permit; withdraw required amount (0.5 mg/ml) from single-use vial, give undiluted over 2-5 min or diluted in 100 ml 0.9% NaCl and give as intermittent infusion, do not give through line with dextrose or any other product
• Store at room temperature for 4 hr or 24 hr refrigerated

ADVERSE EFFECTS
CNS: Depression, dizziness, *fatigue,* fever, headache, insomnia, *peripheral neuropathy*
CV: **QT prolongation**, peripheral edema
GI: Abdominal pain, anorexia, constipation, diarrhea, dyspepsia, nausea, vomiting, weight loss
HEMA: Anemia, neutropenia, thrombocytopenia
INTEG: *Alopecia,* rash, stomatitis, infusion-related reactions
META: Hypokalemia
MS: Arthralgia, myalgia, bone/back pain
RESP: Cough, dyspnea
SYST: Infection

Pharmacokinetics

Absorption	Protein binding, 49%-65%
Distribution	Unknown
Metabolism	Inhibits CYP3A4
Excretion	Feces 82%, urine 9%
Half-life	40 hr, increased levels in renal/hepatic disease

Pharmacodynamics
Unknown

INTERACTIONS
Individual drugs
Arsenic trioxide, bepridil, chloroquine, clarithromycin, dextromethorphan, dronedarone, droperidol, erythromycin, halofantrine, haloperidol, levomethadyl, methadone, pentamidine, pimozide, posaconazole, probucol, propafenone, quiNIDine, saquinavir, sparfloxacin, troleandomycin, and ziprasidone; also to a lesser degree abarelix, alfuzosin, amoxapine, apomorphine, artemether; lumefantrine, asenapine, ofloxacin, cloZAPine, cyclobenzaprine, dasatinib, dolasetron, flecainide, gatifloxacin, gemifloxacin, iloperidone, lapatinib, levofloxacin, lopinavir; ritonavir, magnesium sulfate; potassium sulfate; sodium sulfate, maprotiline, mefloquine, moxifloxacin, nilotinib, norfloxacin, octreotide, ciprofloxacin, OLANZapine, ondansetron, paliperidone, palonosetron, QUEtiapine, ranolazine, risperiDONE, sertindole, SUNItinib, tacrolimus, telavancin, telithromycin,

tetrabenazine, venlafaxine, vardenafil, vorinostat: increased QT prolongation

Drug classifications
Certain phenothiazines (chlorproMAZINE, mesoridazine, thioridazine), class IA antiarrhythmics (disopyramide, procainamide, quiNIDine), class III antiarrhythmics (amiodarone, bretylium, dofetilide, ibutilide, sotalol), also to a lesser degree, beta-agonists, halogenated anesthetics, local anesthetics, some phenothiazines (fluPHENAZine, perphenazine, prochlorperazine, trifluoperazine), tricyclic antidepressants: increased QT prolongation

NURSING CONSIDERATIONS
Assessment
• Peripheral neuropathy: assess for pain, numbness in extremities
• Infection: assess for increased temperature, sore throat, flulike symptoms
• **QT prolongation: assess for drug interactions that may occur; monitor ECG, heart rate**
• **Bone marrow depression: CBC and differential, serum creatinine/bun/electrolytes, liver function tests, baseline and periodically, increased AST/ALT >3 × ULN or total bilirubin >1.5 × ULN are at a greater chance of grade 4 or febrile neutropenia**

Patient/family education
• **Infection: teach patient to notify prescriber of increased temperature, sore throat, fatigue, flu-like symptoms**
• **QT prolongation: teach patient to report extra heartbeats**
• Peripheral neuropathy: teach patient to report tingling, pain in extremities
• Teach patient reason for product and expected results
• Advise patient to report side effects to health care provider
• Advise patient to avoid other medications, supplements unless approved by provider, serious drug interactions may occur
• Discuss hair loss and use of wig or hairpiece
⚠ **Advise patient to notify prescriber if pregnancy is planned or suspected (pregnancy D), avoid breastfeeding**

Evaluation
Positive therapeutic outcome
• Decreasing tumor spread and size

⚠ HIGH ALERT

erlotinib (Rx)
(er-loe′tye-nib)
Tarceva
Func. class.: Misc. antineoplastic
Chem. class.: Epidermal growth factor receptor inhibitor
Pregnancy category D

ACTION: Not fully understood. Inhibits intracellular phosphorylation of cell surface receptors associated with epidermal growth factor receptors.

Therapeutic outcome: Decrease in tumor size

USES: Non–small cell lung cancer (NSCLC) including EGFR exon 19 deletions or exon 21 substitution mutations, pancreatic cancer

CONTRAINDICATIONS
Pregnancy **D**, breastfeeding

Precautions: Renal, hepatic; ocular, pulmonary disorders; children; geriatric, diverticulitis

DOSAGE AND ROUTES
Non–small cell lung cancer (NSCLC)
Adult: PO 150 mg/day
Pancreatic cancer
Adult: PO 100 mg/day in combination with gemcitabine 1000 mg/m^2 cycle 1, days 1, 8, 15, 22, 29, 36, 43 of an 8-wk cycle; cycle 2 and subsequent cycles, days 1, 8, 15 of a 4-wk cycle

CYP3A4 inducers concurrently (such as rifampin or phenytoin)
Dosage increase is advised

CYP3A4 inhibitors (atazanavir, clarithromycin, indinavir, itraconazole, ketoconazole, telithromycin, ritonavir, saquinavir, troleandomycin, nelfinavir)
Dosage reduction may be needed.

Hepatic dose
Adult: PO interrupt if total bilirubin >3 times ULN and/or transaminases >5 times ULN

Available forms: Tabs 25, 100, 150 mg

Implementation
• Administer 1 hr before or 2 hr after food

ADVERSE EFFECTS
CNS: CVA, anxiety, depression, headache, rigors, insomnia
CV: MI/ischemia

EENT: Ocular changes, *conjunctivitis, eye pain,* hypertrichosis

GI: *Nausea, diarrhea, vomiting, anorexia, mouth ulceration,* hepatic failure, GI perforation

GU: Renal impairment/failure

HEMA: DVT, bleeding

INTEG: *Rash,* Stevens-Johnson–like skin reactions, toxic epidermal necrolysis

MISC: *Fatigue, infection*

RESP: Interstitial lung disease, *cough, dyspnea,* ARDS, pulmonary fibrosis

SYST: Hepatorenal syndrome

Pharmacokinetics

Absorption	Slowly absorbed
Distribution	Unknown
Metabolism	Metabolized by CYP3A4
Excretion	Feces (86%), urine (<4%)
Half-life	36 hr elimination

Pharmacodynamics

Onset	Unknown
Peak	3-7 hr
Duration	Unknown

INTERACTIONS

Individual drugs

Metoprolol, warfarin: increased plasma concentrations

Smoking: decreased erlotinib level, dose may need to be increased

Drug classifications

CYP3A4 inducers (phenytoin, rifampin, carBAMazepine, phenobarbital), proton-pump inhibitors: decreased erlotinib levels

CYP3A4 inhibitors (clarithromycin, erythromycin, itraconazole, ketoconazole, telithromycin): increased erlotinib concentrations

HMG-CoA reductase inhibitors: increased myopathy

NSAIDs: GI bleeding may be fatal

Drug/herb

St. John's wort: decreased erlotinib levels

Drug/food

Grapefruit juice: increased effect of erlotinib

Drug/labs

Increase: INR, PT, AST, ALT, bilirubin

NURSING CONSIDERATIONS

Assessment

⚠ **Serious skin toxicities: toxic epidermal necrolysis, Stevens-Johnson syndrome, check for rash, blistering, discontinue treatment, may need corticosteroid**

⚠ **Assess for MI/ischemia, CVA in pancreatic cancer**

⚠ **Assess for pulmonary changes: lung sounds, cough, dyspnea; interstitial lung disease may occur, may be fatal; discontinue therapy if confirmed**

• **Assess for ocular changes:** eye irritation, corneal erosion/ulcer, aberrant eyelash growth

• Assess for GI symptoms: frequency of stools; if diarrhea is poorly tolerated, therapy may be discontinued for up to 14 days; monitor for dehydration, fluid status during period of vomiting and diarrhea

• Monitor blood studies: INR, LFTs, PT

• **Hepatic failure: interrupt dosing if severe changes to liver function occur (total bilirubin >3× ULN and/or transaminases >5× ULN for normal pretreatment LFTs)**

⚠ **GI perforation/bleeding: some cases have been fatal, usually occurs in those using NSAIDs, taxanes, or those with diverticulitis or peptic ulcer disease, discontinue if these occur**

Patient/family education

⚠ **Teach patient to report adverse reactions immediately: SOB, severe abdominal pain, persistent diarrhea or vomiting, ocular changes, skin eruptions (face, upper chest/back pain)**

• Explain reason for treatment, expected results

⚠ **Advise patient to use contraception during treatment; pregnancy D, avoid breastfeeding**

• Instruct patient to avoid use with other products, herbs, or supplements unless approved by provider

• Instruct patient to avoid smoking; decreases effect of this product

Evaluation

Positive therapeutic outcome

• Decrease non–small cell lung cancer cells

---

ertapenem (Rx)

(er-tah-pen'em)

INVanz

Func. class.: Antiinfective, miscellaneous

Chem. class.: Carbapenem

Pregnancy category B

Do not confuse: INVanz/Aninza

ACTION: Interferes with cell wall replication of susceptible organisms

Therapeutic outcome: Bactericidal action against the following organisms: *Bacteroides fragilis, Bacteroides distasonis, Bacteroides*

ovatus, Bacteroides thetaiotaomicron, Bacteroides uniformis; Clostridium clostridioforme, Escherichia coli, Eubacterium lentum, Haemophilus influenzae (β lactamase–negative), *Klebsiella pneumoniae, Moraxella catarrhalis, Peptostreptococcus* sp., *Porphyromonas asaccharolytica, Prevotella bivia, Staphylococcus aureus* (methicillin-susceptible); *Streptococcus agalactiae, Streptococcus pneumoniae* (penicillin-susceptible), *Streptococcus pyogenes*

USES: Bacteremia, *Bacteroides distasonis, Bacteroides fragilis, Bacteroides ovatus, Bacteroides thetaiotaomicron, Bacteroides uniformis, Bacteroides vulgatus, Citrobacter freundii, Citrobacter koseri, Clostridium clostridioforme, Clostridium perfringens,* community-acquired pneumonia, diabetic foot ulcer, endomyometritis, *Enterobacter aerogenes, Enterobacter cloacae, Escherichia coli, Eubacterium lentum, Fusobacterium, Haemophilus influenzae* (beta-lactamase negative), *Haemophilus influenzae* (beta-lactamase positive), *Haemophilus parainfluenzae,* intraabdominal infections, *Klebsiella oxytoca, Klebsiella pneumoniae, Moraxella catarrhalis, Morganella morganii, Peptostreptococcus, Porphyromonas asaccharolytica, Prevotella bivia, Proteus mirabilis, Proteus vulgaris, Providencia rettgeri, Providencia stuartii, Serratia marcescens,* skin infections, *Staphylococcus aureus* (MSSA), *Staphylococcus epidermidis, Streptococcus agalactiae* (group B streptococci), *Streptococcus pneumoniae, Streptococcus pyogenes* (group A beta-hemolytic streptococci), surgical infection prophylaxis, urinary tract infections

CONTRAINDICATIONS
Hypersensitivity to this product or its components, to amide-type local anesthetics (IM only); anaphylactic reactions to β-lactams, other carbapenems

Precautions: Pregnancy **B,** breastfeeding, children, geriatric, renal/hepatic/GI disease, seizures

DOSAGE AND ROUTES
Complicated intraabdominal infections
Adult: IM/**IV** 1 g/day × 5-14 days
Child 3 mo–12 yr: IM/**IV** 15 mg/kg bid (max 1 g/day) × 5-14 days

Complicated skin/skin structure infections
Adult/adolescent: IM/**IV** 1 g/day × 7-14 days
Child 3 mo–12 yr: IM/**IV** 15 mg/kg bid × 7-14 days

Community-acquired pneumonia
Adult/adolescent: IM/**IV** 1 g/day × 10-14 days
Child 3 mo–12 yr: IM/**IV** 15 mg/kg bid × 10-14 days, max 1 g/day

Complicated UTI
Adult/adolescent: IM/**IV** 1 g/day × 10-14 days
Child 3 mo–12 yr: IM/**IV** 15 mg/kg bid × 10-14 days

Acute pelvic infections
Adult/adolescent: IM/**IV** 1 g/day × 3-10 days
Child 3 mo–12 yr: IM/**IV** 15 mg/kg bid × 3-10 days

Surgical infection prophylaxis
Adult: IV 1 g as a single dose 1 hr prior to surgical incision

Renal dose
Adult: IM/IV CCr ≤30 ml/min, 500 mg/day

Available forms: Powder, lyophilized, 1 g

Implementation
IV route
• Visually inspect for particulate matter and discoloration before use: may be colorless to pale yellow; do not mix with other products; dextrose solutions are not compatible
• 1 g vial: For each gram reconstitute with 10 ml of either NS injection, sterile water for injection, or bacteriostatic water for injection to 100 mg/ml, shake
• 1 g dose: immediately transfer contents of the reconstituted vial to 50 ml of NS injection; for a dose <1 g (pediatric patients 3 mo to 12 yr): from the reconstituted vial, immediately withdraw a volume equal to 15 mg/kg of body weight (max 1 g/day) and dilute in NS injection to a concentration of 20 mg/ml or less

IV infusion route
• Complete the infusion within 6 hr of reconstitution, infuse over 30 min; do not co-infuse with other medications
• The reconstituted IV solution may be stored at room temperature if used within 6 hr, or stored under refrigeration for 24 hr and used within 4 hr after removal from refrigeration; do not freeze

IM route
• Reconstitute the 1 g vial of ertapenem with 3.2 ml of 1% lidocaine HCl injection (without EPINEPHrine) (280 mg/ml), agitate well to form a solution; the IM reconstituted formulation is not for IV use
• IM administration may be used as an alternative to IV administration in the treatment of

infections where IM therapy is appropriate; only given via IM injection × 7 days
• For a 1 g dose: immediately withdraw the contents of the vial and inject deeply into a large muscle, aspirate prior to injection to avoid injection into a blood vessel
• For a dose <1 g (i.e., for pediatric patients 3 mo to 12 yr): immediately withdraw a volume equal to 15 mg/kg (max 1 g/day) and inject deeply into a large muscle, aspirate prior to injection to avoid injection into a blood vessel; use the reconstituted IM solution within 1 hour after preparation

Y-site compatibilities: Acyclovir, alfentanil, amifostine, amikacin, aminocaproic acid, aminophylline, amphotericin B lipid complex, amphotericin B liposome, argatroban, arsenic trioxide, atenolol, atracurium, azithromycin, aztreonam, bivalirudin, bleomycin, bumetanide, buprenorphine, busulfan, butorphanol, calcium chloride/gluconate, CARBOplatin, carmustine, chloramphenicol, cimetidine, ciprofloxacin, cisatracurium, CISplatin, cyclophosphamide, cycloSPORINE, cytarabine, dacarbazine, DACTINomycin, DAPTOmycin, dexamethasone, dexmedetomidine, dexrazoxane, digoxin, diltiazem, diphenhydrAMINE, DOCEtaxel, dolasetron, DOPamine, doxacurium, doxycycline, enalaprilat, ePHEDrine, EPINEPHrine, eptifibatide, erythromycin, esmolol, etoposide, etoposide phosphate, famotidine, fenoldopam, fluconazole, fludarabine, fluorouracil, foscarnet, fosphenytoin, furosemide, ganciclovir, gatifloxacin, gemcitabine, gemtuzumab, gentamicin, glycopyrrolate, granisetron, haloperidol, heparin, hydrocortisone, HYDROmorphone, ifosfamide, inamrinone, insulin (regular), irinotecan, isoproterenol, ketorolac, labetalol, lepirudin, leucovorin, levofloxacin, lidocaine, linezolid, LORazepam, magnesium sulfate, mannitol, mechlorethamine, melphalan, meperidine, mesna, metaraminol, methotrexate, methyldopate, methylPREDNISolone, metoclopramide, metroNIDAZOLE, milrinone, mitoMYcin, mivacurium, morphine, moxifloxacin, nalbuphine, naloxone, nesiritide, nitroglycerin, nitroprusside, norepinephrine, octreotide, oxaliplatin, oxytocin, PACLitaxel, pamidronate, pancuronium, pantoprazole, PEMEtrexed, PENTobarbital, PHENobarbital, phentolamine, phenylephrine, polymixin B, potassium acetate/chloride/phosphates, procainamide, propranolol, ranitidine, remifentanil, rocuronium, sodium acetate/bicarbonate/phosphates, streptozocin, succinylcholine, SUFentanil, sulfamethoxazole-trimethoprim, tacrolimus, telavancin, teniposide, theophylline, thiotepa, tigecycline, tirofiban, tobramycin, trimethobenzamide, vancomycin, vasopressin, vecuronium, vinBLAStine, vinCRIStine, vinorelbine, voriconazole, zidovudine, zoledronic acid

ADVERSE EFFECTS
CNS: Insomnia, seizures, dizziness, *headache*, agitation, confusion, somnolence, disorientation, edema, hypotension
CV: Tachycardia, seizures
GI: *Diarrhea, nausea, vomiting*, pseudomembranous colitis, cholelithiasis, jaundice, abdominal pain
GU: *Vaginitis*, dysuria
INTEG: *Rash*, urticaria, *pruritus*, pain at inj site, *infused vein complication, phlebitis/thrombophlebitis*, erythema at inj site, dermatitis
RESP: Dyspnea, cough, pharyngitis, crackles, respiratory distress
SYST: Anaphylaxis, angioedema

Pharmacokinetics
Absorption	Almost completely absorbed (IM); completely absorbed (**IV**)
Distribution	85%-95% plasma protein bound
Metabolism	Liver (IM, **IV**)
Excretion	Urine (80%), feces (10%), breast milk (IM, **IV**)
Half-life	4 hr (**IV**)

Pharmacodynamics
	IM	IV
Onset	Unknown	Immediate
Peak	2.3 hr	Dose-dependent
Duration	Unknown	Unknown

INTERACTIONS
Individual drugs
Probenecid: increased ertapenem plasma levels; do not coadminister
Valproic acid: decreased effect of valproic acid
Warfarin: Increase: INR

Drug/lab test
Increased: hepatic enzymes

NURSING CONSIDERATIONS
Assessment
• Assess for renal disease: lower dose may be required
• **Pseudomembranous colitis: Assess bowel pattern daily: if severe diarrhea occurs, product should be discontinued**
• **Assess for infection:** temp, sputum, characteristics of wound before, during, after treatment

⚠ Assess for allergic reactions, anaphylaxis: rash, urticaria, pruritus may occur a few days after therapy begins; assess for sensitivity to carbapenem antibiotics, other β-lactam antibiotics, penicillins

• Assess for overgrowth of infection: perineal itching, fever, malaise, redness, pain, swelling, drainage, rash, diarrhea, change in cough or sputum

Patient/family education
⚠ Advise patient to report severe diarrhea; may indicate pseudomembranous colitis
⚠ Advise patient to report overgrowth of infection: black, furry tongue, vaginal itching, foul-smelling stools

• Caution patient to avoid breastfeeding; product is excreted in breast milk

Evaluation
Positive therapeutic outcome
• Negative C&S, absence of signs and symptoms of infection

TREATMENT OF OVERDOSE:
Administer EPINEPHrine, antihistamines; resuscitate if needed (anaphylaxis)

---

erythromycin base (Rx)
(eh-rith-roh-my′sin)
Apo Erythro ✦, Ery-Tab, Novo-Rythro Encap ✦, PCE
erythromycin ethylsuccinate (Rx)
Apo-Erythro-ES ✦, EES, Erythro-ES ✦, Ery Ped, Novo-Rythro ✦
erythromycin lactobionate (Rx)
Erythrocin
erythromycin stearate (Rx)
Apo-Erythro-S ✦, Erythrocin, My-E, Novo-Rythro ✦
Func. class.: Antiinfective
Chem. class.: Macrolide
Pregnancy category B

Do not confuse: erythromycin/ azithromycin

ACTION: Binds to 50S ribosomal subunits of susceptible bacteria and suppresses protein synthesis

Therapeutic outcome: Bactericidal action against the following organisms: *Neisseria gonorrhoeae, Streptococcus pneumoniae, Mycoplasma pneumoniae, Corynebacterium diphtheriae, Bordetella pertussis, Borrelia burgdorferi, Listeria monocytogenes, Treponema pallidum;* streptococci, staphylococci; gram-negative pathogens: *Neisseria, Haemophilus influenzae* (when used with sulfonamides), *Legionella pneumophila, Chlamydia trachomatis*

USES: Mild to moderate respiratory tract, skin, soft tissue infections, Legionnaire's disease, syphilis

CONTRAINDICATIONS
Hypersensitivity, preexisting liver disease (estolate)

Precautions: Pregnancy **B,** breastfeeding, geriatric, hepatic/GI disease, QT prolongation, seizure disorder, myasthenia gravis

DOSAGE AND ROUTES
Acne vulgaris
Adult: PO 250 mg qid

Mild to moderately severe upper respiratory tract infections (otitis media, sinusitis) or lower respiratory tract infections (pneumonia, bronchitis) caused by susceptible organisms
Adult: PO 250-500 mg (of base, estolate or stearate) q6hr or 400-800 mg (ethylsuccinate) q6hr; IV 15-20 mg/kg/day in divided doses q4-6 hr, max 4 g/day
Adolescent/child/infant: PO 20-50 mg/kg/day divided q6hr, max adult doses; IV 15-20 mg/kg/day in divided doses q4-6hr, or as a continuous infusion, max dose 4 g/day
Neonate >7 days, weighing ≥1200 g: PO 30 mg/kg/day in divided doses q8hr
Neonate >7 days, weighing <1200 g: PO 20 mg/kg/day in divided doses q12hr
Neonate ≤7 days: PO 20 mg/kg/day PO in divided doses q12hr

Pneumonia caused by *Chlamydia trachomatis* in infants and neonates
Infant/neonate: PO; the CDC recommends 50 mg/kg/day in four divided doses × 14 days (erythromycin base or ethylsuccinate)

***Mycoplasma* infection such as *Mycoplasma pneumoniae* pneumonia**
Adult: PO 250-500 mg tid
Adult/adolescent/child/infant: IV 15-20 mg/kg/day, given in divided doses q4-6hr, or as a continuous infusion, maximum dose 4 g/day; replace by oral dosage as soon as possible

Legionnaire's disease (caused by *Legionella pneumophila*)
Adult: PO/IV 0.5-1 g q6hr × 21 days

Treatment of group A beta-hemolytic streptococcal (GAS) pharyngitis (primary rheumatic fever prophylaxis)

Adult: PO 250-500 mg (base, estolate, or stearate) q6hr or 400-800 mg (ethylsuccinate) q6hr × 10 days

Adolescent/child/infant: PO 20-50 mg/kg/day, divided q6hr × 10 days, max adult dose

Secondary prevention of rheumatic fever (prevention of recurrent attacks of rheumatic fever)

Adult/adolescent/child: PO 250 mg bid in patients allergic to penicillin and sulfADIAZINE for 10 yr or age 40 yr, whichever is longer, secondary prophylaxis (American Heart Association)

Listeriosis

Adult: PO 250-500 mg (base, estolate or stearate) q6hr or 400-800 mg (ethylsuccinate) q6hr

Adolescent/child/infant: PO 20-50 mg/kg/day PO, divided q6hr, max adult doses

Cervicitis caused by *Chlamydia trachomatis*

Adult/adolescent: PO; the CDC recommends erythromycin base 500 mg qid or erythromycin ethylsuccinate 800 mg qid × 7 days as alternatives to first-line agents doxycycline or azithromycin

Pregnant female: As alternatives to first-line agents azithromycin or amoxicillin, the CDC recommends PO base 500 mg qid × 7 days, base 250 mg qid × 14 days, ethylsuccinate 800 mg qid × 7 days, ethylsuccinate PO 400 mg qid × 14 days

Child ≤45 kg: The CDC recommends base or ethylsuccinate PO 50 mg/kg/day in 4 doses × 14 days

Proctitis caused by *Chlamydia trachomatis*

Adult/adolescent: PO base 500 mg qid

Chlamydial conjunctivitis caused by *Chlamydia trachomatis* including trachoma and inclusion conjunctivitis

Pregnant and lactating woman/child <8 yr: PO 250-500 mg qid × 10-14 days

Infant pneumonia caused by *Chlamydia trachomatis*

Infant/neonate: PO (base or ethylsuccinate); the CDC recommends 50 mg/kg/day 4 divided doses × 14 days

Nongonococcal urethritis (NGU) caused by *Chlamydia trachomatis* or *Ureaplasma urealyticum*

Adult/adolescent: PO; the CDC recommends 500 mg (base) qid or 800 mg (ethylsuccinate) qid × 7 days as alternatives to first-line agents doxycycline or azithromycin

Pregnant female: PO; the CDC recommends base 500 mg qid × 7 days

Child <45 kg: PO; the CDC recommends base 50 mg/kg/day in 4 divided doses × 10-14 days, second course of therapy may be required

Ophthalmia neonatorum caused by *Chlamydia trachomatis*

Neonate: PO (erythromycin base or ethylsuccinate); the CDC recommends 50 mg/kg/day in qid × 14 days, may be repeated if condition returns

Lymphogranuloma venereum caused by *Chlamydia trachomatis*

Adult: PO (base); the CDC recommends 500 mg qid × 21 days as an alternative to doxycycline

Adjunctive treatment of diphtheria to prevent establishment of carrier state and to eradicate *Corynebacterium diphtheriae* in carriers

Adult: PO 500 mg q6hr × 10 days

Intestinal amebiasis (unable to take metroNIDAZOLE)

Adult: PO 250 mg q6hr × 10-14 days

Adolescent/child: PO 30-50 mg/kg/day, divided q6hr × 10-14 days, max adult dose

Pertussis (whooping cough) caused by *Bordetella pertussis* or for postexposure pertussis prophylaxis

Adult: PO 500 mg PO qid (2 g total) × 14 days

Adolescent/child/infant: PO 40-50 mg/kg/day (max 2 g/day) in 4 divided doses × 14 days

Primary or secondary syphilis (caused by *Treponema pallidum*) in penicillin-allergic, nonpregnant patients

Adult: PO (CDC) 500 mg qid × 14 days as an alternative therapy

Surgical infection prophylaxis as a bowel preparation in combination with neomycin

Adult: It is generally recommended that if surgery is scheduled for 8 AM, 1 g erythromycin PO with neomycin sulfate PO should be given at 1 PM, 2 PM, and 11 PM on the day before surgery

E

Impetigo/burn wound infection (unlabeled)

Adult: PO 250-500 mg q6hr (base, estolate, stearate) or 400-800 mg (ethylsuccinate) q6hr

Adolescent/child/infant: PO 20-50 mg/kg/day divided q6hr

Available forms: Base: enteric-coated tab 250, 333, 500 mg; film-coated tab 250, 500 mg; enteric-coated caps, 250, 333 mg; stearate: film-coated tabs, 250 mg, granules for oral susp: 200, 400 mg/5 ml powder for inj 500 mg, 1 g (lactobionate); 1 g (as gluceptate)

Implementation

• Store at room temp; store susp in refrigerator
• Adequate intake of fluids (2 L) during diarrhea episodes

PO route

• Give around the clock on an empty stomach, at least 1 hr before or 2 hr after meals; may be taken with food if GI upset occurs; do not take with juices; take dose with a full glass of water; use calibrated measuring device for drops or susp; shake well
• Store susp in refrigerator
• Do not crush or chew enteric-coated tab

IV route

• Add 10 ml of sterile water for inj without preservatives to 250- or 500-mg vials and 20 ml to 1-g vial; sol is stable for 1 wk after reconstitution if refrigerated

Intermittent IV infusion route

• Dilute further in 100-250 ml of 0.9% NaCl or D₅W
• Give over 20-60 min to avoid phlebitis; assess for pain along vein; slow inf if pain occurs; apply ice to site and notify prescriber if unable to relieve pain

Continuous infusion route

• May also be administered as an inf in a dilution of 1 g/L of 0.9% NaCl, D₅W, over 4 hr

Erythromycin lactobionate

Y-site compatibilities: Acyclovir, alfentanil, amikacin, aminocaproic acid, aminophylline, amiodarone, anidulafungin, argatroban, atenolol, atosiban, atracurium, atropine, azaTHIOprine, benztropine, bivalirudin, bleomycin, bumetanide, buprenorphine, butorphanol, calcium chloride/gluconate, CARBOplatin, caspofungin, cefotaxime, cefTAZidime, cefTRIAXone, cefuroxime, chlorproMAZINE, cimetidine, CISplatin, cyanocobalamin, cyclophosphamide, cycloSPORINE, cytarabine, DACTINomycin, DAPTOmycin, dexmedetomidine, digoxin, diltiazem, diphenhydrAMINE, DOBUTamine, DOCEtaxel, DOPamine, doxacurium, doxapram, DOXOrubicin, enalaprilat, ePHEDrine, EPINEPHrine, epirubicin, epoetin alfa, eptifibatide, ertapenem, esmolol, etoposide, famotidine, fenoldopam, fentaNYL, fluconazole, fludarabine, fluorouracil, folic acid, foscarnet, gatifloxacin, gemcitabine, gentamicin, glycopyrrolate, granisetron, hydrocortisone, HYDROmorphone, hydrOXYzine, IDArubicin, ifosfamide, imipenem-cilastatin, insulin (regular), irinotecan, isoproterenol, labetalol, levofloxacin, lidocaine, LORazepam, LR, mannitol, mechlorethamine, meperidine, methicillin, methotrexate, methoxamine, methyldopa, methylPREDNISolone, metoclopramide, metroNIDAZOLE, miconazole, midazolam, milrinone, mitoXANtrone, morphine, multiple vitamins injection, mycophenolate nafcillin, nalbuphine, naloxone, nesiritide, netilmicin, niCARdipine, nitroglycerin, norepinephrine, octreotide, ondansetron, oxacillin, oxaliplatin, oxytocin, PACLitaxel, palonosetron, pamidronate, pancuronium, papaverine, pentamidine, pentazocine, perphenazine, phenylephrine, phytonadione, piperacillin, piperacillin-tazobactam, polymyxin B, procainamide, prochlorperazine, promethazine, propranolol, protamine, pyridoxine, quiNIDine, ranitidine, Ringer's, ritodrine, sodium acetate/bicarbonate, succinylcholine, SUFentanil, tacrolimus, temocillin, teniposide, theophylline, thiamine, thiotepa, tigecycline, tirofiban, TNA, tobramycin, tolazoline, TPN, trimetaphan, urokinase, vancomycin, vasopressin, vecuronium, verapamil, vinCRIStine, vinorelbine, vitamin B complex/C, voriconazole, zidovudine, zoledronic acid

ADVERSE EFFECTS

CNS: Seizures
CV: Dysrhythmias, QT prolongation
EENT: Hearing loss, tinnitus
GI: *Nausea, vomiting, diarrhea,* hepatotoxicity, abdominal pain, stomatitis, heartburn, anorexia, pruritus ani, pseudomembranous colitis, esophagitis, hepatotoxicity
GU: *Vaginitis, moniliasis*
INTEG: Rash, urticaria, pruritus, thrombophlebitis, injection-site reactions (**IV** site)
SYST: Anaphylaxis

Pharmacokinetics

Absorption	Well absorbed (PO)
Distribution	Widely distributed; minimally distributed (CSF); crosses placenta
Metabolism	Liver, partially
Excretion	Bile, unchanged; kidneys (minimal), unchanged
Half-life	1-3 hr

Pharmacodynamics

	PO	IV
Onset	1 hr	Rapid
Peak	1-4 hr	Infusion's end
Duration	Unknown	Unknown

INTERACTIONS
Individual drugs
Alfentanil, ALPRAZolam, bromocriptine, busPI-Rone, carBAMazepine, cilostazol, clindamycin, cloZAPine, cycloSPORINE, diazepam, digoxin, disopyramide, felodipine, ibrutinib, methylPREDNISolone, midazolam, quiNIDine, rifabutin, sildenafil, tacrolimus, tadalafil, theophylline, triazolam, vardenafil, vinBLAStine, warfarin: increased toxicity, increased action

Diltiazem, itraconazole, ketoconazole, nefazodone, pimozide, verapamil: increased serious dysrhythmias, do not use together

Drug classifications
Ergots: increased action, toxicity
HMG-CoA reductase inhibitors: increased action, toxicity
Products that increase QT prolongation: increased QT
Protease inhibitors: serious dysrhythmias

Drug/lab test
Increased: AST/ALT
Decreased: folate assay
False increase: 17-OHCS/17-KS

NURSING CONSIDERATIONS
Assessment
• Assess patient for previous sensitivity reaction
• **Assess patient for signs and symptoms of infection** including characteristics of wounds, sputum, urine, stool, WBC >10,000/mm^3, earache, fever; obtain baseline information before, during treatment
• Obtain C&S test results before beginning product therapy to identify if correct treatment has been initiated
• Assess for allergic reactions: rash, urticaria may occur a few days after therapy begins
• Identify urine output; if decreasing, notify prescriber (may indicate nephrotoxicity); also monitor increases in BUN, creatinine
• Monitor blood studies: AST, ALT, CBC, Hct, bilirubin, LDH, alkaline phosphatase, Coombs' test monthly if patient is on long-term therapy
• Monitor electrolytes: potassium, sodium, chloride monthly if patient is on long-term therapy
• **Assess for overgrowth of infection: perineal itching, fever, malaise, redness, pain, swelling, drainage, rash, diarrhea, change in cough, sputum**

• **Pseudomembranous colitis: assess for diarrhea with blood, mucus, abdominal pain, fever, product should be discontinued immediately**
• **Anaphylaxis: assess for generalized hives, itching, flushing, swelling of lips/tongue/throat, wheezing; have emergency equipment nearby**
• QT prolongation: may occur (IV >15 mg/min), those with electrolyte imbalances, congenital QT prolongation, and the elderly are at greater risk; correct electrolyte imbalances prior to treatment; monitor ECG

Patient/family education
• Teach patient to report sore throat, bruising, bleeding, joint pain; may indicate blood dyscrasias (rare)
• Advise patient to contact prescriber if vaginal itching, loose foul-smelling stools, furry tongue occur; may indicate superinfection
• Instruct patient to take all medication prescribed for the length of time ordered
• Teach patient to avoid use with other products unless approved by prescriber

Evaluation
Positive therapeutic outcome
• Absence of signs/symptoms of infection (WBC <10,000/mm^3, temp WNL, absence of red, draining wounds, earache)
• Reported improvement in symptoms of infection

TREATMENT OF OVERDOSE:
Withdraw product, maintain airway, administer EPINEPHrine, aminophylline, O$_2$, **IV** corticosteroids

erythromycin ophthalmic
See Appendix B

erythromycin topical
See Appendix B

escitalopram (Rx)
(es-sit-tal'oh-pram)
Cipralex ✦, Lexapro
Func. class.: Antidepressant, selective serotonin reuptake inhibitor
Pregnancy category C

ACTION: Inhibits CNS neuron uptake of serotonin but not of norepinephrine

Therapeutic outcome: Decreased symptoms of depression

USES: General anxiety disorder; major depressive disorder in adults/adolescents

Unlabeled uses: Panic disorder, social phobia, autism

CONTRAINDICATIONS

Hypersensitivity to this product or citalopram, MAOIs

Precautions: Pregnancy **C**, breastfeeding, geriatric, renal/hepatic disease, history of seizures, abrupt discontinuation, bleeding, anticoagulants

> **BLACK BOX WARNING:** Children ≤12 yr/adolescents, suicidal ideation

DOSAGE AND ROUTES

Adult: PO 10 mg/day in AM or PM; after 1 wk if no clinical improvement is noted, dosage may be increased to 20 mg/day PM; maintenance 10-20 mg/day; reassess to determine need for treatment
Geriatric/hepatic dose: PO 10 mg/day

Available forms: Tabs 5, 10, 20 mg; oral sol 5 mg (as base)/5 ml (contains sorbitol)

Implementation

• Give with food or milk for GI symptoms; give with full glass of water
• Give crushed if patient is unable to swallow medication whole, scored tabs can be cut
• Give dose at bedtime if oversedation occurs during the day
• Give gum, hard candy, frequent sips of water for dry mouth
• Oral sol: measure with calibrated device
• Store at room temperature; do not freeze
• Provide assistance with ambulation during therapy, because drowsiness, dizziness occur
• Provide safety measures primarily in geriatric
• Check to see if PO medication swallowed

ADVERSE EFFECTS

CNS: *Headache, nervousness, insomnia,* **suicidal ideation,** *drowsiness, anxiety, tremor, dizziness, fatigue, sedation, poor concentration, abnormal dreams, agitation,* **seizures,** apathy, euphoria, hallucinations, delusions, psychosis, **neuroleptic malignant syndrome–like reactions,** ataxia, worsening depression

CV: *Hot flashes, palpitations,* angina pectoris, **hemorrhage,** hypertension, **tachycardia,** 1st-degree AV block, **bradycardia, MI, thrombophlebitis,** postural hypotension

EENT: Visual changes, ear/eye pain, photophobia, tinnitus, pupil dilation, dental pain

GI: *Nausea, diarrhea, dry mouth, anorexia, dyspepsia, constipation, cramps, vomiting, taste changes, flatulence, decreased appetite,* hepatitis

GU: *Dysmenorrhea, decreased libido, urinary frequency, UTI,* amenorrhea, cystitis, impotence, urine retention, ejaculation disorder

HEMA: Impaired platelet aggregation

INTEG: *Sweating, rash, pruritus,* acne, alopecia, urticaria, photosensitivity, bruising

MS: *Pain,* arthritis, twitching, osteopenia

RESP: *Infection, pharyngitis, nasal congestion, sinus headache, sinusitis, cough, dyspnea, bronchitis,* asthma, hyperventilation, pneumonia

SYST: *Asthenia, viral infection, fever, allergy, chills,* **serotonin syndrome, neonatal abstinence syndrome, Stevens-Johnson syndrome**

Pharmacokinetics

Absorption	Unknown
Distribution	Unknown
Metabolism	Liver
Excretion	Urine
Half-life	Unknown

Pharmacodynamics

Unknown

INTERACTIONS
Individual drugs

Alcohol: increased CNS depression
Amantadine, bromocriptine, busPIRone, lithium, traMADol, tryptophan: increased serotonin syndrome
BusPIRone: increased symptoms of OCD
CarBAMazepine, lithium, phenytoin, warfarin: increased levels or toxicity of each specific product
Cyproheptadine: decreased escitalopram effect
Diazepam: increased half-life of diazepam
Haloperidol: increased effect of haloperidol

Drug classifications

Antidepressants, opioids, sedatives: increased CNS depression
Antidysrhythmics, antipsychotics: increased levels, toxicity
Highly protein-bound products: increased side effects of escitalopram
MAOIs: do not use with or 14 days before escitalopram
NSAIDs, salicylates, anticoagulants, SSRIs, platelet inhibitors: increased bleeding risk
Phenothiazines: increased levels of phenothiazines
SSRIs, SNRIs, serotonin-receptor agonists, amphetamines: increased serotonin syndrome
Tricyclics: increased levels of tricyclics

Drug/herb
Kava: increased CNS effect
St. John's wort: do not use together, serotonin syndrome may occur

Drug/food
Grapefruit juice: increased escitalopram effect

Drug/lab test
Increased: serum bilirubin, blood glucose, alkaline phosphatase
Decreased: VMA, 5-HIAA
False increase: urinary catecholamines

NURSING CONSIDERATIONS
Assessment

> **BLACK BOX WARNING:** Assess mental status: mood, sensorium, affect, **suicidal tendencies,** increase in psychiatric symptoms, depression, panic, not approved for use in children

• Assess appetite in bulimia nervosa, weight daily, increase nutritious foods in diet, watch for bingeing and vomiting
⚠ Assess allergic reactions: itching, rash, urticaria; product should be discontinued; may need to give antihistamine
• Monitor B/P (lying/standing), pulse q4hr; if systolic B/P drops 20 mm Hg, hold product, notify prescriber; take VS q4hr in patients with cardiovascular disease
• Monitor blood studies: CBC, leukocytes, differential, cardiac enzymes if patient is receiving long-term therapy; check platelets; bleeding can occur
⚠ Serotonin syndrome: Assess for nausea, vomiting, sedation, dizziness, sweating, facial flushing, mental changes, shivering, increased B/P: discontinue, notify prescriber
• Monitor liver function tests: AST, ALT, bilirubin, creatinine; thyroid function studies
• Monitor weight qwk; appetite may decrease with product
⚠ Monitor ECG for flattening of T wave, bundle branch, AV block, dysrhythmias in cardiac patients
• Monitor alcohol consumption; if alcohol is consumed, hold dose until AM

Patient/family education
• Teach patient that therapeutic effect may take 1-4 wk, may have increased anxiety for first 5-7 days, do not abruptly discontinue
⚠ Serotonin syndrome: To report immediately nausea, vomiting, sedation, dizziness, sweating, facial flushing, mental changes, shivering
• Advise patient to use caution in driving, other activities requiring alertness because of drowsiness, dizziness, blurred vision

• Advise patient to use sunscreen to prevent photosensitivity
• Advise patient to avoid alcohol ingestion, other CNS depressants
• Advise patient to notify prescriber if pregnant or plan to become pregnant or breastfeed, discuss sexual dysfunction
• Advise patient to change positions slowly; orthostatic hypotension may occur
• Teach patient to avoid all OTC products unless approved by prescriber, to take without regard to meals
• Teach patient to report immediately signs of urinary retention

> **BLACK BOX WARNING:** Teach patient that clinical worsening and suicide risk may occur, especially in adolescents and young adults

• Teach patient using MedGuide provided
• Teach patient about drug interactions

Evaluation
Positive therapeutic outcome
• Decreased depression

TREATMENT OF OVERDOSE:
Activated charcoal, supportive care

⚠ HIGH ALERT

eslicarbazepine
(es'lye-kar-bay'ze-peen)
Aptiom
Func. class.: Anticonvulsant, misc
Chem. class.: Voltage-gated sodium channel (VGSC) blocker
Pregnancy category C

ACTION: Exact mechanism unknown; a voltage-gated sodium-channel blocker inhibits repetitive neuronal firing

USES: Partial seizures, adjunctive treatment

CONTRAINDICATIONS
Hypersensitivity to this product or OXcarbazepine

Precautions: Breastfeeding, abrupt discontinuation, depression, driving/operating machinery, ethanol intoxication, hepatic disease, renal disease, hyponatremia, suicidal ideation, pregnancy **C**

DOSAGE AND ROUTES
Adult: PO 400 mg/day, after 1 wk increase to 800 mg/day, max 1600 mg/day

Renal dose
Adult: PO CCr <50 ml/min, 200 mg/day, after 2 wk increase to 400 mg/day, max 600 mg/day

Available forms: Tab 200, 400, 600, 800 mg

Implementation
- May be taken without regard to food
- May be crushed or swallowed whole

ADVERSE EFFECTS

CNS: Drowsiness, dizziness, amnesia, depression, insomnia, lethargy, memory impairment, confusion, fatigue, headache, speech disturbance, suicidal thoughts/behaviors, tremor
CV: Hypertension, peripheral edema
EENT: Blurred vision, nystagmus, diplopia
GI: Nausea, constipation, diarrhea, hypercholesterolemia/hypertriglyceride, vomiting, hepatotoxicity
GU: Cystitis
INTEG: Rash, Stevens-Johnson syndrome, toxic epidermal necrolysis, anaphylaxis, angioedema
META: Hyponatremia
RESP: Cough

Pharmacokinetics

Absorption	Unknown
Distribution	Unknown
Metabolism	Liver
Excretion	Urine, feces
Half-life	Terminal 13-20 hr

Pharmacodynamics

Onset	Unknown
Peak	1-4 hr
Duration	Unknown

INTERACTIONS

Individual drugs

Bedaquiline, bocepevir, bosutinib, carbozantinib, cobicistant, elvitegravir, emtricitubine, crizotinib, cycloSPORINE, dronederone, erlotinib, fosamprenavir, galantamine, gefitinib, HYDROcodone, maraviroc, oxyCODONE, paliperidone, perm panel, pimozide, praziquantel, QUEtiapine, ranolazine, rilpivirine: decreased effects of these agents

CYP1A2, CYP2C19 substrates: decreased eslicarbamazepine effect

Drug classifications

CYP3A inducers: decreased effect of these agents

NURSING CONSIDERATIONS

Assessment
- Seizures: character, location, duration, intensity, frequency, aura
- Hepatic studies: ALT, AST, bilirubin; sodium

BLACK BOX WARNING: Mental status: mood, sensorium, affect, behavioral changes, suicidal thoughts/behaviors; if mental status changes, notify prescriber

- Eye problems: need for ophthalmic examinations before, during, after treatment (slit lamp, funduscopy, tonometry)
- Allergic reaction: purpura, red, raised rash; if these occur; product should be discontinued

Patient/family education
- Instruct patient to carry emergency ID stating patient's name, products taken, condition, prescriber's name and phone number
- Instruct patient to avoid driving, other activities that require alertness, usually for the first 3 days of treatment
- Instruct patient not to discontinue medication quickly after long-term use
- Instruct patient to notify prescriber if pregnancy is planned or suspected, pregnancy **C**, avoid breastfeeding
- Instruct patient to report signs of decreased renal function, dizziness, increased cholesterol, ocular toxicity, suicidal ideation, skin rashes
- Teach patient to take with or without food; tablet can be crushed

Evaluation
Positive therapeutic outcome
- Decreased seizure activity; document on patient's chart

⚠ HIGH ALERT

esmolol (Rx)

(ez′moe-lole)
Brevibloc
Func. class.: β-Adrenergic blocker (antidysrhythmic II)
Pregnancy category C

Do not confuse: esmolol/Osmitrol, Brevibloc/Brevital

ACTION: Competitively blocks stimulation of β_1-adrenergic receptors in the myocardium; produces negative chronotropic, inotropic activity (decreases rate of SA node discharge, increases recovery time), slows conduction of AV node, decreases heart rate, decreases O_2 consumption in myocardium; also decreases renin-aldosterone-angiotensin system at high doses; inhibits β_2-receptors in bronchial system at higher doses

Therapeutic outcome: Decreased supraventricular tachycardia

USES: Supraventricular tachycardias, non-compensatory sinus tachycardia, hypertensive crisis, intraoperative and postoperative tachycardia and hypertension, atrial fibrillation/flutter

Unlabeled uses: Hypertensive crisis/urgency, unstable angina

CONTRAINDICATIONS
Heart block (2nd- or 3rd-degree), cardiogenic shock, CHF, cardiac failure, hypersensitivity, severe bradycardia

Precautions: Pregnancy C, breastfeeding, geriatric patients, hypotension, peripheral vascular disease, diabetes, hypoglycemia, thyrotoxicosis, renal disease, atrial fibrillation, bronchospasms, hyperthyroidism, myasthenia gravis, asthma, COPD, CV disease, pheochromocytoma, abrupt discontinuation

DOSAGE AND ROUTES
Atrial fibrillation/flutter
Adult: IV Loading dose 500 mcg/kg/min over 1 min; maintenance 50 mcg/kg/min for 4 min; if no response in 5 min, give 2nd loading dose; then increase INF to 100 mcg/kg/min for 4 min; if no response, repeat loading dose, then increase maintenance INF by 50 mcg/kg/min (max of 200 mcg/kg/min); titrate to patient response
Child: IV A total loading dose of 600 mcg/kg over 2 min, maintenance IV INF 200 mcg/kg/min, titrate upward by 50-100 mcg/kg/min q5-10min until B/P, heart rate reduced by >10%

Perioperative hypertension/tachycardia
Adult: IV immediate control 80 mg (bolus) over 30 seconds, then 150 mcg/kg/min, adjust to response, max 300 mcg/kg/min

Hypertensive emergency (unlabeled)
Adult: IV 250-500 mcg/kg over 1 min, then IV INF 50-100 mcg/kg/min × 4 min

Available forms: Inj 10 mg, 250 mg/ml

Implementation

IV route
• Check that correct concentration is being given
• The 10 mg/ml inj solution needs no dilution and may be used as an **IV** loading dose using handheld syringe
Continuous IV infusion route
• Ready-to-use bags premixed isotonic sol of 10 mg/ml and 20 mg/ml are available in 100, 250 ml bags; use controlled device, a central line is preferred, rate is based on patient's weight
• Store at room temperature for 24 hr; sol should be clear

Y-site compatibilities: Amikacin, aminophylline, ampicillin, amiodarone, atracurium, butorphanol, calcium chloride, ceFAZolin, cefmetazole, cefoperazone, cefTAZidime, ceftizoxime, chloramphenicol, cimetidine, cisatracurium, clindamycin, diltiazem, DOPamine, enalaprilat, erythromycin, famotidine, fentaNYL, gentamicin, heparin, hydrocortisone, regular insulin, labetalol, magnesium sulfate, methyldopate, metroNIDAZOLE, midazolam, morphine, nafcillin, nitroglycerin, norepinephrine, nitroprusside, pancuronium, penicillin G potassium, phenytoin, piperacillin, polymyxin B, potassium chloride, potassium phosphate, propofol, ranitidine, remifentanil, streptomycin, tacrolimus, tobramycin, trimethoprim/sulfamethoxazole, vancomycin, vecuronium, voriconazole, zoledronic acid

Y-site incompatibilities: Furosemide

ADVERSE EFFECTS
CNS: Confusion, light-headedness, paresthesia, somnolence, fever, dizziness, fatigue, headache, depression, anxiety, seizures
CV: Hypotension, bradycardia, chest pain, peripheral ischemia, shortness of breath, CHF, conduction disturbances 1st-, 2nd-, 3rd-degree heart block
GI: *Nausea,* vomiting, anorexia, gastric pain, flatulence, constipation, heartburn, bloating
GU: Urinary retention, impotence, dysuria
INTEG: *Induration, inflammation at inj site,* discoloration, edema, erythema, burning, pallor, flushing, rash, pruritus, dry skin, alopecia
RESP: Bronchospasm, dyspnea, cough, wheezing, nasal stuffiness, pulmonary edema

Pharmacokinetics

Absorption	Complete
Distribution	Unknown
Metabolism	Liver
Excretion	Kidneys
Half-life	9 min

Pharmacodynamics

Onset	Rapid
Peak	Unknown
Duration	1-2 min

INTERACTIONS
Individual drugs
Amphetamine, ePHEDrine, EPINEPHrine, norepinephrine, phenylephrine, pseudoephedrine: increased α-adrenergic stimulation
Clonidine: possibly fatal increased B/P
Digoxin: increased digoxin levels
Diltiazem, verapamil:

Increase: potentiate suppressive effects of these products

Thyroid hormones: decreased effect of salicylates, esmolol, decreased action of thyroid hormone

Drug classifications
Antidiabetics: Increased: effect of antidiabetic

MAOIs, solatol: avoid use

General anesthetics: increased antihypertensive effect

Drug/herb
Ephedra, hawthorn: decreased antihypertensive effect

Drug/lab test
Interference: glucose/insulin tolerance test

NURSING CONSIDERATIONS
Assessment
• **Dysrhythmias: Monitor B/P during beginning treatment, periodically thereafter; pulse q4hr; note rate, rhythm, quality; apical/radial pulse before administration; notify prescriber of any significant changes (pulse <50 bpm); if severe, slow or stop infusion**

• **Check for baselines in renal, liver function tests before therapy begins**

• **CHF: Assess for edema in feet, legs daily; monitor I&O, daily weight; check for jugular vein distention, crackles bilaterally, dyspnea**

• **Bronchospasm: Assess breath sounds and respiratory patterns**

Patient/family education
• Teach patient need for medication and expected results

• Caution patient to rise slowly to prevent orthostatic hypotension

• Advise patient to notify if pain, swelling occurs at **IV** site

• **Teach patient to notify prescriber if chest pain, shortness of breath, wheezing, low B/P occur**

Evaluation
Positive therapeutic outcome
• Absence of dysrhythmias

TREATMENT OF OVERDOSE:
Defibrillation, vasopressor for hypotension

esomeprazole (Rx)
(es'oh-mep'rah-zohl)
NexIUM
Func. class.: Anti-ulcer, proton pump inhibitor
Chem. class.: Benzimidazole
Pregnancy category B

Do not confuse: NexIUM/NexAVAR

ACTION: Suppresses gastric secretion by inhibiting hydrogen/potassium ATPase enzyme system in the gastric parietal cell; characterized as gastric acid pump inhibitor, since it blocks final step of acid production

Therapeutic outcome: Absence of duodenal ulcers; decreased gastroesophageal reflux

USES: Gastroesophageal reflux disease (GERD), adult/child/infant; severe erosive esophagitis; treatment of active duodenal ulcers in combination with antiinfectives for *Helicobacter pylori* infection; long-term use in hypersecretory conditions

CONTRAINDICATIONS
Hypersensitivity to proton-pump inhibitors (PPIs)

Precautions: Pregnancy **B**, breastfeeding, children, geriatric, hypomagnesemia, osteoporosis

DOSAGE AND ROUTES
Active duodenal ulcers associated with *H. pylori*
Adult: PO 40 mg/day × 10-14 days in combination with clarithromycin 500 mg bid × 10 days and amoxicillin 1000 mg bid × 10 days

Hepatic dose
Adult: PO/IV max 20 mg/day (severe hepatic disease)

GERD/erosive esophagitis
Adult: PO 20 or 40 mg/day × 4-8 wk; no adjustment needed in renal, liver failure, geriatric; **IV** 20 or 40 mg/day up to 10 days

Child and adolescent 12-17 yr: PO 20 or 40 mg/day 1 hr before meals up to 8 wk

Child 1-11 yr and ≥20 kg: PO 10 mg/day 1 hr before meals for up to 8 wk

Infant ≥1 mo: IV 0.5 mg/kg over 10-30 min

Infant 1-11 mo (>7.5-12 kg): PO 10 mg daily up to 6 wk

Infant 1-11 mo (5-7.5 kg): PO 5 mg daily up to 6 wk

Infant 1-11 mo (3-5 kg): PO 2.5 mg daily up to 6 wk

Available forms: Del rel caps 20, 40 mg; powder for **IV** inj 20, 40 mg/vial; del rel powder for oral susp 2.5, 5, 20, 40 mg

Implementation
PO route
• Swallow caps whole; do not crush or chew; cap may be opened and sprinkled over Tbsp of applesauce
• Same time daily, 1 hr before meal
• **Oral susp (del rel):** empty contents of packet into container with 1 Tbsp of water, let stand 2-3 min to thicken, restir, give within 30 min of mixing; any residual product should be flushed with more water, taken immediately
• **NG tube (del rel oral susp):** add 15 ml water to contents of packet in syringe, shake, leave 2-3 min to thicken, shake, inject through NG tube within 30 min

IV, direct route
• Reconstitute each vial with 5 ml 0.9% NaCl, D₅W, LR; give over 3 min
Intermittent IV INF route
• Dilute reconstituted sol to 50 ml, give over 30 min, do not admix, flush line with D₅W, 0.9% NaCl, LR after inf

Solution compatibilities: D_5W, LR, 0.9% NaCl

ADVERSE EFFECTS
CNS: *Headache, dizziness*
GI: *Diarrhea, flatulence,* abdominal pain, constipation, dry mouth, **hepatic failure, hepatitis,** microscopic colitis
INTEG: *Rash,* dry skin
MISC: **Heart failure**
RESP: *Cough,* **pneumonia**
SYST: **Stevens-Johnson syndrome, toxic epidermal necrolysis, exfoliative dermatitis**

Pharmacokinetics
Absorption	Unknown
Distribution	97% plasma protein bound
Metabolism	Liver (metabolites)
Excretion	Urine (metabolites), feces (metabolites); in geriatric, elimination rate decreased, bioavailability increased
Half-life	1-1½ hr

Pharmacodynamics
Onset	Unknown
Peak	1½ hr
Duration	Unknown

INTERACTIONS
Individual drugs
Calcium carbonate, clopidogrel, dapsone, indinavir, iron, itraconazole, ketoconazole, mycophenolate, vitamin B_{12}: decreased effect
Increase: effect of methotrexate, tacrolimus, warfarin
Cilostazol, clozapine, those drugs metabolized by CYP2C19, diazepam, digoxin, penicillins, saquinavir: increased effect, toxicity

Drug/lab test
Interference: sodium, Hgb, WBC, platelets, magnesium

NURSING CONSIDERATIONS
Assessment
• **Assess GI system: bowel sounds, abdomen for pain, swelling, anorexia, bloody stools; pseudomembranous colitis may occur**
• **Hepatic failure, hepatitis: monitor AST, ALT, alkaline phosphatase during treatment**
• **Serious skin disorders: Stevens-Johnson syndrome, toxic epidermal necrolysis, exfoliative dermatitis**

Patient/family education
• Instruct patient to report severe diarrhea; product may have to be discontinued, rash
• Advise diabetic patients that hypoglycemia may occur
• Advise patient to avoid hazardous activities; dizziness may occur
• Advise patient to avoid alcohol, salicylates, ibuprofen; may cause GI irritation
• Teach patient to take ≥1 hr prior to meal; not to crush, chew delayed-release product, if missed, take as soon as remembered if not almost time for next dose
• Teach patient if cap cannot be swallowed whole contents may be mixed with a tablespoon of applesauce

Evaluation
Positive therapeutic outcome
• Absence of epigastric pain, swelling, fullness

estradiol (Rx)
(ess-tra-dye′ole)
Estrace
estradiol cypionate (Rx)
Depo-Estradiol
estradiol topical emulsion (Rx)
Estrasorb
estradiol valerate (Rx)
Delestrogen
estradiol transdermal system (Rx)
Alora, Climara, Estraderm, Minivelle, Vivelle
estradiol vaginal tablet (Rx)
Vagifem Dot
estradiol vaginal ring (Rx)
Estring, Femring
estradiol gel (Rx)
Divigel, Elestrin, Estrogel
estradiol spray (Rx)
Evamist

Func. class.: Estrogen, progestin
Chem. class.: Nonsteroidal synthetic estrogen

Pregnancy category X :star:

ACTION: Needed for adequate functioning of female reproductive system; affects release of pituitary gonadatropins, inhibits ovulation, promotes adequate calcium use in bone structure

Therapeutic outcome: Decreased tumor size in prostatic cancer; increased estrogen levels in menopause, female hypogonadism

USES: Vasomotor symptoms associated with menopause, inoperable breast cancer (selected cases), prostatic cancer, atrophic vaginitis, kraurosis vulvae, hypogonadism, primary ovarian failure, prevention of osteoporosis, castration

CONTRAINDICATIONS
Pregnancy **X**, breastfeeding, reproductive cancer, genital bleeding (abnormal, undiagnosed), protein S or C deficiency, antithrombin deficiency, angioedema, MI, stroke

> **BLACK BOX WARNING:** Breast/endometrial cancer, thromboembolic disorders, MI, stroke

Precautions: Hypertension, asthma, blood dyscrasias, gallbladder disease, CHF, diabetes mellitus, bone disease, depression, migraine headache, seizure disorders, renal/hepatic disease, family history of cancer of breast or reproductive tract, history of smoking, uterine fibroids, vaginal irritation/infection, history of angioedema

> **BLACK BOX WARNING:** Cardiac disease, dementia, accidental exposure pets/children (topical)

DOSAGE AND ROUTES
Hormone replacement/menopause symptoms
Adult: TD 1 patch delivering 0.025, 0.0375, 0.05, 0.075, or 0.1 mg/day 2×/wk (Alora, Estraderm, Vivelle-Dot); 1 patch delivering 0.025, 0.0375, 0.05, 0.06, 0.075, or 0.1 mg/day replace q7 days (Climara); 1 patch delivering 0.025 mg/day replace q7 days, may increase to 2 patches after 4-6 wk; **GEL** apply entire unit dose packet to 5- × 7-inch area of upper thigh/day, alternate thighs; **SPRAY** (Evamist) 1 spray to inner surface of forearm/day in AM

Menopause/hypogonadism/castration/ovarian failure
Adult: PO 0.5-2 mg/day 3 wk on, 1 wk off or continuously; IM 1-5 mg q3-4wk (cypionate), 1-5 mg q3-4wk; 10-20 mg q4wk (valerate); TOP Estraderm 0.05 mg/24 hr applied 2 ×/wk, Climara 0.05 mg/hr applied 1 ×/wk in a cyclic regimen; women with hysterectomy may use continuously

Prostatic cancer
Adult: IM 30 mg q1-2wk (valerate); PO 1-2 mg tid (oral estradiol)

Breast cancer (palliative treatment)
Adult: PO 10 mg tid × 3 mo or longer

Atropic vaginitis/kraurosis vulvae
Adult: VAG cream 2-4 g/day × 1-2 wk, then 1 g 1-3 ×/wk cycled; VAG tab 1/day × 2 wk, maintenance 1 tab 2 ×/wk; VAG ring inserted and left in place continuously for 3 mo

Vasomotor symptoms
Adult: TOP after cleaning and drying skin on left thigh, calf, rub in contents of pouch using both hands until completely absorbed; wash hands

Available forms: Estradiol: tabs 0.5, 1, 2 mg; **valerate:** inj 10, 20, 40 mg/ml; **transdermal** 0.014, 0.025, 0.0375, 0.05, 0.075, 0.1 mg/24-hr release rate; **vag cream** 100 mcg/g; **vag ring** 2 mg/90 days; **vag tab** 10 mcg; **topical emulsion:** 2.5 mg; gel 0.1%, 0.06%, (Divigel); **spray** (Evamist) 1.53 mg/actuation

Implementation
PO route
- Give titrated dose, use lowest effective dose
- Give with food or milk to decrease GI symptoms

IM route
- Administer deeply in large muscle mass; product is painful
- Rotate syringe to mix oil and medication

Transdermal route
- May contain aluminum or other metals in backing of patch, can overheat in MRI scan and burn patients
- Apply to area free of hair to ensure adhesion on trunk of body 2 ×/wk; press firmly and hold in place for 10 sec to ensure good contact; do not apply to breasts
- Start transdermal dose 7 days before last PO dose if routes are to be changed

Topical route spray (Evamist)
- Use daily; spray to inner upper arm; may increase to 2-3 ×/day based on response; let dry for 2 min, avoid secondary exposure to children, pets, caregivers

Vaginal route
- Place cream in applicator by attaching tube to applicator; squeeze cream into tube to mark; insert with patient reclining
- Use a new applicator daily

ADVERSE EFFECTS
CNS: Dizziness, headache, migraine, depression, seizures
CV: Hypertension, thrombophlebitis, edema, thromboembolism, stroke, pulmonary embolism, MI, chest pain
EENT: Contact lens intolerance, increased myopia, astigmatism, throat swelling, eyelid edema
GI: *Nausea*, vomiting, diarrhea, anorexia, pancreatitis, cramps, constipation, increased appetite, increased weight, cholestatic jaundice, hepatic adenoma
GU: Amenorrhea, cervical erosion, breakthrough bleeding, dysmenorrhea, vaginal candidiasis, breast changes, *gynecomastia, testicular atrophy, impotence;* increased risk of breast, endometrial cancer, changes in libido; toxic shock, vaginal wall ulceration/erosion (vag ring)
INTEG: Rash, urticaria, acne, hirsutism, alopecia, oily skin, seborrhea, purpura, erythema, pruritus, melasma; site irritation (transdermal)
META: Folic acid deficiency, hypercalcemia, hyperglycemia

Absorption	Well absorbed
Distribution	Widely distributed, crosses placenta
Metabolism	Unknown
Excretion	Unknown
Half-life	Unknown

Pharmacodynamics

	PO	IM	IV
Onset	Rapid	Slow	Rapid
Peak	Unknown	Unknown	Unknown
Duration	Unknown	Unknown	Unknown

INTERACTIONS
Individual drugs
Calcium, phenylbutazone, rifampin: decreased estradiol action
CycloSPORINE, dantrolene: increased toxicity
Tamoxifen: decreased tamoxifen action

Drug classifications
Anticoagulants: decreased action of anticoagulants
Anticonvulsants, barbiturates: decreased estradiol action
Corticosteroids: increased action of corticosteroids, tricyclics
Hypoglycemics (oral): decreased action of hypoglycemics

Drug/herb
Black cohosh, DHEA: altered estrogen effect
Saw palmetto, St. John's wort: decreased estrogen effect

Drug/food
Grapefruit juice: increased estrogen level

Drug/lab test
Increased: BSP retention test; PBI; T_4; serum sodium; platelet aggregation; thyroxine-binding globulin (TBS); prothrombin; factors VII, VIII, IX, X; triglycerides
Decreased: serum folate, serum triglyceride, T_3 resin uptake test, glucose tolerance test, antithrombin III, pregnanediol, metyrapone test
False positive: LE prep, ANA titer

NURSING CONSIDERATIONS
Assessment

> **BLACK BOX WARNING:** Assess for previous breast/endometrial cancer, thromboembolic disorders, MI, stroke, dementia, use adequate screening for these conditions, estrogen increases the risk

- Monitor blood glucose in patient with diabetes; hyperglycemia may occur
- Monitor B/P q4hr; watch for increase caused by water and sodium retention
- Monitor I&O ratio; be alert for decreasing urinary output and increasing edema; monitor weight daily; notify prescriber if weekly weight gain is >5 lb; if increased, diuretic may be ordered
- Obtain liver function tests baseline, periodically, including AST, ALT, bilirubin, alkaline phosphatase, periodic folic acid level
- Assess edema, hypertension, cardiac symptoms, jaundice
- Assess mental status: affect, mood, behavioral changes, aggression; depression may occur, product may need to be discontinued
- Assess female patient for intact uterus; if so, progesterone should be added to estrogen therapy to decrease risk of endometrial cancer

Patient/family education
- Tell patient to take exactly as prescribed; do not double doses
- ⚠ Advise patient that increased weight gain and symptoms of fluid retention should be reported to prescriber: edema of feet, ankles, sacral area; abnormal vaginal bleeding; breast lumps; hepatic disease (dark urine, clay-colored stools, jaundice of skin, sclera, pruritus); to report dermal rash with transdermal patch
- ⚠ Caution patient that thromboembolic symptoms should be reported: tenderness in legs, chest pain, dyspnea, headaches, blurred vision
- Inform patient to use sunscreen and protective clothing because sunburns may occur
- Advise patient to stop smoking; smokers have a greater chance of thromboembolic disorder
- Teach patient to avoid grapefruit or grapefruit juice (PO)
- Teach patient that smoking increases CV conditions, encourage to stop
- Advise patient to notify prescriber if pregnancy is planned or suspected, and not to become pregnant when using estrogen
- Inform patient to report changes in blood glucose, if diabetic

Evaluation
Positive therapeutic outcome
- Reversal of menopausal symptoms
- Decrease in tumor size in prostatic or breast cancer

- Decrease in itching, inflammation of vagina
- Absence of symptoms of osteoporosis

estrogens, conjugated (Rx)
Cenestin, Premarin
estrogens, conjugated
synthetic B (Rx)
Enjuvia
Pregnancy category X

Do not confuse: Premarin/Provera

ACTION: Needed for adequate functioning of female reproductive system; affects release of pituitary gonadotropins; inhibits ovulation; promotes adequate calcium use in bone structures

Therapeutic outcome: Decreased tumor size in prostatic cancer; increased estrogen levels in menopause, female hypogonadism

USES: Symptoms associated with menopause, inoperable breast cancer, prostatic cancer, abnormal uterine bleeding, hypogonadism, primary ovarian failure, prevention of osteoporosis, castration, atrophic vaginitis

CONTRAINDICATIONS
Pregnancy **X,** breastfeeding, thromboembolic disorders, reproductive cancer, genital bleeding (abnormal, undiagnosed), hypersensitivity, MI, stroke, phlebitis

> **BLACK BOX WARNING:** Endometrial breast cancer, thromboembolic diseases

Precautions: Hypertension, asthma, blood dyscrasias, gallbladder disease, CHF, diabetes mellitus, bone disease, depression, migraine headache, seizure disorders, renal/hepatic disease, family history of cancer of breast or reproductive tract, history of smoking, dementia, hypothyroidism, obesity, SLE

DOSAGE AND ROUTES
>> Estrogens, conjugated
Menopause
Adult: PO 0.3-1.25 mg/day 3 wk on, 1 wk off

Prevention of osteoporosis
Adult: PO 0.3 mg/day or in a cycle

Atrophic vaginitis
Adult: VAG cream 0.5 g/day × 21 days, off 7 days, repeat

Prostatic cancer
Adult: PO 1.25-2.5 mg tid

Advanced inoperable breast cancer
Adult: PO 10 mg tid × 3 mo or longer

Abnormal uterine bleeding
Adult: IV/IM 25 mg, repeat in 6-12 hr

Castration/primary ovarian failure
Adult: PO 1.25 mg/day 3 wk on, 1 wk off

Hypogonadism
Adult: PO 0.3 or 0.625 mg q day/3 wk on, 1 wk off; adjust to response

>> Estrogens, conjugated synthetic B
Menopause
Adult: PO 0.625 mg/day initially, may increase based on response

Available forms: Tabs 0.3, 0.45, 0.625, 0.9, 1.25, 2.5 mg; inj 25 mg/vial; vag cream 0.625 mg/g; synthetic B: tabs 0.625, 1.25 mg

Implementation
PO route
• Give titrated dose, use lowest effective dose
• Give in 1 dose in AM for prostatic cancer, vaginitis, hypogonadism
• Give with food or milk to decrease GI symptoms
IM route
• Reconstitute after withdrawing at least 5 ml of air from container and inject sterile diluent on vial side, rotate to dissolve
• Give IM inj deeply in large muscle
Vaginal route
• Place cream in applicator by attaching tube to applicator, squeeze cream into tube to mark, insert with patient recumbent
• Applicator should be washed after each use

IV, direct route
• Reconstitute as for IM, inject into distal port of running IV line of D$_5$W, 0.9% NaCl, LR, at a rate of 5 mg/min or less

Y-site compatibilities: Heparin/hydrocortisone, potassium chloride, vit B/C

ADVERSE EFFECTS
CNS: Dizziness, headache, migraine, depression, seizures, mood disturbances
CV: Hypertension, thrombophlebitis, edema, thromboembolism, stroke, pulmonary embolism, MI, chest pain
EENT: Contact lens intolerance, increased myopia, astigmatism
GI: *Nausea*, vomiting, diarrhea, anorexia, pancreatitis, cramps, constipation, increased appetite, cholestatic jaundice, hepatic adenoma, weight gain/loss
GU: Amenorrhea, cervical erosion, breakthrough bleeding, dysmenorrhea, vaginal candidiasis, breast changes, *gynecomastia, testicular*

atrophy, impotence, increased risk of breast, endometrial cancer, libido changes
INTEG: Rash, urticaria, acne, hirsutism, alopecia, oily skin, seborrhea, purpura, melasma
META: Folic acid deficiency, hypercalcemia, hyperglycemia

Pharmacokinetics

Absorption	Well absorbed (PO), completely absorbed (**IV**)
Distribution	Widely distributed, crosses placenta
Metabolism	Liver, exclusively; hepatic recirculation
Excretion	Kidney
Half-life	Unknown

Pharmacodynamics

	PO	IM	IV
Onset	Rapid	Slow	Immediate
Peak	Unknown	Unknown	Unknown
Duration	Unknown	Unknown	Unknown

INTERACTIONS
Individual drugs
Bosentan, cycloSPORINE, dantrolene: increased toxicity
Phenylbutazone, rifampin: decreased action of estrogens
Tamoxifen, thyroid: decreased tamoxifen action

Drug classifications
Anticoagulants: decreased action of anticoagulants
Anticonvulsants, barbiturates: decreased action of estrogens
Corticosteroids: increased action of corticosteroids
Oral hypoglycemics: decreased action of hypoglycemics
Tricyclic antidepressants: decreased effect of the antidepressant

Drug/food
Grapefruit juice: increased estrogen level

Drug/lab test
Increased: BSP retention test; PBI, T$_4$; serum sodium; platelet aggregation; thyroxine-binding globulin (TBG); prothrombin; factors VII, VIII, IX, X; triglycerides
Decreased: serum folate, serum triglyceride, T$_3$ resin uptake test, glucose tolerance test, antithrombin III, pregnanediol, metyrapone test
False positive: LE prep, ANA titer

NURSING CONSIDERATIONS
Assessment

> **BLACK BOX WARNING:** Breast, endometrial cancer: estrogens should not be used in known, suspected, or history of these disorders

> **BLACK BOX WARNING:** Stroke, thromboembolic disease of MI: should not be used in these conditions or known protein C deficiency, protein S deficiency or antithrombin in deficiency

- Monitor blood glucose in patient with diabetes; hyperglycemia may occur
- Monitor B/P q4hr; watch for increase caused by water and sodium retention
- Monitor I&O ratio; be alert for decreasing urinary output and increasing edema; monitor weight daily; notify prescriber if weekly weight gain is >5 lb; if increased, diuretic may be ordered
- Obtain liver function tests, including AST, ALT, bilirubin, alkaline phosphatase
- Assess edema, hypertension, cardiac symptoms, jaundice
- Assess mental status: affect, mood, behavioral changes, aggression; depression may occur; product may need to be discontinued
- Assess female patient for intact uterus; if so, progesterone should be added to estrogen therapy to decrease risk of endometrial cancer; abnormal uterine bleeding, breast exam

Patient/family education
- Caution patient to take exactly as prescribed and not to double doses

> **BLACK BOX WARNING:** Advise patient that increased weight gain and symptoms of fluid retention should be reported to prescriber: edema of feet, ankles, sacral area; abnormal vaginal bleeding; breast lumps; hepatic disease (dark urine, clay-colored stools, jaundice of skin, sclera, pruritus)

⚠ Caution patient that thromboembolic symptoms should be reported: pain, redness, tenderness in legs; chest pain, dyspnea, headaches, blurred vision
- Inform patient that sunburns may occur and to use sunscreen and protective clothing
- Advise patient to stop smoking; smokers have a greater chance of thromboembolic disorder
- **Tell patient to use nonhormonal birth control and to notify prescriber if pregnancy is suspected**
- Tell patient that vasomotor symptoms improve in 2 wk, max relief 8 wk

Evaluation
Positive therapeutic outcome
- Reversal of menopause symptoms
- Decrease in tumor size in prostatic, breast cancer
- Decrease in itching, inflammation of vagina
- Absence of symptoms of osteoporosis

⚠ HIGH ALERT

eszopiclone (Rx)
(es-zop'i-klone)
Lunesta
Func. class.: Sedative-hypnotic, non-benzodiazepine
Chem. class.: Cyclopyrrolone
Pregnancy category C
Controlled substance schedule IV

ACTION: Interacts with GABA receptors

Therapeutic outcome: Ability to sleep and stay asleep throughout the night

USES: Insomnia

CONTRAINDICATIONS
Hypersensitivity

Precautions: Pregnancy **C,** breastfeeding, children, geriatric, severe hepatic disease, abrupt discontinuation, COPD, depression, labor, sleep apnea, substance abuse, suicidal ideation, ethanol intoxication

DOSAGE AND ROUTES
Adult: PO 1 mg immediately before bed, may increase to 3 mg if needed

Hepatic dose/CYP3A4 inhibitors
Adult: PO 1 mg immediately before bed in severe hepatic disease, max 2 mg/day

Available forms: Tabs 1, 2, 3 mg

Implementation
- Do not break, crush, or chew tab
- For short-term use only
- Give immediately before bedtime
- Avoid use with a high-fat meal
- Provide assistance with ambulation, nightlight, call bell within reach
- Check to see product is swallowed

ADVERSE EFFECTS
CNS: Worsening depression, hallucinations, headache, daytime drowsiness, **suicidal thoughts/actions,** migraine, restlessness, anxiety, sleep driving, sleep walking
CV: Peripheral edema, chest pain
GI: Dry mouth, bitter taste (dysgeusia)

GU: Gynecomastia, dysmenorrhea
INTEG: Rash, angioedema

Pharmacokinetics

Absorption	Unknown
Distribution	Unknown
Metabolism	Extensively in the liver by CYP3A4, CYP2E1; protein binding 52%-59%
Excretion	Via kidneys
Half-life	6 hr, geriatric 9 hr

Pharmacodynamics

Onset	Rapid
Peak	1 hr
Duration	6 hr

INTERACTIONS
Drug classifications
CNS depressants: increased CNS depression
CYP3A4 inducers (dexamethasome, barbiturates, carBAMazepine, OXcarbazepine, phenytoin, fosphenytoin, ethotoin): Decrease: eszopiclone effect
CYP3A4 inhibitors (clarithromycin, itraconazole, ketoconazole, nefazodone, nelfinavir, ritonavir, troleandomycin): increased toxicity due to decreased eszopiclone elimination

Drug/food
High-fat meal: decreased product action

Drug/herb
• St. John's wort: Decrease: eszopiclone effect

NURSING CONSIDERATIONS
Assessment
• Anaphylaxis, angioedema: monitor during first dose
• **Assess sleep pattern:** ability to go to sleep, stay asleep; early morning awakenings; conservative methods used
• Monitor for abuse of this or other products

Patient/family education
• Caution patient that daytime drowsiness may occur; not to engage in hazardous activities until effect is known, memory problems may occur
• Advise patient that all other medications and supplements should be avoided unless approved by prescriber
• Advise patient to notify prescriber if pregnancy is suspected or planned
• Discuss alternative methods to improve sleep: reading, quiet environment, warm bath, milk
• Teach patient to avoid use after a high-fat meal
• Teach patient to swallow tab whole
• Teach patient not to stop drug abruptly, tolerance may occur

Evaluation
Positive therapeutic outcome
• Ability to sleep and stay asleep throughout the night

etanercept (Rx)
(eh-tan'er-sept)
Enbrel
Func. class.: Antirheumatic agent (disease-modifying) (DMARDs)
Chem. class.: Anti-TNF agent
Pregnancy category B

ACTION: Binds to tumor necrosis factor (TNF), which decreases inflammation and immune response

Therapeutic outcome: Decreased pain, inflammation

USES: Acute, chronic rheumatoid arthritis that has not responded to other disease-modifying agents; polyarticular course juvenile rheumatoid arthritis (JRA), ankylosing spondylitis, plaque psoriasis, psoriatic arthritis

Unlabeled uses: Crohn's disease

CONTRAINDICATIONS
Sepsis

Precautions: Pregnancy **B**, breastfeeding, children <4 yr, geriatric, malignancies, CHF, seizures, multiple sclerosis, latex hypersensitivity

> BLACK BOX WARNING: Infection, lymphoma, neoplastic disease, TB

DOSAGE AND ROUTES
Rheumatoid/psoriatic arthritis, ankylosing spondylitis
Adult: SUBCUT 50 mg qwk or 25 mg 2×/wk, 3-4 days apart; may be used with methotrexate for psoriatic arthitis
Child 2-17 yr: SUBCUT 0.8 mg/kg/wk, max 50 mg/wk

Plaque psoriasis
Adult: SUBCUT 50 mg 2 ×/wk × 3 mo, then 50 mg q wk maintenance
Adolescent and child 4-17 yr (unlabeled): SUBCUT 0.8 mg/kg/wk, max 50 mg/wk

Juvenile rheumatoid arthritis (JRA)
Adolescent and child 2-17 yr: SUBCUT 0.8 mg/kg/wk, max 50 mg/wk

Available forms: Powder for inj 25 mg; inj 50 mg/ml; auto injector, single use

Implementation

• May be administered by the patient or a caregiver after instruction. Assess the patient's or caregiver's ability to inject subcut and observe the first injection

• Administration of one 50 mg/ml prefilled syringe or autoinjector provides a dose equivalent to two, 25 mg prefilled syringes or two, 25 mg vials of lyophilized

• The needle cap on the prefilled syringe and on the SureClick autoinjector contain dry natural rubber (latex) and should not be handled by persons sensitive to this product

Inj route

• Inspect for particulate matter and discoloration prior to use, solution should be clear and colorless, although small white particles may be noted in the autoinjector or prefilled syringe

Subcut route

• Injection sites include front of the thigh; abdomen except the 2 inches around the navel; or outer area of the upper arm. Rotate injection sites. Do not administer where skin is tender, bruised, red, or hard. Also, do not inject directly into any raised, thick, red, or scaly skin patches or lesions related to psoriasis

Reconstitution and administration of the vial

• Do not mix or transfer the contents of one vial into another vial. Also, do not filter reconstituted product during preparation or administration. Do not add other medications to solutions containing etanercept. ONLY use the supplied diluent

• A vial adaptor is supplied for use when reconstituting the powder; however, the adaptor should not be used if multiple doses are going to be withdrawn from the vial. To reconstitute using the vial adaptor, slide the plunger into the flange end of the syringe. Attach the plunger to the gray rubber stopper in the syringe by turning the plunger clockwise until a slight resistance is felt. Remove the twist-off cap from the prefilled diluent syringe by turning counterclockwise. Once the twist-off cap is removed, twist the vial adapter onto the syringe clockwise until a slight resistance is felt. Place the vial adapter over the top of the vial being careful not to bump or touch the plunger; the plastic spike inside the vial adapter should puncture the gray stopper. Push the plunger down until all the liquid from the syringe is in the vial and gently swirl to dissolve the powder. After the diluent is added, some foaming may occur. Do not shake. Generally, dissolution takes less than 10 min; the solution should be clear and colorless. Each reconstituted vial contains 25 mg/ml of

etanercept. Turn the vial upside down and slowly pull the plunger down to the unit markings on the side of the syringe that correspond with the needed dose. Gently tap the syringe to make any air bubbles rise to the top of the syringe, and slowly push the plunger up to remove them. Remove the syringe from the vial adapter by turning the syringe counterclockwise and attach the 27 gauge needle

• If the vial will be used for multiple doses, use a 25-gauge needle for reconstituting and withdrawing the solution. Insert the 25 gauge needle or the vial adapter straight into the center of the gray stopper. A "pop" will be felt. Inject the diluent very slowly. After the diluent is added, some foaming may occur. Do not shake. Swirl contents gently during dissolution. Generally, dissolution takes less than 10 minutes; the solution should be clear and colorless. Write the mixing date on the supplied sticker and attach to the vial. Each reconstituted vial contains 25 mg/ml of etanercept. Withdraw the correct dose of the solution into the syringe; remove any air bubbles. Remove the 25-gauge needle from the syringe. Attach a 27-gauge needle

• Hold the barrel of the syringe with one hand and pull the needle cover straight off. Hold the syringe in one hand like a pencil and use the other hand to gently pinch a fold of skin at the cleaned injection site. Insert the needle at a 45° angle to the skin. Let go of the skin, and hold the syringe near its base to stabilize it. Push the plunger to inject all of the solution at a slow, steady rate. Withdraw the needle at the same angle as insertion. Do NOT rub the site

• Use as soon as possible after reconstitution. Place reconstituted vials for multiple doses in the refrigerator at 2-8° C (36°-46° F) within 4 hr of reconstitution and may be stored up to 14 days. DO NOT FREEZE

Use of the SureClick autoinjector

• Allow to reach room temperature, do not shake. Immediately before use, remove the needle shield by pulling it straight off

• Stretch the skin under and around the prefilled autoinjector, place the open end against the injection site at a 90° angle. Without pushing the purple button on top, push the autoinjector firmly against the skin to unlock. Press the purple button on top once and release the button. Listen for the first click. Wait for the second click or wait 15 seconds, and remove the autoinjector from injection site. Do NOT rub the site

• Look at the inspection window. If it is not purple, call 1-888-436-2735; do not try to reuse the autoinjector

---

Use of the prefilled syringe

• **Single-use:** allow to come to room temperature, do not shake. Remove the needle shield. Check to see if the amount of liquid in the prefilled syringe falls between the two purple fill level indicator lines on the syringe. If bubbles are seen, very gently tap the syringe. Turn the syringe so that the purple horizontal lines on the barrel are directly facing you. Do not use if the syringe does not have the right amount of liquid
• Hold the barrel of the prefilled syringe with one hand and pull the needle cover straight off. Holding the syringe with the needle pointing up, check the syringe for air bubbles. If there are bubbles, gently tap until the air bubbles rise to the top of the syringe. Slowly push the plunger up to force the air bubbles out of the syringe
• Insert the needle at a 45° angle to the pinched skin. Push the plunger to inject all of the solution at a slow, steady rate. Withdraw the needle at the same angle as insertion. Do NOT rub the site

ADVERSE EFFECTS

CNS: Headache, asthenia, dizziness, *seizures*
CV: **Heart failure**
GI: Abdominal pain, dyspepsia, vomiting, **hepatitis,** diarrhea
HEMA: Pancytopenia, **anemia, thrombocytopenia, leukopenia, neutropenia**
INTEG: Rash, *inj site reaction,* keratoderma blenorrhagicum
RESP: Pharyngitis, rhinitis, *cough, URI,* non-URI sinusitis
SYST: **Serious infections, sepsis, death, malignancies, Stevens-Johnson syndrome,** reactivation of hepatitis B virus, lupuslike syndrome

Pharmacokinetics

Absorption	Rapidly absorbed (60%)
Distribution	Unknown
Metabolism	Unknown
Excretion	Unknown
Half-life	115 hr

Pharmacodynamics

Unknown

INTERACTIONS
Individual drugs
Anakinra, cyclophosphamide, rilonacept: avoid use
SulfaSALAzine: increased neutropenia

Drug classifications
Immunizations: should be brought up to date before treatment

Immunizations, live virus vaccines: do not give concurrently

Drug/lab test
Increased: LFTs

NURSING CONSIDERATIONS
Assessment
• **Rheumatoid arthritis:** assess for pain; check ROM, inflammation of joints, characteristics of pain
• Assess inj site for pain, swelling; usually occurs after 2 inj (4-5 days)

> **BLACK BOX WARNING: Infection:** patients using immunosuppressives, corticosteroids, methotrexate are at greater risk, assess for fever, discontinue in those that develop a serious infection, do not use in active infection

> **BLACK BOX WARNING: Hypersensitivity:** to this product, latex needle cap, benzyl alcohol; usual reaction to this product lasts 3-5 days

Patient/family education
• Teach patient that product must be continued for prescribed time to be effective; to avoid aspirin, alcoholic beverages
• Instruct patient to use caution when driving; dizziness may occur
• Teach patient about self-administration, if appropriate: inj should be made in thigh, abdomen, upper arm; rotate sites at least 1 in from old site, check for injection reactions, reactions usually last 3-5 days

Evaluation
Positive therapeutic outcome
• Decreased pain in arthritic conditions
• Decreased inflammation in arthritic conditions

ethambutol (Rx)
(e-tham′byoo-tole)
Etibi 🍁, **Myambutol**
Func. class.: Antitubercular
Chem. class.: Diisopropylethylene diamide derivative
Pregnancy category B

Do not confuse: ethambutol/Ethmozine

ACTION: Inhibits RNA synthesis, decreases tubercle bacilli replication

Therapeutic outcome: Resolution of TB infection

USES: Pulmonary TB, as an adjunct, other mycobacterial infections

CONTRAINDICATIONS

Hypersensitivity, optic neuritis, child <13 yr

Precautions: Pregnancy **B**, breastfeeding, renal disease, diabetic retinopathy, cataracts, ocular defects, hepatic and hematopoietic disorders

DOSAGE AND ROUTES

Adult and child >13 yr: PO 15-25 mg/kg/day as a single dose or (treatment naive) or 25 mg/kg q day (treatment experienced)

Renal dose
Adult: PO CCr 10-50 ml/min dose q24-36hr; CCr <10 ml/min dose q48hr

Retreatment
Adult: PO 25 mg/kg/day as single dose × 2 mo with at least 1 other product, then decrease to 15 mg/kg/day as single dose, max 2.5 g/day
Child: PO 15 mg/kg/day

Available forms: Tabs 100, 400 mg

Implementation
• Give with meals to decrease GI symptoms, at same time each day to maintain blood level
• 4 hr between this product and antacids
• Give antiemetic if vomiting occurs

ADVERSE EFFECTS

CNS: *Headache, confusion,* fever, malaise, dizziness, *disorientation,* hallucinations, peripheral neuropathy
EENT: Blurred vision, optic neuritis, photophobia, decreased visual acuity
GI: *Abdominal distress, anorexia, nausea, vomiting*
INTEG: Dermatitis, pruritus, **toxic epidermal necrolysis,** erythema multiforme
META: *Elevated uric acid, acute gout,* liver function impairment
MISC: **Thrombocytopenia,** joint pain, **anaphylaxis**

Pharmacokinetics

Absorption	Rapidly absorbed
Distribution	Widely distributed, crosses blood-brain barrier, placenta
Metabolism	Liver
Excretion	Kidneys, unchanged
Half-life	3 hr, increased in liver, kidney disease

Pharmacodynamics

Onset	Rapid
Peak	2-4 hr
Duration	Unknown

INTERACTIONS
Drug classifications

Aluminum, antacids: decreased absorption, separate by 4 hr
Neurotoxic agents, other: increased neurotoxicity

NURSING CONSIDERATIONS
Assessment

• Obtain C&S tests including sputum tests before initiating treatment; monitor qmo to detect resistance
• Monitor liver function tests qwk × 2 wk, then q2mo: ALT, AST, bilirubin; renal studies: before, qmo: BUN, creatinine output, specific gravity, urinalysis, uric acid; decreased appetite, jaundice, dark urine, fatigue
• Assess patient's mental status often: affect, mood, behavioral changes; psychosis may occur with hallucinations, confusion
• Assess patient for vision disturbance that may indicate optic neuritis: blurred vision, change in color perception; may lead to blindness
⚠ **Serious skin reaction: toxic epidermal necrolysis**

Patient/family education
• Advise patient that compliance with dosage schedule and duration is necessary to eradicate disease; to keep scheduled appointments, including ophthalmic appointments, or relapse may occur
• Caution patient to report weakness, fatigue, loss of appetite, nausea, vomiting, yellowing of skin or eyes, tingling/numbness of hands/feet, weight gain, or decreased urine output
• Instruct patient to report any vision changes; rash; hot, swollen, painful joints; numbness or tingling of extremities to physician
• Caution patient to inform prescriber if pregnancy is suspected

Evaluation
Positive therapeutic outcome
• Decreased symptoms of TB
• Decrease in acid-fast bacteria

etodolac (Rx)
(ee-toe-doe′lak)
Ultradol ✤
Func. class.: Nonsteroidal antiinflammatory, nonopioid analgesic
Pregnancy category C

Do not confuse: Lodine/codeine/iodine

ACTION: Inhibits COX 1,2; analgesic, antiinflammatory properties

---

Therapeutic outcome: Decreased pain, inflammation

USES: Mild to moderate pain, osteoarthritis, rheumatoid arthritis, arthralgia, myalgia, juvenile rheumatoid arthritis

CONTRAINDICATIONS

Hypersensitivity; patients in whom aspirin, io-dides, or other NSAIDs have produced asthma, rhinitis, urticaria, nasal polyps, angioedema, bronchospasm; avoid in 2nd half of pregnancy

Precautions: Pregnancy **C,** breastfeeding, children, geriatric, bleeding, GI/cardiac/renal/hepatic disorders, bronchospasm, nasal polyps, alcoholism, bone marrow suppression, MI, hemophilia, neutropenia, ulcerative colitis

> BLACK BOX WARNING: GI bleeding, perforation, MI, stroke

DOSAGE AND ROUTES
Osteoarthritis
Adult: PO 300 mg bid-tid, or 400-500 mg bid initially, then adjust to 600-1200 mg/day in divided doses; max 1200 mg/day; ext rel 400-1000 mg/day

Analgesia
Adult: PO 200-400 mg q6-8hr; max 1200 mg/day; patients <60 kg max 20 mg/kg

Available forms: Caps 200, 300 mg; tabs 400, 500 mg; ext rel tabs 400, 600 mg

Implementation
• Do not break, crush, or chew ext rel tabs
• Administer with full glass of water to enhance absorption
• Administer with food or milk to decrease gastric symptoms; food will slow absorption slightly, will not decrease absorption

ADVERSE EFFECTS

CNS: Dizziness, headache, drowsiness, fatigue, tremors, confusion, insomnia, anxiety, depression, light-headedness, vertigo
CV: Tachycardia, peripheral edema, fluid retention, palpitations, dysrhythmias, CHF
EENT: Tinnitus, hearing loss, blurred vision, photophobia
GI: *Nausea, anorexia,* vomiting, diarrhea, jaundice, **cholestatic hepatitis,** constipation, flatulence, cramps, dry mouth, peptic ulcer, dyspepsia, **GI bleeding**
GU: **Nephrotoxicity, dysuria, hematuria, oliguria, azotemia, cystitis, UTI**
HEMA: **Blood dyscrasias**
INTEG: Erythema, urticaria, purpura, rash, pruritus, sweating, **Stevens-Johnson syndrome**
SYST: **Angioedema, anaphylaxis**

Pharmacokinetics
Absorption	Well absorbed
Distribution	Highly bound to plasma protein
Metabolism	Unknown
Excretion	Unknown
Half-life	7 hr

Pharmacodynamics
Onset	½ hr
Peak	1-2 hr
Duration	4-12 hr

INTERACTIONS
Individual drugs

> BLACK BOX WARNING: Aspirin: may increase GI toxicity, NSAIDs

Cidofovir, cycloSPORINE, digoxin, lithium, methotrexate, phenytoin: increased toxicity

Drug classifications
Aminoglycosides: Increased toxicity
Antacids: delayed etodolac effect
β-Adrenergic blockers: decreased effect
Diuretics: decreased effectiveness of diuretics

Drug/herb
Arginine, gossypol: increased gastric irritation
Bearberry, bilberry: increased NSAIDs action
Bogbean, chondroitin, saw palmetto, turmeric: increased bleeding risk
St. John's wort: severe photosensitivity

Drug/Lab
Increased: BUN, creatinine
Decreased: Hgb/Hct, WBC

NURSING CONSIDERATIONS
Assessment
• Assess pain: location, frequency, characteristics; relief after medication
• Assess for GI bleeding: black stools, hematemesis
• **Assess for asthma, aspirin hypersensitivity, nasal polyps that may be hypersensitive to etodolac**
• Monitor blood counts during therapy; watch for decreasing platelets; if low, therapy may need to be discontinued, then restarted after hematologic recovery; watch for blood dyscrasia (thrombocytopenia): bruising, fatigue, bleeding, poor healing

Patient/family education
• Inform patient that product must be continued for prescribed time to be effective

> **BLACK BOX WARNING:** avoid aspirin, alcoholic beverages, NSAIDs

- Caution patient to report bleeding, bruising, fatigue, malaise because blood dyscrasias can occur
- Instruct patient to use caution when driving; drowsiness, dizziness may occur
- Teach patient to take with a full glass of water to enhance absorption

Evaluation
Positive therapeutic outcome
- Decreased pain
- Decreased inflammation
- Increased mobility

⚠ HIGH ALERT

etoposide (Rx)
(e-toe´poe-side)
Toposar, VePesid ✦

etoposide phosphate (Rx)
Etopophos
Func. class.: Antineoplastic—miscellaneous
Chem. class.: Semisynthetic podophyllotoxin
Pregnancy category D

ACTION: Inhibits cells from entering mitosis, depresses DNA, RNA synthesis, cell cycle specific S and G_2, binds to a complex of DNA and topoisomerase II leading to DNA strand breaks

Therapeutic outcome: Prevention of rapid growth of malignant cells

USES: Leukemias, testicular cancer, small cell lung cancer

Unlabeled uses: Lymphomas

CONTRAINDICATIONS
Pregnancy **D**, breastfeeding, hypersensitivity

Precautions: Children, renal/hepatic disease, gout, neutropenia, thrombocytopenia

> **BLACK BOX WARNING:** Bone marrow depression, infection, bleeding, requires an experienced clinician

DOSAGE AND ROUTES
Testicular cancer
Adult: IV 100 mg/m²/day on days 1, 2 in combination with bleomycin and CISplatin (BEP) or 100 mg/m²/day on days 1, 3, 5, repeat q3wk or q4wk

Renal dose
Adult: IV CCr 45-60 ml/min reduce dose by 15%; CCr 30-44 ml/min reduce dose by 20%; CCr <30 ml/min reduce dose by 25%

Hepatic dose
Adult: IV/PO total bilirubin 1.5-3 mg/dl: reduce dose by 50%; total bilirubin 3-5 mg/dl: reduce dose by 75%; total bilirubin >5 mg/dl: hold

Available forms: Inj 20 mg/ml, caps 50 mg; 100 mg powder for injection

Implementation
PO route
- Caps need to be refrigerated
- Give without regard to food
- Increase fluid intake to 2-3 L/day to prevent urate deposits, calculi formation
- Refrigerate oral product, do not freeze

IV route
- Do not use acrylic or ABS plastic devices, may crack, leak

Intermittent IV infusion route (etoposide)
- Use cytotoxic handling procedures
- Dilute 5 ml vial with D_5W or 0.9% NaCl (200-400 mcg/ml); give slowly over 30-60 min; do not give over <30 min, hypotension may occur
- 200 mcg/ml is stable for 96 hr; 400 mcg/ml 48 hr
- Use Luer-Lok tubing to prevent leakage; do not let sol come in contact with skin; if contact occurs, wash well with soap and water

Y-site compatibilities: Acyclovir, alfentanil, allopurinol, amifostine, amikacin, aminocaproic acid, aminophylline, amiodarone, amphotericin B colloidal, amphotericin B lipid complex, amphotericin B liposome, ampicillin, ampicillin-sulbactam, anidulafungin, atenolol, atracurium, aztreonam, bivalirudin, bleomycin, bumetanide, buprenorphine, butorphanol, calcium chloride/gluconate, CARBOplatin, caspofungin, ceFAZolin, cefotaxime, cefoTEtan, cefOXitin, cefTAZidime, ceftizoxime, cefTRIAXone, cefuroxime, chloramphenicol, chlorproMAZINE, cimetidine, ciprofloxacin, cisatracurium, CISplatin, cladribine, clindamycin, codeine, cyclophosphamide, cycloSPORINE, cytarabine, DACTINomycin, DAPTOmycin, DAUNOrubicin, dexamethasone, dexmedetomidine, dexrazoxane, digoxin, diltiazem, diphenhydrAMINE, DOBUTamine, DOCEtaxel, DOPamine, doxacurium, DOXOrubicin, DOXOrubicin HCl, DOXOrubicin liposomal, doxycycline, droperidol, enalaprilat, ePHEDrine, EPINEPHrine, epirubicin, ertapenem, erythromycin, esmolol, famotidine, fenoldopam, fentaNYL, floxuridine, fluconazole, fludarabine, fluorouracil,

---

foscarnet, fosphenytoin, furosemide, ganciclovir, gatifloxacin, gemcitabine, gentamicin, glycopyrrolate, granisetron, haloperidol, heparin, hydrALAZINE, hydrocortisone, HYDROmorphone, hydrOXYzine, ifosfamide, imipenem-cilastatin, inamrinone, insulin (regular), irinotecan, isoproterenol, ketorolac, labetalol, lansoprazole, leucovorin, levofloxacin, levorphanol, lidocaine, linezolid, LORazepam, magnesium sulfate, mannitol, mechlorethamine, melphalan, meperidine, meropenem, mesna, methohexital, methotrexate, methyldopate, methylPREDNISolone, metoclopramide, metoprolol, metroNIDAZOLE, micafungin, midazolam, milrinone, minocycline, mitoXANtrone, mivacurium, morphine, nafcillin, nalbuphine, naloxone, nesiritide, nitroglycerin, nitroprusside, norepinephrine, NS, octreotide, ofloxacin, ondansetron, oxaliplatin, PACLitaxel, palonosetron, pamidronate, pancuronium, PEMEtrexed, pentamidine, pentazocine, PENTobarbital, PHENobarbital, phenylephrine, piperacillin, piperacillin-tazobactam, polymyxin B, potassium chloride/phosphates, procainamide, prochlorperazine, promethazine, propranolol, quinupristin-dalfopristin, ranitidine, remifentanil, rocuronium, sargramostim, sodium acetate/bicarbonate/phosphates, succinylcholine, SUFentanil, sulfamethoxazole-trimethoprim, tacrolimus, teniposide, theophylline, thiotepa, ticarcillin, ticarcillin-clavulanate, tigecycline, tirofiban, tobramycin, topotecan, trimethobenzamide, vancomycin, vasopressin, vecuronium, verapamil, vinBLAStine, vinCRIStine, vinorelbine, voriconazole, zidovudine, zoledronic acid

Y-site incompatibility: IDArubicin

Intermittent IV INF route (etoposide phosphate)
• Reconstitute each vial with 5 or 10 ml of D₅W, 0.9% NaCl for a concentration of 20 mg/ml or 10 mg/ml, respectively; may give diluted or undiluted to concentration of as little as 0.1 mg/ml, give over 5-210 min

Y-site compatibilities: Acyclovir, alfentanil, amifostine, amikacin, aminocaproic acid, aminophylline, amiodarone, ampicillin, ampicillin-sulbactam, anidulafungin, atenolol, atracurium, aztreonam, bivalirudin, bleomycin, bumetanide, buprenorphine, butorphanol, calcium acetate/chloride/gluconate, CARBOplatin, carmustine, caspofungin, ceFAZolin, cefonicid, cefoperazone, cefotaxime, cefoTEtan, cefOXitin, cefTAZidime, ceftizoxime, cefTRIAXone, cefuroxime, chloramphenicol, cimetidine, ciprofloxacin, cisatracurium, CISplatin, clindamycin, codeine, cyclophosphamide, cycloSPORINE, cytarabine, dacarbazine, DACTINomycin, DAPTOmycin, DAUNOrubicin, dexamethasone, digoxin, diltiazem, diphenhydrAMINE, DOBUTamine, DOCEtaxel, DOPamine, doripenem, doxacurium, DOXOrubicin, doxycycline, enalaprilat, ePHEDrine, EPINEPHrine, epirubicin, ertapenem, erythromycin, esmolol, famotidine, fenoldopam, fentaNYL, floxuridine, fluconazole, fludarabine, fluorouracil, foscarnet, fosphenytoin, furosemide, ganciclovir, gatifloxacin, gemcitabine, gentamicin, glycopyrrolate, granisetron, haloperidol, heparin, hydrALAZINE, hydrocortisone, HYDROmorphone, hydrOXYzine, IDArubicin, ifosfamide, inamrinone, insulin (regular), irinotecan, isoproterenol, ketorolac, labetalol, leucovorin, levofloxacin, levorphanol, lidocaine, linezolid, LORazepam, magnesium sulfate, mannitol, mechlorethamine, meperidine, meropenem, mesna, metaraminol, methotrexate, methyldopate, metoclopramide, metoprolol, metroNIDAZOLE, midazolam, milrinone, minocycline, mitoXANtrone, mivacurium, morphine, nafcillin, nalbuphine, naloxone, nesiritide, netilmicin, nitroglycerin, nitroprusside, norepinephrine, octreotide, ofloxacin, ondansetron, oxaliplatin, PACLitaxel, palonosetron, pamidronate, pancuronium, PEMEtrexed, pentamidine, pentazocine, PENTobarbital, PHENobarbital, phenylephrine, piperacillin, piperacillin-tazobactam, plicamycin, polymyxin B, potassium chloride/phosphates, procainamide, promethazine, propranolol, quiNIDine, quinupristin-dalfopristin, ranitidine, remifentanil, riTUXimab, rocuronium, sodium acetate/bicarbonate/phosphates, streptozocin, succinylcholine, SUFentanil, sulfamethoxazole-trimethoprim, tacrolimus, teniposide, theophylline, thiopental, thiotepa, ticarcillin, ticarcillin-clavulanate, tigecycline, tirofiban, tobramycin, tolazoline, trastuzumab, trimethobenzamide, vancomycin, vasopressin, vecuronium, verapamil, vinBLAStine, vinCRIStine, vinorelbine, voriconazole, zidovudine, zoledronic acid

ADVERSE EFFECTS
CNS: Headache, *fever,* peripheral neuropathy, paresthesia, confusion, chills, fever
CV: *Hypotension,* **MI,** dysrhythmia
GI: *Nausea, vomiting, anorexia,* **hepatotoxicity,** dyspepsia, diarrhea, constipation
GU: **Nephrotoxicity**
HEMA: **Thrombocytopenia, leukopenia, myelosuppression, anemia**
INTEG: *Rash, alopecia,* phlebitis at **IV** site, radiation recall, **Stevens-Johnson syndrome**
RESP: **Bronchospasm,** pleural effusion
SYST: **Anaphylaxis, secondary malignancy**

Pharmacokinetics

Absorption	Variably absorbed
Distribution	Rapidly absorbed, 97% protein binding, crosses placenta
Metabolism	Liver, some
Excretion	Kidneys, unchanged 50%; breast milk, feces
Half-life	1/2-2 hr (initial), terminal 5 1/4 hr

Pharmacodynamics

Unknown

INTERACTIONS
Individual drugs

Conivaptan, cycloSPORINE, imatinib, nilotinib, etravirine, telithromycin: increased etoposide effect, toxicity

Filgrastim, sargramostim: decreased etoposide effect, separate ≥24 hr

Radiation: increased bone marrow depression

Drug classifications

Other antineoplastics, immunosuppressives: increased bone marrow depression

Anticoagulants, NSAIDs, platelet inhibitors, thrombolytics, salicylates: increased bleeding risk

Live virus vaccines: increased adverse reactions

Drug/food

Grapefruit juice: decreased etoposide (PO)

Drug/lab test

Decreased: platelets, RBC, WBC, neutrophils, Hgb, calcium, phosphate

Increased: uric acid, potassium

NURSING CONSIDERATIONS
Assessment

• Monitor B/P (baseline and q15min) during administration

> **BLACK BOX WARNING: Bone marrow suppression:** monitor CBC, differential, platelet count weekly; withhold product if WBC is <500/mm³ or platelet count is <75,000/mm³; notify prescriber of results; recovery will take 3 wk, treatment should be delayed

• **Nephrotoxicity: monitor renal function tests: BUN, urine CCr before, during therapy; I&O ratio; report fall in urine output of 30 ml/hr; for decreased hyperuricemia**

> **BLACK BOX WARNING:** Monitor for cold, fever, sore throat (may indicate beginning of infection); notify prescriber if these occur, treat active infection prior to treatment

> **BLACK BOX WARNING:** Assess for bleeding: hematuria, guaiac, bruising or petechiae, mucosa or orifices q8hr; no rectal temp; avoid IM inj; use pressure to venipuncture sites

⚠ Injection site reaction: closely monitor site for infiltration

⚠ Assess for symptoms indicating severe allergic reactions: rash, pruritus, urticaria, itching, flushing, bronchospasm, hypotension; EPINEPHrine and crash cart should be nearby

⚠ Geriatric patients: assess for increased alopecia, GI effects, infection, nephrotoxicity, myelosuppression

> **BLACK BOX WARNING:** Must be administered by a clinician experienced in the use of cytotoxic products

Patient/family education

• Teach patient to avoid use of products containing aspirin or ibuprofen, razors, commercial mouthwash because bleeding may occur; to report symptoms of bleeding (hematuria, tarry stools)

• Instruct patient to report signs of anemia (fatigue, headache, irritability, faintness, shortness of breath)

• Teach patient to report any changes in breathing or coughing even several months after treatment

⚠ Advise patient that contraception will be necessary during treatment because teratogenesis may occur

⚠ Pregnancy: instruct patient to notify prescriber if pregnancy is planned or suspected, pregnancy (D)

• Caution patient that hair loss may occur during treatment; a wig or hairpiece may make patient feel better; new hair will be different in color, texture

• Advise patient to avoid vaccinations during treatment because serious reactions may occur

> **BLACK BOX WARNING: Infection:** teach patient to report signs/symptoms of infection: fever, chills, sore throat; patient should avoid crowds and persons with known infections

• Teach patient to take as prescribed (PO), not to double dose

---

⚠ Nurse Alert   ✴ Key NCLEX® Drug   ›› Drug Specifics

Evaluation
Positive therapeutic outcome
• Decreased spread of malignant, leukemic cells

etravirine (Rx)
(e-tra′veer-een)
Intelence
Func. class.: Antiretroviral
Chem. class.: Non-nucleoside reverse transcriptase inhibitor (NNRTI)
Pregnancy category B

ACTION: Binds directly to reverse transcriptase, blocking the RNA- and DNA-dependent DNA polymerase action, causing a disruption of the enzyme's catalytic site

Therapeutic outcome: Increased CD4 count, decrease viral load

USES: In combination with other antiretroviral agents for HIV infection in treatment-experienced patients with evidence of HIV replication despite ongoing antiretroviral therapy

CONTRAINDICATIONS
Hypersensitivity, breastfeeding

Precautions: Pregnancy **B**, impaired hepatic function, children, antimicrobial resistance, geriatric patients, hepatitis, hypercholesterolemia, hypertriglycerides, immune reconstitution syndrome

DOSAGES AND ROUTES
Adult/child/adolescent ≥6 yr, ≥30 kg: PO 200 mg bid
Child/adolescent ≥6 yr, 25 to 29 kg: 150 mg bid
Child/adolescent ≥6 yr, 20 to 24 kg: 125 mg bid
Child/adolescent ≥6 yr, 16 to 19 kg: 100 mg bid

Available forms: Tabs 100, 200 mg

Implementation
• Give in combination with other antiretrovirals with food
• Store in cool environment; protect from light

ADVERSE EFFECTS
CNS: *Headache, insomnia,* amnesia, anxiety, confusion, fatigue, nightmares, peripheral neuropathy, **seizures, stroke,** tremor
CV: **Atrial fibrillation,** hypertension, MI
EENT: Blurred vision
GI: *Nausea, vomiting, diarrhea, anorexia,* abdominal pain, increased AST/ALT, constipation, flatulence, gastritis, GERD, **hematemesis, hepatitis,** hepatomegaly, **pancreatitis**
GU: **Renal failure**
HEMA: **Hemolytic anemia, neutropenia, thrombocytopenia,** anemia

INTEG: *Rash,* erythema multiforme, **angioedema, Stevens-Johnson syndrome**
MS: **Rhabdomyolysis**
OTHER: Diabetes mellitus, gynecomastia, hyperamylasemia, hypercholesterolemia, hyperglycemia, hyperlipidemia
RESP: Dyspnea, **bronchospasm**
SYST: **DRESS**

Pharmacokinetics

Absorption	Unknown
Distribution	Plasma protein binding 99.9%
Metabolism	By CYP3A4, 2C9, 2C19
Excretion	Feces
Half-life	21-61 hr

Pharmacodynamics
Unknown

INTERACTIONS
Individual drugs
Atazanavir, carBAMazepine, delavirdine, fosamprenavir, fosphenytoin, phenytoin, PHENobarbital, rifapentine, rifampin, tipranavir: do not use concurrently
CycloSPORINE, sirolimus, tacrolimus: altered effect
CYP3A4 inducers: amiodarone, atazanavir, clarithromycin, flecainide, fosamprenavir, lidocaine, mexiletine, propafenone, quiNIDine, sildenafil, tadalafil, vardenafil: decreased levels
CYP3A4 inhibitors: fluconazole, itraconazole, ketoconazole, lopinavir, posaconazole, ritonavir, voriconazole: increased etravirine levels
Darunavir, dexamethasone, disopyramide, efavirenz, nevirapine, ritonavir, tipranavir: decreased etravirine levels
Diazepam, rifampin, voriconazole, warfarin: increased levels
Methadone: increased withdrawal symptoms

Drug classifications
HMG-CoA reductase inhibitors: increased myopathy, rhabdomyolysis

Drug/herb
St. John's wort: decreased etravirine

NURSING CONSIDERATIONS
Assessment
• Assess symptoms of HIV and for possible infections; increased temp
⚠ Monitor for fatal hypersensitivity reactions: fever, rash, nausea, vomiting, fatigue, cough, dyspnea, diarrhea, abdominal discomfort; treatment should be discontinued and not restarted; incidence of rash may be worse in women

- Assess blood dyscrasias (anemia, granulocytopenia): bruising, fatigue, bleeding, poor healing
- Renal failure: monitor renal studies: BUN, serum uric acid, CCr before, during therapy; these may be elevated throughout treatment
- Monitor hepatic studies before, during therapy: bilirubin, AST, ALT, amylase, alk phos, creatine phosphokinase, creatinine, qmo
- **HIV:** monitor blood counts q2wk; monitor viral load and CD4 counts during treatment; watch for decreasing granulocytes, Hgb; if low, therapy may have to be discontinued and restarted after hematologic recovery; blood transfusions may be required; cholesterol/lipid profile

Patient/family education
- Inform patient that product is not a cure but will control symptoms; patient is still infective, may pass AIDS virus on to others
- ⚠ Instruct patient to notify prescriber of sore throat, swollen lymph nodes, malaise, fever; other infections may occur; to stop product and notify prescriber immediately if skin rash, fever, cough, shortness of breath, GI symptoms occur; advise all health care providers that allergic reaction has occurred with etravirine
- Advise patient that follow-up visits must be continued since serious toxicity may occur; blood counts must be done
- ⚠ Instruct patient to use contraception during treatment; still able to transmit disease
- Give patient Medication Guide and Warning Card, discuss points on guide
- Inform patient that other products may be necessary to prevent other infections
- Advise patient to take medication following a meal

Evaluation
Positive therapeutic outcome
- Increased CD4 count, decreased viral load

⚠ HIGH ALERT

everolimus (Rx)

(e-ve-ro′li-mus)

Afinitor, Afinitor Disperz, Zortress

Func. class.: Antineoplastic (miscellaneous)

Chem. class.: Immunosuppressant, macrolide

Pregnancy category D

Do not confuse: everolimus/sirolimus/tacrolimus/temsirolimus

ACTION: Proliferation signal inhibitor that inhibits mammalian target of rapamycin (mTOR); this pathway is dysregulated in cancer

USES: Renal cell cancer in those with failed treatment with suritinib or sorafenib or SUNItinib, kidney transplant rejection prophylaxis with cycloSPORINE, subependymal giant cell astrocytoma, progressive pancreatic neuroendocrine tumor (PNET) with unresectable locally advanced metastatic disease, renal angiomyolipoma, tuberous sclerosis complex, breast cancer hormone receptor positive/HER-2 negative, liver transplant rejection prophylaxis

Therapeutic outcome: Decreasing tumor size, decreasing spread of malignancy

CONTRAINDICATIONS
Breastfeeding; hypersensitivity to this product, Rapamune, and Torisel; pregnancy **D**

Precautions: Children, renal/hepatic disease, diabetes mellitus, infection, hyperlipidemia, pleural effusion

> **BLACK BOX WARNING:** Immunosuppression, infection, renal artery thrombosis, renal impairment, renal vein thrombosis, neoplastic disease, heart transplant

DOSAGE AND ROUTES
Kidney transplant rejection prophylaxis (Zortress)
Adult: PO 0.75 mg q12hr with cycloSPORINE in combination with basiliximab corticosteroids, reduced doses of cycloSPORINE

Liver transplant rejection prophylaxis
Adult: PO 1 mg bid starting at least 30 days after transplant in combination with reduced-dose tacrolimus and corticosteroids

Advanced renal cancer (Afinitor)
Adult: PO 10 mg qd as long as clinically beneficial; with strong CYP3A4 inducers 10 mg qd, may increase by 5-mg increments to 20 mg qd

Progressive neuroendocrine tumor (PNET) (Afinitor only)
Adult: PO 10 mg/day, reduce dose to 5 mg/day if intolerable adverse reactions occur

Subependymal giant cell astrocytoma (SEGA) (Afinitor only)
Adult/adolescent/child ≥3 yr: PO 4.5 mg/m^2, titrate to target trough level of 5-15 ng/ml

Hepatic dose
Adult: PO (Child-Pugh A) Afinitor 7.5 mg/day; (Child-Pugh B) Afinitor 5 mg qd; not to be used in Child-Pugh C

Available forms: Tabs 0.25, 0.5, 0.75, 2.5 (Zortress); 2.5, 5, 7.5, 10 mg (Afinitor)

Implementation
• Swallow tabs whole with a full glass of water; do not chew, crush, or break
• Afinitor: take at same time of day, consistently with or without food; if unable to swallow, disperse in 30 ml of water
• Zortress: must take consistently with or without food, give at same time of day q12h with cycloSPORINE
• Follow procedure for proper handling of antineoplastics
• Give all medications PO if possible, avoiding IM inj; bleeding may occur
• Store protected from light, at room temperature

Afinitor adjustments for toxicity
Noninfectious pneumonitis
Grade 1, asymptomatic with radiographic findings only: No dose change
Grade 2, symptomatic but no interference with activities of daily living (ADL): Consider withholding therapy; resume Afinitor at a lower dose when symptoms improve to ≤ grade 1; discontinue Afinitor if symptoms do not improve within 4 wk
Grade 3, symptomatic and interfering with ADL and oxygen therapy indicated: Hold therapy; consider resuming Afinitor at a lower dose when symptoms improve to ≤ grade 1; consider discontinuing Afinitor if grade 3 toxicity recurs
Grade 4, life-threatening and ventilator support indicated: Discontinue therapy
Stomatitis
Grade 1, minimum symptoms and normal diet: No dose adjustment required
Grade 2, symptomatic but can eat and swallow modified diet: Hold therapy until symptoms improve to ≤ grade 1 and resume Afinitor at the same dose; if grade 2 toxicity recurs, hold therapy and resume Afinitor at a lower dose when symptoms improve to ≤ grade 1
Grade 3, symptomatic and unable to adequately eat or hydrate orally: Hold therapy; resume Afinitor at a lower dose when symptoms improve to ≤ grade 1
Grade 4, symptomatic and life-threatening: Discontinue therapy

Other nonhematologic toxicity (excluding metabolic events)
Grade 1: No dose adjustment required if toxicity is tolerable
Grade 2: No dose adjustment required if toxicity is tolerable; if toxicity is intolerable, hold therapy until symptoms improve to ≤ grade 1 and resume Afinitor at the same dose; if grade 2 toxicity recurs, hold therapy and resume Afinitor at a lower dose when symptoms improve to ≤ grade 1
Grade 3: Hold therapy; consider resuming Afinitor at a lower dose when symptoms improve to ≤ grade 1; if grade 3 toxicity recurs, consider discontinuing therapy
Grade 4: Discontinue Afinitor therapy
Metabolic events (hyperglycemia, dyslipidemia)
Grade 1 or 2: No dose adjustment required
Grade 3: Temporarily withhold therapy; resume Afinitor at a lower dose
Grade 4: Discontinue Afinitor therapy

ADVERSE EFFECTS
CNS: *Headache, insomnia, paresthesia, chills,* fever, seizure, personality changes, dizziness
CV: *Hypertension, CHF, peripheral edema,* chest pain
EENT: Blurred vision, photophobia, eyelid edema, epistaxis, sinusitis, cataracts, conjunctivitis
GI: Nausea, vomiting, diarrhea, constipation, stomatitis, anorexia, abdominal pain, dysgeusia, noninfectious hepatitis
GU: Renal failure, **UTI**, renal tubular necrosis
HEMA: Anemia, leukopenia, thrombocytopenia, hemorrhage
INTEG: *Rash, acne,* leukocytoclastic vasculitis
META: Hyperglycemia, increased creatinine, *hyperlipemia,* hypophosphatemia, weight loss
RESP: Pleural effusion, *dyspnea,* noninfectious pneumonitis, **pneumonitis,** pulmonary alveolar proteinosis

Pharmacokinetics
Absorption	Rapid
Distribution	Protein binding 74%
Metabolism	Extensively by CYP3A4
Excretion	Feces 80%, urine 5%
Half-life	30 hr, reduced by high-fat meal

Adverse effects: *italics* = common; **bold** = life-threatening

Pharmacodynamics

Onset	Unknown
Peak	1-2 hr
Duration	Unknown

INTERACTIONS
Individual drugs
Cimetidine, cycloSPORINE, danazol, erythromycin: increased everolimus effect

CarBAMazepine, PHENobarbital, phenytoin, rifamycin, rifapentine

Drug classifications
Immunosuppressants: increased nephrotoxicity

Antifungals, calcium channel blockers, CYP3A4 inhibitors (strong, moderate), HIV-protease inhibitors: increased everolimus effect

Vaccines: decreased effect of these products

Decrease: everolimus effect: CYP3A4 inducers

Drug/herb
St. John's wort: may decrease the effect of everolimus

Drug/food
Alters bioavailability; use consistently with or without food; do not use with grapefruit juice

Drug/lab test
Increased: bilirubin, calcium, cholesterol, glucose, potassium, lipids, phosphate, triglycerides, uric acid

Decreased: calcium, glucose, potassium, magnesium, phosphate

NURSING CONSIDERATIONS
Assessment
• Monitor lipid profile: cholesterol, triglycerides, a lipid-lowering agent may be needed; blood glucose

> **BLACK BOX WARNING:** Monitor **immunosuppression:** Hgb, WBC, platelets during treatment qmo; if leukocytes <3000/mm³ or platelets <100,000/mm³, product should be discontinued or reduced; decreased hemoglobulin level may indicate bone marrow suppression

• Monitor hepatic studies: alk phos, AST, ALT, amylase, bilirubin, and for hepatotoxicity: dark urine, jaundice, itching, light-colored stools; product should be discontinued

> **BLACK BOX WARNING: Infection:** bacterial/fungal infections can occur and are more common with combination immunosuppression therapy

> **BLACK BOX WARNING: Renal artery/vein thrombosis (Zortress):** may result in graft loss within 30 days after transplantation

Patient/family education

> **BLACK BOX WARNING:** Advise to report fever, rash, severe diarrhea, chills, sore throat, fatigue; serious infections may occur; clay-colored stools, cramping (hepatotoxicity)

• Advise to avoid crowds, persons with known infections to reduce risk of infection

⚠ Teach to use contraception before, during, and 12 wk after product has been discontinued, avoid breastfeeding

⚠ Teach to notify prescriber if pregnancy is planned or suspected; pregnancy (D)

• Advise not to use with grapefruit juice

• Inform to avoid live virus vaccines, that frequent lab tests are required

• Advise to take up to 6 hr after normally scheduled time if dose is missed

• Advise that product may decrease male/female fertility

• Teach that drinking alcohol is not recommended

• Teach patient to take consistently with or without food

• Teach patient to report visual changes, weight gain, edema, shortness of breath, impaired wound healing

Evaluation
Positive therapeutic outcome
• Decreasing size of tumor, decreasing spread of malignancy

exemestane (Rx)
(x-ee-mes´tane)
Aromasin
Func. class.: Antineoplastic
Chem. class.: Aromatase inhibitor
Pregnancy category D

Do not confuse: exemestane/ezetimibe/estramustine

ACTION: Lowers serum estradiol concentrations by irreversibly inhibiting aromatase; many breast cancers have strong estrogen receptors

Therapeutic outcome: Prevention of rapidly growing malignant cells

USES: Advanced breast carcinoma that has not responded to other therapy in estrogen receptor–positive patients (postmenopausal), estrogen receptor-positive early breast cancer that has received tamoxifen

CONTRAINDICATIONS
Pregnancy **X,** breastfeeding, hypersensitivity, premenopausal women

Precautions: Children, geriatric, renal/hepatic disease, osteoporosis, vit D deficiency, hepatic/renal disease

DOSAGE AND ROUTES
Adult: PO 25 mg/day after meals; may need 50 mg/day if taken with a potent CYP3A4 inhibitor

Available forms: Tabs 25 mg

Implementation
• Give after food or fluids for GI upset
• Store in light-resistant container at room temperature

ADVERSE EFFECTS
CNS: Headache, fatigue, depression, insomnia, anxiety, hot flashes, diaphoresis, dizziness, neuropathy
CV: Hypertension, edema, **thrombolism**
GI: Nausea, vomiting, increased appetite, diarrhea, constipation, abdominal pain
HEMA: *Lymphopenia*
MS: Fracture, bone loss, arthralgia, osteoporosis
RESP: Cough, dyspnea
INTEG: Alopecia, hot flashes, sweating

Pharmacokinetics	
Absorption	Rapidly absorbed
Distribution	Unknown
Metabolism	Liver
Excretion	Feces, urine
Half-life	24 hr

Pharmacodynamics
Unknown

INTERACTIONS
Drug classifications
CYP3A4 inducers, estrogens: decreased exemestane action

Drug/lab
Increase: AST, ALT, alk phos, bilirubin, creatinine

NURSING CONSIDERATIONS
Assessment
• Assess B/P; hypertension may occur
• Bone mineral density, x-ray of thoracic or lumbar spine if bone changes are suspected

Patient/family education
• Instruct patient to report any complaints, side effects to prescriber; if dose is missed, do not double next dose, **to immediately report chest pain**
• Advise patient that hot flashes can occur and are reversible after discontinuing treatment
• Inform patient about who should be told about therapy
• Advise patient to use reliable contraception, pregnancy **X**, do not breastfeed

Evaluation
Positive therapeutic outcome
• Decreased spread of malignant cells in breast cancer

▲ HIGH ALERT

exenatide (Rx)
(ex-en′a-tide)
Bydureon, Byetta
Func. class.: Antidiabetic
Chem. class.: Incretin mimetic
Pregnancy category C

ACTION: Binds and activates known human GLP-1 receptor, mimics natural physiology for self-regulating glycemic control

Therapeutic outcome: Decreased polyuria, polydipsia, polyphagia; improved Hgb A1c

USES: Type 2 diabetes mellitus given in combination with metformin, sulfonylurea, or a thiazolidinedione, insulin glargine

CONTRAINDICATIONS
Hypersensitivity

BLACK BOX WARNING: Medullary thyroid carcinoma, multiple endocrine neoplasia syndrome type 2 (MEN-2), thyroid cancer

Precautions: Pregnancy **C,** geriatric, severe renal/hepatic/GI disease, vitamin D deficiency

DOSAGE AND ROUTES
Adult: SUBCUT 5 mcg bid 1 hr before morning and evening meal; may increase to 10 mcg bid after 1 mo of therapy; ext rel subcut (Bydureon) 2 mg q7 days; ext rel inj 2 mg q7 days

Available forms: Inj 5, 10 mcg pen; ext rel powder for susp for inj 2 mg

Implementation
• Store in refrigerator; unopened pen may be stored at room temperature after opening for up to 30 days
Subcut route (regular release—Byetta)
• Give SUBCUT only, do not give **IV/IM**
• Pen needles must be purchased separately and be compatible

- Prime prior to use
- Inject into thigh, abdomen, upper arm

Subcut route (extended release— Bydureon)

- Give 1× wk; the dose can be given at any time of day, without regard to meals
- Available as a single dose tray containing a vial of 2 mg, a prefilled syringe delivering 0.65 ml diluent, a vial connector, and two custom needles (23G, 5/16″) specific to this delivery system (one is a spare needle); do not substitute needles or any other components
- Inject immediately after the white/off-white powder is suspended in the diluent and transferred to the syringe
- Inject subcutaneously into the thigh, abdomen, or upper arm; rotate sites to prevent lipodystrophy
- Give 1 hr before meals, approximately 6 hr apart; if patient is NPO, may need to hold dose to prevent hypoglycemia
- Store in refrigerator; unopened pen may be stored at room temperature after opening for up to 30 days
- If added to insulin glargine, insulin detemir, a dosage reduction in these products may be required

ADVERSE EFFECTS

CNS: *Headache, dizziness,* jittery feeling, restlessness, weakness

ENDO: Hypoglycemia, thyroid hyperplasia

GI: Nausea, vomiting, diarrhea, dyspepsia, anorexia, gastroesophageal reflux, weight loss, pancreatitis

SYST: Angioedema, anaphylaxis

INTEG: Serious injection-site reactions (cellulitis, abscess, skin necrosis)

Pharmacokinetics

Absorption	Unknown
Distribution	Unknown
Metabolism	Unknown
Excretion	Glomerular filtration
Half-life	Unknown

Pharmacodynamics

Onset	Unknown
Peak	Immediate release: 2.1 hr; ext rel: 2 wk
Duration	Unknown

INTERACTIONS
Individual drugs

Acetaminophen: may decrease the effect of acetaminophen

Acetaminophen (elixir), digoxin, lovastatin: decreased action of these products

Alcohol, disopyramide: increased hypoglycemia

Dextrothyroxine, niacin, triamterene: decreased hypoglycemia efficacy

Erythromycin, metoclopramide: do not use with exenatide

Drug classifications

ACE inhibitors, anabolic steroids, androgens, fibric acid derivatives, sulfonylureas: increased hypoglycemia

Corticosteroids, phenothiazines: increased hyperglycemia

Estrogens, MAOIs, oral contraceptives, progestins, thiazide diuretics: decreased hypoglycemia

NURSING CONSIDERATIONS
Assessment

- Monitor fasting blood, glucose, A1c levels, postprandial glucose during treatment to determine diabetes control
- **Pancreatitis: severe abdominal pain, with/without vomiting; product should be discontinued**
- Assess for hypo/hyperglycemic reaction that can occur soon after meals; for severe hypoglycemia give **IV** D₅W, then **IV** dextrose solution
- ⚠ **Anaphylaxis, angioedema: product should be discontinued immediately**
- Assess for nausea, diarrhea, vomiting, ability to tolerate product, may cause dehydration

Patient/family education

- Teach patient symptoms of hypo/hyperglycemia, what to do about each; to have glucagon emergency kit available; to carry a glucose source (candy, sugar cube) to treat hypoglycemia
- Advise patient that product must be continued on daily or weekly basis (ext rel); explain consequences of discontinuing product abruptly
- Teach patient that diabetes is a lifelong illness; product will not cure disease
- Advise patient to carry emergency ID with prescriber and medications
- Advise patient to continue weight control, dietary restrictions, exercise, hygiene
- Inform patient that regular blood glucose monitoring and A1c testing is needed
- Advise patient to notify prescriber if pregnant or intend to become pregnant
- Advise patient to read "Information for the Patient" and "Pen User Manual"; provide education on self-injection
- ⚠ **Pancreatitis: if severe abdominal pain with or without vomiting occurs, seek medical attention immediately**

- Review injection procedure, to store product in refrigerator, room temperature after first use, discard 30 days after first use, do not freeze, protect from light (Byetta)

Evaluation
Positive therapeutic outcome
- Decrease in polyuria, polydipsia, polyphagia, clear sensorium; improved A1c, weight; absence of dizziness, stable gait

ezetimibe (Rx)
(ehz-eh-tim′bee)
Ezetrol ✦, **Zetia**
Func. class.: Antilipemic
Pregnancy category C

ACTION: Inhibits absorption of cholesterol by the small intestine

Therapeutic outcome: Decreased cholesterol levels

USES: Hypercholesterolemia, homozygous familial hypercholesterolemia (HoFH), homozygous sitosterolemia

CONTRAINDICATIONS
Hypersensitivity, severe hepatic disease

Precautions: Pregnancy **C**, breastfeeding, children, hepatic disease

DOSAGE AND ROUTES
Adult: **PO** 10 mg/day; may be given with HMG-CoA reductase inhibitor at same time; may be given with bile acid sequestrant; give ezetimibe 2 hr before or 4 hr after the bile acid sequestrant

Available forms: Tabs 10 mg

Implementation
- Give without regard to meals

ADVERSE EFFECTS
CNS: Fatigue, dizziness, headache
GI: Diarrhea, abdominal pain
MISC: Chest pain
MS: *Myalgias, arthralgias,* back pain, myopathy, **rhabdomyolysis**
RESP: Pharyngitis, sinusitis, cough, URI
EENT: Sinusitis, nasopharyngitis

Pharmacokinetics

Absorption	Unknown
Distribution	Unknown
Metabolism	Small intestine, liver
Excretion	Urine (11%), feces (78%)
Half-life	Unknown

Pharmacodynamics
Unknown

INTERACTIONS
Individual drugs
Cholestyramine: decreased ezetimibe action
CycloSPORINE: increased action of ezetimibe

Drug classifications
Antacids: decreased action of ezetimibe
Fibric acid derivatives, bile acid sequestrants: increased ezetimibe action

Drug/lab test
Increase: LFTs

NURSING CONSIDERATIONS
Assessment
- **Hypercholesterolemia:** obtain diet history; monitor fat content, lipid levels (triglycerides, LDL, HDL, total cholesterol), LFTs baseline and periodically during treatment
- **Myopathy/rhabdomyolysis: monitor for increased CPK; myalgia, muscle cramps, musculoskeletal pain, lethargy, fatigue, fever; more common when combined with statins**

Patient/family education
- Teach patient that compliance is needed
- Advise that risk factors should be decreased: high-fat diet, smoking, alcohol consumption, absence of exercise
- Advise patient to notify prescriber if pregnancy is suspected or planned or if breastfeeding
- Advise patient to notify prescriber if unexplained weakness, or muscle pain is present
- Teach patient to notify prescriber of dietary/herbal supplements

Evaluation
Positive therapeutic outcome
- Decreased cholesterol

ezogabine (Rx)
(e-zog′a-been)
Potiga
Func. class.: Anticonvulsant
Controlled Substance Schedule V

ACTION: The exact mechanism of anticonvulsant effects is not fully known. However, studies indicate that the drug enhances transmembrane potassium currents, which may stabilize the resting membrane potential and reduce brain excitability. May also augment GABA-mediated currents

USES: Partial seizures, migraines

CONTRAINDICATIONS
Hypersensitivity

Precautions: Suicidal ideation/behavior, prostatic hypertrophy, dementia, psychotic disorders, QT prolongation, congestive heart failure, ventricular hypertrophy, hypokalemia, hypomagnesemia, abrupt discontinuation, renal impairment, hepatic disease, geriatrics, pregnancy category C, breastfeeding, neonates, infants, children, adolescents

DOSAGE AND ROUTES
Adult/geriatric patient ≤65 yr: PO Initially, 100 mg tid; increase by ≤50 mg tid per day at weekly intervals depending on response, up to a maintenance dose of 200-400 mg tid depending on response; max is 400 mg tid (1200 mg/day).
Geriatric patient >65 yr: PO Initially, 50 mg tid; increase by ≤50 mg tid per day at weekly intervals depending on response; max 250 mg tid (750 mg/day).

Available forms: Film-coated tabs 50, 200, 300, 400 mg

Implementation
• Tabs should be swallowed whole without regard to meals
• Give in 3 equally divided doses

ADVERSE EFFECTS
CNS: Dizziness, drowsiness, memory impairment, tremor, vertigo, abnormal coordination, disturbance in attention, gait disturbance, aphasia, dysarthria, balance disorder, paresthesias, amnesia, dysphagia, myoclonia, hypokinesia, confusion, anxiety, hallucinations, suicidal thoughts/behaviors, fatigue, asthenia, malaise, euphoria
EENT: *Diplopia, blurred vision,* retinal pigment change
GI: *Nausea, constipation, dyspepsia, xerostomia, constipation, weight gain, appetite stimulation*
GU: *Urinary retention, hydronephrosis, dysuria, urinary hesitation, hematuria, chromaturia*
HEMA: Thrombocytopenia, leukopenia, neutropenia
INTEG: Rash, alopecia, blue skin discoloration
MISC: *Influenza, dyspnea,* QT prolongation
MS: Muscle spasms, weakness

Pharmacokinetics

Pharmacokinetics	
Absorption	Rapid, 60%
Distribution	Extensively in the body, 80% protein binding
Metabolism	Extensive (glucuronidation, acetylation), metabolite (N-glucuronides)
Excretion	Renal 36% (exogabine), 18% (NAMR), 24% (N-glucuronides); fecal 14%
Half-life	Elimination 7 hr, metabolite 11 hr

Pharmacodynamics	
Onset	Unknown
Peak	0.5-2 hr, increased by high-fat food
Duration	Unknown

INTERACTIONS
Individual drugs
Amantadine: increased urinary retention

Arsenic trioxide, chloroquine, chlorproMAZINE, clarithromycin, dextromethorphan; dronedarone, droperidol, erythromycin, grepafloxacin, halofantrine, levomethadyl, mesoridazine, methadone, pentamidine, pimozide, posaconazole, probucol, propafenone, quiNIDine, saquinavir, sparfloxacin, terfenadine, thioridazine, troleandomycin, ziprasidone: increased QT prolongation

Buprenorphine, butorphanol, dronabinol, ethanol, mirtazapine, nabilone, nalbuphine, opiate agonists, pentazocine, pregabalin, traMADol, traZODone, ethanol: increased CNS depression

CarBAMazepine: decreased effect of ezogabine
Digoxin: increased effect of each product
Phenytoin: decreased effect of each product

Drug classifications
Antimuscarinics, H1-blockers: increased urinary retention

Class IA antiarrhythmics (disopyramide, procainamide, quiNIDine), Class III antiarrhythmics (amiodarone, dofetilide, ibutilide, sotalol): increased QT prolongation

Anxiolytics, hypnotics, opiate agonists, sedatives, skeletal muscle relaxants: increased CNS depression

NURSING CONSIDERATIONS
Assessment
• Seizures: Assess for type, duration, location, activity, presence of aura

---

• **QT prolongation:** Monitor in those with known QT prolongation, congestive heart failure, ventricular hypertrophy, hypokalemia, hypomagnesemia, and in patients receiving medications known to cause QT prolongation. QT prolongation can occur within 3 hrs of dose

• **Abrupt withdrawal:** Withdraw gradually to minimize increased seizure frequency

• **Suicidal thoughts/behaviors:** Assess for any unusual changes in moods or behaviors, including emotional lability or emerging or worsening depression and suicidal ideation

Patient/family education

• Instruct patient to avoid driving or operating machinery, or performing other tasks that require mental alertness until reaction is known

• Instruct patient to avoid concurrent use of alcohol

• Instruct patient to avoid abruptly discontinuing this medication

• **Suicidal thought/behaviors:** Advise patient to notify prescriber immediately for suicidal thought/behaviors

• **Teach patient to report vision changes immediately**

E

Adverse effects: *italics* = common; **bold** = life-threatening

factor IX complex (human)
Alpha Nine SD, Bebulin VH, BeneFIX, Mononine, Profilnine SD
Func. class.: Hemostatic
Chem. class.: Factors II, VII, IX, X
Pregnancy category C

Therapeutic outcome: Replacement of factors II, VII, IX, X

USES: Hemophilia B (Christmas disease), factor IX deficiency, anticoagulant reversal, control of bleeding in patients with factor VIII inhibitors; reversal of overdose of anticoagulants in emergencies

CONTRAINDICATIONS
Hypersensitivity to mouse/hamster protein, DIC, mild factor IX deficiency

DOSAGE AND ROUTES
Bleeding in hemophilia A and inhibitors of factor VIII (Proplex T, Konyne 80)
Adult and child: 75 units/kg, repeat in 12 hr

Factor IX complex (human) bleeding in hemophilia B
Adult and child: IV Establish 25% of normal factor IX activity or 60-75 units/kg then 10-20 units/kg/day × 1-2 wk

Prophylaxis of bleeding in hemophilia B
Adult and child: IV 10-20 units/kg 1-2 ×/wk

Reversal of oral anticoagulant
Adult and child: 15 units/kg

Factor VII deficiency (use Proplex T only)
Adult and child: IV 0.5 units/kg × body weight (kg) × desired factor IX increase (in % of normal); repeat q4-6hr if needed

Factor IX (human) minor to moderate hemorrhage
Use only Alpha Nine, Alpha Nine SD
Adult and child: IV Dose to increase plasma factor IX level to 20%-30% in one dose

Serious hemorrhage
Adult and child: IV Dose to increase plasma factor IX level to 30%-50% given as daily INF

Minor hemorrhage (Mononine only)
Adult and child: IV dose to increase plasma factor IX level to 15%-25% (20-30 units/kg), may repeat in 24 hr if needed

Major hemorrhage
Adult and child: IV dose to increase plasma factor IX level to 25%-50% (75 units/kg) q18-30hr for up to 10 days

factor IX Fc fusion protein, recombinant
(fak'tor nine')
Alprolix
Func. class.: Hemostatic
Pregnancy category C

USES: Hemophilia B, surgical bleeding

CONTRAINDICATIONS: Bleeding disorders

DOSAGE AND ROUTES
Hemophilia B
Adult, adolescent, child, infant, and neonate: IV INF infuse dose ≤10 ml/min dose (IU) = body weight (kg) × desired factor IX increase (IU/dl or % of normal) × reciprocal of recovery (IU/kg per IU/dl) *OR* IU/dl (or % of normal) = [total dose (IU)/body weight (kg)] × recovery (IU/dl per IU/kg)

Surgical bleeding control, prevention
Adult, adolescent, child, infant, and neonate: Dose and duration of treatment depend on the severity of the factor IX deficiency, the location and extent of bleeding, and the patient's clinical condition. Refer to hemophilia B for dosage formula

Routine bleeding prophylaxis to prevent/reduce frequency of bleeding episodes
Adult, adolescent, child, infant, and neonate: IV INF initially, 50 IU/kg every week or 100 IU/kg q10d

famciclovir (Rx)
(fam-sye-klo'vir)
Famvir
Func. class.: Antiviral
Chem. class.: Guanosine nucleoside
Pregnancy category B

ACTION: Inhibits DNA polymerase and viral DNA synthesis by conversion of this guanosine nucleoside to penciclovir

Therapeutic outcome: Decreasing size and number of lesions

USES: Treatment of acute herpes zoster (shingles), genital herpes, recurrent mucocutaneous herpes simplex virus (HSV) in HIV patients, initial episodes of herpes genitalis, herpes labialis in the immunocompromised

CONTRAINDICATIONS
Hypersensitivity to this product, penciclovir, acyclovir, ganciclovir, valacyclovir, or valganciclovir

Precautions: Pregnancy **B**, breastfeeding, renal disease

DOSAGE AND ROUTES
Herpes zoster
Adult: PO 500 mg q8hr × 7 days

Renal dose
Adult: PO; 40-59 ml/min 500 mg q12hr; 20-39 ml/min 500 mg q24hr; CCr <20 ml/min 250 mg q24hr

Suppression of recurrent HSV
Adult: PO 250 mg q12hr up to 1 yr

Renal dose
Adult: PO CCr 20-39 ml/min 125 mg q12hr × 5 days; CCr <20 ml/min 125 mg q24hr × 5 days

Recurrent genital herpes
Adult: PO 1000 mg bid in a single dose

Renal dose
Adult: PO CCr 40-59 ml/min 500 mg q12hr × 1 day; CCr 20-39 ml/min 500 mg as a single dose; CCr <20 ml/min 250 mg as a single dose

Suppression of recurrent genital herpes
Adult: PO 250 mg bid for up to a year

Renal dose
Adult: PO CCr 20-39 ml/min 125 mg q12hr; CCr <20 ml/min 125 mg q24hr

Herpes genitalis initial episodes
Adult: PO 250 mg tid × 7-10 days

Available forms: Tabs 125, 250, 500 mg

Implementation
• Give with or without meals; absorption does not appear to be lowered when taken with food
• Give within 72 hr of the appearance of rash in herpes zoster

ADVERSE EFFECTS
CNS: *Headache, fatigue, dizziness,* paresthesia, somnolence, fever
GI: Nausea, vomiting, diarrhea, constipation, abdominal pain, anorexia

GU: Decreased sperm count
INTEG: *Pruritus*
MS: Back pain, arthralgia
RESP: Pharyngitis, sinusitis

Pharmacokinetics

Absorption	Well absorbed, 77%
Distribution	Protein binding 20%
Metabolism	Intestinal tissue, blood, liver
Excretion	Breast milk, kidney, bile
Half-life	Terminal 2-3 hr

Pharmacodynamics

Onset	Unknown
Peak	1 hr
Duration	8 hr

INTERACTIONS
Individual drugs
Probenecid: increased effect of famciclovir
Zoster vaccine: decreased effect of vaccine

NURSING CONSIDERATIONS
Assessment
• **Herpes zoster:** assess number and distribution of lesions; also burning, itching, or pain (early symptoms of herpes infection); neuralgia during, after treatment
• **Acute renal failure: usually in high doses or in those >65 yr; monitor renal function tests: urine CCr, BUN before, during treatment if patient has decreased renal function; dosage may need to be lowered; hepatic studies: LFTs**
• Monitor bowel pattern before, during treatment; diarrhea may occur
• Assess for posttherapeutic neuralgia during and after treatment

Patient/family education
• Teach patient how to recognize signs of beginning of infection
• Teach patient how to prevent the spread of infection to others
• Teach patient reason for medication and expected results
• Advise patient that this medication does not prevent spread of disease to others, that condoms should be used
• Advise women with genital herpes to have yearly Pap smears; cervical cancer is more likely

Evaluation
Positive therapeutic outcome
• Decreased size and spread of lesions
• Prevention of recurrence (genital herpes)
• Decreased time for healing

Adverse effects: *italics* = common; **bold** = life-threatening

famotidine (Rx, OTC)
(fa-moe'ti-deen)
**Acid Control ✦, Pepcid, Pepcid AC,
Peptic Guard ✦, Ulcidine ✦**
Func. class.: H₂-histamine receptor antagonist, antiulcer agent
Pregnancy category B

ACTION: Inhibits histamine at H₂-receptor site in gastric parietal cells, which inhibits gastric acid secretion while pepsin remains at a stable level

Therapeutic outcome: Healing of duodenal ulcers or gastric ulcers; prevention of duodenal ulcers; decreases symptoms of gastroesophageal reflux disease or Zollinger-Ellison syndrome, heartburn

USES: Short-term treatment of duodenal ulcer, maintenance therapy for duodenal ulcer, Zollinger-Ellison syndrome, multiple endocrine adenomas, gastric ulcers, heartburn, gastroesophageal reflux disease

Unlabeled uses: GI disorders in those taking NSAIDs, urticaria, prevention of stress ulcers, aspiration pneumonitis, prevention of paclitaxel hypersensitivity reactions

CONTRAINDICATIONS
Hypersensitivity

Precautions: Pregnancy **B**, breastfeeding, children <12 yr, geriatric, severe renal/hepatic disease

DOSAGE AND ROUTES
Short-term treatment of gastric ulcer
Adult: PO 40 mg/day at bedtime × 4-8 wk, then 20 mg at bedtime if needed (maintenance); IV 20 mg q12hr if unable to take PO
Child 1-16 yr: PO 0.5 mg/kg/day at bedtime or divided bid, max 40 mg/day; IV 1-2 mg/kg/day in 1-2 divided doses

Pathologic hypersecretory conditions
Adult: PO 20 mg q6hr; may give up to 160 mg q6hr if needed; IV 20 mg q12hr if unable to take PO

GERD
Adult: PO 20 mg bid ≤ 6 wk; 40 mg bid ≤ 2 wk (ulcerative esophagitis)

Heartburn relief/prevention
Adult: PO 10 mg with water, 15 min-1 hr before eating

Renal dose
Adult: PO CCr <50 ml/min; give 50% of dose or extend interval to q36-48hr

Available forms: Tabs 10, 20, 40 mg; powder for oral susp 40 mg/5 ml; inj 10 mg/ml, 20 mg/50 ml 0.9% NaCl; orally disintegrating tabs (RPD) 20, 40 mg; chew tabs 10 mg

Implementation
PO route
• Administer oral susp after shaking well; discard unused sol after 1 mo
• Store in cool environment (oral)

Direct IV route
• Give **IV** direct after diluting 2 ml of product (10 mg/ml) in 0.9% NaCl to total volume of 5-10 ml; inject over 2 min to prevent hypotension

Intermittent IV infusion route
• Administer after diluting 20 mg of product in 100 ml of LR, 0.9% NaCl, D₅W, D₁₀W; run over 15-30 min

Continuous IV infusion route
• **Adults:** Dilute 40 mg/250 ml D₅W or NS, infuse over 24 hr, run at 11 ml/hr, use infusion device
• Store in cool environment (oral); **IV** sol is stable for 48 hr at room temperature; do not use discolored sol

Y-site compatibilities: Acyclovir, allopurinol, amifostine, aminophylline, amphotericin, ampicillin, ampicillin/sulbactam, inamrinone, amsacrine, atropine, aztreonam, bretylium, calcium gluconate, ceFAZolin, cefoperazone, cefotaxime, cefoTEtan, cefOXitin, cefTAZidime, ceftizoxime, cefTRIAXone, cefuroxime, cephalothin, cephapirin, chlorproMAZINE, CISplatin, cladribine, cyclophosphamide, cytarabine, dexamethasone, dextran 40, digoxin, diphenhydrAMINE, DOBUTamine, DOPamine, DOXOrubicin, droperidol, enalaprilat, EPINEPHrine, erythromycin lactobionate, esmolol, filgrastim, fluconazole, fludarabine, folic acid, gentamicin, granisetron, haloperidol, heparin, hydrocortisone, HYDROmorphone, hydrOXYzine, imipenem/cilastatin, regular insulin, isoproterenol, labetalol, lidocaine, LORazepam, magnesium sulfate, melphalan, meperidine, methotrexate, methylPREDNISolone, metoclopramide, mezlocillin, midazolam, morphine, nafcillin, nitroglycerin, nitroprusside, norepinephrine, ondansetron, oxacillin, PACLitaxel, perphenazine, phenylephrine, phenytoin, phytonadione, piperacillin, potassium chloride, potassium phosphate, procainamide, propofol, sargramostim, sodium bicarbonate, teniposide, theophylline, thiamine, thiotepa, ticarcillin, ticarcillin-clavulanate, verapamil, vinorelbine

ADVERSE EFFECTS
CNS: *Headache, dizziness,* paresthesia, depression, anxiety, somnolence, insomnia, fever, seizures in renal disease

CV: Dysrhythmias, QT prolongation (impaired renal functioning)
EENT: Taste change, tinnitus, orbital edema
GI: *Constipation,* nausea, vomiting, anorexia, cramps, abnormal liver enzymes, diarrhea
HEMA: Thrombocytopenia, aplastic anemia
INTEG: Rash, toxic epidermal necrolysis, Stevens-Johnson syndrome
MS: Myalgia, arthralgia
RESP: Pneumonia

Pharmacokinetics

Absorption	50% absorbed (PO)
Distribution	Plasma, protein binding (15%-20%)
Metabolism	Liver (30% active metabolizing)
Excretion	Kidneys (70%)
Half-life	2½-3½ hr

Pharmacodynamics

	PO	IV
Onset	60 min	Immediate
Peak	1-3 hr	1-4 hr
Duration	12 hr	12 hr

INTERACTIONS
Individual drugs
Cefditoren, cefpodoxime, itraconazole, ketoconazole: decreased absorption of each specific product
Atazanivir, delavirdine: decreased effects of each specific product

Drug classifications
Antacids: decreased absorption of famotidine

NURSING CONSIDERATIONS
Assessment
• **Assess patient with ulcers or suspected ulcers:** epigastric, abdominal pain, hematemesis, occult blood in stools, blood in gastric aspirate before treatment; throughout treatment, monitor gastric pH (maintain at pH 5)
• Monitor I&O ratio, BUN, creatinine, CBC with differential monthly

Patient/family education
• Caution patient to avoid driving, other hazardous activities until stabilized on this medication; dizziness may occur
• Advise patient to avoid black pepper, caffeine, alcohol, harsh spices, NSAIDs, extremes in temperature of food; tell patient to avoid OTC preparations: aspirin, cough/cold preparations; condition may worsen

• Advise patient to avoid taking OTC and prescription preparations of this product concurrently
• Tell patient that smoking decreases the effectiveness of the product; that smoking cessation should be considered
• Instruct patient that product must be continued for prescribed time to be effective and taken exactly as prescribed; doses are not to be doubled; take missed dose when remembered up to 1 hr before next dose
• Tell patient to report diarrhea, black tarry stools, sore throat, rash, dizziness, confusion, or delirium to prescriber immediately

Evaluation
Positive therapeutic outcome
• Decreased pain in abdomen
• Healing of ulcers

RARELY USED

fat emulsions (Rx)
(fat ee-mul'shuns)
Intralipid 10%, Intralipid 20%, Liposyn II 10%, Liposyn II 20%, Liposyn III 10%, Liposyn III 20%, Soyacal 20%
Func. class.: Caloric
Chem. class.: Fatty acid, long chain
Pregnancy category C

ACTION: Needed for energy, heat production; consists of neutral triglycerides, primarily unsaturated fatty acids

Therapeutic outcome: Increased available calories and fatty acids

USES: Increase calorie intake, prevent fatty acid deficiency

CONTRAINDICATIONS
Hypersensitivity to this product, eggs, soybeans, or legumes; hyperlipemia; lipid necrosis; acute pancreatitis accompanied by hyperlipemia; hyperbilirubinemia of the newborn; renal insufficiency; hepatic damage

DOSAGE AND ROUTES
Deficiency
Adult and child: **IV** 8%-10% of required calorie intake (intralipid)

Adjunct to TPN
Adult: **IV** 1 ml/min over 15-30 min (10%) or 0.5 ml/min over 15-30 min (20%); may increase to 500 ml over 4-8 hr if no adverse reactions occur; max 2.5 g/kg

---

Child: IV 0.1 ml/min over 10-15 min (10%) or 0.05 ml/ min over 10-15 min (20%); may increase to 1 g/kg over 4 hr if no adverse reactions occur; max 4 g/kg

Prevention of deficiency
Adult: IV 500 ml 2 ×/wk (10%), given 1 ml/min for 30 min, max 500 ml over 6 hr
Child: IV 5-10 ml/kg/day (10%), given 0.1 ml/min for 30 min, max 100 ml/hr

Available forms: Inj 10% (50, 100, 200, 250, 500 ml), 20% (50, 100, 200, 250, 500 ml)

febuxostat (Rx)
(feb-ux'oh-stat)
Uloric
Func. class.: Antigout drug, antihyperuricemic
Chem. class.: Xanthine oxidase inhibitor
Pregnancy category C

ACTION: Inhibits the enzyme xanthine oxidase, reducing uric acid synthesis; more selective for xanthine oxidase than allopurinol

Therapeutic outcome: Decreased signs/symptoms of gout, hyperuricemia

USES: Chronic gout, hyperuricemia

CONTRAINDICATIONS
Hypersensitivity

Precautions: Pregnancy **C**, breastfeeding, children, renal/hepatic/cardiac/neoplastic disease, stroke, MI, organ transplant, Lesch-Nyhan syndrome

DOSAGE AND ROUTES
Adult: PO 40 mg daily, may increase to 80 mg daily if uric acid levels are >6 mg/dl after 2 wk of therapy

Available forms: Tabs 40, 80 mg

Implementation
PO route
• Give without regard to meals or antacid; may crush and add to foods or fluids

ADVERSE EFFECTS
CNS: Weakness, flushing
CV: MI, atrial fibrillation, atrial flutter, AV block, bradycardia, hyper/hypotension, palpitations, sinus tachycardia, stroke, angina
EENT: Retinopathy, cataracts, epistaxis
GI: *Nausea, vomiting, anorexia,* constipation, diarrhea, dyspepsia, hematemesis, hepatitis, hepatomegaly, weight gain/loss, cholecystitis, cholelithiasis, melena

GU: Renal failure, urinary urgency/frequency/incontinence, nephrolithiasis, hematuria
HEMA: Thrombocytopenia, anemia, pancytopenia, leukopenia, bone marrow suppression
INTEG: Rash
MISC: Arthralgia, gout flare

Pharmacokinetics
Absorption	Unknown
Distribution	Protein binding 99.2%
Metabolism	Unknown
Excretion	Feces, urine
Half-life	5-8 hr

Pharmacodynamics
Onset	Unknown
Peak	1-1.5 hr
Duration	Unknown

INTERACTIONS
Individual drugs
AzaTHIOprine, didanosine, mercaptopurine: increased toxicity
Rasburicase: increased xanthine nephropathy, calculi

Drug classifications
Antineoplastics: increased xanthine nephropathy, calculi

Drug/lab
Increase: LFTs

NURSING CONSIDERATIONS
Assessment
• **Hyperuricemia:** Monitor uric acid levels q2wk; uric acid levels should be 6 mg/dl or less
• Hepatic studies prior to use, then at 2, 4 mo, and then periodically; assess for fatigue, anorexia, right upper abdominal discomfort, dark urine, jaundice
• Monitor CBC, AST, BUN, creatinine before starting treatment, periodically, flares may occur during first 6 wk of treatment
• **Renal disease:** Monitor I&O ratio; increase fluids to 2 L/day to prevent stone formation and toxicity
• Assess for rash, hypersensitivity reactions; discontinue
• **Assess for gout:** joint pain, swelling; may use with NSAIDs for acute gouty attacks and gout flare (first 6 wk)

Patient/family education
• Inform patient that tabs may be crushed
• Teach patient to take as prescribed; if dose is missed, take as soon as remembered; do not double dose

---

- Teach patient to increase fluid intake to 2 L/day unless contraindicated
- Advise patient to avoid alcohol, caffeine; will increase uric acid levels
- Advise patient to report cardiovascular events to prescriber, immediately
- **Gout:** teach patient that flares may occur during first 6 wk of treatment

Evaluation

Positive therapeutic outcome
- Decreased pain in joints, decreased stone formation in kidneys, decreased uric acid levels

felodipine (Rx)
(feh-loh'dih-peen)
Plendil, Renedil ✦
Func. class.: Calcium-channel blocker, antihypertensive, antianginal
Chem. class.: Dihydropyridine
Pregnancy category C

Do not confuse: Plendil/Pindolol/Pletal/ PriLOSEC/ Prinival/Isordil

ACTION: Inhibits calcium ion influx across cell membrane, resulting in inhibition of excitation/contraction of vascular smooth muscle

Therapeutic outcome: Decreased B/P in hypertension

USES: Essential hypertension, alone or with other antihypertensives

CONTRAINDICATIONS
Hypersensitivity to this product or dihydropyridines, sick sinus syndrome, 2nd- or 3rd-degree heart block, hypotension <90 mm Hg systolic

Precautions: Pregnancy C, breastfeeding, children, geriatric, CHF, hepatic injury, renal disease, coronary artery disease

DOSAGE AND ROUTES
Adult: PO 5 mg/day initially, usual range 2.5-10 mg/day; max 10 mg/day; do not adjust dosage at intervals of <2 wk
Geriatric: PO 2.5 mg/day

Hepatic dose
Adult: PO 2.5-5 mg/day, max 10 mg/day

Available forms: Ext rel tabs 2.5, 5, 10 mg

Implementation
PO route
- Do not break, crush, or chew ext rel tabs
- Give once a day with food for GI symptoms

ADVERSE EFFECTS
CNS: *Headache,* fatigue, drowsiness, dizziness, anxiety, depression, nervousness, insomnia, light-headedness, paresthesia, tinnitus, psychosis, somnolence
CV: **Dysrhythmias,** *edema,* **CHF,** hypotension, palpitations, **MI, pulmonary edema,** tachycardia, syncope, AV block, angina
GI: Nausea, vomiting, diarrhea, **gastric upset,** constipation, increased liver function studies, dry mouth
GU: Nocturia, polyuria, sexual dysfunction, decreased libido
HEMA: Anemia
INTEG: Rash, pruritus, peripheral edema
MISC: Flushing, sexual difficulties, cough, nasal congestion, shortness of breath, wheezing, epistaxis, respiratory infection, chest pain, **angioedema,** gingival hyperplasia, **Stevens-Johnson syndrome**

Pharmacokinetics

Absorption	Well absorbed
Distribution	Unknown; protein binding >99%
Metabolism	Liver, extensively
Excretion	Kidneys
Half-life	11-16 hr

Pharmacodynamics

Onset	2-3 hr
Peak	2½-5 hr
Duration	<24 hr

INTERACTIONS
Individual drugs
Alcohol, carBAMazepine, cimetidine, clarithromycin, conivaptan, cycloSPORINE, dalfopristin, delavirdine, diltiazem, erythromycin, itraconazole, ketoconazole, miconazole, phenytoin, propanolol, quiNIDine, quinupristin, zileuton: increased hypotension
Digoxin, disopyramide, phenytoin: increased bradycardia, increased CHF

Drug classifications
β-Adrenergic blockers: increased bradycardia, CHF
Nitrates: increased hypotension
NSAIDs: decreased antihypertensive effects

Drug/herb
Ginkgo, ginseng, hawthorn: increased antihypertensive effect
Ephedra, St. John's wort: decreased antihypertensive effect

✦ Canada only

Adverse effects: *italics* = common; **bold** = life-threatening

Drug/food
Grapefruit juice: increased felodipine level

NURSING CONSIDERATIONS
Assessment
• CHF: Assess fluid volume status: I&O ratio and record; weight; skin turgor; adequacy of pulses; moist mucous membranes; bilateral lung sounds; peripheral pitting edema; dehydration symptoms of decreasing output, thirst, hypotension, dry mouth, and mucous membranes should be reported; for CHF: weight gain, crackles, dyspnea, edema, jugular venous distention
• Monitor ALT, AST, bilirubin daily if these are elevated
• Monitor cardiac status: B/P, pulse, respiration, ECG, periodically
• **Assess for anginal pain:** duration; intensity; ameliorating, aggravating factors

Patient/family education
• Caution patient to avoid hazardous activities until stabilized on product and dizziness is no longer a problem
• Instruct patient to limit caffeine consumption; to avoid alcohol and OTC products unless directed by prescriber
• Urge patient to comply in all areas of medical regimen: diet, exercise, stress reduction, product therapy; to notify prescriber of irregular heartbeat, shortness of breath, swelling of feet and hands, pronounced dizziness, constipation, nausea, hypotension
• Advise patient to use protective clothing, sunscreen to prevent photosensitivity
• Teach patient to change positions slowly to prevent orthostatic hypotension
• Advise patient to obtain correct pulse; to contact prescriber if pulse is <50 bpm
• Teach patient to use as directed even if feeling better; may be taken with other CV products (nitrates, β-blockers); that capsules may appear in stools but are insignificant
• Teach patient to practice good oral hygiene to prevent gingival hyperplasia
• Advise patient not to stop medication abruptly
• Advise patient to avoid grapefruit juice

Evaluation

Positive therapeutic outcome
• Decreased B/P
• Decreased anginal attacks
• Increase in activity tolerance

fenofibrate (Rx)
(fen-oh-fee′brate)
Antara, Fenoglide ✦, Lipidil EZ ✦, Lipidil Micro ✦, Lipidil Supra ✦, Lipofem, Lipofen, Lofibra, Tricor, Triglide
Func. class.: Antilipemic
Chem. class.: Fibric acid derivative
Pregnancy category C

ACTION: Increases lipolysis and elimination of triglyceride-rich particles from plasma by activating lipoprotein lipase, resulting in triglyceride change in size and composition of LDL, leading to rapid breakdown of LDL; mobilizes triglycerides from tissue; increases excretion of neutral sterols

Therapeutic outcome: Decreasing cholesterol levels and low-density lipoproteins, decreased pruritus

USES: Hypercholesterolemia, patients with types IV, V hyperlipidemia who do not respond to other treatment and who are at risk for pancreatitis; Fredrickson type IV, V hypertriglyceridemia

CONTRAINDICATIONS
Hypersensitivity, severe renal/hepatic disease, primary biliary cirrhosis, preexisting gallbladder disease, breastfeeding

Precautions: Pregnancy **C,** geriatric, peptic ulcer, pancreatitis, renal/hepatic disease, diabetes mellitus

DOSAGE AND ROUTES
Hypertriglyceridemia
Adult: PO (Antara) 43-130 mg/day; (Lofibra) 67-200 mg/day; (Tricor) 48-145 mg/day; (Triglide) 50-160 mg/day

Primary hypercholesterolemia/ mixed hyperlipidemia
Adult: PO (Antara) 130 mg/day; (Lofibra) 200 mg/day; (Tricor) 145 mg/day; (Triglide) 160 mg/day

Renal dose (geriatric)
Adult: PO (Tricor) CCr 30-80 ml/min 48 mg/day; CCr <30 ml/min contraindicated
Adult: PO (Triglide, Lipofem) CCr 11-49 ml/min 50 mg/day; (Antara) 30 mg/day; (Fenoglide) 40 mg/day; (Lofibra) 67 mg/day; (Antara, Lipofem, Lofibra, Triglide) CCr <30 ml/min, contraindicated

Available forms: Cap: Antara 30, 90 mg; Lipofen 50, 150 mg tab: Triglide 50, 160 mg; Lofibra 54, 160 mg; Tricor 48, 145 mg; Fenoglide 40, 120 mg

Implementation

• Do not break, crush, or chew tabs
• Give with evening meal; if dose is increased, give with breakfast and evening meal (Lipofen, Lofibra); Triglide, Antara without regard to food; may increase q4-8wk
• Brands are not interchangeable; therapy should be discontinued if there is not adequate response after 2 mo
• Store in cool environment in tight, light-resistant container

ADVERSE EFFECTS

CNS: Fatigue, weakness, drowsiness, dizziness, insomnia, depression, vertigo
CV: Angina, hypertension, hypotension
GI: Nausea, vomiting, dyspepsia, increased liver enzymes, flatulence, hepatomegaly, gastritis, **pancreatitis, cholelithiasis**
GU: Dysuria, urinary frequency
HEMA: Anemia, *leukopenia*, **thrombosis, pulmonary embolism**
INTEG: *Rash,* urticaria, pruritus, photosensitivity
MISC: Polyphagia, weight gain, infection, flu-like syndrome
MS: Myalgias, arthralgias, *myopathy,* **rhabdomyolysis**
RESP: Pharyngitis, bronchitis, cough

Pharmacokinetics

Absorption	Unknown
Distribution	Protein binding 99%
Metabolism	Liver
Excretion	Urine 60%, feces 25%
Half-life	20 hr

Pharmacodynamics

Onset	Unknown
Peak	6-8 hr
Duration	Unknown

INTERACTIONS
Individual drugs
CycloSPORINE: increased nephrotoxicity

Drug classifications
Anticoagulants (oral): increased effect of anticoagulants

Antidiabetics: increased effect of antidiabetics
Bile acid sequestrants: decreased absorption
HMG-CoA reductase inhibitors: do not use together, rhabdomyolysis may occur

Drug/herb
Red yeast rice: increased effects

Drug/food
Increased absorption

Drug/lab test
Increase: ALT, AST, BUN, CK, creatinine
Decrease: WBC, uric acid, Hgb

NURSING CONSIDERATIONS
Assessment
• **Hypercholesterolemia:** Monitor lipid levels (triglycerides, LDL, HDL, total cholesterol), fat content
• Liver function tests, baseline and periodically during treatment; CPK if muscle pain occurs, CBC, Hct, Hgh, pro-time with anticoagulant therapy
• **Assess for pancreatitis, cholelithiasis, renal failure, rhabdomyolysis (when combined with HMG-CoA reductase inhibitors), myositis; product should be discontinued**
• Assess nutrition: fat, protein, carbohydrates, nutritional analysis should be completed by dietitian

Patient/family education
• Inform patient that compliance is needed
• Instruct patient not to consume chipped or broken tabs (Triglide)
• Teach patient that risk factors—high-fat diet, smoking, alcohol consumption, absence of exercise—should be decreased
• Caution patient to notify prescriber if pregnancy is planned or suspected
• Teach patient to notify prescriber if the GI symptoms of diarrhea, abdominal or epigastric pain, nausea, or vomiting occur
• Instruct patient to report GU symptoms: dysuria, proteinuria, oliguria, decreased libido, impotence
• **Advise patient to notify prescriber of muscle pain, weakness, fever, fatigue, epigastric pain**

Evaluation
Positive therapeutic outcome
• Decrease in cholesterol to desired level after 8 wk

⚠ HIGH ALERT

fentaNYL (Rx)

(fen'ta-nill)

RAN-Fentanyl ✦, Sublimaze

fentaNYL transdermal (Rx)

Duragesic

Func. class.: Opioid analgesic

Chem. class.: Synthetic phenylpiperidine derivative

fentaNYL nasal spray (Rx)

Lazanda

fentaNYL SL spray (Rx)

Subsys

fentaNYL SL

Abstral

fentaNYL buccal

Fentora

fentaNYL lozenge

Actiq

Pregnancy category C

Controlled substance schedule II

Do not confuse: fentaNYL/Sufenta

ACTION: Inhibits ascending pain pathways in CNS, increases pain threshold, alters pain perception by binding to opiate receptors

Therapeutic outcome: Relief of pain, supplement to anesthesia

USES: Controls moderate to severe pain; preoperatively, postoperatively; adjunct to general anesthetic, adjunct to regional anesthesia; **FentaNYL:** for anesthesia as premedication, conscious sedation; **Actiq:** for breakthrough cancer pain

CONTRAINDICATIONS

Hypersensitivity to opiates, myasthenia gravis

> **BLACK BOX WARNING:** headache, migraine (Actiq), Astral, Fentora, Lazanda, Onsolis, emergency dept use (Abstral, Lazanda), outpatient surgeries (Duragesic TD), opioid-naive patients, respiratory disorders, depression

Precautions: Pregnancy **C**, breastfeeding, geriatric, increased ICP, seizure disorders, cardiac dysrhythmias, severe respiratory disorders

> **BLACK BOX WARNING:** Children, accidental exposure, ambient temperature increase, fever, skin abrasion (TD patch), substance abuse, surgery, requires an experienced clinician

DOSAGE AND ROUTES

>> FentaNYL

Anesthetic

Adult: IV 50-100 mcg/kg over 1-2 min, max 150 mcg/kg

Anesthesia supplement

Adult and child >12 yr: IM/IV 2-20 mcg/kg IV INF 0.025-0.25 mcg/kg/min

Induction and maintenance

Child 2-12 yr: IV 2-3 mcg/kg

Preoperatively

Adult and child >12 yr: IM/IV 50-100 mcg q30-60min before surgery

Postoperatively

Adult and child >12 yr: IM/IV 0.05-0.1 mg q1-2hr prn

Moderate/severe pain

Adult: IV/IM 50-100 mcg q1-2hr

>> Actiq

Adult: Transmucosal 200 mcg, redose if needed 15 min after completion of 1st dose, max 2 doses during titration period, max 4 doses/day

>> Fentora

Adult: BUCCAL/SL 100 mcg placed above rear molar between upper cheek and gum, a second 100 mcg dose, if needed, may be started 30 min after first dose

>> ABSTRAL

Adult: SL 100 mcg, another dose may be taken 30 min after first, max 2 doses per episode of breakthrough pain, ≥2 hr must elapse before treating again, titrate stepwise over consecutive episodes

>> FentaNYL transdermal

Adult: 25 mcg/hr; may increase until pain relief occurs; apply patch to flat surface on upper torso and wear for 72 hr; apply new patch to different site for continued relief

>> FentaNYL nasal spray

Adult: 100 mcg (1 spray in 1 nostril), may retreat after ≥2 hr, titrate upward to adequate analgesia, treat a max of 4 episodes q day

>> FentaNYL SL spray

Adult: SL 100 mcg sprayed under the tongue; titrate stepwise carefully

Available forms: Inj 0.05 mg/ml; lozenges 100, 200, 300, 400, 600, 800, 1200, 1600 mcg; lozenges on a stick 200, 400, 600, 800, 1200, 1600 mcg; buccal tab 100, 200, 400, 600, 800 mcg; transdermal patch 12, 25, 50, 75, 100 mcg/hr; SL tab (ABSTRAL) 100, 200, 300, 400, 600, 800 mcg; SL spray: 100, 200, 400, 600, 1200, 1600 mcg/spray; nasal spray 100, 400 mcg/actuation

---

Implementation

- Store in light-resistant area at room temperature
- **Overdose has been fatal when confusing products/dose; recheck both before using**

Transmucosal route

- Remove foil just before administration; instruct patient to place between cheek and lower gum, moving it back and forth and sucking, not chewing (Actiq); place above rear molar (Fentora); place film on the inside of the cheek (Onsolis); all products not used or partially used should be flushed down the toilet; this product may be used SL

Transdermal route

- Apply patch to chest on a flat area with skin intact; for skin preparation, use clear water with no soap; clip hair, skin should be dry before applying patch; apply immediately after removing from package and press firmly in place with palm of hand; flush old patch down toilet immediately upon removal

Use pain dosing

- Dosage is titrated based on patient's report of pain; dosage is determined by calculating the previous 24-hr requirement and converting to equianalgesic morphine dose
- To convert to another opioid analgesic, remove transdermal patch and begin treatment with half the equal pain-controlling dose of the new analgesic in 12-18 hr

SL spray

- Open blister package with scissors immediately prior to use; spray contents under tongue; dispose of unit by placing it into disposable bags provided; seal bag, discard into trash container out of reach of children.

IV route

- Give by inj (IM, **IV**), only with resuscitative equipment available; give slowly to prevent rigidity
- Give **IV** undiluted by anesthesiologist or diluted with 5 ml or more sterile water or 0.9% NaCl given through Y-tube or 3-way stopcock given at 0.1 mg or less/1.2 min
- Muscular rigidity may occur with rapid IV administration

Y-site compatibilities: Abciximab, acyclovir, alemtuzumab, alfentanil, alprostadil, amikacin, aminocaproic acid, aminophylline, amiodarone, amphotericin B cholesteryl, amphotericin B lipid complex, amphotericin B liposome, anidulafungin, argatroban, ascorbic acid injection, atenolol, atracurium, atropine, azaTHIOprine, aztreonam, benztropine, bivalirudin, bleomycin, bumetanide, buprenorphine, butorphanol, calcium chloride/gluconate, CARBOplatin, caspofungin, ceFAZolin, cefmetazole, cefonicid, cefotaxime, cefoTEtan, cefOXitin, cefTAZidime, ceftizoxime, ceftobiprole, cefTRIAXone, cefuroxime, cephalothin, chloramphenicol, chlorproMAZINE, cimetidine, cisatracurium, CISplatin, clindamycin, cloNIDine, cyanocobalamin, cyclophosphamide, cycloSPORINE, cytarabine, DACTINomycin, DAPTOmycin, dexamethasone, dexmedetomidine, digoxin, diltiazem, diphenhydrAMINE, DOBUTamine, DOCEtaxel, DOPamine, doripenem, doxacurium, doxapram, DOXOrubicin, doxycycline, enalaprilat, ePHEDrine, EPINEPHrine, epirubicin, epoetin alfa, eptifibatide, erythromycin, esmolol, etomidate, etoposide, famotidine, fenoldopam, fluconazole, fludarabine, fluorouracil, folic acid, furosemide, ganciclovir, gatifloxacin, gemcitabine, gentamicin, glycopyrrolate, granisetron, heparin, hydrocortisone, HYDROmorphone, hydrOXYzine, IDArubicin, ifosfamide, imipenem-cilastatin, inamrinone, insulin (regular), irinotecan, isoproterenol, ketorolac, labetalol, lansoprazole, levofloxacin, lidocaine, linezolid, LORazepam, LR, magnesium sulfate, mannitol, mechlorethamine, meperidine, metaraminol, methicillin, methotrexate, methotrimeprazine, methoxamine, methyldopate, methylPREDNISolone, metoclopramide, metoprolol, metroNIDAZOLE, mezlocillin, miconazole, midazolam, milrinone, minocycline, mitoXANtrone, mivacurium, morphine, moxalactam, multiple vitamins injection, mycophenolate, nafcillin, nalbuphine, naloxone, nesiritide, netilmicin, niCARdipine, nitroglycerin, nitroprusside, norepinephrine, octreotide, ondansetron, oxacillin, oxaliplatin, oxytocin, PACLitaxel, palonosetron, pamidronate, pancuronium, papaverine, PEMEtrexed, penicillin G potassium/sodium, pentamidine, pentazocine, PENTobarbital, PHENobarbital, phenylephrine, phytonadione, piperacillin, piperacillin-tazobactam, polymyxin B, potassium chloride, procainamide, prochlorperazine, promethazine, propofol, propranolol, protamine, pyridoxine, quiNIDine, quinupristin-dalfopristin, ranitidine, remifentanil, Ringer's, ritodrine, riTUXimab, rocuronium, sargramostim, scopolamine, sodium acetate/bicarbonate, succinylcholine, SUFentanil, tacrolimus, teniposide, theophylline, thiamine, thiopental, thiotepa, ticarcillin, ticarcillin-clavulanate, tigecycline, tirofiban, TNA, tobramycin, tolazoline, TPN, trastuzumab, trimetaphan, urokinase, vancomycin, vasopressin, vecuronium, verapamil, vinCRIStine, vinorelbine, vitamin B complex/C, voriconazole, zoledronic acid

ADVERSE EFFECTS

CNS: Dizziness, delirium, euphoria, sedation, confusion, weakness, dizziness
CV: Bradycardia, cardiac arrest, hypo/hypertension
EENT: Blurred vision, miosis
GI: Nausea, vomiting, constipation
GU: Urinary retention
INTEG: Rash, diaphoresis
MS: Muscle rigidity
RESP: Respiratory depression, arrest, laryngospasm

Pharmacokinetics

Absorption	Well absorbed (IM), completely absorbed (**IV**)
Distribution	Unknown, crosses placenta
Metabolism	Extensively, liver; 80% bound to plasma proteins
Excretion	Kidneys, up to 25% unchanged; breast milk
Half-life	IV 2-4 hr; transdermal 13-22 hr; transmucosal 7 hr; buccal 4-12 hr

Pharmacodynamics

	IM	IV	TD
Onset	7-15 min	Rapid	6 hr
Peak	30 min	3-5 min	12-24 hr
Duration	1-2 hr	½-1 hr	72 hr

INTERACTIONS
Individual drugs
Alcohol: increased respiratory depression, hypotension, increased sedation

> **BLACK BOX WARNING:** Cimetidine, conivaptan, cycloSPORINE, fluconazole, itraconazole, ketoconazole, nefazodone, ranolazine, zafirlukast, zileuton: increased fentaNYL effect, fatal respiratory depression, CYP3A4 inhibitors

Diazepam: increased CV depression
Droperidol: increased hypotension

Drug classifications
Antipsychotics, opioids, skeletal muscle relaxants: effects increased, protease inhibitors
CNS depressants, sedative/hypnotics: increased respiratory depression, hypotension
CYP3A4 inducers (carBAMazepine, PHENobarbital, phenytoin, rifampin): decreased fentaNYL effect
MAOIs: increased fatal reactions

Drug/herb
St. John's wort, valerian: increased fentaNYL action
Echinacea: decreased effect of fentaNYL

Drug/lab test
Increased: amylase, lipase

NURSING CONSIDERATIONS
Assessment
• Monitor VS after parenteral route (B/P, pulse, respiration); note muscle rigidity; take drug history before administering product; check renal/liver function tests

> **BLACK BOX WARNING:** Respiratory depression: Monitor character, rate, rhythm; notify prescriber if respirations <10/min

• Monitor CNS changes: dizziness, drowsiness, hallucinations, euphoria, LOC, pupil reaction
• Monitor allergic reactions: rash, urticaria; product should be discontinued
• **Assess for pain:** intensity, location, duration, type, before and 15 min after IM route or 3-5 min after **IV** route

> **BLACK BOX WARNING: Headache, migraine:** Abstral, Actiq, Fentora, Lazanda, Onsolis are not to be used for this condition; Abstral, Lazanda is not to be used in the ED; DurAgesic TD is not to be used for outpatient surgery patients

> **BLACK BOX WARNING: Apnea, respiratory arrest in opioid-naive patients:** Do not use Abstral, Actiq, Duragesic, Fentora, Lazanda, Onsolis, opioid tolerant are those using ≥60 ml/day oral morphine, ≥30 mg/day oxyCODONE PO, 8 mg/day HYDROmorphone, 25 mcg tid fentaNYL/hr

Patient/family education
• Discuss the dangers of children or pets getting the product
• Advise patient to report any symptoms of CNS changes, allergic reactions
• Instruct patient to avoid CNS depressants: alcohol, sedative-hypnotics for at least 24 hr after taking this product
• Teach patient that dizziness, drowsiness, confusion are common, and to avoid getting up without assistance
• Discuss in detail with patient all aspects of the product
• Teach patient CNS changes: physical dependence; not to use with alcohol, other CNS depressants

Transdermal route

> **BLACK BOX WARNING: Ambient temperature increase:** Discuss with patient that excessive heat may increase absorption; excessive perspiration may alter adhesiveness; do not use with heating pads, electric blankets, heat/tanning lamps, saunas, hot tubs, heated waterbeds, sunbathing

• Discuss with patient that hair may need to be clipped before applying
• Teach patient how to dispose of patch: place sticky sides together and flush in toilet
• May add first aid tape around the edges if there is a problem with adhesion

Evaluation
Positive therapeutic outcome
• Maintenance of anesthesia
• Decreased breakthrough cancer pain
• General pain relief

TREATMENT OF OVERDOSE:
Naloxone 0.2-0.8 **IV**, O_2, **IV** fluids, vasopressors

---

ferrous fumarate (Rx)
Femiron, Feostat, Ferrate, Ferretts, Ferrocite, Hemocyte, Palafer ❧
ferrous gluconate (Rx)
Fergon
ferrous sulfate (Rx) ✪
Feosol, Fer-Gen-Sol, Fer-In-Sol, FeroSul
ferrous sulfate, dried (Rx)
Feosol, Feratab, Slow Fe
carbonyl iron (OTC)
(kar'boh-nil)
ICAR Pediatric, Iron Chews
iron polysaccharide (OTC)
iFerex, Niferex, Nu-Iron
Func. class.: Hematinic
Chem. class.: Iron preparation
Pregnancy category B, C

ACTION: Replaces iron stores needed for red blood cell development, energy and O_2 transport, utilization; fumarate contains 33% elemental iron; gluconate, 12%; sulfate, 20%; iron, 30%; ferrous sulfate exsiccated

Therapeutic outcome: Prevention and correction of iron deficiency

USES: Iron deficiency anemia, prophylaxis for iron deficiency in pregnancy, nutritional supplementation

CONTRAINDICATIONS
Sideroblastic anemia, thalassemia, hemosiderosis/hemochromatosis

Precautions: Pregnancy **B** (ferric gluconate complex), **C** (iron dextran, oral products); anemia (long-term), peptic ulcer disease, hemolytic anemia, cirrhosis, ulcerative colitis/regional enteritis, sulfite sensitivity

> **BLACK BOX WARNING:** Accidental exposure

DOSAGE AND ROUTES
Fumarate
Adult: PO 50-100 mg tid
Child: PO 3 mg/kg/day (elemental iron) tid-qid
Infant: PO 10-25 mg/day (elemental iron) in 3-4 divided doses, max 15 mg/day

Gluconate
Adult: PO 60 mg bid-qid
Child 6-12 yr: PO 3 mg/kg/day divided

Sulfate
Adult: PO 0.750-1.5 g/day in divided doses tid
Child 6-12 yr: 600 mg/day in divided doses

Pregnancy
Adult: PO 300-600 mg/day in divided doses

Iron polysaccharide
Adult: 100-200 mg tid
Child: PO 4-6 mg/kg/day in 3 divided doses (severe iron deficiency)

Available forms: Fumarate: tabs 90, 150, 200, 300, 324, 325 mg; chewable tabs 100 mg; extended release tabs 18 mg; **gluconate:** tabs 225, 240, 324, 325 mg; **sulfate:** tabs 195, 300, 325 mg; elixir 220 mg/5 ml; dried: tabs 200 mg; ext rel tabs 160 mg; ext rel caps 160 mg; **iron polysaccharide:** tabs 50 mg; caps 150 mg; sol 100 mg/5 ml

Implementation
PO route
• Swallow all tabs whole; do not break, crush, or chew
• Give between meals for best absorption; may give with juice; do not give with antacids or milk, delay at least 1 hr; if GI symptoms occur, give after meals even if absorption is decreased; eggs, milk products, chocolate, caffeine interfere with absorption; ferrous gluconate is less GI irritating than ferrous sulfate
• Give **liquid** preparations through plastic straw to avoid discoloration of tooth enamel; dilute thoroughly
• Store in tight, light-resistant container
• Give at least 1 hr before bedtime because corrosion may occur in stomach

---

Adverse effects: *italics* = common; **bold** = life-threatening

- Give for <6 mo for anemia
- Store at room temperature; protect from moisture

ADVERSE EFFECTS
GI: *Nausea, constipation, epigastric pain, black and red tarry stools,* vomiting, diarrhea
INTEG: Temporarily discolored tooth enamel and eyes
SYST: Hypersensitivity reactions (Ferrlecit)

Pharmacokinetics

Absorption	Up to 30%
Distribution	Bound to transferrin, crosses placenta
Metabolism	Recycled
Excretion	Feces, urine, skin, breast milk
Half-life	Unknown

Pharmacodynamics
Unknown

INTERACTIONS
Individual drugs
Chloramphenicol, vit C: increased absorption of iron products
Cholestyramine, L-thyroxine, levodopa, methyldopa, penicillamine, tetracycline, vitamin E: decreased absorption of each product

Drug classifications
Antacids, H_2 antagonists, proton pump inhibitors: decreased absorption of iron preparations
Fluoroquinolones: decreased absorption of fluoroquinolone

Drug/food
Caffeine, dairy products, eggs: decreased absorption

Drug/lab test
False positive: occult blood

NURSING CONSIDERATIONS
Assessment
- Monitor blood studies: Hct, Hgb, reticulocytes, bilirubin before treatment, at least monthly; iron studies (Fe, TIBC, ferritin)
- **Assess for toxicity: nausea, vomiting, diarrhea (green, then tarry stools,) hematemesis, pallor, cyanosis, shock, coma**
- Assess bowel elimination; if constipation occurs, increase water, bulk, activity before laxatives are required
- **Assess nutrition:** amount of iron in diet (meat, dark green leafy vegetables, dried beans, dried fruits, eggs); provide referral to dietitian if indicated

- Identify cause of iron loss or anemia, including salicylates, sulfonamides, antimalarials, quiNIDine

Patient/family education
- Advise patient that iron will make stools black or dark green, stain teeth; that iron poisoning may occur if increased beyond recommended level
- **Accidental exposure: advise patient to keep out of reach of children, pets**
- **Caution patient not to substitute one iron salt for another; elemental iron content differs (e.g., 300 mg ferrous fumarate contains about 100 mg elemental iron, whereas 300 mg ferrous gluconate contains only about 30 mg elemental iron)**
- **Caution patient to avoid reclining position for 15-30 min after taking product to avoid esophageal corrosion; to follow diet high in iron**
- Caution patient to avoid taking iron, dairy products, calcium supplements, vit C together; they compete for absorption

Evaluation

Positive therapeutic outcome
- Decreased fatigue, weakness
- Improvement in Hct, Hgb, reticulocytes

TREATMENT OF OVERDOSE:
Induce vomiting; give eggs, milk until lavage can be done

fesoterodine (Rx)
(fess'oh-ter-oh-deen)
Toviaz
Func. class.: Overactive bladder product
Chem. class.: Muscarinic receptor antagonist
Pregnancy category C

ACTION: Relaxes smooth muscles in urinary tract by inhibiting acetylcholine at postganglionic sites

Therapeutic outcome: Absence of urinary frequency, urgency, incontinence

USES: Overactive bladder (urinary frequency, urgency), urinary incontinence

CONTRAINDICATIONS
GI obstruction, ileus, pyloric stenosis, urinary retention, gastric retention, hypersensitivity, closed-angle glaucoma

Precautions: Pregnancy **C,** breastfeeding, children, renal/hepatic disease, urinary tract obstruction, ambient temperature increase, autonomic neuropathy, constipation, contact lenses, hazardous activity, GERD, gastroparesis, myasthenia gravis, prostatic hypertrophy, toxic megacolon, ulcerative colitis, possible cross-sensitivity with tolterodine

DOSAGE AND ROUTES

Adult and geriatric: PO EXT REL 4 mg/day, may increase to 8 mg/day based on response, max 4 mg/day in those taking potent CYP3A4 inhibitors

Renal dose
Adult: PO EXT REL CCr <30 ml/min max 4 mg/ day in severe renal impairment

Available forms: Ext rel tabs 4, 8 mg

Implementation

• Do not break, crush, or chew ext rel product
• Give without regard to meals
• Store at room temperature; protect from moisture

ADVERSE EFFECTS

CNS: Insomnia
CV: Chest pain, angina, **QT prolongation**, peripheral edema
EENT: Xerophthalmia
GI: *Nausea, vomiting,* abdominal pain, constipation, dry mouth
GU: Dysuria, urinary retention, urinary tract infection
INTEG: Rash, angioedema
MISC: Peripheral edema, insomnia
MS: Back pain
RESP: Cough, upper respiratory infection
SYST: Infection

Pharmacokinetics

Absorption	Rapid
Distribution	Protein binding 50%
Metabolism	Unknown
Excretion	Urine, feces
Half-life	7 hr

Pharmacodynamics

Peak	5 hr

INTERACTIONS

Drug classifications
Anticholinergics, antimuscarinics: increased anticholinergic effect
CYP3A4 inhibitors (antiretroviral protease inhibitors, azole antifungals), macrolide antiinfectives: increased action of fesoterodine
Diuretics: increased urinary frequency

Drug/herb
Caffeine, green tea, guarana: decreased fesoterodine

Drug/food
Grapefruit juice: increased fesoterodine level
Cola, coffee, tea: decreased fesoterodine level

NURSING CONSIDERATIONS
Assessment
• **Assess urinary patterns:** distention, nocturia, frequency, urgency, incontinence
• **Assess for allergic reactions:** rash, angioedema; if this occurs, product should be discontinued

Patient/family education
• Advise patient not to drink liquids before bedtime
• Instruct the patient on the importance of bladder maintenance
• Teach patient not to use new meds, herbs without prescriber approval

Evaluation

Positive therapeutic outcome
• Absence of urinary frequency, urgency, incontinence

---

fexofenadine (Rx, OTC)
(fex-oh-fin′a-deen)
Allegra
Func. class.: Histamine antagonist, 2nd generation
Chem. class.: Piperidine, peripherally selective
Pregnancy category C

Do not confuse: Allegra/Viagra

ACTION: Acts on blood vessels, GI, respiratory system by competing with histamine for H_1-receptor site; decreases allergic response by blocking pharmacologic effects of histamine; less sedation rate than with other antihistamines

Therapeutic outcome: Absence of allergy symptoms and rhinitis

USES: Rhinitis, allergy symptoms, chronic idiopathic urticaria

CONTRAINDICATIONS
Breastfeeding, newborn or premature infants, hypersensitivity

Precautions: Pregnancy **C,** children, geriatric, respiratory disease, closed-angle glaucoma, prostatic hypertrophy, bladder neck obstruction, asthma, renal failure

DOSAGE AND ROUTES
Adult and child >12 yr: PO Rx only 60 mg bid or 180 mg/day; PO OTC only 60 mg bid or 180 mg/day (self-treatment of allergic rhinitis)

Adverse effects: *italics* = common; **bold** = life-threatening

Child 6-11 yr: PO 30 mg bid; Orally disintegrating tab 30 mg bid dissolved on tongue

Renal dose
Adult and child ≥12 yr: PO CCr <80 ml/min 60 mg/day
Child 2-11 yr: PO CCr <80 ml/min 30 mg/day
Child <2 yr: PO CCr <80 ml/min 15 mg/day

Available forms: Caps 60 mg; tabs 30, 60, 180 mg; oral susp 6 mg/ml; orally disintegrating tab 30 mg

Implementation
• Give without regard to meals; caps/tabs should not be given with or right before grapefruit, orange, or apple juice
• **Orally disintegrating tab:** allow to dissolve, swallow
• **Oral susp:** shake well, use calibrated measuring device
• Store in tight, light-resistant container

ADVERSE EFFECTS
CNS: Headache, stimulation, drowsiness, sedation, fatigue, confusion, blurred vision, tinnitus, restlessness, tremors, paradoxical excitation in children or geriatric
CV: Hypotension, palpitations, bradycardia, tachycardia, **dysrhythmias (rare)**
GI: Nausea, diarrhea, abdominal pain, vomiting, constipation
GU: Frequency, dysuria, urinary retention, impotence
HEMA: **Hemolytic anemia, thrombocytopenia, leukopenia, agranulocytosis, pancytopenia**
INTEG: Rash, eczema, photosensitivity, urticaria
RESP: Thickening of bronchial secretions; dry nose, throat

Pharmacokinetics

Absorption	Well absorbed
Distribution	Unknown
Metabolism	Liver
Excretion	Kidneys
Half-life	Unknown

Pharmacodynamics

Onset	1 hr
Peak	2-3 hr
Duration	12-24 hr

INTERACTIONS
Individual drugs
Erythromycin, ketoconazole: increased fexofenadine effect

Rifampin: decreased fexofenadine effect
Aluminum, antacids, magnesium: decreased fexofenadine effect

Drug/food
Apple, orange, grapefruit juice: decreased absorption

Drug/lab test
False negative: skin allergy tests (discontinue antihistamine 3 days before testing)

NURSING CONSIDERATIONS
Assessment
• **Allergy:** assess for itchy, runny, watery eyes; congested nose; before and during treatment
• Assess respiratory status: rate, rhythm, increase in bronchial secretions, wheezing, chest tightness; provide fluids to 2 L/day to decrease secretion thickness
• Monitor I&O ratio: be alert for urinary retention, frequency, dysuria, especially geriatric; product should be discontinued if these occur

Patient/family education
• Teach all aspects of product uses; to notify prescriber if confusion, sedation, hypotension occur; to avoid driving or other hazardous activity if drowsiness occurs; to avoid alcohol or other CNS depressants that may potentiate effect
• Instruct patient to take 1 hr before or 2 hr after meals to facilitate absorption
• **Instruct patient not to exceed recommended dose; dysrhythmias may occur**
• Teach patient that hard candy, gum, frequent rinsing of mouth may be used for dryness

Evaluation
Positive therapeutic outcome
• Absence of running or congested nose, rashes

TREATMENT OF OVERDOSE: Administer lavage, diazepam, vasopressors, **IV** phenytoin

fidaxomicin (Rx)
(fye-dax-oh-mye′sin)
Dificid
Func. class.: Antiinfective-macrolide
Pregnancy category B

ACTION: Bactericidal against *Clostridium difficile;* is a fermentation product obtained from *Dactylosporangium aurantiacum;* inhibits RNA synthesis by inhibiting transcription of bacterial RNA polymerases; may act at the early stages of transcription

Therapeutic outcome: Resolution of *C. difficile* based on stool culture

USES: Pseudomembranous colitis, *C. difficile*-associated diarrhea

CONTRAINDICATIONS
Hypersensitivity

Precautions: Pregnancy **B**, breastfeeding, children

DOSAGE AND ROUTES
Adult: **PO** 200 mg bid × 10 days

Available forms: Tab 200 mg

Implementation:
• Give without regard to food
• Store at room temperature

ADVERSE EFFECTS
GI: Nausea, vomiting, abdominal pain, **GI bleeding**, intestinal obstruction
HEMA: *Anemia, neutropenia*
INTEG: Rash, pruritus
META: *Metabolic acidosis,* hyperglycemia

Pharmacokinetics

Absorption	Minimal
Distribution	GI tract
Metabolism	P-glucoprotein
Excretion	Feces 92%; parent drug
Half-life	12 hr

Pharmacodynamics

Onset	<1 hr
Peak	1 hr
Duration	1-5 hr

INTERACTIONS
Individual drugs
CycloSPORINE: Increased fidaxomicin action

Drug/lab test
Increased: glucose, LFTs, alk phos
Decreased: sodium bicarbonate, platelets

NURSING CONSIDERATIONS
Assessment
⚠ **Pseudomembranous colitis:** Assess for diarrhea, abdominal pain, fever, fatigue, anorexia, possible anemia, elevated WBC and low serum albumin; this product may be used in place of vancomycin; monitor CBC with differential, and stool culture (*C. difficile*); not to be used for systemic infection; obtain C&S prior to use; monitor glucose (diabetic patients); monitor fluid, electrolyte depletion

Patient/family education
• Advise patient to report GI bleeding, severe abdominal pain, continuing diarrhea

• Teach patient to report if pregnancy is planned or suspected or if breastfeeding
• Teach patient to take without regard to food

Evaluation

Positive therapeutic outcome
• Resolution of *C. difficile,* decreased diarrhea

⚠ HIGH ALERT

filgrastim (Rx)
(fill-gras′stim)
G-CSF, granulocyte colony stimulator, Neupogen
Func. class.: Biological modifier
Chem. class.: Granulocyte colony-stimulating factor
Pregnancy category C

ACTION: Stimulates proliferation and differentiation of neutrophils; a glycoprotein

Therapeutic outcome: Absence of infection

USES: To decrease infection in patients receiving antineoplastics that are myelosuppressive; to increase WBC in patients with product-induced neutropenia; bone marrow depression, acute radiation exposure

Unlabeled uses: Neutropenia in HIV infection, aplastic anemia, ganciclovir-induced neutropenia, zidovudine-induced neutropenia

CONTRAINDICATIONS
Hypersensitivity to proteins of *Escherichia coli*

Precautions: Pregnancy **C**, breastfeeding, children, myeloid malignancies, radiation therapy, sepsis, sickle cell disease, chemotherapy, respiratory disease

DOSAGE AND ROUTES
After myelosuppressive chemotherapy
Adult and child: **IV**/SUBCUT 5 mcg/kg/day in a single dose up to 14 days; may increase by 5 mcg/kg in each chemotherapy cycle

After myelosuppresive doses of radiation
Adult and child >7 mo: SUBCUT 10 mcg/kg/day, start as soon as possible after receiving ≥2 gray (Gy)

After bone marrow transplantation
Adult: **IV**/SUBCUT 10 mcg/kg as an INF (**IV**) over 4 or 24 hr, begin 24 hr after chemotherapy and 24 hr after bone marrow transplantation

Peripheral blood progenitor cell collection/therapy

Adult: 10 mcg/kg/day as a BOL or CONT INF × 4 days or more before leukapheresis, continue to last leukapheresis, may alter dose if WBC >100,000/mm^3

Severe neutropenia (chronic), idiopathic/cyclical

Adult: SUBCUT 5 mcg/kg daily

Available forms: Inj 300 mcg/ml, 480 mcg/1.6 ml, 480 mcg/0.8 ml

Implementation
• Store in refrigerator; do not freeze; may store at room temp up to 24 hr
• Given by subcut injection, short IV infusion, continuous SC or IV infusion
• Avoid use within 24 hr before or after chemotherapy
• Do not shake commercial single-dose vials prior to withdrawing the dose. If the vial is shaken and froth or bubbles form, allow the vial to stand undisturbed for a few min until the froth or bubbles dissipate
• Prior to injection, filgrastim may be allowed to reach room temperature for a maximum of 24 hr. Any vial or syringe exposed to room temperature for more than 24 hr should be discarded
• Visually inspect for particulate matter and discoloration prior to use

IV route
• May be diluted with 5% dextrose. Do not dilute with NS; product may precipitate
• May be diluted to concentrations 5-15 mcg/ml; should be protected from absorption to plastic by the addition of albumin to a final albumin concentration of 2 mg/ml. Do not dilute filgrastim to a concentration <5 mcg/ml

IV infusion
• Infuse IV over 15-30 min or as a continuous infusion over 24 hr

SUBCUT route
• May divide into 2 injections if dose is >1 ml
• Subcut injection: no dilution is necessary; inject by rapid subcut injection taking care not to inject intradermally
• Subcut continuous infusion: infuse subcut at a rate not to exceed 2 ml/hour

Y-site compatibilities: Acyclovir, allopurinol, amikacin, aminophylline, ampicillin, ampicillin/sulbactam, aztreonam, bleomycin, bumetanide, buprenorphine, butorphanol, calcium gluconate, CARBOplatin, carmustine, ceFAZolin, cefoTEtan, cefTAZidime, chlorproMAZINE, cimetidine, CISplatin, cyclophosphamide, cytarabine, dacarbazine, DAUNOrubicin, dexamethasone, diphenhydrAMINE, DOXOrubicin, doxycycline, droperidol, enalaprilat, famotidine, floxuridine, fluconazole, fludarabine, gallium, ganciclovir, granisetron, haloperidol, hydrocortisone, hydromorphone, hydrOXYzine, IDArubicin, ifosfamide, leucovorin, LORazepam, mechlorethamine, melphalan, meperidine, mesna, methotrexate, metoclopramide, miconazole, minocycline, mitoXANtrone, morphine, nalbuphine, netilmicin, ondansetron, plicamycin, potassium chloride, promethazine, ranitidine, sodium bicarbonate, streptozocin, ticarcillin, ticarcillin/clavulanate, tobramycin, trimethoprim-sulfamethoxazole, vancomycin, vinBLAStine, vinCRIStine, vinorelbine, zidovudine

ADVERSE EFFECTS

CNS: Fever, headache
GI: Nausea, vomiting, diarrhea, mucositis, anorexia
HEMA: Thrombocytopenia, excessive leukocytosis
INTEG: Alopecia, exacerbation of skin conditions, urticaria, cutaneous vasculitis, allergic reactions
MS: Osteoporosis, skeletal pain
OTHER: Chest pain, hypotension
RESP: Acute respiratory distress syndrome, wheezing, alveolar hemorrhage

Pharmacokinetics

Absorption	Well absorbed (SUBCUT), completely absorbed (**IV**)
Distribution	Unknown
Metabolism	Unknown
Excretion	Unknown
Half-life	Unknown

Pharmacodynamics

	IV	SUBCUT
Onset	5-60 min	5-60 min
Peak	24 hr	2-8 hr
Duration	up to 1 wk	up to 1 wk

INTERACTIONS

Individual drugs
Lithium: do not use concurrently

Drug classifications
Antineoplastics: increased neutrophils, do not use together 24 hr before or after antineoplastics

Drug/lab test
Increased: uric acid, lactate dehydrogenase, alkaline phosphatase, WBC

NURSING CONSIDERATIONS
Assessment
• Monitor blood studies: CBC, platelet count before treatment and twice weekly; neutrophil counts (ANC) drop by 50% if filgrastim is discontinued the next day but treatment should continue until ANC >10,000/mm^3
• Assess for bone pain: frequency, intensity, duration; analgesics may be given; opiates should not be used
• Check B/P, heart rate, respiration; baseline, during treatment
• **Respiratory distress syndrome: fever, dyspnea; withhold product if these occur**
• **Allergic reactions: rash, wheezing, facial edema, dyspnea may occur within 30 min of use; give antihistamines, bronchodilators and EPINEPHrine if needed**

Patient/family education
• Teach patient technique for self-administration: dose, side effects, disposal of containers and needles; provide instruction sheet
• That bone pain is common

Evaluation
Positive therapeutic outcome
• Absence of infection

finasteride (Rx)
(fin-ass′te-ride)
Propecia, Proscar
Func. class.: Androgen hormone inhibitor, hair stimulant
Chem. class.: 5-α-Reductase inhibitor
Pregnancy category X

Do not confuse: Proscar/ProSom/Prozac, finasteride/furosemide

ACTION: Inhibits 5-α-reductase and reduction in dihydrotestosterone (DHT); DHT induces androgenic effects by binding to androgen receptors in the cell nuclei of the prostate gland, liver, skin; prevents development of benign prostatic hypertrophy (BPH)

Therapeutic outcome: Reduced prostate size

USES: Symptomatic BPH; male-pattern baldness (Propecia)

CONTRAINDICATIONS
Pregnancy **X**, breastfeeding, children, women who are pregnant or may become pregnant should not handle tabs, hypersensitivity

Precautions: Large residual urinary volume, severely diminished urinary flow, liver function abnormalities

DOSAGE AND ROUTES
BPH
Adult: PO 5 mg/day × 6-12 mo

Male-pattern baldness
Adult: PO 1 mg/day for 3 mo or more for results

Available forms: Tabs (Propecia) 1 mg, (Proscar) 5 mg

Implementation
• Administer without regard to meals; give for a minimum of 6 mo; not all patients will respond
• Store at temp <86° F (30° C); protect from light; keep container tightly closed

ADVERSE EFFECTS
GU: Impotence, decreased libido, decreased volume of ejaculate, sexual dysfunction
INTEG: Rash
MISC: Breast tenderness, secondary malignancy

Pharmacokinetics
Absorption	63%, readily
Distribution	Plasma protein binding, crosses blood-brain barrier
Metabolism	Liver
Excretion	Kidneys, metabolites (39%); feces (57%)
Half-life	6-15 hr

Pharmacodynamics
Onset	Immediate
Peak	1-2 hr
Duration	14 days

INTERACTIONS
Drug classifications
Anticholinergics, bronchodilators (adrenergic), theophylline: decreased effect of finasteride

Drug/lab test
Decreased: PSA levels (finasteride)

NURSING CONSIDERATIONS
Assessment
• **BPH:** Assess urinary patterns, residual urinary volume, severely diminished urinary flow; PSA levels and digital rectal exam results before initiating therapy and periodically thereafter
• Monitor liver function tests before initiating treatment; extensively metabolized in liver

Patient/family education
• Advise patient that pregnant women or women who may become pregnant should not touch crushed tab or come into contact with semen

Adverse effects: *italics* = common; **bold** = life-threatening

of a patient taking this product; may adversely affect development of male fetus

• Inform patient that volume of ejaculate may be decreased during treatment; impotence and decreased libido may also occur and may continue after discontinuing treatment

• Inform patient that Propecia results may not occur for 3 mo

• Inform patient that Proscar results may not occur for 6-12 mo

Evaluation
Positive therapeutic outcome
• Decreased postvoiding dribbling, frequency, nocturia
• Increased urinary flow
• Regression of prostate size
• Hair growth within 3-6 mo

fingolimod (Rx)
(fin-gol′i-mod)
Gilenya
Func. class.: Biologic response modifier
Chem. class.: Sphingosine 1-phosphate receptor modulator
Pregnancy category C

ACTION: Binds with high affinity to sphingosine 1 phosphate receptors, blocks lymphocyte egress to lymph nodes, reducing the number of peripheral blood lymphocytes, may reduce lymphocyte migration into the CNS

Therapeutic outcome: Improved symptoms of multiple sclerosis and prevention of increasing disability

USES: To reduce frequency of exacerbation, to delay physical disability of relapsing forms of MS

CONTRAINDICATIONS
Hypersensitivity

Precautions: AIDS, asthma, AV block, bradycardia, breastfeeding, dysrhythmias, cardiac disease, children, COPD, diabetes mellitus, heart failure, hepatic disease, HIV, hypertension, immunosuppression, infants, leukemia, lymphoma, neonates, pregnancy **C**, QT prolongation, respiratory insufficiency, sick sinus syndrome, syncope, uveitis

DOSAGE AND ROUTES
Adult: PO 0.5 mg/day

Hepatic dose
Adult: PO Child-Pugh C, total score >10: Closely monitor, fingolimod exposure is doubled

Available forms: Cap 0.5 mg

Implementation
PO route
• Watch patient for 6 hr after initial dose or if product is not given for >2 wk for development of bradycardia. Give without regard to food
• Store at room temperature, protect from moisture

ADVERSE EFFECTS
CNS: Asthenia, depression, fatigue, headache, dizziness, **progressive multifocal leukoencephalopathy**, migraine, paresthesias, **stroke**
CV: **AV block, bradycardia**, chest pain, hypertension, palpitations, **QT prolongation**
EENT: Blurred vision, vision impairment, ocular pain, macular edema
GI: Abdominal pain, anorexia, diarrhea, jaundice, vomiting, weight loss
HEMA: **Leukopenia, lymphopenia, neutropenia**
INTEG: Alopecia, pruritus
MS: Back pain
RESP: Dyspnea, cough
SYST: Infection, influenza, **secondary malignancy**

Pharmacokinetics

Absorption	Protein binding (99.7%)
Distribution	Distributed to RBCs (86%)
Metabolism	Metabolized by CYP4F2 and CYP2D6 to a lesser extent
Excretion	Excreted in urine (81% inactive metabolites)
Half-life	Terminal half-life 6-9 days

Pharmacodynamics

Onset	Unknown
Peak	12-16 hr
Duration	Steady state 1-2 mo

INTERACTIONS
Individual drugs
Digoxin: increased risk of heart block, serious bradycardia
Ketoconazole: increased fingolimod effect

Drug classifications
Class Ia/III antidysrhythmics: increased risk of torsades de pointes
β-blockers, calcium channel blockers: increased risk of heart block, serious bradycardia
Antineoplastics, immunosuppressants, immune modulating therapies: increased immunosuppression
Inactive vaccines, toxoids: decreased effects
Live vaccines: increased infection risk

NURSING CONSIDERATIONS
Assessment
• **Multiple sclerosis:** Assess for improving paresthesia, muscle weakness, clonus, muscle spasms, difficulty in moving, difficulty in coordination in balance, speech, swallowing, vision problems, fatigue; prevention of increasing disability
• **Monitor laboratory values: obtain before initial dose, CBC, LFTs, serum bilirubin, ophthalmologic exam, antibodies to VZV if there is not a history of chickenpox or without vaccination, may give VZV vaccination of antibody-negative patient before giving product, postpone for 1 month after vaccination; obtain ECG for evidence of bradycardia, or AV block**
• **Progressive multifocal leukoencephalopathy (PML):** Assess for confusion, apathy, dizziness, unstable gait; may be fatal; discontinue product; contact prescriber

Bradycardia:
• **Monitor for ≥6 hr after beginning dose, ECG before and after**
• **1st dose, if heart rate <45 bpm or new heart block (2nd degree) occurs, do not use until resolved**
• **Monitor for QT prolongation**

Patient/family education
• Provide med guide to patient and explain use of product and expected results
• Advise patient that continuing follow-up exams and laboratory tests will be required on a regular basis
• Advise patient to use contraception during and for 2 months after conclusion of treatment

Liver dysfunction:
• **Teach patient to report jaundice, nausea, vomiting, anorexia, abdominal pain, fatigue, dark urine**

Cardiac changes:
• **Chest pain, palpitations**

Evaluation
Positive therapeutic outcome
• Improved symptoms of multiple sclerosis and prevention of increasing disability

---

flecainide (Rx)
(flek′a-nide)
Tambocor ❦
Func. class.: Antidysrhythmic (Class IC)
Pregnancy category C

ACTION: Decreases conduction in all parts of the heart, with greatest effect on the His-Purkinje system, which stabilizes the cardiac membrane

Therapeutic outcome: Absence of dysrhythmias

USES: Life-threatening ventricular dysrhythmias, sustained ventricular tachycardia; supraventricular tachydysrhythmias, paroxysmal atrial fibrillation/flutter associated with disabling symptoms

Unlabeled uses: Atrial fibrillation, single dose

CONTRAINDICATIONS
Hypersensitivity, AV bundle branch block, cardiogenic shock, QT prolongation

Precautions: Pregnancy **C**, breastfeeding, children, renal/hepatic disease, CHF, respiratory depression, myasthenia gravis, geriatric, electrolyte abnormalities, atrial fibrillation, sick sinus syndrome, torsades de pointes

> **BLACK BOX WARNING:** MI, cardiac arrhythmias, atrial fibrillation

DOSAGE AND ROUTES
PSVT/PAT
Adult: PO 50 mg q12hr; may increase every 4 days by 50 mg q12hr to desired response; max 300 mg/day

Life-threatening ventricular dysrhythmias
Adult: PO 100 mg q12hr, may increase by 50 mg q12hr q4days; max 400 mg/day

Renal dose
Adult: PO CCr <35 ml/min dose 100 mg daily or 50 mg bid initially

Available forms: Tabs 50, 100, 150 mg

Implementation
PO route
• Give reduced dosage slowly with ECG monitoring; do not increase dose <4 days apart
• Give with meals if GI upset occurs
• Therapeutic trough serum concentrations for adults range from 200-1000 ng/mL (average 500 ng/mL); toxicity is more common with trough serum concentrations >1000 ng/mL; usual therapeutic range in children is 200-500 ng/mL; in some cases, up to 800 ng/mL may be required
• Adjust dosage at intervals of ≥4 days (approximate plateau effects) following dosage adjustments; however, longer intervals are needed in patients with renal or hepatic impairment
• Frequent serum drug concentration monitoring is required for patients with severe renal

(CrCl <35 ml/min) or hepatic disease, and may also be helpful in patients with CHF or in patients with moderate renal disease
• Monitoring of flecainide serum concentrations is strongly recommended in patients receiving amiodarone therapy

ADVERSE EFFECTS

CNS: *Headache, dizziness,* involuntary movement, confusion, psychosis, restlessness, irritability, paresthesias, ataxia, flushing, somnolence, depression, anxiety, malaise, fatigue, asthenia, tremors
CV: *Hypotension,* bradycardia, angina, PVCs, heart block, cardiovascular collapse/arrest, dysrhythmias, CHF, fatal ventricular tachycardia, palpitations, QT prolongation, torsades de pointes
EENT: Tinnitus, *blurred vision,* hearing loss, corneal deposits, dry eyes
GI: Nausea, vomiting, anorexia, constipation, abdominal pain, flatulence, change in taste, diarrhea
GU: Impotence, decreased libido, polyuria, urinary retention
HEMA: Leukopenia, thrombocytopenia
INTEG: Rash, urticaria, edema, swelling
RESP: Dyspnea, respiratory depression

Pharmacokinetics

Absorption	Well absorbed
Distribution	Widely distributed
Metabolism	Liver
Excretion	30% kidneys, unchanged
Half-life	14 hr

Pharmacodynamics

Onset	Unknown
Peak	3 hr
Duration	Unknown

INTERACTIONS
Individual drugs
Amiodarone, cimetidine, ritonavir: increased level of flecainide
Digoxin: increased digoxin levels
Disopyramide, verapamil: increased CV depressant action
Propanolol: increased effects of both products

Drug classifications
Acidifying agents, alkalizing agents: increased or decreased effect
β-Adrenergic blockers: increased CV depressant action
Class IA/III antidysrhythmics, some phenothiazines, β agonists, local anesthetics, tricyclics, haloperidol, chloroquine, droperidol, pentamidine; CYP3A4 inhibitors (amiodarone, clarithromycin, erythromycin, telithromycin, troleandomycin), arsenic trioxide, levomethadyl; CYP3A4 substrates (methadone, pimozide, QUEtiapine, quiNIDine, risperiDONE, ziprasidone): increase QT prolongation

Drug/herb
Hawthorn: do not use concurrently

Drug/lab test
Increased: CPK

NURSING CONSIDERATIONS
Assessment

> **BLACK BOX WARNING:** MI, CHF, cardiogenic shock: should not be used in these conditions

> **BLACK BOX WARNING:** Atrial fibrillation: avoid use, risk of ventricular dysrhythmias

> **BLACK BOX WARNING:** Cardiac dysrhythmias: discontinue in those with prolonged QRS >180 ms, or prolonged PR >300 ms; monitor ECG, B/P, pulse, monitor for QT prolongation, monitor ECG before and during treatment

• Monitor I&O ratio; electrolytes prior to use: potassium, sodium, chloride; check weight daily and for signs of CHF or pulmonary toxicity: dyspnea, fatigue, cough, fever, chest pain, jugular vein distention, crackles; if these occur, product should be discontinued
• Monitor liver function studies: AST, ALT, bilirubin, alkaline phosphatase
• Assess patient for CNS symptoms: confusion, psychosis, numbness, depression, involuntary movements; if these occur, product should be discontinued
• Monitor cardiac rate, respiration: rate, rhythm, character, chest pain; watch for ventricular tachycardia, supraventricular tachycardia, or fibrillation
• **Flecainide level:** Monitor level in those with CHF or renal failure, peak, trough

Patient/family education
• Instruct patient to report side effects immediately to prescriber (chest pain, trouble breathing, sweating)
• Instruct patient to complete follow-up appointment with health care provider, including pulmonary function tests, chest x-ray
• Teach patient to change position slowly from lying or sitting to standing to minimize orthostatic hypotension
• Advise patient not to skip or double doses, take missed dose as soon as remembered (within 6 hr) of next dose

- Advise patient to carry/wear emergency ID with disorder, medications taken, that follow-up will be needed
- Advise patient to avoid hazardous activities that require alertness until response is known

Evaluation
Positive therapeutic outcome
- Absence of dysrhythmias

fluconazole (Rx)
(floo-kon'a-zole)
Diflucan
Func. class.: Antifungal
Chem. class.: Triazole
Pregnancy category C

Do not confuse: Diflucan/Diprivan

ACTION: Inhibits ergosterol biosynthesis, causes direct damage to membrane phospholipids in the cell wall of fungi

Therapeutic outcome: Fungistatic fungicidal against the following susceptible organisms: *Candida, Cryptococcus neoformans*

USES: Oropharyngeal candidiasis; chronic mucocutaneous candidiasis; systemic, vaginal, urinary candidiasis; cryptococcal meningitis; prevention of candidiasis in bone marrow transplant in those who receive chemotherapy and/or radiation therapy, cystitis, fungal prophylaxis, peritonitis, pneumonia, pyelonephritis

CONTRAINDICATIONS
Hypersensitivity to this product or azoles, pregnancy **D**

Precautions: Breastfeeding, renal/hepatic disease, torsades de pointes

DOSAGE AND ROUTES
Vulvovaginal candidiasis
Adult: PO 150 mg as a single dose

Serious fungal infections
Adult: PO/IV 50-400 mg initially, then 200 mg once daily for 4 wk
Child: 6-12 mg/kg/day

Oropharyngeal candidiasis
Adult: PO/IV 200 mg initially, then 100 mg/day for at least 2 wk
Child: PO/IV 6 mg/kg initially, then 3 mg/kg/day for ≥2 wk

Esophageal candidiasis
Adult: PO/IV 200 mg on 1st day, then 100 mg/day × ≥3 wk and for ≥2 wk after resolution of symptoms

Child: PO/IV 6 mg/kg on 1st day, then 3 mg/kg/day × ≥3 wk and for ≥2 wk after resolution of symptoms

Cryptococcal meningitis
Adult: PO/IV 400 mg on 1st day, then 200 mg/day × 10-12 wk after CSF culture negative
Child/infant/neonate >14 days: PO/IV 12 mg/kg on 1st day, then 6-12 mg/kg/day × 10-12 wk after negative CSF culture
Neonate 0-14 days: PO/IV 12 mg/kg on 1st day, then 6-12 mg/kg q72hr × 10-12 wk after negative CSF culture

Prevention of candidiasis in bone marrow transplant
Adult: PO/IV 400 mg/day; those anticipated to have neutrophils <500/mm³, start several days prior to anticipated onset of neutropenia and continue for 7 days after rise of neutrophils >1000/mm³

Renal dose
Adult: PO CCr <50 ml/min after loading dose, give 50% of usual dose

Available forms: Tabs 10, 40, 50, 100, 150, 200 mg; inj 2 mg/ml; powder for oral susp 50, 200 mg/ml

Implementation
- Take with food to reduce GI effects
PO route
- Add water in 2 portions, review manufacturer reconstitution instructions
- Shake oral susp before each use; use within 2 wk

Intermittent IV infusion route
- Give after diluting according to package directions; run at 200 mg/hr or less; do not use plastic containers in connections
- Do not admix
- Administer **IV** using an in-line filter, using distal veins; check for extravasation and necrosis q2hr
- Give product only after C&S confirms organism, product needed to treat condition
- Store protected from moisture and light, diluted sol is stable for 24 hr

Y-site compatibilities: Acyclovir, aldesleukin, alfentanil, allopurinol, amifostine, amikacin, aminocaproic acid, aminophylline, amiodarone, anidulafungin, ascorbic acid injection, atenolol, atracurium, atropine, azaTHIOprine, aztreonam, benztropine, bivalirudin, bleomycin, bumetanide, buprenorphine, butorphanol, calcium chloride, CARBOplatin, caspofungin, ceFAZolin, cefepime, cefmetazole, cefonicid, cefoTEtan, cefOXitin, cefpirome, cefTAZidime, ceftizoxime, ceftobiprole, cephalothin, cephapirin, chlorproMAZINE, cimetidine, cisatracurium, CISplatin, codeine, cyanocobalamin, cyclophosphamide, cycloSPORINE, cytarabine, DACTINomycin, DAPTOmycin, dexamethasone, diltiazem, dimenhyDRINATE, diphenhydrAMINE, DOBUTamine, DOCEtaxel, DOPamine, doripenem, doxacurium, DOXOrubicin, DOXOrubicin liposomal, doxycycline, droperidol, drotrecogin alfa, enalaprilat, ePHEDrine, EPINEPHrine, epirubicin, epoetin alfa, eptifibatide, ertapenem, erythromycin, esmolol, etoposide, famotidine, fenoldopam, fentaNYL, filgrastim, fludarabine, fluorouracil, folic acid, foscarnet, gallium, ganciclovir, gatifloxacin, gemcitabine, gentamicin, glycopyrrolate, granisetron, heparin, hydrocortisone, HYDROmorphone, IDArubicin, ifosfamide, IV immune globulin, inamrinone, indomethacin, insulin (regular), irinotecan, isoproterenol, ketorolac, labetalol, lansoprazole, leucovorin, levofloxacin, lidocaine, linezolid, LORazepam, LR, magnesium sulfate, mannitol, mechlorethamine, melphalan, meperidine, meropenem, metaraminol, methicillin, methotrexate, methoxamine, methyldopate, methylPREDNISolone, metoclopramide, metoprolol, metroNIDAZOLE, mezlocillin, miconazole, midazolam, milrinone, minocycline, mitoXANtrone, morphine, moxalactam, multiple vitamins injection, mycophenolate, nafcillin, nalbuphine, naloxone, nesiritide, nitroglycerin, nitroprusside, norepinephrine, octreotide, ondansetron, oxacillin, oxaliplatin, oxytocin, PACLitaxel, palonosetron, pamidronate, pancuronium, papaverine, PEMEtrexed, penicillin G potassium/sodium, pentazocine, PENTobarbital, PHENobarbital, phenylephrine, phenytoin, phytonadione, piperacillin-tazobactam, polymyxin B, potassium chloride, procainamide, prochlorperazine, promethazine, propofol, propranolol, protamine, pyridoxine, quiNIDine, quinupristin-dalfopristin, ranitidine, remifentanil, Ringer's, ritodrine, riTUXimab, rocuronium, sargramostim, sodium acetate/bicarbonate, succinylcholine, SUFentanil, tacrolimus, temocillin, teniposide, theophylline, thiotepa, ticarcillin-clavulanate, tigecycline, tirofiban, TNA, tobramycin, tolazoline, TPN, trastuzumab, trimetaphan, urokinase, vancomycin, vasopressin, vecuronium, verapamil, vinCRIStine, vinorelbine, voriconazole, zidovudine, zoledronic acid

Y-site incompatibilities: Amphotericin B, ampicillin, calcium gluconate, cefotaxime, cefTRIAXone, cefTAZidime, cefuroxime, chloramphenicol, clindamycin, diazepam, digoxin, erythromycin lactobionate, furosemide, haloperidol, hydrOXYzine, imipenem/cilastatin, pentamidine, ticarcillin, trimethoprim/sulfamethoxazole

ADVERSE EFFECTS
CNS: *Headache,* seizures
CV: QT prolongation, torsades de pointes
GI: *Nausea, vomiting,* diarrhea, cramping, flatus, increased AST, ALT, hepatotoxicity, abdominal pain, cholestasis
HEMA: Agranulocytosis, eosinophilia, leukopenia, neutropenia, thrombocytopenia
INTEG: Stevens-Johnson syndrome, angioedema, anaphylaxis, exfoliative dermatitis, toxic epidermal necrolysis

Pharmacokinetics

Absorption	Well absorbed (PO)
Distribution	Widely distributed (peritoneum, CSF)
Metabolism	<10%, liver
Excretion	80% kidneys (unchanged)
Half-life	30 hr, increased in renal disease

Pharmacodynamics

	PO	IV
Onset	Unknown	Immediate
Peak	1-2 hr	Infusion's end
Duration	Unknown	Unknown

INTERACTIONS
Individual drugs
Alfentanil, buprenorphine, ergot, fentaNYL, methadone, saquinavir, SUFentanil, zidovudine: increased effect of each specific drug
CycloSPORINE, phenytoin, rifabutin, sirolimus, tacrolimus, theophylline, zidovudine, zolpidem: increased plasma concentrations
Lovastatin, simvastatin: increased myopathy, rhabdomyolysis risk
Warfarin: increased anticoagulation

Drug classification
Contraceptives (oral), calcium channel blockers: decreased effect
Oral sulfonylureas (glipiZIDE): hypoglycemia
Proton pump inhibitors: decreased fluconazole

Drug/herb
Gossypol: increased nephrotoxicity

Drug/lab test
Increased: alk phos, LFTs
Decreased: WBC, platelets

NURSING CONSIDERATIONS
Assessment
• **Assess for signs and symptoms of infection:** clearing of CSF culture during treatment, obtain C&S baseline and during treatment, product may be started as soon as culture is taken

---

⚠ Nurse Alert　　　✴ Key NCLEX® Drug　　　>> Drug Specifics

• Monitor for hepatotoxicity: increased AST, ALT, alkaline phosphatase, bilirubin; discontinue product if hepatotoxicity occurs
• Monitor for skin symptoms: color, lesions, injection site reactions; if lesions progress, discontinue product

Patient/family education
• Caution patient that long-term therapy may be needed to clear infection; to take entire course of medication; take in equal intervals (PO), not to add new meds, herbs without prescriber approval
• Teach patient the signs and symptoms of hepatotoxicity: nausea, vomiting, clay-colored stools, dark urine, anorexia, fatigue, jaundice, skin rash; prescriber should be notified immediately, abdominal pain, fever, bruising, bleeding
• Inform patient that medication may be taken with food to reduce GI effects
• Advise patient to consider using alternative contraception if using oral contraceptives, pregnancy D

Evaluation
Positive therapeutic outcome
• Decreasing oral candidiasis, fever, malaise, rash
• Negative C&S for infecting organism

fluidrocortisone (Rx)
(floo-droe-kor′ti-sone)
Func. class.: Synthetic corticosteroid
Pregnancy category C

ACTION: Promotes increased reabsorption of sodium and loss of potassium, water, hydrogen from distal tubules

Therapeutic outcome: Correction of adrenal insufficiency

USES: Adrenal insufficiency, salt-losing adrenogenital syndrome, Addison's disease

CONTRAINDICATIONS
Children <2 yr, hypersensitivity

Precautions: CHF, hypertension, diabetes, acute glomerulonephritis, amebiasis, psychosis, Cushing's syndrome, fungal infections, pregnancy C, breastfeeding, children >2 yrs, osteoporosis

DOSAGE AND ROUTES
Adult: PO 100-200 mcg/day
Child: PO 50-100 mcg/day

Available forms: Tabs 100 mcg (0.1 mg)

Implementation
• Titrate to lowest dose
• Give with food or milk to decrease GI symptoms

ADVERSE EFFECTS
CV: Hypertension, circulatory collapse, thrombophlebitis, embolism, tachycardia, CHF, edema
CNS: Flushing, sweating, headache, paralysis, dizziness, seizure
ENDO: Weight gain, adrenal suppression, hyperglycemia
META: Hypokalemia
MISC: Hypersensitivity, cataracts, GI ulcers, anaphylaxis, infection
MS: Fractures, osteoporosis, weakness

Pharmacokinetics
Absorption	Unknown
Distribution	Unknown
Metabolism	Liver
Excretion	Urine
Half-life	18-36 hr

Pharmacodynamics
Onset	Unknown
Peak	1.5 hr
Duration	Unknown

INTERACTIONS
Drug classifications
Barbiturates: decreased fludrocortisone action
Loop/thiazide diuretics, potassium-wasting products: increased potassium levels
Sodium-containing products: increased B/P

Drug/lab test
Increased: potassium, sodium
Decreased: HCT

NURSING CONSIDERATIONS
Assessment
• Assess weight daily, notify prescriber of weekly gain >5 lb
• Monitor I&O, be alert for decreasing output, increasing edema
• Monitor B/P, pulse, notify prescriber of chest pain
• Potassium depletion: assess for paresthesia, fatigue, nausea, vomiting, dysrhythmias, weakness, depression, polyuria
• Electrolytes: monitor sodium, potassium, chloride; hypokalemia is common

Patient/family education
• Teach patient that emergency ID as corticosteroid user should be carried
• Teach patient not to discontinue abruptly

Adverse effects: *italics* = common; **bold** = life-threatening

- Instruct patient to notify health care provider of muscle cramps, weight gain, edema, nausea, infection, trauma, stress
- Advise patient to avoid exposure to disease, trauma

Evaluation
Positive therapeutic outcome
- Correction of adrenal insufficiency

flumazenil (Rx)
(flu-maz′e-nil)
Anexate ✦, Romazicon
Func. class.: Antidote: Benzodiazepine receptor antagonist
Chem. class.: Imidazobenzodiazepine derivative
Pregnancy category C

ACTION: Antagonizes the actions of benzodiazepines on the CNS, competitively inhibits the activity at the benzodiazepine receptor complex

Therapeutic outcome: Reversed benzodiazepine toxic effects

USES: Reversal of the sedative effects of benzodiazepines

CONTRAINDICATIONS
Hypersensitivity to this product or benzodiazepines, serious tricyclic overdose, patients given benzodiazepine for control of life-threatening condition

Precautions: Pregnancy **C**, breastfeeding, children, geriatric, ambulatory patients, renal/hepatic disease, status epilepticus, head injury, labor and delivery, hypoventilation, panic disorder, drug/alcohol dependency

> **BLACK BOX WARNING:** Benzodiazepine dependence, seizures

DOSAGE AND ROUTES
Reversal of conscious sedation or in general anesthesia
Adult: IV 0.2 mg (2 ml) given over 15 sec; wait 45 sec, then give 0.2 mg (2 ml) if consciousness does not occur; may be repeated at 60-sec intervals as needed (max 3 mg/hr) or 1 mg/5 min
Child: IV 10 mcg (0.01 mg)/kg; cumulative dose of 1 mg or less

Management of suspected benzodiazepine overdose
Adult: IV 0.2 mg (2 ml) given over 30 sec; wait 30 sec, then give 0.3 mg (3 ml) over 30 sec if consciousness does not occur; further doses of 0.5 mg (5 ml) can be given over 30 sec at intervals of 1 min up to cumulative dose of 3 mg

Child: IV 10 mcg (0.01 mg/kg); cumulative dose of less than 1 mg

Available forms: Inj 0.1 mg/ml

Implementation
Direct IV route
- Give directly undiluted or diluted in 0.9% NaCl, D$_5$W, or LR; give over 15-30 sec into running **IV**, check for extravasation
- Use large vein
- Check airway and **IV** access before administration
- Stable for 24 hr if drawn into a syringe or mixed with other solutions

ADVERSE EFFECTS
CNS: Dizziness, agitation, emotional lability, confusion, *seizures,* somnolence, panic attacks
CV: Hypertension, palpitations, cutaneous vasodilatation, *dysrhythmias,* bradycardia, tachycardia, chest pain
EENT: Abnormal vision, blurred vision, tinnitus
GI: Nausea, vomiting, hiccups
SYST: Headache, inj site pain, increased sweating, fatigue, rigors

Pharmacokinetics

Absorption	Complete
Distribution	Unknown
Metabolism	Liver
Excretion	Unknown
Half-life	41-79 min

Pharmacodynamics

Onset	1-2 min
Peak	10 min
Duration	Unknown

INTERACTIONS
Individual drugs
Zaleplon, zolpidem: antagonize action

Drug classifications
Benzodiazepines: antagonize action
Toxicity: mixed product overdosage

NURSING CONSIDERATIONS
Assessment
- Assess cardiac status using continuous monitoring
- Assess for seizures, protect patient from injury; most likely in those who usually experience withdrawal from sedatives
- Assess for GI symptoms: nausea, vomiting; place in side-lying position to prevent aspiration
- **Assess for allergic reactions:** flushing, rash, urticaria, pruritus

---

BLACK BOX WARNING: Seizures/benzodiazepine dependence: Do not use in those who have used these products for interictal psychosis, status epilepticus, use in ICU cautiously where there may be unrecognized benzodiazepine dependence

Evaluation
Positive therapeutic outcome
- Decreased sedation, respiratory depression
- Absence of toxicity

flunisolide nasal agent
See Appendix B

fluocinolone topical
See Appendix B

fluorometholone ophthalmic
See Appendix B

⚠ HIGH ALERT

fluorouracil (Rx)
(flure-oh-yoor′a-sil)
5-FU, Carac, Efudex, Fluoroplex, Tolak
Func. class.: Antineoplastic, antimetabolite
Chem. class.: Pyrimidine antagonist
Pregnancy category X

Do not confuse: fluorouracil/flucytosine/Cara/Kuric

ACTION: Inhibits DNA, RNA synthesis; interferes with cell replication by competitively inhibiting thymidylate synthesis; cell cycle specific (S phase)

Therapeutic outcome: Prevention of rapidly growing malignant cells

USES: Systemic: cancer of breast, colon, rectum, stomach, pancreas; **Topical:** superficial basal cell carcinoma; multiple actinic keratoses

Unlabeled uses: Anal, biliary tract, cervical, head and neck, hepatocellular, and ovarian cancers

CONTRAINDICATIONS
Pregnancy **X**, breastfeeding, hypersensitivity, poor nutritional status, serious infections, dihydropyrimidine dehydrogenase deficiency (DPD)

BLACK BOX WARNING: Bone marrow suppression

Precautions: Children, renal/hepatic disease, angina, stomatitis, diarrhea, sunlight exposure, vaccination, occlusive dressing

BLACK BOX WARNING: GI bleeding

DOSAGE AND ROUTES
Doses vary widely, doses are based on actual body weight, unless obese, then based on lean body weight

Advanced colorectal cancer
Adult: IV bolus 300-500 mg/m^2/day $\times$ 4-5 days q28 days or 600-1500 mg/m^2 qwk or every other wk; continuous IV infusion: 300-1000 mg/m^2/day $\times$ 4-5 days q4wk or 300 mg/m^2/day indefinitely; high dose 3000-3400 mg/m^2 over 24-72 hr

Breast cancer
Adult: IV bolus 400-600 mg/m^2 on days 1 and 8 of every cycle with cyclophosphamide and methotrexate or 600 mg/m^2 on day 1 with cyclophosphamide and methotrexate q21-28 days

Pancreatic cancer
Adult: IV bolus 600 mg/m^2 on day 1, 8, 29, 36 with DOXOrubicin and mitoMYcin q8wk or 600 mg/m2 bolus on days 1, 8, 29, 36 with streptozocin

Actinic/solar keratoses
Adult: TOP 1% cream/solution bid or 2%-5% SOL for hands

Superficial basal cell carcinoma
Adult: TOP 5% cream/solution 2 $\times$/day $\times$ 3-12 wk

Available forms: Inj 50 mg/ml; cream 0.5%, 1%, 4%, 5%; topical solution, 2%, 5%

Implementation
- Avoid contact with skin (very irritating); wash completely to remove
- Give fluids **IV** or PO before chemotherapy to hydrate patient
- Give antiemetic 30-60 min before giving product to prevent vomiting, and prn for several days thereafter; antibiotics for prophylaxis of infection
- Provide liquid diet: carbonated beverages; gelatin may be added if patient is not nauseated or vomiting
- Rinse mouth tid-qid with water, club soda; brush teeth bid-qid with soft brush or cotton-tipped applicators for stomatitis; use unwaxed dental floss

Topical route
- The 1% strength is used on face, other higher strengths are used on other parts of the body
- Wear gloves when applying; may use with a loose dressing; use a plastic or wooden

applicator, do not use occlusive dressings; may use gauze dressing

IV route
• Prepare in biological cabinet using gloves, gown, mask
• **IV** undiluted; may inject through Y-tube or 3-way stopcock; give over 1-3 min
• May be diluted in 0.9% NaCl, D₅W; given as a continuous infusion in plastic containers over 2-8 hr; do not refrigerate/freeze; protect from light; discard unused portion, stable for 24 hr at room temperature; do not use discolored, cloudy solution; solution is pale yellow; for crystals, dissolve by warming slowly and shaking; cool to body temperature before use

Y-site compatibilities: Acyclovir, alatrofloxacin, alfentanil, allopurinol, amifostine, amikacin, amphotericin B lipid complex, amphotericin B liposome, ampicillin, ampicillin-sulbactam, anidulafungin, argatroban, atenolol, atracurium, azithromycin, aztreonam, bivalirudin, bleomycin, bumetanide, butorphanol, calcium gluconate, CARBOplatin, ceFAZolin, cefepime, cefotaxime, cefoTEtan, cefOXitin, cefTAZidime, ceftizoxime, cefTRIAXone, cefuroxime, cimetidine, cisatracurium, CISplatin, clindamycin, codeine, cyclophosphamide, cycloSPORINE, DAPTOmycin, dexamethasone, digoxin, DOCEtaxel, DOPamine, doripenem, DOXOrubicin liposomal, enalaprilat, ePHEDrine, ertapenem, erythromycin, esmolol, etoposide phosphate, famotidine, fenoldopam, fentaNYL, fluconazole, fludarabine, foscarnet, fosphenytoin, furosemide, ganciclovir, gatifloxacin, gemcitabine, gentamicin, granisetron, heparin, hydrocortisone, HYDROmorphone, ifosfamide, imipenem-cilastatin, inamrinone, isoproterenol, ketorolac, labetalol, leucovorin, levorphanol, lidocaine, linezolid, magnesium sulfate, mannitol, melphalan, meperidine, meropenem, mesna, methohexital, methotrexate, methylPREDNISolone, metoprolol, metroNIDAZOLE, milrinone, mitoMYcin, mitoXANtrone, morphine sulfate, nalbuphine, naloxone, nesiritide, nitroglycerin, nitroprusside, octreotide, ofloxacin, PACLitaxel, palonosetron, pamidronate, pancuronium, pantoprazole, PEMEtrexed, PENTobarbital, PHENobarbital, phenylephrine, piperacillin, piperacillin-tazobactam, potassium chloride/phosphates, procainamide, propofol, propranolol, ranitidine, remifentanil, riTUXimab, sargramostim, sodium acetate/bicarbonate/phosphates, succinylcholine, SUFentanil, sulfamethoxazole-trimethoprim, teniposide, theophylline, thiopental, thiotepa, ticarcillin, ticarcillin-clavulanate, tigecycline, tirofiban, tobramycin, trastuzumab, vasopressin, vecuronium, vinBLAStine, vinCRIStine, vitamin B complex/C, voriconazole, zidovudine, zoledronic acid

Y-site incompatibilities: Droperidol, vinorelbine

ADVERSE EFFECTS
SYSTEMIC use
CNS: Lethargy, malaise, weakness, acute cerebellar dysfunction
CV: Myocardial ischemia, angina
EENT: Epistaxis, light intolerance, lacrimation
GI: *Anorexia, stomatitis,* diarrhea, nausea, vomiting, hemorrhage, enteritis, glossitis
HEMA: Thrombocytopenia, leukopenia, myelosuppression, anemia, agranulocytosis
INTEG: *Rash,* fever, photosensitivity, anaphylaxis

Pharmacokinetics

Absorption	Completely bioavailable (**IV**), minimal (topical)
Distribution	Widely distributed, concentration in tumor
Metabolism	Liver, converted to active metabolite
Excretion	Lungs (60%-80%), kidneys (up to 15%)
Half-life	16 min (**IV**)

Pharmacodynamics
Unknown

INTERACTIONS
Individual drugs
Leucovorin: increased toxicity, bone marrow depression
MetroNIDAZOLE: increased toxicity, irinotecan
Phenytoin: decreased effect of phenytoin
Radiation: increased toxicity, bone marrow suppression

Drug classifications
Anticoagulants, NSAIDs, platelet inhibitors, thrombolytics: increased bleeding
Antineoplastics: increased toxicity, bone marrow depression
Live virus vaccines: decreased antibody response

Drug/lab test
Increased: AST, ALT, LDH, serum bilirubin, Hct, Hgb, WBC, platelets, 5-HIAA
Decreased: albumin

NURSING CONSIDERATIONS
Assessment
• Monitor ECG; watch for ST-T wave changes, low QRS and T, possible dysrhythmias (sinus tachycardia, heart block, PVCs)

• Assess buccal cavity q8hr for dryness, sores or ulceration, white patches, oral pain, bleeding, dysphagia; obtain prescription for viscous lidocaine (Xylocaine)

• Assess tachypnea, ECG changes, dyspnea, edema, fatigue; identify dyspnea, crackles, unproductive cough, chest pain, tachypnea

> **BLACK BOX WARNING: Bone marrow suppression:** Monitor daily during IV treatment: monitor CBC, differential, platelet count daily (**IV**); withhold product if WBC is <4000/mm³ or platelet count is <100,000/mm³; notify prescriber of results if WBC <20,000/mm³, platelets <50,000/mm³; nadir of leukopenia within 2 wk, recovery 1 mo; if pretreatment of WBC <2000/mm³ or platelets <100,000/mm³, delay until recovery of counts above this level; nadir usually 9-14 days, recovery 30 days

• **Palmar-plantar erythrodysesthesia:** hand/foot tingling changing to pain, redness

• **Infiltration:** monitor frequently for pain, redness, inflammation at site; if present, stop infusion and start at new site; may use ice at site

• Monitor renal function studies: BUN, creatinine, serum uric acid, urine CCr before, during therapy; I&O ratio; report fall in urine output to <30 ml/hr

• Monitor temp q4hr (may indicate beginning of infection)

• Monitor liver function tests before, during therapy (bilirubin, AST, ALT, LDH) as needed or monthly; jaundice of skin, sclera, dark urine, clay-colored stools, itchy skin, abdominal pain, fever, diarrhea

• **Assess for bleeding:** hematuria, stool guaiac, bruising or petechiae, mucosa or orifices q8hr; inflammation of mucosa, breaks in skin

⚠ Assess for infection: those with current infections should be treated prior to receiving 5-FU, the dose reduced or discontinued if infection occurs

• Toxicity: Assess for hemorrhage, severe vomiting, severe diarrhea, stomatitis, WBC <3500/mm³, platelets <100,000 notify prescriber

• Acute cerebellar dysfunction: Monitor for dizziness, weakness

Patient/family education
⚠ Caution patient that contraceptive measures are recommended during therapy, pregnancy X

• **Bleeding:** Teach patient to avoid using aspirin, NSAIDs, or ibuprofen-containing products, razors, commercial mouthwash because bleeding may occur; to report symptoms of bleeding (hematuria, tarry stools), IM injections if counts are low

• **Instruct patient to report signs of anemia** (fatigue, headache, irritability, faintness, SOB)

• **Instruct patient to report signs of stomatitis** (bleeding, white spots, ulcerations in the mouth); tell patient to examine mouth daily, to report symptoms; viscous lidocaine (Xylocaine) may be used

• Teach patient to avoid crowds, persons with known infections

• Advise patient to avoid vaccinations during therapy, to use sunscreen or stay out of the sun to prevent burns; about hair loss; explore use of wigs or other products until hair regrowth occurs

Evaluation
Positive therapeutic outcome
• Prevention of rapid division of malignant cells

FLUoxetine (Rx)
(floo-ox′uh-teen)
PROzac, PROzac Weekly, Sarafem
Func. class.: Antidepressant, selective serotonin reuptake inhibitor
Pregnancy category C

Do not confuse: PROzac/Proscar/PriLOSEC/Prosom, Sarafem/Serophene

ACTION: Inhibits CNS neuron uptake of serotonin but not of norepinephrine

Therapeutic outcome: Decreased symptoms of depression after 2-3 wk

USES: Major depressive disorder, obsessive-compulsive disorder (OCD), bulimia nervosa; *Sarafem:* premenstrual dysphoric disorder (PMDD), panic disorder

Unlabeled uses: Alcoholism, anorexia nervosa, borderline personality disorder, obesity, posttraumatic stress disorder, social phobia

CONTRAINDICATIONS
Hypersensitivity

Precautions: Pregnancy **C,** breastfeeding, geriatric, diabetes mellitus, narrow-angle glaucoma, cardiac malformations in infants (exposed to FLUoxetine in utero), osteoporosis, QT prolongation

> **BLACK BOX WARNING:** Children, suicidal ideation

DOSAGE AND ROUTES
Depression/OCD
Adult: PO 20 mg/day AM; after 4 wk if no clinical improvement is noted, dosage may be increased to 20 mg bid in AM, afternoon; max 80 mg/day; PO 90 mg weekly
Geriatric: PO 10 mg/day, increase as needed
Child 7-17 yr: PO 5-10 mg/day, max 20 mg/day

Alcoholism (unlabeled)
Adult: PO 20-80 mg/day

Anorexia nervosa (unlabeled)
Adult: PO 10 mg every other day-20 mg/day

Borderline personality disorder (unlabeled)
Adult: PO 20 mg/day, max 80 mg/day

Kleptomania (unlabeled)
Adult: PO 60-80 mg/day

Posttraumatic stress disorder (unlabeled)
Adult: PO 10-80 mg/day

Premenstrual dysphoric disorder (Sarafem)
Adult: PO 20 mg/day, may be taken daily 14 days before menses

Available forms: Caps 10, 20, 40 mg; tabs 10, 20, 60 mg; oral sol 20 mg/5 ml; del rel caps (PROzac Weekly) 90 mg

Implementation
• Give without regard to meals
• Give dose at bedtime if oversedation occurs during day; may take entire dose at bedtime; geriatric may not tolerate once/day dosing, crush if patient unable to swallow whole (tabs only)
• **PROzac Weekly:** Give on same day each week, swallow whole, do not crush, cut, chew
• Store at room temperature; do not freeze

ADVERSE EFFECTS
CNS: *Headache, nervousness, insomnia, drowsiness, anxiety, tremor, dizziness, fatigue, sedation, poor concentration, abnormal dreams, agitation,* seizures, apathy, euphoria, hallucinations, delusions, psychosis, suicidal ideation, neuroleptic malignant syndrome–like reactions, serotonin syndrome
CV: *Hot flashes, palpitations,* angina pectoris, hemorrhage, hypertension, tachycardia, 1st-degree AV block, bradycardia, MI, thrombophlebitis, generalized edema, torsades de pointes
EENT: Visual changes, ear/eye pain, photophobia, tinnitus, increased intraocular pressure
GI: *Nausea, diarrhea, dry mouth, anorexia, dyspepsia, constipation,* taste changes, flatulence, decreased appetite

GU: *Dysmenorrhea, decreased libido, urinary frequency, urinary tract infection,* amenorrhea, cystitis, impotence, urine retention
INTEG: *Sweating, rash, pruritus,* acne, alopecia, urticaria; angioedema, exfoliative dermatitis, Stevens-Johnson syndrome, toxic epidermal necrolysis
MS: *Pain,* arthritis, twitching
RESP: *Pharyngitis, cough, dyspnea, bronchitis,* asthma, hyperventilation, pneumonia
SYST: *Asthenia,* serotonin syndrome, flu-like symptoms, neonatal abstinence syndrome

Pharmacokinetics

Absorption	Well absorbed
Distribution	Crosses blood-brain barrier
Metabolism	Liver, extensively to norfluoxetine
Excretion	Kidneys, unchanged (12%), metabolite (7%); steady state 28-35 days, protein binding 94%
Half-life	1-3 days metabolite up to 1 wk

Pharmacodynamics

Onset	Unknown
Peak	6-8 hr
Duration	Unknown

INTERACTIONS
Individual drugs
Alcohol: increased CNS depression
Antidiabetics: increased levels or toxicity
Bosentan, budesonide, carBAMazepine, darifenacin, diazepam, digoxin, donepezil, lithium, paricalcitol, phenytoin, thioridazine, vinBLAStine, warfarin: increased toxicity
Cyproheptadine: decreased FLUoxetine effect
BusPIRone, haloperidol, loxapine, selegiline, thiothixene, tryptophan: increased serotonin syndrome, do not use concurrently

Drug classifications
Anticoagulants, NSAIDs, platelet inhibitors, salicylates, thrombolytics: increased bleeding risk
Antidepressants, opioids, sedative/hypnotics: increased CNS depression
MAOIs: hypertensive crisis, seizures; do not use with or 14 days prior to FLUoxetine
SSRIs, SNRIs, serotonin-receptor agonists, tricyclics: increased serotonin syndrome, do not use concurrently

Drug/herb
Hops, kava, lavender, valerian: increased CNS effect

St. John's wort, SAM-e: do not use together; increased risk of serotonin syndrome

NURSING CONSIDERATIONS
Assessment
• Monitor B/P (lying, standing), pulse q4hr; if systolic B/P drops 20 mm hg, hold product and notify prescriber; take VS q4hr in patients with CV disease
• Monitor **blood studies:** CBC, leukocytes, differential, cardiac enzymes if patient is receiving long-term therapy; check platelets, bleeding can occur; thyroid growth rate (children)
• Monitor **hepatic studies:** AST, ALT, bilirubin
• Check weight qwk; appetite may increase with product
• **Assess ECG for flattening of T-wave, bundle branch block, AV block, dysrhythmias in cardiac patients**

> **BLACK BOX WARNING:** Assess mental status: mood, sensorium, affect, suicidal tendencies; increase in psychiatric symptoms: depression, panic; monitor for seizures; seizure potential is increased; Sarafem is not approved for children

• Monitor urinary retention, constipation; constipation is more likely to occur in children or geriatric
• Identify patient's alcohol consumption; if alcohol is consumed, hold dose until AM
• **Serotonin syndrome: symptoms can occur anytime after first dose, nausea/vomiting, sedation, dizziness, diaphoresis, mental changes, elevated B/P; if these occur product should be stopped, notify prescriber**
• **Assess appetite in bulimia nervosa,** monitor weight daily, increase nutritious foods in diet, watch for bingeing and vomiting
• **Serious skin reactions: angioedema, exfoliative dermatitis, Stevens-Johnson syndrome, toxic epidermal necrolysis**
• Assess allergic reactions: itching, rash, urticaria, product should be discontinued; may need to give antihistamine

Patient/family education
• Teach patient that therapeutic effects may take 1-4 wk, not to discontinue abruptly, that follow-up will be required
• Instruct patient to use caution in driving or other activities requiring alertness because of drowsiness, dizziness, blurred vision; to avoid rising quickly from sitting to standing, especially geriatric; to use sunscreen to prevent photosensitivity
• Caution patient to avoid alcohol ingestion, other CNS depressants

• Advise patient not to discontinue medication quickly after long-term use: may cause nausea, headache, malaise
• Instruct patient to increase fluids, bulk in diet if constipation, urinary retention occur, especially geriatric
• Advise patient to take gum, hard sugarless candy, or frequent sips of water for dry mouth
• Teach patient to avoid all OTC products unless approved by prescriber
• Advise patient to notify prescriber if allergic reactions occur (rash, trouble breathing, itching)
• Advise patient to change positions slowly, orthostatic hypotension may occur
• **Teach that suicidal thoughts, behavior may occur in young adults, children, usually during early treatment**
• Inform patient to notify prescriber of worsening symptoms or if insomnia, anxiety, or depression continues
• **Serotonin syndrome: Teach patient to report fever, sweating, diarrhea, poor coordination, nausea/vomiting, sedation, flushing, mental changes**

Evaluation
Positive therapeutic outcome
• Decrease in depression
• Absence of suicidal thoughts
• Decreased symptoms of OCD

TREATMENT OF OVERDOSE:
Activated charcoal, supportive care

fluPHENAZine decanoate (Rx)
(floo-fen'ah-zeen)
Modecate ✦
fluPHENAZine hydrochloride (Rx)
Func. class.: Antipsychotic/neuroleptic
Chem. class.: Phenothiazine, piperazine
Pregnancy category C

ACTION: Depresses cerebral cortex, hypothalamus, limbic system, which control activity and aggression; blocks neurotransmission produced by dopamine at synapse; exhibits strong α-adrenergic and anticholinergic blocking action; mechanism for antipsychotic effects is unclear

Therapeutic outcome: Decreased signs and symptoms of psychosis

USES: Schizophrenia

Unlabeled uses: Agitation

CONTRAINDICATIONS
Hypersensitivity, blood dyscrasias, coma, bone marrow depression, closed-angle glaucoma

Precautions: Pregnancy **C**, breastfeeding, children <12 yr, geriatric, seizure disorders, hypertension, hepatic/cardiac disease, abrupt discontinuation, accidental exposure, agranulocytosis, ambient temperature increase, angina, hypersensitivity to benzyl alcohol/parabens/sesame oil/tartrazine dye, QT prolongation, suicidal ideation, renal failure, Parkinson's disease, hypocalcemia, head trauma, prostatic hypertrophy, pulmonary disease, infection, ileus, chemotherapy, breast cancer

> **BLACK BOX WARNING:** Increased mortality in elderly patients with dementia-related psychosis

DOSAGE AND ROUTES
>> Decanoate

Adult and child >12 yr: IM/SUBCUT 12.5-25 mg q1-3wk, may increase slowly, max 100 mg/dose

>> HCl

Adult: PO 2.5-10 mg, in divided doses q6-8hr, max 40 mg/day; IM initially 1.25 mg then 2.5-10 mg in divided doses q6-8hr

Available forms: decanoate: inj 25, 100 ❤ mg/ml; elixir 2.5 mg/5 ml; oral sol 5 mg/ml; **HCl:** tabs 1, 2.5, 5, 10 mg; inj 2.5 mg/ml

Implementation
PO route
• Give with food, milk, or a full glass of water to minimize gastric irritation
• **Oral concentrate:** Give using a calibrated measuring device. Dilute just before use with 120-240 ml of water, saline, milk, 7-Up, carbonated orange beverage, or the following juices: apricot, orange, pineapple, prune, tomato or V-8. Do not mix with beverages containing caffeine (coffee, cola), tannics (tea), or pectinates (apple juice) or with other liquid medications. Avoid spilling the solution on the skin and clothing
• **Oral elixir:** Give using a calibrated measuring device. Avoid spilling the solution on the skin and clothing
Injectable routes
• Visually inspect for particulate matter and discoloration prior to use; slight yellow to amber color does not alter potency, markedly discolored solutions should be discarded, protect from light
IM route (fluPHENAZine HCl only)
• No dilution necessary, if irritation occurs, subsequent IM doses may be diluted with NS for injection or 2% procaine

• Inject slowly and deeply into the upper, outer quadrant of the gluteal muscle using a dry syringe and needle; aspirate prior to injection
• Keep patient in a recumbent position $\geq$ 30 min following injection to minimize hypotensive effects
• Rotate the site of injection to avoid irritation or sterile abscess formation with repeat use
IM injection (fluPHENAZine decanoate)
• Use a dry syringe and needle of at least 21-G; do not dilute
• Inject slowly and deeply into the upper outer quadrant of the gluteal muscle, aspirate
• Keep patient in a recumbent position for at least 30 min following the initial injection to minimize hypotensive effects
• Rotate the site of injection to avoid irritation or sterile abscess formation with repeat administration
Subcut injection route (fluPHENAZine decanoate)
• Use a dry syringe and a needle of at least 21-G; do not dilute
• Inject subcut taking care not to inject intradermally
• Keep patient in a recumbent position for at least 30 min following the initial injection to minimize hypotensive effects. Rotate the injection sites

ADVERSE EFFECTS
CNS: *EPS, pseudoparkinsonism, akathisia, dystonia, tardive dyskinesia, drowsiness, headache,* seizures, neuroleptic malignant syndrome, drowsiness
CV: *Orthostatic hypotension,* hypertension, cardiac arrest, ECG changes, tachycardia
EENT: Blurred vision, glaucoma, dry eyes, nasal congestion
GI: *Dry mouth, nausea, vomiting, anorexia, constipation,* diarrhea, jaundice, weight gain, paralytic ileus, hepatitis, cholecystic jaundice
GU: Urinary retention, urinary frequency, enuresis, impotence, amenorrhea, gynecomastia
HEMA: Anemia, leukopenia, leukocytosis, agranulocytosis, aplastic anemia, thrombocytopenia
INTEG: *Rash,* photosensitivity, dermatitis, hyperpigmentation (long-term use)
RESP: Laryngospasm, dyspnea, respiratory depression

Pharmacokinetics
Absorption	Well absorbed (PO, IM)
Distribution	Widely absorbed, crosses blood-brain barrier, placenta
Metabolism	Liver, extensively, not dialyzable
Excretion	Kidneys (metabolites)
Half-life	HCl-4.7-15.3 hr, enanthate 15 hr, decanoate 7-10 days

Pharmacodynamics

	PO/IM	IM	IM
	HCl	Enanthate	Decanoate
Onset	1 hr	1-2 days	1-3 days
Peak	1½-2 hr	2-3 days	1-2 days
Duration	6-8 hr	1-3 wk	>4 wk

INTERACTIONS
Individual drugs
Alcohol, haloperidol, metyrosine, risperiDONE: increased effects of both products, oversedation

Amiodarone, ARIPiprazole, arsenic trioxide, astemizole, dasatinib, disopyramide, dofetilide, droperidol, erythromycin, flecainide, gatifloxacin, haloperidol, ibutilide, levomethadyl, lurasidone, ondansetron, paliperidone, palonosetron, pimozide, procainamide probucol, ranolazine, quiNIDine, sotalol, sparfloxacin, saquinavir, SUNItinib, vorinostat, ziprasidone: increased QT prolongation, torsades de pointes (at higher doses)

EPINEPHrine: increased toxicity

Levodopa: decreased antiparkinson activity

Lithium: decreased effects of lithium

Drug classifications
Anticholinergics: increased anticholinergic effects

Barbiturates: decreased effect of fluphenazine, oversedation

CNS depressants: oversedation

Smoking: decreased effects of fluphenazine

Drug/herb
Betel palm, kava: increased EPS

Cola tree, hops, kava, nettle, nutmeg: possible increased action

Henbane leaf: increased anticholinergic effect

Drug/lab test
Increased: liver function tests, cardiac enzymes, cholesterol, blood glucose, prolactin, bilirubin, cholinesterase

Decreased: hormones (blood and urine)

False positive: pregnancy tests, PKU, urinary steroids, 17-OHCS

NURSING CONSIDERATIONS
Assessment

> **BLACK BOX WARNING:** Increased mortality in elderly patients with dementia-related psychosis; not approved for this use

• **QT prolongation, torsades de pointes:** ECG for changes

• Assess mental status: orientation, mood, behavior, presence and type of hallucinations before initial administration and monthly; this product should significantly reduce psychotic behavior

• Monitor bilirubin, CBC, liver function tests monthly; ophthalmic exams periodically

• Assess affect, orientation, LOC, reflexes, gait, coordination, sleep pattern disturbances

• Monitor B/P with patient sitting, standing, and lying down; take pulse and respirations q4hr during initial treatment; establish baseline before starting treatment; report drops of 30 mm Hg; obtain baseline ECG, Q-wave and T-wave changes

• Check for dizziness, faintness, palpitations, tachycardia on rising; severe orthostatic hypotension is common

• **Assess for EPS** including akathisia (inability to sit still, no pattern to movements), tardive dyskinesia (bizarre movements of the jaw, mouth, tongue, extremities), pseudoparkinsonism (rigidity, tremors, pill rolling, shuffling gait); an antiparkinson product should be prescribed

• Assess for constipation, urinary retention daily; if these occur, increase bulk, water in diet

Patient/family education
• Caution patient to avoid hazardous activities until product response is determined; dizziness, blurred vision may occur

• Inform patient that orthostatic hypotension occurs often and to rise from sitting or lying position gradually; tell patient to avoid hot tubs, hot showers, tub baths because hypotension may occur; tell patient that in hot weather, heat stroke may occur; extra precautions are necessary to stay cool

• Instruct patient to avoid abrupt withdrawal of this product, or EPS may result; product should be withdrawn slowly

• Advise patient that follow-up lab and ophthalmic exams are needed

• Teach patient to avoid OTC preparations (cough, hay fever, cold) unless approved by physician because serious product interactions may occur; avoid use with alcohol, CNS depressants; increased drowsiness may occur

• Instruct patient to use a sunscreen and sunglasses to prevent burns

• Teach patient about EPS and necessity of meticulous oral hygiene because oral candidiasis may occur

• Instruct patient to take antacids 2 hr before or after this product

• Advise patient to report sore throat, malaise, fever, bleeding, mouth sores; if these occur, CBC should be performed and product discontinued

Evaluation
Positive therapeutic outcome
- Decrease in emotional excitement, hallucinations, delusions, paranoia
- Reorganization of patterns of thought, speech

TREATMENT OF OVERDOSE:
Lavage if orally ingested; provide airway; *do not induce vomiting or use EPINEPHrine*

flurandrenolide topical
See Appendix B

flurbiprofen ophthalmic
See Appendix B

⚠ HIGH ALERT

flutamide (Rx)
(floo′ta-mide)
Euflex ✚
Func. class.: Antineoplastic hormone
Chem. class.: Antiandrogen
Pregnancy category D

ACTION: Interferes with androgen uptake in the nucleus or androgen activity in target tissues; arrests tumor growth in androgen-sensitive tissue (i.e., prostate gland)

Therapeutic outcome: Prevention of rapidly growing malignant cells

USES: Metastatic prostatic carcinoma, stage D₂ in combination with LHRH agonistic analogs (leuprolide), B₂-C in combination with goserelin and radiation

CONTRAINDICATIONS
Pregnancy **D**, hypersensitivity

> **BLACK BOX WARNING:** Severe hepatic disease

Precautions: G6PD deficiency, hemoglobinopathy, lactase deficiency, polycystic ovary syndrome, tobacco smoking

DOSAGE AND ROUTES
Adult: PO 250 mg q8hr for a daily dose of 750 mg

Available forms: Caps 125, 250 ✚ mg

Implementation
- Used in combination with LHRH agonist (leuprolide)
- Give without regard to food with a full glass of water
- Use cytotoxic handling procedures

ADVERSE EFFECTS
CNS: *Hot flashes,* drowsiness, confusion, depression, anxiety, paresthesia
GI: *Diarrhea, nausea, vomiting,* increased liver function studies, **hepatitis**, anorexia, **hepatotoxicity**, abdominal pain, cholestasis, **hepatic necrosis/failure**
GU: *Decreased libido, impotence, gynecomastia*
HEMA: Leukopenia, thrombocytopenia, hemolytic anemia
INTEG: Irritation at site, rash, photosensitivity
MISC: Edema, neuromuscular and pulmonary symptoms, hypertension, **secondary malignancy**

Pharmacokinetics

Absorption	Well absorbed
Distribution	Unknown; protein binding
Metabolism	Liver
Excretion	Unknown
Half-life	6 hr

Pharmacodynamics

Onset	Unknown
Peak	2 hr
Duration	Unknown

INTERACTIONS
Individual drugs
Leuprolide: decreased flutamide action
Warfarin: increased PT

Drug/lab test
Increased: LFTs, BUN, creatinine
Decreased: WBC, platelets

NURSING CONSIDERATIONS
Assessment

> **BLACK BOX WARNING: Severe hepatic disease:** Monitor before start of therapy and q month × 4 months, monitor AST, ALT, alkaline phosphatase, which may be elevated; product may need to be discontinued; CBC, bilirubin, creatinine periodically

- Identify CNS symptoms: drowsiness, confusion, depression, anxiety

Patient/family education
- Tell the patient to report side effects: decreased libido, impotence, breast enlargement, hot flashes, diarrhea, which occur when the two products are given together; **also nausea, vomiting; jaundice in eyes, skin; dark urine, clay-colored stools; hepatotoxicity may occur**

- Inform patient that this product is taken with leuprolide for medical castration; do not change dosing

⚠ Advise patient to use contraception during treatment, pregnancy D

- Teach patient to use with full glass of water, without regard to food

Evaluation

Positive therapeutic outcome
- Prevention of rapid division of malignant cells

---

fluticasone (Rx)

(floo-tic′a-sone)
Flonase, Flovent HFA, Flovent Diskus ♦, Veramyst (nasal spray)
Func. class.: Corticosteroids, inhalation; antiasthmatic
Pregnancy category C

ACTION: Decreases inflammation by inhibiting mast cells, macrophages, and leukotrienes; antiinflammatory and vasoconstrictor properties

Therapeutic outcome: Decreased severity of asthma

USES: Prevention of chronic asthma during maintenance treatment in those requiring oral corticosteroids; nasal symptoms of seasonal/perennial and allergic/nonallergic rhinitis

CONTRAINDICATIONS

Hypersensitivity to this product or milk protein, primary treatment in status asthmaticus, acute bronchospasm

Precautions: Pregnancy **C**, breastfeeding, active infections, glaucoma, diabetes, immunocompromised patients, Cushing syndrome

DOSAGE AND ROUTES

Prevention of chronic asthma during maintenance treatment in those requiring oral corticosteroids

>> **Flovent HFA**

Adult and child ≥12 yr: INH 88-440 mcg bid (in those previously taking bronchodilators alone); INH 88-220 mcg bid, max 440 mcg bid (in those previously taking inhaled corticosteroids); INH 440 mcg bid, max 880 mcg bid (in those previously taking oral corticosteroids)
Child 4-11 yr: INH 88 mg bid

>> **Flovent Diskus ♦**

Adult and child ≥12 yr: INH 100 mcg bid, max 500 mcg bid (in those previously taking bronchodilators alone); INH 100-250 mcg bid, max 500 mcg bid (in those previously taking inhaled corticosteroids); INH 500-1000 mcg bid,

max 1000 mcg bid (in those previously taking oral corticosteroids)
Child 4-11 yr: INH initially 50 mcg bid, max 100 mcg bid (in those previously taking bronchodilators alone or inhaled corticosteroids)

Nasal symptoms of seasonal, perennial allergic, nonallergic rhinitis
>> **Flonase**

Adult: Nasal 2 sprays initially, in each nostril per day or 1 spray bid, when controlled, lower to 1 spray in each nostril per day
Adolescent/child >4 yr: Nasal 1 spray in each nostril per day, may increase to 2 sprays in each nostril per day, when controlled, lower to 1 spray in each nostril per day

>> **Veramyst**

Adult/child ≥12 yr: Nasal 2 sprays in each nostril per day
Child 2-11 yr: Nasal 1 spray in each nostril per day

Available forms: Oral inh aerosol 44, 110, 220 mcg; oral inh powder 50, 100, 250 mcg; nasal spray (Veramyst) 27.5 mcg/actuation, (propionate) 50 mcg/actuation, 27.5 mcg/spray (furoate)

Implementation
- Give at 1 min intervals
- Decrease dose to lowest effective dose after desired effect; decrease dose at 2- to 4-wk intervals
- Blow nose prior to use

Inhalation route: powder for oral inhalation (Flovent Diskus)
- Fill in the "Pouch opened" and "Use by" dates in the blank lines on the label. The "Use by" date for Flovent diskus 50 mcg is 6 wk from the date the pouch is opened. The "Use by" date for diskus 100 mcg and 250 mcg is 2 months from the date pouch is opened
- Open the diskus by holding in one hand and using the thumb of the other to push the thumbgrip away as far as it will go until the mouthpiece shows and snaps into place
- Hold and slide the lever away from the patient as far as it will go until it clicks. The number on the dose counter will count down by 1; the diskus is now ready to use
- Before inhaling the dose, have patient breathe out, hold the diskus level and away from the mouth. Breathe out into the mouthpiece
- Instruct the patient to put the mouthpiece to the lips and breathe in through the mouth quickly and deeply through the diskus. The patient should then remove the diskus from the mouth, hold breath for about 10 sec, and breathe out slowly

---

• After taking a dose, close the diskus by sliding the thumbgrip back as far as it will go. The diskus will click shut. The lever will automatically return to its original position

• The counter displays how many doses are left. The counter number will count down each time the patient uses the diskus. After 55 doses (23 doses from the sample pack), numbers 5 to 0 appear in red to warn that there are only a few doses left

• After use, instruct patient to rinse mouth with water and spit out the water; patient should not swallow it

• To avoid the spread of infection, do not use the inhaler for more than one person

Intranasal

• Prime before first use

• Shake well before each use

• Rinse tip after use, dry with tissue

ADVERSE EFFECTS

CNS: Fever, headache, nervousness, dizziness, fatigue, migraines, numbness in fingers

EENT: *Pharyngitis,* sinusitis, rhinitis, laryngitis, hoarseness, dry eyes, cataracts, nasal discharge, epistaxis, blurred vision

GI: Diarrhea, abdominal pain, nausea, vomiting, *oral candidiasis,* gastroenteritis

GU: UTI

INTEG: Urticaria, dermatitis

META: Hyperglycemia, growth retardation in children, cushingoid features

MISC: Influenza, eosinophilic conditions, angioedema, Churg-Strauss syndrome, adrenal insufficiency (high doses), bone mineral density reduction

MS: Osteoporosis, muscle soreness, joint pain, arthralgia

RESP: *Upper respiratory infection,* dyspnea, cough, bronchitis, bronchospasm

Pharmacokinetics

Absorption	30% aerosol, 13.5% powder
Distribution	Protein binding 91%
Metabolism	In liver after absorption in lung
Excretion	<5% in urine and feces
Half-life	7.8 hr

Pharmacodynamics

	Intranasal	INH
Onset	12 hr	24 hr
Peak	Several days	Several days
Duration	1-2 wk	1-2 wk

INTERACTIONS

Individual drugs

Amprenavir, atazanavir, darunavir, delavirdine, fosamprenavir, nelfinavir, ritonavir, saquinavir: increased fluticasone levels

Isoproterenol (asthma patients): increased cardiac toxicity

Mecasermin: decreased effects of mecasermin

Drug classifications

CYP3A4 inhibitors (ketoconazole, itraconazole): increased fluticasone levels

NURSING CONSIDERATIONS

Assessment

• **Assess respiratory status:** lung sounds, pulmonary function tests during and several months after change from systemic to inhalation corticosteroids

• Assess for withdrawal symptoms from oral corticosteroids: depression, pain in joints, fatigue

⚠ **Monitor adrenal insufficiency: nausea, weakness, fatigue, hypotension, hypoglycemia, anorexia; may occur when changing from systemic to inhalation corticosteroids; may be life-threatening**

• Monitor growth rate in children; blood glucose, serum potassium in all patients

• Monitor adrenal function tests periodically: hypothalamic-pituitary-adrenal axis suppression in long-term treatment

Patient/family education

⚠ **Teach patient to report immediately cushingoid symptoms: no appetite, nausea, weakness, fatigue, decreased B/P**

• Teach patient how to use and when it may be empty

• Advise patient to use bronchodilator first before using inhalation, if taking both

• Caution patient not to use for acute asthmatic attack; acute asthma may require oral corticosteroids

• Advise patient to avoid smoking, smoke-filled rooms, those with URIs, those not immunized against chickenpox or measles

• Advise patient to use medical ID identifying corticosteroid use

Evaluation

Positive therapeutic outcome

• Decreased severity of asthma, COPD, allergies

---

fluticasone topical
See Appendix B

fluvastatin (Rx)
(flu′vah-stay-tin)
Lescol, Lescol XL
Func. class.: Antilipidemic
Chem. class.: HMG-CoA reductase inhibitor
Pregnancy category X

ACTION: Inhibits HMG-CoA reductase enzyme, which reduces cholesterol synthesis

Therapeutic outcome: Decreased cholesterol levels and LDLs, increased HDLs

USES: As an adjunct in primary hypercholesterolemia (types Ia, Ib), coronary atherosclerosis in CAD; secondary prevention of coronary events in patients with CAD; adjunct to diet to reduce LDL, total cholesterol, apo B levels in heterozygous familial hypercholesterolemia (LDL-C $\geq$190 mg/dl) or LDL-C $>$160 mg/dl with history of premature CV disease

CONTRAINDICATIONS
Pregnancy **X**, breastfeeding, hypersensitivity, active liver disease

Precautions: Past liver disease, alcoholism, severe acute infections, trauma, hypotension, uncontrolled seizure disorders, severe metabolic disorders, electrolyte imbalance, myopathy, rhabdomyolysis

DOSAGE AND ROUTES
Adult: PO 20-40 mg/day in PM initially, usual range 20-80 mg, max 80 mg; may be given in 2 doses (40 mg AM, 40 mg PM); dosage adjustments may be made in 4-wk intervals

Heterozygous familial hypercholesterolemia
Adolescent $\geq$1 yr postmenarche (10-16 yr): PO 20 mg daily at bedtime, may increase q6wk, max 40 mg bid (cap) or 80 mg (ext rel)

Available forms: Caps 20, 40 mg; ext rel tab 80 mg

Implementation
• Give without regard to food at any time of day (tab) or in the evening (cap)
• Store at room temperature, protected from light

ADVERSE EFFECTS
CNS: Headache, dizziness, insomnia, confusion
EENT: Lens opacities
GI: *Nausea, constipation, diarrhea, abdominal pain, cramps, dyspepsia, flatus,* liver dysfunction, **pancreatitis**

HEMA: **Thrombocytopenia, hemolytic anemia, leukopenia**
INTEG: Rash, pruritus
MISC: Fatigue, influenza, photosensitivity
MS: Myalgia, *arthritis, arthralgia,* myositis, **rhabdomyolysis**

Pharmacokinetics
Absorption	Unknown
Distribution	Steady state 4-5 wk
Metabolism	Liver
Excretion	Feces, kidneys
Half-life	9 hr

Pharmacodynamics
Unknown

INTERACTIONS
Individual drugs
Alcohol, cimetidine, ranitidine, omeprazole: increased fluvastatin effect, rifampin
Cholestyramine, colestipol: decreased fluvastatin effect; separate by $\geq$4 hr
Colchicine, cycloSPORINE, niacin: increased myopathy
Digoxin, phenytoin, warfarin: increased action, monitor closely
Fluconazole, itraconazole, ketoconazole: increased adverse reactions
TraMADol: increased serotonin syndrome

Drug classifications
Fibric acid derivatives, protease inhibitors: increased myopathy, erythromycin

Drug/herb
Red yeast rice: increased adverse reactions
Gotu kola, St. John's wort: decreased effect

Drug/lab test
Increased: LFTs, CK
Decreased: platelets, WBC

NURSING CONSIDERATIONS
Assessment
• **Hypercholesterolemia:** Assess nutrition: fat, protein, carbohydrates; nutritional analysis should be completed by dietitian before treatment
• Assess fasting lipid profile (cholesterol, LDL, HDL, triglycerides) q4-6wk, then q3-6mo when stable
• Monitor bowel pattern daily; diarrhea may be a problem
• **Hepatotoxicity/pancreatitis:** Monitor liver function studies q1-2mo during the first 1½ yr of treatment; AST, ALT, liver function test results may be increased
• Monitor renal studies in patients with compromised renal system: BUN, I&O ratio, creatinine

• Obtain ophth exam before, 1 mo after treatment begins, annually; lens opacities may occur
• **Myopathy, rhabdomyolysis: Assess for muscle pain, tenderness; obtain baseline CPK, if elevated or if symptoms occur, product should be discontinued**

Patient/family education
• Inform patient that compliance is needed for positive results to occur, not to double doses
• Advise patient to notify prescriber if GI symptoms of diarrhea, abdominal or epigastric pain, nausea, vomiting, or if chills, fever, sore throat occur; also muscle pain, weakness, tenderness
• Advise patient that blood studies and eye exam will be necessary during treatment, that effect may take ≥4 wk
⚠ Instruct patient to report suspected pregnancy, not to use during pregnancy (X)
• Advise patient that previously prescribed regimen will continue, including diet, exercise, smoking cessation
• Instruct patient to notify all health care providers of products taken
• Teach patient to take without regard to meals, to take immediate release product in the evening, to separate by ≥4 hr with bile-acid product

Evaluation
Positive therapeutic outcome
• Decreased LDL, VLDL, total cholesterol levels
• Improved ratio of HDLs

folic acid (vitamin B$_9$) (PO, OTC; IM/IV, Ph)
(foe-lik a'sid)
Apo-Folic ✦, Folvite, Novo-Folacid ✦
Func. class.: Vitamin B-complex group, water-soluble vitamin
Chem. class.: Supplement
Pregnancy category A

ACTION: Needed for erythropoiesis; increases RBC, WBC, and platelet formation in megaloblastic anemias

Therapeutic outcome: Absence of macrocytic, megaloblastic anemias

USES: Megaloblastic or macrocytic anemia caused by folic acid deficiency; liver disease; alcoholism; hemolysis; intestinal obstruction; pregnancy; to reduce risk of neural tube defect

CONTRAINDICATIONS
Hypersensitivity

Precautions: Pregnancy **A**, anemias other than megaloblastic/macrocytic anemia, vit B$_{12}$ deficiency anemia, uncorrected pernicious anemia

DOSAGE AND ROUTES
RDA
Adult (pregnant/breastfeeding): PO 600 mcg/day
Adult and child ≥14 yr: PO 400 mcg
Child 9-13 yr: PO 300 mcg
Child 4-8 yr: PO 200 mcg
Child 1-3 yr: PO 150 mcg
Infant 6 mo-1 yr: PO 80 mcg
Neonate and infant <6 mo: PO 65 mcg

Megaloblastic/macrocytic anemia due to folic acid or nutritional deficiency
Pregnant/lactating: PO 800-1000 mcg

Therapeutic dose
Adult and child: PO/IM/SUBCUT/**IV** up to 1 mg/day

Maintenance dose
Adult and child >4 yr: PO/IM/**IV**/SUBCUT 0.4 mg/day
Child <4 yr: PO/IM/**IV**/SUBCUT up to 0.3 mg/day
Infant: PO/IM/**IV**/SUBCUT up to 0.1 mg/day
Pregnant/lactating: PO/IM/**IV**/SUBCUT 0.8-1 mg/day

Prevention of neural tube defects during pregnancy
Adult: PO 0.6 mg/day

Prevention of megaloblastic anemia during pregnancy
Adult: PO/IM/SUBCUT up to 1 mg/day during pregnancy

Tropical sprue
Adult: PO 3-15 mg/day

Available forms: Tabs 0.1, 0.4, 0.8, 1, 5 mg; inj 5, 10 mg/ml

Implementation
SUBCUT route
• Do not inject intradermally
IM route
• Inject deeply in large muscle mass, aspirate

Direct IV route
• Give **IV** directly, undiluted 5 mg or less over 1 min or more
Continuous IV route
• May be added to most **IV** sol or TPN
• Store in light-resistant container

ADVERSE EFFECTS

CNS: Confusion, depression, excitability, irritability

GI: Anorexia, nausea, bitter taste

INTEG: Flushing, pruritus, rash, erythema

RESP: Bronchospasm

SYST: Anaphylaxis (rare)

Pharmacokinetics

Absorption	Well absorbed
Distribution	Liver, crosses placenta
Metabolism	Liver (converted to active metabolite)
Excretion	Kidneys (unchanged)
Half-life	Unknown

Pharmacodynamics

Onset	Unknown
Peak	½-1 hr
Duration	Unknown

INTERACTIONS

Individual drugs

CarBAMazepine: increased need for folic acid

Fosphenytoin: decreased fosphenytoin levels, may increase seizures

Methotrexate, sulfaSALAzine, trimethoprim: decreased action of folic acid

Phenytoin: decreased phenytoin levels, may increase seizures

Drug classifications

Estrogens, glucocorticoids, hydantoins: increased need for folic acid

Sulfonamides: decreased action of folic acid

NURSING CONSIDERATIONS

Assessment

• **Megaloblastic anemia:** Assess patient for fatigue, dyspnea, weakness, activity intolerance (signs of megaloblastic anemia)

• Monitor Hgb, Hct, and reticulocyte count; folate levels: 6-15 mcg/ml baseline, throughout treatment

• Assess nutritional status: bran, yeast, dried beans, nuts, fruits, fresh vegetables, asparagus; if high folic acid foods are missing from the diet, a referral to a dietitian may be indicated

• Identify products currently taken: alcohol, oral contraceptives, estrogens, glucocorticoids, carBAMazepine, hydantoins, trimethoprim; these products may cause increased folic acid use by the body and contribute to deficiency if taking other neurotoxic products

Patient/family education

• Advise patient to take product exactly as prescribed; not to double doses, toxicity may occur

• Instruct patient to notify prescriber of side effects; rash or fever may indicate hypersensitivity

• Advise patient that urine may become more yellow

• Instruct patient to increase intake of foods rich in folic acid in diet as recommended by dietitian or health care provider

• Advise patient to avoid breastfeeding

Evaluation

Positive therapeutic outcome

• Absence of fatigue, weakness, dyspnea

• Absence of symptoms of megaloblastic anemia

• Increase in reticulocyte count within 5 days

• Absence of neural tube defect

⚠ HIGH ALERT

fondaparinux (Rx)

(fon-dah-pair′ih-nux)

Arixtra

Func. class.: Anticoagulant, antithrombotic

Chem. class.: Synthetic, selective factor Xa inhibitor

Pregnancy category B

Do not confuse: Arixtra/Anti-Xa

ACTION: Inhibits factor Xa; interrupts blood coagulation and inhibits thrombin formation; does not inactivate thrombin (activated factor II) or affect platelets

Therapeutic outcome: Prevention of deep vein thrombosis

USES: Prevention/treatment of deep vein thrombosis, pulmonary emboli in hip and knee replacement, hip fracture or abdominal surgery, acute MI, unstable angina

CONTRAINDICATIONS

Hypersensitivity to this product; hemophilia, leukemia with bleeding, peptic ulcer disease, hemorrhagic stroke, surgery, thrombocytopenic purpura, weight <50 kg, severe renal disease (CCr <30 ml/min), active major bleeding, bacterial endocarditis

Precautions: Pregnancy **B**, breastfeeding, children, geriatric, alcoholism, hepatic disease (severe), blood dyscrasias, heparin-induced thrombocytopenia, uncontrolled severe hypertension, acute nephritis, mild to moderate renal disease

BLACK BOX WARNING: Spinal/epidural anesthesia, lumbar puncture

---

Adverse effects: *italics* = common; **bold** = life-threatening

DOSAGE AND ROUTES
Deep vein thrombosis/PE
Adult <50 kg: SUBCUT 5 mg/day × 5 days or more until INR is 2-3; give warfarin within 72 hr of fondaparinux

Adult 50-100 kg: SUBCUT 7.5 mg/day × 5 days or more until INR is 2-3; give warfarin within 72 hr of fondaparinux

Adult >100 kg: SUBCUT 10 mg/day × 5 days or more until INR is 2-3; give warfarin within 72 hr of fondaparinux

Prevention of deep vein thrombosis
Adult: SUBCUT 2.5 mg/day, given 6 hr after surgery (hemostasis established); continue for 5-9 days; hip surgery up to 32 days; abdominal surgery up to 24 days

Renal disease
Adult: Do not use if CCr <30 ml/min; CCr 30-50 ml/min, use cautiously

Available forms: Inj 2.5 mg/0.5 ml, 5 mg/0.4 ml, 7.5 mg/0.6 ml, 10 mg/0.8 ml pre-filled syringes

Implementation
• Do not mix with other products or solutions; cannot be used interchangeably (unit to unit) with other anticoagulants
• Give only after screening patient for bleeding disorders
• Store at 77° F (25° C); do not freeze
SUBCUT route
• Administer SUBCUT only; do not give IM
• Check for discolored sol or sol with particulate; if present, do not give
• Administer to recumbent patient, rotate inj sites (left/right anterolateral, left/right postero-lateral abdominal wall), administer 6-8 hr after surgery
• Wipe surface of inj site with alcohol swab, twist plunger cap and remove, remove rigid needle guard by pulling straight off needle, do not aspirate, do not expel air bubble from surface
• Insert whole length of needle into skin fold held with thumb and forefinger
• When product is injected, a soft click may be felt or heard
• Give at same time each day to maintain steady blood levels
• Avoid all IM inj that may cause bleeding
⚠ **Administer only this product when ordered; not interchangeable with heparin**

ADVERSE EFFECTS
CNS: *Fever,* confusion, headache, dizziness, *insomnia*

GI: *Nausea, vomiting,* diarrhea, dyspepsia, *constipation,* increased AST, ALT
GU: UTI, urinary retention
HEMA: *Anemia,* minor bleeding, purpura, hematoma, **thrombocytopenia, major bleeding (intracranial, cerebral, retroperitoneal hemorrhage), postoperative hemorrhage, heparin-induced thrombocytopenia**
INTEG: Local reaction—*rash,* pruritus, inj site bleeding, increased wound drainage, bullous eruption
META: Hypokalemia
MISC: Hypotension, pain, *edema*

Pharmacokinetics

Absorption	Rapidly, completely absorbed
Distribution	Blood; does not bind to plasma proteins except 94% to ATIII
Excretion	Eliminated unchanged in 72 hr in normal renal function
Half-life	17-21 hr

Pharmacodynamics

Onset	Unknown
Peak	3 hr
Duration	Unknown

INTERACTIONS
Do not mix with other products or inf fluids

Individual drugs
Abciximab, clopidogrel, dipyridamole, eptifibatide, quiNIDine, tirofiban, valproic acid: increased risk of bleeding

Drug classifications
NSAIDs, salicylates: increased risk of bleeding

Drug/herb
Feverfew, garlic, ginger, ginkgo, ginseng, green tea, horse chestnut, kava: increased risk of bleeding

NURSING CONSIDERATIONS
Assessment

> **BLACK BOX WARNING:** Monitor patients who have received epidural/spinal anesthesia or lumbar puncture for neurological impairment, including spinal hematoma, may lead to permanent disability or paralysis

• **Hemorrhage:** Assess for hemorrhage if coadministered with other products that may cause bleeding
• Assess blood studies (Hct, CBC, coagulation studies, platelets, occult blood in stools), anti-Xa; if platelets <100,000/mm³, treatment

should be discontinued; renal studies: BUN, creatinine
• Assess for bleeding: gums, petechiae, ecchymosis, black tarry stools, hematuria; notify prescriber

Patient/family education
• Advise patient to use soft-bristle toothbrush to avoid bleeding gums, to use electric razor
• Advise patient to report any signs of bleeding: gums, under skin, urine, stools
• Caution patient to avoid OTC products containing aspirin, NSAIDs

Evaluation

Positive therapeutic outcome
• Absence of deep vein thrombosis

formoterol (Rx)
(for-moh′ter-ahl)
Foradil Aerolizer, Oxeze ✿, Performomist
Func. class.: β-Adrenergic agonist
Chem. class.: Sympathomimetic catecholamine
Pregnancy category C

Do not confuse: Foradil/Toradol

ACTION: Has β_1 and β_2 action; relaxes bronchial smooth muscle and dilates the trachea and main bronchi by increasing levels of cyclic AMP, which relaxes smooth muscles; causes increased contractility and heart rate by acting on β-receptors in the heart

Therapeutic outcome: Bronchodilatation, increased heart rate and cardiac output from action on β-receptors in heart

USES: Maintenance, treatment of asthma, COPD, prevention of exercise-induced bronchospasm

CONTRAINDICATIONS
Hypersensitivity to sympathomimetics, monotherapy for asthma, COPD, status asthmaticus

Precautions: Pregnancy C, geriatric, cardiac disorders, hyperthyroidism, diabetes mellitus, prostatic hypertrophy, hypertension, African descendants

> BLACK BOX WARNING: Asthma-related death

DOSAGE AND ROUTES
Maintenance, treatment of asthma
Adult and child ≥5 yr: INH AM and PM long-term, 1 cap (12 mcg) q12hr using aerolizer inhaler

Maintenance of COPD
Adult: INH 12 mcg q12hr

Prevention of exercise-induced bronchospasm
Adult and child ≥12 yr: INH prn 1 cap (12 mcg) at least 15 min before exercise, do not use additional doses for ≥12 hr

Available forms: INH powder in cap 12 mcg; nebulizer sol for inhalation 20 mcg/2 ml

Implementation
• Store at room temperature; protect from heat, moisture
Inhalation route
• Place cap in aerolizer inhaler; the cap is punctured; do not wash aerolizer inhaler
• Pull off cover, twist mouthpiece to open, push buttons in; make sure the four pins are visible; remove cap from blister pack, place cap in chamber; twist to close, press (a click will be heard), release; patient should exhale, place inhaler in mouth, inhale rapidly

ADVERSE EFFECTS
CNS: Tremors, *anxiety*, insomnia, headache, dizziness, stimulation
CV: Palpitations, tachycardia, hypertension, chest pain
GI: Nausea, vomiting, xerostomia
RESP: Bronchial irritation, dryness of oropharynx, **bronchospasms (overuse)**; infection, inflammatory reactions (child)

Pharmacokinetics

Absorption	Rapid (INH)
Distribution	Plasma protein binding 61%-64% at concentrations of 0.1-100 ng/mL; 31%-38% at concentrations of 5-500 ng/mL
Metabolism	Liver, lungs, GI tract
Excretion	Urine, feces
Half-life	10 hr mean terminal elimination half-life

Pharmacodynamics

Onset	Unknown
Peak	5 min (INH)
Duration	Unknown

INTERACTIONS
Amoxapine, arsenic trioxide, chloroquine, clarithromycin, dasatinib, dolasetron, droperidol, erythromycin, halofantrine, levomethadyl, ondansetron, paliperidone,

palonosetron, pentamidine, probucol, ranolazine, SUNItinib, vorinostat, pimozide, risperiDONE, ziprasidone: increased QT prolongation

Drug classifications

Class IA/III antidysrhythmics, phenothiazines, halogenated anesthetics, tricyclics, some quinolones: increase QT prolongation

β-blockers: decreased action of formoterol

MAOIs, antidepressants (tricyclics): serious dysrhythmias

Sympathomimetics, thyroid hormones, tricyclics, some quinolones: increased action of both products

Loop/thiazide diuretics: increased hypokalemia

NURSING CONSIDERATIONS
Assessment

• Assess respiratory function: B/P, pulse, lung sounds, be alert for bronchospasm may occur with this patient
• Cardiac status: Assess for hypertension, palpitations, tachycardia; if CV reactions occur, product may need to be discontinued
• Assess I&O ratio; check for urinary retention, frequency, hesitancy
• Assess for paresthesias and coldness of extremities; peripheral blood flow may decrease

Patient/family education

• Review package insert with patient and inform about all aspects of product
• Teach correct use of inhaler; not to swallow caps
• Teach use of spacer device in children or geriatric
• Advise patient to avoid getting aerosol in eyes
• Instruct patient to rinse mouth after use
• Advise patient to wash inhaler in warm water and dry daily
• Advise patient to avoid smoking, smoke-filled rooms, persons with respiratory infections

> **BLACK BOX WARNING:** Asthma-related death, severe asthma exacerbations: if wheezing worsens and cannot be relieved during an acute asthma attack, immediate medical attention should be sought

Evaluation
Positive therapeutic outcome

• Absence of dyspnea, wheezing
• Improved airway exchange
• Improved ABGs

TREATMENT OF OVERDOSE:
Administer β-blocker

fosamprenavir (Rx)

(fos-am-pren'a-veer)

Lexiva

Func. class.: Antiretroviral
Chem. class.: Protease inhibitor

Pregnancy category C

ACTION: Prodrug of amprenavir; inhibits human immunodeficiency virus (HIV) protease, which prevents maturation of the infectious virus

Therapeutic outcome: Decreasing symptoms of HIV

USES: HIV-1 infection in combination with antiretrovirals

CONTRAINDICATIONS
Hypersensitivity to protease inhibitors

Precautions: Pregnancy **C**, breastfeeding, geriatric, liver disease, hemolytic anemia, diabetes, sulfa sensitivity, autoimmune disease with immune reconstitution

DOSAGE AND ROUTES
Therapy-naïve patients

Adult: PO 1400 mg bid without ritonavir, or fosamprenavir 1400 mg/day and ritonavir 200 mg/day, or fosamprenavir 700 mg bid and ritonavir 100 mg bid

Adolescent/child/infant ≥4 wk: PO 30 mg/kg bid, max 1400 mg/dose, without ritonavir

Protease-experienced patients (PI)

Adult: PO 700 mg bid and ritonavir 100 mg bid

Adolescent/child ≥20 kg: PO 18 mg/kg bid with ritonavir 3 mg/kg bid

Adolescent/child 15 kg to <20 kg: PO 23 mg/kg bid with ritonavir 3 mg/kg bid

Adolescent/child 11 kg to <15 kg: PO 30 mg/kg bid with ritonavir 3 mg/kg bid

Adolescent/child <11 kg: PO 45 mg/kg bid with ritonavir 7 mg/kg bid

Infant ≥6 mo, 15 kg to <20 kg: PO susp 23 mg/kg bid with ritonavir 3 mg/kg bid

Infant ≥6 mo, 11 kg to <15 kg: PO susp 30 mg/kg bid with ritonavir 3 mg/kg bid

Infant ≥6 mo, <11 kg: PO susp 45 mg/kg bid with ritonavir 7 mg/kg bid

Combination with efavirenz

Adult: PO add another 100 mg/day of ritonavir for a total of 300 mg/day when all three products are given

Hepatic dose

Adult: PO (Child-Pugh 5-6) 700 mg bid without ritonavir (treatment-naive patients) or 700 mg bid with ritonavir 100 mg qd

---

(treatment-naive or experienced patients); (Child-Pugh 7-9) 700 mg bid without ritonavir (treatment-naive or experienced patients) or 450 mg bid with ritonavir 100 mg qd (treatment-naive or experienced patients); (Child-Pugh 10-15) 350 mg bid without ritonavir (treatment-naive patients) or 300 mg bid with ritonavir 100 mg qd (treatment-naive or experienced patients)

Available forms: Tabs 700 mg (equivalent to 600 mg amprenavir); oral suspension 50 mg/ml

Implementation
• **Tabs:** Administer without regard to food
• **Oral susp:** *Adult:* give without food; *child:* give with food; if vomiting occurs within 30 min, readminister; shake oral susp vigorously prior to dosing, use calibrated device
• Patients receiving phosphodiesterase type 5 (PDE5) inhibitors may be at increased risk for PDE5 inhibitor adverse effects

ADVERSE EFFECTS
CNS: Headache, fatigue, depression, oral paresthesia
GI: *Nausea, diarrhea, vomiting, abdominal pain*
INTEG: Rash, pruritus
MISC: Redistribution or accumulation of body fat, hyperglycemia, **Stevens-Johnson syndrome**

Pharmacokinetics
Absorption	Unknown
Distribution	90% protein binding
Metabolism	In the liver by CYP3A4
Excretion	Excretion of unchanged product is minimal
Half-life	Unknown

Pharmacodynamics
Onset	Unknown
Peak	1½-4 hr
Duration	Unknown

INTERACTIONS
Individual drugs
⚠ **Amiodarone, flecainide, lidocaine, midazolam, pimozide, propafenone, triazolam: serious life-threatening reactions**
CarBAMazepine, dexamethasone, efavirenz, lopinavir/ritonavir, nevirapine, phenytoin, ranitidine, saquinavir: decreased fosamprenavir levels, avoid concurrent use
ARIPiprazole, itraconazole, ketoconazole, rifabutin, sildenafil, vardenafil: increased effect
Methadone: decreased effect

Warfarin: increased effect of warfarin
Ritonavir with boceprevir or ritonavir with telaprevir not recommended: increased treatment failure
Decreased dose of maraviroc with product is used with ritonavir; do not use maraviroc with unboosted fosamprenavir

Drug classifications
Antacids: decreased fosamprenavir levels
⚠ **Barbiturates, proton-pump inhibitors, calcium channel blockers, ergots, H₂ receptor antagonists: serious life-threatening reactions**
Contraceptives (oral): decreased effect
Estrogens, H₂ receptor antagonists, oral contraceptives, proton-pump inhibitors: avoid use; may lose virologic response and possibly lead to resistance of fosamprenavir
HMG-CoA reductase inhibitors: increased toxicity

Drug/herb
Avoid use with St. John's wort, may lose virologic response and possibly lead to resistance of fosamprenavir

Drug/lab test
Increased: serum glucose, AST, ALT, triglycerides

NURSING CONSIDERATIONS
Assessment
• Assess bowel pattern before, during treatment; monitor hydration
• Assess skin eruptions, rash, urticaria, itching
• **HIV:** Monitor viral load, CD4 cell counts, plasma HIV RNA, serum cholesterol, lipid profile baseline, throughout treatment
⚠ **Stevens-Johnson syndrome: report immediately**
⚠ **Immune reconstitution syndrome: may occur with combination antiretroviral therapy; autoimmune disease may also develop, up to months after treatment starts**

Patient/family education
• Advise patient to avoid taking product with other medications unless directed by provider
• Teach patient that product does not cure, but does manage symptoms; that product does not prevent transmission of HIV to others
• Advise patient to use nonhormonal form of birth control while taking this product
• Instruct patient if dose is missed, take as soon as remembered up to 1 hr before next dose; do not double dose
• Instruct patient not to alter dose or stop therapy without talking to physician
• Advise physician if patient has a sulfa allergy

• Advise patient to report all medications, including herbal supplements, to prescriber

Evaluation
Positive therapeutic outcome
• Decreasing symptoms of HIV

---

foscarnet (Rx)
(foss-kar′net)
Foscavir
Func. class.: Antiviral
Chem. class.: Inorganic pyrophosphate organic analog
Pregnancy category C

ACTION: Antiviral activity is produced by selective inhibition at the pyrophosphate binding site on virus-specific DNA polymerases and reverse transcriptases at concentrations that do not affect cellular DNA polymerases

Therapeutic outcome: Virostatic agents against CMV retinitis

USES: Treatment of CMV, retinitis, herpes simplex virus (HSV) infections; used with ganciclovir for relapsing patients

CONTRAINDICATIONS
Hypersensitivity, CCr <0.4 ml/min/kg

Precautions: Pregnancy C, breastfeeding, children, geriatric, seizure disorders, severe anemia

> **BLACK BOX WARNING:** Renal disease, electrolyte/mineral imbalances

DOSAGE AND ROUTES
Acyclovir-resistant mucocutaneous herpes simplex virus infection (herpes labialis, herpes febrilis, herpes genitalis) in HIV-infected patients
Adult/adolescent (unlabeled): IV 40 mg/kg q8-12hr × 2-3 wk or until lesions are healed

Cytomegalovirus (CMV) encephalitis (unlabeled); cytomegalovirus (CMV) neurological disease (unlabeled) (including encephalitis) in HIV-infected patients
Adult/adolescent: IV 90 mg/kg q12hr or 60 mg/kg q8hr × 3 wk (or until symptomatic improvement) with ganciclovir 5 mg/kg **IV** q12hr × 2-3 wk

Encephalitis (unlabeled) caused by human herpesvirus 6 (HHV-6) in immunocompromised patients
Adult: IV 60 mg/kg q8hr or 90 mg/kg q12hr alone or in combination with ganciclovir 5 mg/kg **IV** q12hr

Cytomegalovirus (CMV) retinitis or disseminated disease (unlabeled) in HIV-infected patients, recurrent or relapsed cytomegalovirus (CMV) retinitis in HIV-infected patients
Adult: IV Induction with 90 mg/kg q12hr or 60 mg/kg **IV** q8hr for 14-21 days, depending upon the clinical response

Renal dose
Adult: HSV induction dosage equivalent to 80 mg/kg/day (40 mg/kg IV q12hr)
Adult: IV CCr >1.4 ml/min/kg: no change; CCr >1-1.4 ml/min/kg: decrease to 30 mg/kg q12hr; CCr >0.8-1 ml/min/kg: decrease to 20 mg/kg q12hr; CCr >0.6-0.8 ml/min/kg: decrease to 35 mg/kg/day; CCr >0.5-0.6 ml/min/kg: decrease to 25 mg/kg/day; CCr ≥0.4-0.5 ml/min/kg: decrease to 20 mg/kg/day; CCr <0.4 ml/min/kg: not recommended

HSV induction dosage equivalent to 120 mg/kg/day (40 mg/kg IV q8hr)
Adult: IV CCr >1.4 ml/min/kg: no change; CCr >1-1.4 ml/min/kg: decrease to 30 mg/kg q8hr; CCr >0.8-1 ml/min/kg: decrease to 35 mg/kg q12hr; CCr >0.6-0.8 ml/min/kg: decrease to 25 mg/kg q12hr; CCr >0.5-0.6 ml/min/kg: decrease to 40 mg/kg/day; CCr ≥0.4-0.5 ml/min/kg: decrease to 35 mg/kg/day; CCr <0.4 ml/min/kg: not recommended

CMV induction dosage equivalent to 180 mg/kg/day (60 mg/kg q8hr)
Adult: IV CCr >1.4 ml/min/kg: no change; CCr >1-1.4 ml/min/kg: decrease to 45 mg/kg q8hr; CCr >0.8-1 ml/min/kg: decrease to 50 mg/kg q12hr; CCr >0.6-0.8 ml/min/kg: decrease to 40 mg/kg q12hr; CCr >0.5-0.6 ml/min/kg: decrease to 60 mg/kg/day; CCr ≥0.4-0.5 ml/min/kg: decrease to 50 mg/kg/day; CCr <0.4 ml/min/kg: not recommended

CMV induction dosage equivalent to 180 mg/kg/day (90 mg/kg IV q12hr)
Adult: IV CCr >1.4 ml/min/kg: no change; CCr >1-1.4 ml/min/kg: decrease to 70 mg/kg q12hr; CCr >0.8-1 ml/min/kg: decrease to 50 mg/kg q12hr; CCrl >0.6-0.8 ml/min/kg: decrease to 80 mg/kg/day; CCr >0.5-0.6 ml/min/kg: decrease to 60 mg/kg/day; CCr ≥0.4-0.5 ml/min/kg: decrease to 50 mg/kg/day; CCr <0.4 ml/min/kg: not recommended

Available forms: Inj 6000 mg/250 ml, 12,000 mg/500 ml (24 mg/ml)

⚠ Nurse Alert   ✳ Key NCLEX® Drug   >> Drug Specifics

Implementation

Intermittent IV infusion route

• Administer increased fluids before, during product administration to induce diuresis and minimize renal toxicity

• Administer via inf pump, at no more than 1 mg/kg/min; do not give by rapid or bolus **IV**; give by central venous line or peripheral vein; standard 24 mg/ml sol may be used without dilution if using by central line; dilute the 24 mg/ml sol to 12 mg/ml with D_5W or 0.9% NaCl if using peripheral vein

• Monitor patient closely during therapy; if tingling, numbness, paresthesias occur, stop inf and obtain lab sample for electrolytes

Y-site incompatibilities: Manufacturer recommends that product not be given with other medications in syringe or admixed

ADVERSE EFFECTS

CNS: *Fever,* dizziness, *headache,* **seizures,** *fatigue,* neuropathy, asthenia, encephalopathy, malaise, meningitis, *paresthesia,* depression, *confusion, anxiety*

CV: ECG abnormalities, 1st-degree AV block, nonspecific ST-T segment changes, cerebrovascular disorder, cardiomyopathy, **cardiac arrest,** atrial fibrillation, CHF, sinus tachycardia

GI: *Nausea, vomiting, diarrhea, anorexia,* abdominal pain, **pancreatitis**

GU: **Acute renal failure,** decreased CCr and increased serum creatinine, azotemia, diabetes mellitus

HEMA: Anemia, **granulocytopenia, leukopenia, thrombocytopenia, thrombosis,** lymphadenopathy, neutropenia

INTEG: *Rash,* sweating, pruritus, skin discoloration

RESP: *Coughing, dyspnea,* pneumonia, **pulmonary infiltration, pneumothorax, hemoptysis**

SYST: *Hypokalemia, hypocalcemia, hypomagnesemia,* hypophosphatemia

Pharmacokinetics

Absorption	Complete (**IV**)
Distribution	14%-17% plasma protein binding
Metabolism	Not metabolized
Excretion	Kidneys (79%-92%) unchanged, breast milk
Half-life	18-88 hr; increased in renal disease

Pharmacodynamics

Onset	48 hr
Peak	2 wk
Duration	Unknown

INTERACTIONS
Individual drugs

Acyclovir, cidofovir, CISplatin, penicillamine, tacrolimus, tenofovir, vancomycin, amphotericin B, cycloSPORINE, lithium: increased nephrotoxicity

Pentamidine: increased hypocalcemia

Drug classifications

> **BLACK BOX WARNING:** Aminoglycosides, gold compounds, NSAIDs: increased nephrotoxicity

NURSING CONSIDERATIONS
Assessment

• **General** culture should be done before treatment with foscarnet is begun; cultures of blood, urine, and throat may all be taken; CMV is not confirmed by this method; the diagnosis is made by an ophth exam

> **BLACK BOX WARNING: Renal tubular disorders:** Assess kidney: BUN, serum creatinine, creatinine clearance, if CCr <0.4 ml/min/kg, discontinue product

• Blood counts should be done q2wk; watch for decreasing granulocytes, Hgb; if low, therapy may have to be discontinued and restarted after hematologic recovery; blood transfusions may be required

• Assess for GI symptoms: severe nausea, vomiting, diarrhea; severe symptoms may necessitate discontinuing product

• Monitor electrolytes and minerals: calcium, phosphorous, magnesium, sodium, potassium; watch closely for tetany during first administration

⚠ **Assess for symptoms of blood dyscrasias (anemia, granulocytopenia); bruising, fatigue, bleeding, poor healing**

• **Assess for symptoms of allergic reactions:** flushing, rash, urticaria, pruritus

CMV retinitis: Culture should be done prior to treatment (blood, urine, throat); a negative culture does not rule out CMV; ophthalmic exam should confirm diagnosis

Patient/family education

• Advise patient to notify prescriber if sore throat, swollen lymph nodes, malaise, fever occur; may indicate presence of other infections

• Advise patient to report perioral tingling, numbness in extremities, and paresthesias; inf should be stopped and electrolytes should be requested

• Caution patient that serious product interactions may occur if OTC products are ingested; check first with prescriber

• Inform patient that product is not a cure but will control symptoms

• Advise patient that ophth exams must be continued

Evaluation
Positive therapeutic outcome
• Improvement in CMV retinitis

fosinopril (Rx)
(foss-in-o′pril)
Monapril
Func. class.: Antihypertensive
Chem. class.: Angiotensin-converting enzyme (ACE) inhibitor
Pregnancy category D

Do not confuse: Monopril/minoxidil/Monurol

ACTION: Selectively suppresses renin-angiotensin-aldosterone system; inhibits ACE; prevents conversion of angiotensin I to angiotensin II; results in dilatation of arterial, venous vessels

Therapeutic outcome: Decreased B/P in hypertension

USES: Hypertension, alone or in combination with thiazide diuretics, systolic CHF

CONTRAINDICATIONS
Breastfeeding, children, hypersensitivity to ACE inhibitors, history of ACE inhibitor–induced angioedema

> **BLACK BOX WARNING:** Pregnancy **D**

Precautions: Geriatric, impaired liver function, hypovolemia, blood dyscrasias, CHF, COPD, asthma, angioedema, hyperkalemia, renal artery stenosis, renal disease, aortic stenosis, autoimmune disorders, collagen vascular disease, febrile illness

DOSAGE AND ROUTES
Hypertension
Adult: PO 5-10 mg/day initially, then 20-40 mg/day divided bid or daily, max 80 mg/day

CHF
Adult: PO 10 mg/day, then up to 40 mg/day, increased over several weeks; use lower dose in those undergoing diuresis before fosinopril

Available forms: Tabs 10, 20, 40 mg
Implementation
• Store in tight container at 86° F (30° C)
• Severe hypotension may occur after 1st dose of this medication; hypotension may be prevented by reducing or discontinuing diuretic therapy 3 days before beginning benzapril therapy

ADVERSE EFFECTS
CNS: *Headache, dizziness,* fatigue, syncope
CV: *Hypotension,* orthostatic hypotension, tachycardia
GI: *Nausea,* constipation, *vomiting,* diarrhea, **hepatotoxicity, cholestatic jaundice, fulminant hepatic necrosis, hepatic failure, death**
GU: Increased BUN, creatinine, azotemia, **renal artery stenosis**
HEMA: Decreased Hct, Hgb, **eosinophilia, leukopenia, neutropenia, agranulocytosis**
META: *Hyperkalemia*
RESP: *Cough*
SYST: **Anaphylaxis, angioedema**

Pharmacokinetics
Absorption	30%
Distribution	Crosses placenta
Metabolism	Liver, converted to fosinoprilat
Excretion	50% kidneys (metabolites), 50% feces
Half-life	12 hr: fosinoprilat

Pharmacodynamics
Onset	1 hr
Peak	2-6 hr
Duration	24 hr

INTERACTIONS
Individual drugs
Alcohol (acute ingestion): increased hypotension (large amounts)
Digoxin, hydrALAZINE, lithium, prazosin: increased toxicity

Drug classifications
Adrenergic blockers, antihypertensives, diuretics, ganglionic blockers, nitrates: increased hypotension
Antacids: decreased absorption
Diuretics (potassium-sparing), sympathomimetics, NSAIDs, vasodilators: increased toxicity
Salicylates: decreased antihypertensive effect

Drug/herb
Hawthorn: increased antihypertensive effect
Ephedra: decreased antihypertensive effect

Drug/lab test
Increased: AST, ALT, alkaline phosphatase, glucose, bilirubin, uric acid
Positive: ANA titer
False positive: urine acetone

NURSING CONSIDERATIONS
Assessment
• **Hypertension:** Monitor B/P, check for orthostatic hypotension, syncope; if changes occur, dosage change may be required
⚠ **Collagen vascular disease: Monitor blood studies: neutrophils, decreased platelets; obtain WBC with differential at baseline and qmo × 6 mo, then q2-3mo × 1 yr; if neutrophils <1000/mm³, discontinue**
• Monitor renal studies: protein, BUN, creatinine; watch for increased levels that may indicate nephrotic syndrome and renal failure; monitor urine daily for protein; monitor renal symptoms: polyuria, oliguria, frequency, dysuria
• Establish baselines in renal, liver function tests before therapy begins
• Check potassium levels throughout treatment although hyperkalemia rarely occurs
• **CHF:** Check for edema in feet, legs daily, monitor weight daily
• **Assess for allergic reactions:** rash, fever, pruritus, urticaria; product should be discontinued if antihistamines fail to help

Patient/family education
• Advise patient not to discontinue product abruptly; warn patient to tell all persons associated with his or her care
• Teach patient not to use OTC products (cough, cold, allergy) unless directed by prescriber because serious side effects can occur; xanthines such as coffee, tea, chocolate, cola can prevent action of product
• Teach patient the importance of complying with dosage schedule, even if feeling better; to continue with medical regimen to decrease B/P: exercise, smoking cessation, decreasing stress, diet modifications
• Emphasize the need to rise slowly to sitting or standing position to minimize orthostatic hypotension; not to exercise in hot weather or increased hypotension can occur
• Advise patient to notify prescriber of mouth sores, sore throat, fever, swelling of hands or feet, irregular heartbeat, chest pain, coughing, shortness of breath
• Instruct patient to report excessive perspiration, dehydration, vomiting, diarrhea; may lead to fall in B/P
• Caution patient that product may cause dizziness, fainting, light-headedness; may occur

during 1st few days of therapy; to avoid activities that may be hazardous
• Teach patient how to take B/P, normal readings for age-group

> **BLACK BOX WARNING:** Advise patient to notify prescriber if pregnancy is planned or suspected, pregnancy **D**, to use contraception during treatment

Evaluation
Positive therapeutic outcome
• Decreased B/P in hypertension

TREATMENT OF OVERDOSE:
0.9% NaCl IV inf, hemodialysis

fosphenytoin (Rx)
(foss-fen´i-toy-in)
Func. class.: Anticonvulsant
Chem. class.: Hydantoin, phosphate phenytoin ester
Pregnancy category D

ACTION: Inhibits spread of seizure activity in motor cortex by altering ion transport; increases AV conduction; prodrug of phenytoin

Therapeutic outcome: Decreased seizures, absence of dysrhythmias

USES: Generalized tonic-clonic seizures, status epilepticus, partial seizures

CONTRAINDICATIONS
Pregnancy **D**, hypersensitivity, bradycardia, SA and AV block, Stokes-Adams syndrome

Precautions: Breastfeeding, allergies, renal/hepatic disease, myocardial insufficiency, hypoalbuminemia, hypothyroidism, Asian patients positive for HLA-B 1502, abrupt discontinuation, agranulocytosis, alcoholism, carBAMazepine/barbiturate hypersensitivity, bone marrow suppression, CAD, geriatrics, hemolytic anemia, hyponatremia, methemoglobinemia, myasthenia gravis, psychosis, suicidal ideation

> **BLACK BOX WARNING:** Rapid IV infusion

DOSAGE AND ROUTES
All doses in PE (phenytoin sodium equivalent)

Status epilepticus
Adult and adolescent: IV 15-20 mg PE/kg

Nonemergency/maintenance dosing
Adult and adolescent >16 yr: IM/IV 10-20 mg PE/kg 10 mg dose; 4-6 mg PE/kg/day (maintenance); start maintenance 12 hr after loading dose; give in 2-3 divided doses

Available forms: Inj 150 mg (100 mg PE), 750 mg (500 mg PE), 50 mg/ml vials

Implementation
Injectable routes

• Give IM/IV; the dosage, concentration, and infusion rate of fosphenytoin should always be expressed, prescribed, and dispensed in phenytoin sodium equivalents (PE); exercise extreme caution when preparing and administering fosphenytoin; the concentration and dosage should be carefully confirmed; fatal overdoses have occurred in children when the per-ml concentration of the product (50 mg PE/mL) was misinterpreted as the total amount of drug in the vial

• Visually inspect for particulate matter and discoloration prior to use

IV infusion route
• Prior to infusion, dilute in 5% dextrose or 0.9% saline solution to a concentration ranging from 1.5-25 mg PE/ml

• Because of the risk of hypotension, do not exceed recommended infusion rates. Continuous monitoring of ECG, B/P, and respiratory function is recommended, especially throughout the period when phenytoin concentrations peak (about 10-20 min after the end of the infusion)

• Loading doses should always be followed by maintenance doses of oral or parenteral phenytoin or parenteral fosphenytoin

• Adult: Infuse IV at a rate max 150 mg PE/min

• Elderly or debilitated adult: infuse IV at a max 3 mg PE/kg/min or 150 mg PE/min, whichever is less

• Child: infuse IV at a rate of 0.5-3 mg PE/kg/min, max 150 mg PE/min, whichever is less

• Infant, neonate: infuse IV at a rate max 0.5-3 mg PE/kg/min

Y-site compatibilities: Aminocaproic acid, amphotericin B lipid complex, amphotericin B liposome, anidulafungin, atenolol, bivalirudin, bleomycin, CARBOplatin, CISplatin, cyclophosphamide, cytarabine, DACTINomycin, DAPTOmycin, dexmedetomidine, diltiazem, DOCEtaxel, doxacurium, eptifibatide, ertapenem, etoposide, fludarabine, fluorouracil, gatifloxacin, gemcitabine, gemtuzumab, granisetron, ifosfamide, levofloxacin, linezolid, LORazepam, mechlorethamine, meperidine, methotrexate, metroNIDAZOLE, nesiritide, octreotide, oxaliplatin, oxytocin, PACLitaxel, palonosetron, pamidronate, pantoprazole, PEMEtrexed, PHENobarbital, piperacillin-tazobactam, rocuronium, sodium acetate, tacrolimus, teniposide, thiotepa, tigecycline, tirofiban, vinCRIStine, vinorelbine, voriconazole, zoledronic acid

Y-site incompatibilities: Caspofungin, DOXOrubicin, epirubicin, fenoldopam, IDArubicin, midazolam, mitoXANtrone, mycophenolate, quinupristin-dalfopristin

ADVERSE EFFECTS
CNS: *Drowsiness,* dizziness, insomnia, paresthesias, depression, **suicidal tendencies,** aggression, headache, confusion, paresthesia, emotional lability, syncope, cerebral edema

CV: Hypotension, hypertension, **CHF, shock, dysrhythmias**

EENT: Nystagmus, diplopia, blurred vision

GI: Nausea, vomiting, diarrhea, constipation, anorexia, weight loss, **hepatitis,** jaundice, gingival hyperplasia

HEMA: **Agranulocytosis, leukopenia, aplastic anemia, thrombocytopenia, megaloblastic anemia**

INTEG: Rash, lupus erythematosus, **Stevens-Johnson syndrome,** hirsutism, hypersensitivity, pruritus

RESP: **Bronchospasm, cough**

SYST: Hyperglycemia, hypokalemia, **toxic epidermal necrolysis (Asian patients positive for HLA-B 1502), DRESS, purple glove syndrome, anaphylaxis**

Pharmacokinetics

Absorption	Unknown
Distribution	Protein binding 99%
Metabolism	Liver: converted to phenytoin
Excretion	Kidneys
Half-life	Unknown

Pharmacodynamics

Unknown

INTERACTIONS
Individual drugs

Alcohol: decreased effects of fosphenytoin (chronic use)

Amiodarone, chloramphenicol, cimetidine: increased fosphenytoin level

CarBAMazepine, folic acid, rifampin, theophylline, tramadol: decreased effects of fosphenytoin

Delavirdine: do not use concurrently; decreased virologic response, resistance

Drug classifications

Antacids, antihistamines, antineoplastics, CYP1A2 inducers: decreased effects of fosphenytoin

Antidepressants (tricyclics), CYP1A2 inhibitors, estrogens, H$_2$-receptor antagonists, phenothiazines, salicylates, sulfonamides: increased fosphenytoin level

---

Drug/herb
Ginseng, valerian: decreased anticonvulsant effect

Ginkgo: increased anticonvulsant effect

Drug/lab test
Increased: glucose, alkaline phosphatase

Decreased: dexamethasone, metyrapone test serum, PBI, urinary steroids, potassium

NURSING CONSIDERATIONS
Assessment
• Assess drug level: target level 10-20 mcg/ml; toxic level 30-50 mcg/ml, wait at least 2 hr after dose before testing, 4 hr after IM dose

• **Assess seizure activity including type, location, duration, and character; provide seizure precaution**

• Assess renal studies: urinalysis, BUN, urine creatinine

• Monitor hepatic studies: ALT, AST, bilirubin, creatinine

• Assess allergic reaction: red raised rash; if this occurs, product should be discontinued

• **Monitor for toxicity: bone marrow depression, nausea, vomiting, ataxia, diplopia, cardiovascular collapse, slurred speech, confusion**

• Assess product level: toxic level 30-50 mcg/ml

⚠ **Assess for rash, discontinue as soon as rash develops, serious adverse reactions such as Stevens-Johnson syndrome can occur**

⚠ **Assess mental status: mood, sensorium, affect, memory (long, short), especially geriatric; suicidal thoughts/behaviors**

⚠ **Serious skin reactions: usually occurring within 28 days of treatment; if a rash develops, patient should be evaluated for DRESS**

• **Assess for blood dyscrasias:** fever, sore throat, bruising, rash, jaundice, epistaxis (long-term treatment only)

• Monitor blood studies: RBC, Hct, Hgb, reticulocyte counts weekly for 4 wk, then monthly; also check thyroid function tests, serum calcium, albumin, phosphorus, potassium

Patient/family education
• Teach patient the reason for and expected outcome of treatment

• Instruct patient not to use machinery or engage in hazardous activity; drowsiness, dizziness may occur

• Advise patient to carry/wear emergency ID identifying product used, name of prescriber

• Advise patient to notify prescriber of rash, bleeding, bruising, slurred speech, jaundice of skin or eyes, joint pain, nausea, vomiting, severe headache, depression, suicidal ideation

• Advise patient to keep all medical appointments, including lab work, physical assessment

• Advise patient to notify prescriber if pregnancy is planned or suspected; to use contraception with this product

Evaluation
Positive therapeutic outcome
• Decreased seizure activity

frovatriptan (Rx)
(froh-vah-trip′tan)
Frova
Func. class.: Antimigraine agent
Chem. class.: 5-HT$_1$ receptor agonist
Pregnancy category C

ACTION: Binds selectively to the vascular 5-HT$_{1B}$, 5-HT$_{1D}$ receptor subtypes, exerts antimigraine effect; binds to benzodiazepine receptor sites, causes vasoconstriction in cranium

Therapeutic outcome: Absence of migraines

USES: Acute treatment of migraine with or without aura

CONTRAINDICATIONS
Angina pectoris, history of MI, documented silent ischemia, Prinzmetal's angina, ischemic heart disease, concurrent ergotamine-containing preparations, uncontrolled hypertension, hypersensitivity, basilar or hemiplegic migraine; ischemic bowel disease; peripheral vascular disease, severe hepatic disease, prophylactic migraine treatment

Precautions: Pregnancy **C**, breastfeeding, children, geriatric, postmenopausal women, men >40 yr, risk factors for CAD, hypercholesterolemia, obesity, diabetes, impaired hepatic function, seizure disorder

DOSAGE AND ROUTES
Adult: PO 2.5 mg; a 2nd dose may be taken after ≥2 hr; max 3 tabs/day (7.5 mg)

Available forms: Tabs 2.5 mg

Implementation
• Ensure that tablets are swallowed whole

• Provide quiet, calm environment with decreased stimulation from noise, bright light, excessive talking

ADVERSE EFFECTS
CNS: *Hot sensation,* paresthesia, *dizziness,* headache, fatigue, cold sensation, insomnia, anxiety, somnolence, **seizures**

CV: *Flushing,* chest pain, palpitation
GI: Dry mouth, dyspepsia, abdominal pain, diarrhea, vomiting, nausea
MS: Skeletal pain

Pharmacokinetics

Absorption	Absolute bioavailability of PO dose ~20% in males, 30% in females
Distribution	Protein binding 15%; reversibly bound to blood cells at equilibrium 60%
Metabolism	Liver, by CYP1A2
Excretion	Urine (32%), feces (62%)
Half-life	25-29 hr

Pharmacodynamics

Onset	10 min-2 hr
Peak	2-4 hr
Duration	Unknown

INTERACTIONS
Individual drugs
Estrogen, propranolol: increased effects of frovatriptan

Drug classifications
CYP1A2 inhibitors (cimetidine, ciprofloxacin, erythromycin), oral contraceptives: increased frovatriptan levels

Selective serotonin reuptake inhibitors, other serotonin agonists (dextromethorphan, antidepressants): increased toxicity, MAOIs

NURSING CONSIDERATIONS
Assessment
• **Migraine:** aura, alleviating/exacerbating factor, diet, character
• Assess for ingestion of tyramine-containing foods (pickled products, beer, wine, aged cheese), food additives, preservatives, colorings, artificial sweeteners, chocolate, caffeine, which may precipitate these types of headaches
• Assess B/P; signs/symptoms of coronary vasospasms
• Assess for stress level, activity, recreation, coping mechanisms
• Assess neurologic status: LOC, paresthesia, hot/cold sensations, dizziness, headache, fatigue

Patient/family education
• Instruct patient to report any side effects to prescriber
• Advise patient to use contraception while taking product
• Advise patient that photosensitivity may occur, to use sunscreen and wear protective clothing when outdoors

• Advise patient to have dark, quiet environment available

Evaluation

Positive therapeutic outcome
• Decrease in frequency, severity of migraine

TREATMENT OF OVERDOSE:
No specific antidote; monitor patient closely for ≥48 hr, treat any symptoms as necessary

> **⚠ HIGH ALERT**
>
> ## fulvestrant (Rx)
> (full-ves′trant)
> **Faslodex**
> *Func. class.:* Antineoplastic
> **Pregnancy category D**

ACTION: Inhibits cell division by binding to competitive cytoplasmic estrogen receptors; resembles normal cell complex but inhibits DNA synthesis and estrogen response of target tissue

Therapeutic outcome: Decreased tumor size, spread of malignancy

USES: Advanced breast carcinoma in estrogen-receptor–positive patients (usually postmenopausal)

CONTRAINDICATIONS
Pregnancy **D**, breastfeeding, children, hypersensitivity

Precautions: Hepatic disease, jaundice, thrombocytopenia, biliary tract disease, coagulopathy

DOSAGE AND ROUTES
Adult: IM 500 mg as two 5-ml inj on days 1, 15, 29 and q mo thereafter

Available forms: Inj 50 mg/ml

Implementation
• Give IM 5 ml as one inj in each buttock slowly, over 1-2 min
• Give antacid before oral agent; give product after evening meal, before bedtime
• Give antiemetic 30-60 min before giving product to prevent vomiting
• Provide liquid diet, if needed, including cola, Jell-O; dry toast or crackers may be added if patient is not nauseated or vomiting
• Increase fluids to 2 L/day unless contraindicated
• Store in refrigerator, protect from light

ADVERSE EFFECTS
CNS: *Headache,* depression, dizziness, insomnia, paresthesia, anxiety

---

GI: *Nausea, vomiting,* anorexia, constipation, diarrhea, abdominal pain, hepatitis, hepatic failure, hyperbilirubinemia
HEMA: Anemia
INTEG: *Rash,* sweating, *hot flashes,* inj site pain
MS: Bone pain, arthritis, back pain
RESP: Pharyngitis, dyspnea, cough
SYST: Angioedema

Pharmacokinetics

Absorption	Unknown
Distribution	Unknown
Metabolism	CYP3A4
Excretion	Feces 90%
Half-life	40 days

Pharmacodynamics

Unknown

INTERACTIONS
Drug classifications
Anticoagulants: do not use concurrently; increased bleeding

Drug/lab test
Increased: LFTs

NURSING CONSIDERATIONS
Assessment
• Monitor for side effects, report to prescriber
• Monitor for anticoagulant use

Patient/family education
• Advise patient to report any complaints, side effects to prescriber
• Teach patient to increase fluids to 2 L/day unless contraindicated
• Advise patient to report vaginal bleeding immediately
• Teach patient that tumor flare—increase in size of tumor, increased bone pain—may occur and will subside rapidly; may take analgesics for pain
• **Teach patient to use contraception, pregnancy D**

Evaluation

Positive therapeutic outcome
• Decreased tumor size, decreased spread of malignancy

furosemide (Rx)
(fur-oh′se-mide)
Lasix
Func. class.: Loop diuretic
Chem. class.: Sulfonamide derivative
Pregnancy category C

Do not confuse: furosemide/torsemide, Lasix/Lanoxin/Lomotil/Losec/Luvox

ACTION: Acts on the ascending loop of Henle in the kidney, inhibiting reabsorption of electrolytes sodium and chloride, causing excretion of sodium, calcium, magnesium, chloride, water, and some potassium; decreases reabsorption of sodium and chloride and increases excretion of potassium in the distal tubule of the kidney; responsible for slight antihypertensive effect and peripheral vasodilatation

Therapeutic outcome: Decreased edema in lung tissue, peripherally; decreased B/P

USES: Pulmonary edema, edema in CHF, nephrotic syndrome, ascites, hepatic disease, hypertension

Unlabeled uses: Hypercalcemia in malignancy

CONTRAINDICATIONS
Anuria, hypovolemia

Precautions: Pregnancy C, diabetes mellitus, dehydration, severe renal disease, cirrhosis, ascites, hypersensitivity to sulfonamides, breastfeeding, infants, electrolyte depletion

DOSAGE AND ROUTES
Adult: PO 20-80 mg/day in AM, may give another dose in 6 hr, up to 600 mg/day; IM/IV 20-40 mg, increased by 20 mg q2hr until desired response
Child: PO/IM/IV 1-2 mg/kg, may increase by 1-2 mg/kg/q6-8hr up to 6 mg/kg

Antihypercalcemia
Adult: IM/IV 80-100 mg q1-4hr or PO 120 mg/day or divided bid
Child: IM/IV 25-50 mg, repeat q4hr if needed

Acute/chronic renal failure
Adult: PO 80 mg/day, increase by 80-120 mg/day to desired response; IV 100-200 mg, max 600-800 mg

Available forms: Tabs 20, 40, 80 mg; oral sol 8 mg/ml, 10 mg/ml; inj IM, IV 10 mg/ml

Implementation
• Give in AM to avoid interference with sleep
• Potassium replacement if potassium level is <3.0 mg/dl; product may be crushed if patient is unable to swallow
PO route
• With food or milk or use oral sol if nausea occurs; absorption may be reduced slightly

IV route
• Do not use sol that is yellow, has a precipitate or crystals

Adverse effects: *italics* = common; **bold** = life-threatening

IV, direct route
- Give undiluted through Y-tube on 3-way stopcock; give 20 mg or less/min

Intermittent IV inf route
- May be added to 0.9% NaCl, D₅W, use within 24 hr to ensure compatibility; give through Y-tube or 3-way stopcock; give at 4 mg/min or less, use inf pump

Y-site compatibilities: Acyclovir, alfentanil, allopurinol, alprostadil, amifostine, amikacin, aminocaproic acid, aminophylline, amphotericin B cholesteryl/lipid complex/liposome, anidulafungin, argatroban, ascorbic acid, atenolol, atropine, azaTHIOprine, aztreonam, bivalirudin, bleomycin, bumetanide, calcium chloride/gluconate, CARBOplatin, cefamandole, ceFAZolin, cefepime, cefonicid, cefotaxime, cefoTEtan, cefOXitin, cefTAZidime, ceftizoxime, ceftobiprole, cefTRIAXone, cefuroxime, chloramphenicol, CISplatin, cladribine, clindamycin, cyanocobalamin, cyclophosphamide, cycloSPORINE, cytarabine, DACTINomycin, DAPTOmycin, dexamethasone, dexmedetomidine, digoxin, DOCEtaxel, doripenem, doxacurium, DOXOrubicin liposome, enalaprilat, ePHEDrine, EPINEPHrine, etoposide, fentaNYL, fludarabine, fluorouracil, folic acid, foscarnet, gallium nitrate, ganciclovir, granisetron, heparin, hydrocortisone, HYDROmorphone, ifosfamide, imipenemcilastatin, indomethacin, insulin (regular), isosorbide, kanamycin, leucovorin, lidocaine, linezolid, LORazepam, LR, mannitol, mechlorethamine, melphalan, meropenem, methicillin, methotrexate, methylPREDNISolone, metoprolol, metroNIDAZOLE, mezlocillin, micafungin, miconazole, mitoMYcin, moxalactam, multiple vitamins injection, nafcillin, naloxone, nitroprusside, octreotide, oxacillin, oxaliplatin, oxytocin, PACLitaxel, palonosetron, pamidronate, pantoprazole, PEMEtrexed, penicillin G, PENTobarbital, PHENobarbital, phytonadione, piperacillin, piperacillin-tazobactam, potassium chloride, procainamide, propofol, propranolol, ranitidine, remifentanil, Ringer's, ritodrine, sargramostim, sodium acetate/bicarbonate, succinylcholine, SUFentanil, temocillin, teniposide, theophylline, thiopental, thiotepa, ticarcillin, ticarcillin-clavulanate, tigecycline, tirofiban, TNA, tobramycin, urokinase, vit B/C, voriconazole, zoledronic acid

Y-site incompatibilities: Amsacrine, bleomycin, DOXOrubicin, droperidol, esmolol, fluconazole, gentamicin, IDArubicin, metoclopramide, milrinone, netilmicin, ondansetron, quiNIDine, vinBLAStine, vinCRIStine

ADVERSE EFFECTS

CNS: Headache, fatigue, weakness, vertigo, paresthesias
CV: Orthostatic hypotension, chest pain, ECG changes, **circulatory collapse**
EENT: *Loss of hearing*, ear pain, tinnitus, blurred vision
ELECT: *Hypokalemia, hypochloremic alkalosis, hypomagnesemia, hyperuricemia, hypocalcemia, hyponatremia,* metabolic alkalosis
ENDO: *Hyperglycemia*
GI: *Nausea*, diarrhea, dry mouth, vomiting, anorexia, cramps, oral or gastric irritations, pancreatitis
GU: *Polyuria*, **renal failure**, *glycosuria*, bladder spasms
HEMA: **Thrombocytopenia, agranulocytosis**, leukopenia, neutropenia, anemia
INTEG: *Rash, pruritus, purpura*, **Stevens-Johnson syndrome**, sweating, photosensitivity, urticaria
MS: Cramps, stiffness
SYST: **Toxic epidermal necrolysis**

Pharmacokinetics

	PO
Absorption	GI tract (60%-70%)
	PO/IM/IV
Distribution	Crosses placenta
Metabolism	Liver (30%-40%)
Excretion	Breast milk, urine, feces
Half-life	½-1 hr

Pharmacodynamics

	PO	IM	IV
Onset	1 hr	½ hr	5 min
Peak	1-2 hr	Unknown	½ hr
Duration	6-8 hr	4-8 hr	2 hr

INTERACTIONS

Individual drugs
CISplatin, vancomycin: increased risk of ototoxicity
Digoxin: increased toxicity
Lithium: decreased renal clearance, causing increased toxicity
Probenecid: decreased furosemide effect

Drug classifications
Aminoglycosides: increased ototoxicity
Anticoagulants, salicylates: increased effects
Antihypertensives: increased antihypertensive effect
Nitrates: increased hypotensive action

Nondepolarizing skeletal muscle relaxants, **salicylates, aminoglycosides, CISplatin:** increased toxicity

Drug/lab test
Interference: GTT
Increase: LDL

NURSING CONSIDERATIONS
Assessment
• **Ototoxicity:** Assess patient for tinnitus, hearing loss, ear pain; periodic testing of hearing is needed when high doses of this product are given by **IV** route

• **Hypokalemia:** acidic urine, reduced urine osmolality, nocturia, polyuria and polydipsia; hypotension, broad T-wave, U-wave, ectopy, tachycardia, weak pulse; muscle weakness, altered LOC, drowsiness, apathy, lethargy, confusion, depression; anorexia, nausea, cramps, constipation, distention, paralytic ileus; hypoventilation, respiratory muscle weakness

• Monitor for CV, GI, neurologic manifestations of hyponatremia: increased B/P, cold, clammy skin, hypovolemia or hypervolemia; anorexia, nausea, vomiting, diarrhea, abdominal cramps; lethargy, increased ICP, confusion, headache, seizures, coma, fatigue, tremors, hyperreflexia

• Monitor for neurologic, respiratory manifestations of hyperchloremia: weakness, lethargy, coma; deep rapid breathing

• **CHF:** Assess fluid volume status: I&O ratios and record, count or weigh diapers as appropriate, weight, distended red veins, crackles in lung, color, quality, and specific gravity of urine, skin turgor, adequacy of pulses, moist mucous membranes, bilateral lung sounds, peripheral pitting edema; dehydration symptoms of decreasing output, thirst, hypotension, dry mouth and mucous membranes should be reported

• Monitor electrolytes: potassium, sodium, chloride, magnesium; also include BUN, blood pH, ABGs, uric acid, CBC, blood glucose

• **Hypertension:** Assess B/P before and during therapy lying, standing, and sitting as appropriate; orthostatic hypotension can occur rapidly

Patient/family education
• Teach patient to take the medication early in the day to prevent nocturia

• Instruct the patient to take with food or milk if GI symptoms of nausea and anorexia occur

• Teach patient to maintain a record of weight on a weekly basis and notify physician of weight loss of >5 lb

• Caution the patient that this product causes a loss of potassium, that food rich in potassium should be added to the diet; refer to a dietitian for assistance in planning

• Caution the patient to rise slowly from sitting or reclining positions, not to exercise in hot weather or stand for prolonged periods because orthostatic hypotension will be enhanced; lie down if dizziness occurs

• Advise patient to wear protective clothing and sunscreen to prevent photosensitivity

• Caution patient not to use alcohol or any OTC medications without physician's approval; serious product reactions may occur

• Emphasize the need to contact physician immediately if muscle cramps, weakness, nausea, dizziness, or numbness occurs

• Teach patient to take and record own B/P and pulse

• Advise patient to continue taking medication even if feeling better; this product controls symptoms but does not cure the condition

• Advise the patient with hypertension to continue other medical treatment (exercise, weight loss, relaxation techniques, cessation of smoking)

Evaluation
Positive therapeutic outcome
• Decreased edema
• Decreased B/P
• Lowered calcium level in malignancy
• Increased diuresis

gabapentin (Rx)

(gab'a-pen-tin)
Gralise, Horizant, Neurontin
Func. class.: Anticonvulsant
Chem. class.: GABA analogue
Pregnancy category C

Do not confuse: Neurontin/Noroxin/Neoral

ACTION: Mechanism unknown; may increase seizure threshold; structurally similar to GABA; gabapentin binding sites in neocortex, hippocampus

Therapeutic outcome: Decreased seizure activity

USES: Adjunct treatment of partial seizures, with or without generalization in patients >12 yr; adjunct in partial seizures in children 3-12 yr, postherpetic neuralgia, primary restless leg syndrome (RLS) in adults

Unlabeled uses: Tremors in multiple sclerosis, neuropathic pain, bipolar disorder, migraine prophylaxis, diabetic neuropathy

CONTRAINDICATIONS

Hypersensitivity to this product

Precautions: Pregnancy **C**, breastfeeding, children <3 yr, geriatric, renal disease, hemodialysis, suicidal thoughts, depression

DOSAGE AND ROUTES

Seizures with or without secondary generalized tonic-clonic seizures (Neurontin only)

Adult and child >12 yr: PO 900-1800 mg/day in 3 divided doses; may titrate to 1800 mg/day
Child 3-12 yr: PO 10-15 mg/kg/day in 3 divided doses, initially titrate dose upward over approximately 3 days; if >5 yr old, 40 mg/kg/day in 3 divided doses; all given in 3 divided doses

Postherpetic neuralgia

Adult: PO (Neurontin) 300 mg on day 1, 600 mg/day divided bid on day 2, 900 mg/day divided tid, may titrate to 1800-3600 mg divided tid if needed; ext rel tab (Gralise only) 300 mg on day 1, then 600 mg on day 2, 900 mg on days 3-6, 1200 mg on days 7-10, 1500 mg on days 11-14, 1800 mg on day 15 and thereafter; Horizant only: 600 mg in AM × 3 days, day 4 give 600 mg bid

Moderate to severe RLS (Horizant only)

Adult: PO ext rel tab 600 mg qd with food at about 5 PM; if dose is missed, take next day at 5 PM

Renal Dose

Adult and child >12 yr PO immediate release: CCr ≥ 60 ml/min: No change; CCr >30-59 ml/min: Total dose range 400-1400 mg/day given divided bid; CCr >15-29 ml/min: Total dose range 200-700 mg/day PO given in a single daily dose; CCr = 15 ml/min: Total dose range 100-300 mg/day given in one daily dose as 100, 125, 150, 200, or 300 mg; CCr <15 ml/min: Reduce daily dose in proportion to CCr (CCr = 7.5 ml/min should receive one-half the dose that patients with CCr of 15 ml/min receive) Adult: PO extended-release tablets (Gralise tablets only): CCr ≥ 60 ml/min: No change; CCr 30-59 ml/min: 600-1800 mg/day as tolerated; CCr <30 ml/min: Do not use; extended-release tablets (Horizant tablets only) CCr ≥ 60 ml/min: No change; before discontinuing reduce the dose to 600 mg q daily × 1 wk before discontinuing; CCr 30-59 ml/min: for RLS, start at 300 mg/day, increase to 600 mg/day as needed; for PHN, start at 300 mg in the AM × 3 days, then increase to 300 mg bid, increase to 600 mg bid as needed; for dose tapering prior to discontinuation, reduce the maintenance dose to q daily in the AM × 1 wk before discontinuing; CCr 15-29 ml/min: for RLS, 300 mg/day; for PHN, 300 mg PO on day 1 and day 3, then 300 mg q day in the AM, increase dose to 300 mg bid as needed; for dose tapering, if dose is 300 mg bid, reduce dose to 300 mg q day in AM ×1 wk before discontinuation; if the dose is 300 q day no taper is required; CCr < 15 ml/min: for RLS and PHN, 300 mg every other day; for PHN, dose can be increased to 300 mg q day in AM; no dose taper is required prior to discontinuing.

Available forms: Caps 100, 300, 400 mg; tabs 600, 800 mg; oral sol 250 mg/5 ml; Horizant: ext rel tab 300, 600 mg (Gralise)

Implementation

• Do not break, crush, or chew caps, ext rel tabs; cap may be opened and contents put in applesauce or dissolved in juice; scored tab may be cut in half
• Gradually withdraw over 7 days; abrupt withdrawal may precipitate seizures
• Give at least 2 hr apart when giving antacids; give without regard to meals; immediate release
• Store at room temperature away from heat and light
• Provide assistance with ambulation during early part of treatment; dizziness occurs
• **Provide seizure precautions:** padded side rails, move objects that may harm patient
• **Oral sol:** measure with calibrated device, refrigerate

- **Ext release:** give with food at about 5 PM, bioavailability is increased with food; **do not interchange Gralise with Horizant**

ADVERSE EFFECTS

CNS: *Drowsiness, confusion,* dizziness, fatigue, anxiety, somnolence, ataxia, amnesia, abnormal thinking, unsteady gait, depression; 3-12 yr old: emotional lability, aggression, thought disorder, hyperkinesia, hostility, **seizures, suicidal ideation,** impaired cognition, euphoria
CV: Vasodilatation, peripheral edema, hypotension, hypertension
EENT: Dry mouth, blurred vision, diplopia, nystagmus, conjunctivitis; otitis media (child 3-12 yr)
GI: Constipation/diarrhea, weight gain, increased appetite, dental abnormalities, nausea, vomiting; diarrhea (Gralise) G
GU: Impotence, bleeding, *UTI*; (Gralise)
HEMA: **Leukopenia, thrombocytopenia,** decreased WBC
INTEG: Pruritus, abrasion, **Stevens-Johnson syndrome,** acne vulgaris
MS: Myalgia, back pain, gout
RESP: Rhinitis, pharyngitis, coughing, upper respiratory infection (child 3-12 yr)
Syst: Drug reaction with eosinophilia and systemic symptoms (**DRESS**); dehydration (child 3-12 yr)

Pharmacokinetics

Absorption	Unknown
Distribution	Unknown
Metabolism	None
Excretion	Urine unchanged
Half-life	5-7 hr

Pharmacodynamics

	IMMEDIATE RELEASE	EXTENDED RELEASE
Onset	Unknown	Unknown
Peak	2 hr	8 hr-Gralise, 5-7 hr-Horizant
Duration	Unknown	Unknown

INTERACTIONS
Individual drugs
Alcohol: increased CNS depression
Cimetidine, sevelamer: decreased gabapentin levels
HYDROcodone: decreased effect of HYDROcodone

Drug classifications
Antacids: decreased gabapentin levels
Antihistamines, sedatives, all other CNS depressants: increased CNS depression

Drug/lab test
False positive: urinary protein using Ames N-multistix SG

NURSING CONSIDERATIONS
Assessment
- **Assess seizures: aura, location, duration, frequency, activity at onset**
- Assess renal studies: urinalysis, BUN, urine creatinine q3mo
- ⚠ **Assess mental status: mood, sensorium, affect, behavioral changes, suicidal thoughts/behaviors; if mental status changes, notify prescriber**
- Assess eye problems, need for ophth exam before, during, after treatment (slit lamp, fundoscopy, tonometry)
- Monitor WBC, gabapentin level (therapeutic 5.9-21 mcg/ml, toxic >85 mcg/ml), serum creatinine/BUN, weight
- Monitor for drug reaction with eosinophilia and systemic symptoms
- Provide increased fluids, bulk in diet for constipation

Patient/family education
- Advise patient to carry/wear emergency ID stating patient's name, products taken, condition, prescriber's name and phone number
- Advise patient to avoid driving, other activities that require alertness
- Teach patient not to discontinue medication quickly after long-term use, withdrawal-precipitated seizures may occur, not to double dose; if dose is missed, take if 2 hr or more before next dose
- Teach patient to gradually withdraw over 7 days; abrupt withdrawal may precipitate seizures
- Teach patient to use hard candy, gum, and frequent rinsing of mouth for dry mouth
- Teach patient to increase fluids, bulk in diet for constipation
- Advise patient to notify prescriber if pregnancy is planned or suspected, avoid breastfeeding
- Advise patient to take extended release product with food
- Advise patient to keep oral solution refrigerated

Evaluation
Positive therapeutic outcome
- Decreased seizure activity; document on patient's chart

TREATMENT OF OVERDOSE:
Lavage, VS

galantamine (Rx)

(gah-lan'tah-meen)
Razadyne, Razadyne ER, Reminyl ✚
Func. class.: Anti-Alzheimer's agent
Chem. class.: Cholinesterase inhibitor
Pregnancy category B

ACTION: Enhances cholinergic functioning by increasing acetylcholine

Therapeutic outcome: Decreased signs and symptoms of Alzheimer's dementia

USES: Mild to moderate dementia of Alzheimer's disease, vascular dementia, dementia with Lewy bodies

CONTRAINDICATIONS

Hypersensitivity to this product, children, GI bleeding, jaundice, renal failure

Precautions: Pregnancy **B**, respiratory/renal/hepatic/cardiac disease, seizure disorder, peptic ulcer, asthma, bradycardia, heart block, geriatric patients, surgery, urinary tract obstruction, breastfeeding

DOSAGE AND ROUTES

Adult: PO 4 mg bid with morning and evening meals; after 4 wk or more may increase to 8 mg bid; after another 4 wk may increase to 12 mg bid; usual dose 16-24 mg/day in 2 divided doses; EXT REL 8 mg/day in AM; may increase to 16 mg/day after 4 wk, and 24 mg/day after another 4 wk

Hepatic dose
Adult: (Child-Pugh 7-9) PO max 16 mg/day
Adult: (Child-Pugh 10-15) avoid PO use

Renal dose
Adult: PO CCr 10-70 ml/min; max 16 mg/day; CCr <9 ml/min: PO avoid use

Available forms: Tabs 4, 8, 12 mg; ext rel caps 8, 16, 24 mg; oral sol 4 mg/ml

Implementation

• Give with meals, morning and evening, ext rel product can be opened and sprinkled on food; do not crush/chew
• Dose increase after minimum of 4 wk at prior dose; if dose is interrupted for several days, restart at lower dose, titrate to current dose
• Provide assistance with ambulation during beginning therapy
• Perform complete suicide assessment
• Oral solution: use pipette provided; put in liquid and have patient consume

ADVERSE EFFECTS

CNS: *Tremors, insomnia,* depression, dizziness, headache, somnolence, fatigue

CV: Bradycardia, chest pain
GI: *Nausea, vomiting, anorexia, abdominal distress, flatulence,* diarrhea
GU: Urinary incontinence, bladder outflow obstruction, hematuria
HEMA: Anemia
META: Weight decrease
MS: Asthenia
RESP: URI, rhinitis

Pharmacokinetics

Absorption	Rapidly and completely absorbed
Distribution	18% protein binding
Metabolism	Liver
Excretion	Kidneys; clearance decreased in geriatric, hepatic/renal disease, females (20% lower)
Half-life	Elimination 7 hr

Pharmacodynamics

Onset	Unknown
Peak	1 hr
Duration	Unknown

INTERACTIONS
Drug classifications

Cholinesterase inhibitors, cholinomimetics: synergistic effect
CYP3A4/CYP2D6 inducers (bosentan, carBAMazepine, fosphenytoin, nevirapine, OXcarbazepine, phenytoin, rifabutin, rifampin, rifapentine, troglitazone), anticholinergics: decreased galantamine effect
CYP3A4/CYP2D6 inhibitors (antiretroviral protease inhibitors, clarithromycin, conivaptan, delaviridine, diltiazem, efavirenz, erythromycin, fluconazole, fluvoxaMINE, imatinib, itraconazole, ketoconazole, nefazodone, niCARdipine, troleandomycin, verapamil, voriconazole, zafirlukast): increased galantamine effect
NSAIDs: increased GI effects

Drug/herb

St. John's wort: decreased galantamine effect

NURSING CONSIDERATIONS
Assessment

• **Alzheimer's disease:** Assess mental status: affect, mood, behavioral changes, depression, memory, attention, confusion, cognitive functioning
• Assess liver function enzymes: AST, ALT, alkaline phosphatase, LDH, bilirubin, CBC
• Assess for severe GI effects: nausea, vomiting, anorexia, weight loss; GU effects: urinary retention, bladder obstruction

- Assess B/P, heart rate, respiration during initial treatment

Patient/family education
- Teach patient or caregiver correct procedure for giving oral sol, using instruction sheet provided
- Instruct patient or caregiver to notify prescriber of severe GI effects
- Instruct patient or caregiver to report hypo/hypertension, slow heart rate
- Teach patient to take with food to minimize side effects

Evaluation

Positive therapeutic outcome
- Decreased symptoms of dementia
- Increased coherence
- Improved cognitive performance (memory, orientation, attention, reasoning, language, praxis)

TREATMENT OF OVERDOSE:
Administer **IV** atropine titrated to effect at an initial dose of 0.5-1 mg, with subsequent doses based on clinical response; provide general supportive measures

ganciclovir (Rx)
(gan-sye′kloe-vir)
Cytovene, Vitrasert, Zirgan
Func. class.: Antiviral
Chem. class.: Synthetic nucleoside analog
Pregnancy category C

Do not confuse: Cytovene/Cytosar

ACTION: Inhibits replication of herpes viruses in vitro; competitively inhibits human cytomegalovirus (CMV) DNA polymerase and is incorporated, resulting in termination of DNA elongation

Therapeutic outcome: Decreased proliferation of virus responsible for CMV retinitis

USES: Cytomegalovirus (CMV) retinitis in immunocompromised persons, including those with AIDS, after indirect ophthalmoscopy confirms diagnosis; prophylaxis of CMV in transplantation

Unlabeled uses: CMV pneumonia in organ transplant patients, CMV gastroenteritis in patients with irritable bowel syndrome, CMV pneumonitis

CONTRAINDICATIONS
Hypersensitivity to acyclovir, famciclovir, penciclovir, valacyclovir, valganciclovir, or ganciclovir

> **BLACK BOX WARNING:** ANC <500/mm³, platelet count <25,000/mm³ (intravitreal)

Precautions: Pregnancy **C**, breastfeeding, children <6 mo, geriatric, preexisting cytopenias, renal function impairment, radiation therapy

> **BLACK BOX WARNING:** Secondary malignancy, bone marrow suppression, anemia, infertility, neutropenia

DOSAGE AND ROUTES
Induction treatment
Adult: IV 5 mg/kg/dose given over 1 hr q12hr × 2-3 wk

Maintenance treatment
Adult: IV INF 5 mg/kg/day given over 1 hr, daily × 7 days/wk; or 6 mg/kg/day × 5 days/wk; PO 1000 mg tid with food or 500 mg q3hr while awake; Intravitreal 4.5-mg implant

Prevention of CMV infection
Adult: IV 5 mg/kg/dose over 1 hr q12hr × 1-2 wk, then 5 mg/kg/day × 7 days/wk, then 6 mg/kg/day × 5 days/wk; PO 1000 mg tid, starting 10 days posttransplant × 14 days

Renal dose
Adult: IV CCr 50-69 ml/min, reduce to 2.5 mg/kg q12hr (induction), 2.5 mg/kg q24hr (maintenance); PO 1500 mg/day or 500 mg tid; IV CCr 25-49 ml/min reduce to 2.5 mg q24hr (induction); 1.25 mg/kg q24hr (maintenance); PO 1000 mg/day or 500 mg bid; IV CCr 10-24 ml/min reduce to 1.25 mg/kg q24hr (induction); 0.625 mg/kg q24hr (maintenance); PO 500 mg/day; IV CCr <10 ml/min reduce to 1.25 mg/kg 3×/wk after hemodialysis (induction); 0.625 mg/kg 3×/wk after hemodialysis (maintenance); PO 500 mg 3×/wk after hemodialysis

Available forms: Powder for inj 500 mg/vial, caps 250, 500 mg; implant, intravitreal 4.5 mg

Implementation
PO route
- Give with food, do not open or crush caps

IV route
- Product should be mixed under strict aseptic conditions using gloves, gown, and mask and using precautions for antineoplastics
Intermittent IV inf route
- Administer **IV** after reconstituting 500 mg/10 ml of sterile water for inj (50 mg/ml); shake; further dilute in 100 ml of D₅W, 0.9% NaCl, LR, Ringer's and run over 1 hr; use inf pump, in-line filter, flush line well before and after product
- Do not give by BOL **IV**, IM, SUBCUT inj
- Use reconstituted sol within 12 hr, do not refrigerate or freeze; do not use sol with

particulate matter or discoloration, fludarabine, sargramostim

Y-site compatibilities: Allopurinol, CISplatin, cyclophosphamide, enalaprilat, etoposide, filgrastim, fluconazole, gatifloxacin, granisetron, linezolid, melphalan, methotrexate, PACLitaxel, propofol, tacrolimus, teniposide, thiotepa

Y-site incompatibilities: Amsacrine, fludarabine, foscarnet, ondansetron, sargramostim, vinorelbine

Intravitreal implant route
• Implanted by surgeon only
• Handle carefully to prevent damage to coating

ADVERSE EFFECTS

CNS: *Fever,* chills, **coma,** *confusion,* abnormal thoughts, dizziness, bizarre dreams, *headache,* psychosis, tremors, somnolence, *paresthesia,* *weakness,* **seizures,** peripheral neuropathy
CV: Dysrhythmia, hypo/hypertension
EENT: Retinal detachment in CMV retinitis, cataracts, ocular hypertension, ocular pain, conjunctival scarring
GI: *Abnormal liver function tests, nausea, vomiting, anorexia, diarrhea, abdominal pain,* hemorrhage, perforation, pancreatitis
GU: Hematuria, *increased creatinine,* BUN
HEMA: **Granulocytopenia, thrombocytopenia, irreversible neutropenia, anemia, eosinophilia, pancytopenia**
INTEG: *Rash,* alopecia, *pruritus,* urticaria, pain at inj site, phlebitis
RESP: Dyspnea

Pharmacokinetics

Absorption	Completely absorbed, increased bioavailability with fatty foods
Distribution	Crosses blood-brain barrier, CSF
Metabolism	Not metabolized
Excretion	Kidneys (90%) unchanged, breast milk
Half-life	3 hr

Pharmacodynamics

Unknown

INTERACTIONS
Individual drugs
Adriamycin, amphotericin B, cycloSPORINE, dapsone, DOXOrubicin, flucytosine, mycophenolate, pentamidine, probenecid, tacrolimus, trimethoprim/sulfa combinations, vinBLAStine, vinCRIStine: increased ganciclovir toxicity

Didanosine: increased didanosine effect
Imipenem with cilastatin: increased risk for seizures
Probenecid: decreased renal clearance of ganciclovir
Radiation, zidovudine: severe granulocytopenia; do not give together
Tenofovir: increased effect

Drug classifications
Antineoplastics: severe granulocytopenia; do not give together
Nucleoside analogs, NSAIDs: increased toxicity

NURSING CONSIDERATIONS
Assessment
• **CMV retinitis:** Culture should be done before treatment with ganciclovir is initiated; cultures of blood, urine, and throat may all be taken; CMV is not confirmed by this method; the diagnosis is made by an ophthalmic exam
• Assess kidney, liver function; increases in hemopoietic studies: BUN, serum creatinine, AST creatinine clearance, ALT, A:G ratio, baseline, and drip treatment; blood counts should be done q2wk; watch for decreasing granulocytes, Hgb; if low, therapy may have to be discontinued and restarted after hematologic recovery; blood transfusions may be required
• Assess for GI symptoms: severe nausea, vomiting, diarrhea; severe symptoms may necessitate discontinuing product
• Monitor electrolytes and minerals: calcium, phosphorus, magnesium, sodium, potassium; watch closely for tetany during 1st administration
• Assess for symptoms of allergic reactions: flushing, rash, urticaria, pruritus

> **BLACK BOX WARNING: Monitor for leukopenia/neutropenia/thrombocytopenia:** WBCs, platelets q2day during 2 ×/day dosing and qwk thereafter; check for leukopenia with daily WBC count in patients with prior leukopenia with other nucleoside analogs or for whom leukopenia counts are <1000 cells/mm^3 at start of treatment; bruising, fatigue, bleeding, poor healing

• Assess for seizures, dysrhythmias

> **BLACK BOX WARNING:** Assess for secondary malignancy; avoid direct contact with powder in caps/solution; if skin contact occurs, wash thoroughly with soap and water; do not get in the eyes

Patient/family education

• Advise patient to notify prescriber if sore throat, swollen lymph nodes, malaise, fever occur; may indicate other infections
• Advise patient to report perioral tingling, numbness in extremities, and paresthesias
• Caution patient that serious product interactions may occur if OTC products are ingested; check first with prescriber
• Inform patient that product is not a cure, but will control symptoms
• Advise patient that regular blood tests, ophth exams must be continued
• Inform patient that major toxicities may necessitate discontinuing product
• **Instruct patient to use contraception during treatment and that infertility may occur; men should use barrier contraception for 90 days after treatment**
• Teach patient to take PO with food
• **Teach patient to report infection: fever, chills, sore throat; blood dyscrasias: bruising, bleeding, petechiae**
• Tell patient to avoid crowds, persons with respiratory infection
• Advise patient to use sunscreen to prevent burns
• Advise patient to report itching, redness, or eye pain

Evaluation

Positive therapeutic outcome
• Decreased symptoms of CMV infection

ganciclovir ophthalmic
See Appendix B

gatifloxacin ophthalmic
See Appendix B

⚠ HIGH ALERT

gemcitabine (Rx)
(gem-sit′a-been)
Gemzar
Func. class.: Antineoplastic—miscellaneous
Chem. class.: Pyrimidine analog
Pregnancy category D

Do not confuse: Gemzar/Zinecard

ACTION: Exhibits antitumor activity by killing cells undergoing DNA synthesis (S phase) and blocking G_1/S-phase boundary

Therapeutic outcome: Prevention of growth of tumor

USES: Adenocarcinoma of the pancreas (nonresectable stage II, III, or metastatic stage IV); in combination with CISplatin for inoperable, advanced, or metastatic non–small cell lung cancer; advanced breast cancer in combination with PACLitaxel; with CARBOplatin for ovarian cancer, biliary tract cancer

CONTRAINDICATIONS
Pregnancy **D**, breastfeeding, hypersensitivity

Precautions: Children, geriatric, myelosuppression, radiation therapy, renal/hepatic disease

DOSAGE AND ROUTES
Pancreatic carcinoma (nonresectable stage II, III, IV)
Adult: IV 1000 mg/m² given over ½ hr qwk × 7 wk, then 1 wk rest period; subsequent cycles should be infused once qwk × 3 wk out of every 4 wk depending on hematologic toxicity

Non–small cell lung cancer

4 wk schedule
Adult: IV 1000 mg/m² given over ½ hr on days 1, 8, 15 of each 28-day cycle; give CISplatin **IV** 100 mg/m² on day 1 after gemcitabine

3 wk schedule
Adult: IV 1250 mg/m² given over ½ hr on days 1, 8 of each 21-day cycle; give CISplatin 100 mg/m² after the INF of gemcitabine on day 1

Advanced breast cancer
Adult: IV 1250 mg/m² over ½ hr on days 1 and 8 of a 21-day cycle; give with PACLitaxel on day 1, 175 mg/m² over 3 hr prior to gemcitabine

Available forms: Lyophilized powder for inj 200 mg, 1 gm, 2 gm; solution for inj 1 gm/26.3 ml, 200 mg/ 5.26 ml, 2 gm/52.6 ml

Implementation
• Give increased fluid intake to 2-3 L/day to prevent dehydration, unless contraindicated
• Provide antiemetic agents before and after treatment

IV route
• Prepare in biological cabinet using gown, mask, gloves
• After reconstituting with 0.9% NaCl 5 ml/200 mg vial of product or 25 ml/1 g of product, shake (38 mg/ml); may be further diluted with 0.9% NaCl to concentrate as low as 0.1 mg/ml; discard unused portion, give over ½ hr, do not admix

Y-site compatibilities: Alemtuzumab, alfenfanil, allopurinol, amifostine, amikacin, aminophylline, ampicillin, anidulafugin, argatroban, aztreonam, bivalirudin, bleomycin, bumetanide,

*Adverse effects: italics = common; **bold** = life-threatening*

butorphanol, calcium gluconate, caspofungin, cefOXitin, cefTAZidime, ceftizoxime, cefTRIAXone, chlorproMAZINE, cimetidine, ciprofloxacin, CISplatin, clindamycin, cyclophosphamide, cytarabine, DACTINomycin, DAUNOrubicin, diphenhydrAMINE, DOBUTamine, DOCEtaxel, DOPamine, DOXOrubicin, droperidol, enalaprilat, etoposide, famotidine, floxuridine, fluconazole, fludarabine, fluorouracil, gentamicin, granisetron, haloperidol, heparin, hydrocortisone, HYDROmorphone, IDArubicin, ifosfamide, leucovorin, linezolid, LORazepam, mannitol, meperidine, mesna, metoclopramide, metroNIDAZOLE, minocycline, mitoXANtrone, morphine, nalbuphine, ondansetron, PACLitaxel, promethazine, ranitidine, streptozocin, teniposide, thiotepa, ticarcillin, tigecycline tobramycin, topotecan, trimethoprim/sulfamethoxazole, vancomycin, vinBLAStine, vinCRIStine, vinorelbine, voriconazole zidovudine, zoledronic acid

Y-site incompatibilities: Acyclovir, amphotericin B colloidal, amphotericin B lipid complex, amphotericin B liposome, cefepime, cefoperazone, cefotaxime, chloramphenicol, dantrolene, DAPTOmycin, diazepam, furosemide, ganciclovir, imipenem-cilastatin, irinotecan, ketorolac, lansoprazole, methotrexate, methylPREDNISolone, mitoMYcin, nafcillin, pantoprazole, PEMEtrexed, phenytoin, piperacillin, prochlorperazine, thiopental

ADVERSE EFFECTS
GI: Diarrhea, nausea, vomiting, anorexia, constipation, stomatitis, diarrhea, hepatotoxicity
GU: Proteinuria, hematuria
HEMA: Leukopenia, anemia, neutropenia, thrombocytopenia
INTEG: Irritation at site, rash, alopecia
MISC: Dyspnea, fever, hemorrhage, infection, flulike syndrome, paresthesia, peripheral edema, myalgia, capillary leak syndrome
RESP: Dyspnea, bronchospasm, pneumonitis

Pharmacokinetics

Absorption	Unknown
Distribution	Crosses placenta
Metabolism	Unknown
Excretion	Unknown
Half-life	42-379 min

Pharmacodynamics
Unknown

INTERACTIONS
Individual drug
Alcohol: increased bleeding

Drug classifications
Anticoagulants, NSAIDs, salicylates: increased bleeding
Antineoplastics, radiation: increased myelosuppression, diarrhea
Live virus vaccines: decreased antibody response

Drug/lab test
Increased: BUN, AST, ALT, alkaline phosphatase, bilirubin, creatinine

NURSING CONSIDERATIONS
Assessment
• **Bone marrow depression: monitor CBC, differential, platelet count before each dose; single agent: absolute granulocyte count >1000, and platelets >100,000, give complete dose; absolute granulocyte count 500-999, platelets 50,000-99,999, give 75%; absolute granulocyte count <500 or platelets <50,000, do not give; combination with PACLitaxel in breast cancer: absolute granulocyte count >1200 and platelets >75,000, give complete dose; absolute granulocyte count 1000-1199 or platelets 50,000-75,000, give 75%; absolute granulocyte 700-999 or platelets ≥50,000, give 50%; granulocyte count <700 or platelets <50,000, do not give; combination with CARBOplatin in ovarian cancer: absolute granulocyte count >1500 and platelet count >100,000, give complete dose; absolute granulocyte count 1000-1499 or platelets 75,000-99,999, give 75%; absolute granulocyte count <1000 or platelets <75,000, do not give**
• **Assess for blood dyscrasias:** bruising, bleeding, petechiae
• Monitor I&O, nutritional intake
• Monitor renal/hepatic studies before, during treatment; may increase AST, ALT, alkaline phosphatase, bilirubin, BUN, creatinine
• Assess food preferences: list likes, dislikes
• Assess buccal cavity for dryness, sores or ulceration, white patches, oral pain, bleeding, dysphagia
• Assess GI symptoms: frequency of stools; cramping
• **Capillary leak syndrome: Monitor for hemoconcentration, decreased albumin, B/P; discontinue**
• Assess signs of dehydration: rapid respirations, poor skin turgor, decreased urine output, dry skin, restlessness, weakness

Patient/family education
• Teach patient to rinse mouth tid-qid with water, club soda; brush teeth bid-tid with soft brush or cotton-tipped applicator for stomatitis; use unwaxed dental floss

---

- Advise patient to avoid foods with citric acid or hot or rough texture if stomatitis is present; to drink adequate fluids
- Advise patient to report stomatitis; any bleeding, white spots, ulcerations in mouth; tell patient to examine mouth daily, report symptoms
- Advise patient to report signs of anemia: fatigue, headache, faintness, shortness of breath, irritability; hematuria, dysuria
- Advise patient to use contraception during therapy and for 4 mo after (pregnancy D)
- Instruct patient to avoid use with NSAIDs, salicylates, alcohol; not to receive vaccinations during treatment
- Teach about possible hair loss and what can be done
- Advise to report flulike symptoms, swelling of feet/legs, bruising; bleeding of gums, blood in urine, stools, emesis
- Teach to avoid crowds, persons with known upper respiratory infections
- Advise patient to use electric razor

Evaluation

Positive therapeutic outcome
- Decrease in tumor size, decrease in spread of cancer, symptom relief

TREATMENT OF OVERDOSE:
Induce vomiting, provide supportive care

gemfibrozil (Rx)
(gem-fye′broe-zil)
Lopid
Func. class.: Antilipemic
Chem. class.: Fibric acid derivative
Pregnancy category C

Do not confuse: Lopid/Levbid/Slo-bid

ACTION: Inhibits biosynthesis of VLDL, decreases triglycerides production in the liver, increases HDLs

Therapeutic outcome: Decreased hepatic triglyceride production, VLDL; accelerates removal of cholesterol from liver

USES: Type IIb, IV, V hyperlipidemia as adjunct with diet therapy, hypertriglyceridemia

CONTRAINDICATIONS
Severe renal/hepatic disease, preexisting gallbladder disease, primary biliary cirrhosis, hypersensitivity

Precautions: Pregnancy **C**, breastfeeding, renal disease, cholelithiasis

DOSAGE AND ROUTES
Adult: PO 600 mg bid 30 min before meals

Hepatic/renal dose
Avoid use

Available forms: Tabs 600 mg; caps 300 mg ✦

Implementation
- Give 30 min before AM and PM meals

ADVERSE EFFECTS
CNS: Fatigue, vertigo, headache, paresthesia, dizziness, somnolence
GI: Nausea, vomiting, *dyspepsia, diarrhea, abdominal pain*
HEMA: Leukopenia, anemia, eosinophilia, thrombocytopenia
INTEG: Rash, urticaria, pruritus
MISC: Task perversion
MS: Myopathy, **rhabdomyolysis**
SYST: Angioedema, exfoliative dermatitis

Pharmacokinetics

Absorption	Well absorbed
Distribution	Unknown, plasma protein binding >95%
Metabolism	Liver, minimal
Excretion	Kidney, unchanged (70%), feces (6%)
Half-life	1½ hr

Pharmacodynamics

Onset	1-2 hr
Peak	1-2 hr
Duration	2-4 months

INTERACTIONS
Individual drugs
Do not use with repaglinide, simvastatin
Repaglinide: increased hypoglycemic effect
Warfarin: increased anticoagulant properties

Drug classifications
Bile acid sequestrants: decreased effect of gemfibrozil, separate by >2 hr
HMG-CoA reductase inhibitors: increased risk of myositis, myalgia, rhabdomyolysis
Sulfonylureas: increased hypoglycemic effect

Drug/lab test
Increased: liver function tests, CK, bilirubin, alkaline phosphatase
Decreased: Hgb, Hct, WBC, potassium

NURSING CONSIDERATIONS
Assessment
- **Hypercholesteremia:** Assess nutrition: fat, protein, carbohydrates; nutritional analysis should be performed by dietitian before treatment is initiated; monitor triglycerides, cholesterol, lipids baseline, during treatment;

Adverse effects: italics = common; **bold** = life-threatening

LDL and VLDL should be watched closely and if increased, product should be discontinued
• Assess renal, liver function tests, CBC, blood glucose if patient is on long-term therapy; if liver function test results increase, product should be discontinued; monitor hematologic and hepatic function
• Monitor bowel pattern daily; diarrhea may be a problem
• **Myopathy, rhabdomyolysis: Assess for muscle pain, tenderness; obtain baseline CPK: if elevated or if these occur, product should be discontinued**

Patient/family education
• Inform patient that compliance is needed for positive results to occur; not to double doses, take missed dose as soon as remembered unless almost time for next dose; that product may be discontinued if no improvement in 3 mo
• Caution patient to decrease risk factors: high-fat diet, smoking, alcohol consumption, lack of exercise
• Advise patient to notify prescriber if GI symptoms of diarrhea, abdominal or epigastric pain, nausea, vomiting occur; or if chills, fever, sore throat occur; also occurrence of muscle cramps, abdominal cramps, severe flatulence

Evaluation
Positive therapeutic outcome
• Decreased cholesterol levels, serum triglyceride and improved ratio with HDLs

gemifloxacin (Rx)
(gem-ah-flox'a-sin)
Factive
Func. class.: Antiinfective
Chem. class.: Fluoroquinolone
Pregnancy category C

ACTION: Inhibits DNA gyrase, which is an enzyme involved in replication, transcription, and repair of bacterial DNA

Therapeutic outcome: Negative C&S, decreasing symptoms of infection

USES: Acute bacterial exacerbation of chronic bronchitis caused by *Streptococcus pneumoniae, Haemophilus influenzae, Haemophilus parainfluenzae, Moraxella catarrhalis;* community-acquired pneumonia caused by *Streptococcus pneumoniae* including multi-product-resistant strains, *H. influenzae, M. catarrhalis, Mycoplasma pneumoniae, Chlamydia pneumoniae, Klebsiella pneumoniae*

CONTRAINDICATIONS
Hypersensitivity to quinolones

Precautions: Pregnancy **C,** breastfeeding, children, geriatric, hypokalemia, hypomagnesemia, renal disease, seizure disorders, excessive exposure to sunlight, psychosis, increased intracranial pressure, history of QT interval prolongation, dysrhythmias, myasthenia gravis, torsades de pointes

> **BLACK BOX WARNING:** Tendon pain/rupture, tendinitis

DOSAGE AND ROUTES
Adult: PO 320 mg/day × 5-7 days depending on type of infection

Renal dose
Adult: PO CCr ≤40 ml/min 160 mg q24hr

Available forms: Tabs 320 mg

Implementation
• Give with or without food
• Theophylline should not be used with this product; toxicity may result
• Administer 2 hr before or 3 hr after antacids, iron, zinc, or buffered products; 2 hr before sucralfate

ADVERSE EFFECTS
CNS: *Dizziness, headache,* somnolence, depression, insomnia, nervousness, confusion, agitation, **seizures, pseudotumor cerebri**
CV: QT prolongation, vasodilatation
EENT: Visual disturbances, retinal detachment
GI: Diarrhea, *nausea,* vomiting, anorexia, flatulence, heartburn, dry mouth; increased AST, ALT; constipation, abdominal pain, **pseudomembranous colitis**
GU: Crystalluria (rare), vaginitis, interstitial nephritis
INTEG: Rash, pruritus, urticaria, *photosensitivity*
SYST: Anaphylaxis, Stevens-Johnson syndrome, toxic epidermal necrolysis, exfoliative dermatitis

Pharmacokinetics
Absorption	Rapidly, bioavailability 71%
Distribution	Unknown
Metabolism	Unknown
Excretion	In urine as active product, metabolites
Half-life	4-12 hr

Pharmacodynamics
Onset	Unknown
Peak	$^1/_2$ hr
Duration	Unknown

INTERACTIONS
Individual drugs
Amoxapine, chloroquine, cloZAPine, dasatinib, dolasetron, dronedarone, droperidol, erythromycin, flecainide, haloperidol, lapatinib, maprotiline, methadone, octreotide, ondansetron, palonosetron, pentamidine, pimozide, propafenone, ranolazine, risperidone, sertindole, SUNItinib, tacrolimus, telithromycin, troleandomycin, vardenafil, vorinostat, ziprasidone: increased QT prolongation

Probenecid: may increase toxicity

Theophylline: toxicity; do not use concurrently

Drug classifications
Antacids containing aluminum, iron, magnesium, sucralfate, zinc: decreased absorption; give 2 hr before or 3 hr after meals

Antiarrhythmics (amiodarone, disopyramide, procainamide, quiNIDine, sotalol), antidepressants (tricyclics), b-blockers, halogenated/local anesthetics: may decrease effect, resulting in life-threatening dysrhythmias, QT prolongation

Drugs that increase QT prolongation: increased QT prolongation

NSAIDs: increased CNS stimulation

NURSING CONSIDERATIONS
Assessment
• Monitor renal, liver function tests: BUN, creatinine, AST, ALT, electrolytes
• Monitor I&O ratio; urine pH, <5.5 is ideal
• Assess CNS symptoms: insomnia, vertigo, headache, agitation, confusion

> **BLACK BOX WARNING: Tendon rupture**
> Assess for tendon pain, inflammation; if present discontinue use; more common with corticosteroids; discontinue immediately if tendon pain, inflammation occurs

⚠ Assess allergic reactions and anaphylaxis: rash, flushing, urticaria, pruritus, chills, fever, joint pain; may occur a few days after therapy begins; EPINEPHrine and resuscitation equipment should be available for anaphylactic reaction

• **Pseudomembranous colitis: Monitor bowel pattern daily; if severe diarrhea, fever, abdominal pain occurs, product should be discontinued**

• **Assess for overgrowth of infection:** perineal itching, fever, malaise, redness, pain, swelling, drainage, rash, diarrhea, change in cough, sputum

• **QT prolongation: Avoid use of quinolones in those with known QT prolongation;** females and those with ongoing proarrhythmic conditions (TdP) are at greater risk; monitor ECG and/or Holter monitoring if product is used

• **Toxic psychosis/pseudotumor cerebri: Assess for headache, blurred vision, neck/shoulder pain, nausea/vomiting, dizziness, tinnitus; discontinue immediately**

Patient/family education
• Advise patient that fluids must be increased to 2 L/day to avoid crystallization in kidneys
• Instruct patient that if dizziness or light-headedness occurs, to ambulate, perform activities with assistance
• Instruct patient to complete full course of product therapy
• Teach patient to contact prescriber if adverse reactions occur
• Teach patient to avoid iron- or mineral-containing supplements or aluminum/magnesium antacids within 2 hr before or 3 hr after dosing
• Advise patient that photosensitivity may occur and sunscreen should be used
• Advise patient to use frequent rinsing of mouth, sugarless candy or gum for dry mouth
• Teach patient to avoid other medication unless approved by prescriber

Evaluation
Positive therapeutic outcome
• Negative C&S, absence of signs/symptoms of infection

gentamicin (Rx)
(jen-ta-mye′sin)
Cidomycin ✹
Func. class.: Antiinfective
Chem. class.: Aminoglycoside
Pregnancy category C

ACTION: Interferes with protein synthesis in bacterial cell by binding to 30S ribosomal subunit, causing misreading of genetic code; inaccurate peptide sequence forms in protein chain, causing bacterial death

Therapeutic outcome: Bactericidal effects for the following organisms: *Pseudomonas aeruginosa, Proteus, Klebsiella, Serratia, Escherichia coli, Enterobacter, Citrobacter, Staphylococcus, Shigella, Salmonella, Acinetobacter, Bacillus anthracis*

USES: Severe systemic infections of CNS; respiratory, GI, and urinary tracts; bone; skin; soft tissues; caused by susceptible strains

CONTRAINDICATIONS
Hypersensitivity to this or other aminoglycosides

> **BLACK BOX WARNING:** Pregnancy **D**

Precautions: Breastfeeding, geriatric, neonates, pseudomembranous colitis

> **BLACK BOX WARNING:** Renal disease, hearing deficits, myasthenia gravis, Parkinson's disease, infant botulism, neuromuscular disease, tinnitus

DOSAGE AND ROUTES
Severe systemic infections
Adult: IV INF 3-6 mg/kg/day in 3 divided doses q8hr; IM 3-5 mg/kg/day in divided doses q8hr
Child: IV/IM 2-2.5 mg/kg q8hr

Neonate and infant: IV/IM 2.5 mg/kg q8-12hr

Neonate <1 wk: 2.5 mg/kg q12hr

Renal dose
Adult: IM/IV CCr 70-100 ml/min reduce dose by multiplying maintenance dose by 0.85, give q8-12hr; CCr 50-69 ml/min reduce dose as above, give q12hr; CCr 25-49 ml/min reduce as above, give q24hr; CCr <25 ml/min reduce as above, give based on serum concentrations

Renal dose: extend interval (unlabeled)
Adult: IV CCr 40-59 ml/min, 5-7 mg/kg q36hr; CCr 20-39 ml/min, 5-7 mg/kg q48hr; CCr <20 ml/min, 5-7 mg/kg once, then base on serial levels

Available forms: Inj 10, 40 mg/ml; premixed inj 40, 60, 70, 80, 90, 100, 120 mg/100 ml NS

Implementation

IM route
• Give inj deeply in large muscle mass; rotate sites
IV route
• Give in even doses around the clock; product must be given for 10-14 days to ensure organism death and prevent superinfection
• After diluting in 50-200 ml normal saline, D₅W, decrease volume of diluent in child; maintain 0.1% solution, run over ½-1 hr (adults), up to 2 hr (child). Give by intermittent inf, flush with 0.9% NaCl or D₅W after inf
• Separate aminoglycosides and penicillins by ≥1 hr
• Store in tight container

IV compatibility of gentamicin sulfate with: Alatrofloxacin, aldesleukin, alemtuzumab, alfentanil, alprostadil, amifostine, amikacin, aminocaproic acid, aminophylline, amiodarone, amsacrine, anidulafungin, argatroban, arsenic trioxide, ascorbic acid injection, asparaginase, atenolol, atracurium, atropine, aztreonam, benztropine, bivalirudin, bleomycin, bumetanide, buprenorphine, butorphanol, calcium chloride/gluconate, CARBOplatin, carmustine, caspofungin, cefamandole, ceFAZolin, cefepime, cefotaxime, cefOXitin, cefpirome, ceftaroline, cefTAZidime, ceftizoxime, cefTRIAXone, cefuroxime, chlorothiazide, chlorpheniramine, chlorproMAZINE, cimetidine, ciprofloxacin, cisatracurium, CISplatin, clarithromycin, clindamycin, cloxacillin, codeine, colistimethate, cyanocobalamin, cyclophosphamide, cycloSPORINE, cytarabine, DACTINomycin, DAPTOmycin, DAUNOrubicin citrate liposome, DAUNOrubicin hydrochloride, dexmedetomidine, dexrazoxane, digoxin, diltiazem, dimenhyDRINATE, diphenhydrAMINE, DOBUTamine, DOCEtaxel, dolasetron, DOPamine, doripenem, doxacurium, doxapram, DOXOrubicin hydrochloride, DOXOrubicin hydrochloride liposomal, doxycycline, edetate calcium disodium, edetate disodium, enalaprilat, EPHEDrine, EPINEPHrine, epirubicin, epoetin alfa, eptifibatide, ergonovine, ertapenem, erythromycin lactobionate, esmolol, etoposide, etoposide phosphate, famotidine, fenoldopam, fenta-NYL, fluconazole, fludarabine, fluorouracil, foscarnet, gallamine, gallium, gatifloxacin, gemcitabine, glycopyrrolate, granisetron, HYDROmorphone, hydrOXYzine, ifosfamide, imipenemcilastatin, irinotecan, isoproterenol, ketamine, ketorolac, labetalol, lactated Ringer's injection, lansoprazole, lepirudin, leucovorin, levofloxacin, lidocaine, lincomycin, linezolid, LORazepam, magnesium sulfate, mannitol, mechlorethamine, melphalan, meperidine, mephentermine sulfate, meropenem, mesna, metaraminol, methyldopa, methylprednisolone sodium succinate, metoclopramide, metoprolol, metroNIDAZOLE, midazolam, milrinone, minocycline, mitoXANtrone, mivacurium, morphine, multiple vitamins injection, mycophenolate mofetil, nafcillin, nalbuphine, nalorphine, naloxone, netilmicin, niCARdipine, nitroglycerin, nitroprusside, norepinephrine, octreotide, ondansetron, oritavancin, oxacillin, oxaliplatin, oxytocin, PACLitaxel (solvent/surfactant), palonosetron, pamidronate, pancuronium, papaverine, penicillin G potassium/sodium, pentazocine, perphenazine, PHENobarbital, phentolamine, phenylephrine, phytonadione, piperacillin, polymyxin B, posaconazole, potassium acetate/chloride, procainamide, prochlorperazine, promazine, promethazine, propranolol, protamine, pyridoxine, quiNIDine gluconate, ranitidine, remifentanil, Ringer's injection, riTUXimab, rocuronium, sargramostim, sodium acetate/bicarbonate/citrate, streptomycin, succinylcholine, SUFentanil, tacrolimus, telavancin, temocillin, teniposide, theophylline, thiamine, thiotepa, ticarcillin, ticarcillin-clavulanate, tigecycline, tirofiban, TNA (3-in-1), tobramycin, tolazoline, topotecan, TPN (2-in-1), trastuzumab, trimetaphan, tubocurarine, urokinase, vancomycin, vasopressin, vecuronium, verapamil, vinBLAStine, vinCRIStine, vinorelbine, vitamin B complex with C, voriconazole, zidovudine, zoledronic acid

ADVERSE EFFECTS

CNS: Confusion, depression, numbness, tremors, seizures, muscle twitching, neurotoxicity, dizziness, vertigo, encephalopathy, fever, headache, lethargy
CV: Hypotension, hypertension, palpitations, edema
EENT: Ototoxicity, deafness, visual disturbances, tinnitus
GI: *Nausea, vomiting, anorexia,* increased ALT, AST, bilirubin, hepatomegaly, hepatic necrosis, splenomegaly
GU: Oliguria, hematuria, renal damage, azotemia, renal failure, nephrotoxicity, proteinuria
HEMA: Agranulocytosis, thrombocytopenia, leukopenia, eosinophilia, anemia
INTEG: *Rash,* burning, urticaria, dermatitis, alopecia, photosensitivity, anaphylaxis
MS: Twitching, myasthenia gravis–like symptoms
RESP: Apnea

Pharmacokinetics

Absorption	Well absorbed (IM)
Distribution	Distributed in extracellular fluids, poorly distributed in CSF; crosses placenta
Metabolism	Liver, minimal
Excretion	Mostly unchanged (79%) kidneys
Half-life	1-2 hr; infants 6-7 hr; increased in renal disease

Pharmacodynamics

	IM	IV
Onset	Rapid	Rapid
Peak	30-90 min	Infusion's end
Duration	Unknown	Unknown

INTERACTIONS
Individual drugs

> **BLACK BOX WARNING:** Acyclovir, amphotericin B, cidofovir, CISplatin, cycloSPORINE, ethacrynic acid, foscarnet, furosemide, ganciclovir, mannitol, methoxyflurane, pamidronate, polymyxin, tacrolimus, vancomycin, zoledronic acid: increased ototoxicity, neurotoxicity, nephrotoxicity

Drug classifications

> **BLACK BOX WARNING:** Aminoglycosides, cephalosporins, penicillins: increased otoxicity, neurotoxicity, nephrotoxicity

Nondepolarizing neuromuscular blockers: increased neuromuscular blockade, respiratory depression
Penicillins: Do not use at the same time as or physically mix with penicillins

Drug/lab test
Increase: LDH, AST, ALT, bilirubin, BUN, creatinine, eosinophils
Decrease: Hgb, WBC, platelets, granulocytes

NURSING CONSIDERATIONS
Assessment
• Assess patient for previous sensitivity reaction
• **Assess patient for signs and symptoms of infection** including characteristics of wounds, sputum, urine, stool, WBC >10,000/mm^3, fever; obtain baseline during treatment

> **BLACK BOX WARNING: Neuromuscular disease (myasthenia gravis, Parkinson's disease, infant botulism):** Assess for paresthesias, tetany, Chvostek's/Trousseau's signs, confusion (adults) tetany, muscle weakness (infants); correct electrolyte imbalance

• Complete C&S before beginning product therapy; this will ensure that correct treatment has been initiated
• **Assess for allergic reactions:** rash, urticaria, pruritus, chills, fever, joint pain may occur a few days after therapy begins

> **BLACK BOX WARNING: Renal disease:** Identify urine output; if decreasing, notify prescriber (may indicate nephrotoxicity); also, increased BUN, creatinine, urine CCr <80 ml/min; monitor I&O ratio; urinalysis daily for proteinuria, cells, casts; report sudden change in urine output; assess urine pH if product is used for UTI; urine should be kept alkaline

G

• Monitor blood studies: AST, ALT, CBC, Hct, bilirubin, LDH, alkaline phosphatase, Coombs' test monthly if patient is on long-term therapy
• Monitor electrolytes: potassium, sodium, chloride, magnesium monthly if patient is on long-term therapy
• Monitor for bleeding: ecchymosis, bleeding gums, hematuria; assess stool guaiac daily if on long-term therapy
• **Assess for overgrowth of infection:** perineal itching, fever, malaise, redness, pain, swelling, drainage, rash, diarrhea, change in cough, sputum
• Obtain weight before treatment; calculation of dosage is usually based on ideal body weight but may be calculated on actual body weight
• Monitor VS during inf, watch for hypotension, change in pulse
• Assess **IV** site for thrombophlebitis including pain, redness, swelling q30min, change site if needed; apply warm compresses to discontinued site
• Obtain serum peak, measured at 30-60 min after **IV** inf or 60 min after IM inj, trough level measured just before next dose; blood level should be 2-4 times bacteriostatic level (based on traditional dosing)

> BLACK BOX WARNING: **Assess for deafness** by audiometric testing, ringing, roaring in ears, vertigo; assess hearing before, during, after treatment

• Assess for dehydration: high specific gravity, decrease in skin turgor, dry mucous membranes, dark urine

Patient/family education
• Teach patient to report sore throat, bruising, bleeding, joint pain; may indicate blood dyscrasias (rare)
• Advise patient to contact prescriber if vaginal itching, loose foul-smelling stools, furry tongue occur; may indicate superimposed infection
• Teach patient to drink adequate fluids
• Teach patient to avoid hazardous activities until reaction is known

> BLACK BOX WARNING: Advise patient to report loss of hearing, ringing, roaring in ears; feeling of fullness in the head

Evaluation
Positive therapeutic outcome
• Absence of signs/symptoms of infection (WBC <10,000/mm^3, temp WNL, absence of red, draining wounds)
• Reported improvement in symptoms of infection

TREATMENT OF OVERDOSE: Withdraw product, hemodialysis

gentamicin ophthalmic
See Appendix B

gentamicin topical
See Appendix B

▲ HIGH ALERT
glatiramer (Rx)
(glah-teer'a-mer)
Copaxone
Func. class.: Multiple sclerosis agent
Pregnancy category B

ACTION: Unknown; may modify the immune responses responsible for multiple sclerosis (MS)

Therapeutic outcome: Decreased symptoms of MS

USES: Reduction of the frequency of relapses in patients with relapsing-remitting MS after first clinical episode with MRI results consistent with MS

CONTRAINDICATIONS
Hypersensitivity to this product or mannitol

Precautions: Pregnancy **B**, breastfeeding, children <18 yr, immune disorders, renal disease

DOSAGE AND ROUTES
Adult: SUBCUT 20 mg/day; **20 mg/ml and 40 mg/ml are not interchangeable** (20 mg/ml solution); 40 mg (40 mg/ml solution) 3 × per wk, give ≥ 48 hr apart

Available forms: Inj premixed 20 mg/ml, 40 mg/ml

Implementation
SUBCUT route
• Refrigerate
• Use a sterile syringe/needle to transfer the supplied diluent into the vial, rotate vial gently, do not shake; withdraw medication using a syringe with 27-G needle; administer SUBCUT into hip, thigh, arm; discard unused portion
• Use SUBCUT route only; do not give IM or **IV**, do not expel air bubble in prefilled syringe
• Do not use sol that contains precipitate or is discolored
• Give 40-mg dose on same 3 days of the week, must be 48 hr apart

ADVERSE EFFECTS
CNS: Anxiety, hypertonia, tremor, vertigo, speech disorder, agitation, confusion, flushing

CV: Migraine, syncope, tachycardia, vasodilatation, chest pain, hypertension
EENT: Ear pain, blurred vision
GI: Nausea, vomiting, diarrhea, anorexia, gastroenteritis
GU: Urgency, dysmenorrhea, vaginal moniliasis
HEMA: Ecchymosis, lymphadenopathy
INTEG: Pruritus, rash, sweating, urticaria, erythema, injection site reaction
META: Edema, weight gain
MS: Arthralgia, back pain, neck pain, increased muscle tone
RESP: Bronchitis, dyspnea, laryngismus, rhinitis

Pharmacokinetics
Unknown

Pharmacodynamics
Unknown

INTERACTIONS
Individual drugs: Denosumab, natalizumab, roflumilast: increased serious infection
Leflunomide: increased toxicity

Drug classifications: Avoid use with live virus vaccines

Drug/Herb
Echinacea: decreased glatiramer effect

NURSING CONSIDERATIONS
Assessment
• Monitor blood, renal, liver function tests before treatment
• Assess for CNS symptoms: anxiety, confusion, vertigo
• Assess GI status: diarrhea, vomiting, abdominal pain, gastroenteritis
• Assess cardiac status: tachycardia, palpitations, vasodilatation, chest pain

Patient/family education
• Give written, detailed instructions about the product; provide initial and return demonstrations on inj procedure; give information on use and disposal of product
• Advise patient that blurred vision, sweating may occur
• Advise patient that irregular menses, dysmenorrhea, or metorrhagia as well as breast pain may occur; use contraception during treatment
• Advise patient to notify prescriber if pregnancy is suspected or if nursing
• Advise patient not to change dosing or to stop taking product without advice of prescriber
• That the 20 mg/ml and 40 mg/ml are not interchangeable

Evaluation
Positive therapeutic outcome
• Decreased symptoms of multiple sclerosis

> **⚠ HIGH ALERT**
>
> **glimepiride (Rx)**
> (gly-meh′pih-ride)
> **Amaryl**
> **glipiZIDE (Rx)**
> (glip-i′zide)
> **Glucotrol, Glucotrol XL**
> *Func. class.:* Antidiabetic
> *Chem. class.:* Sulfonylurea
> (2nd generation)
> **Pregnancy category C**

Do not confuse: glipiZIDE/glucotrol/glyBURIDE

ACTION: Causes functioning β cells in pancreas to release insulin, leading to drop in blood glucose levels; may improve insulin binding to insulin receptors or increase the number of insulin receptors with prolonged administration; may also reduce basal hepatic glucose secretion; not effective if patient lacks functioning β cells

Therapeutic outcome: Decrease in polyuria, polydipsia, polyphagia, clear sensorium, absence of dizziness, stable gait

USES: Type 2 diabetes mellitus

CONTRAINDICATIONS
Hypersensitivity to sulfonylureas/sulfonamides, type 1 diabetes, diabetic ketoacidosis

Precautions: Pregnancy **C**, geriatric, cardiac disease, severe renal/hepatic disease, G6PD deficiency

DOSAGE AND ROUTES
Glimepiride
Adult: PO 1-2 mg/day with breakfast, then increase by ≤2 mg/day at q1-2wk, max 8 mg/day
Geriatric: PO 1 mg/day, may increase if needed

Renal/Hepatic dose
Adult: PO 1 mg/day with breakfast, may titrate upward as needed

GlipiZIDE
Adult: PO 5 mg initially before breakfast, then increase by 2.5-5 mg after several days, to desired response; max 40 mg/day in divided doses or 15 mg/dose; (XL) PO 5 mg/day with breakfast, may increase to 10 mg/day; max 20 mg/day
Geriatric: PO 2.5 mg/day, may increase if needed

Adverse effects: *italics* = common; **bold** = life-threatening

Hepatic dose
Adult: PO 2.5 mg initially, then increase to desired response; max 40 mg/day in divided doses or 15 mg/dose

Available forms: Glimepiride: tabs 1, 2, 4 mg; glipiZIDE: tabs 5, 10 mg scored; EXT REL tabs 2.5, 5, 10 mg

Implementation
- Do not break, crush, or chew ext rel tabs
- Convert from other oral hypoglycemic agents or insulin dosage of <40 units/day; change may be made without gradual dosage change
- Patients taking >40 units/day of insulin convert gradually by receiving oral hypoglycemic agents and 50% of previous insulin dosage for 3-5 days
- Monitor serum or urine glucose and ketones 3 ×/day during conversion
- **GlipiZIDE:** 30 min before meals (regular release); with breakfast (ext rel)
- **Glimepiride:** with breakfast; if patient is NPO, may need to hold dose to prevent hypoglycemia
- Give tab crushed and mixed with meal or fluids for patients with difficulty swallowing
- For severe hypoglycemia give **IV** D$_{50}$W, then **IV** dextrose solution
- Store in tight container in cool environment

ADVERSE EFFECTS
CNS: *Headache, weakness, dizziness, drowsiness,* tinnitus, fatigue, vertigo
ENDO: Hypoglycemia
GI: Hepatotoxicity, cholestatic jaundice, nausea, vomiting, diarrhea, heartburn
HEMA: Leukopenia, thrombocytopenia, agranulocytosis, aplastic anemia, increased AST, ALT, alkaline phosphatase, pancytopenia, hemolytic anemia
INTEG: Rash, allergic reactions, pruritus, urticaria, eczema, photosensitivity, erythema, allergic vasculitis
SYST: Serious hypersensitivity

Pharmacokinetics

Absorption	Completely absorbed, GI tract
Distribution	Unknown
Metabolism	Liver
Excretion	Via kidneys
Half-life	2-4 hr; 5 hr glimepiride

Pharmacodynamics

	glipiZIDE	glimepiride
Onset	1-1½ hr	
Peak	1-2 hr	2-3 hr
Duration	10-12 hr	

INTERACTIONS
Individual drugs
Charcoal, cholestyramine, diazoxide, isoniazid, rifampin: possible decreased action of glipiZIDE

Chloramphenicol, cimetidine, clarithromycin, clofibrate, fenfluramine, fluconazole, gemfibrozil, guanethidine, insulin, methyldopa, phenylbutazone, probenecid, sulfinpyrizine, voriconazole: increased hypoglycemia

Digoxin: increased action of digoxin, cycloSPORINE

Drug classifications
Androgens, anticoagulants, fibric acid derivatives, H$_2$-antagonists, magnesium salts, MAOIs, NSAIDs, salicylates, sulfonamides, tricyclics, urinary acidifiers: increased hypoglycemia
β-Blockers: may mask symptoms of hypoglycemia
Diuretics (thiazide), corticosteroids, hydantoins, colesevelam, urinary alkalinizers: possible decreased action of glipiZIDE
Glycosides: increased action of glycosides

Drug/herb
Garlic, horse chestnut: increased antidiabetic effect
Chromium: decreased antidiabetic effect
Chromium, coenzyme Q10, fenugreek, ginseng: increased or decreased hypoglycemic effect
Green tea: decreased hypoglycemic effect

Drug/lab test
Increase: AST, ALT, LDH, BUN, creatinine

NURSING CONSIDERATIONS
Assessment
- **Assess for hypoglycemic/hyperglycemic reactions** that can occur soon after meals; hypoglycemic reactions (sweating, weakness, dizziness, anxiety, tremors, hunger); hyperglycemic reactions; A1c (baseline, q3mo) during treatment
- **Blood dyscrasias:** Monitor CBC

Patient/family education
- **Teach patient to check for symptoms of cholestatic jaundice: dark urine, pruritus, yellow sclera; if these occur, prescriber should be notified**
- Teach patient to use capillary blood glucose test
- Teach patient to report bleeding, bruising, weight gain, edema, SOB, weakness, sore throat, swelling in ankles, rash
- Teach patient symptoms of hypo/hyperglycemia, what to do about each
- Instruct patient that product must be continued on daily basis; explain consequence of discontinuing product abruptly

• Caution patient to avoid OTC medications unless approved by a prescriber
• Teach patient that diabetes is a lifelong illness; that this product is not a cure
• Teach patient to avoid alcohol; inform about disulfiram reaction (nausea, headache, cramps, flushing, hypoglycemia)
• Instruct patient that all food included in diet plan must be eaten to prevent hypoglycemia
• Advise patient to use sunscreen or stay out of the sun to prevent burns
• Advise patient to carry/wear emergency ID and carry a glucagon emergency kit for emergency purposes; also prescriber name, phone number, and medications taken
• Teach patient ext rel tab may appear in stool

Evaluation

Positive therapeutic outcome
• Decrease in polyuria, polydipsia, polyphagia; clear sensorium; absence of dizziness; stable gait
• Improved serum glucose, A1c

⚠ HIGH ALERT

glyBURIDE (Rx)
(glye´byoor-ide)
DiaBeta, Euglucon ✦, Glynase PresTab
Func. class.: Antidiabetic
Chem. class.: Sulfonylurea (2nd generation)
Pregnancy category C

Do not confuse: glyBURIDE/Glucotrol/ glipiZIDE, DiaBeta/Zebeta

ACTION: Causes functioning β cells in pancreas to release insulin, leading to drop in blood glucose levels; may improve insulin binding to insulin receptors and increase number of insulin receptors with prolonged administration; may also reduce basal hepatic glucose secretion; not effective if patient lacks functioning β cells

Therapeutic outcome: Decrease in polyuria, polydipsia, polyphagia, clear sensorium, absence of dizziness, stable gait

USES: Type 2 diabetes mellitus

CONTRAINDICATIONS
Hypersensitivity to sulfonylureas, type 1 diabetes, diabetic ketoacidosis, renal failure

Precautions: Pregnancy **C**, geriatric, cardiac/thyroid disease, severe renal/hepatic disease, severe hypoglycemic reactions, sulfonamide/sulfonylurea hypersensitivity, G6PD deficiency

DOSAGE AND ROUTES
DiaBeta
Adult: PO 1.25-5 mg initially, then increased to desired response at weekly intervals up to 20 mg/day; may be given as a single or divided dose
Geriatric: PO 1.25 mg initially, then increased to desired response; max 20 mg/day, maintenance 1.25-20 mg/day

Glynase PresTab (micronized)
Adult: PO 1.5-3 mg/day initially, may increase by 1.5 mg/wk, max 12 mg/day
Geriatric: PO 0.75-3 mg/day, may increase by 1.5 mg/wk

Available forms: Tabs (DiaBeta) 1.25, 2.5, 5 mg; tabs micronized (Glynase PresTab) 1.5, 3, 6 mg

Implementation
• Conversion from other oral hypoglycemic agents or insulin dosage of <40 units/day; change may be made without gradual dosage change
• Patients taking >40 units/day of insulin convert gradually by receiving oral hypoglycemic agents and 50% of previous insulin dosage for 3-5 days
• Monitor serum or urine glucose and ketones 3 ×/day during conversion
• Give product 30 min before breakfast; if large dose is required, may be divided into two; give with meals to decrease GI upset and provide best absorption; if patient is NPO, may need to hold dose to avoid hypoglycemia, take at same time each day
• Give tab crushed and mixed with meal or fluids for patients with difficulty swallowing
• For severe hypoglycemia, give **IV** D$_{50}$W, then **IV** dextrose sol
• Store in tight container in cool environment

ADVERSE EFFECTS
CNS: *Headache, weakness,* paresthesia, tinnitus, fatigue, vertigo
EENT: Blurred vision
ENDO: Hypoglycemia
GI: Nausea, fullness, heartburn, **hepatoxicity, cholestatic jaundice,** vomiting, diarrhea, **hepatic failure** (rare)
HEMA: **Leukopenia, thrombocytopenia, agranulocytosis, aplastic anemia,** increased AST, ALT, alkaline phosphatase
INTEG: Rash, allergic reactions, pruritus, urticaria, eczema, photosensitivity, erythema
MS: Joint pains, vasculitis

Pharmacokinetics

Absorption	Completely absorbed GI tract
Distribution	99% plasma protein binding
Metabolism	Liver
Excretion	Urine, feces (metabolites), crosses placenta
Half-life	10 hr

Pharmacodynamics

Onset	2 hr
Peak	2-4 hr
Duration	24 hr

INTERACTIONS
Individual drugs
Bosentan: increased LFTs, avoid concurrent use

Charcoal, cholestyramine, isoniazid, rifampin thyroid: decreased action of glyBURIDE

Clarithromycin, chloramphenicol, fenfluramine, fluconazole, gemfibrozil, guanethidine, insulin, methyldopa, phenylbutazone, probenecid, sulfinpyrazone: increased hypoglycemia

Colesevelam: increased triglyceride levels

CycloSPORINE: increased action of cycloSPORINE

Diazoxide: both products may have action decreased

Digoxin: increased level

Drug classifications
Androgens, anticoagulants, antidepressants (tricyclics), β-blockers, H₂-antagonists, magnesium salts, MAOIs, NSAIDs, salicylates, sulfonamides, urinary acidifiers: increased hypoglycemia, voriconazole

β-Adrenergic blockers: increased masking of symptoms of hypoglycemia

Diuretics (thiazide), hydantoins, urinary alkalinizers, corticosteroids, phenothiazines, oral contraceptives, estrogens: decreased action of glyBURIDE

Drug/herb
Garlic, horse chestnut: increased antidiabetic effect

Green tea: decreased hypoglycemic effect

Drug/lab test
Increased: AST, ALT, LDH, BUN, creatinine, alkaline phosphatase

Decrease: Hgb, sodium, glucose, platelets, WBC

NURSING CONSIDERATIONS
Assessment
• Assess for hypo/hyperglycemic reactions that can occur soon after meals; hypoglycemic reactions (sweating, weakness, dizziness, anxiety, tremors, hunger); hyperglycemic reactions; A1c (baseline, q3mo) during treatment

• Blood dyscrasias: Monitor CBC, check liver function tests periodically, AST, LDH, and renal studies: BUN, creatinine during treatment

Patient/family education
• Teach patient to check for symptoms of cholestatic jaundice: dark urine, pruritus, yellow sclera; if these occur, prescriber should be notified

• Teach patient to use capillary blood glucose test

• Teach patient symptoms of hypo/hyperglycemia, what to do about each

• Instruct patient that product must be continued on daily basis; explain consequence of discontinuing product abruptly

• Teach patient to report bleeding, bruising, weight gain, edema, shortness of breath, weakness, sore throat

• Teach patient to take product in AM to prevent hypoglycemic reactions at night

• Caution patient to avoid OTC medications unless approved by a prescriber

• Teach patient that diabetes is a lifelong illness; that this product is not a cure

• Instruct patient that all food included in diet plan must be eaten to prevent hypoglycemia

• Advise patient to carry/wear emergency ID and carry a glucagon emergency kit for emergency purposes: have sugar packets available; also prescriber name, phone number, and medications

• Advise patient to use sunscreen or stay out of the sun to prevent burns

Evaluation
Positive therapeutic outcome
• Decrease in polyuria, polydipsia, polyphagia; clear sensorium; absence of dizziness; stable gait

• Improved serum glucose, A1c

golimumab (Rx)
(goal-lim'yu-mab)
Simponi, Simponi Aria
Func. class.: Antirheumatic agent (disease modifying), immunomodulator
Chem. class.: Monoclonal antibody, DMARDS, tumor necrosis factor (TNF) modifier
Pregnancy category B

ACTION: Monoclonal antibody specific for human tumor necrosis factor (TNF); elevated levels of TNF are found in patients with rheumatoid arthritis

Therapeutic outcome: Decreased pain, decreased inflammation in joints, better ROM

USES: Rheumatoid arthritis, ankylosing spondylitis, psoriatic arthritis, ulcerative colitis

CONTRAINDICATIONS
Hypersensitivity active infections

Precautions: Pregnancy **B,** breastfeeding, children, geriatric patients, CNS demyelinating disease, Guillain-Barré syndrome, CHF, hepatitis B carriers, blood dyscrasias, surgery, MS, neurological disease, diabetes, immunosuppression

BLACK BOX WARNING: Infection

DOSAGE AND ROUTES
Rheumatoid arthritis
Adult: SUBCUT 50 mg qmo; for RA give with methotrexate; IV (Simponi Aria only) 2 mg/kg over 30 min, repeat in 4 wk, then q8wk; give with methotrexate

Ankylosing spondylitis/psoriatic arthritis
Adult: SUBCUT 50 mg monthly

Ulcerative colitis
Adult: SUBCUT 200 mg for 1 dose, then 100 mg in 2 wk; maintenance 100 mg q4wk starting at wk 6

Available forms: Inj 50 mg/0.5 ml, 100 mg/ml prefilled syringe, SmartJect Auto Injector; inj 50 mg/4 ml single-use vial

Implementation
SUBCUT route
• Refrigerate; do not freeze; allow to warm to room temp before using
• Visually inspect solution for particulate or discoloration, solution should be clear to slightly opalescent and colorless to slightly yellow; there may be tiny white particles; do not shake
• *SmartJect autoinjector:* Allow to reach room temperature for 30 min prior to use, remove cap, inject within 5 min of removing cap, do not put cap back on, place the open end against the inj site at a 90-degree angle, without pushing button, push the injector firmly against the skin, press the button once and release, listen for the first click, wait for the second click or 15 sec, and remove the injector; do not rub site
• *Prefilled syringe:* Allow to warm to room temperature for 30 min, remove needle cover by pulling straight off, do not twist or recap, inject within 5 min of needle cover removal, hold the syringe in one hand like a pencil and use the other to pinch the skin, inject needle at a 45-degree angle, push plunger down as far as it will go, keep pressure on the plunger head and

remove needle from skin, remove pressure from the plunger head, the needle guard will cover the needle, do not rub site

IV route (Simponi Aria)
• Calculate number of vials needed; do not shake; dilute total volume of product in NS to yield 100 ml for infusion, slowly add product, mix gently
• Infuse over 30 min; use infusion set with in-line, sterile, non-pyrogenic, low-protein binding filter (≤0.22 mm pore size)

ADVERSE EFFECTS
CNS: Dizziness, paresthesia, **CNS demyelinating disorder**, weakness
CV: Hypertension, **CHF**
GI: **Hepatitis**
HEMA: **Agranulocytosis, aplastic anemia, leukopenia, polycythemia, thrombocytopenia, pancytopenia**
INTEG: Psoriasis
MISC: **Increased risk of cancer**, antibody development to this drug, **risk of infection (TB, invasive fungal infections, other opportunistic infections); may be fatal**, inj site reactions

Pharmacokinetics

Absorption	Unknown
Distribution	Unknown
Metabolism	Unknown
Excretion	Unknown
Half-life	Terminal 2 wk

Pharmacodynamics
Unknown

INTERACTIONS
Individual drugs
Abatacept, adalimumab, anakinra, etanercept, immunosuppressants, inFLIXimab, rilonacept, riTUXimab: increased infection
Warfarin, cycloSPORINE, theophylline: dosage change may be needed

Drug classifications
Live vaccines: do not give concurrently; immunization should be brought up to date before treatment

Drug/lab tests
Increase: LFTs
Decrease: Platelets, WBC

NURSING CONSIDERATIONS
Assessment
• **Assess for pain,** stiffness, ROM, swelling of joints during treatment

• Check for inj site pain, swelling; usually occur after 2 inj (4-5 days)

> **BLACK BOX WARNING: Check for infections** (fever, flulike symptoms, dyspnea, change in urination, redness/swelling around any wounds), stop treatment if present; some serious infections including sepsis may occur, may be fatal; patients with active infections should not be started on this product

• **Blood dyscrasias:** CBC, differential before and periodically during treatment

> **BLACK BOX WARNING: TB:** Obtain TB skin test before starting treatment; treat latent TB before starting therapy

> **BLACK BOX WARNING: Neoplastic disease:** May occur in those <18 yr; avoid use in those with known malignancies

• **CHF:** Monitor B/P, pulse, edema, shortness of breath
• **Psoriasis:** May occur or worsen; LFTs, hepatitis B serology, may reactivate HBV

Patient/family education
• Teach patient about self-administration if appropriate: inj should be made in thigh, abdomen, upper arm; rotate sites at least 1 inch from old site; do not inject in areas that are bruised, red, hard
• Advise patient that if medication is not taken when due, inject next dose as soon as remembered and inject next dose as scheduled

> **BLACK BOX WARNING:** Teach patient to report signs, symptoms of infection, allergic reaction, or lupuslike syndrome

Evaluation
Positive therapeutic outcome
• Decreased inflammation, pain in joints

goserelin (Rx)
(goe′se-rel-lin)
Zoladex
Func. class.: Gonadotropin-releasing hormone, antineoplastic
Chem. class.: Synthetic decapeptide analog of LHRH
Pregnancy category D (breast cancer), X (endometriosis)

ACTION: Inhibitor of pituitary gonadotropin secretion; initially increases LH and FSH, with increases in testosterone, reduction in sex steroid levels (substitute serum testosterone levels)

Therapeutic outcome: Decrease in tumor size and spread of malignant cells

USES: Advanced prostate cancer Stage B2-C (10.8 mg); endometriosis, advanced breast cancer, endometrial thinning (3.6 mg)

CONTRAINDICATIONS
Pregnancy **D** (breast cancer), **X** (endometriosis), breastfeeding, nondiagnosed vaginal bleeding, children, 10.8 mg dose in women, hypersensitivity to LHRH, LHRH-agonist analogs

Precautions: Spinal cord decompression, renal disease, bone mineral density loss

DOSAGE AND ROUTES
Adult: SUBCUT 3.6 mg q4wk (implant) or 10.8 mg q12wk

Endometrial thinning
Adult: SUBCUT 1-2 depot inj (usually 1 depot, surgery performed at 4 wk); (if 2 depots, surgery performed 2-4 wk after 2nd depot)

Available forms: Depot inj 3.6, 10.8 mg

Implementation
Depot
• Give SUBCUT using implant, inserted by qualified person into upper subcutaneous tissue in abdominal wall q28days or q12wk (10.8 mg), do not attempt to remove air bubbles from syringe

ADVERSE EFFECTS
CNS: Headaches, spinal cord compression, anxiety, depression, dizziness, insomnia, lethargy, hot flashes, emotional lability
CV: Dysrhythmia, cerebrovascular accident, hypertension, MI, chest pain, CHF; sudden cardiac death, stroke (men)
ENDO: Gynecomastia, breast tenderness, hot flashes; hyperglycemia, diabetes (men)
GI: Nausea, vomiting, constipation, diarrhea, ulcer
GU: *Spotting, breakthrough bleeding, decreased libido,* renal insufficiency, urinary obstruction, urinary tract infection, impotence
INTEG: Rash, pain on inj, diaphoresis
MS: Osteoneuralgia
RESP: *COPD, URI*

Pharmacokinetics

Absorption	Well absorbed
Distribution	Unknown
Metabolism	Unknown
Excretion	Unknown
Half-life	4½ hr

Pharmacodynamics

Onset	Unknown
Peak	14-28 days
Duration	Treatment length

INTERACTIONS
Drug/lab test
Increased: alkaline phosphatase, estradiol, FSH, LH
Decreased: progesterone

NURSING CONSIDERATIONS
Assessment
• **Reproductive studies:** monitor pelvic ultrasound, pelvic exam, PSA, serum estradiol/testosterone, pregnancy test prior to therapy
• Monitor I&O ratios; palpate bladder for distention in urinary obstruction
• **Cancer metastases:** monitor for relief of bone pain (back pain), change in motor function
• Blood studies: monitor acid phosphatase; calcium in breast/prostate cancer, hypercalcemia may occur

Patient/family education
• Caution patient that gynecomastia and postmenopausal symptoms may occur but will decrease after treatment is discontinued; that bone pain may increase, then decrease, may use analgesics
• Teach patient to contact prescriber for difficulty urinating, hot flashes occur during treatment
• Advise patient not to breastfeed while taking product; use effective nonhormonal contraception
• **Advise patient to notify prescriber if chest pain, weakness, difficulty breathing occur; may indicate MI or stroke**

Evaluation
Positive therapeutic outcome
• More normal levels of PSA, acid phosphatase, alkaline phosphatase; testosterone level of <25 mg/dl

granisetron (Rx)
(grane-iss′e-tron)
Granisol, Kytril ✦, Sancuso
Func. class.: Antiemetic
Chem. class.: 5-HT$_3$ receptor antagonist
Pregnancy category B

ACTION: Prevents nausea, vomiting by blocking serotonin peripherally, centrally, and in the small intestine

Therapeutic outcome: Absence of nausea and vomiting

USES: Prevention of nausea, vomiting associated with cancer chemotherapy including high-dose CISplatin, radiation

Unlabeled uses: Acute nausea, vomiting after surgery

CONTRAINDICATIONS
Hypersensitivity to this product or benzyl alcohol

Precautions: Pregnancy **B**, breastfeeding, children, geriatric, ondansetron/palonosetron/dolasetron hypersensitivity, cardiac dysrhythmias, cardiac/hepatic disease/GI, electrolyte imbalances

DOSAGE AND ROUTES
Nausea, vomiting in chemotherapy
Adult and child ≥2 yr: IV 10 mcg/kg over 5 min, 30 min before the start of cancer chemotherapy, TD apply 1 patch (3.1 mg/24 hr) to upper arm 24-48 hr before chemotherapy; patch may be worn up to 7 days
Adult: PO 1 mg bid, give 1st dose 1 hr before chemotherapy and next dose 12 hr after 1st or 2 mg as a single dose anytime within 1 hr prior to chemotherapy

Nausea, vomiting in radiation therapy
Adult: PO 2 mg/day 1 hr prior to radiation

Available forms: Inj 0.1 mg/ml, 1 mg/ml; tabs 1 mg, oral sol 2 mg/10 ml; patch TD 3.1 mg/24 hr

Implementation
PO route
• Give dose 1 hr prior to chemotherapy/radiation and another dose 12 hr after the first
• **Transdermal:** Apply to clean, dry skin on upper arm q24-48hr prior to chemotherapy

IV route
• May give undiluted over 30 sec via Y-site
IV intermittent infusion route
• Dilute in 0.9% NaCl for inj or D$_5$W (20-50 ml), give over 5-15 min, ½ hr prior to chemotherapy
• Store at room temp for 24-hr dilution

Y-site compatibilities: Acetaminophen, alemtuzumab, alfentamil, allopurinol, amifostine, amikacin, aminophylline, amphotericin B cholesteryl, ampicillin, ampicillin/sulbactam, amsacrine, aztreonam, bleomycin, bumetanide, buprenorphine, butorphanol, calcium gluconate, CARBOplatin, carmustine, ceFAZolin, cefepime, cefonicid, cefotaxime, cefoTEtan, cefOXitin, cefTAZidime, ceftizoxime, cefTRIAXone, cefuroxime, chlorproMAZINE, cimetidine, ciprofloxacin, CISplatin, cladribine, clindamycin, cyclophosphamide, cytarabine, dacarbazine,

Adverse effects: *italics* = common; **bold** = life-threatening

G

DACTINomycin, DAUNOrubicin, dexamethasone, diphenhydrAMINE, DOBUTamine, DOPamine, DOXOrubicin, DOXOrubicin liposome, doxycycline, droperidol, enalaprilat, etoposide, famotidine, filgrastim, floxuridine, fluconazole, fluorouracil, fludarabine, furosemide, gallium, ganciclovir, gentamicin, haloperidol, heparin, hydrocortisone, HYDROmorphone, hydrOXYzine, IDArubicin, ifosfamide, imipenem-cilastatin, leucovorin, LORazepam, magnesium sulfate, melphalan, meperidine, mesna, methotrexate, methylPREDNISolone, metoclopramide, metroNIDAZOLE, mezlocillin, miconazole, minocycline, mitoMYcin, mitoXANtrone, morphine, nalbuphine, netilmicin, ofloxacin, PACLitaxel, piperacillin, piperacillin/tazobactam, plicamycin, potassium chloride, prochlorperazine, promethazine, propofol, ranitidine, sargramostim, sodium bicarbonate, streptozocin, teniposide, thiotepa, ticarcillin, ticarcillin/clavulanate, tobramycin, trimethoprim/sulfamethoxazole, vancomycin, vinBLAStine, vinCRIStine, vinorelbine, voriconazole, zidovudine, zoledronic acid

Y-site incompatibilities: Amphotericin B coloidal, diazepam, phenytoin

Solution compatibilities: D$_5$W, 0.9% NaCl

Transdermal route
• Apply to dry, clean, intact skin of upper, outer arm 24 hr prior to chemotherapy; firmly press on skin; keep on during chemotherapy; can bathe; avoid swimming, whirlpool; remove ≥24 hr after chemotherapy

ADVERSE EFFECTS
CNS: *Headache, asthenia,* anxiety, dizziness, EPS (rare)
CV: Hypertension, QT prolongation
GI: Diarrhea, *constipation,* increased AST, ALT, *nausea*
HEMA: Leukopenia, anemia, thrombocytopenia
MISC: Rash, bronchospasm

Pharmacokinetics
Absorption	Unknown
Distribution	Unknown
Metabolism	Liver
Excretion	Unknown
Half-life	10-12 hr

Pharmacodynamics
Unknown

INTERACTIONS
Individual drugs
Amoxapine, arsenic, chloroquine, cloZAPine, dasatinib, dolasetron, dronedarone, droperidol, erythromycin, flecainide, fluconazole, haloperidol, lapatinib, maprotiline, methadone, octreotide, ondansetron, palonosetron, pentamidine, pimozide, posaconazole, propafenone, ranolazine, risperiDONE, sertindole, SUNItinib, tacrolimus, telithromycin, troleandomycin, vardenafil, vorconizole, vorinostat, ziprasidone: increased QT prolongation

Drug classifications
Antipsychotics: increased EPS
β-blockers, class I, III antidysrhythmics, halogenated/local anesthetics, phenothiazines, tricyclics: increased QT prolongation

NURSING CONSIDERATIONS
Assessment
• Assess patient for absence of nausea, vomiting during chemotherapy
• **Assess patient for hypersensitive reaction:** rash, bronchospasm

Extrapyramidal symptoms
Grimacing, shuffling gait, tremors, involuntary movements, rare

QT prolongation
Monitor ECG in those with heart disease, renal disease, or the elderly

Patient/family education
• Advise patient to report diarrhea, constipation, rash, or changes in respirations

Evaluation
Positive therapeutic outcome
• Absence of nausea, vomiting during cancer chemotherapy

guaiFENesin (Rx, OTC)

(gwye-fen´e-sin)

Alfen, Altarussin, Balminil ✹, Benylin Chest Congestion Extra Strength ✹, Benylin E ✹, Bismutal ✹, Bronchophan, Expectorant ✹, Calmylin Expectorant ✹, Cough Syrup Expectorant ✹, Diabetic Tussin, Expectorant Syrup ✹, Guiatuss, Jack & Jill ✹, Miltuss EX, Mucinex, Naldecon Senior EX, Organidin NR, Robitussin GuaiFENesin ✹, Scot-Tussin Expectorant, Siltussin DAS, Siltussin SA, Vicks Chest Congestion Relief ✹, Vicks DayQuil Mucus Control ✹

Func. class.: Expectorant

Pregnancy category C

ACTION: Increases the volume and reduces the viscosity of secretions in the trachea and bronchi to facilitate secretion removal

Therapeutic outcome: Decreased cough

USES: Productive and nonproductive cough

CONTRAINDICATIONS

Hypersensitivity, chronic persistent cough

Precautions: Pregnancy **C,** breastfeeding, CHF, asthma, emphysema, fever

DOSAGE AND ROUTES

Adult and child ≥12 yr: PO 200-400 mg q4hr, or EXT REL 600-1200 mg q12hr; max 2.4 g/day
Child 6-11 yr: PO 100-200 mg q4hr or EXT REL 600 mg q12hr; max 1.2 g/day
Child 2-5 yr: PO: 50-100 mg q4hr; max 600 mg/day, EXT REL 300 mg q12hr, max 600 mg/day

Available forms: Tabs 100, 200, 400 mg; ext rel tabs 600, 1200 mg; syr 100 mg/5 ml; oral sol 100 mg/5 ml; oral granules 50, 100 mg/packet; caps 200 mg; liquid 100, 200 mg/5 ml

Implementation

• Store at room temperature; provide room humidification to assist with liquefying secretions
• Avoid fluids for ½ hr after administration

ADVERSE EFFECTS

CNS: Drowsiness, headache, dizziness
GI: Nausea, anorexia, vomiting, diarrhea

Pharmacokinetics

Absorption	Well absorbed
Distribution	Unknown
Metabolism	Unknown
Excretion	Unknown
Half-life	1 hr

Pharmacodynamics

	PO	PO–EXT REL
Onset	½ hr	Unknown
Peak	Unknown	Unknown
Duration	4-6 hr	12 hr

NURSING CONSIDERATIONS

Assessment

• **Assess cough:** type, frequency, character, including characteristics of sputum; lung sounds bilaterally; fluids should be increased to 2 L/day to decrease secretion viscosity (thickness)

Patient/family education

• Caution patient to avoid driving, other hazardous activities if drowsiness occurs (rare)
• Advise patient to avoid smoking, smoke-filled rooms, perfumes, dust, environmental pollutants, cleansers
• Instruct patient to notify prescriber if dry, nonproductive cough lasts over 7 days

Evaluation

Positive therapeutic outcome

• Absence of dry cough
• Thinner, more productive cough that raises secretions

Adverse effects: *italics* = common; **bold** = life-threatening

halcinonide topical
See Appendix B

haloperidol (Rx)
(hal-oh-pehr'ih-dol)
haloperidol decanoate (Rx)
haloperidol lactate (Rx)
Haldol
Func. class.: Antipsychotic/neuroleptic
Chem. class.: Butyrophenone
Pregnancy category C

Do not confuse: haloperidol/Halotestin

ACTION: Depresses cerebral cortex, hypothalamus, limbic system, which control activity and aggression; blocks neurotransmission produced by dopamine at synapse; exhibits strong α-adrenergic, anticholinergic blocking action; mechanism for antipsychotic effects unclear

Therapeutic outcome: Decreased signs and symptoms of psychosis

USES: Psychotic disorders, control of tics, vocal utterances in Tourette's syndrome, short-term treatment of hyperactive children showing excessive motor activity, prolonged parenteral therapy in chronic schizophrenia, organic mental syndrome with psychotic features, emergency sedation of severely agitated or delirious patients, ADHD

Unlabeled uses: Nausea, vomiting in chemotherapy, hiccups, autism, migraine headache

CONTRAINDICATIONS
Children <3 yr, hypersensitivity, coma, Parkinson's disease, CNS depression

Precautions: Pregnancy **C,** breastfeeding, geriatric, seizure disorders, hypertension, hepatic/cardiac/pulmonary disease, prostatic hypertrophy, hyperthyroidism, thyrotoxicosis, blood dyscrasias, brain damage, bone marrow depression, alcohol and barbiturate withdrawal states, angina, epilepsy, urinary retention, closed-angle glaucoma

> **BLACK BOX WARNING:** Dementia; increased mortality in elderly patients with dementia-related psychosis

DOSAGE AND ROUTES
Acute psychosis
Adult: IM/IV (lactate) 2-10 mg, may repeat q1hr, convert to **PO** as soon as possible, **PO** should be 150% of total parenteral dose required

Child 6-12 yr: IM/IV (lactate) (unlabeled) 1-3 mg q4-8hr, max 0.15 mg/kg/day, switch to **PO** as soon as possible

Chronic psychosis
Adult: IM (decanoate) 50-100 mg q4wk, max 100 mg for 1st inj
Child 3-12 yr: PO/IM 0.05-0.15 mg/kg/day

Tourette's syndrome
Adult and adolescent: PO 0.5-2 mg bid-tid, increased until desired response occurs
Elderly: PO 0.5-2 mg bid-tid; may increase gradually
Child 3-12 yr or weighing 15-40 kg: PO 0.25-0.5 mg/day in 2-3 divided doses, increase by 0.25-0.5 mg q5-7days, max 0.15 mg/kg/day

Prevention of chemotherapy related to nausea and vomiting (unlabeled)
Adult: PO 1-2 mg q4-6hr

Hiccups (unlabeled)
Adult: PO 0.5-2 mg bid-tid or SUBCUT 5-10 mg/day

Autism (unlabeled)
Child: PO 0.04 mg/kg/day or 1-3 mg/day, max 4 mg/day

Available forms: Tabs 0.5, 1, 2, 5, 10, 20 mg; **lactate:** oral sol 2 mg/ml; inj 5 mg/ml; **decanoate:** 50 mg/ml, 100 mg/ml

Implementation
PO route—oral liquid
• Give product in liquid form mixed in glass of juice or caffeine-free cola if hoarding is suspected; do not mix in caffeine drinks, tannics, pectins
• Give decreased dosage in geriatric because of slower metabolism
• Give PO with full glass of water, milk; or give with food to decrease GI upset
• Give antacids 2 hr before or after this product
• Store in tight, light-resistant container; oral sol in amber bottle
• Avoid skin contact with oral susp or sol: may cause contact dermatitis
IM route
• Inject in deep muscle mass, do not give SUBCUT; use 21-gauge 2-in needle; do not administer sol with a precipitate; give <3 ml per inj site; give slowly, may be painful
• Patient should remain lying down after IM inj for at least 30 min

IV route (lactate) (unlabeled)
• Give undiluted for psychotic episode at 5 mg/min
• Only use lactate for IV
• Closely monitor ECG for QT prolongation

• Switch to oral as soon as possible if needed; give first PO dose within 12-24 hr of last parenteral dose

Y-site compatibilities: Alcohol 10%, dextrose 5%, alemtuzumab, Amifostine, Aminocaproic acid, amiodarone, amphotericin B liposome (AmBisome), Amsacrine, anidulafungin, argatroban, Arsenic trioxide, Asparaginase, atenolol, azithromycin, bleomycin, Cangrelor, CARBOplatin, carmustine, Caspofungin, ceftaroline, cisatracurium, CISplatin, Cladribine, cloNIDine, codeine phosphate, cyclophosphamide, cytarabine, DACTINomycin, DAPTOmycin, DAUNOrubicin liposome, DAUNOrubicin, Dexmedetomidine, Dexrazoxane, diltiazem, DOCEtaxel, dolasetron, Doxacurium, DOXOrubicin, DOXOrubicin liposomal, epirubicin, eptifibatide, ertapenem, etoposide, etoposide phosphate, fenoldopam, filgrastim, Fludarabine, gatifloxacin, gemcitabine, granisetron, HYDROmorphone, IDArubicin, ifosfamide, irinotecan, Ketamine, lepirudin, leucovorin, levofloxacin, linezolid, LORazepam, mechlorethamine, melphalan, Mesna, methadone, metroNIDAZOLE, milrinone, MitoXANtrone, Mivacurium, morphine, moxifloxacin, mycophenolate mofetil, nesiritide, niCARDipine, octreotide, oritavancin, oxaliplatin, PAClitaxel (solvent/surfactant), palonosetron, pamidronate, pancuronium, PEMEtrexed, potassium acetate, propofol, Quinupristin-Dalfopristin, remifentanil, riTUXimab, rocuronium, Sodium acetate, tacrolimus, Teniposide, Thiotepa, tigecycline, tirofiban, topotecan, TPN (2-in-1), vecuronium, vinBLAStine, vinCRIStine, vinorelbine, voriconazole, zoledronic acid

Y-site incompatibilities: Fluconazole, foscarnet, heparin, sargramostim

ADVERSE EFFECTS
CNS: *EPS, pseudoparkinsonism, akathisia, dystonia, tardive dyskinesia, drowsiness, headache,* **seizures, neuroleptic malignant syndrome,** confusion
CV: *Orthostatic hypotension,* hypertension, **cardiac arrest,** ECG changes, **tachycardia, QT prolongation, sudden death**
EENT: Blurred vision, glaucoma, dry eyes
GI: *Dry mouth, nausea, vomiting, anorexia, constipation,* diarrhea, jaundice, weight gain, **ileus, hepatitis**
GU: Urinary retention, urinary frequency, dysuria, enuresis, impotence, amenorrhea, gynecomastia
INTEG: *Rash,* photosensitivity, dermatitis
RESP: **Laryngospasm,** dyspnea, **respiratory depression**
SYST: **Risk of death (dementia)**

Pharmacokinetics
Absorption	Well absorbed (PO, IM); decanoate (IM) absorbed slowly
Distribution	High concentrations in liver, crosses placenta, protein binding 92%
Metabolism	Liver, extensively
Excretion	Kidneys, breast milk
Half-life	Terminal half-life 12-36 hr (metabolized)

Pharmacodynamics
	PO	IM	IM (decanoate)
Onset	Erratic	½ hr	3-9 days
Peak	2-6 hr	30-45 min	4-11 days
Duration	8-12 hr	4-8 hr	3 wk

INTERACTIONS
Individual drugs
Alcohol: increased effects of both products, oversedation

Amoxapine, chloroquine, cloZAPine, dasatinib, dolasetron, dronedarone, droperidol, erythromycin, flecainide, lapatinib, maprotiline, methadone, octreotide, ondansetron, palonosetron, pentamidine, pimozide, propafenone, ranolazine, risperiDONE, sertindole, SUNItinib, tacrolimus, telithromycin, troleandomycin, vardenafil, vorinostat, ziprasidone: increased QT prolongation, usually with IV use

CarBAMazepine: decreased effects of haloperidol

EPINEPHrine: increased toxicity

Levodopa: decreased effects of levodopa

Lithium: increased toxicity; decreased effects of lithium

PHENobarbital: decreased effects of haloperidol

Drug classifications
Anticholinergics: increased anticholinergic effects

Barbiturate anesthetics: oversedation

β-Adrenergic blockers: increased effects of both products

Class IA, III antidysrhythmics, halogenated/local anesthetics, phenothiazines, tricyclics, β-blockers: increased QT prolongation

CNS depressants: oversedation

SSRIs, SNRIs: increased serotonin syndrome, increased neuroleptic malignant syndrome

Adverse effects: *italics* = common; **bold** = life-threatening

Drug/lab test
Increased: liver function tests

NURSING CONSIDERATIONS
Assessment

> **BLACK BOX WARNING:** Assess for dementia, affect, orientation, LOC, reflexes, gait, coordination, sleep pattern disturbances, risk for death in dementia-related psychosis

• Assess mental status: orientation, mood, behavior, presence and type of hallucinations before initial administration and monthly; this product should significantly reduce psychotic behavior
• Monitor I&O ratio; palpate bladder if low urinary output occurs, especially in geriatric; urinalysis is recommended before, during prolonged therapy
• Monitor bilirubin, CBC, liver function tests monthly
• Assess affect, orientation, LOC, reflexes, gait, coordination, sleep pattern disturbances
• Monitor B/P with patient sitting, standing, and lying; take pulse and respirations q4hr during initial treatment; establish baseline before starting treatment; report drops of ≥30 mm Hg; obtain baseline ECG, Q-wave and T-wave changes
• Check for dizziness, faintness, palpitations, tachycardia on rising; severe orthostatic hypotension is common
• **Assess for neuroleptic malignant syndrome: hyperpyrexia, muscle rigidity, increased CPK, altered mental status; product should be discontinued immediately; if seizures, hypo/hypertension, tachycardia occur, notify prescriber immediately**
• **Assess for EPS** including akathisia (inability to sit still, no pattern to movements), tardive dyskinesia (bizarre movements of the jaw, mouth, tongue, extremities), pseudoparkinsonism (ragged tremors, pill rolling, shuffling gait); an antiparkinsonian product should be prescribed
• Assess for constipation and urinary retention daily; if these occur, increase bulk, water in diet
• **Abrupt discontinuation: Do not withdraw abruptly, taper**
⚠ **QT prolongation: More common with IV use at high doses; monitor ECG in those with CV disease**

Patient/family education
• Teach patient to use good oral hygiene; use frequent rinsing of mouth, sugarless gum for dry mouth; oral candidiasis may occur
• Advise patient to avoid hazardous activities until product response is determined and effects are known; dizziness, blurred vision are common
• Inform patient that orthostatic hypotension occurs often and to rise from sitting or lying position gradually; tell patient that in hot weather heat stroke may occur; take extra precautions to stay cool
• **Instruct patient to avoid abrupt withdrawal of this product, or EPS may result; product should be withdrawn slowly**
• Caution patient to avoid OTC preparations (cough, hay fever, cold) unless approved by prescriber, since serious product interactions may occur; avoid use with alcohol, CNS depressants since increased drowsiness may occur
• Tell patient to report impaired vision, jaundice, muscle twitching

Evaluation
Positive therapeutic outcome
• Decrease in emotional excitement, hallucinations, delusions, paranoia, reorganization of patterns of thought, speech; improvement in specific behaviors

TREATMENT OF OVERDOSE:
Lavage if orally ingested; provide airway; *do not induce vomiting*

⚠ HIGH ALERT

heparin (Rx)
(hep′a-rin)
Hepalean ✦, Heparin Leo ✦, Hep-Lock, Hep-Lock U/P, Monoject Prefill
Func. class.: Anticoagulant, antithrombotic
Pregnancy category C

Do not confuse: heparin/Hespan

ACTION: Prevents conversion of fibrinogen to fibrin and prothrombin to thrombin by enhancing inhibitory effects of antithrombin III

Therapeutic outcome: Prevention of thrombi

USES: Prevention and treatment of MI, open heart surgery, disseminated intravascular clotting syndrome, atrial fibrillation with embolization; as an anticoagulant in transfusion and dialysis procedures; to maintain patency of indwelling venipuncture devices; diagnosis, treatment of disseminated intravascular coagulation (DIC)

CONTRAINDICATIONS
Bleeding, hypersensitivity to this product, corn, porcine protein (pork product)

Precautions: Pregnancy C, children, geriatric, alcoholism, hyperlipidemia, diabetes, renal disease, heparin-induced thrombocytopenia (HIT), hemophilia, leukemia with bleeding, peptic ulcer disease, severe thrombocytopenic purpura, renal/hepatic disease (severe), blood dyscrasias, severe hypertension, subacute bacterial endocarditis, acute nephritis; benzyl alcohol products in neonates, infants, pregnancy, lactation

DOSAGE AND ROUTES
Deep vein thrombosis/pulmonary embolism
Adult: IV BOL 80 international units/kg, then maintenance IV INF 18 international units/kg/hr; if aPTT <35 (1.2×normal), increase IV INF rate by 4 international units/kg/hr and rebolus with 80 international units/kg; if aPTT 35-45 (1.2-1.5 × normal), increase IV INF by 2 international units/kg/hr and rebolus with 40 international units/kg; if aPTT 46-70 (1.5-2.3 × normal), maintain IV INF; if aPTT 71-90 (2.3-3 × normal), decrease IV INF by 2 international units/kg/hr; if aPTT >90 (>3 × normal), hold IV INF for 1 hr, then decrease rate 3 international units/kg/hr
Child/infant/neonate: IV loading dose 75 international units/kg
Child >1 yr: 20 international units/kg/hr, **infant, neonate <1 yr:** 28 international units/kg/hr as initial maintenance dose

Thrombosis prophylaxis (open heart/CV surgery)
Adult: IV ≥150 international units/kg, procedures <60 min up to 300 international units/kg, procedures >60 min up to 400 international units/kg, based on ACT

Thrombosis prophylaxis (PCI, not receiving abciximab)
Adult: IV BOL weight-adjusted with 60-100 international units/kg, maintain ACT within 250-300 sec (HemoTec) or 300-350 sec (Hemochron)
Child/infant/neonate: IV BOL 100-150 international units/kg

Prophylaxis for DVT/PE
Adult: SUBCUT 5000 units q8-12hr

IV catheter occlusion prophylaxis
Adult and child: IV 10-100 units/ml
Infant <10 kg: IV 10 units/ml

Available forms: Sol for inj 10, 100, 1000, 2000, 5000, 7500, 10,000, 20,000, 40,000 units/ml; premixed 1000 units/500 ml, 2000 units/1000 ml, 12,500 units/250 ml, 25,000 units/250 ml, 25,000 units/500 ml; lock flush preparations 10 units/ml

Implementation
• Heparin and low-molecular-weight heparins are not interchangeable
• Give at same time each day to maintain steady blood levels
• Cannot be used interchangeably (unit for unit) with LMWHs or heparinoids
• Store at room temperature
SUBCUT route
• Give SUBCUT with at least 25-G ³/₈-in needle; do not massage area or aspirate fluid when giving SUBCUT inj; give in abdomen between pelvic bones, rotate sites; leave in for 10 sec; apply gentle pressure for 1 min
• Changing needles is not recommended
Heparin lock route
• **Do not mistake heparin sodium injection 10,000 units/ml and Hep-Lock U/P 10 units/ml; they have similar blue labeling; deaths in pediatric patients have occurred when heparin sodium injection vials were confused with heparin flush vials**
• Inject 10-100 units/0.5-1 ml after each inf or q8-12hr

Direct IV route
• Give loading dose undiluted over ≥1 min; use before continuous infusion
Continuous IV infusion route
• Dilute 25,000 units/250-500 ml 0.9% NaCl or D₅W (50-100 units/ml); some solutions are premixed and ready for use
• When product is added to inf sol for cont IV, invert container at least 6 × to ensure adequate mixing

Y-site compatibilities: acetaminophen, acetylcysteine, acyclovir, Alcohol 10%, dextrose 5%, alemtuzumab, alfentanil, allopurinol, Amifostine, Aminocaproic acid, aminophylline, amphotericin B lipid complex, Amphotericin B liposome, anidulafungin, argatroban, Arsenic trioxide, ascorbic acid injection, asparaginase, atenolol, atropine, azaTHIOprine, azithromycin, Aztreonam, Benztropine, Betamethasone, Bivalirudin, bleomycin, Bretylium, bumetanide, buprenorphine, butorphanol, Caffeine, calcium chloride/gluconate, Cangrelor, CARBOplatin, carmustine, Cefamandole, ceFAZolin, Cefoperazone, cefotaxime, cefoTEtan, Cefotiam, cefOXitin, ceftaroline, cefTAZidime, ceftizoxime, Ceftobiprole, cefTRIAXone, cefuroxime, Cephapirin, chloramphenicol succinate, chlordiazePOXIDE, chlorothiazide, chlorpheniramine, cimetidine, CISplatin, Cladribine, clindamycin, Cloxacillin, codeine, Colistimethate, Cyanocobalamin, cyclophosphamide, cycloSPORINE, cytarabine, DACTINomycin, DAPTOmycin, DAUNOrubicin citrate liposome, dexamethasone, Dexmedetomidine, Dexrazoxane, digoxin, DOCEtaxel, DOPamine, doripenem, Doxacurium, Doxapram, DOXOrubicin liposomal, Edetate calcium disodium, Edrophonium, enalaprilat, Ephedrine sulfate, EPINEPHrine, epoetin alfa, eptifibatide, Ergonovine, ertapenem, esmolol, estrogens conjugated, Ethacrynate, etoposide, etoposide phosphate, famotidine, fenoldopam, fentaNYL, flecainide, fluconazole, Fludarabine, fluorouracil, folic acid (as sodium salt), foscarnet, Gallamine, Gallium, ganciclovir, gemcitabine, Gemtuzumab, Glycopyrrolate, granisetron, hydrocortisone, HYDROmorphone, ibuprofen lysine, ifosfamide, imipenem-cilastatin, indomethacin, irinotecan, Isoproterenol, ketorolac, Lactated Ringer's Injection, lansoprazole, leucovorin, lidocaine, Lincomycin, linezolid, LORazepam, magnesium sulfate, mannitol, mechlorethamine, melphalan, Mephentermine, meropenem, Mesna, Metaraminol, methadone, Methohexital, methotrexate, Methoxamine, Methyldopa, methylergonovine, metoclopramide, metoprolol, metroNIDAZOLE, micafungin, midazolam, milrinone, minocycline, mitoMYcin, Mivacurium, morphine, moxifloxacin, Multiple vitamins injection, nafcillin, Nalbuphine, Nalorphine, naloxone, neostigmine, nitroglycerin, nitroprusside, norepinephrine, octreotide, ondansetron, oxacillin, oxaliplatin, oxytocin, PAClitaxel (solvent/surfactant), palonosetron, pamidronate, pancuronium, PEMEtrexed, penicillin G potassium/sodium, PENTobarbital, Phenobarbital, phentolamine, phenylephrine, phytonadione, piperacillin sodium, piperacillin-tazobactam, potassium acetate/chloride, procainamide, prochlorperazine, Promazine, propofol, propranolol, pyridostigmine, pyridoxine, ranitidine, remifentanil, Ringer's injection, riTUXimab, rocuronium, sargramostim, scopolamine, Sodium acetate/Bicarbonate/fusidate, succinylcholine, Sufentanil, tacrolimus, theophylline, thiamine, Thiopental, Thiotepa, Ticarcillin, ticarcillin-clavulanate, tigecycline, tirofiban, Tolazoline, topotecan, TPN (2-in-1), Tranexamic, trastuzumab, Trimetaphan, trimethobenzamide, Tubocurarine, urokinase, vasopressin, vecuronium, verapamil, vinBLAstine, vinCRIStine, voriconazole, warfarin, zidovudine, zoledronic acid.

Y-site incompatibilities: Alteplase, ciprofloxacin, dacarbazine, diazepam, DOBUTamine, DOXOrubicin, ergotamine, gentamicin, haloperidol, IDArubicin, methotrimeprazine, phenytoin, promethazine, tobramycin, triflupromazine

ADVERSE EFFECTS
CNS: *Fever,* chills, headache

GU: Hematuria
HEMA: **Hemorrhage, thrombocytopenia, anemia, HIT**
INTEG: *Rash,* dermatitis, urticaria, pruritus, delayed transient alopecia, hematoma, cutaneous necrosis (SUBCUT), injection site reactions
META: Hyperlipidemia
SYST: Anaphylaxis

Pharmacokinetics

Absorption	Well absorbed (SUBCUT)
Distribution	Unknown
Metabolism	Partially in kidney, liver
Excretion	Lymph, spleen, in urine (<50% unchanged)
Half-life	1-2 hr (dose dependent)

Pharmacodynamics

	SUBCUT	IV
Onset	½-1 hr	5 min
Peak	2 hr	10 min
Duration	8-12 hr	2-6 hr

INTERACTIONS
Individual drugs
Dextran, dipyridole, ticlopidine, clopidogrel, presgrel: increased action of heparin
Digoxin: decreased action of heparin
Nicotine: decreased action of heparin

Drug classifications
Anticoagulants (oral), cephalosporins, NSAIDs, penicillins, platelet inhibitors, salicylates, antineoplastics, SSRIs, SNRIs: increased action of heparin, quinidine, valproic acid
Antihistamines, tetracyclines, cardiac glycosides: decreased action of heparin, nitroglycerin
Corticosteroids: decreased action of corticosteroids

Drug/herb
Anise, arnica, chamomile, clove, dong quai, feverfew, garlic, ginger, ginkgo, green tea, horse chestnut: increased bleeding risk

Drug/lab test
Increased: ALT, AST, INR, pro-time, PTT, potassium
Decreased: platelets

NURSING CONSIDERATIONS
Assessment
• Assess for blood studies (Hct, occult blood in stools) q3mo if patient is on long-term therapy
• Monitor PPT, which should be 1½-2 × control, PTT; often done daily, APTT, ACT
• Monitor platelet count q2-3day; thrombocytopenia may occur on fourth day of treatment and resolve, or continue to eighth day of treatment

---

⚠ Bleeding, hemorrhage: Assess for bleeding gums, petechiae, ecchymosis, black tarry stools, hematuria, epistaxis, decrease in Hct, B/P; notify prescriber immediately; HIT may occur after product discontinuation
• **Monitor for hypersensitivity:** fever, skin rash, urticaria; notify prescriber immediately

Patient/family education
• Advise patient to avoid OTC preparations that may cause serious product interactions unless directed by prescriber; may contain aspirin or other anticoagulants, notify all health care persons of heparin use
• Tell patient that product may be withheld during active bleeding (menstruation), depending on condition
• Caution patient to use soft-bristle toothbrush to avoid bleeding gums; avoid contact sports; use electric razor; avoid IM inj
• Instruct patient to carry/wear emergency ID or other identification identifying product taken and condition treated
• Advise patient to report any signs of bleeding: gums, under skin, urine, stools; or unusual bruising even after discontinuing product

Evaluation
Positive therapeutic outcome
• Prevention of new clots
• PTT of 1.5-2.5 × control
• Free-flowing **IV**, DVT and pulmonary emboli

TREATMENT OF OVERDOSE:
Withdraw product, give protamine sulfate 1 mg protamine/100 units heparin

---

hepatitis B immune globulin (HBIG) (Rx)
(hep-a-tite′iss)
HepaGam B, Hyper HEP B S/D, Nabi-HB
Func. class.: Immune globulin
Pregnancy category C

ACTION: Provides passive immunity to hepatitis B

Therapeutic outcome: Passive immunity to hepatitis B

USES: Prevention of hepatitis B virus in exposed patients, including passive immunity in neonates born to HBsAg-positive mothers, prevention of hepatitis B recurrence after liver transplant in HBsAg-positive patients

CONTRAINDICATIONS
Hypersensitivity to immune globulins, coagulation disorders

Precautions: Pregnancy **C,** breastfeeding, children, geriatric, hemophilia, active infection, IgA deficiency, maltrose sensitivity

DOSAGE AND ROUTES
Hepatitis B exposure in those at high risk
Adult and child: IM 0.06 ml/kg (usual 3-5 ml) within 7 days of exposure; repeat 28 days after exposure, if patient wishes not to receive the hepatitis B vaccine

Prevention of hepatitis B infection recurrence after liver transplant
Adult: IV (HepaGam B only) 20,000 international units concurrent with grafting transplanted liver, then 20,000 international units/day on days 1-7, then 20,000 international units q2wk starting on day 14, then 20,000 international units qmo, starting on month 4

Neonates born to hepatitis B surface antigen–positive mothers: IM 0.5 ml within 12 hr of birth

Available forms: Inj 1-, 4-, 5-ml vials; neonatal syringe 0.5 ml; HepaGam B sol for inj 312, 1560 units/ml; Hyper HEP B S/D 217 units/ml

Implementation
IM route
• After rotating vial, do not shake
• Only with EPINEPHrine 1:1000 on unit to treat laryngospasm
• In deltoid for better absorption (adult)

IV route (Hepa Gam B only)
• Calculate volume needed for each 20,000 international units dose by using measured potency of each lot, HBIG potency is stamped on label
• Promptly use after vial is entered, discard unused product
• Give at 2 ml/min through separate IV line, use inf pump, decrease to 1 ml/min, if infusion-related event occurs, patient becomes uncomfortable
• Do not use HyperHEP B BS/D or Nabi-HB IV

ADVERSE EFFECTS
CNS: Headache, dizziness, fever, chills
GI: Nausea, vomiting
INTEG: Soreness at inj site, urticaria, erythema, swelling
SYST: Induration, **anaphylaxis,** angioedema

Pharmacokinetics

Absorption	Slowly absorbed
Distribution	Unknown
Metabolism	Unknown
Excretion	Unknown
Half-life	3 wk

Pharmacodynamics

Onset	1-7 days
Peak	3-10 days
Duration	2-6 mo

INTERACTIONS
Drug classifications
MMR, rotavirus vaccines, varicella: do not use within 3 mo of hepatitis B immune globulin

NURSING CONSIDERATIONS
Assessment
• Assess for history of allergies, skin conditions (eczema, psoriasis, dermatitis), reactions to vaccinations
• Assess for skin reactions: rash, induration, urticaria
• Assess for sneezing, pruritus, angioedema, dysphagia, vomiting, abdominal pain
⚠ Assess for anaphylaxis: inability to breathe, bronchospasm, hypotension, wheezing, diaphoresis, fever, flushing; epinephrine and emergency equipment should be available
• Can be used with hepatitis B vaccine in cases of direct contact

Patient/family education
• Teach patient purpose of product and expected results
• Give patient a list of adverse reactions that need to be reported immediately: wheezing, vomiting, sneezing, abdominal pain, sweating, tightness in chest
• Advise patient that pain, rash, swelling at inj site can be expected
• Give patient written record of immunization
• Do not obtain MMR or varicella vaccine within 3 months of this product

Evaluation

Positive therapeutic outcome
• Prevention of hepatitis B

homatropine ophthalmic
See Appendix B

hydrALAZINE (Rx)
(hye-dral′a-zeen)
Apresoline ✹
Func. class.: Antihypertensive, direct-acting peripheral vasodilator
Chem. class.: Phthalazine
Pregnancy category C

Do not confuse: hydrALAZINE/hydrOXYzine, **Apresoline**/allopurinol

ACTION: Vasodilates arterioles in smooth muscle by direct relaxation; reduces B/P with reflex increases in heart rate, stroke volume, cardiac output

Therapeutic outcome: Decreased B/P in hypertension, decreased afterload in CHF

USES: Essential hypertension, hypertensive emergency/urgency, preeclampsia

Unlabeled uses: CHF

CONTRAINDICATIONS
Hypersensitivity to hydrALAZINEs, mitral valvular rheumatic heart disease, CAD

Precautions: Pregnancy **C,** breastfeeding, geriatric, CVA, advanced renal disease, liver disease, SLE, dissecting aortic aneurysm

DOSAGE AND ROUTES
Hypertension
Adult: PO 10 mg qid 2-4 days, then 25 mg qid for rest of 1st wk, then 50 mg qid individualized to desired response; max 300 mg/day
Child: PO 0.75-1 mg/kg/day in 2-4 divided doses; max 25 mg/dose, increase over 3-4 wk to max 7.5 mg/kg/day or 200 mg, whichever is less

Hypertensive crisis
Adult: IV BOL 10-20 mg q4-6hr; administer PO as soon as possible; IM 10-50 mg q4-6hr
Child: IV BOL 0.1-0.6 mg/kg q4hr; IM 0.1-0.6 mg/kg q4-6hr, max 1.7-3.5 mg/kg/day

CHF (unlabeled)
Adult: PO 10-25 mg bid, max 75 mg tid

Available forms: Inj 20 mg/ml; tabs 10, 25, 50, 100 mg

Implementation
PO route
• Give with meals to enhance absorption
• Store protected from light and heat
IM route
• Do not admix; switch to PO as soon as possible

Direct IV route
• Give by **IV** undiluted through Y-tube or 3-way stopcock, give each 10 mg over 1 min or more
• Administer with patient in recumbent position; keep in that position for 1 hr after administration

Y-site compatibilities: Heparin, hydrocortisone, potassium chloride, verapamil, vit B/C

Y-site incompatibilities: Aminophylline, ampicillin, diazoxide, furosemide, PACLitaxel

ADVERSE EFFECTS
CNS: *Headache, tremors, dizziness, anxiety,* peripheral neuritis, depression, fever, chills
CV: *Palpitations, reflex tachycardia, angina,* **shock,** rebound hypertension, orthostatic hypotension
GI: *Nausea, vomiting, anorexia, diarrhea,* constipation, paralytic ileus, **hepatotoxicity**
GU: Urinary retention, glomerulonephritis, hematuria
HEMA: **Leukopenia, agranulocytosis,** anemia, **thrombocytopenia**
INTEG: Rash, pruritus, urticaria
MISC: Nasal congestion, muscle cramps, *lupuslike symptoms,* flushing, edema, dyspnea

Pharmacokinetics

Absorption	Rapidly absorbed (PO); well absorbed (IM); completely absorbed (**IV**)
Distribution	Widely distributed; crosses placenta
Metabolism	GI mucosa, liver extensively
Excretion	Kidneys, urine (12%-14%)
Half-life	2-8 hr

Pharmacodynamics

	PO	IM	IV
Onset	½ hr	10-30 min	5-20 min
Peak	1-2 hr	1 hr	10-80 min
Duration	6-12 hr	2-6 hr	Up to 12 hr

INTERACTIONS
Individual drugs
Alcohol: increased hypotension
Indomethacin: decreased effects of hydrALAZINE

Drug classifications
β-**Adrenergic blockers: metoprolol, propranolol; increased effects**
MAOIs: severe hypotension
Other antihypertensives, thiazide diuretics: increased hypotension

Sympathomimetics (EPINEPHrine, norepinephrine): increased tachycardia, angina
NSAIDs, estrogens: decreased hydrALAZINE effects

Drug/Food
Increase: drug absorption; have patient take with food

NURSING CONSIDERATIONS
Assessment
• **Assess cardiac status:** B/P q5min for 2 hr, then qhr for 2 hr, then q4hr; pulse, jugular venous distention q4hr decreased after level
• Monitor electrolytes, blood studies: potassium, sodium, chloride, carbon dioxide, CBC, serum glucose; LE prep, ANA titer before starting treatment
• Monitor weight daily, I&O; check for edema in feet, legs daily; check skin turgor, dryness of mucous membranes for hydration status
• Assess for crackles, dyspnea, orthopnea; peripheral edema, fatigue, weight gain, jugular vein distention (CHF)
• For fever, joint pain, rash, sore throat (lupuslike symptoms), notify prescriber

Patient/family education
• Teach patient to take with food to increase bioavailability (PO)
• Teach patient to avoid OTC preparations unless directed by prescriber
• Advise patient to notify prescriber if chest pain, severe fatigue, fever, muscle or joint pain occur
• Advise patient to rise slowly to prevent orthostatic hypertension
• Advise patient to notify prescriber if pregnancy is suspected

Evaluation
Positive therapeutic outcome
• Decreased B/P, decreased afterload in hypertension

TREATMENT OF OVERDOSE:
Administer vasopressors, volume expanders for shock; if PO, lavage or give activated charcoal, digitalization

---

hydrochlorothiazide (Rx)
(hye-droe-klor-oh-thye′a-zide)
Apo-Hydrol ✦, Neo-Codema ✦, Urozide ✦
Func. class.: Diuretic, antihypertensive
Chem. class.: Thiazide, sulfonamide derivative
Pregnancy category B

ACTION: Acts on the distal tubule in the kidney, increasing excretion of sodium, water, chloride, and potassium

Adverse effects: *italics* = common; **bold** = life-threatening

Therapeutic outcome: Decreased B/P, decreased edema in lung tissues peripherally

USES: Edema, hypertension, diuresis, CHF; idiopathic lower extremity edema therapy

CONTRAINDICATIONS
Hypersensitivity to thiazides or sulfonamides, anuria, renal decompensation, pregnancy (D) preeclampsia

Precautions: Pregnancy **B,** breastfeeding, hypokalemia, renal/hepatic disease, gout, COPD, lupus erythematosus, diabetes mellitus, hyperlipidemia, CCr <30 ml/min, hypomagnesemia

DOSAGE AND ROUTES
Hypertension
Adult/adolescent: PO 12.5-25 mg/day, may increase to 50 mg/day in 1-2 divided doses, max 100 mg/day

Child >6 mo: PO 1-2 mg/kg/day in divided doses; max 37.5 mg/day for 6 mo-2 yr; max 37.5 mg/day

Child <6 mo: PO up to 2-3.3 mg/kg/day in divided doses

Renal dose
Adult: PO CCr <30 ml/min, do not use, not effective

Available forms: Tabs 12.5, 25, 50 mg; caps 12.5 mg

Implementation
PO route
- Give in AM to avoid interference with sleep
- Provide potassium replacement if potassium level is ≤3.0 mg/dl; give whole tab or use oral sol lightly; product may be crushed if patient is unable to swallow, replace magnesium if needed
- Administer with food; if nausea occurs, absorption may be increased

ADVERSE EFFECTS
CNS: Drowsiness, paresthesia, depression, headache, *dizziness, fatigue, weakness,* fever

CV: Irregular pulse, *orthostatic hypotension,* palpitations, volume depletion, allergic myocarditis

EENT: Blurred vision

ELECT: *Hypokalemia,* hypercalcemia, hyponatremia, hypochloremia, hypomagnesemia

GI: *Nausea, vomiting, anorexia,* constipation, diarrhea, cramps, **pancreatitis,** GI irritation, **hepatitis**

GU: *Frequency,* polyuria, **uremia,** glucosuria, hyperuricemia, jaundice, erectile dysfunction

HEMA: Aplastic anemia, hemolytic anemia, leukopenia, agranulocytosis, thrombocytopenia, neutropenia

INTEG: *Rash,* urticaria, purpura, photosensitivity, alopecia, erythema multiforme

META: *Hyperglycemia, hyperuricemia,* **renal failure,** increased creatinine, BUN

SYST: Stevens-Johnson syndrome

Pharmacokinetics
Absorption	Variable
Distribution	Extracellular spaces; crosses placenta
Metabolism	Excreted unchanged in urine
Excretion	Breast milk
Half-life	6-15 hr

Pharmacodynamics
Onset	2 hr
Peak	4 hr
Duration	6-12 hr

INTERACTIONS
Individual drugs
Amphotericin B, piperacillin, ticarcillin: increased hypokalemia

Cholestyramine, colestipol: decreased absorption of hydrochlorothiazide

Diazoxide: increased hyperglycemia, hyperuricemia, hypotension

Lithium: increased toxicity

Drug classifications
Antidiabetics: decreased effect of antidiabetic agent

Cardiac glycosides, nondepolarizing skeletal muscle relaxants: increased toxicity

Diuretics (loop): increased effects of diuretic

Corticosteroids: increased hypokalemia

NSAIDs: decreased thiazide effect

Drug/food
Licorice: increased severe hypokalemia

Drug/lab test
Increased: parathyroid test, uric acid, calcium, glucose, cholesterol, triglycerides

Decreased: potassium, sodium, Hgb, WBC, platelets

NURSING CONSIDERATIONS
Assessment
- Monitor glucose in urine if patient is diabetic
- Assess improvement in CVP q8hr
- Check for rashes, temp elevation daily
- Assess for confusion, especially in geriatric patients; take safety precautions if needed
- Monitor for acidic urine, reduced urine, osmolality, nocturia; hypotension, broad T-wave, U-wave, ectopy, tachycardia, weak pulse; muscle weakness, altered LOC, drowsiness, apathy, lethargy, confusion, depression; anorexia, nausea,

cramps, constipation, distention, paralytic ileus; hypoventilation, respiratory muscle weakness
• Assess fluid volume status: I&O ratios, record, count, or weigh diapers as appropriate; weight; distended red veins; crackles in lungs; color, quality, and specific gravity of urine; skin turgor; adequacy of pulses; moist mucous membranes; bilateral lung sounds; peripheral pitting edema; assess for dehydration: symptoms of decreasing output, thirst, hypotension; dry mouth and mucous membranes should be reported
• Monitor electrolytes: potassium, sodium, calcium, magnesium; also include BUN, blood pH, ABGs, uric acid, CBC, blood glucose, renal function
• Assess **hypertension** B/P before, during therapy with patient lying, standing, and sitting as appropriate; orthostatic hypotension can occur rapidly
• **Hypersensitivity to sulfonamides: rash, discontinue; fatal Stevens-Johnson syndrome may occur**

Patient/family education
• Teach patient to take the medication early in the day at same time of day to prevent nocturia
• Instruct patient to take with food or milk if GI symptoms of nausea and anorexia occur
• Teach patient to maintain a weekly record of weight and notify prescriber of weight loss >5 lb
• Caution patient that this product causes a loss of potassium and that food rich in potassium should be added to the diet; refer to a dietitian for assistance in planning
• Caution patient to rise slowly from sitting or reclining positions, not to exercise in hot weather or stand for prolonged periods since orthostatic hypotension will be enhanced; lie down if dizziness occurs to prevent postural hypotension
• Teach patient not to use alcohol or any OTC medications without prescriber's approval; serious product reactions may occur
• **Emphasize the need to contact prescriber immediately if muscle cramps, weakness, nausea, dizziness, or numbness occurs; rash**
• Teach patient to take own B/P and pulse and record findings
• Teach patient to continue taking medication even if feeling better; this product controls symptoms but does not cure the condition
• Advise patient with hypertension to continue other medical treatment (exercise, weight loss, relaxation techniques, cessation of smoking)
• Teach patient to monitor weight and report changes to prescriber
• Discuss dietary potassium requirements

• Advise patient that follow-ups and routine lab tests will be required
• Teach patient how to take B/P, to continue with other medical regimens (weight loss, exercise)

Evaluation
Positive therapeutic outcome
• Decreased edema
• Decreased B/P
• Increased diuresis

TREATMENT OF OVERDOSE:
Lavage if taken orally, monitor electrolytes, administer dextrose in saline, monitor hydration, CV, renal status

⚠ HIGH ALERT

HYDROcodone (Rx)
(hye-droe-koe'done)
Hycodan ♣, Robidone ♣
HYDROcodone/ acetaminophen (Rx)
Anexsia, Co-Gesic, Dolorex Forte, Duocet, Hycet, Hydrocet, Hydrogesic, Liquicet, Lorcet, Lortab, NorCo, Panlor, Verdrocet, Vicodin, Vicodin ES, Vicodin HP, Xodol, Zydone
HYDROcodone/ibuprofen (Rx)
Ibudone, Reprexain, Vicoprofen, Xylon
Func. class.: Antitussive opioid analgesic/ nonopioid analgesic
Pregnancy category C
Controlled substance schedule II

Do not confuse: HYDROcodone/ hydrocortisone, **Hycodan**/Vicodin

ACTION: Acts directly on cough center in medulla to suppress cough; binds to opiate receptors in the CNS to reduce pain

Therapeutic outcome: Pain relief, decreased cough, decreased diarrhea

USES: Mild to moderate pain

CONTRAINDICATIONS
Acne rosacea/vulgaris, Cushing's, measles, perioral dermatitis, varicella, abrupt discontinuation, hypersensitivity to this product or benzyl

Precautions: Pregnancy **C**, breastfeeding, neonates, addictive personality, increased ICP, MI (acute), severe heart disease, respiratory depression, renal/hepatic disease, bowel impaction, urinary retention, viral infection, ulcerative colitis, seizures, sulfite hypersensitivity, psychosis, hypertension, hyperthyroidism

Dosages and routes
Analgesic
Adult: PO 2.5-10 mg q4-6hr prn, max 60 mg/day

Available forms: HYDROcodone: bulk powder; **HYDROcodone/acetaminophen:** 5 mg HYDROcodone/500 mg acetaminophen (Co-Gesic, Lorcet, Lortab 5/500, Vicodin); 7.5 mg HYDROcodone/400 mg acetaminophen (Zydone), 7.5 mg HYDROcodone/500 mg acetaminophen (Lortab 7.5/500), 7.5 mg HYDROcodone/750 mg acetaminophen (Vicodin ES), 5 mg HYDROcodone/325 acetaminophen, 10 mg HYDROcodone/325 acetaminophen (Norco), 10 mg HYDROcodone/500 mg acetaminophen (Lortab 10/500), 10 mg HYDROcodone/650 mg acetaminophen (Lorcet 10/650, Vicodin HP), 10 mg HYDROcodone/660 acetaminophen (Vicodin HP); caps 5 mg HYDROcodone/500 mg acetaminophen (Stagesic, Zydone); **HYDROcodone/ibuprofen:** tabs 7.5 mg HYDROcodone/200 mg ibuprofen (Vico-profen)

Implementation
Check product carefully before using; fatalities have occurred by using wrong dose, wrong product
- Do not break, crush, or chew tabs; only scored tabs may be broken
- Give with antiemetic if nausea, vomiting occur
- Give when pain is beginning to return; determine dosage interval by patient response; continuous dosing of medication is more effective than given prn
- Medication should be slowly withdrawn after long-term use to prevent withdrawal symptoms

> **BLACK BOX WARNING:** Max 4 g acetaminophen with combination product

- Store in light-resistant container at room temperature
- May be given with food or milk to lessen GI upset

ADVERSE EFFECTS
CNS: *Drowsiness,* dizziness, light-headedness, confusion, headache, sedation, euphoria, dysphoria, weakness, hallucinations, disorientation, mood changes, dependence, seizures
CV: Palpitations, tachycardia, bradycardia, change in B/P, circulatory depression, syncope, cardiac arrest (child)

EENT: Tinnitus, blurred vision, miosis, diplopia
GI: *Nausea, vomiting, anorexia, constipation,* cramps, dry mouth, ulcers
GU: Increased urinary output, dysuria, urinary retention
INTEG: Rash, urticaria, flushing, pruritus
RESP: Respiratory depression, pulmonary edema, bronchopneumonia, respiratory arrest (child)

Pharmacokinetics
Absorption	Well absorbed
Distribution	Unknown; crosses placenta
Metabolism	Liver, extensively
Excretion	Kidneys
Half-life	3½-4½ hr

Pharmacodynamics
	PO (analgesic)	PO (antitussive)
Onset	10-20 min	Unknown
Peak	30-60 min	Unknown
Duration	4-6 hr	4-6 hr

INTERACTIONS
Individual drugs
Alcohol: increased CNS depression

Drug classifications
Antidepressants (tricyclics), CNS depressants, general anesthetics, opioids, phenothiazines, sedative/hypnotics, skeletal muscle relaxants: increased CNS depression
MAOIs: increased severe reactions

Drug/herb
Lavender, valerian: increased CNS depression

Drug/lab test
Increased: amylase, lipase

NURSING CONSIDERATIONS
Assessment
- **Assess pain:** intensity, type, location, duration, precipitating factor before and 1 hr after giving product, titrate upward by 25%; assess need for pain medication, physical dependency
- Monitor VS after parenteral route; note muscle rigidity; product history; liver; renal function tests; cough; and respiratory dysfunction: respiratory depression, character, rate, rhythm; notify prescriber if respirations are <10/min
- **Monitor CNS changes:** dizziness, drowsiness, hallucinations, euphoria, LOC, pupil reaction
- Monitor allergic reactions: rash, urticaria

• **Bowel status:** constipation; provide fluids, fiber in diet, may need stimulant laxative

Patient/family education
• Instruct patient to report any symptoms of CNS changes, allergic reactions; to avoid CNS depressants: alcohol, sedative/hypnotics for at least 24 hr after taking this product
• Teach patient that dizziness, drowsiness, and confusion are common and to avoid getting up without assistance, driving, or other hazardous activities
• Discuss in detail all aspects of the product

Evaluation
Positive therapeutic outcome
• Decreased pain
• Decreased cough
• Teach patient to notify prescriber if pregnancy is planned or suspected
• Advise patient for dry mouth, use sugarless gum, frequent sips of water
• Advise patient to notify prescriber of relief of pain

> **BLACK BOX WARNING:** Advise patient not to exceed 4000 mg in combination product with acetaminophen, check all other products that may contain acetaminophen

TREATMENT OF OVERDOSE:
Naloxone HCl (Narcan) 0.2-0.8 **IV**, O₂, **IV** fluids, vasopressors

hydrocortisone (Rx)
(hy-droh-kor′tih-sone)
Cortef, Colocort, Cortena, Cortifoam
hydrocortisone acetate (Rx)
Anucort, Anusol, Cortifoam, Hemril, Protocort, Rectasol, Rectasol HC
hydrocortisone sodium succinate (Rx)
A-hydroCort, Solu-Cortef
Func. class.: Short-acting glucocorticoid
Chem. class.: Natural nonfluorinated, group IV potency (valerate), group VI potency (acetate and plain)
Pregnancy category C

Do not confuse: hydrocortisone/
HYDROcodone

ACTION: Decreases inflammation by suppressing migration of polymorphonuclear leukocytes and fibroblasts and reversing increased capillary permeability and lysosomal stabilization (systemic); antipruritic, antiinflammatory (topical)

Therapeutic outcome: Decreased inflammation

USES: Severe inflammation, septic shock, adrenal insufficiency, ulcerative colitis, collagen disorders, asthma, COPD, SLE, Stevens-Johnson syndrome, ulcerative colitis, TB

CONTRAINDICATIONS
Hypersensitivity, fungal infections

Precautions: Pregnancy **C**, breastfeeding, diabetes mellitus, glaucoma, osteoporosis, seizure disorders, ulcerative colitis, CHF, myasthenia gravis, renal disease, esophagitis, peptic ulcer, metastatic carcinoma, septic shock, Cushing syndrome, hepatic disease, hypothyroidism, coagulopathy, thromboembolism, children <2 yr, psychosis, idiopathic thrombocytopenia (IM), acute glomerulonephritis, amebiasis, nonasthmatic bronchial disease, AIDS, TB, recent MI (associated with left-ventricular rupture)

DOSAGE AND ROUTES
Adrenal insufficiency/inflammation
Adult: PO 20-240 mg daily in divided doses; IM/IV 100-500 mg (succinate), may repeat q2-6hr, then 50-100 mg IM as needed

Shock prevention
Adult: IM/IV 50 mg/kg repeated q4hr; repeat q24hr as needed (succinate)
Child: IM/IV 0.16-1 mg/kg or 6-30 mg/m² given daily or bid (succinate)

Colitis
Adult: PO 20-240 mg (base)/day in 2-4 divided doses; enema 100 mg nightly for 21 days; susp 1 2-3 × /day × 2 wk; foam 1 applicatorful 1-2 × day × 2-3 wk
Child: PO 2-8 mg (base)/kg/day or 60-240 mg (base)/m²/day in 3-4 divided doses

Topical route
Adult and child >2 yr: Apply to affected area daily-qid

Available forms: Hydrocortisone: enema 100 mg/60 ml; tabs 5, 10, 20 mg; **acetate:** rectal aerosol foam: 10%; **cypionate:** tabs 5, 10, 20 mg; **succinate:** inj 100, 250, 500, 1000 mg vial

Implementation
PO route
• Give with food or milk to decrease GI symptoms
Rectal route
• Use applicator provided
• Clean applicator after each use
• Retain for 1 hr if possible
Topical route
• Apply only to affected areas; do not get in eyes

- Cleanse and dry area before applying medication, then cover with occlusive dressing (only if prescribed); seal to normal skin; change q12hr; systemic absorption may occur; use only on dermatoses; do not use on weeping, denuded, or infected area
- Use for a few days after area has cleared
- Store at room temperature

Nasal route
- Patient should clear nasal passages before administration; use decongestant if needed; shake inhaler, invert, tilt head backward, insert nozzle into nostril, away from septum; hold other nostril closed and depress activator, inhale through nose, exhale through mouth

IM route
- Give deeply in large muscle mass; rotate sites; avoid deltoid; use 21-gauge needle

IV route
- **Succinate:** IV in mix-o-vial or reconstitute 250 mg or less/2 ml bacteriostatic water for injection, mix gently; give direct IV over 1 min or more; may be further diluted in 100, 250, 500, or 1000 ml of D_5W, D_5/0.9% NaCl, 0.9% NaCl given over ordered rate

Sodium succinate preparations

Y-site compatibilities: Acetaminophen, acyclovir, alemtuzumab, alfentanil, allopurinol, amifostine, ampicillin, amphotericin B cholesteryl, inamrinone, amsacrine, atracurium, atropine, aztreonam, betamethasone, calcium gluconate, cefepime, cefmetazole, cephalothin, chlordiazePOXIDE, chlorproMAZINE, cisatracurium, cladribine, cyanocobalamin, cytarabine, dexamethasone, digoxin, diphenhydrAMINE, DOPamine, DOXOrubicin liposome, droperidol, edrophonium, enalaprilat, EPINEPHrine, esmolol, conjugated estrogens, ethacrynate, famotidine, fentaNYL, fentaNYL/droperidol, filgrastim, fludarabine, fluorouracil, foscarnet, furosemide, gallium, granisetron, heparin, hydrALAZINE, regular insulin, isoproterenol, kanamycin, lidocaine, LORazepam, magnesium sulfate, melphalan, menadiol, meperidine, methicillin, methoxamine, methylergonovine, minocycline, morphine, neostigmine, norepinephrine, ondansetron, oxacillin, oxytocin, PACLitaxel, pancuronium, penicillin G potassium, pentazocine, phytonadione, piperacillin/tazobactam, prednisoLONE, procainamide, prochlorperazine, propofol, propranolol, pyridostigmine, remifentanil, scopolamine, sodium bicarbonate, succinylcholine, tacrolimus, teniposide, theophylline, thiotepa, trimethaphan, trimethobenzamide, vecuronium, vinorelbine, zoledronic acid

Y-site incompatibilities: Diazepam, ergotamine tartrate, IDArubicin, phenytoin, sargramostim

ADVERSE EFFECTS

CNS: Depression, flushing, sweating, headache, mood changes, **pseudotumor cerebri**, euphoria, insomnia, **seizures**

CV: Hypertension, **circulatory collapse, thrombophlebitis, embolism,** tachycardia, edema, heart failure

EENT: Fungal infections, increased intraocular pressure, blurred vision, cataracts, glaucoma

GI: Diarrhea, nausea, abdominal distention, **GI hemorrhage,** increased appetite, **pancreatitis,** vomiting

HEMA: **Thrombocytopenia**

INTEG: Acne, poor wound healing, ecchymosis, petechiae

MISC: Adrenal insufficiency (after stress/ withdrawal)

MS: Fractures, osteoporosis, weakness

Pharmacokinetics

Absorption	Well absorbed (PO); systemic (topical)
Distribution	Crosses placenta
Metabolism	Liver, extensively
Excretion	Kidney
Half-life	3-5 hr, adrenal suppression 3-4 days

Pharmacodynamics

	PO	IM	IV	TOPICAL
Onset	1-2 hr	20 min	Rapid	Min to hr
Peak	1 hr	4-8 hr	1-2 hr	Hr to days
Duration	1½ days	1½ days	1½ days	Hr to days

INTERACTIONS

Individual drugs

Alcohol, amphotericin B, cycloSPORINE, digoxin: increased side effects

Bosentan, carBAMazepine, cholestyramine, colestipol, ePHEDrine, phenytoin, rifampin, theophylline: decreased action of hydrocortisone

Drug classifications

Acetaminophen, NSAIDs, salicylates: increased risk of GI bleeding

Anticoagulants, calcium supplements, toxoids, vaccines: decreased action of each specific drug

Anticonvulsants: decreased effects of anticonvulsant

Antidiabetics: decreased effects of antidiabetics

Barbiturates: decreased action of hydrocortisone

Diuretics: increased side effects
Live virus vaccines/toxoids: increased neurologic reactions

Drug/herb
Ephedra: decreased hydrocortisone levels

Drug/lab test
Increased: cholesterol, sodium, blood glucose, uric acid, calcium, urine glucose
Decreased: calcium, potassium, T_4, T_3, thyroid ^{131}I uptake test, urine 17-OHCS, 17-KS
False negative: skin allergy tests

NURSING CONSIDERATIONS
Assessment
• **Adrenal insufficiency (cushingoid symptoms):** nausea, anorexia, shortness of breath, moon face, fatigue, dizziness, weakness, joint pain before and during treatment; monitor plasma cortisol levels during long-term therapy (normal level is 138-635 nmol/L when obtained at 8 AM); check adrenal function periodically for hypothalamic-pituitary-adrenal axis suppression
• Monitor potassium, blood glucose, urine glucose while patient is on long-term therapy; hypokalemia and hyperglycemia may occur
• Monitor I&O ratio; be alert for decreasing urinary output and increasing edema; weigh daily; notify prescriber of weekly gain >5 lb or edema, hypertension, cardiac symptoms
• **Assess for infection:** increased temp, WBC even after withdrawal of medication; product masks infection symptoms; if fever develops, product should be discontinued
• Check for potassium depletion: paresthesias, fatigue, nausea, vomiting, depression, polyuria, dysrhythmias, weakness
• Assess mental status: affect, mood, behavioral changes, aggression
• Check nasal passages during long-term treatment for changes in mucus (nasal)
• Assess for systemic absorption: increased temp, inflammation, irritation (topical)
• GI effects: nausea, vomiting, anorexia or appetite stimulation, diarrhea, constipation, abdominal pain, hiccups, gastritis, pancreatitis, GI bleeding/perforation with long-term treatment

Patient/family education
• Teach patient all aspects of product use, including cushingoid symptoms
• Advise patient to carry/wear emergency ID as corticosteroid user; not to discontinue abruptly; adrenal crisis can result
• Instruct patient to notify prescriber if therapeutic response decreases; dosage adjustment may be needed
• Instruct patient to notify prescriber of signs of infection

• Teach patient that product can mask infections and cause hyperglycemia (diabetic)
• Teach patient to avoid live-virus vaccines if using steroids long term
• **Teach patient not to discontinue abruptly, adrenal crisis can result; product should be tapered**
• Caution patient to avoid OTC products unless directed by prescriber: salicylates, alcohol in cough products, cold preparations
• **Teach patient symptoms of adrenal insufficiency:** nausea, anorexia, fatigue, dizziness, dyspnea, weakness, joint pain; and when to notify prescriber
• Advise patient that long-term therapy may be needed to resolve infection (1-2 mo depending on type of infection)
• **Teach patient to report immediately abdominal pain, black tarry stools, as GI bleeding/perforation can occur**
• **Advise patient not to discontinue abruptly or adrenal crisis can result; product should be tapered**

Nasal route
• Instruct patient to clear nasal passages if sneezing attack occurs, then repeat dose; to continue using product even if mild nasal bleeding occurs; bleeding is usually transient
• Teach method of instillation after providing written instruction from manufacturer on instillation

Evaluation
Positive therapeutic outcome
• Decrease in runny nose (nasal)
• Decreased inflammation
• Absence of severe itching, patches on skin, flaking (top)
• Decreased GI symptoms

---

hydrocortisone topical
See Appendix B

⚠ HIGH ALERT

HYDROmorphone (Rx)
(hye-droe-mor'fone)
Dilaudid, Dilaudid-HP, Exalgo, Hydromorph Contin ✹
Func. class.: Antitussive, opioid analgesic agonist
Chem. class.: Phenanthrene derivative, guaifenesin
Pregnancy category C
Controlled substance schedule II

Do not confuse: HYDROmorphone/ meperidine/morphine, **Dilaudid**/Demerol

ACTION: Inhibits ascending pain pathways in CNS, increases pain threshold, alters pain perception

Therapeutic outcome: Decreased cough, decreased pain

USES: As an antitussive to suppress cough; moderate to severe pain

CONTRAINDICATIONS
Hypersensitivity to this product, sulfite, COPD, cor pulmonale, emphysema, GI obstruction, ileus, increased intracranial pressure, obstetric delivery, status asthmaticus

> **BLACK BOX WARNING:** Respiratory depression, opioid-naive patients

Precautions: Pregnancy **C,** breastfeeding, children <18 yr, increased ICP, addictive personality, renal/hepatic disease, MI (acute), abrupt discontinuation, adrenal insufficiency, angina, asthma, biliary tract disease, bladder obstruction, hypothyroidism, hypovolemia, hypoxemia, IBD, IV use, labor, latex hypersensitivity, myxedema, seizure disorders, sleep apnea

> **BLACK BOX WARNING:** Substance abuse, accidental exposure, potential for overdose/poisoning

DOSAGE AND ROUTES
Analgesic
Adult: **PO** (oral solution) 2.5-10 mg q3-6hr or (tabs) 2-4 mg q4-6hr; ext rel (Exalgo): Convert to ext rel by giving total daily dose of immediate release in one daily dose, titrate if needed ext rel q3-4days until adequate pain relief; use 25%-50% increase for each titration step, if more than 2 doses of rescue medication is needed in 24 hr consider titration; **IV** 0.2-1 mg q2-3hr; give over 2-3 min; **IM/SUBCUT** 1-2 mg q4-6hr prn, may be increased (opioid-naive patients may require lower dose); **RECT** 3 mg q6-8hr prn
Geriatric: PO 1-2 mg q4-6hr

Available forms: Powder of injection 250 mg; inj 1, 2, 4, 10 mg/ml; tabs 2, 4, 8 mg; oral sol 5 mg/5 ml; supp 3 mg, ext rel tab 8, 12, 16, 32 mg

Hepatic dose
Adult: Child- Pugh B or C (oral liquid, immediate-release tab, suppository) give reduced dose based on response, impairment; parenteral give 25%-50% of dose (moderate impairment)

Implementation
• Give with antiemetic if nausea, vomiting occur
• Give when pain is beginning to return; determine dosage interval by patient response; continuous dosing of medication is more effective given prn; explain analgesic effect
• Withdraw medication slowly after long-term use to prevent withdrawal symptoms
• Store in light-resistant container at room temperature

PO route
• May be given with food or milk to lessen GI upset

Extended release

> **BLACK BOX WARNING:** Do not use extended-release products in opioid-naive patients or with other extended-release opioids

• **Converting from oral opioids;** conversion ratios are approximate; initiate ext rel tabs at 50% of calculated total daily equivalent dose of ext rel, give q24hr; max increase q2-3days, consider titration increases of 25%-50% in each step
• **Converting from transdermal patch (fentaNYL)** initiate ext rel tabs 18 hr after removal of patch; for each 25 mcg/hr dose of transdermal fentaNYL the dose is 12 mg q24hr, start dose at 50% of calculated HYDROmorphone ext rel dose q24hr; titrate no more often than q3-4days, consider dose increases of 25%-50% with each step; if more than 2 rescue doses are required in 24 hr, consider titration

SUBCUT route
• Do not give if sol is cloudy or a precipitate has formed; rotate inj sites
• Use short 30-G needle, make sure not to inject intradermally

Direct IV route
• Give after diluting with 5 ml or more of sterile water or 0.9% NaCl for inj
• Give slowly at 2 mg over 3-5 min or less through Y-connector or 3-way stopcock

IV infusion route
• Dilute each 0.1-1 mg/ml in 0.9% NaCl, deliver by opioid syringe infusion; may be diluted in D_5W, D_5/NaCl, 0.45% NaCl or 0.9% NaCl for larger amounts and through an infusion pump

Y-site compatibilities: Acyclovir, allopurinol, amifostine, amikacin, amsacrine, aztreonam, cefamandole, cefepime, cefoperazone, cefotaxime, cefOXitin, cefTAZidime, ceftizoxime, cefuroxime, chloramphenicol, CISplatin, cladribine, clindamycin, cyclophosphamide, cytarabine, diltiazem, DOBUTamine, DOPamine, DOXOrubicin, doxycycline, EPINEPHrine, erythromycin lactobionate, famotidine, fentaNYL, filgrastim, fludarabine, foscarnet, furosemide, gentamicin, granisetron, heparin, kanamycin, labetalol, LORazepam, magnesium sulfate, melphalan, methotrexate, metroNIDAZOLE, midazolam, milrinone, morphine, nafcillin, niCARdipine, nitroglycerin, norepinephrine, ondansetron, oxacillin, PACLitaxel, penicillin G potassium, piperacillin, piperacillin/tazobactam, propofol, ranitidine, teniposide, thiotepa, ticarcillin, tobramycin, trimethoprim/sulfamethoxazole, vancomycin, vecuronium, vinorelbine

Y-site incompatibilities: Ampicillin, diazepam, minocycline, PHENobarbital, phenytoin, sargramostim

Solution compatibilities: D₅W, D₅/0.45% NaCl, D₅/0.9% NaCl, D₅/LR, D₅/Ringer's, 0.45% NaCl, 0.9% NaCl, Ringer's, LR

ADVERSE EFFECTS

CNS: Dizziness, drowsiness, *sedation, confusion,* headache, euphoria, mood changes, **seizures**

CV: *Hypotension, bradycardia,* palpitations, change in B/P, tachycardia, peripheral vasodilatation

EENT: Miosis, diplopia, blurred vision, tinnitus

GI: *Nausea, constipation, vomiting, anorexia,* dry mouth, cramps, paralytic ileus

GU: Increased urinary output, dysuria, urinary retention

INTEG: Urticaria, rash, flushing, bruising, diaphoresis, pruritus

RESP: **Respiratory depression,** dyspnea

Pharmacokinetics

Absorption	Well absorbed (PO), complete (IV)
Distribution	Unknown; crosses placenta
Metabolism	Liver, extensively
Excretion	Kidneys
Half-life	Varied

Pharmacodynamics

	PO/IM/ SUBCUT	IV	RECT
Onset	15-30 min	10-15 min	15-30 min
Peak	30-60 min	15-30 min	30-90 min
Duration	4-5 hr	2-3 hr	4-5 hr

INTERACTIONS
Individual drugs
Alcohol: increased respiratory depression, hypotension, sedation

Drug classifications
Antipsychotics, opiates, sedative/hypnotics, skeletal muscle relaxants: increased effects
MAOIs: increased severe reactions

Opiate antagonists: decreased HYDROmorphone effects

Drug/herb
Chamomile, hops, kava, lavender, St. John's wort, valerian: increased action

Drug/lab test
Increased: amylase

NURSING CONSIDERATIONS
Assessment
• **Assess pain control,** sedation by scoring on 0-10 scale; around-the-clock dosing is best for pain control
• Monitor VS after parenteral route; note muscle rigidity; product history

> **BLACK BOX WARNING:** Respiratory dysfunction; respiratory depression; monitor character, rate, rhythm; notify prescriber if respirations are <10/min

• Monitor CNS changes: dizziness, drowsiness, hallucinations, euphoria, LOC, pupil reaction
• Monitor allergic reactions: rash, urticaria; bowel function, constipation

Patient/family education
• Instruct patient to report any symptoms of CNS changes, allergic reactions; to avoid CNS depressants: alcohol, sedative-hypnotics for at least 24 hr after taking this product
• Advise patient that dizziness, drowsiness, and confusion are common and to avoid getting up without assistance, driving, or other hazardous activities
• Discuss in detail all aspects of the product

> **BLACK BOX WARNING:** Teach patient that extended-release products must be taken whole

Evaluation
Positive therapeutic outcome
• Decreased pain
• Decreased cough

TREATMENT OF OVERDOSE:
Naloxone HCl (Narcan) 0.2-0.8 **IV,** O₂, **IV** fluids, vasopressors

hydroxychloroquine (Rx)
(hye-drox-ee-klor'oh-kwin)
Apo-Hydroxyquine ✦, Plaquenil
Func. class.: Antimalarial, antirheumatic (DMARDs)
Chem. class.: 4-Aminoquinoline derivative
Pregnancy category C

ACTION: Impairs complement-dependent antigen-antibody reactions

Adverse effects: *italics* = common; **bold** = life-threatening

Therapeutic outcome: Resolution of infection

USES: Malaria caused by *Plasmodium vivax, P. malariae, P. ovale, P. falciparum* (some strains); LE, rheumatoid arthritis

CONTRAINDICATIONS
Hypersensitivity to this product or chloroquine, retinal field changes

> **BLACK BOX WARNING:** Children (long-term), ocular disease

Precautions: Pregnancy **C**, breastfeeding, blood dyscrasias, severe GI disease, neurologic disease, alcoholism, hepatic disease, G6PD deficiency, psoriasis, eczema

DOSAGE AND ROUTES
Malaria
Adult: PO **suppression or prevention** 400 mg qwk, begin 1-2 wk before travel, continue 4 wk after returning; **treatment** 800 mg, then 400 mg after 6-8 hr, then 400 mg/day on 2nd and 3rd day, total dose 2 g
Child: PO **suppression or prevention** 6.4 mg/kg (5 mg/kg base) qwk, begin 1-2 wk before travel, continue 4 wk after returning; **treatment** 10 mg/kg, 6.4 mg/kg (5 mg/kg base), at 6, 24, 48 hr after 1st dose

Lupus erythematosus
Adult: PO 400 mg (310 mg base) daily-bid; length depends on patient response; **maintenance** 200-400 mg/day

Rheumatoid arthritis
Adult: PO 400-600 mg/day for 4-12 wk; then 200-300 mg/day after good response

Available forms: Tabs 200 mg

Implementation
PO route
• Give before or after meals with milk, at same time each day to maintain product level
• Tabs may be crushed and mixed with food, fluids
• Malaria prophylaxis should be started 2 wk prior to exposure and 4-6 wk after leaving exposure area
• Store in tight, light-resistant container at room temperature; keep inj in cool environment

ADVERSE EFFECTS
CNS: Headache, stimulation, fatigue, irritability, **seizures,** bad dreams, dizziness, confusion, psychosis, decreased reflexes
CV: Hypotension, heart block, **asystole with syncope**

EENT: *Blurred vision, corneal changes, retinal changes, difficulty focusing,* tinnitus, vertigo, deafness, photophobia, corneal edema
GI: *Nausea, vomiting, anorexia,* diarrhea, cramps
HEMA: Thrombocytopenia, agranulocytosis, leukopenia, aplastic anemia
INTEG: Pruritus, pigmentation changes, skin eruptions, lichen planus–like eruptions, eczema, **exfoliative dermatitis,** alopecia, **Stevens-Johnson syndrome,** photosensitivity

Pharmacokinetics
Absorption	Well absorbed
Distribution	Widely distributed, crosses placenta
Metabolism	Liver
Excretion	Urine/feces
Half-life	3-5 day

Pharmacodynamics
Onset	Rapid
Peak	1-2 hr
Duration	Days-weeks

INTERACTIONS
Individual products
Magnesium, aluminum products: decreased malarial action
Digoxin: increased levels
Methotrexate: decreased levels
Rabies vaccine: increased antibody titer

Drug classifications
Live-virus vaccines, botulinum toxoids: decreased effects

NURSING CONSIDERATIONS
Assessment
• **Assess for lupus erythematosus, malaria symptoms** before treatment and daily
• **Assess for rheumatoid arthritis:** pain, swelling, ROM, temp of joints, for decreased reflexes: knee, ankle
• Assess ophthalmic exam baseline, q6mo if long-term treatment or product dosage >150 mg/day
• Assess hepatic studies qwk: AST, ALT, bilirubin
• **Blood dyscrasias:** Assess blood studies: CBC, platelets; WBC, RBC, platelets may be decreased; if severe, product should be discontinued; malaise, fever, bruising, bleeding (rare)
• Assess for decreased reflexes: knee, ankle
• Assess ECG during therapy
• **Assess for depression of T waves, widening of QRS complex**
• **Assess allergic reactions:** pruritus, rash, urticaria

• **Assess for ototoxicity** (tinnitus, vertigo, change in hearing); audiometric testing should be done before, after treatment

⚠ **Assess for toxicity: blurring vision, difficulty focusing, headache, dizziness, knee, ankle reflexes; product should be discontinued immediately**

Patient/family education
• Teach patient to use sunglasses in bright sunlight to decrease photophobia
• Teach patient that urine may turn rust or brown
• Teach patient to report hearing, vision problems; fever, fatigue, bruising, bleeding, which may indicate blood dyscrasias

Evaluation

Positive therapeutic outcome
• Decreased symptoms of malaria, LE, rheumatoid arthritis

TREATMENT OF OVERDOSE:
Induce vomiting; gastric lavage; administer barbiturate (ultra–short-acting), vasopressor, ammonium chloride; tracheostomy may be necessary

---

⚠ HIGH ALERT

hydroxyurea (Rx)
(hye-drox-ee-yoo-ree′ah)
Droxia, Hydrea
Func. class.: Antineoplastic, antimetabolite
Chem. class.: Synthetic urea analog
Pregnancy category D

Do not confuse: hydroxyurea/ hydrOXYzine

ACTION: Acts by inhibiting DNA synthesis without interfering with RNA or protein synthesis; incorporates thymidine into DNA, causing direct damage to DNA strands; cell cycle specific (S phase)

Therapeutic outcome: Prevention of rapidly growing malignant cells

USES: Melanoma, chronic myelogenous leukemia, recurrent or metastatic ovarian cancer, squamous cell carcinoma of the head and neck, sickle cell anemia

CONTRAINDICATIONS
Pregnancy **D**, breastfeeding, hypersensitivity, leukopenia (<2500/mm³), thrombocytopenia (<100,000/mm³), anemia (severe), bone marrow suppression, dental disease, geriatrics, HIV,

hyperkalemia, hyperphosphatemia, hyperuricemia, hypocalcemia, infection, infertility, IM injection, tumor lysis syndrome, vaccinations

Precautions: Renal disease (severe)

BLACK BOX WARNING: Requires an experienced clinician, secondary malignancy

---

DOSAGE AND ROUTES
Ovarian cancer, malignant melanoma
Adult: PO 80 mg/kg as a single dose q3day or 20-30 mg/kg as a single dose daily

Ovarian cancer in combination with radiation
Adult: PO 80 mg/kg as a single dose q3day; should be started 7 days before irradiation

Sickle cell anemia
Adult: PO 15 mg/kg/day, may increase by 5 mg/kg/day q12wk; max 35 mg/day

Renal disease
Adult: CCr <59 ml/min use 50% of dose

Available forms: Caps 200, 300, 400, 500 mg

Implementation
• Do not crush or chew caps; for difficulty swallowing, caps may be opened and contents mixed with water
• Avoid contact with skin, very irritating; wash completely to remove
• Give fluids **IV** or PO before chemotherapy to hydrate patient
• Give antiemetic 30-60 min before giving product and prn to prevent vomiting; antibiotics for prophylaxis of infection
• Provide liquid diet: carbonated beverages; gelatin may be added if patient is not nauseated or vomiting

ADVERSE EFFECTS
CNS: Headache, confusion, hallucinations, dizziness, **seizures**
CV: Angina, ischemia
GI: Nausea, vomiting, anorexia, diarrhea, stomatitis, constipation, **hepatotoxicity,** pancreatitis
GU: Increased BUN, uric acid, creatinine, temporary renal function impairment
HEMA: Leukopenia, anemia, thrombocytopenia, megaloblastic erythropoiesis
INTEG: *Rash,* urticaria, pruritus, dry skin, facial erythema
MISC: Fever, chills, malaise, secondary cancers, **tumor lysis syndrome**
META: Hyperphosphatemia, hyperuricemia, hypocalcemia

RESP: Pulmonary fibrosis, diffuse pulmonary infiltrates

Pharmacokinetics

Absorption	Well absorbed
Distribution	Crosses blood-brain barrier
Metabolism	Liver (50%)
Excretion	Kidneys, unchanged (50%), eliminated as CO_2
Half-life	Terminal 3.5-4.5 hr

Pharmacodynamics

Onset	Unknown
Peak	1-4 hr
Duration	Unknown

INTERACTIONS
Individual drugs
Didanosine, stavudine: increased pancreatitis/hepatotoxicity

Probenecid, sulfinpyrazone: increased uric acid levels

Radiation: increased toxicity

Drug classifications
Anticoagulants, NSAIDs, thrombolytics, salicylates, platelet inhibitors: increased bleeding

Antineoplastics: increased toxicity

Hematopoietic progenitor cells (sargramostim, filgrastim): do not use within 24 hr before or after antineoplastic

Live-virus vaccines: do not use together

Drug/lab test
Increased: BUN, creatinine, LFTs, uric acid

Decreased: Hgb, WBC, platelets, phosphate, calcium

NURSING CONSIDERATIONS
Assessment
• Assess buccal cavity q8hr for dryness, sores or ulceration, white patches, oral pain, bleeding, dysphagia; obtain prescription for viscous lidocaine (Xylocaine)

• Assess symptoms indicating severe allergic reaction: rash, pruritus, urticaria, purpuric skin lesions, itching, flushing

• **Bone marrow suppression: Determine the hemoglobin concentration, total leukocyte count, and platelet count at least once a week during entire course; if the WBC ≤2500/mm³ or platelets ≤100,000/mm³, interrupt Hydrea until the values rise significantly toward normal concentrations. If severe anemia occurs, manage it without interrupting Hydrea receipt. For Droxia, monitor blood counts q2wk and interrupt drug receipt if neutrophils <2000/mm³,** platelets <80,000/mm³, hemoglobin <4.5 g/dl, or if reticulocytes <80,000/mm³ when the hemoglobin concentration is <9 g/dl. After recovery, Droxia may be resumed at a lower dose; Droxia therapy requires an experienced clinician knowledgeable in the use of this medication for the treatment of sickle cell anemia

⚠ Assess for increased uric acid levels, swelling, joint pain primarily in extremities; patient should be well hydrated to prevent urate deposits

⚠ Monitor renal function studies: BUN, creatinine, serum uric acid, urine CCr before, during therapy; I&O ratio; report fall in urine output to <30 ml/hr

⚠ Monitor temp (may indicate beginning of infection)

⚠ Monitor liver function tests before, during therapy (bilirubin, AST, ALT, LDH) as needed or monthly, pancreatitis may also occur

⚠ Cutaneous vasculitic toxicity and gangrene: more common in those receiving interferon

⚠ Assess for bleeding: hematuria, stool guaiac, bruising or petechiae, mucosa or orifices q8hr

⚠ Assess for tumor lysis syndrome: hyperkalemia, hyperphosphatemia, hyperuricemia, hypocalcemia, uric acid nephropathy, acute renal failure; metabolic acidosis can occur, aggressive alkalinization of urine and allopurinol can prevent this

⚠ Severe allergic reaction: assess for rash, urticaria, itching, flushing

⚠ Neurotoxicity: assess for headaches, hallucinations, seizures, dizziness

⚠ Pulmonary reactions: assess for pulmonary fibrosis, fever, dyspnea, diffuse pulmonary infiltrates

> **BLACK BOX WARNING:** Secondary malignancy: leukemia may occur after extended use

> **BLACK BOX WARNING:** Only experienced clinicians should use this product

Patient/family education
⚠ Teach patient to notify prescriber if pregnancy is planned or suspected, pregnancy (D)

• Teach patient to avoid use of products containing aspirin or ibuprofen, razors, commercial mouthwash, since bleeding may occur; instruct patient to report symptoms of bleeding (hematuria, tarry stools)

⚠ Nurse Alert   ✴ Key NCLEX® Drug   ≫ Drug Specifics

- Teach patient to rinse mouth tid-qid with water, club soda; brush teeth bid-qid with soft brush or cotton-tipped applicators for stomatitis; use unwaxed dental floss
- Instruct patient to report signs of anemia (fatigue, headache, irritability, faintness, shortness of breath)
- Advise patient to report any changes in breathing or coughing even several mo after treatment; to avoid crowds and persons with respiratory tract or other infections
- Caution patient not to have any vaccinations without the advice of the prescriber; serious reactions can occur

⚠ Advise patient to notify prescriber of fever, chills, sore throat, nausea, vomiting, anorexia, diarrhea, bleeding, bruising; may indicate blood dyscrasias; mental status change, pancreatitis, hepatotoxicity

Evaluation
Positive therapeutic outcome
- Prevention of rapid division of malignant cells

hydrOXYzine (Rx)
(hye-drox′i-zeen)
Atarax ✦, Vistaril
Func. class.: Antianxiety, sedative, hypnotic, antihistamine, antiemetic
Chem. class.: Piperazine derivative
Pregnancy category C

Do not confuse: hydrOXYzine/hydrALAZINE, **Vistaril**/Versed

ACTION: Depresses subcortical levels of CNS, including limbic system, reticular formation; anticholinergic, antiemetic, antihistaminic responses; competes with H_1-receptor sites

Therapeutic outcome: Absence of allergy symptoms, rhinitis, pruritus, absence of nausea/vomiting, sedation, absence of anxiety

USES: Anxiety preoperatively; postoperatively to prevent nausea, vomiting; to potentiate opioid analgesics; sedation; pruritus; prevention of alcohol withdrawal

CONTRAINDICATIONS
Pregnancy (1st trimester), breastfeeding, acute asthma, hypersensitivity to this product or cetirizine

Precautions: Pregnancy C (2nd/3rd trimesters), geriatric, debilitated patients, renal/hepatic disease, closed-angle glaucoma, COPD, prostatic hypertrophy, asthma

DOSAGE AND ROUTES
Anxiety
Adult: PO 25-100 mg tid-qid, max 400 mg/day; IM 50-100 mg q4-6hr
Child >6 yr: PO 50-100 mg/day in divided doses, max 100 mg/day or 2 mg/kg/day
Child <6 yr: PO 50 mg/day in divided doses, max 50 mg/day or 2 mg/kg/day

Alcohol withdrawal
Adult: IM 50-100 mg, then q4-6hr

Preoperatively/postoperatively (nausea/vomiting)
Adult: IM 25-100 mg q4-6hr
Child: IM 0.5-1.1 mg/kg as a single dose

Pruritus
Adult: PO 25 mg tid-qid; IM 50-100 mg, then q4-6hr prn, switch to PO as soon as feasible
Child ≥6 yr: PO 50-100 mg/day in divided doses; IM 0.5-1 mg/kg/dose q4-6hr prn, use PO when possible
Child <6 yr: PO 50 mg/day in divided doses

Renal dose
Adult: PO CCr <50 ml/min reduce dose by 50%

Available forms: Tabs 10, 25, 50 mg; caps 25, 50, 100 mg; oral sol 10 mg/5 ml; oral susp 25 mg/5 ml; inj 25, 50 mg/ml

Implementation
PO route
- Give without regard to meals
- May crush tab if patient is unable to swallow whole
- Caps may be opened and product mixed with food/fluids for patients with swallowing difficulties
- Shake oral susp before giving

IM route
- Give IM inj in large muscle mass; aspirate to prevent **IV** administration; use Z-track method; severe necrosis can result with improper technique; never give **IV**/SUBCUT

Syringe compatibilities: Atropine, atropine/meperidine, benzquinamide, bupivacaine, butorphanol, chlorproMAZINE, cimetidine, codeine, diphenhydrAMINE, doxapram, droperidol, fentaNYL, fluPHENAZine, glycopyrrolate, HYDROmorphone, lidocaine, meperidine, meperidine/atropine, methotrimeprazine, metoclopramide, midazolam, morphine, nalbuphine, oxymorphone, pentazocine, perphenazine, procaine, prochlorperazine, promazine, promethazine, remifentanil, scopolamine, SUFentanil, thiothixene

Adverse effects: *italics* = common; **bold** = life-threatening

Syringe incompatibilities: Aminophylline, chloramphenicol, dimenhyDRINATE, heparin, penicillin G potassium, PENTobarbital, PHENobarbital, phenytoin

ADVERSE EFFECTS

CNS: *Dizziness, drowsiness,* confusion, headache, tremors, fatigue, depression, seizures
CV: Hypotension
GI: Dry mouth, nausea, diarrhea, increased appetite, weight gain

Pharmacokinetics

Absorption	Well absorbed
Distribution	Not known
Metabolism	Liver, completely
Excretion	Feces, urine, bile
Half-life	3 hr

Pharmacodynamics

	PO/IM
Onset	15-60 min
Peak	2-4 hr
Duration	4-6 hr

INTERACTIONS
Individual drugs
Alcohol: increased CNS depression
Atropine, disopyramide, haloperidol, quiNIDine: increased anticholinergic reactions

Drug classifications
Analgesics, barbiturates, CNS depressants, opiates, sedative/hypnotics: increased CNS depression
Antidepressants, antihistamines, MAOIs, phenothiazines: increased anticholinergic reactions

Drug/lab test
False negative: skin allergy testing
False increase: 17-hydroxycorticosteroids

NURSING CONSIDERATIONS
Assessment
• Anticholinergic effects: dry mouth, dizziness, confusion, hypotension, increased sedation; monitor B/P
• Assess respiratory status: rate, rhythm, increase in bronchial secretions, wheezing, chest tightness; provide fluids to 2 L/day to decrease secretion thickness
• Monitor I&O ratio: be alert for urinary retention, frequency, dysuria, especially in geriatric; product should be discontinued if these occur
• Observe for drowsiness, dizziness
• Assess cough characteristics including type, frequency, thickness of secretions; evaluate response to this medication if using for cough

Patient/family education
• Caution patient to avoid hazardous activities and activities requiring alertness, since dizziness may occur; instruct patient to request assistance with ambulation
• Advise patient to avoid alcohol, other CNS depressants including cough, cold preparations; CNS depression may occur
• Teach all aspects of product use; to notify prescriber if confusion, sedation, hypotension occur; to avoid driving and other hazardous activity if drowsiness occurs
• Caution patient not to exceed recommended dosage; dysrhythmias may occur
• Tell patient hard candy, gum, frequent rinsing of mouth may be used for dryness

Evaluation
Positive therapeutic outcome
• Absence of nausea, vomiting
• Decreased anxiety

TREATMENT OF OVERDOSE:
Lavage if orally ingested, VS, supportive care, **IV** norepinephrine for hypotension

Hylan G-F 20
Synvisc, Synvisc One
See Appendix A, Selected New Drugs

hyoscyamine (Rx)
(hye-oh-sye′a-meen)
Anaspaz, Colidrops, Colytrol Pediatric, Cystospaz-M, ED-SPAZ, HydroMax-DT, HydroMax-FT, HydroMax-SR, HyoMax, HyoMax SL, Hyosyne, Levsin SL, Medispax, NuLev, Oscimin, Spasdel, Symax
Func. class.: Anticholinergic/antispasmodics
Chem. class.: Belladonna alkaloid
Pregnancy category C

ACTION: Inhibits muscarinic actions of acetylcholine at postganglionic parasympathetic neuroeffector sites, reduces rigidity, tremors, hyperhidrosis of parkinsonism

Therapeutic outcome: Absence of peptic ulcer after treatment

USES: Treatment of peptic ulcer disease in combination with other products; other GI disorders, other spastic disorders, IBS, urinary incontinence

CONTRAINDICATIONS
Hypersensitivity to anticholinergics, closed-angle glaucoma, GI obstruction, myasthenia gravis,

---

paralytic ileus, GI atony, toxic megacolon, prostatic hypertrophy, urinary tract obstruction

Precautions: Pregnancy **C**, geriatric, hyperthyroidism, CAD, dysrhythmias, CHF, ulcerative colitis, hypertension, hiatal hernia, renal/hepatic disease, urinary retention

DOSAGE AND ROUTES
Adult/adolescent/child ≥12 yr: PO/SL 0.125-0.25 mg q4hr; ext rel 0.375-0.75 mg q12hr
Adult: IM/SUBCUT/IV 0.25-0.5 mg single dose or 2-4×/day q6hr
Geriatric: Max 1.5 mg/day in divided doses or max 4 biphasic tabs
Child 2-12 yr: PO SL 0.0625-0.125 q4hr

Available forms: Tabs 0.125, 0.15 mg; ext rel caps 0.375 mg; time rel tabs 0.375 ml; sol 0.125 mg/ml; elix 0.125 mg/ml; inj 0.5 mg/ml, SL tab 0.125 mg, tab biphasic 0.125, 0.375 mg; orally disintegrating tab 0.125 mg

Implementation
PO route
- Do not break, crush, or chew time rel caps
- Give ½ hour before meals for better absorption
- Give decreased dose to geriatric patients; metabolism may be slowed
- Store in tight container protected from light

IV route
- Use undiluted, inject slowly

ADVERSE EFFECTS
CNS: *Confusion, stimulation in geriatric,* headache, insomnia, dizziness, drowsiness, anxiety, weakness, hallucination
CV: *Palpitations,* tachycardia
EENT: *Blurred vision,* photophobia, mydriasis, cycloplegia, increased ocular tension
GI: *Dry mouth, constipation, paralytic ileus,* heartburn, nausea, vomiting, dysphagia, absence of taste
GU: *Urinary hesitancy, retention,* impotence
INTEG: Urticaria, rash, pruritus, anhidrosis, fever, allergic reactions

Pharmacokinetics
Absorption	Well
Distribution	Cross blood-brain barrier, placenta
Metabolism	Liver
Excretion	Urine
Half-life	3½ hr

Pharmacodynamics
	PO	IM/IV/SUBCUT
Onset	30 min	2-3 min
Peak	Unknown	Unknown
Duration	4-6 hr	4-6 hr

INTERACTIONS
Individual drugs
Amantadine: increased anticholinergic effect
Ketoconazole, levodopa: decreased effects

Drug classifications
Antacids: decreased hyoscyamine effect
Antidepressants (tricyclics), antihistamines, H_1, MAOIs: increased anticholinergic effect
Phenothiazines: decreased effect of phenothiazines

NURSING CONSIDERATIONS
Assessment
- Monitor VS, cardiac status: checking for dysrhythmias, increased rate, palpitations
- Monitor I/O ratio; check for urinary retention or hesitancy
- Monitor GI complaints: pain, bleeding (frank or occult), nausea, vomiting, anorexia

Patient/family education
- Teach patient to avoid driving, other hazardous activities until stabilized on medication
- Teach patient to avoid alcohol or other CNS depressants; will enhance sedating properties of this product
- Teach patient to avoid hot environments; heat stroke may occur; product suppresses perspiration
- Teach patient to use sunglasses when outside to prevent photophobia; may cause blurred vision
- Teach patient to use gum, hard candy, frequent rinsing of mouth for dryness of oral cavity
- Teach patient to increase fluids, bulk, exercise to decrease constipation

Evaluation
Positive therapeutic outcome
- Absence of epigastric pain, bleeding, nausea, vomiting

H

ibandronate (Rx)

(eye-ban'dro-nate)

Boniva

Func. class.: Bone-resorption inhibitor, electrolyte modifier

Chem. class.: Bisphosphonate

Pregnancy category C

ACTION: Inhibits bone resorption, apparently without inhibiting bone formation and mineralization; absorbs calcium phosphate crystals in bone and may directly block dissolution of hydroxyapatite crystals of bone; more potent than other products

Therapeutic outcome: Increased bone mineral density

USES: Osteoporosis and prophylaxis

Unlabeled uses: Hypercalcemia, osteolytic metastases, Paget's disease

CONTRAINDICATIONS

Achalasia, esophageal stricture, hypocalcemia, intraarterial administration, renal failure, hypersensitivity to bisphosphonates, inability to stand or sit upright

Precautions: Pregnancy **C**, breastfeeding, children, geriatric, anemia, chemotherapy, coagulopathy, dental disease, diabetes mellitus, dysphagia, GI/renal disease, GERD, hypertension, infection, multiple myeloma, phosphate hypersensitivity, vitamin D deficiency

DOSAGE AND ROUTES

Postmenopausal osteoporosis/ prophylaxis

Adult: PO 150 mg qmo; **IV** BOL 3 mg q3mo

Paget's disease (unlabeled)

Adult: IV 2 mg as a single dose

Bone metastases (unlabeled)

Adult: IV 6 mg over 1 hr × 3 days, repeat q4wk

Hypercalcemia (unlabeled)

Adult: IV INF 2 mg over 2 hr

Renal dose

Adult: PO CCr <30 ml/min, avoid use

Available forms: Tabs 2.5, 150 mg; sol for inj 3 mg/ml

Implementation

PO route

• Give early AM with a glass of water; if qmo, give on same day of each month

• Store at room temperature

Direct IV route

• Use single-dose prefilled syringe; discard unused portion; give over 15-30 sec

• Store at room temperature

• Do not use if discolored or if sol contains particulates

ADVERSE EFFECTS

CNS: Fever, insomnia, dizziness, headache

CV: Hypertension, **atrial fibrillation**

EENT: Ocular pain/inflammation, uveitis

GI: Constipation, nausea, vomiting, diarrhea, dyspepsia

INTEG: Rash, inj site reaction

META: *Hypomagnesemia, hypophosphatemia, hypocalcemia,* hypercholesterolemia

MS: Bone pain, myalgia, osteonecrosis of the jaw

SYST: **Stevens-Johnson syndrome, erythema multiforme, dermatitis bullous**

Pharmacokinetics

Absorption	Poor
Distribution	Taken up primarily by bones, 86%-99% protein binding
Metabolism	Unknown
Excretion	Primarily by kidneys
Half-life	5-60 hr

Pharmacodynamics

Onset	Unknown
Peak	0.5-2 hr
Duration	Up to 1 mo

INTERACTIONS

Individual drugs

Calcium, vitamin D, iron, aluminum, magnesium salts: decreased ibandronate effect, separate by 1 hr

Increased: GI irritation: NSAIDs, salicylates

Drug classifications

Aminoglycosides, NSAIDs, radiopaque contrast agents: possible increased neurotoxicity

Loop diuretics: increased hypocalcemia

Drug/food

• Do not take with food, calcium

Drug/lab test

Increased: cholesterol

Decreased: alk phos, magnesium, calcium, phosphate

Increased: cholesterol

NURSING CONSIDERATIONS

Assessment

• **Anaphylaxis: swelling of face, lips, mouth, rash, sweating, wheezing, trouble breathing, discontinue immediately, provide supportive treatment**

- **Osteoporosis:** before and during treatment; monitor DEXA scan for bone mineral density, correct electrolyte imbalances (calcium, magnesium, phosphate) before starting therapy
- Assess for blood studies: electrolytes, Ca, P, Mg; creatinine/BUN
- Assess for atrial fibrillation
- **Assess dental health; before dental extraction, give antiinfectives; osteonecrosis of the jaw may occur**
- Assess for bone pain; use analgesics; may begin within 24 hr, or even years after treatment, pain usually subsides after treatment is discontinued

Patient/family education
- **Teach patient to report hypercalcemic relapse:** nausea, vomiting, bone pain, thirst; unusual muscle twitching, muscle spasms, severe diarrhea, constipation
- Advise patient to continue with dietary recommendations, including calcium and vit D
- Instruct patient to obtain an analgesic from provider for bone pain
- Advise patient that if nausea/vomiting occur, small, frequent meals may help
- Teach patient to report vision symptoms: blurred vision, edema, inflammation; report to prescriber
- Teach to report if pregnancy is planned or suspected or if planning to breastfeed, pregnancy (C)
- Encourage to exercise regularly, to stop smoking, and decrease alcohol
- Advise to take in AM at least 60 min before other meds, food, beverages, to take monthly dose on same day
- **Teach to sit upright ≥60 min after PO dose**

Evaluation
Positive therapeutic outcome
- Increased bone mineral density

A HIGH ALERT

ibrutinib
(eye-broo′ti-nib)
Imbruvica
Func. class.: Antineoplastic-biologic response modifier
Chem. class.: Signal transduction inhibitor (STI)

Pregnancy category D

ACTION: Irreversible inhibitor of Bruton's tyrosine kinases in B cells responsible for tumor growth

Therapeutic outcome: Decrease in progression of disease

USES: Recurrent mantle cell lymphoma in patients who have received at least 1 prior treatment

CONTRAINDICATIONS
Pregnancy (**D**), breastfeeding, hypersensitivity

Precautions: Children, geriatric patients, active infections, anticoagulant therapy, bleeding, hepatic/renal disease, neutropenia, surgery

DOSAGE AND ROUTES
Adult: PO 560 mg (4×140 mg caps)/day

Dosage adjustment for ≥ grade 3 nonhematologic, ≥ grade 3 neutropenia with infection or fever, or grade 4 hematologic toxicities
Interrupt therapy; resume upon recovery to grade 1 or baseline as indicated here:
- **First occurrence: resume dosing at original dose (daily dose = 560 mg/day)**
- **Second occurrence: reduce dose by 1 capsule (daily dose = 420 mg/day)**
- **Third occurrence: reduce dose by 2 capsules (daily dose = 280 mg/day)**
- **Fourth occurrence: discontinue**

Available forms: Caps 140 mg

Implementation
- Give at same time of day with water; if dose is missed, take as soon as possible on same day; do not double
- Do not open, break, chew cap

ADVERSE EFFECTS
CNS: Fatigue, fever
CV: Hypertension, *atrial fibrillation*, peripheral edema
EENT: Sinusitis
GI: Nausea, vomiting, dyspepsia, anorexia, abdominal pain, constipation, stomatitis, diarrhea, GI bleeding
GU: Increased serum creatinine, UTI
HEMA: *Neutropenia, thrombocytopenia,* anemia, bleeding, epistaxis, transient lymphocytosis
INTEG: Rash, skin infections
MS: Pain, arthralgia, muscle cramps
RESP: Cough, dyspnea
SYST: *Secondary malignancy,* infection

Pharmacokinetics

Absorption	Unknown
Distribution	Protein binding 97.3%
Metabolism	By CYP3A4/CYP2D6
Excretion	Primarily in feces, small amount in urine
Half-life	Terminal 4-8 hr

Adverse effects: *italics* = common; **bold** = life-threatening

Pharmacodynamics

Onset	Unknown
Peak	1-2 hr
Duration	Unknown

INTERACTIONS
Drug classifications
Moderate or strong CYP3A4 inducers: decreased ibrutinib effect; avoid concurrent use
Moderate or strong CYP3A4 inhibitors: increased ibrutinib effect; avoid concurrent use

Drug/food
Grapefruit juice: increased plasma concentrations

Drug/herb
St. John's wort: decreased SUNItinib concentration

NURSING CONSIDERATIONS
Assessment
• **Bleeding:** bruising, grade 3 or higher bleeding events may occur
• Monitor hepatic/renal function, signs/symptoms of infection

Patient/family education
• Instruct patient to report adverse reactions immediately: SOB, bleeding
• Teach patient about reason for treatment, expected result
• Teach patient that many adverse reactions may occur: high B/P, bleeding, mouth swelling
• Teach patient to avoid persons with known upper respiratory infections; that immunosuppression is common
• Teach patient to avoid grapefruit juice or medications, herbs; there are many interactions
• **Teach patient to report if pregnancy is planned or suspected, pregnancy (D)**
• Teach patient to report bleeding, severe infections, renal toxicity (maintain hydration), development of second malignancies, diarrhea (contact physician if it persists)
• Teach patient to take with water (avoid food because increases drug levels) at same time each day; do not open, break, or chew

Evaluation
Positive therapeutic outcome
• Decrease in progression of disease

---

ibuprofen (OTC, Rx)
(eye-byoo-proe'fen)
Advil, Caldolor, Ibuprohm, Ibutab, Midol, Motrin ✹, Motrin IB, Pamprin IB ✹, Profen, Tab-Profen
ibuprofen lysine (Rx)
NeoProfen
Func. class.: NSAID

ACTION: Inhibits COX-1, COX-2 by blocking arachidonate; analgesic, antiinflammatory, antipyretic

Therapeutic outcome: Decreased pain, inflammation, fever

USES: Rheumatoid arthritis, osteoarthritis, primary dysmenorrhea, dental pain, musculoskeletal disorders, fever, migraine, patent ductus arteriosus

CONTRAINDICATIONS
Avoid pregnancy (**D**) 3rd trimester, hypersensitivity to this product, NSAIDs, salicylates, asthma, severe renal/hepatic disease

> **BLACK BOX WARNING:** Perioperative pain in CABG

Precautions: Pregnancy (**C**) (1st and 2nd trimester), breastfeeding, children, geriatric, bleeding disorders, GI disorders, cardiac disorders, hypersensitivity to other antiinflammatory agents, CHF, CCr <25 ml/min

> **BLACK BOX WARNING:** GI bleeding, MI, stroke

DOSAGE AND ROUTES
Self-treatment of minor aches/pain
Adult/adolescent: PO (OTC product) 200 mg q4-6hr, may increase to 400 mg q4-6hr; max 1200 mg/day

Analgesia
Adult: PO 200-400 mg q4-6hr; max 3.2 g/day; OTC use max 1200 mg/day
Child: PO 4-10 mg/kg/dose q6-8hr

Moderate to severe pain (hospitalized patients) (Caldolor)
Adult: IV 400-800 mg q6hr as an adjunct to opiate agonist therapy

Dysmenorrhea
Adult: PO 400 mg q4-6hr; max 1200 mg/day

Antipyretic
Child 6 mo-12 yr: PO 5 mg/kg (temp <102.5° F or 39.2° C), 10 mg/kg (temp >102.5° F), may repeat q6-8hr; max 40 mg/kg/day

Antiinflammatory
Adult: PO 400-800 mg tid-qid; max 3.2 g/day
Child: PO 30-40 mg/kg/day in 3-4 divided doses; max 50 mg/kg/day

Patent ductus arteriosus (PDA) (Neoprofen)
Premature neonate ≤32 wk gestation who weighs 500-1500 g: IV 10 mg/kg initially, then if needed, 2 doses 5 mg/kg at 24 hr intervals; if oliguria occurs, hold dose

Available forms: Tabs 100, 200, 300, 400, 600, 800 mg; liqui-gel caps 200 mg; oral susp 100 mg/5 ml; liquid 100 mg/5 ml; chew tabs 50, 100 mg; drops 50 mg/1.25 ml; inj 10 mg/ml (NeoProfen)

Implementation
PO route
• Administer to patient crushed or whole; 800-mg tab may be dissolved in water
• Give with food or milk to decrease gastric symptoms; give 2 hr before or 30 min after meals; absorption may be slowed
• Shake susp well before use
• Store at room temperature
• Do not use in pregnancy after 30 wk gestation

IV route
• Must be well hydrated prior to administration
• Dilute to ≤4 mg/ml (0.9% NaCl, LR, D_5W); infuse over ≥30 min
• Discard unused portion
Intermittent IV infusion route
• Visually inspect for particulate
• Ibuprofen lysine: dilute with dextrose or saline to appropriate volume (10 mg/ml of ibuprofen is recommended) given within 30 min of preparation: give via port that is nearest insertion site; give over 15 min
• Check for extravasation; do not give in same line with TPN, interrupt TPN for 15 min before and after product administration

ADVERSE EFFECTS
CNS: *Headache,* dizziness, drowsiness, fatigue, tremors, confusion, insomnia, anxiety, depression
CV: Tachycardia, peripheral edema, palpitations, dysrhythmias, **CV thrombotic events, MI, stroke**
EENT: Tinnitus, hearing loss, blurred vision
GI: *Nausea, anorexia,* vomiting, diarrhea, jaundice, **hepatitis,** constipation, flatulence, cramps, dry mouth, peptic ulcer, **GI bleeding, ulceration, necrotizing enterocolitis, GI perforation**
GU: Nephrotoxicity, dysuria, hematuria, oliguria, azotemia
HEMA: Blood dyscrasias, increased bleeding time
INTEG: Purpura, rash, pruritus, sweating, urticaria, **necrotizing fasciitis,** photosensitivity, photophobia
META: Hyperkalemia, hyperuricemia, hypoglycemia, hyponatremia
SYST: Anaphylaxis, Stevens-Johnson syndrome

Pharmacokinetics
Absorption	Well absorbed
Distribution	Not known; crosses placenta
Metabolism	Liver, extensively
Excretion	Kidneys, unchanged (10%)
Half-life	1.8-2 hr

Pharmacodynamics
Onset	½ hr
Peak	1-2 hr
Duration	4-6 hr

INTERACTIONS
Individual drugs
Alcohol, aspirin: increased GI reactions
Aspirin: decreased ibuprofen action
CycloSPORINE, lithium, methotrexate: increased toxicity
Furosemide: decreased effect of furosemide
Radiation: increased risk of blood dyscrasias
Valproic acid, warfarin: increased risk of bleeding

Drug classifications
Anticoagulants, antiplatelet agents, salicylates, thrombolytics: increased risk of bleeding
Anticoagulants (oral): increased toxicity
Antidiabetics (oral): increased hypoglycemia
Antihypertensives: decreased effect of antihypertensives
Antineoplastics: increased risk of blood dyscrasias
Corticosteroids, NSAIDs: increased GI reactions
Diuretics: decreased effectiveness of diuretics (thiazides)

Drug/herb
Feverfew, garlic, ginger, ginkgo, ginseng *(Panax):* increased risk of bleeding

Drug/lab test
Increased: BUN, creatinine, LFTs
Decreased: Hgb/Hct, blood glucose, WBC, platelets

NURSING CONSIDERATIONS
Assessment
- **Assess for infection;** may mask symptoms
- **Assess pain:** location, duration, type, intensity before dose, 1 hr after
- Assess musculoskeletal status: ROM before dose, 1 hr after
- Monitor liver function tests: AST, ALT, bilirubin, creatinine if patient is on long-term therapy, monitor electrolytes as needed

> **BLACK BOX WARNING:** Perioperative pain in CABG: MI and stroke can result for 10-14 days, can be fatal, those taking NSAIDs are at greater risk of MI and stroke, even in first few weeks of therapy

- **Nephrotoxicity:** Monitor renal function tests: BUN, urine creatinine if patient is on long-term therapy
- Assess cardiac status: edema (peripheral), tachycardia, palpitations; monitor B/P, pulse for character, quality, rhythm
- Monitor blood studies: CBC, Hct, Hgb, protime if patient is on long-term therapy
- Check I&O ratio; decreasing output may indicate renal failure if patient is on long-term therapy
- Assess for history of peptic ulcer disorder; asthma, aspirin, hypersensitivity, check closely for hypersensitivity reactions

> **BLACK BOX WARNING:** GI bleeding/perforation: chronic use can cause gastritis with or without bleeding; in those with a prior history of peptic ulcer disease or GI bleeding, initiate treatment at lower dose; geriatrics are at greater risk, as are those who consume >3 alcohol drinks/day

- **Assess for allergic reactions:** rash, urticaria; if these occur, product may have to be discontinued
- Assess for vision changes: blurring, halos; may indicate corneal, retinal damage
- Identify prior product history; there are many product interactions
- Identify fever: length of time in evidence and related symptoms

Patient/family education
- Teach patient to use sunscreen, sunglasses, and protective clothing to prevent photosensitivity, photophobia
- Advise patient to read label on other OTC products
- Inform patient that the therapeutic response takes 1 mo (arthritis)

- Caution patient to avoid alcohol ingestion, salicylates, NSAIDs; GI bleeding may occur
- Advise patient with allergies that allergic reactions may develop
- Advise patient to use sunscreen to prevent photosensitivity
- Advise patient to report use of this product to all health care providers
- **Nephrotoxicity: advise to report change in urinary pattern, weight increase, edema, increased pain in joints, fever, blood in urine; monitor fluid status, BUN, creatinine**
- ⚠ **Pregnancy:** notify prescriber if pregnancy (C) is planned or suspected; avoid during 3rd trimester; pregnancy (D) IV after 30 wk

> **BLACK BOX WARNING:** MI/stroke: Teach patient to report signs/symptoms of MI/stroke immediately and discontinue product

Evaluation
Positive therapeutic outcome
- Decreased pain
- Decreased inflammation
- Decreased fever
- Increased mobility

TREATMENT OF OVERDOSE:
Lavage, activated charcoal, induce diuresis

> **⚠ HIGH ALERT**
>
> # ibutilide (Rx)
> (eye-byoo′te-lide)
> **Corvert**
> *Func. class.:* Antidysrhythmic (Class III)
> *Chem. class.:* Methane sulfonamide
> **Pregnancy category C**

ACTION: Prolongs duration of action potential and effective refractory period

USES: For rapid conversion of atrial fibrillation/flutter occurring within 1 wk of coronary artery bypass or valve surgery

CONTRAINDICATIONS
Hypersensitivity

Precautions: Pregnancy **C**, breastfeeding, children <18 yr; geriatric, sinus node dysfunction, 2nd- or 3rd-degree AV block, electrolyte imbalances, bradycardia, renal/hepatic disease, CHF

> **BLACK BOX WARNING:** QT prolongation, torsades de pointes, ventricular arrhythmias, ventricular tachycardia, cardiac dysrhythmias, atrial fibrillation

DOSAGE AND ROUTES
Atrial fibrillation/flutter
Adult: IV INF (≥60 kg) 1 vial (1 mg) given over 10 min, may repeat same dose in 10 min; **IV** INF (<60 kg) 0.01 mg/kg given over 10 min, may repeat same dose in 10 min

Available forms: Inj 1 mg/10 ml

Implementation

IV route
• Give reduced dosage slowly with ECG monitoring only
• Give undiluted or diluted in 50 ml of 0.9% NaCl or D$_5$W (0.017 mg/ml), give over 10 min
• Solution is stable for 48 hr refrigerated or 24 hr at room temperature
• Do not admix with other solution, products
• **Ice compress after stopping inf for extravasation; remove tubing and attempt to aspirate product, elevate affected areas**
• Stop infusion as soon as arrhythmia is stopped
• Do not use if discolored or if particulate is present

ADVERSE EFFECTS
CNS: *Headache*
CV: *Hypotension, bradycardia,* **sinus arrest, CHF, dysrhythmias,** hypertension, extrasystoles, ventricular tachycardia, bundle branch block, AV block, palpitations, supraventricular extrasystoles, syncope, **prolonged QT interval, torsades de pointes**
GI: Nausea

Pharmacokinetics

Absorption	Unknown
Distribution	Unknown
Metabolism	Liver
Excretion	Kidney
Half-life	6 hr

Pharmacodynamics

Unknown

INTERACTIONS
Individual drugs
Digoxin: masking of cardiotoxicity

Drug classifications
Antidepressants (tricyclics/tetracyclics): prodysrhythmia
Antihistamines, H$_2$-receptor antagonists, antidepressants, tetracyclines, tricyclics, phenothiazines: increased prodysrhythmia
Class Ia antidysrhythmics (disopyramide, quiNIDine, procainamide), class III agents (amiodarone, sotalol): do not use
within 5 hr of ibutilide, QT prolongation may occur

NURSING CONSIDERATIONS
Assessment

> **BLACK BOX WARNING:** ECG continuously for >4 hr to determine product effectiveness; measure PR, QRS, QT intervals, check for PVCs, other dysrhythmias; discontinue if atrial fibrillation/flutter ceases; continue until QT interval corrected for heart rate (QTc) returns to baseline; if used ≥2 days, anticoagulation must be adequate

• Monitor I&O ratio; monitor electrolytes: potassium, sodium, chloride
• Monitor liver function tests: AST, ALT
• Monitor for dehydration or hypovolemia
• Assess for CNS symptoms: confusion, psychosis, numbness, depression, involuntary movements; if these occur product should be discontinued
• Monitor cardiac rate, respiration; rate, rhythm, character, chest pain, ventricular tachycardia, supraventricular tachycardia or fibrillation

Patient/family education
• Instruct patient to report side effects immediately to prescriber

Evaluation
Positive therapeutic outcome
• Decrease in atrial fibrillation/flutter

icosapent
(eye-koe′sa-pent)
Vascepa
Func. class.: Antilipidemic
Chem. class.: Omega-3 fatty acid ethylester
Pregnancy category C

ACTION: Inhibits hepatic very-low-density lipoprotein (VLDL) and triglyceride synthesis; enhances clearance of triglycerides from circulating VLDL particles

Therapeutic outcome: Decrease in triglycerides

USES: As adjunct to diet in adults with severe hypertriglyceridemia (500 mg/dl)

CONTRAINDICATIONS
Hypersensitivity to icosapent ethyl

Precautions: Hepatic disease, bleeding, breastfeeding, children, fish/shellfish hypersensitivity, thrombolytic/anticoagulation therapy, pregnancy (C)

Adverse effects: *italics* = common; **bold** = life-threatening

DOSAGE AND ROUTES
Adult: PO 2 g bid

Available forms: Soft gel cap 1 g

Implementation
- Give with food, swallow whole
- Store at room temperature

ADVERSE EFFECTS
HEMA: Ecchymosis, epistaxis
MS: Arthralgia

Pharmacokinetics	
Absorption	Unknown
Distribution	Protein binding 99%
Metabolism	Unknown
Excretion	Unknown
Half-life	89 hr

Pharmacodynamics	
Onset	Unknown
Peak	5 hr
Duration	Unknown

INTERACTIONS
Drug classifications

Anticoagulants, platelet inhibitors, thrombolytics: increased effects of these agents

Drug/lab test

Increased: bleeding time

NURSING CONSIDERATIONS
Assessment
- **Hypertriglyceridemia:** Obtain diet history including fat, cholesterol in diet; cholesterol, triglyceride levels periodically during treatment
- **Liver disease:** Monitor LFTs baseline, periodically in those with liver disease
- **Bleeding:** Monitor for ecchymosis, epistaxis, bleeding time; use cautiously in anticoagulant/thrombolytic therapy
- **Fish/shellfish hypersensitivity:** Identify fish hypersensitivity, use cautiously

Patient/family education
- Teach patient that blood work may be necessary during treatment
- Advise patient to report bleeding if anticoagulants or thrombolytics are used
- Advise patient not to break, crush, open, or dissolve caps
- Inform patient that previously prescribed regimen will continue: low-cholesterol diet, exercise program, smoking cessation

Evaluation
Positive therapeutic outcome
- Decrease in triglycerides

⚠ HIGH ALERT

IDArubicin (Rx)
(eye-da-roo'bi-sin)
Idamycin PFS
Func. class.: Antineoplastic, antibiotic
Chem. class.: Anthracycline glycoside
Pregnancy category D

Do not confuse: IDArubicin/DOXOrubicin/DAUNOrubicin/epirubicin, Idamycin/Adriamycin

ACTION: Not cell cycle specific; topoisomerase II inhibitor, a vesicant; intercalculating between DNA base pairs, causing shape change, low free radicals

Therapeutic outcome: Prevention of rapidly growing malignant cells

USES: Used in combination with other antineoplastics for acute myelocytic leukemia in adults

CONTRAINDICATIONS
Pregnancy **D**, breastfeeding, hypersensitivity

> **BLACK BOX WARNING:** Myelosuppression, bilirubin >5 mg/dl

Precautions: Children, gout, bone marrow depression, preexisting CV disease

> **BLACK BOX WARNING:** Renal/hepatic disease, heart failure

DOSAGE AND ROUTES
Adult: IV 8-12 mg/m²/day × 3 days in combination with cytarabine (induction)

Renal/hepatic dose

> **BLACK BOX WARNING: Adult: IV** if bilirubin is 2.5-5 mg/dl, give 50% of dose; if bilirubin >5 mg/dl, do not use; if CCr >2.5 mg/dl, reduce dose

Available forms: Inj 1 mg/ml

Implementation
- Store at room temp for 3 days after reconstituting or for 7 days refrigerated

IV route
- Avoid contact with skin; very irritating; wash completely to remove
- Administer antiemetic 30-60 min before giving product and prn to prevent vomiting; administer antibiotics for prophylaxis of infection

---

Intermittent IV infusion route
• Product should be prepared by experienced personnel using proper precautions (biological cabinet, wearing gown, gloves, mask)
• Do not give IM/subcut
• Give after reconstituting 5-mg vial with 5 ml of 0.9% NaCl (1 mg/1 ml); give over 10-15 min through Y-tube or 3-way stopcock of inf of D₅W or 0.9% NaCl; discard unused portion
• Apply ice compress after stopping infusion (extravasation)
• **Use a free-flowing IV, don't give IM/ SUBCUT**
• **A vesicant; monitor for necrosis**

Y-site compatibilities: Amifostine, amikacin, aztreonam, cimetidine, cladribine, cyclophosphamide, cytarabine, diphenhydrAMINE, droperidol, erythromycin, filgrastim, granisetron, imipenem/cilastatin, magnesium sulfate, mannitol, melphalan, metoclopromide, potassium chloride, ranitidine, sargramostim, thiotepa, vinorelbine

Y-site incompatibilities: Acyclovir, ampicillin/sulbactam, ceFAZolin, cefTAZidime, clindamycin, dexamethasone, etoposide, furosemide, gentamicin, hydrocortisone, LORazepam, meperidine, methotrexate, mezlocillin, sargramostim, sodium bicarbonate, vancomycin, vinCRIStine

ADVERSE EFFECTS
CNS: Fever, chills, headache, *seizures*
CV: *Dysrhythmias,* **CHF,** *pericarditis, myocarditis,* peripheral edema, angina, **MI, myocardial toxicity**
GI: Nausea, vomiting, abdominal pain, mucositis, diarrhea, **hepatotoxicity**
GU: Nephrotoxicity, red urine
HEMA: **Thrombocytopenia, leukopenia, anemia**
INTEG: Rash, **extravasation,** dermatitis, reversible alopecia, urticaria, thrombophlebitis, tissue necrosis at inj site, radiation recall
SYST: **Infection,** tumor lysis syndrome

Pharmacokinetics
Absorption	Complete bioavailability
Distribution	Rapidly distributed, protein binding 97%
Metabolism	Liver, extensively
Excretion	Bile
Half-life	22 hr

Pharmacodynamics
Unknown

INTERACTIONS
Individual drugs
Cyclophosphamide: increased cardiotoxicity
Radiation: increased toxicity
Trastuzumab: increased CHF, ventricular dysfunction

Drug classifications
Anticoagulants, salicylates, NSAIDs, thrombolytics: increased bleeding risk, avoid concurrent use
Antineoplastics: increased toxicity
Class IA/III, some phenothiazines, other products that increase QT prolongation: increased ECG changes (QT prolongation, changes in QRS voltage)
Corticosteroids: decreased IDArubicin effect
Live virus vaccines: decreased antibody response

Drug/lab test
Increased: uric acid, phosphate, potassium
Decreased: calcium, platelets, neutrophils

NURSING CONSIDERATIONS
Assessment
• **Assess for tumor lysis syndrome: hyperkalemia, hyperphosphatemia, hyperuricemia, hypocalcemia**
• **Assess symptoms indicating severe allergic reaction: rash, pruritus, urticaria, purpuric skin lesions, itching, flushing; product should be discontinued**
• Assess for tachypnea, dyspnea, edema, fatigue

> **BLACK BOX WARNING: Assess for cardiac toxicity:** CHF, dysrhythmias, cardiomyopathy; cardiac studies should be done before and periodically during treatment; ECG, chest x-ray, MUGA

> **BLACK BOX WARNING:** Monitor CBC, differential, platelet count weekly; severe myelosuppression can occur

• Monitor renal function studies: BUN, uric acid, urine CCr, electrolytes, before, during therapy
• Monitor temp (may indicate beginning of infection)

> **BLACK BOX WARNING:** Monitor liver function tests before, during therapy (bilirubin, AST, ALT, LDH) as needed or monthly; note jaundice of skin and sclera, dark urine, clay-colored stools, itchy skin, abdominal pain, fever, diarrhea; hepatotoxicity can be severe, do not use if bilirubin >5 mg/dl

- Assess for bleeding: hematuria, stool guaiac, bruising or petechiae, mucosa or orifices, assess for inflammation of mucosa, breaks in skin
- Identify effects of alopecia on body image; discuss feelings about body changes

> **BLACK BOX WARNING:** Assess for local irritation, pain, burning at injection site, extravasation, a vesicant

Patient/family education
- Teach patient to avoid use of products containing aspirin or ibuprofen, razors, commercial mouthwash, since bleeding may occur; to report symptoms of bleeding (hematuria, tarry stools)
- Instruct patient to report signs of anemia (fatigue, headache, irritability, faintness, shortness of breath)
- Advise patient that hair may be lost during treatment; a wig or hairpiece may make patient feel better; new hair may be different in color, texture
- Teach patient to rinse mouth tid-qid with water, club soda; brush teeth bid-qid with soft brush or cotton-tipped applicators for stomatitis; use unwaxed dental floss
- Tell patient not to have any vaccinations without the advice of the prescriber; serious reactions can occur
⚠ Teach patient to report if pregnancy is planned or suspected, pregnancy (D)
⚠ Advise patient that contraception is needed during treatment and for several mo after the completion of therapy
⚠ Teach patient to report signs of CHF, cardiac toxicity, beginning infection
- Advise patient to avoid crowds, those with upper respiratory illness
- Advise that all body fluids change color

Evaluation
Positive therapeutic outcome
- Prevention of rapid division of malignant cells

---

idelalisib
(eye-del′a-lis′ib)
Zydelig
Func. class.: Antineoplastic-biologic response modifier
Chem. class.: Signal transduction inhibitor (STI)
Pregnancy category D

ACTION: Selective, small-molecule inhibitor of one kinase (expressed in both normal and malignant B-cells). Induces apoptosis and inhibited proliferation, inhibits several cell signaling pathways.

Therapeutic outcome: Decreased disease progression

USES: Treatment of relapsed chronic lymphocytic leukemia (CLL), in combination with rituximab, in those whom rituximab alone should not be used; non-Hodgkin's lymphoma (NHL), relapsed follicular B-cell NHL in those who have received at least 2 prior systemic therapies

CONTRAINDICATIONS: Infusion-related reaction, serious rash, pregnancy **D**

Precautions: Serious allergic reactions, grade 3 or 4 neutropenia, breastfeeding, hyperglycemia/hypoglycemia

> **BLACK BOX WARNING:** Serious hepatotoxicity, grade 3 or higher diarrhea or colitis, fatal/serious pneumonitis

DOSAGE AND ROUTES
Treatment of relapsed chronic lymphocytic leukemia (CLL)
Adult: PO 150 mg bid until disease progression or unacceptable toxicity, with 8 doses of rituximab (given as 375 mg/m² IV on day 1, then 2 wk later rituximab 500 mg/m² IV q2wk × 3 more doses, followed by rituximab 500 mg/m² IV q4wk × 4 doses)

Treatment of small lymphocytic lymphoma (SLL) in those who have received at least 2 prior systemic therapies
Adult: PO 150 mg bid until disease progression or unacceptable toxicity

Hepatic dose
- AST/ALT >3-5 × ULN: No change; monitor AST/ALT at least every week until ≤1 × ULN
- AST/ALT >5-20 × ULN: Hold doses, monitor AST/ALT at least every week, when AST/ALT are ≤1 × ULN, resume at 100 mg bid
- AST/ALT >20 × ULN: Permanently discontinue
- Bilirubin >1.5-3 × ULN: No change; monitor bilirubin at least every week until ≤1 × ULN
- Bilirubin >3-10 × ULN: Hold treatment; monitor bilirubin at least every week; when bilirubin is ≤1 × ULN, resume treatment at 100 mg bid
- Bilirubin >10 × ULN: Permanently discontinue

Available forms: Tabs 100, 150 mg

Implementation
- Take without regard to food, do not crush or dissolve tabs

• Do not take 2 doses at the same time, if a dose is missed by <6 hr, take the dose, take next dose at usual time

Therapeutic drug monitoring: dosage adjustments due to treatment-related toxicity

• **Moderate diarrhea (4-6 stools/day over baseline):** Continue current dosing; monitor at least every week until diarrhea is resolved
• **Severe diarrhea (≥7 stools/day over baseline) or diarrhea requiring hospitalization:** Hold treatment, and monitor at least every week for resolution. When diarrhea has resolved, resume with 100 mg bid
• **Life-threatening diarrhea:** Permanently discontinue treatment
• **Neutropenia: ANC 1000-1499 cells/mm³:** no change; ANC 500-999 cells/mm³: continue current dosing; monitor ANC at least every week; ANC <500 cells/mm³: hold treatment and monitor ANC at least every week, when ANC ≥500 cells/mm³, resume treatment at 100 mg bid
• **Thrombocytopenia: Platelet count 50,000-75,000 cells/mm³:** no change; platelet count 25,000-49,000 cells/mm³: continue dose; monitor platelet count at least every week; platelet count <25,000 cells/mm³: hold treatment, monitor platelet count at least every week, when platelet count ≥25,000 cells/mm³, resume treatment at 100 mg bid
• **Symptomatic pneumonitis (any severity):** Discontinue treatment
• **Other severe or life-threatening toxicities:** Hold until toxicity is resolved; if resuming treatment, reduce the dose to 100 mg bid; permanently discontinue treatment for any recurrence of severe or life-threatening toxicity after rechallenge

ADVERSE EFFECTS

CNS: Insomnia, fatigue, fever, headache
EENT: Sinusitis
ENDO: Hypoglycemia, hyperglycemia, hyponatremia
GI: Nausea, vomiting, *hepatic failure*, **GI perforation**, stomatitis, colitis, diarrhea, anorexia, abdominal pain
HEMA: Thrombocytopenia, neutropenia, anemia
INTEG: Rash
RESP: Pneumonitis, dyspnea, cough
SYST: Serious/fatal rashes

Pharmacokinetics

Absorption	Unknown
Distribution	84% protein binding
Metabolism	Unknown
Excretion	Unknown
Half-life	Half-life 8.2 hr

Pharmacodynamics

Onset	Unknown
Peak	1.5 hr
Duration	Unknown

INTERACTIONS
Drug classifications:
CYP3A4 inhibitors, inducers, substrates: avoid concurrent use

Drug/lab test:
Increase: LFTs

NURSING CONSIDERATIONS
Assessment
• **Hepatic failure:** Increased LFTs generally occurred within the first 12 wk of treatment and were reversible with dose interruption. Monitor LFTs q2wk × 3 mo of treatment, then q4wk for 3 mo, and q1-3 mo thereafter; monitor weekly if AST or ALT are >3 times the upper limit of normal (ULN) or bilirubin >1.5 × ULN. Hepatotoxicity may require treatment interruption, dose reduction, or discontinuation of therapy.
• **Severe diarrhea/GI perforation:** Generally responds poorly to antimotility agents. The occurrence of ≥7 stools/day over baseline or hospitalization due to diarrhea may result in interruption of therapy, dose reduction, or permanent discontinuation. Assess for new or worsening abdominal pain, chills, fever, or nausea/vomiting. If intestinal perforation occurs, permanently discontinue treatment.
• **Pneumonitis:** Monitor for cough, dyspnea, hypoxia, and bilateral interstitial infiltrates, or a decline in oxygen saturation by >5%. If pneumonitis is suspected, hold therapy. Permanently discontinue treatment for pneumonitis and consider treatment with corticosteroids.

Patient/family education
• Instruct patient to report planned or suspected pregnancy (D), use effective contraception during treatment and for at least 1 month after the last dose
• Instruct patient to avoid breastfeeding
• Instruct patient to report new or worsening side effects

Evaluation
Positive therapeutic outcome
• Decreased disease progression

⚠ HIGH ALERT

ifosfamide (Rx)
(i-foss'fa-mide)

Ifex

Func. class.: Antineoplastic alkylating agent

Chem. class.: Nitrogen mustard

Pregnancy category D

Do not confuse: ifosfamide/cyclophosphamide

ACTION: Alkylates DNA, RNA; inhibits enzymes that allow synthesis of amino acids in proteins; also responsible for cross-linking DNA strands; activity is not cell cycle stage specific

Therapeutic outcome: Prevention of rapidly growing malignant cells

USES: Testicular cancer

Unlabeled uses: Soft-tissue sarcoma, Ewing's sarcoma, non-Hodgkin's lymphoma, lung/pancreatic cancer, sarcoma, bladder, breast, cervical, thymic cancer, desmoid tumor, Ewing sarcoma, rhabdomyosarcoma

CONTRAINDICATIONS
Pregnancy **D**, hypersensitivity

> **BLACK BOX WARNING:** Bone marrow suppression

Precautions: Renal/hepatic disease, breastfeeding, children, accidental exposure, dehydration, dental disease, infection, IM injection, ocular exposure, varicella

> **BLACK BOX WARNING:** Coma, hemorrhagic cystitis

DOSAGE AND ROUTES
Adult: IV 1.2-2 g/m²/day × 5 days; repeat course q3wk; give with mesna, in combination with 1-2 other antineoplastic agents

Renal dose
Adult: IV CCr 31-60 ml/min give 75% of dose; CCr 10-30 ml/min give 50% of dose; CCr <10 ml/min, do not give

Available forms: Inj 1, 3 g vials

Implementation
• Administer antiemetic 30-60 min before product to prevent vomiting
• Visually inspect parenteral products for particulate matter and discoloration prior to use
• Store powder at room temperature

IV route
• Give as an intermittent infusion or continuous infusion
• Well hydrate with at least 2 L/day of oral or IV fluids should be given to prevent bladder toxicity
• Must be given in combination with mesna to prevent hemorrhagic cystitis
• Close hematologic monitoring is recommended. WBC count, platelet count, and hemoglobin should be obtained prior to each use and periodically thereafter
• A urinalysis should be performed prior to each dose to monitor for hematuria

Reconstitution and further dilution
• Reconstitute 1 or 3 g with 20 or 60 ml, respectively, of sterile water for injection or bacteriostatic water for injection containing parabens or benzyl alcohol to give IV solutions containing 50 mg/ml
• Solutions may be diluted further to achieve concentrations of 0.6-20 mg/ml in the following solutions: D₅W, NS, LR
• Infuse slowly over at least 30 min
• Diluted and reconstituted solutions refrigerated and used within 24 hours

Y-site compatibilities: Acyclovir, Alatrofloxacin, alemtuzumab, alfentanil, allopurinol, Amifostine, amikacin, Aminocaproic acid, aminophylline, amiodarone, amphotericin B cholesteryl (Amphotec), amphotericin B conventional colloidal, amphotericin B lipid complex (Abelcet), amphotericin B liposome (AmBisome), ampicillin, ampicillin-sulbactam, anidulafungin, argatroban, Arsenic trioxide, atenolol, Atracurium, azithromycin, Aztreonam, bivalirudin, bleomycin, bumetanide, buprenorphine, Butorphanol, Calcium chloride/gluconate, CARBOplatin, Caspofungin, ceFAZolin, Cefoperazone, cefotaxime, cefoTEtan, cefOXitin, cefTAZidime, cefTAZidime (L-arginine), ceftizoxime, cefTRIAXone, cefuroxime, chlorproMAZINE, cimetidine, ciprofloxacin, cisatracurium, CISplatin, clindamycin, codeine, cycloSPORINE, cytarabine, DACTINomycin, DAPTOmycin, DAUNOrubicin liposome, dexamethasone phosphate, dexmedetomidine, Dexrazoxane, digoxin, diltiazem, diphenhydrAMINE, DOBUTamine, DOCEtaxel, dolasetron, DOPamine, doripenem, Doxacurium, DOXOrubicin, DOXOrubicin liposomal, doxycycline, droperidol, enalaprilat, Ephedrine, EPINEPHrine, epirubicin, ertapenem, erythromycin, esmolol, etoposide, etoposide phosphate, famotidine, fenoldopam, fentaNYL, filgrastim, fluconazole, Fludarabine, fluorouracil, foscarnet, fosphenytoin, furosemide, Gallium nitrate, ganciclovir, gatifloxacin, gemcitabine, Gemtuzumab, gentamicin, granisetron, haloperidol, heparin, hydrocortisone phosphate/succinate, HYDROmorphone, hydrOXYzine, IDArubicin, imipenem-cilastatin, inamrinone, insulin, regular, Isoproterenol, ketorolac, labetalol, lansoprazole, lepirudin, leucovorin, levofloxacin, Levorphanol, lidocaine, linezolid, LORazepam, magnesium sulfate, mannitol, melphalan, meperidine, meropenem, Mesna, Methohexital, methylPREDNISolone, metoclopramide, metoprolol, metroNIDAZOLE, midazolam, milrinone, minocycline, mitoMYcin, mitoXANtrone, Mivacurium, morphine, moxifloxacin, Nalbuphine, naloxone, nesiritide, niCARdipine, nitroglycerin, nitroprusside, norepinephrine, octreotide, ofloxacin, ondansetron, oxaliplatin, PAClitaxel (solvent/surfactant), palonosetron, pamidronate, pancuronium, PEMEtrexed, pentamidine, PENTobarbital, Phenobarbital, phenylephrine, piperacillin, piperacillin-tazobactam, potassium acetate/chloride, procainamide, prochlorperazine, promethazine, propofol, propranolol, Quinupristin-Dalfopristin, ranitidine, Rapacuronium, remifentanil, riTUXimab, rocuronium, sargramostim, sodium acetate/bicarbonate/phosphates, succinylcholine, Sufentanil, sulfamethoxazole-trimethoprim, tacrolimus, Teniposide, theophylline, Thiopental, Thiotepa, ticarcillin, ticarcillin-clavulanate, tigecycline, tirofiban, TNA (3-in-1), tobramycin, topotecan, TPN (2-in-1), trastuzumab, vancomycin, vasopressin, vecuronium, verapamil, vinBLAStine, vinCRIStine, vinorelbine, voriconazole, zidovudine, zoledronic acid

Additive compatibilities: CARBOplatin, CISplatin, epirubicin, etoposide, fluorouracil, mesna

ADVERSE EFFECTS

CNS: Facial paresthesia, fever, malaise, somnolence, confusion, depression, hallucinations, dizziness, disorientation, seizures, coma, cranial nerve dysfunction, encephalopathy

GI: Nausea, vomiting, anorexia, hepatotoxicity, stomatitis, constipation, diarrhea, dyslipidemia, hyperglycemia

GU: Hematuria, nephrotoxicity, hemorrhagic cystitis, dysuria, urinary frequency, retrograde ejaculation

HEMA: Thrombocytopenia, leukopenia, anemia

INTEG: Dermatitis, alopecia, pain at inj site, hyperpigmentation

META: Metabolic acidosis

Pharmacokinetics

Absorption	Complete bioavailability
Distribution	Saturation at high dosages
Metabolism	Liver
Excretion	Breast milk
Half-life	15 hr, depends on dose

Pharmacodynamics

Unknown

INTERACTIONS
Individual drugs
Allopurinol: increased toxicity
Radiation: increased bone marrow suppression

Drug classifications
Anticoagulants, NSAIDs, salicylates, thrombolytics: increased bleeding risk
Antineoplastics: increased bone marrow suppression
CYP3A4 inducers, barbiturates: increased toxicity
CYP3A4 inhibitors: decreased ifosfamide effect
Live virus vaccines: decreased antibody response
Do not use within 24 hr of hematopoietic progenitor cells

NURSING CONSIDERATIONS
Assessment
⚠ **Monitor CBC, differential, platelet count weekly; withhold product if WBC is <2000 or platelet count is <50,000; notify prescriber of results if WBC <10,000/mm³, platelets <100,000/mm³, severe myelosuppression**

• Monitor renal function studies: BUN, serum uric acid, urine CCr before, during therapy; I&O ratio; report fall in urine output of 30 ml/hr
• Monitor for cold, fever, sore throat (may indicate beginning of infection); identify edema in feet and joints, stomach pain, shaking; prescriber should be notified
• Assess for bleeding: hematuria, guaiac, bruising or petechiae, mucosa or orifices; no rect temp

> **BLACK BOX WARNING:** I&O ratio; monitor for hematuria; hemorrhagic cystitis can occur; increase fluids to 3 L/day; urinalysis prior to each dose; do not give at night

• Monitor liver function tests before, during therapy (ALT, AST, LDH); jaundice of skin, sclera, dark urine, clay-colored stools, itching, abdominal pain, fever, diarrhea that may indicate liver involvement

Patient/family education
• Teach patient to avoid use of products containing aspirin or NSAIDs, razors, commercial mouthwash, since bleeding may occur; to report symptoms of bleeding (hematuria, tarry stools)
• Instruct patient to report signs of anemia (fatigue, headache, irritability, faintness, shortness of breath)
• Advise patient to report any changes in breathing or coughing even several mo after treatment; to avoid crowds and persons with respiratory tract or other infections
• Teach patient that hair loss is common; discuss the use of wigs or hairpieces; that hair may be a different texture when regrowth occurs
• Caution patient not to have any live virus vaccinations without the advice of the prescriber; serious reactions can occur for 3 months–1 yr, to discuss encephalopathy, neurotoxicity
• Teach patient to notify prescriber if pregnancy is planned or suspected, pregnancy (D)
• Advise patient that contraception is needed during treatment and for several mo after completion of therapy
• Advise patient to report confusion, hallucinations, extreme drowsiness, numbness, tingling; avoid use of alcohol for ≥4 months after treatment
• Teach patient to avoid driving, hazardous activities until reaction is known
• Instruct patient to drink extra fluids in order to urinate often to prevent hemorrhagic cystitis

Evaluation

Positive therapeutic outcome
• Prevention of rapid division of malignant cells
• Absence of swelling at night
• Increased appetite, increased weight

iloperidone (Rx)
(ill-o-pehr′ih-dohn)
Fanapt
Func. class.: Antipsychotic
Chem. class.: Benzisoxazole derivative
Pregnancy category C

ACTION: Unknown; may be mediated through both dopamine type 2 (D_2) and serotonin type 2 (5-HT_2) antagonism; high receptor binding affinity for norepinephrine (alpha 1)

Therapeutic outcome: Decreased signs/symptoms of schizophrenia

USES: Schizophrenia

CONTRAINDICATIONS
Breastfeeding, hypersensitivity

Precautions: Pregnancy **C,** children, geriatric patients, renal/hepatic disease, breast cancer, Parkinson's disease, dementia with Lewy bodies, seizure disorder, QT prolongation, bundle branch block, acute MI, ambient temperature increase, AV block, stroke, substance abuse, suicidal ideation, tardive dyskinesia, torsades de pointes, blood dyscrasias, dysphagia

> **BLACK BOX WARNING:** Increased mortality in elderly patients with dementia-related psychosis

DOSAGE AND ROUTES
Adult: PO 1 mg bid, may increase to target dose of 6-12 mg bid with daily dose adjustment of max 2 mg bid; titrate slowly; max 24 mg/day in two divided doses; reduce dose by 50% in poor metabolizer of CYP2D6 or when used with strong CYP2D6/CYP3A4 inhibitors

Available forms: Tabs 1, 2, 4, 6, 8, 10, 12 mg; titration pack

Implementation
• Give reduced dose in geriatric patients
• Give anticholinergic agent on order from prescriber, to be used for EPS
• Avoid use with CNS depressants
• Provide decreased stimulus by dimming lights, avoiding loud noises
• Provide supervised ambulation until patient is stabilized on medication; do not involve in strenuous exercise program because fainting is possible; patient should not stand still for a long time
• Give increased fluids to prevent constipation
• Provide sips of water, candy, gum for dry mouth
• Store in tight, light-resistant container (PO); store unopened vials in refrigerator; protect from light; do not freeze

ADVERSE EFFECTS
CNS: *EPS, pseudoparkinsonism, akathisia, dystonia, tardive dyskinesia;* drowsiness, seizures, neuroleptic malignant syndrome, dizziness, delirium, depression, paranoia, fatigue, hostility, lethargy, restlessness, vertigo, tremor, drowsiness
CV: Orthostatic hypotension, heart failure, AV block, QT prolongation, tachycardia
EENT: Blurred vision, cataracts, nystagmus, tinnitus
GI: *Nausea,* vomiting, *anorexia, constipation,* jaundice, weight gain/loss, abdominal pain, stomatitis, xerostomia
GU: Hyperprolactinemia, urinary retention/incontinence, testicular pain, renal failure
MISC: Renal artery occlusion

HEMA: Agranulocytosis, leukopenia, neutropenia

Pharmacokinetics

Absorption	Unknown
Distribution	Unknown
Metabolism	Extensively, liver (major metabolite) CYP2D6, CYP3A4
Excretion	Urine
Half-life	Terminal 18 hr extensive metabolizers; 33 hr poor metabolizers

Pharmacodynamics

Onset	Unknown
Peak	2-4 hr
Duration	Unknown

INTERACTIONS
Individual drugs

Alcohol: increased sedation

Chloroquine, clarithromycin, droperidol, erythromycin, haloperidol, methadone, pentamidine: increased QT prolongation

Drug classifications

CYP2D6, CYP3A4 inducers (carBAMazepine, barbiturates, phenytoins, rifampin): decreased iloperidone action

CYP2D6, CYP3A4 inhibitors (delavirdine, indinavir, itraconazole, dalfopristin, ritonavir, tipranavir): increased iloperidone effect, decreased clearance, reduce dose

Class IA/ III antidysrhythmics, some phenothiazines, β-agonists, local anesthetics, tricyclics: increased QT prolongation

Other CNS depressants: increased sedation

SSRIs, SNRIs, serotonin-agonists: increased serotonin syndrome, neuroleptic malignant syndrome

Drug/lab test

Increased: prolactin levels, cholesterol, glucose, lipids, triglycerides

Decreased: potassium

NURSING CONSIDERATIONS
Assessment

• Assess AIMS assessment, lipid panel, blood glucose, CBC, glycosylated hemoglobin A1C, LFTs, neurologic function, pregnancy test, serum creatinine, electrolytes, prolactin, thyroid function studies, weight

• Assess affect, orientation, LOC, reflexes, gait, coordination, sleep pattern disturbances

• Monitor B/P standing and lying; also pulse, respirations; take these q4hr during initial treatment; establish baseline before starting treatment; report drops of 30 mm Hg; watch for ECG changes; QT prolongation may occur

• Assess for dizziness, faintness, palpitations, tachycardia on rising

• **Assess for EPS,** including akathisia, tardive dyskinesia (bizarre movements of the jaw, mouth, tongue, extremities), pseudoparkinsonism (rigidity, tremors, pill rolling, shuffling gait)

> **BLACK BOX WARNING:** Assess for serious reactions in the geriatric patient: fatal pneumonia, heart failure, sudden death, not to be used in the elderly with dementia

• **Assess for neuroleptic malignant syndrome:** hyperthermia, increased CPK, altered mental status, muscle rigidity

• Assess for constipation, urinary retention daily; if these occur, increase bulk and water in diet

• Monitor weight gain, hyperglycemia, metabolic changes in diabetes

Patient/family education

• Teach that orthostatic hypotension may occur and to rise from sitting or lying position gradually

• Advise to avoid hot tubs, hot showers, tub baths; hypotension may occur

• Teach to avoid abrupt withdrawal of this product; EPS may result; product should be withdrawn slowly; to review symptoms of neuroleptic malignant syndrome

• Teach to avoid OTC preparations (cough, hay fever, cold) unless approved by prescriber; serious product interactions may occur; avoid use of alcohol; increased drowsiness may occur

• Advise to avoid hazardous activities if drowsy or dizzy

• Teach compliance with product regimen

• Teach to report impaired vision, tremors, muscle twitching

• Teach that heat stroke may occur in hot weather; take extra precautions to stay cool

• Advise to use contraception; inform prescriber if pregnancy is planned or suspected

Evaluation

Positive therapeutic outcome

• Decrease in emotional excitement, hallucinations, delusions, paranoia; reorganization of patterns of thought, speech

TREATMENT OF OVERDOSE:
Lavage if orally ingested; provide airway; *do not induce vomiting*

> **⚠ HIGH ALERT**

imatinib (Rx)

(im-ah-tin'ib)

Gleevec

Func. class.: Antineoplastic— miscellaneous

Chem. class.: Protein-tyrosine kinase inhibitor

Pregnancy category D

ACTION: Inhibits Bcr-Abl tyrosine kinase created in chronic myeloid leukemia (CML), also inhibits tyrosine kinases including EGF, FGF, PDGF, SCF, VEGF, NGF

Therapeutic outcome: Decreased tumor size, prevention of spread of cancer

USES: Treatment of chronic myeloid leukemia (CML), Philadelphia chromosome positive in blast cell crisis or chronic failure; gastrointestinal stromal tumors (GIST), positive for C-KIT; chronic eosinophilic leukemia, Philadelphia chromosome positive (PH+), acute lymphocytic leukemia, dermatofibrosarcoma protuberans, myelodysplastic syndrome, systemic mastocytosis

CONTRAINDICATIONS

Pregnancy **D**, hypersensitivity

Precautions: Breastfeeding, children, geriatric, cardiac/renal/hepatic/dental disease, GI bleeding, bone marrow suppression, infection, thrombocytopenia, neutropenia, immunosuppression

DOSAGE AND ROUTES

Treatment of Philadelphia chromosome positive (Ph+) chronic myelogenous leukemia (CML) chronic phase as initial therapy

Adult: PO 400 mg/day, continue as long as is beneficial; may increase to 600 mg/day in the absence of severe adverse reactions and severe non-leukemia–related neutropenia or thrombocytopenia

Adolescent/child >2 yr: PO 340 mg/m²/day, max 600 mg/day; daily dose may be given as a single dose or split into 2 doses given once in the morning and once in the evening

Adult patients with Ph+ CML in chronic phase after failure of interferon-alfa therapy

Adult: PO 400 mg/day; continue as long as is beneficial; may increase to 600 mg/day

Pediatric patients with Ph+ CML in chronic phase whose disease has recurred after hematopoietic stem cell transplant or who are resistant to interferon-alfa therapy

Adolescent/child >3 yr: PO 260 mg/m²/day; may be given as single daily dose or may be divided and given once in the morning and once in the evening; may increase to 340 mg/m²/day

Adult patients with Ph+ CML in accelerated phase or blast crisis

Adult: PO 600 mg/day, continue as long as is beneficial, may increase to 800 mg/day (400 mg bid)

Adult patients with resistant or relapsed Ph+ acute lymphocytic leukemia (ALL)

Adult: PO 600 mg/day, continue as long as is beneficial

Adult patients with *Kit* (CD117) positive unresectable and/or metastatic GIST

Adult: PO 400-600 mg/day, may increase to 400 mg bid

Adjuvant treatment of *Kit* (CD117) positive GIST after complete gross resection

Adult: PO 400 mg/day

Hypereosinophilic syndrome (HES) and/or chronic eosinophilic leukemia (CEL) who have the FIPL1L1-PDGFR alpha fusion kinase (mutational analysis or FISH demonstration of CHIC2 allele deletion) and for patients with HES and/or CEL who are FIPL1L-PDGFR alpha fusion kinase negative or unknown

Adult: PO 400 mg/day in those who are FIPL1L1-PDGFR alpha fusion kinase negative or unknown; for HES/CEL patients with demonstrated FIP1L1-PDGFR alpha fusion kinase, 100 mg/day, may increase to 400 mg

Myelodysplastic syndrome (MDS)/myeloproliferative disease (MPD) associated with the PDGFR (platelet-derived growth factor receptor) gene rearrangements

Adult: PO 400 mg/day

Aggressive systemic mastocytosis (ASM) without D816V c-Kit mutation or with c-Kit mutation status unknown

Adult: PO 400 mg/day in those without the FIP1L1-PDGFR alpha c-Kit mutation. If c-Kit status is unknown or not available, give 400 mg/day

Unresectable, recurrent, and/or metastatic dermatofibrosarcoma protuberans (DFSP)
Adult: PO 400 mg bid (800 mg/day)

Hepatic dose
Adult: PO total bilirubin 1.5-3 × ULN and any AST, decrease initial dose to 400 mg/ day; total bilirubin >3 × ULN and any AST, decrease initial dose to 300 mg/day

Renal dose
Adult: PO CCr 40-59 ml/min, max 600 mg/ day; CCr 20-39 ml/min decrease initial dose by 50%, max 400 mg/day; CCr <20 ml/min use with caution 100 mg/day

Available forms: Tabs 100, 400 mg

Implementation
PO route
- Give with meal and large glass of water to decrease GI symptoms, doses of 800 mg should be given 400 mg bid
- Tab may be dispersed in a glass of water or apple juice, use 50 ml of liquid for 100 mg tab, 200 ml/400 mg
- Store at 25° C (77° F)
- Continue as long as is beneficial

ADVERSE EFFECTS
CNS: CNS hemorrhage, headache, dizziness, insomnia, **subdural hematoma**
CV: Hemorrhage, heart failure, cardiac tamponade, cardiac toxicity
EENT: Blurred vision, conjunctivitis
GI: *Nausea,* hepatotoxicity, *vomiting, dyspepsia,* GI hemorrhage, *anorexia,* abdominal pain, GI perforation, diarrhea
HEMA: Neutropenia, thrombocytopenia, bleeding, hypereosinophilia
INTEG: *Rash, pruritus,* alopecia, photosensitivity
META: Edema, fluid retention, hypokalemia
MISC: Fatigue, epistaxis, pyrexia, night sweats, increased weight, flulike symptoms, hypothyroidism
MS: Cramps, pain, arthralgia, myalgia
RESP: Cough, dyspnea, nasopharyngitis, pneumonia, URI, pleural effusion, edema

Pharmacokinetics

Absorption	Well absorbed; bound to plasma protein (98%)
Distribution	Unknown
Metabolism	Liver (metabolites)
Excretion	Feces, primarily (metabolites)
Half-life	18-40 hr

Pharmacodynamics

Onset	Unknown
Peak	2-4 hr
Duration	24 hr (imatinib), 40 hr (metabolite)

INTERACTIONS
Individual drugs
Acetaminophen: increased hepatotoxicity
Simvastatin: increased plasma concentrations
Warfarin: increased plasma concentration of warfarin; avoid coadministration; use low-molecular-weight anticoagulants instead

Drug classifications
Calcium channel blockers, ergots: increased plasma concentrations
CYP3A4 inducers (carBAMazepine, dexamethasone, PHENobarbital, phenytoin, rifampin): decreased imatinib concentrations
CYP3A4 inhibitors (clarithromycin, erythromycin, ketoconazole, itraconazole): increased imatinib concentrations

Drug/herb
St. John's wort: decreased imatinib concentration

Drug/lab test
Increased: bilirubin, amylase, LFTs
Decreased: albumin, calcium, potassium, sodium, phosphate, platelets, neutrophils, leukocytes, lymphocytes

NURSING CONSIDERATIONS
Assessment
- **Bone marrow suppression: Assess ANC and platelets; in chronic phase if ANC <1 × 10^9/L and/or platelets <50 × 10^9/L, stop until ANC >1.5 × 10^9/L and platelets >75 × 10^9/L; in accelerated phase/blast crisis if ANC <0.5 × 10^9/L and/or platelets <10 × 10^9/L, determine whether cytopenia is related to biopsy/aspirate; if not, reduce dose by 200 mg; if cytopenia continues, reduce dose by another 100 mg; if cytopenia continues for 4 wk, stop product until ANC ≥1 × 10^9/L**
- ⚠ **Assess for hepatotoxicity: monitor liver function tests before treatment, qmo if line transaminases are >5 × IULN, withhold imatinib until transaminase levels return to <2.5 × IULN**
- ⚠ **Renal toxicity: monitor bilirubin, if >3 × IULN, withhold imatinib until bilirubin levels return to <1.5 × IULN**
- Assess GI symptoms: frequency of stools
- Assess signs of fluid retention, edema: weigh, monitor lung sounds, 50-ml fluid retention is dose dependent

⚠ Monitor CBC for first month, biweekly next month, and periodically thereafter; neutropenia (2-3 wk), thrombocytopenia (3-4 wk) and anemia may occur, may need dosage decrease or discontinuation

Patient/family education
• Instruct patient to report adverse reactions immediately: shortness of breath, swelling of extremities, bleeding
• Teach patient reason for treatment, expected result
• Instruct patient to eat a nutritious diet with iron, vit supplement, low fiber, few dairy products
• Teach patient not to stop or change dose; to avoid hazardous activities until response is known, dizziness may occur
• Teach patient to take with food and water; for those unable to swallow tabs, to mix in liquid (30 ml for 100 mg or 200 ml for 400 mg); after dissolved, stir and consume
• Advise patient to avoid OTC products unless approved by prescriber
⚠ Teach patient to notify prescriber if pregnancy is planned or suspected, pregnancy (D), do not breastfeed

Evaluation
Positive therapeutic outcome
• Decrease in leukemic cells, size of tumors

---

imipenem/cilastatin (Rx)
(i-me-pen'em sye-la-stat'in)
Primaxin IM, Primaxin IV
Func. class.: Antiinfective, miscellaneous penicillin
Chem. class.: Carbapenem
Pregnancy category C

Do not confuse: imipenem/Omnipen, Primaxin/Premarin

ACTION: Interferes with cell wall replication of susceptible organisms; osmotically unstable cell wall swells and bursts from osmotic pressure; addition of cilastatin prevents renal inactivation that occurs with high urinary concentrations of imipenem

Therapeutic outcome: Bactericidal action against the following: *Streptococcus pneumoniae,* group A β-hemolytic streptococci, *Staphylococcus aureus,* enterococcus; gram-negative organisms: *Klebsiella, Proteus, Escherichia coli, Acinetobacter, Serratia, Pseudomonas aeruginosa; Salmonella, Shigella, Haemophilus influenzae, Listeria* spp.

USES: Serious infections caused by gram-positive or gram-negative organisms

CONTRAINDICATIONS
Hypersensitivity, IM hypersensitivity to local anesthetics of the amide type, or carbapenems, AV block, shock (IM)

Precautions: Pregnancy C, breastfeeding, children, geriatric, hypersensitivity to cephalosporins, penicillins, seizure disorders, renal disease, head trauma, pseudomembranous colitis, ulcerative colitis, diabetes mellitus

DOSAGE AND ROUTES
Doses based on imipenem content
Intraabdominal infections, gynecologic infections, lower respiratory tract infections, skin and skin structure infections, bone and joint infections, septicemia, endocarditis, febrile neutropenia (unlabeled), and polymicrobial infections for fully susceptible organisms including gram-positive/gram-negative aerobes and anaerobes
Adult ≥70 kg: IV 250 mg q6hr (mild infections); 500 mg q6-8hr (moderate infections); 500 mg q6hr (severe life-threatening infections)
Adult 60-<70 kg: IV 250 mg q8hr (mild infections); 250 mg q6hr (moderate or severe life-threatening infections)
Adult 50-<60 kg: IV 125 mg q6hr (mild infections) 250 mg q6hr (moderate or severe life-threatening infections)
Adult 40-<50 kg: IV 125 mg q6hr (mild infections); 250 mg q6-8hr (moderate infections); 250 mg q6hr (severe life-threatening infections)
Adult 30-<40 kg: IV 125 mg q8hr (mild infections); 125 mg q6hr or 250 mg q8hr (moderate infections); 250 mg q8hr (severe life-threatening infections)
Adolescent/child/infant ≥3 mo: IV 15-25 mg/kg q6hr
Infant 1-3 mo weighing ≥1500 g: IV 25 mg/kg q6hr
Neonate 1-4 wk weighing ≥1500 g: IV 25 mg/kg q8hr
Neonate <7 days weighing ≥1500 g: IV 25 mg/kg q12hr

Moderately susceptible organisms, primarily some strains of *P. aeruginosa*
Adult ≥70 kg: IV 500 mg q6hr (mild infections); 500 mg q6hr or 1 g q8hr (moderate infections); 1 g q6-8hr (life-threatening infections)

Adult 60-≤70 kg: IV 500 mg q8hr (mild infections); 500 mg q8hr or 750 mg q8hr (moderate infections); 0.75-1 g q8hr (life-threatening infections)

Adult 50-≤60 kg: IV 250 mg q6hr (mild infections); 250-500 mg q6hr (moderate infections); 500 mg q6hr or 750 mg q8hr (life-threatening infections)

Adult 40-≤50 kg: IV 250 mg q6hr (mild infections); 250 mg q6hr or 500 mg q8hr (moderate infections); 500 mg q6-8hr (life-threatening infections)

Adult 30-≤40 kg: IV 250 mg q8hr (mild infections); 250 mg q6-8hr; 250 mg q6hr or 500 mg q8hr (life-threatening infections)

Adolescent/child/infant >3 mo: IV 15-25 mg/kg q6hr

Infant 1-3 mo weighing ≥1500 g: IV 25 mg/kg q6hr

Neonate 1-4 wk weighing ≥1500 g: IV 25 mg/kg q8hr

Neonate <7 days weighing ≥1500 g: IV 25 mg/kg q12hr

Mild to moderate lower respiratory tract, skin and skin structure, or gynecologic infections
Adult/adolescent/child ≥12 yr: IM 500 or 750 mg q12hr, max 1.5 g/day

Mild to moderate intraabdominal infections, including acute gangrenous or perforated appendicitis and appendicitis with peritonitis
Adult/adolescent/child ≥12 yr: IM 750 mg q12hr, max 1.5 g/day

Community-acquired pneumonia (CAP) in ICU patients with risk factors for *Pseudomonas* infection
Imipenem; cilastatin in combination with ciprofloxacin or an aminoglycoside plus a respiratory fluoroquinolone or an advanced macrolide

Adult ≥70 kg: IV 500 mg q6-8hr
Adult 60-≤70 kg: IV 250 mg q6hr
Adult 50-≤60 kg: IV 250 mg q6hr
Adult 40-≤50 kg: IV 250 mg q6-8hr
Adult 30-≤40 kg: IV 125 mg q6hr or 250 mg q8hr

Imipenem renal dose
Adults 70 kg or more: IV If 70-kg dose is 1 g/day, reduce dose to: CCr 41 to 70 ml/min/1.73 m²: 250 mg q 8 hr; CCr 6 to 40 ml/min/1.73 m²: 250 mg q 12 hr; CCr 5 ml/min/1.73 m² or less: do not use unless hemodialysis is instituted within 48 hr; If 70-kg dose is 1.5 g/day reduce dose to: CCr 41 to 70 m/min/1.73 m²: 250 mg q 6 hr; CCr 21 to 40 ml/min/1.73 m²: 250 mg q 8 hr; CCr 6 to 20 ml/min/1.73 m²: 250 mg q 12 hr; CCr 5 ml/min/1.73 m² or less: do not use unless hemodialysis is instituted within 48 hr; If 70-kg dose is 2 g/day, reduce dose to: CCr 41 to 70 ml/min/1.73 m²: 500 mg q 8 hr; CCr 21 to 40 ml/min/1.73 m²: 250 mg q 6 hr; CCr 6 to 20 ml/min/1.73 m²: 250 mg q 12 hr; CCr 5 ml/min/1.73 m² or less: do not use unless hemodialysis is instituted within 48 hr; If 70-kg dose is 3 g/day, reduce dose to: CCr 41 to 70 ml/min/1.73 m²: 500 mg q 6 hr; CCr 21 to 40 ml/min/1.73 m²: 500 mg q 8 hr; CCr 6 to 20 ml/min/1.73 m²: 500 mg q 12 hr; CCr 5 ml/min/1.73 m² or less: do not use unless hemodialysis is instituted within 48 hr; If 70-kg dose is 4 g/day, reduce dose to: CCr 41 to 70 ml/min/1.73 m²: 750 mg q 8 hr; CCr 21 to 40 ml/min/1.73 m²: 500 mg q 6 hr; CCr 6 to 20 ml/min/1.73 m²: 500 mg q 12 hr; CCr 5 ml/min/1.73 m² or less: do not use unless hemodialysis is instituted within 48 hr

Available forms: Powder for inj sol 250, 500; powder for inj susp 500 mg

Implementation
IM route
• Reconstitute 500 mg/2 ml lidocaine without epiNEPHrine; shake well, withdraw and administer entire vial; give inj deep in large muscle mass, aspirate, product for IM is not for IV use

Intermittent IV infusion route
• Reconstitute each 250 or 500 mg/10 ml of compatible diluent; shake well; transfer the resulting susp to ≥100 ml of compatible diluent; add 10 ml to each previously reconstituted vial and shake to ensure all medication is used; transfer the remaining contents of the vial to the inf container; do not administer susp by direct inj
• Give each 250- or 500-mg dose over 20-30 min, and each 1-g dose over 40-60 min; administer over 15-20 min for pediatric patients; do not administer direct **IV**; do not admix with other antibiotics

Y-site compatibilities: Acyclovir, alfentanil, amifostine, amikacin, aminocaproic acid, andulafungin, argatroban, ascorbic acid, atenolol, atracurium, atropine, benztropine, bivalirudin, bleomycin, bumetanide, buprenorphine, butorphanol, CARBOplatin, caspofungin, ceFAZolin, cefotaxime, cefoTEtan, cefOXitin, cefTAZidime, ceftizone, cefuroxime, chloramphenicol, cimetidine, CISplatin, clindamycin, codeine, cyanocobalamin, cyclophosphamide, cycloSPORINE, cytarabine, DACTINomycin, dexamethasone, dexrazoxane, digoxin, diltiazem, diphenhydrAMINE, DOCEtaxel, dolasetron, DOPamine, doxacurium, DOXOrubicin, DOXOrubicin liposomal, doxycycline, enalaprilat, famotidine, fludarabine, foscarnet, granisetron, IDArubicin, regular insulin, melphalan, methotrexate, ondansetron, propofol, tacrolimus, teniposide, thiotepa, vinorelbine, zidovudine

Y-site incompatibilities: Fluconazole, meperidine, sargramostim

ADVERSE EFFECTS

CNS: Fever, somnolence, seizures, confusion, dizziness, weakness, myoclonus, drowsiness
CV: Hypotension, palpitations, tachycardia
GI: Diarrhea, nausea, vomiting, pseudomembranous colitis, hepatitis, glossitis, gastroenteritis, abdominal pain, jaundice
GU: Renal toxicity/failure
HEMA: Agranulocytosis, eosinophilia, neutropenia, decreased Hgb, Hct
INTEG: Rash, urticaria, pruritus, pain at inj site, phlebitis, erythema at inj site, erythema multiforme
MISC: Hearing loss, tinnitus, electrolyte abnormalities
RESP: Chest discomfort, dyspnea, hyperventilation
SYST: Anaphylaxis, Stevens-Johnson syndrome, toxic epidermal necrolysis, angioedema

Pharmacokinetics

Absorption	Complete bioavailability (IV)
Distribution	Widely distributed; crosses placenta
Metabolism	Liver
Excretion	Kidneys, unchanged (70%-80%); breast milk
Half-life	1 hr; increased in renal disease

Pharmacodynamics

	IM	IV
Onset	Unknown	Rapid
Peak	Unknown	20 min-1 hr

INTERACTIONS
Individual drugs
Aminophylline, cycloSPORINE, ganciclovir, theophylline: increased risk of seizures
Probenecid: increased imipenem plasma levels
Valproic acid: decreased effect of valproic acid

Drug classifications
β-Lactam antibiotics: increased antagonistic effect

Drug/lab test
Increased: AST, ALT, LDH, BUN, alkaline phosphatase, bilirubin, creatinine, potassium, chloride

Decreased: sodium
False positive: direct Coombs' test

NURSING CONSIDERATIONS
Assessment
• Assess patient for previous penicillin sensitivity reaction or sensitivity to other β-lactams, may have sensitivity to this product
• **Assess patient for signs and symptoms of infection,** including characteristics of wounds, sputum, urine, stool, WBC >10,000/mm³, fever; obtain baseline information before, during treatment
• Complete C&S tests before beginning product therapy to identify if correct treatment has been initiated
• **Assess for allergic reactions, anaphylaxis: rash, urticaria, pruritus, chills, wheezing, laryngeal edema, fever, joint pain; angioedema may occur a few days after therapy begins; epiNEPHrine, resuscitation equipment should be available for anaphylactic reaction**
• Identify urine output; if decreasing, notify prescriber (may indicate nephrotoxicity); also check for increased BUN, creatinine, electrolytes
• Monitor blood studies: AST, ALT, CBC, Hct, bilirubin, LDH, alkaline phosphatase, Coombs' test monthly if patient is on long-term therapy
• Monitor electrolytes: potassium, sodium, chloride monthly if patient is on long-term therapy
• Assess bowel pattern daily; if severe diarrhea occurs, product should be discontinued; may indicate pseudomembranous colitis
• **Monitor for bleeding:** ecchymosis, bleeding gums, hematuria, stool guaiac daily if patient is on long-term therapy
• Assess for overgrowth of infection: perineal itching, fever, malaise, redness, pain, swelling, drainage, rash, diarrhea, change in cough, sputum

Patient/family education
• Advise patient to report sore throat, bruising, bleeding, joint pain; may indicate blood dyscrasias (rare)
• Advise patient to contact prescriber if vaginal itching, loose foul-smelling stools, furry tongue occur; may indicate superinfection
• **Advise patient to notify prescriber of diarrhea with blood or pus; may indicate pseudomembranous colitis**
⚠ Instruct patient to report seizures immediately

Evaluation
Positive therapeutic outcome
• Absence of signs/symptoms of infection (WBC <10,000/mm³, temp WNL, absence of red, draining wounds)

- Reported improvement in symptoms of infection

Treatment of anaphylaxis: EPINEPHrine, antihistamines, resuscitate if needed

---

imipramine (Rx)
(im-ip′ra-meen)
Impril ♣, Novo-Pramine ♣, Tofranil, Tofranil PM
Func. class.: Antidepressant, tricyclic
Chem. class.: Dibenzazepine, tertiary amine
Pregnancy category D

Do not confuse: imipramine/desipramine

ACTION: Blocks reuptake of norepinephrine and serotonin into nerve endings, increasing action of norepinephrine and serotonin in nerve cells; has anticholinergic effects

Therapeutic outcome: Decreased symptoms of depression after 2-3 wk; decreased bedwetting in children

USES: Depression, enuresis in children

Unlabeled uses: Chronic pain, migraine headaches, cluster headaches as adjunct, incontinence

CONTRAINDICATIONS

Pregnancy **D**, hypersensitivity to this product or carBAMazepine; acute MI

Precautions: Suicidal patients, severe depression, increased intraocular pressure, closed-angle glaucoma, urinary retention, cardiac/hepatic disease, hyperthyroidism, electroshock therapy, elective surgery, breastfeeding, geriatric, seizure disorders, prostatic hypertrophy, MI, hypersensitivity to tricyclics, AV block, bundle-branch block, ileus, QT prolongation

> **BLACK BOX WARNING:** Children other than for enuresis; suicidal ideation

DOSAGE AND ROUTES
Depression
Adult: PO 75-100 mg/day in divided doses; may increase by 25-50 mg up to 200 mg, 200 mg/day (outpatients); 300 mg/day (inpatients); may give daily dose at bedtime
Geriatric: PO 30-40 mg at bedtime, may increase to 100 mg/day in divided doses
Child ≥6 yr (unlabeled): PO 1.5 mg/kg/day in divided doses; max 2.5 mg/kg/day

Enuresis
Child 6-12 yr: PO 10-25 mg at bedtime, max 50 mg

Available forms: Tabs 10, 25, 50 mg; caps 75, 100, 125, 150 mg

Implementation
PO route
- Do not break, crush, or chew caps
- Give with food or milk
- Store in tight container at room temp; do not freeze

ADVERSE EFFECTS

CNS: *Dizziness, drowsiness,* confusion, headache, anxiety, tremors, stimulation, weakness, insomnia, nightmares, EPS (geriatric), increased psychiatric symptoms, paresthesia, **seizures**, ataxia
CV: *Orthostatic hypotension, ECG changes, tachycardia,* hypertension, palpitations, **dysrhythmias**
EENT: Blurred vision, tinnitus, mydriasis
ENDO: Hyperglycemia, hypothyroidism/hyperthyroidism, goiter, SIADH
GI: *Diarrhea, dry mouth,* nausea, vomiting, **paralytic ileus,** increased appetite, cramps, epigastric distress, jaundice, **hepatitis,** stomatitis, constipation, taste change, weight gain
GU: *Retention,* **acute renal failure,** impotence, decreased libido
HEMA: **Agranulocytosis, thrombocytopenia, eosinophilia, leukopenia**
INTEG: Rash, urticaria, sweating, pruritus, photosensitivity, hyperpigmentation (rare)

Pharmacokinetics

Absorption	Well absorbed
Distribution	Widely distributed; crosses placenta
Metabolism	Liver, extensively
Excretion	Kidneys, breast milk
Half-life	6-20 hr

Pharmacodynamics

	PO
Onset	1 hr
Peak	Unknown
Duration	Unknown

INTERACTIONS
Individual drugs
Alcohol: increased effects
CloNIDine: hyperpyretic crisis, seizures, hypertensive episode
CloNIDine, guanethidine: decreased effects
Gatifloxacin, levofloxacin, moxifloxacin, ziprasidone: increased QT interval

Drug classifications
MAOIs: hyperpyretic crisis, hypertensive episode, seizures

SSRIs, SNRIs, serotonin-receptor agonists: increased serotonin syndrome, increased neuroleptic malignant syndrome; avoid concurrent use

Sympathomimetics (direct acting [EPINEPH-rine]), barbiturates, benzodiazepines, CNS depressants: increased effects

Sympathomimetics (indirect acting [ePHED-rine]): decreased effects

Tricyclic antidepressants, class IA/III anti-dysrhythmics: increased QT interval

Drug/herb
St. John's wort: serotonin syndrome

Drug/lab test
Increased: serum bilirubin, blood glucose, alkaline phosphatase, LFTs

Decreased: VMA, 5-HIAA, urinary catecholamines

NURSING CONSIDERATIONS
Assessment
• Monitor B/P (with patient lying, standing), pulse q4hr; if systolic B/P drops 20 mm Hg, hold product, notify prescriber; take vital signs q4hr in patients with CV disease

• Monitor blood studies: CBC, leukocytes, differential, cardiac enzymes if patient is receiving long-term therapy

• Monitor hepatic studies: AST, ALT, bilirubin

• Check weight weekly; appetite may increase with product

• QT prolongation: Assess ECG for flattening of T wave, bundle branch block, AV block, dysrhythmias in cardiac patients

• Assess for EPS primarily in geriatric: rigidity, dystonia, akathisia

> **BLACK BOX WARNING:** Assess mental status: mood, sensorium, affect, suicidal tendencies especially in children, young adults; increase in psychiatric symptoms: depression, panic

• Monitor urinary retention, constipation; constipation is more likely to occur in children or geriatric

⚠ Assess for withdrawal symptoms: headache, nausea, vomiting, muscle pain, weakness, diarrhea, insomnia, restlessness; do not usually occur unless product was discontinued abruptly

• Identify alcohol consumption; if alcohol is consumed, hold dose until AM

Patient/family education

> **BLACK BOX WARNING:** Teach patient to report suicidal thoughts, behaviors immediately; more common in children, young adults

• Teach patient that therapeutic effects may take 2-3 wk

• Teach patient to use caution in driving and other activities requiring alertness because of drowsiness, dizziness, blurred vision; to avoid rising quickly from sitting position, especially geriatric; orthostatic hypotension may occur

• Teach patient to avoid alcohol ingestion, other CNS depressants during treatment

• Teach patient not to discontinue medication quickly after long-term use: may cause nausea, headache, malaise

• Teach patient to wear sunscreen or large hat, since photosensitivity occurs

• Teach patient to increase fluids, bulk in diet if constipation, urinary retention occur, especially geriatric

• Teach patient to take gum, hard sugarless candy, frequent sips of water for dry mouth

Evaluation
Positive therapeutic outcome
• Decreased depression
• Absence of suicidal thoughts
• Decreased enuresis in children
• Decreased pain

TREATMENT OF OVERDOSE:
ECG monitoring, lavage, activated charcoal, administer anticonvulsant

---

immune globulin IM (IMIg, IgIM) (Rx)
Bay Gam 15%, Flebogamma 5%, Flebogamma DIF 5%, Gama STAN S/D, Gamunex 10%, Privigen 10%, Vivaglobin 10%

immune globulin IV (IGIV, IVIG) (Rx)
Bay Gam 15%, Carimune DF, Flebogamma 5%, Flebogamma 10% DIF, Gammaked, Gammaplex, Gammar-P IV, Gammagard S/D, Gamunex, Iveegam EN, Octagam, Polygam S/D, Privigen, Vivaglobin

immune globulin SC (SCIG, IGSC) (Rx)
Bay Gam 15%, Flebogamma 5%, Flebogamma DIF 5%, Gammagard Liquid 10%, Gammaked, Gammaplex, Gamunex 10%, Hizentra, Privigen 10%, Vivaglobin

Func. class.: Immune serum
Chem. class.: IgG
Pregnancy category C

Do not confuse: Iveegam/Invega

ACTION: Provides passive immunity to hepatitis A, measles, varicella, rubella, immune globulin deficiency; contains γ-globulin antibodies (IgG)

Therapeutic outcome: Absence of infection

USES: Immunodeficiency syndrome, B-cell chronic lymphocytic leukemia, Kawasaki's syndrome, bone marrow transplantation, pediatric HIV infection, agammaglobulinemia, hepatitis A, B exposure, measles exposure, measles vaccine complications, purpura, rubella exposure, chickenpox exposure, chronic inflammatory demyelinating polyneuropathy, multifocal motor neuropathy

Unlabeled uses: **IV** posttransfusion purpura, Guillain-Barré syndrome

CONTRAINDICATIONS
Coagulopathy, hemophilia, IgA deficiency, thrombocytopenia, hypersensitivity

Precautions: Pregnancy **C,** breastfeeding, children, agammaglobulinemia, bleeding, hypogammaglobulinemia, infection, IV, viral infection

DOSAGE AND ROUTES
>> Immune globulin IM (IMIg, IgIM)
Hepatitis A prophylaxis
Adult, geriatric, adolescent, child, infant (unlabeled): IM 0.02 ml/kg for those who have not received Hepatitis A vaccine and have been exposed in the last 2 wk

Measles prophylaxis (exposed in last 6 days)
Adult: IM 0.25 ml/kg (immunocompetent)
Child (unlabeled): IM 0.5 ml/kg as a single dose, max 15 ml (immunocompromised)

Varicella prophylaxis
Adult: IM 0.6-1.2 ml/kg as soon as possible and if varicella-zoster immune globulin is not available

Rubella prophylaxis in exposed/ susceptible who will not consider a therapeutic abortion
Adult: Pregnant women IM 0.55 ml/kg

Immunoglobulin deficiency
Adult: 1.32 ml/kg, then 0.66 ml/kg (at least 100 mg/kg) q3-4wk

>> Immune globulin IV (IVIG, IGIV)
Primary immunodeficiency
Gammagard S/D
Adult/adolescent/child: IV 300-600 mg/kg q3-4wk

Polygam S/D
Adult/adolescent/child: IV 100 mg/kg qmo; initially 200-400 mg/kg may be used

Gammar-P IV
Adult: IV 200-400 mg/kg q3-4wk
Adolescent/child: IV 200 mg/kg q3-4wk

Gamunex
Adult/adolescent/child: IV INF 300-600 mg/kg (3-6 ml/kg) q3-4wk; initial infusion rate 1 mg/kg/min (max 8 mg/kg/min)

Iveegam EN
Adult/adolescent/child: IV 200 mg/kg qmo; max 800 mg/kg qmo

Gammagard Liquid/Flebogamma 5%
Adult/adolescent/child: IV 300-600 mg/kg q3-4wk

Privigen
Adult/adolescent/child ≥3 yr: IV 200-800 mg q3-4wk

Idiopathic thrombocytopenic purpura (ITP)
Carimune NF
Adult/child: IV 400 mg/kg qd × 2-5 days; in acute ITP of childhood, only 2 of the 5 days are needed if initial platelets are 30,000-50,000 mcl after 2 doses

Gammagard S/D/Polygam S/D
Adult/adolescent/child: IV 1000 mg/kg as a single dose; may give on alternate days for up to 3 doses

Gamunex
Adult/adolescent/child: IV INF total dose of 2000 mg/kg, divided as 1000 mg/kg (10 ml/kg) given on 2 consecutive days; initial rate is 1 mg/kg/min (max 8 mg/kg/min), if after 1st dose adequate platelets are observed after 24 hr, may withhold 2nd dose

Privigen
Adult/adolescent ≥15 yr: 1 g/kg/day × 2 days

Kawasaki disease
Iveegam EN
Child: IV 400 mg/kg qd × 4 consecutive days or a single dose of 2000 mg/kg over 10 hr; give with aspirin 100 mg/kg/day through 14th day of illness, then 3-5 mg/kg each day thereafter for 5 wk

Gammagard S/D/Polygam S/D
Infant/child: IV 1000 mg/kg (single dose) or 400 mg/kg/day × 4 days beginning within 7 days of fever onset, with aspirin 80-100 mg/kg/day × 4 divided doses

Immune globulin SC (SCIG/IgSC)
Adult/child >2 yr: SC infusion 100-200 mg/kg qwk; **Vivaglobin** brand of SGIG 160 mg IgG/ml, SC inj; max 15 ml for injection, given at max of 20 ml/hr

Hizentra
Adult/child: 1.53 × previous IGIV dose in g divided by number of wk between IGIV dose; multiply dose in g × 5 for dose in ml, adjust by 1.3 trough before last IGIV treatment, give by subcut infusion qwk

Available forms: IM (Bay Gam) inj 2, 10 ml vial; **IV** (Gamimune N) 5%, 10% sol; powder for inj (Carimune NF) 1-, 3-, 6-, 12-g vials; (Gammagard S/D) 50 mg protein/ml in 2.5-, 5-, 10-g vials; (Gammar-P IV) 1-, 2.5-, 5-, 10-g vials; (Iveegam) 500 mg, 1-, 2.5-, 5-g vials; (Panglobulin) 6-, 12-g vials; (Polygam S/D) 2.5-, 5-, 10-g vials; sol for inj (Gamunex) 1-, 2.5-, 5-, 10-, 20-g vials; human sol for inj: Flebogamma 5%, 10% DIF; subcut inj 10%, 16%, 20% single use

Implementation
IM route
• Give IM (IGIM) inj in deltoid or anterolateral thigh in adults or anterolateral thigh in young children; if large amounts are given, several injections may be needed
• Do not give the IM preparation **IV**, SUBCUT, or intradermally
• Sol should be transparent and clear or slightly colored
• Store at 36°-46° F (2°-8° C)

IV route
• Warm to room temperature before administration (diluent, powder for inj)
• A transfer device is provided by manufacturer; this product should not be agitated or shaken
• Do not give the **IV** preparation SUBCUT, IM, or intradermally
• Check for adverse reaction during inf; stop inf if adverse reactions occur

Y-site compatibilities: Fluconazole, sargramostim

Gamimune N: Dilute **IV** with D₅W; give 0.01 ml/kg/min; may increase to 0.02-0.04 ml/kg/min if no adverse reactions occur; may increase to 0.08 ml/kg/hr; sol should be refrigerated; do not freeze

Gammagard S/D: Reconstitute with sterile water for inj (50 mg protein/ml); give within 2 hr of reconstitution; give 0.5 ml/kg/hr; may increase to 4 ml/kg/hr if no adverse reactions occur; use inf set provided

Gammar-P IV: Give 0.01 ml/kg/min (50 mg/ml sol) over 15-30 min; may increase to 0.02 ml/kg/min; if adverse reactions are not present, may increase to 0.03-0.06 ml/kg/min; do not freeze; store at room temperature

Iveegam (5%): Give 1-2 ml/min; refrigerate, do not freeze

ADVERSE EFFECTS
CNS: Headache, fatigue, malaise
GI: Abdominal pain
HEMA: Thromboembolism (Vivaglobin)
INTEG: Pain at inj site, rash, pruritus, chills
MS: Arthralgia, chest pain
SYST: Lymphadenopathy, **anaphylaxis; life-threatening hypoglycemia (Octagam 5%, 10%)**

Pharmacokinetics

Absorption	Well absorbed (IM); completely absorbed (**IV**)
Distribution	Rapidly
Metabolism	Liver, catabolism
Excretion	Kidneys
Half-life	3-4 wk

Pharmacodynamics

	IM	IV
Onset	Unknown	Rapid
Peak	Unknown	Unknown
Duration	Unknown	Unknown

INTERACTIONS
Drug classifications
Live virus vaccines: do not give within 3 mo

Drug/lab test
Interference: glucose testing system

NURSING CONSIDERATIONS
Assessment
• Assess for exposure date: this product should be given within 6 days of measles, 1 wk of hepatitis B, 14 days of hepatitis A; if the date of exposure is outside these limits, immune globulin will not be effective
• Monitor blood studies in leukemia, idiopathic thrombocytopenic purpura: WBCs (leukemia), platelets
• Identify the number of inj of this product patient has received; multiple inj may lead to sensitization (diaphoresis, fever, chills, malaise)
• **Assess for anaphylaxis in patient receiving IV immune globulin: diaphoresis, flushing, nausea, vomiting, wheezing, difficulty**

breathing, hypotension, chest tightness, fever, weakness, sneezing, abdominal pain; VS should be monitored during inf and 1 hr after beginning inf; emergency equipment should be available with epinephrine and antihistamines to treat anaphylaxis

Patient/family education
• Advise patient that passive immunity is temporary; explain reason for and expected results of this product
• Advise patient that pain and tenderness may occur at inj site

Evaluation
Positive therapeutic outcome
• Prevention of infection
• Increased platelets

TREATMENT OF ANAPHYLAXIS: EPINEPHrine, diphenhydrAMINE, O_2, vasopressors, corticosteroids

---

indacaterol
(in-da-kat'er-ol)
Arcapta Neohaler
Func. class.: β_2-agonist, long-acting
Pregnancy category C

ACTION: An agonist at β_2-receptors. These receptors are present in large numbers in the lungs and are located on bronchiolar smooth muscle. Stimulation of β_2-receptors in the lung causes relaxation of bronchial smooth muscle, which produces bronchodilation and an increase in bronchial airflow. These effects may be mediated, in part, by increased activity of adenyl cyclase, an intracellular enzyme responsible for the formation of cyclic-3′,5′-adenosine monophosphate (cAMP); has >24 times greater agonist activity at β_2-receptors (primarily in the lung) than at β_1-receptors (primarily in the heart)

USES: Bronchitis, chronic obstructive pulmonary disease (COPD), emphysema

CONTRAINDICATIONS
Acute bronchospasm, acute asthma attack, status asthmaticus, acute respiratory insufficiency, monotherapy of asthma

Precautions: Cardiac arrhythmias, congenital long QT syndrome, diabetes mellitus, hypertension, hyperthyroidism (thyrotoxicosis, thyroid disease), hypokalemia, ischemic cardiac disease (coronary artery disease), milk protein hypersensitivity, pheochromocytoma, QT prolongation, seizure disorder, severe hepatic disease, tachycardia, torsades de pointes history, unusual responsiveness to other sympathomimetic amines; not indicated for neonates, infants, children, or adolescents under the age of 18 years, pregnancy C, breastfeeding

> **BLACK BOX WARNING:** Asthma-related deaths

DOSAGE AND ROUTES
Adult: INH 75 mcg (contents of 1 capsule) inhaled once daily; administer at the same time every day, max 1 dose in 24 hours

Available forms:
Powder for inhalation: 75 mcg

Implementation
Inhalation route
• For oral inhalation use only; *not* to swallow the capsules; always use the Neohaler inhaler; this inhaler should not be used with any other products; do *not* use with a spacer
• To administer, use dry hands to remove a capsule from the blister pack immediately before use and place into the capsule chamber of the Neohaler inhaler; click the inhaler closed; do not place capsule into the mouthpiece; then, holding upright, depress buttons fully one time to pierce capsule; a click will be heard; have patient breathe out fully away from inhaler; place inhaler in the mouth with lips closed around the mouthpiece and buttons positioned to the left and right (not up and down), then breathe deeply, rapidly, steadily in through the inhaler. A whirring sound should be heard; if no sound is heard, check the chamber—capsule may be stuck. Gently tap the base of the device to loosen capsule if necessary. After inhalation, the patient should hold breath as long as comfortable while removing inhaler from the mouth; check the chamber to see if any powder remains in the capsule; repeat inhalation steps until no powder remains. Most patients can empty the capsule in one or two inhalations. After administration, open the chamber and discard the empty capsule
• The gelatin capsule might break into very small pieces, which can pass through the inhaler screen and reach the mouth. Accidental inhalation or ingestion of these pieces is harmless; piercing the capsule more than once increases the risk of shattering capsule; do not wash inhaler; keep it dry. A clean, dry, lint-free cloth may be used to wipe out the inhaler
• Use the new inhaler provided with each new prescription
• To avoid the spread of infection, do not share the inhaler

Adverse effects: *italics* = common; **bold** = life-threatening

ADVERSE EFFECTS

CNS: Headache, tremor

CV: Sinus tachycardia, hypertension, QT prolongation and ST-T wave changes, prolonged QTc (an increase of >60 ms from baseline), nonsustained ventricular tachycardia, supraventricular tachycardia (SVT) episodes, intermittent ectopic atrial rhythm

ENDO: Hyperglycemia

GI: Nausea, dry mouth (xerostomia)

META: Hypokalemia

MS: Muscle cramps/spasm, musculoskeletal pain

RESP: Paradoxical bronchospasm, cough, dyspnea, sputum purulence or volume, wheezing, nasopharyngitis, pneumonia, sinusitis and upper respiratory tract infection

Pharmacokinetics

Absorption	Unknown
Distribution	Steady state 12-15 days protein binding 94%-96%
Metabolism	By CYP3A4, CYP1A1, CYP2D6, UTG1A1
Excretion	Renal 2%-6%, fecally >90%
Half-life	Terminal 45.5-126 hrs

Pharmacodynamics

Onset	5 min
Peak	15 min
Duration	Unknown

INTERACTIONS

Individual drugs

Amoxapine, some antipsychotics (phenothiazines, pimozide, haloperidol risperiDONE, sertindole ziprasidone), arsenic trioxide, astemizole, bepridil, cisapride, citalopram, chloroquine, clarithromycin, dasatinib, dolasetron, dronedarone, droperidol, erythromycin, flecainide, halofantrine, levomethadyl, maprotiline, methadone, ondansetron, paliperidone, palonosetron, pentamidine, probucol, propafenone, some quinolones (ofloxacin, gatifloxacin, gemifloxacin, grepafloxacin, levofloxacin, moxifloxacin, sparfloxacin), ranolazine, sunitinib, terfenadine, thioridazine, troleandomycin, vorinostat, tetrabenazine: increased QT prolongation

Aminophylline, theophylline: increased hypokalemia

Furazolidone, procarbazine, rasagiline: increased cardiovascular reactions

Drug classifications

Class IA/III antiarrhythmics, halogenated anesthetics, tricyclic antidepressants: increased QT prolongation

Corticosteroids: increased hypokalemia

MAOIs: increased cardiovascular reactions

NURSING CONSIDERATIONS

Assessment

> **BLACK BOX WARNING:** Asthma-related death; not to be used in asthma

• **COPD, emphysema, bronchospasm:** Monitor pulmonary function tests

⚠ **QT prolongation:** Monitor ECG, ejection fraction for QT prolongation

• **Paradoxical bronchospasm:** If paradoxical bronchospasm occurs, discontinue this medication immediately, use a short-acting beta-agonist for rescue therapy, as appropriate

Patient/family education

• Teach patient/family to report dyspnea, wheezing, bronchospasm

• Teach patient/family not to use with other products unless approved by prescriber; there are many interactions

> **BLACK BOX WARNING:** Not to use for asthma

---

indapamide (Rx)

(in-dap′a-mide)

Lozide ✦

Func. class.: Diuretic, thiazide-like, antihypertensive

Chem. class.: Thiazide-like sulfonamide derivative

Pregnancy category D

ACTION: Acts on proximal section of distal renal tubule by inhibiting reabsorption of sodium, may act by direct vasodilatation caused by blocking of calcium channels

Therapeutic outcome: Decreased B/P; decreased edema in lung tissues, peripherally

USES: Edema of CHF, hypertension, diuresis

CONTRAINDICATIONS

Hypersensitivity to this product or sulfonamides, anuria, hepatic coma

Precautions: Breastfeeding, hypokalemia, severe renal disease, hepatic disease, ascites, dehydration, CCr <30 ml/min (not effective), diabetes mellitus, gout, pregnancy (**B**), cardiac dysrhythmias

---

DOSAGE AND ROUTES
Edema
Adult: PO 2.5 mg/day in AM; may be increased to 5 mg/day if needed after 1 wk

Antihypertensive
Adult: PO 1.25-5 mg/day; may increase to 5 mg/day over 8 wk

Available forms: Tabs 1.25, 2.5 mg

Implementation
• Give in AM to avoid interference with sleep
• Provide potassium replacement if potassium level is <3.0 mg/dl; give whole
• Give with food and milk if nausea occurs, absorption may be increased

ADVERSE EFFECTS
CNS: Depression, *headache, dizziness, fatigue, weakness, nervousness, agitation,* extremity numbness
CV: Orthostatic hypotension, palpitations, volume depletion, PVCs, dysrhythmias, vasculitis
EENT: Blurred vision, nasal congestion, increased intraocular pressure
ELECT: *Hypokalemia, hypercalcemia, hyponatremia, hypochloremic alkalosis, hypomagnesemia,* hyperuricemia, hyperglycemia
GI: *Nausea,* vomiting, anorexia, constipation, diarrhea, cramps, abdominal pain, dry mouth, hypercholesterolemia
GU: *Frequency, polyuria, nocturia,* impotence
HEMA: Agranulocytosis, anemia
INTEG: Rash, *pruritus,* Stevens-Johnson syndrome
MS: Cramps

Pharmacokinetics
Absorption	Well absorbed
Distribution	Widely distributed
Metabolism	Liver, 7%
Excretion	Unchanged (urine)
Half-life	14-18 hr

Pharmacodynamics
Onset	1-2 hr
Peak	2 hr
Duration	Up to 36 hr

INTERACTIONS
Individual drugs
Amphotericin B: decreased potassium
Cholestyramine, colestipol: decreased absorption
Diazoxide: hyperglycemia
Digoxin, lithium: increased toxicity
Indomethacin: decreased hypotensive effect

Drug classifications
Anticoagulants, antidiabetics, antigout agents: decreased effects
Diuretics (other), steroids: decreased potassium
Muscle relaxants, steroids: increased toxicity
NSAIDs: decreased hypotensive effects

Drug/food
Licorice: increased severe hypokalemia

Drug/herb
Hawthorn: increased antihypertensive effect

Drug/lab test
Increased: calcium, parathyroid test, glucose, uric acid

NURSING CONSIDERATIONS
Assessment
• Check for rashes, temp elevation daily
• Monitor patients that receive cardiac glycosides for increased hypokalemia, toxicity
• Monitor for hypokalemia: acidic or reduced urine, osmolality, nocturia; hypotension, broad T-wave, U-wave, ectopy, tachycardia, weak pulse; muscle weakness, altered LOC, drowsiness, apathy, lethargy, confusion, depression; anorexia, nausea, cramps, constipation, distention, paralytic ileus; hypoventilation, respiratory muscle weakness
• Monitor for hypomagnesemia: agitation, muscle twitching, paresthesias, hyperactive reflexes, positive Babinski reflex, dysphagia, nystagmus, seizures, tetany; nausea, vomiting, diarrhea, anorexia, abdominal distention; ectopy, tachycardia, broad, flat- or inverted T-waves, depressed ST segment, prolonged QT interval, decreased cardiac output, hypotension
• Monitor for hyponatremia: increased B/P, cold, clammy skin, hypo/hypervolemia; anorexia, nausea, vomiting, diarrhea, abdominal cramps; lethargy, increased ICP, confusion, headache, seizures, coma, fatigue, tremors, hyperreflexia
• Monitor for manifestations of hyperchloremia: weakness, lethargy, coma, deep rapid breathing
• Assess fluid volume status: I&O ratios and record, weight, distended red veins, crackles in lung, color, quality and specific gravity of urine, skin turgor, adequacy of pulses, moist mucous membranes, bilateral lung sounds, peripheral pitting edema; dehydration symptoms of decreasing output, thirst, hypotension, dry mouth and mucous membranes should be reported
• Monitor electrolytes: potassium, sodium, calcium, magnesium; also include BUN, blood pH, ABGs, uric acid, CBC, blood glucose
• Assess B/P before, during therapy with patient lying, standing, and sitting as appropriate; orthostatic hypotension can occur rapidly

Patient/family education
• Teach patient to take the medication early in the day to prevent nocturia, to avoid alcohol
• Instruct the patient to take with food or milk if GI symptoms of nausea and anorexia occur
• Teach patient to maintain weekly record of weight and notify prescriber of weight loss >5 lb
• Caution the patient that this product causes a loss of potassium, so food rich in potassium should be added to the diet; refer to a dietitian for assistance in planning
• Caution the patient to rise slowly from sitting or reclining positions, not to exercise in hot weather or stand for prolonged periods, since orthostatic hypotension will be enhanced; lie down if dizziness occurs
• Teach patient not to use alcohol or any OTC medications without prescriber's approval; serious product reactions may occur
• Emphasize the need to contact prescriber immediately if muscle cramps, weakness, nausea, dizziness, or numbness occur
• Teach patient to take own B/P and pulse and record findings
• Instruct patient to continue taking medication even if feeling better; this product controls symptoms but does not cure the condition
• Advise the patient with hypertension to continue other medical treatment (exercise, weight loss, relaxation techniques, cessation of smoking)
• Do not stop product abruptly

Evaluation
Positive therapeutic outcome
• Decreased edema
• Decreased B/P
• Increased diuresis

TREATMENT OF OVERDOSE:
Lavage, monitor electrolytes, administer IV fluids, monitor hydration, CV, renal status

---

⚠ HIGH ALERT

indinavir (Rx)
(en-den'a-veer)
Crixivan
Func. class.: Antiretroviral
Chem. class.: Protease inhibitor
Pregnancy category C

Do not confuse: indinavir/Denavir

ACTION: Inhibits HIV-1 protease; this prevents maturation of the infectious virus

Therapeutic outcome: Decreased signs/symptoms of HIV-1 infection

USES: HIV-1 in combination with other antiretrovirals

Unlabeled uses: Prevention of HIV-1 after exposure

CONTRAINDICATIONS
Hypersensitivity, breastfeeding

Precautions: Pregnancy C, children, renal/hepatic disease, history of renal stones, diabetes, hypercholesterolemia, hemophilia, autoimmune disease, immune reconstitution syndrome

DOSAGE AND ROUTES
Adult: PO 800 mg q8hr; 600 mg q8hr with delaviridine 400 mg tid; 600 mg q8hr with itraconazole 200 mg bid or ketoconazole

Hepatic dose
Adult: PO 600 mg q8hr

Available forms: Caps 200, 400 mg

Implementation
• Do not break, crush, or chew caps
• Give with water 1 hr before or 2 hr after meals; may be given with other liquids or small meal; do not give with high-fat, high-protein meals
• Give in equal intervals around the clock
• Dosage adjustment will need to be considered when given with other antiretrovials
• Give water to 1.5 L/day minimum, to prevent nephrolithiasis

ADVERSE EFFECTS
CNS: *Headache, insomnia,* dizziness, somnolence
GI: *Diarrhea, abdominal pain, nausea, vomiting,* anorexia, dry mouth
GU: Nephrolithiasis
INTEG: Rash
MISC: Asthenia, insulin-resistant hyperglycemia, hyperlipidemia, ketoacidosis, lipodystrophy
MS: Pain

Pharmacokinetics

Absorption	Unknown
Distribution	Unknown
Metabolism	60% protein binding; liver
Excretion	<20% unchanged, urine; 83% feces
Half-life	Terminal 2 hr

Pharmacodynamics
Unknown

INTERACTIONS
Individual drugs
Amiodarone, alfuzosin, pimozide: life-threatening dysrhythmias

Clarithromycin, zidovudine: increased levels of both products

Isoniazid: increased isoniazid level

Midazolam, rifampin, triazolam: increased life-threatening dysrhythmias

Drug classifications
Anticonvulsants: decreased effect of both products

CYP3A4 inducers (barbiturates, carBAMazepine, efavirenz, fluconazole, modafinil, nevirapine, nonnucleoside reverse transcriptase inhibitors, phenytoin, rifamycins): decreased indinavir levels

CYP3A4 inhibitors (aprepitant, azole antifungals, delavirdine, itraconazole, ketoconazole, nefazodone, protease inhibitors, verapamil); phosphotriesterases: increased indinavir levels

CYP3A4 substrates (azole antifungals, benzodiazepines, calcium channel blockers, immunosuppressants, macrolides, sildenafil, SSRIs, statins, tadalafil, vardenafil): decreased effect of these substrates

Ergots: increased life-threatening dysrhythmias

Oral contraceptives: increased levels of oral contraceptives

Statins (atorvastatin, lovastatin, simvastatin): increased myopathy

Drug/herb
St. John's wort: decreased indinavir level, avoid use

Drug/food
High fat, high protein, grapefruit juice: decreased absorption

Drug/lab test
Increased: AST, ALT, amylase, total bilirubin

NURSING CONSIDERATIONS
Assessment
• Assess for lower back, flank pain: indicates kidney stones
• Monitor signs of infection, anemia
• Monitor liver studies: ALT, AST; total bilirubin, amylase; all may be elevated
• Determine the presence of other STDs
• Assess bowel pattern before, during treatment; if severe abdominal pain with bleeding occurs, product should be discontinued; monitor hydration
• Assess skin eruptions: rash, urticaria, itching
• Assess allergies before treatment, reaction to each medication; place allergies on chart
• Monitor viral load CD4 during treatment

Evaluate:
• Therapeutic response: decreasing viral load, symptoms of HIV

Patient/family education
• Advise to take as prescribed; if dose is missed, take as soon as remembered up to 1 hr before next dose; do not double dose
• Advise that product must be taken in equal intervals around the clock to maintain blood levels for duration of therapy
• Instruct patient to increase fluids to prevent kidney stones; if stone formation occurs, treatment may need to be interrupted
• Inform patient that product does not cure AIDS, controls symptoms only; not to donate blood
• Advise patient that hyperglycemia may occur; watch for symptoms (thirst, hunger, dry, itchy skin); notify prescriber

Evaluation
Positive therapeutic outcome
• Decreased signs/symptoms of infection, HIV

---

indomethacin (Rx)
(in-doe-meth'a-sin)
Indocin, Nu-Indo ✦
Func. class.: NSAID (nonsteroidal antiinflammatory), antirheumatic
Chem. class.: Acetic acid derivative
Pregnancy category B (1st trimester), D (2nd/3rd trimesters)

Do not confuse: Indocin/Endocet, minocin/Vicodin

ACTION: Inhibits prostaglandin synthesis by decreasing enzyme needed for biosynthesis; analgesic, antiinflammatory, antipyretic

Therapeutic outcome: Decreased pain, inflammation; closure of patent ductus arteriosus (premature infants)

USES: Rheumatoid arthritis, ankylosing spondylitis, osteoarthritis, bursitis, tendinitis, acute gouty arthritis; closure of patent ductus arteriosus in premature infants (**IV**)

CONTRAINDICATIONS
Pregnancy **D** (3rd trimester) hypersensitivity, asthma, aortic coarctation, bleeding, salicylate/NSAID hypersensitivity, GI bleeding

> **BLACK BOX WARNING:** Perioperative pain in CABG

Precautions: Pregnancy **B** (1st trimester), breastfeeding, children, bleeding disorders, GI disorders, cardiac disorders, asthma, diabetes, acute bronchospasm, ulcerative colitis, seizures, Parkinson's disease, renal/hepatic disease, depression, neonates

> **BLACK BOX WARNING:** Stroke, GI bleeding, MI, those taking NSAIDs are at greater risk of MI and stroke, even in first few weeks of therapy

DOSAGE AND ROUTES
Arthritis/antiinflammatory
Adult: PO 25-50 mg bid-tid, max 200 mg/day; SUS REL 75 mg daily; may increase to 75 mg bid

Acute gouty arthritis
Adult: PO 50 mg tid; use only for acute attack, then reduce dosage

Patent ductus arteriosus
Longer or repeated treatment courses may be necessary for very premature infants
Infant <2 days: IV 0.2 mg/kg, then 0.1 mg/kg × 2 doses at 12, 24 hr
Infant 2-7 days: IV 0.2 mg/kg, then 0.2 mg/kg × 2 doses at 12, 24 hr
Infant >7 days: IV 0.2 mg/kg, then 0.25 mg/kg × 2 doses at 12, 24 hr

Available forms: Caps 25, 50 mg; sus rel caps 75 mg; oral susp 5 mg/ ml; inj 1-mg vials; supp 50 mg

Implementation
PO route
• Swallow sus rel cap whole; do not break, crush, or chew sus rel cap
• Give with food or milk to decrease gastric symptoms and prevent ulceration
• Shake susp; do not mix with other liquids
Rectal route
• Have patient retain rect supp for 1 hr after insertion
• Store at room temperature

IV route
• Give after diluting 1 mg with 1 or 2 ml saline or sterile water for inj without preservative; give 1 or 0.5 mg/ml, respectively, do not dilute further; give over 5-35 sec to avoid dramatic shift in cerebral blood flow; avoid extravasation
• Hold dose in patent ductus arterious in oliguria <0.6 ml/kg/hr

ADVERSE EFFECTS
CNS: Dizziness, drowsiness, fatigue, confusion, insomnia, anxiety, depression, *headache*
CV: Tachycardia, peripheral edema, palpitations, dysrhythmias, hypertension, **CV thrombotic events, MI, stroke**
EENT: Tinnitus, hearing loss, blurred vision

GI: *Nausea,* anorexia, *vomiting,* diarrhea, jaundice, **cholestatic hepatitis,** *constipation,* flatulence, cramps, dry mouth, peptic ulcer, **ulceration, perforation, GI bleeding**
GU: Nephrotoxicity (dysuria, hematuria, oliguria, azotemia)
HEMA: Blood dyscrasias, prolonged bleeding
INTEG: Purpura, rash, pruritus, sweating

Pharmacokinetics

Absorption	Well absorbed (PO); erratic (RECT); complete (**IV**)
Distribution	Crosses blood-brain barrier; placenta, 99% plasma protein binding
Metabolism	Liver, extensively
Excretion	Breast milk; urine 60%, feces 33%
Half-life	1 hr first pass, 2.6-11.2 hr second pass

Pharmacodynamics

	PO	PO–ext rel	IV
Onset	30 min	½ hr	2 day
Peak	2 hr	Unknown	Unknown
Duration	4-6 hr	4-6 hr	Unknown

INTERACTIONS
Individual drugs
Abciximab, aspirin, clopidogrel, eptifibatide, plicamycin, ticlodipine, tirofiban: increased bleeding risk
Cidofovir, cycloSPORINE, lithium, methotrexate, probenecid: increased toxicity
Digoxin, penicillamine, phentoin: increased effect of each specific product

Drug classifications
Aminoglycosides: increased effects of aminoglycosides
Anticoagulants, SNRIs, SSRIs, thrombolytics: increased risk of bleeding
Antihypertensives: decreased effect of antihypertensives
Diuretics (potassium sparing): increased hyperkalemia

NURSING CONSIDERATIONS
Assessment
• Assess for patent ductus arteriosus: respiratory rate, character, heart sounds
• Assess for joint pain (duration, intensity, ROM), baseline and during treatment
• Assess for confusion, mood changes, hallucinations, especially in geriatric

• Assess renal, liver, blood studies: BUN, creatinine, AST, ALT, Hgb before treatment, periodically thereafter; if renal function decreases, do not give subsequent doses

BLACK BOX WARNING: Assess for cardiac disease, CV, thrombotic events (MI, stroke) prior to administration, not to be used for perioperative pain in CABG surgery

BLACK BOX WARNING: GI bleeding/perforation: chronic use can lead to GI bleeding: use cautiously in those with a history of active GI disease

BLACK BOX WARNING: MI, stroke: risk may be greater with longer-term use and in those with CV risk factors

Patient/family education
• Advise patient to report change in vision, blurring, rash, tinnitus, black stools
• Tell patient not to use for any other condition than prescribed
• Advise patient to avoid use with OTC medications for pain unless approved by prescriber, to report use to all providers
• Advise patient to avoid hazardous activities, since dizziness or drowsiness can occur
• Instruct patient to use sunscreen to prevent photosensitivity

BLACK BOX WARNING: MI/stroke: Teach patient to immediately report and seek medical attention for signs/symptoms of MI/stroke, discontinue product

Evaluation
Positive therapeutic outcome
• Decreased stiffness
• Increased joint mobility
• Decreased pain

inFLIXimab (Rx)
(in-fliks′ih-mab)
Remicade
Func. class.: Monoclonal antibody
Chem. class.: Tumor necrosis factor modifiers
Pregnancy category B

Do not confuse: inFLIXimab/riTUXimab, Remicade/Renacidin

ACTION: Monoclonal antibody that neutralizes the activity of tumor necrosis factor α (TNFα) that has been found in Crohn's disease; decreased infiltration of inflammatory cells

Therapeutic outcome: Decreased cramping and blood in stools

USES: Crohn's disease, fistulizing, moderate to severe; rheumatoid arthritis given with methotrexate, plaque psoriasis, ankylosing spondylitis, ulcerative colitis, psoriatic arthritis, psoriasis

Unlabeled uses: Behçet's syndrome, uveitis, juvenile arthritis

CONTRAINDICATIONS
Hypersensitivity to murines, moderate to severe CHF (NYHA class III/IV)

Precautions: Pregnancy **B,** breastfeeding, children, geriatric, COPD, hepatotoxicity, hematologic abnormalities, hepatitis B, Guillain-Barré syndrome, seizures, multiple sclerosis

BLACK BOX WARNING: Infection, neoplastic disease, TB

DOSAGE AND ROUTES
Crohn's disease (moderate to severe/fistulizing)/ankylosing spondylitis
Adult/adolescent/child ≥6 yr: IV INF 5 mg/kg initially, then repeat dose 2, 6 wk, then q8wk; may increase to 10 mg/kg if needed (adults)

Ulcerative colitis/plaque psoriasis
Adult/adolescent/child ≥ 6 yr: IV infusion 5 mg/kg initially and at 2, 4 wk, then 5 mg/kg q8wk

Rheumatoid arthritis
Adult: IV 3 mg/kg initially, and 2, 6 wk and q8wk thereafter, max 10 mg/kg/dose

Available forms: Powder for inj 100 mg

Implementation
Intermittent IV infusion route
• Administer immediately after reconstitution; reconstitute each vial with 10 ml of sterile water for inj, further dilute total dose/250 ml of 0.9% NaCl inj to a total conc of between 0.4 and 4 mg/ml; use 21-G or smaller needle for reconstitution, direct sterile water at glass wall of vial, gently swirl, do not shake, may foam; allow to stand for 5 min, give within 3 hr
• Give over ≥2 hr, use polyethylene-lined inf with in-line, sterile, low-protein-bind filter
• Do not admix
• Provide refrigerated storage, do not freeze

ADVERSE EFFECTS
CNS: *Headache, dizziness, depression, vertigo, fatigue, anxiety, fever,* seizures, *chills, flulike symptoms,* demyelinating disease
CV: Chest pain, hypo/hypertension, tachycardia,

CHF, acute coronary syndrome
GI: *Nausea, vomiting, abdominal pain, stomatitis, constipation, dyspepsia, flatulence*
GU: Dysuria, frequency
HEMA: Anemia, leukopenia, thrombocytopenia, pancytopenia
INTEG: *Rash, dermatitis, urticaria,* dry skin, sweating, flushing, hematoma, pruritus, keratoderma blennorrhagicum
MS: Myalgia, back pain, arthralgia
RESP: URI, pharyngitis, bronchitis, cough, dyspnea, sinusitis
SYST: Anaphylaxis, fatal infections, sepsis, malignancies, immunogenicity, Stevens-Johnson syndrome, toxic epidermal necrolysis

Pharmacokinetics

Absorption	Unknown
Distribution	Vascular compartment
Metabolism	Unknown
Excretion	Unknown
Half-life	9½ days

Pharmacodynamics

Unknown

INTERACTIONS
Drug classifications
Live virus vaccines: do not administer live vaccines concurrently
TNF blockers (abatacept, anakinra, golimumab, rilonacept): increased infections, neutropenia; avoid concurrent use

NURSING CONSIDERATIONS
Assessment
• Assess GI symptoms: nausea, vomiting, abdominal pain
• Take periodic blood counts: CBC
• Assess CV status: B/P, pulse, chest pain
⚠ Assess for allergic reaction, anaphylaxis: rash, dermatitis, urticaria, fever, chills, dyspnea, hypotension; discontinue if severe; administer epinephrine, corticosteroids, antihistamines; assess for allergy to murine proteins before starting therapy

> **BLACK BOX WARNING:** Fatal infections: discontinue if infection occurs, do not administer to patients with active infections; identify TB before beginning treatment, a TB test should be obtained; if present, TB should be treated before giving inFLIXimab; exercise caution when switching one DMARD to another

• Report suspected adverse reactions to the FDA (1-800-FDA-1088)

> **BLACK BOX WARNING:** Assess for neoplastic disease in those <18 yr, including heptosplenic T-cell lymphoma, usually occurs in those with inflammatory bowel disease

Patient/family education
• Instruct patient to report infusion reaction immediately
• Instruct patient to notify prescriber immediately if infection occurs
• Advise patient not to breastfeed while taking this product
• Advise patient to notify prescriber of GI symptoms, hypersensitivity reactions
• Advise patient not to operate machinery or drive if dizziness, vertigo occurs
• Teach patient to avoid live virus vaccinations, bring up to date prior to use

Evaluation
Positive therapeutic outcome
• Absence of blood in stool
• Reported improvement in comfort
• Weight gain

---

insulin, inhaled
(in'su-lin)
Afrezza
Func. class.: Antidiabetic—insulin
Pregnancy category C

ACTION: Endogenous insulin regulates carbohydrate, fat, and protein metabolism by the storage of and inhibiting the breakdown of glucose, fat, and amino acids. Insulin decreases glucose concentrations by the uptake of glucose in muscle and adipose tissue, and by inhibiting hepatic glucose production. Insulin also regulates fat metabolism by the storage of fat and inhibiting the mobilization of fat for energy in adipose tissues (lipolysis and free fatty acid oxidation).

Therapeutic outcome: Decrease in blood glucose levels

USES: Diabetes mellitus types 1 and 2

CONTRAINDICATIONS: Hypersensitivity, lung cancer, asthma, COPD, hypoglycemia, smoking

Precautions: Hepatic disease, renal impairment, renal failure, diabetic ketoacidosis (DKA), hypokalemia, pregnancy **C**, breastfeeding, child <18 yr

DOSAGE AND ROUTES
Adult: INH: (type 1) the average initial dose is 0.5-0.6 unit/kg/day, usually ≥3 administrations/day;

(type 2) the average initial dose is 0.2-0.6 unit/kg/day. When used in combination with oral hypoglycemic agents, may only need a single dose of a longer-acting insulin at a dosage of 10 units or 0.2 units/kg/day.

Available forms: 4 units powder for inh

Implementation

• Give by inhalation only; use at beginning of a meal (blue cartridge = 4 units of regular insulin, green cartridge = 8 units of regular insulin); multiple cartridges may be needed; for single-use only; inhaler should be discarded after 15 days; store unopened cartridge packages in refrigerator, if not refrigerated, use within 10 days

• Sealed (unopened) blister cards and strips must be used within 10 days. Cartridges left over in an opened strip must be used within 3 days. Remove a blister card from the foil package. Tear along a perforation to remove one strip. Press the clear side of the strip to push the cartridge out. To load the cartridge, hold the inhaler level in one hand with the white mouthpiece on the top and purple base on the bottom; open the inhaler by lifting the white mouthpiece to a vertical position. Before placing the cartridge in the inhaler, both the cartridge and the inhaler should be at room temperature for 10 minutes. Hold the cartridge with the cup facing down, and line up the cartridge with the opening in the inhaler. The pointed end of the cartridge should line up with the pointed end in the inhaler. The cartridge can be placed into the inhaler; ensure that the cartridge lies flat in the inhaler. Once the cartridge is loaded, keep level.

• Remove the purple mouthpiece cover. Hold the inhaler away from the mouth and fully exhale. While keeping the head level, place the mouthpiece in the mouth and tilt the inhaler down toward the chin. Close lips around the mouthpiece to form a seal. Inhale deeply through the inhaler. Hold breath for as long as is comfortable, and at the same time remove the inhaler from the mouth. Exhale and continue to breathe normally.

ADVERSE EFFECTS

CNS: Headache, fatigue
ENDO: Hypoglycemia
GI: Nausea, diarrhea
MISC: Urinary tract infection, weight gain, hypokalemia, peripheral edema
RESP: Cough, throat irritation/pain, productive cough, decreased pulmonary function tests, bronchitis, **acute bronchospasm**

Pharmacokinetics

Absorption	Unknown
Distribution	Unknown
Metabolism	Unknown
Excretion	Unknown
Half-life	Unknown

Pharmacodynamics

Onset	Unknown
Peak	Unknown
Duration	Unknown

INTERACTIONS
Drug classifications

ACE inhibitors, angiotensin II receptor antagonists, β-blockers: increased hypoglycemia

Bronchodilators, other inhaled products, agonists, MAOIs, salicylates: increased inhaled insulin effect

Testosterone derivatives, or anabolic steroids: increased or decreased hypoglycemic effects

Thiazide diuretics; thyroid hormones, estrogens, progestins, or oral contraceptives, corticosteroids: decreased hypoglycemic effects

Individual drugs

Alcohol, fenfluramine: increased inhaled insulin effect

Bumetanide, furosemide, niacin (nicotinic acid), torsemide: increased hyperglycemia

cloNIDine, metoclopramide, tegaserod: increased or decreased hypoglycemic effects

Danazol, dextrothyroxine, EPINEPHrine, triamterene: decreased hypoglycemic effects

Disopyramide, guanethidine, octreotide: increased hypoglycemia

Pioglitazone, troglitazone: increased heart failure, ischemic events

NURSING CONSIDERATIONS
Assessment

• Monitor fasting blood glucose, A1c may be drawn to identify treatment effectiveness

• Monitor urine ketones during illness, insulin requirements may increase during times of stress, trauma, illness, surgery

• Assess for hypoglycemic reaction; can occur during peak times (sweating, weakness, dizziness, chills, confusion, headache, nausea, rapid, weak pulse)

• Assess for hyperglycemia: acetone breath, polyuria, fatigue, polydipsia, flushed dry skin, lethargy

Patient/family education

• Teach patient that blurred vision occurs; patient should not operate machinery until effect

is known and should not change corrective lens for at least 1 mo
• Teach patient to keep all insulin equipment available at all times
• Inform patient that product does not cure, but controls symptoms
• Advise patient to carry ID as diabetic
• Teach patient about the symptoms of hypoglycemia, hyperglycemia, ketoacidosis
• Teach patient about dosage and how to use product, that the rest of the plan must be followed

Evaluation
Positive therapeutic outcome
• Decrease in blood glucose levels

⚠ HIGH ALERT

INSULINS

RAPID ACTING
insulin glulisine (Rx)
Apidra, Apidra SoloStar
insulin aspart (Rx)
NovoLOG, NovoLOG Flexpen, NovoLOG PenFill, NovoMix 30 ✦, NovoRapid ✦
insulin lispro (Rx)
HumaLOG, HumaLOG U-200 KwikPen

SHORT ACTING
insulin, regular (OTC)
Humulin R ✦, NovoLIN R, ReliOn R
insulin, regular concentrated (Rx)
Humulin RU-500

INTERMEDIATE ACTING
insulin, isophane suspension (NPH) (OTC)
Humulin N, NovoLIN ge NPH ✦, NovoLIN N, NovoLIN N Prefilled, ReliOn N

LONG ACTING
insulin detemir (Rx)
Levemir
insulin glargine (Rx)
Lantus, Toujeo Solostar

MIXTURES
insulin, isophane suspension and regular insulin (Rx)
HumaLIN 70/30, HumaLIN 30/70 ✦, NovoLIN 70/30, NovoLIN 70/30 Prefilled, ReliOn 70/30

isophane insulin suspension (NPH) and insulin mixtures (Rx)
Humulin 50/50
insulin lispro mixture (Rx)
HumaLOG KwikPen Mix 50/50, HumaLOG Mix 25 ✦, HumaLOG Mix 50 ✦, HumaLOG Mix 75/25, HumaLOG Mix 50/50
insulin aspart mixture (Rx)
NovoLOG 70/30, Novolog Mix Flexpen Prefilled Syringe 70/30
Func. class.: Antidiabetic, pancreatic hormone
Chem. class.: Modified structures of endogenous human insulin
Pregnancy category B, C

Do not confuse: Lantus/lente

ACTION: Decreases blood glucose; by transport of glucose into cells and the conversion of glucose to glycogen, indirectly increases blood pyruvate and lactate, decreases phosphate and potassium; insulin may be human (processed by recombinant DNA technologies)

Therapeutic outcome: Decreased blood glucose levels in diabetes mellitus

USES: Type 1 diabetes mellitus, type 2 diabetes mellitus, gestational diabetes, insulin lispro may be used in combination with sulfonylureas in children >3 yr

CONTRAINDICATIONS
Hypersensitivity to protamine; creosol (aspart)

Precautions: Pregnancy **B** (lispro, detemir, aspart, regular), **C** (all others)

DOSAGE AND ROUTES
>> Insulin glulisine
Adult/adolescent/child ≥4 yr: SUBCUT dosage individualized, give within 15 min before or 20 min after starting a meal
Adult: IV dilute to 1 unit/ml in INF systems with 0.9% NaCl, using PVC Viaflex INF bags and PVC tubing, use dedicated line

>> Insulin aspart
Adult/adolescent/child ≥6 yr: Intermittent SUBCUT total daily dose is given as 2-4 inj/day just prior to beginning of a meal; in general, 50%-70% of total daily insulin may be given as insulin aspart, the remainder should be intermediate or long-acting insulin; CONTINUOUS SUBCUT used with external insulin pump via cont SUBCUT insulin INF (CSII), the insulin dose should be based on the insulin dose from the previous regimen

>> Insulin lispro
Adult/adolescent/child ≥3 yr: SUBCUT 15 min before meals; **continuous subcut infusion (external insulin pump)** the total daily dose should be based on the insulin dose in previous regimen, 50% of total dose can be given as meal-related boluses and the remainder as basal infusion

>> Human regular
Adult: SUBCUT ½-1 hr before meals

Insulin, isophane suspension
Adult: SUBCUT dosage individualized by blood, urine glucose; usual dose 7-26 units; may increase by 2-10 units/day if needed

>> Insulin detemir
Adult/adolescent/child ≥2 yr: SUBCUT 1 or 2 times/day; if 1 time, give with evening meal

>> Insulin glargine
Adult and child ≥6 yr: SUBCUT 10 international units/day, range 2-100 international units/day

>> Regular insulin (ketoacidosis)
Adult: IV 5-10 units, then 5-10 units/hr until desired response, then switch to SUBCUT dose; **IV/INF** 2-12 units (50 units/500 ml of normal saline)
Child: IV 0.1 units/kg

>> Replacement
Adult and child: SUBCUT 0.5-1 units/kg/day qid given 30 min before meals
Adolescent: SUBCUT 0.8-1.2 mg/kg/day; this dosage is used during rapid growth

Available forms: NPH inj 100 units/ml; **regular** inj 100 units/ml, cartridges 100 units/ml; **insulin analog** inj 100 units/ml; **isophane insulin** inj 100 units/ml, cartridges 100 units/ml; **insulin lispro** 100 units/ml, 1.5-ml cartridges; insulin lispro Humalog KwikPen sol for inj 100 units/ml, Humalog KwikPen 200 U/ml prefilled pen solution for injection; **insulin glulisine** inj 100 units/ml; **insulin glargine** inj 100, 300 units/ml; **insulin detemir** inj 100 units/ml in 10 vials, 3-ml cartridges; **insulin aspart** inj 100 mg/ml (Flexpen, PenFill)

Implementation
• Store at room temperature for <1 mo (some insulins); keep away from heat and sunlight; refrigerate all other supply; NPH, premixed insulins are cloudy; regular, rapid-acting analogs, long-acting analogs are clear; do not freeze—**IV** route, regular only

SUBCUT route
• Give after warming to room temperature by rotating in palms to prevent injecting cold insulin; use only insulin syringes with markings or syringe matching units/ml; rotate inj sites within one area: abdomen, upper back, thighs, upper arm, buttocks; keep record of sites
• Give increased dosages if tolerance occurs
• Premixed insulins and NPH are cloudy suspensions
• Regular human insulin, rapid-acting analogs, and long-acting analogs are clear; do not use if cloudy, thick, or discolored

CONT SUBCUT route (insulin infusion CSII)
• Do not mix with other insulins when using a pump
• Insulin lispro 3 ml cartridges are to be used in Disetronic H-TRON plus V100 pump using Disetronic rapid inf sets; the inf set and the cartridge adapter should be changed q3day; replace 3 ml cartridge q6days

IV route (insulin glulisine only)
• Dilute to 1 international unit/ml in infusion systems with 0.9% NaCl using PVC viaflex inf bags and PVC tubing; use dedicated line; do not admix

IV route (regular only)
⚠ When regular insulin is administered IV, monitor glucose, potassium often to prevent fatal hypoglycemia, hypokalemia
• **IV** direct, undiluted via vein, Y-site, 3-way stopcock; give at 50 units/min or less
• Give by cont inf after diluting with **IV** sol and run at prescribed rate; use **IV** inf pump for correct dosing; give reduced dose at serum glucose level of 250 mg/100 ml

Additive compatibilities: Bretylium, cimetidine, lidocaine, meropenem, ranitidine, verapamil

Additive incompatibilities: Aminophylline, amobarbital, chlorothiazide, cytarabine, DOBUTamine, PENTobarbital, PHENobarbital, phenytoin, secobarbital, sodium bicarbonate, thiopental

Y-site compatibilities: Amiodarone, ampicillin, ampicillin/sulbactam, aztreonam, ceFAZolin, cefoTEtan, DOBUTamine, esmolol, famotidine, gentamicin, heparin, heparin/hydrocortisone, imipenem/cilastatin, indomethacin, magnesium sulfate, meperidine, meropenem, midazolam, morphine, nitroglycerin, oxytocin, PENTobarbital, potassium chloride, propofol, ritodrine, sodium bicarbonate, sodium nitroprusside, tacrolimus, terbutaline, ticarcillin, ticarcillin/clavulanate, tobramycin, vancomycin, vit B/C

Y-site incompatibilities: Nafcillin

ADVERSE EFFECTS
EENT: Blurred vision, dry mouth

INTEG: Flushing, rash, urticaria, warmth, *lipodystrophy*, lipohypertrophy, swelling, redness
META: *Hypoglycemia,* rebound hyperglycemia (Somogyi effect 12-72 hr or longer)
MISC: Peripheral edema
SYST: Anaphylaxis

Pharmacokinetics

Absorption	Rapidly absorbed (SUBCUT)
Distribution	Widely distributed
Metabolism	Liver, muscle, kidney
Excretion	Kidneys
Half-life	Regular 3-5 min; NPH 10 min

Pharmacodynamics

Rapid acting	
Insulin glulisine	Onset 15-30 min, peak ½-1½ hr, duration 3-4 hr
Insulin aspart	Onset 10-20 min, peak 1-3 hr, duration 3-5 hr
Insulin lispro	Onset 15-30 min, peak ½-1½ hr, duration 3-4 hr
Short acting	
Insulin regular	Onset 30 min, peak 2.5-5 hr, duration up to 6 hr
Intermediate acting	
Insulin, isophane suspension (NPH)	Onset 1.5-4 hr, peak 4-12 hr, duration up to 24 hr
Long acting	
Insulin detemir	Onset 0.8-2 hr, peak unknown, duration up to 24 hr (concentration dependent)
Insulin glargine	Onset 1.5 hr, no peak identified, duration ≥ 24 hr
Mixtures	
Insulin, isophane suspension and regular insulin (70/30)	Onset 10-20 hr, peak 2.4 hr, duration up to 24 hr
Isophane insulin suspension (NPH) and insulin mixtures (50/50)	Onset ½-1 hr, peak dual, duration 10-16 hr

INTERACTIONS
Individual drugs
Alcohol: increased hypoglycemia
DOBUTamine: increased insulin need
EPINEPHrine: decreased hypoglycemia
Sulfinpyrazone, tetracycline: decreased insulin need

Drug classifications
Anabolic steroids, β-adrenergic blockers, hypoglycemics (oral), salicylates: increased hypoglycemia
Contraceptives (oral), corticosteroids, diuretics (thiazide), thyroid hormones: decreased hypoglycemia
Estrogens: increased insulin need
MAOIs: decreased insulin need

Drug/lab test
Increased: VMA
Decreased: potassium, calcium
Interference: liver, thyroid function tests

NURSING CONSIDERATIONS
Assessment
• Fasting blood glucose, also Hgb A1c may be tested to identify treatment effectiveness q3mo
• Urine ketones during illness; insulin requirements may increase during stress, illness, surgery
• For hypoglycemic reaction that can occur during peak time (sweating, weakness, dizziness, chills, confusion, headache, nausea, rapid weak pulse, fatigue, tachycardia, memory lapses, slurred speech, staggering gait, anxiety, tremors, hunger)
• For hyperglycemia: acetone breath, polyuria, fatigue, polydipsia, flushed, dry skin, lethargy

Patient/family education
• Advise patient that blurred vision occurs; not to change corrective lens until vision is stabilized 1-2 mo
• **Advise patient to keep insulin, equipment available at all times; carry a glucagon kit, candy, or lump sugar to treat hypoglycemia**

- Inform patient that product does not cure diabetes but controls symptoms
- Advise patient to carry emergency ID as diabetic
- Instruct patient to recognize hypoglycemia reaction: headache, tremors, fatigue, weakness
- Instruct patient to recognize hyperglycemia reaction: frequent urination, thirst, fatigue, hunger
- Teach patient the dosage, route, mixing instructions, any diet restrictions, disease process
- **Teach patient the symptoms of ketoacidosis: nausea, thirst, polyuria, dry mouth, decreased B/P, dry, flushed skin, acetone breath, drowsiness, Kussmaul respirations**
- Advise patient that a plan is necessary for diet, exercise; all food on diet should be eaten; exercise routine should not vary
- Teach patient about blood glucose testing; make sure patient is able to determine glucose level
- Advise patient to avoid OTC products unless directed by prescriber

Evaluation

Positive therapeutic outcome
- Decrease in polyuria, polydipsia, polyphagia; clear sensorium; absence of dizziness; stable gait
- Blood glucose level under control

TREATMENT OF OVERDOSE:
Glucose 25 g **IV,** via dextrose 50% sol, 50 ml, or glucagon 1 mg

---

interferon alfacon-1 (Rx)
(in-ter-feer′on al′fa-kon)
Infergen
Func. class.: Recombinant type 1 interferon
Pregnancy category C

ACTION: Induces biologic responses and has antiviral, antiproliferative, and immunomodulatory effects

Therapeutic outcome: Decreased signs/ symptoms of hepatitis C

USES: Chronic hepatitis C infections in those 18 yr and older with compensated liver disease who have anti-HCV antibodies or HCV RNA, may use in combination with ribavirin

CONTRAINDICATIONS
Hypersensitivity to α-interferons, or products from *Escherichia coli,* uncompensated hepatic disease, autoimmune hepatitis

Precautions: Pregnancy **C,** breastfeeding, children <18 yr, thyroid disorders, myelosuppression, hepatic disease, alcoholism, geriatric patients, seizure disorder, hepatitis

> **BLACK BOX WARNING:** Cardiac disease, autoimmune disorder, infection, depression

DOSAGE AND ROUTES
Adult: Monotherapy: SUBCUT 9 mcg as a single inj 3 times per week × 24 wk; leave at least 48 hr between injections; those who did not respond or relapsed after discontinuation, give 15 mcg 3 times per week × 48 wk; **combination:** subcut 15 mcg/day with ribavirin 1000 mg/day PO (<75 kg), 1200 mg/day PO (≥75 kg) give in 2 divided doses for up to 48 wks, use stepwise dose reduction in the interferon dose from 15 mcg to 9 mcg to 6 mcg for serious adverse reactions

Available forms: Inj 9 mcg/0.3 ml, 15 mcg/0.5 ml

Implementation
- Do not shake vial; use 1 dose per vial; discard unused portion; use proper inj sites; rotate sites, discard unused product, give at bedtime for better tolerance

ADVERSE EFFECTS
CNS: Headache, fatigue, fever, rigors, insomnia, dizziness, agitation, nervousness, anxiety, lability, abnormal thinking, depression
CV: Hypertension, palpitation, tachycardia
EENT: Tinnitus, earache, conjunctivitis, eye pain
GI: Abdominal pain, nausea, diarrhea, anorexia, dyspepsia, vomiting, constipation, flatulence, hemorrhoids, decreased salivation
GU: Dysmenorrhea, vaginitis, menstrual disorders
HEMA: Granulocytopenia, thrombocytopenia, leukopenia, ecchymosis, **aplastic anemia**
INTEG: Alopecia, pruritus, rash, erythema, dry skin
MISC: Anaphylaxis, angioedema, flulike illness
MS: Back, limb, neck, skeletal pain, rigors
RESP: Pharyngitis, upper respiratory infection, cough, sinusitis, rhinitis, respiratory tract congestion, epistaxis, dyspnea, bronchitis

Pharmacokinetics

Unknown

Adverse effects: *italics* = common; **bold** = life-threatening

Pharmacodynamics

Onset	Unknown
Peak	24-36 hr
Duration	Unknown

INTERACTIONS
Individual drugs
Eflornithine (systemic): increased hearing loss, consider serial audiograms

Drug classifications
NRTIs: increased effect, use together cautiously

NURSING CONSIDERATIONS
Assessment
⚠ Pregnancy: determine if patient is pregnant before use with ribavirin, pregnancy (X) when used with ribavirin
• Assess CBC, liver function tests, ECG, platelet counts, heme concentration, ANC, serum creatinine concentration, albumin, bilirubin, TSH, T_4

> **BLACK BOX WARNING: Hemolytic anemia:** ribavirin may be used with this product and cause hemolytic anemia, cardiac symptoms

• Assess for myelosuppression, low dose if neutrophil count is <500 × 10-6/L or if platelets are <50 × 10-9/L, monitor for infection
• Assess for hypersensitivity; discontinue immediately if hypersensitivity occurs

Patient/family education
• Provide patient or family member with written, detailed instructions about the product
• Caution patient to use contraception during treatment
⚠ Teach patient to report if pregnancy is planned or suspected; pregnancy (C), when combined with ribavirin pregnancy (X)
• Teach patient to use OTC analgesics to decrease flulike symptoms
• If patient will be self-administering injection, teach all aspects of product use, administration, disposal; provide med guide

Evaluation
Positive therapeutic outcome
• Decreased hepatitis C signs/symptoms

interferon beta-1a (Rx)
(in-ter-feer'on)
Avonex, Rebif
interferon beta-1b (Rx)
Betaseron, Extavia
Func. class.: Multiple sclerosis agent, immune modifier
Chem. class.: Interferon, *Escherichia coli* derivative
Pregnancy category C

ACTION: Antiviral, immunoregulatory; action not clearly understood; biologic response-modifying properties mediated through specific receptors on cells, inducing expression of interferon-induced gene products

Therapeutic outcome: Decreased symptoms of multiple sclerosis

USES: Ambulatory patients with relapsing or remitting multiple sclerosis

CONTRAINDICATIONS
Hypersensitivity to natural or recombinant interferon-beta or human albumin, hamster protein, rotavirus vaccine

Precautions: Pregnancy **C**, breastfeeding, children <18 yr, chronic progressive multiple sclerosis, depression, mental disorders, seizure disorders, latex allergy, autoimmune disorders, bone marrow suppression, hepatotoxicity, cardiac disease, alcoholism, chickenpox, herpes zoster

DOSAGE AND ROUTES
>> Interferon beta-1a
Remitting-relapsing multiple sclerosis
Adult: IM (Avonex) 30 mcg qwk; SUBCUT (Rebif) 22 or 44 mcg 3 ×/wk with each dose 48 hr apart, titrate to full dose over 4-wk period

>> Interferon beta-1b
Relapsing/remitting multiple sclerosis
Adult: SUBCUT 0.0625 mg every other day for wk 1 and 2; then 0.125 mg every other day for wk 3 and 4; then 0.1875 mg every other day for wk 5 and 6; then 0.25 mg every other day thereafter; higher doses should not be used

Available forms: Beta-1a (Avonex): 33 mcg (6.6 million international units/vial) (auto-injector pen); (Rebif) 22 mcg, 44 mcg/0.5 ml; beta-1b: powder for inj 0.3 mg (9.6 m international units)

Implementation

• Reconstitute 0.3 mg (9.6 million international units)/1.2 ml of supplied diluent (0.2 mg or 8 million international units concentration); rotate vial gently, do not shake; withdraw 1 ml using a syringe with 27-G needle; administer SUBCUT only into hip, thigh, arm; discard unused portion

>> Interferon beta-1a

• Reconstitute with 1.1 ml of diluent, swirl, give within 6 hr
• Store in refrigerator; do not freeze
• Visually inspect parenteral products for particulate matter and discoloration prior to use

IM route

• Premedication with acetaminophen or ibuprofen and give at bedtime to lessen flulike symptoms
• Interferon beta-1a (Avonex) 30 mcg is equivalent to 6 million IU
• If a dose is missed, give it as soon as possible; continue the regular schedule but do not give 2 injections within 2 days of each other; all products are for single-use only. Do not re-use needles, syringes, prefilled syringes, or autoinjectors, rotate injection sites
• Check site to minimize injection site reactions
• Do not inject into an area of the body where skin is irritated, reddened, bruised, infected, or scarred
• The injection site should be checked after 2 hours for redness, edema, or tenderness
• The manufacturer of Avonex offers free training on IM use for patients and health care partners. Contact MS ActiveSource for more information (800-456-2255)

Reconstitution and administration of Avonex lyophilized powder for IM route

• Use aseptic technique for preparation of solution
• Sites for injection include the thigh or upper arm
• Slowly add 1.1 ml sterile water for injection, preservative-free (supplied by manufacturer) to the vial. Rapid addition of the diluent may cause foaming
• Gently swirl; do not shake. Final concentration should be 30 mcg/ml (6 million IU/ml)
• The solution should be clear to slightly yellow without particles. Discard if the reconstituted product contains particulate matter or is discolored
• Withdraw 1 ml of reconstituted solution into a syringe. Attach the sterile needle and inject IM
• A 25 gauge, 1″ needle for IM may be substituted for the 23 gauge, 1¼″ needle provided

• *Storage:* Use within 6 hours of reconstitution; store reconstituted solution refrigerated; do NOT freeze. Discard any unused solution; both drug and diluent vials are single-use only

Administration of Avonex prefilled syringe

• Patients may self-inject only if provider determines that it is appropriate, and with medical follow-up, and after proper training in IM injection technique
• The first injection should be performed under the supervision of an appropriately qualified person
• If self-injecting, rotate between thighs. With help from another person, may rotate between thighs and upper arms
• Wash hands prior to handling the Dose Pack
• Remove prefilled syringe from the refrigerator to warm to room temperature (usually 30 min before use). Do not use external heat sources such as hot water to warm the syringe
• Hold the syringe so the cap is facing down and the 0.5 mL mark is at eye level. Be sure the amount of liquid in the syringe is the same or very close to the 0.5 mL mark. If the correct amount of liquid is not in the syringe, do not use it and call the pharmacist
• Hold syringe upright so that the rubber cap faces up. Remove the cap by bending it at a 90 degree angle until it snaps free
• Attach the needle by pressing it onto the syringe and turning it clockwise until it locks in place. Be careful not to push the plunger while attaching the needle
• Use the alcohol wipe to clean the skin at the injection site you choose. Then, pull the protective cover straight off the needle; do not twist the cover off
• Inject intramuscularly at a 90 degree angle into the thigh or upper arm as directed by the provider
• Use gauze pad to apply pressure for a few seconds after the injection
• Dispose of used needles and syringes in a puncture-resistant container and discard appropriately
• Instruct patients to contact the health care provider if a skin reaction occurs that does not resolve in a few days
• A 25 gauge, 1″ needle for intramuscular injection may be substituted for the 23 gauge, 1¼″ needle provided by the manufacturer, if deemed appropriate by the physician
• Refer to the Patient Medication Guide for detailed instructions for preparing and giving a dose
• *Storage:* Store refrigerated, if refrigeration is unavailable, may store at 77 degrees F or less

for up to 7 days; after removal from refrigerator, do not store product above 25 degrees C. If the product has been exposed to conditions other than recommended, discard the product. Do not expose to high temperatures. Do not freeze. Protect from light

Administration of Avonex prefilled autoinjector

• Patients may self-inject only if their provider determines that it is appropriate, and with medical follow-up, and after proper training in IM technique

• The first injection should be performed under the supervision of provider

• Remove one Administration Dose Pack from the refrigerator to warm to room temperature (about 30 min before use). Do not use external heat sources such as hot water to warm the syringe Dose Pack

• Wash hands prior to handling Dose Pack contents

• Ensure tamper-evident cap has not been removed or is loose. Then grasp the cap and bend it at a 90-degree angle until it snaps off. Pull off the sterile foil from the needle cover

• Hold the Avonex pen with the glass syringe tip pointing up. Press the needle onto the glass syringe tip. Gently turn the needle clockwise until firmly attached. Do not remove plastic cover from the needle

• Hold Pen with one hand and using other hand, hold onto the injector shield (grooved area) tightly and quickly pull up on the injector shield until the injector shield covers the needle all the way. The plastic needle cover will pop off after the injector shield has been fully extended

• When the injector shield is extended the right way, there will be a small blue rectangular area next to the oval medication display window. Check the display window and make sure the Avonex is clear and colorless

• Do not use the injection if the liquid is colored, cloudy, or has lumps or particles. Air bubbles will not affect your dose

• Do not push down on the injector shield and the blue activation button at the same time until you are ready to give injection

• Avonex pen should be injected into the upper, outer thigh

• Use the alcohol wipe to clean the skin at the injection site you choose and allow it to dry prior to injection

• Hold Pen at 90-degree angle to the injection site. Firmly push the body of the pen down against the thigh to release the safety lock. Safety lock is released when blue rectangle area above the oval medication display window is gone.

Push down on blue activation button with thumb and count to 10. You will hear a click if the injection is given the right way

• After counting to 10, pull the pen straight out of the skin. Use gauze pad to apply pressure for a few seconds

• The circular display window on the pen will be yellow if you have received the full dose

• Cover exposed needle with pen cover. Do not hold the pen cover with your hands while inserting the needle

• Dispose of used needles and syringes in a puncture-resistant container and discard appropriately

• Instruct patients to contact the health care provider if a skin reaction occurs that does not resolve in a few days

• Refer to the Patient Medication Guide for detailed instructions for preparing and giving a dose

• *Storage:* Store at 36°-46° F (2°-8° C). If refrigeration is unavailable, may store at 77° F (25° C) or less for up to 7 days. After removal from refrigerator, do not store product above 77° F (25° C). If the product has been exposed to conditions other than recommended, discard the product and do not use. Do not expose to high temperatures. Do not freeze. Protect from light

Subcutaneous administration

• Give at the same time (preferably late in the afternoon or evening) on the same days of the week at least 48 hr apart

• Do not give on two consecutive days. If a dose is missed, administer the dose as soon as possible then skip the following day. Return to the regular schedule the following week

• Premedication with acetaminophen or ibuprofen may lessen the severity of flulike symptoms

• Interferon beta-1a (Rebif) 44 mcg is equivalent to 12 million IU

• Rotate injection sites. Appropriate injection sites include thigh, outer surface of upper arm, stomach, or buttocks. Do not inject into an area where the skin is irritated, reddened, bruised, or infected

• A "Starter Pack" containing a lower dose of Rebif syringes is available for the initial titration period. Patients and/or caregivers should be trained and understand appropriate preparation and administration

• The manufacturer offers complimentary services including injection training and reimbursement support. Contact MS LifeLines at 877-44-REBIF

Injection (Rebif)
• Interferon beta-1a (Rebif) is available in a prefilled syringe with a 29-gauge needle
• Inject subcutaneously into the outer surface of the upper arm, abdomen, thigh, or buttock. Do not inject the area near the navel or waistline. Take care not to inject intradermally
• Discard any unused solution. Prefilled syringes do not contain preservatives and are single-use only

>> Interferon beta-1b
• Reconstitute by injecting diluent provided (1.2 ml) into vial, swirl (8 milli-international units/ml), use 27-G needle for inj
• Give acetaminophen for fever, headache; use SUBCUT route only; do not give IM or **IV**
• Store reconstituted sol in refrigerator; do not freeze; do not use sol that contains precipitate or is discolored

Subcut route
• The manufacturers of Betaseron and of Extavia offer materials to assist with training on subcut use: call 1-800-788-1467 (Betaseron), 1-888-669-6682 (Extavia)
• Premedication with acetaminophen or ibuprofen and use of product at bedtime may lessen the severity of flulike symptoms
• Visually inspect parenteral products for particulate matter and discoloration prior to use. Do not use if particulate matter is present

Reconstitution
• Add 1.2 ml of 0.54% sodium chloride injection (supplied by the manufacturer) to the vial by using the vial adapter to attach the prefilled syringe that contains the diluent. Keep the plunger depressed, and gently swirl; do not shake. If you take your thumb off the plunger, the solution may come back into the syringe before the product is fully reconstituted. If foaming occurs, allow the vial to sit until the foam settles; final concentration (250 mcg interferon beta-1b/ml, which corresponds to 8 million International Units/ml)
• If not used immediately, store in the refrigerator for up to 3 hr; do not freeze; discard any unused portion after 3 hr

Injection
• Withdraw the desired amount of the reconstituted solution into the syringe by turning the vial and syringe to get the vial on top. Pull the plunger back to get the desired amount of product; turn the syringe to point the needle upward, and tap the syringe and release any air bubbles. Twist the vial adapter to remove it and the vial
• Choose an injection site on the upper, back arms; abdomen; buttocks; or front thighs. Do

not inject within 2 in of the navel or in a site where the skin is red, bruised, infected, broken, painful, uneven, or scabbed; rotate injection sites to minimize injection site reactions such as necrosis or localized infection
• Inject subcutaneously. Take care not to inject intradermally

ADVERSE EFFECTS
CNS: *Headache, fever, pain, chills, mental changes,* depression, hypertonia, **suicide attempts, seizures**
CV: *Migraine, palpitations, hypertension,* tachycardia, peripheral vascular disorders
EENT: Conjunctivitis, blurred vision
GI: *Diarrhea, constipation, vomiting, abdominal pain*
GU: *Dysmenorrhea, irregular menses, metrorrhagia,* cystitis, breast pain
HEMA: Decreased lymphocytes, ANC, WBC, *lymphadenopathy,* anemia
INTEG: *Sweating, inj site reaction*
MS: *Myalgia,* myasthenia
RESP: *Sinusitis,* dyspnea

Pharmacokinetics
Absorption	50% is absorbed
Distribution	Unknown
Metabolism	Unknown
Excretion	Unknown
Half-life	8 min–4½ hr (beta-1b), 8.6 hr (beta-1a)

Pharmacodynamics
	Beta-1a	Beta-1b
Onset	Up to 12 hr	Rapid
Peak	16 hr	2-8 hr
Duration	4 days	Unknown

INTERACTIONS
Individual drugs
Zidovudine: decreased clearance

Drug classifications
Antiretrovirals (NNRTIs, NRTIs, protease inhibitors): increased hepatic damage
Antineoplastics: increased myelosuppression

Drug/herb
Astragalus, echinacea, melatonin: change in immunomodulation

Drug/lab test
Increased: liver function tests
Interference: vaccines, toxoids; avoid concurrent use

Adverse effects: *italics* = common; **bold** = life-threatening

NURSING CONSIDERATIONS
Assessment
• Monitor blood, renal, liver function tests: CBC, differential, platelet counts, BUN, creatinine, ALT, urinalysis; if neutrophil count is $<750/mm^3$, or if AST, ALT is $10 \times$ greater than ULN, or if bilirubin is $5 \times$ greater than ULN, discontinue product; when neutrophil count exceeds $750/mm^3$ and liver function or renal studies return to normal, treatment may resume at 50% original dosage
• Assess for CNS symptoms: headache, fatigue, depression; if depression occurs and is severe, product should be discontinued
• Assess for multiple sclerosis symptoms
• Assess mental status: depression, depersonalization, suicidal thoughts, insomnia
• Monitor GI status: diarrhea or constipation, vomiting, abdominal pain
• Monitor cardiac status: increased B/P, tachycardia

Patient/family education
• Provide patient or family member with written, detailed instructions about the product; provide initial and return demonstrations on inj procedure; give information on use and disposal of product
• Inform patient that blurred vision, hearing loss, sweating may occur
• Advise female patients that irregular menses, dysmenorrhea, or metrorrhagia as well as breast pain may occur; use contraception during treatment; product may cause spontaneous abortion
• Teach patient to use sunscreen to prevent photosensitivity
• Instruct patient to notify prescriber if pregnancy is suspected
• Teach patient inj technique and care of equipment
• Instruct patient to notify prescriber of increased temp, chills, muscle soreness, fatigue

Evaluation
Positive therapeutic outcome
• Decreased symptoms of multiple sclerosis

interferon gamma-1b (Rx)
(in-ter-feer′on)
Actimmune
Func. class.: Biologic response modifier
Chem. class.: Lymphokine, interleukin type
Pregnancy category C

ACTION: Species-specific protein synthesized in response to viruses; potent phagocyte-activating effects; capable of mediating the killing of *Staphylococcus aureus, Toxoplasma gondii,* *Leishmania donovani, Listeria monocytogenes, Mycobacterium avium-intracellulare;* enhances oxidative metabolism of macrophages; enhances antibody-dependent cellular cytotoxicity

Therapeutic outcome: Decreased signs/symptoms of infection (serious) in chronic granulomatous disease

USES: Serious infections associated with chronic granulomatous disease, osteopetrosis

Unlabeled uses: Osteoporosis, *Mycobacterium avium* complex (MAC), ovarian cancer

CONTRAINDICATIONS
Hypersensitivity to interferon γ, *Escherichia coli*–derived products

Precautions: Pregnancy **C**, breastfeeding, children <1 yr, cardiac disease, seizure/CNS disorders, myelosuppression

DOSAGE AND ROUTES
Adult: SUBCUT 50 mcg/m² (1.5 million units/m²) for patient with a surface area of >0.5 m²; 1.5 mcg/kg/dose for patient with a surface area of $<0.5/m^2$; give on Monday, Wednesday, Friday for 3 ×/wk dosing

Available forms: Inj 100 mcg (2 million units)/single-dose vial

Implementation
• Give at bedtime to minimize adverse reactions; administer acetaminophen for fever, headache; use 50% of the dosage prescribed if severe reactions occur or discontinue treatment until reactions subside
• Give in right or left deltoid and anterior thigh; warm to room temperature before use; do not leave at room temperature >12 hr (unopened vial); does not contain preservatives
• Store in refrigerator upon receipt; do not freeze; do not shake

ADVERSE EFFECTS
CNS: *Headache, fatigue,* depression, fever, chills
GI: *Nausea, anorexia,* abdominal pain, weight loss, diarrhea, vomiting, colitis
HEMA: Leukopenia, thrombocytopenia, neutropenia
INTEG: Rash, pain at inj site, Stevens-Johnson syndrome
MS: Myalgia, arthralgia

Pharmacokinetics

Absorption	Slowly absorbed 89%
Distribution	Unknown
Metabolism	Unknown
Excretion	Unknown
Half-life	5.9 hr

Pharmacodynamics

Onset	Unknown
Peak	7 hr
Duration	Unknown

INTERACTIONS
Individual drugs
Aminophylline, theophylline: increased levels

Drug classifications
Myelosuppressive agents: increased myelosuppression

Protease inhibitors, nucleoside reverse transcriptase inhibitors (NRTIs), nonnucleoside reverse transcriptase inhibitors (NNRTIs): increased liver toxicity

NURSING CONSIDERATIONS
Assessment
• Monitor blood, renal, hepatic studies: CBC with differential, platelet count, BUN, creatinine, ALT, urinalysis before, q3mo during treatment
• Assess for infection: headache, fever, chills, fatigue; these are common adverse reactions
• Monitor CNS symptoms: headache, fatigue, depression

Patient/family education
• Provide patient or family member with written, detailed instructions about the product; provide initial and return demonstrations on inj procedure; give information on use and disposal of product
• Caution patient to use contraception during treatment

Evaluation
Positive therapeutic outcome
• Decreased serious infections
• Improvement in existing infections and inflammatory conditions

⚠ HIGH ALERT

ipilimumab
(ip-i-lim′ue-mab)
Yervoy
Func. class.: Antineoplastic; biologic response modifier
Pregnancy category C

ACTION: A recombinant, human monoclonal antibody that binds to the cytotoxic T-lymphocyte–associated antigen 4 (CTLA-4); action is indirect, possibly through T-cell–mediated antitumor immune responses

Therapeutic outcome: Decreased spread of malignant cells

USES: Treatment of unresectable or metastatic malignant melanoma

CONTRAINDICATIONS
Hypersensitivity

Precautions: Pregnancy, breastfeeding, Crohn's disease, hepatitis, immunosuppression, inflammatory bowel disease, iritis, ocular disease, organ transplant, pancreatitis, renal disease, rheumatoid arthritis, sarcoidosis, systemic lupus erythematosus, thyroid disease, ulcerative colitis, uveitis

DOSAGE AND ROUTES
Adult and geriatric: IV 3 mg/kg over 90 min q3wk × 4 doses. Permanently discontinue if the full treatment course is not completed within 16 wk from first dose or for severe or life-threatening adverse reactions; withhold a dose for any moderate endocrine or immune-mediated adverse reactions; if the moderate adverse reaction completely or partially resolves (Grade 0-1) and if the patient is receiving less than 7.5 mg predniSONE or equivalent per day, resume at a dose of 3 mg/kg IV every 3 wk until all 4 planned doses or 16 wk from first dose, whichever occurs earlier; if moderate adverse reactions are persistent or if the corticosteroid dose cannot be reduced to 7.5 mg predniSONE or equivalent per day, permanently discontinue

Available forms: Solution for inj 50 mg/10 ml, 200 mg/40 ml

Implementation
Intermittent IV infusion route
• Visually inspect parenteral products for particulate matter and discoloration before using whenever solution and container permit; solution may have a pale yellow color and have translucent-to-white, amorphous particles; discard the vial if the solution is cloudy, if there is pronounced discoloration, or if particulate matter is present
• Allow vials to stand at room temperature for 5 min before infusion preparation; withdraw the required volume and transfer into an IV bag. Discard partially used vials or empty vials; dilute with 0.9% sodium chloride injection, or 5% dextrose injection, to a final concentration (1-2 mg/ml); mix diluted solution by gentle inversion; do not admix
• Give infusion over 90 min through an IV line with a low-protein binding in-line filter, do not give with other products; after each infusion, flush the line with 0.9% sodium chloride Injection, or 0.5% dextrose injection
• Store once diluted, store for no more than 24 hr refrigerated or at room temperature

Adverse effects: *italics* = common; **bold** = life-threatening

ADVERSE EFFECTS

CNS: Severe and fatal immune-mediated neuropathies, fatigue, fever, headache
EENT: Episcleritis, iritis, Uveitis
ENDO: Severe and fatal immune-mediated endocrinopathies
GI: Severe and fatal immune-mediated enterocolitis, hepatitis; pancreatitis, abdominal pain, colitis, constipation, decreased appetite, diarrhea, nausea, vomiting
INTEG: Severe and fatal immune-mediated dermatitis, pruritus, rash, urticaria
MISC: Anemia, cough, dyspnea, eosinophilia, nephritis
SYST: Antibody formation, Stevens-Johnson syndrome, toxic epidermal necrolysis

> **BLACK BOX WARNING:** Adrenal insufficiency, diarrhea, Gullain-Barré syndrome, hepatic disease, myasthenia gravis, hyperhypothyroidism, hypopituitarism, peripheral neuropathy, serious rash

Pharmacokinetics

Absorption	Unknown
Distribution	Steady state (end of 3rd dose)
Metabolism	Unknown
Excretion	Unknown
Half-life	Terminal 15.4 days

Pharmacodynamics

Onset	Unknown
Peak	Unknown
Duration	Unknown

NURSING CONSIDERATIONS

Assessment

• **Serious skin disorders:** Stevens-Johnson syndrome, toxic epidermal necrolysis: permanently discontinue in these or rash complicated by full thickness dermal ulceration or necrotic, bullous, or hemorrhagic manifestations like bullous rash; give systemic corticosteroids at a dose of 1-2 mg/kg/day of predniSONE or equivalent; when dermatitis is controlled, taper corticosteroids over a period of at least 1 month. Withhold in those with moderate to severe reactions; for mild to moderate dermatitis (localized rash and pruritus), give topical or systemic corticosteroids
• **Hepatotoxicity:** Baseline and before each dose; rule out infectious or malignant causes and increase the frequency of liver function test monitoring until resolution;

permanently discontinue in those with Grade 3-5 give systemic corticosteroids at a dose of 1-2 mg/kg/day of prednisone or equivalent
• **Neuropathy:** Monitor for motor or sensory neuropathy (unilateral or bilateral weakness, sensory alterations, or paresthesias) before each dose; permanently discontinue if severe neuropathy (interfering with daily activities) such as Guillain-Barré-like syndromes occur
• **Endocrinopathy:** Monitor thyroid function tests at baseline and before each dose; monitor hypophysitis, adrenal insufficiency, adrenal crisis, hyperthyroidism, hypothyroidism (fatigue, headache, mental status changes, abdominal pain, unusual bowel habits, hypotension, or nonspecific symptoms that may resemble other causes)

Patient/family education

⚠ Instruct patient/family to report immediately allergic reaction, skin rash, severe abdominal pain, yellowing of skin, eyes; tingling of extremities, change in bowel habits
⚠ Discuss reason for treatment and expected results

Evaluation

Positive therapeutic outcome
• Decreasing spread of malignant melanoma

ipratropium (Rx)

(i-pra-troe′pee-um)
Atrovent HFA
Func. class.: Anticholinergic, bronchodilator
Chem. class.: Synthetic quaternary ammonium compound
Pregnancy category B

Do not confuse: Atrovent/Alupent

ACTION: Inhibits interaction of acetylcholine at receptor sites on the bronchial smooth muscle, resulting in decreased cyclic guanosine monophosphate (cyclic GMP) and bronchodilatation

Therapeutic outcome: Bronchodilatation

USES: Bronchospasm, COPD; rhinorrhea (nasal spray)

CONTRAINDICATIONS

Hypersensitivity to this product, atropine, bromide, soybean, or peanut products

Precautions: Pregnancy **B**, breastfeeding, children <12 yr, angioedema, heart failure, surgery, acute bronchospasm, closed-angle glaucoma, prostatic hypertrophy, bladder neck obstruction, urinary retention

DOSAGE AND ROUTES
Bronchospasm in chronic bronchitis/emphysema
Adult: INH 2 sprays (17 mcg/spray) 3-4×/day, max 12 INH/24 hr, SOL 500 mcg (1 unit dose) given 3-4×/day by nebulizer; nasal spray: 2 sprays (42 mcg/spray) 3-4×/day
Child 5-12 yr: NASAL 2 sprays in each nostril 3×/day

Rhinorrhea perennial rhinitis
Adult/child ≥6 yr: INTRANASAL 2 sprays (43 mcg)/nostril bid or tid
Child 5-12 yr: INTRANASAL 2 sprays (0.03%) in each nostril 3×/day

Available forms: Aerosol 17 mcg/actuation; nasal spray 0.03%, 0.06%; sol for inh 0.0125% ✚, 0.02%

Implementation
• Give after shaking container; have patient exhale, place mouthpiece in mouth, inhale slowly, hold breath, remove, exhale slowly; allow at least 1 min between inhalations
• Give this medication before other medications and allow at least 5 min between each
Nebulizer route
• Use solution in nebulizer with a mouthpiece rather than a face mask
Intranasal route
• Prime pump, initially requires 7 actuations of the pump, priming again is not necessary if used regularly; tilt head backward after dose
• Store in light-resistant container; do not expose to temperature over 86° F (30° C)

ADVERSE EFFECTS
CNS: *Anxiety, dizziness, headache,* nervousness
CV: Palpitations
EENT: Dry mouth, blurred vision, nasal congestion
GI: *Nausea, vomiting, cramps*
INTEG: Rash
RESP: *Cough, worsening of symptoms,* **bronchospasm**

Pharmacokinetics

Absorption	Minimal
Distribution	Does not cross blood-brain barrier
Metabolism	Liver, minimal
Excretion	Unknown
Half-life	2 hr

Pharmacodynamics

Onset	5-15 min
Peak	1-1½ hr
Duration	3-6 hr

INTERACTIONS
Individual drugs
Disopyramide: increased anticholinergic action

Drug classifications
Antihistamines, phenothiazines: increased anticholinergic action
Bronchodilators (other): increased toxicity

Drug/herb
Belladonna: increased anticholinergic effect
Green tea (large amounts), guarana: increased bronchodilator effect

NURSING CONSIDERATIONS
Assessment
• Monitor respiratory function: vital capacity, FEV, ABGs, lung sounds, heart rate, rhythm (baseline, during treatment); if severe bronchospasm is present, a more rapid medication is required
• Monitor for evidence of allergic reactions, paradoxical bronchospasm; withhold dose and notify prescriber; identify if patient is allergic to belladonna products or atropine; allergy to this product may occur

Patient/family education
• Advise patient not to use OTC medications unless approved by prescriber; extra stimulation may occur; to use this medication before other medications and allow at least 5 min between each to prevent overstimulation
• Teach patient that compliance is necessary with number of inhalations/24 hr, or overdose may occur
• Instruct geriatric patients to use spacer device
• Teach patient the proper use of the inhaler; review package insert with patient; to avoid getting aerosol in eyes: blurring may result; to wash inhaler in warm water daily and dry; to avoid smoking, smoke-filled rooms, persons with respiratory tract infections
• Teach patient if paradoxical bronchospasm occurs to stop product immediately and notify prescriber; to limit caffeine products such as chocolate, coffee, tea, and colas
• Instruct patient on administration of dose, not to use more than prescribed; serious side effects may occur; if dose is missed, take when remembered; space other doses on new time schedule; do not double doses
• Instruct patient to "prime" the inhaler before using for the first time by releasing 2 test sprays into the air, away from the face, rinse after use

Adverse effects: *italics* = common; **bold** = life-threatening

- Teach patient that each inhaler has 200 actuations or sprays
- Use spacer to improve drug use if required

Evaluation

Positive therapeutic outcome
- Absence of dyspnea, wheezing after 1 hr
- Improved airway exchange
- Improved ABGs

irbesartan (Rx)
(er-be-sar'tan)

Avapro

Func. class.: Antihypertensive
Chem. class.: Angiotensin II receptor
(type AT_1)

Pregnancy category C (1st trimester), D (2nd/3rd trimesters)

Do not confuse: Avapro/Anaprox

ACTION: Blocks the vasoconstrictor and aldosterone-secreting effects of angiotensin II; selectively blocks the binding of angiotensin II to the AT_1 receptor found in tissues

Therapeutic outcome: Decreased B/P

USES: Hypertension, alone or in combination, nephropathy in patients with type 2 diabetes mellitus; proteinuria

Unlabeled uses: Heart failure

CONTRAINDICATIONS
Hypersensitivity

> **BLACK BOX WARNING:** Pregnancy **D** (2nd/3rd trimesters)

Precautions: Pregnancy **C** (1st trimester), breastfeeding, children <6 yr, geriatric, renal/hepatic disease, renal artery stenosis, hypersensitivity to ACE inhibitors, African descent, angioedema

DOSAGE AND ROUTES
Hypertension
Adult: PO 150 mg/day; may be increased to 300 mg/day; volume-depleted patients: start with 75 mg/day

Nephropathy in patients with type 2 diabetes mellitus
Adult: PO maintenance dose 300 mg/day, start 75 mg/day

Available forms: Tabs 75, 150, 300 mg

Implementation
- Administer without regard to meals
- May be used with other antihypertensives, diuretic

ADVERSE EFFECTS
CNS: Dizziness, anxiety, *headache, fatigue,* syncope
CV: Hypotension
GI: *Diarrhea, dyspepsia,* hepatitis, cholestasis
HEMA: Thrombocytopenia
MISC: Edema, chest pain, rash, tachycardia, UTI, **angioedema,** hyperkalemia
RESP: *Cough, upper respiratory infection,* rhinitis, pharyngitis, sinus disorder

Pharmacokinetics

Absorption	Well absorbed
Distribution	Bound to plasma proteins (90%)
Metabolism	Liver (minimal) by CYP2C9
Excretion	Feces, urine
Half-life	11-15 hr

Pharmacodynamics

Unknown

INTERACTIONS
Drug classifications
CYP2C9 inhibitors (amiodarone, delavirdine, fluconazole, FLUoxetine, fluvastatin, fluvoxaMINE, imatinib, sulfonamides, sulfinpyrazone, voriconazole, zafirlukast): increased irbesartan level
Diuretics (potassium sparing), ACE inhibitors, potassium salt substitutes: increased hyperkalemia
NSAIDs: decreased antihypertensive effect

Drug/herb
Astragalus, cola tree: increased or decreased antihypertensive effect
Black cohosh, goldenseal, hawthorn, kelp: increased antihypertensive effect
Guarana, khat, licorice, yohimbe: decreased antihypertensive effect

NURSING CONSIDERATIONS
Assessment
- Hypotension: For severe hypotension, place in supine position and give IV infusion of NS; drug may be continued after B/P is restored
- Assess B/P, pulse q4hr; note rate, rhythm, quality
- Monitor electrolytes: potassium, sodium, chloride
- Obtain baselines for renal, liver function tests before therapy begins
- Monitor for edema in feet, legs daily
- Assess for skin turgor, dryness of mucous membranes for hydration status

Patient/family education
• Advise patient to comply with dosage schedule, even if feeling better
• Inform patient that product may cause dizziness, fainting, light-headedness
• Caution patient to rise slowly to sitting or standing position to minimize orthostatic hypotension

> **BLACK BOX WARNING:** Advise patient to notify prescriber if pregnancy is suspected; pregnancy (D) 2nd/3rd trimester, (C) 1st trimester

• Teach patient not to stop product abruptly
• Teach patient to take without regard to food

Evaluation
Positive therapeutic outcome
• Decreased B/P

⚠ HIGH ALERT

irinotecan (Rx)
(ear-een-oh-tee′kan)
Camptosar
Func. class.: Antineoplastic hormone
Chem. class.: Topoisomerase inhibitor
Pregnancy category D

ACTION: Cytotoxic by producing damage to single-strand DNA during DNA synthesis, binds to topoisomerase I

Therapeutic outcome: Prevention in growth of tumor

USES: Metastatic carcinoma of colon or rectum, or 1st-line treatment in combination with fluorouracil (5-FU) and leucovorin for metastatic carcinoma of colon or rectum

CONTRAINDICATIONS
Pregnancy **D**, hypersensitivity

Precautions: Breastfeeding, children, geriatric, irradiation, hepatic disease

> **BLACK BOX WARNING:** Myelosuppression, diarrhea

DOSAGE AND ROUTES
First-line treatment of colorectal cancer in combination with 5-fluorouracil: IV dosage (with bolus 5-FU/leucovorin)
Adult: IV 125 mg/m^2 over 90 min followed by leucovorin (20 mg/m^2 IV bolus) and then 5-FU (500 mg/m^2 IV bolus) on days 1, 8, 15, and 22; the next course begins on day 43 or when toxicity has recovered to NCI grade 1 or less

Intravenous dosage (with infusional 5-FU/leucovorin)
Adult: IV 180 mg/m^2 over 90 min followed by leucovorin (200 mg/m^2 IV over 2 hr) then 5-FU bolus and continuous infusion (400 mg/m^2 IV bolus, then 600 mg/m^2 IV infusion over 22 hr); give days 1, 15, and 29, while leucovorin and 5-FU are given on days 1, 2, 15, 16, 29, and 30; the next course begins on day 43 or when toxicity has recovered to NCI grade 1 or less

Available forms: Inj 20 mg/ml

Implementation
• Use cytotoxic handling precautions

IV route
• Premedicate with antiemetic, dexamethasone plus another antiemetic agent, such as a 5-HT$_3$ blocker, given at least 30 min before use
• Prior to beginning a course of therapy, the granulocyte count should be ≥1500, the platelet count ≥100,000 and treatment-related diarrhea should be fully resolved
Dilution
• Dilute appropriate dose in D$_5$W (preferred) or NS injection to a final concentration of 0.12-2.8 mg/ml
• Store up to 24 hr at room temperature and room lighting; because of possible microbial contamination during preparation, an admixture prepared with D$_5$W or NS should be used within 6 hr; solutions prepared with D$_5$W, refrigerated and protected from light, can be stored for up to 48 hr; avoid refrigeration if prepared with NS
Intravenous infusion
• Infuse intravenously over 90 min

ADVERSE EFFECTS
CNS: Fever, headache, chills, dizziness
CV: Vasodilatation, edema, **thromboembolism**
GI: Severe diarrhea, *nausea, vomiting,* anorexia, constipation, cramps, flatus, stomatitis, dyspepsia, **hepatotoxicity**
HEMA: Leukopenia, anemia, neutropenia
INTEG: Irritation at site, rash, sweating, alopecia
MISC: Asthenia, weight loss, back pain
RESP: Dyspnea, increased cough, rhinitis

Pharmacokinetics

Absorption	Complete
Distribution	Widely, 30%-68% bound to plasma proteins, increased risk of toxicity in those homozygous for UGT1A128
Metabolism	Unknown
Excretion	Urine/bile
Half-life	6-12 hr

Adverse effects: *italics* = common; **bold** = life-threatening

Pharmacodynamics

Unknown

INTERACTIONS
Individual products
CarBAMazepine, PHENobarbital, phenytoin: decreased irinotecan levels

Dexamethasone: increased lymphocytopenia, hyperglycemia

Fluorouracil: increased toxicity

Prochlorperazine: increased akathisia

Radiation: increased myelosuppression, diarrhea

Drug classifications
Anticoagulants, NSAIDs: increased bleeding risk

Antineoplastics: increased myelosuppression, diarrhea

CYP3A4 inhibitors (ketoconazole): increased irinotecan levels

CYP3A4 inducers (phenytoin, carBAMazepine, PENTobarbital): decreased irinotecan levels

Diuretics: increased dehydration

Drug/herb
St. John's wort: decreased product level; avoid concurrent use

Drug/lab test
Increased: ALK phos, AST, LFTs, bilirubin

Decreased: platelets, WBC, neutrophils, Hgb/Hct

NURSING CONSIDERATIONS
Assessment
• Assess for CNS symptoms: fever, headache, chills, dizziness

> **BLACK BOX WARNING:** Assess CBC, differential, platelet count weekly; use colony-stimulating factor if WBC is <2000/mm³, platelet count is <100,000/mm³, Hgb ≤9 g/dl, neutrophils ≤1000/mm³; notify prescriber of these results, product should be discontinued

• Assess buccal cavity for dryness, sores or ulceration, white patches, oral pain, bleeding, dysphagia

> **BLACK BOX WARNING:** Assess GI symptoms: frequency of stools; cramping; severe life-threatening diarrhea may occur with fluid and electrolyte imbalances; treat diarrhea within 24 hr of use with 0.25-1 mg atropine IV; treat diarrhea >24 hr of use with loperamide; diarrhea >24 hr (late diarrhea) can be fatal

• Assess early diarrhea and other cholinergic symptoms, treat with atropine; late diarrhea can be life threatening, must be treated promptly with loperamide

• Assess signs of dehydration: rapid respirations, poor skin turgor, decreased urine output; dry skin, restlessness, weakness

• Assess for bone marrow depression: bruising, bleeding, blood in stools, urine, sputum, emesis

Patient/family education
• Advise patient to avoid foods with citric acid or hot or rough texture if stomatitis is present; to drink adequate fluids

• Advise patient to report stomatitis; any bleeding, white spots, ulcerations in mouth; tell patient to examine mouth daily, report symptoms

• Advise patient to report signs of anemia: fatigue, headache, faintness, shortness of breath, irritability, infection, rash

• **Advise patient to use contraception during therapy; to report if pregnancy is planned or suspected, pregnancy (D)**

• Advise patient to avoid vaccinations while taking this product

• **Instruct patient to report diarrhea that occurs 24 hr after administration; severe dehydration can occur rapidly**

• Teach patient to avoid salicylates, NSAIDs, alcohol; bleeding may occur; to avoid all of these products unless approved by prescriber

Evaluation
Positive therapeutic outcome
• Decrease in tumor size, decrease in spread of cancer

iron, carbonyl
See ferrous fumarate

iron dextran (Rx)
DexFerrum, InFed

Func. class.: Hematinic

Chem. class.: Ferric hydroxide complex with dextran

Pregnancy category C

Do not confuse: Imferon/Imuran/Roferon-A/Interferon

ACTION: Iron is carried by transferrin to the bone marrow, where it is incorporated into hemoglobin

Therapeutic outcome: Prevention and resolution of iron-deficiency anemia

USES: Iron-deficiency anemia

CONTRAINDICATIONS

> **BLACK BOX WARNING:** Hypersensitivity

Precautions: Pregnancy **C,** breastfeeding, infants <4 mo, children, acute renal disease, asthma, rheumatoid arthritis (**IV**), all anemias excluding iron-deficiency anemia, hepatic/cardiac/renal disease, neonates, ankylosing spondylitis, lupus, hypotension

DOSAGE AND ROUTES

Adult and child: IM 0.5 ml as a test dose by Z-track, then no more than the following total dose including test dose per day:

Adult/adolescent/child (>15 kg):

Total iron dextran dose in ml =

$[0.0442 \times (\text{Desired Hb} - \text{observed Hb}) \times \text{LBW}]$
$+ (0.26 \times \text{LBW}),$

max of undiluted is 100 mg (2 ml)/day

Child (10-15 kg):

Total iron dextran dose in ml =

$[0.0442 \times (\text{Desired Hb} - \text{observed Hb}) \times \text{LBW}]$
$+ (0.26 \times \text{ABW}),$

max of undiluted iron dextran is 100 mg (2 ml)/day

Child/Infant >4 mo (5-9.9 kg):

Total iron dextran dose in ml =

$[0.0442 \times (\text{Desired Hb} - \text{observed Hb}) \times \text{LBW}]$
$+ (0.26 \times \text{ABW})$

Infants >4 mo (<5 kg):

Total iron dextran dose in ml =

$[0.0442 \times (\text{Desired Hb} - \text{observed Hb}) \times \text{LBW}]$
$+ (0.26 \times \text{ABW})$

Available forms: Inj IM/**IV** 50 mg/ml (2 ml, 10 ml vials)

Implementation
IM route
• Discontinue oral iron before parenteral; give only after test dose of 25 mg by preferred route; wait at least 1 hr before giving remaining portion
• Give IM inj deep in large muscle mass; use Z-track method and 19-G, 20-G 2-, 3-inch needle; ensure needle is long enough to place product deep in muscle; change needles after withdrawing medication and injecting to prevent skin and tissue staining

IV route
• Give **IV** after flushing tubing with 10 ml of 0.9% NaCl; give undiluted; give 1 ml (50 mg) or less over 1 min or more; flush line after use with 10 ml of 0.9% NaCl; patient should remain recumbent for 30-60 min to prevent orthostatic hypotension
• **IV** inj requires single-dose vial without preservative; verify on label **IV** use is approved
• Give by cont inf after diluting in 50-250 ml of 0.9% NaCl for inf; administer over 4-5 hr
• Give only with epinephrine available in case of anaphylactic reaction during dose

• Store at room temperature in cool environment

ADVERSE EFFECTS
CNS: Headache, paresthesia, dizziness, shivering, weakness, seizures
CV: Chest pain, shock, hypotension, tachycardia
GI: *Nausea,* vomiting, metallic taste, abdominal pain
HEMA: Leukocytosis
INTEG: Rash, pruritus, urticaria, fever, sweating, chills, brown skin discoloration, pain at inj site, necrosis, sterile abscesses, phlebitis
MISC: Anaphylaxis
RESP: Dyspnea

Pharmacokinetics

Absorption	Well absorbed; lymphatics over wk or mo
Distribution	Crosses placenta
Metabolism	Slow; blood loss, desquamation
Excretion	Breast milk, feces, urine, bile
Half-life	6 hr

Pharmacodynamics

Unknown

INTERACTIONS
Individual drugs
Chloramphenicol: decreased reticulocyte response
Oral iron: do not use together, increased toxicity

Drug/lab test
False increase: serum bilirubin
False decrease: serum calcium
False positive: ^{99m}Tc diphosphate bone scan, iron test (large doses >2 ml)

NURSING CONSIDERATIONS
Assessment
• Observe for 1 hr after test dose
• Monitor blood studies: Hct, Hgb, reticulocytes, transferrin, plasma iron concentrations, ferritin, total iron-binding bilirubin before treatment, at least monthly

> **BLACK BOX WARNING:** Assess for allergic reaction and anaphylaxis; rash, pruritus, fever, chills, wheezing; notify prescriber immediately, keep emergency equipment available

• Assess cardiac status: anginal pain, hypotension, tachycardia
• Assess for nutrition: amount of iron in diet (meat, dark green leafy vegetables, dried fruits, eggs); cause of iron loss or anemia, including salicylates, sulfonamides

Adverse effects: *italics* = common; **bold** = life-threatening

- Monitor pulse, B/P during **IV** administration
- Assess for toxicity: nausea, vomiting, diarrhea, fever, abdominal pain (early symptoms); cyanotic lips, nailbeds, seizures, CV collapse (late symptoms)

Patient/family education

- **Caution patient that iron poisoning may occur if increased beyond recommended level; to not take oral iron preparation or vitamins containing iron unless approved by prescriber**
- **Advise patient that delayed reaction may occur 1-2 days after administration and last 3-4 days (IV) or 3-7 days (IM); report fever, chills, malaise, muscle/joint aches, nausea, vomiting, backache**
- Advise patient to avoid breastfeeding
- Advise patient that stools may become dark

Evaluation

Positive therapeutic outcome
- Increased serum iron levels, Hct, Hgb

TREATMENT OF OVERDOSE:

Discontinue product, treat allergic reaction, give diphenhydrAMINE or EPINEPHrine as needed for anaphylaxis; give iron-chelating product in acute poisoning

iron polysaccharide
See ferrous fumarate

iron sucrose (Rx)
Velphro, Venofer
Func. class.: Hematinic
Chem. class.: Ferric hydroxide complex with dextran
Pregnancy category B

ACTION: Iron is carried by transferrin to the bone marrow, where it is incorporated into hemoglobin

Therapeutic outcome: Improved signs/symptoms of iron deficiency anemia; iron levels improved

USES: Iron deficiency anemia, hyperphosphatemia in chronic kidney disease on dialysis

Unlabeled uses: Dystrophic epidermolysis bullosa (DEB)

CONTRAINDICATIONS

Hypersensitivity, all anemias excluding iron deficiency anemia, iron overload

Precautions: Pregnancy **B**, breastfeeding (**IV**), children, geriatric, abdominal pain, anaphylactic shock, arthralgia, chest pain, cough, diarrhea, dizziness, dyspnea, edema, increased LFTs, fever, headache, heart failure, hyper/ hypotension, infection, MS pain, nausea/vomiting, seizures, weakness

DOSAGE AND ROUTES

Adult: **IV** 5 ml (100 mg of elemental iron) given during dialysis, most will need 1000 mg of elemental iron over 10 sequential dialysis sessions

Hyperphosphatemia in chronic kidney disease
Adult: PO 500 mg tid

Available forms: Inj 20 mg/ml; chew tab 500 mg

Implementation

⚠ Give only with epinephrine, Solu-MEDROL in case of anaphylactic reaction during dose
- Do not use if particulate is present, or if sol is discolored

IV route
- Give directly in dialysis line by slow inj or inf; give by slow inj at 1 ml/min (5 min/vial); inf dilute each vial exclusively in a maximum of 100 ml of 0.9% NaCl, give at rate of 100 mg of iron/15 min, discard unused portions
- Store at room temperature in cool environment, do not freeze
- Do not use with other IV products

ADVERSE EFFECTS

CNS: Headache, dizziness
CV: Chest pain, hypo/hypertension, hypervolemia, heart failure
GI: *Nausea, vomiting, abdominal pain*
INTEG: Rash, pruritus, urticaria, fever, sweating, chills
MISC: Anaphylaxis, hyperglycemia
RESP: Dyspnea, pneumonia, cough

Pharmacokinetics

Absorption	Unknown
Distribution	Unknown
Metabolism	Unknown
Excretion	Urine
Half-life	6 hr

Pharmacodynamics

Unknown

INTERACTIONS
Individual drugs
Chloramphenicol: decreased iron sucrose
Dimercaprol, iron (oral): increased toxicity; do not use together

Drug/lab test
Increased: glucose

NURSING CONSIDERATIONS
Assessment
• Monitor blood studies: Hct, Hgb, reticulocytes, transferrin, plasma iron concentrations, ferritin, total iron binding, bilirubin before treatment, at least monthly
• Assess for allergy: anaphylaxis, rash, pruritus, fever, chills, wheezing; notify prescriber immediately, keep emergency equipment available
• Assess cardiac status: hypotension, hypertension, hypervolemia
• Assess for toxicity: nausea, vomiting, diarrhea, fever, abdominal pain (early symptoms), cyanotic-looking lips and nailbeds, seizures, CV collapse (late symptoms)

Patient/family education
• Teach patient that iron poisoning may occur if increased beyond recommended level; not to take oral iron preparations
• Teach patient to report itching, rash, chest pain, headache, vertigo, nausea, vomiting, abdominal pain, joint/muscle pain, numbness, tingling

Evaluation
Positive therapeutic outcome
• Increased serum iron levels, Hct, Hgb

TREATMENT OF OVERDOSE:
Discontinue product, treat allergic reaction, give diphenhydrAMINE or epinephrine as needed, give iron-chelating product in acute poisoning

isoniazid (Rx)
(eye-soe-nye′a-zid)
Isotamine ✦
Func. class.: Antitubercular
Chem. class.: Isonicotinic acid hydrazide
Pregnancy category C

ACTION: Bactericidal interference with lipid, nucleic acid biosynthesis

Therapeutic outcome: Resolution of TB infection

USES: Treatment, prevention of TB

CONTRAINDICATIONS
Hypersensitivity

| BLACK BOX WARNING: Acute liver disease |

Precautions: Pregnancy **C**, diabetic retinopathy, cataracts, ocular defects, renal disease, **IV** drug users, people >35 yr, postpartum period, HIV, neuropathy

| BLACK BOX WARNING: Female (African descent, Hispanic), alcoholism |

DOSAGE AND ROUTES
Treatment
Adult/adolescent with or without HIV: PO/IM 5 mg/kg/day up to 300 mg/day or 15 mg/kg 2-3 times per week, max 900 mg 2-3 times per week
Child and infant HIV positive: PO/IM 10-15 mg/kg/day; max 300 mg/day

Available forms: Tabs 100, 300 mg; inj 100 mg/ml; oral sol 10 mg/ml

Implementation
• Give antiemetic for vomiting
• Provide a list of foods to avoid while taking this product
PO route
• Give with meals to decrease GI symptoms; absorption is better when taken on empty stomach, 1 hr before or 2 hr after meals
IM route
• Give inj deep in large muscle mass, massage; rotate inj sites, warm inj to room temperature to dissolve crystals

ADVERSE EFFECTS

Hypersensitivity: Fever, skin eruptions, lymphadenopathy, vasculitis
CNS: *Peripheral neuropathy, dizziness,* memory impairment, **toxic encephalopathy,** seizures, psychosis, slurred speech
EENT: Blurred vision, optic neuritis
GI: *Nausea, vomiting,* epigastric distress, **jaundice, fatal hepatitis**
HEMA: **Agranulocytosis, hemolytic anemia, aplastic anemia, thrombocytopenia, eosinophilia, methemoglobinemia**
MISC: Dyspnea, vit B$_6$ deficiency, pellagra, hyperglycemia, metabolic acidosis, gynecomastia, rheumatic syndrome, systemic lupus erythematosus–like syndrome

Pharmacokinetics

Absorption	Well absorbed
Distribution	Widely
Metabolism	Liver
Excretion	Kidneys
Half-life	1-4 hr

Pharmacodynamics

	PO	IM
Onset	Rapid	Rapid
Peak	1-2 hr	45-60 min
Duration	6-8 hr	6-8 hr

INTERACTIONS
Individual drugs
Alcohol, carBAMazepine, cycloSERINE, ethionamide, meperidine, phenytoin, rifampin, warfarin: increased toxicity

BCG vaccine, ketoconazole: decreased effectiveness

Drug classifications
Antacids, aluminum: decreased absorption

Benzodiazepines: increased toxicity

SSRIs, SNRIs: increased serotonin syndrome

Drug/food
Tyramine foods: increased toxicity

Drug/lab test
Increased: LFTs, bilirubin, glucose

Decreased: platelets, granulocytes

NURSING CONSIDERATIONS
Assessment
• Obtain C&S tests, including sputum tests, before treatment; monitor every mo to detect resistance

> **BLACK BOX WARNING:** Monitor liver function tests weekly; obtain baseline in all patients, those >35 yr and all women should be monitored periodically; monitor ALT, AST, bilirubin; increased results may indicate hepatitis; renal studies during treatment, monthly: BUN, creatinine, output, specific gravity, urinalysis, uric acid; those with fast acetylation (genetic) may metabolize product more than 5 times faster (Black, Asian, and some Caucasians are at greater risk); fatal hepatitis is a greater risk in Blacks/Hispanics after birth

• Assess mental status often: affect, mood, behavioral changes; psychosis may occur with hallucinations, confusion
• Assess hepatic status: decreased appetite, jaundice, dark urine, fatigue
• Assess for visual disturbance that may indicate optic neuritis: blurred vision, change in color perception; may lead to blindness

Patient/family education
• Instruct patient that compliance with dosage schedule for duration is necessary; not to skip or double doses; that scheduled appointments must be kept or relapse may occur

• Caution patient to avoid alcohol while taking product or hepatotoxicity may result; to avoid ingestion of aged cheeses, fish or hypertensive crisis may result; give patient written directions on which foods to avoid while taking this medication
• Tell patient to report peripheral neuritis: weakness, tingling/numbness of hands/feet, fatigue; hepatotoxicity: loss of appetite, nausea, vomiting, jaundice of skin or eyes

> **BLACK BOX WARNING: Fatal hepatitis:** teach patient to notify prescriber immediately of yellow skin/eyes, dark urine, loss of appetite

Evaluation
Positive therapeutic outcome
• Decreased symptoms of TB
• Culture negative for TB

TREATMENT OF OVERDOSE:
Pyridoxine

> ## isosorbide dinitrate (Rx)
> (eye-soe-sor'bide)
> **Apo-ISDN ✤, Dilatrate-SR, Isochron, IsoDitrate, Isordil**
> ## isosorbide mononitrate (Rx)
> **Apo-ISMN ✤, Imdur**
> *Func. class.:* Antianginal, vasodilator
> *Chem. class.:* Nitrate
> **Pregnancy category C**

Do not confuse: Imdur/Imuran/Inderal/K-Dur

ACTION: Relaxation of vascular smooth muscle, which leads to decreased preload, afterload, thus decreasing left ventricular end-diastolic pressure, and systemic vascular resistance and reducing cardiac O_2 demand

Therapeutic outcome: Relief and prevention of angina pectoris

USES: Treatment, prevention of chronic stable angina pectoris

CONTRAINDICATIONS
Hypersensitivity to this product or nitrates, severe anemia, closed-angle glaucoma

Precautions: Pregnancy **C**, breastfeeding, children, orthostatic hypotension, MI, CHF, severe renal/hepatic disease, increased ICP, cerebral hemorrhage, acute MI, geriatrics, GI disease, syncope

DOSAGE AND ROUTES
Dinitrate
Adult: PO 5-20 mg bid-tid, initially, maintenance 10-40 mg bid-tid; SL buccal tab 2.5-5 mg; may repeat q5-10min × 3 doses; ext rel 40-80 mg q8-12hr, max 160 mg/day

Mononitrate
Adult: PO (Monoket) 10-20 mg bid, 7 hr apart; (Imdur) initiate at 30-60 mg/day as a single dose, increase q3day as needed; may increase to 120 mg/day; max 240 mg/day

Available forms: Dinitrate: sus rel caps 40 mg; SR tabs 40 mg; tabs 5, 10, 20, 30, 40 mg; SL tabs 2.5, 5 mg; chew tabs 5, 10 mg; mononitrate: tabs (Monoket) 10, 20 mg; ext rel tabs (Imdur) 30, 60, 120 mg

Implementation
PO route
• Swallow sus rel cap and ext rel tab whole; do not break, crush, or chew
• Do not swallow SL tab; tab should be dissolved under tongue
• Chew tab should be chewed thoroughly
• Give 1 hr before or 2 hr after meals with 8 oz of water
SL route
• Hold SL tab under tongue until dissolved (a few min); do not take anything PO when SL tab is in place
• Sustained release cap/tab: allow dosing interval >18 hr

ADVERSE EFFECTS
CNS: *Vascular headache, flushing, dizziness,* weakness
CV: *Orthostatic hypotension,* tachycardia, **collapse,** syncope
GI: Nausea, vomiting
INTEG: Pallor, sweating, rash
MISC: Twitching, hemolytic anemia, **methemoglobinemia,** tolerance, xerostomia

Pharmacokinetics

Absorption	Well absorbed
Distribution	Unknown
Metabolism	Liver
Excretion	Urine, metabolites
Half-life	Dinitrate 1 hr, mononitrate 5 hr

Pharmacodynamics

	Sus rel	SL	PO
Onset	Up to 4 hr	2-5 min	15-30 min
Peak	Unknown	Unknown	Unknown
Duration	5 hr	2 hr	5-6 hr

INTERACTIONS
Individual drugs
Alcohol: increased hypotension
Rosiglitazone: increased myocardial ischemia; avoid concurrent use
⚠ Sildenafil, tadalafil, vardenafil: fatal hypotension, do not use together

Drug classifications
Antihypertensives, β-adrenergic blockers, calcium channel blockers, diuretics, phenothiazines: increased hypotension
Sympathomimetics: increased heart rate, B/P

NURSING CONSIDERATIONS
Assessment
• **Assess for pain:** duration, time started, activity being performed, character, intensity
⚠ Methemoglobinemia (rare): assess for cyanosis of lips, nausea/vomiting, coma, shock; usually caused by high dose of product, but may occur with normal dosing
• Monitor for orthostatic B/P, pulse at baseline, during treatment and periodically thereafter

Patient/family education
• Teach patient that tolerance may occur if taken over long periods; to prevent, allow intervals of 12-14 hr/day without product
• Advise patient to treat headache with OTC analgesics
• Instruct patient to not skip or double doses; if dose is missed take when remembered if 2 hr before next dose (dinitrate), 6 hr before next dose (sus rel), or 8 hr before next dose (mononitrate)
• Caution patient to avoid alcohol and OTC medications unless approved by prescriber
• Inform patient that product may be taken before stressful activity: exercise, sexual activity
• Advise patient that SL tab may sting mucous membranes
• Caution patient to avoid driving and hazardous activities if dizziness occurs
• Advise patient to comply with complete medical regimen
• Caution patient to make position changes slowly to prevent orthostatic hypotension
⚠ Teach patient not to use with sildenafil, tadalafil, vardenafil with nitrates; may cause serious drop in B/P
⚠ Teach patient not to discontinue abruptly; may cause heart attack
⚠ Teach patient to use at beginning of angina symptoms, may repeat every 15 min; if no relief seek medical attention immediately

Evaluation
Positive therapeutic outcome
• Decrease in, prevention of anginal pain

itraconazole (Rx)
(it-tra-kon'a-zol)
Onmel, Sporanox
Func. class.: Antifungal (systemic)
Chem. class.: Triazole derivative
Pregnancy category C

ACTION: Alters cell membranes and inhibits several fungal enzymes

Therapeutic outcome: Fungistatic against *Histoplasma capsulatum, Blastomyces dermatitis, Cryptococcus neoformans, Aspergillus fumigatus, Candida*

USES: Histoplasmosis, blastomycosis (pulmonary and extrapulmonary), aspergillosis onychomycosis of toenail/fingernail

Unlabeled uses: Dermatomycosis, chromoblastomycosis, coccidioidomycosis, pityriasis versicolor, sebopsoriasis, vaginal candidiasis, cryptococcal, subcutaneous mycoses, dimorphic infections, fungal keratitis, alternariosis, zygomycosis

CONTRAINDICATIONS
Hypersensitivity, fungal meningitis, onychomycosis, or dermatomycosis in cardiac dysfunction; in pregnant women (pregnancy **C**)

> BLACK BOX WARNING: Heart failure, ventricular dysfunction, coadministration with other drugs

Precautions: Pregnancy **C**, breastfeeding, children, cardiac/renal/hepatic disease, achlorhydria or hypochlorhydria (product-induced), dialysis, hearing loss, cystic fibrosis neuropathy

DOSAGE AND ROUTES
Dose varies with type of infection
Adult: PO 200 mg/day with food; may increase to 400 mg/day if needed; life-threatening infections may require a loading dose of 200 mg tid × 3 days

Available forms: Caps 100 mg; oral sol 10 mg/ml; tab 200 mg

Implementation
PO route
• Swallow caps whole; do not break, crush, or chew
• Give caps after full meal to ensure absorption
• Give with food or milk to prevent nausea and vomiting

• Take 2 hr before administration of other products that increase gastric pH
• Store in tight container at room temperature; do not freeze
• *Oral sol and caps are not interchangeable on a mg/mg basis*
• **Oral sol:** patient should swish in mouth vigorously

ADVERSE EFFECTS
CNS: Headache, dizziness, insomnia, somnolence, depression
CV: Hypertension, CHF
GI: Nausea, vomiting, anorexia, diarrhea, cramps, *abdominal pain,* flatulence, GI bleeding, hepatotoxicity
GU: Gynecomastia, impotence, decreased libido
INTEG: Pruritus, fever, rash, toxic epidermal necrolysis, Stevens-Johnson syndrome
MISC: Edema, fatigue, malaise, hypokalemia, tinnitus, rhabdomyolysis
RESP: Rhinitis, sinusitis, upper respiratory infection, pulmonary edema

Pharmacokinetics
Absorption	Variable
Distribution	Tissue, plasma, CSF, 99.8% protein bound
Metabolism	Liver, extensively, inhibits CYP4503A enzyme
Excretion	Feces, breast milk
Half-life	IV 35.4 hr; terminal 29.4 hr; PO 64 hr; pediatric 35.8 hr

Pharmacodynamics
Onset	Unknown
Peak	4 hr
Duration	Unknown

INTERACTIONS
Individual drugs
BusPIRone: increased busPIRone levels, toxicity
Busulfan, clarithromycin, cycloSPORINE, atorvastatin, carBAMazepine, disopyramide, QUEtiapine, diazepam, digoxin, felodipine, fentaNYL, indinavir, isradipine, niCARdipine, NIFEdipine, nimoldipine, phenytoin, ritonavir, saquinavir, tacrolimus, warfarin: increased toxicity
CarBAMazepine, isoniazid: decreased itraconazole action
Didanosine: decreased antifungal action
Dofetilide, dronedarone, levomethadyl, pimozide, quiNIDine: life-threatening CV reaction

---

ALPRAZolam, clorazepate, clorazepine, diazepam, estazolam, flurazepam, midazolam (oral), triazolam: increased sedation
QuiNIDine: increased tinnitus, hearing loss, increased toxicity
Rifamycins: decreased action of itraconazole

Drug classifications
Antacids, H₂-receptor antagonists: decreased action of itraconazole
Calcium channel blockers: increased edema
Contraceptives (oral): decreased effect
Proton pump inhibitors: decreased itraconazole action
Hepatotoxic products: hepatotoxicity
Oral hypoglycemics: increased effects of oral hypoglycemics

Drug/food
Increased: absorption

Drug/lab test
Increased: LFTs, alk phos, bilirubin, triglyceride, GGT

NURSING CONSIDERATIONS
Assessment
• Assess for infection: WBC, sputum baseline, periodically, may start treatment before obtaining results
⚠ Monitor for hepatotoxicity: increasing AST, ALT, alkaline phosphatase, bilirubin
• Monitor for allergic reaction: dermatitis, rash; product should be discontinued, antihistamines (mild reaction) or epinephrine (severe reaction) administered; check inj site for thrombophlebitis
• Monitor for hypokalemia, check potassium level: anorexia, drowsiness, weakness, decreased reflexes, dizziness, increased urinary output, increased thirst, paresthesias; if these occur, product should be decreased or discontinued and potassium administered

Patient/family education
• Advise patient that long-term therapy may be needed to clear infection (1 wk-6 mo depending on type of infection)
• Teach patient side effects and when to notify prescriber
• Instruct patient to avoid hazardous activities if dizziness occurs
• Instruct patient to take 2 hr before administration of other products that increase gastric pH (antacids, H₂-blockers, omeprazole, sucralfate, anticholinergics)
• Teach patient importance of compliance with product regimen
• **Instruct patient to notify prescriber of GI symptoms, signs of liver dysfunction**

(fatigue, jaundice, nausea, anorexia, vomiting, dark urine, pale stools)

Evaluation
Positive therapeutic outcome
• Decreased fever, malaise, rash
• Negative C&S for infectious organism

RARELY USED

ivacaftor
(eye′va-kaf′tor)
Kalydeco
Func. class.: Respiratory agent
Pregnancy category B

USES: Cystic fibrosis in those with G551D, G1244E, G1349D, G178R, G551S, S1255P, S549N, S549R mutation in the *CFTR* gene

DOSAGE AND ROUTES
Renal dose
Adult/adolescent/child ≥6 yr: PO 150 mg every 12 hr with fat-containing food
Child 2-5 yr ≥ 14 kg: PO 75 mg q12hr with fat-containing food
Child 2-5 yr <14 kg: PO 50 mg q12hr with fat-containing food

⚠ HIGH ALERT

ixabepilone (Rx)
(ix-ab-ep′i-lone)
Ixempra
Func. class.: Antineoplastic— miscellaneous
Chem. class.: Epothilone
Pregnancy category D

ACTION: Microtubule stabilizing agent; micotubules are needed for cell division

Therapeutic outcome: Decreased tumor size, decreased spread of malignancy

USES: Breast cancer

CONTRAINDICATIONS
Pregnancy **D**, hypersensitivity to products with polyoxyethylated castor oil, breastfeeding, neutropenia <1500/mm³, thrombocytopenia <100,000/mm³

BLACK BOX WARNING: Hepatic disease

Precautions: Children, geriatric, alcoholism, bone marrow suppression, cardiac dysrhythmias, cardiac/renal disease, diabetes mellitus, peripheral neuropathy, ventricular dysfunction

---

DOSAGE AND ROUTES
Breast cancer, metastatic or locally advanced given with capecitabine, and resistant to anthracycline, taxane
Adult: IV INF 40 mg/m² over 3 hr q3wk plus capecitabine PO 2000 mg/m²/day in 2 divided doses on days 1-14 q21day; in those with BSA >2.2 m², dose should be calculated for a BSA of 2.2 m²

Breast cancer, metastatic or locally advanced resistant/refractory to anthracyclines, taxanes, capecitabine
Adult: IV INF 40 mg/m² over 3 hr q3wk; in those with BSA >2.2 m², dose should be calculated for a BSA of 2.2 m²

Dosage reduction in those taking a strong CYP3A4 inhibitor
Adult: IV INF 20 mg/m² over 3 hr q3wk

Available forms: Powder for inj 15, 45 mg

Implementation
• Premedicate with histamine antagonists 1 hr prior to use, prevents hypersensitivity
• Give antiemetic 30-60 min before giving product and prn

IV route
• Let kit stand at room temperature for 30 min; to reconstitute, withdraw supplied diluent (8 ml for 15 mg vials, 23.5 ml for 45 mg vials); slowly inject solution into vial; gently swirl and invert to mix, final conc 2 mg/ml; further dilute in LR in DEHP-free bags; final conc should be 0.2-0.6 mg/ml; after added, mix by manual rotation
• Diluted sol is stable for 6 hr at room temperature; inf must be completed within 6 hr
• Use in-line filter 0.2-1.2 mcm
• Give over 3 hr

ADVERSE EFFECTS
CNS: *Peripheral neuropathy,* chills, fatigue, fever, flushing, headache, insomnia, impaired cognition, asthenia
CV: Bradycardia, *hypotension,* abnormal ECG, angina, atrial flutter, cardiomyopathy, chest pain, edema, MI, vasculitis
GI: *Nausea, vomiting, diarrhea,* abdominal pain, anorexia, colitis, constipation, gastritis, jaundice, GERD, hepatic failure, trismus
GU: Renal failure
HEMA: Neutropenia, thrombocytopenia, anemia, infections, coagulopathy
INTEG: *Alopecia,* rash, hot flashes
META: Hypokalemia, metabolic acidosis
MS: *Arthralgia, myalgia*
RESP: Bronchospasm, cough, dyspnea

SYST: *Hypersensitivity reactions,* anaphylaxis, dehydration, radiation recall reaction

Pharmacokinetics
Absorption	Unknown
Distribution	Unknown
Metabolism	Liver by CYP3A4
Excretion	Feces 65%, urine 21%
Half-life	Terminal 52 hr

Pharmacodynamics
Unknown

INTERACTIONS
Drug classifications
CYP3A4 inducers (aminoglutethimide, barbiturates, bexarotene, bosentan, carBAMazepine, dexamethasone, efavirenz, griseofulvin, modafinil, nafcillin, nevirapine, OXcarbazepine, phenytoin, rifamycin, topiramate): decreased ixabepilone levels
CYP3A4 inhibitors (amiodarone, amprenavir, aprepitant, atazanavir, chloramphenicol, clarithromycin, conivaptan, cycloSPORINE, danazol, darunavir, dalforpristan, delavirdine, diltiazem, erythromycin, estradiol, fluconazole, fluvoxaMINE, fosamprenavir, imatinib, indinavir, isoniazid, itraconazole, ketoconazole, lopinavir, miconazole, nefazodone, nelfinavir, propoxyphene, ritonavir, RU-486, saquinavir, tamoxifen, telithromycin, troleandomycin, verapamil, voriconazole, zafirlukast): increased ixabepilone level

Drug/herb
St. John's wort: avoid use

Drug/food
Grapefruit products: avoid use

Drug/lab test
Increased: LFTs, bilirubin
Decreased: platelets, neutrophils, RBC, potassium

NURSING CONSIDERATIONS
Assessment
• Monitor CBC, differential, platelet count prior to therapy, qwk; withhold product if WBC is <1500/mm³ or platelet count is <100,000/mm³, notify prescriber
• Monitor temp q4hr (may indicate beginning infection)

> **BLACK BOX WARNING:** Monitor liver function tests before, during therapy (bilirubin, AST, ALT, LDH) prn or qmo; check for jaundiced skin and sclera, dark urine, clay-colored stools, itchy skin, abdominal pain, fever, diarrhea

• Monitor VS during 1st hr of inf; check IV site for signs of infiltration

• **Cardiac ischemia:** Monitor cardiac function in those with cardiac function that is impaired; chest pain, ECG changes may occur

⚠ **Assess for hypersensitive reactions, anaphylaxis including hypotension, dyspnea, angioedema, generalized urticaria; discontinue inf immediately; keep emergency equipment available**

• Assess effects of alopecia on body image; discuss feelings about body changes

Patient/family education

• Teach patient to report signs of infection: fever, sore throat, flulike symptoms

• Teach patient to report signs of anemia: fatigue, headache, faintness, shortness of breath

• Teach patient to report any complaints or side effects to nurse or prescriber

• Caution patient that hair may be lost during treatment; a wig or hairpiece may make patient feel better; new hair may be different in color, texture

• Advise patient that pain in muscles and joints 2-5 days after inf is common

• **Advise patient to use nonhormonal type of contraception**

• Instruct patient to avoid receiving vaccinations while on this product

Evaluation

Positive therapeutic outcome

• Decreased tumor size, decreased spread of malignancy

ketoconazole (Rx)

(kee-toe-koe′na-zole)
Func. class.: Antifungal
Chem. class.: Imidazole derivative
Pregnancy category C

Therapeutic outcome: Fungistatic/fungicidal against susceptible organisms: *Blastomycoses, Candida, Coccidioides, Cryptococcus, Histoplasma;* topical route: tinea cruris, tinea corporis, tinea versicolor, *Pityrosporum ovale*

USES: Systemic candidiasis, chronic mucocandidiasis, oral thrush, candiduria, coccidioidomycosis, histoplasmosis, chromomycosis, paracoccidioidomycosis, blastomycosis, tinea cruris, tinea corporis, tinea versicolor, *Pityrosporum ovale*

CONTRAINDICATIONS

Breastfeeding, hypersensitivity, fungal meningitis

> **BLACK BOX WARNING:** Coadministration with other drugs; ergot derivatives, cisapride, or triazolam may cause fatal cardiac arrhythmias due to inhibition of CYP3A4 enzyme system

> **BLACK BOX WARNING:** Hepatic disease

DOSAGE AND ROUTES

Adult: PO 200-400 mg once/day for 1-2 wk (candidiasis), 6 wk (other infections); 400 mg tid (prostate cancer, unlabeled)
Child >2 yr: PO 3.3-6.6 mg/kg/day as single daily dose

ketoconazole topical

See Appendix B

ketoprofen (OTC, Rx)

(ke-to-proe′fen)
Apo-Keto ✿
Func. class.: NSAID; nonopioid analgesic, antirheumatic
Chem. class.: Propionic acid derivative
**Pregnancy category C (1st trimester),
D (2nd/3rd trimesters)**

ACTION: Inhibits COX-1, COX-2; analgesic, antiinflammatory, antipyretic

Therapeutic outcome: Decreased pain, inflammation

USES: Mild to moderate pain; osteoarthritis; rheumatoid arthritis; dysmenorrhea; OTC relief of minor aches, pains

CONTRAINDICATIONS

Pregnancy **D**, 2nd/3rd trimesters; hypersensitivity to this product, NSAIDs, salicylates

> **BLACK BOX WARNING:** Perioperative pain in CABG

Precautions: Pregnancy (**C**) (1st trimester), breastfeeding, children, geriatric, bleeding/GI/cardiac disorders, hypersensitivity to other antiinflammatory agents, asthma, severe renal/hepatic disease, ulcer disease

> **BLACK BOX WARNING:** GI bleeding, MI, stroke

DOSAGE AND ROUTES
Antiinflammatory
Adult: PO 50 mg qid or 75 mg tid, max 300 mg/day or ext rel 200 mg/day

Analgesic
Adult: PO 25-50 mg q6-8hr, max 300 mg/day

Available forms: Caps 50, 75 mg; ext rel caps 200 mg

Implementation
• Store at room temperature
• Give with antacids, milk, or food for GI upset
• Swallow whole; do not break, crush, chew, or open ext rel cap
• Give with 8 oz of water and sit upright for 30 min after dose to prevent ulceration
• Give with food or milk to decrease gastric symptoms; give 30 min before or 2 hr after meals; absorption may be slowed

ADVERSE EFFECTS

CNS: Dizziness, drowsiness, fatigue, confusion, insomnia, depression, headache
CV: Tachycardia, peripheral edema, palpitations, dysrhythmias, hypertension, **CV thrombotic events, MI, stroke**
EENT: Tinnitus, hearing loss, blurred vision
GI: *Nausea, anorexia, vomiting, diarrhea,* jaundice, **hepatitis,** constipation, flatulence, cramps, dry mouth, peptic ulcer, **GI bleeding**
GU: Nephrotoxicity: **dysuria, hematuria, oliguria, azotemia**
HEMA: **Blood dyscrasias**
INTEG: Purpura, rash, pruritus, sweating
SYST: Anaphylaxis

Pharmacokinetics

Absorption	Well absorbed
Distribution	Not known
Metabolism	Liver
Excretion	Kidneys
Half-life	2-4 hr; 5.4 hr (ext rel)

Pharmacodynamics

Onset	Unknown
Peak	1.2 hr; 6.8 hr (ext rel)
Duration	Unknown

INTERACTIONS
Individual drugs
Alcohol, cidofovir: increased adverse GI reactions, toxicity

Aspirin: increased ketoprofen levels, increased adverse GI reactions

Clopidogrel, eptifibatide, ticlopidine, tirofiban: increased risk of bleeding

CycloSPORINE, lithium, methotrexate, phenytoin: increased ketoprofen levels, increased toxicity

Insulin: increased hypoglycemia

Probenecid: increased ketoconazole levels

Drug classifications
Anticoagulants, thrombolytics: increased risk of bleeding

Antihypertensives: decreased effect of antihypertensives

Antineoplastics: increased hematologic toxicity

Corticosteroids: increased adverse GI reactions

Diuretics: decreased effectiveness of diuretics

NSAIDs: increased adverse GI reactions

Sulfonylureas: increased hypoglycemia

Drug/herb
Feverfew, garlic, ginger, ginkgo, ginseng *(Panax):* increased risk of bleeding

Drug/lab test
Increased: bleeding time, BUN, alkaline phosphatase, AST, ALT, creatinine, LDH

NURSING CONSIDERATIONS
Assessment
• **Assess for pain:** type, location, intensity; ROM before and 1-2 hr after treatment

• Monitor renal, liver function tests: AST, ALT, bilirubin, creatinine, BUN, urine creatinine, CBC Hct, Hgb, pro-time if patient is on long-term therapy

• Check I&O ratio; decreasing output may indicate renal failure (long-term therapy)

• **Assess hepatotoxicity:** dark urine, clay-colored stools, jaundice of skin and sclera, itching, abdominal pain, fever, diarrhea if patient is on long-term therapy

• Assess for allergic reactions: rash, urticaria; if these occur, product may have to be discontinued

• Assess for ototoxicity: tinnitus, ringing, roaring in ears; audiometric testing needed before, after long-term therapy

• Assess for vision changes: blurring, halos; may indicate corneal, retinal damage

• Check edema in feet, ankles, legs

• Identify prior product history; there are many product interactions

> **BLACK BOX WARNING:** Assess for CV thrombotic events: MI, stroke

> **BLACK BOX WARNING:** For GI bleeding: blood in sputum, emesis, stools

Patient/family education
• Teach patient to report any symptoms of hepatotoxicity, renal toxicity, vision changes, ototoxicity, allergic reactions, bleeding (long-term therapy)

• Advise patient to take with 8 oz of water and sit upright for 30 min after dose to prevent ulceration, not to crush or chew ext rel products

• Caution patient not to exceed recommended dosage, acute poisoning may result; to take as prescribed; do not double dose

• Advise patient to read label on other OTC products; many contain other antiinflammatories

• Advise patient to use sunscreen, protective clothing to prevent photosensitivity

• Inform patient that the therapeutic response takes 2 wk (arthritis)

• Teach patient to report tinnitus, confusion, diarrhea, sweating, hyperventilation, blurred vision, fever, joint aches

• Caution patient to avoid alcohol ingestion; GI bleeding may occur

• Teach patient to report use to all providers

• Teach patient to report planned or suspected pregnancy, D (2nd/3rd trimester)/C (1st trimester); avoid breastfeeding

Evaluation
Positive therapeutic outcome
• Decreased pain
• Decreased inflammation
• Increased mobility
• Decreased fever

K

ketorolac (systemic, nasal) (Rx)

(kee'toe-role-ak)

Acular, Sprix, Toradol ✦

Func. class.: Nonsteroidal antiinflammatory (NSAID), nonopioid analgesic

Chem. class.: Acetic acid

Pregnancy category C; D (third trimester)

ACTION: Inhibits prostaglandin synthesis by decreasing an enzyme needed for biosynthesis; analgesic, antiinflammatory, antipyretic effects

Therapeutic outcome: Decreased pain, inflammation, ocular itching

USES: Mild to moderate pain (short term); decreased ocular itching in seasonal allergic conjunctivitis (ophthalmic)

CONTRAINDICATIONS

Pregnancy **D** (3rd trimester), hypersensitivity, asthma, hepatic disease, peptic ulcer disease, CV bleeding

> **BLACK BOX WARNING:** Breastfeeding, severe renal disease, labor and delivery, perioperative pain in CABG, prior to major surgery, epidural/intrathecal administration, GI bleeding, hypovolemia

Precautions: Pregnancy **C**, GI/cardiac disorders, hypersensitivity to other antiinflammatory agents, CCr <25 ml/min

> **BLACK BOX WARNING:** Children, geriatric, bleeding, MI, stroke

DOSAGE AND ROUTES

Adult/adolescent >17 yr and ≥50 kg: PO continuation from **IM/IV** only 20 mg, then 10 mg q4-6hr prn, max 40 mg/day; nasal 1 spray (15.75 mg/spray) in each nostril (31.5 mg/spray) q6-8hr, max 4 doses/day × 5 days

Adult/adolescent >17 yr and <50 kg: IM (single dose) 30-60 mg, **IV** 15-30 mg; **IM/IV** (multiple dosing) 15-30 mg q6hr, max 60 mg/day × 5 day combined either **PO/IM/IV;** nasal 1 spray (15.75 mg/spray) in one nostril q6-8hr, max 4 doses/day × 5 days

Renal dose
Do not use in advanced renal disease

Ophthalmic route

Adult: 1 gtt (0.25 mg) qid × 7 days
Child: IV 1 mg/kg, then 0.5 mg/kg q6hr

Available forms: Inj 15, 30 mg/ml (prefilled syringes); ophth 0.5% sol; tabs 10 mg; nasal spray 15.75 mg/spray

Implementation

PO route

• Administer to patient crushed or whole
• Max 5 days
• Give with full glass of water; give with food or milk to decrease gastric symptoms; give 30 min before or 2 hr after meals; absorption may be slowed

Nasal route

• Prime pump before using for the first time, point away from person/pets, pump activator 5 times, no need to re-prime
• For single use only, discard 24 hr after opening if not used
• Do not share with others
• Have patient blow nose, sit upright to spray

IM/IV route

• IV give undiluted ≥15 sec
• Give IM inj deeply into large muscle mass
• Store at room temperature, protect from light

Y-site compatibilities: Cisatracurium, remifentanil, SUFentanil

Syringe incompatibilities: Morphine, meperidine, promethazine, hydrOXYzine

Solution compatibilities: D₅W, 0.9% NaCl, LR, D₅, plasmalate

ADVERSE EFFECTS

CNS: Dizziness, *drowsiness*, tremors, **seizures**

CV: Hypertension, flushing, syncope, pallor, edema, vasodilatation, **CV thrombotic events, MI, stroke**

EENT: Tinnitus, hearing loss, blurred vision, transient burning/stinging

GI: Nausea, anorexia, vomiting, diarrhea, constipation, flatulence, cramps, dry mouth, peptic ulcer, **GI bleeding, perforation,** taste change, **hepatitis, hepatic failure**

GU: Nephrotoxicity: dysuria, hematuria, oliguria, azotemia

HEMA: Blood dyscrasias, prolonged bleeding

INTEG: Purpura, rash, pruritus, sweating, **angioedema, Stevens-Johnson syndrome, toxic epidermal necrolysis**

Pharmacokinetics

Absorption	Rapidly, completely absorbed
Distribution	Bound to plasma proteins (99%)
Metabolism	Liver (<50%)
Excretion	Kidney, metabolites (92%); breast milk (6%); feces
Half-life	6 hr (IM); increased in renal disease

Pharmacodynamics

	IM	Ophth/PO
Onset	Up to 10 min	Unknown
Peak	50 min IM; 2-3 hr PO; 0.5-2 hr nasal	Unknown; 6-8 hr nasal
Duration	4-6 hr PO	Unknown

INTERACTIONS
Individual drugs
Alcohol, aspirin: increased GI effects

Aspirin: increased ketorolac levels, contraindicated

Cefamandole, cefoperazone, cefoTEtan, clopidogrel, eptifibatide, plicamycin, ticlopidine, tirofiban, valproic acid: increased risk of bleeding

CycloSPORINE, lithium, methotrexate, pentoxifylline, probenecid: increased toxicity

Drug classifications
ACE inhibitors: increased renal impairment

Anticoagulants: increased effects

Antihypertensives: decreased antihypertensive effect

Salicylates, SNRIs, SSRIs, thrombolytics: increased risk of bleeding

Corticosteroids, NSAIDs, potassium products, steroids: increased GI effects

Diuretics: decreased diuretic effect

NSAIDs (other): increased ketorolac levels; contraindicated

Drug/lab test
Increased: AST, ALT, LDH, bleeding time

NURSING CONSIDERATIONS
Assessment

> **BLACK BOX WARNING:** Monitor renal, hepatic, blood studies: BUN, creatinine, AST, ALT, Hgb before treatment, periodically thereafter, check for dehydration

• **Monitor for aspirin sensitivity,** asthma; these patients may be more likely to develop hypersensitivity to NSAIDs

• Assess patient's eyes: redness, swelling, tearing, itching

• **Monitor for pain:** type, location, intensity, ROM before and 1 hr after treatment

> **BLACK BOX WARNING:** Assess for GI bleeding: blood in sputum, emesis, stools

> **BLACK BOX WARNING:** Do not use epidurally, intrathecally; alcohol is present in the solution

> **BLACK BOX WARNING:** Assess for CV thrombotic events: MI, stroke; do not use for perioperative pain in CABG

Patient/family education
• Teach patient that product must be continued for prescribed time to be effective; to avoid aspirin, alcoholic beverages, other NSAIDs, acetaminophen

• Caution patient to report bleeding, bruising, fatigue, malaise, since blood dyscrasias do occur

• Instruct patient to use caution when driving; drowsiness, dizziness may occur

• Instruct patient to take with a full glass of water to enhance absorption

• Caution patient that this product may cause eye redness, burning if soft contact lenses are worn

• Advise to report use to all health care providers, not to use with other products unless approved by prescriber; use for ≤5 days

• Instruct patient to report change in urine pattern, weight increase, pain in joints, fever, blood in urine (indicates nephrotoxicity); bruising, black tarry stools (indicates bleeding)

• Caution patient not to breastfeed

• Instruct patient to report if pregnancy is planned or suspected, pregnancy (C) systemic

• **Nasal:** Instruct patient to discard within 24 hr of opening; may cause irritation; may drink water after dose

> **BLACK BOX WARNING:** Instruct patient to report change in urine pattern, weight increase, edema, increased joint pain, fever, blood in urine (indicates nephrotoxicity); bruising, black tarry stools (indicates bleeding); pruritus, jaundice, nausea, right upper quadrant pain, abdominal pain (hepatotoxicity); to notify prescriber immediately

Evaluation
Positive therapeutic outcome
- Decreased pain
- Decreased inflammatory response
- Increased mobility
- Decreased ocular itching

ketorolac ophthalmic
See Appendix B

ketotifen ophthalmic
See Appendix B

⚠ HIGH ALERT

labetalol (Rx)
(la-bet'a-lole)

Trandate

Func. class.: Antihypertensive, antianginal
Chem. class.: α- and β-blocker
Pregnancy category C

Do not confuse: Trandate/Tridate

ACTION: Produces decreases in B/P without reflex tachycardia or significant reduction in heart rate through mixture of α-blocking, β-blocking effects; elevated plasma resins are reduced

Therapeutic outcome: Decreased B/P

USES: Mild to moderate hypertension; treatment of severe hypertension (**IV**)

Unlabeled uses: Hypertension in patients with pheochromocytoma, hypertension in clonidine withdrawal

CONTRAINDICATIONS

Hypersensitivity to β-blockers, cardiogenic shock, heart block (2nd or 3rd degree), sinus bradycardia, CHF, bronchial asthma

Precautions: Pregnancy **C**, breastfeeding, geriatric, major surgery, diabetes mellitus, thyroid/renal/hepatic disease, COPD, well-compensated heart failure, CAD, nonallergic bronchospasm, peripheral vascular disease

> **BLACK BOX WARNING:** Abrupt discontinuation

DOSAGE AND ROUTES
Hypertension
Adult: PO 100 mg bid; may be given with a diuretic; may increase to 200 mg bid after 2 days; may continue to increase q1-3days; max 2400 mg/day in divided doses

Hypertensive crisis
Adult: **IV** intermittent 20 mg over 2 min, may repeat 20-80 mg over 2 min q10min, 200 mg

Available forms: Tabs 100, 200, 300 mg; inj 5 mg/ml in 20, 40 ml vials

Implementation
• Store in dry area at room temp; do not freeze
PO route
• Give before meals, at bedtime; tab may be crushed or swallowed whole; give with food to prevent GI upset, increase absorption
• **Do not discontinue prior to surgery**
• Store protected from light, moisture; place in cool environment

Direct IV route
• Give undiluted (5 mg/ml) over 2 min
Continuous IV infusion route
• Give after diluting in LR, D₅W, D₅ in 0.2%, 0.9%, 0.33% NaCl or Ringer's; infusion is titrated to patient's response; 200 mg of product/160 ml sol (1 mg/ml); 300 mg of product/240 ml sol (1 mg/ml); 200 mg of product/250 ml sol (2 mg/3 ml); use inf pump
• Keep patient recumbent during and for 3 hr after inf, monitor VS q5-15min

Y-site compatibilities: Amikacin, aminophylline, amiodarone, ampicillin, butorphanol, calcium gluconate, cefTAZidime, ceftizoxime, cimetidine, diltiazem, DOBUTamine, DOPamine, enalaprilat, EPINEPHrine, erythromycin, esmolol, famotidine, fentaNYL, gentamicin, HYDROmorphone, lidocaine, LORazepam, magnesium sulfate, meperidine, metroNIDAZOLE, midazolam, milrinone, morphine, niCARdipine, nitroglycerin, nitroprusside, norepinephrine, oxacillin, potassium chloride, potassium phosphate, propofol, ranitidine, sodium acetate, tobramycin, vancomycin, vecuronium

Y-site incompatibilities: Cefoperazone, nafcillin

ADVERSE EFFECTS
CNS: *Dizziness,* mental changes, drowsiness, *fatigue,* headache, catatonia, depression, anxiety, nightmares, paresthesias, lethargy
CV: *Orthostatic hypotension,* **bradycardia,** **CHF,** chest pain, **ventricular dysrhythmias,** AV block, scalp tingling
EENT: *Tinnitus,* vision changes, sore throat, double vision, dry burning eyes, floppy iris syndrome, nasal congestion
ENDO: Hyperkalemia
GI: *Nausea, vomiting, diarrhea,* dyspepsia, taste distortion, **hepatotoxicity**
GU: Impotence, dysuria, ejaculatory failure
HEMA: **Agranulocytosis, thrombocytopenia, purpura** (rare)
INTEG: Rash, alopecia, urticaria, pruritus, fever, **exfoliative dermatitis**
RESP: **Bronchospasm,** dyspnea, wheezing

Pharmacokinetics

Absorption	Bioavailability 25% (PO); complete (**IV**)
Distribution	Crosses placenta, CNS
Metabolism	Liver, extensively
Excretion	Breast milk, kidneys, bile
Half-life	6-8 hr

Pharmacodynamics

	PO	IV
Onset	30 min	2-5 min
Peak	1 hr	5-15 min
Duration	24 hr	2-4 hr

INTERACTIONS
Individual drugs
Alcohol (large amounts), cimetidine, nitroglycerin: increased hypotension

Lidocaine: decreased effect

Verapamil: increased myocardial depression

Drug classifications
Antidepressants, tricyclics: increased tremor

Antidiabetics: increased or decreased effect

Antihypertensives: increased hypotension

β-Blockers, bronchodilators, sympathomimetics, xanthines: decreased effects

Diuretics: increased hypotension

General anesthetics, hydantoins, class IC antidysrhythmics: increased myocardial depression

MAOIs: do not use within 2 wk

NSAIDs, salicylates: decreased antihypertensive effect

Theophyllines: decreased bronchodilatation

Drug/herb
Hawthorn: increased antihypertensive effect

Ephedra: decreased antihypertensive effect

Drug/lab test
Increased: ANA titer, blood glucose, alkaline phosphatase, LDH, AST, ALT, BUN, potassium, triglycerides, uric acid, serum lipoprotein

False increase: urinary catecholamines

NURSING CONSIDERATIONS
Assessment
• **Hypertension:** monitor B/P at beginning of treatment, periodically thereafter; pulse q4hr; note rate, rhythm, quality: apical/radial pulse before administration; notify prescriber of any significant changes (pulse <50 bpm)

• Check for baselines in renal, liver function tests before therapy begins

• **CHF: assess for edema in feet, legs daily, monitor I&O, daily weight; check for jugular vein distention, crackles bilaterally, dyspnea**

> **BLACK BOX WARNING:** Abrupt discontinuation: Product should be tapered to prevent adverse reactions

Patient/family education

> **BLACK BOX WARNING:** Teach patient not to discontinue product abruptly, precipitate angina might occur; taper over 2 wk

• Teach patient not to use OTC products containing α-adrenergic stimulants (such as nasal decongestants, cold preparations); to avoid alcohol, smoking; to limit sodium intake as prescribed

• Teach patient that product may mask symptoms of hypoglycemia; monitor blood glucose closely

• Teach patient how to take pulse and B/P at home; advise when to notify prescriber

• Instruct patient to comply with weight control, dietary adjustments, modified exercise program

• Advise patient to carry/wear emergency ID to identify products being taken, allergies; that product controls symptoms but does not cure the condition

• **Teach patient to report symptoms of CHF: difficulty breathing, especially on exertion or when lying down, night cough, swelling of extremities, bradycardia, dizziness, confusion, depression, fever**

• Teach patient to take product as prescribed, not to double or skip doses; take any missed doses as soon as remembered if at least 4 hr until next dose

• Advise patient to avoid driving or other hazardous activities until response is known; dizziness, drowsiness occurs

• Teach patient to take product at bedtime for 1 dose

Evaluation
Positive therapeutic outcome
• Decreased B/P in hypertension (after 1-2 wk)

• Absence of dysrhythmias

TREATMENT OF OVERDOSE:
Lavage, **IV** glucagon or atropine for bradycardia, **IV** theophylline for bronchospasm, digoxin, O_2, diuretic for cardiac failure, hemodialysis, **IV** glucose for hyperglycemia, **IV** diazepam (or phenytoin) for seizures

lacosamide (Rx)
(la-koe′sa-mide)

Vimpat

Func. class.: Anticonvulsant

Chem. class.: Functionalized amino acid

Pregnancy category C

Controlled substance schedule V

ACTION: May act through action at sodium channels; exact action is unknown

---

Therapeutic outcome: Decrease in severity of seizures

USES: Partial seizures

CONTRAINDICATIONS
Hypersensitivity

Precautions: Pregnancy **C,** breastfeeding, allergies, renal/hepatic disease, geriatric patients, child <17 yr, acute MI, atrial fibrillation/flutter, AV block, bradycardia, cardiac disease, congenital heart disease, dehydration, depression, dialysis, hazardous activity, electrolyte imbalance, heart failure, labor, PR prolongation, sick sinus syndrome, substance abuse, suicidal ideation, syncope, torsades de pointes

DOSAGE AND ROUTES
Adult and child ≥17 yr: PO 50 mg bid, may increase qwk by 100 mg bid to 200-400 mg/day; **IV** 50 mg 2 ×/day, infuse over 30-60 min, may be increased 100 mg/day weekly, up to 200-400 mg/day maintenance

Renal/hepatic dose
Adult: PO/IV max 300 mg/day in mild to moderate hepatic disease or CCr ≤30 ml/min

Available forms: Film-coated tabs 50, 100, 150, 200 mg; **IV** 20 ml single-use vials (200 mg/20 ml), oral sol 10 mg/ml

Implementation
• Store PO products/IV vials at room temp; sol is stable for 24 hr when mixed with compatible diluents in glass or PVC bags at room temp
PO route
• **Tablet:** give without regard to meals
• **Oral sol:** measure with calibrated measuring device

IV route
• May give undiluted or mixed in 0.9% NaCl, D₅W, or LR
• Infuse over 30-60 min, stable for 24 hr at room temperature
• Do not use if discolored or particulates are present; discard unused portions

ADVERSE EFFECTS
CNS: Dizziness, syncope, tremor, vertigo, ataxia, drowsiness, fever, hypoesthesia, paresthesias, depression, fatigue, headache, confusion, irritability, psychological dependence, **suicidal ideation,** euphoria
CV: *Atrial fibrillation/flutter, AV block,* bradycardia, myocarditis, orthostatic hypotension, palpitations, **PR prolongation**
EENT: Diplopia, blurred vision, nystagmus, tinnitus

GI: Nausea, constipation, vomiting, **hepatitis,** diarrhea, dyspepsia
HEMA: Anemia, neutropenia, agranulocytosis
INTEG: Rash, erythema, inj site reaction, pruritus, xerostomia
MS: Asthenia, dysarthria, muscle cramps
SYST: Drug reaction with eosinophilia and systemic symptoms (DRESS)

Pharmacokinetics

Absorption	Unknown
Distribution	Protein binding <15%
Metabolism	Liver
Excretion	Kidneys (95%)
Half-life	13 hr (PO), elimination half-life 15-23 hr

Pharmacodynamics

	PO	IV
Onset	Unknown	Unknown
Peak	1-4 hr (PO)	30-60 min
Duration	Unknown	Unknown

INTERACTIONS
Individual drugs
Atazanavir, dronedarone, digoxin, lopinavir, ritonavir: increase PR prolongation

Drug classifications
β-blockers, calcium-channel blockers: increase PR prolongation
CYP2C19 inhibitors (fluconazole, isoniazid, miconazole): increase lacosamide effect

Drug/lab test
Increased: LFTs

NURSING CONSIDERATIONS
Assessment
⚠ **Assess for seizures: duration, type, intensity, precipitating factors**
• Monitor for renal function: albumin concentration
• Assess CV status: orthostatic hypotension, PR prolongation; monitor cardiac status throughout treatment
⚠ **Assess mental status: mood, sensorium, affect, memory (long, short), depression, suicidal ideation, psychological dependence**
• Assess for rash, hypersensitivity reactions
⚠ **Pregnancy: Enroll in UCB Antiepileptic Drugs Registry 888-537-7734**

Patient/family education
⚠ **Caution patient not to discontinue product abruptly, taper over 1 wk; seizures may occur**

- Advise patient to avoid hazardous activities until stabilized on product
- Instruct patient to carry emergency ID stating product use

⚠ **Advise patient to notify prescriber of suicidal thoughts or actions, syncope, cardiac changes**
- Instruct patient to notify prescriber if pregnancy is planned or suspected
- Teach patient that interactions with other medications may occur
- Give patient MediGuide for proper use and risks

Evaluation
Positive therapeutic outcome
- Decrease in severity of seizures

lactulose (Rx)
(lak′tyoo-lose)
Constulose, Enulose, Generlac, Kristalose
Func. class.: Laxative (hyperosmotic/ammonia detoxicant)
Chem. class.: Lactose synthetic derivative
Pregnancy category B

Do not confuse: lactulose/lactose

ACTION: Prevents absorption of ammonia in colon by acidifying stool; increases water, softens stool

Therapeutic outcome: Decreased constipation, decreased blood ammonia level

USES: Chronic constipation, portal-systemic encephalopathy in patients with hepatic disease

CONTRAINDICATIONS
Hypersensitivity, low-galactose diet

Precautions: Pregnancy **B**, breastfeeding, geriatric and debilitated patient, diabetes mellitus

DOSAGE AND ROUTES
Constipation
Adult: PO 15-30 ml/day (10-20 g), may increase to 60 ml/day prn
Child (unlabeled): PO 7.5 ml/day

Hepatic encephalopathy
Adult: PO 30-45 ml (20-30 g) tid or qid until stools are soft; retention enema 300 ml diluted
Infant: PO 2.5-10 ml/day in divided doses
Child: PO 40-90 ml/day in divided doses given 3-4 ×/day

Available forms: Oral sol 10 g/15 ml; packets: 10, 20 g; rectal sol: 10 g/15 ml

Implementation
PO route
- Give with full glass of fruit juice, water, milk to increase palatability of oral form; for rapid effect, give on empty stomach; increase fluids by 2 L/day; do not give with other laxatives; if diarrhea occurs, reduce dosage
- Kristalose: dissolve contents of packet in 4 oz of water

Rectal route
- **Administer retention enema** by diluting 300 ml of lactulose/700 ml of water or of 0.9% NaCl; administer by rect balloon catheter; retain for 30-60 min; repeat if evacuated too quickly

ADVERSE EFFECTS
GI: *Nausea, vomiting, anorexia, abdominal cramps, diarrhea,* flatulence, *distention, belching*
META: Hypernatremia

Pharmacokinetics
Absorption	Poorly absorbed
Distribution	Not known
Metabolism	Colonic bacteria to acids
Half-life	Unknown

Pharmacodynamics
Unknown

INTERACTIONS
Individual drugs
Neomycin: decreased lactulose effect
NIFEdipine extended release tab: increased GI obstruction

Drug classifications
Antiinfectives (oral), antacids: decreased lactulose effect
Laxatives: do not use together (hepatic encephalopathy)

Drug/herb
Flax, senna: increased laxative effect

Drug/lab test
Blood glucose (diabetic patients): increase
Blood ammonia: decrease

NURSING CONSIDERATIONS
Assessment
- **Stool:** Assess for amount, color, consistency
- Monitor glucose levels in diabetic patients (increases)
- **Cause of constipation:** Determine whether fluids, bulk, or exercise is missing from lifestyle
- Monitor blood, urine, electrolytes if used often by patient; may cause diarrhea, hypokalemia, hypernatremia; check I&O ratio to identify fluid loss

- Assess cramping, rectal bleeding, nausea, vomiting; if these symptoms occur, product should be discontinued; identify cause of constipation: identify whether fluids, bulk, or exercise is missing from lifestyle, replace any loss
- **Hepatic encephalopathy: Monitor blood ammonia level (30-70 mg/100 ml); monitor for clearing of confusion, lethargy, restlessness, irritability (hepatic encephalopathy); may decrease ammonia level by 50%, monitor sodium in higher doses**

Patient/family education
- Discuss with patient that adequate fluid consumption is necessary
- Teach patient that normal bowel movements do not always occur daily
- **Teach patient not to use in presence of abdominal pain, nausea, vomiting; tell patient to notify prescriber of unrelieved constipation or if symptoms of electrolyte imbalance occur: muscle cramps, pain, weakness, dizziness, excessive thirst**
- Teach patient not to use laxatives for long-term therapy; bowel tone will be lost
- Do not give at bedtime as a laxative; may interfere with sleep
- Notify prescriber if diarrhea occurs; may indicate overdosage

Evaluation
Positive therapeutic outcome
- Decreased constipation
- Decreased blood ammonia level
- Clearing of mental state

lamiVUDine (3TC) (Rx)
(lam-i'vue-dine)
Epivir, Epivir-HBV, Heptovir ✦
Func. class.: Antiretroviral
Chem. class.: Nucleoside reverse transcriptase inhibitor (NRTI)
Pregnancy category C

Do not confuse: lamiVUDine/ LamoTRIgine

ACTION: Inhibits replication of HIV virus by incorporating into cellular DNA by viral reverse transcriptase, thereby terminating the cellular DNA chain

Therapeutic outcome: Improved symptoms of HIV infection

USES: HIV infection in combination with at least 2 other antiretrovirals; chronic hepatitis B (Epivir-HBV)

Unlabeled uses: Prophylaxis of HIV postexposure with indinavir and zidovudine

CONTRAINDICATIONS
Hypersensitivity

Precautions: Pregnancy **C**, breastfeeding, children, geriatric, granulocyte count <1000/mm^3 or Hgb <9.5 g/dl, renal disease, pancreatitis, peripheral neuropathy

BLACK BOX WARNING: Severe hepatic dysfunction, lactic acidosis

DOSAGE AND ROUTES
HIV infection
Adult and adolescent >16 yr: PO 150 mg bid or 300 mg/day
Child 3 mo-16 yr: PO 4 mg/kg bid; max 150 mg bid

Renal dose
Adult: PO CCr 30-49 ml/min: Epivir 150 mg/day; Epivir HBV 100 mg 1st dose, then 50 mg/day; CCr 15-29 ml/min: Epivir 150 mg 1st dose, then 100 mg/day; Epivir HBV 100 mg 1st dose, then 25 mg/day; CCr 5-14 ml/min: Epivir 150 mg 1st dose, then 50 mg/day; Epivir HBV 35 mg 1st dose, then 15 mg/day; CCr <5 ml/min: Epivir 50 mg 1st dose, then 25 mg/day; Epivir HBV 35 mg 1st dose, then 10 mg/day

Chronic hepatitis B
Adult: PO 100 mg/day
Child/adolescent 2-17 yr: PO 3 mg/kg/day, max 100 mg

Available forms: Oral sol (**Epivir**) 10 mg/ml, tabs 150, 300/mg; oral sol (**Epivir-HBV**) 5 mg/ml, tabs 100 mg

Implementation
- **Epivir and Epivir-HBV are not interchangeable**
- Administer PO daily, bid without regard to meals
- **Give with other antiretrovirals only**
- Store in cool environment; protect from light

ADVERSE EFFECTS
CNS: *Fever, headache, malaise, dizziness, insomnia, depression, fatigue, chills,* **seizures,** peripheral neuropathy, paresthesia
EENT: Taste change, hearing loss, photophobia
GI: *Nausea, vomiting, diarrhea,* anorexia, cramps, dyspepsia, **hepatomegaly with steatosis, pancreatitis**
HEMA: **Neutropenia,** anemia, **thrombocytopenia**
INTEG: *Rash*
MS: *Myalgia, arthralgia, pain*
RESP: *Cough*

SYST: Lactic acidosis, anaphylaxis, Stevens-Johnson syndrome

Pharmacokinetics

Absorption	Rapidly absorbed
Distribution	Extravascular space
Metabolism	Protein binding <36%
Excretion	Unchanged in urine
Half-life	Terminal half-life 5-7 hr

Pharmacodynamics

Unknown

INTERACTIONS
Individual drugs

AMILoride, dofetilide, entecavir, metFORMIN, memantine, procainamide, trospium, trimethoprim/sulfamethoxazole: increased level of lamiVUDine

Emtricitabine: do not combine, duplication

Zalcitabine: decreased both products, avoid concurrent use

Drug classifications

Interferons: decrease lamiVUDine

Drug/lab test

Increased: ALT, bilirubin

Decreased: Hgb, neutrophil, platelet count

NURSING CONSIDERATIONS
Assessment

• **HIV:** Test for HIV before starting treatment; monitor blood counts q2wk; watch for neutropenia, thrombocytopenia, Hgb, CD4, viral load, lipase, triglycerides periodically during treatment; if low, therapy may have to be discontinued and restarted after hematologic recovery; blood transfusions may be required; assess for lessening of symptoms; if HBV is present, a higher dose of Epivir-HBV is needed

• **Hepatitis B: Assess for fatigue, anorexia, pruritus, jaundice during and for several months after discontinuation; monitor liver function tests: AST, ALT, bilirubin; amylase; bilirubin, triglycerides, lipase**

• **Monitor children for pancreatitis: abdominal pain, nausea, vomiting, neuropathy**

> BLACK BOX WARNING: **Assess for lactic acidosis, severe hepatomegaly with steatosis:** obtain baseline liver function tests; if elevated, discontinue treatment; discontinue even if liver function tests are normal and symptoms of lactic acidosis, severe hepatomegaly develops; may be fatal

Patient/family education

• Teach patient that GI complaints and insomnia resolve after 3-4 wk of treatment

• Tell patient that product is not a cure for AIDS but will control symptoms; compliance is needed, take as directed, to complete full course of treatment even if feeling better

• **Teach patient to notify prescriber of sore throat, swollen lymph nodes, malaise, fever, peripheral neuropathy; other infections may occur**

• Teach patient that virus is still infective, may pass AIDS virus to others

• **Encourage patient to continue follow-up visits since serious toxicity may occur; blood counts must be done q2wk**

• Tell patient that other products may be necessary to prevent other infections

• Teach patient that product may cause fainting or dizziness

• **Teach patient not to breastfeed; lamiVUDine is excreted in breast milk**

Evaluation

Positive therapeutic outcome

• Absence of infection, symptoms of HIV infection

---

lamoTRIgine (Rx)
(lam-o-trye′geen)
LaMICtal, Lamictal CD, Lamictal ODT, Lamictal XR
Func. class.: Anticonvulsant—miscellaneous
Chem. class.: Phenyltriazine
Pregnancy category C

Do not confuse: lamoTRIgine/lamiVUDine, **LaMICtal**/LamISIL/Lomotil

ACTION: May inhibit voltage-sensitive sodium channels, decreasing seizures

Therapeutic outcome: Decrease in intensity and number of seizures

USES: Adjunct in the treatment of partial, tonic-clonic seizures, children with Lennox-Gastaut syndrome, bipolar disorder

Unlabeled uses: Absence seizures

CONTRAINDICATIONS
Hypersensitivity

Precautions: Pregnancy C (cleft lip/palate in 1st trimester), breastfeeding, geriatric, renal/hepatic/cardiac disease, severe depression, suicidal ideation, blood dyscrasias, children <16 yr, serious rash

DOSAGE AND ROUTES
Seizures: monotherapy

Adult and adolescent ≥16 yr: PO 50 mg/day for wk 1 and 2, then increase to 100 mg divided bid for wk 3 and 4; maintenance 300-500 mg/day; receiving enzyme inducing AEDs (carBAMazepine, PHENobarbital, phenytoin, primidone but not valproic acid); ext rel 50 mg/day × 1-2 wks, then 100 mg/day during wk 3-4, then 200 mg/day during wk 5, then 300 mg/day during wk 6, then 400 mg/day during wk 7; after wk 7 range is 400-600 mg/day

Adolescent <16 yr and child: PO 0.3 mg/kg/day wk 1 and 2, then 0.6 mg/kg/day wk 3 and 4; depends on use of AED; usual dosage 4.5-7.5 mg/kg/day, max 300 mg/day

Monotherapy for patients taking valproate

Adult/adolescent ≥16 yr: receiving lamoTRIgine and valproate, without enzyme-inducing drug PO (immediate-release) stabilize on valproate and target dose of 200 mg/day lamoTRIgine; if patient is not taking lamoTRIgine 200 mg/day, increase dose by 25-50 mg/day q1-2wk to reach 200 mg/day; while maintaining lamoTRIgine 200 mg/day, decrease valproate to 500 mg/day by ≤500 mg/day/wk, maintain valproate at 500 mg/day × 1 wk, then increase lamoTRIgine to 300 mg/day, while decreasing valproate 250 mg/day × 1 wk, then discontinue valproate and increase lamoTRIgine by 100 mg/day qwk to maintenance dosage of 500 mg/day

Seizures: multiple therapy with valproate

Adult and adolescent ≥16 yr: PO 25 mg every other day, then 25 mg/day wk 3-4, increase by 25-50 mg q1-2wk; maintenance 100-500 mg/day
Adolescent <16 yr and child: PO 0.1-0.2 mg/kg/day initially, then increase q2wk as needed to 1.5 mg/kg/day or 200 mg/day

Bipolar disorder (Escalation regimen in those not taking carBAMazepine, or other enzyme-inducing drugs or valproate)

Adult and adolescent ≥16 yr: PO wk 1-2 25 mg/day; wk 3-4 50 mg/day; wk 5 100 mg/day; wk 6-7 200 mg/day; for patients taking valproic acid: wk 1-2 25 mg every other day; wk 3-4 25 mg/day; wk 5 50 mg/day; wk 6 100 mg/day; wk 7 100 mg/day

Hepatic dose
Adult (moderate hepatic impairment or severe without ascites): PO reduce by 25%
Adult (severe hepatic impairment with ascites): PO reduce by 50%

Available forms: Tabs 25, 100, 150, 200 mg; chew tabs 5, 25 mg; oral disintegrating tab 25, 50, 100, 200 mg; oral disintegrating 25-50, 50-100, 25-50-100 mg titration kit; PO ext rel 25-50-100, 50-100-200 mg titration kit; PO 25-100 mg starter kit, ext rel 25, 50, 100, 250, 300 mg

Implementation
PO route
• **Orange Starter Kit:** for those **NOT** taking carBAMazepine, phenytoin, PHENobarbital, primidone, rifampin, or valproate
• **Green Starter Kit:** for those taking carBAMazepine, phenytoin, PHENobarbital, primidone, rifampin but **NOT** valproate
• **Blue Starter Kit: for those taking valproate**
• Discontinue all products gradually ≥2 wk, abrupt discontinuation can increase seizures
• All forms may be given without regard to meals
• **Chewable dispersible tab:** may be swallowed whole, chewed, mixed in water or fruit juice; to mix add to small amount of liquid in a glass or spoon, tabs will dissolve in 1 min, then mix in more liquid and swirl and swallow immediately
• **Orally disintegrating tabs:** place on tongue, move around in mouth, when disintegrated, swallow; examine blister pack before use, do not use if blisters are torn or missing; do not cut tabs in half
• **Extended-release tabs:** swallow whole, do not cut, break, chew
• Give correct starter kit: **severe side effects have occurred from incorrect starter kit**
• Give in divided doses with or after meals to decrease adverse effects

ADVERSE EFFECTS
CNS: Fever, insomnia, tremor, depression, anxiety, *dizziness*, ataxia, *headache*, **suicidal ideation, seizures, poor concentration**
EENT: Nystagmus, *diplopia, blurred vision*
GI: *Nausea, vomiting, anorexia*, abdominal pain, **hepatotoxicity**
GU: *Dysmenorrhea*
HEMA: Anemia, **DIC**, leukopenia, **thrombocytopenia**
INTEG: **Rash (potentially life-threatening)**, alopecia, photosensitivity
CV: chest pain, palpitations
MS: neck pain, myalgias
SYST: **Stevens-Johnson syndrome, angioedema, toxic epidermal necrolysis, DRESS**

Pharmacokinetics

Absorption	Well absorbed, rapid
Distribution	Protein binding 55%, crosses placenta
Metabolism	Glucuronic acid conjunction
Excretion	Excreted in breast milk
Half-life	Terminal 24 hr; 15 hr with enzyme inducers

Pharmacodynamics

Onset	Unknown
Peak	1.4-2.3 hr
Duration	Unknown

INTERACTIONS
Individual drugs
Acetaminophen, carBAMazepine, OXcarbaze-pine, PHENobarbital, phenytoin, primidone: decreased lamoTRIgine serum concentration

Valproic acid: decreased metabolic clearance of lamoTRIgine

Drug classifications
CYP3A4 inhibitors: decreased metabolic clearance of lamoTRIgine

Contraceptives (oral), estrogens, succinimides, rifamycins: decreased lamoTRIgine serum concentration

Drug/herb
Ginkgo: increased anticonvulsant effect

Ginseng, santonica: decreased anticonvulsant effect

NURSING CONSIDERATIONS
Assessment
⚠ **Assess for rash (Stevens-Johnson syndrome or toxic epidermal necrolysis) in pediatric patients; product should be discontinued at first sign of rash**
• **Assess for seizure activity:** duration, type, intensity, halo before seizure
• Assess for hypersensitive reactions
⚠ **Bipolar disorder: suicidal thoughts/behaviors**

Patient/family education
• Caution patient not to discontinue product abruptly; seizures may occur
• Caution patient to avoid hazardous activities until stabilized on product
• Advise patient to notify prescriber of skin rash or increased seizure activity
• Instruct patient to report to prescriber if pregnancy is suspected or planned
• Teach patient to use sunscreen and protective clothing; photosensitivity occurs

• Advise patient to carry/wear emergency ID stating product use
⚠ **Advise patient to notify prescriber immediately of suicidal thoughts, behaviors**
⚠ **Teach patient to notify prescriber if pregnancy is planned or suspected, pregnancy (C), product decreases folate; avoid breastfeeding**

Evaluation
Positive therapeutic outcome
• Decrease in severity of seizures or severity of bipolar symptoms

lansoprazole (Rx, OTC)
(lan-soe′prah-zole)
Prevacid, Prevacid SoluTab
Func. class.: Proton-pump inhibitor
Chem. class.: Benzimidazole
Pregnancy category B

Do not confuse: Prevacid/Pravachol/Prinivil

ACTION: Suppresses gastric secretion by inhibiting hydrogen/potassium ATPase enzyme system in gastric parietal cell; characterized as gastric acid pump inhibitor since it blocks final step of acid production

Therapeutic outcome: Reduction in gastric pain, swelling, fullness

USES: Gastroesophageal reflux disease (GERD), severe erosive esophagitis, poorly responsive systemic GERD, pathologic hypersecretory conditions (Zollinger-Ellison syndrome, systemic mastocytosis, multiple endocrine adenomas); possibly effective for treatment of duodenal, gastric ulcers, maintenance of healed duodenal ulcers

CONTRAINDICATIONS
Hypersensitivity

Precautions: Pregnancy **B,** breastfeeding, children, hypomagnesemia, osteoporosis

DOSAGE AND ROUTES
Frequent heartburn
Adult: PO 15 mg qd up to 14 days

Duodenal ulcer
Adult: PO 15 mg/day before meals for 4 wk, then 15 mg/day to maintain healing of ulcers; ulcers associated with *Helicobacter pylori:* 30 mg lansoprazole, 500 mg clarithromycin, 1 g amoxicillin bid × 14 days or 30 mg lansoprazole, 1 g amoxicillin tid × 14 days

---

Pathologic hypersecretory conditions
Adult: PO 60 mg/day, may give up to 90 mg bid, administer >120 mg/day in divided doses

GERD/esophagitis
Adult/adolescent: PO 15-30 mg/day × 8 wk
Child 1-11 yr (>30 kg): PO 30 mg/day ≤12 wk
Child 1-11 yr (≤30 kg): 15 mg/day ≤12 wk

Stress gastric prophylaxis
Adult: NG use 30 mg oral cap or 300 mg disintegrating tab

Available forms: del rel caps 15, 30 mg; oral powder; orally disintegrating tabs 15, 30 mg

Implementation
PO route
• Swallow del rel cap whole; do not break, crush, chew, or open
• Administer before eating
• **Oral cap:** Open cap and pour ¼ of granules into NG feeding syringe with plunger removed, slowly add water and depress plunger, repeat until all granules are used, flush tube with 15 ml water
• Place on tongue, allow to dissolve, use without regard to water
• **Oral syringe:** Dissolve 15 mg/4 ml or 30 mg/10 ml water; use extra water in syringe to remove all of the product
NG tube
• **Oral disintegrating tab:** Mix 30 mg tab in 10 ml water, give via NG tube, flush tube with 10 ml sterile water, clamp for 60 min

ADVERSE EFFECTS
CNS: *Headache*
GI: Diarrhea, abdominal pain, vomiting, nausea, *constipation,* flatulence, acid regurgitation, anorexia, irritable colon, microscopic colitis
GU: Hematuria, glycosuria, impotence, kidney calculus, breast enlargement

Pharmacokinetics
Absorption	Rapid after granules leave stomach
Distribution	Protein binding 97%
Metabolism	Liver extensively
Excretion	Urine, feces; clearance decreased in geriatric, renal/hepatic disease
Half-life	Plasma 1.5 hr

Pharmacodynamics
Unknown

INTERACTIONS
Individual products
Octreotide, misoprostol: decreased lansoprazole effect

Extended release amphetamine/dextroamphetamine: decreased release of extended-release product

Calcium carbonate, iron salts, itraconazole, ketoconazole, atazanavir, ampicillin: decreased absorption of each specific product

FluvoxaMINE, voriconazole: increased lansoprazole toxicity

Warfarin: increased bleeding risk
Sucralfate: delayed absorption of lansoprazole
Clopidogrel: decreased antiplatelet effect

Drug/herb
• Avoid use with red yeast rice, St. John's wort

Drug/food
• Food decreases rate of absorption; use before food

Drug classifications
Loop/thiazide diuretics: increased hypomagnesemia

Antimuscarinics, H_2 blockers: decreased lansoprazole effect

NURSING CONSIDERATIONS
Assessment
• Assess GI system; bowel sounds q8hr, abdomen for pain, swelling, anorexia, blood in stool, emesis
• Monitor liver enzymes (AST, ALT, alkaline phosphatase) during treatment
• Monitor INR and pro-time when taking warfarin
• Low magnesium may occur

Patient/family education
• **Instruct patient to report severe diarrhea; product may have to be discontinued**
• Inform diabetic patient that hypoglycemia may occur
• Encourage patient to avoid hazardous activities; dizziness may occur
• Tell patient to avoid alcohol, salicylates, ibuprofen; may cause GI irritation
• Teach patient that if using OTC for heartburn, it may take 1-4 days to see full benefit

Evaluation
Positive therapeutic outcome
• Absence of gastric pain, swelling, fullness

lapatinib (Rx)
(la-pa′tin-ib)
Tykerb
Func. class.: Antineoplastic—miscellaneous
Chem. class.: Biologic response modifier, signal transduction inhibitor (STIs)
Pregnancy category D

Therapeutic outcome: Decrease in breast cancer progression

USES: Advanced/metastatic breast cancer patients with tumor that overexpresses HER2 protein and who have received previous chemotherapy

CONTRAINDICATIONS
Pregnancy **D**, hypersensitivity, breastfeeding

DOSAGE AND ROUTES
Advanced/metastatic breast cancer with HER2 overexpression who have received previous therapy
Adult: PO 1250 mg (5 tabs)/day 1 hr before or after food on days 1-21 plus capecitabine 2000 mg/m^2/day in 2 divided doses on days 1-14 in a repeating 21-day cycle; continue until therapeutic response or toxicity occurs

Metastatic breast cancer with HER2 overexpression for whom hormonal therapy is indicated
Adult: PO 1500 mg (6 tabs) 1 hr before food with letrozole 2.5/day

Hepatic dose
Adult (Child-Pugh C): PO 750 mg/day (with capecitabine); 1000 mg/day (with letrozole)

latanoprost ophthalmic
See Appendix B

ledipasvir/sofosbuvir
(le-dip′as-vir/soe-fos′bue-veer)
Harvoni
Func. class.: Antiviral antihepatitis agent
Pregnancy category B

ACTION: A combination product with a HCV NS5A inhibitor (ledipasvir) and a nucleotide analog HCV NS5B polymerase inhibitor (sofosbuvir)

Therapeutic outcome: Hepatitis C RNA reduction

USES: Chronic hepatitis C virus (HCV) genotype 1 infection in patients with compensated liver disease

CONTRAINDICATIONS: Hypersensitivity

Precautions: Decompensated hepatic disease, decompensated cirrhosis, severe renal impairment (eGFR <30 ml/min/1.73 m^2), end-stage renal failure requiring dialysis, pregnancy (**B**), breastfeeding

DOSAGE AND ROUTES
Adults with or without cirrhosis who are treatment-naive: PO one tab (90 mg ledipasvir; 400 mg sofosbuvir) every day with or without food for 12 wk; 8 wk can be considered for those patients with a baseline HCV RNA <6 million IU/ml
Adults without cirrhosis who are treatment-experienced: PO one tab (90 mg ledipasvir; 400 mg sofosbuvir) every day with or without food for 12 wk
Adults with cirrhosis who are treatment-experienced: PO one tab (90 mg ledipasvir; 400 mg sofosbuvir) every day with or without food for 24 wk

Available forms: Tab 90/400 mg

Implementation
• Without regard to food

ADVERSE EFFECTS
CNS: Fatigue, headache, insomnia
GI: Nausea, vomiting, diarrhea

Pharmacokinetics

Absorption	Unknown
Distribution	Ledipasvir: >99.8% protein binding, Sofosbuvir: 61%-65% protein binding
Metabolism	Unknown
Excretion	Ledipasvir: biliary; Sofosbuvir: kidneys 80% recovered in the urine
Half-life	Terminal half-life 47 hr

Pharmacodynamics

Onset	Unknown
Peak	Ledipasvir peak 4-5 hr, Sofosbuvir peak 0.8-1 hr
Duration	Unknown

INTERACTIONS
Drug classifications
Avoid use with products that increase P-glycoprotein

Drug/lab test
Increased: bilirubin

NURSING CONSIDERATIONS
Assessment
• Hepatitis C: monitor hepatitis C RNA, serum bilirubin, creatinine

Patient/family education
• Instruct patient to report effects to the prescriber

Evaluation
Positive therapeutic outcome
• Hepatitis C RNA reduction

leflunomide (Rx)
(leh-floo′noh-mide)
Arava
Func. class.: Antirheumatic (DMARDs)
Chem. class.: Immune modulator, pyrimidine synthesis inhibitor
Pregnancy category X

ACTION: Inhibits an enzyme involved in pyrimidine synthesis and has antiproliferative, antiinflammatory effect

Therapeutic outcome: Decreased pain, joint swelling, increased mobility

USES: Rheumatoid arthritis, to reduce disease process as well as symptoms

Unlabeled uses: Juvenile rheumatoid arthritis

CONTRAINDICATIONS
Breastfeeding, hypersensitivity

> BLACK BOX WARNING: Pregnancy **X**

Precautions: Children, renal disorders, vaccinations, infection, alcoholism, immunosuppression, jaundice, lactase deficiency, hepatic disease

DOSAGE AND ROUTES
Adult: PO loading dose 100 mg/day × 3 days, maintenance 20 mg/day; may be decreased to 10 mg/day if not well tolerated

Juvenile rheumatoid arthritis (unlabeled)
Adolescent and child >40 kg: PO 20 mg/day
Adolescent and child 20-40 kg: PO 15 mg/day
Adolescent and child 10-19.9 kg: PO 10 mg/day

Available forms: Tabs 10, 20, 100 mg
Implementation
• Give with full glass of water to enhance absorption
• Give PO with food, milk, or antacids for GI upset, give same time each day; loading dose is recommended
• **Drug elimination:** to eliminate product give cholestyramine 8 g tid × 11 days, check levels

ADVERSE EFFECTS
CNS: Dizziness, insomnia, depression, paresthesia, anxiety, migraine, neuralgia, headache
CV: Palpitations, hypertension, chest pain, angina pectoris, peripheral edema
EENT: Pharyngitis, oral candidiasis, stomatitis, dry mouth, blurred vision
GI: *Nausea, anorexia, vomiting, constipation, flatulence, diarrhea, increased liver function tests,* **hepatotoxicity,** weight loss
HEMA: Anemia, ecchymosis, hyperlipidemia
INTEG: Rash, pruritus, alopecia, acne, hematoma, herpes infections
RESP: Pharyngitis, rhinitis, bronchitis, cough, respiratory infection, pneumonia, sinusitis, **interstitial lung disease**
SYST: **Opportunistic/fatal infections, Stevens-Johnson syndrome**

Pharmacokinetics
Absorption	Unknown
Distribution	Unknown
Metabolism	Liver
Excretion	Kidneys
Half-life	Unknown

Pharmacodynamics
Unknown

INTERACTIONS
Individual drugs
Activated charcoal, cholestyramine: decreased effect of leflunomide, use for overdose
Methotrexate: increased hepatotoxicity
Rifampin: increased leflunomide levels

Drug classifications
Hepatotoxic agents: increased side effects of leflunomide
Live virus vaccines: decreased antibody reaction
NSAIDs: increased NSAID effect

NURSING CONSIDERATIONS
Assessment

> BLACK BOX WARNING: **Hepatic studies:** If ALT elevations are >2× ULN, reduce dose to 10 mg/day, monitor monthly or more frequently

- Screen for latent TB before starting treatment; if TB is present, treat before using this product
- **Interstitial lung disease: assess for worsening cough, dyspnea, fever; may need to be discontinued**
- Monitor liver function tests: if ALT elevations are >2 times baseline, reduce dosage to 10 mg/day
- Obtain CBC with differential qmo × 6 mo, then q6-8wk thereafter, pregnancy test, electrolytes
- **Assess arthritic symptoms:** ROM, mobility, swelling of joints, baseline, during treatment
- **Assess for infection:** fatal opportunistic infections can occur

> **BLACK BOX WARNING: Pregnancy (X):** Determine that patient is not pregnant before treatment; not to be given to women of child-bearing potential who are not using reliable contraception

Patient/family education
- Teach patient that product must be continued for prescribed time to be effective, that up to a month may be required for improvement
- Instruct patient to take with food, milk, or antacids to avoid GI upset, take at same time of day
- Advise patient to use caution when driving; drowsiness, dizziness may occur
- Advise patient to take with a full glass of water to enhance absorption, may continue with correct prescribed treatment with other antiinflammatories

> **BLACK BOX WARNING:** Advise patient not to become pregnant (**X**) while taking this product

- Inform patient that hair may be lost, review alternatives
- Advise patient to avoid live virus vaccinations during treatment

Evaluation
Positive therapeutic outcome
- Increased joint mobility without pain
- Decreased joint swelling

TREATMENT OF OVERDOSE:
Give cholestyramine 8 g tid × 11 days

⚠ HIGH ALERT

letrozole (Rx)
(let′tro-zohl)
Femara
Func. class.: Antineoplastic, nonsteroidal aromatase inhibitor
Pregnancy category D

ACTION: Binds to the heme group of aromatase; inhibits conversion of androgens to estrogens to reduce plasma estrogen levels

Therapeutic outcome: Decreased spread of malignancy

USES: Early, advanced, or metastatic breast cancer in postmenopausal women who are hormone receptor positive

CONTRAINDICATIONS
Pregnancy **D**, hypersensitivity, premenopausal females

Precautions: Hepatic disease, respiratory disease, osteoporosis

DOSAGE AND ROUTES
Adult: PO 2.5 mg/day

Available forms: Tabs 2.5 mg

Implementation
- May administer bisphosphates to increase bone density
- Give with food or fluids for GI upset
- Give in equal intervals q6hr

ADVERSE EFFECTS
CNS: Somnolence, dizziness, depression, anxiety, *headache, lethargy*
CV: Angina, **MI, CVA, thromboembolic events,** peripheral edema, hypertension
GI: *Nausea, vomiting, anorexia,* constipation, heartburn, diarrhea
GU: Endometrial cancer, vaginal bleeding, endometrial proliferation disorder
INTEG: *Rash, pruritus,* alopecia, sweating
MISC: Hot flashes, night sweats, **second malignancies, anaphylaxis, angioedema**
MS: Arthralgia, arthritis, bone fracture, myalgia, osteoporosis
RESP: Dyspnea, cough

Pharmacokinetics
Absorption	Well absorbed
Distribution	Widely distributed, steady state 2-6 wk
Metabolism	Liver
Excretion	Kidneys
Half-life	Terminal 48 hr

Pharmacodynamics
Onset	Unknown
Peak	2 days
Duration	Unknown

INTERACTIONS
Drug classifications
Estrogens, oral contraceptives: decreased letrozole effect

NURSING CONSIDERATIONS
Assessment
- Monitor temperature q4hr; may indicate beginning of infection
- Monitor LFTs before, during therapy (bilirubin, AST, ALT, LDH) as needed or monthly

Patient/family education
- Advise patient to avoid use of alcohol, which potentiates this product
- Tell patient that product may be taken without regard to meals
- **Teach patient to report vaginal bleeding, diarrhea, chest/bone pain**
- **Advise patient to use adequate contraception in perimenopausal, recently menopausal women, pregnancy D**

Evaluation
Positive therapeutic outcome
- Prevention of rapid division of malignant cells, postmenopausal cancer, prostate cancer

TREATMENT OF OVERDOSE:
Induce vomiting, provide supportive care

RARELY USED

leucovorin (Rx)
(loo-koe-vor'in)
Func. class.: Vitamin/folic acid antagonist antidote
Chem. class.: Tetrahydrofolic acid derivative
Pregnancy category C

USES: Megaloblastic or macrocytic anemia caused by folic acid deficiency, overdose of folic acid antagonist, methotrexate toxicity, toxicity caused by pyrimethamine/trimethoprim/trimetrexate, pneumocystosis, toxoplasmosis

CONTRAINDICATIONS
Hypersensitivity to this product or folic acid, benzyl alcohol, anemias other than megaloblastic not associated with vit B_{12} deficiency

DOSAGE AND ROUTES
Megaloblastic anemia caused by enzyme deficiency
Adult and child: PO/IM/**IV** up to 6 mg/day

Megaloblastic anemia caused by deficiency of folate
Adult and child: IM 1 mg or less/day until adequate response

Advanced colorectal cancer
Adult: IV 200 mg/m², then 5-fluorouracil 370 mg/m²; or leucovorin 20 mg/m², then 5-fluorouracil 425 mg/m²; give daily × 5 days q4-5wk

Methotrexate toxicity—leucovorin rescue
Adult and child: PO/IM/**IV (normal elimination)** given 6 hr after dose of methotrexate 10 mg/m² until methotrexate is $<5 \times 10^{-8}$ m, CCr has increased 50% above prior level, or methotrexate level is 5×10^{-8} m at 24 hr or at 48 hr level is $>9 \times 10^{-8}$ m; give leucovorin 100 mg/m² q3hr until level drops to $<10^{-8}$ m

Pyrimethamine/trimethoprim toxicity
Adult and child: PO/IM 5-15 mg/day

⚠ HIGH ALERT

leuprolide (Rx)
(loo-proe'lide)
Eligard, Lupron Depo, Lupron Depot-Ped
Func. class.: Antineoplastic hormone
Chem. class.: Gonadotropin-releasing hormone
Pregnancy category X

Do not confuse: Lupron/Lopurin/Nuprin

ACTION: Causes initial increase in circulating levels of LH, FSH; continuous administration results in decreased LH, FSH; in men testosterone is reduced to castration levels; in premenopausal women estrogen is reduced to menopausal levels

Therapeutic outcome: Prevention of rapidly growing malignant cells in prostate cancer, decreased pain in endometriosis, resolution of central precocious puberty (CPP)

USES: Metastatic prostate cancer (inj implant), management of endometriosis (depot), CPP, uterine leiomyomata (fibroids)

CONTRAINDICATIONS
Pregnancy **X,** breastfeeding, hypersensitivity to GnRH or analogs, thromboembolic disorders, undiagnosed vaginal bleeding; Viadur implant or Eligard should not be used in women or children

Precautions: Edema, hepatic disease, CVA, MI, seizures, hypertension, diabetes mellitus, CHF, depression, osteoporosis, spinal cord compression, urinary tract obstruction

DOSAGE AND ROUTES
Prostate cancer
Adult: SUBCUT 1 mg/day; IM 7.5 mg/dose qmo; Viadur implant (72 mg) qyr; or IM 22.5 mg q3mo; or IM 30 mg q4mo; or IM 45 mg q6mo

---

Adverse effects: *italics* = common; **bold** = life-threatening

Endometriosis/fibroids
Adult: IM 3.75 mg qmo for 6 mo, 11.25 mg q3mo for 6 mo, or IM 30 mg q4mo

Central precocious puberty
Child: SUBCUT 50 mcg/kg/day; increase as needed by 10 mcg/kg/day
Child >37.5 kg: IM 15 mg q4wk
Child 25-37.5 kg: IM 11.25 mg q4wk
Child ≤25 kg: 7.5 mg q4wk

Available forms: Depot inj: 3.75, 7.5, 11.25, 15, 22.5, 30, 45 mg; Inj: 5 mg/ml (2.8 ml multidose vials)

Implementation
- Store in tight container at room temp
- Use depot only IM; never give SUBCUT
- Unused vials may be stored at room temperature

Subcut route
- No dilution needed; if patient is self-administering make sure patient uses syringes provided by manufacturer
- **Viadur Duros implant:** Insert in inner aspect of arm, remove after 12 mo
- **Eligard subcut:** Bring to room temp, once mixed give within 30 min; prepare the 2 syringes for mixing, join the 2 syringes by pushing in and twisting until secure; mix the product by pushing the contents of both syringes back and forth between syringes until uniform, should be light tan to tan; hold syringes vertically with syringe B on the bottom, draw entire mixed product into syringe B (short, wide syringe) by depressing the syringe A plunger and slightly withdrawing syringe B plunger, uncouple syringe A while pushing down on syringe A plunger, small air bubbles will remain; hold syringe B upright, remove pink cap, attach needle cartridge to the end of syringe B, remove needle cover, give by subcut route

IM route
- **Give monthly:** reconstitute single-use vial with 1 ml of diluent; if multiple vials are used, withdraw 0.5 ml and inject into each vial (1 ml), withdraw all and inject at 90-degree angle (3.75 mg)
- **Give 3 month:** reconstitute microspheres using 1.5 ml of diluent and inject in vial, shake, withdraw and inject
- **12-month:** inserted into upper arm; at the end of 12 months, implant must be removed
- Use syringe and product packaged together; give deep in large muscle mass; rotate sites

ADVERSE EFFECTS
CNS: Memory impairment, depression, seizures
CV: MI, pulmonary emboli, dysrhythmias, peripheral edema

GI: Anorexia, diarrhea, GI bleeding, nausea, vomiting
GU: Edema, hot flashes, impotence, decreased libido, amenorrhea, vaginal dryness, gynecomastia, profuse vaginal bleeding
INTEG: Alopecia
MS: Bone pain
Prostate cancer: Increased bone pain for the first 4 wk of treatment, those with metastases in spinal column might have severe back pain
RESP: Dyspnea, pulmonary fibrosis, interstitial lung disease

Pharmacokinetics

Absorption	Rapidly absorbed (SUBCUT); slowly absorbed (IM depot)
Distribution	Unknown
Metabolism	Unknown
Excretion	Unknown
Half-life	3-4 hr

Pharmacodynamics

Onset	Unknown
Peak	4 hr
Duration	Unknown

INTERACTIONS
Individual drugs
Flutamide, megestrol: increased antineoplastic action

Drug/herb
Do not confuse with black cohosh or chaste tree fruit, may interfere with treatment

NURSING CONSIDERATIONS
Assessment
- **Assess for symptoms of endometriosis/ fibroids** including lower abdominal pain, excessive vaginal bleeding, bloating if product is given for the diagnosis of endometriosis
- **For central precocious puberty (CPP):** the diagnosis should have been confirmed by development of secondary sex characteristics in children <9 yr; also included to confirm the diagnosis of CPP is estradiol/testosterone, GnRH test, tomography of head, adrenal steroid, chorionic gonadotropin, wrist x-ray, height, weight; patients with CPP display the signs of testicular growth, facial, body hair (boys), breast development, menses (girls)
- Monitor liver function tests before, during therapy (bilirubin, AST, ALT, LDH) as needed or monthly; prostate-specific antigen in prostate cancer; calcium, testosterone, bone mineral density, blood glucose, HbA1c

---

• Monitor pituitary gonadotropic and gonadal function during therapy and 4-8 wk after therapy is decreased; check LH, FSH, acid phosphate at beginning of treatment

• **Tumor flare: monitor worsening of signs and symptoms (normal during beginning therapy): fatigue, increased pulse, pallor, lethargy, edema in feet, joints, stomach pain, shaking**

• Monitor renal status: I&O ratio, check for bladder distention daily during beginning therapy (renal obstruction)

• **Severe allergic reaction: rash, pruritus, urticaria, purpuric skin lesions, itching, flushing**

Patient/family education

• Advise patient to notify prescriber if menstruation continues (menstruation should stop); to use a nonhormonal method of contraception during therapy

⚠ **Teach patient to notify prescriber if pregnancy is planned or suspected (X), avoid breastfeeding**

• Instruct patient to report any complaints, side effects to nurse or prescriber; hot flashes may occur; record weight, report gain of 2 lb/day

• Teach patient how to prepare, administer; to rotate sites for SUBCUT/IM inj; to keep accurate records of dosing (prostate cancer)

• Instruct patient that tumor flare may occur: increase in size of tumor, increased bone pain; tell patient that bone pain disappears after 1 wk; may take analgesics for pain

• Advise the patient not to breastfeed while taking this product

• Inform patient that voiding problems may increase in beginning of therapy, but will decrease in several weeks

Evaluation
Positive therapeutic outcome

• Decreased size, spread of malignancy
• Decreased pain in endometriosis, fibroids
• Decreased signs of CPP
• Increased follicle maturation

levalbuterol (Rx)

(lev-al-bute′er-ole)
Xopenex, Xopenex HFA
Func. class.: Bronchodilator
Chem. class.: Adrenergic β₂-agonist
Pregnancy category C

ACTION: Causes bronchodilatation by action on β_2 (pulmonary) receptors by increasing levels of cyclic adenosine monophosphate (AMP), which relaxes smooth muscle; produces bronchodilatation; CNS, cardiac stimulation, increased diuresis, and increased gastric acid secretion

Therapeutic outcome: Increased ability to breathe because of bronchodilatation

USES: Treatment or prevention of bronchospasm (reversible obstructive airway disease), asthma

CONTRAINDICATIONS

Hypersensitivity to sympathomimetics, this product, or albuterol

Precautions: Pregnancy **C**, breastfeeding, hyperthyroidism, diabetes mellitus, hypertension, prostatic hypertrophy, closed-angle glaucoma, seizures, renal disease, QT prolongation, tachydysrhythmias, severe cardiac disease, hypokalemia, children

DOSAGE AND ROUTES
Bronchospasm

Adult and child ≥12 yr: INH 0.63 mg tid, q6-8hr by nebulization; may increase to 1.25 mg q8hr

Adult/adolescent/child >4 yr: (HFA, metered dose) 90 mcg (2 INH) q4-6hr

Child 6-11 yr: INH 0.31 mg tid via nebulization, max 0.63 mg tid

Asthma, relief (unlabeled)

Child <4 yr: nebulizer solution 0.31-1.25 in Nebsol 3 ml q4-6hr prn, or 0.075 mg/kg in Nebsol q20min × 3 doses, then 0.075-0.15 mg/kg up to 5 mg q1-4hr

Available forms: Inh pediatric 0.31 mg/3 ml; sol 0.63/3 ml, 1.25 mg/3 ml, 125 mg/0.5 ml, 45 mcg per actuation (HFA)

Implementation

• Give by nebulization q6-8hr; wait at least 1 min between inhalation of aerosols

• Use this medication before other medications and allow 5 min between each to prevent overstimulation

Inhalation route

• Shake well before use, use a spacer device, prime with 4 test sprays in new canister or when not used for >3 days

Nebulizer route

• Dilute conc sol with normal sterile saline (1.25 mg/0.5ml) before use

ADVERSE EFFECTS

CNS: *Tremors, anxiety,* insomnia, headache, dizziness, stimulation, *restlessness,* weakness, irritability

CV: Palpitations, tachycardia, hypertension, angina, hypotension, dysrhythmias, **QT prolongation**

EENT: Dry nose, irritation of nose and throat
GI: Heartburn, nausea, vomiting, diarrhea, rhinitis
INTEG: Rash
META: Hypokalemia, hyperglycemia
MS: Muscle cramps
RESP: Cough, dyspnea
SYST: Anaphylaxis, angioedema

Pharmacokinetics

Absorption	Unknown
Distribution	Unknown
Metabolism	Liver extensively, tissues
Excretion	Unknown, breast milk
Half-life	Unknown

Pharmacodynamics

	INH SOL	INH AEROSOL
Onset	5-15 min	4.5-10.2 min
Peak	1½ hr	76-78 min
Duration	5-6 hr	6 hr

INTERACTIONS
Individual drugs
Haloperidol, chloroquine, droperidol, pentamidine, arsenic trioxide, levomethadyl: increased QT prolongation, Increase: hypokalemia: loop/thiazide diuretics

Drug classifications
Adrenergics: increased levalbuterol action
β-Adrenergic blockers: decreased levalbuterol action, severe bronchospasm may occur
Bronchodilators (aerosol): increased action of bronchodilator
Class IA/III antidysrhythmics, some phenothiazines, beta agonists, local anesthetics, tricyclics, CYP3A4 inhibitors (amiodarone, clarithromycin, erythromycin, telithromycin, troleandomycin), CYP3A4 substrates (methadone, pimozide, QUEtiapine, quiNIDine, risperiDONE, ziprasidone): increased QT prolongation
Loop/thiazide diuretics: increased hypokalemia
MAOIs: increased levalbuterol action

Drug/herb
Cola nut, guarana, tea (black/green), coffee, yerba maté: increased stimulation

NURSING CONSIDERATIONS
Assessment
• Assess cardiac status: palpitations, increased or decreased B/P, dysrhythmias
• **QT prolongation:** Monitor ECG for QT prolongation, ejection fraction; assess for chest pain, palpitations, dyspnea

• **Assess respiratory function:** vital capacity, forced expiratory volume, ABGs, lung sounds, heart rate, rhythm (baseline, during therapy); character of sputum: color, consistency, amount
• Determine that patient has not received theophylline therapy before giving dose, to prevent additive effect; client's ability to self-medicate
• **Monitor for evidence of allergic reactions; paradoxic bronchospasm, anaphylaxis, angioedema; withhold dose; notify prescriber**

Patient/family education
• Tell patient not to use OTC medications before consulting prescriber; extra stimulation may occur; instruct patient to use this medication before other medications and allow at least 5 min between each to prevent overstimulation; to limit caffeine products such as chocolate, coffee, tea, and cola or herbs such as cola nut, guarana, yerba maté
⚠ **Teach patient that if paradoxical bronchospasm occurs to stop product immediately and notify prescriber**
• Teach patient to use this product first, if using other inhalers, wait 5 min or more between products; rinse mouth with water after each dose to prevent dry mouth

Evaluation
Positive therapeutic outcome
• Absence of dyspnea and wheezing after 1 hr
• Improved airway exchange
• Improved ABGs

TREATMENT OF OVERDOSE:
Administer a β₁-adrenergic blocker

---

levETIRAcetam (Rx)
(lev-ee-tye′ra-see-tam)
Keppra, Keppra XR
Func. class.: Anticonvulsant
Pregnancy category C

ACTION: Unknown; may inhibit nerve impulses by limiting influx of sodium ions across cell membrane in motor cortex

Therapeutic outcome: Absence of seizures

USES: Adjunctive therapy in partial-onset seizures, primary generalized tonic-clonic seizures, myoclonic seizures in juvenile patients

CONTRAINDICATIONS
Hypersensitivity, breastfeeding

Precautions: Pregnancy C, children, geriatric, cardiac/renal disease, psychosis

---

DOSAGE AND ROUTES
Adjunctive treatment of partial seizures
Adult and adolescent ≥16 yr: IV 500 mg bid, may titrate by 1000 mg/day q2wk; max 3000 mg/day in divided doses; ext rel 1000 mg/day, may increase q2wk, max 3000 mg/day
Adolescent <16 yr/child/infant: PO 10 mg/kg bid, increase the daily dose q2wk, by 20 mg/kg to 30 mg/kg bid; if unable to tolerate, may reduce dose

Myoclonic seizures/tonic-clonic seizures/partial seizures
Adult and adolescent >16 yr: PO/IV 500 mg bid, may increase by 1000 mg/day q2wk; max 3000 mg/day

Renal dose
Adult: PO CCr 50-80 ml/min, 500-1000 mg q12hr, ext rel 1000-2000 q24hr, max 2000 mg/day; CCr 30-49 ml/min, 250-750 mg q12hr, ext rel 500-1500 mg q24hr, max 1500 mg/day; CCr <30 ml/min 250-500 mg q12hr, ext rel 500-1000 mg q24hr, max 1000 mg/day

Available forms: Tabs 250, 500, 750, 1000; oral sol 100 mg/ml; SOL for inj 100 mg, 5 ml, ext rel tab 500, 750 mg; 1000 mg/100 ml 0.75% NaCl, 1500 mg/100 ml 0.54% NaCl, 500 mg/100 ml 0.82% NaCl

Implementation
PO route
- Ext rel product should not be used in dialysis patients
- Give with food, milk to decrease GI symptoms (rare)
- **Child <20 kg:** give oral sol, use calibrated device
- Store at room temperature (PO); diluted preparation stable for 24 hr at room temperature in polyvinyl bags

Intermittent IV route
- Single-use vials: dilute in 100 mg of 0.9% NaCl, D₅W, LR; give over 15 min, discard unused vial contents, do not use product with particulates or discoloration

Additive compatibilities: Diazepam, LORazepam, valproate

ADVERSE EFFECTS
CNS: Dizziness, somnolence, asthenia, psychosis, **suicidal ideation,** non-psychotic behavioral symptoms, headache, ataxia
EENT: Diplopia, conjunctivitis
GI: Nausea, vomiting, anorexia, diarrhea, constipation, **hepatitis**
HEMA: Infection, leukopenia

INTEG: Pruritus, rash
MISC: Abdominal pain, pharyngitis, infection
SYST: **Stevens-Johnson syndrome, toxic epidermal necrolysis,** dehydration (child <4 yr)

Pharmacokinetics
Absorption	Rapidly absorbed
Distribution	Widely distributed, not protein bound
Metabolism	Liver, small amount
Excretion	Kidneys, 66% unchanged
Half-life	6-8 hr, longer in renal disease/geriatric

Pharmacodynamics
Unknown

INTERACTIONS
Individual drugs
CarBAMazepine: increased carBAMazepine toxicity
Sevelamer: decreased levetiracetam absorption; separate by 1 hr before, 3 hr after sevelamer

Drug classifications
TCAs, antihistamines, benzodiazepines, other CNS depressants: increased sedation

Drug/lab test
Decreased: Hct/Hgb, WBC, RBC

NURSING CONSIDERATIONS
Assessment
- Monitor urine function tests (BUN, urine protein) periodically during treatments
- ⚠ Assess seizure activity including type, location, duration, and character; provide seizure precautions
- Assess blood studies: CBC, LFTs
- ⚠ Assess mental status: mood, sensorium, affect, behavioral changes, suicidal thoughts/behaviors

Patient/family education
- Teach patient to carry/wear emergency ID stating patient's name, products taken, condition, prescriber's name, phone number
- Caution patient to avoid driving, other activities that require alertness until stabilized on medication, until response is known, drowsiness occurs during first month
- Teach patient not to discontinue medication quickly after long-term use
- ⚠ Instruct patient to report suicidal thoughts
- Teach patient to use a nonhormonal type of contraception to prevent harm to the fetus
- Teach patient to take exactly as prescribed, do not double or omit doses
- Advise not to breastfeed, excreted in breast milk

Adverse effects: *italics* = common; **bold** = life-threatening

Evaluation
Positive therapeutic outcome
• Decreased seizure activity

levobetaxolol ophthalmic
See Appendix B

levobunolol ophthalmic
See Appendix B

levocabastine ophthalmic
See Appendix B

levocetirizine (Rx)
(lee-voh-she-teer′ah-zeen)
Xyzal
Func. class.: Antihistamine, low sedating
Chem. class.: H₁-histamine blocker
Pregnancy category B

ACTION: Acts on blood vessels, GI, respiratory system by competing with histamine for H₁-receptor site; decreases allergic response by blocking pharmacologic effects of histamine; minimal anticholinergic action

Therapeutic outcome: Absence of running or congested nose or rashes

USES: Perennial or seasonal rhinitis, allergy symptoms, chronic idiopathic urticaria

CONTRAINDICATIONS
Breastfeeding; end-stage renal disease; dialysis; child 6-11 yr with renal disease; hypersensitivity to this product, cetrizine, hydroxyzine

Precautions: Pregnancy **B**, driving, renal disease

DOSAGE AND ROUTES
Adult and child ≥12 yr: PO 2.5-5 mg/day in the evening
Child 6-11 yr: PO (oral SOL) 2.5 mg/day in the evening
Child 2-5 yr: PO (oral SOL) 1.25 mg/day in the evening
Geriatric: PO 2.5-5 mg/day in the evening

Renal dose
Adult: PO CCr 50-80 ml/min 2.5 mg/day; CCr 30-50 ml/min 2.5 mg every other day; CCr 10-30 ml/min 2.5 mg 2 ×/wk; CCr <10 ml/min, do not use

Available forms: Tabs 5 mg; oral sol 2.5 mg/5 ml

Implementation
• Give without regard to meals in the evening; tabs are scored and may be broken in half
• Store in tight, light-resistant container

ADVERSE EFFECTS
CNS: *Drowsiness, fatigue,* asthenia, dizziness
RESP: Pneumonia, cough

Pharmacokinetics

Absorption	Rapid
Distribution	Unknown
Metabolism	Protein binding 91%-92%
Excretion	Urine 85.4%, feces 12.9%
Half-life	8 hr

Pharmacodynamics

Onset	Unknown
Peak	0.9 hr
Duration	Unknown

INTERACTIONS
Individual drugs
Alcohol: increased CNS depression
Ritonavir: increased half-life; decreased clearance of levocetirizine

Drug classifications
MAOIs, phenothiazines, tricyclics: increased anticholinergic/sedative effect
Other CNS depressants: increased CNS depression

Drug/lab test
False negative: skin allergy tests

NURSING CONSIDERATIONS
Assessment
• Allergy symptoms: pruritus, urticaria, watering eyes, baseline, during treatment
• Respiratory status: rate, rhythm, increase in bronchial secretions, wheezing, chest tightness
• Liver function tests, serum creatinine, BUN

Patient/family education
• Teach patient all aspects of product use; to notify prescriber if confusion, sedation, hypotension occur, not to exceed recommended dose
• Advise patient to avoid driving, other hazardous activities if drowsiness occurs
• Advise patient to avoid alcohol, other CNS depressants
• Inform patient that product is not recommended during breastfeeding

Evaluation
Positive therapeutic outcome
• Absence of running or congested nose or rashes

TREATMENT OF OVERDOSE:
Administer diazepam, vasopressors, IV phenytoin

---

levodopa-carbidopa (Rx)

(lee-voe-doe′pa kar-bi-doe′pa)

Apo-Levocarb ✹, Duodopa ✹, Rytary, Sinemet, Sinemet CR

Func. class.: Antiparkinsonism agent
Chem. class.: Catecholamine
Pregnancy category C

ACTION: Decarboxylation of levodopa in periphery is inhibited by carbidopa; more levodopa is made available for transport to brain and conversion to dopamine in the brain

Therapeutic outcome: Absence of involuntary movements

USES: Parkinson's disease, parkinsonism resulting from carbon monoxide, chronic manganese intoxication, cerebral arteriosclerosis

Unlabeled uses: Restless legs syndrome

CONTRAINDICATIONS

Hypersensitivity, malignant melanoma, history of malignant melanoma, or undiagnosed skin lesions resembling melanoma

Precautions: Pregnancy **C**, breastfeeding, diabetes, renal/cardiac/hepatic/respiratory disease, MI with dysrhythmias, open-angle glaucoma, seizures, peptic ulcer, depression

DOSAGE AND ROUTES
Beginning therapy for those not taking levodopa

Adult: PO 25 mg carbidopa/100 mg levodopa tid, may increase daily or every other day by 1 tab to desired response (8 tabs/day); ext rel tabs (Sinemet CR) carbidopa 50 mg/levodopa 200 mg bid; ext rel caps (Rytary) 23.75 mg/95 mg tid × 3 days then 36.25 mg/145 mg tid on day 4, may increase to 97.5 mg/390 mg tid

For those not taking levodopa ER

Adult: PO 50 mg carbidopa/200 mg levodopa bid

For those taking levodopa ER

Adult: Begin treatment with 10% more levodopa/day given PO q4-8hr, may increase or decrease dose q3days

For those taking levodopa <1.5 g/day

Adult: PO 25 mg carbidopa/100 mg levodopa tid-qid, may increase daily to desired response

For those taking levodopa >1.5 g/day

Adult: PO 25 mg carbidopa/250 mg levodopa tid-qid, may increase daily to desired response

Restless legs syndrome (RLS) (unlabeled)

Adult: PO carbidopa 25 mg/levodopa 100 mg, 1 tab at bedtime, may repeat if awakening within 2 hr or 50 mg carbidopa/200 mg levodopa SUS REL tab 1-2 tabs 1 hr before bedtime

Available forms: Tabs 10 mg carbidopa/100 mg levodopa, 25 mg carbidopa/100 mg levodopa, 25 mg carbidopa/250 mg levodopa; ext rel tab 25 mg/100 mg, 50 mg/200 mg carbidopa/levodopa (Sinemet CR); oral disintegrating tab (Parcopa) 10 mg carbidopa/100 mg levodopa, 25 mg carbidopa/100 mg levodopa, 25 mg carbidopa/250 mg levodopa; ext rel caps (Rytary) 23.75 mg/95 mg, 36.25 mg/145 mg, 48.75/195 mg, 61.25/245 mg

Implementation
PO route

• Swallow **ext rel tabs** whole; do not break, crush, or chew

• **Oral disintegrating tab:** gently remove from bottle, place on tongue, swallow with saliva; after it dissolves, liquid is not necessary

• Give product until NPO before surgery; check with prescriber for continuing product

• Adjust dosage depending on patient response

• Give with meals or after meals to prevent GI symptoms; limit protein taken with product

• Give only after MAOIs have been discontinued for 2 wk; if previously on levodopa, discontinue for at least 8 hr before change to levodopa-carbidopa

ADVERSE EFFECTS

CNS: *Involuntary choreiform movements, hand tremors, fatigue, headache, anxiety, twitching, numbness, weakness, confusion, agitation, insomnia, nightmares,* psychosis, hallucination, hypomania, severe depression, dizziness, impulsive behaviors, **neuroleptic malignant syndrome**

CV: *Orthostatic hypotension,* tachycardia, hypertension, palpitation

EENT: Blurred vision, diplopia, dilated pupils

GI: *Nausea, vomiting, anorexia, abdominal distress, dry mouth, flatulence, dysphagia, bitter taste, diarrhea, constipation*

HEMA: **Hemolytic anemia, leukopenia, agranulocytosis**

INTEG: Rash, sweating, alopecia

MISC: Urinary retention, incontinence, weight change, dark urine

Pharmacokinetics

Absorption	Well absorbed (PO); ER dose slowly absorbed
Distribution	Widely distributed
Metabolism	Liver, extensively
Excretion	Kidneys, metabolites
Half-life	Levodopa (1 hr); carbidopa (1-2 hr)

Pharmacodynamics

	PO	PO-ER
Onset	Unknown	Unknown
Peak	1 hr	2½ hr
Duration	6-24 hr	Unknown

INTERACTIONS
Individual drugs
Metoclopramide: increased effects of levodopa
Papaverine, pyridoxine: decreased effects of levodopa

Drug classifications
Antacids: increased effects of levodopa
Anticholinergics, antipsychotics, benzodiazepines, hydantoins: decreased effects of levodopa
MAOIs: hypertensive crisis

Drug/food
Protein: decreased absorption of levodopa

Drug/lab test
Increased: AST, ALT, bilirubin, LDH, alkaline phosphatase, BUN, serum glucose
Decreased: BUN, creatinine, uric acid
False increase: urine protein
False positive: urine ketones (dipstick), Coombs' test
False negative: urine glucose

NURSING CONSIDERATIONS
Assessment
• Assess for **parkinsonism:** shuffling gait, muscle rigidity, involuntary movements, pill rolling, muscle spasms, drooling before and during treatment
• Assess B/P, respiration, orthostatic B/P
• Monitor I&O ratio; retention commonly causes decreased urinary output, distention, frequency, incontinence; palpate bladder if retention occurs
• Assess for muscle twitching, blepharospasm that may indicate toxicity
• Monitor renal, liver, hematopoietic studies; also for diabetes, acromegaly during long-term therapy
• Monitor for constipation, cramping, pain in abdomen, abdominal distention; increase fluids, bulk, exercise if this occurs
• Assess for tolerance over long-term therapy; dose may have to be increased or changed
• Assess for mental status: affect, mood, CNS depression, worsening of mental symptoms during early therapy

Patient/family education
• Teach patient to change positions slowly to prevent orthostatic hypotension
• Teach patient to report side effects: twitching, eye spasms, grimacing, protrusion of tongue, personality changes that indicate overdose
• Instruct patient to use product exactly as prescribed; if product is discontinued abruptly, parkinsonian crisis may occur; do not double doses; take missed dose as soon as remembered up to 2 hr before next dose
• Teach patient that urine, sweat may darken and is harmless
• Advise patient to use physical activities to maintain mobility and lessen spasms
• Instruct patient that OTC medications should not be used unless approved by prescriber
• Advise patient that drowsiness, dizziness are common; to avoid hazardous activities until response is known
• Explain that sips of water, hard candy, or gum may lessen dry mouth
• Teach patient to take with meals to prevent GI symptoms; to limit protein intake, which impairs product's absorption

Evaluation
Positive therapeutic outcome
• Decrease in akathisia
• Improved mood
• Decreased involuntary movements

levofloxacin (Rx)
(lev-o-floks′a-sin)
Levaquin
Func. class.: Antiinfective
Chem. class.: Fluoroquinolone antibacterial
Pregnancy category C

ACTION: Interferes with conversion of intermediate DNA fragments into high molecular weight DNA in bacteria; DNA gyrase inhibitor; inhibits topoisomerase IV

Therapeutic outcome: Bacteriocidal action against the following: *Streptococcus pneumoniae, Streptococcus pyogenes, Haemophilus influenzae, Haemophilus parainfluenzae, Moraxella catarrhalis, Klebsiella pneumoniae, Mycoplasma pneumoniae, Escherichia coli, Serratia marcescens,*

Chlamydia pneumoniae, Legionella pneumophilia, Enterococcus faecalis, Staphylococcus epidermidis, Staphylococcus pyogenes, Staphylococcus aureus, Bacillusanthracis

USES: Acute sinusitis, acute chronic bronchitis, community-acquired pneumonia, uncomplicated skin infections, UTI, cellulitis, prostatitis, inhalational anthrax (postexposure), acute pyelonephritis, inhalation anthrax in children

CONTRAINDICATIONS
Hypersensitivity to quinolones

Precautions: Pregnancy **C**, breastfeeding, children; photosensitivity, acute MI, atrial fibrillation, colitis, dehydration, diabetes, QT prolongation, myasthenia gravis, renal disease, seizure disorder, syphilis

> **BLACK BOX WARNING:** Tendon pain/rupture, tendinitis

DOSAGE AND ROUTES
Acute bacterial exacerbation of chronic bronchitis
Adult: PO/IV 500 mg q24hr × 7 days

Acute bacterial sinusitis
Adult: PO 500 mg q24hr × 10-14 days or 750 mg q24hr × 5 days

Mild-moderate UTI/acute pyelonephritis
Adult: PO/IV 750 mg q24hr × 5 days or 250 mg q24hr × 10 days

Chronic bacterial prostatitis
Adult: PO 500 mg q24hr × 28 days

Postexposure inhalational anthrax
Adult/adolescent/child >50 kg: PO/IV 500 mg q24hr × 60 days
Infant >6 mo and child <50 kg: IV 8 mg/kg q12hr × 60 days, max 250 mg/dose

Pneumonia, community acquired
Adult: PO/IV 500 mg q24hr × 7-14 days or 750 mg q24hr × 5 days

Pneumonia, nosocomial
Adult: PO/IV 750 mg q24hr × 7-14 days

SSSI, complicated
Adult: PO/IV 750 mg q24hr × 7-14 days

SSSI, uncomplicated
Adult: PO 500 mg q24hr × 7-10 days

UTI, complicated
Adult: PO/IV 750 mg q24hr × 5 days or 250 mg q24hr × 10 days

UTI, uncomplicated
Adult: PO 250 mg q24hr × 3 days

Plague *(Yersinia pestis)*
Adult: PO/IV 500 mg q24hr × 10-14 days (with pneumonia, 750 mg q24hr)
Adolescent/child <50 kg: PO/IV 8 mg/kg (max 250 mg/dose) q12hr × 10-14 days

Renal disease
Adult: PO/IV CCr 20-49 ml/min: for 750-mg dose, give 750 mg q48hr; for 500-mg dose, give 500 mg once, then 250 mg q24hr; for 250-mg dose, no adjustment; CCr 10-19 ml/min: for 750-mg dose, give 750 mg once, then 500 mg q48hr; for 500-mg dose, give 500 mg once, then 250 mg q48hr; for 250-mg dose, give 250 mg q48hr, except when treating complicated UTI, then no dose adjustment

Available forms: Single-use vials (500, 750 mg), premixed flexible container; 250 mg/50 ml D$_5$W, 500 mg/100 ml D$_5$W, 750 mg/150 ml D$_5$W; tabs 250, 500, 750 mg; oral sol 25 mg/ml

Implementation
• Obtain C&S before treatment and periodically
• Give PO 2 hr before or 2 hr after antacids, iron, calcium, zinc; give fluids
• Check for irritation, extravasation, phlebitis daily

Oral solution
• Give 1 hr prior to or 2 hr after food

Intermittent IV infusion route
• Discard any unused sol in the single-dose vial
• Visually inspect for particulate matter/discoloration prior to use
IV (single use vial)
• **500 mg/20 ml vials:** To prepare a dose of 500 mg, withdraw 10 ml from a 20-ml vial and dilute with a compatible IV solution (D$_5$W, NS) to a total volume of 50 ml. To prepare a 500-mg dosage, withdraw all 20 ml from the vial and dilute with a compatible IV solution to a total volume of 100 ml
• **750 mg/30 ml vials:** To prepare a dose of 750 mg, withdraw 30 ml from a 30-ml vial and dilute with a compatible intravenous solution (D$_5$W, NS) to a total volume of 150 ml
• The concentration of the diluted solution should be 5 mg/ml prior to administration. Solutions contain no preservatives; any unused portions must be discarded
• **Storage:** The diluted solution may be stored for up to 72 hours when stored at or below 25° C (77° F) or for 14 days when stored under refrigeration at 5° C (41° F) in plastic containers. Solutions may be frozen for up to 6 months (−20° C or −4° F) in glass bottles or plastic containers. Thaw frozen solutions at room temperature (25° C or 77° F) or in a

refrigerator (8° C or 46° F). Do not force thaw by microwave or water bath immersion. Do not refreeze after initial thawing

Premixed IV solution

• No dilution is necessary

Intermittent IV injection

• Infuse doses of ≤500 mg IV over 60 minutes and doses of 750 mg IV over 90 minutes. Shorter infusions or bolus injections should be avoided because of the risk of hypotension

Y-site compatibilities: Alemtuzumab, alfentanil, amifostine, amikacin, aminocaproic acid, aminophylline, ampicillin, ampicillin-sulbactam, anidulafungin, argatroban, atenolol, atracurium, aztreonam, bivalirudin, bleomycin, bumetanide, buprenorphine, busulfan, butorphanol, caffeine citrate, calcium gluconate, CARBOplatin, carmustine, caspofungin, cefepime, cefoTEtan, ceftaroline, cefTAZidime, ceftizoxime, cefTRIAXone, cefuroxime, chlorproMAZINE, cimetidine, cisatracurium, CISplatin, clindamycin, codeine, cyclophosphamide, cycloSPORINE, cytarabine, dacarbazine, DACTINomycin, DAPTOmycin, DAUNOrubicin liposomal, dexamethasone, dexrazoxane, digoxin, diltiazem, diphenhydrAMINE, DOBUTamine, DOCEtaxel, dolasetron, DOPamine, doripenem, doxacurium, doxycycline, droperidol, enalaprilat, ePHEDrine, EPINEPHrine, epirubicin, ertapenem, erythromycin, esmolol, etoposide, etoposide phosphate, famotidine, fenoldopam, fentaNYL, filgrastim, floxuridine, fluconazole, fludarabine, foscarnet, fosphenytoin, gallium, gemcitabine, gemtuzumab, gentamicin, granisetron, haloperidol, hydrocortisone, HYDROmorphone, IDArubicin, ifosfamide, imipenem-cilastatin, irinotecan, isoproterenol, labetalol, lepirudin, leucovorin, levorphanol, lidocaine, linezolid, mannitol, mechlorethamine, meperidine, mesna, methylPREDNISolone, metoclopramide, metroNIDAZOLE, midazolam, milrinone, minocycline, mitoMYcin, mitoXANtrone, mivacurium, morphine, mycophenolate mofetil, nalbuphine, naloxone, nesiritide, netilmicin, niCARdipine, octreotide, ondansetron, oxacillin, oxaliplatin, oxytocin, PACLitaxel, palonosetron, pamidronate, pancuronium, PEMEtrexed, penicillin G sodium, pentamidine, phenylephrine, plicamycin, potassium acetate/chloride, promethazine, propranolol, quinupristin-dalfopristin, ranitidine, remifentanil, rocuronium, sargramostim, sodium bicarbonate, succinylcholine, SUFentanil, sulfamethoxazole-trimethoprim, tacrolimus, teniposide, theophylline, thiotepa, ticarcillin, ticarcillin-clavulanate, tigecycline, tirofiban, tobramycin, topotecan, trimethobenzamide, vancomycin, vasopressin, vecuronium, verapamil, vinBLAStine, vinCRIStine, vinorelbine, voriconazole, zidovudine, zoledronic acid

Solution compatibilities: 0.9% NaCl, D_5W, $D_5/0.9\%$ NaCl, D_5LR, $D_5/0.45\%$ NaCl, sodium lactate, plasma-lyte 56/D_5W

ADVERSE EFFECTS

CNS: *Headache,* dizziness, *insomnia,* anxiety, **seizures,** *encephalopathy,* paresthesia, **pseudotumor cerebri**
CV: Chest pain, palpitations, vasodilatation, **QT prolongation (rapid infusion),** hypotension
EENT: Dry mouth, visual impairment, tinnitus
GI: *Nausea,* flatulence, *vomiting,* diarrhea, abdominal pain, **pseudomembranous colitis, hepatotoxicity, esophagitis, pancreatitis**
GU: Vaginitis, crystalluria
HEMA: Eosinophilia, **hemolytic anemia,** lymphophemia
INTEG: Rash, pruritus, photosensitivity, **epidermal necrolysis,** injection site reaction, edema
MISC: Hypoglycemia, hypersensitivity, tendon rupture, **rhabdomyolysis**
RESP: Pneumonitis
SYST: Anaphylaxis, multisystem organ failure, Stevens-Johnson syndrome, angioedema, toxic epidermal necrolysis

Pharmacokinetics

Absorption	Unknown
Distribution	Unknown
Excretion	Kidneys unchanged
Half-life	6-8 hr

Pharmacodynamics

Onset	Immediate
Peak	Infusion's end
Duration	Unknown

INTERACTIONS

Individual drugs

Calcium, iron, sucralfate, zinc: decreased absorption of levofloxacin
Foscarnet: increased CNS stimulation, seizures
Haloperidol, chloroquine, droperidol, pentamidine, arsenic trioxide, levomethadyl: increased QT prolongation
Magnesium: decreased levofloxacin absorption; do not use in same **IV** line
Probenecid: increased levofloxacin levels
Theophylline: decreased theophylline clearance; toxicity may result
Warfarin: increased bleeding

Drug classifications

Antacids (magnesium, aluminum): decreased absorption of levofloxacin

> **BLACK BOX WARNING:** Corticosteroids: increased tendon rupture

Class IA/III antidysrhythmics, some phenothiazines, beta agonists, local anesthetics, tricyclics, CYP3A4 inhibitors (amiodarone, clarithromycin, erythromycin, telithromycin, troleandomycin), CYP3A4 substrates (methadone, pimozide, QUEtiapine, quiNIDine, risperiDONE, ziprasidone): increased QT prolongation

NSAIDs, cycloSPORINE: increased CNS stimulation, seizures

Drug/lab test

Increased: PT, INR
Decreased: glucose, lymphocytes

NURSING CONSIDERATIONS
Assessment

• Assess patient for previous sensitivity reaction to quinolones
• **Assess patient for signs and symptoms of infection,** including characteristics of wounds, sputum, urine, stool, WBC >10,000/mm³, fever; baseline, during treatment
• Obtain C&S before beginning product therapy to identify if correct treatment has been initiated
• **QT prolongation: Monitor for QT prolongation, ejection fraction; assess for chest pain, palpitations, dyspnea**
• **Pseudomembranous colitis: Assess for diarrhea, abdominal pain, fever, fatigue, anorexia; possible anemia, elevated WBC and low serum albumin; stop product and give usually either vancomycin or IV metroNIDAZOLE**
• **Assess for allergic reactions and anaphylaxis: rash, urticaria, pruritus, chills, fever, joint pain; may occur a few days after therapy begins; EPINEPHrine and resuscitation equipment should be available for anaphylactic reaction**
• Determine urine output; if decreasing, notify prescriber (may indicate nephrotoxicity); also check for increased BUN, creatinine
• Monitor blood tests: AST, ALT, CBC, Hct, bilirubin, LDH, alkaline phosphatase, Coombs' test monthly if patient is on long-term therapy
• Monitor electrolytes: potassium, sodium, chloride monthly if patient is on long-term therapy

• Monitor for bleeding: ecchymosis, bleeding gums, hematuria, stool guaiac daily if on long-term therapy
• **Assess for overgrowth of infection: perineal itching, fever, malaise, redness, pain, swelling, drainage, rash, diarrhea, change in cough, sputum**

> **BLACK BOX WARNING: Tendon rupture:**
> Discontinue product at first sign of tendon pain or inflammation; usually the Achilles tendon is affected, can occur up to a few months after treatment and may require surgical repair; steroids may increase risk

Patient/family education

• Teach patient to report sore throat, bruising, bleeding, joint pain; may indicate **blood dyscrasias (rare)**
• Advise patient to contact prescriber if vaginal itching, loose foul-smelling stools, furry tongue occur, may indicate superinfection; report itching, rash, pruritus, urticaria
• Instruct patient to take all medication prescribed for the length of time ordered; product must be taken around the clock to maintain blood levels; do not give medication to others
• Advise patient to notify prescriber of diarrhea with blood or pus
• Instruct patient to take 2 hr before antacids, iron, calcium, zinc products
• Tell patient to complete full course of therapy; to increase fluid intake to 2 L/day to prevent crystalluria
• Advise patient to avoid hazardous activities until response to product is known
• Instruct patient to rinse mouth frequently and use sugarless candy or gum for dry mouth
• Instruct patient to avoid taking other medications unless approved by prescriber
• Teach patient to monitor glucose (diabetes)
• Advise patient to avoid sun exposure or use sunscreen to prevent phototoxicity

> **BLACK BOX WARNING:** Teach patient to notify prescriber of tendon pain, inflammation, avoid corticosteroids with this product

Evaluation
Positive therapeutic outcome

• Absence of signs/symptoms of infection (WBC <10,000/mm³, temp WNL)
• Reported improvement in symptoms of infection

levofloxacin ophthalmic
See Appendix B

levomilnacipran

(lee′voe-mil-na′si-pran)

Fetzima

Chem. class.: Antidepressant

Func. class.: Serotonin

Pregnancy category C

ACTION: May potentiate serotonergic, andrenergic activity in the CNS; is a potent inhibitor of adrenal serotonin and norepinephrine reuptake

Therapeutic outcome: Decreased depression

USES: Major depressive disorder in adults

CONTRAINDICATIONS

Alcohol intoxication, alcoholism, closed angle glaucoma, hepatic disease, hepatitis, jaundice, hypersensitivity

Precautions: Pregnancy **C**, breastfeeding, geriatric patients, mania, hypertension, renal/cardiac disease, seizures, increased intraocular pressure, anorexia, bleeding, dehydration, diabetes, hypotension, hypovolemia, orthostatic hypotension, abrupt product withdrawal

> **BLACK BOX WARNING:** Children, suicidal ideation

DOSAGE AND ROUTES

Adult: PO 20 mg/day × 2 days, then 40 mg/day, may increase in increments of 40 mg at intervals of at least 2 days, max 120 mg/day; max 80 mg/day (strong CYP3A4 inhibitors therapy)

Renal dose

Adult: PO CCr 30-59 ml/min, max 80 mg/day; 15-29 ml/min, max 40 mg/day; <15 ml/min, avoid use

Available forms: Ext rel caps 20, 40, 80, 120 mg

Implementation

• Swallow cap whole; do not break, crush, or chew; do not sprinkle on food or mix with liquid
• Give without regard to food
• Give at the same time of day

ADVERSE EFFECTS

CNS: Dizziness, agitation, hallucinations, seizures, drowsiness, mania, migraine, paresthesias, serotonin syndrome, suicidal ideation, syncope

CV: Hypertension, palpitations, dysrhythmia, sinus tachycardia

EENT: Teeth grinding, blurred vision

GI: Constipation, diarrhea, nausea, vomiting, anorexia, dry mouth, abdominal pain

GU: Urinary retention

SYST: Serotonin syndrome, **Stevens-Johnson syndrome**

Pharmacokinetics

Absorption	Unknown
Distribution	22% protein binding
Metabolism	By CYP2D6 in the liver
Excretion	Unknown
Half-life	12 hr

Pharmacodynamics

Onset	Unknown
Peak	6-8 hr
Duration	Unknown

INTERACTIONS

Individual drugs

Linezolid, methylene blue IV: do not use concurrently

Drug classifications

Anticoagulants, antiplatelets, NSAIDs, salicylates: increased bleeding risk

CYP34A inhibitors: increased levomilnacipran effect

MAOIs: Coadministration contraindicated within 14 days of MAOI

SSRIs, serotonin receptor agonists, SNRIs: increased serotonin syndrome

NURSING CONSIDERATIONS

Assessment

• Serotonin syndrome: assess for nausea/vomiting, dizziness, facial flush, shivering, sweating

> **BLACK BOX WARNING: Depression:** assess mood, sensorium, affect, suicidal tendencies, increase in psychiatric symptoms, depression, panic; monitor children qwk face to face during first 4 wk or dosage change, then every other week for the next 4 wk, then at 12 wk

• Monitor B/P lying, standing; pulse q4hr; if systolic B/P drops 20 mm Hg, hold product, notify prescriber; take VS q4hr in patients with CV disease
• Hepatic studies: monitor AST ALT, bilirubin
• Withdrawal symptoms: assess for headache, nausea, vomiting, muscle pain, weakness; not common unless product is discontinued abruptly

Patient/family education

• Teach patient signs and symptoms of bleeding (GI bleeding, nosebleed, ecchymoses, bruising)

- Instruct patient to use caution when driving and in other activities requiring alertness because of drowsiness and blurred vision
- Instruct patient to avoid alcohol ingestion, MAOIs, other CNS depressants
- Instruct patient not to discontinue medication quickly after long-term use; may cause headache, malaise; taper

BLACK BOX WARNING: Teach patient that clinical worsening and suicidal risk may occur

- Teach patient to notify prescriber if pregnancy is planned or suspected, or if breastfeeding
- Teach patient improvement may occur in 4-8 wk or up to 12 wk (geriatric patients)

Evaluation
Positive therapeutic outcome
- Decreased depression

levothyroxine (Rx)
(lee-voe-thye-rox′een)
Eltroxin ✦, Levothroid, Levoxyl, Synthroid, Tirosint, Unithroid
Func. class.: Thyroid hormone
Chem. class.: Levoisomer of thyroxine
Pregnancy category A

Do not confuse: Synthroid/Symmetrel

ACTION: Controls protein synthesis; increases metabolic rate, cardiac output, renal blood flow, O_2 consumption, body temp, blood volume, growth, development at cellular level via action on thyroid hormone receptors

Therapeutic outcome: Correction of lack of thyroid hormone

USES: Hypothyroidism, myxedema coma, thyroid hormone replacement, thyrotoxicosis, congenital hypothyroidism, some types of thyroid cancer, pituitary TSH suppression

CONTRAINDICATIONS
Adrenal insufficiency, recent MI, thyrotoxicosis, hypersensitivity to beef, alcohol intolerance (inj only)

BLACK BOX WARNING: Obesity treatment

Precautions: Pregnancy **A**, breastfeeding, geriatric, angina pectoris, hypertension, ischemia, cardiac disease, diabetes

DOSAGE AND ROUTES
Severe hypothyroidism
Adult ≤50 yr: PO 1.7 mcg/kg/day, 6-8 wk, average dose 100-200 mcg/day; IM/IV 50-100 mcg/day as a single dose or 50% of usual oral dosage

Adult >50 yr without heart disease or <50 yr with heart disease: PO 25-50 mcg/day, titrate q6-8wk
Adult >50 yr with heart disease: PO 12.5-25 mcg/day, titrate by 12.5-25 mcg q6-8wk
Child >12 yr: PO 2-3 mcg/kg/day given as a single dose AM
Child 6-12 yr: PO 4-5 mcg/kg/day given as a single dose AM
Child 1-5 yr: PO 5-6 mcg/kg/day given as a single dose AM
Child 6-12 mo: PO 6-8 mcg/kg/day given as a single dose AM
Child <6 mo: PO 8-10 mcg/kg/day given as a single dose AM

Myxedema coma
Adult: IV 200-500 mcg; may increase by 100-300 mcg after 24 hr; give oral medication as soon as possible

Subclinical hypothyroidism
Adult: PO 1 mcg/kg/day may be sufficient

Available forms: Powder for inj 100, 200, 500 mcg/vial; tabs 25, 50, 88, 100, 112, 125, 137, 150, 175, 200, 300; cap (liquid filled) 13, 25, 50, 75, 88, 100, 112, 125, 137, 150 mcg

Implementation
- Store in tight, light-resistant container; sol should be discarded if not used immediately
- Withdraw medication 4 wk before RAIU test
PO route
- Give in AM if possible as a single dose to decrease sleeplessness; give at same time each day to maintain product level
- Give crushed and mixed with water, nonsoy formula, or breast milk for infants/children
- Give only for hormone imbalances; not to be used for obesity, male infertility, menstrual conditions, lethargy; give lowest dosage that relieves symptoms; lower dosage for geriatric and in cardiac disease
- Separate antacids, iron, calcium products by 4 hr

Direct IV route
- Give IV after diluting with provided diluent (0.9% NaCl), 500 mcg/5 ml, 200 mcg/2 ml; shake well; give through Y-tube or 3-way stopcock; give 100 mcg or less over 1 min; do not add to IV infusion; considered incompatible in syringe with all other products

ADVERSE EFFECTS
CNS: *Anxiety, insomnia, tremors,* headache, **thyroid storm,** excitability
CV: *Tachycardia, palpitations, angina, dysrhythmias,* hypertension, **cardiac arrest**

Adverse effects: *italics* = common; **bold** = life-threatening

GI: Nausea, diarrhea, increased or decreased appetite, cramps

MISC: Menstrual irregularities, weight loss, sweating, heat intolerance, fever, alopecia, decreased bone mineral density

Pharmacokinetics

Absorption	Erratic (PO); complete (**IV**)
Distribution	Widely distributed
Metabolism	Liver; enterohepatic recirculation
Excretion	Feces via bile; breast milk (small amounts)
Half-life	6-7 days

Pharmacodynamics

	PO	IV
Onset	24 hr	
Peak	12-48 hr	12-48 hr
Duration	Unknown	Unknown

INTERACTIONS
Individual drugs
Aluminum, calcium, iron, magnesium, sucralfate, rifampin, rifabutin: decreased levothyroxine effects

Orlistat, ferrous sulfate: decreased absorption of levothyroxine

Drug classifications
Antacids: decreased levothyroxine effects

Anticoagulants (oral): increased anticoagulant effect

Antidepressants (tricyclics): increased tricyclic effect

Bile acid sequestrants: decreased levothyroxine absorption

EPINEPHrine products: increased cardiac insufficiency risk

Estrogens: decreased thyroid hormone effects

Selective serotonin reuptake inhibitors: decreased levothyroxine effects

Sympathomimetics: increased sympathomimetic effect

Drug/herb
Soy: decreased thyroid hormone effect

Drug/lab test
Increased: CPK, LDH, AST, blood glucose
Decreased: thyroid function tests

NURSING CONSIDERATIONS
Assessment
• Determine if the patient is taking anticoagulants, antidiabetic agents; document on chart

• Take B/P, pulse before each dose; monitor I&O ratio and weight every day in same clothing, using same scale, at same time of day

• Monitor height, weight, psychomotor development, and growth rate if given to a child

• Monitor T_3, T_4, which are decreased; radioimmunoassay of TSH, which is increased; radioactive iodine uptake (RAIU), which is increased if patient's dosage of medication is too low

• Monitor pro-time (may require decreased anticoagulant); check for bleeding, bruising

• Assess for increased nervousness, excitability, irritability, which may indicate a too-high dosage of medication, usually after 1-3 wk of treatment

• Assess cardiac status: angina, palpitations, chest pain, change in VS; the geriatric patient may have undetected cardiac problems and baseline ECG should be completed before treatment

Patient/family education
• Teach patient that product is not a cure but controls symptoms and that treatment is long term

• Instruct patient to report excitability, irritability, anxiety, sweating, heat intolerance, chest pain, palpitations, which indicate overdose

• Advise patient not to switch brands unless approved by prescriber; bioavailability may differ; do not take with food; absorption will be decreased

• Teach patient that product may be discontinued after giving birth; thyroid panel will be evaluated after 1-2 mo

• Teach patient or parent that hyperthyroid child will show almost immediate behavior/personality change; that hair loss will occur in child but is temporary

• Caution patient that product is not to be taken to reduce weight

• Caution patient to avoid OTC preparations with iodine; read labels; other medications should not be used unless approved by prescriber

• Teach patient to avoid iodine-rich food: iodized salt, soybeans, tofu, turnips, high-iodine seafood, some bread

Evaluation
Positive therapeutic outcome
• Absence of depression

• Weight loss, increased diuresis, pulse, appetite

• Absence of constipation, peripheral edema, cold intolerance, pale, cool dry skin, brittle nails, alopecia, coarse hair, menorrhagia, night blindness, paresthesias, syncope, stupor, coma, rosy cheeks

• Improved levels of T_3, T_4 by laboratory tests

• Child: age-appropriate weight, height, and psychomotor development

TREATMENT OF OVERDOSE:
Withhold dose for up to 1 wk; acute overdose: gastric lavage or induced emesis, activated charcoal; provide supportive treatment to control symptoms

⚠ HIGH ALERT

lidocaine, parenteral (Rx)
(lye′doe-kane)
LidoPen Auto-Injector, Xylocaine, Xylocard ✦
Func. class.: Antidysrhythmic (class IB)
Chem. class.: Aminoacyl amide
Pregnancy category B

ACTION: Increases electrical stimulation threshold of ventricle and His-Purkinje system, which stabilizes cardiac membrane and decreases automaticity

Therapeutic outcome: Decreased ventricular dysrhythmia

USES: Ventricular tachycardia, ventricular dysrhythmias during cardiac surgery, MI, digoxin toxicity, cardiac catheterization

CONTRAINDICATIONS
Hypersensitivity to amides, severe heart block, supraventricular dysrhythmias, Adams-Stokes syndrome, Wolff-Parkinson-White syndrome

Precautions: Pregnancy **B**, breastfeeding, children, geriatric, renal/hepatic disease, CHF, respiratory depression, malignant hyperthermia, myasthenia gravis, weight <50 kg

DOSAGE AND ROUTES
Adult: IV BOL 50-100 mg (1-1.5 mg/kg) 25-50 mg/min, repeat q3-5min, max 300 mg in 1 hr; begin **IV** INF 1-4 mg/min (20-50 mcg/kg/min)

Available forms: IV inf 0.2% (2 mg/ml), 0.4% (4 mg/ml), 0.8% (8 mg/ml); **IV admixture** 4% (40 mg/ml), 10% (100 mg/ml), 20% (200 mg/ml); **IV direct** 1% (10 mg/ml), 2% (20 mg/ml); inj (to IV admixture) 20% (200 mg/ml)

Implementation
IM route
• Administer in deltoid, aspirate to prevent **IV** administration
• Check site daily for extravasation

Direct IV route
• Give undiluted (1%, 2% only); give 6 mg or less over 1 min; if using an **IV** line, use port near insertion site, flush with 0.9% NaCl (50 ml)
• Store at room temperature; sol should be clear

Continuous IV infusion route
• Give after adding 1 g/250-1000 ml of D₅W; give 1-4 mg/min; use infusion pump for correct dosage; pediatric inf is 120 mg of lidocaine/100 ml of D₅W; 1-2.5 ml/kg/hr = 20-50 mcg/kg/min; use only 1%, 2% sol

Solution compatibilities: D₅W, D₅/0.9% NaCl, D₅/0.45% NaCl, D₅/LR, LR, 0.9% NaCl, 0.45% NaCl

Y-site compatibilities: Acetaminophen, alemtuzumab, alfentanil, alteplase, amikacin, aminocaproic acid, aminophylline, amiodarone, amphotericin B lipid/liposome, anidulafungin, argatroban, ascorbic acid injection, atenolol, atracurium, atropine, azithromycin, aztreonam, benztropine, bivalirudin, bleomycin, bumetanide, buprenorphine, butorphanol, calcium chloride/gluconate, CARBOplatin, carmustine, ceFAZolin, cefotaxime, cefoTEtan, cefOXitin, ceftaroline, cefTAZidime, ceftizoxime, cefTRIAXone, cefuroxime, chloramphenicol, chlorproMAZINE, cimetidine, ciprofloxacin, cisatracurium, CISplatin, clarithromycin, clindamycin, cyanocobalamin, cyclophosphamide, cycloSPORINE, cytarabine, DACTINomycin, DAPTOmycin, DAUNOrubicin, dexamethasone, dexmedetomidine, dexrazoxane, digoxin, diltiazem, diphenhydrAMINE, DOBUTamine, DOCEtaxel, dolasetron, DOPamine, doxacurium, DOXOrubicin, DOXOrubicin liposomal, doxycycline, enalaprilat, EPINEPHrine, epirubicin, epoetin alfa, eptifibatide, ertapenem, erythromycin, esmolol, etomidate, etoposide, etoposide phosphate, famotidine, fenoldopam, fentaNYL, fluconazole, fludarabine, fluorouracil, folic acid, furosemide, gentamicin, granisetron, haloperidol, heparin, hydrocortisone, imipenem/cilastatin, inamrinone, insulin, isoproterenol, ketorolac, labetalol, levofloxacin, linezolid, LORazepam, magnesium sulfate, meperidine, methylPREDNISolone, metoclopramide, metoprolol, metroNIDAZOLE, micafungin, midazolam, morphine, nafcillin, niCARDipine, nitroglycerin, nitroprusside, norepinephrine, ondansetron, palonosetron, penicillin G potassium, phenylephrine, phytonadione, piperacillin/tazobactam, potassium chloride, procainamide, prochlorperazine, promethazine, propofol, propranolol, protamine, quinupristin/dalfopristin, ranitidine, remifentanil, sodium bicarbonate, tacrolimus, theophylline, ticarcillin/clavulanate, tigecycline, tirofiban, tobramycin, vancomycin, vasopressin, verapamil, vitamin B complex with C, voriconazole, warfarin

Y-site incompatibilities: Acyclovir, amphotericin B cholesteryl sulfate complex/colloidal, azaTHIOprine, caspofungin, diazepam, ganciclovir, lansoprazole, pantoprazole, phenytoin, thiopental, trimethoprim/sulfamethoxazole

ADVERSE EFFECTS

CNS: *Headache, dizziness,* involuntary movement, confusion, tremor, *drowsiness,* euphoria, seizures, shivering
CV: *Hypotension, bradycardia,* heart block, cardiovascular collapse, arrest
EENT: Tinnitus, blurred vision
GI: Nausea, vomiting, anorexia
HEMA: Methemoglobinemia
INTEG: Rash, urticaria, edema, swelling, petechiae, pruritus
MISC: Febrile response, phlebitis at inj site
RESP: Dyspnea, respiratory depression

Pharmacokinetics

Absorption	Complete bioavailability (**IV**)
Distribution	Erythrocytes, cardiovascular endothelium
Metabolism	Liver
Excretion	Kidneys
Half-life	Biphasic 8 min, 1-2 hr

Pharmacodynamics

	IV	IM
Onset	2 min	5-15 min
Peak	Unknown	½ hr
Duration	20 min	1½ hr

INTERACTIONS

Individual drugs

Amiodarone, phenytoin, procainamide, propranolol: increase cardiac depression, toxicity
Cimetidine, metoprolol, phenytoin: increased lidocaine effects
CycloSPORINE: decreased effect of cycloSPORINE
Tubocurarine: increased neuromuscular blockade

Drug classifications

Antihypertensives, MAOIs: increased hypotensive effects
β-blockers, protease inhibitors: increased lidocaine effects, toxicity
Barbiturates: decreased lidocaine effects
Neuromuscular blockers: increased neuromuscular blockade

Drug/lab test

Increased: CPK

NURSING CONSIDERATIONS

Assessment

• Assess for oxygenation or perfusion deficit: decreased B/P, chest pain, dizziness, loss of consciousness
• Assess respiratory status: auscultate lung fields for bibasilar crackles in patients with advanced CHF
• Assess for urinary retention: check for pain, abdominal absorption, palpate bladder; check males with benign prostatic hypertrophy; anticholinergic reaction may cause retention
• Monitor I&O ratio, electrolytes (potassium, sodium, chloride); watch for decreasing urinary output, possible retention
• Monitor liver function tests: AST, ALT, bilirubin, alk phos
• **Monitor ECG continuously to determine product effectiveness, measure PR, QRS, QT intervals, check for PVCs, other dysrhythmias; monitor B/P continuously for hypo/hypertension; check for rebound hypertension after 1-2 hr, prolonged PR/QT intervals, QRS complex; if QT or QRS increases by 50% or more, withhold next dose, notify prescriber**
• Monitor for CNS symptoms: confusion, numbness, depression, involuntary movements; if these occur, product should be discontinued
• Monitor blood levels (therapeutic level 1.5-5 mcg/ml), notify prescriber of abnormal results

Patient/family education

• Teach patient or family reason for use of medication and expected results
⚠ Instruct patient in at-home use of Lidopen Auto-Injector; patient should call prescriber before use if heart attack is imminent

Evaluation

Positive therapeutic outcome

• Decreased B/P, dysrhythmias
• Decreased heart rate
• Normal sinus rhythm

TREATMENT OF OVERDOSE:

Oxygen, artificial ventilation, ECG, administer DOPamine for circulatory depression, diazepam or thiopental for seizures; decreased product or discontinuation may be required

lidocaine topical

See Appendix B

linaclotide
(lin'a-kloe'tide)
Linzess
Func. class.: Functional GI disorder agent
Chem. class.: Selective guanylate cyclase C agonist
Pregnancy category C

Therapeutic outcome: Decreased constipation in IBS

USES: Irritable bowel syndrome (IBS) with constipation, chronic constipation not associated with IBS

CONTRAINDICATIONS
Hypersensitivity, urticaria, infection, sinusitis, GI obstruction

> **BLACK BOX WARNING:** Children <6 yr, infants, neonates

DOSAGE AND ROUTES
Constipation
Adult: PO 145 mcg/day on empty stomach, AM

Irritable bowel syndrome
Adult: PO 290 mcg/day on empty stomach, AM

⚠ HIGH ALERT

linagliptin
(lin-a-glip'tin)
Tradjenta
Func. class.: Antidiabetic
Chem. class.: Dipeptidyl peptidase-4 inhibitor
Pregnancy category B

ACTION: Slows the inactivation of incretin hormones. Concentrations of the active, intact hormones are increased by linagliptin, thereby increasing and prolonging the action of these hormones. Incretin hormones are released by the intestine throughout the day, and levels are increased in response to a meal.

Therapeutic outcome: Decreasing blood glucose level, A1C; decreasing polydipsia, polyphagia

USES: Type 2 diabetes mellitus

CONTRAINDICATIONS
Hypersensitivity to linagliptin, type 1 diabetes mellitus, diabetic ketoacidosis (DKA)

Precautions: Pregnancy category **B**, breastfeeding, adolescents or children <18 years old, debilitated physical condition, malnutrition, uncontrolled adrenal insufficiency, pituitary insufficiency, hypothyroidism, diarrhea, gastroparesis, GI obstruction, ileus, female hormonal changes, high fever, severe psychological stress, uncontrolled hypercortisolism, hyperthyroidism

DOSAGE AND ROUTES
Adult: PO 5 mg/day; when used with a sulfonylurea, a lower dose of the sulfonylurea or insulin may be necessary to minimize the risk of hypoglycemia

Available forms: Tab 5 mg
Implementation
• Given once daily; may give without regard to food
• Store at room temperature

ADVERSE EFFECTS
CNS: Headache
EENT: Nasopharyngitis
ENDO: Hyperuricemia, hypoglycemia
GI: Body weight loss, **pancreatitis**
INTEG: **Serious angioedema, exfoliative dermatitis, hypersensitivity reactions,** urticaria
MISC: Arthralgia, back pain
RESP: Bronchial hyperreactivity (with **bronchospasm**), cough, nasopharyngitis

Pharmacokinetics
Absorption	Rapidly, bioavailability 30%
Distribution	Extensive, tissues; protein binding concentration dependent
Metabolism	Weak CYP3A4 inhibitor
Excretion	90% unchanged, 80% enterohepatic, urine 5%
Half-life	Terminal >100 hr, effective 12 hr

Pharmacodynamics
Onset	Unknown
Peak	Unknown
Duration	Unknown

INTERACTIONS
Individual drugs
Alcohol, cisapride, lithium, metoclopramide, tegaserod: increased need for dosing change
Bumetanide, dextrothyroxine, ethacrynic acid, ethotoin, fosphenytoin, furosemide, glucagon, niacin (nicotinic acid), phenothiazine, phenytoin, torsemide, triamterene: decreased hypoglycemic effect
CloNIDine, dexfenfluramine, disopyramide, fenfluramine, FLUoxetine, guanethidine, octreotide: increased hypoglycemia

Adverse effects: *italics* = common; **bold** = life-threatening

Reserpine, β-blockers: increased masking the signs and symptoms of hypoglycemia

Drug classifications
Beta blockers, ACE inhibitors, angiotensin II receptor antagonists, fibric acid derivatives, monoamine oxidase inhibitors (MAOIs), salicylates, sulfonylureas: increased or prolonged hypoglycemia

Atypical antipsychotics (ARIPiprazole, cloZAPine, OLANZapine, QUEtiapine, risperiDONE, and ziprasidone), carbonic anhydrase inhibitors, estrogens, glucocorticoids, oral contraceptives, progestins, thiazide diuretics, thyroid hormones: decreased hypoglycemic effect

Androgens, quinolones: increased need for dosing change

CYP3A4 inducers (topiramate, rifabutin, pioglitazone, OXcarbazepine, carBAMazepine, nevirapine, modafinil, metyrapone, etravirine, efavirenz, bosentan, barbiturates, aprepitant, fosaprepitant): decreased effect of linagliptin

Drug/lab test
Increased: uric acid

NURSING CONSIDERATIONS
Assessment
• Monitor blood glucose, A1C, during treatment to determine diabetes control
• Monitor CBC baseline and periodically during treatment, report decreased blood counts

Patient/family education
• Teach patient the symptoms of hypo/hyperglycemia and what to do about each; to have glucagon emergency kit available, carry sugar packets
• Advise patient that product must be continued on a daily basis, explain consequences of discontinuing product abruptly; to take only as directed
• Direct patient to avoid OTC products unless approved by prescriber
• Teach patient that diabetes is a life-long illness, product will not cure diabetes
• Advise patient to carry emergency ID with prescriber, condition and medications taken
⚠ Report immediately, skin disorders, swelling, difficulty breathing, or severe abdominal pain

Evaluation
Positive therapeutic outcome
• Improving blood glucose level, A1C; decreasing polydipsia, polyphagia, polyuria, clear sensorium, absence of dizziness

lindane (OTC)
(lin-dane)
Hexit ✦
Func. class.: Scabicide/pediculicide
Chem. class.: Chlorinated hydrocarbon (synthetic)
Pregnancy category C

ACTION: Stimulates nervous system of arthropods, resulting in seizures, death of organism

Therapeutic outcome: Resolution of infestation

USES: Scabies, lice (head/pubic/body), nits in those intolerant to or who do not respond to other agents

CONTRAINDICATIONS
Hypersensitivity; patients with known seizure disorders; Norwegian (crusted) scabies

> **BLACK BOX WARNING:** Premature neonate; inflammation of skin, abrasions, or breaks in skin; seizure disorder

Precautions: Pregnancy **C**, breastfeeding, infants, children <10 yr; avoid contact with eyes

DOSAGE AND ROUTES
Lice
Adult and child: Shampoo using 30 ml, work into lather, rub for 5 min, rinse, dry with towel; use fine-toothed comb to remove nits; most require 1 oz, max 2 oz

Scabies
Adult and child: TOP cream/lotion wash area with soap and water, remove visible crusts; apply to skin surfaces; remove with soap, water 8-12 hr after application; may reapply in 1 wk if needed; TOP apply 1% cream/lotion to skin from neck to bottom of feet, toes; repeat in 1 wk if necessary; most require 1 oz, max 2 oz

Available forms: Lotion, shampoo, cream (1%)

Implementation
• Apply to body areas, scalp only; do not apply to face, lips, mouth, eyes, any mucous membrane, anus, or meatus
• Give topical corticosteroids as ordered to decrease contact dermatitis; provide antihistamines
• Apply menthol or phenol lotions to control itching
• Give topical antibiotics for infection

• Provide isolation until areas on skin, scalp have cleared and treatment is completed
• Remove nits by using a fine-toothed comb rinsed in vinegar after treatment; use gloves
• Caregivers applying these products to another person should wear gloves less permeable to lindane, thoroughly clean hands after application, avoid natural latex gloves

Cream/ointment/lotion
• Use for scabies only; skin should be clean without other products on it, wait 1 hr after bathing or showering before application, shake well, apply under fingernails after trimming, a toothbrush can be used to apply; after application wrap toothbrush in paper and discard, use only a single application, apply as a thin layer over all skin from neck down, close bottle with leftover and discard
• Do not cover, wash off after 8-12 hr using warm (not hot) water, do not leave on >12 hr

Shampoo
• For lice only, do not use other hair products before use, shake well, hair should be completely dry, use only enough shampoo to lightly wet the hair and scalp, work into hair, do not use water, allow to remain only 4 min, rinse and lather away, towel briskly

ADVERSE EFFECTS

CNS: Seizures, stimulation, dizziness
INTEG: *Pruritus, rash, irritation, contact dermatitis*

Pharmacokinetics	
Absorption	20%
Distribution	Fat
Metabolism	Liver
Excretion	Kidneys
Half-life	18 hr

Pharmacodynamics	
Onset	3 hr
Peak	Rapid
Duration	3 hr

INTERACTIONS

Oil-based hair dressing: increased absorption; wash, rinse, and dry hair before using lindane

NURSING CONSIDERATIONS
Assessment

> **BLACK BOX WARNING:** Skin with abrasions, breaks, inflammation; do not use on these areas

• **Infestation:** Assess head, hair for lice and nits before, after treatment; if scabies are present, check all skin surfaces

• Identify source of infection: school, family members, sexual contacts

Patient/family education
• Advise patient to wash all inhabitants' clothing, using insecticide; preventive treatment may be required for all persons living in same house, using lotion or shampoo to decrease spread of infection; use rubber gloves when applying product
• Instruct patient that itching may continue for 4-6 wk; that product must be reapplied if accidently washed off, or treatment will be ineffective; remove after specified time to prevent toxicity
• **Advise patient not to apply to face; if contact with eyes occurs, flush with water**
• Advise patient that sexual contacts should be treated simultaneously
⚠ **Inform the patient of CNS toxicity: dizziness, cramps, anxiety, nausea, vomiting, seizures**

Evaluation
Positive therapeutic outcome
• Decreased crusts, nits, brownish trails on skin, itching papules in skinfolds
• Decreased itching after several wk

TREATMENT OF INGESTION:
Gastric lavage, saline laxatives, **IV** diazepam (Valium) for seizures (if taken orally)

---

linezolid (Rx)
(lih-nee'zoh-lid)
Zyvox
Func. class.: Broad-spectrum antiinfective
Chem. class.: Oxazolidinone
Pregnancy category C

Do not confuse: Zyvox/Ziox/Zosyn

ACTION: Inhibits protein synthesis by interfering with translation; binds to bacterial 23S ribosomal RNA of the 50S subunit, preventing formation of the bacterial translation process in primarily gram-positive organisms

Therapeutic outcome: Negative blood cultures, absence of signs/symptoms of infection

USES: Vancomycin-resistant *Enterococcus faecium* infections, nosocomial pneumonia caused by *Staphylococcus aureus* or *Streptococcus pneumoniae*, uncomplicated or complicated skin and skin structure infections, community-acquired pneumonia, *Pasteurella multocida*, viridans Streptococcus, *E. faecium* infections *S. aureus, S. pyogenes;* can be used for MSSA/MSRA/MDRSP/ strains

---

Adverse effects: *italics* = common; **bold** = life-threatening

CONTRAINDICATIONS
Hypersensitivity

Precautions: Pregnancy **C,** breastfeeding, children, thrombocytopenia, bone marrow suppression, hypertension, hyperthyroidism, pheochromocytoma, seizure disorder, ulcerative colitis, MI, PKU, renal/GI disease

DOSAGE AND ROUTES
Vancomycin-resistant *E. faecium* infections
Adult/adolescent/child ≥12 yr: IV/PO 600 mg q12hr × 14-28 days; max 1200 mg/day
Child <12 yr/infant/term neonate: IV/PO 10 mg/kg q8hr × 14-28 days

Nosocomial pneumonia/complicated skin infections/community-acquired pneumonia/concurrent bacterial infection
Adult: IV/PO 600 mg q12hr × 10-14 days; max 1200 mg/day
Child birth-11 yr: PO 10 mg/kg q8hr × 10-14 days

Uncomplicated skin infections
Adult: IV/PO 400 mg q12hr × 10-14 days; max 1200 mg/day
Adolescent: PO 600 mg q12hr × 10-14 days, max 1200 mg/day
Infant, preterm <7 days old: PO 10 mg/kg q12hr × 10-14 days

Available forms: Tabs 600 mg; oral susp 100 mg/5 ml; inj 2 mg/ml

Implementation
PO route
• Store reconstituted oral susp at room temperature, use within 3 wk
• Give over 30-120 min; do not use **IV** inf bag in series connections, do not use with additives in sol, do not use with another product, administer separately, flush line before and after use

Intermittent IV infusion route
• Do not use if particulate is present; yellow color is normal
• Premixed solutions are ready to use (2 mg/ml)

Y-site compatibilities: Acyclovir, alfentanil, amikacin, aminophylline, ampicillin, aztreonam, bretylium, buprenorphine, butorphanol, calcium gluconate, CARBOplatin, ceFAZolin, cefoperazone, cefoTEtan, cefOXitin, cefTAZidime, ceftizoxime, cefTRIAXone, cefuroxime, cimetidine, ciprofloxacin, cisatracurium, CISplatin, clindamycin, cyclophosphamide, cycloSPORINE, cytarabine, HYDROmorphone, ifosfamide, labetalol, leucovorin, levofloxacin, lidocaine, LORazepam, magnesium sulfate, mannitol, meperidine, meropenem, mesna, methotrexate, methylPREDNISolone, metoclopramide, metroNIDAZOLE, midazolam, minocycline, mitoXANtrone, morphine, nalbuphine, naloxone, nitroglycerin, ofloxacin, ondansetron, PACLitaxel, PENTobarbital, piperacillin, potassium chloride, prochlorperazine, promethazine, propranolol, ranitidine, remifentanil, theophylline, ticarcillin, tobramycin, vancomycin, vecuronium, verapamil, vinCRIStine, zidovudine

Solution compatibilities: D₅W, 0.9% NaCl, LR

ADVERSE EFFECTS
CNS: *Headache,* dizziness, insomnia
GI: *Nausea, diarrhea,* increased ALT, AST, *vomiting,* taste change, tongue color change, **pseudomembranous colitis**
HEMA: **Myelosuppression**
MISC: Vaginal moniliasis, fungal infection, oral moniliasis, **lactic acidosis,** anaphylaxis, angioedema, **Stevens-Johnson syndrome**

Pharmacokinetics

Absorption	Rapid, excessive
Distribution	Protein binding 31%
Metabolism	Oxidation of the morpholine ring
Excretion	Unknown
Half-life	Unknown

Pharmacodynamics

Unknown

INTERACTIONS
Individual drugs
Amoxapine, cyclobenzaprine, maprotiline, methyldopa, mirtazapine, traZODone: increased hypertensive crisis, seizures, coma

Drug classifications
Adrenergic blockers: increased effects of adrenergics
Antidepressants (tricyclics): increased hypertensive crisis, seizures, coma
MAOIs or those that possess MAOI-like action (flurazolidone, isoniazid, procarbazine): do not use together; hypertensive crisis may occur
SSRIs, SNRIs: increased serotonin syndrome
Serotoninergic agents: increased effect

Drug/herb
Green tea, valerian, ginseng, yohimbe, kava: avoid use

Drug/food
Tyramine foods: avoid; increased pressor response

NURSING CONSIDERATIONS
Assessment
- Assess CNS symptoms: headache, dizziness
- Monitor liver function tests: AST, ALT
- Monitor CBC weekly, assess for myelosuppression (anemia, leukopenia, pancytopenia, thrombocytopenia)

⚠ **Pseudomembranous colitis: Assess for diarrhea, abdominal pain, fever, fatigue, anorexia; possible anemia, elevated WBC, and low serum albumin; stop product and usually give either vancomycin or IV metroNIDAZOLE**

⚠ **Serotonin syndrome: at least 2 wk should elapse between continuing linezolid and start of serotonergic agents; assess for increased heart rate, shivering, sweating, dilated pupils, tremor, high B/P, hyperthermia, headache, confusion; if these occur stop linezolid; administer a serotonin antagonist if needed**

⚠ **Lactic acidosis: repeated nausea/vomiting, unexplained acidosis, low bicarbonate level: notify prescriber immediately**

⚠ **Anaphylaxis/angioedema/Stevens-Johnson syndrome: rash, pruritus, difficulty breathing, fever: have emergency equipment nearby**

- **Diabetes mellitus:** Monitor those receiving insulin or oral antidiabetics for increased hypoglycemia

Patient/family education
- Advise patient if dizziness occurs, to ambulate and perform activities with assistance
- Advise patient to complete full course of product therapy
- Advise patient to contact prescriber if adverse reaction occurs
- Advise patient to avoid large amounts of tyramine-containing foods (give list)

Evaluation
Positive therapeutic outcome
- Decreased symptoms of infection, blood cultures negative

RARELY USED

liothyronine (T₃) (Rx)
(lye-oh-thye′roe-neen)
Cytomel, Triostat
Func. class.: Thyroid hormone
Chem. class.: Synthetic T₃
Pregnancy category A

Therapeutic outcome: Correction of lack of thyroid hormone

USES: Hypothyroidism, myxedema coma, thyroid hormone replacement, nontoxic goiter, T_3 suppression test, congenital hypothyroidism

CONTRAINDICATIONS
Adrenal insufficiency, MI, thyrotoxicosis, untreated hypertension

> **BLACK BOX WARNING:** Obesity treatment

DOSAGE AND ROUTES
Adult: PO 25 mcg/day, increase by 12.5-25 mcg q1-2wk until desired response; maintenance dose 25-75 mcg/day; max 100 mcg/day
Geriatric: PO 5 mcg/day, increase by 5 mcg/day q1-2wk, maintenance 25-75 mcg/day

Congenital hypothyroidism
Child >3 yr: PO 50-100 mcg/day
Child <3 yr: PO 5 mcg/day, increase by 5 mcg q3-4day titrated to response; infant maintenance 20 mcg/day; 1-3 yr 50 mcg/day

Myxedema, severe hypothyroidism
Adult: PO 25-50 mcg, then may increase by 5-10 mcg q1-2wk; maintenance dose 50-100 mcg/day

Myxedema coma/precoma
Adult: IV 25-50 mcg initially; 5 mcg in geriatric; 10-20 mcg in cardiac disease; give doses q4-12hr

Nontoxic goiter
Adult: PO 5 mcg/day, increase by 12.5-25 mcg q1-2wk; maintenance dose 75 mcg/day

Suppression test (T₃)
Adult: PO 75-100 mcg daily × 1 wk; ^{131}I is given before and after 1st wk dose

---

RARELY USED

liotrix (Rx)
(lye′oh-trix)
T₃/T₄, Thyrolar
Func. class.: Thyroid hormone
Chem. class.: Levothyroxine/liothyronine (synthetic T₄, T₃)
Pregnancy category A

USES: Hypothyroidism, thyroid hormone replacement

CONTRAINDICATIONS
Adrenal insufficiency, MI, thyrotoxicosis

> **BLACK BOX WARNING:** Obesity treatment

DOSAGE AND ROUTES
Adult: PO a single dose of Thyrolar ¼ or ½ adult dose, adjust as needed at 2-wk intervals
Geriatric: PO ¼ tab initially, adjust q6-8wk

Adverse effects: *italics* = common; **bold** = life-threatening

⚠ HIGH ALERT

liraglutide (Rx)
(lir′a-gloo′tide)
Saxenda, Victoza
Func. class.: Antidiabetic agent
Chem. class.: Incretin mimetics
Pregnancy category C

ACTION: Improved glycemic control and potential weight loss via activation of the glucagon-like peptide-1 (GLP-1) receptor

Therapeutic outcome: Stable and improved serum glucose, HbA1C, weight loss

USES: Type 2 diabetes mellitus in combination with diet and exercise, obesity

CONTRAINDICATIONS
Hypersensitivity, pancreatitis

Precautions: Alcoholism, breastfeeding, children, cholelithiasis, ketoacidosis, diarrhea, elderly, fever, gastroparesis, hepatic disease, hypoglycemia, infection, renal disease, surgery, thyroid disease, trauma, vomiting, pregnancy **C**

> **BLACK BOX WARNING:** Medullary thyroid carcinoma (MTC), multiple endocrine neoplasia syndrome type 2 (MEN 2), thyroid cancer

DOSAGE AND ROUTES
Adult: SUBCUT 0.6 mg/day × 1 wk, then increase to 1.2 mg/day, max 1.8 mg/day

Available forms: Solution for injection 18mg/3 ml prefilled pen

Implementation
SUBCUT route
• Give by SUBCUT only, inspect for particulate matter or discoloration, do not use if unusually viscous, cloudy, discolored, or if particles are present; give daily at any time without regard to meals; pen needles must be purchased separately, use Novo Nordisk needles, prime before first use, see manual for directions; give in thigh, abdomen, or upper arm; lightly pinch fold of skin, insert needle at 90-degree angle or 45-degree angle if thin, release skin, aspiration is not needed, give over 6 seconds, rotate injection sites
• Storage: do not store pen with needle attached; avoid direct heat and sunlight, discard 30 days after first use, after first use may be stored at room temperature or refrigerated, do not freeze; if >3 days have elapsed since last dose, reinitiate at 0.6 mg, titrate
• If dose is missed, resume once daily dosing at next scheduled dose

ADVERSE EFFECTS
CNS: Dizziness, headache
CV: Hypertension
ENDO: Hypoglycemia
EENT: Sinusitis
GI: Abdominal pain, anorexia, constipation, diarrhea, dyspepsia, nausea, vomiting, **pancreatitis**
INTEG: **Angioedema,** erythema, injection site reaction, urticaria
MS: Back pain
SYST: Antibody formation, infection, influenza, **secondary thyroid malignancy, anaphylaxis, angioedema**

Pharmacokinetics

Absorption	Protein binding (98%)
Distribution	Binds to albumin, then released into circulation
Metabolism	Unknown
Excretion	Unknown
Half-life	12-13 hr

Pharmacodynamics

Onset	Unknown
Peak	Peak 8-12 hr
Duration	Unknown

INTERACTIONS
Individual drugs
Atorvastatin, acetaminophen, griseofulvin: increased or decreased effects of each specific drug

Baclofen, cycloSPORINE, tacrolimus, dextrothyroxine, diazoxide, phenytoin, fosphenytoin, ethotoin, isoniazid, niacin, nicotine: increased hyperglycemic reactions

Bortezomib, cloNIDine, alcohol, lithium, pentamidine: increased or decreased hypoglycemic reactions

Dexfenfluramine, fenfluramine, disopyramide, FLUoxetine, mecasermin, octreotide, pegvisomant, salicylates: increased hypoglycemic reactions

Digoxin: decreased digoxin levels

Drug classifications
Angiotensin II receptor antagonists, ACE inhibitors, other antidiabetics, β-blockers, fibric acid derivatives, MAOIs, salicylates: increased hypoglycemic reactions

Protease inhibitors, phenothiazines, atypical antipsychotics, corticosteroids, carbonic anhydrase inhibitors, estrogens, progestins, oral contraceptives, growth hormones, sympathomimetics: increased hyperglycemic reactions

Androgens, quinolones: decreased liraglutide effect

⚠ Nurse Alert   ✴ Key NCLEX® Drug   ≫ Drug Specifics

NURSING CONSIDERATIONS

> **BLACK BOX WARNING:** Thyroid C-cell tumors: monitor during treatment

Assessment
• Watch for hypoglycemic reactions that can occur soon after meals: hunger, sweating, weakness, dizziness, tremors, restlessness, tachycardia
• Assess for hypersensitivity to this product
• Monitor serum glucose, A1C, CBC during treatment
• **Assess for stress:** diabetic patients exposed to stress, surgery, fever, infections may require insulin administration temporarily
• **Assess for serious skin reactions: angioedema; also pancreatitis, secondary thyroid malignancy**

Patient/family education
• Teach patient the symptoms of hypo/hyperglycemia and what to do about each, to have glucagon emergency kit available, carry a carbohydrate source at all times
• Teach patient about side effects associated with therapy such as nausea and vomiting; upward dose titration can be delayed or ignored depending on tolerance
• Teach patient that diabetes is a lifelong illness, product does not cure disease and must be continued on a daily basis
• Instruct patient to carry emergency ID with prescriber's phone number and medications taken
• Advise patient to continue with other recommendations: diet, exercise, hygiene
• Teach patient to test blood glucose using a blood glucose meter
• Advise patient to avoid other medications, herbs, supplements unless approved by prescriber
• **Advise patient to report serious skin effects, abdominal pain with nausea/vomiting**
• Provide patient with written instructions if self-administration is ordered

Evaluation
Positive therapeutic outcome
• Stable and improved serum glucose, A1C, weight loss

lisdexamfetamine (Rx)
(lis-dex'am-fet'a-meen)
Vyvanse
Func. class.: CNS stimulant
Chem. class.: Amphetamine
Pregnancy category C
Controlled substance schedule II

ACTION: Increases release of norepinephrine, DOPamine in cerebral cortex to reticular activating system

Therapeutic outcome: Ability to focus, decreased hyperactivity

USES: Attention-deficit disorder with hyperactivity (ADHD), binge eating disorder

CONTRAINDICATIONS
Hyperthyroidism, hypertension, glaucoma, severe arteriosclerosis, CV disease, anxiety, breastfeeding, hypersensitivity to sympathomimetic amines

Precautions: Pregnancy **C**, children <6 yr, Tourette's syndrome, depression, anorexia nervosa, psychosis, seizure disorder, suicidal ideation, MI, heart failure, alcoholism, aortic stenosis, bipolar disorder

> **BLACK BOX WARNING:** Substance abuse

DOSAGE AND ROUTES
Adult/Child 6-12 yr: PO 30 mg/day in the AM, may increase by 20 mg/day at weekly intervals; max 70 mg/day

Available forms: Caps 10, 20, 30, 40, 50, 60, 70 mg

Implementation
• Provide gum, hard candy, frequent sips of water for dry mouth

> **BLACK BOX WARNING:** Before giving this product, identify substance abuse; there is a high potential for abuse

ADVERSE EFFECTS
CNS: *Hyperactivity, insomnia, restlessness, talkativeness,* dizziness, headache, dysphoria, irritability, aggressiveness, CNS tumor, dependence, addiction, mild euphoria, somnolence, lability, psychosis, mania, hallucinations, aggression, movement disorders, psychiatric events (child)
CV: *Palpitations, tachycardia,* hypertension, decrease in heart rate, **dysrhythmias,** MI, **cardiomyopathy**
EENT: Blurred vision, mydriasis, diplopia
ENDO: Growth inhibition
GI: *Anorexia,* dry mouth, diarrhea, weight loss
GU: Impotence, change in libido
INTEG: Urticaria, **angioedema, Stevens-Johnson syndrome, toxic epidermal necrolysis**
MISC: **Rhabdomyolysis**

Pharmacokinetics

Absorption	Unknown
Distribution	Crosses placenta, breast milk
Metabolism	Liver
Excretion	Urine pH dependent
Half-life	<1 hr

Adverse effects: *italics* = common; **bold** = life-threatening

Pharmacodynamics

Unknown

INTERACTIONS
Individual drugs
AcetaZOLAMIDE, sodium bicarbonate: increased lisdexamfetamine effect

Ascorbic acid, ammonium chloride: decreased lisdexamfetamine effect

Haloperidol, meperidine, modafinil, PHENobarbital, phenytoin: increased CNS effect

Melatonin: increased CNS stimulation

Phenytoin: decreased absorption

Drug classifications
Adrenergic blockers, antidiabetics: decreased effect

Antacids: increased lisdexamfetamine effect

⚠ **MAOIs or within 14 days of MAOIs: hypertensive crisis**

Phenothiazines, tricyclics: increased CNS effect

Urinary acidifiers: decreased lisdexamfetamine effect

Urinary alkalinizers: increased lisdexamfetamine effect

Drug/herb
Eucalyptus: decreased stimulant effect

Green tea, guarana, khat, melatonin: increased stimulant effect

St. John's wort: serotonin syndrome

Drug/food
Caffeine: increased amine effect

NURSING CONSIDERATIONS
Assessment
• Monitor VS, B/P; this product may reverse antihypertensives; check patients with cardiac disease often

• Monitor CBC, urinalysis; in diabetes: blood glucose; insulin changes may be required, since eating may decrease

• **Serotonin syndrome, neuroleptic malignant syndrome: Assess for increased heart rate, shivering, sweating, dilated pupils, tremors, high B/P, hyperthermia, headache, confusion; if these occur, stop product, administer a serotonin antagonist if needed; at least 2 wk should elapse between discontinuation of serotonergic agents and start of this product**

• Monitor height, growth rate in children; growth rate may be decreased

• Assess mental status: mood, sensorium, affect, stimulation, insomnia, irritability

• Assess for tolerance or dependency: an increased amount may be used to get same effect; will develop after long-term use

• Assess for overdose: pain, fever, dehydration, insomnia, hyperactivity

Patient/family education
• Advise patient to decrease caffeine consumption (coffee, tea, cola, chocolate); may increase irritability, stimulation

• Advise patient to avoid OTC preparations unless approved by prescriber

• Teach patient to taper product over several weeks; depression, increased sleeping, lethargy

• Advise to take every day in AM

• Give without regard to meals

• Caps: may take whole or opened with contents dissolved in water and taken

• Avoid breastfeeding

• Advise to use as part of a comprehensive treatment program

• Caution patient to avoid alcohol ingestion

• Advise patient to avoid hazardous activities until stabilized on medication

• Instruct patient to get needed rest; patient will feel more tired at end of day

⚠ **Seizures: Product may decrease seizure threshold; those with a seizure disorder should notify prescriber if seizure occurs**

• Teach patient to report CNS changes, blurred vision, dose may need decreasing

> **BLACK BOX WARNING:** Serious CV effects may occur from increasing dose

Evaluation
Positive therapeutic outcome
• Ability to stay on task, decreased hyperactivity

TREATMENT OF OVERDOSE:
Administer fluids, antihypertensive for increased B/P, ammonium chloride for increased excretion, chlorproMAZINE to antagonize CNS effect

lisinopril (Rx)
(lyse-in'oh-pril)

Zestril

Func. class.: Antihypertensive, angiotensin converting enzyme (ACE) I inhibitor

Chem. class.: Enalaprilat lysine analog

Pregnancy category D

Do not confuse: lisinopril/Risperdal/ Lipitor, Zestril/Zetia/Zipexa

ACTION: Selectively suppresses renin-angiotensin-aldosterone system; inhibits ACE; prevents conversion of angiotensin I to angiotensin II

Therapeutic outcome: Decreased B/P in hypertension, decreased preload, afterload in CHF

USES: Mild to moderate hypertension, adjunctive therapy of systolic CHF, acute MI

Unlabeled uses: Diabetic nephropathy/retinopathy, proteinuria, post MI

CONTRAINDICATIONS
Hypersensitivity, angioedema

> **BLACK BOX WARNING:** Pregnancy **D** (2nd/3rd trimesters)

Precautions: Pregnancy **C** (1st trimester), breastfeeding, renal disease, hyperkalemia, renal artery stenosis, CHF, aortic stenosis

DOSAGE AND ROUTES
Hypertension
Adult: PO initially 10 mg, 10-40 mg/day; may increase to 80 mg/day if required
Child ≥6 yr: PO 0.7 mg/kg/day, up to 5 mg/day; titrate q1-2wk up to 0.6 mg/kg/day or 40 mg/day
Geriatric: PO 2.5-5 mg/day, increase q7day

CHF
Adult: PO 5 mg initially with diuretics/digoxin, range 5-40 mg

Acute myocardial infarction
Adults who are hemodynamically stable: PO give 5 mg within 24 hr of onset of symptoms, then 5 mg after 24 hr, 10 mg after 48 hr, then 10 mg/day

Renal dose
Adult: PO CCr <30 ml/min reduce dose by 50%, initially 5 mg/day, max 40 mg/day; CCr <10 ml/min 2.5 mg/day, max 40 mg/day

Available forms: Tabs 2.5, 5, 10, 20, 30 40 mg

Implementation
• Store in airtight container at 86° F (30° C) or less
• Severe hypotension may occur after 1st dose of this medication; may be prevented by reducing or discontinuing diuretic therapy 3 days before beginning lisinopril therapy
• Without regard to food

ADVERSE EFFECTS
CNS: *Vertigo,* depression, **stroke,** insomnia, paresthesias, *headache,* fatigue, asthenia, *dizziness*
CV: Chest pain, *hypotension,* sinus tachycardia
EENT: Blurred vision, nasal congestion
GI: Nausea, vomiting, anorexia, constipation, flatulence, GI irritation, diarrhea, **hepatic failure, hepatic necrosis, pancreatitis**
GU: **Proteinuria, renal insufficiency,** sexual dysfunction, impotence
HEMA: **Neutropenia, agranulocytosis**

INTEG: Rash, pruritus
MISC: Muscle cramps, *hyperkalemia*
RESP: Dry cough, dyspnea
SYST: **Angioedema, anaphylaxis, toxic epidermal necrolysis**

Pharmacokinetics
Absorption	Variable
Distribution	Unknown
Metabolism	Not metabolized
Excretion	Kidneys, unchanged
Half-life	12 hr

Pharmacodynamics
Onset	1 hr
Peak	6-8 hr
Duration	24 hr

INTERACTIONS
Individual drugs
Alcohol (large amounts), probenecid: increased hypotension
Allopurinol: increased hypersensitivity
Aspirin: decreased lisinopril effect
CycloSPORINE: increased hyperkalemia
Indomethacin: decreased antihypertensive effect
Lithium: increased levels of lithium, toxicity

Drug classifications
Antihypertensives, diuretics, nitrates, phenothiazines: increased hypotension
Diuretics, potassium-sparing, potassium salt substitutes, potassium supplements: increased hyperkalemia
NSAIDs: decreased lisinopril effect

Drug/food
High-potassium diet (bananas, orange juice, avocados, broccoli, nuts, spinach) should be avoided; hyperkalemia may occur

Drug/lab test
Interference: glucose/insulin tolerance tests, ANA titer

NURSING CONSIDERATIONS
Assessment
• Assess blood studies: platelets, WBC with differential: baseline, q3mo; if neutrophils are <1000/mm^3, discontinue treatment
• **Hypertension:** monitor B/P, check for orthostatic hypotension, syncope; if changes occur, dosage change may be required

> **BLACK BOX WARNING:** Assess for pregnancy before starting, pregnancy **(D)**

• Establish baselines in renal/liver function tests before therapy begins

Adverse effects: *italics* = common; **bold** = life-threatening

• Monitor renal/liver function tests: protein, BUN, creatinine; watch for increased levels that may indicate nephrotic syndrome and renal failure; monitor renal symptoms: polyuria, oliguria, frequency, dysuria

• Check potassium levels throughout treatment, although hyperkalemia rarely occurs

• **CHF:** check for edema in feet, legs daily, weight daily, dyspnea, wet crackles

• **Assess for anaphylaxis, toxic epidermal necrolysis, angioedema, allergic reactions: rash, fever, pruritus, urticaria; facial swelling, dyspnea, tongue swelling (rare); product should be discontinued if antihistamines fail to help**

Patient/family education

• Caution patient not to discontinue product abruptly; advise patient to inform all health care providers about taking this product

• Teach patient not to use OTC products (cough, cold, allergy) unless directed by prescriber; serious side effects can occur

• Teach patient the importance of complying with dosage schedule, even if feeling better; to continue with medical regimen to decrease B/P: exercise, cessation of smoking, decreasing stress, diet modifications

• Teach patient to notify prescriber of mouth sores, sore throat, fever, swelling of hands or feet, irregular heartbeat, chest pain, coughing, shortness of breath

• Caution patient to report excessive perspiration, dehydration, vomiting, diarrhea; may lead to fall in B/P

• Emphasize the need to rise slowly to sitting or standing position to minimize orthostatic hypotension; not to exercise in hot weather or increased hypotension can occur

• Caution patient that product may cause dizziness, fainting, light-headedness; may occur during 1st few days of therapy; to avoid activities that may be hazardous

• Teach patient how to take B/P, and normal readings for age-group; advise patient to take B/P regularly

• Instruct patient to avoid increasing potassium in the diet

> **BLACK BOX WARNING:** Advise patient to report if pregnancy is planned or suspected (pregnancy **D**), 2nd/3rd trimesters

Evaluation
Positive therapeutic outcome
• Decreased B/P in hypertension
• Decreased CHF symptoms

TREATMENT OF OVERDOSE: 0.9% NaCl **IV** inf, hemodialysis

lithium (Rx)
(li'thee-um)
Carbolith ✲, Lithane ✲, Lithobid
Func. class.: Antimanic, antipsychotic
Chem. class.: Alkali metal ion salt
Pregnancy category D

ACTION: May alter sodium, potassium ion transport across cell membrane in nerve, muscle cells; may balance biogenic amines of norepinephrine, serotonin in CNS areas involved in emotional responses

Therapeutic outcome: Stable mood

USES: Bipolar disorder (manic phase), prevention of bipolar manic-depressive psychosis

CONTRAINDICATIONS
Pregnancy **D**, breastfeeding, children <12 yr, hepatic disease, brain trauma, organic brain syndrome, schizophrenia, severe cardiac/renal disease, severe dehydration

Precautions: Geriatric, thyroid disease, seizure disorders, diabetes mellitus, systemic infection, urinary retention, QT prolongation

> **BLACK BOX WARNING:** Lithium level >1.5 mmol/L

DOSAGE AND ROUTES
Bipolar disorder (mania)
Adult: PO 300-600 mg tid; maintenance 300 mg tid or qid; EXT REL 900 mg q12hr; dosage should be individualized to maintain blood levels at 0.5-1.5 mEq/L or 0.6-1.2 mEq/L (maintenance)

Geriatric: PO 300 mg bid, increase q7day by 300 mg to desired dose

Child: PO 15-20 mg/kg/day in 3-4 divided doses; increase as needed; do not exceed adult doses; maintain blood levels at 0.4-0.5 mEq/L

Renal dose
Adult: PO CCr 10-50 ml/min 50%-75% of dose; CCr <10 ml/min 25%-50% of dose

Available forms: Caps 150, 300, 600 mg; tabs 300 mg; ext rel tabs 300, 450 mg; syr 300 mg/5 ml (8 mEq/5 ml)

Implementation
• Do not break, crush, or chew caps and slow rel caps
• Administer reduced dosage to geriatric; give with meals to avoid GI upset

---

- Provide adequate fluids (2-3 L/day) to prevent dehydration during initial treatment, 1-2 L/day during maintenance
- Give list of products that interact with lithium

ADVERSE EFFECTS

CNS: *Headache, drowsiness, dizziness, tremors,* twitching, ataxia, **seizures,** slurred speech, restlessness, *confusion,* stupor, memory loss, clonic movements, *fatigue*
CV: *Hypotension,* ECG changes, **dysrhythmias, circulatory collapse, edema,** Brugada syndrome, QT prolongation
EENT: Tinnitus, blurred vision
ENDO: Hypothyroidism, goiter, hyperglycemia, hyperthyroidism, hyponatremia
GI: *Dry mouth, anorexia, nausea, vomiting, diarrhea,* incontinence, abdominal pain, metallic taste
GU: **Polyuria, glycosuria, proteinuria, albuminuria,** urinary incontinence, polydipsia
HEMA: **Leukocytosis**
INTEG: Drying of hair, alopecia, rash, pruritus, hyperkeratosis, *acneiform rash, folliculitis*
MS: *Muscle weakness*

Pharmacokinetics

Absorption	Completely absorbed
Distribution	Reabsorbed by renal tubules (80%); crosses blood-brain barrier; crosses placenta
Metabolism	Unknown
Excretion	Urine, unchanged
Half-life	18-36 hr depending on age

Pharmacodynamics

Onset	Rapid
Peak	½-3 hr
Duration	Unknown

INTERACTIONS
Individual drugs
AcetaZOLAMIDE, aminophylline, mannitol, sodium bicarbonate: increased renal clearance
Calcium iodide, iodinated glycerol, potassium iodide: increased hypothyroid effect
CarBAMazepine, FLUoxetine, methyldopa, probenecid: increased lithium effect/ toxicity
Haloperidol: increased neurotoxicity
Indomethacin, losartan: increased toxicity
Thioridazine: brain damage
Urea: decreased lithium effect

Drug classifications
Antithyroid agents: increased hypothyroid effects
β-Blockers used for lithium tremor: increase masking of lithium toxicity

Neuromuscular blocking agents: increased effect of neuromuscular blocking effects
NSAIDs, thiazides: increased lithium toxicity
Phenothiazines: increased effect of phenothiazines
Theophyllines, urinary alkalinizers: decreased effect of lithium

Drug/herb
Guarana, tea (black/green): decreased lithium effect
- Avoid use with kava, St. John's wort, valerian

Drug/food
Significant changes in sodium intake will alter lithium excretion

Drug/lab test
Increased: potassium excretion, urine glucose, blood glucose, protein, BUN
Decreased: VMA, T_3, T_4, PBI, ^{131}I

NURSING CONSIDERATIONS
Assessment
- **Bipolar disorder:** manic symptoms, mood, behavior before and during treatment
- Assess for lithium toxicity: Vomiting, diarrhea, poor coordination, fine motor tremors, weakness, lassitude; major toxicity: coarse tremors, severe thirst, tinnitus, dilute urine

> **BLACK BOX WARNING:** Monitor serum lithium levels weekly initially, then q2mo (therapeutic level: 0.5-1.5 mEq/L); toxic level >1.5 mcg/L; twitching; toxicity and therapeutic levels are very close; toxicity may occur rapidly; blood levels are measured before the AM dose

- Assess weight daily; check for edema in legs, ankles, wrists; report if present; check skin turgor at least daily
- Monitor sodium intake; decreased sodium intake with decreased fluid intake may lead to lithium retention; increased sodium and fluids may decrease lithium retention
- Monitor urine for albuminuria, glycosuria, uric acid during beginning treatment, q2mo thereafter
- Assess neurologic status: LOC, gait, motor reflexes, hand tremors
- ECG in those >50 yr with CV disease; cardiology consult is recommended in those with risk factors, QT prolongation may occur

Patient/family education
- Provide patient with written information on symptoms of minor toxicity: vomiting, diarrhea, poor coordination, fine motor tremors, weakness, lassitude; major

toxicity: **coarse tremors, severe thirst, tinnitus, dilute urine**
• Advise patient to monitor urine specific gravity; emphasize need for follow-up care to determine lithium effects
⚠ **Advise patient that contraception is necessary, since lithium may harm fetus, pregnancy D**
• Caution patient not to operate machinery until lithium levels are stable and response determined; that beneficial effects may take 1-3 wk
• Provide to the patient a list of products that interact with lithium and discuss need for adequate, stable intake of salt and fluid
• Advise patient to have lithium levels monitored to ensure effectiveness

Evaluation

Positive therapeutic outcome
• Decrease in excitement, poor judgment, insomnia (manic phase)
• Decreased mood swings and lability

TREATMENT OF OVERDOSE:
Induce emesis or lavage, maintain airway, respiratory function; dialysis for severe intoxication

Iodoxamide ophthalmic
See Appendix B

loperamide (OTC, Rx)
(loe-per'a-mide)
Diamode, Imodium, Imodium A-D,
Func. class.: Antidiarrheal
Chem. class.: Piperidine derivative
Pregnancy category C

Do not confuse: Imodium/Indocin, Loperamide/furosemide

ACTION: Direct action on intestinal muscles to decrease GI peristalsis; reduces volume, increases bulk; electrolytes are not lost

Therapeutic outcome: Absence of diarrhea

USES: Diarrhea (cause undetermined), chronic diarrhea, to decrease amount of ileostomy discharge, traveler's diarrhea

CONTRAINDICATIONS
Hypersensitivity, pseudomembranous colitis, constipation, dysentery, GI bleeding/obstruction/perforation, ileus, vomiting

Precautions: Pregnancy **C**, breastfeeding, children <2 yr, hepatic disease, gastroenteritis, toxic megacolon, geriatric patients, dehydration, bacterial disease, AIDS, severe ulcerative colitis

DOSAGE AND ROUTES
Adult: PO 4 mg, then 2 mg after each loose stool, max 16 mg/24 hr
Child 9-11 yr: PO 2 mg, then 1 mg after each loose stool, max 6 mg/24 hr
Child 6-8 yr: PO 2 mg, then 0.1 mg/kg after each loose stool, max 4 mg/day
Child 2-5 yr: PO 1 mg, then 0.1 mg/kg after each loose stool, max 4 mg/24 hr

Traveler's diarrhea (unlabeled)
Adult: PO 4 mg, then 2 mg after each diarrhea stool, max 16 mg/day

Available forms: Caps 2 mg; liquid 1 mg/5 ml; tabs 2 mg; chew tabs 2 mg

Implementation
• Do not break, crush, or chew caps
• Store in airtight containers
• Do not mix oral sol with other sol

ADVERSE EFFECTS
CNS: Dizziness, drowsiness, fatigue
GI: *Nausea, dry mouth, vomiting, constipation,* abdominal pain, anorexia, **toxic megacolon**, bacterial enterocolitis, flatulence
INTEG: Rash
MISC: Hyperglycemia
SYST: **Anaphylaxis, angioedema, toxic epidermal necrolysis**

Pharmacokinetics

Absorption	Poor
Distribution	Unknown
Metabolism	Liver
Excretion	Feces, unchanged; small amount in urine
Half-life	9-14 hr

Pharmacodynamics

Onset	½-1 hr
Peak	Unknown
Duration	24 hr

INTERACTIONS
Individual drugs
Alcohol: increased CNS depression

Drug classifications
Antihistamines, analgesics (opioids), sedative/hypnotics: increased CNS depression

Drug/herb
Chamomile, hops, kava, skullcap, valerian: increased CNS depression
Nutmeg: increased antidiarrheal effect

NURSING CONSIDERATIONS
Assessment
• Monitor electrolytes (potassium, sodium, chloride) if patient is on long-term therapy; check fluid status, skin turgor
• **Stools:** Assess bowel pattern before, during treatment; check for rebound constipation after termination of medication; check bowel sounds
• Check response after 48 hr; if no response, product should be discontinued and other treatment initiated
• **Assess for abdominal distention, toxic megacolon, which may occur in ulcerative colitis**
• **Assess for dehydration, CNS symptoms in children or those with hepatic disease**

Patient/family education
• Caution patient to avoid alcohol and OTC products unless directed by prescriber; may cause increased CNS depression
• Advise patient not to exceed recommended dosage; product may be habit forming; ileostomy patient may take this product for extended time
• Advise patient that product may cause drowsiness and to avoid hazardous activities until response to product is determined
• Teach patient that dry mouth can be decreased by frequent sips of water, hard candy, sugarless gum

Evaluation
Positive therapeutic outcome
• Decreased diarrhea

---

loratadine (Rx, OTC)
(lor-a′ti-deen)
Alavert, Claritin, Children's Claritin RediTabs, Dimetapp, Triaminic Allerchews
Func. class.: Antihistamine (2nd generation)
Chem. class.: Selective histamine (H_1) receptor antagonist
Pregnancy category B

Do not confuse: loratadine/lovastatin/LORazepam/losartan

ACTION: Binds to peripheral histamine receptors, which provides antihistamine action without sedation

Therapeutic outcome: Decreased nasal stuffiness, itching, swollen eyes

USES: Seasonal rhinitis, chronic idiopathic urticaria for those ≥2 yr

CONTRAINDICATIONS
Hypersensitivity, acute asthma attacks, lower respiratory tract disease

Precautions: Pregnancy **B**, increased intraocular pressure, bronchial asthma, breastfeeding, hepatic/renal disease

DOSAGE AND ROUTES
Adult and child ≥6 yr: PO 10 mg/day
Child 2-5 yr: PO 5 mg/day

Renal dose
Adult: PO CCr <30 ml/min 10 mg every other day

Hepatic dose
Adult: PO 10 mg every other day

Available forms: Tabs 10 mg; rapid-disintegrating tabs 10 mg; orally disintegrating tabs 10 mg; syr 1 mg/ml; susp 5 mg/ml; ext rel tabs 10 mg

Implementation
• Give on an empty stomach, 1 hr before or 2 hr after meals to facilitate absorption
• **Rapid-disintegrating tabs:** Place rapidly disintegrating tabs on tongue, then swallow after disintegrated with or without water
• Use within 6 mo of opening pouch; immediately after opening blister pack
• Store in airtight, light-resistant container
• **Ext rel tab:** Do not break, crush, or chew

ADVERSE EFFECTS
CNS: Sedation (more common with increased dosages), headache, fatigue, restlessness
EENT: Dry mouth

Pharmacokinetics
Absorption	Well absorbed
Distribution	Unknown
Metabolism	Liver, extensively, to active metabolite desloratadine
Excretion	Kidneys
Half-life	17-28 hr

Pharmacodynamics
Peak	1.3-2.5 hr
Duration	>24 hr

INTERACTIONS
Individual drugs
Alcohol: increased CNS depression
Cimetidine, ketoconazole: increased loratadine level

Drug classifications
Antidepressants, antihistamines (other), sedative-hypnotics: increased CNS depression

---

Adverse effects: *italics* = common; **bold** = life-threatening

Macrolides (clarithromycin, erythromycin): increased loratadine level

Drug/lab test
False negative: skin allergy tests (discontinue antihistamine 3 days before testing)

NURSING CONSIDERATIONS
Assessment
• **Assess allergy:** hives, rash, rhinitis
• Assess respiratory status: rate, rhythm, increase in bronchial secretions, wheezing, chest tightness

Patient/family education
• Teach all aspects of product uses; to notify prescriber if confusion, sedation, hypotension occur; to avoid driving and other hazardous activity if drowsiness occurs; to avoid alcohol and other CNS depressants that may potentiate effect
• Teach patient to take 1 hr before or 2 hr after meals to facilitate absorption
• Advise patient to use sunscreen or stay out of the sun to prevent burns
• Caution patient not to exceed recommended dosage; dysrhythmias may occur
• Teach patient that hard candy, gum, frequent rinsing of mouth may be used for dryness

Evaluation
Positive therapeutic outcome
• Absence of runny or congested nose, other allergy symptoms

▲ HIGH ALERT

LORazepam (Rx)
(lor-az'e-pam)
Ativan
Func. class.: Sedative-hypnotic, antianxiety agent
Chem. class.: Benzodiazepine, short acting
Pregnancy category D
Controlled substance schedule IV

Do not confuse: LORazepam/ALPRAZolam/clonazePAM

ACTION: Potentiates the actions of GABA, an inhibitory neurotransmitter, especially in the limbic system and reticular formation, which depresses the CNS

Therapeutic outcome: Decreased anxiety, relaxation

USES: Anxiety, irritability in psychiatric or organic disorders, preoperatively; adjunct in endoscopic procedures, status epilepticus

Unlabeled uses: Antiemetic before chemotherapy, rectal use, insomnia

CONTRAINDICATIONS
Pregnancy **D**, breastfeeding, hypersensitivity to benzodiazepines/benzyl alcohol, closed-angle glaucoma, psychosis, history of drug abuse, COPD, sleep apnea

Precautions: Geriatric, debilitated patients, children <12 yr, renal/hepatic disease, addiction, suicidal ideation, abrupt discontinuation

DOSAGE AND ROUTES
Anxiety
Adult/adolescent: PO 2-3 mg/day in divided doses, max 10 mg/day
Geriatric: PO 1-2 mg/day in divided doses, or 0.5-1 mg at bedtime

Insomnia (unlabeled)
Adult: PO 2-4 mg at bedtime; only minimally effective after 2 wk continuous therapy
Geriatric: PO 0.5-1 mg initially

Preoperatively
Adult: IM 50 mcg/kg 2 hr before surgery; **IV** 44 mcg/kg 15-20 min before surgery, max 2 mg 15-20 min before surgery
Child ≥12 yr: IV 0.05 mg/kg

Status epilepticus
Neonate: IV 0.05 mg/kg
Child: IV 0.1 mg/kg up to 4 mg/dose; RECT (unlabeled) 0.05-0.1 mg × 2; wait 7 min before giving 2nd dose

Sedation in mechanically ventilated patients (unlabeled)
Adult/adolescent (intermittent): IV 0.044 mg/kg q2-4hr, prn, max 4 mg

Single-dose IV (infusion)
Adult/adolescent: 0.5-8 mg/hr titrate, use loading dose of 2-4 mg

Available forms: Tabs 0.5, 1, 2 mg; inj 2, 4 mg/ml; conc sol 2 mg/ml

Implementation
PO route
• Give largest dose before bedtime if giving in divided dose
• **Concentrate:** use calibrated dropper; add to food/drink, consume immediately
• Give with food or milk for GI symptoms; crush tab if patient is unable to swallow medication whole; provide sugarless gum, hard candy, frequent sips of water for dry mouth
SUBCUT route
• Use by SUBCUT route for rapid response (investigational use)
IM route
• Give deep in muscle mass; if using for preoperative sedation, give 2 hr or more before surgical procedure
• Use this route when IV route is not feasible

Direct IV route
- Prepare immediately before use; short stability time
- Dilute with sterile water for inj, 0.9% NaCl, or D₅W just before using; give by Y-site or 3-way stopcock at 2 mg/min
- Do not use sol that is discolored or contains a precipitate
- **Do not use in neonates (benzyl alcohol)**

Y-site compatibilities: Acetaminophen, acyclovir, albumin, allopurinol, amifostine, amikacin, amoxicillin, amoxicillin/clavulanate, amphotericin B cholesteryl, amsacrine, atenolol, atracurium, bivalirudin, bleomycin, bumetanide, butorphanol, calcium chloride/gluconate, CARBOplatin, ceFAZolin, cefepime, cefotaxime, cefoTEtan, cefOXitin, cefTAZidime, ceftizoxime, ceftobiprole, cefTRIAXone, cefuroxime, chloramphenicol, chlorproMAZINE, cimetidine, ciprofloxacin, cisatracurium, CISplatin, cladribine, clindamycin, cloNIDine, cyclophosphamide, cycloSPORINE, cytarabine, DACTINomycin, DAPTOmycin, dexamethasone, dexmedetomidine, diltiazem, DOBUTamine, DOCEtaxel, DOPamine, doripenem, DOXOrubicin, DOXOrubicin liposomal, droperidol, enalaprilat, ePHEDrine, EPINEPHrine, epirubicin, eptifibatide, erythromycin, esmolol, etomidate, famotidine, fenoldopam, fentaNYL, filgrastim, fluconazole, fludarabine, fosphenytoin, furosemide, ganciclovir, gatifloxacin, gemcitabine, gentamicin, glycopyrrolate, granisetron, haloperidol, heparin, hydrocortisone, HYDROmorphone, hydrOXYzine, ifosfamide, inamrinone, insulin (regular), irinotecan, isoproterenol, ketorolac, labetalol, lidocaine, linezolid, magnesium sulfate, mannitol, mechlorethamine, melphalan, meropenem, metaraminol, methadone, methotrexate, methyldopate, methylPREDNISolone, metoclopramide, metoprolol, metroNIDAZOLE, micafungin, midazolam, milrinone, minocycline, mitoXANtrone, morphine, mycophenolate, nafcillin, nalbuphine, naloxone, nesiritide, niCARdipine, nitroglycerin, nitroprusside, norepinephrine, octreotide, oxaliplatin, oxytocin, PACLitaxel, palonosetron, pamidronate, pancuronium, PEMEtrexed, pentamidine, PENTobarbital, PHENobarbital, piperacillin, piperacillin-tazobactam, polymyxin B, potassium chloride, propofol, ranitidine, remifentanil, tacrolimus, teniposide, theophylline, thiotepa, ticarcillin, ticarcillin-clavulanate, tigecycline, tirofiban, tobramycin, TPN, trastuzumab, trimethobenzamide, trimethoprim-sulfamethoxazole, vancomycin, vasopressin, vecuronium, verapamil, vinCRIStine, vinorelbine, voriconazole, zidovudine

Y-site incompatibilities: IDArubicin, ondansetron, sargramostim

ADVERSE EFFECTS
CNS: *Dizziness, drowsiness,* confusion, headache, anxiety, tremors, stimulation, fatigue, depression, insomnia, hallucinations, weakness, unsteadiness
CV: *Orthostatic hypotension,* **ECG changes, tachycardia,** hypotension, **apnea, cardiac arrest (IV, rapid)**
EENT: *Blurred vision,* tinnitus, mydriasis
GI: Constipation, dry mouth, nausea, vomiting, anorexia, diarrhea
INTEG: Rash, dermatitis, itching
MISC: Acidosis

Pharmacokinetics

Absorption	Well absorbed (PO); completely absorbed (IM)
Distribution	Widely distributed; crosses placenta, blood-brain barrier
Metabolism	Liver, extensively
Excretion	Kidneys, breast milk
Half-life	42 hr (neonates), 10.5 hr (older child), 12 hr (adult), 91% protein bound

Pharmacodynamics

	PO	IM	IV
Onset	1 hr	15-30 min	
Peak	1-2 hr	1-1½ hr	1-1.5 hr
Duration	12-24 hr	6-8 hr	6-8 hr

INTERACTIONS
Individual drugs
Alcohol: increased CNS depression
Disulfiram: increased LORazepam effects
Oral contraceptives, valproic acid: decreased LORazepam effects

Drug classifications
CNS depressants: increased LORazepam effects

Drug/herb
Chamomile, hops, kava, lavender, valerian: increased CNS depression

Drug/lab test
Increased: AST, ALT

NURSING CONSIDERATIONS
Assessment
- **Assess degree of anxiety; what precipitates anxiety and whether product controls symptoms; other signs of anxiety: dilated**

Adverse effects: *italics* = common; **bold** = life-threatening

pupils, inability to sleep, restlessness, inability to focus
• Assess for alcohol withdrawal symptoms, including hallucinations (visual, auditory), delirium, irritability, agitation, fine to coarse tremors
• Monitor B/P (with patient lying/standing), pulse; check respiratory rate; if systolic B/P drops 20 mm Hg, hold product, notify prescriber; respirations q5-15min if given **IV**
• Monitor CBC during long-term therapy; blood dyscrasias have occurred (rare)
• Monitor for seizure control; type, duration, and intensity of seizures; what precipitates seizures
• Monitor hepatic studies: AST, ALT, bilirubin, creatinine, LDH, alkaline phosphatase
• Assess mental status: mood, sensorium, affect, sleeping pattern, drowsiness, dizziness, suicidal tendencies, and ability of product to control these symptoms; check for tolerance, withdrawal symptoms: headache, nausea, vomiting, muscle pain, weakness after long-term use

Patient/family education
⚠ Teach patient to notify prescriber if pregnancy is planned or suspected; pregnancy (D), do not breastfeed
• Advise patient that product may be taken with food; that product is not to be used for everyday stress or used longer than 4 mo unless directed by a prescriber; to take no more than prescribed amount; may be habit forming
• Caution patient to avoid OTC preparations unless approved by prescriber; to avoid alcohol, other psychotropic medications unless prescribed by physician; not to discontinue medication abruptly after long-term use
• Inform patient to avoid driving and activities that require alertness; drowsiness may occur; to rise slowly or fainting may occur, especially in geriatric
• Inform patient that drowsiness may worsen at beginning of treatment
• Teach patient/family to report suicidal ideation

Evaluation

Positive therapeutic outcome
• Decreased anxiety, restlessness, insomnia

TREATMENT OF OVERDOSE:
Lavage, VS, supportive care

lorcaserin
(lor-ca-ser′in)
Belviq
Func. class.: Weight-control agent (anorexiant)
Chem. class.: Serotonin 2C (5-HT$_{2C}$) receptor agonist
Pregnancy category X
Controlled substance IV

ACTION: Decreases food consumption and decreases hunger by selectively activating 5-HT$_{2C}$ receptors

Therapeutic outcome: Decrease in weight

USES: Obesity management

CONTRAINDICATIONS
Pregnancy (**X**), breastfeeding, hypersensitivity, severe renal impairment

Precautions: Children, other organic causes of obesity, anemia, AV block, bradycardia, bundle branch block, depression, dialysis, liver/kidney disease, multiple myeloma, neutropenia, suicidal ideation, Peyronie's disease, pulmonary hypertension, sick sinus syndrome

DOSAGE AND ROUTES
Renal dose
Adult: PO 10 mg bid; do not exceed recommended dosage

Available forms: Tabs, film-coated 10 mg

Implementation
• Identify obesity if patient is on weight reduction program that includes dietary changes, exercise
• May give without regard to food

ADVERSE EFFECTS
CNS: Insomnia, depression, serotonin syndrome, anxiety, suicidal ideation, dizziness, headache, fatigue
CV: Bradycardia, hypertension
GI: Diarrhea, constipation, nausea
HEMA: Neutropenia, leukopenia, lymphopenia
INTEG: Rash
MS: Back pain

Pharmacokinetics

Absorption	Unknown
Distribution	70% protein binding
Metabolism	Unknown
Excretion	Unknown
Half-life	11 hr

Pharmacodynamics

Onset	Unknown
Peak	Unknown
Duration	Unknown

INTERACTIONS
Individual drugs
Linezolid, buPROPion, lithium, sibutramine, traMADol: increased life-threatening serotonin syndrome

Insulin: increased risk of hypoglycemia with this product

Drug classifications
SSRIs, SNRIs, serotonin receptor agonists, MAOIs, tricyclic antidepressants: increased life-threatening serotonin syndrome

Sulfonylureas: increased risk of hypoglycemia with this product

Drug/herb
St. John's wort: increased serotonin syndrome

NURSING CONSIDERATIONS
Assessment
• Monitor weight weekly; oral hypoglycemic dosage might need to be reduced in diabetic patients
• Monitor blood glucose, CBC with differential, Hct/Hgb, serum prolactin
• Pregnancy (X): do not use in pregnancy
• **Suicidal ideation: use caution in psychiatric disorders with emotional lability; assess for depression, suicidal thoughts/ behaviors**

Patient/family education
• Advise patient to avoid hazardous activities until stabilized on medication
• Inform patient to discuss unpleasant side effects
• **Teach patient to notify prescriber if pregnancy is planned or suspected, pregnancy X**

Evaluation
Positive therapeutic outcome
• Decrease in weight

losartan (Rx)
(low-sar'tan)
Cozaar
Func. class.: Antihypertensive
Chem. class.: Angiotensin II receptor (type AT_1)

**Pregnancy category C (1st trimester),
D (2nd/3rd trimesters)**

Do not confuse: losartan/valsartan,
Cozaar/Zocor

ACTION: Blocks the vasoconstrictor and aldosterone-secreting effects of angiotensin II; selectively blocks the binding of angiotensin II to the AT_1 receptor found in tissues

Therapeutic outcome: Decreased B/P

USES: Hypertension, alone or in combination; nephropathy in type 2 diabetes, proteinuria, stroke prophylaxis in hypertensive patients with left ventricular hypertrophy

CONTRAINDICATIONS
Hypersensitivity

> **BLACK BOX WARNING:** Pregnancy **D** (2nd/3rd trimesters)

Precautions: Pregnancy **C** (1st trimester), breastfeeding, children, geriatric, hypersensitivity to ACE inhibitors, hepatic disease, angioedema, renal artery stenosis, African descent, hyperkalemia, hypotension

DOSAGE AND ROUTES
Hypertension
Adult: PO 50 mg/day alone or 25 mg/day when used in combination with diuretic; maintenance 25-100 mg/day
Child ≥6 yr: PO 0.7 mg/kg/day, max 50 mg/day

Hepatic dose
Adult: PO 25 mg/day as starting dose/volume depletion

Hypertension with left ventricular hypertrophy (benefit does not apply to those of African descent)
Adult: PO 50 mg/day, add hydrochlorothiazide 12.5 mg/day and/or increase losartan to 100 mg/day, then increase hydrochlorothiazide to 25 mg/day

Nephropathy in type 2 diabetes patients
Adult: PO 50 mg/day, may increase to 100 mg/ day

Available forms: Tabs 25, 50, 100 mg

Implementation
• Administer without regard to meals

ADVERSE EFFECTS
CNS: *Dizziness, insomnia,* anxiety, confusion, abnormal dreams, migraine, tremor, vertigo, headache, malaise, depression, fatigue
CV: Angina pectoris, 2nd-degree AV block, **CVA,** *hypotension,* **MI, dysrhythmias**
EENT: Blurred vision, burning eyes, conjunctivitis
GI: *Diarrhea, dyspepsia,* anorexia, constipation, dry mouth, flatulence, gastritis, vomiting

Adverse effects: *italics* = common; **bold** = life-threatening

GU: Impotence, nocturia, urinary frequency, urinary tract infection, **renal failure**
HEMA: Anemia, **thrombocytopenia**
INTEG: Alopecia, dermatitis, dry skin, flushing, photosensitivity, rash, pruritus, sweating **angioedema**
META: Gout, hyperkalemia, hypoglycemia
MS: Cramps, myalgia, pain, stiffness
RESP: *Cough, upper respiratory infection,* congestion, dyspnea, bronchitis

Pharmacokinetics

Absorption	Well absorbed
Distribution	Bound to plasma proteins
Metabolism	Extensive
Excretion	Feces, urine
Half-life	Biphasic, 2 hr, 6-9 hr

Pharmacodynamics

Unknown

INTERACTIONS
Individual drugs
Fluconazole: increased antihypertensive effect
Lithium: increased toxicity
PHENobarbital, rifamycin: decreased antihypertensive effect

Drug classifications
ACE inhibitors, diuretics (potassium-sparing), potassium supplements: increased hyperkalemia
NSAIDs, salicylates: decreased antihypertensive effect

NURSING CONSIDERATIONS
Assessment
• Assess B/P with position changes, pulse q4hr; note rate, rhythm, quality
• Monitor electrolytes: potassium, sodium, chloride
• Obtain baselines for renal, electrolyte, liver function tests before therapy begins
• **CHF:** assess for jugular vein distention, weight daily, edema in feet, legs daily
• **Angioedema: facial swelling, dyspnea, wheezing, may occur rapidly, tongue swelling (rare)**
• **Blood dyscrasias: thrombocytopenia, anemia (rare)**

Patient/family education
• Teach patient to avoid sunlight or wear sunscreen if in sunlight; photosensitivity may occur
• Advise patient to comply with dosage schedule, even if feeling better
• Teach patient to notify prescriber of mouth sores, fever, swelling of hands or feet, irregular heartbeat, chest pain

• Advise patient that excessive perspiration, dehydration, vomiting, diarrhea may lead to fall in blood pressure, consult prescriber if these occur
• Inform patient that product may cause dizziness, fainting; light-headedness may occur, to avoid hazardous activities until reaction is known
• Caution patient to rise slowly to sitting or standing position to minimize orthostatic hypotension

> **BLACK BOX WARNING:** Advise patient to use contraception while taking this product, pregnancy **D** 2nd/3rd trimesters

Evaluation
Positive therapeutic outcome
• Decreased B/P

loteprednol ophthalmic
See Appendix B

lovastatin (Rx)
(loe′va-sta-tin)
Altoprev, Mevacor
Func. class.: Antilipemic
Chem. class.: HMG-CoA reductase inhibitor
Pregnancy category X

Do not confuse: lovastatin/Lotensin/Leustatin, **Mevacor**/mivacron

ACTION: By inhibiting HMG-CoA reductase, which reduces cholesterol synthesis

Therapeutic outcome: Decreased cholesterol levels and LDL, increased HDL

USES: As an adjunct in primary hypercholesterolemia (types IIa, IIb), atherosclerosis, heterozygous familial hypercholesterolemia (adolescents)

CONTRAINDICATIONS
Pregnancy **X,** breastfeeding, hypersensitivity, active liver disease

Precautions: Past liver disease, alcoholism, severe acute infections, trauma, hypotension, uncontrolled seizure disorders, severe metabolic disorders, electrolyte imbalances, visual condition, children

DOSAGE AND ROUTES
Adult: PO 20 mg/day with evening meal; may increase to 20-40 mg/day in single or divided doses; max 40 mg/day; ext rel 20-60 mg/day at bedtime; max 40 mg/day

---

Heterozygous familial hypercholesterolemia

Adolescent 10-17 yr: PO 10-40 mg with evening meal

Renal dose
Adult: PO CCr <30 mg/min max 20 mg/day unless titrated

Available forms: Tabs 10, 20, 40 mg; ext rel tab 10, 20, 40, 60 mg

Implementation

• Give with evening meal; if dosage is increased, take with breakfast and evening meal
• Altroprev is not equivalent to Mevacor
• Store in cool environment in airtight, light-resistant container
• Do not crush or chew ext rel tab

ADVERSE EFFECTS

CNS: Dizziness, headache, tremor, insomnia, paresthesia

EENT: Blurred vision, lens opacities

GI: Nausea, constipation, diarrhea, dyspepsia, *flatus,* abdominal pain, heartburn, **liver dysfunction,** vomiting, acid regurgitation, dry mouth, dysgeusia

HEMA: **Thrombocytopenia, hemolytic anemia, leukopenia**

INTEG: Rash, pruritus, photosensitivity

MS: Muscle cramps, myalgia, **myositis, rhabdomyolysis;** leg, shoulder, or localized pain

Pharmacokinetics

Absorption	Poorly absorbed, erratic
Distribution	Crosses placenta, blood-brain barrier
Metabolism	Liver, extensively
Excretion	Feces (83%); kidneys, urine (10%)
Half-life	3-4 hr

Pharmacodynamics

Onset	Unknown
Peak	2-4 hr
Duration	Unknown

INTERACTIONS
Individual drugs

Bosentan, exonatide: decreased action of lovastatin

Clarithromycin, clofibrate, cycloSPORINE, danazol, diltiazem, erythromycin, gemfibrozil, niacin, quinupristin-dalfopristin, telithromycin, verapamil: increased myalgia, myositis, rhabdomyolysis; avoid concurrent use

Diltiazem: increased lovastatin effects
Warfarin: increased bleeding

Drug classifications

Azole antifungals, protease inhibitors: increased myositis, myalgia, rhabdomyolysis
Bile acid sequestrants: decreased lovastatin effects

Drug/herb

Pectin, St. John's wort: decreased effect
Red yeast rice: increased adverse reactions

Drug/food

Increased levels of lovastatin with food, must be taken with food
Grapefruit juice: increased toxicity
Oat bran: decreased absorption

Drug/lab test

Increased: CPK, liver function tests

NURSING CONSIDERATIONS
Assessment

• Assess nutrition: fat, protein, carbohydrates; nutritional analysis should be completed by dietitian before treatment
• Monitor bowel pattern daily; diarrhea may be a problem
• Monitor triglycerides, fasting cholesterol LDL, HDL at baseline, throughout treatment; watch LDL and VLDL closely; if increased, product should be discontinued
• Assess for muscle pain, tenderness, obtain CPK; if these occur, product may need to be discontinued
• **Rhabdomyolysis: muscle pain, increased CPK, weakness, swelling of affected muscles; if these occur and if confirmed by CPK, product should be discontinued**

Patient/family education

• Inform patient that compliance is needed for positive results to occur; not to double doses
• Inform patient that blood work and ophthalmic exam will be necessary during treatment
• Teach patient that risk factors should be decreased: high-fat diet, smoking, alcohol consumption, absence of exercise
⚠ **Advise patient to report if pregnancy is suspected, pregnancy X, do not breastfeed**
• Advise patient to notify prescriber if the GI symptoms of diarrhea, abdominal or epigastric pain, nausea, vomiting occur; or if chills, fever, sore throat, blurred vision, dizziness, headache, muscle pain, weakness occur
• Advise patient to stay out of the sun or use sunscreen to prevent burns
• Instruct patient that product should be taken with food, not to crush, chew ext rel product

Evaluation
Positive therapeutic outcome
- Decreased cholesterol, serum triglyceride levels
- Improved level of HDL

RARELY USED

loxapine (Rx)
(lox'a-peen)
Adasuve, Loxapac ✦
Func. class.: Antipsychotic/neuroleptic
Chem. class.: Dibenzoxazepine
Pregnancy category C

Therapeutic outcome: Decreased psychotic behavior

USES: Schizophrenia, bipolar disorder

Unlabeled uses: Depression, anxiety

CONTRAINDICATIONS
Hypersensitivity, coma

> **BLACK BOX WARNING:** Acute bronchospasm, asthma, COPD, emphysema

DOSAGE AND ROUTES
Adult: PO 10 mg bid-qid initially; may be rapidly increased depending on severity of condition; maintenance 60-100 mg/day; inhalation powder 10 mg as a single dose in 24 hr
Geriatric: PO 5-10 mg/day bid, increase q4-7day by 5-10 mg, max 250 mg/day

Evaluation
Positive therapeutic outcome
- Decrease in emotional excitement, hallucinations, delusions, paranoia
- Reorganization of patterns of thought, speech

TREATMENT OF OVERDOSE:
Lavage; barbiturates; provide airway, **IV** fluids; do not use EPINEPHrine, which may increase hypotension

---

RARELY USED

lubiprostone (Rx)
(loo-bee-pros'tone)
Amitiza
Func. class.: Miscellaneous gastrointestinal agent
Pregnancy category C

USES: Chronic idiopathic constipation, constipation-predominant irritable bowel syndrome in women >18 yr, opiate agonist–induced constipation with chronic noncancer pain

CONTRAINDICATIONS
Hypersensitivity, GI obstruction

DOSAGE AND ROUTES
Chronic idiopathic constipation/opiate agonist–induced constipation
Adult: PO 24 mcg bid with food/water

IBS with constipation (women)
Adult and adolescent ≥18 yr: PO 8 mcg bid with food and water

Hepatic dosage
Adult: For chronic constipation 16 mcg bid (Child-Pugh B); 8 mcg bid (Child-Pugh C); for irritable bowel: 8 mcg daily (Child-Pugh C), may be increased if tolerated

---

RARELY USED

lucinactant
(loo'sin-ak'tant)
Surfaxin
Func. class.: Synthetic lung surfactant

USES: Prevention of respiratory distress syndrome (RDS) in premature neonates

DOSAGE AND ROUTES
Premature neonate
Intratracheal 5.8 ml/kg birth weight divided in 4 doses; give each dose with neonate in a different position; provide positive pressure ventilation when stable; dosage may be repeated 4 times in first 48 hr

---

lurasidone (Rx)
(loo-ras'i-done)
Latuda
Func. class.: Atypical antipsychotic
Chem. class.: Benzoisothiazol derivative
Pregnancy category B

ACTION: May modulate central dopaminergic and serotoninergic activity, high affinity for dopamine-D_2 receptors, serotonin 5-HT_{2A} receptors, and partial agonist at serotonin 5-HT_{1A} receptor

Therapeutic outcome: Decreasing hallucinations, delusions, agitation, social withdrawal

USES: Schizophrenia, depression associated with bipolar disorder I

CONTRAINDICATIONS
Hypersensitivity

Precautions: Abrupt discontinuation, ambient temperature increase, breast cancer, breastfeeding, cardiac disease, children, dehydration, diabetes, ketoacidosis, driving/operating machinery, dysphagia, geriatrics, heart failure, hematological/hepatic/renal disease, hypotension, hypovolemia, MI, infertility, obesity, Parkinson's disease, pregnancy **B**, seizures, strenuous exercise, stroke, substance abuse, suicidal ideation, syncope, tardive dyskinesia

BLACK BOX WARNING: Dementia: antipsychotics, such as lurasidone, are not approved for the treatment of dementia-related psychosis in geriatric patients and may increase the risk of death in this population

DOSAGE AND ROUTES
Schizophrenia
Adult: PO 40 mg/day, range 40-160 mg/day, those receiving CYP3A4 inhibitors (max 80 mg/day), do not use with strong CYP3A4 inducers/inhibitors

Bipolar disorder I
Adult: PO 20 mg qday, max 120 mg/day

Hepatic/renal dose
Adult: PO Child-Pugh class B/C, CCr ≥10 ml/min-<50 ml/min max 40 mg/day

Available forms: 20, 40, 80, 120 mg tabs

Implementation
• Give with a meal of at least 350 calories
• Store at room temperature, protect from moisture

ADVERSE EFFECTS
CNS: Agitation, akathisia, anxiety, dizziness, drowsiness, fatigue, hyperthermia, insomnia, dystonic reactions; **neuroleptic malignant syndrome (rare)**, pseudoparkinsonism, restlessness, **seizures, suicidal ideation**, syncope, tardive dyskinesia, vertigo
CV: Angina, **AV block, bradycardia**, hypertension, orthostatic hypotension, **sinus tachycardia, stroke**
EENT: Blurred vision
ENDO: Diabetes mellitus, ketoacidosis, hyperglycemia, hyperprolactimemia
GI: Abdominal pain, diarrhea, dyspepsia, nausea, vomiting, gastritis, weight gain/loss
GU: Amenorrhea, breast enlargement, dysmenorrhea, impotence, dysuria, renal failure
HEMA: **Agranulocytosis, anemia, leucopenia, neutropenia**
INTEG: Pruritus, rash
MS: Back pain, dysarthria; **rhabdomyolysis (rare)**
SYST: **Angioedema**

Pharmacokinetics
Absorption	9%-19%
Distribution	99% protein binding
Metabolism	Unknown
Excretion	80% feces, 9% urine
Half-life	18 hr

Pharmacodynamics
Onset	Unknown
Peak	1-3 hr
Duration	Steady state 7 days

INTERACTIONS
Individual drugs
Metoclopramide: do not use concurrently

Drug classifications
Other CNS depressants, alcohol: increased sedation
Strong CYP3A4 inhibitors: increased lurasidone effect, do not use concurrently
SSRIs, SNRIs: increased serotonin syndrome, neuroleptic malignant syndrome

NURSING CONSIDERATIONS
Assessment
• **Assess for schizophrenia:** hallucinations, delusions, agitation, social withdrawal; monitor orientation, behavior, mood prior to and periodically during therapy
• **Assess for neuroleptic malignant syndrome (rare): fever, dyspnea, tachycardia, seizures, sweating, hypertension, hypotension, muscle stiffness, pallor, report immediately**
• **Monitor for blood dyscrasias: CBC periodically, blood dyscrasias may occur**
• **Monitor for serious cardiac symptoms: AV block, stroke, bradycardia may occur**
• Assess AIMS assessment, thyroid function tests, LFTs, lipid panel, electrolytes
• **Assess for EPS:** restlessness, difficulty speaking, loss of balance, pill rolling, masklike face, shuffling gait, rigidity, tremors, muscle spasms; monitor prior to and periodically during therapy; report tardive dyskinesia immediately

BLACK BOX WARNING: Dementia: This product is not approved for the elderly with dementia-related psychosis

• Monitor for weight gain, hyperglycemia, metabolic changes in diabetes

Patient/family education
• Explain reason for treatment and expected results

    Adverse effects: *italics* = common; **bold** = life-threatening

- Teach patient to report EPS, blood dyscrasias: sore throat, fever, unusual bleeding/bruising
- Teach patient that lab work will be needed regularly
- Advise patient to avoid hazardous activities until response is known
- Teach patient to avoid OTC products unless approved by prescriber
- Teach patient to report fast heartbeat, extra beats

Evaluation

Positive therapeutic outcome
- Decreasing hallucinations, delusions, agitation, social withdrawal

luliconazole topical
See Appendix B

lymphocyte immune globulin (antithymocyte) (Rx)
Atgam
Func. class.: Immune globulin immunosuppressant
Pregnancy category C

ACTION: Produces immunosuppression by inhibiting the function of T lymphocytes

Therapeutic outcome: Absence of transplant rejection; hematologic remission (aplastic anemia)

USES: Renal organ transplants to prevent rejection, aplastic anemia

Unlabeled uses: Immunosuppressant in liver, bone marrow, heart and other organ transplants, stem cell transplant preparations

CONTRAINDICATIONS
Hypersensitivity to this product or equine/porcine protein, acute illness

Precautions: Pregnancy **C**, breastfeeding, children, severe renal/hepatic disease, leukopenia, thrombocytopenia

> **BLACK BOX WARNING:** Infection, neoplastic disease

DOSAGE AND ROUTES
Renal allograft
Adult/child: **IV** 10-15 mg/kg/day × 14 days, then every other day for 14 more days if needed up to 21 days total

Delay of renal allograft rejection
Adult: **IV** 15 mg/kg/day × 7-14 days, then every other day × 14 days for a total of 21 doses in 28 days

Aplastic anemia
Adult: **IV** 10-20 mg/kg/day × 8-14 days, then every other day for up to 21 total doses

Available forms: Inj 50 mg horse gamma globulin/ml

Implementation

IV route
- Use 0.2-1 micron in-line filter
- Do not infuse <4 hr
- Keep emergency equipment nearby for severe allergic reactions
- **Aplastic anemia:** Skin testing must be completed before treatment; use intradermal inj of 0.1 ml of a 1:1000 dilution (5 mcg of horse IgG) in 0.9% NaCl; if a wheal or rash or both >10 mm, use caution during inf
- Dilute in saline sol before inf; invert **IV** bag, so undiluted product does not contact the air inside; concentration should not be >4 mg/ml

ADVERSE EFFECTS
Renal transplant
CNS: Fever, chills, headache, dizziness, weakness, faintness, **seizures**
CV: Chest pain, hypo/hypertension, tachycardia
GI: Diarrhea, nausea, vomiting, epigastric pain, **GI bleeding**
INTEG: Rash, pruritus, urticaria, wheal, injection site reactions
SYST: Anaphylaxis

Aplastic anemia
CNS: Fever, chills, headache, **seizures**, lightheadedness, encephalitis, postviral encephalopathy
CV: Bradycardia, myocarditis, irregularity
GI: Nausea, liver function test abnormality
HEMA: Thrombocytopenia

Pharmacokinetics

Absorption	Unknown
Distribution	Unknown
Metabolism	Unknown
Excretion	Unknown
Half-life	5.7 days

Pharmacodynamics

Onset	Rapid
Peak	Unknown
Duration	Unknown

NURSING CONSIDERATIONS
Assessment
• Assess for infection; if infection occurs, evaluation will be needed to continue treatment
• Monitor renal function tests: BUN, creatinine at least monthly during treatment, 3 mo after treatment
• Monitor liver function tests: alkaline phosphatase, AST, ALT, bilirubin

Patient/family education
• Advise patient to report fever, rash, chills, sore throat, fatigue, since serious infections may occur
• **Caution patient to use contraceptive measures during treatment and for 12 wk after ending therapy; product is teratogenic**
• Caution patient to avoid crowds and persons with known infections to reduce risk of infection

Evaluation
Positive therapeutic outcome
• Absence of graft rejection
• Hematologic recovery (aplastic anemia)

L

macitentan

(ma'si-ten'tan)

Opsumit

Func. class.: Antihypertensive

Chem. class.: Vasodilator/endothelin receptor antagonist

Pregnancy category X

ACTION: Prevents the binding of ET-1 to ETA and ETB receptors on human pulmonary arterial smooth muscle

USES: Pulmonary arterial hypertension; WHO Group 1 to delay disease progression

CONTRAINDICATIONS

Breastfeeding, hypersensitivity, (pregnancy category **X**)

Precautions: Anemia, hepatic disease, pulmonary edema

DOSAGE AND ROUTES

Adult: PO 10 mg/day

Available forms: Tabs 10 mg

Implementation

• Do not break, crush, chew tabs; take without regard to food; if a dose is missed, then take when remembered (do not take more than 1 tab/day)

• Do not discontinue abruptly

ADVERSE EFFECTS

CNS: Headache

GI: Hepatotoxicity

GU: Decreased sperm counts

HEMA: Anemia

RESP: Pharyngitis, pulmonary edema, bronchitis

Pharmacokinetics

Absorption	Rapid
Distribution	Unknown
Metabolism	By CYP3A4, CYP2C19
Excretion	Unknown
Half-life	Terminal: 15 hr; effective: 9 hr

Pharmacodynamics

Onset	Unknown
Peak	2 hr
Duration	Unknown

INTERACTIONS

Drug classifications

CYP3A4 inhibitors: increased macitentan effect

Drug/herb

St. John's wort, ephedra (ma huang): require macitentan dosage change

NURSING CONSIDERATIONS

Assessment

• **Pulmonary status:** improvement in breathing, ability to exercise; pulmonary edema that may indicate venoocclusive disease

• Blood studies: CBC with differential; Hct, Hgb may be decreased

• Liver function tests: AST, ALT, bilirubin

> **BLACK BOX WARNING:** Assess pregnancy status before giving this product; pregnancy category **X**

Patient/family education

• Teach patient the importance of complying with dosage schedule even if feeling better

> **BLACK BOX WARNING:** Instruct patient to notify prescriber if pregnancy is planned or suspected (if pregnant, product will need to be discontinued; pregnancy test done monthly); to use 2 contraception methods while taking this product

• Instruct patient not to use OTC products including herbs, supplements, unless approved by prescriber

• Instruct patient to report to prescriber immediately: dizziness, faintness, chest pain, palpitations, uneven or rapid heart rate, headache, edema, weight gain

• Instruct patient not to split, crush, or chew tabs; if a dose is missed, take as soon as remembered (do not take more than 1 tab per day); there are many drug interactions

• Teach patient the signs and symptoms of hepatotoxicity

Evaluation

Positive therapeutic outcome

• Decrease in B/P, decreased shortness of breath

mafenide topical

See Appendix B

magaldrate (OTC)

(mag'al-drate)

Isopan, Losapan ✦, Riopan, Riopan Extra Strength ✦

Func. class.: Antacid

Chem. class.: Aluminum/magnesium hydroxide

Pregnancy category C

ACTION: Neutralizes gastric acidity; product is dissolved in gastric contents; this product is a combination of aluminum and magnesium

Therapeutic outcome: Decreased pain of ulcers

USES: Antacid, hiatal hernia, indigestion/heartburn, hyperacidity

Unlabeled uses: Duodenal and gastric ulcers, peptic ulcer disease (adjunct), reflex esophagitis

CONTRAINDICATIONS
Hypersensitivity to this product or benzyl alcohol

Precautions: Pregnancy **C,** geriatric, fluid restriction, decreased GI motility, GI obstruction, dehydration, renal disease, sodium-restricted diets, bone disease, hypertension, appendicitis, diverticulitis, ulcerative colitis, neonates/infants, hypermagnesemia, hypophosphatemia

DOSAGE AND ROUTES
Adult/child/geriatric: SUSP 5-10 ml (480-1080 mg) with water between meals, at bedtime

Available forms: SUSP 540 mg/5 ml

Implementation
• Take antacids 2 hr before or 2 hr after taking enteric-coated products
• Give laxatives or stool softeners if constipation occurs
• Give SUSP after shaking; give between meals and at bedtime
• Give when stomach is empty after meals and at bedtime

ADVERSE EFFECTS
GI: Constipation, diarrhea, anorexia
META: Hypermagnesemia, hypophosphatemia

Pharmacokinetics

Absorption	Not absorbed
Distribution	Not distributed
Metabolism	Not metabolized
Excretion	Kidneys
Half-life	Unknown

Pharmacodynamics

Onset	Unknown
Peak	½ hr
Duration	1 hr

INTERACTIONS
Individual drugs
ChlordiazePOXIDE, cimetidine, isoniazid, ketoconazole, phenytoin, tetracycline: decreased absorption of each specific product
Flecainide, quiNIDine: increased action when taken in large amounts

Drug classifications
Amphetamines: increased action when taken in large amounts

Anticholinergics, corticosteroids, fluoroquinolones, iron salts, phenothiazines, salicylates: decreased absorption of each specific product
Salicylates: decreased action when taken in large amounts

NURSING CONSIDERATIONS
Assessment
• **Antacid:** location of pain, intensity, characteristics, what aggravates, ameliorates pain; heartburn/indigestion; hematemesis
• Monitor serum magnesium, calcium, phosphate, potassium if using long term or with impaired renal function
• Assess for constipation: increase bulk in diet if needed or obtain order for stool softener

Patient/family education
• Advise patient to separate ingestion of enteric-coated products and antacid by 2 hr
• Advise patient to use product 2 wk or less; product should not be used for long periods
• Teach patient to notify prescriber immediately if coffee-ground emesis, emesis with frank blood, or black tarry stools occur

Evaluation
Positive therapeutic outcome
• Absence of abdominal pain
• Decreased acidity

---

magnesium salts
(mag-neez′ee-um)
magnesium chloride (Rx)
Mag-64
magnesium citrate (OTC)
magnesium gluconate (OTC)
Magtrate
magnesium hydroxide (OTC)
Dulcolax, Phillips Milk of Magnesia, MOM
magnesium oxide (OTC)
Mag-Ox 400, Uro-Mag

⚠ HIGH ALERT

magnesium sulfate (OTC, Rx)
(IV)— HIGH ALERT
Func. class.: Electrolyte; anticonvulsant, laxative, saline; antacid
Pregnancy category A, B

ACTION: Increases osmotic pressure, draws fluid into colon, neutralizes HCl

Therapeutic outcome: Magnesium levels WNL, absence of constipation

USES: Constipation, dyspepsia, bowel preparation before surgery or exam, electrolyte, anticonvulsant, in preeclampsia, eclampsia (magnesium sulfate); cardiac glycoside-induced arrhythmias, nutritional supplement

CONTRAINDICATIONS
Hypersensitivity, abdominal pain, nausea/vomiting, obstruction, acute surgical abdomen, rectal bleeding, heart block, myocardial damage

Precautions: Pregnancy **A, B** (magnesium sulfate), renal disease/cardiac disease

DOSAGE AND ROUTES
Laxative
Adult: PO 15-60 ml at bedtime (Milk of Magnesia)
Adult and child >12 yr: PO 15 g in 8 oz of H_2O (magnesium sulfate); PO 5-30 ml (Concentrated Milk of Magnesia); PO 5-10 oz at bedtime (magnesium citrate)
Child 2-6 yr: 5-15 ml/day (Milk of Magnesia)

Prevention of magnesium deficiency
Adult and child ≥10 yr: PO (male): 350-400 mg/day; (female): 280-300 mg/day; (breastfeeding): 335-350 mg/day; (pregnancy): 320 mg/day
Child 8-10 yr: PO 170 mg/day
Child 4-7 yr: PO 120 mg/day

Magnesium sulfate deficiency
Adult: PO 200-400 mg in divided doses tid-qid; IM 1 g q6hr × 4 doses; **IV** 5 g (severe)
Child 6-12 yr: 3-6 mg/kg/day in divided doses tid-qid

Preeclampsia/eclampsia magnesium sulfate
Adult: IM/IV INF 4-5 g; with 5 g IM in each gluteus, then 5 g q4hr or 4 g **IV** INF, then 1-3 g/hr cont INF, max 40 g/day or 20 g/48 hr in severe renal disease

Available forms: Chloride: sus rel tabs 535 mg (64 mg Mg); enteric tabs 833 mg (100 mg Mg); **hydroxide:** liquid 400 mg/5 ml (164 mg Mg/5 ml); conc liquid 800 mg/5 ml (328 mg Mg/5 ml); chew tabs 300, 600 mg; **Gluconate:** tabs 500 mg; liquid 54 mg/5 ml; **oxide:** tabs 400 mg (241.3 mg Mg); caps 140 mg (84.5 mg Mg); **sulfate:** 500 mg/ml; premixed infusion 1g/100 ml, 2 g/100 ml, 4 g/50 ml, 4 g/100 ml, 20 g/500 ml, 40 g/1000 ml; **citrate:** oral sol 240, 296, 300 ml bottles (77 mEq/100 ml)

Implementation
PO route
• Administer with 8 oz of water

• Refrigerate magnesium citrate before administration
• Shake susp before using
• Administer to patient crushed or whole; chewable tablets may be chewed
• Administer with food or milk to decrease gastric symptoms; give 30 min before or 2 hr after antacids
• Tablets should be chewed thoroughly before swallowing, give 4 oz of water afterward
• **Laxative:** give on empty stomach

IM route (magnesium sulfate)
• Give deeply in gluteal site

IV route (magnesium sulfate)
• Only when calcium gluconate available for magnesium toxicity
Direct IV route
• Dilute 50% solution to 20% or less give at ≤150 mg/min
Continuous IV INF route
• May dilute to 20% sol, infuse over 3 hr
• IV at less than 125 mg/kg/hr; circulatory collapse may occur; use inf pump

Y-site compatibilities: Acyclovir, aldesleukin, alemtuzumab, alfentanil, amifostine, amikacin, aminocaproic acid, argatroban, arsenic trioxide, ascorbic acid injection, asparaginase, atenolol, atosiban, atracurium, atropine, azithromycin, aztreonam, benztropine, bivalirudin, bleomycin, bumetanide, buprenorphine, butorphanol, calcium gluconate, cangrelor, CARBOplatin, carmustine, caspofungin, cefotaxime, cefoTEtan, cefOXitin, cefTAZidime, ceftizoxime, cephapirin, chloramphenicol, chlorproMAZINE, cimetidine, cisatracurium, CISplatin, clindamycin, cloNIDine, codeine, cyanocobalamin, cyclophosphamide, cytarabine, DACTINomycin, DAPTOmycin, DAUNOrubicin liposome, DAUNOrubicin, dexmedetomidine, dexrazoxane, digoxin, diltiazem, dimenhyDRINATE, diphenhydrAMINE, DOBUTamine, DOCEtaxel, dolasetron, DOPamine, doripenem, doxacurium chloride, DOXOrubicin liposomal, doxycycline, enalaprilat, EPHEDrine, EPINEPHrine, epoetin alfa, eptifibatide, ertapenem, esmolol, etoposide, etoposide phosphate, famotidine, fenoldopam, fentaNYL, fluconazole, fludarabine, fluorouracil, folic acid (as sodium salt), foscarnet, gallium, gatifloxacin, gemcitabine, gemtuzumab, gentamicin, glycopyrrolate, granisetron, heparin, HYDROmorphone, hydrOXYzine, IDArubicin, ifosfamide, imipenem-cilastatin, insulin, regular, irinotecan, isoproterenol, kanamycin, ketamine, ketorolac, labetalol, lactated ringer's injection, lepirudin, leucovorin, lidocaine, linezolid, LORazepam, mannitol, mechlorethamine, mesna,

---

⚠ Nurse Alert   ✹ Key NCLEX® Drug   ≫ Drug Specifics

metaraminol, methotrexate, methyldopa, metoclopramide, metoprolol, metroNIDAZOLE, micafungin, midazolam, milrinone, minocycline, mitoMYcin, mitoXANtrone, mivacurium, morphine, moxifloxacin, multiple vitamins injection, mycophenolate mofetil, nafcillin, nalbuphine, nesiritide, netilmicin, niCARdipine, nitroglycerin, nitroprusside, norepinephrine, octreotide, ondansetron, oxaliplatin, oxytocin, PACLitaxel, palonosetron, pamidronate, pancuronium, papaverine, PEMEtrexed, penicillin G potassium/sodium, pentazocine, PENTobarbital, PHENobarbital, phentolamine, phenylephrine, piperacillin, piperacillin tazobactam, polymyxin B, potassium acetate/chloride, procainamide, prochlorperazine, promethazine, propranolol, protamine, pyridoxine, quiNIDine, quinupristin-dalfopristin, ranitidine, remifentanil, ringer's injection, riTUXimab, rocuronium, sargramostim, sodium acetate/bicarbonate, succinylcholine, SUFentanil, tacrolimus, telavancin, teniposide, theophylline, thiamine, thiotepa, ticarcillin, ticarcillin-clavulanate, tigecycline, tirofiban, TNA (3-in-1), tobramycin, tolazoline, topotecan, TPN (2-in-1), trastuzumab, urokinase, vancomycin, vasopressin, vecuronium, verapamil, vinBLAStine, vinCRIStine, vinorelbine, vitamin B complex with C, voriconazole, zoledronic acid

ADVERSE EFFECTS

CNS: Muscle weakness, flushing, sweating, confusion, sedation, depressed reflexes, **flaccid paralysis, hypothermia**
CV: Hypotension, heart block, **circulatory collapse**, vasodilatation
GI: *Nausea, vomiting, anorexia, cramps,* diarrhea
HEMA: Prolonged bleeding time
META: Electrolyte, fluid imbalances
RESP: **Respiratory depression/paralysis**

Pharmacokinetics

Absorption	Unknown
Distribution	Unknown
Metabolism	Unknown
Excretion	Kidneys
Half-life	Unknown
	effective anticonvulsant levels 2.5-7.5 mEq/L

Pharmacodynamics

	PO	IM	IV
Onset	3-6 hr	1 hr	Unknown
Peak	Unknown	Unknown	Unknown
Duration	Unknown	4 hr	½ hr

INTERACTIONS
Individual products
Digoxin: decreased effect of digoxin
Nitrofurantoin: decreased absorption

Drug classifications
Antihypertensives: increased hypotension, calcium channel blockers
Antiinfectives (fluoroquinolones), tetracyclines: decreased absorption
Neuromuscular blockers: increased effect

NURSING CONSIDERATIONS
Assessment
• Assess I&O ratio; check for decrease in urinary output
• **Laxative:** assess cause of constipation; lack of fluids, bulk, exercise
• Assess cramping, rectal bleeding, nausea, vomiting; product should be discontinued
⚠ **Assess magnesium toxicity: thirst, confusion, decrease in reflexes**
• Assess visual changes: blurring, halos, corneal and retinal damage
• Assess edema in feet, ankles, legs
• Assess prior product history; there are many product interactions
• **Eclampsia:** seizure precautions, BP, ECG (magnesium sulfate)

Patient/family education
• Teach not to use laxatives for long-term therapy; bowel tone will be lost
• Teach that chilling helps the taste of magnesium citrate
• Teach to shake suspension well
• Teach to not use at bedtime as a laxative; may interfere with sleep; MOM is usually given at bedtime
• Teach to give citrus fruit after administering to counteract unpleasant taste
• Teach reason for product, expected result

Evaluation

Positive therapeutic outcome
• Decreased constipation; absence of seizures (eclampsia), normal serum calcium levels

mannitol (Rx)
(man'i-tole)
Osmitrol, Resectisol
Func. class.: Diuretic-osmotic
Chem. class.: Hexahydric alcohol
Pregnancy category C

ACTION: Increases osmolarity of glomerular filtrate, which raises osmotic pressure of fluid in renal tubules; there is a decrease in reabsorption of water, electrolytes; increases in urinary

M

output, sodium, chloride, potassium, calcium, phosphorus, uric acid, urea, magnesium

USES: Edema; promote systemic diuresis in cerebral edema, decrease intraocular pressure, improve renal function in acute renal failure, chemical poisoning, urinary bladder irrigation, kidney transplant

Unlabeled uses: traumatic brain injury

CONTRAINDICATIONS

Active intracranial bleeding, hypersensitivity, anuria, severe pulmonary congestion, edema, severe dehydration, progressive heart disease, renal failure, acute MI, aneurysm, stroke

Precautions: Pregnancy **C,** breastfeeding, geriatric, dehydration, severe renal disease, CHF, electrolyte imbalances

DOSAGE AND ROUTES
Oliguria, prevention
Adult: IV after initial test dose and if urine output is 30-50 mg/hr × 2 hr, give 20-100 g of a 15% or 20% SOL in a 24-hr period

Oliguria, treatment
Adult: IV after initial test dose, give balance of 50 g of a 20% SOL over 1 hr, then 5% via CONT IV INF to maintain output at 50 ml/hr
Child (unlabeled): IV 0.5-2 g/kg as a 15%-20% SOL, run over 30-60 min; maintenance 0.25-0.5 g/kg q4-6hr

Edema
Adult: IV after dose, use product 10%-20% at a rate of 25-75 ml/hr, give loop diuretics prior to mannitol
Child: IV (unlabeled) 0.5-2 g/kg of 15%-20% mannitol over 2-6 hr

Intraocular pressure
Adult: IV 1.5-2 g/kg of a 15%-20% SOL over 30-60 min

ICP
Adult: IV 1-2 g/kg, then 0.25-1 g/kg q4hr

Diuresis in product intoxication
Adult and child >12 yr: 5%-25% SOL continuously up to 200 g **IV,** while maintaining 100-500 ml urine output/hr

Kidney transplant
Adult: Donor **IV** 12.5 g prior to nephrectomy, with adequate hydration, may repeat
Recipient: 50 g prior to revascularization

Traumatic brain injury (unlabeled)
Adult: IV 1.4 g/kg prior to neurosurgery with fluid replacement

Available forms: Inj 5%, 10%, 15%, 20%, 25%; GU irrigation 5%

Implementation
Irrigation
• Use 100 ml of 25%/900 ml of sterile water for inj (2.5% sol)
• Administer potassium replacement if potassium level is <3 mg/ml

Intermittent/continuous IV route
• Change IV set q24hr
• May warm solution to dissolve crystals
• Precipitate may occur with PVC
• Use an in-line filter for 15%, 20%, 25%; give with inf pump; check **IV** patency at inf site before, during administration; do not use sol that is yellow or has a precipitate or crystals, use in-line filter, do not give as direct injection; to redissolve, run bottle under hot water and shake vigorously; cool to body temp before giving
• Run at 30-50 ml/hr in oliguria; run over 30-60 min in increased ICP; run over 30 min for intraocular pressure; 60-90 min after surgery
• Monitor for infiltration
• **Test dose** with severe oliguria, 0.2 g/kg over 3-5 mins; if continued oliguria give 2nd test dose; if no response, reassess patient

Y-site compatibilities: Acetaminophen, acyclovir, alemtuzumab, amifostine, amikacin, ampicillin, atropine, asparaginase, aztreonam, bivalirudin, bumetanide, calcium gluconate, caspofungin, ceFAZolin, cefotaxime, cefOXitin, cefTAZidime, ceftizoxime, chloramphenicol, cimetidine, cisatracurium, clindamycin, DAPTOmycin, dexmedetomidine, digoxin, diltiazem, diphenhydrAMINE, DOBUTamine, DOPamine, DOXOrubicin liposome, doxycycline, enalaprilat, EPINEPHrine, ertapenem, esmolol, famotidine, fenoldopam, fentaNYL, fluconazole, fludarabine, gentamicin, granisetron, heparin, HYDROmorphone, hydrOXYzine, IDArubicin, imipenem/cilastatin, insulin, isoproterenol, ketorolac, labetalol, levofloxacin, lidocaine, linezolid, LORazepam, meperidine, metoclopramide, metoprolol, metroNIDAZOLE, micafungin, midazolam, milrinone, morphine, nafcillin, niCARdipine, nitroglycerin, nitroprusside, norepinephrine, ondansetron, oxaliplatin, PACLitaxel, palonosetron, pantoprazole, penicillin G potassium, phenylephrine, piperacillin/tazobactam, potassium chloride, procainamide, prochlorperazine, promethazine, propofol, propranolol, protamine, quinupristin/dalfopristin, ranitidine, remifentanil, sargramostim, sodium bicarbonate, tacrolimus, thiotepa, ticarcillin/clavulanate, tirofiban, tobramycin, trimethoprim/sulfamethoxazole, vancomycin, vasopressin, verapamil, vinCRIStine, vitamin B complex with C, voriconazole, zoledronic acid

Y-site incompatibilities: Aminophylline, amphotericin B cholesteryl sulfate complex, calcium chloride, cefepime, cefTRIAXone, cefuroxime, ciprofloxacin, dexamethasone sodium phosphate, diazepam, drotrecogin, haloperidol, lansoprazole, methylPREDNISolone sodium succinate, phenytoin, phytonadione

ADVERSE EFFECTS

CNS: *Dizziness, headache, seizures, rebound increased ICP,* confusion
CV: Edema, hypotension, hypertension, **tachycardia, CHF,** thrombophlebitis, angina-like chest pains, fever, chills, **circulatory overload,** PVCs
EENT: Loss of hearing, blurred vision, nasal congestion, decreased intraocular pressure
ELECT: Fluid, electrolyte imbalances, **acidosis,** electrolyte loss, dehydration, hyper/hypokalemia
GI: *Nausea, vomiting,* dry mouth, diarrhea
GU: Marked diuresis, urinary retention, thirst
RESP: Pulmonary congestion, *cough,* dyspnea
INTEG: Injection site reaction

Pharmacokinetics

Absorption	Complete
Distribution	Extracellular spaces
Metabolism	Minimal
Excretion	Renal
Half-life	100 min

Pharmacodynamics

Onset	½-1 hr
Peak	1 hr
Duration	6-8 hr

INTERACTIONS
Individual drugs
Lithium: increased elimination of mannitol
Imipramine: increased excretion of imipramine
Arsenic trioxide, levomethadyl: increased hypokalemia

Drug classifications
Salicylates, barbiturates, bromides: increased excretion of each specific product

Drug/food
Potassium foods: increased hyperkalemia

Drug/lab test
Interference: inorganic phosphorus, ethylene glycol

NURSING CONSIDERATIONS
Assessment
• Assess neurologic status: LOC, ICP reading, pupil size and reaction when product is given for increased ICP

• Assess for vision changes or eye discomfort or pain before, during treatment (increases intraocular pressure); neurologic checks, ICP during treatment (increased ICP)
• Assess patient for tinnitus, hearing loss, ear pain; periodic testing of hearing is needed when high doses of this product are given by **IV** route
• Assess fluid volume status: check I&O ratios and record hourly urine values, CVP, breath sounds, weight, distended red veins, crackles in lungs, color, quality, and specific gravity of urine, skin turgor, adequacy of pulses, moist mucous membranes (provide adequate fluids), bilateral lung sounds, peripheral pitting edema
• Assess for dehydration; symptoms of decreasing output, thirst, hypotension, dry mouth and mucous membranes should be reported
• Monitor electrolytes: potassium, sodium, calcium, magnesium; also include BUN, ABGs, CVP, PAP, CBC; regularly monitor serum and urine levels of sodium and potassium
• Assess B/P before, during therapy with patient lying, standing, and sitting as appropriate; orthostatic hypotension can occur rapidly
• Monitor for rebound ICP: headache, confusion

Patient/family education
• Teach patient reason for and method of treatment, pain at injection site, hearing loss, blurred vision

Evaluation
Positive therapeutic outcome
• Decreased intraocular pressure
• Prevention of hypokalemia (diuretic use)
• Decreased edema
• Decreased ICP
• Increased diuresis of >30 ml/hr
• Increased excretion of toxic substances

TREATMENT OF OVERDOSE:
Discontinue infusion; correct fluid, electrolyte imbalances; hemodialysis; monitor hydration, CV, renal function

maraviroc (Rx)
(mah-rav′er-rock)
Selzentry
Func. class.: Antiretroviral
Chem. class.: Fusion inhibitor, CCR5-receptor antagonist
Pregnancy category B

ACTION: Interferes with entry into HIV-1 by inhibiting the fusion of the virus and cell membrane

M

Therapeutic outcome: Improvement in CD4, viral load, T-cell count

USES: CCR5-tropic HIV in combination with other antiretroviral agents in treating experienced patients

CONTRAINDICATIONS
Hypersensitivity, dialysis, renal impairment

Precautions: Pregnancy **B**, breastfeeding, Asian patients, renal/hepatic/cardiac disease, electrolyte imbalance, dehydration, immune reconstitution syndrome, infection, MI, orthostatic hypotension, children, geriatric

> **BLACK BOX WARNING:** Hepatitis/hepatotoxicity, fever, serious rash; eosinophilia, or elevated IgE prior to hepatotoxicity may occur

DOSAGE AND ROUTES
Those not taking CYP3A inducers/inhibitors
Adult/adolescent ≥16 yr: PO 300 mg bid

Those taking CYP3A4 inhibitors with/without a CYP3A inducer
Adult/adolescent ≥16 yr: PO 150 mg bid

Those taking CYP3A4 inducers without a strong CYP3A inhibitor
Adult/adolescent ≥16 yr: PO 600 mg bid

Renal dose
Adult: PO ≤30 ml/min, reduce dose to 150 mg bid

Available forms: Tabs 150, 300 mg

Implementation
• May give without regard to meals, with 8 oz of water
• Store at room temperature

ADVERSE EFFECTS
CNS: Dizziness, depression, viral meningitis, disturbances in consciousness, peripheral neuropathy, paresthesia, dysesthesia, fever
CV: MI, cardiac ischemia, orthostatic hypotension
EENT: Gingival hyperplasia, visual changes
GI: Diarrhea, constipation, dyspepsia, pseudomembranous colitis, hepatotoxicity
INTEG: Rash, urticaria, pruritus, folliculitis
MS: Joint pain, leg pain, muscle cramps
RESP: Cough, URI, sinusitis, bronchitis, pneumonia, bronchospasm, obstruction, dyspnea
SYST: Herpes virus, lipodystrophy, malignancy

Pharmacokinetics

Absorption	Unknown
Distribution	Unknown
Metabolism	By P450 system, CYP3A metabolism
Excretion	Urine 20%, feces 76%
Half-life	Unknown

Pharmacodynamics
Unknown

INTERACTIONS
Drug classifications
CYP3A inhibitors (amiodarone, aprepitant, chloramphenicol, clarithromycin, conivaptan, cycloSPORINE, dalfopristin, danazol, diltiazem, erythromycin, estradiol, fluconazole, fluvoxaMINE, imatinib, isoniazid, itraconazole, ketoconazole, miconazole, nefazodone, niCARdipine, propoxyphene, RU-486, tamoxifen, telithromycin, troleandomycin, verapamil, voriconazole, zafirlukast); reduce dose: increased maraviroc levels
CYP3A4 inducers (aminoglutethimide, barbiturates, bexaroten, bosentan, carBAMazepine, dexamethasone, efavirenz, fosphenytoin, griseofulvin, modafinil, nafcillin, OXcarbazepine, phenytoin, rifabutin, rifampin, rifapentine, topiramate, tipranavir): increase dose; decreased maraviroc effect

Drug/food
High-fat meal: decreased absorption 33%

Drug/herb
St. John's wort: decreased maraviroc effect

Drug/lab test
Increase: AST, ALT, bilirubin, amylase, lipase

NURSING CONSIDERATIONS
Assessment
• **HIV:** CD4, T-cell count, plasma HIV RNA, CCR5-tropic HIV-1; assess for change in symptoms, other infections during treatment
• Monitor renal tests: serum creatinine
• Assess bowel pattern before, during treatment
• **Allergies:** skin eruptions: rash, urticaria, itching; assess allergies before treatment and before each dose

> **BLACK BOX WARNING: Hepatitis:** assess for dark urine, abdominal pain, vomiting, yellowing of skin/eyes, hepatomegaly: if present, discontinue product; monitor LFTs

Patient/family education
• Advise patient to take as prescribed; if dose is missed, take as soon as remembered up to 1 hr before next dose; do not double dose

---

• Teach patient that product does not cure infection, just controls symptoms, and does not prevent infecting others

⚠ Teach patient to report sore throat, fever, fatigue; may indicate superinfection; yellow skin/eyes, abdominal pain, vomiting (hepatitis); itching, dyspnea (allergic reaction)

• Advise patient that product must be taken in equal intervals around the clock to maintain blood levels for duration of therapy

• Instruct patient to notify prescriber of side effects

• Advise patient to avoid driving or other hazardous activities until reaction is known; dizziness may occur

• Teach patient to make position changes slowly to prevent postural hypotension

⚠ Inform patient to notify prescriber if pregnancy is planned or suspected, not to breastfeed

Evaluation

Positive therapeutic outcome
• Improvement in CD4, viral load, T-cell count

---

mecasermin (Rx)

(mec-a′sir-men)
Increlex
Func. class.: Biologic response modifier; insulin-like growth factor
Pregnancy category C

ACTION: Stimulates growth; IGF-1 is the principal hormonal mediator of statural growth; GH binds to its receptor in the liver and other tissues

Therapeutic outcome: Increased height

USES: Growth failure in children with severe primary insulin-like growth factor-1 (IGF-1) deficiency (primary IGFD) or with growth hormone (GH) gene deletion who have developed neutralizing antibodies to GH

Unlabeled uses: ALS

CONTRAINDICATIONS

Hypersensitivity, benzyl alcohol, closed epiphyses, active/suspected neoplasia, **IV** use

Precautions: Pregnancy **C**, breastfeeding, children <2 yr, diabetes mellitus, hypothyroidism, lymphoid tissue hypertrophy, increased ICP, malnutrition, scoliosis, sleep apnea

DOSAGE AND ROUTES

Child ≥2 yr: SUBCUT 0.04-0.08 mg/kg (40-80 mcg/kg) bid; if well tolerated for 1 wk, may increase by 0.04 mg/kg/dose, max 0.12 mg/kg bid

Available forms: Inj 10 mg/ml

Implementation
SUBCUT route

• Give within 20 min of a meal or snack; do not give if unable to eat or if vomiting

• Rotate inj site; use sterile, disposable syringe/needles; use small-volume syringe for accurate measurement

• Store in refrigerator before opening, avoid freezing; after opening, stable for 30 days after initial vial entry, store in refrigerator, do not use if particulate matter is present, avoid direct light, do not use after expiration date

• Do not double dose if a dose is missed

ADVERSE EFFECTS

CNS: Headache, seizures, dizziness, cardiac valvulopathy, increased intracranial pressure
CV: Cardiac murmur
EENT: Ear pain, otitis media, abnormal tympanometry, papilledema, visual impairment, tonsillar hypertrophy, sinusitis
ENDO: Hypoglycemia, ketosis, hypothyroidism, hypercholesterolemia, hypertriglyceridemia
GI: Vomiting, nausea
HEMA: Thymus hypertrophy, lymphadenopathy
INTEG: Pruritus, urticaria, anaphylaxis, angioedema
MISC: Bruising, lipohypertrophy, hypersensitivity reactions, inj site reaction
MS: Arthralgia, joint pain, slipped upper femoral epiphysis
RESP: Snoring, apnea
SYST: Antibodies to growth hormone, secondary malignancy

Pharmacokinetics

Absorption	Near 100%
Distribution	Unknown
Metabolism	Liver/kidneys
Excretion	Unknown
Half-life	5.8 hr

Pharmacodynamics

Unknown

INTERACTIONS
Drug classifications

Antidiabetics, corticosteroids: increased hypoglycemia
Psychostimulants: decrease in growth suppression possible

NURSING CONSIDERATIONS
Assessment

• Monitor preprandial glucose at beginning of treatment and until well tolerated

---

Adverse effects: *italics* = common; **bold** = life-threatening

M

- Monitor by funduscopic exam at beginning, periodically during treatment
- Assess for **allergic reactions;** if present, interrupt treatment and notify prescriber
- Assess growth rate of child at intervals during treatment

⚠ Serious skin disorders: angioedema; anaphylaxis

Patient/family education

- Teach patient that treatment may continue for years; regular assessments are required
- Advise patient to avoid hazardous activities, driving within 2-3 hr of dosing
- Teach patient correct administration and needle disposal, rotation of injection sites

Evaluation

Positive therapeutic outcome
- Growth in children

---

meclizine (OTC, Rx)

(mek´li-zeen)
Antivert, Bonine, Dramamine Less Drowsy Formula
Func. class.: Antiemetic, antihistamine, anticholinergic
Chem. class.: H$_1$-receptor antagonist, piperazine derivative
Pregnancy category B

ACTION: Acts centrally by blocking chemoreceptor trigger zone, which in turn acts on vomiting center

Therapeutic outcome: Decreased nausea in motion sickness; decreased vertigo

USES: Vertigo, motion sickness

CONTRAINDICATIONS

Hypersensitivity to cyclizines, shock

Precautions: Pregnancy **B,** breastfeeding, children, geriatric, closed-angle glaucoma, glaucoma, prostatic hypertrophy, hypertension, urinary retention, GI obstruction, contact lenses

DOSAGE AND ROUTES
Vertigo
Adult/adolescent: PO 25-100 mg/day in divided doses

Motion sickness
Adult/adolescent: PO 25-50 mg 1 hr before traveling; repeat dose q24hr prn

Available forms: Tabs 12.5, 25, 50 mg

Implementation
- May give without regard to food

- **Chew tab:** Give without regard to water or may be swallowed whole with water
- Give lowest possible dose in geriatric, anticholinergic effects

ADVERSE EFFECTS

CNS: *Drowsiness,* fatigue, restlessness, headache, insomnia
CV: Hypotension
EENT: Dry mouth, blurred vision
GI: Nausea, anorexia, constipation, increased appetite
GU: Urinary retention

Pharmacokinetics

Absorption	Well absorbed
Distribution	Unknown
Metabolism	Unknown
Excretion	Unknown
Half-life	6 hr

Pharmacodynamics

Onset	1 hr
Peak	Unknown
Duration	8-24 hr

INTERACTIONS
Individual drugs
Alcohol: increased effects
Atropine: increased anticholinergic effects

Drug classifications
Antihistamines, antidepressants, phenothiazines: increased anticholinergic effect
CNS depressants, opioids: increased CNS depression

Drug/herb
Hops, valerian, kava: increased sedative effect

Drug/lab test
False negative: allergy skin testing (allergen extracts)

NURSING CONSIDERATIONS
Assessment
- **Vertigo/motion sickness:** nausea, vomiting after 1 hr, assess vertigo periodically
- Monitor VS, B/P

⚠ Assess for signs of toxicity of other products or masking of symptoms of disease: brain tumor, intestinal obstruction
- Observe for drowsiness, dizziness, LOC

Patient/family education
- Teach patient that a false-negative result may occur with skin testing for allergies; these procedures should not be scheduled for 4 days after discontinuing use

---

• Teach patient to avoid hazardous activities, activities requiring alertness; dizziness may occur; instruct patient to request assistance with ambulation
• Teach patient to avoid alcohol, other depressants, breastfeeding, report severe side effects

Evaluation

Positive therapeutic outcome
• Absence of dizziness, vomiting

---

medroxyPROGESTERone (Rx)

(me-drox-ee-proe-jess'te-rone)
Depo-Provera, Depo-subQ Provera, Gen-Medroxy ✤, Provera
Func. class.: Hormone: progestogen, contraceptive, antineoplastic
Chem. class.: Progesterone derivative
Pregnancy category X

Do not confuse: medroxyPROGESTERone/methylPREDNISolone, **Provera**/Premarin/Covera

ACTION: Inhibits secretion of pituitary gonadotropins, which prevents follicular maturation and ovulation; antineoplastic action against endometrial cancer

Therapeutic outcome: Decreased abnormal uterine bleeding, absence of amenorrhea

USES: Uterine bleeding (abnormal), secondary amenorrhea, contraceptive, prevention of endometrial changes associated with estrogen replacement therapy (ERT), inoperable, recurrent, metastatic endometrial/renal cancer

CONTRAINDICATIONS

Pregnancy **X**, hypersensitivity, reproductive cancer, genital bleeding (abnormal, undiagnosed), missed abortion, stroke, cerebrovascular disease, cervical cancer, hepatic disease, uterine/vaginal cancer

> **BLACK BOX WARNING:** Breast cancer, MI, stroke, thromboembolic disease, thrombophlebitis

Precautions: Breastfeeding, hypertension, asthma, blood dyscrasias, gallbladder disease, CHF, diabetes mellitus, bone disease, depression, migraine headache, seizure disorders, renal/hepatic disease, family history of cancer of breast or reproductive tract, bone mineral density loss, ocular disorders, AIDS/HIV, alcoholism, children, hyperlipidemia

> **BLACK BOX WARNING:** Use of this product has been shown to increase dementia in women ≥65 yr old; use may increase osteoporosis in long-term treatment, those at greater risk also smoke, adequate calcium and vitamin D should be taken

DOSAGE AND ROUTES
Secondary amenorrhea
Adult: PO 5-10 mg/day × 5-10 days

Uterine bleeding
Adult: PO 5-10 mg/day × 5-10 days starting on 16th or 21st day of menstrual cycle

With ERT
Adult: PO 5-10 mg qd × 10-14 or more days/mo (sequential estrogen); 2.5-5 mg qd (continuous estrogen)

Contraceptive
Adult: IM 150 mg q12wk; SUBCUT (depot SUBCUT Provera 104 inj) 104 mg q3mo

Endometrial/renal cancer
Adult: IM 400 mg-1 g (using 400 mg/ml depot inj susp) qwk

Available forms: Tabs 2.5, 5, 10 mg; inj susp 50, 150, 400 mg/ml; depot SUBCUT inj: 104 mg/0.65 ml

Implementation
PO route
• Give without regard to food
IM route
• Visually inspect particulate matter and discoloration prior to use
• Give titrated dose; use lowest effective dose; give oil sol deep in large muscle mass (IM); rotate sites; use after warming to dissolve crystals
Depo-Provera Contraceptive injection suspension:
• IM only, NEVER IV
• Instruct patient on risks and warnings associated with hormonal contraceptives (see Patient Information)
• The possibility of pregnancy should be excluded prior to giving the first dose of medroxyprogesterone or whenever more than 14 weeks have passed since the last dose
• Do not dilute
• Shake vigorously immediately before administration
• Inject deeply into the gluteal or deltoid muscle. Aspirate prior to injection to avoid injection into a blood vessel
Depo-Provera Sterile Aqueous Suspension, preserved:
• IM only, NEVER IV

M

- Instruct patient on risks and warnings associated with progestin use (see Patient Information)
- Shake vigorously immediately before use
- When multidose vials are used, take special care to prevent contamination
- Inject deeply into the gluteal or deltoid muscle. Aspirate prior to injection

SUBCUT route

Depo-subQ Provera 104 Contraceptive Injection Suspension ONLY:
- For SUBCUT use only; NEVER give IM or IV
- Instruct patient on risks and warnings associated with hormonal contraceptives (see Patient Information)
- Shake vigorously for at least 1 min before use
- Inject the entire contents of the prefilled syringe subcut into the anterior thigh or abdomen, avoiding boney areas and the umbilicus. Gently grasp and squeeze a large area of skin in the chosen injection area, ensuring that the skin is pulled away from the body. Insert the needle at a 45-degree angle. Inject until the syringe is empty; this usually requires 5-7 seconds. Following use, press lightly on the injection site with a clean cotton pad for a few seconds; do not rub the area

ADVERSE EFFECTS

CNS: Dizziness, headache, migraine, depression, fatigue, nervousness
CV: Hypotension, thrombophlebitis, edema, thromboembolism, stroke, pulmonary embolism, MI
EENT: Diplopia
GI: *Nausea*, vomiting, anorexia, cramps, increased weight, cholestatic jaundice, abdominal pain
GU: Amenorrhea, cervical erosion, breakthrough bleeding, dysmenorrhea, vaginal candidiasis, breast changes, *gynecomastia, testicular atrophy, impotence,* endometriosis, spontaneous abortion, vaginitis, increased/decreased libido
INTEG: Rash, urticaria, acne, hirsutism, alopecia, oily skin, seborrhea, purpura, melasma, photosensitivity, injection site reaction
META: Hyperglycemia
MS: Decreased bone density
SYST: Angioedema, anaphylaxis

Pharmacokinetics
Unknown

Pharmacodynamics

	PO	IM
Onset	Unknown	Unknown
Peak	Unknown	Unknown
Duration	2-4 hr	Unknown

INTERACTIONS
Individual drugs
Aminoglutethimide, carBAMazepine, phenytoin, PHENobarbital, rifampin: decreased contraceptive effect

Drug categories
Anticoagulants, corticosteroids: decreased bone mineral density

Drug/lab test
Increased: LFTs, HDL, triglycerides, coagulation tests
Decreased: GTT

NURSING CONSIDERATIONS
Assessment
- Assess for symptoms indicating severe allergic reaction, angioedema; have EPINEPHrine and resuscitative equipment available
- Monitor B/P at beginning of treatment and periodically; check weight daily; notify prescriber of weekly weight gain >5 lb; bone mineral density
- Monitor I&O ratio: be alert for decreasing urinary output, increasing edema, hypertension
- Assess liver function tests: ALT, AST, bilirubin, periodically during long-term therapy
- **Bone mineral density loss:** in those taking anticoagulants, corticosteroids with Depo-Provera or Depo-subQ Provera
- Assess for edema, hypertension, cardiac symptoms, jaundice
- Assess mental status: affect, mood, behavioral changes, depression

Patient/family education
- Advise patients to avoid sunlight or use sunscreen; photosensitivity and melasma (brown patches on the face) can occur
- Teach patient about cushingoid symptoms: weight gain, moon face, buffalo hump, acne
- Teach women patients to report breast lumps, vaginal bleeding, edema, jaundice, dark urine, clay-colored stools, dyspnea, headache, blurred vision, abdominal pain, sudden changes in speech/coordination, numbness or stiffness in legs, chest pain; teach men to report impotence or gynecomastia
- ⚠ Teach patient to report suspected pregnancy (X) immediately; fertility returns in 6-12 mo after discontinuing

> **BLACK BOX WARNING:** Long-term use decreases bone density; exercise, calcium supplements can help lessen osteoporosis

Evaluation
Positive therapeutic outcome
- Decreased abnormal uterine bleeding
- Absence of amenorrhea

- Prevention of pregnancy
- Arrested spread of malignant cells

⚠ HIGH ALERT

megestrol (Rx)

(me-jess′trole)

Megace, Megace ES

Func. class.: Antineoplastic hormone
Chem. class.: Progestin

Pregnancy category D (tabs), X (susp)

Do not confuse: Megace/Reglan

ACTION: Affects endometrium by antiluteinizing effect; this is thought to bring about cell death, stimulates appetite by unknown action

Therapeutic outcome: Prevention of rapidly growing malignant cells; weight gain, increased appetite in AIDS

USES: Breast, endometrial cancer; increased weight, decreased cachexia and anorexia associated with AIDS

Unlabeled uses: Hot flashes, prostate cancer

CONTRAINDICATIONS

Pregnancy **X** (susp), **D** (tabs), hypersensitivity

Precautions: Diabetes, thrombosis, adrenal insufficiency

DOSAGE AND ROUTES

Endometrial/ovarian carcinoma
Adult: PO 40-320 mg/day in divided doses

Breast carcinoma
Adult: PO 40 mg qid or 160 mg/day

AIDS
Adult: PO 800 mg/day (oral SUSP) or 625 mg/day (ES)

Hot flashes (unlabeled)
Adult: PO 20 mg bid

Available forms: Tabs 20, 40 mg; oral susp 40, 125 mg/ml

Implementation
- Administer with meals for GI symptoms
- Oral susp is usually used for AIDS patients; shake well
- Give tablets for carcinoma
- Give without regard to food

ADVERSE EFFECTS

CNS: Mood swings, insomnia, fever, lethargy, depression
CV: **Thrombophlebitis, thromboembolism,** hypertension

ENDO: Adrenal insufficiency
GI: Nausea, vomiting, diarrhea, abdominal cramps, weight gain, flatus, indigestion
GU: Gynecomastia, fluid retention, hypercalcemia, vaginal bleeding, discharge, impotence, decreased libido, menstruation disorders
INTEG: Alopecia, rash, pruritus, purpura, itching, sweating
META: Hyperglycemia
MISC: **Tumor flare**
RESP: Dyspnea

Pharmacokinetics

Absorption	Well absorbed; food increases oral sol
Distribution	Unknown
Metabolism	Liver, completely
Excretion	Feces, urine
Half-life	13-105 hr

Pharmacodynamics

Onset	Several wk to mo
Peak	Unknown

INTERACTIONS

Individual drugs
Dofetilide: do not use with megestrol

Drug/lab test
Increased: glucose

NURSING CONSIDERATIONS

Assessment
- PSA levels in men (prostate cancer); blood glucose, liver function studies, serum calcium, weight
- Monitor effects of alopecia on body image; discuss feelings about body changes
- In AIDS patients monitor calorie counts, weight, appetite
- **Assess for thrombophlebitis: Homan's sign, pain, redness, swelling in calf, thigh; notify prescriber immediately if these occur**

Patient/family education
- Teach patient to report any complaints or side effects to prescriber
- **Advise patient that contraceptive measures must be used during and 4 mo after treatment; product is teratogenic: pregnancy D tabs, pregnancy X susp**
- Explore with patient the need for wig or a hairpiece for hair loss
- Caution patient to report vaginal bleeding to prescriber
- Review with patient the need to comply with dosage schedule, not to miss or double doses; missed doses may be taken up to 1 hr before next dose

M

- Teach patient how to recognize signs of fluid retention, thromboembolism and report immediately
- Teach that gynecomastia and alopecia can occur; reversible after discontinuing treatment
- Advise to monitor blood glucose if diabetic

Evaluation

Positive therapeutic outcome
- Decreased spread of malignant cells
- Weight gain, increased appetite in AIDS patients
- Resolved dysfunctional uterine bleeding

⚠ HIGH ALERT

melphalan (Rx)
(mel'fa-lan)
Alkeran
Func. class.: Antineoplastic, alkylating agent
Chem. class.: Nitrogen mustard
Pregnancy category D

Do not confuse: melphalan/myleran, Alkeran/Alferon

ACTION: Responsible for cross-linking DNA strands leading to cell death; activity is not cell cycle phase specific

Therapeutic outcome: Prevention of rapidly growing malignant cells

USES: Multiple myeloma, advanced ovarian cancer

Unlabeled uses: Breast, testicular, prostate carcinoma; osteogenic sarcoma, amyloidosis, chronic myelogenous leukemia, non-Hodgkin's lymphoma

CONTRAINDICATIONS
Pregnancy **D**, breastfeeding

> **BLACK BOX WARNING:** Hypersensitivity to this product

Precautions: Children, radiation therapy, infection, renal disease

> **BLACK BOX WARNING:** Bone marrow depression, secondary malignancy, radiation therapy: requires an experienced clinician

DOSAGE AND ROUTES
Multiple myeloma
Adult: PO 6 mg qd × 2-3 wk, adjust dose based on blood counts or 10 mg qd × 7-10 days
Adult: IV INF 16 mg/m²; reduce in renal insufficiency; give over 15-20 min; give at 2-wk intervals × 4 doses, then at 4-wk intervals

Ovarian carcinoma
Adult: PO 200 mcg/kg/day × 5 days q4-5wk

Available forms: Tabs 2 mg; powder for inj 50 mg

Implementation
- Give fluids **IV** or PO before chemotherapy to hydrate patient
- Give antacid before oral agent; give product after evening meal, before bedtime; provide antiemetic 30-60 min before giving product and prn to prevent vomiting; give antibiotics for prophylaxis of infection
- Give in AM so product can be eliminated before bedtime
- Use a liquid diet: carbonated beverages; gelatin may be added if patient is not nauseated or vomiting

PO route
- Give 1 hr before or 2 hr after meals to prevent nausea/vomiting
- Protect from light, store refrigerated

Intermittent IV INF route
- Use gloves during administration; if skin exposure occurs, wash immediately with soap and water, use cytotoxic handling procedures
- Reconstitute with provided diluent (10 ml) to 5 mg/ml; shake until clear; further dilute with 0.9% NaCl to <0.45 mg/ml; give over 15-20 min; give within 1 hr, degrading of product occurs rapidly; make sure infusion is completed in time specified

Y-site compatibilities: Acyclovir, amikacin, aminophylline, ampicillin, aztreonam, bleomycin, bumetanide, buprenorphine, butorphanol, calcium gluconate, CARBOplatin, carmustine, ceFAZolin, cefepime, cefoperazone, cefotaxime, cefoTEtan, cefTAZidime, ceftizoxime, cefTRIAXone, cefuroxime, cimetidine, CISplatin, clindamycin, cyclophosphamide, cytarabine, dacarbazine, DACTINomycin, DAUNOrubicin, dexamethasone, diphenhydrAMINE, DOXOrubicin, doxycycline, droperidol, enalaprilat, etoposide, famotidine, floxuridine, fluconazole, fludarabine, fluorouracil, furosemide, gallium, ganciclovir, gentamicin, granisetron, haloperidol, heparin, hydrocortisone sodium phosphate, hydromorphone, hydrOXYzine, IDArubicin, ifosfamide, imipenem-cilastatin, LORazepam, mannitol, mechlorethamine, meperidine, mesna, methylPREDNISolone, metoclopramide, methotrexate, metroNIDAZOLE, miconazole, minocycline, mitoMYcin, mitoXANtrone, morphine, nalbuphine, netilmicin, ondansetron, pentostatin, piperacillin, plicamycin, potassium chloride, prochlorperazine, promethazine, ranitidine, sodium bicarbonate, streptozocin, teniposide, thiotepa, ticarcillin, ticarcillin/clavulanate, to-bramycin, trimethoprim/sulfamethoxazole, van-comycin, vinBLAStine, vinCRIStine, vinorelbine, zidovudine

ADVERSE EFFECTS

GI: *Nausea, vomiting,* stomatitis, diarrhea, **hepatotoxicity**
GU: Amenorrhea, hyperuricemia, gonadal suppression
HEMA: Thrombocytopenia, neutropenia, leukopenia, anemia
INTEG: Rash, urticaria, alopecia, pruritus, necrosis, extravasation
RESP: Fibrosis, dysplasia, dyspnea, pneumonitis
SYST: Anaphylaxis, allergic reaction, **secondary malignancies,** edema

Pharmacokinetics

Absorption	Variable; incompletely absorbed
Distribution	Rapidly distributed, protein binding ≤ 30%-90%
Metabolism	Bloodstream
Excretion	Kidneys, unchanged (10%)
Half-life	2 hr

Pharmacodynamics

Unknown

INTERACTIONS
Individual drugs

Sargramostim, GM-CSF, filgrastim, G-CSF: avoid administration 24 hr before or 24 hr after this product
Carmustine: increased pulmonary toxicity
CycloSPORINE: increased renal failure risk
Nalidixic acid: increased enterocolitis risk
Radiation: increased toxicity

Drug classifications

Anticoagulants, NSAIDs, salicylates, thrombolytics, platelet inhibitors: increased bleeding risk
Antineoplastics: increased toxicity
Live virus vaccines: increased adverse reactions; decreased antibody reaction

Drug/lab test

Decrease: Hgb, RBC, WBC, platelets
False-positive: direct Coombs test

NURSING CONSIDERATIONS
Assessment

BLACK BOX WARNING: Monitor full nadir 2-3 wk; CBC, differential, platelet count weekly; notify prescriber; withhold product if WBC is <3000/mm³ or platelet count is <100,000/mm³; notify prescriber; recovery usually occurs in 6 wk

• **Hyperuricemia:** assess for increased uric acid levels, swelling, joint pain primarily in extremities; patient should be well hydrated to prevent urate deposits, monitor uric acid levels
• **Infection:** monitor for cold, fever, chills, sore throat
• **Assess for bleeding:** hematuria, guaiac, bruising or petechiae, from mucosa or orifices q8hr; no rectal temp
• **Assess for symptoms indicating severe allergic reaction: rash, pruritus, urticaria, purpuric skin lesions, itching, flushing; assess allergy to chlorambucil; cross-sensitivity may occur**

Patient/family education

• Teach patient to avoid use of products containing aspirin or ibuprofen, nausea/vomiting, dehydration, decreased urine output; to report symptoms of bleeding (hematuria, tarry stools)
• Instruct patient to report signs of anemia (fatigue, headache, irritability, faintness, shortness of breath)
• Instruct patient to report any changes in breathing or coughing even several mo after treatment; to avoid crowds and persons with respiratory tract or other infections
• Tell patient hair loss is common; discuss the use of wigs or hairpieces
• Caution patient not to have any vaccinations without the advice of the prescriber, serious reactions can occur
⚠ Advise patient to report suspected pregnancy, that contraception is needed during treatment and for several mo after the completion of therapy, pregnancy D
• Teach patient to rinse mouth tid-qid with water, club soda; brush teeth bid-qid with soft brush or cotton-tipped applicators for stomatitis, use unwaxed dental floss

Evaluation
Positive therapeutic outcome

• Decreased size of tumor
• Decreased spread of malignancy

---

memantine (Rx)
(me-man′teen)
Ebixa ✚, **Namenda, Namenda XR**
Func. class.: Anti–Alzheimer's disease agent
Chem. class.: NMDA receptor antagonist
Pregnancy category B

ACTION: Antagonist action of CNS NMDA receptors that may contribute to the symptoms of Alzheimer's disease

Therapeutic outcome: Improved mood, orientation, decreasing confusion

USES: Moderate to severe dementia in Alzheimer's disease

Unlabeled uses: Vascular dementia

CONTRAINDICATIONS
Hypersensitivity, children

Precautions: Pregnancy **B**, breastfeeding, renal disease, seizures, severe hepatic disease, GU conditions that raise urine pH, renal failure

DOSAGE AND ROUTES
Adult: PO 5 mg/day, may increase dose in 5-mg increments ≥1-wk intervals over a 3-wk period; recommended target dose as 10 mg bid at week 4; ext rel 7 mg/day, increased by 7 mg ≥1 wk up to target dose of 28 mg/day

Available forms: Tabs 5, 10 mg; tab titration pak 5, 10 mg; oral sol 2 mg/ml, 10 mg/5 ml; cap ext rel 7, 14, 21, 28 mg

Implementation
• Can be taken without regard to meals
• Give twice a day if dose >5 mg
• Dosage is adjusted to response no more than q1wk
• Provide assistance with ambulation during beginning therapy; dizziness may occur
• **Extended Release Caps:** Do not crush, chew, divide; swallow whole or open and sprinkle on applesauce
• When switching from immediate release product begin the ext rel the day after the last dose of immediate release product. Those on 10 mg bid should be switched to ext rel 28 mg q day

ADVERSE EFFECTS
CNS: *Dizziness, confusion,* somnolence, headache, hallucinations, stroke, insomnia, depression, anxiety
CV: Hypertension, heart failure, CHF
GI: Vomiting, constipation
INTEG: Rash
MISC: Back pain, fatigue, pain, influenzalike symptoms
RESP: Coughing, dyspnea

Pharmacokinetics

Absorption	Rapidly absorbed PO
Distribution	44% protein binding
Metabolism	Very little
Excretion	57%-82% excreted unchanged in urine
Half-life	Terminal elimination half-life 60-80 hr

Pharmacodynamics
Unknown

INTERACTIONS
Individual drugs
Cimetidine, hydrochlorothiazide, nicotine, quiNIDine, ranitidine, triamterene: increased/decreased levels of both products
Ergot, levodopa: increased effect of each

Drug classifications
Drugs that make the urine alkaline (sodium bicarbonate, carbonic anhydrase inhibitors): decreased clearance
Use cautiously with amantadine, dextromethorphan, ketamine: reaction unknown

Drug/lab test
Increase: alkaline phosphatase

NURSING CONSIDERATIONS
Assessment
• Alzheimer's dementia: affect, mood, behavioral changes; hallucinations, confusion, attention, orientation, memory; monitor serum creatinine

Patient/family education
• Advise to report side effects: restlessness, psychosis, visual hallucinations, stupor, loss of consciousness; indicate overdose
• Advise patient to avoid alcohol, nicotine
• Advise to use product exactly as prescribed; product is not a cure
• Teach patient to avoid OTC, herbal products unless approved by prescriber

Evaluation
Positive therapeutic outcome
• Decrease in confusion, improved mood or ability to maintain function, even with no improvement in symptoms

---

⚠ HIGH ALERT

meperidine (Rx)
(me-per'i-deen)
Demerol, Meperitab
Func. class.: Opioid analgesic
Chem. class.: Phenylpiperidine derivative
Pregnancy category C
Controlled substance schedule II

Do not confuse: meperidine/ HYDROmorphone/meprobamate/morphine, Demerol/Dilaudid/Desyrel/Demulen

ACTION: Depresses pain impulse transmission at the spinal cord level by interacting with opioid receptors

Therapeutic outcome: Relief of pain

USES: Moderate to severe pain, preoperatively, postoperatively, general anesthesia maintenance, sedation induction

CONTRAINDICATIONS
Hypersensitivity, severe respiratory insufficiency

Precautions: Pregnancy **C**, breastfeeding, children, geriatric, addictive personality, increased ICP, respiratory depression, renal/hepatic disease, seizure disorder, abrupt discontinuation, chronic pain, cardiac disease, adrenal insufficiency, alcoholism, angina, anticoagulant therapy, asthma, atrial flutter, biliary tract disease, bladder obstruction, cardiac dysrhythmias, COPD, CNS depression, coagulopathy, constipation, cor pulmonale, dehydration, diarrhea, driving epidural use, geriatrics, GI obstruction, head trauma, heart failure, hypotension, hypothyroidism, ileus, IBS, IM/intrathecal/IV use, labor, myxedema/thrombocytopenia, MAOI therapy

DOSAGE AND ROUTES
Moderate to severe pain
Adult: PO/SUBCUT/IM 50-150 mg q3-4hr prn
Child: PO/SUBCUT/IM 1-1.8 mg/kg q3-4hr prn, max single dose 150 mg

Preoperatively
Adult: IM/SUBCUT 50-100 mg 30-90 min before surgery
Child: IM/SUBCUT 1-2 mg/kg 30-90 min before surgery, max 100 mg

Renal dose
Adult: PO/SUBCUT/IM/IV, CCr 10-50 ml/min give 75% of dose; CCr <10 ml/min give 25%-50% of dose

Labor analgesia
Adult: SUBCUT/IM 50-100 mg given when contractions are regulary spaced, repeat q1-3hr prn

Available forms: Inj 10, 25, 50, 75, 100 mg/ml; tabs 50, 100 mg; syr 50 mg/5 ml

Implementation
• Give with antiemetic if nausea, vomiting occur
• Administer when pain is beginning to return; determine dosage interval by patient response; continuous dosing of medication is more effective given prn
• Medication should be slowly withdrawn after long-term use to prevent withdrawal symptoms
• Store in light-resistant container at room temperature
PO route
• May be given with food or milk to lessen GI upset

• Syr should be mixed with 4 oz of water
• **Oral liquid:** dilute in 4 oz water
IM/SUBCUT route
• Do not give if cloudy or a precipitate has formed
• Patient should remain recumbent for 1 hr after administration
• Inject IM into a large muscle mass; IM is preferred route for multiple injections

Direct IV route
• Give after diluting to 10 mg/ml with sterile water, 0.9% NaCl for inj; give slowly at ≤25 mg/min; rapid administration may cause respiratory depression, hypotension, circulatory collapse
• Have emergency equipment and opiate antagonist on hand
Continuous IV infusion route
• Give after diluting to 1 mg/ml with D_5W, $D_{10}W$, dextrose/saline combinations, dextrose/Ringer's, inj combinations, 0.45% NaCl, 0.9% NaCl, Ringer's, LR; give by inf pump; titrate according to response

Syringe compatibilities: Acetaminophen, butorphanol, chlorproMAZINE, cimetidine, dimenhyDRINATE, diphenhydrAMINE, droperidol, fentaNYL, glycopyrrolate, hydrOXYzine, ketamine, metoclopramide, midazolam, ondansetron, pentazocine, perphenazine, prochlorperazine, promazine, ranitidine, scopolamine

Syringe incompatibilities: Heparin, morphine, PENTobarbital

Y-site compatibilities: Abelcet, acetaminophen, amifostine, amikacin, anidulafungin, atenolol, aztreonam, bumetanide, cefamandole, ceFAZolin, cefmetazole, cefotaxime, cefOXitin, cefTAZidime, ceftizoxime, cefTRIAXone, cefuroxime, cladribine, clindamycin, diltiazem, diphenhydrAMINE, DOBUTamine, DOPamine, doxycycline, droperidol, erythromycin lactobionate, famotidine, filgrastim, fluconazole, fludarabine, gallium, gentamicin, granisetron, hydrocortisone, regular insulin, kanamycin, labetalol, lidocaine, melphalan, methyldopate, metoclopramide, metoprolol, metroNIDAZOLE, ondansetron, oxytocin, PACLitaxel, penicillin G potassium, piperacillin, potassium chloride, propofol, propranolol, ranitidine, sargramostim, teniposide, thiotepa, ticarcillin, ticarcillin/clavulanate, tobramycin, vancomycin, verapamil, vinorelbine

Y-site incompatibilities: Cefoperazone, IDArubicin, imipenem/cilastatin, mezlocillin, minocycline
Continuous intrathecal infusion route
• Use controlled-infusion device, an implantable controlled-microinfusion device is used

M

Adverse effects: *italics* = common; **bold** = life-threatening

for highly concentrated infusion, monitor for several days after implantation
• Infusion reservoir should only be filled by those fully qualified
• To prevent pain, depletion of reservoir should be avoided

ADVERSE EFFECTS
CNS: Drowsiness, dizziness, confusion, headache, sedation, euphoria, increased ICP, seizures, serotonin syndrome
CV: Palpitations, bradycardia, hypotension, change in B/P, tachycardia (IV)
EENT: Tinnitus, blurred vision, miosis, diplopia, depressed corneal reflex
GI: Nausea, vomiting, anorexia, constipation, cramps, biliary spasm, paralytic ileus
GU: Urinary retention, dysuria
INTEG: Rash, urticaria, bruising, flushing, diaphoresis, pruritus
RESP: Respiratory depression
SYST: Anaphylaxis

Pharmacokinetics

Absorption	Well absorbed (IM, SUBCUT); 50% (PO)
Distribution	Widely distributed; crosses placenta; protein binding 65%-75%; toxic by-product accumulation can result from regular use or in renal disease
Metabolism	Liver, extensively to active/ inactive metabolites
Excretion	Kidneys; breast milk
Half-life	3-4 hr

Pharmacodynamics

	PO	IM/SUBCUT	IV
Onset	15 min	10 min	immediate, peak 5-7 min
Peak		½-1 hr	5-7 min
Duration	2-4 hr	2-4 hr	2 hr

INTERACTIONS
Individual drugs
Alcohol: increased respiratory depression, hypotension, sedation
Phenytoin: decreased meperidine effect
Procarbazine: fatal reaction, do not use together

Drug classifications
CNS depressants, opioids, sedative/hypnotics, antipsychotics, skeletal muscle relaxants: increased effects

SSRIs, SNRIs, serotonin-receptor agonists: increased serotonin syndrome, increased neuroleptic malignant syndrome
MAOIs: do not use for 2 wk before taking meperidine; may cause fatal reaction
Protease inhibitor antiretrovirals: increased adverse reactions

Drug/herb
St. John's wort: increased CNS depression

Drug/lab test
Increased: amylase, lipase

NURSING CONSIDERATIONS
Assessment
• **Assess pain:** location, duration, intensity before and 1 hr (IM, SUBCUT, PO), 5-10 min (IV) after administration
• Assess renal function before initiating therapy; poor renal function can lead to accumulation of toxic metabolite and seizures
• Monitor VS after parenteral route; note muscle rigidity, product history, liver, kidney function tests, respiratory dysfunction: respiratory depression, character, rate, rhythm; notify prescriber if respirations are <10/min
• Monitor CNS changes: dizziness, drowsiness, hallucinations, euphoria, LOC, pupil reaction; these are due to metabolite produced; CNS stimulation occurs with chronic or high doses
• Monitor allergic reactions: rash, urticaria
• Assess for constipation; increase fluids, bulk in diet; give stimulant laxatives if needed

Patient/family education
• Advise patients to avoid CNS depressants (alcohol, sedative/hypnotics) for at least 24 hr after taking this product
• Discuss with patient that dizziness, drowsiness, and confusion are common; to avoid getting up without assistance
• Discuss in detail with patient all aspects of the product, including its purpose and what to expect
• Caution patient to make position changes carefully to lessen orthostatic hypotension

Evaluation
Positive therapeutic outcome
• Decreased pain

TREATMENT OF OVERDOSE:
Naloxone 0.2-0.8 mg IV (caution in physically dependent patients), O_2, IV fluids, vasopressors

> **⚠ HIGH ALERT**
>
> # mercaptopurine (6-MP) (Rx)
>
> (mer-kap-toe-pyoor´een)
> **Purinethol, Purixan**
> *Func. class.:* Antineoplastic, antimetabolite
> *Chem. class.:* Purine analog
> **Pregnancy category D**

ACTION: Inhibits purine metabolism at multiple sites, which inhibits DNA and RNA synthesis S phase of cell cycle

Therapeutic outcome: Prevention of rapidly growing malignant cells

USES: Acute lymphocytic leukemia

Unlabeled uses: Ulcerative colitis; Crohn's disease

CONTRAINDICATIONS
Pregnancy **D**, hypersensitivity, breastfeeding, patients with prior product resistance

Precautions: Renal/hepatic disease, tumor lysis syndrome, dental disease, herpes, radiation therapy, leukopenia, thrombocytopenia, anemia, requires an experienced clinician, secondary malignancy, infection, hypocalcemia, hyperuricemia, hyperphosphatemia, hyperkalemia

DOSAGE AND ROUTES
Acute lymphocytic leukemia
Adult: PO 2.5-5 mg/kg/day or 80-100 mg/m²/day, maintenance 1.5-2.5 mg/kg/day
Child: PO 2.5-5 mg/kg/day, maintenance 1.5-2.5 mg/kg/day or 70-100 mg/m²/day

Available forms: Tabs 50 mg; susp 2000 mg/100 ml

Implementation
• Give fluids **IV** or PO before chemotherapy to hydrate patient
• Give antiemetic 30-60 min before giving product and prn to prevent vomiting
• Give in PM on empty stomach
• Give entire dose at one time
• Provide liquid diet: carbonated beverages; gelatin may be added if patient is not nauseated or vomiting
• Tab may be crushed and added to fluids or food to facilitate swallowing
• **Suspension:** Shake well; wash syringe with warm, soapy water; rinse; move plunger up and down several times; use only after dry; after opening, use within 6 wk

ADVERSE EFFECTS
CNS: Weakness
GI: *Nausea, vomiting, anorexia, diarrhea, stomatitis,* **hepatotoxicity** (with high doses), jaundice, gastritis, **pancreatitis**
GU: **Renal failure,** hyperuricemia, **oliguria,** crystalluria, **hematuria**
HEMA: **Thrombocytopenia, leukopenia, myelosuppression, anemia**
INTEG: *Rash,* dry skin, urticaria, alopecia

Pharmacokinetics
Absorption	Variable
Distribution	Widely, body water
Metabolism	Liver, extensively
Excretion	Kidneys unchanged (small amounts)
Half-life	Terminal 47 min (adult) 21 min (child)

Pharmacodynamics
Onset	Unknown
Peak	1-2 hr
Duration	Unknown

INTERACTIONS
Individual products
Allopurinol: increased effects of this agent; avoid use or decrease dose
Azathioprine, sulfamethoxazole-trimethoprim: avoid concurrent use—increased bone marrow depression
Balsalazide, mesalamine, olsalazine, sulfaSALAzine: decreased TPMT, rapid bone marrow suppression; use cautiously
Radiation: increased effects
Warfarin: increased effect of warfarin

Drug classifications
Anticoagulants, NSAIDs, platelet inhibitors, salicylates, thrombolytics: increased bleeding risk
Antineoplastics, immunosuppressants: increased effects
Live virus vaccines: decreased antibodies

NURSING CONSIDERATIONS
Assessment
• Assess buccal cavity for dryness, sores or ulceration, white patches, oral pain, bleeding, dysphagia; obtain prescription for viscous lidocaine (Xylocaine)
⚠ Assess symptoms indicating severe allergic reaction: rash, pruritus, urticaria, purpuric skin lesions, itching, flushing, laryngeal edema

- Bone marrow suppression: monitor CBC, differential, platelet count weekly; withhold product if WBC is <4000/mm³ or platelet count is <100,000/mm³; notify prescriber of results if WBC <20,000/mm³, platelets <150,000/mm³ or at first sign of abnormally large decrease in blood counts, unless bone marrow aplasia is the goal

⚠ Thiopurine methyltransferase (TPMT) deficiency: individuals are prone to rapid bone marrow suppression; dosage reduction may be required in homozygous TPMT-deficient persons

- Assess for increased uric acid levels, swelling, joint pain primarily in extremities; patient should be well hydrated to prevent urate deposits
- Monitor renal function tests: BUN, creatinine, serum uric acid, urine CCr before, during therapy; check I&O ratio; report fall in urine output to <30 ml/hr

⚠ Tumor lysis syndrome: monitor for increased potassium, uric acid, phosphate, decreased urine output, calcium

- Monitor temp q4hr (may indicate beginning of infection)

⚠ Monitor liver function tests before, during therapy (bilirubin, AST, ALT, LDH) as needed or monthly; check for yellowing of skin or sclera, dark urine, clay-colored stools, itchy skin, abdominal pain, fever, diarrhea; hepatic encephalopathy, toxic hepatitis, ascites: can be fatal

- **Assess for bleeding:** hematuria, stool guaiac, bruising or petechiae, mucosa or orifices q8hr; check for inflammation of mucosa, breaks in skin, avoid IM injections if platelets are low; blood transfusions may be needed

Patient/family education

- Encourage patient to rinse mouth tid-qid with water, club soda; brush teeth bid-qid with soft brush or cotton-tipped applicators for stomatitis; use unwaxed dental floss

⚠ Pregnancy: advise patient that contraceptive measures are recommended during therapy (D); serious teratogenic effects may occur, to avoid breast-feeding

- Teach patient to avoid use of products containing aspirin or NSAIDs, razors, commercial mouthwash, since bleeding may occur; to report symptoms of bleeding (hematuria, tarry stools)
- Instruct patient to report signs of anemia (fatigue, headache, irritability, faintness, shortness of breath)
- Instruct patient to report any changes in breathing or coughing even several mo after treatment; to avoid crowds and persons with respiratory tract or other infections
- Caution patient not to have any vaccinations without the advice of the prescriber; serious reactions can occur
- Advise patient to take entire dose at one time

⚠ Teach patient to notify prescriber of fever, chills, sore throat, nausea, vomiting, anorexia, diarrhea, bleeding, or bruising, which may indicate blood dyscrasias/infection

Evaluation

Positive therapeutic outcome
- Prevention of rapid division of malignant cells

---

meropenem (Rx)

(mer-oh-pen′em)

Merrem IV

Func. class.: Antiinfective—miscellaneous

Pregnancy category B

ACTION: Interferes with cell wall replication of susceptible organisms

Therapeutic outcome: Bactericidal action against the following: *Streptococcus pneumoniae,* group A β-hemolytic streptococci, *viridans* group streptococci, enterococcus; gram-negative organisms *Klebsiella, Proteus, Escherichia coli, Pseudomonas aeruginosa, Bacteroides fragilis, Bacteroides thetaiotamicron,* bacterial meningitis (>3 mo old)

USES: *Acinetobacter, Aeromonas hydrophila, Bacteroides distasonis, Bacteroides fragilis, Bacteroides ovatus, Bacteroides thetaiotaomicron, Bacteroides uniformis, Bacteroides ureolyticus, Bacteroides vulgatus, Campylobacter jejuni, Citrobacter diversus, Citrobacter freundii, Clostridium difficile, Clostridium perfringens, Enterobacter cloacae, Enterococcus faecalis, Escherichia coli, Eubacterium lentum, Fusobacterium, Haemophilus influenzae* (beta-lactamase negative), *Haemophilus influenzae* (beta-lactamase positive), *Hafnia alvei, Klebsiella oxytoca, Klebsiella pneumoniae, Moraxella catarrhalis, Morganella morganii, Neisseria meningitidis, Pasteurella multocida, Peptostreptococcus, Porphyromonas asaccharolytica, Prevotella bivia, Prevotella intermedia, Prevotella melaninogenica, Propionibacterium acnes, Proteus mirabilis, Proteus vulgaris, Pseudomonas aeruginosa, Salmonella, Serratia marcescens, Shigella, Staphylococcus aureus* (MSSA), *Staphylococcus epidermidis,*

Streptococcus agalactiae (group B streptococci), *Streptococcus pneumoniae, Streptococcus pyogenes* (group A beta-hemolytic streptococci), *Viridans streptococci, Yersinia enterocolitica;* appendicitis, bacteremia, intraabdominal infections, meningitis, peritonitis, skin/skin structure infections

Unlabeled uses: Febrile neutropenic, community-acquired pneumonia

CONTRAINDICATIONS
Hypersensitivity to meropenem, carbapenems: hypersensitivity to cephalosporins, penicillins

Precautions: Pregnancy **B**, breastfeeding, geriatric, renal disease, seizure disorder, gram-negative infection, pneumonia, hypersensitivity to pneumonia

DOSAGE AND ROUTES
Intraabdominal infections (complicated appendicitis, peritonitis)
Adult/adolescent/child >50 kg: IV 1 g q8hr or 500 mg q6hr
Adolescent/child ≤50 kg/infant ≥3 mo: IV 20 mg/kg q8hr

Complicated skin and skin structure infections
Adult/adolescent/child >50 kg: IV 500 mg q8hr
Adolescent/child ≤50 kg/infant ≥3 mo: IV 10 mg/kg q8hr

Bacterial meningitis
Adult: IV 2 g q8hr
Adolescent/child ≤50 kg/infant: IV 40 mg/kg q8hr

Renal dose
Adult: IV CCr 26-50 ml/min give dose q12hr; CCr 10-25 ml/min give ½ dose q12hr; CCr <10 ml/min give ½ dose q24hr

Available forms: Powder for inj 500 mg, 1 g

Implementation
Direct IV route
• Reconstitute 500 mg or 1 g vials with 10, 20 ml of sterile water for inj respectively, shake to dissolve and let stand until clear (average conc 50 mg/ml) reconstituted sol may be stored for 3 hr at room temperature or 13 hr refrigerated, inject up to 1 g in 5-20 ml over 3-5 min
Intermittent IV infusion route
• Vials may be directly constituted with compatible inf fluid (NS, D₅W) to 2.5-50 mg/ml vials; vials with 0.9% NaCl can be stored up to 2 hr at room temperature, or 18 hr refrigerated, D₅W may be stored up to 1 hr at room temperature

or up to 15 hr refrigerated, infuse over 15-30 min
Continuous IV infusion route (unlabeled)
• **3 g/day continuous IV infusion:** Constitute a 1 g vial according to manufacturer's recommendations; further dilute in 50 ml or 250 ml of NS and run over 8 hr for cont inf, administer a new infusion bag q8hr
• **4 g/day continuous IV infusion:** Constitute a 1 g vial according to manufacturer recommendations. Further dilute in 100 ml of NS and administer over 6 hr. For cont inf, administer a new infusion bag q6hr
• **3 g/day IV continuous infusion in ambulatory infusion pump with freezer packs:** Reconstitute 1 g vial according to manufacturer recommendations by adding 20 ml of NS into each vial. Add 3 g (60 ml) to a 100-ml medication cassette reservoir and bring the final volume to 100 ml (final concentration, 30 mg/ml) run over 24 hr

Y-site compatibilities: Alemtuzumab, aminocaproic acid, aminophylline, anidulafungin, argatroban, atenolol, atropine, azithromycin, bivalirudin, bleomycin, CARBOplatin, carmustine, caspofungin, cimetidine, CISplatin, cyclophosphamide, cycloSPORINE, cytarabine, DACTINomycin, DAPTOmycin, dexamethasone, dexmedetomidine, dexrazoxane, digoxin, diltiazem, diphenhydrAMINE, DOCEtaxel, doxacurium, DOXOrubicin liposomal, enalaprilat, eptifibatide, etoposide, etoposide phosphate, fluconazole, fludarabine, fluorouracil, foscarnet, furosemide, gallium, gatifloxacin, gemcitabine, gemtuzumab, gentamicin, granisetron, heparin sodium, HYDROmorphone, ifosfamide, insulin (regular), irinotecan, lepirudin, leucovorin, linezolid injection, LORazepam, mechlorethamine, methotrexate, metoclopramide, metroNIDAZOLE, milrinone, mitoXANtrone, morphine, nesiritide, norepinephrine, octreotide, oxaliplatin, oxytocin, PACLitaxel, palonosetron, pamidronate, pancuronium, PEMEtrexed, PHENobarbital, potassium acetate/chloride, rocuronium, teniposide, thiotepa, tigecycline, tirofiban, TNA (3-in-1) Total Nutrient Admixture, vancomycin, vasopressin, vecuronium, vinBLAStine, vinCRIStine, vinorelbine, voriconazole, zoledronic acid

Additive compatibilities: Aminophylline, atropine, cimetidine, dexamethasone, DOBUTamine, DOPamine, enalaprilat, fluconazole, furosemide, gentamicin, heparin, insulin (regular), magnesium sulfate, metoclopramide, morphine, norepinephrine, PHENobarbital, ranitidine, vancomycin

M

ADVERSE EFFECTS

CNS: Fever, somnolence, *seizures,* dizziness, weakness, *headache,* myoclonia, confusion, insomnia, agitation, confusion, drowsiness

CV: Hypotension, tachycardia

ENDO: Hypoglycemia

GI: Diarrhea, nausea, vomiting, **pseudomembranous colitis, hepatitis,** glossitis, jaundice

HEMA: **Eosinophilia, neutropenia,** decreased Hgb, Hct, **agranulocytosis**

INTEG: *Rash,* urticaria, *pruritus,* pain at inj site, phlebitis, erythema at inj site

RESP: Chest discomfort, dyspnea, hyperventilation, **pulmonary embolism**

SYST: Anaphylaxis, Stevens-Johnson syndrome, angioedema

Pharmacokinetics

Absorption	Complete bioavailability
Distribution	Widely distributed
Metabolism	Liver
Excretion	Kidneys
Half-life	1 hr; increased in renal disease

Pharmacodynamics

Onset	Rapid
Peak	Dose dependent
Duration	Unknown

INTERACTIONS

Individual drugs

Probenecid: increased meropenem levels

Valproic acid: decreased effect of valproic acid

Drug/herb

Do not use acidophilus with antiinfectives; separate by several hours

Drug/lab test

Increased: AST, ALT, LDH, BUN, alkaline phosphatase, bilirubin, creatinine

Decreased: prothrombin time

False positive: direct Coombs' test

NURSING CONSIDERATIONS

Assessment

• Assess patient for previous sensitivity reaction to carbapenem antiinfectives, penicillins, cephalosporins

• **Assess patient for signs and symptoms of infection,** including characteristics of wounds, sputum, urine, stool, WBC $>10,000/100$ mm^3, fever; obtain baseline information before, during treatment

• Complete C&S tests before beginning product therapy to identify if correct treatment has been initiated

⚠ Seizures: may occur in those with brain lesions, seizure disorder, bacterial meningitis, or renal disease; stop product, notify prescriber if seizures occur

• **Assess for allergic reactions, anaphylaxis:** rash, urticaria, pruritus, chills, fever, joint pain; angioedema may occur a few days after therapy begins; EPINEPHrine and resuscitation equipment should be available for anaphylactic reaction; identify if there has been hypersensitivity to penicillins, cephalosporins, beta-lactams: cross-sensitivity may occur

• Identify urine output; if decreasing, notify prescriber (may indicate nephrotoxicity); also check for increased BUN, creatinine

• Monitor blood studies: AST, ALT, CBC, Hct, bilirubin, LDH, alkaline phosphatase, Coombs' test monthly if patient is on long-term therapy

• Monitor electrolytes: potassium, sodium, chloride monthly if patient is on long-term therapy

⚠ Assess bowel pattern daily; if severe diarrhea occurs, product should be discontinued; may indicate pseudomembranous colitis

• Monitor for bleeding: ecchymosis, bleeding gums, hematuria, stool guaiac daily if on long-term therapy

⚠ Assess for overgrowth of infection: perineal itching, fever, malaise, redness, pain, swelling, drainage, rash, diarrhea, change in cough, sputum

Patient/family education

• Teach patient to report sore throat, bruising, bleeding, joint pain; may indicate blood dyscrasias (rare)

• Advise patient to contact prescriber if vaginal itching, loose foul-smelling stools, furry tongue occur; may indicate superinfection; seizures

• Advise patient to avoid breastfeeding; product is excreted in breast milk

⚠ Advise patient to notify prescriber of diarrhea with blood or pus; may indicate pseudomembranous colitis

Evaluation

Positive therapeutic outcome

• Absence of signs/symptoms of infection (WBC $<10,000/$mm^3, temp WNL, absence of red draining wounds)

• Reported improvement in symptoms of infection

TREATMENT OF ANAPHYLAXIS: EPINEPHrine, antihistamines, resuscitate if needed

mesalamine, 5-ASA (Rx)

(mez-al'a-meen)
Apriso, Asacol, Asacol HD, Canasa, Delzicol, Lialda, Pentasa, Rowasa
Func class.: GI antiinflammatory
Chem. class.: 5-Aminosalicylic acid
Pregnancy category B

Do not confuse: Asacol/Ansaid/Os-Cal

ACTION: May diminish inflammation by blocking cyclooxygenase, inhibiting prostaglandin production in colon, local action only

Therapeutic outcome: Decreased cramping, pain in GI conditions

USES: Mild to moderate active distal ulcerative colitis, proctitis

Unlabeled uses: Crohn's disease

CONTRAINDICATIONS

Hypersensitivity to this product or salicylates, 5-aminosalicylates

Precautions: Pregnancy **B**, breastfeeding, children, geriatric, renal disease, sulfite sensitivity, pyloric stenosis, GI obstruction

DOSAGE AND ROUTES
Treatment of ulcerative colitis

Adult: RECT 60 ml (4 g) at bedtime, retained for 8 hr × 3-6 wk; del rel tab (Lialda) 2.4-4.8 g/day × 8 wk; del rel tab (Asacol) 1.6 g × 6 wk; cont rel cap (Pentasa) 1 g qid up to 8 wk; RECT SUPP 500 mg bid retained for 1-3 hr × 3-6 wk until remission, may increase to tid if needed; del rel cap (Delzicol) 800 mg tid ×6 wk

Maintenance of remission

Adult: PO (delayed release tabs: Asacol) 800 mg bid or 400 mg qid; (delayed release caps: Apriso) 1500 mg (4 caps) each AM; (delayed release tabs: Lialda) 2.4 g (2 tab)/day with a meal; del rel cap (Delzicol) 800 mg bid

Available forms: Rectal Susp 4 g/60 ml (Rowasa, ss Rowasa); del rel tabs 400 mg (Asacol); 800 mg (Asacol HD); ext rel tab 500 mg; ext rel cap 250 mg, 500 mg (Pentasa); del rel tab (Lialda) 1.2 g; 0.375 g (Apriso); rect supp 1000 mg; del rel cap (Delzicol) 400 mg

Implementation
PO route

- Do not break, crush, or chew del rel tabs
- **Lialda:** take with a meal
- **Apriso caps:** without regard to meals in AM
- **Delzicol caps:** give ≥1 hr before a meal or 2 hr after a meal

Rectal route (susp)

- Give at bedtime, retained until AM; empty bowel before insertion
- Store at room temperature
- Usual course of therapy is 3-6 wk
- Give after shaking bottle well

ADVERSE EFFECTS

CNS: *Headache, fever, dizziness,* insomnia, asthenia, weakness, fatigue
CV: Pericarditis, myocarditis, chest pain, palpitations
EENT: Sore throat, cough, pharyngitis, rhinitis
GI: *Cramps, gas, nausea, diarrhea,* rectal pain, constipation
GU: Nephrotoxicity, interstitial nephritis
INTEG: *Rash, itching,* acne
SYST: *Flulike symptoms, malaise,* back pain, peripheral edema, leg and joint pain, arthralgia, dysmenorrhea, **anaphylaxis**, acute intolerance syndrome

Pharmacokinetics

Absorption	20%-30% (PO), 10%-25% (RECT)
Distribution	Unknown
Metabolism	Unknown
Excretion	Feces
Half-life	1 hr; metabolite 5-10 hr

Pharmacodynamics

Unknown

INTERACTIONS
Individual drugs

Azathioprine, mercaptopurine: increased action of each product
Lactulose: decreased mesalamine absorption
Omeprazole: increased mesalamine absorption
Warfarin: decreased effect of warfarin

Drug classifications

H_2 blockers: do not give with Apriso
NSAIDs: increased nephrotoxicity
Antacids: decreased mesalamine absorption

Drug/lab test

Increased: AST, ALT, alkaline phosphatase, LDH, GGTP, amylase, lipase

NURSING CONSIDERATIONS
Assessment

- Assess for GI symptoms: cramping, gas, nausea, diarrhea, rectal pain, abdominal pain; if severe, the product should be discontinued
- Assess for allergy to salicylates, sulfonamides; if allergic reactions occur, discontinue product
- Assess renal function before, during treatment: BUN, creatinine periodically

M

Adverse effects: *italics* = common; **bold** = life-threatening

Patient/family education

• Advise patient to notify prescriber if abdominal pain, cramping, diarrhea with blood, headache, fever, rash, chest pain occur; product should be discontinued
• Teach correct administration for PO or enema

Evaluation

Positive therapeutic outcome

• Absence of pain, bleeding from GI tract

⚠ HIGH ALERT

metFORMIN (Rx)

(met-for'min)

Fortamet, Glucophage, Glucophage XR, Glumetza, Glycon ✦, Riomet

Func. class.: Antidiabetic, oral
Chem. class.: Biguanide

Pregnancy category B

ACTION: Inhibits hepatic glucose production and increases sensitivity of peripheral tissue to insulin

Therapeutic outcome: Blood glucose at normal levels

USES: Type 2 diabetes mellitus

CONTRAINDICATIONS

Creatinine ≥1.5 mg/ml (males); diabetic ketoacidosis, metabolic acidosis, renal failure, radiographic contrast use

Precautions: Pregnancy **B**, breastfeeding, geriatric, thyroid disease, previous CHF, hypersensitivity; hepatic disease; creatinine ≥1.4 (females); alcoholism; cardiopulmonary disease; acidemia; acute MI; cardiogenic shock; renal disease, heart failure

> **BLACK BOX WARNING:** History of lactic acidosis

DOSAGE AND ROUTES
Type 2 diabetes mellitus

Adult: PO 500 mg bid or 850 mg/day initially, then 500 mg weekly or 850 mg q2wk up to 2000 mg/day in divided doses; dosage adjustment q2-3wk or 850 mg/day with morning meal with dosage increased every other week, max 2550 mg/day; ext rel (Glucophage XR) 500 mg qd with evening meal; may increase by 500 mg qwk, max 2000 mg/day; (Glumetza) 1000 mg qd with food, preferably with the PM meal, may increase by 500 mg qwk, max 2000 mg/day; (Fortamet) 500-1000 mg qd with PM meal, may increase by 500 mg qwk, max 2550 mg/day

Geriatric: PO use lowest effective dose

Available forms: Tabs 500, 850, 1000 mg; ext rel tabs 500, 750, 850, 1000 mg; oral sol (Riomet) 500 mg/5 ml

Implementation

• Conversion from other oral hypoglycemic agents; change may be made without gradual dosage change; monitor serum or urine glucose and ketones tid during conversion
• **Immediate rel:** give twice a day with meals to decrease GI upset and provide best absorption
• Give immediate rel tabs crushed and mixed with meal or fluids for patients with difficulty swallowing
• **Extended release product:** may also be taken as a single dose; titrate slowly to therapeutic response, side-effect tolerance
• Do not break, crush, or chew ext rel tabs
• Give in AM to prevent hypoglycemic reactions in PM
• Store in tight container in cool environment

ADVERSE EFFECTS

CNS: *Headache, weakness, dizziness, drowsiness,* tinnitus, fatigue, vertigo, *agitation*
CV: Heart failure
ENDO: Lactic acidosis, hypoglycemia
GI: Nausea, vomiting, diarrhea, heartburn, anorexia, metallic taste
HEMA: Thrombocytopenia, decreased vit B_{12} levels
INTEG: Rash

Pharmacokinetics

Absorption	Unknown
Distribution	Unknown
Metabolism	Unknown
Excretion	Kidneys, unchanged (35%-50%)
Half-life	1½-6 hr

Pharmacodynamics

Onset	Unknown
Peak	1-2 hr (immediate rel); 7 hr (ext rel); 2.5 hr (sol)
Duration	Unknown

INTERACTIONS
Individual drugs

Cimetidine, digoxin, morphine, procainamide, quiNIDine, ranitidine, triamterone, vancomycin: increased metFORMIN level
β-blockers, phenytoin: increased hyperglycemia
Digoxin: increased digoxin levels
Dofetilide: increased lactic acidosis, do not use together

Radiologic contrast media: do not give together; may cause renal failure

Drug classifications
Calcium channel blockers, contraceptives (oral), corticosteroids, diuretics, estrogens, phenothiazines, sympathomimetics: increased hypoglycemia

Drug/herb
Garlic, green tea: increased hypoglycemia
Glucosamine: increased hyperglycemia

Drug/lab test
Decreased: vitamin B_{12}

NURSING CONSIDERATIONS
Assessment
• Assess for hypoglycemic reactions (sweating, weakness, dizziness, anxiety, tremors, hunger), hyperglycemic reactions soon after meals; these occur rarely with this product
• Monitor CBC (baseline, q3mo) during treatment; check liver function tests (AST, LDH) and renal tests (BUN, creatinine) periodically during treatment; glucose, A1c; folic acid, vitamin B_{12} q1-2yr
• **Surgery:** product should be discontinued temporarily for surgical procedures when patient is NPO, or if contrast media is used; resume when patient is eating

> BLACK BOX WARNING: Monitor for lactic acidosis: malaise, myalgia, abdominal distress; risk increases with age, poor renal function; monitor electrolytes, lactate, pyruvate, blood pH, ketones, glucose; suspect in any diabetic patient with metabolic acidosis, with ketoacidosis; immediately stop product if hypoxemia, or significant renal dysfunction occurs

Patient/family education
• Teach patient to regularly self-monitor blood glucose using blood glucose meter
• Teach patient symptoms of hypo/hyperglycemia, what to do about each (rare)
• Advise patient that product must be continued on daily basis; explain consequence of discontinuing product abruptly
• Advise patient to take product in morning to prevent hypoglycemic reactions at night
• Advise patient to avoid OTC medications, alcohol unless approved by the prescriber
• Teach patient that diabetes is a lifelong illness; that this product controls symptoms, but does not cure the condition

> BLACK BOX WARNING: **Teach patient symptoms of lactic acidosis**—hyperventilation, fatigue, malaise, myalgia, chills, somnolence—and to stop product/notify prescriber immediately

• Teach patient to carry/wear emergency ID and glucagon emergency kit for emergencies
• Advise patient that glucophage XR tab may appear in stool
• Advise patient to take with meals, not to break, crush, chew ext rel product

Evaluation
Positive therapeutic outcome
• Decrease in polyuria, polydipsia, polyphagia; clear sensorium; absence of dizziness; stable gait; blood glucose, A1C at normal level

▲ HIGH ALERT

methadone (Rx)
(meth'a-done)
Dolophine, Metadol ✦, Methadose
Func. class.: Opioid analgesic
Chem. class.: Synthetic diphenylheptane derivative
Pregnancy category C
Controlled substance schedule II

Do not confuse: methadone/methylphenidate

ACTION: Depresses pain impulse transmission at the spinal cord level by interacting with opioid receptors; produces CNS depression

Therapeutic outcome: Relief of pain; successful opioid withdrawal

USES: Severe pain, opiate withdrawal

Unlabeled uses: Bone pain

CONTRAINDICATIONS
Hypersensitivity to this product, or hypersensitivity to chlorobutanol (inj route), asthma, ileus

> BLACK BOX WARNING: Respiratory depression

Precautions: Pregnancy **C,** breastfeeding, children <18 yr, geriatric, addictive personality, increased ICP, MI (acute), severe heart disease, respiratory depression, renal/hepatic disease, respiratory insufficiency, torsades de pointes, pulmonary disease, COPD, seizures

BLACK BOX WARNING: QT prolongation, pain

DOSAGE AND ROUTES
Severe pain
Adult: PO 2.5 mg q8-12hr in opioid-naive, titrate; IV/IM/SUBCUT 2.5-10 mg q8-12hr in opioid-naive

Opiate withdrawal
Adult including pregnant women: PO 20-30 mg initially, unless low opioid tolerance is expected, additional 5-10 mg q2-4hr as needed after initial dose, if symptoms continue may give for up to 5 days

Renal/hepatic dose
Adult: PO may need to be modified

Available forms: Inj 10 mg/ml; tabs 5, 10 mg; oral sol 5, 10 mg/5 ml/(concentrate); 10 mg/ml/(concentrate); dispersible tabs 40 mg

Implementation
• Medication should be slowly withdrawn after long-term use to prevent withdrawal symptoms
PO route
• When using during a methadone maintenance program, use only PO according to NATA guidelines
• May be given with food or milk to lessen GI upset
• Store in light-resistant container at room temperature
IM/SUBCUT route
• Do not give if cloudy or a precipitate has formed
• Give deeply in large muscle mass (IM); rotate inj sites
• Pain and induration may occur at site

ADVERSE EFFECTS
CNS: *Drowsiness, dizziness, confusion, headache, sedation,* euphoria, seizures
CV: Palpitations, bradycardia, change in B/P, cardiac arrest, shock, hypotension, torsades de pointes, QT prolongation
EENT: Tinnitus, blurred vision, miosis, diplopia
GI: *Nausea, vomiting, anorexia, constipation, cramps,* biliary tract spasm
GU: Increased urinary output, dysuria, urinary retention, impotence
INTEG: *Rash,* urticaria, bruising, flushing, diaphoresis, pruritus
RESP: Respiratory depression, respiratory arrest

Pharmacokinetics
Absorption	Well absorbed (PO, SUBCUT, IM)
Distribution	Widely distributed; crosses placenta, half as active PO, as inj
Metabolism	Liver, extensively
Excretion	Kidneys, breast milk
Half-life	2-3 hr; extended interval with continued dosing

Pharmacodynamics
	PO	IM/SUBCUT
Onset	½-1 hr	20 min
Peak	1-1.5 hr	1½-2 hr
Duration	4-12 hr	4-6 hr

INTERACTIONS
Individual drugs
Alcohol: increased respiratory depression, hypotension, sedation
Nalbuphine, pentazine, phenytoin, rifampin: decreased analgesia
Selegiline: do not use within 2 wk of methadone

Drug classifications
Antipsychotics, opiates, sedative/hypnotics, skeletal muscle relaxants: increased respiratory depression, hypotension
Class IA antiarrhythmics (disopyramide, procainamide, quiNIDine), class III antiarrhythmics (amiodarone, bretylium, dofetilide, ibutilide, sotalol), astemizole, arsenic trioxide, bepridil, cisapride, chloroquine, clarithromycin, levomethadyl, pentamidine, some phenothiazines, pimozide, probucol, sparfloxacin, terfenadine: increased QT prolongation
CYP3A4 inducers (barbiturates, bosentan, carBAMazepine, efavirenz, phenytoins, nevirapine, rifabutin, rifampin): decreased methadone effect, withdrawal symptoms may occur
CYP3A4 inhibitors (aprepitant, antiretroviral protease inhibitors, clarithromycin, danazol, delavirdine, diltiazem, erythromycin, fluconazole, FLUoxetine, fluvoxaMINE, imatinib, ketoconazole, mibefradil, nefazodone, telithromycin, voriconazole): increased toxicity
MAOIs: do not use for 2 wk before taking methadone: unpredictable reactions

Drug/food
Avoid use with grapefruit juice

🔺 Nurse Alert   ✴ Key NCLEX® Drug   ≫ Drug Specifics

Drug/herb
Chamomile, hops, kava, valerian: increased CNS depression

St. John's wort: avoid use, withdrawal may result

Drug/lab test
Increased: amylase, lipase

NURSING CONSIDERATIONS
Assessment
• **Assess for pain:** type, location, intensity, grimacing before and 1½-2 hr after administration; use pain scoring

• Monitor VS after parenteral route; note muscle rigidity, product history, liver, kidney function tests

• Monitor CNS changes: dizziness, drowsiness, hallucinations, euphoria, LOC, pupil reaction

• Monitor allergic reactions: rash, urticaria

• Monitor opioid detoxification: no analgesia occurs, only prevention of withdrawal symptoms

> **BLACK BOX WARNING:** Monitor B/P, pulse, ECG: hypotension, palpitations may occur

• Monitor bowel changes; bulk, fluids, laxatives should be used for constipation

> **BLACK BOX WARNING:** Respiratory dysfunction: respiratory depression, character, rate, rhythm; notify prescriber if respirations <10/min

> **BLACK BOX WARNING: QT prolongation:** may be dose related or use with other products that increase QT

> **BLACK BOX WARNING: Accidental exposure:** make sure product is not accessible to children, pets

> **BLACK BOX WARNING: Overdose, poisoning:** advise persons involved in correct use

> **BLACK BOX WARNING: Substance abuse:** may occur but has less psychological dependence than other opiate agonists

Patient/family education
• Instruct patient to report any symptoms of CNS changes, allergic reactions; to avoid CNS depressants (alcohol, sedative-hypnotics) for at least 24 hr after taking this product

• Discuss with patient that dizziness, drowsiness, and confusion are common; to avoid getting up without assistance

• Discuss in detail with patient all aspects of the product

• Caution patient to make position changes slowly to prevent orthostatic hypotension

• Teach patient withdrawal symptoms may occur: nausea, vomiting, cramps, fever, faintness, anorexia

• Advise patient to maintain proper hydration, avoid alcohol use

• Teach patient to avoid use with other products without approval of prescriber; many drug interactions

Evaluation
Positive therapeutic outcome
• Decreased pain
• Successful opioid withdrawal

TREATMENT OF OVERDOSE:
Naloxone (Narcan) 0.2-0.8 mg **IV**, O₂, **IV** fluids, vasopressors

---

methimazole (Rx)
(meth-im′a-zole)
Tapazole
Func. class.: Thyroid hormone antagonist (antithyroid)
Chem. class.: Thioamide
Pregnancy category D

M

Do not confuse: methimazole/metoprolol/minoxidil

ACTION: Inhibits synthesis of thyroid hormones by decreasing iodine use in the manufacture of thyroglobin and iodothyronine; does not affect already formed hormones, does not affect circulatory T_4, T_3

Therapeutic outcome: Decreased T_4 levels, hyperthyroid symptoms

USES: Hyperthyroidism, preparation for thyroidectomy

CONTRAINDICATIONS
Pregnancy **D**, breastfeeding, hypersensitivity

Precautions: Infection, bone marrow depression, hepatic disease, bleeding disorders

DOSAGE AND ROUTES
Hyperthyroidism
Adult: PO 15 mg/day (mild hyperthyroidism); 30-40 mg/day (moderate-severe); 60 mg/day (severe); maintenance dosage 5-15 mg/day, may be divided

Child: PO 0.4 mg/kg/day in divided doses q8hr; continue until euthyroid; maintenance dosage 0.2 mg/kg/day in divided doses q8hr, max 30 mg/24 hr, may be divided

---

Adverse effects: *italics* = common; **bold** = life-threatening

Preparation for thyroidectomy

Adult and child: PO same as above; iodine may be added for 10 days before surgery

Thyrotoxic crisis

Adult and child: PO same as hyperthyroidism with iodine and propranolol

Available forms: Tabs 5, 10, 15, 20 mg

Implementation

- Give with meals to decrease GI upset; give at same time each day to maintain product level
- Give lowest dosage that relieves symptoms
- Store in light-resistant container
- Increase fluids to 3-4 L/day, unless contraindicated

ADVERSE EFFECTS

CNS: *Drowsiness, headache, vertigo, fever,* paresthesias, neuritis
ENDO: *Enlarged thyroid*
GI: *Nausea, diarrhea, vomiting, jaundice, hepatitis,* loss of taste
GU: Nephritis
HEMA: Agranulocytosis, leukopenia, thrombocytopenia, hypothrombinemia, lymphadenopathy, bleeding, vasculitis
INTEG: *Rash, urticaria, pruritus, alopecia, hyperpigmentation,* lupuslike syndrome
MS: Myalgia, arthralgia, nocturnal muscle cramps

Pharmacokinetics

Absorption	Rapidly absorbed
Distribution	Crosses placenta
Metabolism	Liver, extensively
Excretion	Kidneys, unchanged; breast milk
Half-life	5-13 hr

Pharmacodynamics

Onset	Rapid
Peak	Peak 30-60 min
Duration	2-4 hr

INTERACTIONS

Individual drugs

Amiodarone, potassium iodide: decreased effectiveness
Digoxin: increased response
Radiation: increased bone marrow depression
Warfarin: decreased anticoagulant effect

Drug classifications

Antineoplastics: increased bone marrow depression

Drug/lab test

Increased: pro-time, AST, ALT, alkaline phosphatase

NURSING CONSIDERATIONS

Assessment

- **Hyperthyroidism:** palpitations, nervousness/loss of hair, insomnia, heat intolerance, weight loss, diarrhea
- **Hypothyroidism:** constipation, dry skin, weakness, fatigue, headache, intolerance to cold, weight gain; adjustment may be needed
- Monitor pulse, B/P, temp; check I&O ratio; check for edema (puffy hands, feet, periorbititis); indicates hypothyroidism
- Check weight daily; same clothing, scale, time of day
- Monitor T_3, T_4, which are increased; serum TSH, which is decreased; free thyroxine index, which is increased if dosage is too low; discontinue product 3-4 wk before radioactive iodine uptake
- ⚠ Monitor blood studies: CBC for blood dyscrasias (leukopenia, thrombocytopenia, agranulocytosis); if these occur, product should be discontinued and other treatment initiated; LFTs, may occur at higher doses
- **Assess for hypersensitivity** (rash, enlarged cervical lymph nodes); product may have to be discontinued
- **Assess for hypoprothrombinemia** (bleeding, petechiae, ecchymosis)
- Monitor clinical response: after 3 wk should include increased weight, pulse, decreased T_4
- ⚠ Assess for bone marrow depression: sore throat, fever, fatigue

Patient/family education

- Advise patient to abstain from breastfeeding after delivery; product appears in breast milk
- Instruct patient to take pulse daily; to keep graph of weight, pulse, mood
- Advise patient to report redness, swelling, sore throat, mouth lesions, which indicate blood dyscrasias
- Caution patient to avoid OTC products that contain iodine; that seafood and other iodine-containing products may be restricted by prescriber
- Caution patient not to discontinue this medication abruptly; thyroid crisis may occur; stress patient compliance
- Advise patient that response may take several mo if thyroid is large
- Teach patient symptoms/signs of overdose: periorbital edema, cold intolerance, mental depression; notify prescriber at once
- **Teach patient symptoms of inadequate dosage**: tachycardia, diarrhea, fever, irritability; prescriber should be notified to adjust
- Teach patient to take medication exactly as prescribed, not to skip or double doses; missed

doses should be taken when remembered up to 1 hr before next dose
• Instruct patient to carry ID describing medication taken and condition being treated

Evaluation

Positive therapeutic outcome
• Decreased weight gain
• Decreased pulse
• Decreased T_4
• Decreased B/P

⚠ HIGH ALERT

methotrexate (Rx)
(meth-oh-trex'ate)
Rheumatrex, Trexall
Func. class.: Antineoplastic, antimetabolite
Chem. class.: Folic acid antagonist
Pregnancy category X

Do not confuse: methotrexate/metolazone/mitoxantene

ACTION: Inhibits an enzyme that reduces folic acid, which is needed for nucleic acid synthesis in all cells; cell cycle specific (S phase); immunosuppressive

Therapeutic outcome: Prevention of rapidly growing malignant cells; immunosuppression

USES: Acute lymphocytic leukemia, in combination for breast, lung, head, neck carcinoma, lymphoma, sarcoma, gestational choriocarcinoma, hydatidiform mole, psoriasis, rheumatoid arthritis, mycosis fungoides, osteosarcoma

CONTRAINDICATIONS
Hypersensitivity, leukopenia ($<3500/mm^3$), thrombocytopenia ($<100,000/mm^3$), anemia, psoriatic patients with severe renal disease, alcoholism, HIV infection, AIDS

BLACK BOX WARNING: Pregnancy **X**, hepatic disease

Precautions: Breastfeeding, children

BLACK BOX WARNING: Renal disease, ascites, diarrhea, exfoliative dermatitis, infection, intrathecal administration, lymphoma, pleural effusion, pulmonary disease, radiation therapy, stomatitis, tumor lysis syndrome, ascites, renal impairment, stomatitis

DOSAGE AND ROUTES
Acute lymphocytic leukemia
Adult and child: PO/IM/**IV** 3.3 mg/m²/day × 4-6 wk until remission, then 20-30 mg/m² PO/IM qwk in 2 divided doses or 2.5 mg/kg **IV** q2wk

Burkitt's lymphoma (stages I, II, III) (unlabeled)
Adult: PO 10-25 mg/day × 4-8 days with 7-day rest period
Child ≥3 yr: intrathecally 12 mg q2-5days; child 2-3 yr 10 mg q2-5days; child 1-2 yr: 8 mg q2-5days

Meningeal leukemia
Adult: 12 mg/m² IT q2-5days until CSF is normal, then one additional dose, max 15 mg

Choriocarcinoma
Adult and child: PO/IM 15-30 mg/kg/day × 5 days, then off 1 wk; may repeat

Breast cancer
Adult: **IV** 40-60 mg/m² on day 1 of every 21-28 days with other antineoplastics

Epidermal head/neck cancer
Adult/child: **IV** 40 mg/m² on days 1 and 15, q21 days alone or in combination with bleomycin, CISplatin
Adult: PO 25-50 mg/m² q7 days
Child: PO 7.5-30 mg/m² q7-14 days

Rheumatoid arthritis
Adult: PO 7.5 mg/wk or divided doses of 2.5 mg q12hr × 3 dose qwk, max 20 mg/wk

Polyarticular-course juvenile RA
Child: PO/IM 10 mg/m² qwk

Osteosarcoma
Adult and child: **IV** 12 g/m² given over 4 hr, then leucovorin rescue is given

Mycosis fungoides
Adult: PO 2.5-10 mg/day until cleared (may be many mo); IM 50 mg qwk or 15-37.5 mg 2 ×/wk

Psoriasis
Adult: PO/IM/**IV** 10-25 mg qwk or 2.5 mg PO q12hr × 3 doses qwk; may increase to 25 mg qwk, max 30 mg/wk

Available forms: Tabs 2.5, 5, 7.5, 10, 15 mg; inj 25 mg/ml (2, 4, 8, 10, 20, 40 vials); 25 mg/ml (2,10 ml vials with benzyl alcohol); powder for inj 1 g

Implementation
• Avoid contact with skin, since product is very irritating; wash completely to remove
⚠ Leucovorin rescue: Administer leucovorin calcium within 24 hr of giving this

M

product to prevent tissue damage; check agency policy; continue until methotrexate level <10⁻⁸ m

• Give antiemetic 30-60 min before giving product and prn to prevent vomiting; administer antibiotics for infection prophylaxis
• Give in AM so product can be eliminated before bedtime
• Provide liquid diet: carbonated beverages; gelatin may be added if patient is not nauseated or vomiting

PO route
• Give 1 hr before or 2 hr after meals to prevent vomiting
• Make sure product is taken weekly in RA, JRA

IM route
• Give deeply in large muscle mass
• Store in tightly closed container in cool environment; store inj, powder for inj in dark, dry area

Direct IV route
• Give **IV** reconstitute to ≤ 25 mg/ml of sterile water for inj; give through **Y**-tube or 3-way stopcock

Intermittent/continuous IV route
• Further dilute in D₅W, D₅/0.9% NaCl, 0.9% NaCl; prior to infusion check patency of vein, flush with 5-10 ml of D₅W, 0.9% NaCl, infuse at 4-20 mg/hr or prescribed rate

IV infusion
• Intermediate or high dose: 500 mg/m² over <4 hr or >1 g/m² over >4 hr; confirm WBC >15 mm³, neutrophils >200 mm³, platelets > 75,000/mm³, serum bilirubin <1.2 mg/dl, serum creatinine WNL, SGPT <450 U, creatinine clearance >60 ml/min
⚠ **Give sodium bicarbonate tabs or IV fluids to prevent precipitation of product at high doses; urine pH should be >7; may need to reduce dose if BUN is 20-30 mg/dl or creatinine is 1.2-2 mg/dl; stop product if BUN >30 mg/dl or creatitine is >2 mg/dl**

Syringe incompatibilities: Droperidol, ranitidine

Y-site compatibilities: Acyclovir, alemtuzumab, alfentanye, allopurinol, amifostine, aminophylline, asparaginase, aztreonam, bleomycin, cefepime, cefTRIAXone, cimetidine, CISplatin, cyclophosphamide, cytarabine, DAUNOrubicin, dexchlorpheniramine, diphenhydrAMINE, doripenem, DOXOrubicin, etoposide, famotidine, filgrastim, fludarabine, fluorouracil, furosemide, gallium, ganciclovir, granisetron, heparin, HYDROmorphone, imipenem-cilastatin, leucovorin, LORazepam, melphalan, mesna,

methylPREDNISolone, metoclopramide, mitoMYcin, morphine, ondansetron, oxacillin, PACLitaxel, piperacillin/tazobactam, prochlorperazine, ranitidine, sargramostim, teniposide, thiotepa, vinBLAStine, vinCRIStine, vinorelbine, zolendronic acid

Y-site incompatibilities: Droperidol, IDArubicin

Additive compatibilities: Cephalothin, cyclophosphamide, cytarabine, fluorouracil, hydrOXYzine, mercaptopurine, ondansetron, sodium bicarbonate, vinCRIStine

Additive incompatibilities: Bleomycin, prednisoLONE

Solution compatibilities: Amino acids, 4.25%/D₂₅, D₅W, sodium bicarbonate 0.05 mol/L, 0.9% NaCl

> **BLACK BOX WARNING: Intrathecal route:** use preservative-free solutions, reconstitute with normal saline, the dose should be drawn into a 5-10 ml syringe after lumbar puncture, the volume of CSF should be withdrawn equal to volume of methotrexate, allow CSF to flow into syringe and mix, inject over 15-30 sec with bevel of needle upward

ADVERSE EFFECTS

CNS: Dizziness, seizures, headache, confusion, encephalopathy, hemiparesis, malaise, fatigue, chills, fever, leukoencephalopathy; arachnoiditis (intrathecal)
EENT: Blurred vision, optic neuropathy
GI: *Nausea, vomiting, anorexia, diarrhea, ulcerative stomatitis,* hepatotoxicity, cramps, ulcer, gastritis, GI hemorrhage, abdominal pain, hematemesis, hepatic fibrosis, acute toxicity
GU: Urinary retention, renal failure, menstrual irregularities, defective spermatogenesis, hematuria, azotemia, uric acid nephropathy
HEMA: Leukopenia, thrombocytopenia, myelosuppression, anemia
INTEG: *Rash, alopecia,* dry skin, urticaria, photosensitivity, folliculitis, vasculitis, petechiae, ecchymosis, acne, alopecia, severe fatal skin reactions
RESP: Methotrexate-induced lung disease
SYST: Sudden death, *Pneumocystis jiroveci* pneumonia, tumor lysis syndrome, secondary malignancy

---

⚠ Nurse Alert   ✳ Key NCLEX® Drug   >> Drug Specifics

Pharmacokinetics

Absorption	Well absorbed (GI)
Distribution	Widely distributed; crosses placenta
Metabolism	Not metabolized
Excretion	Kidneys, unchanged; breast milk (minimal)
Half-life	Terminal 10-12 hr; increased in renal disease

Pharmacodynamics

	PO	IM/IV	IT
Onset	Unknown	Unknown	Unknown
Peak	1-4 hr	½-2 hr	Unknown
Duration	Unknown	Unknown	Unknown

INTERACTIONS
Individual drugs
Acitretin: increased hepatitis; avoid concurrent use

Alcohol, phenylbutazone, probenecid, radiation, theophylline: increased toxicity

Digoxin (PO), fosphenytoin, phenytoin: decreased effect of each specific product

Folic acid: decreased effect of methotrexate, asparaginase

Radiation: increased bone marrow suppression

Drug classifications
Anticoagulants (oral): increased hypoprothrombinemia

Antineoplastics, NSAIDs, penicillins, salicylates, sulfa products: increased toxicity

Live virus vaccines: decreased antibodies

Proton pump inhibitors: do not use concurrently

NURSING CONSIDERATIONS
Assessment
• Assess buccal cavity q8hr for dryness, sores or ulceration, white patches, oral pain, bleeding, dysphagia; obtain prescription for viscous lidocaine (Xylocaine)

• **Assess symptoms indicating severe allergic reaction: rash, pruritus, urticaria, purpuric skin lesions, itching, flushing**

• Assess tachypnea, ECG changes, dyspnea, edema, fatigue; identify dyspnea, crackles, unproductive cough, chest pain, tachypnea

BLACK BOX WARNING: **Infection:** those with active infections should be treated for infection prior to product use; monitor temperature, fever may indicate beginning of infection

• **Monitor CBC, differential, platelet count weekly; avoid use until WBC is** >1500/mm^3

or platelet count is >75,000/mm^3, neutrophils >200/mm^3, notify prescriber of results if WBC <20,000/mm^3, platelets <150,000/mm^3; WBC, platelet nadirs occur on day 7; monitor

• Assess for increased uric acid levels, swelling, joint pain primarily in extremities; patient should be well hydrated to prevent urate deposits

• Make sure drug-drug interacting products are discontinued prior to therapy, and do not resume until methotrexate level is safe

BLACK BOX WARNING: Renal disease: avoid use in renal failure; monitor renal function studies: BUN, creatinine, serum uric acid, urine CCr before, during therapy; check I&O ratio; report fall in urine output to <30 ml/hr

BLACK BOX WARNING: **Hepatotoxicity:** monitor liver function tests before, during therapy (bilirubin, AST, ALT, LDH) as needed or monthly; check for jaundice of skin and sclera, dark urine, clay-colored stools, itchy skin, abdominal pain, fever, diarrhea (hepatotoxicity)

• Assess for bleeding: hematuria, stool guaiac, bruising or petechiae, mucosa or orifices; check for inflammation of mucosa, breaks in skin

• Identify effects of alopecia on body image; discuss feelings about body changes

• Identify edema in feet, joint and stomach pain, shaking; prescriber should be notified

• Monitor methotrexate levels, adjust leucovorin dose based on the level

BLACK BOX WARNING: Pulmonary toxicity: those with ascites or pleural effusions are at greater risk for toxicity, fluid should be removed before treatment, monitor plasma methotrexate level

BLACK BOX WARNING: Tumor lysis syndrome: hyperkalemia, hyperphosphatemia, hyperuricemia, hypocalcemia, decreased urine output; use aggressive hydration and allopurinol to correct severe electrolyte imbalances, renal toxicity

BLACK BOX WARNING: **Serious skin reaction:** Stevens-Johnson syndrome, exfoliative dermatitis, skin necrosis, erythema multiforme may occur within days of receiving product by any route; product should be discontinued

⚠ **Strokelike encephalopathy: common in high-dose therapy; assess for confusion, hemiparesis, seizures, coma; usually transient**

M

Adverse effects: *italics* = common; **bold** = life-threatening

• **Rheumatoid arthritis:** ROM, pain, joint swelling, prior to and during treatment
• **Psoriasis:** assess skin lesions prior to and during treatment

Patient/family education
• Encourage patient to rinse mouth tid-qid with water, club soda; brush teeth bid-qid with soft brush or cotton-tipped applicators for stomatitis; use unwaxed dental floss

> **BLACK BOX WARNING:** Advise patient that contraceptive measures for women and men are recommended during therapy; product is teratogenic; contraception should be used for 3 mo (male) and 4-6 wk (female); to discontinue breastfeeding; toxicity to infant may occur (X)

> **BLACK BOX WARNING:** Teach patient to avoid use of products containing aspirin or NSAIDs, razors, commercial mouthwash, since bleeding may occur; to report symptoms of bleeding (hematuria, tarry stools)

• Caution patient to report signs of anemia (fatigue, headache, irritability, faintness, shortness of breath); seizures
• Advise patient to report any changes in breathing or coughing even several mo after treatment; to avoid crowds and persons with respiratory tract or other infections
• Advise patient to report stomatitis: any bleeding, white spots, ulcerations in mouth to prescriber; tell patient to examine mouth daily, report symptoms, use good oral hygiene
• Teach patient that hair may be lost during treatment; a wig or hairpiece may make patient feel better; new hair may be different in color, texture
• Caution patient not to have any vaccinations without the advice of the prescriber; serious reactions can occur
• Advise patient to use sunblock or protective clothing to prevent burns
• Teach patient to use good dental care, to prevent overgrowth of infection in the mouth
• Teach patient how to use this product with leucovorin rescue
• Teach patient to continue leucovorin until told it is safe to stop
• Teach patient to report CNS symptoms, vision changes
• Teach patient to report fever, other symptoms of infection
• Teach patient to report decreased urine output

Evaluation
Positive therapeutic outcome
• Prevention of rapid division of malignant cells
• Decreased joint inflammation in RA

⚠ HIGH ALERT

methyldopa/methyldopate (Rx)
(meth-ill-doe′pa)
Func. class.: Antihypertensive
Chem. class.: Centrally acting α-adrenergic inhibitor
Pregnancy category B (PO) C (IV)

Do not confuse: methyldopa/L-dopa (levodopa)

ACTION: Stimulates central inhibitory α₂-adrenergic receptors or acts as false transmitter, resulting in reduction of arterial pressure

Therapeutic outcome: Decreased B/P in hypertension

USES: Hypertension, hypertensive crisis

CONTRAINDICATIONS
Active hepatic disease, hypersensitivity, MAOI therapy

Precautions: Pregnancy **B**, geriatric patients, cardiac disease, autoimmune disease, depression, dialysis, hemolytic anemia, Parkinson's disease, pheochromocytoma, sulfite hypersensitivity

DOSAGE AND ROUTES
Adult: PO 250-500 mg bid or tid, then adjusted q2day prn, 0.5-2 g/day in 2-4 divided doses (maintenance), max 3 g/day; **IV** 250-500 mg in 100 ml D₅W q6hr, run over 30-60 min, max 1 g q6hr, switch to PO as soon as possible
Child: PO 10 mg/kg/day in 2-4 divided doses, max 65 mg/kg or 3 g/day, whichever is less; **IV** 20-40 mg/kg/day in 4 divided doses, max 65 mg/kg or 3 g, whichever is less

Renal dose
Adult: PO CCr 10-50 ml/min dose q8-12hr; CCr <10 ml/min dose q12-24hr

Available forms: Methyldopa: tabs 250, 500 mg; methyldopate: inj 50 mg/ml (250 mg/5 ml)

Implementation
PO route
• Give before meals
• Shake susp before using
• Store in airtight container at room temperature
• Increase in dose should be done in the evening to minimize drowsiness

Intermittent IV infusion route
- Give after diluting in 100 ml of 0.9% NaCl, D₅W, D₅/0.9% NaCl, 5% sodium bicarbonate, Ringer's; administer over 30-60 min

Y-site compatibilities: Alemtuzumab, alfentanil, amikacin, aminophylline, anidulafungin, ascorbic acid, atenolol, atracurium, atropine, aztreonam, benztropine, bivalirudin, bleomycin, bumetanide, buprenorphine, butorphanol, calcium chloride/gluconate, caspofungin, cefamandole, ceFAZolin, cefmetazole, cefonicid, cefotaxime, cefoTEtan, cefOXitin, cefTAZidime, ceftizoxime, cefTRIAXone, cefuroxime, cephalothin, chlorproMAZINE, cimetidine, clindamycin, cyanocobalamin, cycloSPORINE, DACTINomycin, DAPTOmycin, dexamethasone, digoxin, diltiazem, diphenhydrAMINE, DOCEtaxel, DOPamine, doxycycline, enalaprilat, ePHEDrine, EPINEPHrine, epoetin alfa, ertapenem, erythromycin, esmolol, etoposide, etoposide phosphate, famotidine, fenoldopam, fentaNYL, fluconazole, fludarabine, gatifloxacin, gemcitabine, gentamicin, glycopyrrolate, granisetron, heparin, hydrocortisone, HYDROmorphone, hydrOXYzine, IDArubicin, insulin(regular), irinotecan, isoproterenol, labetalol, lidocaine, linezolid, LORazepam, magnesium sulfate, mannitol, mechlorethamine, meperidine, metaraminol, methicillin, methoxamine, methylPREDNISolone, metoclopramide, metoprolol, metroNIDAZOLE, mezlocillin, miconazole, midazolam, milrinone, minocycline, mitoXANtrone, morphine, moxalactam, multiple vitamins, mycophenolate mofetil, nafcillin, nalbuphine, naloxone, netilmicin, nitroglycerin, nitroprusside, norepinephrine, octreotide, ondansetron, oxacillin, oxaliplatin, oxytocin, PACLitaxel, palonosetron, pamidronate, pancuronium, pantoprazole, papaverine, PEMEtrexed, penicillin G potassium/sodium, pentazocine, phentolamine, phenylephrine, phytonadione, piperacillin, polymyxin B, potassium chloride, procainamide, prochlorperazine, promethazine, propranolol, protamine, pyridoxine, quiNIDine, ranitidine, ritodrine, sodium bicarbonate, succinylcholine, SUFentanil, tacrolimus, teniposide, theophylline, thiamine, thiotepa, ticarcillin, ticarcillin-clavulanate, tigecycline, tirofiban, tobramycin, tolazoline, trimetaphan, urokinase, vancomycin, vasopressin, vecuronium, verapamil, vinorelbine, voriconazole, zoledronic acid

Additive compatibilities: Aminophylline, ascorbic acid, chloramphenicol, diphenhydrAMINE, heparin, magnesium sulfate, multivitamins, netilmicin, potassium chloride, promazine, sodium bicarbonate, succinylcholine, verapamil, vit B/C

Additive incompatibilities: Amphotericin B, barbiturates, methohexital, sulfonamides

Solution compatibilities: D₅W, D₅/0.9% NaCl, Ringer's, sodium bicarbonate 5%, 0.9% NaCl, amino acids 4.25%/D₂₅, Dextran₆/0.9% NaCl, Normosol R, Normosol M/D₅W

ADVERSE EFFECTS

CNS: *Drowsiness, weakness, dizziness, sedation, headache,* depression, psychosis, paresthesias, parkinsonism, Bell's palsy, nightmares, **drug fever**

CV: Bradycardia, **myocarditis**, orthostatic hypotension, angina, edema, weight gain, **CHF**, paradoxical pressor response (**IV** use)

EENT: Nasal congestion

ENDO: Breast enlargement, gynecomastia, amenorrhea

GI: Nausea, vomiting, diarrhea, constipation, **hepatic dysfunction**, sore or "black" tongue, **pancreatitis**, colitis, flatulence

GU: Impotence, failure to ejaculate

HEMA: **Leukopenia, thrombocytopenia, hemolytic anemia, granulocytopenia**, positive Coombs' test

INTEG: Lupuslike syndrome, rash, **toxic epidural necrolysis**

Pharmacokinetics

Absorption	50% (PO)
Distribution	Crosses placenta, blood-brain barrier
Metabolism	Liver, moderately
Excretion	Kidneys, unchanged (partially)
Half-life	1½ hr

Pharmacodynamics

	PO	IV
Onset	Onset 4-6 hr	Unknown
Peak	4-6 hr	Onset 4-6 hr
Duration	24-48 hr	10-16 hr

INTERACTIONS
Individual drugs
Alcohol: CNS depression
Haloperidol: increased psychosis
Iron: decreased methyldopa absorption
Levodopa: increased CNS toxicity, hypotension
Lithium: increased lithium toxicity
TOLBUTamide: increased hypoglycemia

Drug classifications
Amphetamines, antidepressants (tricyclics), barbiturates, NSAIDs, phenothiazines: decreased antihypertensive effect

M

Analgesics, antidepressants, antihistamines, sedative/hypnotics: increased CNS depression

Antihypertensives, diuretics: increased hypotension

β-Adrenergic blockers: increased B/P

MAOIs: increased pressor effect, do not use concurrently

Sympathomimetic amines: increased pressor effect

Drug/lab test

Increased: creatinine, LFTs

Decreased: platelets, WBC, Hgb/Hct

Interference: urinary uric acid, serum creatinine, AST

False increase: urinary catecholamines

NURSING CONSIDERATIONS
Assessment

• **Hemolytic anemia: monitor blood tests: CBC, neutrophils, decreased platelets; direct Coombs' test before, after 6, 12 mo of therapy; a positive test may indicate hemolytic anemia; usually reverses within weeks to months after discontinuing treatment, monitor Hgb/Hct and RBC, do not start therapy in those with hemolytic anemia**

• Monitor renal studies: protein, BUN, creatinine; watch for increased levels that may indicate nephrotic syndrome: polyuria, oliguria, frequency; report weight gain >5 lb

• **Drug-induced hepatitis/drug fever: usually subsides within 3 months of discontinuing therapy**

• **Product tolerance:** may occur within 3 mo of starting treatment; dosage change and other products may be needed

• Obtain baselines in renal, liver function tests before therapy begins; check potassium levels, although hyperkalemia rarely occurs

• Monitor B/P, pulse if the product is being used for hypertension; notify prescriber of changes

• Monitor edema in feet, legs daily; monitor I&O; check weight for decreasing output

• Assess for allergic reaction: rash, fever, pruritus, urticaria; product should be discontinued if antihistamines fail to help

• Monitor CNS symptoms, especially in the geriatric; depression; change in mental status

Patient/family education

• Instruct patient not to discontinue product abruptly, or withdrawal symptoms may occur: anxiety, increased B/P, headache, insomnia, increased pulse, tremors, nausea, sweating

• Caution patient not to use OTC (cough, cold, or allergy) products unless directed by prescriber

• Teach patient about excessive perspiration, dehydration, vomiting, diarrhea; may lead to fall in B/P; consult prescriber if these occur

• Advise patient that product may cause dizziness, fainting; light-headedness may occur during 1st few days of therapy; that product may cause dry mouth, use hard candy, saliva product, or frequent rinsing of mouth; caution patient to change position slowly, to rise slowly to sitting or standing position to minimize orthostatic hypotension, especially geriatric

• Caution patient that compliance is necessary; not to skip or stop product unless directed by prescriber

• Teach patient that product may cause skin rash

• Teach patient to avoid hazardous activities, since product may cause drowsiness, dizziness

Evaluation

Positive therapeutic outcome
• Decreased B/P

TREATMENT OF OVERDOSE:
Gastric evacuation, sympathomimetics may be indicated if severe; hemodialysis

methylergonovine (Rx)
(meth-ill-er-goe-noe′veen)
Methergine
Func. class.: Oxytocic
Chem. class.: Ergot alkaloid
Pregnancy category C

ACTION: Stimulates uterine and vascular smooth muscle, causing contractions, decreased bleeding, arterial vasoconstriction

Therapeutic outcome: Absence of hemorrhage

USES: Prevention, treatment of hemorrhage postpartum or after abortion, uterine contractions

CONTRAINDICATIONS
Pregnancy (4th stage of labor [other than obstetric delivery/abortion]), hypersensitivity to ergot preparations, preeclampsia, eclampsia, elective induction of labor

Precautions: Severe renal/hepatic disease, jaundice, diabetes mellitus, seizure disorders, sepsis, CAD, last stage of labor

DOSAGE AND ROUTES
Adult: PO 200 mcg tid-qid up to 7 days; IM/IV 200 mcg q2-4hr for 1-5 doses

Available forms: Inj 200 mcg/ml; tabs 200 mcg

Implementation
PO route
- PO is the preferred route
- Do not exceed dosage limits
- Store tabs at room temperature
- Give with water

IM route
- Give inj deeply in large muscle mass, aspirate
- Protect from light

Direct IV route
- Give by this route for severe, life-threatening hemorrhage
- Give directly undiluted or diluted with 5 ml of 0.9% NaCl given through Y-site or 3-way stopcock; give 0.2 mg/min; use clear, colorless sol
- Store up to 2 mo if unused

Y-site compatibilities: Heparin, hydrocortisone sodium succinate, potassium chloride, vit B/C

ADVERSE EFFECTS
CNS: *Headache, dizziness,* seizures, hallucinations, **stroke (IV)**
CV: *Hypotension,* chest pain, palpitations, *hypertension,* dysrhythmias; **CVA (IV)**
EENT: Tinnitus
GI: *Nausea, vomiting*
GU: Cramping
INTEG: Sweating, rash, allergic reactions
MS: Leg cramps
RESP: *Dyspnea*

Pharmacokinetics

Absorption	Well absorbed (PO, IM)
Distribution	Unknown
Metabolism	Liver, possibly
Excretion	Unknown
Half-life	½-2 hr

Pharmacodynamics

	PO	IM	IV
Onset	5-15 min	5 min	Immediate
Peak	Unknown	Unknown	Unknown
Duration	3 hr	3 hr	Unknown

INTERACTIONS
Individual drugs
Smoking: increased vasoconstriction

Drug classifications
CYP3A4 inhibitors: increased ergot toxicity, do not use together
Vasopressors, ergots, anesthetics (regional): increased vasoconstriction

NURSING CONSIDERATIONS
Assessment
- Monitor B/P, pulse; watch for change that may indicate hemorrhage
- Assess fundal tone, nonphasic contractions; check for relaxation or severe cramping
- **Assess for ergotism or overdose:** nausea, vomiting, weakness, muscular pain, insensitivity to cold, paresthesia of extremities; product should be decreased or infusion discontinued
- Before administering ergonovine, check calcium levels; if hypocalcemia is present, correction should be made to increase effectiveness of this product
- Monitor prolactin levels and for decreased breast milk production

Patient/family education
- Inform patient that abdominal cramps are a side effect of this medication
- Instruct patient to notify prescriber if chest pain, nausea, vomiting, headache, muscle pain, weakness, or cold, numb extremities occur

Evaluation
Positive therapeutic outcome
- Prevention of hemorrhage

M

methylnaltrexone (Rx)
(meth-il-nal-trex′one)
Relistor
Func. class.: Opioid antagonist
Pregnancy category B

ACTION: Peripheral mu-opioid receptor antagonist that reduces constipation associated with opiate agonists

Therapeutic outcome: Decreased constipation

USES: Treatment of opioid-induced constipation in patients with advanced illness who are receiving palliative care when response to laxative therapy has been insufficient

CONTRAINDICATIONS
Hypersensitivity, GI obstruction, **IV** route

Precautions: Pregnancy **B,** breastfeeding, renal disease, children, diarrhea, driving, operating machinery, geriatric patients, neoplastic disease, Crohn's disease, peptic ulcer, ulcerative colitis

DOSAGE AND ROUTES
Opiate-agonist induced constipation
Adult >114 kg: SUBCUT 0.15 mg/kg every other day prn

Adverse effects: *italics* = common; **bold** = life-threatening

Adult 62-114 kg: SUBCUT 12 mg every other day prn, max 12 mg/24 hr
Adult 38-62 kg: SUBCUT 8 mg every other day prn, max 8 mg/24 hr
Adult <38 kg: SUBCUT 0.15 mg/kg every other day prn, max 0.15 mg/kg/24 hr

Renal dose
Adult: SUBCUT CCr <30 ml/min, reduce normal adult dose by 50%

Available forms: Solution for inj 12 mg/0.6 ml, 8 mg/0.4 ml

Implementation
• Give SUBCUT only; oral dose is investigational and not currently available
• Do not give **IV; IV** dosing for urinary retention is investigational
• Store at 15°-30° C (59°-86° F); do not freeze
• Store away from light
SUBCUT route
• Inspect the solution before use; it should be a clear, colorless to pale yellow aqueous solution; do not use if particulate matter or discoloration are present
• Withdraw the needed amount of solution into a sterile syringe; if immediate administration is impossible, the syringe may be kept at room temperature for up to 24 hr; the syringe does not need to be kept away from light during the 24-hr period; immediately discard any unused portion in the vial; no preservatives are present
• Administer into the upper arm, abdomen, or thigh no more than 1 ×/24 hr; rotate inj sites; do not inject the same spot each time; do not inject into areas where skin is tender, bruised, red, or hard; avoid areas with scars or stretch marks
• If using with retractable needle, slowly push down on the plunger past the resistance point until the syringe is empty and a click is heard

ADVERSE EFFECTS
CNS: Dizziness
GI: Nausea, vomiting, diarrhea, flatulence, abdominal pain, **GI perforation**
INTEG: Hyperhidrosis

Pharmacokinetics

Absorption	Unknown
Distribution	Protein binding 11%-15.3%
Metabolism	Unknown
Excretion	Unknown
Half-life	Terminal 8 hr

Pharmacodynamics

Onset	Unknown
Peak	30 min (SUBCUT)
Duration	Unknown

NURSING CONSIDERATIONS
Assessment
• Monitor serum creatinine
• **Opioid-induced constipation:** assess for stool characteristics: amount, consistency; bowel sounds during treatment

Patient/family education
• Teach patient that after 30 min, toilet facilities should be nearby, bowel relaxation occurs, not to use more than one dose in 24 hr
• Advise patient to notify prescriber of abdominal pain, continuous or severe diarrhea, nausea or vomiting
• Teach patient to avoid use in pregnancy unless absolutely necessary; avoid in breastfeeding

Evaluation
Positive therapeutic outcome
• Decreased constipation

methylphenidate (Rx)
(meth-ill-fen'i-date)
Biphentin ✦, Concerta, Daytrana, Metadate CD, Methidate, Methylin, Quillivant XR, Ritalin, Ritalin LA, Ritalin SR
Func. class.: Cerebral stimulant
Chem. class.: Piperidine derivative
Pregnancy category C
Controlled substance schedule II

Do not confuse: methylphenidate/methadone

ACTION: Increases release of norepinephrine and dopamine in cerebral cortex to reticular activating system; exact action not known

Therapeutic outcome: Increased alertness, decreased fatigue, ability to stay awake (narcolepsy), increased attention span, decreased hyperactivity (ADHD)

USES: Attention deficit disorder with hyperactivity (ADHD), narcolepsy (except Concerta, Metadate CD, Ritalin LA), attention deficit disorder (ADD)

CONTRAINDICATIONS
Hypersensitivity, anxiety, history of Tourette's syndrome, children <6 yr, glaucoma, anorexia nervosa, tartrazine dye hypersensitivity, glaucoma

Precautions: Pregnancy **C,** breastfeeding, hypertension, depression, seizures

BLACK BOX WARNING: Substance abuse

DOSAGE AND ROUTES
Attention-deficit/hyperactivity disorder (ADHD) initial treatment (not currently on methylphenidate)
>> Regular release: Ritalin, Methylin, Methylin oral sol, Methylin chew tabs

Adult: PO 20-30 mg/day, range 10-60 mg/day in 2-3 divided doses, 30-45 min before meals
Child ≥6 yr: PO 5 mg bid initially, increase 5-10 mg/day qwk, usual dose 0.3-2 mg/kg/day, max 60 mg/day

>> Extended release: Ritalin SR, Metadate ER, Methylin ER
Adult/adolescent/child ≥6 yr: PO max 20-30 mg tid

>> Extended-release once-daily tabs: Concerta
Adult: PO 18-36 mg/day initially, then adjust by 18 mg q wk, max 72 mg/day
Adolescent: PO 18 mg/day initially, then adjust by 18 mg q wk, max 72 mg/day
Child ≥6 yr: PO 18 mg/day initially, then adjust by 18 mg q wk, max 54 mg/day

>> Extended-release once-daily capsules: Ritalin LA
Adult/adolescent/child ≥6 yr: PO 10-20 mg/day in AM initially, adjust by 10 mg qwk, max 60 mg/day

>> Extended-release once-daily capsules: Metadate CD
Adult/adolescent/child ≥6 yr: PO 20 mg/day in AM, adjust by 10-20 mg qwk, max 60 mg/day

>> Transdermal: Daytrana
Adolescent/child ≥6 yr: TD wk 1: 10 mg/day (9-hr patch); wk 2: 15 mg/day (9-hr patch); wk 3: 20 mg/day (9-hr patch); wk 4: 30 mg/day (9-hr patch)

Conversion to once-daily from other forms for ADHD
>> Extended-release once-daily capsules: Metadate CD
Adult/adolescent/child ≥6 yr: PO give no more than total daily dose of other forms, may adjust by 20 mg qwk, max 60 mg/day

>> Extended-release once-daily capsules: Ritalin LA
Adult/adolescent/child ≥6 yr: PO give no more than total daily dose of other forms, may adjust by 10 mg qwk, max 60 mg/day

>> Extended-release once-daily tablets: Concerta
Adult/adolescent/child ≥6 yr (currently receiving 10-15 mg/day): PO 18 mg q AM initially, adjust by 18 mg qwk, max 72 mg/day (adult); max 72 mg/day, 2 mg/kg/day (adolescent); 54 mg/day (child)
Adult/adolescent/child ≥6 yr (currently receiving 20-30 mg/day): PO 36 mg q AM, adjust by 18 mg qwk, max 72 mg/day (adult); 72 mg/day, 2 mg/kg/day (adolescent); 54 mg/day (child)
Adult/adolescent/child ≥6 yr (currently receiving 30-45 mg/day): PO 54 mg q AM, adjust by 18 mg qwk, max 72 mg/day (adult); 72 mg/day, 2 mg/kg/day (adolescent); 54 mg/day (child)
Adult/adolescent/child ≥6 yr (currently receiving 40-60 mg/day): PO 72 mg q AM, 72 mg/day

>> Extended-release once daily tabs: Quillivant XR
Child > 6 yr/adolescent: PO 20 mg/day in AM, may increase by 10-20 mg qwk

>> Transdermal: Daytrana
Adolescent and child ≥6 yr: TD wk 1: 10 mg/day (9-hr patch); wk 2: 15 mg/day (9-hr patch); wk 3: 20 mg/day (9-hr patch); wk 4: 30 mg/day (9-hr patch)

Narcolepsy
>> Immediate release: Ritalin, Methylin oral sol, Methylin chew tabs
Adult: PO 20-30 mg/day, range 10-60 mg/day in 2-3 divided doses
Child ≥6 yr: PO 5 mg bid, may increase by 5-10 mg qwk, max 60 mg/day

>> Extended-release tabs: Ritalin SR, Metadate ER
Adult/adolescent/child ≥6 yr: PO max 20 mg tid

Poststroke depression; major depression (unlabeled)
Adult and geriatric: PO (immediate rel tabs) 2.5 mg bid morning/noon, may increase by 2.5-5 mg q2-3days

Available forms: Tabs 5, 10, 20 mg; ext rel tabs 10, 20, mg; ext rel tabs (Concerta) 18, 27, 36, 54 mg; ext rel caps 10, 20, 30, 40 mg; oral sol 5 mg, 10 mg/ml; chew tabs (Methylin) 2.5, 5, 10 mg; transdermal patch 12.5 cm^2 (10 mg), 18.75 cm^2 (15 mg), 25 cm^2 (20 mg), 37.5 cm^2 (30 mg)

Implementation
PO route
• Do not chew, crush time rel tabs; caps may be opened and beads sprinkled over spoonful of applesauce

---

• Give at least 6 hr before bedtime (regular release); at least 10 hr (ext rel) to avoid sleeplessness; titrate to patient's response; lowest dosage should be used to control symptoms
• Give gum, hard candy, frequent sips of water for dry mouth at beginning of treatment; these symptoms tend to lessen with time
• Avoid Metadate CD on day of surgery

Transdermal route
• Place on clean, dry area of the hip; avoid waist; removal is 9 hr after application; fold after removal and flush down toilet
• If patch falls off, apply a new patch to a different site; total wear time should be 9 hr

ADVERSE EFFECTS

CNS: *Hyperactivity, insomnia, restlessness, talkativeness,* dizziness, headache, akathisia, dyskinesia, masking or worsening of Tourette's syndrome, **seizures,** drowsiness, toxic psychosis, hallucinations, **neuroleptic malignant syndrome, aggression, cerebral vasculitis, hemorrhage, stroke (rare)**
CV: *Palpitations, tachycardia,* B/P changes, angina, **dysrhythmias**
ENDO: Growth retardation
GI: Nausea, anorexia, dry mouth, weight loss, abdominal pain
HEMA: **Leukopenia, anemia, thrombocytopenic purpura**
INTEG: **Exfoliative dermatitis,** urticaria, rash, erythema multiforme, **hypersensitivity reactions;** patch: permanent loss of skin color
MISC: Fever, arthralgia, scalp hair loss, **rhabdomyolysis**

Pharmacokinetics

Absorption	Well absorbed (PO); delayed (ext rel)
Distribution	Widely distributed; crosses placenta
Metabolism	Liver
Excretion	Kidneys
Half-life	1-3 hr

Pharmacodynamics

	PO	PO–ext rel
Onset	Varies with formulation	2 hr
Peak	1-3 hr	4 hr
Duration		6-8 hr

INTERACTIONS
Individual drugs
Guanethidine: decreased effect of guanethidine

Drug classifications
Anticonvulsants, antidepressants (tricyclics), SNRIs, CNS stimulants, selective serotonin reuptake inhibitors (SSRIs): increased effects
MAOIs (or within 14 days of MAOIs), vasopressors: hypertensive crisis
Antihypertensives: decreased effects of antihypertensives

Drug/herb
Cola nut, guarana, horsetail, yerba maté, yohimbe: increased CNS stimulation
Melatonin: synergistic effect

Drug/food
Caffeine: increased stimulation

NURSING CONSIDERATIONS
Assessment
• **ADHD:** In children or adults with ADHD, monitor for improved organizational skills, attention span, attending to tasks, impulse control, socialization, and ability to get along better with others

> **BLACK BOX WARNING: Substance abuse:** there is a high potential for abuse, use caution in those with history of substance abuse

• Monitor VS, B/P, since this product may reverse antihypertensives; check patients with cardiac disease more often for increased B/P
• Perform CBC, urinalysis; for diabetic patients monitor blood glucose, urine glucose; insulin changes may be required, since eating will decrease, but decreased growth will resume when product is discontinued
• Monitor height and weight q3mo since growth rate in children may be decreased; appetite is suppressed, weight loss is common during the first few mo of treatment
• Monitor mental status: mood, sensorium, affect, stimulation, insomnia; aggressiveness may occur; depression with crying spells may occur after product has worn off
• Assess for tolerance; should not be used for extended time except in ADHD; dosage should be discontinued gradually to prevent withdrawal symptoms
• **Assess for narcoleptic symptoms before medication and after; ability to stay awake should increase significantly**
⚠ Assess for withdrawal symptoms: headache, nausea, vomiting, muscle pain, weakness; product tolerance will develop after long-term use; dosage should not be increased if tolerance develops, usually not associated with drug holidays
• Assess appetite, sleep, speech patterns

Patient/family education
• Teach patient to decrease caffeine consumption (coffee, tea, cola, chocolate); not to use guarana, cola nut, yerba maté, which may increase irritability and stimulation; to avoid OTC preparations unless approved by prescriber; to avoid alcohol ingestion; these may cause serious product interactions
• Advise patient to taper off product over several wk; or depression, increased sleeping, lethargy may occur
• Notify prescriber if skin irritation or rash occurs
• Caution patient to avoid hazardous activities until stabilized on medication
• Instruct patient not to double doses if medication is missed; prescriber may suggest product holidays (ADHD) during the school year to assess progress and determine continued product necessity
• Instruct patient/family to notify prescriber if significant side effects occur: tremors, insomnia, palpitations, restlessness; product changes may be needed
• Inform patient that if dry mouth occurs to use frequent sips of water, sugarless gum, hard candy during beginning therapy; dry mouth lessens with continued treatment
• Encourage patient to get needed rest; patient will feel more tired at end of day; to take last dose at least 6 hr before bedtime to avoid insomnia
• Advise patient that shell of Concerta tab may appear in stools

Evaluation
Positive therapeutic outcome
• Decreased hyperactivity in ADHD
• Improved attention span in ADHD
• Absence of sleeping during day in narcolepsy

TREATMENT OF OVERDOSE:
Administer fluids, hemodialysis, peritoneal dialysis, antihypertensives for increased B/P; administer short-acting barbiturate before lavage

---

methylPREDNISolone (Rx)
(meth-ill-pred-niss′oh-lone)
A-Methapred, Depo-Medrol, Medrol, Solu-MEDROL
Func. class.: Corticosteroid, synthetic
Chem. class.: Glucocorticoid, immediate acting
Pregnancy category C

Do not confuse: methylPREDNISolone/
medroxyPROGESTERone/predniSONE/
methylTESTOSTERone

ACTION: Decreases inflammation by suppression of migration of polymorphonuclear leukocytes, fibroblasts; reverses increased capillary permeability and lysosomal stabilization

Therapeutic outcome: Decreased inflammation

USES: Severe inflammation, shock, adrenal insufficiency, collagen disorders, management of acute spinal cord injury, multiple sclerosis

CONTRAINDICATIONS
Hypersensitivity, intrathecal use, neonates

Precautions: Pregnancy **C**, breastfeeding, diabetes mellitus, glaucoma, osteoporosis, seizure disorders, ulcerative colitis, CHF, myasthenia gravis, renal disease, esophagitis, peptic ulcer, tartrazine, benzyl alcohol, corticosteroid hypersensitivity, viral infection, TB, traumatic brain injury, Cushing's syndrome, measles, varicella, fungal infections

DOSAGE AND ROUTES
Adrenal insufficiency/inflammation
Adult: PO 4-48 mg in 4 divided doses; IM 10-120 mg (acetate); IM/IV 10-40 mg (succinate); intraarticular 4-80 mg (acetate)
Child: IV 0.5-1.7 mg/kg in 3-4 divided doses (succinate)

Multiple sclerosis
Adult: PO 160 mg/day × 1 wk, then 64 mg every other day × 30 days

Available forms: Tabs 2, 4, 6, 8, 16, 32 mg; inj 20, 40, 80 mg/ml acetate; inj 40, 125, 500, 1000, 2000 mg/vial succinate

Implementation
PO route
• Give with food or milk to decrease GI symptoms
• Single daily dose should be given in AM to coincide with body's normal cortisol secretion
IM route
• Give IM inj deep in large muscle mass; rotate sites; avoid deltoid; use 21-G needle; injection site reaction may occur (induration, pain at site, atrophy)
• Give in one dose in AM to prevent adrenal suppression; avoid SUBCUT administration; may damage tissue

IV route
• Use only methylPREDNISolone sodium succinate (Solu-MEDROL) IV, never use methylPREDNISolone acetate suspension IV
• Give after diluting with provided diluent, agitate slowly; give directly over 3-15 min; doses ≥2 mg/kg or 250 mg should be given by

M

intermittent IV infusion unless potential benefits outweigh potential risks

Intermittent/continuous IV infusion route
- Dilute further in D₅W, 0.9% NaCl, D₅NS, haze may form, give over 15-60 min, large doses (≥500 mg) give over 30-60 min
- Give after shaking susp (parenteral)
- Give titrated dosage; use lowest effective dosage

Y-site compatibilities: Acetaminophen, acyclovir, amifostine, aztreonam, cefepime, CISplatin, cladribine, cyclophosphamide, cytarabine, DOPamine, DOXOrubicin, enalaprilat, famotidine, fludarabine, granisetron, heparin, inamrinone, melphalan, meperidine, methotrexate, metroNIDAZOLE, midazolam, morphine, piperacillin/tazobactam, sodium bicarbonate, tacrolimus, teniposide, theophylline, thiotepa, vit B with C

Y-site incompatibilities: Ondansetron, PACLitaxel, sargramostim, vinorelbine

Inhalation route
- Give inh with water to decrease possibility of fungal infections
- Give titrated dosage; use lowest effective dosage
- Clean aerosol topically daily with warm water; dry thoroughly
- Store in cool environment; do not puncture or incinerate container

Topical route
- Cleanse area before applying product
- Apply only to affected areas; do not get in eyes
- Apply medication, then cover with occlusive dressing (only if prescribed); seal to normal skin; change q12hr; systemic absorption may occur
- Apply only to dermatoses; do not use on weeping, denuded, or infected area
- Apply treatment for a few days after area has cleared
- Store at room temperature

ADVERSE EFFECTS
CNS: Depression, flushing, sweating, headache, mood changes
CV: Hypertension, circulatory collapse, thrombophlebitis, embolism, tachycardia
EENT: Fungal infections, increased intraocular pressure, blurred vision, cataracts
GI: Diarrhea, nausea, abdominal distention, GI hemorrhage, increased appetite, pancreatitis
HEMA: Thrombocytopenia
INTEG: Acne, poor wound healing, ecchymosis, petechiae
MS: Fractures, osteoporosis, weakness

Pharmacokinetics

Absorption	Well absorbed (PO); systemic (topical)
Distribution	Crosses placenta
Metabolism	Liver, extensively
Excretion	Kidney
Half-life	3-5 hr (plasma) 18-36 hr (tissue); adrenal suppression 3-4 days

Pharmacodynamics

	PO	IM	IV	Topical
Onset	Unknown	Unknown	Rapid	Min to hr
Peak	2 hr	4-8 days	Unknown	Hr to days
Duration	1½ days	1-4 wk	Unknown	Hr to days

INTERACTIONS
Individual drugs
Amphotericin B: increased side effects
Insulin: increased need for insulin
Phenytoin, rifampin: decreased action; increased metabolism
Somatrem: decreased effect

Drug classifications
Contraceptives, oral: increased methylPREDNISolone action
CYP3A4 inducers (barbiturates, bosentan, carBAMazepine, efavirenz, phenytoins, nevirapine, rifabutin, rifampin): decreased methylPREDNISolone effect
CYP3A4 inhibitors (aprepitant, antiretroviral protease inhibitors, clarithromycin, danazol, delavirdine, diltiazem, erythromycin, fluconazole, FLUoxetine, fluvoxaMINE, imatinib, ketoconazole, mibefradil, nefazodone, telithromycin, voriconazole): increased adrenal suppression
Diuretics: increased side effects
Hypoglycemic agents: increased need for hypoglycemic agents
Vaccines: decreased effects of vaccines

Drug/herb
St. John's wort: avoid use

Drug/food
Grapefruit juice: increased methylPREDNISolone level; do not use concurrently

Drug/lab test
Increased: cholesterol, blood glucose
Decreased: calcium, potassium, T₄, T₃, thyroid radioactive iodine uptake test, urine 17-OHCS, 17-KS
False negative: skin allergy tests

NURSING CONSIDERATIONS
Assessment
• **Adrenal insufficiency:** assess for weight loss, nausea, vomiting, confusion, anxiety, hypotension, weakness
• Monitor plasma cortisol levels during long-term therapy (normal level 138-635 nmol/L when drawn at 8 AM)
• Monitor potassium, blood glucose, urine glucose while patient is on long-term therapy; hypokalemia and hyperglycemia
• Monitor weight daily; notify prescriber of weekly gain >5 lb
• Monitor B/P q4hr, pulse; notify prescriber if chest pain occurs
• Monitor I&O ratio; be alert for decreasing urinary output and increasing edema
• Monitor adrenal function periodically for hypothalamic-pituitary-adrenal axis suppression
• **Assess for infection:** increased temp, WBC even after withdrawal of medication; product masks infection symptoms
• Assess for potassium depletion: paresthesias, fatigue, nausea, vomiting, depression, polyuria, dysrhythmias, weakness
• Assess for edema, hypertension, cardiac symptoms
• Assess mental status: affect, mood, behavioral changes, aggression
• Check temp; if fever develops, product should be discontinued
• Assess for systemic absorption: increased temp, inflammation, irritation (topical)

Patient/family education
• Teach patient that emergency ID as corticosteroid user should be carried/worn
• Advise patient to notify prescriber if therapeutic response decreases; dosage adjustment may be needed
⚠ **Caution patient not to discontinue abruptly; adrenal crisis can result**
• Teach patient to take PO with food, milk, to decrease GI symptoms
• Caution patient to avoid OTC products: salicylates, alcohol in cough products, cold preparations unless directed by prescriber
• Teach patient all aspects of product use including cushingoid symptoms
• Teach patient symptoms of **adrenal insufficiency:** nausea, anorexia, fatigue, dizziness, dyspnea, weakness, joint pain
• Inform patient that long-term therapy may be needed to clear infection (1-2 mo depending on type of infection)
Nasal route
• Advise patient to clear nasal passages if sneezing attack occurs; repeat dose

• Advise patient to continue using product even if mild nasal bleeding occurs; is usually transient
• Teach patient method of instillation after providing written instructions from manufacturer
• Teach patient to recognize **cushingoid symptoms:** buffalo hump, moon face, rapid weight gain, excess sweating
• **Infection:** Teach patient to avoid persons with known infections; corticosteroids can mask symptoms of infection
Topical route
• Advise patient to avoid sunlight on affected area; burns may occur

Evaluation
Positive therapeutic outcome
• Ease of respirations, decreased inflammation
• Absence of severe itching, patches on skin, flaking (top)

metipranolol ophthalmic
See Appendix B

metoclopramide (Rx)
(met-oh-kloe-pra′mide)
Apo-Metoclop ♣, Metozolv ODT, Reglan
Func. class.: Cholinergic, antiemetic
Chem. class.: Central dopamine receptor antagonist
Pregnancy category B

M

Do not confuse: metoclopramide/metolazone, **Reglan**/Megace/Renagel

ACTION: Enhances response to acetylcholine of tissue in upper GI tract, which causes contraction of gastric muscle, relaxes pyloric, duodenal segments, increases peristalsis without stimulating secretions, blocks dopamine in chemoreceptor trigger zone of CNS

Therapeutic outcome: Decreased symptoms of delayed gastric emptying, decreased nausea, vomiting

USES: Prevention of nausea, vomiting induced by chemotherapy, radiation; delayed gastric emptying, gastroesophageal reflux

CONTRAINDICATIONS
Hypersensitivity to this product or procaine or procainamide, seizure disorder, pheochromocytoma, breast cancer (prolactin dependent), GI obstruction

Precautions: Pregnancy **B**, breastfeeding, GI hemorrhage, CHF, Parkinson's disease

| BLACK BOX WARNING: Tardive dyskinesia |

Adverse effects: *italics* = common; **bold** = life-threatening

DOSAGE AND ROUTES
Nausea/vomiting (chemotherapy)
Adult: **IV** 1-2 mg/kg 30 min before administration of chemotherapy, then q2hr × 2 doses, then q3hr × 3 doses
Child (unlabeled): **IV** 1-2 mg/kg/dose

Facilitation of small bowel intubation in radiologic exams
Adult and child >14 yr: **IV** 10 mg over 1-2 min
Child 6-14 yr: **IV** 2.5-5 mg
Child <6 yr: **IV** 0.1 mg/kg

Diabetic gastroparesis
Adult: **PO** 10 mg 30 min before meals, at bedtime × 2-8 wk
Geriatric: **PO** 5 mg ½ hr before meals, at bedtime, increase to 10 mg if needed

Gastroesophageal reflux
Adult: **PO** 10-15 mg qid 30 min before meals and at bedtime
Child: **PO** 0.4-0.8 mg/kg/day divided in 4 doses

Renal dose
Adult: **IV** CCr <40 ml/min 50% of dose

Available forms: Tabs 5, 10 mg; syr 5 mg/5 ml; inj 5 mg/ml; orally disintegrating tab 5, 10 mg; oral sol 5 mg/5 ml

Implementation
PO route
• Use gum, hard candy, frequent rinsing of mouth for dryness of oral cavity
• Give ½-1 hr before meals for better absorption
• **Oral disintegrating:** place on tongue, allow to dissolve, swallow, remove from bottle immediately before use
IM route
• Give for postop nausea and vomiting before end of surgery

Direct IV route
• Give **IV** undiluted if dose is ≤10 mg; give over 2 min
• Give diphenhydrAMINE **IV** or benztropine IM for EPS
• Discard open ampules
Intermittent IV infusion route
• Dilute more than 10 mg in 50 ml or more D₅W, NaCl, Ringer's, LR and give over 15 min or more

Y-site compatibilities: Acetaminophen, acyclovir, aldesleukin, alfentanil, amifostine, amikacin, aminophylline, ascorbic acid, atracurium, atropine, azaTHIOprine, aztreonam, bivalirudin, bleomycin, bumetanide, buprenorphine, butorphanol, calcium chloride/gluconate, CARBOplatin, caspofungin, ceFAZolin, cefonicid, cefoperazone, cefotaxime, cefoTEtan, cefOXitin, cefTAZidime, ceftizoxime, cefTRIAXone, cefuroxime, chloramphenicol, chlorproMAZINE, cimetidine, ciprofloxacin, cisatracurium, CISplatin, cladribine, clindamycin, cyanocobalamin, cyclophosphamide, cycloSPORINE, cytarabine, DACTINomycin, DAPTOmycin, dexamethasone, dexmedetomidine, digoxin, diltiazem, diphenhydrAMINE, DOBUTamine, DOCEtaxel, DOPamine, doripenem, doxapram, DOXOrubicin hydrochloride, doxycycline, droperidol, enalaprilat, ePHEDrine, EPINEPHrine, epirubicin, epoetin alfa, ertapenem, erythromycin, esmolol, etoposide, etoposide phosphate, famotidine, fenoldopam, fentaNYL, filgrastim, fluconazole, fludarabine, folic acid, foscarnet, gallium nitrate, gemcitabine, gentamicin, glycopyrrolate, granisetron, heparin, hydrocortisone, HYDROmorphone, IDArubicin, ifosfamide, imipenem/cilastatin, indomethacin, insulin, isoproterenol, ketorolac, labetalol, leucovorin, levofloxacin, lidocaine, linezolid, LORazepam, magnesium sulfate, mannitol, mechlorethamine, melphalan, meperidine, meropenem, metaraminol, methadone, methotrexate, methoxamine, methyldopate, methylPREDNISolone, metoprolol, metroNIDAZOLE, miconazole, midazolam, milrinone, minocycline, mitoMYcin, morphine, moxalactam, multiple vitamins, nafcillin, nalbuphine, naloxone, nesiritide, nitroglycerin, nitroprusside, norepinephrine, octreotide, ondansetron, oxaliplatin, oxytocin, PACLitaxel, palonosetron, pantoprazole, papaverine, PEMEtrexed, penicillin G, pentamidine, pentazocine, PENTobarbital, PHENobarbital, phentolamine, phenylephrine, phytonadione, piperacillin/tazobactam, potassium chloride, procainamide, prochlorperazine, promethazine, propranolol, protamine, pyridoxine, quinupristin/dalfopristin, ranitidine, remifentanil, riTUXimab, rocuronium, sargramostim, sodium acetate/bicarbonate, succinylcholine, SUFentanil, tacrolimus, teniposide, theophylline, thiamine, thiotepa, ticarcillin/clavulanate, tigecycline, tirofiban, tobramycin, tolazoline, topotecan, trastuzumab, trimethaphan, urokinase, vancomycin, vasopressin, vecuronium, verapamil, vinBLAStine, vinCRIStine, vinorelbine, voriconazole, zidovudine

Y-site incompatibilities: Amphotericin B cholesteryl/colloidal, amphotericin B liposome, amsacrine, cefepime, dantrolene, diazepam, diazoxide, DOXOrubicin liposome, ganciclovir, inamrinone, phenytoin, propofol, trimethoprim/sulfamethoxazole

---

ADVERSE EFFECTS

CNS: *Sedation, fatigue, restlessness, headache, sleeplessness, dystonia,* dizziness, drowsiness, **suicidal ideation, seizures, EPS, neuroleptic malignant syndrome; tardive dyskinesia** (>3 mo, high doses)

CV: Hypotension, **supraventricular tachycardia**

GI: Dry mouth, constipation, nausea, anorexia, vomiting, diarrhea

GU: Decreased libido, prolactin secretion, amenorrhea, galactorrhea

HEMA: **Neutropenia, leukopenia, agranulocytosis**

INTEG: Urticaria, rash

Pharmacokinetics

Absorption	Well absorbed (PO)
Distribution	Widely distributed; crosses blood-brain barrier, placenta
Metabolism	Liver, minimally
Excretion	Kidneys, breast milk
Half-life	2.5-6 hr

Pharmacodynamics

	PO	IM	IV
Onset	½-1 hr	10-15 min	1-3 min
Peak	Unknown	Unknown	Unknown
Duration	1-2 hr	1-2 hr	1-2 hr

INTERACTIONS
Individual drugs
Alcohol: increased sedation
Haloperidol: increased extrapyramidal reaction

Drug classifications
Anticholinergics, opiates: decreased action of metoclopramide
CNS depressants: increased sedation
MAOIs: avoid use
Phenothiazines: increased extrapyramidal reaction

Drug/lab test
Increased: prolactin, aldosterone, thyrotropin

NURSING CONSIDERATIONS
Assessment
• Assess GI complaints: nausea, vomiting, anorexia, constipation, abdominal distention before, after administration

BLACK BOX WARNING: Assess for EPS and tardive dyskinesia (more likely to occur in treatment >3 mo, geriatric): rigidity, grimacing, shuffling gait, tremors, rhythmic involuntary movements of tongue, mouth, jaw, feet, hands; these side effects should be reported to prescriber immediately; some effects may be irreversible; assess for involuntary movements frequently

• Assess mental status: depression, anxiety, irritability during treatment

⚠ **Neuroleptic malignant syndrome: assess for hyperthermia, change in B/P, pulse, tachycardia, sweating, rigidity, altered consciousness**

Patient/family education
• Instruct patient to avoid driving, other hazardous activities until stabilized on this medication
• Advise patient to avoid alcohol and other CNS depressants that enhance sedating properties of this product
• Advise patient to notify prescriber if involuntary movements occur

Evaluation
Positive therapeutic outcome
• Absence of nausea, vomiting, anorexia, fullness

metolazone (Rx)
(me-tole′a-zone)
Zaroxolyn
Func. class.: Diuretic, antihypertensive
Chem. class.: Thiazide-like quinazoline derivative
Pregnancy category B

Do not confuse: metolazone/methotrexate/metoclopramide

ACTION: Acts on the distal tubule and cortical thick ascending limb of the loop of Henle in the kidney, increasing excretion of sodium, water, chloride, magnesium, potassium, and bicarbonate, decreases GFR

Therapeutic outcome: Decreased B/P, decreased edema in lung tissue and peripherally

USES: Edema, hypertension

CONTRAINDICATIONS
Pregnancy (**D**) (preeclampsia, intrauterine growth retardation), hypersensitivity to thiazides or sulfonamides, anuria, coma, hepatic encephalopathy

M

Precautions: Pregnancy **B,** breastfeeding, geriatric, hypokalemia, renal/hepatic disease, gout, COPD, lupus erythematosus, diabetes mellitus, hypotension, history of pancreatitis, hypersensitivity to sulfonamides, thiazides, electrolyte imbalance

DOSAGE AND ROUTES
Edema
Adult: PO 5-10 mg/day; max 20 mg/day

Hypertension
Adult: PO 2.5-5 mg/day
Child: PO 0.2-0.4 mg/kg/day in divided doses q12-24hr

Available forms: Tabs 2.5, 5, 10 mg

Implementation
• Give in AM to avoid interference with sleep
• Provide potassium replacement if potassium level is 3.0; product may be crushed if patient is unable to swallow
• Give with food; if nausea occurs, absorption may be increased

ADVERSE EFFECTS
CNS: Anxiety, depression, headache, *dizziness, fatigue, weakness*
CV: *Orthostatic hypotension,* palpitations, volume depletion, chest pain, hypotension
EENT: Blurred vision
ELECT: *Hypokalemia,* hypercalcemia, hyponatremia
GI: *Nausea, vomiting, anorexia,* constipation, diarrhea, cramps, pancreatitis, GI irritation, dry mouth, jaundice, hepatitis
GU: *Frequency,* polyuria, uremia, glucosuria, nocturia, impotence
HEMA: Aplastic anemia, hemolytic anemia, leukopenia, agranulocytosis, neutropenia
INTEG: *Rash,* urticaria, purpura, photosensitivity, fever, dry skin, toxic epidermal necrolysis, Stevens-Johnson syndrome
META: *Hyperglycemia,* increased creatinine, BUN
MS: Muscle cramps, joint pain, swelling

Pharmacokinetics
Absorption	GI tract (10%-20%)
Distribution	Crosses placenta; protein binding 33%
Metabolism	Urine, unchanged
Excretion	Breast milk
Half-life	8 hr (extended); 14 hr (prompt)

Pharmacodynamics
Onset	Unknown
Peak	8 hr
Duration	12-24 hr

INTERACTIONS
Individual drugs
Alcohol: increased hypotension (large amounts)
Amphotericin B, digoxin, mezlocillin, piperacillin: increased hypokalemia
Lithium: increased toxicity

Drug classifications
Antidiabetics: increased hyperglycemia
Antihypertensives: increased antihypertensive effect
Barbiturates, nitrates, opioids: increased hypotension
Diuretics (loop): increased metolazone effect
Glucocorticoids, laxatives (stimulant): increased hypokalemia
NSAIDs, salicylates: decreased action of metolazone

Drug/food
Licorice: increased severe hypokalemia

Drug/herb
Ephedra (ma huang): decreased antihypertensive effect
Hawthorn: increased antihypertensive effect

Drug/lab test
Increased: calcium, cholesterol, glucose, triglycerides
Decreased: potassium, sodium, chloride, magnesium

NURSING CONSIDERATIONS
Assessment
• **Hypertension:** assess B/P before, during therapy with patient lying, standing, and sitting as appropriate; orthostatic hypotension can occur rapidly
• Monitor blood glucose if patient is diabetic
• **CHF:** assess for improvement in feet, legs, sacral area daily if medication is being used
• Check for rashes, temp elevation daily
• Monitor patients receiving cardiac glycosides for increased hypokalemia
• **Hypokalemia:** assess for postural hypotension, malaise, fatigue, tachycardia, leg cramps, weakness

> **BLACK BOX WARNING:** Hepatic encephalopathy: do not use in hepatic coma or precoma, fluctuations in electrolytes can occur rapidly and precipitate hepatic coma, use caution in those with impaired hepatic function

• Assess and record fluid volume status: I&O ratios; monitor weight, distended red veins, crackles in lung, color, quality, and specific gravity of urine; skin turgor, adequacy of pulses, moist mucous membranes, bilateral lung sounds, peripheral pitting edema; dehydration symptoms of decreasing output, thirst, hypotension, dry mouth and mucous membranes should be reported

• Monitor electrolytes: potassium, sodium, calcium, magnesium; also include BUN, blood pH, ABGs, uric acid, CBC, blood glucose

Patient/family education

• Teach patient to take the medication early in the day to prevent nocturia

• Instruct patient to take with food or milk if GI symptoms of nausea and anorexia occur

• Teach patient to maintain a weekly record of weight and notify prescriber of weight loss >5 lb

• Caution patient that this product causes a loss of potassium, so foods rich in potassium should be added to the diet; refer to a dietitian for assistance in planning

• Caution the patient to rise slowly from sitting or reclining positions, not to exercise in hot weather or stand for prolonged periods, since orthostatic hypotension will be enhanced; lie down if dizziness occurs

• Teach patient not to use alcohol or any OTC medications without prescriber's approval; **serious product reactions may occur**

• **Emphasize the need to contact prescriber immediately if muscle cramps, weakness, nausea, dizziness, or numbness occur**

• Teach patient to take own B/P and pulse and record

• Advise patient to use sunscreen to prevent burns

• Teach patient to continue taking medication even if feeling better; this product controls symptoms but does not cure the condition

• Advise patient with hypertension to continue other medical regimen (exercise, weight loss, relaxation techniques, smoking cessation)

• Do not stop product abruptly

Evaluation

Positive therapeutic outcome
• Decreased edema
• Decreased B/P

TREATMENT OF OVERDOSE:
Lavage if taken orally, monitor electrolytes; administer dextrose in saline; monitor hydration, CV, renal status

---

metoprolol (Rx)
(met-oh-proe′lole)
Lopressor, Nu-Metop ✢, Toprol-XL
Func. class.: Antihypertensive, antianginal
Chem. class.: β_1-Adrenergic blocker
Pregnancy category C

Do not confuse: metoprolol/misoprostol

ACTION: Lowers B/P by β-blocking effects; reduces elevated renin plasma levels; blocks β_2-adrenergic receptors in bronchial, vascular smooth muscle only at high doses, negative chronotropic effect

Therapeutic outcome: Decreased B/P, heart rate, AV conduction

USES: Mild to moderate hypertension, acute MI to reduce cardiovascular mortality, angina pectoris, New York Heart Association class II, III heart failure, cardiomyopathy

CONTRAINDICATIONS
Hypersensitivity to β-blockers, cardiogenic shock, heart block (2nd and 3rd degree), sinus bradycardia, pheochromocytoma, sick sinus syndrome

Precautions: Pregnancy **C**, breastfeeding, geriatric, major surgery, diabetes mellitus, thyroid/renal/hepatic disease, COPD, CAD, nonallergic bronchospasm, CHF, bronchial asthma, CVA, children, depression, vasospastic angina

> **BLACK BOX WARNING:** Abrupt discontinuation

DOSAGE AND ROUTES
Hypertension
Adult: PO 50 mg bid, or 100 mg/day; may give 100-450 mg in divided doses; ext rel 25-100 mg qd, titrate at weekly intervals, max 400 mg/day
Child/adolescent 6-16 yr: PO ext rel 1 mg/kg up to 50 mg qd
Geriatric: PO 25 mg/day initially, increase weekly as needed

Myocardial infarction
Adult: IV BOL (early treatment) 5 mg q2min × 3 doses, then 50 mg PO 15 min after last dose and q6hr × 48 hr (late treatment); PO maintenance 50-100 mg bid for 1-3 yr

Heart failure (NYHA class II/III)
Adult: PO ext rel 25 mg qd × 2 wk (class II); 12.5 mg qd (class III)

Angina
Adult: PO 100 mg/day as a single dose or in 2 divided doses, increase qwk as needed, or 100 mg ext rel tab daily, max 400 mg/day ext rel

---

Migraine prevention (unlabeled)
Adult: PO 25-100 mg bid-qid; 50-200 mg daily (XL)

Available forms: Tabs 25, 50, 100 mg; inj 1 mg/ml; ext rel tabs (tartrate) 100 mg; ext rel tabs (succinate) (XL) 25, 50, 100, 200 mg

Implementation
PO route
- Do not break, crush, or chew ext rel tabs
- Give regular release tab before meals, at bedtime; tab may be crushed or swallowed whole; give with food to prevent GI upset; reduced dosage in renal dysfunction; give at same time each day
- Store in dry area at room temp; do not freeze

Direct IV route
- Give 5 mg/2 min or more × 3 doses at 2 min intervals, start PO 15 min after last **IV** dose

Y-site compatibilities: Abciximab, acyclovir, alemtuzumab, alfentanil, alteplase, amikacin, aminophylline, amiodarone, amphotericin B liposome, anidulafungin, argatroban, ascorbic acid, atracurium, atropine, azaTHIOprine, aztreonam, benztropine, bivalirudin, bleomycin, bumetanide, buprenorphine, butorphanol, calcium chloride/gluconate, CARBOplatin, caspofungin, ceFAZolin, cefonicid, cefoperazone, cefotaxime, cefoTEtan, cefOXitin, cefTAZidime, ceftizoxime, cefTRIAXone, cefuroxime, chloramphenicol, chlorproMAZINE, cimetidine, CISplatin, clindamycin, cyanocobalamin, cyclophosphamide, cycloSPORINE, cytarabine, DACTINomycin, DAPTOmycin, dexamethasone, dexmedetomidine, digoxin, diltiazem, diphenhydrAMINE, DOBUTamine, DOCEtaxel, DOPamine, doxacurium, DOXOrubicin, doxycycline, enalaprilat, ePHEDrine, EPINEPHrine, epirubicin, epoetin alfa, eptifibatide, esmolol, etoposide, etoposide phosphate, famotidine, fenoldopam, fentaNYL, fluconazole, fludarabine, fluorouracil, folic acid, furosemide, ganciclovir, gemcitabine, gentamicin, glycopyrrolate, granisetron, heparin, hydrocortisone, HYDROmorphone, IDArubicin, ifosfamide, imipenem/cilastatin, indomethacin, insulin, isoproterenol, ketorolac, labetalol, linezolid, LORazepam, magnesium sulfate, mannitol, mechlorethamine, meperidine, metaraminol, methotrexate, methoxamine, methyldopate, methylPREDNISolone, metoclopramide, metroNIDAZOLE, midazolam, milrinone, mitoXANtrone, morphine, multivitamins, nafcillin, nalbuphine, naloxone, nitroprusside, norepinephrine, octreotide, ondansetron, oxacillin, oxaliplatin, oxytocin, PACLitaxel, palonosetron, pancuronium, papaverine, PEMEtrexed, penicillin G, pentamidine, pentazocine, PENTobarbital, PHENobarbital, phentolamine, phenylephrine, phytonadione, piperacillin/tazobactam, potassium chloride, procainamide, prochlorperazine, promethazine, propranolol, protamine, pyridoxime, quinupristin/dalfopristin, ranitidine, rocuronium, sodium bicarbonate, succinylcholine, SUFentanil, tacrolimus, teniposide, theophylline, thiamine, thiotepa, ticarcillin/clavulanate, tigecycline, tirofiban, tobramycin, tolazoline, trimetaphan, urokinase, vancomycin, vasopressin, vecuronium, verapamil, vinCRIStine, vinorelbine, voriconazole

Y-site incompatibilities: Allopurinol, amphotericin B cholesteryl/colloidal/lipid complex, dantrolene, diazepam, diazoxide, lepirudin, pantoprazole, phenytoin, trimethoprim/sulfamethoxazole

ADVERSE EFFECTS
CNS: *Insomnia, dizziness,* mental changes, hallucinations, depression, anxiety, headaches, nightmares, confusion, fatigue
CV: CHF, *palpitations,* dysrhythmias, cardiac arrest, AV block, *hypotension,* bradycardia, pulmonary/peripheral edema, chest pain
EENT: Sore throat, dry burning eyes
GI: *Nausea, vomiting,* colitis, cramps, *diarrhea,* constipation, flatulence, dry mouth, *hiccups*
GU: Impotence
HEMA: Agranulocytosis, eosinophilia, thrombocytopenic purpura
INTEG: Rash, purpura, alopecia, dry skin, urticaria, pruritus
RESP: Bronchospasm, dyspnea, wheezing

Pharmacokinetics
Absorption	Well absorbed (PO); completely absorbed (**IV**)
Distribution	Crosses blood-brain barrier, placenta
Metabolism	Liver, extensively
Excretion	Kidneys, breast milk
Half-life	3-4 hr

Pharmacodynamics
	PO	IV
Onset	15 min	Immediate
Peak	2-4 hr	20 min
Duration	6-19 hr	5-8 hr

INTERACTIONS
Individual drugs
Cimetidine: increased metoprolol level
EPINEPHrine, hydrALAZINE, methyldopa prazosin, reserpine: increased hypotension, bradycardia
Insulin: increased hypoglycemia

Drug classifications

Antidiabetics (oral): increased hypoglycemia

Amphetamines, calcium channel blockers, histamine H$_2$ antagonists: increased hypotension, bradycardia

Barbiturates: decreased metoprolol level

MAOIs: do not use together

NSAIDs, salicylates: decreased antihypertensive effect

Xanthines: decreased effects of xanthines

Drug/food

Increased: absorption with food

Drug/lab test

Increased: BUN, potassium, ANA titer, serum lipoprotein, triglycerides, uric acid, alkaline phosphatase, LDH, AST, ALT

NURSING CONSIDERATIONS
Assessment

> **BLACK BOX WARNING:** Abrupt withdrawal: may cause MI, ventricular dysrhythmias, myocardial ischemia; taper dose over 7-14 days

• **Hypertension/angina:** monitor ECG directly when giving IV during initial treatment

• Monitor B/P during beginning treatment, periodically thereafter; pulse q4hr; note rate, rhythm, quality; check apical/radial pulse before administration; notify prescriber of any significant changes (pulse <60 bpm)

• Check for baselines in renal, liver function tests before therapy begins and periodically thereafter

• Assess for edema in feet, legs daily; monitor I&O, daily weight; check for jugular vein distention, crackles bilaterally, dyspnea (CHF)

Patient/family education

> **BLACK BOX WARNING:** Teach patient not to discontinue product abruptly; taper over 2 wk; may cause precipitate angina if stopped abruptly

• Teach patient not to use OTC products containing α-adrenergic stimulants (such as nasal decongestants, cold preparations); to avoid alcohol, smoking and to limit sodium intake as prescribed

• Teach patient how to take pulse and B/P at home; advise when to notify prescriber

• Instruct patient to comply with weight control, dietary adjustments, modified exercise program

• Tell patient to carry/wear emergency ID to identify product being taken, allergies; tell patient product controls symptoms but does not cure

• Caution patient to avoid hazardous activities if dizziness, drowsiness is present, to avoid driving until product response is known

• Teach patient to report symptoms of CHF; difficult breathing, especially with exertion or when lying down, night cough, swelling of extremities or bradycardia, dizziness, confusion, depression, fever, decreased vision

• Teach patient to take product as prescribed, not to double doses or skip doses; take any missed doses as soon as remembered if at least 4 hr until next dose

• Advise to monitor blood glucose closely if diabetic

• Advise to report Raynaud's symptoms

Evaluation

Positive therapeutic outcome

• Decreased B/P in hypertension (after 1-2 wk)

• Absence of dysrhythmias

• Decreased anginal pain

TREATMENT OF OVERDOSE:

Lavage, **IV** atropine for bradycardia, **IV** theophylline for bronchospasm, digoxin, O$_2$, diuretic for cardiac failure, hemodialysis, **IV** glucose for hyperglycemia, **IV** diazepam (or phenytoin) for seizures

M

metroNIDAZOLE (Rx)

(me-troe-ni′da-zole)

Flagyl, Flagyl ER, Flagyl IV, Flagyl IV RTU, Florazone ER ✦, Novonidazole ✦

Func. class.: Antiinfective, miscellaneous

Chem. class.: Nitroimidazole derivative

Pregnancy category B (2nd, 3rd trimesters)

ACTION: Direct-acting amebicide/trichomonacide; binds, degrades DNA structure, inhibiting bacterial nucleic acid synthesis

Therapeutic outcome: Trichomonacidal, amebicidal, bactericidal for the following susceptible organisms: *Bacteroides, Clostridium, Trichomonas vaginalis, Giardia lamblia, Entamoeba histolytica*

USES: Intestinal amebiasis, amebic abscess, trichomoniasis, refractory trichomoniasis, bacterial anaerobic infections, giardiasis; septicemia, endocarditis, bone, joint, and lower respiratory tract infections, rosacea

Unlabeled uses: Crohn's disease

CONTRAINDICATIONS

Pregnancy (1st trimester), breastfeeding, hypersensitivity to this product

Precautions: Pregnancy **B** (2nd/3rd trimesters), candidal infections, heart failure, fungal infection, geriatric, dental disease, bone marrow suppression, hematologic disease, renal/hepatic/GI disease, contracted visual or color fields, blood dyscrasias, CNS disorders

> **BLACK BOX WARNING:** Secondary malignancy

DOSAGE AND ROUTES
Trichomoniasis
Adult: PO 500 mg bid × 7 days or 2 g in single dose; do not repeat treatment for 4-6 wk
Child ≥45 kg (unlabeled): PO 2 g once
Child <45 kg (unlabeled): PO 15 mg/kg/day divided in 3 doses × 7-10 days

Amebic hepatic abscess
Adult: PO 750 mg tid × 7-10 days
Child: PO 35-50 mg/kg/day in 3 divided doses × 7-10 days

Intestinal amebiasis
Adult: PO 750 mg tid × 7-10 days
Child: PO 35-50 mg/kg/day in 3 divided doses × 7-10 days; then oral iodoquinol

Anaerobic bacterial infections
Adult: IV INF 15 mg/kg/over 1 hr, then 7.5 mg/kg **IV** or PO q6hr, max 4 g/day; first maintenance dose should be administered 6 hr after loading dose

Bacterial vaginosis
Adult: PO reg rel 500 mg bid or 250 mg tid × 7 days; ext rel 750 mg/day × 7 days

Giardiasis (unlabeled)
Adult: PO 250 mg tid × 5-7 days
Child: PO 5 mg/kg divided tid × 5 days

Antibiotic-associated pseudomembranous colitis
Adult (unlabeled): PO 250-500 mg 3 times per day × 10-14 days
Child: PO 20 mg/kg/day (max 2 g) divided q6hr

Available forms: Tabs 250, 500 mg; ext rel tabs 750 mg; caps 375 mg; inj sol 5 mg/ml

Implementation
• Store in light-resistant container; do not refrigerate
PO route
• Give with or after a meal to avoid GI symptoms, metallic taste; crush tab if needed, give on empty stomach
Topical route
• A thin coating should be applied to affected area after cleaning with soap and water and patting dry

IV route
• Give intermittent **IV** prediluted; for Flagyl **IV** dilute with 4.4 ml of sterile water or 0.9% NaCl; must be diluted further with ≤8 mg/ml 0.9% NaCl, D_5W, or LR; must neutralize with 5 mEq of $NaCO_3/500$ mg; CO_2 gas will be generated and may require venting; run over 1 hr or more; primary **IV** must be discontinued; may be given as cont inf; do not use aluminum products; **IV** may require venting

Y-site compatibilities: Acyclovir, alemtuzumab, alfentanil, allopurinol, amifostene, amikacin, aminophylline, amiodarone, ampicillin, ampicillin/sulbactam, anidulafungin, atracurium, bivalirudin, bumetanide, buprenorphine, busulfan, butorphanol, calcium acetate/chloride/gluconate, CARBOplatin, ceFAZolin, cefepime, cefoperazone, cefoTEtan, cefotaxime, cefTRIAXone, cefuroxime, chloramphenicol, chlorproMAZINE, cimetidine, ciprofloxacin, cisatracurium, CISplatin, clindamycin, codeine, cyclophosphamide, cycloSPORINE, cytarabine, DACTINomycin, dexamethasone, dexmedetomidine, dexrazoxane, digoxin, diltiazem, dimenhyDRINATE, diphenhydrAMINE, DOBUTamine, DOCEtaxel, DOPamine, doripenem, doxacurium, doxapram, DOXOrubicin, DOXOrubicin liposome, doxycycline, droperidol, enalaprilat, ePHEDrine, EPINEPHrine, epirubicin, eptifibatide, ertapenem, erythromycin, esmolol, etoposide, etoposide phosphate, famotidine, fenoldopam, fentaNYL, fluconazole, fludarabine, fluorouracil, foscarnet, fosphenytoin, furosemide, gemcitabine, gentamicin, glycopyrrolate, granisetron, haloperidol, heparin, hydrALAZINE, hydrocortisone, HYDROmorphone, IDArubicin, ifosfamide, imipenem/cilastatin, inamrinone, insulin, isoproterenol, ketorolac, labetalol, leucovorin, levofloxacin, lidocaine, linezolid, LORazepam, magnesium sulfate, mannitol, mechlorethamine, melphalan, meperidine, meropenem, mesna, metaraminol, methotrexate, methyldopate, methylPREDNISolone, metoclopramide, metoprolol, midazolam, milrinone, mitoXANtrone, morphine, nafcillin, nalbuphine, naloxone, nesiritide, niCARdipine, nitroglycerin, nitroprusside, norepinephrine, octreotide, ondansetron, oxaliplatin, oxytocin, PACLitaxel, palonosetron, pancuronium, pentamidine, pentazocine, PENTobarbital, perphenazine, PHENobarbital, phentolamine, phenylephrine, piperacillin/tazobactam, potassium chloride/phosphates, prochlorperazine, promethazine, propranolol, ranitidine, remifentanil, riTUXimab, rocuronium, sargramostim, sodium acetate/bicarbonate/phosphates, streptozocin, succinylcholine, SUFentanil, tacrolimus, teniposide,

---

⚠ Nurse Alert · ✳ Key NCLEX® Drug · ≫ Drug Specifics

theophylline, thiopental, thiotepa, ticarcillin/clavulanate, tigecycline, tirofiban, tobramycin, trastuzumab, trimethobenzamide, trimethoprim/sulfamethoxazole, vancomycin, vasopressin, vecuronium, verapamil, vinCRIStine, vinorelbine, voriconazole, zidovudine, zoledronic acid

Y-site incompatibilities: Amphotericin B cholesteryl/colloidal/liposome, aztreonam, dantrolene, DAPTOmycin, diazepam, drotrecogin, filgrastim, ganciclovir, pantoprazole, PEMEtrexed, phenytoin, procainamide, quinupristin/dalfopristin

ADVERSE EFFECTS
CNS: *Headache, dizziness,* confusion, irritability, restlessness, ataxia, depression, fatigue, drowsiness, insomnia, paresthesia, peripheral neuropathy, seizures, incoordination, depression, encephalopathy, aseptic meningitis
CV: Flat T-waves
EENT: Blurred vision, sore throat, retinal edema, dry mouth, metallic taste, furry tongue, glossitis, stomatitis, photophobia, optic neuritis
GI: *Nausea, vomiting, diarrhea,* epigastric distress, *anorexia,* constipation, *abdominal cramps,* pseudomembranous colitis, xerostomia, metallic taste, abdominal pain, pancreatitis
GU: Darkened urine, vaginal dryness, polyuria, albuminuria, dysuria, cystitis, decreased libido, nephrotoxicity, incontinence, dyspareunia, candidiasis, increased urinary frequency
HEMA: Leukopenia, bone marrow depression, aplasia, thrombocytopenia
INTEG: Rash, pruritus, urticaria, flushing, phlebitis at injection site, toxic epidermal necrolysis

Pharmacokinetics

Absorption	80% (PO)
Distribution	Widely distributed, crosses placenta
Metabolism	Liver
Excretion	Urine, unchanged; feces
Half-life	6-11 hr

Pharmacodynamics

	PO	IV
Onset	Rapid	Immediate
Peak	1-2 hr	Infusion's end
Duration	Unknown	Unknown

INTERACTIONS
Individual drugs
Alcohol, oral ritonavir, any product with alcohol: increased disulfiram-like reaction

AzaTHIOprine, fluorouracil: increased leukopenia
Amprenavir, disulfiram: do not use bortezomib; norfloxacin, zalcitabine: avoid use
Busulfan: increased busulfan toxicity, avoid concurrent use
Cholestyramine: decreased metroNIDAZOLE, toxicity
Fosphenytoin, lithium, phenytoin, warfarin: increased action of these drugs

Drug classifications
Barbiturates: decreased metroNIDAZOLE half-life
CYP3A4 substrates: increased levels

Drug/lab test
Altered: AST, ALT, LDH
Decrease: WBC, neutrophils
False decrease: triglycerides

NURSING CONSIDERATIONS
Assessment
• **Assess patient for signs and symptoms of infection** including characteristics of wounds, WBC >10,000/mm^3, vaginal secretions, fever; obtain baseline information and during treatment
• Obtain C&S before beginning product therapy to identify if correct treatment has been initiated
• **Assess for allergic reactions:** rash, urticaria, pruritus
• Identify urine output; if decreasing, notify prescriber **(may indicate nephrotoxicity)**; also check for increased BUN, creatinine
• Assess bowel pattern daily; if severe diarrhea occurs, product should be discontinued
• Assess for overgrowth of infection: perineal itching, fever, malaise, redness, pain, swelling, drainage, rash, diarrhea, change in cough, sputum
• Teach patient to notify prescriber if pregnancy is planned or suspected, pregnancy (B) 2nd/3rd trimester in trichomoniasis

> **BLACK BOX WARNING: Secondary malignancy:** use only when indicated, avoid unnecessary use

Patient/family education
• Teach patient to report sore throat, bruising, bleeding, joint pain; may indicate blood dyscrasias (rare)
• Advise patient to contact prescriber if vaginal itching, loose foul-smelling stools, furry tongue occur; may indicate superinfection
• Advise patient to notify physician of numbness or tingling of extremities
• Teach trichomoniasis patient that both partners need to be treated; condoms should be used during intercourse to prevent reinfection

- Advise patient of disulfiramlike reaction to alcohol ingestion; alcohol should not be used within 48 hr of this product
- Inform patient product has a metallic taste and urine may turn dark
- Advise patient to contact prescriber if pregnancy is suspected
- Advise patient to use sips of water, sugarless gum, candy for dry mouth

Evaluation

Positive therapeutic outcome
- Decreased symptoms of infection

metroNIDAZOLE topical
See Appendix B

micafungin (Rx)
(my-ca-fun'gin)
Mycamine
Func. class.: Antifungal, systemic
Chem. class.: Echinocandin
Pregnancy category C

ACTION: Inhibits an essential component in fungal cell walls; causes direct damage to fungal cell wall

Therapeutic outcome: Prevention of *Candida* infection in hematopoietic stem cell transplantation (HSCT); or decreased symptoms of *Candida* infection, negative culture

USES: Treatment of esophageal candidiasis; prophylaxis of *Candida* infections in patients undergoing HSCT; susceptible *Candida* species: *C. albicans, C. glabrata, C. krusei, C. parapsilosis, C. tropicalis,* prophylaxis of HIV-related esophageal candidiasis

CONTRAINDICATIONS
Hypersensitivity to this product or other echinocandins

Precautions: Pregnancy **C**, breastfeeding, children, geriatric, severe hepatic disease, renal impairment, hemolytic anemia

DOSAGE AND ROUTES
Candidemia/acute disseminated candidiasis, abscess, peritonitis
Adult: IV 100 mg/day over 1 hr

Esophageal candidiasis
Adult: IV 150 mg/day, given over 1 hr

Prophylaxis of *Candida* infections
Adult: IV 50 mg/day, given over 1 hr

Available forms: Powder for injection 50 mg, in single-dose vials; 50, 100 mg vial

Implementation
- Protect diluted sol from light
- Do not use if cloudy or precipitated; do not admix product
- Flush line before, after administration with 0.9% NaCl

IV route
- For *Candida* prevention: reconstitute with provided diluent 0.9% NaCl without bacteriostatic product; 50 mg vial/5 ml (10 mg/ml), swirl to dissolve, do not shake; further dilute with 100 ml 0.9% NaCl, only; run over 1 hr
- For *Candida* infection: reconstitute with provided diluent 50 mg/5 ml (10 mg/ml); further dilute 3 reconstituted vials in 100 ml of 0.9% NaCl, run over 1 hr
- Store at room temperature, away from light; do not freeze; discard unused solution

Y-site compatibilities: Aminophylline, bumetanide, calcium chloride/gluconate, cyclo-SPORINE, DOPamine, eptifibatide, esmolol, fenoldopam, furosemide, heparin, HYDROmorphone, lidocaine, LORazepam, magnesium sulfate, milrinone, nitroglycerin, nitroprusside, norepinephrine, phenylephrine, potassium chloride, potassium phosphate, tacrolimus, vasopressin

Y-site incompatibilities: Albumin, amiodarone, cisatracurium, diltiazem, DOBUTamine, EPINEPHrine, insulin, labetalol, meperidine, midazolam, morphine, mycophenolate mofetil, nesiritide, niCARdipine, octreotide, ondansetron, phenytoin, telavancin, vecuronium

ADVERSE EFFECTS
CNS: Convulsions, dizziness, *headache, somnolence,* fever, anxiety
CV: Flushing, hypertension, phlebitis, tachycardia, atrial fibrillation
GI: Abdominal pain, *nausea, anorexia, vomiting, diarrhea,* hepatitis
GU: Renal failure
HEMA: Neutropenia, thrombocytopenia, leukopenia, coagulopathy, anemia, hemolytic anemia
INTEG: *Rash, pruritus, inj site pain*
META: Hypokalemia, hypocalcemia, hypomagnesemia
MS: *Rigors*

Pharmacokinetics	
Absorption	Unknown
Distribution	Protein binding 99%
Metabolism	Liver
Excretion	Feces, urine
Half-life	Terminal 14-17.2 hr

Pharmacodynamics
Unknown

INTERACTIONS
Individual drugs
Itraconazole, sirolimus, NIFEdipine: increased plasma concentrations; may need dosage reduction

Drug/lab test
Increased: ALT/AST, alk phos, bilirubin
Decreased: blood glucose, potassium sodium

NURSING CONSIDERATIONS
Assessment
• Assess for signs and symptoms of infection, clearing of cultures during treatment; obtain culture baseline, throughout; product may be started as soon as culture is taken (esophageal candidiasis); monitor cultures during HSCT, for prevention of *Candida* infections
• Monitor CBC (RBC, Hct, Hgb), differential, platelet count periodically; notify prescriber of results
• Monitor renal studies: BUN, urine CCr, electrolytes before, during therapy
• Monitor hepatic studies before, during treatment: bilirubin, AST, ALT, alkaline phosphatase, as needed
• Assess for bleeding: hematuria, heme-positive stools, bruising or petechiae of mucosa or orifices; blood dyscrasias can occur
• Assess for hypersensitivity: rash, pruritus, facial swelling; also for phlebitis
• Assess for hemolytic anemia
• Assess **GI symptoms:** frequency of stools, cramping; if severe diarrhea occurs, electrolytes may need to be given

Patient/family education
• Advise patient to notify prescriber if pregnancy is suspected or planned
• Teach patient to avoid breastfeeding while taking this product
• Teach patient to inform prescriber of renal or hepatic disease
• **Teach patient to report bleeding, facial swelling, wheezing, difficulty breathing, itching, rash, hives, increasing warmth, flushing**
• Instruct patient to report signs of infection: increased temp, sore throat, flulike symptoms
• **Advise patient to notify prescriber of nausea, vomiting, diarrhea, jaundice, anorexia, clay-colored stools, dark urine; hepatotoxicity may occur**

Evaluation
Positive therapeutic outcome
• Prevention of *Candida* infection in HSCT; decreased symptoms of *Candida* infection, negative culture

---

miconazole (Rx, OTC)
(mi-kon'a-zole)
Oravig
miconazole nitrate
Femizole-M ✦, Monistat, Monistat 3, Monistat 7, Monistat-Derm, Monistat Dual-Pak, Dual Pack; topical: Micatin, Micatin Liquid, Vagistat 3
Func. class.: Antifungal
Chem. class.: Imidazole
Pregnancy category C

ACTION: Alters cell membranes, inhibits fungal enzymes, inhibits sterols so intracellular contents are lost, prevents biosynthesis of phospholipids/triglycerides

Therapeutic outcome: Fungistatic/fungicidal against *Aspergillus, Coccidioides, Cryptococcus, Candida, Dermatophytes, Histoplasma*

USES: Coccidioidomycosis, candidiasis, cryptococcosis, paracoccidioidomycosis, chronic mucocutaneous candidiasis, fungal meningitis; **IV** used for severe infections only; topical for tinea pedis, tinea cruris, tinea corporis, tinea versicolor, vaginal or vulva candidal infections

CONTRAINDICATIONS
Hypersensitivity

Precautions: Pregnancy **C,** renal/hepatic disease

DOSAGE AND ROUTES
Oropharyngeal candidiasis (thrush)
Adult/adolescent ≥16 yr: Buccal apply 1 tab (50 mg) to upper gum region just above incisor tooth q day × 14 days
Adult: **IV** INF 200-3600 mg/day; may be divided in 3 INF at 200-1200 mg/INF; may have to repeat course; IT 20 mg given simultaneously with **IV** for fungal meningitis q1-2day
Child: **IV** 20-40 mg/kg/day, max 15 mg/kg/day
Adult and child: TOP apply to affected area bid × 2-4 wk
Adult: Intravaginal 200 mg SUPP at bedtime × 3 days or 100 mg SUPP × 1 wk

Available forms: Inj 10 mg/ml; aerosol 2%; cream 2%; lotion 2%; powder 2%; spray 2%; vag cream 2%; vag supp 100, 200 mg; buccal tab 50 mg

Implementation
• Have adrenalin, suction, tracheostomy set, endotracheal intubation equipment available
Transmucosal use (adhesive buccal tablet)
• Apply tab in the morning after brushing the teeth; use dry hands

---

Adverse effects: *italics* = common; **bold** = life-threatening

• Place the rounded surface of the tab against the upper gum just above the incisor tooth; hold in place with a slight pressure over the upper lip for 30 seconds to ensure adhesion
• Although the tab is rounded on one side for comfort, the flat side may also be applied to the gum
• The tab will gradually dissolve
• Administration of subsequent tabs should be made to alternating sides of the mouth
• Before applying the next tab, clear away any remaining tab material
• Do not crush, chew or swallow; food and drink can be taken normally; avoid chewing gum
• If tab does not adhere or falls off within the first 6 hr, the same tab should be repositioned immediately. If the tab still does not adhere, a new tab should be used
• If the tab falls off or is swallowed after it was in place for 6 hr or more, a new tab should not be applied until the next regularly scheduled dose

Topical route
• Apply after cleansing area with soap and water before each application; use enough medication to cover lesions completely; dry well
• Store at room temperature in dry place

Vaginal route
• Administer 1 applicator full every night high into the vagina
• Store at room temperature in dry place

IV route
• Give 200 mg initially to prevent severe hypersensitive reaction
• Give **IV** after diluting in ≤1 g/10 ml of sterile water, D₅W, or 0.45% NaCl over 3-5 min
• Give by intermittent **IV** after diluting in 200 ml or more D₅W or 0.9% NaCl; give over 30-60 min
• Store at room temperature; reconstituted sol is stable for 24 hr refrigerated

Y-site compatibilities: Allopurinol, filgrastim, foscarnet, granisetron, melphalan, ondansetron, propofol, sargramostim, teniposide, thiotepa, vinorelbine

Y-site incompatibilities: Fludarabine

ADVERSE EFFECTS
CNS: Drowsiness, headache, lethargy
CV: Tachycardia, dysrhythmias (rapid **IV**)
GI: Nausea, vomiting, anorexia, diarrhea, cramps
GU: Vulvovaginal burning, itching, hyponatremia, pelvic cramps (topical forms)
HEMA: Decreased Hct, thrombocytopenia, hyperlipidemia
INTEG: Pruritus, rash, fever, flushing, hives
SYST: Anaphylaxis

Absorption	Poorly absorbed (PO)
Distribution	Widely distributed (IV); bound to serum proteins (90%)
Metabolism	Liver, extensively
Excretion	Unknown
Half-life	Triphasic: 0.4, 2.1, 24 hr

Pharmacodynamics

	IV	Topical	Vag
Onset	Rapid	Unknown	Unknown
Peak	Infusion's end	Unknown	Unknown
Duration	Unknown	Unknown	Unknown

INTERACTIONS
Individual drugs
Amphotericin B: decreased effect of amphotericin B
Amphotericin B, isoniazid, rifampin: decreased effect of miconazole
Phenytoin: increased effect
Warfarin: increased anticoagulant effect

Drug classifications
Sulfonylureas: increased effect

Drug/lab test
False positive: urine glucose, urine protein

NURSING CONSIDERATIONS
Assessment
• Assess for signs and symptoms of infection: drainage, sore throat, urinary pain, hematuria, fever
• Obtain C&S before beginning treatment; therapy may be started after culture is taken; monitor signs of infection before, throughout treatment
• Monitor bowel pattern before, during treatment; diarrhea may occur
• Monitor cardiac system: B/P, pulse; watch for increasing pulse, cardiac dysrhythmias; product should be discontinued
• Monitor blood studies: WBC, RBC, Hgb, Hct, bleeding time; patients taking anticoagulants may need a decreased dosage; monitor liver and renal studies periodically for patients on longterm therapy
• Monitor I&O ratio; watch for decreasing urinary output, change in specific gravity; discontinue product to prevent renal damage; patients with renal disease may require lowered dose

• Monitor **IV** site for thrombophlebitis; site should be changed q48-72hr
• Monitor for allergies before initiation of treatment and reaction to each medication; highlight allergies on chart; check for allergic reaction: burning, stinging, swelling, redness (topical); observe for skin eruptions after administration of product to 1 wk after discontinuing product

Patient/family education
• Inform patient that culture may be performed after completed course of medication
• Advise patient to notify nurse of diarrhea, symptoms of candidal vaginitis

Topical route
• Teach patient to use medical asepsis (hand washing) before, after each application; to apply with glove to prevent further infection; to avoid contact with eyes; not to use occlusive dressings
• Caution patient to avoid use of OTC creams, ointments, lotions unless directed by prescriber
• Instruct patient to notify prescriber if condition does not improve in 4 wk or if symptoms return in 2 mo; pregnancy or a serious medical condition may be the cause
• Teach patient to use for full prescribed treatment time, or reinfection may occur

Vaginal route
• Instruct patient in asepsis (hand washing) before, after each application
• Teach patient to apply with applicator only; to avoid use of any other vaginal product unless directed by prescriber; sanitary napkin may prevent soiling of undergarments; to abstain from sexual intercourse until treatment is completed or reinfection and irritation may occur; not to use tampons, douches, spermicides; not to engage in sexual activity; product may damage condoms, diaphragms, cervical caps
• Instruct patient to notify prescriber if symptoms persist

Evaluation

Positive therapeutic outcome
• Decreasing oral candidiasis, fever, malaise, rash
• Negative C&S for infectious organism
• Decrease in size, number of lesions
• Decrease in itching or white discharge (vaginal)

TREATMENT OF OVERDOSE:
Withdraw product; maintain airway; administer EPINEPHrine, aminophylline, O₂, **IV** corticosteroids for anaphylaxis

---

miconazole topical
See Appendix B

miconazole vaginal antifungal
See Appendix B

⚠ HIGH ALERT

midazolam (Rx)
(mid'ay-zoe-lam)
Func. class.: Sedative/hypnotic, antianxiety
Chem. class.: Benzodiazepine, short-acting
Pregnancy category D
Controlled substance schedule IV

ACTION: Depresses subcortical levels in CNS; may act on limbic system, reticular formation; may potentiate GABA by binding to specific benzodiazepine receptors

Therapeutic outcome: Sedation for anesthesia induction and procedures

USES: Preoperative sedation, general anesthesia induction, sedation for diagnostic endoscopic procedures, intubation, anxiety

Unlabeled uses: Refractory status epilepticus, alcohol withdrawal, agitation

CONTRAINDICATIONS
Pregnancy **D**, hypersensitivity to benzodiazepines, acute closed-angle glaucoma, epidural/intrathecal use

Precautions: Breastfeeding, children, geriatric, COPD, CHF, chronic renal failure, chills, debilitated, hepatic disease, shock, coma, alcohol intoxication, status asthmaticus

> **BLACK BOX WARNING:** Neonates (contains benzyl alcohol), **IV** administration, respiratory depression/insufficiency, specialized care setting, experienced clinician

DOSAGE AND ROUTES
Preoperative sedation/amnesia induction
Adult and child ≥12 yr: IM 0.07-0.08 mg/kg 30-60 min before general anesthesia
Child 6 mo-5 yr: IV 0.05-0.1 mg/kg, a total dose of 0.6 mg/kg may be needed
Child 6-12 yr: IV 0.025-0.05 mg/kg, a total dose of 0.4 mg/kg may be needed

Induction of general anesthesia
Adult >55 yr: (ASA I/II) IV 150-300 mcg/kg over 30 sec; (ASA III/IV) limit dose to 250 mcg/kg

(nonpremedicated) or 150 mcg/kg (premedicated)

Adult <55 yr: IV 200-350 mcg/kg over 20-30 sec; if patient has not received premedication, may repeat by giving 20% of original dose; if patient has received premedication reduce dosage by 50 mcg/kg

Child: No safe and effective dosage is established; however, doses of 50-200 mcg/kg **IV** have been used

Continuous infusion for mechanical ventilation (critical care)

Adult: IV 0.01-0.05 mg/kg over several min; repeat at 10-15 min intervals until adequate sedation, then 0.02-0.10 mg/kg/hr maintenance; adjust as needed

Child: IV 0.05-0.2 mg/kg over 2-3 min, then 0.06-0.12 mg/kg/hr by CONT INF; adjust as needed

Neonate: IV 0.03 mg/kg/hr titrate using lowest dose

Alcohol withdrawal (unlabeled)

Adult: IV 1-5 mg q1-2hr (mild-moderate symptoms); cont IV inf 1-20 mg q1-2hr (delirium tremens)

Available forms: Inj 1, 5 mg/ml, 25 mg/5 ml, 50 mg/10 ml; syr 2 mg/ml

Implementation

• Store at room temperature; protect from light

PO route

• Remove cap of press-in bottle adaptor and push adaptor into neck of bottle; close with cap, remove cap, and insert tip of dispenser and insert into adaptor; turn upside-down and withdraw correct dose; place in mouth

IM route

• Give inj deep into large muscle mass

IV route

• Give **IV** undiluted or after diluting with D₅W or 0.9% NaCl to a conc of 0.25 mg/ml; give over 2 min (conscious sedation) or over 30 sec (anesthesia induction)

• Ensure immediate availability of resuscitation equipment, O₂ to support airway; do not give by rapid bol

Syringe compatibilities: Alfentanil, atracurium, atropine, benzquinamide, buprenorphine, butorphanol, chlorproMAZINE, cimetidine, cisatracurium, diphenhyDRAMINE, droperidol, fentaNYL, glycopyrrolate, hydromorphine, hydrOXYzine, ketamine, meperidine, metoclopramide, morphine, nalbuphine, promazine, promethazine, remifentanil, scopolamine, SUFentanil, thiethylperazine, trimethobenzamide

Syringe incompatibilities: DimenhyDRINATE, PENTobarbital, perphenazine, prochlorperazine, ranitidine

Y-site compatibilities: Abciximab, acetaminophen, alemtuzumab, alfentamil, amikacin, amiodarone, anidulafungin, argatroban, atracurium, atropine, aztreonam, benzotropine, calcium gluconate, ceFAZolin, cefotaxime, cefOXitine, cefTRIAXone, cimetidine, ciprofloxacin, CISplatin, clindamycin, cloNIDine, cyanocobalamin, cycloSPORINE, DACTINomycin, digoxin, diltiazem, diphenhydrAMINE, DOCEtaxal, DOPamine, doxycycline, enalaprilat, EPINEPHrine, erythromycin, esmolol, etomidate, etoposide, famotidine, fentaNYL, fluconazole, folic acid, gatifloxacin, gemcitabine, gentamicin, glycopyrrolate, granisetron, heparin, hetastarch, HYDROmorphone, hydrOXYzine, inamrinone, isoproterenol, labetalol, lactated Ringer's, levofloxacin, lidocaine, linezolid, LORazepam, magnesium, mannitol, meperidine, methadone, methyldopa, methylPREDNISolone, metoclopromide, metomolol, metroNIDAZOLE, milrinone, morphine, nalbuphine, naloxone, niCARdipine, nitroglycerin, nitroprusside, norepinephrine, ondansetron, oxacillin, oxytocin, PACLitaxel, palonosetron, pancuronium, papaverin, phentolamine, phytonadione, piperacillin, potassium chloride, propanolol, protamine, pyridoxine, ranitidine, remifentanil, sodium nitroprusside, streptokinase, succinylcholine, SUFentanil, teniposide, theophylline, thiotepa, ticarcillin, tobramycin, vancomycin, vasopressin, vecuronium, verapamil, voriconazole, zolendronic acid

Y-site incompatibilities: Foscarnet

ADVERSE EFFECTS

CNS: Retrograde amnesia, euphoria, confusion, headache, anxiety, insomnia, slurred speech, paresthesia, tremors, weakness, chills, agitation, paradoxical reactions

CV: Hypotension, PVCs, tachycardia, bigeminy, nodal rhythm, **cardiac arrest**

EENT: Blurred vision, nystagmus, diplopia, loss of balance

GI: *Nausea, vomiting,* increased salivation, hiccups

INTEG: Urticaria, pain at injection site, swelling at inj site, rash, pruritus at injection site

RESP: Coughing, **apnea, bronchospasm, laryngospasm,** dyspnea, **respiratory depression**

Pharmacokinetics

Absorption	Well absorbed
Distribution	Crosses placenta, blood-brain barrier; protein binding 97%
Metabolism	Liver; by CYP3A4 to metabolites excreted in urine
Excretion	Kidneys, breast milk
Half-life	1-5 hr

Pharmacodynamics

	PO	IM	IV
Onset	10-30 min	15 min	1.5-5 min
Peak	Unknown	½-1 hr	Unknown
Duration	Unknown	2-3 hr	<2 hr

INTERACTIONS
Individual drugs
Alcohol: increased respiratory depression

Cimetidine, erythromycin, ranitidine, theophylline: decreased midazolam metabolism

FluvoxaMINE, indinavir, ritonavir, verapamil, protease inhibitors: increased respiratory depression

Drug classifications
Antihypertensives, nitrates, opiates: increase in hypotension

Barbiturates, opiate analgesics, other CNS depressants: increased respiratory depression

CYP3A4 inducers (azole antifungals, theophylline): increased half-life of midazolam

CYP3A4 inhibitors: increased levels of midazolam

Drug/herb
Kava, valerian: increased sedation

St. John's wort: decreased midazolam

Drug/food
Grapefruit juice: increased midazolam effect (PO)

NURSING CONSIDERATIONS
Assessment
• Monitor B/P, pulse, respiration during **IV**; O₂ and emergency equipment should be nearby

• Monitor inj site for redness, pain, swelling

• Assess degree of amnesia in geriatric; may be increased

• Assess anterograde amnesia

• Assess vital signs for recovery period in obese patient, since half-life may be extended

• **Respiratory depression/insufficiency: assess for apnea, respiratory depression, which may be increased in the geriatric**

Patient/family education
• Inform patient that amnesia occurs; events might not be remembered

• Caution patient to avoid CNS depressants including alcohol for 24 hr after taking this product

Evaluation
Positive therapeutic outcome
• Induction of sedation, amnesia

TREATMENT OF OVERDOSE:
O₂, flumazenil

miglitol (Rx)
(mig′le-tol)
Glyset
Func. class.: Oral hypoglycemic
Chem. class.: α-Glucosidase inhibitor
Pregnancy category B

ACTION: Delays the digestion/absorption of ingested carbohydrates, results in a smaller rise in blood glucose after meals; does not increase insulin production

Therapeutic outcome: Decreased blood glucose levels in diabetes mellitus

USES: Type 2 diabetes mellitus

Unlabeled uses: Type 1 diabetes mellitus

CONTRAINDICATIONS
Hypersensitivity, diabetic ketoacidosis, cirrhosis, IBD, colonic ulceration, partial intestinal obstruction, chronic intestinal disease, ileus

Precautions: Pregnancy **B**, breastfeeding, children, diarrhea, hiatal hernia, hypoglycemia, renal disease, Type 1 diabetes, vomiting

DOSAGE AND ROUTES
Initial dose
Adult: PO 25 mg tid initially, with first bite of meal

Maintenance dose
Adult: PO may be increased to 50 mg tid; may increase to 100 mg tid if needed with dosage adjustment at 4-8 wk intervals

Available forms: Tabs 25, 50, 100 mg

Implementation
• Give tid with first bite of each meal

• Provide storage in airtight container at room temperature

ADVERSE EFFECTS
GI: *Abdominal pain, diarrhea, flatulence,* **hepatotoxicity**
HEMA: Low iron
INTEG: Rash

Pharmacokinetics

Absorption	Unknown
Distribution	Unknown
Metabolism	Not metabolized
Excretion	Kidneys, unchanged product
Half-life	2 hr

Pharmacodynamics

Onset	Unknown
Peak	2-3 hr
Duration	Unknown

INTERACTIONS
Individual drugs
Digoxin: decreased levels of digoxin
Propranolol: decreased levels of propranolol
Ranitidine: decreased levels of ranitidine

Drug classifications
Adsorbents (intestinal), enzymes (digestive): decreased miglitol levels; do not use together

Drug/food
Carbohydrates: increased diarrhea

NURSING CONSIDERATIONS
Assessment
• Assess for hypo/hyperglycemia; even though this product does not cause hypoglycemia, if taking a sulfonylurea or insulin, hypoglycemia may be additive (rare)
• Monitor blood glucose levels, A1c, liver function tests; if hypoglycemia occurs with monotherapy, treat with glucose

Patient/family education
• Teach patient the symptoms of hypo/hyperglycemia and what to do about each
• Instruct that medication must be taken as prescribed; explain consequences of discontinuing the medication abruptly; that during periods of stress, infection, surgery, insulin may be required
• Tell patient to avoid OTC medications unless approved by prescriber
• Teach patient that diabetes is a lifelong illness; product will not cure condition
• Instruct patient to carry/wear emergency ID as diabetic
• Teach patient that diet and exercise regimen must be followed
• Teach patient GI side effects and what to do about them

Evaluation
Positive therapeutic outcome
• Decreased signs, symptoms of diabetes mellitus (polyuria, polydipsia, polyphagia, clear sensorium, absence of dizziness, stable gait)
• Improved blood glucose, A1c

⚠ HIGH ALERT

milrinone (Rx)
(mill-re′none)
Func. class.: Inotropic/vasodilator agent with phosphodiesterase activity
Chem. class.: Bipyridine derivative
Pregnancy category C

ACTION: Positive inotropic agent with vasodilator properties; increases contractility of cardiac muscle; reduces preload and afterload by direct relaxation of vascular smooth muscle; increases myocardial contractility

Therapeutic outcome: Increased inotropic effect resulting in increased cardiac output

USES: Short-term management of advanced CHF that has not responded to other medication

CONTRAINDICATIONS
Hypersensitivity to this product, severe aortic disease, severe pulmonic valvular disease, acute MI

Precautions: Pregnancy **C**, breastfeeding, children, geriatric, renal/hepatic disease, atrial flutter/fibrillation

DOSAGE AND ROUTES
Adult: IV BOL 50 mcg/kg given over 10 min; start INF of 0.375-0.75 mcg/kg/min; reduce dosage in renal impairment

Renal dose
Adult: IV CCr 41-50 ml/min 0.43 mcg/kg/min, titrate up; CCr 31-40 ml/min 0.38 mcg/kg/min, titrate up; CCr 21-30 ml/min 0.33 mcg/kg/min, titrate up; CCr 11-20 ml/min 0.28 mcg/kg/min; CCr 6-10 ml/min 0.23 mcg/kg/min; CCr <6 ml/min 0.20 mcg/kg/min; max all dosages 0.75 mcg/kg/min

Available forms: Inj 1 mg/ml; premixed inj 200 mcg/ml in D₅W

Implementation
Direct IV route
• Give **IV** loading dose undiluted over 10 min; use controlled-rate device
• Administer by direct **IV** into inf through Y-connector or directly into tubing
Continuous IV infusion route
• Dilute 20 mg vial with 80, 112, 180 ml of 0.45% NaCl, 0.9% NaCl, or D₅W to a concentration of 200, 150, 100 mcg/ml respectively
• Do not mix directly with glucose sol (chemical reaction occurs over 24 hr) precipitate

---

forms if milrinone and furosemide come into contact
• Titrate rate based on hemodynamic and clinical response, use controlled device
• Administer potassium supplements if ordered for potassium levels <3.0 mg/dl

Y-site compatibilities: Acyclovir, alfentanil, allopurinol, amifostine, amikacin, aminocaproic acid, aminophylline, amiodarone, amphotericin B liposome, ampicillin, ampicillin-sulbactam, anidulafungin, argatroban, atenolol, atracurium, aztreonam, bivalirudin, bleomycin, bumetanide, buprenorphine, busulfan, butorphanol, calcium chloride/gluconate, CARBOplatin, caspofungin, ceFAZolin, cefepime, cefotaxime, cefoTEtan, cefOXitin, cefTAZidime, ceftizoxime, cefTRIAXone, cefuroxime, chloramphenicol, chlorproMAZINE, cimetidine, ciprofloxacin, cisatracurium, CISplatin, clindamycin, cyclophosphamide, cycloSPORINE, cytarabine, DACTINomycin, DAPTOmycin, dexamethasone, digoxin, diltiazem, DOBUTamine, DOCEtaxel, DOPamine, doripenem, doxacurium, DOXOrubicin, doxycycline, droperidol, enalaprilat, ePHEDrine, EPINEPHrine, epirubicin, eptifibatide, ertapenem, erythromycin, etoposide, famotidine, fenoldopam, fentaNYL, fluconazole, fludarabine, fluorouracil, gallium, ganciclovir, gatifloxacin, gemcitabine, gentamicin, glycopyrrolate, granisetron, haloperidol, heparin, hydrALAZINE, hydrocortisone, HYDROmorphone, IDArubicin, ifosfamide, insulin (regular), irinotecan, isoproterenol, ketorolac, labetalol, levofloxacin, linezolid, LORazepam, magnesium sulfate, mannitol, mechlorethamine, melphalan, meperidine, meropenem, methohexital, methotrexate, methyldopate, methylPREDNISolone, metoclopramide, metoprolol, metroNIDAZOLE, micafungin, midazolam, mitoXANtrone, morphine, mycophenolate, nafcillin, nalbuphine, naloxone, nesiritide, norepinephrine, octreotide, oxacillin, oxaliplatin, oxytocin, PACLitaxel, palonosetron, pamidronate, pancuronium, PEMEtrexed, pentamidine, pentazocine, PENTobarbital, PHENobarbital, phenylephrine, piperacillin, piperacillin-tazobactam, polymyxin B, potassium chloride/phosphates, prochlorperazine, promethazine, propofol, propranolol, quiNIDine, quinupristin-dalfopristin, ranitidine, remifentanil, rocuronium, sodium acetate/bicarbonate/phosphates, streptozocin, succinylcholine, SUFentanil, sulfamethoxazole-trimethoprim, tacrolimus, teniposide, theophylline, thiopental, thiotepa, ticarcillin, ticarcillin-clavulanate, tigecycline, tirofiban, tobramycin, torsemide, vancomycin, vasopressin, vecuronium, verapamil, vinCRIStine, vinorelbine, voriconazole, zidovudine, zoledronic acid

ADVERSE EFFECTS
CV: *Dysrhythmias,* hypotension, chest pain, PVCs
GI: Nausea, vomiting, anorexia, abdominal pain, **hepatotoxicity,** jaundice
HEMA: Thrombocytopenia
MISC: Headache, hypokalemia, tremor, injection site reactions

Pharmacokinetics

Absorption	Completely absorbed
Distribution	Unknown
Metabolism	Liver (50%)
Excretion	Kidney, unchanged (83%), metabolites (12%)
Half-life	2.4 hr; increased in CHF

Pharmacodynamics

Onset	2-5 min
Peak	10 min
Duration	Variable

INTERACTIONS
Drug classifications
Antihypertensives, diuretics: increased effects

NURSING CONSIDERATIONS
Assessment
• Monitor for hypokalemia: acidic urine, reduced urine, osmolality, nocturia; hypotension, broad T-wave, U-wave, ectopy, tachycardia, weak pulse; muscle weakness, altered LOC, drowsiness, apathy, lethargy, confusion, depression; anorexia, nausea, cramps, constipation, distention, paralytic ileus; hypoventilation, respiratory muscle weakness
• Assess fluid volume status: complete I&O ratio and record; note weight, distended red veins, crackles in lung; color, quality, and specific gravity of urine; skin turgor, adequacy of pulses, moist mucous membranes, bilateral lung sounds, peripheral pitting edema; dehydration symptoms of decreasing output, thirst, hypotension, dry mouth and mucous membranes should be reported
• Monitor electrolytes: potassium, sodium, calcium, magnesium; also include BUN, blood pH, ABGs
⚠ Monitor B/P and pulse, ECG continuously during IV; ventricular dysrhythmia can occur; PCWP, CVP, index often during inf; if B/P drops 30 mm Hg, stop inf and call prescriber
• Monitor ALT, AST, bilirubin daily; if these are elevated, hepatotoxicity is suspected
• Monitor platelets; if <150,000/mm³, product is usually discontinued and another product started
• Assess for extravasation: change site q48hr

M

Patient/family education
- Teach patient reason for medication and expected results
- Instruct patient to make position changes slowly; orthostatic hypotension may occur
- Teach patient signs and symptoms of hypersensitivity reactions and hypokalemia

Evaluation

Positive therapeutic outcome
- Increased cardiac output
- Decreased PCWP, adequate CVP
- Decreased dyspnea, fatigue, edema, ECG

TREATMENT OF OVERDOSE:
Discontinue product, support circulation

minocycline (Rx)
(min-oh-sye′kleen)
Arestin, Dynacin, Minocin, Solodyn
Func. class.: Broad-spectrum antiinfective
Chem. class.: Tetracycline
Pregnancy category D

ACTION: Inhibits protein synthesis and phosphorylation in microorganisms by binding to 30S ribosomal subunits and reversibly binding to 50S ribosomal subunits; bacteriostatic

Therapeutic outcome: Bactericidal action against susceptible organisms, including *Neisseria meningitidis, Neisseria gonorrhoeae, Treponema pallidum, Chlamydia trachomatis, Ureaplasma urealyticum, Mycoplasma pneumoniae, Nocardia, Rickettsia*

USES: Syphilis, chlamydial infection, gonorrhea, lymphogranuloma venereum, rickettsial infections, inflammatory acne, meningitis carriers, periodontitis, methicillin-resistant *Staphylococcus aureus* (MRSA) infections, nonnodular moderate to severe acne vulgaris, *Rickettsia* sp.

Unlabeled uses: Rheumatoid arthritis

CONTRAINDICATIONS
Pregnancy **D**, hypersensitivity to tetracyclines, children <8 yr

Precautions: Breastfeeding, hepatic disease

DOSAGE AND ROUTES
Adult: PO/IV 200 mg, then 100 mg q12hr, max 400 mg/24 hr **IV**; subgingival insert into periodontal pocket
Child >8 yr: PO/IV 4 mg/kg then 4 mg/kg/day PO in divided doses q12hr

Rickettsial infections
Adult: PO/IV 200 mg, then 100 mg q12hr

Adolescent/child ≥8 yr: PO/IV 4 mg/kg, then 2 mg kg q12hr, max adult dose

Gonorrhea
Adult: PO 200 mg, then 100 mg q12hr × 4 days or more

Syphilis
Adult: PO 200 mg, then 100 mg q12hr × 10-15 days

Uncomplicated gonococcal urethritis in men
Adult: PO 100 mg q12hr × 5 days

Rheumatoid arthritis (unlabeled)
Adult: PO 100 mg bid for ≤48 wk

Acne vulgaris (solodyn only)
Adult/adolescent/child ≥12 yr: ext rel 1 mg/kg/day × 12 wk or those weighing 126-136 kg: 135 mg/day; 111-125 kg: 115 mg/day; 97-110 kg: 105 mg/day; 85-96 kg: 90 mg/day; 72-84 kg: 80 mg/day; 60-71 kg: 65 mg/day; 50-59 kg: 55 mg/day; 45-49 kg: 45 mg/day

Acne vulgaris (all except solodyn)
Adult/adolescent/child ≥12 yr: ext rel 1 mg/kg × 12 wk or 91-136 kg/135 mg/day; 60-90 kg 90 mg/day; 45-59 kg 45 mg/day

Available forms: Caps 50, 75, 100 mg; powder for inj 100 mg; pellet-filled caps 50, 100 mg; tabs 50, 75, 100 mg; ext rel tabs 45, 55, 65, 80, 90, 105, 115, 135 mg

Implementation
- Store in airtight, light-resistant container at room temp
PO route
- Give around the clock to maintain proper blood levels; give with food to increase absorption of product; do not give within 3 hr of other agents; product interactions may occur
- Give with 8 oz of water 1 hr before bedtime to prevent ulceration
- Shake liquid preparation well before giving; use calibrated device for proper dosing
- Do not give with iron, calcium, magnesium products, or antacids, which decrease absorption and form insoluble chelate

IV route
- Check for irritation, extravasation, phlebitis daily; change site q72hr
- For intermittent inf, dilute each 100 mg/10 ml of 0.9% NaCl, sterile water for inj; further dilute in 500-1000 ml of 0.9% NaCl, D₅W, Ringer's, LR, D₅/LR; give over 6 hr

Y-site compatibilities: Alfentanil, amikacin, atracurium, benztropine, bretylium, buprenorphine, butorphanol, calcium chloride,

CARBOplatin, caspofungin, cefonicid, chlorproMAZINE, cimetidine, codeine, cyclophosphamide, cycloSPORINE, cytarabine, DACTINomycin, dexmedetomidine, diltiazem, diphenhydrAMINE, DOBUTamine, DOCEtaxel, doxacurium, doxycycline, enalaprilat, ePHEDrine, EPINEPHrine, eptifibatide, etoposide, fenoldopam, fentaNYL, fludarabine, gatifloxacin, gemcitabine, gentamicin, glycopyrrolate, granisetron, heparin, hetastarch, IDArubicin, ifosfamide, inamrinone, isoproterenol, labetalol, levofloxacin, lidocaine, linezolid, LORazepam, magnesium sulfate, mannitol, melphalan, metaraminol, methotrexate, methyldopa, metoclopramide, metoprolol, midazolam, mitoXANtrone, nalbuphine, naloxone, perphenazine, potassium chloride, sargramostim, sodium succinate, vinorelbine, vit B/C

Y-site incompatibilities: Aztreonam, filgrastim, HYDROmorphone, meperidine, morphine, teniposide

ADVERSE EFFECTS

CNS: *Dizziness,* fever, light-headedness, vertigo, seizures, increased intracranial pressure
CV: Pericarditis
EENT: Dysphagia, glossitis, decreased calcification, permanent discoloration of teeth, oral candidiasis
GI: *Nausea,* abdominal pain, *vomiting, diarrhea,* anorexia, enterocolitis, hepatotoxicity, flatulence, abdominal cramps, epigastric burning, stomatitis, pseudomembranous colitis
GU: Increased BUN, polyuria, polydipsia, renal failure, nephrotoxicity
HEMA: Eosinophilia, neutropenia, thrombocytopenia, hemolytic anemia, pancytopenia
INTEG: *Rash, urticaria, photosensitivity, increased pigmentation,* exfoliative dermatitis, pruritus, blue-gray color of skin and mucous membranes
MS: Myalgia, arthritis, bone discoloration, joint stiffness
SYST: Angioedema, Stevens-Johnson syndrome

Pharmacokinetics

Absorption	Well absorbed (PO)
Distribution	Widely distributed; some distribution in CSF, crosses placenta
Metabolism	Liver, some
Excretion	Kidneys, unchanged (20%), bile, feces
Half-life	11-17 hr

Pharmacodynamics

	PO	IV
Onset	Rapid	Rapid
Peak	2-3 hr	Infusion's end
Duration	Unknown	Unknown

INTERACTIONS
Individual drugs
Calcium: forms chelates, decreased absorption
CarBAMazepine, phenytoin: decreased effect
Digoxin: increased effect
Insulin: increased effect
Kaolin/pectin, sodium bicarbonate, cimetidine, quinapril, sucralfate, iron: decreased minocycline effect
Theophylline: increased effect
Warfarin: increased effect

Drug classifications
Alkali products, antacids: decreased minocycline effect
Anticoagulants (oral neuromuscular blockers): increased effect
Barbiturates, penicillins: decreased effect
Retinoids: increased chance of pseudomotor cerebri, do not use concurrently

Drug/lab test
False negative: urine glucose with Clinistix, Tes-Tape

NURSING CONSIDERATIONS
Assessment
• Assess patient for previous sensitivity reaction
• **Assess patient for signs and symptoms of infection** including characteristics of wounds, sputum, urine, stool, WBC >10,000/mm³, fever; obtain baseline information before, during treatment
• Obtain C&S before beginning product therapy to identify if correct treatment has been initiated
• **Assess for allergic reactions:** rash, urticaria, pruritus, angioedema
• Monitor blood studies: AST, ALT, CBC, Hct, bilirubin, alkaline phosphatase, amylase monthly if patient is on long-term therapy
• **Pseudomembranous colitis: assess bowel pattern daily; if severe diarrhea occurs, product should be discontinued**
• Monitor for bleeding: ecchymosis, bleeding gums, hematuria, stool guaiac daily if on long-term therapy; blood dyscrasias may occur
• **Assess for overgrowth of infection:** perineal itching, fever, malaise, redness, pain, swelling, drainage, rash, diarrhea, change in cough, sputum; black, furry tongue

M

Patient/family education
• Teach patient to use sunscreen when outdoors to decrease photosensitivity reaction
• Teach patient to report sore throat, bruising, bleeding, joint pain; may indicate blood dyscrasias (rare)
• Advise patient to contact prescriber if vaginal itching, loose foul-smelling stools, furry tongue occur; may indicate superinfection; report itching, rash, pruritus, urticaria
• Instruct patient to take all medication prescribed for the length of time ordered; product must be taken around the clock to maintain blood levels; do not give medication to others; take with a full glass of water; may take with food; not to use outdated product, Fanconi's syndrome may occur

Evaluation

Positive therapeutic outcome
• Absence of signs/symptoms of infection (WBC $<10,000/mm^3$, temp WNL, absence of red, draining wounds)
• Reported improvement in symptoms of infection

minoxidil (Rx, OTC)
(mi-nox'i-dill)
Rogaine (TOP)
Func. class.: Antihypertensive, hair growth stimulant
Chem. class.: Vasodilator, peripheral
Pregnancy category C

Do not confuse: minoxidil/Monopril

ACTION: Directly relaxes arteriolar smooth muscle, causing vasodilatation; reduces peripheral vascular resistance, decreases B/P; increased cutaneous blood flow; stimulation of hair follicles

Therapeutic outcome: Decreased B/P in hypertension; hair growth

USES: Severe hypertension unresponsive to other therapy (use with diuretic and β-blocker); topically to treat alopecia, anal fissures

CONTRAINDICATIONS
Dissecting aortic aneurysm, hypersensitivity, pheochromocytoma

> BLACK BOX WARNING: Acute MI

Precautions: Pregnancy **C**, breastfeeding, children, geriatric, renal disease, CVD

> BLACK BOX WARNING: CAD, CHF, cardiac disease, cardiac tamponade, edema, hypotension, orthostatic hypotension, pericardial effusion

DOSAGE AND ROUTES
Severe hypertension
Adult: PO 5 mg/day in 1-2 divided doses, max 100 mg/day; usual range 10-40 mg/day divided in 1-2 doses
Geriatric: PO 2.5 mg/day, may be increased gradually
Child <12 yr: PO initial 0.1-0.2 mg/kg/day; effective range, 0.25-1 mg/kg/day; max, 50 mg/day

Alopecia
Adult: TOP 1 ml bid, rub into scalp daily, max 2 ml/day

Renal dose
Adult: PO CCr 10-15 ml/min extend interval to q24hr; CCr <10 ml/min not recommended

Anal fissures (unlabeled)
Adult/adolescent: TOP (0.5% minoxidil in white paraffin base) 0.5 g each compounded minoxidil and lignocaine ointment q8hr

Available forms: Tabs 2.5, 10 mg; topical 2%, 5% sol, topical foam 5%

Implementation
PO route
• Administer without regard to meals
• Give with β-blockers and/or diuretic for hypertension
• Store protected from light and heat
Topical route
• Administer 1 ml dose no matter how much balding has occurred; increasing dose does not speed hair growth
• Treatment must continue long term or new hair will be lost again

ADVERSE EFFECTS
Systemic
CNS: Headache, fatigue
CV: *Severe rebound hypertension (on withdrawal in children)*, tachycardia, angina, increased T-wave, **CHF, pulmonary edema, pericardial effusion,** edema, sodium retention, water retention, *hypotension*
GI: Nausea, vomiting
GU: Breast tenderness
HEMA: Hct, Hgb, erythrocyte count may decrease initially, leukopenia
INTEG: Pruritus, **Stevens-Johnson syndrome,** rash, hirsutism, contact dermatitis

---

Pharmacokinetics

Absorption	Well absorbed (PO); minimally absorbed (topical)
Distribution	Widely distributed, protein binding minimal
Metabolism	Liver
Excretion	Kidneys, breast milk
Half-life	4.2 hr

Pharmacodynamics

	PO	Topical
Onset	½ hr	4 mo
Peak	2-3 hr	Unknown
Duration	75 hr	4 mo

INTERACTIONS

Individual
Guanethidine, nitroprusside: increased hypotension

Drug classifications
Antihypertensives, MAOIs, nitrates: increased hypotension

Estrogens, NSAIDs, salicylates: decreased antihypertensive effect

Drug/herb
Hawthorn: increased antihypertensive effect

Drug/lab test
Increased: renal function tests
Decreased: Hgb, Hct, RBC

NURSING CONSIDERATIONS

Assessment
⚠ Monitor closely; usually given with β-blocker to prevent tachycardia and increased myocardial workload; usually given with diuretic to prevent serious fluid accumulation; patient should be hospitalized during beginning treatment
• Monitor B/P, pulse, jugular venous distention periodically throughout treatment
• Monitor electrolytes, blood studies: potassium, sodium, chloride, CBC, serum glucose
⚠ Monitor weight daily, I&O; assess edema in feet, legs daily; check skin turgor, dryness of mucous membranes for hydration status
• Assess for crackles, dyspnea, orthopnea, peripheral edema, fatigue, weight gain, jugular vein distention (CHF)
• Assess for signs of hyperglycemia: acetone breath, increased urinary output, severe thirst, lethargy, dizziness

Patient/family education
Topical route
• Teach patient that new hair will be soft and hardly visible, use on clean, dry scalp before styling aids, wash hands after each use
• Caution patient not to use on other parts of the body; product is to be used on the scalp only
• Instruct patient that hair should be clean before applying medication; do not get on clothing
• Caution patient not to get medication near mucous membranes (mouth, nose, eyes) and to contact prescriber if burning, stinging, or rash occurs

Evaluation

Positive therapeutic outcome
• Decreased B/P in hypertension
• Hair growth (TOP)

mipomersen
(mye′poe-mer-sen)
Kynamro
Func. class.: Antilipemic
Chem. class.: Antisense oligonucleotide
Pregnancy category B

ACTION: Inhibits synthesis of the principal apoliprotein of LDL, VLDL, binds to messenger ribonucleic acid (mRNA)

Therapeutic outcome: Decreasing LDL, total cholesterol, apolipoprotein B, non-high density lipoprotein cholesterol

USES: Reduction of LDL, total cholesterol, apolipoprotein B, non-high density lipoprotein cholesterol (homozygous familial hypercholesterolemia)

CONTRAINDICATIONS

> BLACK BOX WARNING: Hepatic disease

Precautions: Pregnancy (**B**), breastfeeding, dialysis, alcohol ingestion, geriatrics, proteinuria, renal disease, low density lipoprotein apheresis

DOSAGE AND ROUTES

Homozygous familial hypercholesterolemia
Adult: SUBCUT 200 mg qwk

Renal/hepatic dose
Adult: Do not use in severe renal, hepatic disease

Dose adjustments for elevated transaminases during treatment
• ALT or AST ≥ 3× and < 5× ULN: confirm elevation with a repeat test within 1 wk. If

M

confirmed, withhold product, obtain other tests if not already obtained (total bilirubin, alkaline phosphatase, INR) to identify the probable cause. If resuming product after transaminases resolve to <3× ULN, consider monitoring liver-related tests more frequently.

• ALT or AST ≥ 5× ULN: withhold, obtain additional liver-related tests if not already obtained (total bilirubin, alkaline phosphatase, INR) and identify the probable cause. If resuming product after transaminases resolve to < 3× ULN, monitor liver-related tests more frequently.

Available forms: Sol for injection 200 mg/ml

Implementation
• Give on the same day each wk; if a dose is missed, give ≥3 days from the next weekly dose
• Monitor ALT, AST, alkaline phosphatase, and total bilirubin prior to start of therapy; monitor lipid levels ≥q3-4 mo for the first year.
• Monitor LDL-C level after 6 mo

ADVERSE EFFECTS
CNS: Fatigue, headache, fever
CV: Hypertension, palpitations
GI: Abdominal pain, vomiting
GU: Glomerulonephritis, proteinuria
MS: Musculoskeletal pain
SYST: Angioedema

Pharmacokinetics

Absorption	Unknown
Distribution	Protein binding >90%
Metabolism	Unknown
Excretion	Unknown
Half-life	1-2 mo

Pharmacodynamics

Onset	Unknown
Peak	Unknown
Duration	Unknown

INTERACTIONS
Individual drugs
Acetaminophen, methotrexate, tamoxifen, tetracyclines: increased hepatotoxicity risk

NURSING CONSIDERATIONS
Assessment
• Determine if the LDL-C reduction achieved is sufficient to warrant the potential risk of liver toxicity
• Assess geriatric patients: increased risk for hypertension, peripheral edema, hepatic steatosis

• Hypercholesterolemia: diet history: fat content, lipid levels (triglycerides, LDL, HDL, cholesterol); LFTs at baseline, periodically during treatment

Patient/family education
• Teach patient/family that compliance is needed
• Instruct patient to decrease risk factors: high fat diet, smoking, alcohol consumption, absence of exercise
• Instruct patient to notify prescriber if pregnancy is suspected or planned, or if breastfeeding
• Instruct patient to notify prescriber of dietary/herbal supplements

Evaluation
Positive therapeutic outcome
• Decreasing LDL, total cholesterol, apolipoprotein B, non-high density lipoprotein cholesterol

mirabegron
(mir'a-beg'ron)
Myrbetriq
Func. class.: Bladder antispasmodic
Chem. class.: β_2-Adrenergic receptor agonist
Pregnancy category C

ACTION: Relaxes smooth muscles in urinary tract

Therapeutic outcome: Decreasing dysuria, frequency, nocturia, incontinence

USES: Overactive bladder (urinary frequency, urgency), urinary incontinence

CONTRAINDICATIONS
Hypersensitivity

Precautions: Pregnancy (**C**), breastfeeding, children, kidney/liver disease, bladder obstruction, dialysis, hypertension

DOSAGE AND ROUTES
Adult: PO 25 mg/day, may increase to 50 mg/day if needed

Hepatic/renal dose
Adult: PO Child–Pugh B or (CCr 15-29 ml/min, max 25 mg/day; Child–Pugh C or CCr 15 ml/min, not recommended

Available forms: Tabs ext rel 25, 50 mg

Implementation
• Give whole; take with liquids; do not crush, chew, or break ext rel product; use without regard to meals

ADVERSE EFFECTS
CNS: Fatigue, dizziness, headache
CV: Hypertension
EENT: Xerophthalmia, blurred vision
GI: Nausea, vomiting, anorexia, abdominal pain, constipation, diarrhea, dyspepsia
GU: Dysuria, urinary retention, frequency, UTI, bladder discomfort
INTEG: Rash, pruritus
MISC: Arthralgia, back pain
RESP: Pharyngitis
SYST: Stevens–Johnson syndrome

Pharmacokinetics

Absorption	Unknown
Distribution	71% protein binding
Metabolism	Unknown
Excretion	25% unchanged in urine
Half-life	Terminal 50 hr

Pharmacodynamics

Onset	Unknown
Peak	3.5 hr
Duration	Unknown

INTERACTIONS
Individual drugs
CYP3A4 inhibitors: increased mirabegron effect
CYP2D6 substrates: increased effect of these substrates
Digoxin, warfarin, desipramine, thioridazine, flecainide, propafenone: increased effect of these agents

Drug classifications
Antimuscarinic agents (e.g., atropine, scopolamine): increased risk of urinary retention

NURSING CONSIDERATIONS
Assessment
• Urinary patterns: Assess for distention, nocturia, frequency, urgency, incontinence
• Monitor LFTs at baseline, periodically
• Monitor B/P

Patient/family education
• Teach patient to avoid hazardous activities; dizziness can occur
• Advise patient not to drink liquids before bedtime
• Inform patient about the importance of bladder maintenance

Evaluation

Positive therapeutic outcome
• Decreasing dysuria, frequency, nocturia, incontinence

mirtazapine (Rx)
(mer-ta′za-peen)
Remeron, Remeron Soltab
Func. class.: Antidepressant
Chem. class.: Tetracyclic
Pregnancy category C

ACTION: Blocks reuptake of norepinephrine, serotonin into nerve endings, increasing action of norepinephrine, serotonin in nerve cells; antagonist of central α_2-receptors, blocks histamine receptors; has anticholinergic action

Therapeutic outcome: Decreased symptoms of depression after 2-3 wk

USES: Depression, dysthymic disorder, bipolar disorder: depression, agitated depression

CONTRAINDICATIONS
Hypersensitivity to tricyclics, recovery phase of MI, agranulocytosis, jaundice

Precautions: Pregnancy C, geriatric, suicidal patients, severe depression, increased intraocular pressure, closed-angle glaucoma, urinary retention, cardiac/renal/hepatic disease, hypo/hyperthyroidism, electroshock therapy, elective surgery, seizure disorder, bone marrow suppression, thrombocytopenia

> **BLACK BOX WARNING:** Suicidal ideation, children

DOSAGE AND ROUTES
Adult: PO 15 mg/day at bedtime, maintenance to continue for 6 mo, titrate up to 45 mg/day; orally disintegrating tabs open blister pack, place tab on tongue, allow to disintegrate, swallow
Geriatric: PO 7.5 mg nightly, increase by 7.5 mg q1-2wk to desired dose, max 45 mg/day

Available forms: Tabs 15, 30, 45 mg; orally disintegrating tabs (Soltab) 15, 30, 45 mg

Implementation
• Administer without regard to meals; crush if patient is unable to swallow medication whole
• Give dose at bedtime if oversedation occurs during day; may take entire dose at bedtime; geriatric may not tolerate once/day dosing
• Store in tight container at room temperature; do not freeze
• Allow **orally disintegrating tablets** to dissolve on tongue; no water needed; do not split; contain phenylalanine
• **Serotonin syndrome, neuroleptic malignant syndrome: assess for increased heart rate, shivering, sweating, dilated pupils, tremors, high B/P, hyperthermia, headache,**

confusion; if these occur, stop product, administer a serotonin antagonist if needed; at least 2 wk should elapse between discontinuation of serotoninergic agents and start of this product

ADVERSE EFFECTS

CNS: *Dizziness, drowsiness,* confusion, headache, anxiety, tremors, stimulation, weakness, nightmares, EPS (geriatric), increased psychiatric symptoms, **seizures,** abnormal dreams
CV: *Orthostatic hypotension, ECG changes, tachycardia, hypertension,* palpitations
EENT: *Blurred vision,* tinnitus, mydriasis
GI: *Diarrhea, dry mouth,* nausea, vomiting, **paralytic ileus,** increased appetite, cramps, epigastric distress, **jaundice, hepatitis,** stomatitis, constipation, weight gain
GU: *Retention,* **acute renal failure,** urinary frequency
HEMA: **Agranulocytosis, thrombocytopenia, eosinophilia, leukopenia**
INTEG: Rash, urticaria, sweating, pruritus, photosensitivity
MS: Back pain, myalgia
RESP: Cough
SYST: Flulike symptoms, increased lipid levels

Pharmacokinetics

Absorption	Slow, complete
Distribution	Widely distributed; crosses placenta
Metabolism	Liver, extensively
Excretion	Feces; breast milk
Half-life	20-40 hr

Pharmacodynamics

Onset	Unknown
Peak	2 hr
Duration	Unknown

INTERACTIONS
Individual drugs
Alcohol: increased CNS depression
CloNIDine: decreased effects
Fenfluramine, dexfenfluramine, sibutramine, nefazodone: increased serotonin syndrome

Drug classifications
Barbiturates, benzodiazepines, CNS depressants (other): increased effects
MAOIs: hypertensive episode, seizures, hyperpyretic crisis
Sympathomimetics, indirect acting (ePHEDrine): decreased effects
SSRIs, SNRIs, serotonin-receptor agonists: increased serotonin syndrome

Drug/herb
Kava: increased CNS depression
St. John's wort, SAM-e: serotonin syndrome

Drug/lab test
Increased: serum bilirubin, blood glucose, alkaline phosphatase
Decreased: VMA, 5-HIAA
False increase: urinary catecholamines

NURSING CONSIDERATIONS
Assessment
• Monitor B/P (with patient lying, standing), pulse q4hr during beginning treatment; if systolic B/P drops 20 mm Hg, hold product, notify prescriber; take VS q4hr in patients with CV disease
• Monitor blood studies: CBC, leukocytes, differential, cardiac enzymes if patient is receiving long-term therapy, LFTs, serum creatinine/BUN
• Monitor liver function tests: AST, ALT, bilirubin
• Check weight weekly; product may increase appetite
⚠ **Assess ECG for flattening of T wave, bundle branch block, AV block, dysrhythmias in cardiac patients**
• Assess for EPS primarily in geriatric: rigidity, dystonia, akathisia
• Assess mental status: mood, sensorium, affect, suicidal tendencies; assess increase in psychiatric symptoms: depression, panic
• Identify alcohol consumption; if alcohol is consumed, hold dose until AM

Patient/family education
• Inform patient that therapeutic effects may take 2-3 wk; take at bedtime, do not discontinue abruptly
• Advise patient to use caution in driving and other activities requiring alertness because of drowsiness, dizziness, blurred vision; to avoid rising quickly from sitting to standing, especially geriatric
• Caution patient to avoid alcohol ingestion, other CNS depressants
• Teach patient to increase fluids, bulk in diet if constipation, urinary retention occur, especially geriatric
• Teach patient to use gum, hard sugarless candy, or frequent sips of water for dry mouth
• Advise not to use within 14 days of MAOIs

> **BLACK BOX WARNING:** Notify prescriber of suicidal thoughts, behavior

Evaluation
Positive therapeutic outcome
• Decrease in depression
• Absence of suicidal thoughts

⚠ Nurse Alert　　　★ Key NCLEX® Drug　　　≫ Drug Specifics

TREATMENT OF OVERDOSE:
ECG monitoring, lavage, activated charcoal, administer anticonvulsant

misoprostol (Rx)
(mye-soe-prost'ole)
Cytotec
Func. class.: Gastric mucosa protectant; antiulcer
Chem. class.: Prostaglandin E₁ analog
Pregnancy category X

Do not confuse: misoprostol/metoprolol, Cytotec/Cytoxan

ACTION: Inhibits gastric acid secretion; may protect gastric mucosa; can increase bicarbonate, mucus production

Therapeutic outcome: Prevention of gastric ulcers

USES: Prevention of NSAID-induced gastric ulcers

CONTRAINDICATIONS
Hypersensitivity to this product or prostaglandins

BLACK BOX WARNING: Pregnancy **X**, females

Precautions: Breastfeeding, children, geriatric, renal disease, CV disease, abnormal fetal position, cardiac/renal/inflammatory bowel disease, C-section, dehydration, diarrhea, fever, ectopic pregnancy, fetal distress, sepsis, vaginal bleeding

DOSAGE AND ROUTES
Adult: PO 200 mcg qid with food for duration of NSAID therapy with last dose at bedtime; if 200 mcg is not tolerated, 100 mcg may be given

Available forms: Tabs 100, 200 mcg

Implementation
• Give with meals for prolonged product effect; avoid use of magnesium antacids
• Store at room temp

ADVERSE EFFECTS
GI: *Diarrhea,* nausea, vomiting, flatulence, constipation, dyspepsia, abdominal pain
GU: Spotting, cramps, hypermenorrhea, menstrual disorders

Pharmacokinetics

Absorption	Well absorbed
Distribution	Unknown
Metabolism	Liver
Excretion	Kidneys
Half-life	½-1 hr

Pharmacodynamics

Onset	½ hr
Peak	Unknown
Duration	3 hr

INTERACTIONS
Drug/food
Maximum concentrations when taken with food

NURSING CONSIDERATIONS
Assessment
• **NSAID-induced ulcer prophylaxis:** monitor patient for GI symptoms: hematemesis, occult or frank blood in stools, also severe abdominal pain, cramping, severe diarrhea

BLACK BOX WARNING: Pregnancy **X**: obtain a negative pregnancy test in women of childbearing age before starting medication; miscarriages are common

Patient/family education
• Advise patient to avoid black pepper, caffeine, alcohol, harsh spices, extremes in temperature of food, which may aggravate condition
• Caution patient to avoid OTC preparations: aspirin, cough, cold preparations; condition may worsen
• Teach patient that product must be continued for prescribed time to be effective and taken exactly as prescribed; doses are not to be doubled
• Instruct patient to report to prescriber diarrhea, black tarry stools, abdominal pain, cramping, menstrual disorders

BLACK BOX WARNING: Caution patient to prevent pregnancy while taking this product; spontaneous abortion may occur, pregnancy **X**

Evaluation
Positive therapeutic outcome
• Prevention of ulcers

⚠ HIGH ALERT
mitoMYcin (Rx)
(mye-toe-mye'sin)
Mitosyl
Func. class.: Antineoplastic, antibiotic
Pregnancy category D

Do not confuse: mitoMYcin/mithramycin/mitotane/mitoXANtrone

ACTION: Inhibits DNA synthesis, primarily; derived from *Streptomyces caespitosus;* appears to cause cross-linking of DNA; a vesicant

Therapeutic outcome: Prevention of rapidly growing malignant cells

Adverse effects: *italics* = common; **bold** = life-threatening

USES: Pancreas, stomach, colorectal, bladder cancer

CONTRAINDICATIONS

Pregnancy **D** (1st trimester), breastfeeding, hypersensitivity, as a single agent, coagulation disorders

> **BLACK BOX WARNING:** Thrombocytopenia

Precautions: Accidental exposure, acute bronchospasm, anemia, children, dental disease/work, extravasation, females, hemolytic-uremic syndrome, infection, radiation therapy, surgery, vaccines, renal/respiratory disease

> **BLACK BOX WARNING:** Bone marrow suppression, hemolytic uremic syndrome

DOSAGE AND ROUTES
Adult: IV 10-20 mg/m² q6-8wk

Available forms: Inj 5, 20, 40 mg/vial

Implementation

Direct IV route
• Use cytotoxic handling procedures
• Give antiemetic 30-60 min before product to prevent vomiting
• Use port or central line if possible, product is very irritating to tissues
• Reconstitute 5 mg/10 ml; 20 mg/40 ml; 40 mg/80 ml of sterile water for injection (0.5 mg/ml); shake to dissolve, let stand until completely dissolved; stable for 1 wk at room temperature, 2 wk refrigerated, can be further diluted to 20-40 mcg/ml
• Inject reconstituted injection slowly over 5-10 min **IV** push into free-flowing **IV** infusion of 0.9% NaCl or D₅W
• Avoid excessive heat, store reconstituted product in refrigerator, discard after 2 wk, store unreconstituted product at room temp

Syringe compatibilities: Bleomycin, CISplatin, cyclophosphamide, DOXOrubicin, droperidol, fluorouracil, furosemide, heparin, leucovorin, methotrexate, metoclopramide, vinBLAStine, vinCRIStine

Y-site compatibilities: Allopurinol, amifostine, amphotericin B lipid complex, amphotericin B liposome, anidulafungin, argatroban, atenolol, bivalirudin, bleomycin, caspofungin, CISplatin, cyclophosphamide, DACTINomycin, dolasetron, DOXOrubicin, droperidol, epirubicin, ertapenem, fluorouracil, furosemide, granisetron, heparin, leucovorin, melphalan, methotrexate, metoclopramide, nesiritide, octreotide, ondansetron, oxaliplatin, PACLitaxel, palonosetron,

PEMEtrexed, riTUXimab, teniposide, thiotepa, tigecycline, tirofiban, trastuzumab, vinBLAStine, vinCRIStine, voriconazole, zoledronic acid

Y-site incompatibilities: Sargramostim, vinorelbine

ADVERSE EFFECTS
CNS: Fever, headache, confusion, drowsiness, syncope, fatigue
EENT: Blurred vision
GI: *Nausea, vomiting, anorexia, stomatitis,* hepatotoxicity, diarrhea
GU: Urinary retention, renal failure, edema
HEMA: Thrombocytopenia, leukopenia, anemia
INTEG: *Rash,* alopecia, extravasation, nail discoloration
MISC: Hemolytic uremic syndrome, CHF
RESP: Fibrosis, pulmonary infiltrate, dyspnea

Pharmacokinetics

Absorption	Complete bioavailability
Distribution	Widely distributed; concentrates in tumor
Metabolism	Liver, extensively
Excretion	Kidneys, unchanged
Half-life	1 hr

Pharmacodynamics

Unknown

INTERACTIONS
Individual drugs
Radiation: increased toxicity

Drug classifications
Anticoagulants, NSAIDs: increased bleeding risk
Antineoplastics: increased toxicity
Vaccines: avoid concurrent use

Drug/herb
Black cohosh: avoid use

NURSING CONSIDERATIONS
Assessment

> **BLACK BOX WARNING:** Assess for fatal hemolytic uremic syndrome: hypertension, thrombocytopenia, microangiopathic hemolytic anemia; occurs during long-term therapy

• Assess buccal cavity q8hr for dryness, sores or ulceration, white patches, oral pain, bleeding, dysphagia; obtain prescription for viscous lidocaine (Xylocaine)
• Assess symptoms indicating severe allergic reaction: rash, pruritus, urticaria, purpuric skin lesions, itching, flushing

---

BLACK BOX WARNING: Bone marrow suppression: Monitor CBC, differential, platelet count weekly; withhold product if WBC is <4000/mm³ or platelet count is <100,000/mm³ or serum creatinine >1.7 mg/dl; notify prescriber; bleeding: hematuria, guaiac, bruising, petechiae, mucosa, or orifices

• Monitor renal function tests: BUN, creatinine, serum uric acid, urine CCr before, during therapy; check I&O ratio; report fall in urine output to <30 ml/hr; adjust dose based on renal function

⚠ Assess for pulmonary fibrosis, bronchospasm, dyspnea, crackles, unproductive cough, chest pain, tachypnea, fatigue, increased pulse, pallor, lethargy

• Monitor temp q4hr (may indicate beginning of infection)

• Monitor liver function tests before, during therapy (bilirubin, AST, ALT, LDH) as needed or monthly; check for jaundiced skin and sclera, dark urine, clay-colored stools, itchy skin, abdominal pain, fever, diarrhea

• Assess for bleeding: hematuria, stool guaiac, bruising or petechiae, mucosa or orifices q8hr

• Identify effects of alopecia on body image; discuss feelings about body changes

• Identify edema in feet, joint pain, stomach pain, shaking; check for inflammation of mucosa, breaks in skin

Patient/family education

• Advise patient to get adequate fluids 2-3 L/day unless contraindicated

• Encourage patient to rinse mouth tid-qid with water, club soda, brush teeth bid-qid with soft brush or cotton-tipped applicators for stomatitis, use unwaxed dental floss

• Teach patient to avoid use of products containing aspirin or ibuprofen, razors, commercial mouthwash, since bleeding may occur; to report symptoms of bleeding (hematuria, tarry stools)

• Caution patient to report signs of anemia (fatigue, headache, irritability, faintness, shortness of breath)

• Advise patient to report any changes in breathing or coughing even several mo after treatment; to avoid crowds and persons with respiratory tract or other infections

⚠ Teach patient to report signs of IV site reaction, redness, inflammation, burning, pain

• Inform patient that hair may be lost during treatment; a wig or hairpiece may make patient feel better; new hair may be different in color, texture

⚠ Infection: teach patient to report fever, flulike symptoms, sore throat

• Advise patient not to have any vaccinations without the advice of the prescriber; serious reactions can occur

• Teach patient that contraception is needed during treatment and for several mo after completion of therapy

• Teach patient to report immediately urine retention, absence of urine, dyspnea, bleeding, jaundice, signs of pulmonary toxicity

Evaluation

Positive therapeutic outcome

• Prevention of rapid division of malignant cells

⚠ **HIGH ALERT**

mitoXANtrone (Rx)

(mye-toe-zan'trone)
Novantrone
Func. class.: Antineoplastic-antibiotic, immunomodulator
Chem. class.: Synthetic anthraquinone
Pregnancy category D

M

Do not confuse: mitoXANtrone/mitoMYcin/mithramycin/mitotane

ACTION: DNA reactive agent; cytocidal effect on both proliferating and nonproliferating cells; topoisomerase II inhibitor; a vesicant

Therapeutic outcome: Prevention of rapidly growing malignant cells

USES: Acute myelogenous leukemia (adult), relapsed leukemia, breast cancer, multiple sclerosis; used with steroids to treat bone pain (advanced prostate cancer); multiple sclerosis

Unlabeled uses: Liver malignancies, non-Hodgkin's lymphoma, breast cancer, ALL, bone marrow ablation, CLL, hepatocellular cancer, ovarian cancer, pleural effusion, stem cell transplant preparation

CONTRAINDICATIONS

Pregnancy **D**, hypersensitivity

Precautions: Breastfeeding, children, myelosuppression, cardiac/renal/hepatic disease, gout

BLACK BOX WARNING: Secondary malignancy, neutropenia, intrathecal administration, extravasation, heart failure

---

DOSAGE AND ROUTES
Acute nonlymphatic leukemia/induction
Adult: IV INF 12 mg/m²/day on days 1-3, and 100 mg/m² cytosine arabinoside × 7 days as a CONT 24-hr INF

Consolidation
Adult: IV INF 12 mg/m² given as a short 5-15 min INF for 2 days with cytarabine × 5 days

Advanced prostate cancer
Adult: IV 12-14 mg/m² as a single dose or short INF q21day

Multiple sclerosis, relapsing
Adult: IV INF 12 mg/m² as a 5-15 min INF q3mo, cumulative lifetime dose 140 mg/m²

Available forms: Inj 2, 10, 12.5, 15 mg/ml

Implementation
⚠ Do not mix with any other product
• Avoid contact with skin, since medication is very irritating; wash completely to remove
• Give fluids **IV** or PO before chemotherapy to hydrate patient
• Give antacid before oral agent; give product after evening meal, before bedtime; provide antiemetic 30-60 min before giving product and prn to prevent vomiting; administer antibiotics for prophylaxis of infection
• Give topical or systemic analgesics for pain
• Liquid diet: carbonated beverages; gelatin may be added if patient is not nauseated or vomiting
• Sol should be prepared by qualified personnel only under controlled conditions in a biological cabinet using mask, gloves, gown
• Use Luer-Lok tubing to prevent leakage; do not let sol come in contact with skin; if contact occurs, wash well with soap and water

Direct IV route
• Give after diluting with 50 ml or more of 0.9% NaCl or D₅W; give over 3-5 min into running **IV** of D₅W or 0.9% NaCl
Intermittent IV infusion route
• May be diluted further in D₅W, 0.9% NaCl and run over 15-30 min; check for extravasation
Continuous IV infusion route
• Give over 24 hr

Y-site compatibilities: Acyclovir, alemtuzumab, alfentanil, allopurinol, amikacin, aminocaproic acid, aminophylline, amiodarone, anidulafungin, argatroban, arsenic trioxide, atracurium, bivalirudin, bleomycin, bretylium, bumetanide, buprenorphine, butorphanol, calcium chloride, calcium gluconate, CARBOplatin, carmustine, caspofungin, cefoTEtan, ceftizoxime, chloramphenicol, chlorproMAZINE, cimetidine, ciprofloxacin, cisatracurium, CISplatin, cladribine, codeine, cyclophosphamide, cycloSPORINE, cytarabine, DACTINomycin, DAPTOmycin, DAUNOrubicin citrate liposome, dexmedetomidine, dexrazoxane, diltiazem, diphenhydrAMINE, DOBUTamine, DOCEtaxel, dolasetron, DOPamine, doxacurium, doxycycline, droperidol, enalaprilat, ePHEDrine, EPINEPHrine, erythromycin l, esmolol, etoposide, etoposide phosphate, famotidine, fenoldopam, fentaNYL, filgrastim, fluconazole, fludarabine, fluorouracil, ganciclovir, gatifloxacin, gemcitabine, gentamicin, glycopyrrolate, granisetron, haloperidol, hydrALAZINE, hydrocortisone sodium succinate, HYDROmorphone, hydrOXYzine, ifosfamide, imipenemcilastatin, inamrinone, insulin, regular, irinotecan, isoproterenol, ketorolac, labetalol, leucovorin, levofloxacin, levorphanol, lidocaine, linezolid, LORazepam, magnesium sulfate, mannitol, melphalan, meperidine, meropenem, mesna, metaraminol, methohexital, methotrexate, methyldopate, metoclopramide, metoprolol, metroNIDAZOLE, midazolam, milrinone, minocycline, mivacurium, morphine sulfate, nalbuphine, naloxone, nesiritide, niCARdipine, nitroglycerin, norepinephrine, octreotide, ondansetron, oxaliplatin, palonosetron, pamidronate, pancuronium, pentamidine, pentazocine, PENTobarbital, PHENobarbital, phentolamine, phenylephrine, polymyxin B, potassium acetate, potassium chloride, procainamide, prochlorperazine, promethazine hydrochloride, propranolol, quiNIDine gluconate, quinupristin-dalfopristin, ranitidine, remifentanil, riTUXimab, rocuronium, sargramostim, sodium acetate, sodium bicarbonate, succinylcholine, SUFentanil, sulfamethoxazole-trimethoprim, tacrolimus, teniposide, theophylline, thiopental, thiotepa, tigecycline, tirofiban, tobramycin, tolazoline, trastuzumab, trimethobenzamide, vancomycin, vasopressin, vecuronium, verapamil, vinCRIStine, vinorelbine, zidovudine, zoledronic acid

Y-site incompatibilities: PACLitaxel

Additive compatibilities: Cyclophosphamide, cytarabine, fluorouracil, hydrocortisone, potassium chloride

Additive incompatibilities: Heparin

Solution compatibilities: D₅/0.9 NaCl, D₅W, 0.9% NaCl

ADVERSE EFFECTS
CNS: Headache, seizures, fatigue
CV: CHF, cardiomyopathy, dysrhythmias
EENT: Conjunctivitis, blue-green sclera, blurred vision

GI: *Nausea, vomiting, diarrhea, anorexia, mucositis,* hepatotoxicity, abdominal pain, constipation, jaundice
GU: Amenorrhea, menstrual disorders
HEMA: Thrombocytopenia, leukopenia, myelosuppression, anemia, secondary leukemia
INTEG: *Rash,* necrosis at inj site, alopecia, dermatitis, thrombophlebitis at inj site
MISC: Fever, hyperuricemia, infections
RESP: Cough, dyspnea
SYST: Tumor lysis syndrome, sepsis

Pharmacokinetics

Absorption	Completely absorbed
Distribution	Widely distributed, protein binding 78%
Excretion	Bile; kidneys, unchanged (<10%)
Half-life	23-215 hr

Pharmacodynamics

Unknown

INTERACTIONS
Individual drugs
Digoxin, phenytoin: increased mitoXANtrone effects
Radiation: increased toxicity, bone marrow suppression
Trastuzumab: increased adverse reactions

Drug classifications
Anticoagulants, NSAIDs: increased bleeding risk
Antineoplastics: increased toxicity, bone marrow suppression
Live virus vaccines: increased adverse reactions

Drug/herb
Black cohosh, dong quai: avoid use

Drug/lab test
Increased: LFTs, uric acid
Decreased: Hct/Hgb, platelets, WBC

NURSING CONSIDERATIONS
Assessment
• **Multiple sclerosis:** obtain baseline multigated angiogram, left ventricular ejection fraction (LVEF) if symptoms of CHF occur, repeat LVEF or if cumulative dose is >100 mg/m²; do not administer to patients who have received a lifetime dose of ≥140 mg/m² or if LVEF is <50% or significant decrease in LVEF
• Do not administer in multiple sclerosis if neutrophils <1500/mm³
• Obtain pregnancy test in all women of childbearing age

BLACK BOX WARNING: Monitor ECG; watch for ST-T wave changes, low QRS and T, possible dysrhythmias (sinus tachycardia, heart block, PVCs); also monitor ECHO, MUGA, chest x-ray, RAI angiography to assess ejection fraction before, during treatment; product is cardiotoxic: may develop during treatment or months to years after treatment

• Assess buccal cavity q8hr for dryness, sores or ulceration, white patches, oral pain, bleeding, dysphagia; obtain prescription for viscous lidocaine (Xylocaine)
• **Assess symptoms indicating severe allergic reaction: rash, pruritus, urticaria, purpuric skin lesions, itching, flushing**
• Assess tachypnea, ECG changes, dyspnea, edema, fatigue
• Monitor CBC, differential, platelet count weekly; withhold product if WBC is <1500/mm³; leukopenia, neutropenia, thrombocytopenia are expected—leukocyte nadir 10-14 days, recovery in 2-3 wk
• Assess for increased uric acid levels, swelling, joint pain primarily in extremities; patient should be well hydrated to prevent urate deposits
• Monitor renal function tests: BUN, creatinine, urine CCr before, during therapy; determine I&O ratio
• Monitor temp q4hr: may indicate beginning of infection
• **Hepatotoxicity: monitor liver function tests before, during therapy (bilirubin, AST, ALT, LDH) as needed or monthly; dose reduction needed in hepatic disease; check for jaundiced skin and sclera, dark urine, clay-colored stools, itchy skin, abdominal pain, fever, diarrhea**
• **Assess for bleeding:** hematuria, stool guaiac, bruising or petechiae, mucosa or orifices q8hr; check for inflammation of mucosa, breaks in skin
• Identify effects of alopecia on body image; discuss feelings about body changes
⚠ Assess for multiple sclerosis: obtain MUGA, LVEF baselines; repeat LVEF if symptoms of CHF occur or if cumulative dose is >100 mg/m²; do not give to patients who have received a lifetime dose of ≥140 mg/m² or if LVEF is <50% or significant LVEF

BLACK BOX WARNING: Assess for secondary acute myelogenous leukemia (AML), which can develop after taking this product

M

Patient/family education

• Encourage patient to rinse mouth tid-qid with water, club soda; brush teeth bid-qid with soft brush or cotton-tipped applicators for stomatitis; use unwaxed dental floss

• Teach patient to avoid use of products containing aspirin or NSAIDs, razors, commercial mouthwash, since bleeding may occur; to report symptoms of bleeding (hematuria, tarry stools)

• Caution patient to report signs of anemia (fatigue, headache, irritability, faintness, shortness of breath)

• Inform patient that hair may be lost during treatment; a wig or hairpiece may make patient feel better; new hair may be different in color, texture

• Caution patient not to have any vaccinations without the advice of the prescriber; serious reactions can occur

• **Advise patient that contraception is needed during treatment and for several mo after completion of therapy**

> BLACK BOX WARNING: Teach patient to notify prescriber if pregnancy is planned or suspected

• Advise patient that sclera, urine may turn blue or green

• Advise patient to increase fluids to 2-3 L/day unless contraindicated

• Teach patient to avoid crowds, persons with infections

• **Teach patient to report immediately bleeding, dyspnea, possible infections, seizure, jaundice, fever, cough or dyspnea**

Evaluation

Positive therapeutic outcome

• Prevention of rapid division of malignant cells

modafinil (Rx)

(mo-daf′i-nil)

Alertec ✲, Provigil

Func. class.: CNS stimulant
Chem. class.: Racemic compound

Pregnancy category C
Controlled substance IV

ACTION: Similar action as sympathomimetics; does not alter release of dopamine, norepinephrine

Therapeutic outcome: Ability to stay awake

USES: Narcolepsy, shift work sleep disturbance, obstructive sleep apnea

Unlabeled uses: Fatigue in MS, ADHD, symptoms of major depression

CONTRAINDICATIONS

Hypersensitivity, ischemic heart disease, left ventricular hypertrophy, chest pain, dysrhythmias

Precautions: Pregnancy **C**, breastfeeding, child <16 yr, geriatric, unstable angina, history of MI, severe hepatic disease

DOSAGE AND ROUTES

To improve wakefulness with daytime sleepiness

Adult/adolescent ≥16 yr: PO 200 mg qd

Hepatic dose (severe hepatic disease)

Adult: PO 100 mg qd

Multiple sclerosis fatigue (unlabeled)

Adult/elderly/child ≥6 yr: PO 200-400 mg/day in the AM

Major depression symptoms (unlabeled)

Adult: PO 100 mg/day, max 400 mg/day

Available forms: Tabs 100, 200 mg

Implementation

• Give 1 hr before start of shift work, or in the AM for those with narcolepsy or sleep apnea

• Store at room temperature

ADVERSE EFFECTS

CNS: *Headache,* anxiety, cataplexy, depression, dizziness, insomnia, amnesia, confusion, ataxia, tremors, paresthesia, dyskinesia, **suicidal ideation**

CV: Dysrhythmias, hyper/hypotension, chest pain, vasodilation

EENT: Change in vision, *rhinitis,* pharyngitis, epistaxis

GI: Nausea, vomiting, changes in LFTs, anorexia, diarrhea, thirst, mouth ulcers

GU: Ejaculation disorder, urinary retention, albuminuria

HEMA: Eosinophilia

INTEG: Rash, dry skin, herpes simplex, Stevens-Johnson syndrome

MISC: Infection, hyperglycemia, neck pain

RESP: *Dyspnea,* lung changes

Pharmacokinetics

Absorption	Rapid
Distribution	60% protein binding
Metabolism	Liver (90%)
Excretion	Unknown
Half-life	15 hr

Pharmacodynamics

Onset	Unknown
Peak	2-4 hr
Duration	Unknown

INTERACTIONS
Individual drugs
CycloSPORINE, theophylline: decreased effects of these drugs

Methylphenidate: delayed effect of modafinil by 1 hr

Drug classifications
Antidepressants (tricyclics): increased effects

CYP3A4 inhibitors (azole antibiotics, some SSRIs): altered levels of these agents, reaction difficult to predict

CYP2C19 substrates (diazepam, phenytoin, some tricyclics): increased levels of these agents

CYP3A4 inducers (carBAMazepine, phenytoin, rifampin; cycloSPORINE, theophylline): altered levels of these agents

Hormonal contraceptives: decreased effects

Drug/herb
Coffee, cola nut, guarana, mate, tea: increased stimulation

Drug/lab test
Increased: eosinophils, glucose, LFTs

NURSING CONSIDERATIONS
Assessment
• For narcolepsy, shift work, history of sleep apnea
• For depression, suicidal ideation
• Monitor B/P in those with hypertension

Patient/family education
• Advise patient to take only as directed; may be taken with or without food

⚠ Advise patient to use other form of contraception during and at least 30 days after discontinuing medication, if using hormonal birth control; advise patient to notify prescriber if pregnancy is planned or suspected or if breastfeeding

• Advise patient to notify prescriber of allergic reaction, tremors, confusion
• Teach patient to avoid all OTC medications unless approved by prescriber
• Teach patient to avoid hazardous activities until drug effect is known

Evaluation

Positive therapeutic outcome
• Ability to stay awake

montelukast (Rx)
(mon-teh-loo′kast)
Singulair
Func. class.: Bronchodilator
Chem. class.: Leukotriene antagonist, cysteinyl
Pregnancy category B

ACTION: Inhibits leukotriene (LTD$_4$) formation; leukotrienes exert their effects by increasing neutrophil, eosinophil migration; aggregation of neutrophils, monocytes; smooth muscle contraction, capillary permeability; these actions further lead to bronchoconstriction, inflammation, edema

Therapeutic outcome: Ability to breathe with ease

USES: Chronic asthma in adults and children, seasonal allergic rhinitis, bronchospasm prophylaxis

Unlabeled uses: Chronic urticaria

CONTRAINDICATIONS
Hypersensitivity

Precautions: Pregnancy **B**, breastfeeding, children <6 yr, acute attacks of asthma, alcohol consumption, severe hepatic disease, corticosteroid withdrawal, phenylketonuria, suicidal ideation, depression

DOSAGE AND ROUTES
Asthma
Adult and child ≥15 yr: PO 10 mg/day PM
Child 6-14 yr: PO 5 mg chew tabs/day PM
Child 2-5 yr: PO (chew tabs, granules) 4 mg/day
Child 12-23 mo: PO 1 packet of granules taken PM

Exercise-induced bronchoconstriction
Adult/child ≥6 yr: PO 10 mg 2 hr prior to exercise; do not take another dose within 24 hr

Available forms: Tabs 10 mg; chewable tabs 4, 5 mg; oral granules 4 mg/packet

Implementation
PO route
• Give PO in PM daily for all uses except exercise-induced bronchoconstriction; then take 2 hr prior to exercise
• Do not open packet until ready to use; mix whole dose, give within 15 min
• Granules may be given directly in mouth or mixed with a spoonful of soft food (carrots, applesauce, ice cream, rice)

M

ADVERSE EFFECTS

CNS: Dizziness, fatigue, headache, behavior changes, **seizures,** agitation, anxiety, depression, fever, hallucinations, drowsiness, **suicidal ideation,** memory impairment, hostility, somnambulism

GI: Abdominal pain, dyspepsia, nausea, vomiting, diarrhea, **pancreatitis**

HEMA: Thrombocytopenia

INTEG: Rash, pruritus, erythema

MS: Asthenia, myalgia, muscle cramps

RESP: Influenza, cough, nasal congestion

SYST: Anaphylaxis, angioedema, Churg-Strauss syndrome, Stevens-Johnson syndrome, toxic epidermal necrolysis

Pharmacokinetics

Absorption	Rapidly absorbed
Distribution	Protein binding 99%
Metabolism	Liver
Excretion	Bile
Half-life	2.7-5.5 hr

Pharmacodynamics

Onset	Unknown
Peak	3-4 hr
Duration	Unknown

INTERACTIONS

Individual drugs

Rifabutin, rifapentine, carBAMazepine, fosphenytoin, phenytoin, rifampin: decreased montelukast levels

Drug classifications

Barbiturates: decreased montelukast levels

Drug/herb

Tea (green, black), guarana: increased stimulation

Drug/lab test

Increased: ALT, AST

NURSING CONSIDERATIONS

Assessment

⚠ Assess adult patients carefully for symptoms of Churg-Strauss syndrome (rare), including eosinophilia, vasculitic rash, worsening pulmonary symptoms, cardiac complications and/or neuropathy

• Monitor CBC, blood chemistry during treatment

• Assess allergic reactions: rash, urticaria; product should be discontinued

• Assess for behavior changes and suicidal ideation, other neuropsychiatric reactions

• Severe hepatic disease: use cautiously

Patient/family education

• Advise patient to avoid hazardous activities; dizziness may occur

• Teach patient that product is not to be used for acute asthma attacks

• Advise patient to avoid NSAIDs if sensitive to aspirin

• Advise patient to continue to use inhaled β-agonists if exercise-induced asthma occurs

• **Granules:** instruct patient to take directly by mouth or mixed in a spoonful of room temperature soft food (use only applesauce, carrots, rice, or ice cream); use within 15 min of opening packet, discard used portions

Evaluation

Positive therapeutic outcome

• Increased ease of breathing

• Decreased bronchospasm

⚠ HIGH ALERT

morphine (Rx)

(mor´feen)

Astramorph PF, AVINza, Depo Dur, Infumorph PF, Kadian, M.O.S. ✦, MS Contin, MSIR ✦, Oramorph SR

Func. class.: Opioid analgesic

Chem. class.: Alkaloid

Pregnancy category C

Controlled substance schedule II 🔲

Do not confuse: morphine/HYDROmorphone, **MS Contin/oxyCONTIN**

ACTION: Depresses pain impulse transmission at the spinal cord level by interacting with opioid receptors

Therapeutic outcome: Decreased pain

USES: Moderate to severe pain

Unlabeled uses: Agitation, bone/dental pain, dyspnea in end-stage cancer or pulmonary disease, sedation induction, rapid-sequence intubation

CONTRAINDICATIONS

Hypersensitivity, addiction (opioid/alcohol), hemorrhage, bronchial asthma, increased ICP, paralytic ileus, hypovolemic shock, MAOI therapy

> BLACK BOX WARNING: Respiratory depression

Precautions: Pregnancy **C**, breastfeeding, children <18 yr, geriatric, addictive personality, acute MI, severe heart disease, renal/hepatic

---

disease, bowel impaction, abrupt discontinuation, seizures

> **BLACK BOX WARNING:** Accidental exposure, epidural/intrathecal/IM/subcut administration, opioid-naive patients, substance abuse

DOSAGE AND ROUTES
Acute moderate to severe pain
>> PO regular-release
Adult ≥50 kg: Initially, 10-30 mg q3-4hr as needed

Adult <50 kg/geriatric patient: May require lower doses and/or extended dosing intervals; doses should be titrated carefully

Child/infant ≥6 mo: 0.2-0.5 mg/kg q4-6hr as needed

Infant <6 mo/neonate: 0.1 mg/kg PO q3-4hr

>> IV/IM/subcut
Adult ≥50 kg: 2.5-15 mg q2-6hr as needed, titrate or a loading dose of 0.05-0.1 mg/kg **IV**, followed by 0.8-10 mg/hr **IV**, titrate

Adult <50 kg/geriatric patient: May require lower doses and/or extended dosing intervals 0.1 mg/kg q3-4hr, titrate

Child/infant ≥6 mo: 0.05-0.2 mg/kg q2-4hr, titrate to relief max initial doses 15 mg/dose

Neonate/infant <6 mo: 0.03-0.05 mg/kg q3-8hr, titrate to relief

>> Epidural (morphine sulfate injection, but NOT DepoDur)
Adult: Initially, 5 mg in the lumbar region; if pain relief does not occur in 1 hr, give 1-2 mg epidurally; max 10 mg/24 hr; **continuous epidural infusion,** 2-4 mg/24 hr; may give another 1-2 mg

>> Intrathecal dosage (morphine sulfate injection, but NOT DepoDur)
Do not inject >2 ml of the 0.5 mg/ml or 1 ml of the 1 mg/ml ampule

Adult: 0.2-1 mg in the lumbar area as a single dose or to establish dosage for continuous intrathecal infusion; repeated injections are not recommended

>> Rectal dosage
Adult: 10-20 mg PR q4hr, as needed

Child: Individualize

Chronic moderate and severe pain
⚠ Do not use extended-release cap or tab as prn analgesics, for acute pain, or if the pain is mild or not expected to persist for an extended period of time. Use for postoperative pain only if the patient is receiving chronic opioid therapy prior to surgery or if the postoperative pain is expected to be moderate to severe and persist for an extended period of time. Do not use controlled-release tablets (MS Contin) immediately after surgery (for the first 24 hr) in patients not previously taking the drug

⚠ Do not use in opioid-naive patients: 90 mg, 120 mg morphine biphasic-release capsules (AVINza); 100 mg, 130 mg, 150 mg, 200 mg morphine extended-release capsules (Kadian), 100 mg, 200 mg morphine controlrelease tablets (MS Contin); patients considered opioid tolerant are those who are taking at least 60 mg/day oral morphine, 30 mg/day of oral oxyCODONE, 8 mg/day oral HYDROmorphone, or an equal dose of another opioid, for a wk or longer

>> PO [extended-release tab (MS Contin, Oramorph SR) or caps (Kadian, AVINza)] (opiate naïve)
Adult: 15-30 mg q12hr (tabls); 10 mg bid or 20 mg/day (Kadian); or 30 mg/day (AVINza), titrate; AVINza should be adjusted in increments ≤30 mg q4 days; Kadian should be increased ≤20 mg q1-2 days, taper gradually; to discontinue, gradually decrease AVINza, and Kadian over 2-4 days

Child (unlabeled): 0.3-0.6 mg/kg q12hr (tablets)

>> IV/subcut route (opiate naïve)
Adult: IV 2-10 mg loading dose, then 0.8-10 mg/hour **IV**, titrate; maintenance 0.8-80 mg/hour **IV**

Child/infant ≥6 mo: IV Initially, 0.04-0.07 mg/kg/hr (range: 0.025-2.6 mg/kg/hr), **Subcut inf** 0.025-1.79 mg/kg/hr

Infant <6 mo/neonate: IV 0.01 mg/kg/hour **IV**, initially, infusion rates max 0.015-0.02 mg/kg/hour **IV**

Breakthrough pain in patients receiving long-acting or continuous infusion morphine
>> PO (regular-release)
Adult/child: The dose is usually one-fourth to one-third the 8- to 12-hour extended-release dose q4-6hr as needed

Adult/child: For PCA, intermittent dose is usually 25%-30% of the hourly rate IV/SC q6-15min as needed; intermittent IV injection dosage is 25%-30% of the hourly rate given IV/SC q1-2hr as needed

Available forms: HCL: suppositories 10, 20, 30 mg; syrup 1, 5, 10, 20, 50 mg/ml; tabs 10, 20, 40, 60 mg; **Sulfate:** caps ext rel microgranules 10, 15, 30, 60, 100, 200 mg; cap ext rel pellets (Avinza): 30, 45, 60, 75, 90, 120 mg; caps

M

ext rel pellets (Kadian) 10, 20, 30, 40, 50, 60, 70, 80, 100, 130, 150, 200 mg; drops: 20, 50 mg/ml; injection epidural: 0.5, 1, 10, 15 mg/ml; injection (Preservative): 0.5, 1, 2, 10, 15, 25, 50 mg/ml; injection (Corpuject/prefilled syringes): 2, 4, 8, 10, 15 mg/ml; oral solution 10, 20 mg/ml, 20 mg/ml (concentrate); suppositories 5, 10, 20, 30 mg; syrup 1, 5, 10 mg/ml; tab 5, 10, 15, 25, 30, 50 mg; tabs ext rel 15, 30, 60, 100, 200 mg

Implementation

>> PO route

• Give with food or milk to minimize GI effects

Immediate-release cap

• May swallow whole, or opened and contents sprinkled on cool food (pudding or applesauce), or added to juice (given immediately) or delivered via gastric or NG tube by either adding to or following with liquid

Extended-release and controlled-release tabs

• Swallow whole; do not crush, break, dissolve, or chew.

• The use of MS Contin 100 mg or 200 mg tabs should be limited to opioid-tolerant patients requiring oral doses equivalent to $\geq$200 mg/day. Use of the 100 mg or 200 mg tablet is only recommended for patients who have already been titrated to a stable analgesic regimen using lower strengths of MS Contin or other opioids

Sustained-release caps

• Swallow; do not chew, crush, or dissolve

• Caps may be opened and contents sprinkled on applesauce (at room temperature or cooler) immediately prior to ingestion. Do not chew, crush, or dissolve the pellets/beads inside the cap. The applesauce should be swallowed without chewing. If the pellets/beads are chewed, an immediate release of a potentially fatal morphine dose may be delivered. Rinse mouth to ensure all the pellets/beads have been swallowed. Do not separate applesauce into separate doses; the entire portion should be taken. Discard unused portion

• Kadian caps may be given through a 16 French gastrostomy tube; flush with water, and sprinkle the cap contents into 10 ml of water. Using a funnel and a swirling motion, pour the pellets and water into the tube. Rinse the beaker with 10 ml of water, and pour the water into the funnel. Repeat until no pellets remain in the beaker

⚠ Do NOT administer AVINza tabs through a gastrostomy tube. Do NOT administer Kadian or AVINza through a nasogastric tube

⚠ Avoid concurrent administration of AVINza with prescription or nonprescription medications that contain alcohol. Consumption of alcohol while taking the ext rel capsules may result in the rapid release and absorption of a potentially fatal dose of morphine

⚠ AVINza $\geq$90 mg or Kadian 100 mg, 130 mg, 150 mg or 200 mg caps should be given only to opioid tolerant patients

• Begin with immediate release products and titrate to correct dose and convert to a sustained release product

Oral liquid

• Check dose prior to use; many concentrations of oral sol are available; may be diluted in fruit juice; protect from light

>> Injectable administration

• Visually inspect for particulate matter and discoloration before use; do not use if a precipitate is present after shaking; do not use the Duramorph solution if a precipitate is present or if the color is darker than pale yellow

IV route

• Prior to or to use, an opiate antagonist and emergency facilities should be available

⚠ Do not use the highly concentrated morphine injections (i.e., 10-25 mg/ml) for IV, IM, or SC administration of single doses. These injection solutions are intended for use via continuous, controlled-microinfusion devices

Direct IV route

• Dilute dose with $\geq$5 ml of sterile water for injection or NS injection

• Inject 2.5-15 mg directly into a vein or into the tubing of a freely flowing IV solution over 4-5 min; do not give rapidly

Continuous IV infusion

• Dilute in 5% dextrose; use a controlled-infusion device

• Adjust dose and rate based on patient response

Patient-controlled analgesia (PCA)

• A compatible patient-controlled infusion device must be used

• Dilute solutions to obtain a concentration of 1 or 10 mg/ml for ease in calculations and programming of PCA pumps

• Adjust dose and rate based on patient response. Consult the patient-controlled infusion device manual for directions on rate of infusion

Subcut route

• Inject taking care not to inject intradermally

Continuous SC infusion

• Morphine is not approved by the FDA for subcut use

- Dilute to an appropriate concentration in D$_5$W; administer using a portable, controlled, subcut device; adjust rate based on patient response and tolerance
- Max subcut rate 2 ml/hr/site

Intrathecal/epidural route

⚠ Morphine sulfate injection is not interchangeable with morphine sulfate extended-release liposome injection (DepoDur), DepoDur is only for epidural administration

⚠ Do not use Infumorph (10 mg/ml or 25 mg/ml) for single-dose neuraxial injection because lower doses can be more reliably administered with Duramorph (0.5 mg/ml or 1 mg/ml)

>> Rectal route

- Moisten the suppository with water prior to insertion. If suppository is too soft, chill in the refrigerator for 30 min or run cold water over it before removing the wrapper

>> Oral solid formulations

Immediate-release capsules administration

- May be swallowed whole or opened and the contents sprinkled on cool food such as pudding or applesauce
- Capsule contents may be added to juice and administered immediately or delivered via gastric or NG tube by either adding to or following with liquid

>> Extended-release and controlled-release tablets administration

- Swallow whole; do not crush, break, dissolve, or chew
- The use of MS Contin 100 mg or 200 mg tablets should be limited to opioid-tolerant patients requiring oral doses equivalent to ≥200 mg/day. Use of the 100 mg or 200 mg tablet is only recommended for patients who have already been titrated to a stable analgesic regimen using lower strengths of MS Contin or other opioids

Sustained-release capsule administration

- Capsules should be swallowed; do not chew, crush, or dissolve
- Capsules may be opened and the contents sprinkled on applesauce (at room temperature or cooler) immediately prior to ingestion; no other food has been tested. Do not chew, crush, or dissolve the pellets/beads inside the capsule. The applesauce needs to be swallowed without chewing. If the pellets/beads are chewed, an immediate release of a potentially fatal morphine dose may be delivered. Rinse mouth to ensure all the pellets/beads have been swallowed. Do not separate applesauce into separate doses; the entire portion should be taken. Discard any

unused portion of the capsules after the contents have been sprinkled on the applesauce
- Kadian capsules may be administered through a 16 French gastrostomy tube. Flush the tube with water, and sprinkle the capsule contents into 10 ml of water. Using a funnel and a swirling motion, pour the pellets and water into the tube. Rinse the beaker with 10 ml of water, and pour the water into the funnel. Repeat until no pellets remain in the beaker

⚠ Do NOT administer AVINza tablets through a gastrostomy tube. Do NOT administer Kadian or AVINza through a nasogastric tube

⚠ Avoid concurrent administration of AVINza with prescription or non-prescription medications that contain alcohol. Consumption of alcohol while taking the extended-release capsules may result in the rapid release and absorption of a potentially fatal dose of morphine

⚠ The use of AVINza ≥90 mg or Kadian 100 mg, 130 mg, 150 mg or 200 mg capsules should be limited to opioid tolerant patients

>> Oral liquid formulations

Oral solution administration

- Carefully check dose prior to dispensing medication as many concentrations of morphine oral solution are available
- May be diluted in fruit juice prior to administration
- Protect from light

Injectable administration

- Visually inspect parenteral products for particulate matter and discoloration prior to administration whenever solution and container permit. Unopened solutions should be discarded if a precipitate is present that does not disappear with shaking. Do not use the Duramorph solution if a precipitate is present or if the color is darker than pale yellow

>> Intravenous administration

- Prior to administration, an opiate antagonist and facilities for administration of oxygen and control of respiration should be available

⚠ Do not use the highly concentrated morphine injections (i.e., 10-25 mg/ml) for IV, IM, or SC administration of single doses. These injection solutions are intended for use via continuous, controlled-microinfusion devices

Direct IV injection

- Dilute appropriate dose with at least 5 ml of sterile water for injection or NS injection
- Inject 2.5-15 mg directly into a vein or into the tubing of a freely flowing IV solution over 4-5 minutes. Rapid IV injection of morphine

M

may result in an increased frequency of adverse effects. For example, the maximum CNS effects occur 30 minutes after administration. Rapid intravenous administration could result in an overdose

Continuous IV infusion
• Dilute in 5% dextrose
• Administer using a controlled-infusion device
• Adjust dose and rate based on patient response

Patient-controlled analgesia (PCA)
• A compatible patient-controlled infusion device must be used
• Dilute solutions to obtain morphine concentration of 1 or 10 mg/ml for ease in calculations and programming of PCA pumps
• Adjust dose and rate based on patient response. Consult the patient-controlled infusion device operator's manual for directions on administering the drug at the desired rate of infusion

>> Subcutaneous administration
• Inject subcutaneously taking care not to inject intradermally

Continuous SC infusion
• Morphine is not approved by the FDA for subcutaneous administration
• Dilute to an appropriate concentration in D_5W and administer using a portable, controlled, subcutaneous infusion device. Adjust rate based on patient response and tolerance
• Maximum SC rate of infusion is 2 ml/hour/site

>> Intrathecal administration
⚠ Intrathecal dose is approximately one-tenth (1/10) the epidural dose
⚠ Morphine sulfate injection is not interchangeable with morphine sulfate extended-release liposome injection (Depo-Dur). DepoDur is only for epidural administration (see below)
⚠ Do not use Infumorph (10 mg/ml or 25 mg/ml) for single-dose neuraxial injection because lower doses can be more reliably administered with Duramorph (0.5 mg/ml or 1 mg/ml)
• Epidural or intrathecal administration should only be used by specially trained healthcare professionals
• May be given as intermittent bolus, continuous infusion, or as patient-controlled epidural analgesia. Infumorph is only indicated for intrathecal or epidural infusion; Infumorph is not recommended for single-dose intravenous, intramuscular, or subcutaneous administration because of the very large amount of morphine in the ampul and the associated overdosage risk

• Prior to administration, an opiate antagonist and facilities for administration of oxygen and control of respiration should be available. The patient should be in a setting where adequate monitoring is possible. Immediate availability of naloxone injection and resuscitative equipment is also needed during Infumorph reservoir refilling or reservoir manipulation
• Placement of epidural catheter and administration should be at a site near the dermatomes covering the field of pain to decrease dose requirements and increase specificity. For example, for thoracic surgery placement at T2-T8, upper abdominal surgery, T4-L1, lower abdominal surgery, T10-L3, upper extremity surgery, C2-C8 and lower extremity surgery, T12-L3
• Visually inspect parenteral products for particulate matter and discoloration prior to administration whenever solution and container permit. Unopened Infumorph solution should be discarded if a precipitate is present that does not disappear with shaking or if it is not colorless or pale yellow. Do not use the Duramorph solution if a precipitate is present or if the color is darker than pale yellow

Intrathecal injection (morphine sulfate injection)
• No more than 2 or 1 ml of the injection containing 0.5 or 1 mg/ml, respectively, should be injected intrathecally
• After ensuring proper placement of the needle or catheter, inject appropriate dose intrathecally. Monitor patient in a fully equipped and staffed environment for at least 24 hr after each dose, as severe respiratory depression may occur up to 24 hr after drug administration. Repeated intrathecal injections are not recommended other than for establishing initial intrathecal dosage for continuous intrathecal infusion

Continuous intrathecal infusion (morphine sulfate injection)
⚠ Intrathecal dose is approximately one-tenth (1/10) the epidural dose. Epidural dose is usually considered to be one-tenth (1/10) the IV dose
• A controlled-infusion device must be used. For highly concentrated injections, an implantable controlled-microinfusion device is used. Patients should be monitored in a fully equipped and staffed environment for several days following implantation of the device
• If dilution of the injection is necessary, NS injection is recommended
• The infusion device reservoir should only be filled by fully trained and qualified healthcare professionals. Strict aseptic technique must be used. Withdraw dose from the ampul through a 5-μm (or smaller pore diameter) microfilter

to avoid contamination with glass or other particles. Ensure proper placement of the needle when filling the reservoir to avoid accidental overdosage

• To avoid exacerbation of severe pain and/or reflux of CSF into the reservoir, depletion of the reservoir should be avoided

>> Other injectable administration
Epidural administration
⚠ Intrathecal dose is approximately one-tenth (1/10) the epidural dose. Epidural dose is usually considered to be one-tenth (1/10) the IV dose
⚠ Morphine sulfate injection is not interchangeable with morphine sulfate extended-release liposome injection (DepoDur). DepoDur is only for epidural administration (see below)
⚠ Do not use Infumorph (10 mg/ml or 25 mg/ml) for single-dose neuraxial injection because lower doses can be more reliably administered with Duramorph (0.5 mg/ml or 1 mg/ml)

• Epidural administration should only be used by specially trained healthcare professionals
• May be given as intermittent bolus, cont inf, or as patient-controlled epidural analgesia. Infumorph is only indicated for intrathecal or epidural infusion; Infumorph is not recommended for single-dose intravenous, intramuscular, or subcutaneous administration because of the very large amount of morphine in the ampul and the associated overdosage risk
• Prior to administration, an opiate antagonist and facilities for administration of oxygen and control of respiration should be available. The patient should be in a setting where adequate monitoring is possible. Immediate availability of naloxone injection and resuscitative equipment is also needed during Infumorph reservoir refilling or reservoir manipulation
• Placement of epidural catheter and administration should be at a site near the dermatomes covering the field of pain to decrease dose requirements and increase specificity. For example, for thoracic surgery placement at T2-T8, upper abdominal surgery, T4-L1, lower abdominal surgery, T10-L3, upper extremity surgery, C2-C8 and lower extremity surgery, T12-L3

Epidural injection (morphine sulfate injection)
• After ensuring proper placement of the needle or catheter, inject appropriate dose into the epidural space. Monitor patient in a fully equipped and staffed environment for at least 24 hr after each dose, as severe respiratory depression may occur up to 24 hr after drug administration

Continuous epidural infusion (morphine sulfate injection)
⚠ Intrathecal dose is approximately one-tenth (1/10) the epidural dose. Epidural dose is usually considered to be one-tenth (1/10) the IV dose
• A controlled-infusion device must be used. For highly concentrated injections, an implantable controlled-microinfusion device is used. Patients should be monitored in a fully equipped and staffed environment for several days following implantation of the device
• If dilution of the injection is necessary, NS injection is recommended
• The infusion device reservoir should only be filled by fully trained and qualified healthcare professionals. Strict aseptic technique must be used. Withdraw dose from the ampul through a 5-µm (or smaller pore diameter) microfilter to avoid contamination with glass or other particles. Ensure proper placement of the needle when filling the reservoir to avoid accidental overdosage
• To avoid exacerbation of severe pain and/or reflux of CSF into the reservoir, depletion of the reservoir should be avoided

>> Epidural administration (morphine sulfate extended-release liposome injection [DepoDur] ONLY)
⚠ Morphine sulfate ext rel liposome injection (DepoDur) is not interchangeable with other morphine sulfate injections
• DepoDur is only for epidural administration. Do not administer by any other parenteral route
• Epidural administration should only be used by specially trained healthcare professionals
• Prior to administration, an opiate antagonist and facilities for administration of oxygen and control of respiration should be available. The patient should be in a setting where adequate monitoring is possible. Monitor patient in a fully equipped and staffed environment for at least 48 hr after each dose, as severe respiratory depression may occur
• Invert the vial to resuspend particles immediately before withdrawal. Administer DepoDur within 4 hr after withdrawal from the vial when kept at controlled room temperature 59-86° F (15-30° C). The product does not contain any bacteriostatic agents or preservatives. Do not heat- or gas-sterilize

Epidural injection [morphine sulfate extended-release liposome injection (DepoDur)]
• Placement of epidural needle or catheter and administration should be at the lumbar level.

M

Adverse effects: *italics* = common; **bold** = life-threatening

Due to lack of study data, administration of DepoDur at the thoracic level or higher is not recommended

• Determine proper needle or catheter placement by aspiration to check for blood or cerebrospinal fluid and/or by administration of a test dose of 3 ml of 1.5% preservative-free lidocaine and EPINEPHrine (1:200,000). If tachycardia or sudden onset of segmental anesthesia occurs, the needle or catheter is in the intrathecal space and thus, needs to be repositioned. If a test dose is given, flush the catheter with 1 ml of preservative-free normal saline injection and wait at least 15 minutes after test dose administration before administration of DepoDur

• Inject DepoDur at the lumbar level undiluted or diluted up to 5 ml total volume with preservative-free normal saline. During administration, do not use an inline filter or mix DepoDur with any medication. Additionally, do not administer any medication into the epidural space within 48 hr of DepoDur receipt

>> Rectal administration

• Instruct patient on proper use of suppository (see Patient Information)

• Moisten the suppository with water prior to insertion. If suppository is too soft because of storage in a warm place, chill in the refrigerator for 30 minutes or run cold water over it before removing the wrapper

Syringe incompatibilities: Meperidine, thiopental

Y-site compatibilities: Acetaminophen, aldesleukin, allopurinol, amifostine, amikacin, aminophylline, amiodarone, atenolol, atracurium, aztreonam, bumetanide, calcium chloride, cefamandole, ceFAZolin, cefotaxime, cefoTEtan, cefOXitin, cefTAZidime, ceftizoxime, cefTRIAXone, cefuroxime, cephalothin, chloramphenicol, cladribine, clindamycin, cyclophosphamide, cytarabine, dexamethasone, digoxin, diltiazem, DOBUTamine, DOPamine, doxycycline, enalaprilat, EPINEPHrine, erythromycin, esmolol, etomidate, famotidine, fentaNYL, filgrastim, fluconazole, fludarabine, foscarnet, gentamicin, granisetron, heparin, hydrocortisone, HYDROmorphone, kanamycin, labetalol, lidocaine, LORazepam, magnesium sulfate, melphalan, meropenem, methotrexate, methyldopate, methylPREDNISolone, metoclopramide, metoprolol, metroNIDAZOLE, midazolam, milrinone, nafcillin, niCARdipine, nitroglycerin, norepinephrine, ondansetron, oxacillin, oxytocin, PAClitaxel, pancuronium, penicillin G potassium, piperacillin, piperacillin/tazobactam, potassium chloride, propranolol, ranitidine, sodium bicarbonate, teniposide, thiotepa, ticarcillin, ticarcillin/clavulanate, tigecycline, tobramycin, vancomycin, vecuronium, vinorelbine, vit B/C, warfarin, zidovudine, zolendronic acid

Y-site incompatibilities: Furosemide, minocycline, tetracycline

ADVERSE EFFECTS

CNS: Drowsiness, dizziness, *confusion*, headache, *sedation,* euphoria, insomnia, seizures

CV: Palpitations, bradycardia, change in B/P, shock, cardiac arrest, chest pain, hyper/hypotension, edema, tachycardia

EENT: Blurred vision, miosis, diplopia

ENDO: Gynecomastia

GI: Nausea, vomiting, anorexia, *constipation,* cramps, biliary tract pressure

GU: Urinary retention, impotence, gonadal suppression

HEMA: Thrombocytopenia

INTEG: Rash, urticaria, bruising, flushing, diaphoresis, pruritus

RESP: Respiratory depression, respiratory arrest, apnea

Pharmacokinetics

Absorption	Variably absorbed (PO); well absorbed (IM, SUBCUT, RECT); completely absorbed (**IV**)
Distribution	Widely distributed; crosses placenta
Metabolism	Liver, extensively
Excretion	Kidneys
Half-life	1½-2 hr; IM 3-4 hr; AVINza 24 hr; Kadian 11-13 hr

Pharmacodynamics

	PO	PO EXT REL	IM	SUBCUT	RECT	IV	IT
Onset	Variable	Unknown	10-30 min	20 min	Unknown	Rapid	Rapid
Peak	1 hr	Unknown	30-60 min	1-1½ hr	½-1 hr	20 min	Unknown
Duration	4-5 hr	8-12 hr	4-5 hr	4-5 hr	3-7 hr	4-5 hr	Ext

INTERACTIONS
Individual drugs
Alcohol: increased effects with other CNS depressants
Rifampin: decreased analgesic action

Drug classifications
Antipsychotics, opiates, sedative-hypnotics, skeletal muscle relaxants: increased effects with other CNS depressants
MAOIs: unpredictable reaction may occur; avoid use

Drug/herb
Chamomile, hops, kava, St. John's wort, valerian: increased CNS depression

Drug/lab test
Increased: amylase

NURSING CONSIDERATIONS
Assessment
• Assess pain: location, type, character, intensity; give dose before pain becomes extreme
• Monitor I&O ratio; check for decreasing output; may indicate urinary retention; check for constipation; increase fluids, bulk in diet if needed, or stimulant laxatives may be prescribed; monitor serum sodium

> **BLACK BOX WARNING:** Abrupt discontinuation: gradually taper to prevent withdrawal symptoms; decrease by 50% q1-2 days, avoid use of narcotic antagonist

• Monitor CNS changes: dizziness, drowsiness, hallucinations, euphoria, LOC, pupil reactions
• Monitor allergic reactions: rash, urticaria

> **BLACK BOX WARNING:** Accidental exposure: if Duramorph or Infamorph gets on skin, remove contaminated clothing and rinse affected area with water

> **BLACK BOX WARNING:** Assess respiratory dysfunction: depression, character, rate, rhythm; notify prescriber if respirations are <12/min; accidental overdose has occurred with high-potency oral sol

Patient/family education
• Advise patient to report any symptoms of CNS changes, allergic reactions
• Caution patients to avoid CNS depressants (alcohol, sedative/hypnotics) for at least 24 hr after taking this product
• Discuss with patient that dizziness, drowsiness, and confusion are common; to avoid getting up without assistance
• Discuss in detail all aspects of the product and expected response

Evaluation
Positive therapeutic outcome
• Decreased pain

TREATMENT OF OVERDOSE:
Naloxone (Narcan) 0.2-0.8 **IV** (caution with opioid-tolerant individuals), O_2, **IV** fluids, vasopressors

moxifloxacin (Rx)
(mox-i-floks'a-sin)
Avelox, Avelox IV
Func. class.: Antiinfective
Chem. class.: Fluoroquinolone
Pregnancy category C

ACTION: Interferes with conversion of intermediate DNA fragments into high molecular weight DNA in bacteria; DNA gyrase inhibitor

Therapeutic outcome: Bactericidal action against the following: *Staphylococcus aureus, Streptococcus pneumoniae, Haemophilus influenzae, Haemophilus parainfluenzae, Moraxella catarrhalis, Klebsiella pneumoniae, Mycoplasma pneumoniae, Chlamydia pneumoniae; Streptococcus pyogenes, Escherichia coli, Bacteroides fragilis, Streptococcus arginosus, Streptococcus constellatus, Enterococcus faecalis, Proteus mirabilis, Clostridium perfringens, Bacteroides thetalomicron, Peptostreptococcus, Enterobacter cloacae*

USES: Acute bacterial sinusitis, acute bacterial exacerbation of chronic bronchitis, community-acquired pneumonia (mild to moderate), uncomplicated skin/skin structure infections, complicated intraabdominal infections including polymicrobial infections, complicated skin/skin structure infections

Unlabeled uses: Anthrax treatment/prophylaxis, gastroenteritis, MAC, nongonococcal urethritis, shigellosis, surgical infection prophylaxis, TB

CONTRAINDICATIONS
Hypersensitivity to quinolones

Precautions: Pregnancy **C**, breastfeeding, children, renal/hepatic/cardiac disease, epilepsy, uncorrected hypokalemia, prolonged QT interval, patients receiving class IA, III antidsyrhythmics, GI disease, seizure disorder, pseudomembranous colitis, diabetes mellitus

> **BLACK BOX WARNING:** Tendon pain/rupture, tendinitis, myasthenia gravis

Adverse effects: *italics* = common; **bold** = life-threatening

DOSAGE AND ROUTES
Acute bacterial sinusitis
Adult: PO/IV 400 mg q24hr × 10 days

Acute bacterial exacerbation of chronic bronchitis
Adult: PO/IV 400 mg q24hr × 5 days

Community-acquired pneumonia
Adult: PO/IV 400 mg q24hr × 7-14 days

Uncomplicated skin/skin structure infections
Adult: PO/IV 400 mg q24hr × 7 days

Complicated intraabdominal infections
Adult: IV 400 mg/day × 5-14 days

Complicated skin/skin structure infections
Adult: PO/IV 400 mg/day × 7-21 days

Available forms: Tabs 400 mg; inj premix 400 mg/250 ml

Implementation
• Do not use theophylline with this product; may cause toxicity
PO route
• Give once a day for 5-10 days depending on condition
• Give without regard to food
• Store at room temperature

IV route
• Discontinue primary **IV** while administering moxifloxacin, give over 60 min
• Do not give SUBCUT, IM
• Available as premixed sol, may be diluted at ratios from 1:10 to 10:1, do not refrigerate, give by direct infusion or through **Y**-type infusion set, do not add other medications to sol or infuse through same IV line at same time
• Do not refrigerate
• Flush line with compatible sol before and after use
• Do not admix

Solution compatibilities: 0.9% NaCl, D_5, D_{10}, LR, sterile water for inj

ADVERSE EFFECTS
CNS: Headache, dizziness, fatigue, insomnia, depression, restlessness, seizures, confusion, increased intracranial pressure, peripheral neuropathy, pseudotumor cerebri, fever
CV: Prolonged QT interval, dysrhythmias, torsades de pointes, tachycardia
EENT: Blurred vision, tinnitus, taste changes
GI: Nausea, increased ALT, AST, flatulence, heartburn, vomiting, diarrhea, oral candidiasis, dysphagia, pseudomembranous colitis, abdominal pain, dyspepsia, constipation, gastroenteritis, xerostomia
GU: Renal failure
INTEG: Rash, pruritus, urticaria, photosensitivity, flushing, fever, chills, injection site reactions
MISC: Candidiasis vaginitis
MS: Tremor, arthralgia, tendon rupture, myalgia
SYST: Anaphylaxis, Stevens-Johnson syndrome, angioedema, toxic epidermal necrolysis

Pharmacokinetics

Absorption	Well absorbed (75%) (PO)
Distribution	Widely distributed
Metabolism	Liver
Excretion	Kidneys
Half-life	Increased in renal disease

Pharmacodynamics

	PO
Onset	Rapid
Peak	1 hr
Duration	Unknown

INTERACTIONS
Individual drugs
Aluminum hydroxide, calcium, didanosine, iron, sucralfate, zinc sulfate: decreased absorption of moxifloxacin
CycloSPORINE: increased cycloSPORINE effect
Haloperidol, chloroquine, droperidol, pentamidine; arsenic trioxide, levomethadyl: increased QT prolongation
Probenecid: increased blood levels
Warfarin: increased warfarin effect

Drug classifications
Antacids (magnesium), iron salts: decreased absorption of moxifloxacin
Class IA/III antidysrhythmics, some phenothiazines, β-agonists, local anesthetics, tricyclics, CYP3A4 inhibitors (amiodarone, clarithromycin, erythromycin, telithromycin, troleandomycin), CYP3A4 substrates (methadone, pimozide, QUEtiapine, quiNIDine, risperiDONE, ziprasidone): increased QT prolongation
NSAIDs: increased seizure risk

BLACK BOX WARNING: Corticosteroids: increased tendon rupture

Drug/food
Enteral feeding: decreased absorption of moxifloxacin

Drug/lab test
Increased: glucose, amylase, lipids, triglycerides, uric acid, LDH
Decreased: potassium

NURSING CONSIDERATIONS
Assessment
• Assess patient for previous sensitivity reaction
• Assess patient for signs and symptoms of infection including characteristics of wounds, sputum, urine, stool, WBC >10,000/mm³, fever baseline, during treatment
• Obtain C&S before beginning product therapy to identify if correct treatment has been initiated
• **Assess for allergic reactions, Stevens-Johnson syndrome, toxic epidermal necrolysis, and anaphylaxis: rash, urticaria, pruritus, chills, fever, joint pain; may occur a few days after therapy begins; EPINEPHrine and resuscitation equipment should be available for anaphylactic reaction**
• Assess for CNS symptoms: headache, dizziness, fatigue, insomnia, depression, **seizures**
• Identify urine output; if decreasing, notify prescriber (may indicate nephrotoxicity); also check for increased BUN, creatinine, electrolytes
• Monitor blood tests: AST, ALT, CBC, Hct, bilirubin, LDH, alkaline phosphatase, Coombs' test monthly if patient is on long-term therapy
• Monitor electrolytes: potassium, sodium chloride monthly if patient is on long-term therapy
• **Pseudomembranous colitis: assess for diarrhea, abdominal pain, fever, fatigue, anorexia; possible anemia, elevated WBC and low serum albumin; stop product and usually give either vancomycin or IV metro-NIDAZOLE**
• Monitor for bleeding: ecchymosis, bleeding gums, hematuria, stool guaiac daily if on long-term therapy
• Assess for overgrowth of infection: perineal itching, fever, malaise, redness, pain, swelling, drainage, rash, diarrhea, change in cough, sputum

> **BLACK BOX WARNING:** Assess for tendon pain, rupture, tendinitis; if tendon becomes inflamed, drug should be discontinued, more common in achilles tendon

⚠ **QT prolongation: Monitor ECG for QT prolongation, ejection fraction; assess for chest pain, palpitations, dyspnea**

Patient/family education

> **BLACK BOX WARNING:** Notify prescriber of tendon pain, inflammation, stop drug

• Teach patient to report sore throat, bruising, bleeding, joint pain; may indicate blood dyscrasias (rare)
• Advise patient to contact prescriber if vaginal itching, loose foul-smelling stools, furry tongue occur; may indicate superinfection; report itching, rash, pruritus, urticaria
• Instruct patient to take all medication prescribed for the length of time ordered; not to give medication to others
• Advise patient to notify prescriber of diarrhea with blood or pus
• Advise patient to rinse mouth frequently, use sugarless candy or gum for dry mouth
• Advise patient to take as prescribed, not to double or miss doses

Evaluation
Positive therapeutic outcome
• Absence of signs/symptoms of infection (WBC <10,000/mm³, temp WNL)
• Reported improvement in symptoms of infection

moxifloxacin ophthalmic
See Appendix B

M

mupirocin topical
See Appendix B

mycophenolate (Rx)
(mie-koe-feen′oh-late)
Mycophenolate Mofetil CellCept, Myfortic (Rx)
Func. class.: Immunosuppressant
Pregnancy category C

ACTION: Inhibits inflammatory responses that are mediated by the immune system; prolongs survival of allogenic transplants

Therapeutic outcome: Absence of graft rejection

USES: Organ transplants to prevent rejection (renal); prophylaxis of rejection in allogenic cardiac, hepatic, renal transplants

Unlabeled uses: Refractory uveitis, 2nd-line therapy for Churg-Strauss syndrome, diffuse proliferative lupus nephritis (in combination), rheumatoid arthritis, psoriasis

CONTRAINDICATIONS
Hypersensitivity to this product or mycophenolic acid

> **BLACK BOX WARNING:** Pregnancy **D**

Adverse effects: *italics* = common; **bold** = life-threatening

Precautions: Breastfeeding, lymphomas, neutropenia, renal disease, accidental exposure, anemia

> **BLACK BOX WARNING:** Infection, neoplastic disease

DOSAGE AND ROUTES
Renal transplant (to prevent organ rejection)
Adult: PO 1 g or 720 mg bid given to renal transplant patients in combination with corticosteroids and cycloSPORINE; mycophenolate mofetil 1 g or 720 mg mycophenolate sodium
Child: SUSP 600 mg bid or PO cap 750 mg bid body surface area (BSA) of 1.25 to 1.5 m² or 1 g bid BSA >1.5 m²

Renal dose
Adult: PO/IV GFR <25 ml/min, max 2 g/day

Cardiac transplant (to prevent organ rejection)
Adult: PO/IV 1.5 g bid, IV can be started ≤24 hr after transplant, switch to PO when able

Hepatic transplant (to prevent organ rejection)
Adult: PO 1.5 g bid, IV 1 g over ≥2 hr

Available forms: Caps 250 mg; tabs 500 mg; inj (powder) 500 mg/20 ml vial; powder for oral susp 200 mg/ml; ext rel tab (Myfortic) 180, 360 mg

Implementation
• May be given in combination with corticosteroids and cycloSPORINE
PO route
• Do not crush, chew tabs; do not open caps; avoid inhalation or direct contact with skin, mucous membranes; tetratogenic in animals
• Give alone for better absorption
• Delayed rel tabs and caps; oral **susp** and tab are not interchangeable

Intermittent IV infusion route
• Reconstitute each vial with 14 ml D₅W, shake gently, further dilute to 6 mg/ml, dilute 1-g doses in 140 ml D₅W, and 1.5-g doses in 210 ml D₅W, give by slow **IV** infusion ≥2 hr, never give by bolus or rapid **IV** injection
• Do not give with other medications or solutions

Y-site compatibilities: Alemtuzumab, alfentanil, amikacin, anidulafungin, argatroban, bivalirudin, caspofungin, cefepime, DAPTOmycin, DOPamine, norepinephrine, octreotide, oxytocin, tacrolimus, tigecycline, tirofiban, vancomycin, zolendronic acid

Y-site incompatibilities: Acyclovir, allopurinol, amifostine, aminocaproic acid, aminophylline, amphotericin B, colloidal/lipid complex/liposome, ampicillin, atenolol, azithromycin, aztreonam

ADVERSE EFFECTS
CNS: *Tremor, dizziness, insomnia, headache, fever,* progressive multifocal leukoencephalopathy, asthenia, paresthesia, anxiety, pain
CV: *Hypertension, chest pain,* hypotension, edema
GI: *Nausea, vomiting,* stomatitis, *diarrhea, constipation,* GI bleeding, abdominal pain, anorexia, dyspepsia
GU: *UTI, hematuria,* renal tubular necrosis, polyomavirus-associated nephropathy
HEMA: Leukopenia, thrombocytopenia, anemia, pancytopenia, pure red cell aplasia, neutropenia
INTEG: *Rash*
META: *Peripheral edema, hypercholesterolemia, hypophosphatemia, edema, hypo/hyperkalemia, hyperglycemia,* hypocalcemia, hypomagnesemia
MS: Arthralgia, muscle wasting, back pain, weakness
RESP: *Dyspnea, respiratory infection, increased cough, pharyngitis, bronchitis, pneumonia,* pleural effusion, pulmonary fibrosis
SYST: Lymphoma, nonmelanoma skin carcinoma, sepsis

Pharmacokinetics
Absorption	Rapid and complete
Distribution	Unknown
Metabolism	To active metabolite (MPA)
Excretion	Urine, feces
Half-life	Unknown

Pharmacodynamics
Unknown

INTERACTIONS
Individual drugs
Acyclovir, ganciclovir, valcyclovir: increased toxicity
AzaTHIOprine: increased bone marrow suppression
Cholestyramine, cycloSPORINE, rifamycin: decreased levels of mycophenolate
Phenytoin: increased effects; decreased protein binding of phenytoin
Probenecid: increased levels of mycophenolate
Theophylline: increased effects; decreased protein binding of theophylline

---

Drug classifications

Antacids (magnesium, aluminum): decreased levels of mycophenolate

Anticoagulants, NSAIDs, thrombolytics, salicylates: increased risk of bleeding

Contraceptives (oral), live attenuated vaccines: decreased effects

Immunosuppressives, salicylates: increased levels of mycophenolate

Drug/herb

Astragalus, echinacea, melatonin: interferes with immunosuppression

Drug/food

Decreased absorption if taken with food

Drug/lab test

Increased: serum creatinine, BUN, potassium, cholesterol, glucose, abnormal LFTs

Decreased: WBC, platelets, neutrophils

NURSING CONSIDERATIONS

Assessment

• **Progressive multifocal leukoencephalopathy; may be fatal:** ataxia, confusion, apathy, hemiparesis, visual problems, weakness; side effects should be reported to the FDA

> **BLACK BOX WARNING: Infection/lymphoma:** may occur from immunosuppressives, increased infections including BK virus, and may cause kidney graft loss

• Monitor blood tests: CBC monthly during treatment

• Monitor liver function tests: alkaline phosphatase, AST, ALT, bilirubin

• Monitor renal studies: BUN, CCr, electrolytes

⚠ **Obtain pregnancy test within 1 wk prior to initiation of treatment; confirm negative pregnancy test**

Patient/family education

⚠ **Teach patient to report fever, rash, severe diarrhea, chills, sore throat, fatigue, since serious infections may occur**

• Instruct patient to avoid crowds to reduce risk of infection

• Advise patient that repeated lab tests are necessary

⚠ **Instruct patient to notify prescriber if pregnancy is planned or suspected (D), to use two forms of contraception before, during, and 6 wk after therapy**

> **BLACK BOX WARNING:** Advise patient that infection and lymphomas may occur

• Teach patient to take on empty stomach, not to crush, chew, break ext rel caps

Evaluation

Positive therapeutic outcome

• Absence of graft rejection

nabumetone (Rx)

(na-byoo'me-tone)

Relafen ✤

Func. class.: Nonsteroidal antiinflammatory

Chem. class.: Acetic acid derivative

Pregnancy category C

ACTION: Metabolite inhibits COX-1, COX-2 by blocking arachidonate; analgesic, antiinflammatory, antipyretic

Therapeutic outcome: Decreased pain, swelling of joints

USES: Osteoarthritis, rheumatoid arthritis, acute or chronic treatment

CONTRAINDICATIONS

Hypersensitivity to this product or aspirin, NSAIDs

> **BLACK BOX WARNING:** Perioperative pain in CABG surgery

Precautions: Pregnancy **C**, breastfeeding, children, geriatric, bleeding disorders, GI/cardiac/renal disorders, hepatic dysfunction, asthma, bone marrow suppression, lupus (SLE), ulcerative colitis, blood dyscrasias

> **BLACK BOX WARNING:** MI, stroke, GI bleeding

DOSAGE AND ROUTES

Adult: PO 1 g as a single dose or divided bid; may increase to 2 g/day if needed; max 2 g/day if needed (as a divided dose)

Renal dose

Adult: PO CCr 31-49 ml/min, 750 mg daily, max 1500 mg/day; CCr <30 ml/min, 500 mg daily, max 1000 mg/day

Available forms: Tabs 500, 750 mg

Implementation

- Administer tab to patient crushed or whole
- Give with food or milk to decrease gastric symptoms
- Patient should take with a full glass of water and sit upright
- Store at room temp

ADVERSE EFFECTS

CNS: Dizziness, headache, drowsiness, fatigue, tremors, confusion, insomnia, anxiety, depression, nervousness

CV: Tachycardia, peripheral edema, palpitations, **dysrhythmias, CHF, MI, stroke**

EENT: Tinnitus

GI: Nausea, anorexia, vomiting, diarrhea, jaundice, cholestatic hepatitis, constipation, flatulence, cramps, dry mouth, peptic ulcer, gastritis, ulceration, perforation, bleeding

GU: Nephrotoxicity, dysuria, hematuria, azotemia, cystitis

HEMA: Thrombocytopenia

INTEG: Purpura, rash, pruritus, sweating, photosensitivity

RESP: Dyspnea, pharyngitis, bronchospasm

SYST: Anaphylaxis, angioedema, Stevens-Johnson syndrome

Pharmacokinetics

Absorption	Well absorbed
Distribution	Protein binding >99%
Metabolism	Liver, extensively, to inactive metabolite
Excretion	Unknown
Half-life	24 hr

Pharmacodynamics

Onset	Unknown
Peak	2½-4 hr
Duration	Unknown

INTERACTIONS

Individual drugs

Alcohol, potassium: increased GI reactions

Cidofovir, lithium, methotrexate: increased effect of each

Clopidogrel, eptifibatide, ticlopidine: increased risk of bleeding

Radiation: increased risk of hematologic reactions

Drug classifications

Anticoagulants, thrombolytics, SSRIs, SNRIs: increased risk of bleeding

Antihypertensives: decreased effect of antihypertensives

Antineoplastics: increased risk of hematologic reactions

Corticosteroids, NSAIDs, potassium supplements, salicylates: increased GI reactions

Diuretics: decreased effectiveness of diuretics

Drug/herb

Arginine, gossypol: increased gastric irritation

Bearberry, bilberry: increased NSAID effect

Garlic, ginger, ginkgo: increased bleeding risk

Drug/lab test

Increased: bleeding time, K, BUN, AST, ALT, LDH, alkaline phosphatase, creatinine

Decreased: CCr, blood glucose, Hct, Hgb

⚠ Nurse Alert   🔆 Key NCLEX® Drug   >> Drug Specifics

NURSING CONSIDERATIONS
Assessment

> **BLACK BOX WARNING: Cardiac status:** CV thrombic events, MI, stroke; may be fatal, not to be used in perioperative pain after CABG

> **BLACK BOX WARNING: GI status:** ulceration, bleeding, perforation; may be fatal

• **Assess for pain:** frequency, characteristics, location, duration, intensity, relief of pain after medication; and for inflammation of joints, ROM
• Monitor blood counts during therapy; watch for decreasing platelets; if low, therapy may need to be discontinued, restarted after hematologic recovery; check for blood dyscrasias (thrombocytopenia): bruising, fatigue, bleeding, poor healing; monitor liver function tests: AST, ALT, alkaline phosphatase; LDH, blood glucose, WBC, CCr
• Assess for asthma, aspirin sensitivity, nasal polyps; increased hypersensitivity reactions

Patient/family education
• Tell patient that product must be continued for prescribed time to be effective; to avoid aspirin, alcoholic beverages, NSAIDs, and OTC medications unless approved by prescriber
• Caution patient to report bleeding, bruising, fatigue, malaise, since blood dyscrasias do occur
• Instruct patient to use caution when driving; drowsiness, dizziness may occur
• Advise patient to use sunscreen, hat, and other protective clothing to prevent burns
• Advise patient to report dark stools, a change in urine pattern, increased weight, edema, increased pain in joints, fever, blood in urine, blurred vision, ringing or roaring in ears
• Advise to report use to all health care providers

Evaluation
Positive therapeutic outcome
• Decreased pain
• Decreased inflammation
• Increased mobility

nadolol (Rx)
(nay-doe′lole)
Corgard, Syn-Nadol ✦
Func. class.: Antihypertensive, antianginal
Chem. class.: β-Adrenergic receptor blocker
Pregnancy category C

Do not confuse: Corgard/Cognex/Coreg

ACTION: Long-acting, nonselective β-adrenergic receptor blocking agent, blocks β_1 in the heart and β_2 in the lungs, uterus, and circulatory system; mechanism is similar to that of propranolol

Therapeutic outcome: Decreased B/P, heart rate

USES: Chronic stable angina pectoris, mild to moderate hypertension, atrial fibrillation

Unlabeled uses: Tachydysrhythmias, anxiety, tremors, esophageal varices (rebleeding only), prophylaxis of migraine headaches

CONTRAINDICATIONS
Hypersensitivity to this product, cardiac failure, cardiogenic shock, 2nd- or 3rd-degree heart block, bronchospastic disease, sinus bradycardia, CHF, COPD

Precautions: Pregnancy **C**, breastfeeding, diabetes mellitus, renal disease, hyperthyroidism, peripheral vascular disease, myasthenia gravis, major surgery, nonallergic bronchospasm

> **BLACK BOX WARNING:** Abrupt discontinuation

DOSAGE AND ROUTES
Adult: PO 40 mg/day; increase by 40-80 mg q2-14 days; maintenance 40-240 mg/day for angina, 40-320 mg/day for hypertension
Geriatric: PO 20 mg/day, may increase by 20 mg until desired dose

Renal dose
Adult: PO CCr 31-50 ml/min give q24-36hr; CCr 10-30 ml/min give q24-48hr; CCr <10 ml/min give q40-60hr

Migraine prevention (unlabeled)
Adult: PO 40-240 mg/day × 2-18 mo

Available forms: Tabs 20, 40, 80 mg

Implementation
• Give at bedtime; tab may be crushed or swallowed whole; give with food to prevent GI upset; give reduced dosage in renal dysfunction; check apical pulse prior to use, if <50 bpm, withhold dose and notify prescriber
• Store protected from light, moisture; place in cool environment
• Give without regard to food
• Discontinue other antihypertensives gradually

ADVERSE EFFECTS
CNS: Depression, *dizziness*, fatigue, lethargy, paresthesia, headache, *weakness*, insomnia, memory loss, nightmares
CV: *Bradycardia, hypotension*, **CHF**, palpitations, AV block, chest pain, peripheral ischemia,

Adverse effects: *italics* = common; **bold** = life-threatening

flushing, edema, vasodilatation, conduction disturbances

EENT: Blurred vision, dry eyes, nasal congestion

ENDO: Hyperglycemia, hypoglycemia

GI: Nausea, vomiting, diarrhea, colitis, constipation, cramps, dry mouth, flatulence, hepatomegaly, **pancreatitis**, taste distortion

GU: *Impotence,* decreased libido

HEMA: Agranulocytosis, thrombocytopenia

INTEG: Rash, pruritus, fever, alopecia

RESP: Dyspnea, respiratory dysfunction, **bronchospasm,** cough, wheezing, pharyngitis, **laryngospasm, pulmonary edema**

Pharmacokinetics

Absorption	Variably absorbed
Distribution	Crosses placenta; minimal concentration in CNS, protein binding 30%
Metabolism	Unknown
Excretion	Kidneys, unchanged
Half-life	10-24 hr; increased in renal disease

Pharmacodynamics

Onset	Variable
Peak	3-4 hr
Duration	10-24 hr

INTERACTIONS
Individual drugs
CloNIDine, EPINEPHrine: increased hypotension, bradycardia
Digoxin: increased bradycardia
Thyroid: decreased β-blocking effect

Drug classifications
Antihypertensives: increased hypotension
Ergots: peripheral ischemia
MAOIs: increased bradycardia; do not use together
NSAIDs: decreased antihypertensive effect
Phenothiazines: increased hypotensive effects

Drug/lab test
Increased: serum potassium, serum uric acid, ALT, AST, alkaline phosphatase, LDH, blood glucose, cholesterol, ANA, triglycerides

NURSING CONSIDERATIONS
Assessment
• **Pain:** assess for duration, time started, activity being performed, location, character
• **Hypertension:** check that prescriptions have been filled

• **Angina:** monitor frequency of angina, alleviating factors
• Monitor B/P at beginning of treatment, periodically thereafter; note rate, rhythm, quality of apical/radial pulse before administration; notify prescriber of any significant changes (pulse <60 bpm), orthostatic hypotension
• Check for baselines in renal, liver function tests before therapy begins
• Assess for edema in feet, legs daily; monitor I&O, daily weight; check for jugular vein distention and crackles bilaterally, dyspnea **(CHF)**
• Headache, light-headedness, decreased B/P, may indicate a need for decreased dosage

> **BLACK BOX WARNING:** Abrupt discontinuation: can result in MI, myocardial ischemia, ventricular dysrhythmias, severe hypertension, withdraw slowly by tapering over 2 wk

Patient/family education
• Teach patient not to discontinue product abruptly; taper over 2 wk; may cause precipitate angina, serious dysrhythmias if stopped abruptly
• Teach patient not to use OTC products containing α-adrenergic stimulants (such as nasal decongestants, cold preparations); to avoid alcohol and smoking and to limit sodium intake as prescribed, to take as prescribed at same time each day; do not double; take missed dose as soon as remembered if before 8 hr prior to next dose
• Teach patient how to take pulse and B/P at home; to hold dose if pulse is ≤50 bpm, systolic B/P <90 mm Hg; advise when to notify prescriber; to take missed dose as soon as possible if less than 8 hr
• **Hypertension:** instruct patient to comply with weight control, dietary adjustments, modified exercise program; to report weight gain >5 lb, swelling, unusual bruising, bleeding
• Advise patient to carry/wear emergency ID to identify product being taken, allergies; teach patient product controls symptoms but does not cure condition
• Caution patient to avoid hazardous activities if dizziness, drowsiness are present; to rise slowly to prevent orthostatic hypotension
• **Teach patient to report symptoms of CHF:** difficult breathing, especially on exertion or when lying down, night cough, swelling of extremities or bradycardia, dizziness, confusion, depression, fever
• Teach patient to take product as prescribed, not to double doses, skip doses; take any missed doses as soon as remembered if at least 4 hr until next dose

Evaluation

Positive therapeutic outcome
• Decreased B/P in hypertension

nafcillin (Rx)
(naf-sill'in)
Func. class.: Antiinfective, broad-spectrum
Chem. class.: Penicillinase-resistant penicillin
Pregnancy category B

ACTION: Interferes with cell wall replication of susceptible organisms; osmotically unstable cell wall swells, bursts from osmotic pressure

Therapeutic outcome: Bactericidal effects for gram-positive cocci *Staphylococcus aureus, Streptococcus viridans, Streptococcus pneumoniae* and infections caused by penicillinase-producing *Staphylococcus*

USES: Infections caused by penicillinase-producing staphylococci, streptococci; respiratory tract, skin, skin structure, urinary tract, bone, joint infections; sinusitis; endocarditis; septicemia; meningitis

CONTRAINDICATIONS
Hypersensitivity to penicillins or corn

Precautions: Pregnancy **B**, breastfeeding, neonates, GI disease, asthma, hypersensitivity to cephalosporins or carbapenems, electrolyte imbalances, hepatic/renal disease, pseudomembranous colitis

DOSAGE AND ROUTES
Adult: IV 500-2000 mg q4hr; IM 500 mg q6-8hr, max 12 g/day
Infant and child >1 mo: IV 150-200 mg/kg/day in divided doses q4-6hr
Neonate >7 days (weight >2 kg): IV 25 mg/kg q6hr
Neonate ≤7 days (weight ≤2 kg): IV 25 mg/kg q8hr

Available forms: Powder for inj 1 premixed or Add-Vantage vials (1 g)

Implementation
IM route
• Give deep in large muscle mass

IV route
• Reconstitute vials: add 1.7 (1.8 nafcil), 3, 4, or 6.4 ml (6.6 ml NaCl) sterile water for inj, 0.9% NaCl, bacteriostatic water for inj with benzyl alcohol or parabens to vials with 500 mg, 1 g, 2 g of nafcillin, respectively (250 mg/ml); pharmacy bulk pack reconstitute 10 g/93 ml sterile water inj or 0.9% NaCl (100 mg/ml)
• **Nallpen piggyback units:** reconstitute 1 or 2 g with 50-100 ml or 99 ml, respectively, of sterile water for inj, 0.45% NaCl, 0.9% NaCl
• **Unipen piggyback units:** reconstitute according to manufacturer
Direct intermittent IV INJ route
• Further dilute the reconstituted sol in 15-30 ml of sterile water for inj, 0.45% NaCl, 0.9% NaCl; inj slowly over 5-10 min into the tubing of a free-flowing compatible IV solution
Intermittent IV infusion route
• Vials, further dilute reconstituted solution to 2-40 mg/ml, for peripheral vein inf ≤20 mg/ml (preferred); piggyback unit no further dilution needed; infuse ≥30-60 min, make sure entire dose is given before 10% or more of solution is inactivated
• Extravasation management: stop infusion and disconnect; gently aspirate extravasated solution; do not flush line; use hyaluronidase; remove cannula/needle; apply dry cold compresses; elevate extremity

Y-site compatibilities: Acyclovir, alfentanil, amikacin, aminophylline, amphotericin B lipid complex (Abelcet), anidulafungin, argatroban, ascorbic acid injection, atenolol, atracurium, atropine, aztreonam, benztropine, bivalirudin, bleomycin, bretylium, bumetanide, buprenorphine, butorphanol, calcium chloride/gluconate, CARBOplatin, carmustine, cefamandole, ceFAZolin, cefoperazone, cefotaxime, cefoTEtan, cefOXitin, cefTAZidime, ceftizoxime, cefTRIAXone, cefuroxime, chlorproMAZINE, cimetidine, CISplatin, clindamycin, cyanocobalamin, cyclophosphamide, cycloSPORINE, DACTINomycin, DAPTOmycin, DAUNOrubicin liposome, dexamethasone, digoxin, DOBUTamine, DOCEtaxel, DOPamine, DOXOrubicin liposomal, enalaprilat, ePHEDrine, EPINEPHrine, epoetin alfa, erythromycin, etoposide, etoposide phosphate, famotidine, fenoldopam, fentaNYL, fluconazole, fludarabine, foscarnet, furosemide, gallium, ganciclovir, gatifloxacin, gemtuzumab, gentamicin, glycopyrrolate, granisetron, heparin, hydrocortisone, HYDROmorphone, imipenemcilastatin, indomethacin, isoproterenol, ketorolac, lactated Ringer's, lepirudin, leucovorin, lidocaine, linezolid injection, LORazepam, magnesium sulfate, mannitol, methyldopate, methylPREDNISolone, metoclopramide, metoprolol, metroNIDAZOLE, milrinone, morphine, multiple vitamins injection, naloxone, niCARdipine, nitroglycerin, nitroprusside, norepinephrine, octreotide, ondansetron, oxacillin, oxaliplatin, oxytocin,

N

Adverse effects: *italics* = common; **bold** = life-threatening

PACLitaxel (solvent/surfactant), pamidronate, pancuronium, pantoprazole, PEMEtrexed, penicillin G potassium/sodium, PENTobarbital, perphenazine, PHENobarbital, phentolamine, phenylephrine, phytonadione, piperacillin, polymyxin B, potassium acetate/chloride, procainamide, prochlorperazine, propofol, propranolol, ranitidine, ringer's injection, sodium bicarbonate, SUFentanil, tacrolimus, teniposide, theophylline, thiamine, thiotepa, ticarcillin, ticarcillin clavulanate, tigecycline, tirofiban, TNA (3-in-1), tobramycin, tolazoline, TPN (2-in-1), urokinase, vasopressin, vinBLAStine, voriconazole, zidovudine, zoledronic acid

Y-site incompatibilities: Droperidol, fentaNYL/droperidol, labetalol, nalbuphine, pentazocine, regular insulin, verapamil

ADVERSE EFFECTS

CNS: Lethargy, hallucinations, anxiety, depression, muscle twitching, coma, seizures
GI: *Nausea, vomiting, diarrhea,* increased AST, ALT, abdominal pain, glossitis, pseudomembranous colitis
GU: Oliguria, proteinuria, hematuria, vaginitis, moniliasis, glomerulonephritis, interstitial nephritis
HEMA: Anemia, increased bleeding time, bone marrow depression, neutropenia, agranulocytosis
INTEG: Tissue necrosis, extravasation injury at injection site
SYST: Anaphylaxis, serum sickness, Stevens-Johnson syndrome

Pharmacokinetics

Absorption	Well absorbed (IM); erratic (PO)
Distribution	Widely distributed; crosses placenta, 90% protein bound
Metabolism	Liver; 70%
Excretion	Kidneys, unchanged; breast milk
Half-life	30-90 min; increased in renal disease

Pharmacodynamics

	PO	IM	IV
Onset	½ hr	½ hr	Immediate
Peak	1-2 hr	1-2 hr	Infusion end
Duration	Unknown	Unknown	Unknown

INTERACTIONS
Individual drugs
CycloSPORINE: decreased effect of cycloSPORINE
Probenecid: increased nafcillin levels

Drug classifications
Tetracyclines, aminoglycosides: avoid use

Drug/food
Food, carbonated drinks, citrus fruit juices: decreased absorption

Drug/lab test
False positive: urine glucose, urine protein
Decreased: potassium, Hgb/Hct, neutrophils

NURSING CONSIDERATIONS
Assessment
• Assess patient for previous sensitivity reaction to penicillins or other cephalosporins; cross-sensitivity between penicillins and cephalosporins is common
• Assess patient for signs and symptoms of infection including characteristics of wounds, sputum, urine, stool, WBC >10,000/mm³, earache, fever; obtain information baseline, during treatment
• Obtain C&S before beginning product therapy to identify if correct treatment has been initiated
• Assess for allergic reactions, anaphylaxis: rash, urticaria, pruritus, chills, fever, dyspnea, laryngeal edema, joint pain; angioedema may occur a few days after therapy begins; cross-sensitivity with cephalosporins may occur; EPINEPHrine, resuscitation equipment should be available for anaphylactic reaction
• Assess renal function tests: urinalysis, protein, blood, BUN, creatinine; abnormal urinalysis may indicate nephrotoxicity
⚠ Identify urine output; if decreasing, notify prescriber (may indicate nephrotoxicity)
• Monitor blood studies: AST, ALT, CBC, Hct, bilirubin, LDH, alkaline phosphatase, Coombs' test monthly if patient is on long-term therapy, electrolytes
• Monitor electrolytes: potassium, sodium, chloride monthly if patient is on long-term therapy
• Pseudomembranous colitis: assess for diarrhea, abdominal pain, fever, fatigue, anorexia; possible anemia, elevated WBC and low serum albumin; stop product and usually give either vancomycin or IV metroNIDAZOLE
• Monitor for bleeding: ecchymosis, bleeding gums, hematuria, stool guaiac daily if on long-term therapy
• Assess for overgrowth of infection: perineal itching, fever, malaise, redness, pain, swelling,

drainage, rash, diarrhea, change in cough, sputum
• **IV site:** assess for redness, swelling, pain at site

Patient/family education
• Teach patient to report sore throat, bruising, bleeding, joint pain; may indicate blood dyscrasias (rare)
• Advise patient to contact prescriber if vaginal itching, loose foul-smelling stools, furry tongue occur; may indicate superinfection
• Instruct patient to take all medication prescribed for the length of time ordered
• Advise patient to notify prescriber of diarrhea with blood or pus, which may indicate pseudomembranous colitis
• Advise patient to carry/wear emergency ID if allergic to penicillins
• Teach patient to avoid use with other products unless approved by prescriber

Evaluation

Positive therapeutic outcome
• Absence of signs/symptoms of infection (WBC <10,000/mm^3, temp WNL, absence of red, draining wounds, earache)
• Reported improvement in symptoms of infection

TREATMENT OF ANAPHYLAXIS: Withdraw product, maintain airway, administer EPINEPHrine, aminophylline, O$_2$, IV corticosteroids

---

⚠ HIGH ALERT

nalbuphine (Rx)
(nal′byoo-feen)
Nubain ✦
Func. class.: Opioid analgesic
Chem. class.: Synthetic opioid agonist/antagonist
Pregnancy category C

ACTION: Depresses pain impulse transmission at the spinal cord level by interacting with opioid receptors

Therapeutic outcome: Relief of pain

USES: Moderate to severe pain, supplement to anesthesia

CONTRAINDICATIONS
Hypersensitivity to this product or parabens, addiction (opioid)

Precautions: Pregnancy **B,** breastfeeding, addictive personality, increased ICP, MI (acute),

severe heart disease, respiratory depression, renal/hepatic disease, bowel impaction, abrupt discontinuation

DOSAGE AND ROUTES
Analgesic
Adult: SUBCUT/IM/IV max 10 mg q3-6hr prn, max 160 mg/day

Balanced anesthesia adjunct
Adult: IV 0.3-3 mg/kg given over 10-15 min; may give 0.25-0.5 mg/kg as needed (maintenance)

Available forms: Inj 10, 20 mg/ml

Implementation
• Give by inj (IM, **IV**), only with resuscitative equipment available; give slowly to prevent rigidity
• Store in light-resistant area at room temperature
IM route
• Give inj deeply in large muscle mass; rotate inj sites; protect vial from light

Direct IV route
• Give direct **IV** undiluted 10 mg or less over 3-5 min or more into free-flowing IV line of D$_5$W, NS, LR

Syringe compatibilities: Atropine, cimetidine, diphenhydrAMINE, droperidol, glycopyrrolate, hydrOXYzine, lidocaine, midazolam, prochlorperazine, promethazine, ranitidine, scopolamine, trimethobenzamide

Syringe incompatibilities: Diazepam, PENTobarbital

Y-site compatibilities: Amifostine, aztreonam, cladribine, filgrastim, fludarabine, granisetron, melphalan, PACLitaxel, propofol, teniposide, thiotepa, vinorelbine

Y-site incompatibilities: Nafcillin, sargramostim

ADVERSE EFFECTS
CNS: *Drowsiness, dizziness, confusion, headache, sedation, euphoria,* dysphoria (high doses), hallucinations, increased dreaming, tolerance, physical and psychological dependency
CV: Bradycardia, change in B/P, **cardiac arrest**
EENT: Blurred vision, miosis, diplopia
GI: *Nausea, vomiting, anorexia, constipation, cramps,* abdominal pain, dyspepsia, xerostomia, bitter taste
GU: Urinary urgency
INTEG: *Rash,* urticaria, flushing, *diaphoresis,* pruritus
RESP: **Respiratory depression/arrest,** pulmonary edema

Adverse effects: *italics* = common; **bold** = life-threatening

N

Pharmacokinetics

Absorption	Well absorbed (SUBCUT, IM); completely absorbed (**IV**)
Distribution	Crosses placenta
Metabolism	Liver, extensively
Excretion	Feces, kidneys, unchanged (small amounts); breast milk
Half-life	3-6 hr

Pharmacodynamics

	IM	SUBCUT	IV
Onset	Up to 15 min	Up to 15 min	2-3 min
Peak	1 hr	Unknown	½ hr
Duration	3-6 hr	3-6 hr	3-6 hr

INTERACTIONS
Individual drugs
Alcohol: increased respiratory depression, hypotension, sedation

Drug classifications
Antipsychotics, CNS depressants, sedative/hypnotics, skeletal muscle relaxants: increased respiratory depression, hypotension
Opiates: increased effects with other CNS depressants
MAOIs: increase: severe reactions

Drug/herb
Increase: CNS depression, kava, valerian, hops, chamomile

NURSING CONSIDERATIONS
Assessment
• **Assess pain characteristics** (location, intensity, type) before medication administration, 30-60 min after treatment, titrate upward by 25%-50% until pain is reduced by 50%
• Assess bowel status; constipation is common, may need laxative or stool softener
• Monitor VS after parenteral route; note muscle rigidity, product history, liver, kidney function tests; respiratory dysfunction: respiratory depression, character, rate, rhythm; notify prescriber if respirations are <10/min
• **Monitor CNS changes:** dizziness, drowsiness, hallucinations, euphoria, LOC, pupil reaction
• Monitor allergic reactions: rash, urticaria

Patient/family education
• Instruct patient to report any symptoms of CNS changes, allergic reactions
• Teach patient that physical dependency can result from long-term use, although there is a low potential for dependency, profuse sweating,

twitching; without treatment, symptoms resolve in 5-14 days; chronic abstinence syndrome may last 2-6 mo
• Caution patients to avoid CNS depressants: alcohol, sedative/hypnotics for at least 24 hr after taking this product
• Discuss with patient that dizziness, drowsiness, confusion are common; to avoid getting up without assistance
• Discuss in detail all aspects of the product: reason for taking product and expected results
• Instruct patient to change position slowly to prevent orthostatic hypotension

Evaluation
Positive therapeutic outcome
• Relief of pain without respiratory depression

TREATMENT OF OVERDOSE:
Naloxone (Narcan) 0.2-0.8 **IV**, O$_2$, **IV** fluids, vasopressors

naloxone (Rx)
(nal-oks′one)
Evzio, Narcan
Func. class.: Opioid antagonist, antidote
Chem. class.: Thebaine derivative
Pregnancy category C

Do not confuse: naloxone/naltrexone

ACTION: Competes with opioids at opioid-receptor sites

Therapeutic outcome: Absence of opioid overdose

USES: Respiratory depression induced by opioids; refractory circulatory shock, asphyxia neonatorum, coma, hypotension, opiate agonist overdose

Unlabeled uses: IBS, opiate agonist dependence, opiate agonist-induced constipation, pruritus

CONTRAINDICATIONS
Hypersensitivity

Precautions: Pregnancy **B**, breastfeeding, neonates, children, CV disease, opioid dependency, seizure disorder, drug dependency, hepatic disease

DOSAGE AND ROUTES
Opioid-induced respiratory depression (known or suspected opiate agonist overdose)
Adult: IV/SUBCUT/IM 0.4-2 mg; repeat q2-3min if needed, max 10 mg; **IV** infusion loading dose 0.005 mg/kg, then 0.0025 mg/kg/hr; nasal spray 1 spray, may repeat q2-3min in alternate nostril if needed

Child <5 yr or ≤20 kg: **IV**/intraosseous 0.01 mg/kg slowly followed by 0.1 mg/kg if needed; **IV** infusion (PALS) 0.04-0.16 mg/kg/hr, titrate; nasal spray 1 spray, may repeat q2-3min in alternate nostril if needed

Postoperative opioid-induced respiratory depression
Adult: **IV** 0.1-0.2 mg q2-3min prn
Child: **IV** 0.005-0.01 mg/kg q2-3min prn

Nausea/vomiting from continuous morphine infusion/urinary retention (unlabeled)
Adult: **IV** 0.2 mg

Available forms: Inj 0.4, 1 mg/ml; nasal spray 4 mg/0.1 ml

Implementation
• Store at room temperature and protect from light
• Double-check dose; those taking opioids longer term are sensitive to this product

Direct IV route
• Give undiluted (suspected opioid overdose); give 0.4 mg or less over 15 sec or titrate inf to response

Continuous IV infusion route
• Dilute 2 mg/500 ml 0.9% NaCl or D$_5$W (4 mcg/ml), titrate to response
• Give only with resuscitative equipment, O$_2$ nearby
• Use only sol prepared within 24 hr

Y-site compatibilities: Acyclovir, alfentanil, amikacin, aminocaproic acid, aminophylline, anidulafungin, ascorbic acid, atenolol, atracurium, atropine, azaTHIOprine, aztreonam, benztropine, bivalirudin, bleomycin, bumetanide, buprenorphine, butorphanol, calcium chloride/gluconate, CARBOplatin, caspofungin, cefamandole, ceFAZolin, cefmetazole, cefonicid, cefoperazone, cefotaxime, cefoTEtan, cefOXitin, cefTAZidime, ceftizoxime, cefTRIAXone, cefuroxime, cephalothin, cephapirin, chloramphenicol, chlorproMAZINE, cimetidine, CISplatin, clindamycin, cyanocobalamin, cyclophosphamide, cycloSPORINE, cytarabine, DACTINomycin, DAPTOmycin, dexamethasone, digoxin, diltiazem, diphenhydrAMINE, DOBUTamine, DOCEtaxel, DOPamine, doxacurium, DOXOrubicin, doxycycline, enalaprilat, ePHEDrine, EPINEPHrine, epirubicin, epoetin alfa, eptifibatide, ertapenem, erythromycin, esmolol, etoposide, etoposide phosphate, famotidine, fenoldopam, fentaNYL, fluconazole, fludarabine, fluorouracil, folic acid, furosemide, ganciclovir, gatifloxacin, gemcitabine, gentamicin, glycopyrrolate, granisetron, heparin, hydrocortisone, hydrOXYzine, IDArubicin, ifosfamide, imipenem-cilastatin, inamrinone, indomethacin, insulin (regular), irinotecan, isoproterenol, ketorolac, labetalol, levofloxacin, lidocaine, linezolid, LORazepam, mannitol, mechlorethamine, meperidine, metaraminol, methicillin, methotrexate, methyldopate, methylPREDNISolone, metoclopramide, metoprolol, metroNIDAZOLE, mezlocillin, miconazole, midazolam, milrinone, minocycline, mitoXANtrone, morphine, multiple vitamins, mycophenolate, nafcillin, nalbuphine, nesiritide, netilmicin, nitroglycerin, nitroprusside, norepinephrine, octreotide, ondansetron, oxacillin, oxaliplatin, oxytocin, PACLitaxel, palonosetron, pamidronate, pancuronium, papaverine, PEMEtrexed, penicillin G potassium/sodium, pentamidine, pentazocine, PENTobarbital, PHENobarbital, phentolamine, phenylephrine, phytonadione, piperacillin, piperacillin-tazobactam, polymyxin B, potassium chloride, procainamide, prochlorperazine, promethazine, propofol, propranolol, protamine, pyridoxine, quiNIDine, quinupristin-dalfopristin, ranitidine, rocuronium, sodium acetate/bicarbonate, succinylcholine, SUFentanil, tacrolimus, teniposide, theophylline, thiamine, ticarcillin, ticarcillin-clavulanate, tigecycline, tirofiban, tobramycin, tolazoline, urokinase, vancomycin, vasopressin, vecuronium, verapamil, vinCRIStine, vinorelbine, voriconazole, zoledronic acid

ADVERSE EFFECTS
CNS: Nervousness, *seizures*, tremor, opioid withdrawal symptoms
CV: Rapid pulse, **ventricular tachycardia, fibrillation**, increased systolic B/P (high doses), hypo/hypertension, **cardiac arrest, sinus tachycardia**
GI: Nausea, vomiting
RESP: **Pulmonary edema**, dyspnea

Pharmacokinetics

Absorption	Well absorbed (SUBCUT, IM); completely absorbed (**IV**)
Distribution	Rapidly distributed; crosses placenta
Metabolism	Liver
Excretion	Kidneys
Half-life	1 hr; up to 3 hr (neonates)

Pharmacodynamics

	IV	IM/SUBCUT
Onset	1 min	2-5 min
Peak	Unknown	Unknown
Duration	45 min	30-81 min

INTERACTIONS
Individual drugs
TraMADol: increased seizures, overdose

Adverse effects: *italics* = common; **bold** = life-threatening

Drug classifications
Analgesics (opioids): decreased effects of opioid analgesics

Drug/lab test
Interference: urine VMA, 5-HIAA, urine glucose

NURSING CONSIDERATIONS
Assessment
• **Assess for signs of opioid withdrawal** in drug-dependent individuals: cramping, hypertension, anxiety, vomiting; may occur up to 2 hr after administration
• Monitor VS q3-5min; ABGs including Po_2, Pco_2
• Assess cardiac status: tachycardia, hypertension; monitor ECG
• **Assess for pain:** duration, intensity, location before, after administration; may be used for respiratory depression
• **Assess for respiratory dysfunction: respiratory depression, character, rate, rhythm; if respirations are <10/min, probably due to opioid overdose, administer naloxone; monitor LOC**

Patient/family education
• Explain reason for and expected results of medication when patient is alert

Evaluation
Positive therapeutic outcome
• Reversal of respiratory depression
• LOC: alert

---

naphazoline ophthalmic
See Appendix B

---

naproxen
(na-prox′en)
Aleve, Anaprox, Anaprox DS, Apo-Napro-Na ✦, Midol Extended Relief, Nu-Naprox ✦, TH Naproxen
Func. class.: Nonsteroidal antiinflammatory, nonopioid analgesic
Chem. class.: Propionic acid derivative
Pregnancy category B (1st trimester), D (2nd/3rd trimesters) ✷

Do not confuse: Naprosyn/Natacyn/Naprelan

ACTION: Completely inhibits COX-1, COX-2 by blocking arachidonate; analgesic, antiinflammatory, antipyretic

Therapeutic outcome: Decreased pain, inflammation

USES: Mild to moderate pain, osteoarthritis, rheumatoid arthritis, gouty arthritis, primary dysmenorrhea, tendinitis, ankylosing spondylitis, bursitis, myalgia, dental pain, juvenile rheumatoid arthritis

CONTRAINDICATIONS
Pregnancy **C** (2nd/3rd trimesters), hypersensitivity to NSAIDs, salicylates

> **BLACK BOX WARNING:** Perioperative pain in CABG surgery

Precautions: Pregnancy **C** (1st trimester), breastfeeding, children <2 yr, geriatric, bleeding disorders, GI/cardiac disorders, hypersensitivity to other antiinflammatory agents, CCr <30 ml/min, asthma, renal failure, hepatic disease

> **BLACK BOX WARNING:** MI, GI bleeding, stroke

DOSAGE AND ROUTES
200 mg base = 220 mg naproxen sodium

Antiinflammatory/analgesic/antidysmenorrheal
Adult: PO 250-500 mg bid, max 1250 mg/day; DEL REL TAB 375-500 mg bid
Child ≥2 yr: PO 7 mg/kg/12 hr

Antigout
Adult: PO 750 mg, then 250 mg q8hr

OTC use
Adult: PO 220 mg q8-12hr or 440 mg, then 220 mg q12hr, max 660 mg/24 hr, taken no longer than 10 days
Geriatric >65 yr: PO max 220 mg q12hr

Available forms: Naproxen: tabs: 250, 375, 500 mg; del rel tabs (EC-Naprosyn, Naprosyn-E) 250✦, 375, 500 mg; oral susp 125 mg/5 ml; ext rel tabs (CR) 375, 500, 750 mg✦; **naproxen sodium;** tabs 220, 275, 550 mg; ext rel tab 220 mg

Implementation
• Store at room temp
• Administer to patient crushed or whole **(regular release)**; do not crush, break, or chew **extended rel tab**
• Give OTC for 10 days or less unless approved by prescriber
• Adequately hydrate those taking angiotensin receptor blockers/angiotensin-converting enzyme inhibitors
• Give with food or milk to decrease gastric symptoms; give ½ hr before or 2 hr after meals for better absorption
• Patient should take with 8 oz of water and sit upright for 30 min after dose to prevent ulceration

---

ADVERSE EFFECTS

CNS: Dizziness, drowsiness, fatigue, tremors, confusion, insomnia, anxiety, depression
CV: Tachycardia, peripheral edema, palpitations, **dysrhythmias, MI, stroke**
EENT: Tinnitus, hearing loss, blurred vision
GI: Nausea, anorexia, vomiting, diarrhea, jaundice, **hepatitis**, constipation, flatulence, cramps, peptic ulcer, **GI ulceration, bleeding, perforation**
GU: *Nephrotoxicity: dysuria, hematuria, oliguria, azotemia*
HEMA: *Blood dyscrasias*
INTEG: Purpura, rash, pruritus, sweating
SYST: *Anaphylaxis, Stevens-Johnson syndrome*

Pharmacokinetics

Absorption	Completely absorbed
Distribution	Crosses placenta, 99% protein binding
Metabolism	Liver, extensively
Excretion	Breast milk
Half-life	10-20 hr

Pharmacodynamics

Onset	1 hr
Peak	2-4 hr
Duration	<7 hr

INTERACTIONS
Individual drugs

Adefovir, cidofovir: increased nephrotoxicity, avoid concurrent use
Alcohol, aspirin: increased risk of GI side effects
Clopidogrel, eptifibatide, plicamycin, ticlopidine, tirofiban: increased bleeding risk
Lithium, methotrexate, probenecid, radiation: increased toxicity
Cholestyramine, sucralfate: decreased/delayed absorption of naproxen

Drug classifications

ACE inhibitors: possible renal impairment
Antacids: decreased/delayed absorption of naproxen
Anticoagulants, SSRIs, SNRIs, thrombolytics, tricyclics: increased risk of bleeding
Antihypertensives: decreased effect of antihypertensives
Antineoplastics: increased risk of hematologic toxicity
Corticosteroids, NSAIDs: increased risk of GI adverse reactions
Diuretics: decreased effectiveness of diuretics

Drug/herb

Fenugreek, feverfew, garlic, ginger, ginkgo, ginseng *(Panax),* licorice: increased bleeding risk

Drug/lab test

Increased: BUN, alkaline phosphatase, LFTs, potassium, glucose, cholesterol
Decreased: potassium, sodium
False: increased 5-HIAA, 17KS

NURSING CONSIDERATIONS
Assessment

> **BLACK BOX WARNING: Cardiac status:** CV thrombotic events, MI, stroke; may be fatal; not to be used in CABG

> **BLACK BOX WARNING: GI status:** ulceration, bleeding, perforation; may be fatal

• Monitor liver function, renal function, other blood tests: AST, ALT, bilirubin, creatinine, BUN, CBC, Hct, Hgb, pro-time, LDH, blood glucose, WBC, platelets; if patient is on long-term therapy
• Check I&O ratio; decreasing output may indicate renal failure (long-term therapy)
• **Assess hepatotoxicity: dark urine, clay-colored stools, yellowing of the skin and sclera, itching, abdominal pain, fever, diarrhea if patient is on long-term therapy**
• Assess for allergic reactions: rash, urticaria; if these occur, product may have to be discontinued
• **Assess for ototoxicity:** tinnitus, ringing, roaring in ears; audiometric testing needed before, after long-term therapy
• Assess for vision changes: blurring, halos if taking long term; may indicate corneal, retinal damage
• Check for edema in feet, ankles, legs
• Identify prior product history; there are many product interactions
• **Monitor pain:** location, frequency, duration, characteristics, type, intensity before dose and 1 hour after
• **Arthritis:** Assess ROM, pain, swelling before and 1-2 hr after use
• **Fever:** Assess before use and 1 hr after use
• Assess for asthma, aspirin hypersensitivity, or nasal polyps, increased risk of hypersensitivity

Patient/family education

• Teach patient to report any symptoms of renal/hepatic toxicity, vision changes, ototoxicity, allergic reactions, bleeding (long-term therapy); to report use to all health care providers, **signs of MI, stroke**

- Caution patient not to exceed recommended dosage; acute poisoning may result; to take as prescribed, do not double dose
- Teach patient to read label on other OTC products; many contain other antiinflammatories; caution patient to avoid alcohol ingestion; GI bleeding may occur
- Inform patient that the therapeutic response takes 2 wk (arthritis)
- Teach patient to report tinnitus, confusion, diarrhea, sweating, hyperventilation, blurred vision, fever, joint aches, black stools, flulike symptoms
- **Teach patient to notify prescriber if pregnancy is planned or suspected, pregnancy (C), avoid breastfeeding**

Evaluation

Positive therapeutic outcome
- Decreased pain
- Decreased inflammation
- Increased mobility

---

naratriptan (Rx)

(nair'ah-trip-tan)

Amerge

Func. class.: Antimigraine agent

Chem. class.: 5-HT₁-like receptor agonist

Pregnancy category C

Do not confuse: Amerge/Altace/Amaryl

ACTION: Binds selectively to the vascular 5-HT$_1$ receptor subtype, exerts antimigraine effect; causes vasoconstriction in cranial arteries

Therapeutic outcome: Decreased intensity and incidence of migraines

USES: Acute treatment of migraine with or without aura

CONTRAINDICATIONS

Angina pectoris, history of MI, documented silent ischemia, ischemic heart disease, concurrent ergotamine-containing preparations, uncontrolled hypertension, hypersensitivity, severe renal disease (CCr <15 ml/min), severe hepatic disease (Child-Pugh grade C), CV syndromes, hemiplegic or basilar migraines

Precautions: Pregnancy C, breastfeeding, children, geriatric, postmenopausal women, men >40 yr, risk factors for CAD, hypercholesterolemia, obesity, diabetes, impaired renal/hepatic function, peripheral vascular disease

DOSAGE AND ROUTES

Adult: PO 1 or 2.5 mg with fluids; if headache returns, repeat once after 4 hr, max 5 mg/24 hr

Renal/hepatic dose

Adult: PO CCr 15-39 ml/min Max 2.5 mg/24 hr

Available forms: Tabs 1, 2.5 mg

Implementation

- Do not use product if another 5-HT$_1$ agonist or an ergot preparation has been used in past 24 hr
- Give with fluids as soon as symptoms appear; may take another dose after 4 hr; max 5 mg in any 24-hr period
- Provide a quiet, calm environment with decreased stimulation, including noise, bright light, excessive talking

ADVERSE EFFECTS

CNS: Dizziness, sedation, fatigue

CV: Increased B/P, palpitations, tachydysrhythmias, PR and QT$_C$ prolongation, ST/T wave changes, PVCs, atrial flutter, fibrillation, coronary vasospasm

EENT: EENT infections, photophobia

GI: *Nausea, vomiting*

MISC: Temp change sensations, tightness, pressure sensations

MS: *Weakness, neck stiffness,* myalgia

Pharmacokinetics

Absorption	Unknown
Distribution	28%-31% protein binding
Metabolism	Liver (metabolite)
Excretion	Urine/feces
Half-life	6 hr

Pharmacodynamics

Onset	Unknown
Peak	2-3 hr
Duration	Unknown

INTERACTIONS

Individual drugs

Sibutramine: increased serotonin syndrome risk

Drug classifications

5-HT$_1$ agonists, ergot derivatives: increased vasospastic effect

MAOIs: increased risk of adverse reactions, do not use together

SSRIs (FLUoxetine, fluvoxaMINE, PARoxetine, sertraline), SNRIs, serotonin receptor agonists, sibutramine: increased serotonin syndrome, neuroleptic malignant syndrome

Drug/herb

SAMe, St. John's wort: increased serotonin syndrome

NURSING CONSIDERATIONS
Assessment
• Serotonin syndrome, neuroleptic malignant syndrome: assess for increased heart rate, shivering, sweating, dilated pupils, tremors, high B/P, hyperthermia, headache, confusion; if these occur, stop product, administer a serotonin antagonist if needed; at least 2 wk should elapse between discontinuing serotoninergic agents and starting this product
• **Migraines:** assess for aura, duration, effect of lifestyle, aggravating/alleviating factors
• Cardiac status: ECG, increased B/P, dysrhythmias, monitor for PR, QT prolongation, ST-T wave changes, PVCs in those with cardiac disease
• Assess for stress level, activity, recreation, coping mechanisms
• Assess neurologic status: LOC, blurred vision, nausea, tics preceding headache

Patient/family education
• Teach patient to report pain, tightness in chest, neck, throat, or jaw; notify prescriber immediately if sudden, severe abdominal pain occurs
• Teach patient to use contraception while taking product, to notify prescriber if pregnancy is planned or suspected
• Teach patient not to use if another 5-HT$_1$ agonist or an ergot preparation has been used in the past 24 hr; avoid using >2 days/wk, rebound headache may occur

Evaluation
Positive therapeutic outcome
• Absence of migraine headaches

natamycin ophthalmic
See Appendix B

nebivolol (Rx)
(ne-biv'oh-lol)
Bystolic
Func. class.: Antihypertensive
Chem. class.: β$_1$-Blocker
Pregnancy category C

ACTION: Competitively blocks stimulation of β-adrenergic receptors within vascular smooth muscle; decreases rate of SA node discharge, increases recovery time, slows conduction of AV node resulting in decreased heart rate (negative chronotropic effect), which decreases O$_2$ consumption in myocardium due to β$_1$-receptor antagonism; also decreases renin-aldosterone-angiotensin system at high doses, inhibits β$_2$-receptors in bronchial system (high doses)

Therapeutic outcome: Decreased B/P after 1-2 wk

USES: Hypertension alone or in combination
Unlabeled uses: Heart failure

CONTRAINDICATIONS
Cardiogenic shock, acute sick sinus syndrome, AV heart block, hypersensitivity to this agent or β-blockers, heart failure, severe hepatic disease, severe bradycardia

Precautions: Pregnancy C, breastfeeding, children, major surgery, peripheral vascular disease, diabetes mellitus, thyrotoxicosis, COPD, asthma, well-compensated heart failure, renal/hepatic disease, abrupt discontinuation, acute bronchospasm

DOSAGE AND ROUTES
Hypertension
Adult: PO 5 mg/day, may be increased to desired response q2wk; max 40 mg/day
Geriatric: PO max 40 mg/day

Renal dose
Adult: PO CCr <30 ml/min, 2.5 mg/day; may increase cautiously

Hepatic dose
Adult: PO (Child-Pugh class B) 2.5 mg qd; use dose escalation cautiously

Heart failure (unlabeled)
Adult: PO 1.25 mg titrated to max 10 mg/day

Available forms: Tabs 2.5, 5, 10, 20 mg

Implementation
PO route
• Give without regard for meals; tab may be crushed or swallowed whole; give with food to prevent GI upset
• Taper over 1-2 wk when discontinuing; minimize physical exertion; if angina recurs give nebivolol
• Store protected from light, moisture; place in cool environment

ADVERSE EFFECTS
CNS: *Insomnia, fatigue, dizziness, mental changes,* drowsiness, *headache*
CV: **Bradycardia, MI,** AV heart block, edema
GI: *Nausea, diarrhea,* vomiting, abdominal pain
GU: *Impotence*
HEMA: **Thrombocytopenia**
INTEG: Rash, pruritus, vasculitis, urticaria, psoriasis, **angioedema**
MISC: **Renal failure, pulmonary edema,** hyperuricemia, hypercholesterolemia, withdrawal symptoms
RESP: **Bronchospasm,** dyspnea

Absorption	Unknown
Distribution	Unknown
Metabolism	In liver by CYP2D6
Excretion	38% excreted in urine, 44% in feces
Half-life	12 hr

Pharmacodynamics

Onset	Unknown
Peak	1.5-4 hr
Duration	Unknown

INTERACTIONS
Individual drugs
Cimetidine: increased nebivolol action
Mefloquine: do not give
Sildenafil: decreased nebivolol action

Drug classifications
β-blockers, others: do not use concurrently
Calcium channel blockers (nondihydropyri-
dine), CYP2D6 inhibitors (amiodarone, bu-
PROPion, chloroquine, chlorpheniramine,
chlorproMAZINE, cinacalcet, diphenhydrA-
MINE, DULoxetine, FLUoxetine, haloperidol,
imatinib, PARoxetine, promethazine, propoxyphene, quiNIDine, quiNINE, ritonavir, terbinafine, thioridazine): increased nebivolol action
CYP2D6 inducers (rifampin): decreased nebivolol action

Drug/herb
Hawthorn: may increase nebivolol effect
Ephedra: decreased nebivolol effect

Drug/lab test
Increased: serum lipoprotein levels, BUN, potassium, triglyceride, uric acid, LDH, AST, ALT,
alkaline phosphatase
Decreased: platelets

NURSING CONSIDERATIONS
Assessment
• **Hypertension:** monitor B/P during beginning treatment, periodically thereafter; assess
apical/radial pulse before administration; notify
prescriber of any significant changes (pulse
<50 bpm); **signs of CHF** (dyspnea, crackles,
weight gain, jugular vein distention)
• Assess baselines in renal/hepatic studies
before therapy begins and periodically, do not
use in Child-Pugh class >B
• Monitor I&O, edema in feet, legs daily
• Monitor skin turgor, dryness of mucous membranes for hydration status, especially geriatric
patients
• Assess blood glucose in diabetics

Patient/family education
⚠ Caution patient not to discontinue product abruptly; severe cardiac reactions may
occur; taper over 2 wk; do not double dose;
if a dose is missed, take as soon as remembered up to 4 hr before next dose
• Inform patient product may mask signs of
hypoglycemia or alter blood glucose levels
• Advise patient not to use OTC products containing α-adrenergic stimulants (such as nasal
decongestants, OTC cold preparations) unless
directed by prescriber
• Instruct patient to report low pulse, dizziness,
confusion, depression, fever
• Teach patient to take pulse, B/P at home;
advise when to notify prescriber
• Advise patient to comply with weight control,
dietary adjustments, modified exercise program
• Instruct patient to carry emergency ID to
identify product, allergies
• Caution patient to avoid hazardous activities if
dizziness, drowsiness are present
• **Instruct patient to report symptoms of
CHF:** difficulty breathing, especially on exertion
or when lying down, night cough, swelling of
extremities
• Teach patient to continue with required lifestyle changes (exercise, diet, weight loss, stress
reduction)

Evaluation
Positive therapeutic outcome
• Decreased B/P after 1-2 wk
• Decreased dysrhythmias

TREATMENT OF OVERDOSE:
Lavage, **IV** atropine for bradycardia, **IV** theophylline for bronchospasm, digoxin, O₂, diuretic for
cardiac failure, **IV** glucose for hypoglycemia, **IV**
diazepam (or phenytoin) for seizures, **IV** fluids,
IV pressors

---

nelfinavir (Rx)
(nell-fin′a-veer)
Viracept
Func. class.: Antiretroviral
Chem. class.: Protease inhibitor
Pregnancy category B

ACTION: Inhibits HIV-1 protease, which
prevents maturation of the infectious virus

USES: HIV-1 in combination with other antiretrovirals

CONTRAINDICATIONS
Hypersensitivity to protease inhibitors

Precautions: Pregnancy **B,** breastfeeding, hemophilia, PKU, renal/hepatic disease, pancreatitis, diabetes, infection

DOSAGE AND ROUTES
HIV infection
Adult and child >13 yr: PO 750 mg tid or 1250 mg bid, max 2500 mg/day
Child 2-13 yr: PO 25-30 mg/kg tid, max 2500 mg/day

Prevention of HIV infection after exposure (unlabeled)
Adult: PO 1250 mg bid with two other antiretroviral agents $\times$ 4 wk

Available forms: Tabs 250, 625 mg; oral powder 50 mg/g/scoop

Implementation
• Administer with food
• Oral powder can be mixed with fluids; do not mix with juice or acidic fluids; stable mixed for 6 hr, may use in child unable to take tabs; do not mix with water in original bottle

ADVERSE EFFECTS
CNS: Headache, asthenia, poor concentration, seizures, suicidal ideation
CV: Bleeding
ENDO: Hyperglycemia, hyperlipidemia
GI: Diarrhea, nausea, anorexia, dyspepsia, *flatulence,* hepatitis, pancreatitis
HEMA: Anemia, leukopenia, thrombocytopenia, Hgb abnormalities
INTEG: Rash, dermatitis, anaphylaxis
MS: Pain, arthralgia, myalgia, myopathy
OTHER: Hypoglycemia, redistribution/accumulation of body fat, immune reconstitution syndrome

Pharmacokinetics

Absorption	Unknown
Distribution	98% protein binding
Metabolism	Liver (minimal)
Excretion	Feces/urine
Half-life	3½-5 hr

Pharmacodynamics

Onset	Unknown
Peak	2-4 hr
Duration	Unknown

INTERACTIONS
Individual drugs
Amiodarone, lovastatin, midazolam, pimozide, quiNIDine, salmeterol, simvastatin, triazolam: increased serious dysrhythmias

Alfentanil, alosetron, atorvastatin, azithromycin, bortezomib, buprenorphine, busPIRone, cilostazol, cycloSPORINE, disopyramide, DOCEtaxel, dofetilide, donepezil, ethosuximide, fentaNYL, galantamine, gefitinib, halofantrine, indinavir, levomethadyl, systemic lidocaine, PACLitaxel, rifabutin, saquinavir, sibutramine, sildenafil, sirolimus, SUFentanil, tacrolimus, traZODone, ziprasidone, zonisamide: increased effect of each product

CarBAMazepine, nevirapine, PHENobarbital, phenytoin, rifamycin: decreased nelfinavir levels

Delavirdine: increased protease inhibitor levels

Didanosine, methadone, phenytoin: decreased effect

Indinavir, ketoconazole, ritonavir: increased nelfinavir levels

Drug classifications
Calcium channel blockers, tricyclic antidepressants, vinca alkaloids: increased effects
Contraceptives (oral): decreased effect
Ergots: increased serious dysrhythmias
HIV protease inhibitors: increased protease inhibitor levels

Drug/herb
St. John's wort: decreased antiretroviral effect, do not use concurrently

Drug/food
Increased: absorption with food

Drug/lab test
Increased: AST, ALT, alkaline phosphatase, total bilirubin, CPK, LDH, lipids, uric acid
Decreased: WBC, platelets

NURSING CONSIDERATIONS
Assessment
• Assess resistance testing at initiation and failure of treatment
• Assess signs of infection, anemia
• Monitor liver function tests: ALT, AST
• Assess bowel pattern before, during treatment; if severe abdominal pain with bleeding occurs, product should be discontinued; monitor hydration
• Anaphylaxis, hypersensitivity reaction: assess for wheezing, flushing, swelling of lips, tongue, throat, skin eruptions, rash, urticaria, itching
• HIV: Monitor blood studies: serum lipid profile, plasma HIV RNA, blood glucose, viral load, CD4 cell counts baseline, throughout treatment
• Immune reconstitution syndrome: occurs with combination therapy; includes MAC, CMV, PCP, TB that require treatment

• **Phenylketonuria:** powder contains phenylalanine

Patient/family education
• Advise patient to take with meal or snack; if dose is missed, take as soon as remembered up to 1 hr before next dose; do not double dose
• Advise patient to avoid taking with other medications, unless directed by prescriber
• Teach patient that diarrhea is the most common side effect; may use loperamide to control
• Teach patient that product does not cure, but manages symptoms; does not prevent transmission of HIV to others
• Teach patient to use nonhormonal form of contraception while taking this product if using contraceptives
• Teach to report symptoms of hyperglycemia

Evaluation
Positive therapeutic outcome
• Decreasing symptoms of HIV
• Improving viral load and CD4 cell counts

nepafenac ophthalmic
See Appendix B

⚠ HIGH ALERT
nesiritide (Rx)
(nes-eer′ih-tide)
Natrecor
Func. class.: Vasodilator
Chem. class.: Human B-type natriuretic peptide
Pregnancy category C

ACTION: Uses DNA technology; human B-type natriuretic peptide binds to the receptor in vascular smooth muscle and endothelial cells, leading to smooth muscle relaxation

Therapeutic outcome: Improvement in symptoms of CHF

USES: Acutely decompensated CHF

CONTRAINDICATIONS
Hypersensitivity to this product or *E. coli* protein, cardiogenic shock or B/P <90 mm Hg as primary therapy

Precautions: Pregnancy **C,** breastfeeding, children, mitral stenosis; significant valvular stenosis, restriction, or obstructive cardiomyopathy, or any condition that depends on venous return; renal disease, constrictive pericarditis

DOSAGE AND ROUTES
Adult: BOL **IV** 2 mcg/kg, then CONT **IV** INF 0.01 mcg/kg/min

Available forms: Powder for inj, 1.5 mg single-use vial

Implementation
IV route
• Do not administer nesiritide through a central heparin-coated catheter; heparin should be administered through a separate catheter
• Reconstitute one 1.5 mg vial/5 ml of diluent from prefilled 250 ml plastic **IV** bag with diluent of choice (D₅, 0.9% NaCl, D₅/0.9% NaCl, D₅/0.2% NaCl); do not shake vial, roll gently; use only clear sol
• Withdraw all contents of reconstituted vial and add to the 250-ml plastic **IV** bag (6 mcg/ml); invert bag several times
• Use within 24 hr of reconstituting
Direct IV route
• Prime tubing with 5 ml of inf sol, calculate dose based on patients' weight, 0.33 × patient weight (kg) = bolus vol (ml) (6 mcg/ml), withdraw prescribed bolus dose (volume) from prepared inf bag; give over 1 min through IV port
Intermittent IV INF route
• After bolus dose, use inf, give at 0.1 ml/kg/hr (0.01 mcg/kg/min)

Y-site compatibilities: Acyclovir, alfentanil, allopurinol, amifostine, aminocaproic acid, aminophylline, amiodarone, amphotericin B colloidal, amphotericin B lipid complex, amphotericin B liposome, anidulafungin, argatroban, atenolol, atracurium, azithromycin, aztreonam, bivalirudin, bleomycin, buprenorphine, busulfan, butorphanol, calcium acetate/chloride/gluconate, CARBOplatin, carmustine, ceFAZolin, cefotaxime, cefoTEtan, cefOXitin, cefTAZidime, ceftizoxime, cefTRIAXone, cefuroxime, chloramphenicol, cimetidine, ciprofloxacin, cisatracurium, CISplatin, clindamycin, cyclophosphamide, cycloSPORINE, cytarabine, dacarbazine, DACTINomycin, DAUNOrubicin, digoxin, diltiazem, diphenhydrAMINE, DOCEtaxel, dolasetron, doxacurium, DOXOrubicin, doxycycline, droperidol, ePHEDrine, epirubicin, ertapenem, erythromycin, esmolol, etoposide, etoposide phosphate, famotidine, fenoldopam, fentaNYL, filgrastim, fluconazole, fludarabine, fluorouracil, foscarnet, fosphenytoin, ganciclovir, gatifloxacin, gemcitabine, gemtuzumab, glycopyrrolate, granisetron, haloperidol, hydrocortisone, HYDROmorphone, hydrOXYzine, IDArubicin, ifosfamide, imipenem-cilastatin, irinotecan, ketorolac, leucovorin, levofloxacin, lidocaine, linezolid, LORazepam, magnesium sulfate, mannitol, mechlorethamine, melphalan, meropenem, mesna, metaraminol, methohexital, methotrexate, methylPREDNISolone, metoclopramide, metroNIDAZOLE, midazolam, milrinone, minocycline, mitoMYcin, mitoXANtrone, mivacurium, moxifloxacin, mycophenolate, nalbuphine, naloxone, niCARdipine, nitroglycerin, nitroprusside, octreotide, ondansetron, oxaliplatin, oxytocin, PACLitaxel, palonosetron, pamidronate, pancuronium, PEMEtrexed, pentamidine, PENTobarbital, PHENobarbital, phentolamine, phenylephrine, polymyxin B sulfate, potassium chloride/phosphates, prochlorperazine, propranolol, quiNIDine, quinupristin-dalfopristin, ranitidine, remifentanil, rocuronium, sodium acetate/bicarbonate/phosphates, streptozocin, succinylcholine, SUFentanil, tacrolimus, teniposide, theophylline, thiotepa, ticarcillin, tigecycline, tirofiban, tolazoline, topotecan, torsemide, trimethobenzamide, vancomycin, vasopressin, vecuronium, verapamil, vinBLAStine, vinCRIStine, vinorelbine, zidovudine, zoledronic acid

ADVERSE EFFECTS

CNS: Headache, insomnia, dizziness, anxiety, confusion, paresthesia, tremor
CV: *Hypotension,* tachycardia, dysrhythmias, bradycardia, ventricular tachycardia, ventricular extrasystoles, atrial fibrillation
GI: Vomiting, nausea
INTEG: Rash, sweating, pruritus, inj site reaction
MISC: Back pain, abdominal pain
RESP: Increased cough, hemoptysis, apnea

Pharmacokinetics

Absorption	Vascular smooth muscle and endothelial cells
Distribution	Unknown
Metabolism	Unknown
Excretion	Bound to cell surfaces, internalized, and proteolyzed; cleaved by endopeptidases on vascular lumenal surface; renal filtration
Half-life	18 min

Pharmacodynamics

Onset	15 min
Peak	1 hr
Duration	Unknown

INTERACTIONS
Drug classifications
ACE inhibitors, antihypertensives, **IV** nitrates: increased symptomatic hypotension

NURSING CONSIDERATIONS
Assessment
• Assess PCWP, RAP, cardiac index, MPAP, respiratory rate, CUP, B/P, pulse during treatment until stable
• Monitor I&O, daily weight, serum creatinine, BUN
• **Assess for CHF:** weight gain, dyspnea, crackles, I&O ratios, peripheral edema
• **Allergic reactions to peptides: rash, pruritis, wheezing; discontinue immediately; keep emergency equipment available**

Patient/family education
• Explain purpose of medication and expected results, allergic reaction
• Instruct patient to report pain at IV site

Evaluation
Positive therapeutic outcome
• Improvement in CHF with improved PCWP, RAP, MPAP

---

nevirapine (Rx)
(ne-veer′a-peen)
Viramune, Viramune XR
Func. class.: Antiretroviral
Chem. class.: Non-nucleoside reverse transcriptase inhibitor (NNRTI)
Pregnancy category B

Do not confuse: nevirapine/nelfinavir, Viramune/Viracept

ACTION: Binds directly to reverse transcriptase and blocks RNA, DNA, causing a disruption of the enzyme's site

Therapeutic outcome: Improvement of HIV-1 infection

USES: HIV-1 in combination with other highly active antiretroviral treatments (HAART)

CONTRAINDICATIONS

> **BLACK BOX WARNING:** Hypersensitivity, hepatic disease

Precautions: Pregnancy **B,** breastfeeding, children, renal disease, Hispanic patients

> **BLACK BOX WARNING:** Females, hepatitis

DOSAGE AND ROUTES
Treatment of HIV infection in combination with other antiretrovirals
Adult and adolescent: PO 200 mg/day × 2 wk, then 200 mg bid in combination; ext rel tab (adults not currently taking immediate release

nevirapine) 200 mg/day (immediate rel tab) × 14 days with other antiretrovirals; if rash develops during lead-in period and persists beyond 14 days, do not use ext rel tab; if no consistent rash is present then give 400 mg/day ext rel tab with other antiretrovirals; if interrupted > 7 days, restart 14-day lead-in dosing; adults switched from immediate-release tab, 400 mg/day ext rel tab
Neonate ≥15 days old/infant/child: PO 150 mg/m²/day × 14 days, then 150 mg/m² bid; max 400 mg/day

Perinatal transmission prophylaxis (unlabeled)
Females with no previous antiretroviral therapy: PO 200 mg as a single dose at onset of labor with zidovudine 2 mg/kg over 1 hr followed by zidovudine 1 mg/kg/hr until delivery
Neonate ≥34 wk gestation: PO nevirapine 2 mg/kg as a single dose at age 48-72 hr and PO zidovudine 2 mg/kg q6hr for 6 wk

Hepatic dose
Adult: PO do not use in Child-Pugh B or C

Available forms: Tabs 200 mg; oral susp 50 mg/5 ml; ext rel tabs: 400 mg

Implementation
• **Do not initiate treatment in females when CD4 counts >250 cells/mm³, or in males when >400 cells/mm³ unless benefit outweighs risks**
• Give without regard to meals
• Use in combination with at least 1 other antiretroviral
• Give at equal intervals around the clock to maintain blood levels

ADVERSE EFFECTS
CNS: *Paresthesia, headache, fever, peripheral neuropathy*
GI: *Diarrhea,* abdominal pain, *nausea, stomatitis,* hepatotoxicity, hepatic failure
HEMA: Neutropenia, anemia, thrombocytopenia
INTEG: *Rash,* toxic epidermal necrolysis
MISC: Stevens-Johnson syndrome, anaphylaxis
MS: Pain, myalgia, rhabdomyolysis

Pharmacokinetics
Absorption	Rapid
Distribution	Protein binding 60%
Metabolism	Liver, by P450 enzyme system
Excretion	91% urine
Half-life	25-30 hr 50% removed by peritoneal dialysis; slower clearance rate in Hispanics, African Americans

Pharmacodynamics
Onset	Unknown
Peak	4 hr
Duration	Unknown

INTERACTIONS
Individual drugs
Cimetidine: increased nevirapine levels
ClonazePAM, diazepam, warfarin: decreased nevirapine level
Itraconazole: decreased effect of itraconazole
Ketoconazole: decreased effect of ketoconazole
Methadone: decreased effect of methadone

Drug classifications
Anticonvulsants, rifamycins: decreased nevirapine levels
Antiinfectives, macrolides: increased nevirapine levels
Oral contraceptives, protease inhibitors: decreased action

Drug/herb
St. John's wort: decreased nevirapine levels, do not use together

Drug/lab test
Increased: ALT, AST, GGT, bilirubin, Hgb
Decreased: neutrophil count

NURSING CONSIDERATIONS
Assessment
• Use resistance testing before starting and when therapy fails
• **Assess signs of infection,** anemia, hepatotoxicity, immune reconstitution syndrome
• **HIV:** Assess liver, renal, blood tests: ALT, AST, viral load, CD4, plasma HIV RNA, glucose levels in diabetic patients; if liver function tests are elevated significantly, product should be withheld; if treatment is interrupted by >1 wk, restart at initial dose
• Assess bowel pattern before, during treatment; if severe abdominal pain with bleeding occurs, product should be discontinued; monitor hydration
⚠ **Assess skin eruptions; rash, urticaria, itching; if rash is severe or systemic symptoms occur, discontinue immediately**
• Assess allergies before treatment, reaction to each medication
• **Rhabdomyolysis:** assess for pain, tenderness, weakness, edema; product should be discontinued
⚠ **Stevens-Johnson syndrome, toxic epidermal necrolysis, assess for allergies before treatment, reaction to each medication; skin eruptions; rash, urticaria, itching; if rash is severe or systemic symptoms occur, discontinue immediately**

Patient/family education
• Instruct patient to report immediately any right quadrant pain, yellowing of eyes/skin, dark urine, nausea, anorexia, muscle pain/tenderness, rash
• Inform patient that product may be taken with food, antacids
• Advise patient to take as prescribed; if dose is missed, take as soon as remembered up to 1 hr before next dose; do not double dose
• Advise patient that product must be taken in equal intervals around the clock to maintain blood levels for duration of therapy
• Advise patient that product is not a cure, controls symptoms of HIV, does not prevent transmission
• Instruct patient to avoid OTC agents unless approved by prescriber
• Advise patients who are using contraceptives to use a nonhormonal form of contraception during treatment

Evaluation
Positive therapeutic outcome
• Improving viral load and CD4 cell counts
• Absence of AIDS-defining symptoms
• Improvement in quality of life

RARELY USED
niacin (Rx, OTC)
(nye′a-sin)
Equaline Niacin, Niaspan, Ni-Odan ✿, Slo-Niacin
niacinamide (Rx, OTC)
(nye-a-sin′a-mide)
Func. class.: Vitamin B_3 lipid-lowering product
Chem. class.: Water-soluble vitamin
Pregnancy category C

Therapeutic outcome: Decreasing cholesterol and LDL levels, B_3 supplementation

USES: Pellagra, hyperlipidemias (types IV, V), peripheral vascular disease that presents a risk for pancreatitis

CONTRAINDICATIONS
Breastfeeding, hypersensitivity, peptic ulcer, hepatic disease, hemorrhage, severe hypotension

DOSAGE AND ROUTES
Niacin deficiency
Adult: PO 100-500 mg/day in divided doses; IM/SUBCUT 5-100 mg 5 or more times a day; IV 25-100 mg bid or tid
Child: PO up to 300 mg/day in divided doses

Adjunct in hyperlipidemia
Adult: 250 mg after evening meal, may increase dosage at 1-4 wk intervals to 1-2 g tid, max 6 g/day; ext rel 500 mg at bedtime, ×4 wk, then 1000 mg at bedtime for wk 5-8, do not increase by more than 500 mg q4wk, max 2000 mg/day

Pellagra
Adult: PO 300-500 mg/day in divided doses, IM 50-100 mg 5 ×/day or IV 25-100 mg bid by slow IV INF
Child: PO 100-300 mg/day in divided doses; IV up to 300 mg/day by slow IV/INF

Peripheral vascular disease (unlabeled)
Adult: PO 250-800 mg/day in 3-5 divided doses

niCARdipine (Rx)
(nye-card′i-peen)
Cardene, Cardene IV, Cardene SR
Func. class.: Calcium channel blocker, antianginal, antihypertensive
Chem. class.: Dihydropyridine
Pregnancy category C

Do not confuse: niCARdipine/NIFEdipine, Cardene/Cardizem, **Cardene SR**/Cardizem SR

ACTION: Inhibits calcium ion influx across cell membrane during cardiac depolarization, produces relaxation of coronary vascular smooth muscle and peripheral vascular smooth muscle, dilates coronary arteries, increases myocardial oxygen delivery in patients with vasospastic angina

Therapeutic outcome: Decreased angina pectoris, decreased B/P in hypertension

USES: Chronic stable angina pectoris, hypertension

CONTRAINDICATIONS
Sick sinus syndrome, 2nd- or 3rd-degree heart block, hypersensitivity to this product or dihydropyridine, advanced aortic stenosis

Precautions: Pregnancy **C**, breastfeeding, children, geriatric, CHF, hypotension, hepatic injury, renal disease

DOSAGE AND ROUTES
Hypertension
Adult: PO 20 mg tid initially; may increase after 3 days (range 20-40 mg tid) or SUS REL 30 mg bid; may increase to 60 mg bid **IV** 5 mg/hr; may increase by 2.5 mg/hr q15min; max 15 mg/hr

*Adverse effects: *italics* = common; **bold** = life-threatening*

Angina
Adult: PO 20 mg tid, may be adjusted q3day, may use 20-40 mg tid

Renal dose
Adult: PO 20 mg tid or SUS REL 30 mg bid

Hepatic dose
Adult: PO 20 mg bid

Available forms: Caps 20, 30 mg; sus rel caps 30, 45, 60 mg; inj 2.5 mg/ml, premixed 20 mg/200 ml, 40 mg/200 ml

Implementation
PO route
- Do not break, crush, chew, or open sus rel caps
- Give without regard to meals
- Store in airtight container at room temperature

IV route
- Dilute each 25 mg/240 ml of compatible sol (0.1 mg/ml), give slowly, titrate to patient's response, stable for 24 hr at room temperature, change IV site q12 hrs

Solution   compatibilities: D_5W, D_5/0.45% NaCl, D_5/0.9% NaCl

Y-site   compatibilities: Alemtuzumab, amikacin, aminophylline, aztreonam, bivalirudin, butorphanol, calcium gluconate, CARBOplatin, caspofungin, ceFAZolin, ceftizoxime, chloramphenicol, cimetidine, CISplatin, clindamycin, cytarabine, DAPTOmycin, dexmedetomidine, diltiazem, DOBUTamine, DOCEtaxel, DOPamine, DOXOrubicin hydrochloride, enalaprilat, EPINEPHrine, epirubicin, erythromycin, esmolol, famotidine, fenoldopam, fentaNYL, gentamicin, hydrocortisone, HYDROmorphone, labetalol, lidocaine, linezolid, LORazepam, magnesium sulfate, mechlorethamine, methylPREDNISolone, metroNIDAZOLE, midazolam, milrinone, morphine, nafcillin, nesiritide, nitroglycerin, nitroprusside, norepinephrine, octreotide, oxaliplatin, oxytocin, palonosetron, penicillin G potassium, potassium chloride/phosphate, quinupristin-dalfopristin, ranitidine, rocuronium, tacrolimus, tirofiban, tobramycin, trimethoprim/sulfamethoxazole, vancomycin, vasopressin, vecuronium, vinCRIStine, voriconazole, zoledronic acid

Y-site incompatibilities: Amphotericin B liposome/lipid complex, ampicillin, ampicillin/sulbactam, cefepime, cefoperazone, ertapenem, fluorouracil, furosemide, methotrexate, micafungin, pantoprazole, PEMEtrexed, thiopental, thiotepa, tigecycline

ADVERSE EFFECTS
CNS: *Headache, dizziness,* anxiety, depression, confusion, paresthesia, somnolence, *flushing*
CV: Edema, bradycardia, hypotension, palpitations, **pulmonary edema,** chest pain, tachycardia, increased angina, **arrhythmias, CHF**
GI: Nausea, vomiting, gastric upset, constipation, **hepatitis,** abdominal cramps, dry mouth, sore throat
GU: Nocturia, polyuria
INTEG: Rash, infusion site discomfort, **Stevens-Johnson syndrome**
MISC: Blurred vision, flushing, sweating, SOB, impotence

Pharmacokinetics

Absorption	Well absorbed (PO); bioavailability poor
Distribution	Unknown
Metabolism	Liver, extensively
Excretion	Kidneys 60%, feces 35%
Half-life	2-5 hr

Pharmacodynamics

	PO	PO SUS REL	IV
Onset	20 min	Unknown	1 min
Peak	1-2 hr		45 min
Duration	8 hr	10-12 hr	

INTERACTIONS
Individual drugs
Alcohol: increased hypotension
CarBAMazepine, cycloSPORIINE, prazosin, propranolol, quiNIDine: increased risk of toxicity
Cimetidine: increased niCARdipine effects
Digoxin, quiNIDine, theophylline: increased effects
Rifampin: decreased antihypertensive effect

Drug classifications
Antihypertensives, neuromuscular blocking agents, nitrates: increased hypotension
NSAIDs: decreased antihypertensive effect

Drug/herb
Ginkgo, ginseng, hawthorn: increased effect
Ephedra, melatonin, St. John's wort, yohimbe: decreased effect

Drug/food
Grapefruit juice: increased hypotensive effect

Drug/lab test
Increased: LFTs
Decreased: potassium (IV), phosphate, platelets

⚠ Nurse Alert   ✳ Key NCLEX® Drug   ≫ Drug Specifics

NURSING CONSIDERATIONS
Assessment
• Assess fluid volume status (I&O ratio) and record weight, color, quality, and specific gravity of urine, skin turgor, adequacy of pulses, moist mucous membranes, bilateral lung sounds, peripheral pitting edema; dehydration symptoms of decreasing output, thirst, hypotension, dry mouth, and mucous membranes should be reported
• **Monitor for CHF:** weight gain, crackles, jugular venous distention, dyspnea
• **Allergic reactions (Stevens-Johnson syndrome):** If rash is severe and accompanied by joint aches, mouth lesions, discontinue immediately
• **Hypertension:** assess for decreasing B/P; salt in diet, smoking, exercise, diet, weight, monitor B/P often
• **Assess anginal pain:** intensity, location, duration, alleviating factors
• Monitor potassium, renal/liver function tests, periodically

Patient/family education
• Advise patient to avoid hazardous activities until stabilized on product and dizziness is no longer a problem
• Instruct patient to limit caffeine consumption; to avoid alcohol and OTC products unless directed by a prescriber, to take without regard to food, avoid high-fat foods, to swallow sus rel product whole
⚠ **Hypertension: instruct patient to comply with all areas of medical regimen: diet, exercise, stress reduction, product therapy**
• Instruct patient to notify prescriber of irregular heartbeat, shortness of breath, swelling of feet and hands, pronounced dizziness, constipation, nausea, hypotension, change in severity/pattern/incidence of angina
• Teach patient to use medication as directed even if feeling better; may be taken with other cardiovascular products (nitrates, β-blockers)
• Teach patient to take medication exactly as prescribed
• Advise patient to contact prescriber if anginal attacks continue or become worse

Evaluation

Positive therapeutic outcome
• Decreased angina attacks
• Decreased B/P

TREATMENT OF OVERDOSE:
Defibrillation, atropine for AV block, vasopressor for hypotension

---

nicotinamide
See niacin

nicotine
(nik′o-teen)
nicotine chewing gum
Thrive
nicotine inhaler (OTC, Rx)
Nicotrol Inhaler
nicotine lozenge (OTC)
Commit, Nicorette
nicotine nasal spray (Rx)
Nicotrol NS
nicotine transdermal (OTC, Rx)
Nicoderm CQ
Func. class.: Smoking deterrent
Chem. class.: Ganglionic cholinergic agonist
Pregnancy category D (transdermal), C (gum)

ACTION: Agonist at nicotinic receptors in the peripheral and central nervous systems; acts at sympathetic ganglia, on chemoreceptors of the aorta and carotid bodies; also affects adrenaline-releasing catecholamines

Therapeutic outcome: Decreased withdrawal effects when smoking cessation is attempted

USES: Deter cigarette smoking

Unlabeled uses: Tourette's syndrome

CONTRAINDICATIONS
Pregnancy **D** (transdermal, inhaler), hypersensitivity, immediate post-MI recovery period, severe angina pectoris

Precautions: Pregnancy **C** (gum), breastfeeding, vasospastic disease, dysrhythmias, diabetes mellitus, hyperthyroidism, pheochromocytoma, coronary disease, esophagitis, peptic ulcer, renal/hepatic disease; MRI (patch); soy hypersensitivity (mint lozenge)

DOSAGE AND ROUTES
Nicotine chewing gum
Adult: If patient smokes ≤25 cigarettes/day, start with 2 mg gum; if >25 cigarettes/day, start with 4 mg gum; then 1 piece of gum q1-2hr × 6 wk, then 1 piece of gum q2-4hr × 2 wk, then 1 piece of gum q4-8hr × 2 wk, then discontinue; max 24/day

Nicotine inhaler
Adult: Inhale 6 cartridges/day for first 3-6 wk, max 16/day × 12 wk

---

Nicotine lozenge
Adult: If cigarette is desired >30 min after awakening, start with 1-2–mg lozenge; if <30 min after awakening, start with 4-mg lozenge; then 1 q1-2hr, max 20 lozenges/day or 5 lozenges/6 hr × 6 wk, then 1 lozenge q2-4hr × 2 wk, then 1 lozenge q4-8hr × 2 wk, then discontinue

Nicotine nasal spray
Adult: 1 spray in each nostril 1-2 ×/hr, max 5 ×/hr or 40 ×/day, max 3 mo

Nicotine transdermal/inhaler system

NicoDerm
Adult: 21 mg/day × 4-8 wk; 14 mg/day × 2-4 wk; 7 mg/day × 2-4 wk

Nicotrol
Adult: 15 mg/day × 12 wk; 10 mg/day × 2 wk; 5 mg/day × 2 wk

Nicotrol inhaler
Adult: Delivers 30% of what a smoker receives from an actual cigarette

Tourette's syndrome (unlabeled)
Adult and child: Chewing gum 2 mg chewed × ½ hr bid × 1-6 mo; transdermal 7 or 10 mg patch daily × 2 days

Available forms: Gum: 2, 4 mg/piece; nicotine transdermal system (NicoDerm, Nicotine Transdermal System); 7, 14, 21 mg/day delivered; (NicoDerm) 5, 10, 15 mg/day; nicotine inhaler: 4 mg delivered; nasal spray: 0.5 mg of nicotine/actuation; lozenge: 2 mg, 4 mg

Implementation
• Give only prescribed amount, or toxicity may occur
• **Gum:** chew gum slowly for 30 min to promote buccal absorption of the product; do not chew > 45 min
• Begin product withdrawal after 3 mo of use; do not exceed 6 mo
• **Transdermal patch:** apply once a day to a nonhairy, clean, dry area of skin on upper body or upper outer arm; rotate sites to prevent skin irritation
• **Inhaler:** puffing on mouthpiece delivers nicotine through the mouth

ADVERSE EFFECTS
CNS: Dizziness, vertigo, insomnia, headache, confusion, seizures, depression, euphoria, numbness, tinnitus, strange dreams
CV: Dysrhythmias, tachycardia, palpitations, edema, flushing, hypertension
EENT: Jaw ache, irritation in buccal cavity
GI: *Nausea, vomiting, anorexia, indigestion,* diarrhea, abdominal pain, constipation, eructation, irritation
RESP: Breathing difficulty, cough, hoarseness, sneezing, wheezing, bronchial spasm

Pharmacokinetics
Absorption	Slowly absorbed, buccal cavity
Distribution	Unknown
Metabolism	Liver; some by lungs, kidneys
Excretion	Kidneys, unchanged (20%); breast milk
Half-life	1-2 hr

Pharmacodynamics
Onset	Rapid
Peak	½ hr
Duration	Unknown

INTERACTIONS
Individual drugs
Bromocriptine, cabergoline: increased vasoconstriction
Adenosine: increased effects
BuPROPion: increased B/P
Insulin: decreased effect
Cimetidine: decreased nicotine clearance

Drug classifications
Ergots: increased vasoconstriction
α-Blockers: decreased effect

Drug/food
Acidic foods (colas, coffee): avoid use of gum with and for 15 min after

NURSING CONSIDERATIONS
Assessment
• **Assess for adverse reaction to gum:** irritation of buccal cavity, dislike of taste, jaw ache
• **Assess for withdrawal symptoms:** headache, fatigue, drowsiness, restlessness, irritability, severe cravings for nicotine products before, during, and after treatment
• **Smoking:** obtain a nicotine assessment: brand of cigarettes, chewing tobacco, cigars, number of each used per day; what increases need or activities performed when each is used
• Gum should not be used if temporomandibular condition exists
• Assess for nicotine toxicity: GI symptoms (nausea, vomiting, diarrhea), cardiopulmonary symptoms (decreased B/P, dyspnea, change in pulse), weakness, abdominal cramping, headache, blurred vision, tinnitus; product should be discontinued

Patient/family education
- Advise patient to begin product withdrawal after 3 mo use; max 6 mo
- Teach patient all aspects of product; give package insert to patient and explain; caution patient not to exceed prescribed dose
- Caution patient not to use during pregnancy; birth defects may occur

Gum
- Advise patient to chew gum slowly for 30 min to promote buccal absorption of the product; do not chew over 45 min
- Inform patient that gum will not stick to dentures, dental appliances
- Caution patient that gum is as toxic as cigarettes; it is to be used only to deter smoking

Transdermal patch
- Caution patient that patch is as toxic as cigarettes; to be used only to deter smoking
- Caution patient not to use during pregnancy; birth defects may occur
- Instruct patient to keep used and unused system out of reach of children and pets
- Instruct patient to apply once a day to a non-hairy, clean, dry area of skin on upper body or upper outer arm; to rotate sites to prevent skin irritation
- Instruct patient to stop smoking immediately when beginning patch treatment
- Teach patient to apply promptly after removing from protective pouch; system may lose strength
- **Nasal spray:** tilt head back, do not swallow or inhale during administration; after smoking is stopped, use spray up to 8 wk, then discontinue over 6 wk by tapering
- **Lozenges:** allow to dissolve, avoid swallowing
- **Inhalation:** use the inhaler for 20 min
- Advise patient that puffing on mouthpiece delivers nicotine through the mouth lining

Evaluation

Positive therapeutic outcome
- Decrease in urge to smoke
- Decreased need for gum after 3-6 mo

NIFEdipine (Rx)
(nye-fed′i-peen)
Adalat CC, Adalat XL ✦, Afeditab CR, Procardia, Procardia XL
Func. class.: Calcium channel blocker, antianginal, antihypertensive
Chem. class.: Dihydropyridine
Pregnancy category C

Do not confuse: NIFEdipine/niCARdipine/niMODipine

ACTION: Inhibits calcium ion influx across cell membrane during cardiac depolarization, produces relaxation of coronary vascular smooth muscle, dilates coronary vascular arteries, increases myocardial oxygen delivery in patients with vasospastic angina, dilates peripheral arteries

Therapeutic outcome: Decreased angina pectoris, decreased B/P in hypertension

USES: Chronic stable angina pectoris, variant angina, hypertension, migraine prophylaxis

CONTRAINDICATIONS
Hypersensitivity to this product or dihydropyridine, cardiogenic shock

Precautions: Pregnancy **C**, breastfeeding, children, hypotension, sick sinus syndrome, 2nd- or 3rd-degree heart block, hypotension less than 90 mm Hg systolic, hepatic injury, renal disease, acute MI, aortic stenosis, GERD, heart failure

DOSAGE AND ROUTES
Adult: PO immediate release, 10 mg tid; increase in 10-mg increments q7-14day, max 180 mg/24 hr or single dose of 30 mg; sus rel 30-60 mg/day; may increase q7-14day; doses >120 mg not recommended

Hypertension
Adult: PO ext rel 30-60 mg qd, titrate upward as needed; max 90 mg/day (Adalat CC); 120 mg/day (Procardia XL)
Adolescent/child (unlabeled): PO ext rel 0.25-0.5 mg/kg/day, max 3 mg/kg/day

Hiccups (unlabeled)
Adult: PO 10-20 mg tid

Available forms: Caps 10, 20 mg; ext rel tabs (CC, XL) 30, 60, 90 mg

Implementation
PO route
- Do not use immediate release caps within 7 days of MI, coronary syndrome
- Give without regard to meals
- Store in airtight container at room temperature
- Protect caps from direct light, keep in dry area, do not freeze

Sublingual route
- Using a sterile needle, puncture the cap and squeeze medication in buccal/sublingual area (not an FDA-approved use)

ADVERSE EFFECTS
CNS: *Headache*, fatigue, drowsiness, *dizziness*, anxiety, depression, weakness, insomnia,

N

light-headedness, paresthesia, tinnitus, blurred vision, nervousness, tremor, flushing
CV: Dysrhythmias, edema, hypotension, palpitations, tachycardia
GI: *Nausea,* vomiting, diarrhea, gastric upset, constipation, increased LFTs, dry mouth, flatulence, gingival hyperplasia
GU: Nocturia, polyuria
HEMA: Bruising, bleeding, petechiae
INTEG: Rash, pruritus, *flushing,* hair loss, Stevens-Johnson syndrome, toxic epidermal necrolysis, exfoliative dermatitis
MISC: Sexual difficulties, cough, fever, chills

Pharmacokinetics

Absorption	Well absorbed (PO)
Distribution	Protein binding 92%
Metabolism	Liver, extensively
Excretion	Unknown
Half-life	2-5 hr

Pharmacodynamics

	PO	PO EXT REL
Onset	20 min	Unknown
Peak	30 min-1 hr	6 hr
Duration	6-8 hr	24 hr

INTERACTIONS
Individual drugs
Cimetidine, ranitidine: increased risk of toxicity
CarBAMazepine, cycloSPORINE, phenytoin, prazosin, digoxin: increased levels of each product
QuiNIDine: decreased effects
Smoking: decreased NIFEdipine level

Drug classifications
Strong CYP3A4 inducers: use is contraindicated
Antihypertensives, β-adrenergic blockers: increased effects
NSAIDs: decreased antihypertensive effect

Drug/herb
Ginkgo biloba, ginseng, hawthorn: increased effect
Ephedra, melatonin, St. John's wort, yohimbe: decreased effect

Drug/food
Grapefruit juice: increased NIFEdipine level

Drug/lab test
Positive: ANA titer, direct Coombs' test
Increased: CPK, LDH, AST

NURSING CONSIDERATIONS
Assessment
• **Assess anginal pain:** location, intensity, duration, character, alleviating, aggravating factors
• Assess for bruising, petechiae, bleeding
• Monitor potassium, renal/liver function tests periodically during treatment; in those taking antihypertensives, beta blockers, monitor B/P often
• **Serious skin disorders: rash starts suddenly, assess for fever, cutaneous lesions, may have pustules; discontinue product**
• Assess fluid volume status (I&O ratio) and record weight, distended red veins, crackles in lung, color, quality, and specific gravity of urine, skin turgor, adequacy of pulses, moist mucous membranes, bilateral lung sounds, peripheral pitting edema; dehydration symptoms of decreasing output, thirst, hypotension, dry mouth, and mucous membranes should be reported
• Monitor cardiac status: B/P, pulse, respirations, ECG
⚠ **GI obstruction: ext rel products have been associated with rare reports of obstruction in those with strictures, and no known GI disease**

Patient/family education
• Advise patient to avoid hazardous activities until stabilized on product and dizziness is no longer a problem
• Instruct patient to limit caffeine consumption; to avoid alcohol and OTC products unless directed by prescriber
• Advise patient that empty tab shells may appear in stools and are not significant
• Give without regard to meals (exception: Adelat CC should be taken on empty stomach)
• **Hypertension:** instruct patient to comply in all areas of medical regimen: diet, exercise, stress reduction, product therapy
• Tell patient to notify prescriber of irregular heartbeat, SOB, swelling of feet and hands, pronounced dizziness, constipation, nausea, hypotension, severe rash, changes in pattern/frequency/severity of angina
• Teach patient to use as directed even if feeling better; may be taken with other cardiovascular products (nitrates, β-blockers)
• Advise patient to increase fluid intake to prevent constipation
• Teach patient to check for gingival hyperplasia and report promptly
• Teach patient not to discontinue abruptly; gradually taper

Evaluation
Positive therapeutic outcome
• Decreased angina attacks
• Decreased B/P

TREATMENT OF OVERDOSE:
Defibrillation, atropine for AV block, vasopressor for hypotension

---

⚠ HIGH ALERT

nilotinib (Rx)
(nye-loe′ti-nib)

Tasigna

Func. class.: Antineoplastic—miscellaneous

Chem. class.: Protein-tyrosine kinase inhibitor

Pregnancy category D

ACTION: Inhibits BCR-ABL tyrosine kinase created in chronic myeloid leukemia (CML)

Therapeutic outcome: Decrease in progression of disease

USES: Chronic phase/accelerated phase Philadelphia chromosome–positive chronic myelogenous leukemia that is resistant/intolerant to imatinib

CONTRAINDICATIONS
Pregnancy **D**, breastfeeding, hypersensitivity

> **BLACK BOX WARNING:** Hypokalemia, hypomagnesemia, QT prolongation

Precautions: Children, women, geriatric patients, active infections, anemia, cardiac disease, bone marrow suppression, cholestasis, diabetes, gelatin hypersensitivity, infertility, galactose-free diet, lactase deficiency, neutropenia, pancreatitis, thrombocytopenia

> **BLACK BOX WARNING:** Hepatic disease

DOSAGE AND ROUTES
Adult: PO 400 mg q12h; continue until disease progression or unacceptable toxicity

Escalation regimen for those taking a strong CYP3A4 inducer
Adult: PO increase dose as required

Adjustment following discontinuation of a strong CYP3A4 inducer
Adult: PO reduce to 400 mg/bid

For those taking a strong CYP3A4 inhibitor
Adult: PO reduce dose to 400 mg/day

QT prolongation
QTcF >480 msec: Withhold dose

Myelosuppression
ANC 1 × 10⁹/L or platelets <50 × 10⁹/L: Withhold dose

Hepatic Dose
Adult: PO (Child-Pugh classes A-C): newly diagnosed CML 200 mg bid, then escalation to 300 mg bid initially

Available forms: Caps 150, 200 mg

Implementation
• Do not break, crush, or chew caps; if a whole capsule cannot be swallowed, disperse capsule contents in 1 tsp of applesauce
• Give without regard to meals; separate doses by 12 hr; a make-up dose should not be taken if a dose is missed
• Store at 15°-30° C (59°-86° F)

ADVERSE EFFECTS
CNS: Headache, dizziness, fatigue, fever, flushing, paresthesia
CV: **QT prolongation**, palpitations, **torsades de pointes**, AV block
GI: *Nausea,* **hepatotoxicity,** vomiting, dyspepsia, *anorexia, abdominal pain,* constipation, **pancreatitis,** diarrhea, xerostomia
HEMA: **Neutropenia, thrombocytopenia, anemia, pancytopenia**
INTEG: *Rash,* alopecia, erythema
META: Hyperamylasemia, hyperbilirubinemia, hyperglycemia, hyperkalemia, hypocalcemia, hyponatremia, hypomagnesemia
MISC: Diaphoresis, anxiety
MS: Arthralgia, myalgia, back/bone pain, muscle cramps
RESP: Cough, dyspnea
SYST: **Bleeding, tumor lysis syndrome**

Pharmacokinetics

Absorption	Unknown
Distribution	Protein binding 98%, plasma levels 3 hr
Metabolism	By CYP3A4
Excretion	Unknown
Half-life	Elimination 17 hr

Pharmacodynamics

Unknown

INTERACTIONS
Individual drugs
• Product interactions are numerous
Acetaminophen: increased hepatotoxicity
CarBAMazepine, dexamethasone, PHENobarbital, phenytoin, rifampin: decreased concentrations

---

Adverse effects: *italics* = common; **bold** = life-threatening

Clarithromycin, erythromycin, itraconazole, ketoconazole: increased concentrations

Haloperidol, chloroquine, droperidol, pentamidine, arsenic trioxide, levomethadyl: increased QT prolongation

Pimozide, ziprasidone: do not use concurrently

Simvastatin: increased plasma concentrations

Warfarin: increased plasma concentration; avoid use with warfarin, use low-molecular-weight anticoagulants instead

Drug classifications

Class IA/III antidysrhythmics, some phenothiazines, β-agonists, local anesthetics, tricyclics, CYP3A4 inhibitors (amiodarone, clarithromycin, erythromycin, telithromycin, troleandomycin), CYP3A4 substrates (methadone, pimozide, QUEtiapine, quiNIDine, risperiDONE, ziprasidone): increased QT prolongation

Calcium channel blockers: increased plasma concentrations

Phenothiazines: do not use concurrently

Drug/herb

St. John's wort: decreased concentration

Drug/food

Grapefruit juice: increased plasma concentrations

NURSING CONSIDERATIONS
Assessment

• **Assess ANC and platelets; if ANC <1 × 10^9/L and/or platelets <50 × 10^9/L, stop until ANC >1.5 × 10^9/L and platelets >75 × 10^9/L**

• **Monitor CV status: hypertension, QT prolongation can occur; monitor left ventricular ejection fraction (LVEF) baseline periodically**

• **Assess for renal toxicity: if bilirubin >3 × IULN, withhold until bilirubin levels return to <1.5 × IULN**

• **Assess for hepatotoxicity: monitor hepatic function tests, before treatment and qmo; if liver transaminases >5 × IULN, withhold until transaminase levels return to <2.5 × IULN**

• **Myelosuppression: Monitor CBC × 2 mo and then monthly; differential, platelet count weekly; withhold product if WBC is <3500/mm³ or platelet count <100,000/mm³; notify prescriber of these results; product should be discontinued**

• Monitor for bleeding: epistaxis, rectal, gingival, upper GI, genital, and wound bleeding; tumor-related hemorrhage may occur rapidly

⚠ **Tumor lysis syndrome: maintain hydration, correct uric acid prior to use of this product**

• **Monitor electrolytes:** calcium, potassium, magnesium, sodium; lipase, phosphate; hypokalemia, hypomagnesemia should be corrected prior to use

• AST/ALT/bilirubin/lipase/amylase if increased to grade 3, withhold product; resume at 400 mg qd when levels return to grade 1 or below

• **QT prolongation: ECG for QT prolongation, ejection fraction; assess for chest pain, palpitations, dyspnea**

Patient/family education

• Instruct patient to report adverse reactions immediately: SOB, bleeding

• Inform patient reason for treatment, expected result

• Advise patient that many adverse reactions may occur

• Teach patient to avoid persons with known upper respiratory infections; immunosuppression is common

• Instruct in signs/symptoms of low potassium or magnesium

Evaluation
Positive therapeutic outcome

• Decrease in progression of disease

---

niMODipine (Rx)
(ni-moe′dip-een)
Nimotop
Func. class.: Calcium channel blocker
Chem. class.: Dihydropyridine
Pregnancy category C

ACTION: Unknown, may have greater effect on cerebral arteries

Therapeutic outcome: Prevention of vascular spasm (subarachnoid hemorrhage)

USES: Prevention of cerebrovascular spasm in subarachnoid hemorrhage

CONTRAINDICATIONS
Sick sinus syndrome, 2nd- or 3rd-degree heart block, hypotension less than 90 mm Hg systolic, hypersensitivity

Precautions: Pregnancy **C**, breastfeeding, children, geriatric, CHF, hypotension, hepatic injury, renal disease

DOSAGE AND ROUTES
Adult: PO begin therapy within 96 hr, 60 mg q4hr × 21 days

Available forms: Caps 30 mg

Implementation

• May puncture cap and dilute in water and give through nasogastric tube; flush tube with 0.9% NaCl

---

• Store in airtight container at room temperature

ADVERSE EFFECTS

CNS: Headache, fatigue, drowsiness, dizziness, anxiety, depression, weakness, insomnia, confusion, paresthesia, somnolence

CV: Dysrhythmia, edema, CHF, bradycardia, hypotension, palpitations, **MI, pulmonary edema**

GI: Nausea, vomiting, diarrhea, gastric upset, constipation, *hepatitis*, abdominal cramps

GU: Nocturia, polyuria, **acute renal failure**

INTEG: Rash, pruritus, urticaria, photosensitivity, hair loss

MISC: Blurred vision, flushing, nasal congestion, sweating, shortness of breath, gynecomastia, hyperglycemia, sexual difficulties

Pharmacokinetics

Absorption	Well absorbed, poor bioavailability
Distribution	Crosses blood-brain barrier
Metabolism	Liver, extensively
Excretion	Kidneys
Half-life	1-2 hr

Pharmacodynamics

Onset	Unknown
Peak	1 hr
Duration	Unknown

INTERACTIONS

Individual drugs

Alcohol: increased hypotension
Digoxin: increased digoxin levels, bradycardia
PHENobarbital, phenytoin: decreased effectiveness
Propranolol: increased toxicity

Drug classifications

Antihypertensives: increased hypotension
β-Adrenergic blockers: increased bradycardia
Nitrates: increased nitrates

Drug/herb

Barberry, betel palm, burdock, goldenseal, khat, khella, lily of the valley, plantain: increased effect
Yohimbe: decreased effect

NURSING CONSIDERATIONS

Assessment

• Assess fluid volume status (I&O ratio) and record weight; distended red veins; crackles in lung; color, quality, and specific gravity of urine; skin turgor; adequacy of pulses; moist mucous membranes; bilateral lung sounds; peripheral pitting edema; dehydration symptoms of decreasing output, thirst, hypotension, dry mouth and mucous membranes should be reported

• Monitor B/P and pulse; if B/P drops 30 mm Hg, call prescriber

• Monitor ALT, AST, bilirubin daily; if these are elevated, hepatotoxicity is suspected

Nursing diagnoses

• Injury, risk for (uses)
• Knowledge, deficient (teaching)

Evaluation

Positive therapeutic outcome

• Prevention of neurologic damage from subarachnoid hemorrhage

nisoldipine (Rx)

(nye'sol-dye-peen)
Sular
Func. class.: Antihypertensive, calcium channel blocker
Chem. class.: Dihydropyridine
Pregnancy category C

Do not confuse: nisoldipine/NIFEdipine/niMODipine

ACTION: Inhibits calcium ion influx across cell membrane, resulting in dilatation of peripheral arteries

Therapeutic outcome: Decreased B/P in hypertension

USES: Essential hypertension, alone or with other antihypertensives

CONTRAINDICATIONS

Hypersensitivity to this product or dihydropyridines, sick sinus syndrome, 2nd- or 3rd-degree heart block, aortic stenosis

Precautions: Pregnancy C, breastfeeding, children, geriatric, CHF, hypotension <90 mm Hg systolic, hepatic injury, renal disease, acute MI, unstable angina, CAD, cardiogenic shock

DOSAGE AND ROUTES

Adult: PO 17 mg/day initially, may increase by 8.5 mg/wk, usual dose 17-34 mg/day, max 34 mg/day

Geriatric dose: PO 8.5 mg/day, increase based on response

Hepatic dose
Adult: PO 8.5 mg/day

Available forms: Ext rel tabs 8.5, 17, 20, 25.5, 30, 34, 40 mg

Implementation

PO route

• Give once a day, with food to decrease GI symptoms; avoid high-fat foods, grapefruit

ADVERSE EFFECTS

CNS: Headache, fatigue, drowsiness, dizziness, anxiety, depression, nervousness, insomnia, light-headedness, paresthesia, tinnitus, psychosis, somnolence, ataxia, confusion, malaise, migraine, flushing

CV: Dysrhythmias, edema, CHF, hypotension, palpitations, MI, pulmonary edema, tachycardia, syncope, AV block, angina, chest pain, ECG abnormalities

GI: Nausea, vomiting, diarrhea, gastric upset, constipation, elevated liver function tests, dry mouth, dyspepsia, dysphagia, flatulence

GU: Nocturia, hematuria, dysuria

HEMA: Anemia, leukopenia, petechiae

INTEG: Rash, pruritus

MISC: Sexual difficulties, gingival hyperplasia, chills, fever, gout, sweating, cough, nasal congestion, shortness of breath, wheezing, epistaxis, dyspnea

Pharmacokinetics

Absorption	Well absorbed
Distribution	Highly protein bound
Metabolism	Liver
Excretion	Kidneys
Half-life	Unknown

Pharmacodynamics

Onset	Unknown
Peak	6-12 hr
Duration	Unknown

INTERACTIONS

Individual drugs

Cimetidine, ranitidine: increased nisoldipine level

Digoxin: increased effects

Drug classifications

Antifungals (azole), CYP3A4 inhibitors: increased nisoldipine level

Antihypertensives: increased hypotension

β-Adrenergic blockers: increased effects

Hydantoins, CYP3A4 inducers: decreased nisoldipine effect

Drug/herb

Ephedra, melatonin: increased B/P

Hawthorn: decreased B/P

St. John's wort, ginseng, ginkgo biloba: decreased effect

Drug/food

Grapefruit juice: increased hypotension

High-fat foods: increased nisoldipine level

NURSING CONSIDERATIONS

Assessment

• Assess fluid volume status: I&O ratio and record; weight; skin turgor; adequacy of pulses; moist mucous membranes; bilateral lung sounds; peripheral pitting edema; dehydration symptoms of decreasing output, thirst, hypotension, dry mouth and mucous membranes should be reported

• **Angina:** assess frequency, severity of attacks; if angina worsens, report immediately

• Monitor ALT, AST, bilirubin daily if these are elevated and hepatotoxicity is suspected

• Monitor cardiac status: B/P, pulse, respiration, ECG

Patient/family education

• Caution patient to avoid hazardous activities until stabilized on product and dizziness is no longer a problem

• Instruct patient to limit caffeine consumption; to avoid alcohol and OTC products unless directed by prescriber

• Urge patient to comply in all areas of medical regimen: diet, exercise, stress reduction, product therapy; to notify prescriber of irregular heartbeat, SOB, swelling of feet and hands, pronounced dizziness, constipation, nausea, hypotension

• Teach patient to use as directed even if feeling better; may be taken with other cardiovascular products (nitrates, β-blockers)

• Advise patient to rise slowly to prevent orthostatic hypotension

• Teach patient to report nausea, dizziness, edema, SOB, palpitations

Evaluation

Positive therapeutic outcome
• Decreased B/P

RARELY USED

nitazoxanide (Rx)

(nye-taz-ox′a-nide)

Alinia

Func. class.: Antiprotozoal

Pregnancy category B

Therapeutic outcome: C&S negative for organism

USES: Diarrhea caused by *Cryptosporidium parvum* or *Giardia lamblia*

CONTRAINDICATIONS

Hypersensitivity

DOSAGE AND ROUTES

Adult: PO 500 mg q12hr × 3 days
Child 4-11 yr: PO 10 ml (200 mg) q12hr × 3 days
Child 12-47 mo: PO 5 ml (100 mg) q12hr × 3 days

nitrofurantoin (Rx)

(nye-troe-fyoor′an-toyn)

Furadantin, Macrobid, Macrodantin, Novo-Furantoin ✿

Func. class.: Urinary tract antiinfective
Chem. class.: Synthetic nitrofuran derivative

Pregnancy category B

ACTION: Inhibits bacterial acetyl-CoA from interfering with carbohydrate metabolism

Therapeutic outcome: Resolution of infection

USES: Urinary tract infections caused by *Escherichia coli, Klebsiella, Pseudomonas, Proteus vulgaris, Proteus morganii, Serratia, Citrobacter, Staphylococcus aureus, Staphylococcus epidermidis, Enterococcus, Salmonella, Shigella*

CONTRAINDICATIONS

Infants <1 mo, hypersensitivity, anuria, severe renal disease, CCr <60 ml/min, at term pregnancy (38-42 wk), labor, delivery, cholestatic jaundice due to nitrofurantoin therapy

Precautions: Pregnancy **B**, breastfeeding, geriatric, G6PD deficiency, GI disease, diabetes

DOSAGE AND ROUTES
Active infections

Adult: PO 50-100 mg qid after meals or 50-100 mg at bedtime for long-term treatment
Child: PO 5-7 mg/kg/day in 4 divided doses; 1-2 mg/kg/day for long-term treatment; max 7 mg/kg/day

Chronic suppression

Adult: PO 50-100 mg qPM
Child: PO 2 mg/kg/day qPM or 0.5-1 mg/kg q12hr if dose is not well tolerated

Available forms: Caps 25, 50, 100 mg; susp 25 mg/ml; macrocrystal caps (Macrodantin) 25, 50, 100 mg; cap (Macrobid) 100 mg (25 macrocrystals, 75 monohydrate)

Implementation

• Give with meals
• Do not break, crush, chew, or open tabs, caps; store in original container
• Give after clean-catch urine for C&S
• Give two daily doses if urine output is high or if patient has diabetes

ADVERSE EFFECTS

CNS: *Dizziness, headache,* drowsiness, peripheral neuropathy, chills, confusion, vertigo
CV: **Bundle branch block,** chest pain
GI: *Nausea, vomiting, abdominal pain, diarrhea,* **cholestatic jaundice,** loss of appetite, **pseudomembranous colitis, hepatitis,** pancreatitis
HEMA: **Anemia, agranulocytosis, hemolytic anemia, leukopenia, thrombocytopenia**
INTEG: Pruritus, rash, urticaria, **angioedema,** alopecia, tooth staining, **exfoliative dermatitis**
MS: Arthralgia, myalgia, numbness, peripheral neuropathy
RESP: Cough, dyspnea, pneumonitis, pulmonary fibrosis/infiltrate
SYST: **Stevens-Johnson syndrome, superinfection,** SLE-like syndrome

Pharmacokinetics

Absorption	Readily absorbed
Distribution	Crosses placenta, excreted in breast milk
Metabolism	Liver, partially
Excretion	Kidneys, 30%-50% unchanged
Half-life	20-60 min

Pharmacodynamics

Onset	Unknown
Peak	30 min
Duration	6-12 hr

INTERACTIONS
Individual products

Magnesium trisilicate: decreased absorption
Norfloxacin: antagonist effect
Probenecid: increased nitrofurantoin levels

Drug/lab test

Increased: BUN, alkaline phosphatase, bilirubin, creatinine, blood glucose

NURSING CONSIDERATIONS
Assessment

• Monitor blood count during chronic therapy
• Assess CNS symptoms: insomnia, vertigo, headache, drowsiness, seizures

N

- Assess allergy: fever, flushing, rash, urticaria, pruritus
- **Urinary tract infection:** assess for burning, pain on urination, fever; cloudy, foul-smelling urine; I&O ratio; C&S before treatment, after completion; serum creatinine, BUN
- **Hepatotoxicity: assess for yellowing of skin, eyes, dark urine, clay-colored stools; monitor AST, ALT**
- **Pulmonary fibrosis, pneumonitis: assess for dyspnea, tachypnea, persistent cough**
- **Serious skin disorders: assess for fever, flushing, rash, urticaria, pruritus**
- **Peripheral neuropathy:** assess for paresthesias (more common in diabetes mellitus, electrolyte imbalances, vit B deficiency, debilitated patients)
- **Pseudomembranous colitis: assess for diarrhea, abdominal pain, fever, fatigue, anorexia; possible anemia, elevated WBC and low serum albumin; stop product and usually give either vancomycin or IV metro-NIDAZOLE**

Patient/family education
- Teach patient to take with food or milk; avoid alcohol
- Teach patient to protect susp from freezing and shake well before taking
- Teach patient that product may cause drowsiness; instruct client to seek aid in walking and other activities; advise patient not to drive or operate machinery while on medication
- Teach patient that diabetics should monitor blood glucose level
- Teach patient that product may turn urine rust-yellow to brown
- **A Teach patient to notify prescriber of symptoms of pseudomembranous colitis: fever, diarrhea with mucous, pus, or blood; report immediately**

Evaluation

Positive therapeutic outcome
- Decreased dysuria, fever; negative C&S

A HIGH ALERT

nitroglycerin (Rx)
(nye-troe-gli′ser-in)
extended release caps (Rx)
Nitrogard SR ✹, Nitro-Time
translingual spray (Rx)
Nitrolingual, Nitromist
sublingual (Rx)
Nitrostat
rectal ointment
Rectiv
topical ointment (Rx)
Nitro-Bid
transdermal (Rx)
Minitran, Nitro-Dur
Func. class.: Coronary vasodilator, antianginal
Chem. class.: Nitrate
Pregnancy category C

Do not confuse: Nitro-Bid/Nicobid

ACTION: Decreases preload and afterload, which thus decreases left ventricular end-diastolic pressure and systemic vascular resistance; dilates coronary arteries and improves blood flow through coronary vasculature, dilates arterial, venous beds systemically

Therapeutic outcome: Prevention of anginal attack

USES: Chronic stable angina pectoris, prophylaxis of angina pain, CHF associated with acute MI, controlled hypotension in surgical procedures, anal fissures

CONTRAINDICATIONS
Hypersensitivity to this product or nitrites, severe anemia, increased ICP, cerebral hemorrhage, closed-angle glaucoma, cardiac tamponade, cardiomyopathy, constrictive pericarditis

Precautions: Pregnancy **C**, breastfeeding, children, postural hypotension, severe renal/hepatic disease, acute MI, abrupt discontinuation, hyperthyroidism

DOSAGE AND ROUTES
Adult: **SL** dissolve tab under tongue when pain begins; may repeat q5min until relief occurs; take no more than 3 tab/15 min; use 1 tab prophylactically 5-10 min before activities; **SUS REL** cap q6-12hr on empty stomach; **TOP** 1-2 in q8hr; increase to 4 in q4hr as needed; **IV** 5 mcg/min, then increase by 5 mcg/min q3-5min; if no response after 20 mcg/min, increase by 10-20 mcg/min until desired response; **transdermal**

---

apply a patch daily to a site free from hair; remove patch at bedtime to provide 10-12 hr nitrate-free interval to avoid tolerance

Child: IV initial 0.25-0.5 mcg/kg/min, titrate to patient response, usual dose 1-3 mcg/kg/min transmucosal

Anal fisures (Rectiv)

Adult: rectal apply 1 in of 0.4% ointment q12hr × 3 wk

Available forms: Translingual aerosol 0.4 mg/m spray; sus rel tabs 2.5, 6.5, 9 mg; SL tabs 0.3, 0.4, 0.6 mg; topical joint 2%; trans syst 0.1, 0.2, 0.3, 0.4, 0.6, 0.8 mg/hr; inj 25 mg/250 ml, 50 mg/250 ml, 100 mg/250 ml, 50 mg/500 ml, 100 mg/500 ml, 200 mg/500 ml; rectal ointment 0.4% (Rectiv)

Implementation

PO route

• Swallow sus rel tabs whole; do not break, crush, or chew sus rel tabs

• Give 1 hr before or 2 hr after meals with 8 oz of water

SL route

• Should be dissolved under tongue, not swallowed

Aerosol route

• Sprayed under tongue (nitrolingual); not inhaled, prime before 1st-time use or if product has not been used in > 6 wk; press valve head with forefinger

Transmucosal route

• Tab should be placed between cheek and gum line

• Do not take anything PO when tab is in place

Topical ointment route

• Apply ointment using dose-measuring papers supplied; apply to an area without hair; ointment should cover 2-3–inch area; may apply an occlusive dressing as directed

Transdermal route

• Apply transdermal patches to area without hair; press hard to adhere; if patch becomes dislodged, apply a new one

SL route

• Keep tab in original container

• If 3 SL tab in 15 min do not relieve pain, consider diagnosis of MI

• SL tab should be held under tongue until dissolved (a few min); do not take anything by mouth when SL tab is in place

Rectal route

• Cover finger with plastic wrap, disposable glove or finger cot, lay finger alongside 1 inch dosing line on carton, squeeze tube until equal to 1 inch dosing line, insert covered finger no further than 1st finger joint gently into anal

canal and on sides, wash hands thoroughly, if too painful, apply directly to outside of anus

Continuous IV infusion route

• Diluted in D_5, D_5W, 0.9% NaCl for inf to 200-400 mcg/ml depending on patient's fluid status, common dilution is 50 mg/250 ml, use controlled inf device; use glass inf bottles, non–polyvinyl chloride inf tubing; titrate to patient response; do not use filters

Y-site compatibilities: Acyclovir, alfentanil, amikacin, aminocaproic acid, aminophylline, amiodarone, amphotericin B lipid complex, amphotericin B liposome, anidulafungin, argatroban, ascorbic acid, atenolol, atracurium, atropine, azaTHIOprine, aztreonam, benztropine, bivalirudin, bleomycin, bumetanide, buprenorphine, butorphanol, calcium chloride/gluconate, CARBOplatin, caspofungin, cefamandole, ceFAZolin, cefmetazole, cefonicid, cefoperazone, cefotaxime, cefoTEtan, cefOXitin, cefTAZidime, ceftizoxime, cefTRIAXone, cefuroxime, cephalothin, cephapirin, chloramphenicol, chlorproMAZINE, cimetidine, cisatracurium, CISplatin, clindamycin, cloNIDine, cyanocobalamin, cyclophosphamide, cycloSPORINE, cytarabine, DACTINomycin, dexamethasone, digoxin, diltiazem, diphenhydrAMINE, DOBUTamine, DOCEtaxel, DOPamine, doxacurium, DOXOrubicin, doxycycline, drotrecogin alfa, enalaprilat, ePHEDrine, EPINEPHrine, epirubicin, epoetin alfa, eptifibatide, ertapenem, erythromycin, esmolol, etoposide, famotidine, fenoldopam, fentaNYL, fluconazole, fludarabine, fluorouracil, folic acid, ganciclovir, gatifloxacin, gemcitabine, gemtuzumab, gentamicin, glycopyrrolate, granisetron, heparin, hydrocortisone, HYDROmorphone, hydrOXYzine, IDArubicin, ifosfamide, imipenem-cilastatin, indomethacin, insulin (regular), irinotecan, isoproterenol, ketorolac, labetalol, lidocaine, linezolid, LORazepam, magnesium sulfate, mannitol, mechlorethamine, meperidine, metaraminol, methicillin, methotrexate, methoxamine, methyldopate, methylPREDNISolone, metoclopramide, metroNIDAZOLE, mezlocillin, micafungin, miconazole, midazolam, milrinone, minocycline, mitoXANtrone, morphine, moxalactam, mycophenolate, nafcillin, nalbuphine, naloxone, nesiritide, netilmicin, niCARdipine, nitroprusside, norepinephrine, octreotide, ondansetron, oxacillin, oxaliplatin, oxytocin, PACLitaxel, palonosetron, pamidronate, pancuronium, pantoprazole, papaverine, PEMEtrexed, penicillin G potassium/sodium, pentamidine, pentazocine, PENTobarbital, PHENobarbital, phentolamine, phenylephrine, phytonadione, piperacillin, piperacillin-tazobactam, polymyxin B, potassium chloride, procainamide, prochlorperazine, promethazine, propofol, propranolol, protamine, pyridoxine, quiNIDine, quinupristin-dalfopristin, ranitidine, remifentanil, ritodrine, rocuronium, sodium bicarbonate, succinylcholine, SUFentanil, tacrolimus, teniposide, theophylline, thiamine, thiopental, thiotepa, ticarcillin, ticarcillin-clavulanate, tigecycline, tirofiban, tobramycin, tolazoline, trimetaphan, urokinase, vancomycin, vasopressin, vecuronium, verapamil, vinCRIStine, vinorelbine, voriconazole, warfarin, zoledronic acid

Y-site incompatibilities: Alteplase

ADVERSE EFFECTS
CNS: *Headache, flushing, dizziness*
CV: *Postural hypotension,* tachycardia, collapse, syncope, palpitations
GI: Nausea, vomiting
INTEG: Pallor, sweating, rash

Pharmacokinetics

Absorption	Well absorbed (PO, buccal, SL)
Distribution	Unknown
Metabolism	Liver, extensively
Excretion	Kidney
Half-life	1-4 min

Pharmacodynamics

	SUS REL	SL	TD	IV	TRANS-MUCOSAL	AEROSOL	TOPICAL OINT
Onset	20-45 min	1-3 min	½-1 hr	1-2 min	1-2 min	2 min	½-1 hr
Peak	Unknown	Unknown	Unknown	Unknown	Unknown	Unknown	Unknown
Duration	3-8 hr	½ hr	12-24 hr	3-5 min	3-5 hr	½-1 hr	2-12 hr

INTERACTIONS
Individual drugs
Alcohol: increased hypotension, CV collapse
Aspirin: increased nitrate level
Heparin: decreased effects (with IV nitroglycerin)
Sildenafil, tadalafil, vardenafil: increased fatal hypotension, do not use together

Drug classifications
Antihypertensives, β-adrenergic blockers, calcium channel blockers, diuretics: increased hypotension

Drug/lab test
Increased: urine catecholamine, urine VMA
False increase: cholesterol

NURSING CONSIDERATIONS
Assessment
• Monitor orthostatic B/P, pulse
• **Assess pain:** duration, time started, activity being performed, character; check for tolerance if taken over long period
• Monitor for headache, light-headedness, decreased B/P; may indicate a need for decreased dosage

Patient/family education
• Instruct patient to avoid alcohol
• Advise patient that product may cause headache; tolerance usually develops; use nonopioid analgesic
• Teach patient that product may be taken before stressful activity, exercise, sexual activity
• Inform patient that SL tab may sting when product comes in contact with mucous membranes
• Caution patient to avoid hazardous activities if dizziness occurs
• Instruct patient to comply with complete medical regimen
• Advise patient to make position changes slowly to prevent fainting
⚠ Advise patient to never use erectile dysfunction products (sildenafil, tadalafil, vardenafil); may cause severe hypotension, death

Evaluation
Positive therapeutic outcome
• Decreased, prevention of anginal pain

⚠ HIGH ALERT

nitroprusside (Rx)
(nye-troe-pruss'ide)
Nitropress
Func. class.: Antihypertensive, vasodilator
Pregnancy category C

ACTION: Directly relaxes arteriolar, venous smooth muscle, resulting in reduction in cardiac preload, afterload

Therapeutic outcome: Decreased B/P in hypertensive crisis, decreased preload, afterload

---

USES: Hypertensive crisis/urgency/induction, to decrease bleeding by creating hypotension during surgery, acute CHF

CONTRAINDICATIONS

Hypersensitivity, hypertension (compensatory) due to aortic coarctation or AV shunting, acute CHF associated with reduced peripheral vascular resistance, AV shunt, Leber's disease, toxic amblyopia

> **BLACK BOX WARNING:** Cyanide toxicity, do not use in hypothyroidism

Precautions: Pregnancy **C,** breastfeeding, children, geriatric, fluid, electrolyte imbalances, renal/hepatic disease, hypothyroidism, anemia, increased intracranial pressure, hypovolemia

> **BLACK BOX WARNING:** Hypotension

DOSAGE AND ROUTES
Adult and child: IV INF 0.25-1.0 mcg/kg/min; max 10 mcg/kg/min

Renal dose
Adult: IV INF CCr <60 ml/min maintain doses <3 mcg/kg/min to reduce thiocyanate accumulation

Available forms: Inj 50 mg 12 ml

Implementation

Continuous IV infusion route
• Depending on B/P reading q15min
• Reconstitute 50 mg/2-3 ml of D_5W, further dilute in 250, 500, or 1000 ml of D_5W to 200, 100, 50 mcg/ml respectively; use an infusion pump only; wrap bottle with aluminum foil to protect from light; observe for color change in the inf; discard if highly discolored (blue, green, dark red); titrate to patient response, protect from light

Y-site compatibilities: Alfentanil, alprostadil, amikacin, aminocaproic acid, aminophylline, amphotericin B lipid complex, amphotericin B liposome, anidulafungin, argatroban, atenolol, atropine, aztreonam, benztropine, bivalirudin, bleomycin, bumetanide, buprenorphine, butorphanol, calcium chloride/gluconate, CARBOplatin, cefamandole, ceFAZolin, cefmetazole, cefonicid, cefoperazone, cefotaxime, cefoTEtan, cefOXitin, cefTAZidime, ceftizoxime, cefTRIAXone, cefuroxime, cephalothin, chloramphenicol, cimetidine, CISplatin, clindamycin, cyanocobalamin, cyclophosphamide, cycloSPORINE, cytarabine, DACTINomycin, DAPTOmycin, dexamethasone, digoxin, diltiazem, DOCEtaxel, DOPamine, doxacurium, DOXOrubicin, doxycycline, enalaprilat, ePHEDrine, EPINEPHrine, epirubicin, epoetin alfa, eptifibatide, ertapenem, esmolol, etoposide, famotidine, fenoldopam, fentaNYL, fluconazole, fludarabine, fluorouracil, folic acid, furosemide, ganciclovir, gatifloxacin, gemcitabine, gemtuzumab, gentamicin, glycopyrrolate, granisetron, heparin, hydrocortisone, HYDROmorphone, IDArubicin, ifosfamide, inamrinone, indomethacin, insulin (regular), isoproterenol, ketorolac, labetalol, lidocaine, linezolid, LORazepam, magnesium sulfate, mannitol, mechlorethamine, meperidine, metaraminol, methicillin, methoxamine, methyldopate, methylPREDNISolone, metoclopramide, metoprolol, metroNIDAZOLE, mezlocillin, micafungin, miconazole, midazolam, milrinone, minocycline, morphine, moxalactam, multiple vitamins injection, nafcillin, nalbuphine, naloxone, nesiritide, netilmicin, niCARdipine, nitroglycerin, norepinephrine, octreotide, ondansetron, oxacillin, oxaliplatin, oxytocin, PACLitaxel, palonosetron, pamidronate, pancuronium, pantoprazole, penicillin G potassium/sodium, pentamidine, PENTobarbital, PHENobarbital, phentolamine, phenylephrine, phytonadione, piperacillin, piperacillin-tazobactam, polymyxin B, potassium chloride/phosphates, procainamide, propofol, propranolol, protamine, pyridoxine, ranitidine, ritodrine, rocuronium, sodium acetate/bicarbonate, succinylcholine, SUFentanil, tacrolimus, teniposide, theophylline, thiamine, ticarcillin, ticarcillin-clavulanate, tigecycline, tirofiban, tobramycin, tolazoline, trimetaphan, urokinase, vancomycin, vasopressin, vecuronium, verapamil, vinCRIStine, zoledronic acid

ADVERSE EFFECTS
CNS: *Dizziness, headache,* agitation, twitching, decreased reflexes, *restlessness*
CV: *Bradycardia,* ECG changes, tachycardia, *hypotension*
GI: Nausea, vomiting, abdominal pain
INTEG: Pain, irritation at inj site, sweating
MISC: **Cyanide, thiocyanate toxicity,** flushing, hypothyroidism

Pharmacokinetics

Absorption	Complete bioavailability
Distribution	Not known
Metabolism	RBCs, tissues
Excretion	Kidneys
Half-life	2 min

Pharmacodynamics

Onset	1-2 min
Peak	Rapid
Duration	1-10 min

Adverse effects: *italics* = common; **bold** = life-threatening

INTERACTIONS
Individual drugs
Enflurane, halothane; severe hypotension

Drug classifications
Circulatory depressants, ganglionic blockers, volatile liquid anesthetics: severe hypotension

Drug/herb
Hawthorn: increased antihypertensive effect

NURSING CONSIDERATIONS
Assessment

> **BLACK BOX WARNING: Hypotension:** monitor B/P q5min × 2 hr, then qhr × 2 hr; monitor pulse q4hr; monitor jugular venous distention q4hr; ECG should be monitored continuously; monitor PCWP; rebound hypertension may occur after nitroprusside is discontinued, give only with emergency equipment nearby, rapid decrease in B/P may occur

• Monitor electrolytes, blood studies: potassium, sodium, chloride, CO_2, CBC, serum glucose, serum methemoglobin if pulmonary oxygen levels are decreased, ABGs
• Check weight, I&O, edema in feet and legs daily; assess skin turgor, dryness of mucous membranes for hydration status
• Assess for signs of CHF: dyspnea, edema, wet crackles
⚠ Monitor for increased lactate, cyanide, thiocyanate levels if on long-term treatment; thiocyanate toxicity occurs at plasma levels of ≥50 mcg/ml
• Monitor for decrease in bicarbonate, P_{CO_2}, and blood pH; acidosis may occur with this product

Patient/family education
• Teach patient to report headache, dizziness, loss of hearing, blurred vision, dyspnea, faintness; may indicate adverse reactions, pain at IV site

Evaluation
Positive therapeutic outcome
• Decreased B/P in hypertension
• Absence of bleeding in surgery

TREATMENT OF OVERDOSE:
Administer amyl nitrate inh until 3% sodium nitrate sol can be prepared for **IV** administration, then inject sodium thiosulfate **IV**; correct drop in B/P with vasopressor

---

> **⚠ HIGH ALERT**

norepinephrine
(nor-ep-i-nef′rin)
Levophed
Func. class.: Adrenergic
Chem. class.: Catecholamine
Pregnancy category C

Do not confuse: norepinephrine/EPINEPHrine

ACTION: Causes increased contractility and heart rate by acting on β-receptors in heart; also acts on a-receptors, thereby causing vasoconstriction in blood vessels; B/P is elevated, coronary blood flow improves, and cardiac output increases

Therapeutic outcome: Increased B/P with stabilization; adequate tissue perfusion

USES: Acute hypotension, shock

CONTRAINDICATIONS
Hypersensitivity to this product or cyclopropane/halothane anesthesia; ventricular fibrillation, tachydysrhythmias, pheochromocytoma, hypotension, hypovolemia

> **BLACK BOX WARNING:** Extravasation

Precautions: Pregnancy **C**, breastfeeding, geriatric patients, arterial embolism, peripheral vascular disease, hypertension, hyperthyroidism, cardiac disease

DOSAGE AND ROUTES
Adult: IV INF 0.5-1 mcg/min titrated to B/P; maintenance 2-4 mcg/min; max 30 mcg/min
Child: IV INF 0.1 mcg/kg/min titrated to B/P; max 2 mcg/kg/min

Available forms: Inj 1 mg/ml

Implementation
CONT IV INF route
• Dilute with 500-1000 ml D_5W or D_5/0.9% NaCl; average dilution 4 mg/1000 ml diluent (4 mcg base/ml); give as inf 2-3 ml/min; titrate to response
• Store reconstituted sol in refrigerator <24 hr, protect from light, store unopened product at room temp, do not use discolored sol

Y-site compatibilities: Alemtuzumab, alfentanil, amikacin, amiodarone, anidulafungin, argatroban, ascorbic acid, atenolol, atracurium, atropine, aztreonam, benztropine, bivalirudin,

---

bleomycin, bumetanide, buprenorphine, butorphanol, calcium chloride/gluconate, CARBOplatin, caspofungin, cefamandole, ceFAZolin, cefmetazole, cefonicid, cefoperazone, cefotaxime, cefoTEtan, cefOXitin, cefTAZidime, ceftizoxime, ceftobiprole, cefTRIAXone, cefuroxime, cephalothin, chloramphenicol, chlorproMAZINE, cimetidine, cisatracurium, CISplatin, clindamycin, cloNIDine, cyanocobalamin, cyclophosphamide, cycloSPORINE, cytarabine, DAPTOmycin, dexamethasone, digoxin, diltiazem, diphenhydrAMINE, DOBUTamine, DOCEtaxel, DOPamine, doripenem, doxycycline, enalaprilat, ePHEDrine, EPINEPHrine, epirubicin, epoetin alfa, ertapenem, erythromycin, esmolol, etoposide, famotidine, fenoldopam, fentaNYL, fluconazole, fludarabine, gatifloxacin, gemcitabine, gentamicin, glycopyrrolate, granisetron, heparin, hydrocortisone, HYDROmorphone, hydrOXYzine, IDArubicin, ifosfamide, imipenem-cilastatin, irinotecan, isoproterenol, ketorolac, labetalol, lidocaine, linezolid, LORazepam, magnesium sulfate, mannitol, mechlorethamine, meperidine, meropenem, metaraminol, methicillin, methotrexate, methoxamine, methyldopate, methylPREDNISolone, metoclopramide, metoprolol, metroNIDAZOLE, mezlocillin, micafungin, miconazole, midazolam, milrinone, minocycline, mitoXANtrone, morphine, moxalactam, multiple vitamins injection, mycophenolate, nafcillin, nalbuphine, naloxone, netilmicin, niCARdipine, nitroglycerin, nitroprusside, octreotide, ondansetron, oxacillin, oxaliplatin, oxytocin, PACLitaxel, palonosetron, pamidronate, pancuronium, papaverine, PEMEtrexed, penicillin G potassium/sodium, pentamidine, pentazocine, phenylephrine, phytonadione, piperacillin, piperacillin-tazobactam, polymyxin B, potassium chloride, procainamide, prochlorperazine, promethazine, propofol, propranolol, protamine, pyridoxine, quiNIDine, ranitidine, remifentanil, ritodrine, succinylcholine, SUFentanil, tacrolimus, teniposide, theophylline, thiamine, thiotepa, ticarcillin, ticarcillin-clavulanate, tigecycline, tirofiban, tobramycin, tolazoline, trimetaphan, urokinase, vancomycin, vasopressin, vecuronium, verapamil, vinCRIStine, vinorelbine, vitamin B complex with C, voriconazole, zoledronic acid

ADVERSE EFFECTS
CNS: *Headache,* anxiety, dizziness, insomnia, restlessness, tremor, **cerebral hemorrhage**
CV: *Palpitations, tachycardia, hypertension, ectopic beats, angina*
GI: *Nausea, vomiting*
GU: Decreased urine output
INTEG: Necrosis, tissue sloughing with extravasation, **gangrene**

RESP: Dyspnea
SYST: **Anaphylaxis**

Pharmacokinetics
Absorption	Complete
Distribution	Crosses placenta
Metabolism	Liver
Excretion	Urine

Pharmacodynamics
Onset	Immediate
Peak	Rapid
Duration	1 min

INTERACTIONS
Individual drugs
Bicarbonate, sodium: incompatible with alkaline solutions
⚠ Guanethidine, methyldopa: do not use norepinephrine within 2 wk of using these drugs because hypertensive crisis may result

Drug classifications
α-blockers: decreased norepinephrine action
⚠ Antihistamines, ergots, MAOIs, oxytocics, tricyclics: do not use norepinephrine within 2 wk of using these drugs because hypertensive crisis may result
Oxytocics: Increased B/P
MAOIs, tricyclics: increased pressor effect

NURSING CONSIDERATIONS
Assessment
• Assess I&O ratio; notify prescriber if output <30 ml/hr
• Assess B/P, pulse q2-3min after parenteral route, ECG during administration continuously; if B/P increases, product is decreased, CVP or PWP during inf if possible
• Assess paresthesias and coldness of extremities; peripheral blood flow may decrease

BLACK BOX WARNING: Extravasation: inj site: tissue sloughing

• Assess for sulfite sensitivity, which may be life-threatening

Patient/family education
• Teach patient about the reason for product administration
• Advise family to report dyspnea, dizziness, chest pain

Evaluation
Positive therapeutic outcome
• Increased B/P with stabilization
• Adequate tissue perfusion

TREATMENT OF OVERDOSE:
Administer fluids, electrolyte replacement

nortriptyline (Rx)
(nor-trip'ti-leen)
Aventyl ✦, Pamelor
Func. class.: Antidepressant, tricyclic
Chem. class.: Dibenzocycloheptene, secondary amine
Pregnancy category D

Do not confuse: nortriptyline/
amitriptyline

ACTION: Blocks reuptake of norepinephrine, serotonin into nerve endings, increasing action of norepinephrine, serotonin in nerve cells; has anticholinergic effects

Therapeutic outcome: Decreased symptoms of depression after 2-3 wk

USES: Major depression

Unlabeled uses: Chronic pain management

CONTRAINDICATIONS
Hypersensitivity to tricyclics, recovery phase of MI, seizure disorders, prostatic hypertrophy

Precautions: Breastfeeding, suicidal ideation, severe depression, increased intraocular pressure, closed-angle glaucoma, urinary retention, cardiac/hepatic disease, hyperthyroidism, electroshock therapy, elective surgery, pregnancy (**C**), carBAMazepine hypersensitivity

> **BLACK BOX WARNING:** Children, suicidal ideation

DOSAGE AND ROUTES
Adult: PO 25 mg tid or qid; may increase to 150 mg/day; may give daily dose at bedtime
Adolescent: PO 1-3 mg/kg/day in 3-4 divided doses or qd at bedtime; max 150 mg/day
Geriatric: PO 10-25 mg nightly, increase by 10-25 mg at weekly intervals to desired dose; usual maintenance 75 mg/day, max 150 mg/day

Available forms: Caps 10, 25, 50, 75 mg; sol 10 mg/5 ml

Implementation
• Give with food or milk to decrease GI symptoms; mix conc with water, milk, fruit juice to disguise taste
• Give dose at bedtime if oversedation occurs during day; may take entire dose at bedtime; geriatric may not tolerate once/day dosing
• Store in tight, light-resistant container at room temp; do not freeze

ADVERSE EFFECTS
CNS: *Dizziness, drowsiness,* confusion, headache, anxiety, tremors, stimulation, weakness, insomnia, nightmares, EPS (geriatric), increased psychiatric symptoms, **seizures**
CV: *Orthostatic hypotension,* **ECG changes,** *tachycardia,* **hypertension,** palpitations, **dysrhythmias**
EENT: Blurred vision, tinnitus, mydriasis, dry eyes
ENDO: SIADH, hyponatremia, hypothyroidism
GI: *Constipation, dry mouth,* nausea, vomiting, **paralytic ileus,** increased appetite, cramps, epigastric distress, jaundice, **hepatitis,** stomatitis, weight gain
GU: *Retention,* **acute renal failure,** sexual dysfunction
HEMA: **Agranulocytosis, thrombocytopenia, eosinophilia, leukopenia**
INTEG: Rash, urticaria, sweating, pruritus, photosensitivity
SYST: **Serotonin syndrome**

Pharmacokinetics

Absorption	Well absorbed
Distribution	Widely distributed; crosses placenta
Metabolism	Liver, extensively
Excretion	Kidneys, breast milk
Half-life	18-28 hr; steady state 4-19 days

Pharmacodynamics

Unknown

INTERACTIONS
Individual drugs
Alcohol: increased CNS depression
CloNIDine, guanethidine: decreased effects
Smoking (heavy): decreased product effect
Haloperidol, chloroquine, droperidol, pentamidine, arsenic trioxide, levomethadyl: increased QT prolongation

Drug classifications
Barbiturates, benzodiazepines, CNS depressants: increased effects
MAOIs: hypertensive episode, hyperpyretic crisis, seizures
SSRIs, SNRIs, serotonin-receptor agonists: increased serotonin syndrome, neuroleptic malignant syndrome
Class IA/III antidysrhythmics, some phenothiazines, β-agonists, local anesthetics, tricyclics, CYP3A4 inhibitors (amiodarone, clarithromycin, erythromycin, telithromycin, troleandomycin), CYP3A4

substrates (methadone, pimozide, QUE-
tiapine, quiNIDine, risperiDONE, ziprasidone): increased QT prolongation
Sympathomimetics (direct-acting), products increasing QT interval: increased effects
Sympathomimetics (indirect-acting): decreased
effects

Drug/herb
Kava, valerian: increased CNS effect
St. John's wort: decreased nortriptyline level

Drug/lab test
Increased: serum bilirubin, blood glucose, alka-
line phosphatase
Decreased: VMA, 5-HIAA
False increase: urinary catecholamines

NURSING CONSIDERATIONS
Assessment

> **BLACK BOX WARNING: Suicidal thoughts/
> behaviors in children/young adults:** not
> approved for children; monitor for suicidal ide-
> ation in depression, adolescents, young adults

• Monitor B/P (with patient lying, standing),
pulse q4hr; if systolic B/P drops 20 mm Hg,
hold product, notify prescriber; take VS q4hr of
patients with CV disease
• Monitor blood studies: thyroid function tests,
LFTs, serum nortriptyline level/target 50-150 ng/
ml if patient is receiving long-term therapy
• Monitor liver function tests: AST, ALT, bilirubin
• Check weight weekly; appetite may increase
• **QT prolongation: assess for chest pain,
palpitations, dyspnea**
• Assess ECG for flattening of T-wave, bundle
branch block, AV block, dysrhythmias in cardiac
patients
• Assess for EPS primarily in geriatric: rigidity,
dystonia, akathisia
• Assess mental status: mood, sensorium, affect,
suicidal tendencies; increase in psychiatric
symptoms: depression, panic
• Monitor urinary retention, constipation;
constipation is more likely to occur in children
or geriatric
⚠ **Assess for withdrawal symptoms: headache, nausea, vomiting, muscle pain,
weakness; do not usually occur unless
product was discontinued abruptly**
• Monitor for glaucoma exacerbation and
paralytic ileus
• Identify alcohol consumption; if alcohol is
consumed, hold dose until AM
• **Serotonin syndrome, neuroleptic malignant syndrome: assess for increased heart
rate, shivering, sweating, dilated pupils,**
**tremors, high B/P, hyperthermia, headache,
confusion; if these occur, stop product,
administer a serotonin antagonist if needed
(rare)**

Patient/family education
• Teach patient that therapeutic effects may take
2-3 wk
• Teach patient to use caution in driving and
other activities requiring alertness because of
drowsiness, dizziness, blurred vision; to avoid
rising quickly from sitting to standing, especially
geriatric
• Teach patient to avoid alcohol ingestion,
MAOIs within 14 days, other CNS depressants;
teach patient not to discontinue medication
quickly after long-term use; may cause nausea,
headache, malaise
• Teach patient to wear sunscreen or large hat
to avoid burns, because photosensitivity occurs
• Teach patient to increase fluids, bulk in diet
if constipation, urinary retention occur, especially geriatric, worsening depression, suicidal
thoughts/behavior
• Teach patient to take gum, hard sugarless
candy, or frequent sips of water for dry mouth

Evaluation
Positive therapeutic outcome
• Decrease in depression
• Absence of suicidal thoughts

TREATMENT OF OVERDOSE:
ECG monitoring, lavage, activated charcoal, administer anticonvulsant

nystatin (Rx, OTC)
(nis'ta-tin)
**Bio-Statin, Mycostatin, Nadostine ✦,
Nilstat, Pedi-Dri, PMS-Nystatin ✦**
Func. class.: Antifungal
Chem. class.: Amphoteric polyene
Pregnancy category C

ACTION: Interferes with fungal DNA replication; binds sterols in fungal cell membrane,
which increases permeability, resulting in leaking of cell nutrients

Therapeutic outcome: Fungistatic/fungi-
cidal against *Candida* organisms

USES: *Candida* species causing oral, intestinal infections

CONTRAINDICATIONS
Hypersensitivity

Precautions: Pregnancy C

DOSAGE AND ROUTES
Oral infection
Adult/adolescent/child: SUSP 400,000-600,000 units qid, use ½ dose in each side of mouth, swish and swallow, use for at least 48 hr after symptoms are resolved

Infant: SUSP 200,000 units qid (100,000 units in each side of mouth)

Newborn and premature infant: SUSP 100,000 units qid

Adult and child: Troches 200,000-400,000 units qid × up to 2 wk

GI infection
Adult: PO 500,000-1,000,000 units tid

Cutaneous candidiasis
Adult/child:
Top cream/ointment
Apply to affected area bid
Powder
Apply to affected area bid-tid

Available forms: Tabs 500,000 units; oral caps 500,000, 1,000,000 units, bulk powder; susp 1,000,000 unit/ml

Implementation
• Store oral susp at room temp; store tabs in tight, light-resistant containers at room temp
PO route
• Give oral susp dose by placing ½ in each cheek, swish for several min, then swallow; shake susp before use
• Store oral susp at room temp, tab in airtight, light-resistant containers at room temp
Topical route
• Administer by moistening lesions with a swab coated with cream or ointment; use enough medication to cover lesions completely; give after cleansing with soap, water before each application; dry well; very moist lesions are best treated with topical powder

ADVERSE EFFECTS
GI: Nausea, vomiting, anorexia, diarrhea, cramps
INTEG: Rash, urticaria (rare)

Pharmacokinetics

Absorption	Poorly absorbed
Distribution	Unknown
Metabolism	Not metabolized
Excretion	Feces, unchanged
Half-life	Unknown

Pharmacodynamics

Onset	Rapid
Peak	Unknown
Duration	6-12 hr

NURSING CONSIDERATIONS
Assessment
• **Assess for allergic reaction:** rash, urticaria; product may have to be discontinued
• Assess for predisposing factors for candidal infection: antibiotic therapy, pregnancy, diabetes mellitus, sexual partner infection (vag infections), AIDS
• Obtain culture and histologic tests to confirm organism

Patient/family education
• Instruct patient that long-term therapy may be needed to clear infection; to complete entire course of medication
• Teach patient proper hygiene: use no commercial mouthwashes for mouth infection
• Advise patient to avoid getting preparation on hands
• Instruct patient to notify prescriber if irritation occurs; product may have to be discontinued
• Inform patient that relief from itching may occur after 24-72 hr
Topical route
• Advise patient to discontinue use and notify prescriber if irritation occurs
• Teach patient to apply with glove to prevent further infection; product may stain
• Caution patient not to use occlusive dressings; to avoid use of OTC creams, ointments, lotions unless directed by prescriber

Evaluation
Positive therapeutic outcome
• Culture negative for *Candida*
• Decrease in size, number of lesions

nystatin topical
See Appendix B

obinutuzumab

(oh'bi-nue-tooz'ue-mab)

Gazyva

Func. class.: Antineoplastic

Chem. class.: Biologic response modifier

Pregnancy category C

ACTION: A recombinant human monoclonal antibody that binds to the gastric B-lymphocyte–associated antibody, action is indirect, possible through T-cell–mediated anti-tumor responses

Therapeutic outcome: Decreased disease progression

USES: Chronic lymphocytic leukemia

CONTRAINDICATIONS

Hypersensitivity

Precautions: Pregnancy **C**, breastfeeding, cardiac disease, children, human antichimeric antibody (HACA), human antimurine antibody (HAMA), infection, infusion-related reactions, neutropenia, pulmonary disease, thrombocytopenia, tumor lysis syndrome, vaccination

> **BLACK BOX WARNING:** Hepatitis, progressive multifocal leukoencephalopathy

DOSAGE AND ROUTES

Adult: IV **Cycle 1** 100 mg over 4 hr (day 1); then 900 mg (50 mg/hr, increased by 50 mg/hr q30min, to max 400 mg/hr) (day 2); then 1000 mg (100 mg/hr, increased by 100 mg/hr q30min to max 400 mg/hr (day 8, day 115); **Cycle 2-6** 1000 mg (100 mg/hr increased by 100 mg/hr q30min to max 400 mg/hr (day 1 repeat q28 days)

Available forms: Sol for inj 1000 mg/40 ml

Implementation

IV intermittent infusion route

• Due to the risk of hypotension, consider withholding antihypertensive medications for 12 hr before, during, and for the 1st hr after use until B/P is stable

• Give antimicrobial prophylaxis to neutropenic patients throughout treatment; consider antiviral and antifungal prophylaxis as needed

• **Premedication for cycle 1, days 1 and 2:** acetaminophen 650-1000 mg, and diphenhydrAMINE 50 mg at least 30 min prior to infusion, dexamethasone 20 mg IV or methylPREDNISolone 80 mg IV at least 1 hr before infusion

• **Premedication for cycle 1, days 8 and 15 and cycles 2-6, day 1:** acetaminophen 650-1000 mg at least 30 min prior to the infusion; those with any infusion-related reaction with the previous infusion should also receive diphenhydrAMINE 50 mg at least 30 min before the infusion; if the patient had a grade 3 infusion-related reaction with the previous dose or has a lymphocyte count $> 25 \times 10^9/L$, additionally administer dexamethasone 20 mg IV or methylPREDNISolone 80 mg IV at least 1 hr before infusion

• Use in a facility to adequately monitor and treat infusion reactions

• Visually inspect parenteral products for particulate matter and discoloration prior to use

• Prepare all doses in 0.9% NaCl; do not admix; use a final concentration of 0.4-4 mg/ml; give as an IV infusion only

Reconstitution

Cycle 1, day 1 and 2

• Withdraw 4 ml (100 mg) from the vial and dilute into 100 ml 0.9% NaCl; use on day 1; mix by gentle inversion; do not shake, use immediately

• Withdraw the remaining 36 ml (900 mg) and dilute into 250 ml 0.9% NaCl for use on day 2; mix by gentle inversion; do not shake

Cycle 1, day 8 and 15; cycles 2-6

• Withdraw 40 ml (1000 mg) from the vial and dilute into 250 ml 0.9% NaCl mix by gentle inversion; do not shake.

• Storage following reconstitution: Store at 2-8 °C (36-46 °F) for up to 24 hr. Do not freeze. Allow to come to room temperature before administration, use a dedicated line.

• **Day 1 (100-mg dose):** Give at an initial rate of 25 mg/hr over 4 hr. Do not increase the infusion rate.

• **Day 2 (900-mg dose):** Give at an initial rate of 50 mg/hr $\times$ 30 min; if no hypersensitivity or infusion-related events occur, increase the infusion rate by 50 mg/hr q30min to a max rate of 400 mg/hr. If a grade 1-2 infusion-related reaction occurs, the infusion should be temporarily interrupted or the rate reduced. The infusion may be resumed or continued at a reduced rate upon improvement of the patient's symptoms; if the reaction does not recur, the rate may be increased as appropriate for the current cycle and dose. If a grade 3 hypersensitivity or infusion-related event develops, the infusion should be temporarily interrupted. Upon improvement of the patient's symptoms, the infusion can be resumed at half the rate being used at the time that the reaction occurred; if the reaction does not recur, the rate may be increased as appropriate for the current cycle and dose. If a grade 4 hypersensitivity or infusion-related

Adverse effects: *italics* = common; **bold** = life-threatening

O

event develops, discontinue the infusion and do not resume.

• **Subsequent infusions (1000-mg dose):** Give at an initial rate of 100 mg/hr for 30 min; if no hypersensitivity or infusion-related events occur, increase the infusion rate by 100 mg/hr q30min to a max rate of 400 mg/hr; if a grade 1-2 infusion-related reaction occurs, the infusion should be temporarily interrupted or the rate reduced. The infusion may be resumed or continued at a reduced rate upon improvement of the patient's symptoms; if the reaction does not recur, the rate may be increased as appropriate for the current cycle and dose. If a grade 3 hypersensitivity or infusion-related event develops, the infusion should be temporarily interrupted. Upon improvement of the patient's symptoms, the infusion can be resumed at half the rate being used at the time that the reaction occurred; if the reaction does not recur, the rate may be increased as appropriate for the current cycle and dose. If a grade 4 hypersensitivity or infusion-related event develops, discontinue the infusion and do not resume.

ADVERSE EFFECTS

CNS: Headache, fever, chills, flushing
CV: Cardiac arrest, MI, sinus tachycardia, hypertension
GI: Constipation, decreased appetite, diarrhea, hepatitis/hepatic failure nausea, vomiting
HEMA: Neutropenia, thrombocytopenia, lymphopenia, leukopenia
META: Lower potassium/sodium/calcium, aluminum, higher potassium/uric acid
RESP: Wheezing, dyspnea
SYST: Tumor lysis syndrome

Pharmacokinetics

Absorption	Unknown
Distribution	Unknown
Metabolism	Unknown
Excretion	Unknown
Half-life	Terminal half-life 28.4 days

Pharmacodynamics

Onset	Unknown
Peak	Unknown
Duration	Unknown

NURSING CONSIDERATIONS
Assessment

BLACK BOX WARNING: Hepatitis B: reactivation of HBV in those who are HBsAg positive, HBsAg negative, and core antibody anti-HBc positive; may result in fulminant hepatitis, hepatic failure, and death

BLACK BOX WARNING: Progressive multifocal leukoencephalopathy (PML): Notify prescriber of any new or worsening neurologic signs/symptoms (ataxia, visual changes, confusion)

⚠ **Tumor lysis syndrome:** Can occur within 24 hr of 1st infusion, those with high tumor burden or lymphocyte count $>25\times10^9/L$ are at increased risk; monitor serum creatinine, potassium, calcium, uric acid, phosphate closely

BLACK BOX WARNING: Severe/life-threatening infusion reactions: 2/3 of patients have a reaction to 1st dose; consider withholding antihypertensives for 12 hr prior to, during, and after 1st hr of infusion

Patient/family education
• Teach patient about the reason for treatment and expected results

Evaluation
Positive therapeutic outcome
• Decreased disease progression

octreotide (Rx)
(ok-tree′o-tide)
SandoSTATIN, Sandostatin LAR Depot
Func. class.: Growth hormone, antidiarrheal
Chem. class.: Synthetic octapeptide
Pregnancy category B

ACTION: A potent growth hormone similar to somatostatin

Therapeutic outcome: Decreased diarrhea; decreased symptoms of acromegaly, carcinoid tumors, vasoactive intestinal peptide tumors (VIPomas)

USES: Sandostatin: acromegaly, carcinoid tumors, VIPomas; **LAR Depot:** long-term maintenance of acromegaly, carcinoid tumors, VIPomas, short bowel syndrome, insulinoma, hepatorenal syndrome

Unlabeled uses: GI fistula, variceal bleeding, diarrheal conditions, pancreatic fistula, IBS, dumping syndrome

CONTRAINDICATIONS
Hypersensitivity

Precautions: Pregnancy **B,** breastfeeding, children, geriatric, diabetes mellitus, hypothyroidism, renal disease

DOSAGE AND ROUTES
Acromegaly
Adult: SUBCUT/IV 50-100 mcg bid-tid, adjust q2wk based on growth hormone levels (Sandostatin) or IM 20 mg q4wk × 3 mo, adjust by growth hormone levels (Sandostatin LAR)

VIPomas
Adult: SUBCUT/IV 200-300 mcg/day in 2-4 doses for 2 wk, max 450 mcg/day; (Sandostatin) or IM 20 mg q2wk × 2 mo, adjust dose (Sandostatin LAR)

Flushing/diarrhea in carcinoid tumors
Adult: SUBCUT/IV 100-600 mcg/day in 2-4 doses for 2 wk, titrated to patient response (Sandostatin) or IM 20 mg q4wk × 2 mo, adjust dose (Sandostatin LAR)

GI fistula
Adult: SUBCUT 50-200 mcg q8hr

Antidiarrheal in AIDS patients (unlabeled)
Adult: SUBCUT 50 mcg q8h PRN, increase to 500 mcg q8h

Irritable bowel syndrome (unlabeled)
Adult: SUBCUT 100 mcg single dose to 125 mcg bid

Dumping syndrome (unlabeled)
Adult: SUBCUT 50-150 mcg/day

Variceal bleeding (unlabeled)
Adult: IV 25-50 mcg/hr CONT IV INF for 18 hr-5 days

Available forms: Sandostatin: inj 0.05, 0.1, 0.2, 0.5, 1 mg/ml; LAR Depot: inj powder for susp 10 mg, 20, 30 mg/5 ml

Implementation
• Store in refrigerator for unopened amps, vials, or at room temp for 2 wk; protect from light; do not use discolored or cloudy sol
• Do not use if discolored or if particulates are present

IM route
• Reconstitute with diluent provided; give into gluteal, rotate injection sites

SUBCUT route
• Rotate inj sites; use hip, thigh, abdomen
• Avoid using medication that is cold; allow to reach room temperature; do not use LAR Depot, do not use if discolored or if particulates are present

Direct IV route
• Give over 3 min; in an emergency carcinoid crisis, give rapid bolus

Intermittent IV INF route
• Dilute in 50-200 ml D₅W, 0.9% NaCl; give over 15-30 min
• Solution is stable for 24 hr

Y-site compatibilities: Acyclovir, alfentanil, allopurinol, amifostine, amikacin, aminocaproic acid, aminophylline, amiodarone, amphotericin B colloidal, amphotericin B lipid complex, amphotericin B liposome, ampicillin, ampicillin-sulbactam, anidulafungin, argatroban, arsenic trioxide, atenolol, atracurium, azithromycin, aztreonam, bivalirudin, bleomycin, bumetanide, buprenorphine, busulfan, butorphanol, calcium chloride/gluconate, capreomycin, CARBOplatin, carmustine, caspofungin, ceFAZolin, cefepime, cefotaxime, cefoTEtan, cefOXitin, cefTAZidime, ceftizoxime, cefTRIAXone, cefuroxime, chloramphenicol, chlorproMAZINE, ciprofloxacin, cisatracurium, CISplatin, clindamycin, cyclophosphamide, cycloSPORINE, cytarabine, dacarbazine, DACTINomycin, DAPTOmycin, DAUNOrubicin, DAUNOrubicin liposome, dexamethasone, digoxin, diltiazem, diphenhydrAMINE, DOBUTamine, DOCEtaxel, dolasetron, DOPamine, DOXOrubicin, DOXOrubicin liposomal, doxycycline, droperidol, enalaprilat, ePHEDrine, EPINEPHrine, epirubicin, eptifibatide, ertapenem, erythromycin, esmolol, etoposide, famotidine, fenoldopam, fentaNYL, fluconazole, fludarabine, fluorouracil, foscarnet, fosphenytoin, furosemide, gallium nitrate, ganciclovir, gatifloxacin, gemcitabine, gentamicin, glycopyrrolate, granisetron, haloperidol, heparin, hydrALAZINE, hydrocortisone, HYDROmorphone, hydrOXYzine, IDArubicin, ifosfamide, imipenem-cilastatin, insulin (regular), irinotecan, isoproterenol, ketorolac, labetalol, lansoprazole, leucovorin, levofloxacin, lidocaine, linezolid, LORazepam, magnesium sulfate, mannitol, mechlorethamine, melphalan, meperidine, meropenem, mesna, methohexital, methotrexate, methyldopate, methylPREDNISolone, metoclopramide, metoprolol, metroNIDAZOLE, midazolam, milrinone, minocycline, mitoMYcin, mitoXANtrone, mivacurium, morphine, moxifloxacin, mycophenolate, nafcillin, nalbuphine, naloxone, nesiritide, niCARdipine, nitroglycerin, nitroprusside, norepinephrine, ondansetron, oxaliplatin, PACLitaxel, palonosetron, pamidronate, pancuronium, PEMEtrexed, pentamidine, pentazocine, PENTobarbital, PHENobarbital, phenylephrine, piperacillin, piperacillin-tazobactam, polymyxin B, potassium acetate/chloride/phosphates, procainamide, prochlorperazine, promethazine, propranolol, quiNIDine, quinupristin-dalfopristin, ranitidine, remifentanil, rocuronium, sodium acetate/bicarbonate/phosphates, streptozocin, succinylcholine, SUFentanil,

Adverse effects: *italics* = common; **bold** = life-threatening

O

sulfamethoxazole-trimethoprim, tacrolimus, teniposide, thiopental, thiotepa, ticarcillin, ticarcillin-clavulanate, tigecycline, tirofiban, tobramycin, topotecan, vancomycin, vasopressin, vecuronium, verapamil, vinBLAStine, vinCRIStine, vinorelbine, voriconazole, zidovudine, zoledronic acid

ADVERSE EFFECTS

CNS: *Headache, dizziness, fatigue, weakness,* depression, anxiety, tremors, seizures, paranoia

CV: *Sinus bradycardia, conduction abnormalities,* dysrhythmias, chest pain, shortness of breath, thrombophlebitis, ischemia, CHF, hypertension, palpitations, QT prolongation, ST-T wave changes

ENDO: *Hypo/hyperglycemia, ketosis, hypothyroidism,* galactorrhea, diabetes insipidus

GI: *Diarrhea, nausea, abdominal pain, vomiting, flatulence, distension, constipation,* hepatitis, elevated liver function tests, GI bleeding, pancreatitis, cholelithiasis, ileus

GU: UTI

HEMA: Hematoma of inj site, bruise

INTEG: Rash, urticaria, pain, inflammation at inj site

MS: Joint and muscle pain

Pharmacokinetics

Absorption	Rapidly, completely absorbed
Distribution	Unknown
Metabolism	Little
Excretion	Urine, unchanged
Half-life	1.7 hr

Pharmacodynamics

	Subcut/IV	IM
Onset	Unknown	Unknown
Peak	½ hr	2-4 wk
Duration	12 hr	Unknown

INTERACTIONS

Individual drugs

Bromocriptine: decreased: effect of bromocriptine

CycloSPORINE: decreased effect of cycloSPORINE

Haloperidol, chloroquine, droperidol, pentamidine, arsenic trioxide, levomethadyl: increased QT prolongation

Drug classifications

Class IA/III antidysrhythmics, some phenothiazines, β-agonists, local anesthetics, tricyclics, CYP3A4 inhibitors (amiodarone, clarithromycin, erythromycin, telithromycin, troleandomycin), CYP3A4 substrates (methadone, pimozide,

QUEtiapine, quiNIDine, risperiDONE, ziprasidone): increased QT prolongation

Oral antidiabetics: decreased: effect of the oral antidiabetics; monitor blood glucose

CYP3A4 metabolized products: decreased: excretion of these products; reduction of dose may be required

Drug/food

Decreased: absorption of dietary fat, vit B_{12} levels

Drug/lab test

Increased: glucose

Decreased: T_4, thyroid function tests, vit B_{12}, glucose

NURSING CONSIDERATIONS

Assessment

• Identify growth hormone antibodies, IGF-1, 1-4 hr intervals for 8-12 hr after dose in acromegaly; 5-HIAA; blood glucose, serotonin levels (carcinoid tumors), plasma substance P, plasma vasoactive intestinal peptide (VIP) (VIPomas)

• Monitor for fecal fat, serum carotene, somatomedin-C q14 days, glucose; plasma serotonin levels (carcinoid tumors); plasma vasoactive intestinal peptide levels (VIPoma); serum growth hormone, serum IGF-1 baseline and periodically, diabetes to monitor blood glucose

• Monitor thyroid function tests: T_3, T_4, T_7, TSH to identify hypothyroidism

• Assess for allergic reaction: rash, itching, fever, nausea, wheezing

• Assess for cardiac status: bradycardia, conduction abnormalities, dysrhythmias; monitor ECG for QT prolongation, low voltage, axis shifts, early repolarization, R/S transition, early wave progression

• **Allergic reaction:** assess for rash, itching, fever, nausea, wheezing

• Gallbladder disease, pancreatitis: monitor closely

Patient/family education

• Explain reason for medication and expected results

• Advise patient that routine follow-up is needed

• Instruct parents on procedure for medication preparation and inj use; request demonstration; return demonstration; provide written instructions

• Advise patient that dizziness, drowsiness, weakness may occur; to avoid hazardous activities if these occur; to report abdominal pain immediately

• Teach patient that pregnancy may occur in acromegaly since fertility may be restored

• Teach diabetic patients to monitor glucose regularly

Evaluation
Positive therapeutic outcome
• Decreased symptoms of acromegaly, carcinoid, VIPoma
• Decreased diarrhea in AIDS

---

ofloxacin (Rx)
(o-flox′a-sin)
Func. class.: Antiinfective
Chem. class.: Fluoroquinolone
Pregnancy category C

ACTION: Interferes with conversion of intermediate DNA fragments into high molecular weight DNA in bacteria, inhibits DNA gyrase

Therapeutic outcome: Bactericidal action against gram-positive pathogens *Staphylococcus epidermidis,* methicillin-resistant strains of *Staphylococcus aureus, Streptococcus pyogenes, Streptococcus pneumoniae;* gram-negative pathogens *Escherichia coli, Klebsiella* species, *Enterobacter, Salmonella, Shigella, Proteus vulgaris, Proteus rettgeri, Providencia stuartii, Morganella morganii, Pseudomonas aeruginosa, Serratia, Haemophilus* species, *Acinetobacter, Neisseria gonorrhoeae, Neisseria meningitidis, Yersinia, Vibrio, Brucella, Campylobacter,* and *Aeromonas* species; anaerobic pathogens *Bacteroides fragilis intermedius, Clostridium perfringens, Gardnerella vaginalis, Peptococcus niger, Peptostreptococcus* species; *Chlamydia pneumoniae, Chlamydia trachomatis, Legionella pneumoniae, Mycobacterium tuberculosis, Mycoplasma pneumoniae*

USES: Treatment of lower respiratory tract infections (pneumonia, bronchitis), genitourinary infections (prostatitis, UTIs), skin and skin structure infections, gonorrhea, otitis media, conjunctivitis (ophth)

CONTRAINDICATIONS
Hypersensitivity to quinolones, QT prolongation, TB

Precautions: Pregnancy **C,** breastfeeding, children, geriatric, renal disease, seizure disorders, excessive sunlight, hypokalemia, colitis

> **BLACK BOX WARNING:** Tendon pain/rupture, tendinitis, myasthenia gravis

DOSAGE AND ROUTES
Lower respiratory tract infection/ skin and skin structure infections
Adult: PO 400 mg q12hr × 10 days

Prostatitis from *E. Coli*
Adult: PO 300 mg q12hr × 6 wk

Urinary tract infection
Adult: PO 200 mg q12hr × 10 days

Pelvic inflammatory disease
Adult: PO 400 mg q12hr with metroNIDAZOLE × 10-14 days

Traveler's diarrhea (unlabeled)
Adult: PO 200 mg bid × 3 days

Epididymitis (unlabeled)
Adult: PO 300 mg bid × 10 days

Spontaneous bacterial peritonitis (unlabeled)
Adult: PO 400 mg bid

Renal dose
Adult: PO CCr 20-50 ml/min give q24hr; CCr <20 ml/min give ½ of dose q24hr

Hepatic dose
Adult (Child-Pugh class C): PO max 400 mg/day

Available forms: Tabs 200, 300, 400 mg

Implementation
• Store at room temp, protect from light
PO route
• Give in equal intervals q12hr around the clock to maintain proper blood levels; do not give within 2 hr of other agents, since product interactions are possible: give with 8 oz of water
• Do not give with iron, aluminum, zinc products or antacids, which decrease absorption and form insoluble chelate

ADVERSE EFFECTS
CNS: Dizziness, headache, fatigue, somnolence, depression, insomnia, lethargy, malaise, seizures, vertigo
CV: QT prolongation, dysrhythmias, chest pain
EENT: Visual disturbances, pharyngitis
GI: Diarrhea, nausea, vomiting, anorexia, flatulence, heartburn, dry mouth, increased AST, ALT, abdominal pain, constipation, pseudomembranous colitis, abnormal taste, xerostomia
HEMA: Blood dyscrasias
INTEG: Rash, pruritus, photosensitivity
MS: Tendinitis, tendon rupture, rhabdomyolysis
SYST: Anaphylaxis, Stevens-Johnson syndrome, toxic epidermal necrosis

Pharmacokinetics

Absorption	Well absorbed (PO)
Distribution	Widely distributed
Metabolism	Unknown
Excretion	Kidneys, unchanged; breast milk
Half-life	5-9 hr; increased in renal disease

Pharmacodynamics

	PO	Ophth
Onset	Rapid	Unknown
Peak	1-2 hr	Unknown
Duration	Unknown	Unknown

INTERACTIONS
Individual drugs
Chloroquine, clarithromycin, droperidol, erythromycin, haloperidol, methadone, pentamidine: increased QT prolongation
Sevelamer: decreased ofloxacin effect
Sucralfate, zinc sulfate: decreased absorption of ofloxacin, separate by 2 hr
Theophylline: possible toxicity
Warfarin: increased anticoagulation

Drug classifications
Antacids with aluminum, iron salts, magnesium: decreased absorption of ofloxacin, separate by 2 hr
Antidiabetics: altered blood glucose levels
β-agonists, class IA/III antidysrhythmics, local anesthetics, some phenothiazines, tricyclics: increased QT prolongation

> **BLACK BOX WARNING: Corticosteroids:** Increased tendon rupture/tendinitis

NSAIDs: increased CNS stimulation, seizures

Drug/lab test
Increased: INR

NURSING CONSIDERATIONS
Assessment
• Assess patient for previous sensitivity reaction
• Assess patient for signs and symptoms of infection including characteristics of wounds, sputum, urine, stool, WBC >10,000/mm^3, fever; obtain baselines and monitor during treatment
• Obtain C&S before beginning product therapy to identify if correct treatment has been initiated
• **QT prolongation: assess ECG for QT prolongation, ejection fraction; assess for chest pain, palpitations, dyspnea**
• **Pseudomembranous colitis: assess for diarrhea, abdominal pain, fever, fatigue, anorexia; possible anemia, elevated WBC and low serum albumin; stop product and usually give either vancomycin or IV metroNIDAZOLE**

> **BLACK BOX WARNING: Rhabdomyolysis:** assess muscle pain, increased CPK, weakness, swelling of affected muscles; if these occur and if confirmed by CPK, product should be discontinued

• Assess for allergic reactions: rash, urticaria, pruritus; stop product if these occur

• Monitor blood studies: AST, ALT, CBC, serum glucose monthly if patient is on long-term therapy; INR (warfarin use)
• Assess for overgrowth of infection in long-term treatment: perineal itching, fever, malaise, redness, pain, swelling, drainage, rash, diarrhea, change in cough, sputum
• Assess for CNS symptoms: seizures, vertigo, drowsiness, agitation, confusion, tremors

> **BLACK BOX WARNING: Myasthenia gravis:** product may increase weakness; avoid use

Patient/family education
• Instruct patient to take all medication prescribed for the length of time ordered; product must be taken around the clock to maintain blood levels; do not give medication to others
• Teach patient to use sunscreen when outdoors to decrease phototoxicity
• Teach patient that allergic reactions usually occur after first dose, but may occur later; stop product if a reaction occurs
• Advise patient to increase fluids to 2 L/day to prevent crystalluria
• Caution patient to avoid driving and other hazardous activities until response is known; dizziness, confusion, drowsiness may occur
• Teach patient to take without regard to meals
• Teach patient to avoid use with other products unless approved by prescriber
• Teach patient to notify prescriber immediately if tingling, pain in extremities occur

Evaluation
Positive therapeutic outcome
• Absence of signs/symptoms of infection
• Reported improvement in symptoms of infection
• Absence of red or itching eyes (ophth)

ofloxacin ophthalmic
See Appendix B

OLANZapine (Rx)
(oh-lanz′a-peen)
ZyPREXA, Zyprexa Relprevv, Zyprexa Zydis
Func. class.: Antipsychotic/neuroleptic
Chem. class.: Thienobenzodiazepine
Pregnancy category C

Do not confuse: OLANZapine/osalazine, Zyprexa/Celexa/Zyrtec

ACTION: May mediate antipsychotic activity by both DOPamine and serotonin type 2 (5-HT$_2$) antagonism; also, may antagonize muscarinic, histaminic (H$_1$), and α-adrenergic receptors

Therapeutic outcome: Decreased psychotic symptoms

USES: Schizophrenia, acute manic episodes in bipolar disorder, acute agitation

Unlabeled uses: Dementia related to Alzheimer's disease, OCD, acute psychosis

CONTRAINDICATIONS
Hypersensitivity

Precautions: Pregnancy **C**, breastfeeding, geriatric, hypertension, cardiac/renal/hepatic disease, diabetes, agranulocytosis, abrupt discontinuation, Asian patients, closed-angle glaucoma, coma, leukopenia, QT prolongation, tardive dyskinesia, torsades de pointes, suicidal ideation, stroke history, TIA

> **BLACK BOX WARNING:** Dementia, postinjection delirium/sedation syndrome

DOSAGE AND ROUTES
Schizophrenia
Adult: PO 5-10 mg/day initially, may increase dosage by 5 mg at ≥1 wk intervals; orally disintegrating tabs: open blister pack, place tab on tongue, let disintegrate, swallow; max 20 mg/day; ext rel inj (Zyprexa Relprev) IM 150-300 mg q2wk or 405 mg q4wk
Geriatric: PO 5 mg, may increase cautiously at 1 wk intervals, max 20 mg/day
Adolescent: PO 2.5 mg or 5 mg/day, target 10 mg/day

Bipolar mania
Adult: PO 10-15 mg/day, may increase dose after 24 hr by 5 mg, max 20 mg/day
Adolescent: PO 2.5 or 5 mg/day, target 10 mg/day

Agitation associated with schizophrenia, bipolar I mania
Adult: IM (reg rel) 10 mg once
Geriatric: IM (reg rel) 2.5-5 mg once

Available forms: Tabs 2.5, 5, 7.5, 10, 15, 20 mg; **orally disintegrating tabs** 5, 10, 15, 20 mg (Zyprexa Zydis); **powder for injection** 10 mg

Implementation
• Give antiparkinsonian agent for EPS
• Give decreased dose in geriatric
PO route
• Give with full glass of water/milk or with food to decrease GI upset
• **Orally disintegrating tabs:** open blister pack; place tab on tongue until dissolved; swallow; no water needed, do not break, crush, chew
• Store in tight, light-resistant container
IM route (Zyprexa Intramuscular)
• Dissolve contents of vials with 2.1 ml sterile water for injection (5 mg/ml), use immediately

• Do not use IV or SUBCUT
• Inject slowly, deep into muscle mass
IM route (Zyprexa Relprev)

> **BLACK BOX WARNING:** Available only through restricted distribution program due to postinjection delirium/sedation syndrome; give at a facility with emergency services

• Use deep IM gluteal inj only
• Use only diluent provided in kit; give q2-4wk using 19G 1.5-inch needle in kit, in obesity use 19G 2-inch or larger needle
• Provide supervised ambulation until stabilized on medication; do not involve in strenuous exercise program because fainting is possible; patients should not stand still for long periods
• Give increased fluids to prevent constipation
• Give sips of water, candy, gum for dry mouth
• Store in airtight, light-resistant container
• Give orally disintegrating tabs: open blister pack, place tab on tongue until dissolved, swallow; no water needed

ADVERSE EFFECTS
CNS: EPS (pseudoparkinsonism, akathisia, dystonia, tardive dyskinesia), seizures, headache, neuroleptic malignant syndrome (rare), agitation, nervousness, hostility, dizziness, hypertonia, tremor, euphoria, confusion, *drowsiness*, fatigue, *abnormal gait, insomnia, fever*
CV: Hypotension, tachycardia, chest pain, heart failure, sudden death (geriatric, IM), orthostatic hypotension, peripheral edema
ENDO: Increased prolactin levels, hyperglycemia, hypoglycemia
GI: Dry mouth, nausea, vomiting, anorexia, constipation, abdominal pain, weight gain, appetite, dyspepsia, jaundice, hepatitis
GU: Urinary retention, urinary frequency, enuresis, impotence, amenorrhea, gynecomastia, breast engorgement, premenstrual syndrome
HEMA: Neutropenia
INTEG: Rash
MISC: Peripheral edema, accidental injury, hypertonia, hyperlipidemia
MS: Joint pain, twitching
RESP: *Cough, pharyngitis,* fatal pneumonia (geriatric, IM)

Pharmacokinetics
Absorption	Well absorbed
Distribution	93% plasma protein binding
Metabolism	Liver
Excretion	Kidneys
Half-life	Unknown

Adverse effects: *italics* = common; **bold** = life-threatening

Pharmacodynamics

Onset	Unknown
Peak	PO 6 hr, IM 15-45 min
Duration	Unknown

INTERACTIONS
Individual drugs
Alcohol: increased sedation, hypotension

Bromocriptine, levodopa: decreased antiparkinson activity

CarBAMazepine, omeprazole, rifampin: decreased levels of OLANZapine

Diazepam: increased hypotension

FluvoxaMINE: increased OLANZapine levels

Drug classifications
SSRIs, SNRIs: increased serotonin syndrome, increased neuroleptic malignant syndrome

Anesthetics (barbiturates), antidepressants, antihistamines, CNS depressants, sedative/hypnotics: increased sedation

Anticholinergics: increased anticholinergic effects

Antihypertensives: increased hypotension

DOPamine agonists: decreased antiparkinson activity

Drug/lab test
Increased: liver function tests, prolactin, CPK

NURSING CONSIDERATIONS
Assessment

> **BLACK BOX WARNING:** Postinjection delirium/sedation syndrome (Zyprexa Relprevv): monitor continuously for ≥3 hr after injection; this patient must be accompanied when leaving: sedation, coma, delirium, EPS, slurred speech, altered gait, aggression, dizziness, weakness, hypertension, seizures; before leaving, confirm the patient is alert, oriented, and free of any other symptoms

• Assess mental status, orientation, mood, behavior, presence of hallucinations and type before initial administration and monthly

• Monitor I&O ratio; palpate bladder if low urinary output occurs, especially in geriatric

• Monitor bilirubin, CBC

• Monitor urinalysis; recommended before, during prolonged therapy

• Assess affect, orientation, LOC, reflexes, gait, coordination, sleep pattern disturbances

• Monitor B/P sitting, standing, lying; take pulse and respirations q4hr during initial treatment; establish baseline before starting treatment; report drops of 30 mm Hg; obtain baseline ECG

• **Serotonin syndrome:** assess for increased heart rate, shivering, sweating, dilated pupils, tremors, high B/P, hyperthermia, headache, confusion; if these occur, stop product, administer a serotonin antagonist if needed

• Assess dizziness, faintness, palpitations, tachycardia on rising

• Assess for neuroleptic malignant syndrome: hyperpyrexia, muscle rigidity, increased CPK, altered mental status, for acute dystonia (cheek chewing, swallowing, eyes, pill rolling)

• **EPS** including akathisia (inability to sit still, no pattern to movements), tardive dyskinesia (bizarre movements of the jaw, mouth, tongue, extremities), pseudoparkinsonism (rigidity, tremors, pill rolling, shuffling gait)

• Monitor constipation, urinary retention daily; increase bulk, water in diet

Patient/family education

> **BLACK BOX WARNING:** Teach patient about postinjection delirium/sedation syndrome; teach about all symptoms

• Teach patient to use good oral hygiene; frequent rinsing of mouth, candy, ice chips, sugarless gum for dry mouth

• Advise patient to avoid hazardous activities until product response is determined

• Advise patient that orthostatic hypotension occurs often and to rise from sitting or lying position gradually

• Advise patient to avoid hot tubs, hot showers, tub baths, since hypotension may occur

• Advise patient to avoid abrupt withdrawal of this product, or EPS may result; product should be withdrawn slowly

• Advise patient to avoid OTC preparations (cough, hay fever, cold) unless approved by prescriber, since serious product interactions may occur; avoid use with alcohol, CNS depressants, increased drowsiness may occur

• Advise patient that in hot weather, heat stroke may occur; take extra precautions to stay cool

Evaluation
Positive therapeutic outcome
• Decrease in emotional excitement, hallucinations, delusions, paranoia, reorganization of patterns of thought, speech

TREATMENT OF OVERDOSE:
Lavage if orally ingested; provide airway; do not induce vomiting or use epinephrine

olaparib
(oh-lap′a-rib)
Lynparza
Func. class.: Antineoplastic-PARP
Pregnancy category D

USES: Treatment of deleterious or suspected deleterious germline BRCA-mutated advanced ovarian cancer in patients who have not responded successfully to ≥3 prior courses of chemotherapy, as monotherapy

CONTRAINDICATIONS: Hypersensitivity, pregnancy **D**

DOSAGE AND ROUTES
Adult female: PO 400 mg bid until disease progression or unacceptable toxicity. Avoid use of concomitant strong and moderate CYP3A4 inhibitors if possible.

olmesartan (Rx)
(ol-meh-sar′tan)
Benicar
Func. class.: Antihypertensive
Chem. class.: Angiotensin II receptor (type AT$_1$) antagonist
Pregnancy category C (1st trimester), D (2nd/3rd trimesters)

Do not confuse: Benicar/Mevacor

ACTION: Blocks the vasoconstrictor and aldosterone-secreting effects of angiotensin II; selectively blocks the binding of angiotensin II to the AT$_1$ receptor found in tissues

Therapeutic outcome: Decreased B/P

USES: Hypertension, alone or in combination with other antihypertensives

CONTRAINDICATIONS
Hypersensitivity, pregnancy **D** (2nd/3rd trimesters)

Precautions: Breastfeeding, children, geriatric, hepatic disease, CHF, renal artery stenosis, African descent, hyperkalemia

DOSAGE AND ROUTES
Adult: PO single agent 20 mg/day initially in patients who are not volume depleted; may be increased to 40 mg/day if needed after 2 wk
Adolescent ≤16 yr/child ≥6 yr weighing ≥35 kg: PO 20 mg/day, may increase to max 40 mg/day after 2 wk

Adolescent ≤16 yr/child ≥6 yr weighing 20-<35 kg: PO 10 mg/day, may increase to max 20 mg/day after 2 wk

Available forms: Tabs 5, 20, 40 mg

Implementation
• Give without regard to meals
• Compounded suspension may be made in the pharmacy; refrigerate; shake well before use

ADVERSE EFFECTS
CNS: *Dizziness,* fatigue, insomnia, syncope
CV: Chest pain, peripheral edema, tachycardia, *hypotension*
EENT: Sinusitis, rhinitis, pharyngitis
GI: *Diarrhea,* abdominal pain
META: Hyperkalemia
MS: Arthralgia, pain, rhabdomyolysis
RESP: *Upper respiratory infection,* bronchitis
SYST: Angioedema

Pharmacokinetics

Absorption	Unknown
Distribution	Unknown
Metabolism	Unknown
Excretion	Urine, feces
Half-life	Unknown

Pharmacodynamics

Onset	Unknown
Peak	1-2 hr
Duration	Unknown

INTERACTIONS
Individual drugs
Lithium, ACE inhibitors: increased effect

Drug classifications
Antihypertensives (other), diuretics: increased antihypertensive effects
NSAIDs: decreased antihypertensive effect
Antioxidants: increased effects
Potassium supplements, potassium-sparing diuretics: increased hyperkalemia

Drug/herb
Aconite: increased toxicity, death
Astragalus, cola tree: increased or decreased antihypertensive effect
Hawthorn: increased antihypertensive effect
Ephedra: decreased antihypertensive effect

NURSING CONSIDERATIONS
Assessment

BLACK BOX WARNING: Assess for pregnancy; this product can cause fetal death when given in pregnancy, 2nd/3rd trimester

• Assess response and adverse reactions, especially in renal disease, monitor renal function
• Monitor B/P, pulse q4hr; note rate, rhythm, quality; electrolytes: sodium, potassium, chloride; baselines in renal, liver function tests before therapy begins
• Hypotension: place supine; may occur with hyponatremia or in those with volume depletion; more common in those also taking a diuretic

Patient/family education
• Advise to comply with dosage schedule, even if feeling better
• Advise patient to notify prescriber of mouth sores, fever, swelling of hands or feet, irregular heartbeat, chest pain
• Teach that excessive perspiration, dehydration, vomiting, diarrhea may lead to fall in B/P; to consult prescriber if these occur, maintain adequate hydration
• Teach that product may cause dizziness, fainting; light-headedness may occur, avoid hazardous activities
• Advise to rise slowly to sitting or standing position to minimize orthostatic hypotension

> **BLACK BOX WARNING:** Teach to notify prescriber immediately if pregnant; not to use during breastfeeding

• Advise to avoid all OTC medications, unless approved by prescriber
• Teach patient that blood glucose may increase and antidiabetic product may need dosage change
• Advise to inform all health care providers of medication use
• Advise to use proper technique for obtaining B/P and acceptable parameters

Evaluation
Positive therapeutic outcome
• Decreased B/P

---

olopatadine ophthalmic
See Appendix B

olsalazine (Rx)
(ohl-sal'ah-zeen)
Dipentum
Func. class.: Antiinflammatory
Chem. class.: Salicylate derivative
Pregnancy category C

Do not confuse: olsalazine/OLANZapine

ACTION: Bioconverted to 5-aminosalicylic acid, which decreases inflammation

Therapeutic outcome: Lessening of loose diarrhea stools and cramping

USES: Maintenance of remission of ulcerative colitis in patients intolerant to sulfasalazine

CONTRAINDICATIONS
Hypersensitivity to this product or salicylates

Precautions: Pregnancy **C,** breastfeeding, children <14 yr, impaired renal/hepatic function, severe allergy, bronchial asthma

DOSAGE AND ROUTES
Adult: PO 500 mg bid, max 3 g/day

Available forms: Caps 250 mg

Implementation
• Give total daily dose evenly spaced to minimize GI intolerance, give with food
• Store in tight, light-resistant container at room temperature

ADVERSE EFFECTS
CNS: Headache, hallucinations, depression, vertigo, fatigue, dizziness
GI: Nausea, vomiting, abdominal pain, **hepatitis,** diarrhea, bloating, **pancreatitis**
HEMA: Leukopenia, neutropenia, thrombocytopenia, agranulocytosis, anemia
INTEG: Rash, dermatitis, urticaria

Pharmacokinetics
Absorption	Colon 99% converted to mesalamine
Distribution	Colon
Metabolism	Liver
Excretion	Feces
Half-life	0.9 hr

Pharmacodynamics
Onset	Unknown
Peak	1 hr
Duration	12 hr

INTERACTIONS
Individual drugs
AzaTHIOprine: increased toxicity
Mercaptopurine, thioguanine: increased myelosuppression
Warfarin: increased pro-time, INR

Drug/lab test
Increased: AST, ALT

NURSING CONSIDERATIONS
Assessment
⚠ Assess for blood dyscrasias: skin rash, fever, sore throat, bruising, bleeding, fatigue, joint pain (rare)

• **Assess for allergic reaction:** rash, dermatitis, urticaria, pruritus, dyspnea, bronchospasm
• **Colitis:** assess bowel pattern, number of stools, consistency, frequency, pain, mucus before treatment and periodically

Patient/family education
• Advise patient to take as prescribed, take missed dose as soon as remembered
• Inform patient not to operate machinery or drive until effects are known, may cause dizziness
• Advise patient to notify prescriber if symptoms do not improve or if allergic reaction or sore throat occurs
• Teach patient to report diarrhea, rash, bleeding, bruising, fever, hallucinations
• BUN, creatinine in those with renal disease; LFTs (liver disease)

Evaluation
Positive therapeutic outcome
• Absence of fever, mucus in stools

RARELY USED

omacetaxine
(oh′ma-set-ax′een)
Synribo
Func. class.: Antineoplastic miscellaneous
Chem. class.: Cephalotaxine ester (derived from the evergreen tree *Cephalotaxus harringtonia*)
Pregnancy category D

Therapeutic outcome: Decreased CML, positive hematologic response

USES: Chronic or accelerated phase chronic myelogenous leukemia (CML) with resistance or/and intolerance to 2 or more tyrosine kinase inhibitors

CONTRAINDICATIONS
Pregnancy (**D**), breastfeeding, hypersensitivity

DOSAGE AND ROUTES
Adult: SUBCUT 1.25 mg/m² bid × 14 days every 28 days
Grade 4 neutropenia (absolute neutrophil count [ANC] < 0.5 × 10⁹/L) or grade 3 thrombocytopenia (platelet count < 50 × 10⁹/L): Do not start the next cycle until the ANC is ≥1 × 10⁹/L and platelets are 50 × 10⁹/L; when therapy is resumed, reduce the number of dosing days by 2 days/cycle (initial cycles, from 14 to 12 days; maintenance cycles, from 7 to 5 days)

Evaluation
Positive therapeutic outcome
• Decreased CML, positive hematologic response

---

omalizumab (Rx)
(oh-mah-lye-zoo′mab)
Xolair
Func. class.: Antiasthmatic
Chem. class.: Monoclonal antibody
Pregnancy category B

ACTION: Recombinant DNA-derived humanized IgG murine monoclonal antibody that selectively binds to IgE to limit the release of mediators in the allergic response

Therapeutic outcome: Ability to breathe more easily

USES: Moderate to severe persistent asthma

Unlabeled uses: Seasonal allergic rhinitis, food allergy

CONTRAINDICATIONS
Hypersensitivity to hamster protein

BLACK BOX WARNING: Hypersensitivity to this product

Precautions: Pregnancy **B**, breastfeeding, children <12 yr, acute attacks of asthma, lymphoma, nephrotic disease, bronchospasm, neoplastic disease, status asthmaticus

DOSAGE AND ROUTES
Adult/adolescent/child ≥12 yr: SUBCUT 150-375 mg × 2-4 wk, divide inj into 2 sites, if dose is >150 mg; dose is adjusted based on IgE levels and significant changes in body weight

Available forms: Powder for inj, lyophilized 202.5 mg (150 mg/1.2 ml after reconstitution)

Implementation
SUBCUT route
• Reconstitute using 1.4 ml sterile water for inj (150 mg/1.2 ml or 125 mg/ml); gently swirl to dissolve; allow vial to stand and q5min gently swirl for 5-10 sec to dissolve, some vials take ≥20 min, do not use if contents do not dissolve within 40 min, should be clear or slightly opalescent; use large-bore needle to withdraw medication; replace needle with small-bore needle
• Given q2-4wk; product is viscous; if >150 mg is given, divide into two sites; the inj may take 5-10 sec to administer
• Do not give more than 150 mg/inj site

ADVERSE EFFECTS

CV: **Heart failure,** cardiomyopathy, hypotension

HEMA: Serious systemic eosinophilia

INTEG: Pruritus, dermatitis, inj site reactions, rash

MISC: Earache, dizziness, fatigue, pain, **malignancies,** viral infections, **anaphylaxis, thrombocytopenia,** headache

MS: Arthralgia, fracture, leg, arm pain

RESP: Sinusitis, upper respiratory tract infections, pharyngitis, pulmonary hypertension, **bronchospasm**

Pharmacokinetics

Absorption	Slow
Distribution	Unknown
Metabolism	Degradation by liver
Excretion	In bile
Half-life	26 days

Pharmacodynamics

Onset	Unknown
Peak	7-8 days
Duration	Unknown

INTERACTIONS

Drug classifications

Vaccines (live virus): use cautiously

Drug/lab test

Increased: IgE

NURSING CONSIDERATIONS

Assessment

• Monitor respiratory rate, rhythm, depth; auscultate lung fields bilaterally; notify prescriber of abnormalities; monitor pulmonary function tests; serum IgE

> **BLACK BOX WARNING: Assess for anaphylaxis, allergic reactions:** rash, urticaria, inability to breathe, edema of throat; observe for 2 hr, reaction can occur up to 24 hr; have emergency equipment available; product should be discontinued

Patient/family education

• Advise patient that improvement will not be immediate

• Teach patient not to stop taking or decrease current asthma medications unless instructed by prescriber

> **BLACK BOX WARNING:** Instruct patient to report signs of allergic reaction immediately, can be life-threatening

Evaluation

Positive therapeutic outcome

• Ability to breathe more easily

---

omeprazole (Rx, OTC)

(oh-mep′ra-zole)

Losec ✦, PriLOSEC, PriLOSEC OTC

Func. class.: Antiulcer, proton pump inhibitor

Chem. class.: Benzimidazole

Pregnancy category C ✴

Do not confuse: PriLOSEC/Prinivil/predniSONE/PROzac

ACTION: Suppresses gastric secretion by inhibiting hydrogen/potassium ATPase enzyme system in the gastric parietal cell; characterized as a gastric acid pump inhibitor, since it blocks the final step of acid production

Therapeutic outcome: Absence of duodenal ulcers; decreased gastroesophageal reflux

USES: Gastroesophageal reflux disease (GERD), severe erosive esophagitis, poorly responsive systemic GERD, pathologic hypersecretory conditions (Zollinger-Ellison syndrome, systemic mastocytosis, multiple endocrine adenomas); possibly effective for treatment of duodenal ulcers with or without antiinfectives for *Helicobacter pylori*

CONTRAINDICATIONS

Hypersensitivity

Precautions: Pregnancy **C**, breastfeeding, children

DOSAGE AND ROUTES

Active duodenal ulcers

Adult: PO 20 mg/day × 4-8 wk; associated with *H. pylori* 40 mg qAM and clarithromycin 500 mg tid on days 1-14, then 20 mg/day days 15-28

Severe erosive esophagitis/poorly responsive GERD

Adult: PO (DEL REL cap/SUSP) 20 mg/day × 4-8 wk

Pathologic hypersecretory conditions

Adult: PO 60 mg/day; may increase to 120 mg tid; daily doses >80 mg should be divided

Gastric ulcer

Adult: PO 40 mg/day × 4-8 wk

Geriatric: PO max 20 mg/day

Heartburn (OTC)

Adult: PO 1 DEL REL tab (20 mg) daily before AM meal with glass of water

---

Available forms: Del rel caps 10, 20, 40 mg, del rel tabs (PriLOSEC OTC) 20 mg; granules for oral susp 2.5, 10 mg (del rel)

Implementation
• Swallow sus rel caps whole; do not break, crush, chew, or open
• Give before patient eats; may give with antacids

ADVERSE EFFECTS
CNS: *Headache, dizziness, asthenia*
GI: *Diarrhea, abdominal pain, vomiting, nausea, constipation, flatulence, acid regurgitation,* abdominal swelling, anorexia, irritable colon, esophageal candidiasis, dry mouth, **hepatic failure**
INTEG: Rash, dry skin, urticaria, pruritus, alopecia
MISC: *Back pain,* fever, fatigue, malaise
RESP: *Upper respiratory tract infections, cough,* epistaxis, **pneumonia**

Pharmacokinetics

Absorption	Rapidly absorbed
Distribution	Protein binding (95%); gastric parietal cells
Metabolism	Liver, extensively; by CYP450 enzyme system
Excretion	Kidneys, feces
Half-life	½-1 hr; increased in the geriatric, hepatic disease

Pharmacodynamics

Onset	1 hr
Peak	½-3½ hr
Duration	3-4 days

INTERACTIONS
Individual drugs
Ampicillin: decreased effect of ampicillin
Calcium carbonate: decreased absorption of calcium carbonate
Cyanocobalamin: decreased absorption of cyanocobalamin
CycloSPORINE: increased cycloSPORINE levels
Diazepam: increased serum levels of diazepam
Digoxin: increased serum levels, delayed absorption of digoxin
Disulfiram: increased disulfiram levels
Flurazepam: increased flurazepam level
Gefitinib: decreased effect of gefitinib
Indinavir: decreased effect of indinavir
Iron salts: decreased absorption
Ketoconazole: decreased absorption of ketoconazole
Phenytoin: increased serum levels of phenytoin
Triazolam: increased triazolam level
Warfarin: increased bleeding tendencies

Drug classifications
Iron products: decreased absorption of iron

Drug/lab test
Increased: alkaline phosphatase, AST, ALT, bilirubin, gastrin

NURSING CONSIDERATIONS
Assessment
• **Electrolyte imbalances:** hyponatremia, hypomagnesemia in those using this product 3 mo-1 yr; if hypomagnesemia occurs, use of magnesium supplement may be sufficient; if severe, discontinue use
• Assess GI system: bowel sounds q8hr, abdomen for pain and swelling, anorexia
• **Monitor hepatic enzymes:** AST, ALT, increased alkaline phosphatase during treatment; blood studies; CBC, differential during treatment, blood dyscrasias may occur; vitamin B_{12} in long-term treatment
• Teach patient to take as directed, even if feeling better; to take missed dose as soon as remembered; not to double; PriLOSEC OTC can take up to 4 days for full effect

Patient/family education
• Advise patient to report severe diarrhea; black, tarry stools; abdominal cramps/pain, continuing headache; product may have to be discontinued
• Caution patient to avoid driving and other hazardous activities until response to product is known
• Caution patient to avoid alcohol, salicylates, ibuprofen; may cause GI irritation

Evaluation
Positive therapeutic outcome
• Absence of epigastric pain, swelling, fullness

ondansetron (Rx)
(on-dan'sa-tron)
Zofran, Zofran ODT, Zuplenz
Func. class.: Antiemetic
Chem. class.: 5-HT receptor antagonist
Pregnancy category B

Do not confuse: Zofran/Zantac

ACTION: Prevents nausea, vomiting by blocking serotonin (5-HT) peripherally, centrally, and in the small intestine

Therapeutic outcome: Control of nausea, vomiting

USES: Prevention of nausea, vomiting associated with cancer chemotherapy, radiotherapy, and prevention of postoperative nausea, vomiting

Unlabeled uses: Bulimia, pruritus (rectal use), alcoholism, hyperemesis gravidarum

CONTRAINDICATIONS
Hypersensitivity; phenylketonuric hypersensitivity (oral disintegrating tab), torsades de pointes

Precautions: Pregnancy **B**, breastfeeding, children, geriatric, granisetron hypersensitivity, QT prolongation, torsades de pointes

DOSAGE AND ROUTES
Prevention of nausea/vomiting (cancer chemotherapy)
Adult and child 4-18 yr: IV 0.15 mg/kg infused over 15 min, 30 min before start of cancer chemotherapy, max 16 mg/dose; 0.15 mg/kg is given 4 hr and 8 hr after first dose or 16 mg as a single dose; dilute in 50 ml of D_5 or 0.9% NaCl before giving; RECT (unlabeled) 16 mg daily 2 hr before chemotherapy; PO 8 mg ½ hr prior to chemotherapy, repeat 4, 8 hr after 1st dose
Child ≥4 yr: PO 4 mg ½ hr prior to chemotherapy

Prevention of nausea/vomiting (radiotherapy)
Adult: PO 8 mg tid, may repeat q8hr

Prevention of postoperative nausea/vomiting
Adult: IV/IM 4 mg undiluted over >30 sec prior to induction of anesthesia
Child 2-12 yr: IV 0.1 mg/kg (≤40 kg); 4 mg (≥40 kg), give ≥30 sec

Hepatic dose
Adult: PO/IM/IV max dose 8 mg daily

Hyperemesis gravidarum (unlabeled)
Adult: PO/IV 4-8 mg bid-tid

Pruritus (unlabeled)
Adult: PO 4 mg bid

Alcoholism (unlabeled)
Adult: PO 4 mcg/kg bid

Available forms: Inj 2 mg/ml, 32 mg/50 ml (premixed); tabs 4, 8 mg; oral sol 4 mg/5 ml; oral disintegrating tabs 4, 8 mg; oral dissolving film 4.8 mg

Implementation
PO route
• **Oral disintegrating tab:** do not push through foil; gently remove and immediately place on tongue to dissolve, swallow with saliva
• **Oral dissolving film:** fold pouch along dotted line to expose near notch; while folded, tear and remove film, place film on tongue until dissolved, swallow after dissolved; to reach desired dose, administer successive films, allowing each to dissolve before using another
• Check for discoloration or particulate; if particulate is present, shake to dissolve
IM route
• Visually inspect for particulate or discoloration
• May give 4 mg undiluted IM; inject deeply in large muscle mass, aspirate

Direct IV route
• Give **IV** after diluting a single dose in 50 ml of 0.9% NaCl or D_5W, 0.45% NaCl; give over 15 min
• Store at room temperature for 48 hr after dilution
• Do not use IV 32-mg dose in chemotherapy; nausea/vomiting due to QT prolongation, max 16 mg/dose (adult)

Y-site compatibilities: Aldesleukin, amifostine, amikacin, aztreonam, bleomycin, CARBOplatin, carmustine, ceFAZolin, ceforanide, cefotazime, cefOXitin, cefTAZidime, ceftizoxime, cefuroxime, chlorproMAZINE, cimetidine, cisatracurium, CISplatin, cladribine, clindamycin, cyclophosphamide, cytarabine, dacarbazine, DACTINomycin, DAUNOrubicin, dexamethasone, diphenhydrAMINE, DOXOrubicin, DOXOrubicin liposome, doxycycline, droperidol, etoposide, famotidine, filgrastim, floxuridine, fluconazole, fludarabine, gentamicin, haloperidol, heparin, hydrocortisone, HYDROmorphone, hydrOXYzine, ifosfamide, imipenem/cilastatin, magnesium sulfate, mannitol, mechlorethamine, melphalan, meperidine, mesna, methotrexate, metoclopramide, miconazole, mitoMYcin, mitoXANtrone, morphine, PACLitaxel, pentostatin, potassium chloride, prochlorperazine, ranitidine, remifentanil, streptozocin, teniposide, thiotepa, ticarcillin, ticarcillin/clavulanate, vancomycin, vinBLAStine, vinCRIStine, vinorelbine, zidovudine

Y-site incompatibilities: Acyclovir, aminophylline, amphotericin B, ampicillin, ampicillin/sulbactam, cefoperazone, furosemide, ganciclovir, LORazepam, methylPREDNISolone, mezlocillin, piperacillin, sargramostim, sodium bicarbonate

ADVERSE EFFECTS
CNS: *Headache,* dizziness, drowsiness, fatigue, EPS
GI: *Diarrhea, constipation, abdominal pain,* dry mouth
MISC: Rash, bronchospasm (rare), *musculoskeletal pain, wound problems, shivering, fever, hypoxia, urinary retention*

Pharmacokinetics

Absorption	Completely absorbed (**IV**)
Distribution	Unknown
Metabolism	Liver, extensively
Excretion	Kidneys
Half-life	3.5-4.7 hr

Pharmacodynamics

Unknown

INTERACTIONS
Individual drugs
Apomorphine: increased unconsciousness, hypotension: do not use together

CarBAMazepine, phenytoin, rifampin: decreased ondansetron effect

Drug classifications
Increased QT prolongation with other products that prolong QT

Drug/lab test
Increased: LFTs

NURSING CONSIDERATIONS
Assessment
• Assess for absence of nausea, vomiting during chemotherapy
• Assess for hypersensitivity reaction: rash, bronchospasm
• **Assess for EPS** shuffling gait, tremors, grimacing, rigidity
• QT prolongation: monitor ECG in those with cardiac disease and those receiving other products that increase QT

Patient/family education
• Instruct patient to report diarrhea, constipation, rash, changes in respirations, or discomfort at insertion site
• Teach patient reason for medication and expected results

Evaluation
Positive therapeutic outcome
• Absence of nausea, vomiting during cancer chemotherapy

oritavancin
(or-it'a-van'sin)
Orbactiv
Func. class.: Antiinfective agent
Chem. class.: Glycopeptide
Pregnancy category C

ACTION: Inhibits bacterial cell-wall biosynthesis by preventing transglycosylation (polymerization) by binding to precursors, as well as by preventing cross-linking by binding to the peptide bridging segments of the cell wall; also disrupts the bacterial cell membrane integrity, resulting in depolarization, increased permeability, and eventual cell death

Therapeutic outcome: Resolution of infection

USES: *Enterococcus faecalis, Enterococcus faecium, Staphylococcus aureus* (MRSA), *Staphylococcus aureus* (MSSA), *Streptococcus agalactiae* (group B streptococci), *Streptococcus anginosus, Streptococcus constellatus, Streptococcus dysgalactiae, Streptococcus intermedius, Streptococcus pyogenes* (group A β-hemolytic streptococci); treatment of acute bacterial skin and skin structure infections (ABSSSI) due to gram-positive organisms, including cellulitis/erysipelas, major cutaneous abscesses, and wound infections

CONTRAINDICATIONS: Hypersensitivity

Precautions: Anticoagulant therapy, antimicrobial resistance, breastfeeding, colitis, diarrhea, inflammatory bowel disease, infusion reactions, pregnancy (**C**), pseudomembranous colitis, vancomycin hypersensitivity, viral infection

DOSAGE AND ROUTES
Adult: IV 1200 mg once

Available forms: Powder for injection: 400 mg

Implementation
• Visually inspect for particulate matter and discoloration beforehand; the reconstituted solution is clear, colorless to pale yellow
• Reconstitution: Reconstitute each 400-mg vial with 40 ml sterile water for injection. Three vials are necessary for a single dose; gently swirl until dissolved.
• Dilution: Withdraw and discard 120 ml from a 1000-ml intravenous bag of D_5W, transfer 40 ml solution from each of the 3 reconstituted vials to the D_5W IV bag (1.2 mg/ml)
• Storage: Refrigerate or store at room temperature. The combined storage time (from reconstitution to dilution) and 3-hour infusion time should not exceed 6 hr at room temperature or 12 hr if refrigerated.

Intermittent IV INF
• Infuse over 3 hr, do not infuse with other medications or electrolytes, do not use saline-based solution

ADVERSE EFFECTS
CNS: Dizziness, flushing, headache
CV: Sinus tachycardia, phlebitis

Adverse effects: *italics* = common; **bold** = life-threatening

GI: Nausea, vomiting, diarrhea
HEMA: Anemia, eosinophilia
INTEG: Rash, vasculitis, pruritus, **angio-edema,** infusion-related reaction
MISC: Wheezing, bronchospasm
MS: Myalgia, osteomyelitis

Pharmacokinetics

Absorption	Unknown
Distribution	85% protein binding
Metabolism	Unknown
Excretion	Unknown
Half-life	Terminal half-life 245 hr

Pharmacodynamics

Onset	Unknown
Peak	Unknown
Duration	Unknown

INTERACTIONS
Drug classifications
Products metabolized by CYP2D6 and CYP3A4: Increased toxicity

Drug/lab test
Increased: LFTs

NURSING CONSIDERATIONS
Assessment
• Monitor CBC and differential
• Assess for diarrhea, bloody stools, cramping

Patient/family education
• Teach patient reason for product, expected result
• Advise patient product is used only once to resolve infection

Evaluation
Positive therapeutic outcome
• Resolution of infection

orlistat (Rx, OTC)
(or-li′stat)
Alli, Xenical
Chem. class.: Weight control agent, lipase inhibitor
Pregnancy category B

Do not confuse: Xenical/Xeloda

ACTION: Inhibits the absorption of dietary fat

Therapeutic outcome: Decrease in weight

USES: Obesity management

CONTRAINDICATIONS
Hypersensitivity, chronic malabsorption syndrome, cholestasis, pregnancy (**X**)

Precautions: Children, hypothyroidism, other organic causes of obesity, anorexia nervosa, bulimia, nephrolithiasis, GI disease, diabetes, fat-soluble vitamin deficiency, breastfeeding

DOSAGE AND ROUTES
Adult: PO 60 mg (Alli)-120 mg (Xenical) tid with each main meal containing fat, max 360 mg/day

Available forms: Caps 60 mg (Alli), 120 mg (Xenical)

Implementation
• Patient should be on a diet with 30% of calories from fat; omit dose of orlistat if a meal contains no fat

ADVERSE EFFECTS
CNS: *Insomnia,* dizziness, headache, depression, anxiety, fatigue
GI: *Oily spotting, flatus with discharge, fecal urgency, fatty/oily stool, oily evacuation, fecal incontinence,* frequent defecation, nausea, vomiting, abdominal pain, infectious diarrhea, rectal pain, tooth disorder, hypovitaminosis, hepatic failure, hepatitis, pancreatitis
GU: UTI, vaginitis, menstrual irregularity
INTEG: Dry skin, rash
MS: Back pain, arthritis, myalgia, tendinitis
RESP: Influenza, upper, lower respiratory tract infection, EENT symptoms

Pharmacokinetics

Absorption	Minimal
Distribution	99% protein binding
Metabolism	Unknown
Excretion	Feces
Half-life	1-2 hr

Pharmacodynamics

Onset	Unknown
Peak	8 hr
Duration	Unknown

INTERACTIONS
Individual drugs
CycloSPORINE: decreased absorption
Pravastatin: increased lipid-lowering effect
Warfarin: increased effects of warfarin

Drug classifications
Fat-soluble vitamins: decreased absorption

NURSING CONSIDERATIONS
Assessment
• **Weight status:** before starting therapy, obtain testing to rule out physiologic reactions for weight; obtain thyroid testing, BMI, glucose
• Monitor weight weekly, diabetic patients may need reduction in oral hypoglycemics

---

- Assess for misuse in certain populations (anorexia nervosa, bulimia)
- **Hepatotoxicity/pancreatitis: assess for liver injury: jaundice, weakness, abdominal pain (rare)**

Patient/family education
- Advise patient that 60 mg cap can be obtained OTC; 60 mg tid is the highest OTC dose
- Warn patient that safety and effectiveness beyond 2 yr have not been determined
- Instruct patient to read patient's information sheet, discuss unpleasant GI side effects
- Advise patient to avoid hazardous activities until stabilized on medication
- Instruct patient to take a multivitamin containing fat-soluble vitamins, take 2 hr before or after orlistat; psyllium taken with each dose or at bedtime may decrease GI symptoms
- Instruct patient/family to notify prescriber if significant side effects occur
⚠ **Advise prescriber if pregnancy is planned or suspected; pregnancy (X), if breastfeeding, take proper fat-soluble vitamins**
- **Hepatotoxicity/pancreatitis:** advise patient to report yellowing skin/eyes, dark urine, weakness, abdominal pain

Evaluation
Positive therapeutic outcome
- Decreased weight

oseltamivir (Rx)
(oh-sell-tam′ih-ver)
Tamiflu
Func. class.: Antiviral
Chem. class.: Neuramidase inhibitor
Pregnancy category C

ACTION: Inhibits influenza virus neuraminidase with possible alteration of virus particle aggregation and release

Therapeutic outcome: Decreased symptoms of influenza type A

USES: Prevention/treatment of influenza type A or B

Unlabeled uses: Avian influenzae (H5N1), swine flu (H1N1), encephalitis

CONTRAINDICATIONS
Hypersensitivity

Precautions: Pregnancy **C,** geriatric, renal/hepatic/pulmonary/cardiac disease, infants, children, neonates, psychosis, viral infection, breastfeeding

DOSAGE AND ROUTES
Treatment
Adult and child >40 kg: PO 75 bid mg × 5 days, begin treatment within 2 days of onset of symptoms
Child 23-40 kg and ≥1 yr: PO 60 mg bid
Child 15-23 kg and ≥1 yr: PO 45 mg bid
Child ≤15 kg and ≥1 yr: PO 30 mg bid

Prevention
Adult and child ≥13 yr: PO 75 mg/day × ≥7 days; begin treatment within 2 days of contact, max use 6 wk

Renal dose
Adult: PO CCr 10-30 ml/min 75 mg/day × 5 days (treatment); 75 mg every other day or 30 mg/day (prophylaxis)

H1N1 influenzae A virus (unlabeled)
Adult/adolescent/child >40 kg: PO 75 mg bid × 5 days
Child/adolescent 24-40 kg: PO 60 mg bid × 5 days
Child >1 yr and 15-23 kg: PO 45 mg bid × 5 days
Child >1 yr and <15 kg: PO 30 mg bid × 5 days

Available forms: Caps 30, 45, 75 mg; powder for oral susp 6 mg/ml

Implementation
- Give within 2 days of symptoms of influenza; continue for 5 days
- Give at least 4 hr before bedtime to prevent insomnia
- 12 mg/ml concentration will be available for a limited time, new product is 6 mg/ml concentration, take care to give correct dose
- Give without regard to food, give with food for GI upset, take with full glass of water
- **Oral susp:** loosen powder from side of bottle 55 ml shake well (6 mg/ml); remove child-resistant cap and push bottle adapter into neck of bottle, close tightly with child-resistant cap to ensure sealing; use within 17 days of preparation when refrigerated or 10 days at room temperature, write expiration date on bottle, shake well before use, use oral syringe provided but only with markings for 30, 45, 60 mg, confirm dosing instructions are in same units as syringe provided
- Store in airtight, dry container

ADVERSE EFFECTS
CNS: Headache, fatigue, insomnia, dizziness, delirium, **self-injury (children)**
ENDO: Hyperglycemia
GI: *Nausea, vomiting,* diarrhea, abdominal pain
INTEG: Toxic epidermal necrolysis, Stevens-Johnson syndrome, erythema multiforme
RESP: Cough

Absorption	Rapidly absorbed
Distribution	Protein binding 3%
Metabolism	Converted to oseltamivir carboxylate (active form)
Excretion	Eliminated by conversion, urine 99%
Half-life	1-3 hr (active form)

Pharmacodynamics

Unknown

INTERACTIONS
Avoid use with H1N1 virus vaccine, intranasal influenza vaccine

NURSING CONSIDERATIONS
Assessment
• **Influenza:** assess for symptoms of influenza A: increased temperature, malaise, aches and pains

Patient/family education
• Teach patient about aspects of product therapy
• Teach patient to avoid hazardous activities if dizziness occurs
• Advise patient to take as soon as symptoms appear, to take full course, even if feeling better
• Advise patient to take missed dose as soon as remembered if within 2 hr of next dose
• **Teach patient to stop product immediately and report to prescriber skin rash, delirium, psychosis, hallucinations (child)**
• Advise patient that product is not a substitute for a flu shot
• Inform patient to avoid other products without approval of prescriber

Evaluation
Positive therapeutic outcome
• Absence of fever, malaise, cough, dyspnea in influenza A

> ⚠ **HIGH ALERT**
>
> ## oxaliplatin (Rx)
> (ox-al-i′plat-in)
> **Eloxatin**
> *Func. class.:* Antineoplastic
> *Chem. class.:* 3rd-generation platinum analog
> **Pregnancy category D**

ACTION: Forms cross links, inhibiting DNA replication and transcription, cell-cycle nonspecific

Therapeutic outcome: Decreased size of tumor, spread of malignancy

USES: Metastatic carcinoma of the colon or rectum in combination with 5-FU/leucovorin

Unlabeled uses: Relapsed or refractory non-Hodgkin's lymphoma, advanced ovarian cancer

CONTRAINDICATIONS
Pregnancy **D**, breastfeeding, radiation therapy or chemotherapy within 1 mo, thrombocytopenia, smallpox vaccination

> **BLACK BOX WARNING:** Hypersensitivity to this product or other platinum products

Precautions: Children, geriatric, pneumococcus vaccination, renal disease

DOSAGE AND ROUTES
Colorectal cancer
Dosage protocols may vary
Adult: IV INF *Day 1:* oxaliplatin 85 mg/m^2 in 250-500 ml D$_5$W and leucovorin 200 mg/m^2 in D$_5$W, give both over 2 hr at the same time in separate bags using a Y-line, followed by 5-FU 400 mg/m^2 IV BOL over 2-4 min, then 5-FU 600 mg/m^2 IV INF in 500 ml D$_5$W as a 22-hr CONT INF; *Day 2:* leucovorin 200 mg/m^2 IV INF over 2 hr, then 5-FU 400 mg/m^2 IV BOL over 2-4 min, then 5-FU 600 mg/m^2 IV INF in 500 ml D$_5$W as a 22-hr CONT INF; repeat cycle q2wk

Renal dose
Adult: IV CCr <30 ml/min: reduce starting dose to 65 mg/m^2

Available forms: Powder for inj 50, 100 mg single-use vials (5 mg/ml); solution for inj 50 mg/10 ml, 100 mg/20 ml, 200 mg/40 ml

Implementation
Intermittent IV INF route
• Premedicate with antiemetics including 5-HT$_3$ blockers, with or without dexamethasone, prehydration is not needed
• Do not reconstitute or dilute with sodium chloride or any chloride-containing solutions, do not use aluminum equipment during any preparation or administration, will degrade platinum; do not refrigerate unopened powder or solution; do not freeze; protect from light
• Use cytotoxic handling procedures; prepare in biological cabinet using gown, gloves, mask; do not allow product to come in contact with skin; use soap and water if contact occurs
• EPINEPHrine, antihistamines, corticosteroids for hypersensitivity reaction
• **Lyophilized powder:** reconstitute vial 50 mg/10 ml, or 100 mg/20 ml sterile water for

inj or D$_5$W, after reconstitution, solution may be stored for ≤24 hr in refrigerator, after dilution in 250-500 ml D$_5$W, may store ≤24 hr in refrigerator or 6 hr at room temp, infuse over 2 hr
• **Aqueous solution:** dilute in 250-500 ml of D$_5$W, after dilution may store ≤24 hr refrigerator, 6 hr at room temp, infuse over 2 hr

Y-site compatibilities: Alfentanil, amifostine, amikacin, aminocaproic acid, amiodarone, amphotericin B colloidal, amphotericin B lipid complex, amphotericin B liposome, ampicillin, ampicillin-sulbactam, anidulafungin, atenolol, atracurium, azithromycin, aztreonam, bivalirudin, bleomycin, bumetanide, buprenorphine, butorphanol, calcium chloride/gluconate, CARBOplatin, caspofungin, ce-FAZolin, cefotaxime, cefoTEtan, cefOXitin, cefTAZidime, ceftizoxime, cefTRIAXone, cefuroxime, chloramphenicol, chlorproMAZINE, cimetidine, ciprofloxacin, cisatracurium, CISplatin, clindamycin, cyclophosphamide, cycloSPORINE, cytarabine, dacarbazine, DACTINomycin, DAPTOmycin, DAUNOrubicin, dexamethasone, digoxin, diltiazem, diphenhydrAMINE, DOBUTamine, DOCEtaxel, dolasetron, DOPamine, doxacurium, DOXOrubicin, doxycycline, droperidol, enalaprilat, ePHEDrine, EPINEPHrine, epirubicin, ertapenem, erythromycin, esmolol, etoposide, famotidine, fenoldopam, fentaNYL, fluconazole, fludarabine, foscarnet, fosphenytoin, furosemide, gatifloxacin, gemcitabine, gemtuzumab, gentamicin, glycopyrrolate, granisetron, haloperidol, heparin, hydrALAZINE, hydrocortisone, HYDROmorphone, hydrOXYzine, IDArubicin, ifosfamide, imipenem-cilastatin, inamrinone, insulin (regular), irinotecan, isoproterenol, ketorolac, labetalol, leucovorin, levofloxacin, levorphanol, lidocaine, linezolid, LORazepam, magnesium sulfate, mannitol, meperidine, meropenem, mesna, metaraminol, methyldopate, methylPREDNISolone, metoclopramide, metoprolol, metroNIDAZOLE, midazolam, milrinone, minocycline, mitoMYcin, mitoXANtrone, mivacurium, morphine, nafcillin, nalbuphine, naloxone, nesiritide, niCARdipine, nitroglycerin, nitroprusside, norepinephrine, octreotide, ondansetron, PACLitaxel, palonosetron, pancuronium, PEMEtrexed, pentamidine, pentazocine, phenylephrine, piperacillin, polymyxin B, potassium chloride/phosphates, procainamide, prochlorperazine, promethazine, propranolol, quiNIDine, quinupristin-dalfopristin, ranitidine, rocuronium, sodium acetate/phosphates, succinylcholine, SUFentanil, sulfamethoxazole-trimethoprim, tacrolimus, teniposide, theophylline, thiotepa, ticarcillin, ticarcillin-clavulanate, tigecycline, tirofiban, tobramycin, tolazoline, topotecan, trimethobenzamide, vancomycin, vasopressin, vecuronium, verapamil, vinBLAStine, vinCRIStine, vinorelbine, voriconazole, zidovudine, zoledronic acid

ADVERSE EFFECTS
CNS: Peripheral neuropathy, fatigue, headache, dizziness, insomnia
CV: Cardiac abnormalities, **thromboembolism**
EENT: *Decreased visual acuity, tinnitus, hearing loss*
GI: *Severe nausea, vomiting, diarrhea, weight loss,* stomatitis, anorexia, gastroesophageal reflux, constipation, dyspepsia, mucositis, flatulence
GU: Hematuria, dysuria, creatinine
HEMA: **Thrombocytopenia, leukopenia, pancytopenia, neutropenia, anemia, hemolytic uremic syndrome**
INTEG: *Alopecia,* rash, flushing, extravasation, redness, swelling, pain at inj site
META: Hypokalemia
RESP: **Fibrosis,** dyspnea, cough, rhinitis, URI, pharyngitis
SYST: Anaphylaxis, angioedema

Pharmacokinetics

Absorption	Unknown
Distribution	15% of platinum in systemic circulation; 85% is either in tissues or being eliminated in urine
Metabolism	Liver
Excretion	Urine
Half-life	40 days

Pharmacodynamics
Unknown

INTERACTIONS
Individual drugs
Alcohol, aspirin: increased risk of bleeding
Radiation: increased myelosuppression

Drug classifications
Aminoglycosides, diuretics (loop): increased nephrotoxicity
Anticoagulants, NSAIDs, platelet inhibitors, thrombolytics, salicylates: increased risk of bleeding
Live virus vaccines: decreased antibody response
Myelosuppressives: increased myelosuppression
Tannins: increased oxaliplatin toxicity

Drug/lab test
Increased: ALT, AST, bilirubin, creatinine
Decreased: potassium, neutrophils, WBC, platelets

NURSING CONSIDERATIONS
Assessment
• **Bone marrow depression:** monitor CBC, differential, platelet count weekly; withhold product if WBC is <4000 or platelet count is <100,000; notify prescriber of results

• Monitor renal function tests: BUN, creatinine, serum uric acid, urine CCr before, electrolytes during therapy; dose should not be given if BUN >19 mg/dl; creatinine <1.5 mg/dl; I&O ratio; report fall in urine output of <30 ml/hr

> **BLACK BOX WARNING: Assess for anaphylaxis:** wheezing, tachycardia, facial swelling, fainting; discontinue product and report to prescriber; resuscitation equipment should be nearby

• Monitor temp (may indicate beginning infection)
• Monitor liver function tests before, during therapy (bilirubin, AST, ALT, LDH) as needed or monthly
• **Assess for bleeding:** hematuria, guaiac, bruising or petechiae, mucosa or orifices q8hr; obtain prescription for viscous lidocaine (Xylocaine)
• Assess effects of alopecia on body image; discuss feelings about body changes
• Assess for jaundice of skin, sclera; dark urine; clay-colored stools; itchy skin; abdominal pain; fever; diarrhea
• Assess for edema in feet, joint pain, stomach pain, shaking
• **Pulmonary fibrosis: assess for cough, crackles, dyspnea, pulmonary infiltrate; discontinue immediately; may be fatal**

Patient/family education
• **Advise patient to report signs of infection: increased temp, sore throat, flulike symptoms**
• **Advise patient to report signs of anemia:** fatigue, headache, faintness, shortness of breath, irritability
• **Advise patient to report bleeding;** avoid use of razors, commercial mouthwash
• Advise patient to avoid aspirin, ibuprofen, NSAIDs, alcohol; may cause GI bleeding
• **Advise patient to report any changes in breathing, coughing**
• Advise patient that hair may be lost during treatment; a wig or hairpiece may make patient feel better; new hair may be different in color, texture
• Advise patient to report numbness, tingling in face or extremities, poor hearing or joint pain, swelling
• Advise patient not to receive vaccines during treatment
• **Advise patient to use contraception during treatment and 4 mo after; this product may cause infertility, pregnancy D**
• Teach patient to avoid contact with cold (air, ice, liquid); causes acute dysesthesias

Evaluation
Positive therapeutic outcome
• Decreased tumor size, spread of malignancy

> **⚠ HIGH ALERT**

oxazepam (Rx)
(ox-az′e-pam)
Func. class.: Sedative-hypnotic; antianxiety
Chem. class.: Benzodiazepine, short-acting
Pregnancy category D
Controlled substance schedule IV

ACTION: Depresses subcortical levels of CNS, including limbic system, reticular formation; potentiates GABA

Therapeutic outcome: Decreased anxiety, successful alcohol withdrawal, relaxation

USES: Anxiety, alcohol withdrawal

Unlabeled uses: Insomnia

CONTRAINDICATIONS
Pregnancy **D**, breastfeeding, children <6 yr, hypersensitivity to benzodiazepines, closed-angle glaucoma, psychosis

Precautions: Geriatric, debilitated, renal/hepatic disease, depression, suicidal ideation, dementia, sleep apnea, seizure disorder, respiratory depression

DOSAGE AND ROUTES
Anxiety
Adult: PO 15-30 mg tid-qid, max 120 mg/day
Geriatric: PO 10 mg daily bid-tid, max 60 mg/day

Alcohol withdrawal
Adult: PO 15-30 mg tid-qid

Available forms: Caps 10, 15, 30 mg

Implementation
• Give with food or milk for GI symptoms; tab may be crushed if patient is unable to swallow medication whole

ADVERSE EFFECTS
CNS: *Dizziness, drowsiness,* confusion, headache, anxiety, tremors, fatigue, depression, insomnia, hallucinations, paradoxical excitement, transient amnesia
CV: *Orthostatic hypotension,* ECG changes, tachycardia, hypotension
EENT: *Blurred vision,* tinnitus, mydriasis
GI: Nausea, vomiting, anorexia
HEMA: Leukopenia

INTEG: Rash, dermatitis, itching
SYST: Dependence

Pharmacokinetics

Absorption	Well absorbed
Distribution	Widely distributed; crosses placenta, blood-brain barrier
Metabolism	Liver
Excretion	Kidneys, breast milk
Half-life	5-15 hr

Pharmacodynamics

Onset	½-1½ hr
Peak	Unknown
Duration	6-12 hr

INTERACTIONS
Individual drugs
Alcohol: increased CNS depression
Disulfiram: increased oxazepam effects
Levodopa: decreased effects of levodopa
Phenytoin, theophylline, valproic acid: decreased oxazepam effects

Drug classifications
CNS depressants: increased oxazepam effects
Oral contraceptives: increased or decreased oxazepam effect

Drug/herb
Kava, melatonin, valerian: increased CNS depression

Drug/lab test
Increased: AST, ALT, serum bilirubin
Decreased: WBC

NURSING CONSIDERATIONS
Assessment
• **Assess mental status: mood, sensorium, anxiety, affect, sleeping pattern, drowsiness, dizziness, suicidal thoughts, behavior; physical dependency, withdrawal symptoms: anxiety, panic attacks, agitation, seizures, headache, nausea, vomiting, muscle pain, weakness; suicidal thoughts, behavior; indications of increasing tolerance and abuse**
• Monitor B/P with patient lying, standing; pulse; if systolic B/P drops 20 mm Hg, hold product, notify prescriber

Patient/family education
• Teach patient that product may be taken without regard to food or fluids; tab may be crushed or swallowed whole
• Caution patient not to use for everyday stress or longer than 4 mo unless directed by prescriber; not to take more than prescribed amount; not to double doses or skip doses
• Advise patient to avoid OTC preparations unless approved by prescriber; alcohol and CNS depressants will increase CNS depression
• Caution patient to avoid driving and activities that require alertness, since drowsiness may occur; to avoid alcohol and other psychotropic medications; to rise slowly or fainting may occur, especially geriatric; that drowsiness may worsen at beginning of treatment
• Caution patient not to discontinue medication abruptly after long-term use; withdrawal symptoms include vomiting, cramping, tremors, seizures
• Advise patient to use sugarless gum, hard candy, frequent sips of water for dry mouth
• Teach patient that drowsiness may worsen at beginning of treatment
⚠ **Teach patient to notify prescriber if pregnancy is planned or suspected, pregnancy (D)**

Evaluation
Positive therapeutic outcome
• Decreased anxiety, restlessness, sleeplessness (short-term treatment only)

TREATMENT OF OVERDOSE:
Lavage, VS, supportive care

O

OXcarbazepine (Rx)
(ox′kar-baz′uh-peen)
Oxtellar XR, Trileptal
Func. class.: Anticonvulsant
Pregnancy category C

ACTION: May inhibit nerve impulses by limiting influx of sodium ions across cell membrane in motor cortex

Therapeutic outcome: Absence of seizures

USES: Partial seizures

Unlabeled uses: Trigeminal neuralgia, atypical panic disorder, bipolar disorder

CONTRAINDICATIONS
Hypersensitivity

Precautions: Pregnancy **C**, breastfeeding, children <4 yr, hypersensitivity to carbamazepine, renal disease, fluid restriction, hyponatremia, abrupt discontinuation, suicidal ideation

DOSAGE AND ROUTES
Seizures adjunctive therapy
Adult: PO 300 mg bid, may be increased by 600 mg/day in divided doses bid at weekly intervals; maintenance 1200 mg/day; ext rel 600 mg/day × 1 wk,

increase weekly in 600 mg/day increments to 1200-2400 mg/day

Child 4-16 yr: PO 8-10 mg/kg/day divided bid, dose is determined by weight, increase by 5 mg/kg/day q3 days, max doses are weight dependent

Conversion to monotherapy in partial seizures

Adult: PO 300 mg bid with reduction in other anticonvulsants, increase OXcarbazepine by 600 mg/day qwk over 2-4 wk; withdraw other anticonvulsants over 3-6 wk, max 2400 mg/day

Initiation of monotherapy in partial seizures

Adult: PO 300 mg bid, increase by 300 mg/day q3day to 1200 mg divided bid, max 2400 mg/day

Renal dose

Adult: PO CCr <30 ml/min 150 mg bid and increase slowly

Available forms: Film-coated tabs 150, 300, 600 mg; oral susp 300 mg/5 ml; ext rel tab 150, 300, 600 mg

Implementation

- Store product at room temperature
- Provide assistance with ambulation during early part of treatment; dizziness may occur
- Give product with food, milk to decrease GI symptoms
- **Oral susp:** shake well, use calibrated oral syringe provided, use or discard within 7 days of opening
- **Ext rel:** do not crush, break, or chew

ADVERSE EFFECTS

CNS: *Headache, dizziness, confusion, fatigue,* feeling sleepy, ataxia, abnormal gait, tremors, anxiety, agitation, worsening of seizures, suicidal ideation/behavior
CV: *Hypotension,* chest pain, edema, bradycardia, syncope
EENT: *Blurred vision, diplopia, nystagmus,* rhinitis, sinusitis
ENDO: Hypothyroidism, hot flashes
GI: *Nausea, constipation, diarrhea,* anorexia, vomiting, abdominal pain, gastritis
GU: Urinary frequency, hematuria, menses change
INTEG: Purpura, rash, acne
META: Hyponatremia
RESP: Flulike symptoms
SYST: Angioedema, anaphylaxis, Stevens-Johnson syndrome, toxic epidermal necrolysis, drug reaction with eosinophilia and systemic symptoms (DRESS)

Pharmacokinetics

Absorption	Unknown
Distribution	Unknown
Metabolism	Liver; 95% renal extraction
Excretion	Unknown
Half-life	Unknown

Pharmacodynamics

Onset	Unknown
Peak	4-6 hr
Duration	Unknown

INTERACTIONS
Individual products

Alcohol: increased CNS depression
CarBAMazepine: decreased carBAMazepine level, decreased OXcarbazepine levels
Felodipine: decreased effects of felodipine
Nisoldipine, ranolazine: do not use concurrently
PHENobarbital, valproic acid, verapamil: decreased OXcarbazepine level
Phenytoin: decreased OXcarbazepine level

Drug classifications

Contraceptives (oral): decreased oral contraceptive level
MAOIs: do not use concurrently

Drug/herb

Ginkgo: increased anticonvulsant effect
Ginseng, santonica: decreased anticonvulsant effect

Drug/lab test

Decreased: sodium

NURSING CONSIDERATIONS
Assessment

- **Assess seizure activity,** including frequency, duration, and aura; provide seizure precautions
- Assess mental status including mood, sensorium, affect, behavioral changes, suicidal thoughts, behavior; if mental status changes, notify prescriber; usually occurs within the first 3 mo of treatment, but may occur ≤1 yr; if this product is being used with other products that decrease sodium, monitor sodium levels
- Assess eye problems: ophthalmic examinations (slit lamp, funduscopy, tonometry) are needed before, during, after treatment
- Assess patient for hypersensitivity to carBAMazepine
- Assess for serious skin reactions: angioedema, anaphylaxis, Stevens-Johnson syndrome
- Pregnancy: lack of seizure control due to MHD, a metabolite of OXcarbazepine; monitor seizure control

- May monitor target serum level 12-30 mcg/ml to identify compliance/toxicity

Patient/family education
- Caution patient to avoid driving, other activities that require alertness
- Instruct patient to take twice a day at same intervals
- Advise patient not to discontinue medication quickly after long-term use, seizures may increase
- Instruct patient to avoid use of alcohol while taking this medication
- Instruct patient to use alternative contraception if using hormonal method, to report if pregnancy is planned or suspected, pregnancy (**C**)
- ⚠ Teach patient to report skin rashes immediately; serious skin reactions can occur
- Instruct patient to inform prescriber if allergic to carBAMazepine; multisystem hypersensitivity may occur, to report fever, other allergic symptoms
- ⚠ Instruct patient to report suicidal thoughts/behavior immediately

Evaluation
Positive therapeutic outcome
- Decreased seizure activity

TREATMENT OF OVERDOSE:
Activated charcoal, give 0.9% NaCl (hypotensive state), atropine (bradycardia); use benzodiazepines, barbiturates for seizures

oxybutynin (Rx, OTC)
(ox-i-byoo′ti-nin)
Ditropan, Ditropan XL, Gelnique, Oxytrol ✦, Oxytrol Transdermal, Uromax ✦
Func. class.: Anticholinergic
Chem. class.: Synthetic tertiary amine
Pregnancy category B

Do not confuse: Ditropan/diazepam

ACTION: Relaxes smooth muscles in urinary tract by inhibiting acetylcholine at postganglionic sites

Therapeutic outcome: Decreased symptoms of urgency, nocturia, incontinence

USES: Antispasmodic for neurogenic bladder, overactive bladder in females (OTC)

CONTRAINDICATIONS
Hypersensitivity, GI obstruction, urinary retention, glaucoma, severe colitis, myasthenia gravis, unstable CV, infants

Precautions: Pregnancy **B**, breastfeeding, children <12 yr, geriatric, suspected glaucoma, cardiac disease, dementia

DOSAGE AND ROUTES
Adult: PO 5 mg bid-tid, max 5 mg qid; ext rel tabs 5-10 mg/day, may increase by 5 mg, max 30 mg/day; transdermal apply one patch to abdomen, hip, buttock 2 ×/wk (q3-4day); GEL apply contents of 1 packet to abdomen, upper arms, shoulders, thighs daily
Geriatric: PO 2.5-5 mg bid-tid, increase by 2.5 mg q several days
Child ≥6 yr: PO 5 mg bid, not to exceed 5 mg tid; ext rel 5 mg/day, max 20 mg/day
Child 1-5 yr: PO 0.2 mg/kg/dose 2-3 ×/day

Available forms: Syr 5 mg/5 ml; tabs 5 mg; ext rel tabs 5, 10, 15 mg; transdermal 3.9 mg/day; top gel 10% (Gelnique)

Implementation
PO route
- Do not break, crush, or chew ext rel tabs
- May be given with meals or fluids or on an empty stomach

Topical route
- Wash hands, apply to clean, dry, intact skin on abdomen, upper arms/shoulders, thighs, avoid navel, rotate sites
- Squeeze contents in palm of hand or directly on this site, rub gently
- Do not bathe, exercise, swim for 1 hr after application
- Allow to dry before putting on clothing
- Do not be near flame, fire, or smoke until gel has dried
- Delivers 100 mg

Transdermal route
- Apply to clean, dry, intact skin on the abdomen, hip, buttock, use firm pressure, not affected by showering/bathing; rotate sites
- Delivers 3.9 mg/day

ADVERSE EFFECTS
CNS: *Anxiety, restlessness, dizziness,* somnolence, insomnia, nervousness, **seizures,** headache, drowsiness, confusion
CV: *Palpitations, sinus tachycardia,* hypertension, peripheral edema, **QT prolongation**
EENT: Blurred vision, increased intraocular tension; dry mouth, throat, dry eyes
GI: *Nausea, vomiting, anorexia,* abdominal pain, constipation, *dyspepsia,* diarrhea, taste perversion, GERD
GU: Dysuria, impotence, retention, hesitancy
MISC: **Hyperthermia, anaphylaxis, angioedema**

Pharmacokinetics

Absorption	Rapidly absorbed
Distribution	Unknown
Metabolism	Liver
Excretion	Unknown
Half-life	Unknown

Pharmacodynamics

Onset	½-1 hr
Peak	3-4 hr
Duration	6-10 hr

INTERACTIONS
Individual drugs
Acetaminophen: decreased levels of acetaminophen

Amantadine: increased anticholinergic effects

Atenolol: increased levels of atenolol

Digoxin: increased levels of digoxin

Haloperidol, chloroquine, droperidol, pentamidine, arsenic trioxide, levomethadyl: increased QT prolongation

Levodopa: decreased levels of levodopa

Nitrofurantoin: increased levels of nitrofurantoin

Drug classifications
Antihistamines, other anticholinergics: increased anticholinergic effects

Benzodiazepines, sedatives, hypnotics, opioids: increased CNS depression

Class IA/III antidysrhythmics, some phenothiazines, β-agonists, local anesthetics, tricyclics, CYP3A4 inhibitors (amiodarone, clarithromycin, erythromycin, telithromycin, troleandomycin), CYP3A4 substrates (methadone, pimozide, QUEtiapine, quiNIDine, risperiDONE, ziprasidone): increased QT prolongation

NURSING CONSIDERATIONS
Assessment
• **Assess for allergic reactions:** rash, urticaria; if these occur, product should be discontinued

• **Assess urinary patterns:** distention, nocturia, frequency, urgency, incontinence; catheterization may be required to remove residual urine; urinary tract infections should be treated

• **QT prolongation: assess ECG for QT prolongation, ejection fraction; assess for chest pain, palpitations, dyspnea**

Patient/family education
• Advise patient to avoid hazardous activities until response to product is known; dizziness, blurred vision may occur

• Caution patient to avoid OTC medication with alcohol or other CNS depressants

• Teach patient to use frequent rinsing of mouth, sips of water for dry mouth

• Teach patient to stay cool; avoid hot weather, strenuous activity since overheating may occur; product decreases perspiration

• Advise patient to report CNS effects: confusion, anxiety, anticholinergic effect in the geriatric

Transdermal

• Instruct patient to change patch 2×/wk and not to use same site within 7 days

• Instruct patient to use container that is not accessible to pets/children and to dispose of container after use

• Instruct patient to open patch immediately before using

• Instruct patient to remove patch during MRI

Topical gel

• **Instruct patient to rotate sites**

• Instruct patient to apply to clean, dry skin on abdomen, upper arm/shoulders/thighs

• Teach patient that gel is flammable

Evaluation
Positive therapeutic outcome

• Absence of dysuria, frequency, nocturia, incontinence

⚠ HIGH ALERT

oxyCODONE (Rx)
(ox-i-koe′done)

Oxecta, OxyCONTIN, Oxy IR ✦, Roxicodone, Supeudol ✦

oxyCODONE/ acetaminophen (Rx)
Oxycet, Percocet, Primalev, Roxicet, Roxilox, Tylox, Xartemis XR

oxyCODONE/aspirin (Rx)
Endodan ✦, Percodan

oxyCODONE/ibuprofen (Rx)

Func. class.: Opiate analgesic

Chem. class.: Semisynthetic derivative

Pregnancy category B

Controlled substance schedule II

Do not confuse: oxyCODONE/ HYDROcodone/OxyCONTIN, Percodan/ Decadron, **Roxicet**/Roxanol, **Roxicodone**/ Roxanol, **Tylox**/Trimox/Wymox/Xanax

ACTION: Inhibits ascending pain pathways in CNS, increases pain threshold, alters pain perception

Therapeutic outcome: Decreased pain

USES: Moderate to severe pain

Unlabeled uses: Postherpetic neuralgia (cont rel)

CONTRAINDICATIONS
Hypersensitivity, addiction (opiate), asthma, ileus

> **BLACK BOX WARNING:** Respiratory depression

Precautions: Pregnancy **B**, breastfeeding, children <18 yr, addictive personality, increased ICP, MI (acute), severe heart disease, renal/hepatic disease, bowel impaction

> **BLACK BOX WARNING:** Opioid-naïve patients, substance abuse, accidental exposure, potential for overdose/poisoning, status asthmaticus

DOSAGE AND ROUTES
Adult: PO 10-30 mg q4hr (5-15 mg q4-6hr for opiate naive patients); **OxyFast CONC SOL is extremely concentrated, do not use interchangeably;** CONT REL 10 mg q12hr in opiate-naïve patients

Available forms: OxyCODONE: cont rel tabs (OxyCONTIN) 10, 15, 20, 30, 40, 80, 160 mg; immediate rel tabs 5, 7.5, 10, 15, 20, 30 mg; immediate rel caps 5 mg; oral sol 5 mg/5 ml, 20 mg/ml; oxyCODONE with acetaminophen: 2.5 mg/325 mg, 5 mg/325 mg; 7.5 mg/325 mg, 7.5 mg/500 mg, 10 mg/325 mg; oral sol 5 mg/325 mg/5 ml; oxyCODONE with aspirin: 4.88 mg/325 mg oxyCODONE with ibuprofen: 5 mg/400 mg

Implementation
• OxyCODONE should be titrated from the initial recommended dosage to the dose required to relieve pain
• There is no maximum dose of oxyCODONE; however, careful titration is required until tolerance develops to some of the side effects (drowsiness and respiratory depression)
• Store in light-resistant area at room temp
Immediate-release tablets
• May be administered with food or milk to minimize GI irritation
• Oxecta brand tablets: Swallow whole; do not crush or dissolve. Due to the nature of this formulation do not presoak, lick, or otherwise wet tablet prior to dose administration. Administer 1 tablet at a time; allow patient to swallow each tablet separately with sufficient liquid to ensure prompt and complete transit through the esophagus. Do not use this brand for administration via nasogastric, gastric, or other feeding tubes as it may cause obstruction of feeding tubes

Controlled-release tablets (OxyCONTIN)
• Administer whole; do not crush, chew, or break in half. Taking chewed, broken, or crushed controlled-release tabs could lead to the rapid release and absorption of a potentially toxic dose of oxyCODONE
• OxyCONTIN brand tablets: Due to hydro-gelling nature of the 2010 reformulation, do not presoak, lick, or otherwise wet tab prior to dose administration. Administer 1 tab at a time; allow patient to swallow each tab separately with sufficient liquid to ensure prompt and complete transit through the esophagus
• OxyCODONE controlled-release (OxyCONTIN) 60 mg and 80 mg tablets are for use ONLY in opioid-tolerant patients
• May be administered with or without food
Oral concentrate solution route
• As OxyFast is a highly concentrated solution (20 mg oxyCODONE/ml), care should be taken in dispensing and administering this medication. For ease of administration, the solution may be added to 30 ml of a liquid or semisolid food. If the medication is placed in liquid or food, the patient needs to consume immediately; do not store diluted oxyCODONE for future use
PO route
• Do not break, crush, or chew cont rel tabs; give q12hr, no more frequently
• May be given with food or milk to lessen GI upset
• Use 80, 160 mg cont rel tabs (oxyCONTIN) only in opioid-tolerant patients

ADVERSE EFFECTS
CNS: *Drowsiness, dizziness, confusion, headache, sedation, euphoria,* fatigue, abnormal dreams, thoughts, hallucinations
CV: Palpitations, bradycardia, change in B/P
EENT: Tinnitus, blurred vision, miosis, diplopia
GI: *Nausea, vomiting, anorexia, constipation, cramps,* gastritis, dyspepsia, biliary spasms
GU: Increased urinary output, dysuria, urinary retention
INTEG: *Rash,* urticaria, bruising, flushing, diaphoresis, pruritus
RESP: **Respiratory depression**

Pharmacokinetics
Absorption	Well absorbed
Distribution	Widely distributed; crosses placenta, protein binding 45%
Metabolism	Liver, extensively
Excretion	Kidneys, breast milk
Half-life	3-5 hr

Adverse effects: *italics* = common; **bold** = life-threatening

Pharmacodynamics

	PO	RECT
Onset	15-30 min	Unknown
Peak	½-1 hr	Unknown
Duration	Reg rel 2-6 hr, cont rel 12 hr	4-6 hr

INTERACTIONS
Individual drugs
Alcohol: increased respiratory depression, hypotension, sedation

Cimetidine: increased toxicity

Drug classifications
Antipsychotics, CNS depressants, opioids, sedative/hypnotics, skeletal muscle relaxants: increased respiratory depression, hypotension

CYP3A4 inhibitors: increased oxyCODONE level

MAOIs: increased toxicity

Drug/herb
St. John's wort, valerian: increased sedative effect

Drug/lab test
Increased: amylase, lipase

NURSING CONSIDERATIONS
Assessment
• **Pain:** assess intensity, location, type, characteristics; need for pain medication by pain/sedation scoring; physical dependence

• Monitor I&O ratio; check for decreasing output; may indicate urinary retention

• **CNS changes:** assess for dizziness, drowsiness, hallucinations, euphoria, LOC, pupil reaction

• **Allergic reactions:** assess for rash, urticaria

> **BLACK BOX WARNING: Respiratory dysfunction:** assess for respiratory depression, character, rate, rhythm; notify prescriber if respirations are <10/min; also B/P, pulse

• **Bowel status:** assess for constipation; stimulate laxative may be needed with fluids, fiber

• Monitor VS after parenteral route; note muscle rigidity, product history, renal, liver function tests, respiratory dysfunction: respiratory depression, character, rate, rhythm; notify prescriber if respirations are <10/min

> **BLACK BOX WARNING: Substance abuse:** assess for substance abuse in patient/family/friends before prescribing; monitor for abuse

> **BLACK BOX WARNING: Accidental exposure:** dispose of properly away from pets, children

Patient/family education
• Advise patients to avoid CNS depressants: alcohol, sedative/hypnotics

• Discuss with patient that dizziness, drowsiness, and confusion are common; to avoid getting up without assistance

• Discuss in detail all aspects of the product, including purpose and what to expect

• Advise patient to make position changes slowly to lessen orthostatic hypotension

• Advise patient to avoid CNS depressants, alcohol

• Advise patient to avoid operating machinery, driving if drowsiness occurs

• Teach patient that withdrawal symptoms may occur after long-term use: nausea, vomiting, cramps, fever, faintness, anorexia

Evaluation
Positive therapeutic outcome
• Decreased pain

TREATMENT OF OVERDOSE:
Naloxone 0.2-0.8 **IV**, O₂, **IV** fluids, vasopressors; caution with patients physically dependent on opioids

---

oxymetazoline nasal agent
See Appendix B

oxymetazoline ophthalmic
See Appendix B

> **⚠ HIGH ALERT**

oxymorphone (Rx)
(ox-i-mor′fone)

Opana, Opana ER

Func. class.: Opiate analgesic

Chem. class.: Semisynthetic phenanthrene derivative

Pregnancy category B

Controlled substance schedule II

Do not confuse: oxymorphone/oxyCODONE

ACTION: Depresses pain impulse transmission at the spinal cord level by interacting with opioid receptors, increases pain threshold, alters pain perception

Therapeutic outcome: Decreased pain

USES: Moderate to severe pain

CONTRAINDICATIONS
Hypersensitivity, addiction (opioid), asthma, hepatic disease, ileus, intrathecal use, surgery

---

Precautions: Pregnancy **B** (short-term), breastfeeding, children <18 yr, addictive personality, increased ICP, MI (acute), severe heart disease, respiratory depression, renal/hepatic disease, bowel impaction

DOSAGE AND ROUTES
Adult: IM/SUBCUT 1 mg q4-6hr prn; **IV** 0.5 mg q4-6hr prn; PO (immediate release only) 5-20 mg q4-6hr prn; PO-ER 5 mg q12hr in those requiring around the clock dosing

Labor analgesia
Adult: IM 0.5-1 mg

Available forms: Inj 1 mg/ml; supp 5 mg; ER tab, crush resistant 5, 7.5, 10, 15, 20, 30, 40 mg; tabs 5, 10 mg

Implementation
• Give 1 hr before or 2 hr after food (PO)
• Give with antiemetic if nausea, vomiting occur
• Do not break, crush, chew ER product
• Give when pain is beginning to return; determine dosage interval by patient response; continuous dosing of medication is more effective than when given prn
• Medication should be slowly withdrawn after long-term use to prevent withdrawal symptoms
• Store in light-resistant area at room temp
CONTROLLED REL
• **Opiate naive:** start with lowest dose, titrate upward in 5-10 mg q12hr q3-7days to therapeutic response
• **When converting from immediate release to ext rel,** give ½ daily dose of ER product q12hr

Direct IV route
• Give undiluted over 2-3 min, may be diluted in normal saline solution

Syringe compatibilities: Glycopyrrolate, hydrOXYzine, ranitidine

ADVERSE EFFECTS
CNS: *Drowsiness, dizziness, confusion, headache, sedation, euphoria (geriatric),* **seizures,** hallucinations, **increased ICP**
CV: Palpitations, **bradycardia,** change in B/P, hypotension
EENT: Tinnitus, blurred vision, miosis, diplopia
GI: *Nausea, vomiting, anorexia, constipation, cramps*
GU: Dysuria, urinary retention

INTEG: *Rash,* urticaria, bruising, flushing, diaphoresis, pruritus
RESP: Respiratory depression

Pharmacokinetics
Absorption	Well absorbed (RECT, IM, SUBCUT); completely absorbed (**IV**)
Distribution	Widely distributed; crosses placenta
Metabolism	Liver, extensively
Excretion	Kidneys
Half-life	PO: 7-9 hr, ER: 9-11 hr

Pharmacodynamics
	IM/SUBCUT	IV	RECT
Onset	15 min	10 min	30 min
Peak	1-1½ hr	15-30 min	Unknown
Duration	3-6 hr	3-4 hr	3-6 hr

INTERACTIONS
Individual drugs
Alcohol: increased respiratory depression, hypotension, sedation

Drug classifications
CNS depressants, opiates, antipsychotics, skeletal muscle relaxants, sedative/hypnotics: increased respiratory depression, hypotension
MAOIs: do not use 2 wk before oxymorphone; unpredictable effects

Drug/herb
Kava, St. John's wort, valerian: increased sedative effect

Drug/lab test
Increased: amylase

NURSING CONSIDERATIONS
Assessment
• **Pain:** assess location, intensity, type, other characteristics, before and 1 hr after (IM) IV 30 min; need for pain medication, physical dependence, give 25%-50% until there is pain reduction of 50% on pain rating scale, repeat dose may be given at time of peak, if previous dose does not control pain, and respiratory depression has not occurred; give short-acting opioids for breakthrough pain if on controlled rel product

> **BLACK BOX WARNING: Accidental exposure:** Dispose of properly, away from children/pets

> **BLACK BOX WARNING: Overdose/poisoning:** Avoid alcohol ingestion; do not crush, chew, snort, or inject tabs, high abuse potential

> **BLACK BOX WARNING: Opioid-naive patients:** Ext rel tabs are not to be used immediately post-op (12-24 hr after surgery) in these patients

- **Assess bowel/bladder status:** constipation, may need stimulant laxative; I&O ratio for decreasing output, may indicate urinary retention
- Monitor VS after parenteral route; note muscle rigidity, product history, liver, kidney function tests
- Monitor CNS changes: dizziness, drowsiness, hallucinations, euphoria, LOC, pupil reaction
- Monitor allergic reactions: rash, urticaria

Patient/family education
- **Advise patient not to use other CNS depressants: alcohol, sedative/hypnotics**
- Discuss with patient that dizziness, drowsiness, and confusion are common; to avoid getting up without assistance
- Discuss in detail all aspects of the product, including purpose and what to expect
- Advise patient to make position changes slowly to lessen orthostatic hypotension
- Advise patient not to drive, operate machinery if drowsiness occurs

Evaluation
Positive therapeutic outcome
- Decreased pain

TREATMENT OF OVERDOSE:
Naloxone (Narcan) 0.2-0.8 mg **IV**, O₂, **IV** fluids, vasopressors (caution with patients physically dependent on opioids)

> **⚠ HIGH ALERT**
>
> ## oxytocin (Rx)
> (ox-i-toe′sin)
> **Pitocin**
> *Func. class.:* Oxytocic hormone
> **Pregnancy category N/A**

ACTION: Acts directly on myofibrils, producing uterine contraction; stimulates breast milk letdown, vasoactive antidiuretic effect

Therapeutic outcome: Stimulation of labor, control of bleeding; stimulation of milk letdown

USES: Stimulation, induction of labor; missed or incomplete abortion; postpartum bleeding

CONTRAINDICATIONS
Hypersensitivity, serum toxemia, cephalopelvic disproportion, fetal distress, hypertonic uterus, prolapsed umbilical cord, active genital herpes

Precautions: Cervical/uterine surgery, uterine sepsis, primipara >35 yr, 1st/2nd stage of labor

> **BLACK BOX WARNING:** Elective induction of labor

DOSAGE AND ROUTES
Labor induction
Adult: IV 1-2 milliunit/min, increase by 1-2 milliunit q15-60min until regular contractions occur, then decrease dosage

Postpartum hemorrhage
Adult: IV 10-40 units in 1000 ml nonhydrating diluent infused at 20-40 milliunit/min
Adult: IM 3-10 units after placenta delivery

Incomplete abortion
Adult: IV INF 10 units/500 ml D₅W or 0.9% NaCl run at 10-20 milliunit/min; max 30 units/12 hr

Fetal stress test
Adult: IV 0.5 milliunit/min; increase q20min until 3 contractions occur at 10 min

Available forms: Inj 10 units/ml

Implementation

IV route
- Use an inf pump; rotate sol for mixing; have magnesium sulfate available
Labor induction
- Give after diluting 10 units/1000 ml of 0.9% NS or D₅ NS run at 1-2 mU/min at 15-30 min intervals to begin normal labor; dilute 10-40 mU/min; titrate to control postpartum bleeding; dilute 10 units/500 ml sol; run 10 units-20 mU/ml; administer by only 1 route at a time; use inf pump; rotate inf to provide mixing; do not shake
Control of postpartum bleeding
- Dilute 10-40 units/1000 ml of sol; run at 10-20 mU/min; adjust rate as needed
- Have crash cart available on unit (magnesium sulfate at bedside)
Incomplete, inevitable, elective abortion
- Dilute 10 units/500 ml compatible IV solution

Y-site compatibilities: Heparin, hydrocortisone, insulin (regular), meperidine, morphine, potassium chloride, vit B/C, warfarin

---

⚠ Nurse Alert   ✴ Key NCLEX® Drug   ≫ Drug Specifics

ADVERSE EFFECTS

CNS: Seizures, tetanic contractions
CV: Hypo/hypertension, dysrhythmias, increased pulse, bradycardia, tachycardia, premature ventricular contractions
FETUS: Dysrhythmias, jaundice, hypoxia, intracranial hemorrhage
GI: Anorexia, nausea, vomiting, constipation
GU: Abruptio placentae, decreased uterine blood flow
HEMA: Increased hyperbilirubinemia
INTEG: Rash
RESP: Asphyxia
SYST: Water intoxication of mother

Pharmacokinetics

Absorption	Well absorbed (nasal); completely absorbed (**IV**)
Distribution	Widely distributed (extracellular fluid)
Metabolism	Liver, rapidly
Excretion	Kidneys
Half-life	3-12 min

Pharmacodynamics

	Nasal	IV	IM
Onset	5 min	Rapid	3-7 min
Peak	Unknown	Unknown	Unknown
Duration	20 min	1 hr	1 hr

INTERACTIONS

Drug classifications
Vasopressors: increased hypertension

Drug/herb
Ephedra: hypertension

NURSING CONSIDERATIONS

Assessment
• Assess labor contractions: fetal heart tones, frequency, duration, intensity of contractions; if fetal heart tones increase or decrease significantly or if contractions are longer than 1 min, notify prescriber; turn patient on left side to increase oxygen to fetus
⚠ Assess for water intoxication: confusion, anuria, drowsiness, headache; notify prescriber
• Watch for fetal distress, acceleration, deceleration, fetal presentation, pelvic dimensions
• Monitor B/P, pulse, respiratory rate, rhythm, depth
• Monitor I&O ratio
• Provide an environment conducive to letdown reflex

Patient/family education
• Teach patient to report increased blood loss, abdominal cramps, increased temp or foul-smelling lochia
• Advise patient that contractions will be similar to menstrual cramps, gradually increasing in intensity

> **BLACK BOX WARNING:** Elective induction of labor; use only for induction when medically necessary

Evaluation
Positive therapeutic outcome
• Stimulation of milk letdown (nasal)
• Induction of labor
• Decreased postpartum bleeding

⚠ HIGH ALERT

PACLitaxel (Rx)
(pa-kli-tax'el)
PACLitaxel protein-bound particles (Rx)
Abraxane
Func. class.: Antineoplastic—miscellaneous
Chem. class.: Taxane
Pregnancy category D

Do not confuse: PACLitaxel/PARoxetine/Paxil

ACTION: Inhibits the reorganization of the microtubule network needed for interphase and mitotic cellular functions; also causes abnormal bundles of microtubules during cell cycle and multiple esters of microtubules during mitosis

Therapeutic outcome: Prevention of rapidly growing malignant cells

USES: Taxol: metastatic carcinoma of the ovary, breast carcinoma, AIDS-related Kaposi's sarcoma (second line), non–small cell lung cancer (first line), adjuvant treatment for node-positive breast cancer

Unlabeled uses: Advanced head, neck, small cell lung cancer; non-Hodgkin's lymphoma, adenocarcinoma of the upper GI tract, hormone-refractory prostate cancer

CONTRAINDICATIONS
Pregnancy **D**, hypersensitivity to paclitaxel or other products with polyoxyethylated castor oil, albumin

> **BLACK BOX WARNING:** Neutropenia (neutrophils <1500/mm³)

Precautions: Breastfeeding, children, CV/hepatic disease, CNS disorder, renal disease, bone marrow suppression, dental disease/work, extravasation, females, geriatric patients, herpes, infection, infertility, jaundice, ocular exposure, radiation therapy, thrombocytopenia, vaccination

> **BLACK BOX WARNING:** Taxane hypersensitivity, requires a specialized care setting and an experienced clinician

DOSAGE AND ROUTES
>> PACLitaxel
Ovarian carcinoma
Adult: IV INF 135 mg/m² given over 24 hr q3wk, then CISplatin 75 mg/m² or 175 mg/m²
over 3 hr q3wk (refractory or metastatic) or 175 mg/m² over 3 hr

Advanced ovarian carcinoma
Adult: IV INF 175 mg/m² with CISplatin 75 mg/m² over 3 hr q3wk

Breast carcinoma
Adult: IV INF 175 mg/m² over 3 hr q3wk × 4 courses

AIDS-related Kaposi's sarcoma
Adult: IV INF 135 mg/m² over 3 hr q3wk or 100 mg/m² over 3 hr q2wk

1st line non–small cell lung cancer
Adult: IV INF 135 mg/m²/24 hr with CISplatin 75 mg/m² × 3 wk

>> PACLitaxel protein-bound particles
Adult: IV 260 mg/m² q3wk

Hepatic dose
Adult, for 135 mg/m² 24 hr IV inf: AST/ALT 2-10 × ULN, total bilirubin ≤1.5 mg/dl: 100 mg/m²; AST/ALT <10 × ULN, total bilirubin 1.6-7.5 mg/dl: 50 mg/m²; AST/ALT ≥10 × ULN or total bilirubin >7.5 mg/dl: avoid use
Adult, for 175 mg/m² 3 hr IV inf: AST/ALT <10 × ULN, total bilirubin 1.26-2 × ULN: 135 mg/m²; AST/ALT <10 × ULN, total bilirubin 2.01-5 × ULN: 90 mg/m²; AST/ALT ≥10 × ULN or total bilirubin >5 × ULN: avoid use

Available forms: Inj 6 mg/ml, 30 mg/5-ml vial, 100 mg/16.7-ml vial, 150 mg/25-ml vial, 300 mg/50-ml vials; powder for inj, lyophilized 100 mg in single-use vials (Abraxane)

Implementation

> **BLACK BOX WARNING:** Monitor CBC, differential, platelet count weekly; withhold product if WBC is <1500/mm³ or platelet count is <100,000/mm³, notify prescriber of results

• If CISplatin is given, use after taxane

Continuous IV INF route
• After premedicating with dexamethasone 20 mg PO 12 hr and 6 hr before paclitaxel, diphenhydrAMINE 50 mg IV ½-1 hr before PACLitaxel and cimetidine 300 mg or ranitidine 50 mg IV ½-1 hr before PACLitaxel
• For extravasation if given by regular IV, not port

>> PACLitaxel
• After diluting in 0.9% NaCl, D₅, D₅ and 0.9% NaCl, D₅LR (0.3-1.2 mg/ml) chemo dispensing pin or similar devices with spikes should not be used in vials of Taxol, use in-line filter ≤0.22 micron, give as 3 hr or 24 hr inf

• Use only glass bottles, polypropylene, polyolefin bags and administration sets; do not use PVC inf bags or sets

Y-site compatibilities: Acyclovir, amikacin, aminophylline, ampicillin/sulbactam, bleomycin, butorphanol, calcium chloride, CARBOplatin, cefepime, cefoTEtan, cefTAZidime, cefTRIAXone, cimetidine, CISplatin, cladribine, cyclophosphamide, cytarabine, dacarbazine, dexamethasone, diphenhydrAMINE, DOXOrubicin, droperidol, etoposide, famotidine, floxuridine, fluconazole, fluorouracil, furosemide, ganciclovir, gentamicin, granisetron, haloperidol, heparin, hydrocortisone, HYDROmorphone, ifosfamide, LORazepam, magnesium sulfate, mannitol, meperidine, mesna, methotrexate, metoclopramide, morphine, nalbuphine, ondansetron, pentostatin, potassium chloride, prochlorperazine, propofol, ranitidine, sodium bicarbonate, thiotepa, vancomycin, vinBLAStine, vinCRIStine, zidovudine

>> Abraxane

Intermittent IV INF route

• Reconstitute vial by injecting 20 ml of 0.9% NaCl; slowly inject the 20 ml of 0.9% NaCl over at least 1 min to direct the sol flow on wall of vial; do not inject 0.9% NaCl directly onto lyophilized cake (foaming will occur); allow vial to sit for at least 5 min to ensure proper wetting of lyophilized cake; gently swirl or invert vial slowly for at least 2 min until completely dissolved

• Calculate dosing by dosing vol/ml = total dose (mg) ÷ 5 (mg/ml)

ADVERSE EFFECTS

CNS: Peripheral neuropathy
CV: *Bradycardia, hypotension, abnormal ECG,* supraventricular tachycardia (SVT)
GI: *Nausea, vomiting, diarrhea, mucositis; increased bilirubin, alkaline phosphatase, AST*
HEMA: **Neutropenia, leukopenia, thrombocytopenia, anemia,** bleeding, infections
INTEG: Alopecia, tissue necrosis, generalized urticaria, flushing
MS: *Arthralgia, myalgia*
RESP: **Pulmonary embolism,** dyspnea
SYST: *Hypersensitivity reactions,* **anaphylaxis, Stevens-Johnson syndrome, toxic epidermal necrolysis, angioedema**

Pharmacokinetics

Absorption	Completely absorbed
Distribution	89%-98% protein binding
Metabolism	Liver, extensively
Excretion	Unknown
Half-life	5-17 hr

Pharmacodynamics

Onset	Unknown
Peak	1-2 wk
Duration	3 wk

INTERACTIONS
Individual drugs

CycloSPORINE, dexamethasone, diazepam, etoposide, quiNIDine, teniposide, testosterone, verapamil, vinCRIStine: decreased metabolism of PACLitaxel
DOXOrubicin: increased levels of DOXOrubicin
Ketoconazole: increased toxicity, decreased metabolism; avoid concurrent use
Radiation: increased myelosuppression

Drug classifications

Anticoagulants, NSAIDs: increased bleeding risk
Antineoplastics: increased myelosuppression
CYP2C8, CYP2C9 inducers: decreased PACLitaxel level
Vaccines (live virus): decreased immune response

Drug/lab test

Increased: AST/ALT, alk phos, triglycerides
Decreased: neutrophils, platelets, WBCs, Hgb

NURSING CONSIDERATIONS
Assessment

• Assess CNS changes: confusion, paresthesias, psychosis, tremors, seizures, neuropathies; product should be discontinued
• Check buccal cavity q8hr for dryness, sores or ulceration, white patches, oral pain, bleeding, dysphagia; obtain prescription for viscous lidocaine (Xylocaine) to use in mouth

> **BLACK BOX WARNING:** Requires a specialized care setting such as a hospital or facility capable of managing complications; should be used by a clinician experienced in cytotoxic agents

• **Cardiovascular status:** monitor ECG continuously in CV conditions; monitor for hypotension, sinus bradycardia/tachycardia
• **Peripheral neuropathy:** assess for paresthesias, numbness; during inf use ice packs on extremities to lessen continued neuropathy; use ice on extremities when infusing
• **Arthralgia, myalgia:** may begin 2-3 days after infusion and continue for 4-5 days, may use analgesics
• **Nausea, vomiting:** premedicate with antiemetics, nausea and vomiting occur often
• Monitor renal function tests: BUN, creatinine, serum uric acid, urine CCr before, during

Adverse effects: *italics* = common; **bold** = life-threatening

therapy; check I&O ratio; report fall in urine output to <30 ml/hr
- Monitor temp q4hr (may indicate beginning of infection)
- Monitor liver function tests before, during therapy (bilirubin, AST, ALT, LDH) as needed or monthly; check for jaundice of skin and sclera, dark urine, clay-colored stools, itchy skin, abdominal pain, fever, diarrhea
- Assess for bleeding: hematuria, stool guaiac, bruising or petechiae, mucosa or orifices q8hr; check for inflammation of mucosa, breaks in skin
- Assess effects of alopecia on body image; discuss feelings about body changes
- VS during 1st hr of inf, check IV site for signs of infiltration
⚠ **Hypersensitive reactions, anaphylaxis, hypotension, dyspnea, angioedema, generalized urticaria; discontinue inf immediately; keep emergency equipment available, monitor continuously during first 30-60 min, then periodically**
- **Flush:** for mild to moderate flush, may continue diphenhydrAMINE for up to 48 hr
- Effects of alopecia on body image; discuss feelings about body changes

Patient/family education
⚠ **Teach patient to notify prescriber if pregnancy is planned or suspected (D), do not breastfeed**
- Teach patient to avoid use of products containing aspirin or ibuprofen, razors, commercial mouthwash, since bleeding may occur; to report symptoms of bleeding (hematuria, tarry stools)
- Instruct patient to report signs of anemia (fatigue, headache, irritability, faintness, shortness of breath) and CNS reactions (confusion, psychosis, nightmares, seizures, severe headaches)
- Teach patient to rinse mouth tid-qid with water, club soda; brush teeth bid-qid with soft brush or cotton-tipped applicators for stomatitis; use unwaxed dental floss
- Inform patient that hair may be lost during treatment; a wig or hairpiece may make patient feel better; new hair may be different in color, texture
- Inform patient that receiving vaccinations during therapy may cause serious reactions

Evaluation

Positive therapeutic outcome
- Prevention of rapid division of malignant cells

⚠ HIGH ALERT

palbociclib
(pal-boe-sye′klib)
Ibrance
Func. class.: Antineoplastic
Chem. class.: Signal transduction inhibitor
Pregnancy category Unknown

ACTION: Inhibits progression of the cell cycle from G_1 into S phase, decreased proliferation of ER-positive breast cancer cell lines. When combined with antiestrogen therapy (letrozole), decreases retinoblastoma protein (Rb) phosphorylation, reducing E2F expression and signaling, and increasing growth arrest

Therapeutic outcome: Decreased progression of disease

USES: Treatment of estrogen receptor (ER)–positive, HER2-negative advanced breast cancer in postmenopausal women, in combination with letrozole as initial endocrine-based therapy

CONTRAINDICATIONS: Hypersensitivity

Precautions: Breastfeeding, children, fungal/viral infection, infants, infertility, neutropenia, pregnancy, testicular failure, thromboembolic disease

DOSAGE AND ROUTES
Adult female: PO 125 mg daily with food × 21 days, followed by 7 days off, repeat q28 days with letrozole 2.5 mg daily, given continuously through each 28-day cycle until progressive disease or unacceptable toxicity occurs

Available forms: Caps 75, 100, 125 mg

Implementation
Treatment-related hepatotoxicity:
- Grade 1 or 2 hepatotoxicity: No dosage change
- Grade ≥3 hepatotoxicity (AST or ALT >5 × ULN or total bilirubin >3 × ULN) that persists despite medical treatment: Hold until toxicity resolves to grade ≤2 (AST or ALT ≤5 × ULN or total bilirubin ≤3 × ULN), resume treatment at the next lower dose level if not considered a safety risk for the patient; discontinue if grade ≥3 toxicity occurs at a dose of 75 mg/day
Treatment-related nephrotoxicity:
- Grade 1 or 2 nephrotoxicity: No change
- Grade ≥3 nephrotoxicity (CCr >3 × baseline or >4 mg/dl, or requiring hospitalization or dialysis) that persists despite

---

⚠ Nurse Alert　　　　✦ Key NCLEX® Drug　　　　>> Drug Specifics

medical treatment: Hold therapy. When toxicity resolves to grade ≤2 (CCr <3 × baseline or <4 mg/dl) resume at the next lower dose level if not considered a safety risk for the patient, discontinue if grade ≥3 toxicity occurs at a dose of 75 mg/day.
Other dosage adjustments
• Strong CYP3A4 inhibitors: Avoid concomitant use. If a strong CYP3A4 inhibitor is needed, consider reducing the dose to 75 mg daily; if the strong CYP3A4 inhibitor is discontinued, increase the dose upward to the previously tolerated/recommended dose after a washout period of 3-5 half-lives of the inhibitor.
• Strong CYP3A4 inducers: Avoid use

ADVERSE EFFECTS
CNS: Weakness, fever, fatigue
EENT: Stomatitis, oral ulceration, glossitis, pharyngitis, sinusitis, epistaxis
GI: Vomiting, nausea, anorexia, diarrhea,
HEMA: Thrombocytopenia, neutropenia, leukopenia, lymphopenia, anemia
MISC: Peripheral neuropathy, alopecia, infection, pulmonary embolism, thromboembolism

Pharmacokinetics

Absorption	Unknown
Distribution	85% protein bound
Metabolism	Metabolized by CYP3A
Excretion	Unknown
Half-life	Elimination half-life was 24-34 hr

Pharmacodynamics

Onset	Unknown
Peak	Peak 6-12 hr
Duration	Unknown

INTERACTIONS
Drug classifications
CYP3A inhibitors and inducers: avoid concurrent use

Drug/herb
St. John's wort: Avoid concurrent use

Drug/food
Avoid use with grapefruit juice

NURSING CONSIDERATIONS
Assessment
• Pregnancy: Product can cause fetal harm; identify if the patient is pregnant or if pregnancy is planned
• Pulmonary embolism/thromboembolic events: Assess for dyspnea/shortness of

breath, chest pain, arm or leg swelling, sudden numbness or weakness, severe headache or confusion, or problems with vision, speech, or balance
• Blood dyscrasias: Monitor CBC/differential

Patient/family education
• Identify if pregnancy is planned or suspected. Discuss the need for contraception due to possible fetal harm; avoid breastfeeding
• Advise patient laboratory testing will be needed during treatment
• Pulmonary/thromboembolic events: Instruct patient to seek medical attention if dyspnea/shortness of breath, chest pain, arm or leg swelling, sudden numbness or weakness, severe headache or confusion, or problems with vision, speech, or balance develop

Evaluation
Positive therapeutic outcome
• Decreased progression of disease

paliperidone (Rx)
(pal-ee-per'i-done)
Invega, Invega Sustenna
Func. class.: Antipsychotic
Chem. class.: Benzisoxazole derivative
Pregnancy category C

Do not confuse: Invega/Iveegan, paliperidone/risperidone

ACTION: Mediated through both dopamine type 2 (D_2) and serotonin type 2 (5-HT_2) antagonism

Therapeutic outcome: Decrease in emotional excitement, hallucinations, delusions, paranoia; reorganization of patterns of thought, speech

USES: Schizophrenia, schizoaffective disorder

Unlabeled uses: Agitation

CONTRAINDICATIONS
Breastfeeding, seizure disorders, AV block, geriatric, QT prolongation, torsades de pointes, hypersensitivity to this product or risperidone

Precautions: Pregnancy C, children, renal/hepatic disease, obesity, Parkinson's disease, suicidal ideation, diabetes mellitus, hematologic disease

> **BLACK BOX WARNING:** Mortality-related psychosis in dementia

DOSAGE AND ROUTES
Adult: PO 6 mg/day; max 12 mg/day; IM 234 mg on day 1, then 156 mg 1 wk later; after 2nd dose, give 117 mg qmo, range 39-234 mg
Child/adolescent ≥12 yr and ≥51 kg: PO 3 mg/day, may increase if needed by 3 mg/day in intervals >5 days up to max 12 mg/day; <51 kg max 6 mg/day

Renal dose
Adult: PO CCr 50-79 ml/min, 3 mg/day, max 6 mg/day; ext rel/IM 156 mg on day 1, 117 mg 1 wk later, then 78 mg each mo CCr 10-49 ml/min, 1.5 mg/day, max 3 mg/day; IM not recommended

Available forms: Ext rel tabs 1.5, 3, 6, 9 mg; ext rel susp for inj 39 mg/0.25 ml, 78 mg/0.5 ml, 117 mg/0.75 ml, 156 mg/1 ml, 234 mg/1.5 ml

Implementation
PO route
- Do not break, crush, or chew ext rel tabs, use plenty of water
- Give without regard for food
- Give a reduced dose to the geriatric patient
- Give antiparkinsonian agent on order from prescriber; to be used for EPS
- Avoid use with CNS depressants
- Supervise ambulation until patient is stabilized on medication; do not involve in strenuous exercise program, because fainting is possible; patient should not stand still for a long time
- Increase fluids to prevent constipation
- Decrease stimulus by dimming lights, avoiding loud noise
- Provide sips of water, candy, gum for dry mouth
- Store in airtight, light-resistant container

IM route
- Use for IM only, do not use IV or SUBCUT, injection kits contain a prefilled syringe and 2 safety needles, for single use only, shake for 10 secs
- **Deltoid injection:** ≥ 90 kg use 1.5 inch, 22 G needle; < 90 kg use 1 inch, 23 G needle, alternate injections between deltoid muscles
- **Gluteal injection:** use 1.5 inch, 22 G needle; attach needle to luer connection in clockwise motion, pull needle sheath away using straight pull, bring syringe with attached needle upright to de-aerate, de-aerate, inject; after injection, use finger, thumb or flat surface to activate needle protection system, until click heard, use deltoid × 2 dosages

ADVERSE EFFECTS
CNS: *EPS, pseudoparkinsonism, akathisia, dystonia, tardive dyskinesia; drowsiness, insomnia, agitation, anxiety, headache,* seizures, neuroleptic malignant syndrome, dizziness
CV: Orthostatic hypotension, tachycardia, heart failure, QT prolongation, heart block, dysrhythmias
EENT: Blurred vision, cough
ENDO: Insulin increase, hyperinsulinemia, diabetes mellitus, weight gain, hyperglycemia, dyslipidemia
GI: *Nausea,* vomiting, *anorexia, constipation,* weight gain in adolescents, xerostomia
GU: Menstrual irregularities
HEMA: Agranulocytosis

Pharmacokinetics
Absorption	Unknown
Distribution	Unknown, protein binding >74%
Metabolism	Unknown
Excretion	80% urine, 11% feces
Half-life	Elimination 23 hr

Pharmacodynamics
Onset	Unknown
Peak	24 hr
Duration	Unknown

INTERACTIONS
Individual drugs
Abarelix, alfuzosin, amoxapine, apomorphine, chloroquine, dasatinib, dolasetron, droperidol, flecainide, pimozide: increased QT prolongation
Alcohol: increased sedation
Levodopa: decreased levodopa effect
Lithium: increased neurotoxicity
Paliperidone: decreased effect

Drug classifications
Azole antifungals; β-blockers; class IA, III antidysrhythmics; halogenated anesthetics; some antipsychotics; some phenothiazines; tricyclics (high doses): increased QT prolongation
SSRIs, SNRIs: increased serotonin syndrome, increased neuroleptic malignant syndrome
Other antipsychotics: increased EPS
Other CNS depressants, sedatives/hypnotics, opiates: increased sedation

Drug/herb
Betel palm, kava: increased EPS
Cola tree, hops, nettle, nutmeg: increased action
Kava: increased CNS depression

Drug/lab test
Increased: prolactin levels

NURSING CONSIDERATIONS
Assessment

> **BLACK BOX WARNING:** Assess mental status; mood, behavior, confusion, orientation, suicidal thoughts/behaviors; dementia especially in geriatric patients before initial administration and periodically

• **QT prolongation: monitor ECG for QT prolongation, ejection fraction; assess for chest pain, palpitations, dyspnea**
• Assess AIMS assessment, blood glucose, CBC, glycosylated hemoglobulin A1C (HbA1C), LFTs, neurologic function, pregnancy testing, serum creatinine/electrolytes/lipid profile/prolactin, thyroid function tests, weight
• Monitor for swallowing of PO medication; check for hoarding or giving of medication to other patients
• Monitor I&O ratio; palpate bladder if urinary output is low
• Assess affect, orientation, LOC, reflexes, gait, coordination, sleep pattern disturbances
• Monitor B/P standing and lying; also pulse, respirations; take these q4hr during initial treatment; establish baseline before starting treatment; report drops of 30 mm Hg; watch for ECG changes
• Assess for dizziness, faintness, palpitations, tachycardia on rising
• **Hyperprolactinemia:** assess for sexual dysfunction, decreased menstruation, breast pain
• **Assess for EPS,** including akathisia, tardive dyskinesia (bizarre movements of the jaw, mouth, tongue, extremities), pseudoparkinsonism (rigidity, tremors, pill rolling, shuffling gait)
⚠ **Assess for serious reactions in the geriatric patient**
⚠ **Serotonin syndrome, neuroleptic malignant syndrome: assess for increased heart rate, shivering, sweating, dilated pupils, tremors, high B/P, hyperthermia, headache, confusion; if these occur, stop product, administer a serotonin antagonist if needed**
• Assess skin turgor daily
• Assess for constipation, urinary retention daily; if these occur, increase bulk and water in diet; monitor for weight gain in adolescents

Patient/family education
• Advise patient that orthostatic hypotension may occur and to rise from sitting or lying position gradually
• **Advise patient to avoid hot tubs, hot showers, tub baths; hypotension may occur**

• Caution patient to avoid abrupt withdrawal of this product; EPS may result; product should be withdrawn slowly
• Teach patient to avoid OTC preparations (cough, hay fever, cold) unless approved by prescriber; serious product interactions may occur; avoid use of alcohol; increased drowsiness may occur
• Advise patient to avoid hazardous activities if drowsy or dizzy
• Teach patient compliance with product regimen; non-absorbable tab shell is expelled in stool
• Teach patient to report impaired vision, tremors, muscle twitching
• Caution patient that heat stroke may occur in hot weather; take extra precautions to stay cool
• **Teach patient to use contraception, inform prescriber if pregnancy is planned or suspected**

> **BLACK BOX WARNING:** Teach patient to notify prescriber of suicidal thoughts, behaviors, or other changes in behavior; identify dementia in the elderly

Evaluation
Positive therapeutic outcome
• Decrease in emotional excitement, hallucinations, delusions, paranoia; reorganization of patterns of thought, speech

TREATMENT OF OVERDOSE:
Lavage if orally ingested; provide airway; *do not induce vomiting*

palonosetron (Rx)
(pa-lone-o′se-tron)
Aloxi
Func. class.: Antiemetic
Chem. class.: 5-HT₃ receptor antagonist
Pregnancy category B

ACTION: Prevents nausea, vomiting by blocking serotonin peripherally, centrally, and in the small intestine at the 5-HT₃ receptor

Therapeutic outcome: Decreased nausea, vomiting during chemotherapy

USES: Prevention of nausea, vomiting associated with cancer chemotherapy; postoperative nausea/vomiting

CONTRAINDICATIONS
Hypersensitivity

Precautions: Pregnancy **B,** breastfeeding, children, geriatric, with hypokalemia, hypomagnesemia, patients taking diuretics

DOSAGE AND ROUTES

Adult: IV 0.25 mg as a single dose over 30 sec, 30 min prior to chemotherapy, max 0.25 mg IV over q 7 days

Postoperative nausea/vomiting prophylaxis for up to 24 hr after surgery

Adult: IV 0.075 mg given over 10 sec immediately before induction

Available forms: Inj 0.25 mg/5 ml

Implementation

Direct IV route
- Do not mix with other products; flush IV line before, after administration
- Store at room temperature
- **Chemotherapy nausea/vomiting:** give as a single dose over 30 seconds
- **Postoperative nausea/vomiting:** give over 10 seconds immediately prior to anesthesia induction

Syringe compatibilities: Dexamethasone

Y-site compatibilities: Alemtuzumab, alfentanil, amikacin, aminocaproic acid, aminophylline, amiodarone, amphotericin B liposome, ampicillin, ampicillin/sulbactam, atracurium, atropine, azithromycin, aztreonam, bivalirudin, bleomycin, bumetanide, buprenorphine, busulfan, butorphanol, calcium acetate/chloride/gluconate, CARBOplatin, carmustine, caspofungin, ceFAZolin, cefepime, cefotaxime, cefoTEtan, cefOXitin, cefTAZidime, ceftizoxime, cefTRIAXone, cefuroxime, chloramphenicol, chlorproMAZINE, cimetidine, ciprofloxacin, cisatracurium, CISplatin, clindamycin, cyclophosphamide, cycloSPORINE, cytarabine, dacarbazine, DACTINomycin, dantrolene, DAPTOmycin, DAUNOrubicin, dexamethasone, dexmedetomidine, dexrazoxane, digoxin, diltiazem, diphenhydrAMINE, DOBUTamine, DOCEtaxel, DOPamine, doxacurium, DOXOrubicin hydrochloride, droperidol, enalaprilat, ePHEDrine, EPINEPHrine, epirubicin, eptifibatide, erythromycin, esmolol, etoposide, etoposide phosphate, famotidine, fenoldopam, fentaNYL, fluconazole, fludarabine, fluorouracil, foscarnet, fosphenytoin, furosemide, gemcitabine, gentamicin, glycopyrrolate, haloperidol, heparin, hydrALAZINE, hydrocortisone, HYDROmorphone, IDArubicin, ifosfamide, inamrinone, insulin, irinotecan, isoproterenol, ketorolac, labetalol, leucovorin, levofloxacin, lidocaine, linezolid, LORazepam, magnesium sulfate, mannitol, mechlorethamine, melphalan, meperidine, meropenem, mesna, metaraminol, methotrexate, methyldopa, metoclopramide, metoprolol, metroNIDAZOLE, midazolam, milrinone, mitoMYcin, mitoXANtrone, mivacurium, morphine, nalbuphine, naloxone, neostigmine, nesiritide, niCARdipine, nitroglycerin, nitroprusside, norepinephrine, octreotide, oxaliplatin, oxytocin, PACLitaxel, pamidronate, pancuronium, pentazocine, PHENobarbital, phentolamine, phenylephrine, piperacillin/tazobactam, potassium acetate/chloride/phosphates, procainamide, prochlorperazine, promethazine, propranolol, quinupristin/dalfopristin, ranitidine, remifentanil, rocuronium, sodium acetate/bicarbonate/phosphates, streptozocin, succinylcholine, SUFentanil, tacrolimus, teniposide, theophylline, thiotepa, ticarcillin/clavulanate, tigecycline, tirofiban, tobramycin, topotecan, trimethobenzamide, trimethoprim/sulfamethoxazole, vancomycin, vasopressin, vecuronium, verapamil, vinBLAStine, vinCRIStine, vinorelbine, zidovudine

Y-site incompatibilities: Acyclovir, allopurinol, amphotericin B colloidal, diazepam, doxycycline, ganciclovir, imipenem/cilastatin, methylPREDNISolone, minocycline, nafcillin, pantoprazole, pentamidine, PENTobarbital, phenytoin, thiopental

ADVERSE EFFECTS

CNS: *Headache, dizziness, drowsiness, fatigue, insomnia*
GI: *Diarrhea, constipation,* abdominal pain
MISC: Weakness, hyperkalemia, anxiety, rash, bronchospasm (rare), arthralgia, *fever, urinary retention*

Pharmacokinetics

Absorption	Unknown
Distribution	62% protein bound
Metabolism	Liver
Excretion	Unchanged product and metabolites excreted by kidney
Half-life	40 hr

Pharmacodynamics

Unknown

INTERACTIONS

Individual drugs

Chloroquine, clarithromycin, droperidol, erythromycin, grepafloxacin, halofantrine, haloperidol, levomethadyl, methadone, pentamidine: possible QT prolongation
Apomorphine: increased: hypotension, severe

Drug classifications
Class 1A antidysrhythmics (disopyramide, procainamide, quiNIDine), class III anti-dysrhythmics (amiodarone, dofetilide, ibutilide), diuretics (except potassium sparing), some phenothiazines: possible QT prolongation

Drug/lab test
Increase: potassium

NURSING CONSIDERATIONS
Assessment
⚠ Monitor for absence of nausea, vomiting during chemotherapy
⚠ Assess hypersensitivity reaction: rash, bronchospasm
• Cardiac disease: check ECG before use
• Hyperkalemia: monitor potassium baseline and periodically

Patient/family education
• Teach to report diarrhea, constipation, rash, or changes in respirations or discomfort at insertion site
• Advise patient to avoid alcohol, barbiturates
• Teach patient to use other antiemetics if nausea occurs

Evaluation
Positive therapeutic outcome
• Absence of nausea, vomiting during cancer chemotherapy

pamidronate (Rx)
(pam-i-drone'ate)
Aredia
Func. class.: Bone resorption inhibitor, electrolyte modifier
Chem. class.: Bisphosphonate
Pregnancy category D

Do not confuse: Aredia/Adriamycin

ACTION: Inhibits bone resorption, apparently without inhibiting bone formation and mineralization; absorbs calcium phosphate crystals in bone and may directly block dissolution of hydroxyapatite crystals of bone

Therapeutic outcome: Serum calcium at normal level

USES: Moderate to severe Paget's disease, hypercalcemia, osteolytic bone metastases in breast cancer patients, multiple myeloma

Unlabeled uses: Postmenopausal osteoporosis, hyperparathyroidism

CONTRAINDICATIONS
Pregnancy **D**, hypersensitivity to bisphosphonates

Precautions: Children, nursing mothers, renal dysfunction, poor dentition

DOSAGE AND ROUTES
Hypercalcemia of malignancy
Adult: IV INF 60-90 mg as a single dose in moderate hypercalcemia, 90 mg in severe hypercalcemia given over 2-24 hr; dose should be diluted in 1000 ml 0.45% NaCl, 0.9% NaCl, or D_5W; wait 7 days before 2nd course

Osteolytic lesions
Adult: IV 90 mg/500 ml of D_5W, 0.45% NaCl, or 0.9% NaCl given over 4 hr on a monthly basis (multiple myeloma) or over 2 hr q3-4wk (breast carcinoma)

Paget's disease
Adult: IV INF 30 mg/day given over 4 hr × 3 days

Available forms: Powder for inj 30, 90 mg/vial; inj 3, 6, 9 mg/ml

Implementation
IV route
• After reconstituting by adding 10 ml of sterile water for inj to each vial (30 mg/10 ml or 90 mg/10 ml depending on vial used); add to 1000 ml of sterile 0.45%, 0.9% NaCl, D_5W, run over 2-24 hr **(hypercalcemia)**; dilute reconstituted sol in 500 ml of 0.9% NaCl, 0.45% NaCl, or D_5W, give over 4 hr **(multiple myeloma, Paget's disease)**; dilute reconstituted sol in 250 ml of 0.9% NaCl, 0.45% NaCl or D_5W, give over 2 hr **(osteolytic bone metastases of breast cancer)**
• Store inf sol for up to 24 hr at room temperature
• Reconstituted sol with sterile water may be stored under refrigeration for up to 24 hr
• Do not mix with calcium-containing inf sol such as Ringer's sol

Y-site compatibilities: Acyclovir, alfentanil, allopurinol, amifostine, amikacin, aminocaproic acid, aminophylline, amphotericin B lipid complex, amphotericin B liposome, ampicillin, anidulafungin, atenolol, atracurium, azithromycin, aztreonam, bivalirudin, bleomycin, bumetanide, buprenorphine, butorphanol, CARBOplatin, carmustine, ceFAZolin, cefepime, cefoperazone, cefotaxime, cefoTEtan, cefOXitin, cefTAZidime, ceftizoxime, cefTRIAXone, cefuroxime, chloramphenicol, chlorproMAZINE, cimetidine, ciprofloxacin, cisatracurium, CISplatin, clindamycin, cyclophosphamide, cycloSPORINE, cytarabine, dacarbazine, DAPTOmycin, dexamethasone, dexmedetomidine, dexrazoxane, digoxin, diltiazem, diphenhydrAMINE, DOBUTamine, DOCEtaxel, dolasetron, DOPamine, doxacurium, DOXOrubicin, doxycycline, droperidol, enalaprilat, ePHEDrine, EPINEPHrine, epirubicin, ertapenem, erythromycin, esmolol, etoposide, famotidine, fenoldopam, fentaNYL, fluconazole, fludarabine, fluorouracil, foscarnet, fosphenytoin, furosemide, gallium, ganciclovir, gatifloxacin, gemcitabine, gentamicin, glycopyrrolate, granisetron, haloperidol, heparin, hetastarch 6%, hydrALAZINE, hydrocortisone, HYDROmorphone, hydrOXYzine, ifosfamide, imipenem-cilastatin, inamrinone, insulin (regular), isoproterenol, ketorolac, labetalol, levofloxacin, levorphanol, lidocaine, linezolid, LORazepam, magnesium sulfate, mannitol, mechlorethamine, melphalan, meperidine, meropenem, mesna, metaraminol, methotrexate, methyldopate, methylPREDNISolone, metoclopramide, metoprolol, metroNIDAZOLE, midazolam, milrinone, minocycline, mitoXANtrone, mivacurium, morphine, mycophenolate, nafcillin, nalbuphine, naloxone, nesiritide, niCARdipine, nitroglycerin, nitroprusside, norepinephrine, octreotide, ondansetron, oxytocin, PACLitaxel, palonosetron, pancuronium, PEMEtrexed, pentamidine, pentazocine, PENTobarbital, PHENobarbital, phenylephrine, piperacillin, polymyxin B, potassium chloride/phosphates, procainamide, prochlorperazine, promethazine, propranolol, quiNIDine, quinupristin-dalfopristin, ranitidine, remifentanil, rocuronium, sodium acetate/bicarbonate/phosphates, succinylcholine, SUFentanil, sulfamethoxazole-trimethoprim, teniposide, theophylline, thiopental, thiotepa, ticarcillin, ticarcillin-clavulanate, tigecycline, tirofiban, tobramycin, tolazoline, topotecan, trimethobenzamide, vancomycin, vasopressin, vecuronium, verapamil, vinBLAStine, vinCRIStine, vinorelbine, voriconazole, zidovudine

ADVERSE EFFECTS

CNS: Fatigue, *fever*
CV: *Hypertension*, atrial fibrillation
EENT: Ocular pain, inflammation, vision impairment
GI: *Abdominal pain, anorexia, constipation, nausea, vomiting,* dyspepsia
GU: Renal failure
HEMA: Thrombocytopenia, anemia, leukopenia
INTEG: Redness, swelling, induration, pain on palpation at site of catheter insertion
META: Hypokalemia, hypomagnesemia, hypophosphatemia, hypocalcemia, hypothyroidism

MS: *Severe bone pain,* myalgia, osteonecrosis of the jaw
RESP: Coughing, dyspnea, URI
SYST: Angioedema, anaphylaxis

Pharmacokinetics

Absorption	Rapidly cleared from circulation
Distribution	Mainly to bones, primarily in areas of high bone turnover
Metabolism	Unknown
Excretion	Kidneys, unchanged (50%)
Half-life	Biphasic 27 hr; from bone to 300 days

Pharmacodynamics

Onset	1 day
Peak	1 wk
Duration	Unknown

INTERACTIONS
Individual drugs
Calcium, vitamin D: decreased pamidronate effect
CycloSPORINE, tacrolimus, vancomycin: increased nephrotoxicity
Entecavir: increased effect of entecavir

Drug classifications
Aminoglycosides, NSAIDs, radiopaque contrast agents: increased nephrotoxicity
Loop diuretics: increased hypokalemia

Drug/lab test
Increased: creatinine
Decreased: potassium, magnesium, phosphate, calcium, WBC, platelets

NURSING CONSIDERATIONS
Assessment
• **Dental health:** give antiinfectives for dental extractions
• Monitor WBCs, platelets, electrolytes, creatinine, BUN, Hgb/Hct prior to beginning treatment
• Temperature may be elevated during the first 3 days after a dose; risk of fever increases as dose increases
⚠ Renal disease: max 90 mg single dose, longer infusions >2 hr may increase risk for renal toxicity
• **Hypocalcemia:** assess for nausea, vomiting, constipation, thirst, dysrhythmias, hypocalcemia, paresthesia, twitching, laryngospasm, Chvostek's, Trousseau's signs; **hypercalcemia:** thirst, nausea, vomiting, dysrhythmias
• **Dehydration/hypovolemia:** should be corrected during treatment of hypercalcemia, prior to therapy; maintain adequate urine output

---

⚠ Nurse Alert   ✴ Key NCLEX® Drug   >> Drug Specifics

- Assess for atrial fibrillation
- Assess fluid volume status: check I&O ratio and record, assess for distended red veins, crackles in lung, color, quality, and specific gravity of urine, skin turgor, adequacy of pulses, moist mucous membranes, bilateral lung sounds, peripheral pitting edema
- Monitor electrolytes: phosphorus, potassium, sodium, calcium, magnesium; also include BUN, creatinine, CBC, platelets, hemoglobin
- Assess B/P before, during therapy
- Assess for pain: in joints or on exertion, duration and characteristics; analgesics may be ordered
- Assess for phlebitis at **IV** site: swelling, redness, pain, warmth

Patient/family education
- Advise patient to report hypercalcemic relapse: nausea, vomiting, bone pain, thirst; unusual muscle twitching, muscle spasms, severe diarrhea, constipation, ocular symptoms
- Advise patient to continue with dietary recommendations, including calcium and vit D
- To obtain an analgesic from provider for bone pain
- Advise patient that small, frequent meals may help nausea/vomiting
⚠ Teach patient to notify prescriber if pregnancy (D) is planned or suspected

Evaluation

Positive therapeutic outcome
- Decreased calcium levels to normal

---

pancrelipase (Rx)
(pan-kre-li′pase)
Creon, DMH ✦, Pancrease ✦, Pancreaze, Pancrecarb MS, Ultrase MT, VioKase, Zenpep
Func. class.: Digestant
Chem. class.: Pancreatic enzyme (bovine/porcine)
Pregnancy category B

ACTION: Pancreatic enzyme needed for breakdown of substances released from the pancreas

Therapeutic outcome: Increases protein, fat, carbohydrate digestion

USES: Exocrine pancreatic secretion insufficiency, cystic fibrosis (digestive aid), steatorrhea, pancreatic enzyme deficiency

CONTRAINDICATIONS
Allergy to pork

Precautions: Pregnancy **B**, ileus, pancreatitis, Crohn's disease, diabetes mellitus

DOSAGE AND ROUTES
Many products listed above are not interchangeable

Del rel caps—Creon caps, Zenpep caps, Pancreaze caps
Adult/adolescent/child ≥4 yr: PO 500 lipase units/kg/meal, titrate based on response, max 2500 lipase units/kg/meal
Child 1<4 yr: PO 1000 lipase units/kg/meal, titrate based on response, max 2500 lipase units/kg/meal

Available forms: Tabs (VioKase) 10, 20 units; cap, del rel 4, 8, 16 units (Pancrecarb MS), 12, 18, 20 units (Ultrase MT), Ultrase; cap 3000, 4200, 5000, 6000, 8000, 10,500, 12,000, 15,000, 16,000, 16,800, 24,000, 25,000 units

Implementation
- Give after antacid or cimetidine; decreased pH inactivates product
- Administer low-fat diet to decrease GI symptoms
- Provide adequate hydration
- Store in airtight container at room temperature
- Do not crush, chew del rel products, caps

ADVERSE EFFECTS
ENDO: Hyperglycemia, hypoglycemia
GI: Anorexia, nausea, vomiting, diarrhea, cramping, bloating
GU: Hyperuricuria, hyperuricemia

Pharmacokinetics
Unknown

Pharmacodynamics
Unknown

INTERACTIONS
Individual drugs
Acarbose, miglitol: decreased effects of each specific drug
Cimetidine, iron (oral): decreased absorption of pancrelipase

Drug classifications
Antacids: decreased absorption of pancrelipase

NURSING CONSIDERATIONS
Assessment
- Monitor I&O ratio; watch for increasing urinary output
- Monitor fecal fat, nitrogen, pro-time during treatment

Adverse effects: *italics* = common; **bold** = life-threatening

• Monitor for polyuria, polydipsia, polyphagia (may indicate diabetes mellitus); monitor glucose level more frequently
• Assess for allergy to pork; patient may also be sensitive to this product
• Assess for appropriate weight, height, development; there may be a developmental lag
• Check stools for steatorrhea, which signifies undigested fat content

Patient/family education
• Teach patient to always take with food, not to crush, chew del rel product, caps
• Instruct patient to store at room temperature, away from moisture
• Teach patient to take tab with 8 oz or more water, not to let tab sit in mouth; have patient take tab sitting up only
• Advise patient to notify prescriber of allergic reactions, abdominal pain, cramping, or hematuria

Evaluation

Positive therapeutic outcome
• Absence of steatorrhea
• Improved digestion of carbohydrates, proteins, fat

⚠ HIGH ALERT

pancuronium (Rx)
(pan-cure-oh′nee-yum)
Func. class.: Neuromuscular blocker (nondepolarizing)
Chem. class.: Synthetic curariform
Pregnancy category C

ACTION: Inhibits transmission of nerve impulses by binding with cholinergic receptor sites, antagonizing action of acetylcholine

Therapeutic outcome: Paralysis of all skeletal muscles

USES: Facilitation of endotracheal intubation, skeletal muscle relaxation during mechanical ventilation, surgery, or general anesthesia

CONTRAINDICATIONS
Hypersensitivity to bromide ion

Precautions: Pregnancy **C**, breastfeeding, children <2 yr, renal/hepatic/cardiac/neuromuscular disease, electrolyte imbalances, dehydration, previous anaphylactic reactions (other neuromuscular blockers)

BLACK BOX WARNING: Respiratory insufficiency

DOSAGE AND ROUTES
Adult/child/infant >1 mo: IV 0.04-0.1 mg/kg initially or 0.05 mg/kg after initial dose of succinylcholine; maintenance 0.01 mg/kg 60-100 min after initial dose, then 0.01 mg/kg q25-60min as needed; in obese patients, use ideal body weight

Neonate <1 mo: IV test dose 0.02 mg/kg, then 0.03 mg/kg/dose initially, repeat 2 × as needed at 5-10 min intervals; maintenance 0.03-0.09 mg/kg/dose q30min-4hr as needed

Available forms: Inj 1, 2 mg/ml

Implementation
• Use peripheral nerve stimulator (anesthesiologist) to determine neuromuscular blockade; deep tendon reflexes should be monitored during extended periods

Direct IV route
• Give undiluted over 1-2 min (1 mg/ml [10 ml vial], 2 mg/ml [2, 5 ml vial])
Intermittent IV infusion route
• Add 100 mg of product to 250 ml D₅W, 0.9% NaCl, or LR (0.4 mg/ml)
• Store in light-resistant area
• Give anticholinesterase to reverse neuromuscular blockade

Y-site compatibilities: Aminophylline, ceFAZolin, cefuroxime, cimetidine, DOBUTamine, DOPamine, EPINEPHrine, esmolol, fentaNYL, fluconazole, gentamicin, heparin, hydrocortisone, isoproterenol, LORazepam, midazolam, morphine, nitroglycerin, nitroprusside, ranitidine, sulfamethoxazole/trimethoprim, vancomycin

Y-site incompatibilities: Diazepam

Additive compatibilities: Verapamil

Additive incompatibilities: Barbiturates

ADVERSE EFFECTS
CV: Bradycardia, tachycardia, increased, decreased B/P, ventricular extrasystoles, edema, hypotension
EENT: Increased secretions
INTEG: Rash, flushing, pruritus, urticaria, sweating, salivation
MS: Weakness to prolonged skeletal muscle relaxation
RESP: Prolonged apnea, bronchospasm, cyanosis, respiratory depression, dyspnea
SYST: Anaphylaxis

Pharmacokinetics

Absorption	Complete bioavailability
Distribution	Extracellular space; crosses placenta
Metabolism	Plasma
Excretion	Kidneys, unchanged
Half-life	2 hr

Pharmacodynamics

Onset	3-5 min, dose dependent
Peak	3-5 min
Duration	35-40 min

INTERACTIONS
Individual products
Clindamycin, enflurane, isoflurane, lincomycin, lithium, quiNIDine: increased neuromuscular blockade
Theophylline: dysrhythmias

Drug classifications
Aminoglycosides, anesthetics (local), analgesics (opioid), polymyxin antiinfectives, thiazides: increased neuromuscular blockade

Drug/lab test
Decreased: cholinesterase

NURSING CONSIDERATIONS
Assessment
• Monitor vital signs (B/P, pulse, respirations, airway) until fully recovered; note rate, depth, pattern of respirations, strength of hand grip; patient should be intubated before use
• Monitor for electrolyte imbalances (potassium, magnesium) before product is used; electrolyte imbalances may lead to increased action of this product
• **Monitor for recovery:** decreased paralysis of face, diaphragm, leg, arm, rest of body; residual weakness and respiratory problems may occur during recovery period
⚠ Assess for hypersensitive reactions, anaphylaxis: rash, fever, respiratory distress, pruritus; product should be discontinued

Patient/family education
• Provide reassurance if communication is difficult during recovery from neuromuscular blockade
• Provide explanation to patients regarding all procedures or treatments; patient will remain conscious if anesthesia is not given also

Evaluation
Positive therapeutic outcome
• Paralysis of jaw, eyelid, head, neck, rest of body as evaluated by peripheral nerve stimulator

TREATMENT OF OVERDOSE:
Neostigmine, atropine; monitor VS; may require mechanical ventilation

⚠ HIGH ALERT

panitumumab (Rx)
(pan-i-tue′moo-mab)
Vectibix
Func. class.: Antineoplastic—miscellaneous
Chem. class.: Multikinase inhibitor, signal transduction inhibitor
Pregnancy category C

ACTION: Decreases growth and survival of cancer cells by competitive inhibition of EGF receptor

Therapeutic outcome: Decrease in colon carcinoma progression

USES: EGFR expressing metastatic colorectal cancer, not beneficial in *KRAS* mutations in codon 12 or 13

CONTRAINDICATIONS
Hypersensitivity

Precautions: Pregnancy **C,** breastfeeding, children, hepatic disease, acute bronchospasm, diarrhea, hamster protein allergy, hypomagnesemia, hypotension, pulmonary fibrosis, sepsis, *KRAS* mutations, soft-tissue toxicities

BLACK BOX WARNING: Exfoliative dermatitis, infusion-related reactions

DOSAGE AND ROUTES
Adult: IV INF 6 mg/kg over 60 min q2wk; doses > 1000 mg over 90 min

Available forms: Sol for inj 20 mg/ml (100 mg/5 ml, 400 mg/20 ml)

Implementation
Intermittent IV infusion route
• Give in hospital or clinic setting with full resuscitation equipment
• Give only as IV inf using controlled IV inf pump; do not give **IV** push or bolus; use low-protein binding 0.2 or 0.22 micron in-line filter; flush line with 0.9% NaCl before, after administration
• Give over 60 min through a peripheral line or in-dwelling catheter; inf doses of >1000 mg over 90 min
• Dilute in 100 ml of 0.9% NaCl; dilute doses >1000 mg in 150 ml of 0.9% NaCl; mix by

inverting; max 10 mg/ml; use within 6 hr if stored at room temperature; can be stored between 2°-8° C for up to 24 hr
• Store unopened vials in refrigerator; do not shake; protect from direct sunlight; do not freeze

Dosage adjustment for infusion/ dermatologic reaction
⚠ Grade 1/2: reduce infusion by 50%; Grade 3/4: terminate, permanently discontinue depending on severity/resistance

ADVERSE EFFECTS
CNS: Fatigue
CV: Peripheral edema
EENT: Ocular irritation, ocular toxicity
GI: *Nausea, diarrhea, vomiting,* anorexia, mouth ulceration, abdominal pain, constipation
HEMA: Thrombophlebitis
INTEG: *Rash,* pruritus, exfoliative dermatitis, skin fissure, angioedema, severe/fatal infusion reactions
META: Hypocalcemia, hypomagnesemia, antibody formation
RESP: Bronchospasm, cough, dyspnea, hypoxia, pulmonary fibrosis/embolism, pneumonitis, wheezing, interstitial lung disease

Pharmacokinetics

Absorption	38%-49%, high-fat meal decreases absorption
Distribution	Protein binding 99.5%
Metabolism	Liver, oxidative metabolism by CYP3A4, glucuronidation by UGT1A9, some Asian patients (15%-20%) are poor metabolizers
Excretion	Feces 77%
Half-life	Elimination 7.5 day

Pharmacodynamics

Onset	Unknown
Peak	3 hr
Duration	Unknown

INTERACTIONS
Drug classifications
Antineoplastics, other: do not use with other products

NURSING CONSIDERATIONS
Assessment
• **Pulmonary fibrosis:** assess for dyspnea, cough, wheezing, may need to discontinue

BLACK BOX WARNING: Serious skin disorders: assess for fever, sore throat, fatigue, then lesions in mouth, lips; withhold product, notify prescriber

• Monitor serum electrolytes periodically (calcium, magnesium)
• Assess for signs of infection: increased temperature

BLACK BOX WARNING: Assess for signs of infusion reactions: bronchospasm, fever, chills, hypotension; may require discontinuation; have emergency equipment available

• **Assess for signs of ocular toxicity:** ocular irritation, hyperemia

Patient/family education
⚠ Instruct patient to report adverse reactions immediately: difficulty breathing, mouth sores, skin rash, ocular toxicity
• Teach patient reason for treatment, expected results, adverse reactions
• **Teach males/females to use contraception while taking this product and for 6 mo after treatment; do not breastfeed for at least 2 mo after treatment, enroll in Amgen's Pregnancy Surveillance Program (800-772-6436)**
• Advise to use sunscreen while taking, 2 mo after

Evaluation
Positive therapeutic outcome
• Decrease in colon carcinoma progression

pantoprazole (Rx)
(pan-toe-pray′zole)
Panto ✳, Pantoloc ✳, Protonix, Protonix IV, Tecta
Func. class.: Proton pump inhibitor
Chem. class.: Benzimidazole
Pregnancy category C

ACTION: Suppresses gastric secretion by inhibiting hydrogen/potassium ATPase enzyme system in gastric parietal cell; characterized as gastric acid pump inhibitor, since it blocks final step of acid production

Therapeutic outcome: Absence of epigastric fullness, pain, swelling

USES: Gastroesophageal reflux disease (GERD), severe erosive esophagitis, maintenance, long-term pathological hypersecretory conditions including Zollinger-Ellison syndrome

CONTRAINDICATIONS
Hypersensitivity to this product or benzimidazole

Precautions: Pregnancy **C,** breastfeeding, children, proton pump hypersensitivity

DOSAGE AND ROUTES
GERD
Adult: PO 40 mg/day × 8 wk, may repeat course

Erosive esophagitis
Adult: IV 40 mg/day × 7-10 days; PO 40 mg/ day × 8 wk; may repeat PO course

Pathologic hypersecretory conditions
Adult: PO 40 mg bid; IV 80 mg q12hr; max 240 mg/day

Available forms: Del rel tabs 20, 40 mg; powder for inj 40 mg/vial; del rel granules for susp 40 mg

Implementation
• Swallow del rel tabs whole; do not break, crush, or chew
• May take with or without food
• **Suspension:** give in apple juice 30 min before a meal or sprinkled on 1 tbsp of applesauce
• **NG tube:** empty contents of packet of granules into barrel of a 60-ml catheter tip syringe (plunger removed) connected to ≥16F NG tube; add 10 ml apple juice and tap or shake barrel of syringe to empty into the tube; add another 10 ml of apple juice; rinse with additional apple juice until syringe is clear

IV route
• **Use of Protonix IV vials with spiked IV system adaptors is not recommended**
• Visually inspect for particulate matter and discoloration prior to use
• Give as an IV infusion over 15 min either through a dedicated line or a Y-site; a 2-min slow injection regimen is also approved; do not give fast IV push
• When using a Y-site, immediately stop use if a precipitation or discoloration occurs
Reconstitution of vial:
• Use 40 mg vial/10 ml NS; do not freeze
2-minute slow intravenous (IV) infusion injection:
• Dilute one or two 40-mg vials with 10 ml NS per vial to 4 mg/ml, store up to 24 hr at room temperature prior to use; infuse slowly over at least 2 min; do not give with other IV fluids or medications; flush line with D_5W, NS, or LR before and after each dose

15-minute intravenous (IV) infusion:
• Dilute each 40 mg dose with 10 ml NS; the reconstituted vial should be further admixed with 100 ml (for one vial) or 80 ml (for 2 vials) of D_5W, NS, or LR (to 0.4 mg/ml or 0.8 mg/ml, respectively), store up to 6 hr at room temperature prior to further dilution; the admixed solution (0.4 mg/ml or 0.8 mg/ml) may be stored at room temperature and must be used within 24 hr from the time of initial reconstitution; infuse over 15 min at 7 ml/min; do not administer with other IV fluids or medications; flush the IV line with D_5W, NS, or LR before and after each dose

ADVERSE EFFECTS
CNS: *Headache,* insomnia, asthenia, fatigue, malaise, insomnia, somnolence
GI: *Diarrhea, abdominal pain,* flatulence, pancreatitis, weight changes
INTEG: *Rash*
META: Hyperglycemia, weight gain/loss, hyponatremia, hypomagnesemia
MS: Rhabdomyolysis, myalgia
RESP: Pneumonia
SYST: Stevens-Johnson syndrome, toxic epidermal necrolysis, anaphylaxis, angioedema

Pharmacokinetics
Absorption	Unknown
Distribution	Protein binding 97%
Metabolism	Unknown
Excretion	Urine-metabolites, feces, decreased rate in geriatric
Half-life	1½ hr

Pharmacodynamics
Onset	Unknown
Peak	2.4 hr
Duration	>24 hr

INTERACTIONS
Individual drugs
Calcium carbonate, sucralfate, vit B_{12}, ketoconazole, itraconazole, atazanair, ampicillin, iron salts: decreased absorption of these products
Clarithromycin, diazepam, flurazepam, phenytoin, triazolam: increased levels of pantoprazole
Clopidogrel: decreased clopidogrel effect
Warfarin: increased risk of bleeding

Drug/herb
St. John's wort: decreased effect of pantoprazole

NURSING CONSIDERATIONS
Assessment
• **Rhabdomyolysis: muscle pain, increased CPK, weakness, swelling of affected**

muscles; if these occur and if confirmed by CPK, product should be discontinued
• Assess GI system: bowel sounds q8hr, abdomen for pain, swelling, anorexia
• Monitor hepatic enzymes: AST, ALT, alkaline phosphatase during treatment
• **Serious skin reactions: assess for toxic epidermal necrolysis, Stevens-Johnson syndrome, exfoliative dermatitis; fever, sore throat, fatigue, thin ulcers, lesions in the mouth, lips**
• **Electrolyte imbalances:** hyponatremia; hypomagnesemia in those using this product (3 mo-1 yr) if hypomagnesemia occurs, use of magnesium supplements may be sufficient; if severe, discontinuation of this product may be required

Patient/family education
• Advise patient to report severe diarrhea; product may have to be discontinued
• Advise patient with diabetes that hyperglycemia may occur
• Advise patient to avoid hazardous activities; dizziness may occur
• Advise patient to avoid alcohol, salicylates, ibuprofen; may cause GI irritation

Evaluation
Positive therapeutic outcome
• Absence of epigastric pain, swelling, fullness

PARoxetine (Rx)
(par-ox′e-teen)
Paxil, Paxil CR, Pexeva, PMS
Func. class.: Antidepressant, selective serotonin reuptake inhibitor (SSRI)
Chem. class.: Phenylpiperidine derivative
Pregnancy category D

Do not confuse: PARoxetine/PACLitaxel, Paxil/PACLitaxel/Taxol

ACTION: Inhibits CNS neuron reuptake of serotonin but not of norepinephrine or DOPamine

Therapeutic outcome: Relief of depression

USES: Major depressive disorder, obsessive-compulsive disorder, panic disorder, generalized anxiety disorder, posttraumatic stress disorder, premenstrual disorders, social anxiety disorder

Unlabeled uses: Premature ejaculation

CONTRAINDICATIONS
Pregnancy **D**, hypersensitivity, MAOI use, alcohol use

Precautions: Breastfeeding, geriatric, seizure history, patients with history of mania, renal/hepatic disease

BLACK BOX WARNING: Children, suicidal ideation

DOSAGE AND ROUTES
Depression
Adult: PO 20 mg/day in AM; after 4 wk if no clinical improvement is noted, dosage may be increased by 10 mg/day weekly to desired response; max 50 mg/day; or CONT REL 25 mg/day, may increase by 12.5 mg/day weekly up to 62.5 mg/day
Geriatric: PO 10 mg/day, increase by 10 mg to desired dose, max 40 mg/day

Obsessive-compulsive disorder
Adult: PO 40 mg/day in AM; start with 20 mg/day, increase 10 mg/day increments, max 60 mg/day

Panic disorder
Adult: Start with 10 mg/day and increase in 10 mg/day increments to 40 mg/day, max 60 mg/day; or CONT REL 12.5 mg/day max 75 mg/day

Generalized anxiety disorder
Adult: PO 20 mg/day in AM, range 20-50 mg/day

Posttraumatic stress disorder
Adult: PO 20 mg/day, range 20-60 mg/day

Premenstrual disorders
Adult: CONT REL 12.5 mg/day in AM

Renal dose
Adult: PO CCr 30-60 ml/min lower doses may be needed, CCr <30 ml/min 10 mg/day in AM, may increase by 10 mg/day qwk, max 40 mg/day; or CONT REL 12.5 mg/day max 50 mg/day

Hepatic dose
Adult: PO 10 mg/day initially, max 40 mg regular release, CONT REL 12.5 mg/day initially, max 50 mg/day

Available forms: Tabs 10, 20, 30, 40 mg; oral susp 10 mg/5 ml; cont rel 12.5, 25, 37.5 mg

Implementation
• Give with food or milk for GI symptoms; store at room temperature; do not freeze
• Give crushed if patient is unable to swallow whole, regular release only
• Use gum, hard candy, frequent sips of water for dry mouth
• Avoid use with other CNS depressants
• **Oral susp:** shake, measure with oral syringe or calibrated measuring device
• **Cont rel tab:** do not cut, chew, crush; do not give concurrently with antacids

ADVERSE EFFECTS

CNS: *Headache, nervousness, insomnia, drowsiness, anxiety, tremor, dizziness, fatigue, sedation,* abnormal dreams, agitation, apathy, euphoria, hallucinations, delusions, psychosis, **seizures, malignant neuroleptic syndrome–like reactions,** restless legs syndrome
CV: Vasodilatation, postural hypotension, palpitations, bleeding
EENT: Visual changes
GI: *Nausea, diarrhea, constipation, dry mouth, anorexia,* dyspepsia, vomiting, taste changes, flatulence, decreased appetite, cramps
GU: Dysmenorrhea, decreased libido, urinary frequency, UTI, amenorrhea, cystitis, impotence, decreased sperm quality, decreased fertility, *abnormal ejaculation* (male)
INTEG: *Sweating,* rash
MS: Pain, arthritis, myalgia, myopathy, myasthenia
RESP: Infection, pharyngitis, nasal congestion, sinus headache, sinusitis, cough, dyspnea, yawning
SYST: Asthenia, fever, abrupt withdrawal syndrome

Pharmacokinetics

Absorption	Well absorbed
Distribution	Widely distributed; crosses blood-brain barrier, protein-binding 95%
Metabolism	Liver, mostly by CYP2D6 enzyme system
Excretion	Kidneys, unchanged (2%); breast milk
Half-life	21 hr (reg rel); 15-20 hr (cont rel)

Pharmacodynamics

Onset	Unknown
Peak	5.2 hr
Duration	Unknown

INTERACTIONS
Individual drugs

Methylphenidate, traMADol: increased serotonin syndrome
Cimetidine: increased PARoxetine levels
Digoxin: decreased effect of digoxin
L-tryptophan: increased agitation
PHENobarbital: decreased PARoxetine levels
Phenytoin: decreased effect of PARoxetine
⚠ **Pimozide: potentially fatal reactions**
Theophylline: increased theophylline levels
⚠ **Thioridazine: do not use with PARoxetine; hypertensive crisis, seizures, potentially fatal reactions can occur**
Warfarin: increased bleeding

Drug classifications

CYP2D6 inhibitors (aprepitant, delavirdine, imatinib, nefazodone): increased toxicity
Highly protein-bound products: increased side effects
⚠ **MAOIs: hypertensive crisis, seizures; do not use together; potentially fatal reactions can occur**
SSRIs, SNRIs, atypical antipsychotics, serotonin-receptor agonists, tricyclics, amphetamines: increased serotonin syndrome
NSAIDs, thrombolytics, salicylates, platelet inhibitors, anticoagulants: increased bleeding

Drug/herb
Ephedra: hypertensive crisis
Kava: avoid use
St. John's wort: possible serotonin syndrome, avoid use

NURSING CONSIDERATIONS
Assessment

> **BLACK BOX WARNING: Depression/OCD/anxiety/panic attacks:** assess mental status: mood, sensorium, affect, suicidal tendencies (especially in child/young adult), increase in psychiatric symptoms, increasing obsessive thoughts, compulsive behaviors, restrict amount available

P

• **Postural hypotension:** monitor B/P (lying/standing), pulse q4hr; if systolic B/P drops 20 mm Hg, hold product, notify prescriber; take vital signs q4hr in patients with CV disease
• **Renal status:** monitor BUN, creatinine, urinary retention
• **Withdrawal symptoms:** assess for headache, nausea, vomiting, muscle pain, weakness; not usual unless product discontinued abruptly, taper over 1-2 wk
⚠ **Serotonin, neuroleptic malignant syndrome: assess for hallucinations, coma, headache, agitation, shivering/sweating, tachycardia, diarrhea, tremor, hypertension, hyperthermia, rigidity, delirium, coma, myoclonus, agitation, nausea, vomiting**
• Monitor blood studies: CBC, leukocytes, differential, cardiac enzymes if patient is receiving long-term therapy
• Monitor hepatic studies: AST, ALT, bilirubin
• Check weight weekly; appetite may increase with product
• Assess ECG for flattening of T-wave, bundle branch block, AV block, dysrhythmias in cardiac patients
• Assess for EPS primarily in geriatric: rigidity, dystonia, akathisia

• Monitor urinary retention, constipation; constipation is more likely to occur in children or geriatric
• Identify alcohol consumption; if alcohol is consumed, hold dose until AM

Patient/family education
• Advise patient that therapeutic effects may take 1-4 wk
• Teach patient to use caution in driving and other activities requiring alertness because of drowsiness, dizziness, blurred vision; to avoid rising quickly from sitting to standing, especially geriatric
• Caution patient to avoid alcohol ingestion, other CNS depressants, and OTC medication unless prescribed
• Caution patient not to discontinue medication quickly after long-term use; may cause nausea, anxiety, headache, malaise; do not double doses if one is missed
• Advise patient to use gum, hard sugarless candy, or frequent sips of water for dry mouth; if dry mouth continues an artificial saliva product may be used

> BLACK BOX WARNING: Advise patient that depression may worsen, suicidal thoughts/ behavior may occur (especially in child/young adult), to notify prescriber

• Advise patient to discuss sexual side effects: impotence, possible male infertility while taking this product

Evaluation

Positive therapeutic outcome
• Decrease in depression
• Absence of suicidal thoughts

TREATMENT OF OVERDOSE:
Activated charcoal, gastric lavage, maintain airway; for seizures give diazepam, symptomatic treatment

---

⚠ HIGH ALERT

pazopanib
(paz-oh'pa-nib)
Votrient
Func. class.: Antineoplastic biologic response modifier/multikinase angiogenesis inhibitor
Chem. class.: Kinase inhibitor
Pregnancy category D

ACTION: Targets vascular endothelial growth factor receptors; a multikinase angiogenesis inhibitor

Therapeutic outcome: Decrease in size, spread of tumor

USES: Advanced renal cell carcinoma; soft-tissue sarcoma patients who have received prior chemotherapy

CONTRAINDICATIONS
Pregnancy (D), hypothyroidism, QT prolongation, MI, wound dehiscence, hypertension

Precautions: Breastfeeding, children, cardiac/renal/hepatic/dental disease, GI bleeding

> BLACK BOX WARNING: Hepatic disease

DOSAGE AND ROUTES
Adult: PO 800 mg/day without food (1 hr before, 2 hr after a meal), may decrease to 400 mg/day if not tolerated (renal cell cancer); or adjust in 200-mg increments based on toxicity (soft-tissue sarcoma)

Available forms: Tabs 200 mg

Implementation
• Give on an empty stomach (1 hr before or 2 hr after a meal); separate doses by 24 hr
• Do not crush tablets, can lead to an increased rate of absorption, which can affect systemic exposure; only intact, whole tablets should be used
• If a dose is missed, it should not be taken if it is ≤12 hr until the next dose
• Store at 77°F (25°C)

ADVERSE EFFECTS
CNS: Intracranial bleeding, headache
CV: Heart failure, hypertension, hypertensive crisis, chest pain, MI, QT prolongation, torsades de pointes
GI: Nausea, hepatotoxicity, vomiting, dyspepsia, GI hemorrhage, anorexia, abdominal pain, GI perforation, pancreatitis, diarrhea; hepatotoxicity (geriatric)
HEMA: Neutropenia, thrombocytopenia, bleeding
INTEG: Rash, alopecia
MISC: Fatigue, epistaxis, pyrexia, hot sweats, increased weight, flulike symptoms, hypothyroidism, hand–foot syndrome, retinal tear/detachment

Pharmacokinetics

Absorption	Unknown
Distribution	Protein binding 99%
Metabolism	Unknown
Excretion	Unknown
Half-life	31 hr

Pharmacodynamics

Onset	Unknown
Peak	2-4 hr
Duration	24 hr

INTERACTIONS
Individual drugs

Arsenic trioxide, levomethadyl, haloperidol, chloroquine, droperidol, pentamidine: increased QT prolongation, pazopanib concentrations

Simvastatin: increased plasma concentrations of this agent

Warfarin: avoid use with warfarin; use low-molecular-weight anticoagulants instead; increased plasma concentration of warfarin

Drug classifications

Class IA/III antidysrhythmics, some phenothiazines, Beta-agonists, local anesthetics, tricyclics, CYP3A4 inhibitors (amiodarone, clarithromycin, erythromycin, telithromycin, ketoconazole, troleandomycin); CYP3A4 substrates (methadone, pimozide, QUEtiapine, quiNIDine, risperiDONE, ziprasidone): increased QT prolongation, increased pazopanib concentrations

Calcium-channel blockers, ergots: increased plasma concentrations of these agents

CYP3A4 inducers (dexamethasone, phenytoin, carBAMazepine, rifampin, PHENobarbital): decreased pazopanib concentrations

Drug/food

Grapefruit juice: avoid use; increased pazopanib effect

Drug/herb

St. John's wort: decreased pazopanib concentration

NURSING CONSIDERATIONS
Assessment

> **BLACK BOX WARNING:** Hepatic disease: fatal hepatotoxicity can occur; obtain LFTs baseline and at least every 2 wk × 2 mo, then monthly

> **BLACK BOX WARNING:** Fatal bleeding: from GI, respiratory, GU tracts, permanently discontinue in those with severe bleeding

⚠ **Palmar-plantar erythrodysesthesia (hand–foot syndrome):** more common in those previously treated; assess for swelling, numbness, desquamation on palms and soles

⚠ **GI perforation/fistula:** discontinue if this occurs, assess for pain in epigastric area, dyspepsia, flatulence, fever, chills

⚠ **Hypertension/hypertensive crisis:** hypertension usually occurs in the first cycle; in those with preexisting hypertension, do not start treatment until B/P is controlled; monitor B/P every wk × 6 wk, then at start of each cycle or more often if needed, temporarily or permanently discontinue for severe uncontrolled hypertension

Patient/family education

• Advise patient to report adverse reactions immediately: bleeding
• Teach patient about reason for treatment, expected results
• Inform patient that effect on male fertility is unknown

Evaluation

Positive therapeutic outcome
• Decrease in size, spread of tumor

pegaptanib (Rx)
(peg-ap′ta-nib)
Macugen
Func. class: Ophthalmic agent—miscellaneous
Pregnancy category B

ACTION: Binds to vascular endothelial growth factor (VEGF), thereby inhibiting angiogenesis

Therapeutic outcome: Stabilization of vision in macular degeneration

USES: Treatment of neovascular (wet) age-related macular degeneration; may be used alone or with photodynamic therapy (PDT)

CONTRAINDICATIONS
Hypersensitivity, ocular or periocular infections

Precautions: Pregnancy **B**, inflammatory eye disease, ocular hypertension

DOSAGE AND ROUTES
Adult: Intravitreal inj 0.3 mg inj q6wk

Available forms: Inj 0.3 mg, single glass syringes

Implementation

• Administer anesthesia and a broad-spectrum antiinfective prior to injection
• The inj should be done under aseptic conditions
• Remove all air bubbles prior to use
• Store at 36°-46° F, do not freeze or shake vigorously

ADVERSE EFFECTS

EENT: *Anterior chamber inflammation, blurred vision, conjunctival hemorrhage, corneal edema, cataract, eye discharge, eye pain, increased intraocular pressure, punctate keratitis, reduced visual acuity, vitreous floaters, vitreous opacities, blepharitis, conjunctivitis, photophobia,* retinal detachment, iatrogenic traumatic cataract

Pharmacokinetics

Absorption	Unknown
Distribution	Unknown
Metabolism	Unknown
Excretion	Unknown
Half-life	87-100 hr in vitreous humor of the monkey

Pharmacodynamics

Onset	Unknown
Peak	Unknown
Duration	May remain fully active in the eye for 7-28 days

NURSING CONSIDERATIONS
Assessment
- Test visual acuity periodically
- Assess treated eye for increased intraocular pressure, infection, endophthalmitis
- Monitor perfusion of the optic nerve head immediately after injection, tonometry ½ hr after inj, biomicroscopy 2-7 days after inj

Patient/family education
- Instruct patient to report any inflammation, bleeding, eye discharge, opacities to prescriber
- Instruct patient to continue with follow-up care during treatment

Evaluation

Positive therapeutic outcome
- Macular degeneration stabilized

⚠ **HIGH ALERT**

pegfilgrastim (Rx)
(peg-fill-grass'stim)
Neulasta
Func. class.: Hematopoietic agent
Pregnancy category C

ACTION: Stimulates proliferation and differentiation of neutrophils

Therapeutic outcome: Absence of infection

USES: To decrease infection in patients receiving antineoplastics that are myelosuppressive; to increase WBC in patients with product-induced neutropenia

CONTRAINDICATIONS
Hypersensitivity to proteins of *E. coli,* filgrastim

Precautions: Pregnancy **C**, breastfeeding, child <45 kg, adolescents, myeloid malignancies, sickle cell disease, leukocytosis, splenic rupture, allergic-type reactions, ARDS, peripheral blood stem cell mobilization (PBSC)

DOSAGE AND ROUTES
Adult: SUBCUT 6 mg per chemotherapy cycle

Available forms: Sol for inj 10 mg/0.6 ml

Implementation
SUBCUT route
- Give using single-use vials; after dose is withdrawn, do not reenter vial
- Do not use 6-mg fixed dose in infants, children, or others <45 kg
- Inspect sol for discoloration, particulates; if present, do not use
- Do not administer in the period 14 days before and 24 hr after cytotoxic chemotherapy
- Store in refrigerator; do not freeze; may store at room temp up to 6 hr, avoid shaking, protect from light

ADVERSE EFFECTS
CNS: Fever, fatigue, headache, dizziness, insomnia, peripheral edema
GI: *Nausea,* vomiting, diarrhea, mucositis, anorexia, constipation, dyspepsia, abdominal pain, stomatitis, splenic rupture
HEMA: Leukocytosis, granulocytopenia, sickle cell crisis, hemoglobin S disease with crisis
INTEG: Alopecia
MISC: Chest pain, hyperuricemia, anaphylaxis, flulike syndrome, angioedema, antibody formation
MS: Skeletal pain
RESP: Respiratory distress syndrome

Pharmacokinetics

Absorption	Unknown
Distribution	Unknown
Metabolism	Unknown
Excretion	Unknown
Half-life	15-80 hr; 20-38 hr (child)

Pharmacodynamics
Unknown

INTERACTIONS
Individual drug
Lithium: increased release of neutrophils

Drug classifications
Cytotoxic chemotherapy agents: do not use this product concomitantly or 2 wk before or 24 hr after administration of cytotoxics

Drug/lab test
Increased: uric acid, LDH, alkaline phosphatase

NURSING CONSIDERATIONS
Assessment
• **Assess for allergic reactions, anaphylaxis: rash, urticaria; discontinue this product, have emergency equipment nearby**
• Monitor blood studies: CBC, platelet count before treatment and twice weekly; neutrophil counts may be increased for 2 days after therapy
• **ARDS: assess for dyspnea, fever, tachypnea, occasional confusion; obtain ABGs, chest x-ray, product may need to be discontinued**
• Monitor B/P, respirations, pulse before, during therapy
• **Assess for bone pain,** give mild analgesics

Patient/family education
• Teach the technique for self-administration: dose, side effects, disposal of containers and needles; provide instruction sheet
⚠ **Teach patient to notify prescriber immediately of allergic reaction, trouble breathing, abdominal pain**

Evaluation
Positive therapeutic outcome
• Absence of infection

⚠ HIGH ALERT

PEMEtrexed (Rx)
(pem-ah-trex'ed)
Alimta
Func. class.: Antineoplastic-antimetabolite
Chem. class.: Folic acid antagonist
Pregnancy category D

ACTION: Inhibits multiple enzymes that reduce folic acid, which is needed for cell replication

Therapeutic outcome: Decreased spread of mesothelioma, decreased tumor size

USES: Malignant pleural mesothelioma in combination with CISplatin; non–small cell lung cancer as a single agent; non-squamous non–small cell lung cancer (first-line treatment)

CONTRAINDICATIONS
Pregnancy **D**, hypersensitivity, ANC <1500 cells/mm³, CCr <45 ml/min, thrombocytopenia (<100,000/mm³), anemia

Precautions: Breastfeeding, children, renal/hepatic disease

DOSAGE AND ROUTES
Adult: **IV** INF 500-600 mg/m² given over 10 min on day 1 of a 21-day cycle with CISplatin 75 mg/m² INF over 2 hr beginning ½ hr after end of PEMEtrexed INF

Renal dose
Adult: IV infusion CCr <45 ml/min, not recommended

Available forms: Inj, single-use vials, 100, 500 mg

Implementation
• Administer vit B_{12} and low-dose folic acid as a prophylactic measure to treat related hematologic, GI toxicity; at least 5 daily doses of folic acid must be taken in the 7 days preceding first dose
• Premedicate with a corticosteroid (dexamethasone) given PO bid the day before, day of, and day after administration of PEMEtrexed
• **Neurotoxicity: assess for CTC grade 2: withhold until resolution to at least pretherapy value/condition, reduce CISplatin by 50%; CTC grade 3/4; immediately discontinue this product and CISplatin if given in combination**
• **Mucositis: assess for CTC 3-4; withhold until resolution to at least pretherapy value/condition, reduce dose by 50%, if grade 3-4 occurs after 2 dosage reductions, discontinue this product and CISplatin**
• **Bleeding:** assess for bleeding time, coagulation time during treatment; bleeding; hematuria, guaiac, bruising or petechiae, mucosa or orifices q8hr
• Use a liquid diet: carbonated beverage, gelatin; dry toast, crackers may be added when patient is not nauseated or vomiting
• Assist patient with rinsing of mouth tid-qid with water, club soda; brushing of teeth bid-tid with soft brush or cotton-tipped applicators for stomatitis; use unwaxed dental floss

IV route
• **Use cytotoxic handling procedures**
• Reconstitute 500-mg vial/20 ml 0.9% NaCl inj (preservative free) = 25 mg/ml, swirl until dissolved, further dilute with 100 ml 0.9% NaCl inj (preservative free), give as IV inf over 10 min
• Use only 0.9% NaCl inj (preservative free) for reconstitution, dilution
• Store at 77° F, excursions permitted 59°-86°F, not light sensitive, discard unused portions

Dosage adjustments
Do not begin a new cycle unless neutrophils (ANC) ≥1500 cells/mm³, platelets ≥100,000 cells/mm³, CCr is ≥45 ml/min

P

• Platelet nadir <50,000/mm³ regardless of the ANC: If necessary, delay until platelet count recovery, reduce PEMEtrexed and CISplatin, by 50%; if grade 3/4 toxicity occurs after 2 reductions, discontinue both products
• ANC nadir <500/mm³ when platelet nadir is ≥50,000/mm³: If necessary, delay until ANC recovery, reduce PEMEtrexed and CISplatin, by 75%; if grade 3/4 toxicity occurs after 2 reductions, discontinue both products
• CTC Grade 3/4 nonhematologic toxicity including diarrhea requiring hospitalization and excluding neurotoxicity, mucositis, and grade 3 transaminase elevations: Withhold therapy until pre-therapy value or condition, reduce by 75% both products, if grade 3 or 4 toxicity occurs after 2 reductions, discontinue both products
• CTC grade 3/4 mucositis: Withhold therapy until pre-therapy condition, reduce 50% of PEMEtrexed, if grade 3 or 4 mucositis occurs after 2 dosage reductions, discontinue both products
• CTC grade 2 neurotoxicity: Withhold therapy until pre-therapy value or condition, reduce dose of CISplatin by 50%
• CTC grade 3/4 neurotoxicity: discontinue both products

Y-site compatibilities: Acyclovir sodium, alfentanil, allopurinol, amifostine, amikacin, aminocaproic acid, aminophylline, amiodarone, amphotericin B lipid complex, amphotericin B liposome, ampicillin, ampicillin-sulbactam, atenolol, atracurium, azithromycin, aztreonam, bivalirudin, bleomycin, bumetanide, buprenorphine, butorphanol, CARBOplatin, carmustine, ceftizoxime, cefTRIAXone, cefuroxime, cimetidine, cisatracurium, CISplatin, clindamycin, cyclophosphamide, cycloSPORINE, cytarabine, DACTINomycin, DAPTOmycin, dexamethasone, digoxin, diltiazem, diphenhydrAMINE, DOCEtaxel, dolasetron, DOPamine, doxacurium, enalaprilat, ePHEDrine, EPINEPHrine, eptifibatide, ertapenem, esmolol, etoposide, famotidine, fenoldopam, fentaNYL, fluconazole, fludarabine, fluorouracil, foscarnet, fosphenytoin, furosemide, ganciclovir, gatifloxacin, glycopyrrolate, granisetron, haloperidol, heparin, hydrocortisone, HYDROmorphone, hydrOXYzine, ifosfamide, imipenem-cilastatin, insulin (regular), isoproterenol, ketorolac, labetalol, leucovorin, levofloxacin, lidocaine, linezolid, LORazepam, magnesium, mannitol, meperidine, meropenem, mesna, methyldopate, methylPREDNISolone, metoclopramide, metoprolol, midazolam, milrinone, mitoMYcin, mivacurium, morphine, moxifloxacin, nafcillin, naloxone, nesiritide, nitroglycerin, norepinephrine, octreotide, oxaliplatin, PACLitaxel, pamidronate, pancuronium, PENTobarbital, PHENobarbital, piperacillin-tazobactam, polymyxin B, potassium chloride/phosphates, procainamide, promethazine, propranolol, ranitidine, remifentanil, rocuronium, sodium acetate/bicarbonate/phosphates, succinylcholine, SUFentanil, sulfamethoxazole-trimethoprim, tacrolimus, theophylline, thiopental, thiotepa, ticarcillin, ticarcillin-clavulanate, tigecycline, tirofiban, trimethobenzamide, vancomycin, vecuronium, verapamil, vinBLAStine, vinCRIStine, vinorelbine, zidovudine, zoledronic acid

ADVERSE EFFECTS
CNS: *Fatigue, fever, mood alteration, neuropathy*
CV: Thrombosis/embolism, *chest pain*, arrhythmia exacerbation
GI: *Nausea, vomiting, anorexia, diarrhea, ulcerative stomatitis, constipation, dysphagia, dehydration*
GU: Renal failure, *creatinine elevation*
HEMA: Neutropenia, leukopenia, thrombocytopenia, myelosuppression, anemia
INTEG: *Rash, desquamation*
RESP: *Dyspnea*
SYST: Infection with/without neutropenia, radiation recall reaction

Pharmacokinetics
Absorption	Unknown
Distribution	81% protein binding
Metabolism	Not metabolized
Excretion	Excreted in urine (unchanged 70%-90%) Not known if it is excreted in breast milk
Half-life	3.5 hr

Pharmacodynamics
Unknown

INTERACTIONS
Drug classifications
Anticoagulants, NSAIDs, platelet inhibitors, salicylates, thrombolytics: increased bleeding risk
Nephrotoxic products (NSAIDs): decreased PEMEtrexed clearance

NURSING CONSIDERATIONS
Assessment
⚠ Bone marrow depression: monitor CBC, differential, platelet count; monitor for nadir and recovery; a new cycle should not begin if ANC < 1500 cells/mm³, platelets are < 100,000 cells/mm³, creatinine clearance < 45 ml/min

- Monitor renal tests: BUN, serum uric acid, urine CCr, electrolytes before, during therapy
- For previous radiation treatments; radiation recall reactions have occurred (erythema, exfoliative dermatitis, pain, burning)
- Monitor I&O ratio; report fall in urine output to <30 ml/hr
- Monitor temp q4hr; fever may indicate beginning infection; no rectal temps
- Assess bleeding time, coagulation time during treatment; bleeding: hematuria, guaiac, bruising or petechiae, mucosa or orifices q8hr
- Assess buccal cavity q8hr for dryness, sores, ulceration, white patches, oral pain, bleeding, dysphagia
⚠ Assess for symptoms indicating severe allergic reaction/toxic epidermal necrolysis: rash, urticaria, itching, flushing

Patient/family education
- Instruct patient to report any complaints, side effects to nurse or prescriber: black tarry stools, chills, fever, sore throat, bleeding, bruising, cough, shortness of breath, dark or bloody urine
- Instruct patient to avoid foods with citric acid, hot or rough texture if stomatitis is present
- Instruct patient to report stomatitis: any bleeding, white spots, ulcerations in mouth to prescriber; tell patient to examine mouth daily, report symptoms to nurse, use good oral hygiene
- Advise patient that contraceptive measures are recommended during therapy and for at least 8 wk following cessation of therapy, to discontinue breastfeeding; toxicity to infant may occur
- Advise patient to avoid alcohol, salicylates, live vaccines
- Advise patient to avoid use of razors, commercial mouthwash
- Teach to eat foods high in folic acid and take supplements as prescribed

Evaluation

Positive therapeutic outcome
- Decreased spread of malignancy

⚠ HIGH ALERT

pembrolizumab
(pem′broe-liz′ue-mab)
Keytruda
Func. class.: Antineoplastic, biologic response modifier
Chem. class.: Monoclonal antibody
Pregnancy category D

ACTION: A human monoclonal antibody that binds to the programmed death receptor-1 (PD-1) found on T cells and blocks the interaction of PD-1 with its ligands, PD-L1 and PD-L2, on the tumor cell

Therapeutic outcome: Decreased progression of multiple myeloma

USES: Treatment of unresectable or metastatic malignant melanoma in those who have disease progression after ipilimumab or in BRAF V600 mutation–positive patients who have disease progression after ipilimumab and a BRAF inhibitor

CONTRAINDICATIONS: Hypersensitivity, pregnancy **D**, breastfeeding

Precautions: Immune-mediated colitis, immune-mediated hepatitis, immune-mediated hyperthyroidism/hypothyroidism; immune-mediated nephritis, acute interstitial nephritis, and renal failure; immune-mediated pneumonitis, adrenocortical insufficiency, arthritis, exfoliative dermatitis, hemolytic anemia, hypophysitis, myasthenia syndrome, myositis, optic neuritis, pancreatitis, partial seizures after inflammatory foci identified in brain parenchyma, rhabdomyolysis, uveitis, incidence of abortion/stillbirths

DOSAGE AND ROUTES
Adult: IV INF: 2 mg/kg over 30 min q3wk until disease progression

Available forms: Powder for injection 50 mg

Implementation

IV INF route
- Add 2.3 ml of sterile water for injection, 50-mg vial (25 mg/ml); inject sterile water along the walls of the vial and not directly on the powder
- Gently swirl and allow up to 5 min for bubbles to clear, do not shake, solution will be clear to slightly opalescent, colorless to slightly yellow
- Add the required amount of product to a bag of normal saline (0.9% sodium chloride injection) to a final diluted concentration between 1 and 10 mg/ml; mix by gentle inversion
- Discard any unused solution left in the vial
- Storage after reconstitution and dilution: Store at room temperature up to 4 hr or refrigerate up to 24 hr (includes reconstitution, dilution, and administration time). If refrigerated, allow the diluted solution to warm to room temperature before use, give over 30 min.
- Use a sterile, nonpyrogenic, low-protein binding 0.2- to 5-micron in-line or add-on filter
- Do not use with other drugs through the same infusion line

- Grade 2 or 3 toxicity: Withhold and give corticosteroids; resume when the adverse event recovers to grade ≤1. Permanently discontinue if there is no recovery within 12 wk, if the corticosteroid dose cannot be reduced to ≤10 mg/day of predniSONE (or equivalent) within 12 wk, or for recurrent severe or grade 3 colitis.
- Grade 4 toxicity: Permanently discontinue, give corticosteroids

Hepatitis:
- Grade 2 toxicity (AST or ALT >3-5 × upper limit of normal [ULN] or total bilirubin >1.5-3 × ULN): Withhold and give corticosteroids; resume when adverse event recovers to grade 1 or less. Permanently discontinue if there is no recovery within 12 wks or if the corticosteroid dose cannot be reduced to ≤10 mg/day of predniSONE (or equivalent) within 12 wks.
- Grade 3 or 4 toxicity (AST or ALT >5 × ULN or total bilirubin >3 × ULN): Permanently discontinue, give corticosteroids
- Liver metastases and grade 2 elevated transaminase levels at baseline: Permanently discontinue if AST/ALT levels increase by ≥50% over baseline and transaminase level elevations persist for at least 1 wk

ADVERSE EFFECTS

CNS: Seizures, myasthenia gravis, headache, fever, insomnia, chills, dizziness, fatigue
EENT: Optic neuritis
ENDO: Hyponatremia, hypothyroidism/hyperthyroidism, hyperglycemia, hypocalcemia
GI: Nausea, vomiting, abdominal pain, pancreatitis, colitis, diarrhea, hepatitis, constipation
GU: Interstitial nephritis, renal failure
INTEG: Rash, pruritus, skin discoloration
MS: Myalgia, rhabdomyolysis
RESP: Cough, dyspnea, pneumonitis
SYST: Exfoliative dermatitis

Pharmacokinetics

Absorption	Unknown
Distribution	Unknown
Metabolism	Unknown
Excretion	Unknown
Half-life	Unknown

Pharmacodynamics

Onset	Unknown
Peak	Unknown
Duration	Unknown

INTERACTIONS
Drug/lab test
Increased: LFTs, renal function studies

NURSING CONSIDERATIONS
Assessment
- For hyperthyroidism/hypothyroidism, renal function studies baseline, periodically during therapy, temporarily withheld or permanently discontinued
- For pneumonitis (new or worsening cough, chest pain, shortness of breath), confirm with radiographic imaging
- Liver function tests and hepatitis (e.g., jaundice, severe nausea/vomiting, easy bleeding or bruising; withhold and give corticosteroids if grade 2 hepatitis (AST or ALT >3-5 × ULN or total bilirubin >1.5-3 × ULN)

Patient/family education
- Instruct patient to use highly effective contraceptive methods during and for 4 months after treatment, to contact their health care provider if pregnancy is suspected or confirmed (pregnancy D)

Evaluation

Positive therapeutic outcome
- Decreased progression of multiple myeloma

---

penciclovir topical

See Appendix B

PENICILLINS

penicillin G benzathine (Rx)
(pen-i-sill′in)
Bicillin L-A
penicillin G Potassium (Rx)
Pfizerpen
penicillin G procaine (Rx)
penicillin V (Rx)
Apo-Pen-VK ✦, Penicillin VK
Func. class.: Broad-spectrum antiinfective
Chem. class.: Natural penicillin
Pregnancy category B

ACTION: Interferes with cell wall replication of susceptible organisms; osmotically unstable cell wall swells and bursts from osmotic pressure, resulting in cell death

Therapeutic outcome: Bactericidal effects on the gram-positive cocci *Staphylococcus, Streptococcus pyogenes, Streptococcus viridans, Streptococcus faecalis, Streptococcus*

bovis, Streptococcus pneumoniae; gram-negative cocci *Neisseria gonorrhoeae;* gram-positive bacilli *Actinomyces, Bacillus anthracis, Clostridium perfringens, Clostridium tetani, Corynebacterium diphtheriae, Listeria monocytogenes;* gram-negative bacilli *Escherichia coli, Proteus mirabilis, Salmonella, Shigella, Enterobacter, Streptobacillus moniliformis;* spirochete *Treponema pallidum*

USES: Respiratory tract infections, scarlet fever, erysipelas, otitis media, pneumonia, skin and soft tissue infections, gonorrhea

CONTRAINDICATIONS
Hypersensitivity to penicillins, corn

Precautions: Pregnancy **B**, breastfeeding, hypersensitivity to cephalosporins/carbapenem/sulfite, severe renal disease, GI disease, asthma

DOSAGE AND ROUTES
>> Penicillin G benzathine
Early syphilis
Adult: IM 2.4 million units in single dose
Congenital syphilis
Child <2 yr: IM 50,000 units/kg in single dose, max 2.4 million units as a single inj
Prophylaxis of rheumatic fever, glomerulonephritis
Adult and child: IM 1.2 million units in single dose
Upper respiratory tract infections (group A streptococcal)
Adult: IM 1.2 million units in single dose
Child >27 kg: IM 900,000 units in single dose
Child <27 kg: IM 300,000-600,000 units in single dose

Available forms: Inj 300,000 units/ml; 600,000 units/ml

>> Penicillin G
Pneumococcal/streptococcal infections (serious)
Adult: IM/IV 5-24 million units in divided doses q4-6hr
Child <12 yr: IV 150,000-300,000 units/kg/day in 4-6 divided doses; max 24 million units/day
Renal dose
CCr <10 ml/min, give full loading dose, then ½ of loading dose q8-10hr

Available forms: Inj 1, 2, 3 million units/50 ml; powder for inj 1, 5, 20 million units/vial

>> Penicillin G procaine
Moderate to severe pneumococcal infections
Adult and child: IM 600,000-1.2 million units in 1 or 2 doses/day for 10 days to 2 wk

Newborn: Avoid use in newborns
Pneumococcal pneumonia
Adult and child >12 yr: IM 600,000-1.2 million units/day × 7-10 days

Available forms: Inj 600,000, 1,200,000 units/dose

Moderately severe group A streptococcal/staphylococcal pneumonia
Adult, adolescent, child ≥60 lb: IM 600,000-1 million units/day
Adolescent and child <60 lb: IM 300,000 units/day

>> Penicillin V
Pneumococcal/staphylococcal infections
Adult: PO 250-500 mg q6hr
Child <12 yr/adolescent/child >12 yr: PO 25-50 mg/kg/day in divided doses q6-8hr, max 3 g/day

Streptococcal infections
Adult/adolescent/child >12 yr: PO 125 mg q6-8hr × 10 days
Child <12 yr and >27 kg: PO 500 mg q8hr or 12hr × 10 days
Child <12 yr and ≤27 kg: PO 250 mg q8hr or q12hr or 40 mg/kg/day in 3 divided doses × 10 days

Prevention of recurrence of rheumatic fever/chorea
Adult: PO 125-250 mg bid continuously

Vincent's gingivitis/pharyngitis
Adult: PO 250 mg q6-8hr

Renal dose
CCr <50 ml/min dosage reduction indicated based on clinical response, degree of impairment

Available forms: Tabs 250, 500 mg; powder for oral sol 125, 250 mg/5 ml

Implementation
>> Penicillin G benzathine
IM route
• No dilution needed, shake well, give deeply IM in large muscle mass, avoid intravascular inj; aspirate; do not give **IV**

>> Penicillin G
• Penicillin G sodium or potassium can be given IM or IV, vials containing 10 or 20 million units are not for IM use

Intermittent IV infusion route
• Vials/bulk packages; dilute according to manufacturer's directions

---

Adverse effects: *italics* = common; **bold** = life-threatening

• Frozen bags: thaw at room temp, do not force thaw, no reconstitution needed
• Final conc (100,000-500,000 units/ml, adults; 50,000 units/ml, neonate/infant)
• Total daily dose divided q4-6hr and given over 1-2 hr (adult), 15 min (infant/neonate)

>> Penicillin G potassium

Y-site compatibilities: Acyclovir, amiodarone, cyclophosphamide, diltiazem, enalaprilat, esmolol, fluconazole, foscarnet, heparin, HYDROmorphone, labetalol, magnesium sulfate, meperidine, morphine, perphenazine, potassium chloride, tacrolimus, theophylline, verapamil, vit B/C

>> Penicillin G procaine

• No dilution needed, give deep IM inj; avoid intravascular inj; aspirate; do not give IV
• Do not give **IV**
• Give deeply in large muscle mass
• Reconstitute with 0.9% NaCl, sterile water for inj, D₅W; refrigerate unused portion
• Shake medication before administering
• IM route may include procaine reactions: fear of death, depression, seizures, anxiety, confusion, hallucinations

>> Penicillin V

• Orally on empty stomach for best absorption
• Oral susp: tap bottle to loosen, add ½ total amount of water, shake, add remaining water, shake; final conc (125 or 250); store in refrigerator after reconstitution, discard after 14 days
• Give in even doses around the clock; if GI upset occurs, give with food; product must be given for 10-14 days to ensure organism death and prevent superinfection; store in tight container
• Shake susp; store in refrigerator for 2 wk or for 1 wk at room temperature

ADVERSE EFFECTS

CNS: Lethargy, hallucinations, anxiety, depression, twitching, **coma, seizures,** hyperreflexia
GI: *Nausea, vomiting, diarrhea,* increased AST, ALT, abdominal pain, glossitis, colitis, **pseudomembranous colitis**
GU: Oliguria, proteinuria, hematuria, *vaginitis, moniliasis, glomerulonephritis,* renal tubular damage
HEMA: Anemia, increased bleeding time, **bone marrow depression, granulocytopenia,** hemolytic anemia
META: Hyperkalemia, hypokalemia, alkalosis, hypernatremia
MISC: Local pain, tenderness and fever with IM inj, **anaphylaxis serum sickness, Stevens-Johnson syndrome**

>> Penicillin G benzathine

Pharmacokinetics

Absorption	Delayed; prolonged drug levels
Distribution	Widely distributed; crosses placenta
Metabolism	Liver, minimally
Excretion	Kidneys, unchanged; breast milk
Half-life	½-1 hr

Pharmacodynamics

Onset	Slow
Peak	12-24 hr
Duration	1-4 wk

>> Penicillin G

Pharmacokinetics

Absorption	Variably absorbed (PO); well absorbed (IM)
Distribution	Widely distributed; crosses placenta
Metabolism	Liver, minimally
Excretion	Kidneys, unchanged; breast milk
Half-life	½-1 hr

Pharmacodynamics

	PO	IM	IV
Onset	Rapid	Rapid	Rapid
Peak	1 hr	¼-½ hr	Immediate
Duration	Unknown	Unknown	Unknown

>> Penicillin G procaine

Pharmacokinetics

Absorption	Delayed; prolonged drug levels
Distribution	Widely distributed; crosses placenta
Metabolism	Liver, minimally
Excretion	Kidneys, unchanged; breast milk
Half-life	½-1 hr

Pharmacodynamics

Onset	Slow
Peak	1-4 hr
Duration	15 hr

>> Penicillin V

Pharmacokinetics

Absorption	Widely absorbed
Distribution	Widely distributed; crosses placenta
Metabolism	Liver, minimally
Excretion	Kidneys, unchanged; breast milk
Half-life	½-1 hr

Pharmacodynamics

Onset	Rapid
Peak	½ hr
Duration	Unknown

INTERACTIONS
Individual drugs
Aspirin, probenecid: increased penicillin levels
Heparin: increased effect of heparin
Methotrexate: increased effect of methotrexate
Typhoid vaccine: decreased effect of toxoid vaccine

Drug classifications
Contraceptives (oral): decreased contraceptive effectiveness
Tetracyclines: decreased antimicrobial effectiveness of penicillin

Drug/lab test
False positive: urine glucose, urine protein

NURSING CONSIDERATIONS
Assessment
• Assess patient for previous sensitivity reaction to penicillins or cephalosporins; cross-sensitivity between penicillins and cephalosporins is common
• **Assess patient for signs and symptoms of infection** including characteristics of wounds, sputum, urine, stool, WBC >10,000/mm^3, earache, fever; obtain information baseline, during treatment
• Obtain C&S before beginning drug therapy to identify if correct treatment has been initiated
⚠ Assess for allergic reactions: rash, urticaria, pruritus, chills, fever, joint pain; angioedema may occur a few days after therapy begins; EPINEPHrine, resuscitation equipment should be available for anaphylactic reaction
⚠ Pseudomembranous colitis: Assess for diarrhea, abdominal pain, fever, fatigue, anorexia; possible anemia, elevated WBC and low serum albumin; stop product and usually give either vancomycin or IV metroNIDAZOLE

⚠ Identify urine output; if decreasing, notify prescriber (may indicate nephrotoxicity); also check for increased BUN, creatinine
• Monitor blood studies: AST, ALT, CBC, Hct, bilirubin, LDH, alkaline phosphatase, Coombs' test monthly if patient is on long-term therapy
• Monitor electrolytes: potassium, sodium, chloride monthly if patient is on long-term therapy
• Assess bowel pattern daily; if severe diarrhea occurs, product should be discontinued; may indicate pseudomembranous colitis
• Monitor for bleeding: ecchymosis, bleeding gums, hematuria, stool guaiac daily if on long-term therapy
• Assess for overgrowth of infection: perineal itching, fever, malaise, redness, pain, swelling, drainage, rash, diarrhea, change in cough, sputum

Patient/family education
• Teach patient to report sore throat, bruising, bleeding, joint pain; may indicate **blood dyscrasias (rare)**
• Advise patient to contact prescriber if vaginal itching, loose foul-smelling stools, furry tongue occur; may indicate **superinfection**
• Instruct patient to take all medication prescribed for the length of time ordered
• Advise patient to notify prescriber of diarrhea with blood or pus, which may indicate pseudomembranous colitis

Evaluation

Positive therapeutic outcome
• Absence of signs/symptoms of infection (WBC <10,000/mm^3, temp WNL, absence of red, draining wounds, earache)
• Reported improvement in symptoms of infection

TREATMENT OF ANAPHYLAXIS: Withdraw product, maintain airway, administer EPINEPHrine, aminophylline, O$_2$, **IV** corticosteroids

pentamidine (Rx)
(pen-tam′i-deen)
Nebupent, Pentam 300
Func. class.: Antiprotozoal
Chem. class.: Aromatic diamide derivative
Pregnancy category C

ACTION: Interferes with DNA/RNA synthesis in protozoa; has direct effect on islet cells in the pancreas

Therapeutic outcome: Protozoa death

USES: Treatment/prevention of *Pneumocystis jiroveci* infections

Unlabeled uses: Leishmaniasis, African trypanosomiasis

CONTRAINDICATIONS
Hypersensitivity

Precautions: Pregnancy **C**, breastfeeding, children, blood dyscrasias, cardiac/renal/hepatic disease, diabetes mellitus, hypocalcemia, hyper/hypotension, anemia

DOSAGE AND ROUTES
Adult and child ≥4 mo: IV/IM 4 mg/kg/day × 2-3 wk; NEB 300 mg via specific nebulizer given q4wk for prevention

Available forms: Inj; aerosol 300 mg/vial; sol for aerosol 60 mg/vial ✹

Implementation
Inhalation route
• Through nebulizer, using Raspirgard II jet nebulizer; mix contents in 6 ml of sterile water; do not use low pressure (<20 psi); flow rate should be 5-7 L/min (40-50 psi) air or O_2 source over 30-45 min until chamber is empty
IM route
• 300 mg diluted in 3 ml sterile water; give deep IM by Z-track; painful by this route, rotate inj site

Intermittent IV infusion route
• 300 mg/3-5 ml of sterile water for inj, D_5W; withdraw dose and further dilute in 50-250 ml of D_5W; diluted sol is stable for 48 hr; discard unused sol; give over 1 hr or more

Y-site compatibilities: Alfentanil, atracurium, atropine, benztropine, buprenorphine, calcium gluconate, CARBOplatin, caspofungin, chlorpromazine, cimetidine, CISplatin, cyclophosphamide, cycloSPORINE, cytarabine, DACTINomycin, diltiazem, gatifloxacin, zidovudine

Y-site incompatibilities: Foscarnet, fluconazole

ADVERSE EFFECTS
CNS: Disorientation, hallucinations, dizziness, confusion, drowsiness
CV: Hypotension, ventricular tachycardia, QT prolongation, dysrhythmias
GI: *Nausea, vomiting, anorexia,* increased AST, ALT, acute pancreatitis, metallic taste
GU: Acute renal failure, increased serum creatinine, renal toxicity, decreased urination
HEMA: Anemia, leukopenia, thrombocytopenia

INTEG: Sterile abscess, pain at inj site, pruritus, urticaria, rash
META: Hyperkalemia, hypocalcemia, *hypoglycemia,* hypomagnesemia
MISC: Fatigue, fever, chills, night sweats, anaphylaxis, Stevens-Johnson syndrome
RESP: Cough, shortness of breath, bronchospasm (with aerosol), sore throat

Pharmacokinetics

Absorption	Well absorbed (IM); minimally absorbed (INH); completely absorbed (**IV**)
Distribution	Widely distributed; does not appear in CSF
Metabolism	Not known
Excretion	Kidneys, unchanged (up to 30%)
Half-life	6½-9½ hr; increased in renal disease

Pharmacodynamics

	IM	IV	INH
Onset	Unknown	Unknown	Unknown
Peak	½-1 hr	Inf end	Unknown
Duration	Unknown	Unknown	Unknown

INTERACTIONS
Individual drugs
Amphotericin B, CISplatin, vancomycin: increased nephrotoxicity
⚠ Erythromycin IV: fatal dysrhythmias
Haloperidol, chloroquine, droperidol, pentamidine; arsenic trioxide, levomethadyl: increased QT prolongation
Radiation: bone marrow suppression

Drug classifications
Aminoglycosides NSAIDs: increased nephrotoxicity
Antineoplastics: increased bone marrow depression
Class IA/III antidysrhythmics, some phenothiazines, β-agonists, local anesthetics, tricyclics, CYP3A4 inhibitors (amiodarone, clarithromycin, erythromycin, telithromycin, troleandomycin), CYP3A4 substrates (methadone, pimozide, QUEtiapine, quiNIDine, risperiDONE, ziprasidone): increased QT prolongation

Drug/lab test
Decrease: WBC, platelets, Hbg, Hct
Increase: BUN, creatinine

NURSING CONSIDERATIONS
Assessment
⚠ Assess any patient with compromised renal system: product is excreted slowly in poor renal system function; toxicity may occur rapidly

- QT prolongation: ECG for QT prolongation, ejection fraction; assess for chest pain, palpitations, dyspnea
- **Assess patient for infection,** including increased temp, thick sputum, WBC >10,000/mm^3; monitor these signs of infection throughout treatment; obtain C&S before beginning therapy; treatment may begin after culture is obtained
- Assess respiratory system including rate, rhythm, bilateral lung sounds, SOB, wheezing, dyspnea
- Monitor ECG for cardiac dysrhythmias; ECG and pulse should be checked frequently during treatment, since cardiotoxicity can occur
- Assess for hypoglycemia including nausea, tremors, anxiety, chills, diaphoresis, headache, hunger, cold, pale skin; this side effect can last for several mo after treatment is completed
- Monitor for hyperglycemia including flushed, dry skin, acetone breath, thirst, anorexia, drowsiness, polyuria; this side effect can last for several mo after treatment is completed
- Monitor renal function tests including BUN, urinalysis, creatinine; obtain at baseline and frequently during treatment; nephrotoxicity may occur; check I&O, report hematuria, oliguria
- Monitor blood studies including blood glucose, CBC, platelets; blood glucose fluctuations are common; anemia, leukopenia, thrombocytopenia can occur
- Monitor liver function studies including AST, ALT, alkaline phosphatase, bilirubin before beginning treatment and every 3 days during therapy
- Monitor calcium and magnesium before beginning treatment and every 3 days during therapy; hypocalcemia may occur

Patient/family education
- Teach patient to report sore throat, fever, fatigue; could indicate superinfection
- Advise patient not to drink alcohol or take aspirin, since gastric bleeding may occur
- Teach patient to make position changes slowly to prevent orthostatic hypotension
- Advise patient to maintain adequate fluid intake
- Teach patient to complete entire course of medication

Evaluation
Positive therapeutic outcome
- Decreased signs and symptoms of protozoan infections
- Decreased signs and symptoms of *P. jiroveci* pneumonia in HIV infections

⚠ HIGH ALERT
pentazocine (Rx)
(pen-taz′oh-seen)
Talwin, Talwin NX
Func. class.: Opiate analgesic
Chem. class.: Synthetic benzomorphan (agonist/antagonist)
Pregnancy category C
Controlled substance schedule IV

ACTION: Inhibits ascending pain pathways in limbic system, thalamus, midbrain, hypothalamus by binding to opiate receptor sites, altering pain perception and response

Therapeutic outcome: Relief of pain

USES: Moderate to severe pain

CONTRAINDICATIONS
Hypersensitivity to this product or sulfites, addiction (opioid)

Precautions: Pregnancy C, breastfeeding, child <18 yr, addictive personality, increased ICP, MI (acute), severe heart disease, respiratory depression, renal/hepatic disease, seizure disorder, head trauma, bowel impaction, geriatric patients

DOSAGE AND ROUTES
Adult: IV/IM/SUBCUT 30 mg q3-4hr prn, max 360 mg/day

Labor
Adult: IM 30 mg as a single dose; IV 20 mg q2-3hr when contractions are regular, max 2-3 times

Renal dose
Adult: CCr 10-50 ml/min reduce dose by 25%; CCr <10 ml/min reduce dose by 50%

Available forms: Inj 30 mg/ml

Implementation
- Give by inj (IM, IV), only when resuscitative equipment available; give slowly to prevent rigidity
- Store in light-resistant area at room temperature

PO route
- Tabs made in the United States contain naloxone 0.5 mg to prevent abuse if the PO preparation is used IV

IM/SUBCUT route
• Give IM inj deeply in large muscle mass; rotate inj sites; repeated SUBCUT inj may cause necrosis

Direct IV route
• Give after diluting 5 mg/ml of sterile water for inj; give 5 mg or less over 1 min

Syringe compatibilities: Atropine, benzquinamide, butorphanol, chlorproMAZINE, cimetidine, dimenhyDRINATE, diphenhydrAMINE, droperidol, fentaNYL, HYDROmorphone, hydrOXYzine, meperidine, metoclopramide, morphine, perphenazine, prochlorperazine, promazine, promethazine, propiomazine, ranitidine, scopolamine

Syringe incompatibilities: Glycopyrrolate, heparin, PENTobarbital, other barbiturates

Y-site compatibilities: Heparin, hydrocortisone, potassium chloride, vit B/C

Y-site incompatibilities: Nafcillin

Additive incompatibilities: Aminophylline, amobarbital, PENTobarbital, PHENobarbital, secobarbital, sodium bicarbonate

ADVERSE EFFECTS
CNS: *Drowsiness, dizziness, confusion, headache, sedation, euphoria, hallucinations,* dreaming, insomnia, light-headedness
CV: Palpitations, bradycardia, change in B/P, tachycardia, increased B/P (high doses), hypotension, syncope, flushing
EENT: Tinnitus, blurred vision, miosis, diplopia
GI: *Nausea,* vomiting, anorexia, constipation, cramps, dry mouth
GU: Urinary retention, increased urinary output, dysuria
HEMA: Eosinophilia, decreased WBC
INTEG: *Rash,* urticaria, bruising, flushing, diaphoresis, pruritus, severe irritation at inj sites, Stevens-Johnson syndrome
RESP: Respiratory depression

Pharmacokinetics

Absorption	Well absorbed (PO, SUBCUT, IM); completely absorbed (**IV**)
Distribution	Widely distributed; crosses placenta
Metabolism	Liver, extensively
Excretion	Kidneys, small amounts (unchanged)
Half-life	2-3 hr

Pharmacodynamics

	PO	SUBCUT/ IM	IV
Onset	15-30 min	15-30 min	Rapid
Peak	1-3 hr	1-2 hr	15 min
Duration	3 hr	2-4 hr	1 hr

INTERACTIONS
Individual drugs
Alcohol: increased effects

Drug classifications
Antipsychotics, CNS depressants, sedative-hypnotics, skeletal muscle relaxants: increased effects
MAOIs: use cautiously; results are unpredictable
Opiates: decreased effects

Drug/lab test
Increased: amylase

NURSING CONSIDERATIONS
Assessment
• **Assess pain:** location, intensity, type of pain before, after treatment
• Assess bowel status: constipation; may need stimulant laxative/stool softener
• Monitor VS after parenteral route; note muscle rigidity, product history, liver, kidney function tests, respiratory dysfunction: respiratory depression, character, rate, rhythm; notify prescriber if respirations are <10/min
• Monitor CNS changes: dizziness, drowsiness, hallucinations, euphoria, LOC, pupil reaction
• **Monitor allergic reactions:** rash, urticaria
• Assess for withdrawal symptoms in opiate-dependent patients

Patient/family education
• Teach patient to report any symptoms of CNS changes, allergic reactions
• Advise patients to avoid CNS depressants: alcohol, sedative-hypnotics for at least 24 hr after taking this product
• Discuss with patient that dizziness, drowsiness, and confusion are common; to avoid getting up without assistance
• Discuss in detail all aspects of the product
• Instruct patient to change position slowly to prevent orthostatic hypotension
• Teach patient to turn, cough, breathe deeply after surgery to prevent atelectasis
• Teach patient to avoid operating machinery if drowsiness occurs

Evaluation

Positive therapeutic outcome
• Relief of pain

TREATMENT OF OVERDOSE:
Naloxone (Narcan) 0.2-0.8 mg **IV**, O₂, **IV** fluids, vasopressors

peramivir
(per-am′i-vir)
Rapivab
Func. class.: Antiviral
Pregnancy category C

ACTION: Competitively binds to the active site of the influenza virus, inhibits the activity of strains of influenza A and B viruses

Therapeutic outcome: Absence of developing influenza A or B

USES: Treatment of uncomplicated acute influenza (seasonal influenza A virus infection or seasonal influenza B virus infection)

Unlabeled uses: Treatment of H1N1 influenza A virus (swine influenza) infection in pediatric patients requiring hospitalization

CONTRAINDICATIONS: Hypersensitivity

Precautions: Breastfeeding, children, dialysis, infants, infection, pregnancy, psychosis, renal impairment

DOSAGE AND ROUTES
Influenza
Adult: **IV** 600 mg as a single dose infused over 15-30 min, give within 48 hr of onset of influenza symptoms

Available forms: Solution for injection 200 mg/20 ml

Implementation
• For IV use only, do not give IM, visually inspect parenteral products for particulate matter and discoloration
• Dilute the 10 mg/ml to a max volume of 100 ml, use only 0.9% or 0.45% NaCl, 5% dextrose, or LR
• Storage of diluted solution: Use immediately or refrigerate up to 24 hr. Refrigerated solution should be allowed to reach room temperature before administration. Discard any unused diluted solution after 24 hr.
• Give over 15-30 min, do not mix or coadminister with other IV products

ADVERSE EFFECTS
CNS: Delirium, psychosis, hallucinations, insomnia
GI: Constipation, diarrhea, vomiting
MISC: Rash, **Stevens-Johnson syndrome**

Pharmacokinetics
Absorption	Unknown
Distribution	Protein binding <30%
Metabolism	Unknown
Excretion	Unknown
Half-life	Unknown

Pharmacodynamics
Onset	Unknown
Peak	Unknown
Duration	Unknown

INTERACTIONS
Drug classifications:
Intranasal influenza vaccines, H1N1 vaccines: avoid concurrent use

NURSING CONSIDERATIONS
Assessment
• **Assess for hypersensitivity reactions/ Stevens-Johnson syndrome**
• Neuropsychiatric reactions: Assess for delirium, psychosis, hallucinations

Patient/family education
• Teach patient that product is only for use within 48 hr of infection

Evaluation
Therapeutic response
Absence of developing influenza A or B

perindopril (Rx)
(per-in′doe-pril)
Aceon, Coversyl ✦
Func. class.: Antihypertensive
Chem. class.: Angiotensin-converting enzyme (ACE) inhibitor
Pregnancy category D

ACTION: Selectively suppresses renin-angiotensin-aldosterone system; inhibits ACE; prevents conversion of angiotensin I to angiotensin II, resulting in dilatation of arterial and venous vessels

Therapeutic outcome: Decreased B/P in hypertension

USES: Hypertension alone or in combination, MI prophylaxis

Unlabeled uses: MI

CONTRAINDICATIONS
Hypersensitivity, history of angioedema

> **BLACK BOX WARNING:** Pregnancy **D**

Adverse effects: *italics* = common; **bold** = life-threatening

Precautions: Breastfeeding, renal disease, hyperkalemia, hepatic failure, dehydration, bilateral renal artery stenosis, cough, severe CHF, aortic stenosis, African descent

DOSAGE AND ROUTES
Hypertension
Adult: PO 4 mg/day, may increase or decrease to desired response; range 4-8 mg/day may give in 2 divided doses or as a single dose; max 16 mg/day

Patients taking diuretics
Adult: PO 2-4 mg/day in 1-2 divided doses, range 4-8 mg/day

Stable CAD
Adult: PO 4 mg/day × 2 wk, then increase as tolerated to 8 mg/day

Renal dose
Adult: PO CCr 16-29 ml/min, 2 mg every other day; CCr 30-59 ml/min 2 mg/day; CCr ≤15 ml/min 2 mg on dialysis days only

Available forms: Tabs, scored 2, 4, 8 mg

Implementation
• Store in airtight container at 86° F (30° C) or less
• Severe hypotension may occur after 1st dose of this medication; decreased hypotension may be prevented by reducing or discontinuing diuretic therapy 3 days before beginning perindopril therapy
• Give by IV inf of 0.9% NaCl (as ordered) to expand fluid volume if severe hypotension occurs

ADVERSE EFFECTS
CNS: *Insomnia, dizziness,* paresthesias, *headache,* fatigue, anxiety, depression
CV: *Hypotension,* chest pain, tachycardia, dysrhythmias, syncope, cardiac arrest
EENT: *Tinnitus,* visual changes, sore throat, double vision, dry burning eyes
GI: Nausea, vomiting, colitis, cramps, diarrhea, constipation, flatulence, dry mouth, loss of taste, liver failure
GU: Proteinuria, renal failure, increased frequency of polyuria or oliguria
HEMA: Agranulocytosis, neutropenia, bone marrow suppression
INTEG: Rash, purpura, alopecia, hyperhidrosis
META: *Hyperkalemia*
RESP: Dyspnea, dry cough, crackles
SYST: Angioedema

Pharmacokinetics

Absorption	Well absorbed
Distribution	Unknown
Metabolism	Liver
Excretion	Kidneys
Half-life	Unknown

Pharmacodynamics
Unknown

INTERACTIONS
Individual drugs
Allopurinol, NSAIDs: increased hypersensitivity
Lithium: increased serum levels

Drug classifications
Angiotensin II receptor antagonists, antihypertensives, diuretics: increased hypotension
Antihypertensives, neuromuscular blocking agents: increased effects
Diuretics (potassium-sparing), potassium supplements, salt substitutes: hyperkalemia
NSAIDs: decreased effects
NSAIDs, salicylates: decreased antihypertensive effect

Drug/herb
Hawthorn: increased antihypertensive effect
Ephedra: decreased antihypertensive effect

Drug/lab test
Increase: ALT, alk phos, cholesterol, uric acid
Decrease: Hgb/Hct
Interference: glucose/insulin tolerance tests

NURSING CONSIDERATIONS
Assessment
• **Hypertension:** monitor B/P, orthostatic hypotension, syncope; if changes occur dosage change may be required
• Monitor blood studies: neutrophils, decreased platelets
• **CHF:** Check for edema in feet, legs daily
• Monitor renal studies: protein, BUN, creatinine; increased levels may indicate nephrotic syndrome and renal failure
• Monitor renal symptoms: polyuria, oliguria, frequency, dysuria
• Establish baselines in renal, liver function tests before therapy begins
• Check potassium levels throughout treatment, although hyperkalemia rarely occurs
• Assess for allergic reactions: rash, fever, pruritus, urticaria; product should be discontinued if antihistamines fail to help; angioedema: facial swelling, urticaria, product should be discontinued, may be more common in African-Americans

Patient/family education
• Advise patient not to discontinue product abruptly; advise patient to tell all persons associated with health care
• Teach patient not to use OTC products (cough, cold, allergy medications) unless directed by physician; serious side effects can occur; xanthines, such as coffee, tea, chocolate, cola can prevent action of product

• Instruct patient on the importance of complying with dosage schedule, even if feeling better; to continue with medical regimen to decrease B/P: exercise, cessation of smoking, decreasing stress, diet modifications

• Emphasize the need to rise slowly to sitting or standing position to minimize orthostatic hypotension; not to exercise in hot weather, which can cause increased hypotension

• Advise patient to notify prescriber of mouth sores, sore throat, fever, swelling of hands or feet, irregular heartbeat, chest pain, coughing, shortness of breath

• Caution patient to report excessive perspiration, dehydration, vomiting, diarrhea; may lead to fall in B/P

• Caution patient that product may cause dizziness, fainting, light-headedness; may occur during 1st few days of therapy; to avoid activities that may be hazardous

• Teach patient how to take B/P, normal readings for age-group

• Teach patient to report persistent, sustained cough

• Teach patient to avoid potassium supplements, salt substitutes

> **BLACK BOX WARNING:** Notify prescriber if pregnancy is planned or suspected, pregnancy category **D**

Evaluation
Positive therapeutic outcome
• Decreased B/P in hypertension

TREATMENT OF OVERDOSE:
Lavage, **IV** atropine for bradycardia, **IV** theophylline for bronchospasm, digoxin, O_2; diuretic for cardiac failure, hemodialysis

---

⚠ **HIGH ALERT**

pertuzumab
(per-too′zoo-mab)
Perjeta
Func. class.: Antineoplastic biologic response modifier
Chem. class.: Monoclonal antibody, antineoplastic
Pregnancy category D

ACTION: Blocks liquid-dependent action of human epidermal growth factor-2 (HER2), inhibiting signal pathways

Therapeutic outcome: Decreased size, spread of tumor

USES: First-line treatment of (HER2) positive metastatic breast cancer with trastuzumab and DOCEtaxel

CONTRAINDICATIONS

> **BLACK BOX WARNING:** Pregnancy **(D)**

Precautions: Breastfeeding, children, infants, neonates, cardiac arrhythmias, MI, cardiac disease, heart failure, hypertension, infusion-related reactions

DOSAGE AND ROUTES
Adult: **IV** 840 mg over 60 min, then after 3 wk 420 mg over 30–60 min every 3 wk; give with trastuzumab 8 mg/kg **IV** over 90 min, then after 3 wk 6 mg/kg over 30–90 min every 3 wk and DOCEtaxel 75 mg/m 2 IV every 3 wk; dosage may be escalated to 100 mg/m^2

Available forms: Solution for inj 420 mg/14 ml (single-use vials)

Implementation
• Visually inspect for particulate matter and discoloration
Dilution and preparation
• Withdraw the calculated dose from the vial and add to 250 ml 0.9% sodium chloride to PVC or non-PVC polyolefin infusion bag; do not dilute with dextrose 5% solution
• Dilute in normal saline only; do not mix or dilute with other drugs or dextrose solutions
• Mix the diluted solution by gentle inversion; do not shake

IV infusion
• Administer the diluted solution immediately
• Do not administer as an IV push or bolus
• Give the first dose of 840 mg over 60 min and subsequent 420-mg doses over 30–60 min
• If the diluted solution is not used immediately, store at 2°–8° C for up to 24 hr
Delayed or missed doses
• If time since previous dose is 6 wk, give 420 mg IV (do not wait for next scheduled dose)
• If time since previous dose is 6 wk, give 840 mg IV over 60 min, followed 3 wk later by 420 mg IV over 30–60 min repeated every 3 wk
• If DOCEtaxel is discontinued, this product and trastuzumab may continue

ADVERSE EFFECTS
CNS: Headache, fever, peripheral neuropathy, chills, fatigue, asthenia
CV: Heart failure
EENT: Lacrimation, stomatitis
GI: Nausea, vomiting, diarrhea, dysgeusia
HEMA: Anemia, neutropenia
MS: Myalgia
RESP: Upper respiratory infection
SYST: Anaphylaxis, infection, antibody formation

Pharmacokinetics

Absorption	Unknown
Distribution	Unknown
Metabolism	Unknown
Excretion	Unknown
Half-life	Median 18 days

Pharmacodynamics

Onset	Unknown
Peak	Unknown
Duration	Unknown

NURSING CONSIDERATIONS
Assessment
• **HER2 overexpression**: Testing should be done to identify HER2 overexpression before using this product
⚠ **Decreased left ventricular ejection fraction (LVEF): Can occur and is increased in those with a history of prior anthracycline use or radiotherapy to the chest; evaluate LVEF at baseline and every 3 mo; withhold therapy × 3 wk if LVEF is <40% or LVEF is 40%–45% with a 10% or greater absolute decrease from baseline; resume therapy if the LVEF is recovered to >45% or to 40%–45% with <10% absolute decrease at reassessment; if the LVEF has not improved or has declined further, consider permanently discontinuing pertuzumab and trastuzumab after a risk/benefit assessment**
⚠ **Infusion-related reactions/hypersensitivity: Assess anaphylactoid reaction, acute infusion reaction, cytokine-release syndrome 60 min after the first infusion, 30 min after other infusions; monitor for pyrexia, chills, fatigue, headache, asthenia, hypersensitivity, and vomiting; if a significant reaction occurs, slow or interrupt the infusion; permanent discontinuation may be needed in severe reactions**

> **BLACK BOX WARNING: Pregnancy:** Determine if pregnancy is planned or suspected; patients who become pregnant during therapy should report exposure to the Genentech Adverse Event line at 888-835-2555 and enroll in the MOTHER pregnancy registry at 800-690-6720

⚠ **Neutropenia: Can occur, but occurs more commonly when trastuzumab is also used**
• Upper respiratory infection: Monitor for dyspnea, shortness of breath, fever

Patient/family education

> **BLACK BOX WARNING:** Counsel women of childbearing age on the need for contraception during and for 6 mo after therapy; advise patients who suspect pregnancy to contact their health care provider immediately; discontinue breastfeeding

Evaluation
Positive therapeutic outcome
• Decreased size, spread of tumor

RARELY USED

phentolamine (Rx)
(fen-tole′a-meen)
Func. class.: Antihypertensive
Chem. class.: α-Adrenergic blocker
Pregnancy category C

Therapeutic outcome: Decreased B/P, reversal of vasoconstriction (dermal necrosis)

USES: Hypertension; pheochromocytoma; prevention, treatment of dermal necrosis after extravasation of norepinephrine, DOPamine, EPINEPHrine

CONTRAINDICATIONS
Hypersensitivity, MI, coronary insufficiency, angina, hypotension

DOSAGE AND ROUTES
Treatment of hypertensive episodes in pheochromocytoma
Adult: IV/IM 5 mg; repeat if necessary
Child: IV 0.05-0.1 mg/kg; repeat if necessary, max 5 mg

Diagnosis of pheochromocytoma
Adult: IV 5 mg
Child: IV 0.05 mg/kg; if negative, repeat with 0.1 mg/kg IV

Treatment of necrosis
Adult: 5-10 mg/10 ml 0.9% NaCl injected into area of extravasation within 12 hr
Child: 0.1-0.2 mg/kg; max 5 mg

Prevention of dermal necrosis
Adult: IV 10 mg/L of norepinephrine-containing sol
Child: IV 0.1-0.2 mg/kg, max 5 mg

⚠ Nurse Alert   ✱ Key NCLEX® Drug   ≫ Drug Specifics

phenylephrine nasal agent
See Appendix B

phenylephrine ophthalmic
See Appendix B

phenytoin (Rx)
(fen′i-toyn)
Dilantin, Dilantin Infatabs, Phenytek
Func. class.: Anticonvulsant/
antidysrhythmic (class IB)
Chem. class.: Hydantoin
Pregnancy category D

ACTION: Inhibits spread of seizure activity in motor cortex by altering ion transport; increases AV conduction to decrease dysrhythmias

Therapeutic outcome: Decreased seizures, absence of dysrhythmias

USES: Generalized tonic-clonic seizures, status epilepticus, nonepileptic seizures associated with Reye's syndrome or after head trauma, complex/partial seizures

CONTRAINDICATIONS
Pregnancy **D,** hypersensitivity, psychiatric condition, bradycardia, SA and AV block, Stokes-Adams syndrome

Precautions: Geriatric, allergies, renal/hepatic disease, petit mal seizures, hypotension, myocardial insufficiency, Asian patients positive for HLA-B 1502, hepatic failure, acute intermittent porphyria

> BLACK BOX WARNING: IV use

DOSAGE AND ROUTES
Seizures
Adult: PO 15-20 mg/kg (EXT REL) in 3-4 divided doses given q2hr or 400 mg, then 300 mg q2hr × 2 doses, maintenance 4-7 mg/kg/day; max 600 mg/day; **IV** 15-20 mg/kg, max 25-50 mg/min then 100 mg q6-8hr
Child: PO 5 mg/kg/day in 2-3 divided doses, maintenance 4-8 mg/kg/day in 2-3 divided doses, max 300 mg/day; **IV** 15-20 mg/kg at 1-3 mg/kg/min

Status epilepticus
Adult: **IV** 15-20 mg/kg, max 25-50 mg/min; may give 100 mg q6-8hr thereafter

Child: **IV** 15-20 mg/kg, max in divided doses 1-3 mg/kg/min

Ventricular dysrhythmias
Adult: PO loading dose 1 g divided over 24 hr, then 500 mg/day × 2 days; **IV** 250 mg given over 5 min until dysrhythmias subside or 1 g is given, or 100 mg q15min until dysrhythmias subside or 1 g is given
Child: PO 3-8 mg/kg or 250 mg/m^2/day as single dose or divided in 2 doses; **IV** 3-8 mg/kg given over several min, or 250 mg/m^2/day as single dose or divided in 2 doses

Renal dose
Adult: Do not use loading dose if CCr <10 ml/min or hepatic failure

Available forms: Susp 25 mg/5 ml; chew tabs 50 mg; inj 50 mg/ml; ext rel caps 100, 200, 300 mg; prompt rel caps 100 mg

Implementation
PO route
• Do not interchange chewable product with caps, not equivalent; only ext rel caps are to be used for once-a-day dosing
• Give with meals to decrease GI upset
• Chew tab can be crushed or chewed; cap can be opened and mixed with foods or fluids; cap and tab are not interchangeable, only ext rel cap is to be used for once a day dosing
• Do not take antacids or antidiarrheals within 2-3 hr of taking phenytoin
• **Oral suspension:** shake well before each dose G tube/NG tube; dilute susp prior to administration; flush tube with 20 ml water after dose; hold tube feedings 1 hr before and 1 hr after dose
• Allow 7-10 days between dosage changes
• Divided PO doses with or after meals to decrease adverse effects
• 2 hr before or after antacid, enteral feeding
• Shake oral susp well; use measuring device for correct dose

Direct IV route

> BLACK BOX WARNING: Give undiluted at ≤50 mg/min (adult) 1-3 mg/kg/min (neonates); 0.5-1 mg/kg/min

Intermittent IV INF route

> BLACK BOX WARNING: Dilute dose in NS to ≤6.7 mg/ml, complete inf within 1 hr of preparation, use 0.22 or 0.55 micron in-line particulate final filter between **IV** catheter and tubing, flush the **IV** line or catheter with NS before and after use, give at ≤50 mg/min (adult), 0.5-1 mg/kg/min (child, infant, neonate)

P

Additive compatibilities: Bleomycin, verapamil

Y-site compatibilities: Esmolol, famotidine, fluconazole, foscarnet, tacrolimus

Y-site incompatibilities: Enalaprilat, potassium chloride, vit B/C

IV compatibility of phenytoin sodium with: CISplatin, Temocillin

ADVERSE EFFECTS
CNS: Dizziness, insomnia, paresthesias, depression, suicidal tendencies, aggression, headache, confusion, slurred speech, peripheral neuropathy
CV: Hypotension, ventricular fibrillation, bradycardia, cardiac arrest
EENT: Nystagmus, diplopia, blurred vision
ENDO: Diabetes insipidus
GI: Nausea, vomiting, constipation, anorexia, weight loss, hepatitis, jaundice, gingival hyperplasia, abdominal pain
GU: Nephritis, urine discoloration, sexual dysfunction
HEMA: Agranulocytosis, leukopenia, aplastic anemia, thrombocytopenia, megaloblastic anemia
INTEG: Rash, lupus erythematosus, Stevens-Johnson syndrome, hirsutism, toxic epidermal necrolysis
SYST: Hypocalcemia, purple glove syndrome (IV), exacerbation of myasthenia gravis

Pharmacokinetics

Absorption	Slowly absorbed from GI tract; erratic (IM)
Distribution	Crosses placenta, 90%-95% protein binding
Metabolism	Liver, extensively
Excretion	Kidneys, minimally; enters breast milk
Half-life	7-42 hr, dose dependent

Pharmacodynamics

	PO	PO-EXT REL	IM	IV
Onset	2-24 hr	2-24 hr	Erratic	1-2 hr
Peak	1½-3 hr	4-12 hr	Erratic	Unknown
Duration	6-12 hr	12-36 hr	12-24 hr	12-24 hr

INTERACTIONS
Individual drugs
Alcohol (chronic use), calcium (high dose), carBAMazepine, folic acid, rifampin: decreased effects of phenytoin

Chloramphenicol, cimetidine, cycloSERINE, disulfiram, alcohol, amiodarone, FLUoxetine, gabapentin, methylphenidate, felbamate, traZODone, diazepam, valproate: increased phenytoin effect

Delavirdine: decreased response, resistance, do not use together

Drug classifications
Antacids, barbiturates: decreased effect of phenytoin

Antidepressants (tricyclics), benzodiazepines, sulfonamides, H₂ antagonists, azole antifungals, estrogens, succinimides, phenothiazines, salicylates: increased phenytoin level

Drug/food
Enteral tube feeding: may decrease absorption of oral product, do not use enteral feedings 2 hr before and after dose

Drug/lab test
Increased: glucose, alkaline phosphatase, BSP
Decreased: dexamethasone, metyrapone test serum, urinary steroids

NURSING CONSIDERATIONS
Assessment
• Assess product level: toxic level 30-50 mcg/ml; therapeutic level 7.5-20 mcg/ml, wait ≥1 wk to determine level

⚠ Assess mental status: mood, sensorium, affect, memory (long, short), especially geriatric; suicidal thoughts/behaviors

⚠ Phenytoin hypersensitivity syndrome: assess 3-12 wk after start of treatment: rash, temp, lymphadenopathy; may cause hepatotoxicity, renal failure, rhabdomyolysis

⚠ Serious skin disorders: assess for beginning rash that may lead to Stevens-Johnson syndrome or toxic epidermal necrolysis; phenytoin should not be used again, may occur more often in Asian patients with HLA-B 1502

⚠ Purple glove syndrome: with IV use
• Phenytoin level: toxic level 30-50 mcg/ml, therapeutic level: 7.5-20 mcg/ml, wait ≥1 wk to draw levels
• Seizures: assess for duration, type, intensity precipitating factors, obtain EEG periodically, monitor therapeutic level
• Blood studies: CBC, platelets q2wk until stabilized, then qmo × 12, then q3mo; discontinue

product if neutrophils <1600/m³; renal function: albumin conc; folic acid levels, LFTs

• **Blood dyscrasias:** assess fever, sore throat, bruising, rash, jaundice, epistaxis (long-term treatment only)

• Assess renal studies: urinalysis, BUN, urine creatinine

• Monitor blood studies: RBC, Hct, Hgb, reticulocyte counts weekly for 4 wk then monthly; also check thyroid function tests, serum calcium

• Monitor ECG, B/P, respiratory function during IV loading dose; verify potency of IV access port prior to IV infusion

• Monitor EEG function and serum levels periodically

• Monitor liver function tests for renal failure: ALT, AST, bilirubin, creatinine

• Assess for signs of physical withdrawal if medication suddenly discontinued

• Assess eye problems: need for ophth exam before, during, after treatment (slit lamp, funduscopy, tonometry)

• **Monitor for toxicity: bone marrow depression, nausea, vomiting, ataxia, diplopia, CV collapse, slurred speech, confusion**

Patient/family education

• Teach patient to carry/wear emergency ID stating name, products taken, condition, prescriber's name and phone number

• Advise patient to avoid driving and other activities that require alertness until product response is known; dizziness, drowsiness can occur

• Advise patient to avoid alcohol ingestion and CNS depressants unless approved by prescriber; increased sedation may occur

• **Teach patient not to discontinue medication quickly after long-term use; taper off over several wk**

• Advise patient that urine may turn pink, red, or brown

• Caution patient to avoid antacids or antidiarrheals within 2-3 hr of taking phenytoin

• Instruct patient in proper oral hygiene to prevent gingival hyperplasia; to visit dentist routinely

• **Teach patient to use nonhormonal contraception, to notify prescriber if pregnancy is planned or suspected, pregnancy D**

• **Teach patient to notify prescriber of unusual bleeding, bruising, petechiae (bleeding), clay-colored stools, abdominal pain, dark urine, yellowing of skin/eyes (hepatotoxicity); slurred speech, headache, drowsiness**

⚠ **Teach patient to report suicidal thoughts/behaviors immediately**

Evaluation

Positive therapeutic outcome

• Decreased seizure activity

• Decreased dysrhythmias

• Relief of pain

physostigmine ophthalmic
See Appendix B

phytonadione (vit K₁) (Rx)
(fye-toe-na-dye′one)
Mephyton
Func. class.: Vitamin K₁, fat-soluble vitamin
Pregnancy category C

ACTION: Needed for adequate blood clotting (factors II, VII, IX, X)

Therapeutic outcome: Prevention of bleeding

USES: Vitamin K malabsorption, hypoprothrombinemia, prevention of hypoprothrombinemia caused by oral anticoagulants, prevention of hemorrhagic disease of the newborn

CONTRAINDICATIONS
Hypersensitivity, severe hepatic disease, last few wk of pregnancy

Precautions: Pregnancy **C,** neonates, hepatic disease

> **BLACK BOX WARNING: IV** use

DOSAGE AND ROUTES
Hypoprothrombinemia caused by vitamin K malabsorption
Adult: PO/IM 2.5-25 mg; may repeat or increase to 50 mg
Child: PO 2.5-5 mg
Infant: PO/IM 2 mg

Prevention of hemorrhagic disease of the newborn
Neonate: IM 0.5-1 mg within 1 hr after birth; repeat in 2-3 wk if required

Hypoprothrombinemia caused by oral anticoagulants
Adult and child: PO/SUBCUT/IM 1-10 mg, may repeat 12-48 hr after PO dose or 6-8 hr after SUBCUT/IM dose, based on INR

Available forms: Tabs 5 mg; inj 10 mg/ml, 1 mg/0.5 ml

Adverse effects: *italics* = common; **bold** = life-threatening

Implementation

Intermittent IV infusion route
- Give **IV** after diluting with D₅ NS 10 ml or more; give max 1 mg/min
- Give **IV** only when other routes not possible (deaths have occurred)
- Store in airtight, light-resistant container

Y-site compatibilities: Alfentanil, amikacin, aminophylline, ascorbic acid, atracurium, atropine, azaTHIOprine, aztreonam, bumetanide, buprenorphine, butorphanol, calcium chloride/gluconate, ceFAZolin, cefonicid, cefoperazone, cefotaxime, cefoTEtan, cefOXitin, cefTAZidime, ceftizoxime, cefTRIAXone, cefuroxime, chloramphenicol, chlorproMAZINE, cimetidine, clindamycin, cyanocobalamin, cycloSPORINE, dexamethasone, digoxin, diphenhydrAMINE, DOPamine, doxycycline, enalaprilat, ePHEDrine, EPINEPHrine, epoetin alfa, erythromycin, esmolol, famotidine, fentaNYL, fluconazole, folic acid, furosemide, ganciclovir, gentamicin, glycopyrrolate, heparin, hydrocortisone, imipenem-cilastatin, indomethacin, insulin, isoproterenol, ketorolac, labetalol, lidocaine, mannitol, meperidine, metaraminol, methoxamine, methyldopate, metoclopramide, metoprolol, metroNIDAZOLE, midazolam, morphine, multivitamins, nafcillin, nalbuphine, naloxone, nitroglycerin, nitroprusside, norepinephrine, ondansetron, oxacillin, oxytocin, papaverine, penicillin G potassium, pentamidine, pentazocine, PENTobarbital, PHENobarbital, phentolamine, phenylephrine, potassium chloride, procainamide, prochlorperazine, propranolol, pyridoxime, ranitidine, sodium bicarbonate, succinylcholine, SUFentanil, theophylline, thiamine, ticarcillin/clavulanate, tobramycin, tolazoline, trimethaphan, urokinase, vancomycin, vasopressin, verapamil, vitamin B with C

Y-site incompatibilities: Dantrolene, diazepam, diazoxide, magnesium sulfate, phenytoin, trimethoprim/sulfamethoxazole

ADVERSE EFFECTS

CNS: Headache, brain damage (large doses)
GI: Nausea, decreased liver function tests
HEMA: Hemolytic anemia, hemoglobinuria, hyperbilirubinemia
INTEG: Rash, urticaria
RESP: Bronchospasm, dyspnea, chest constriction, respiratory arrest

Pharmacokinetics

Absorption	Well absorbed (PO, IM, SUBCUT)
Distribution	Crosses placenta
Metabolism	Liver, rapidly
Excretion	Breast milk
Half-life	Unknown

Pharmacodynamics

	PO	SUBCUT/IM
Onset	6-12 hr	1-2 hr
Peak	Unknown	6 hr
Duration	Unknown	14 hr

INTERACTIONS

Individual drugs
Sucralfate, mineral oil: decreased action of phytonadione
Warfarin: decreased action of warfarin (large dose of this product)

Drug classifications
Oral anticoagulants: decreased anticoagulant effect
Bile acid sequestrants, antiinfectives, salicylates: decreased action of phytonadione

Drug/food
Olestra: decreased vit K levels

NURSING CONSIDERATIONS

Assessment
- Monitor pro-time during treatment (2-sec deviation from control time, bleeding time, and clotting time)
- Monitor for bleeding, INR pulse, and B/P
- Assess nutritional status: liver (beef), spinach, tomatoes, coffee, asparagus, broccoli, cabbage, lettuce, greens
- Assess for bleeding or bruising: hematuria, black tarry stools, hematemesis

Patient/family education
- Teach patient not to take other supplements unless directed by prescriber; to take this medication as directed
- Teach patient necessary foods high in vit K to be included in diet
- Advise patient to avoid IM inj, hard toothbrush, flossing; use electric razor until treatment is terminated
- Instruct patient to report symptoms of bleeding: bruising, nosebleeds, blood in urine, heavy menstruation, black tarry stools
- Caution patient not to use OTC medications unless approved by prescriber
- Stress the need for periodic lab tests to monitor coagulation levels
- Stress the need for patient to carry/wear emergency ID with condition, treatment, and medications taken

Evaluation

Positive therapeutic outcome
- Decreased bleeding tendencies
- Decreased pro-time
- Decreased clotting time

pilocarpine ophthalmic
See Appendix B

pimecrolimus topical
See Appendix B

⚠ HIGH ALERT

pioglitazone (Rx)
(pie-oh-glye'ta-zone)
Actos
Func. class.: Antidiabetic, oral
Chem. class.: Thiazolidinedione
Pregnancy category C

ACTION: Specifically targets insulin resistance, an insulin sensitizer; regulates the transcription of a number of insulin-responsive genes

Therapeutic outcome: Decreased symptoms of diabetes mellitus

USES: Type 2 diabetes mellitus

CONTRAINDICATIONS
Breastfeeding, children, hypersensitivity to thiazolidinediones, diabetic ketoacidosis

> **BLACK BOX WARNING:** NYHA Class III/IV heart failure

Precautions: Pregnancy **C**, thyroid/renal/hepatic disease, edema, geriatric patients with CV disease, polycystic ovary syndrome, bladder cancer, osteoporosis, pulmonary disease, secondary malignancy

DOSAGE AND ROUTES
Monotherapy
Adult: PO 15-30 mg/day, may increase to 45 mg/day; with strong CYP2C8 max 15 mg/day; those with NYHA class I/II heart failure max 15 mg/day

Combination therapy
Adult: PO 15-30 mg/day with a sulfonylurea, metformin, or insulin; decrease sulfonylurea dose if hypoglycemia occurs; decrease insulin dose by 10%-25% if hypoglycemia occurs or if plasma glucose is <100 mg/dl; max 45 mg/day

Hepatic dose
Do not use in active liver disease or if ALT >2.5 × ULN

Available forms: Tabs 15, 30, 45 mg

Implementation
• Convert from other oral hypoglycemic agents; change may be made with gradual dosage

change; monitor serum glucose during conversion
• Give once a day without regard to meals
• Give tabs crushed and mixed with meal or fluids for patients with difficulty swallowing
• Store in airtight container in cool environment

ADVERSE EFFECTS
CNS: *Headache*
CV: **MI, heart failure, death** (geriatric patients)
ENDO: Hyper/hypoglycemia
MISC: *Myalgia, sinusitis, upper respiratory tract infection, pharyngitis,* **hepatotoxicity,** edema, weight gain, anemia, macular edema; **risk of bladder cancer (use >1 yr),** peripheral/pulmonary edema
MS: Fractures (females), **rhabdomyolysis,** myalgia

Pharmacokinetics
Absorption	Unknown
Distribution	Protein binding >99%
Metabolism	Unknown
Excretion	Kidneys
Half-life	3-7 hr, terminal 16-24 hr

Pharmacodynamics
Onset	Unknown
Peak	6-12 wk
Duration	Unknown

INTERACTIONS
Individual drugs
Atorvastatin: decreased effect of this product
Fluconazole, itraconazole, ketoconazole, miconazole, voriconazole: decreased pioglitazone effect

Drug classifications
CYP2C8 inducers: decreased pioglitazone effect
Oral contraceptives: decreased effect, use an alternative contraceptive method

Drug/herb
Garlic, green tea, horse chestnut: increased hypoglycemia

Drug/lab test
Increased: CPK, LFTs, HDL, cholesterol
Decreased: glucose, Hct/Hgb

NURSING CONSIDERATIONS
Assessment

> **BLACK BOX WARNING: Heart failure:** do not use in NYHA Class III/IV; excessive/rapid weight gain > 5 lb, dyspnea, edema; may need to be reduced or discontinued

• **Hypoglycemic reactions:** assess for hypoglycemic reactions (sweating, weakness, dizziness, anxiety, tremors, hunger), hyperglycemic reactions soon after meals (rare)

• **Bladder cancer: Avoid use in patients with history of bladder cancer; use of pioglitazone >1 yr has been correlated with an increase in bladder cancer; may occur more often with insulin or other antidiabetics**

• **Hepatic disease: check LFTs periodically: AST, LDH; do not start treatment in active heart disease or if ALT >2.5× upper limit of normal; if treatment has already begun, follow closely with continuing ALT levels; if ALT increases to >3× upper limit of normal, recheck ALT as soon as possible, if ALT remains >3× upper limit of normal, discontinue**

• Monitor FBS, glycosylated HbA1c, plasma lipids/lipoproteins, B/P, body weight during treatment

• Monitor CBC with differential prior to and during therapy, more necessary in those with anemia, Hct/Hgb (may be decreased in first few months of treatment)

Patient/family education

• Teach patient to self-monitor using a blood glucose meter

• Teach patient symptoms of hypo/hyperglycemia, what to do about each (rare)

• Advise patient that product must be continued on daily basis; explain consequence of discontinuing product abruptly

• Advise patient to avoid OTC medications or herbal preparations unless approved by prescriber; to report weight gain, edema

• Advise patient that diabetes is lifelong illness; that this product is not a cure, only controls symptoms

⚠ **Instruct patient to notify prescriber if oral contraceptives are used, effect may be decreased**

• Teach patient not to use if breastfeeding

• Teach patient that lab work, eye exams will be needed periodically

Evaluation

Positive therapeutic outcome

• Decrease in polyuria, polydipsia, polyphagia; clear sensorium; absence of dizziness; stable gait; blood glucose, A1c improvement

piperacillin/tazobactam (Rx)

(pip′er-ah-sill′in/ta-zoe-bak′tam)

Tazocin ✦, Zosyn

Func. class.: Broad-spectrum antiinfective
Chem. class.: Extended-spectrum penicillin

Pregnancy category B

ACTION: Interferes with cell wall replication of susceptible organisms; tazobactam is a β-lactamase inhibitor, protects piperacillin from enzymatic degradation

Therapeutic outcome: Bactericidal effects for piperacillin-resistant β-lactamase, *Escherichia coli, Staphylococcus aureus, Bacteroides fragilis, Bacteroides ovatus, Bacteroides thetaiotaomicron, Bacteroides vulgatus, Haemophilus influenzae*

USES: Moderate to severe infections: piperacillin-resistant, β-lactamase strains causing infections in respiratory tract, skin, skin structure, urinary tract, bone, and joint; gonorrhea, pneumonia, infections from penicillinase-producing staphylococci, streptococci

Unlabeled uses: Endocarditis

CONTRAINDICATIONS

Hypersensitivity to penicillins; neonates, carbapenem allergy

Precautions: Pregnancy **B,** breastfeeding, CHF, seizures, hypersensitivity to cephalosporins, renal insufficiency in neonates, GI disease, electrolyte imbalances, biliary obstruction

DOSAGE AND ROUTES

Nosocomial pneumonia

Adult: IV 4.5 g q6hr or 3.375 g q4hr with an aminoglycoside or antipseudomonal fluoroquinolone × 1-2 wk

Appendicitis/peritonitis

Child ≥40 kg (88 lb): IV 3.375 g q6hr × 7-10 days

Child ≥9 mo and <40 g: IV 100 mg (piperacillin)/kg q8hr × 7-10 days

Infant 2 mo to <9 mo: IV 80 mg/kg (piperacillin) q8hr × 7-10 days

Renal dose

Adult: IV CCr 20-40 ml/min give 3.375 g q6hr (nosocomial pneumonia); give 2.25 g q6hr (all other indications); CCr <20 ml/min, give 2.25 g q6hr (nosocomial pneumonia); give 2.25 g q8hr (all other indications)

Available forms: Powder for inj 2 g piperacillin/0.25 g tazobactam, 3 g piperacillin/0.375 g

---

⚠ Nurse Alert   ✱ Key NCLEX® Drug   >> Drug Specifics

tazobactam, 4 g piperacillin/0.5 g tazobactam, 36 g piperacillin/4.5 g tazobactam

Implementation
- **Separate aminoglycoside from piperacillin to avoid inactivation**
- Product after C&S is complete

Intermittent IV infusion route
- Reconstitute each 1 g of product/5 ml 0.9% NaCl for inj or sterile water for inj, dextrose 5%; shake well; further dilute in at least 50 ml compatible IV sol and run as int inf over at least 30 min

ADD-Vantage IV solution: reconstitution
- Reconstitute with 0.9% NaCl or D₅W in the appropriate flexible diluent container provided; for 500 mg vials, use at least a 100 ml diluent container and for 750 mg and 1 g vials, use only the 250 ml diluent container
- Remove the protective covers from the top of the vial and vial port. Remove vial cap (do not access with a syringe) and vial port cover. Screw the vial into the vial port until it will go no further to assure a seal. Once vial is sealed to the port, do not remove. To activate the contents of the vial, squeeze the bottom of the diluent container gently to inflate the portion of the container surrounding the end of the drug vial. With the other hand, push the drug vial down into the container telescoping walls of the container and grasp the inner cap of the vial through the walls of the container. Pull the inner cap from the drug vial. Verify the rubber stopper has been pulled out, allowing the drug and diluent to mix. Mix the container contents thoroughly
- *Storage after reconstitution:* The admixture solution may be stored for up to 24 hr at room temperature. Do not refrigerate or freeze after reconstitution
- Do not use in series connections with flexible containers

Pre-mixed Galaxy IV solution
- Thaw frozen containers at room temperature (20-25° C or 68-77° F) or under refrigeration (2-8° C or 36-46° F). Do not force thaw by immersion in water baths or by microwaving. Check for leaks by squeezing bag firmly
- Do not admix
- Contents of the solution may precipitate in the frozen state and should dissolve with little or no agitation once the solution has reached room temperature
- *Storage:* The thawed solution is stable for 24 hours at room temperature or for 14 days under refrigeration. Do not refreeze thawed product
- Do not use plastic containers in series connections as this could result in an embolism due to residual air being drawn from the primary

container before administration of the fluid from the secondary container is complete

IV infusion
- Infuse IV over at least 30 min. Ambulatory intravenous infusion pumps can be used; the solution is stable for up to 12 hr at room temperature

Y-site compatibilities: Alfentanil, allopurinol, amifostine, amikacin, aminocaproic acid, aminophylline, amphotericin B lipid complex, amphotericin B liposome, anidulafungin, argatroban, ascorbate, aztreonam, bivalirudin, bleomycin, bumetanide, buprenorphine, busulfan, butorphanol, calcium acetate/chloride/gluconate, CARBOplatin, carmustine, cefepime, chloramphenicol, cimetidine, clindamycin, cyclophosphamide, cycloSPORINE, cytarabine, DACTINomycin, DAPTOmycin, dexamethasone, dexrazoxane, diazepam, digoxin, diphenhydrAMINE, DOCEtaxel, DOPamine, doxacurium, enalaprilat, ePHEDrine, EPINEPHrine, eptifibatide, erythromycin, esmolol, etoposide, fenoldopam, fentaNYL, floxuridine, fluconazole, fludarabine, fluorouracil, foscarnet, fosphenytoin, furosemide, gallium, granisetron, heparin, hydrocortisone, HYDROmorphone, ifosfamide, isoproterenol, ketorolac, lansoprazole, lepirudin, leucovorin, lidocaine, linezolid, LORazepam, magnesium sulfate, mannitol, mechlorethamine, melphalan, meperidine, mesna, metaraminol, methotrexate, methylPREDNISolone, metoclopramide, metoprolol, metroNIDAZOLE, milrinone, morphine, naloxone, nitroglycerin, nitroprusside, norepinephrine, octreotide, ondansetron, oxytocin, PACLitaxel, palonosetron, pamidronate, pancuronium, PEMEtrexed, PENTobarbital, PHENobarbital, phentolamine, phenylephrine, plicamycin, potassium chloride/phosphates, procainamide, ranitidine, remifentanil, riTUXimab, sargramostim, sodium acetate/bicarbonate/phosphates, succinylcholine, SUFentanil, sulfamethoxazole-trimethoprim, tacrolimus, telavancin, teniposide, theophylline, thiotepa, tigecycline, tirofiban, trimethobenzamide, vasopressin, vinBLAStine, vinCRIStine, voriconazole, zidovudine, zoledronic acid

Y-site incompatibilities: Fluconazole, ondansetron, sargramostim, vinorelbine

ADVERSE EFFECTS
CNS: Headache, insomnia, dizziness, fever, lethargy, hallucinations, anxiety, depression, twitching, **seizures**, vertigo
CV: Cardiac toxicity, edema
GI: *Nausea, vomiting, diarrhea,* increased AST, ALT, abdominal pain, glossitis, constipation, **pseudomembranous colitis, pancreatitis**

P

GU: Oliguria, proteinuria, hematuria, *vaginitis, moniliasis,* glomerulonephritis, renal failure

HEMA: Anemia, increased bleeding time, bone marrow depression, agranulocytosis, hemolytic anemia

INTEG: Rash, pruritus, exfoliative dermatitis

META: Hypokalemia, hypernatremia

SYST: Serum sickness, anaphylaxis, Stevens-Johnson syndrome

Pharmacokinetics

Absorption	Well absorbed (80%)
Distribution	Widely distributed; crosses placenta
Metabolism	Not metabolized
Excretion	Kidneys, unchanged (90%); bile (10%); breast milk
Half-life	0.7-1.3 hr

Pharmacodynamics

Onset	Rapid
Peak	Inf end
Duration	Unknown

INTERACTIONS
Individual drugs
Aspirin, probenecid: increased piperacillin levels
Methotrexate: increased effect of methotrexate

Drug classifications
Aminoglycosides (**IV**): decreased piperacillin effect
Anticoagulants (oral): increased effect of anticoagulants
Contraceptives (oral): decreased contraceptive effectiveness
Neuromuscular blockers: increased effects
Tetracyclines: decreased antimicrobial effectiveness of piperacillin

Drug/lab test
Increased: eosinophilia, neutropenia, leucopenia, serum creatinine, PTT, AST, ALT, alkaline phosphatase, bilirubin, BUN, electrolytes
Decreased: Hct, Hgb, electrolytes
False positive: urine glucose, urine protein, Coombs' test

NURSING CONSIDERATIONS
Assessment
• Assess patient for previous sensitivity reaction to penicillins or other cephalosporins; cross-sensitivity between penicillins and cephalosporins is common
• Assess patient for signs and symptoms of infection, including characteristics of wounds,
sputum, urine, stool, WBC >10,000/mm^3, fever; obtain information baseline, during treatment
• Obtain C&S before beginning product therapy to identify if correct treatment has been initiated
• **Assess for allergic reactions: rash, urticaria, pruritus, chills, fever, joint pain; angioedema may occur a few days after therapy begins; EPINEPHrine, resuscitation equipment should be available for anaphylactic reaction**
⚠ **Identify urine output; if decreasing, notify prescriber (may indicate nephrotoxicity); also check for increased BUN, creatinine**
• Monitor blood studies: AST, ALT, CBC, Hct, bilirubin, LDH, alkaline phosphatase, Coombs' test monthly if patient is on long-term therapy
• Monitor electrolytes: potassium, sodium, chloride monthly if patient is on long-term therapy
• **Pseudomembranous colitis: assess for diarrhea, abdominal pain, fever, fatigue, anorexia; possible anemia, elevated WBC and low serum albumin; stop product and usually give either vancomycin or IV metroNIDAZOLE**
• Monitor for bleeding: ecchymosis, bleeding gums, hematuria, stool guaiac daily if on long-term therapy
• **Assess for overgrowth of infection:** perineal itching, fever, malaise, redness, pain, swelling, drainage, rash, diarrhea, change in cough, sputum

Patient/family education
• **Teach patient to report sore throat, bruising, bleeding, joint pain; may indicate blood dyscrasias (rare)**
• Advise patient to contact prescriber if vaginal itching, loose foul-smelling stools, furry tongue occur; may indicate **superinfection**
• **Advise patient to notify prescriber of diarrhea with blood or pus, which may indicate pseudomembranous colitis**

Evaluation
Positive therapeutic outcome
• Absence of signs/symptoms of infection (WBC <10,000/mm^3, temp WNL, absence of red, draining wounds)
• Reported improvement in symptoms of infection

TREATMENT OF ANAPHYLAXIS: Withdraw product, maintain airway, administer EPINEPHrine, aminophylline, O$_2$, **IV** corticosteroids

---

pirfenidone
(pir-fen'i-done)
Esbriet
Func. class.: Respiratory agent
Pregnancy category C

USES: Pulmonary fibrosis

CONTRAINDICATIONS: Hypersensitivity

DOSAGE AND ROUTES
Adult: PO Titrate over 2 wk to a maintenance dose of 801 mg tid. Give 267 mg tid on days 1-7, 534 mg tid on days 8-14, and 801 mg tid from day 15 onward

Available forms: Cap 267 mg

pitavastatin (Rx)
(pit'a-va-stat'in)
Livalo
Func. class.: Antilipidemic
Chem. class.: HMG-CoA reductase inhibitor
Pregnancy category X

Do not confuse: pitavastatin/pravastatin

ACTION: Inhibits HMG-CoA reductase enzyme, which reduces cholesterol synthesis, high doses lead to plaque regression

Therapeutic outcome: Decreased cholesterol levels and LDLs, increased HDLs

USES: As an adjunct in primary hypercholesterolemia (types Ia, Ib), dysbetalipoproteinemia, elevated triglyceride levels; prevention of cardiovascular disease by reduction of heart risk in those with mildly elevated cholesterol

CONTRAINDICATIONS
Pregnancy **X**, breastfeeding, hypersensitivity, active liver disease, cholestasis

Precautions: Past liver disease, alcoholism, severe acute infections, trauma, severe metabolic disorders, electrolyte imbalance, seizures, surgery, organ transplant, endocrine disease, females, hypotension, renal disease

DOSAGE AND ROUTES
Adult: PO 2 mg/day, usual range 1-4, max 4 mg/day

Renal dose
Adult: PO CCr 30-60 ml/min 1 mg qd, max 2 mg qd; CCr <30 ml/min on hemodialysis 1 mg qd, max 2 mg qd; CCr <30 ml/min not on hemodialysis—not recommended

Available forms: Tabs 1, 2, 4 mg

Implementation
• Administer total daily dose at any time of day
• Store in cool environment in tight container protected from light

ADVERSE EFFECTS
CNS: Headache
GI: Constipation, diarrhea
INTEG: Rash, pruritus, alopecia
MS: Myalgia, **rhabdomyolysis**, arthralgia
RESP: Pharyngitis

Pharmacokinetics

Absorption	Unknown
Distribution	Concentrations are lower in healthy African Americans
Metabolism	Liver
Excretion	Urine, feces
Half-life	12 hr

Pharmacodynamics

Unknown

INTERACTIONS
Individual drugs
Clofibrate, cycloSPORINE, erythromycin, gemfibrozil, niacin: increased risk of rhabdomyolysis
Colestipol: decreased action of atorvastatin
Erythromycin: increased levels of atorvastatin

Drug classifications
Antifungals (azole): possible rhabdomyolysis

Drug/herb
Red yeast rice: increased pitavastatin effect

Drug/lab test
Increased: bilirubin, alkaline phosphatase, ALT, AST
Interference: thyroid function tests

NURSING CONSIDERATIONS
Assessment
• Assess nutrition: fat, protein, carbohydrates; nutritional analysis should be completed by dietitian before treatment
• **Rhabdomyolysis: assess for muscle pain, tenderness; obtain CPK if these occur; product may need to be discontinued**
• Monitor bowel pattern daily; diarrhea may be a problem
• Monitor triglycerides, cholesterol at baseline, throughout treatment; LDL and VLDL should be watched closely; if increased, product should be discontinued

Adverse effects: *italics* = common; **bold** = life-threatening

- Monitor liver function studies q1-2mo during the first 1½ yr of treatment; AST, ALT, liver function tests may be increased
- Monitor renal studies in patients with compromised renal system: BUN, I&O ratio, creatinine
- Assess eyes via ophthalmic exam 1 mo after treatment begins, annually

Patient/family education
- Inform patient that compliance is needed for positive results to occur, not to double doses
- Teach patient that risk factors should be decreased: high-fat diet, smoking, alcohol consumption, absence of exercise
- Advise patient to notify prescriber if the GI symptoms of diarrhea, abdominal or epigastric pain, nausea, vomiting; chills, fever, sore throat; muscle pain, weakness occur
- Advise patient that treatment will take several years
- Advise patient that blood work will be necessary during treatment
- **Advise patient not to take if pregnant, pregnancy X, avoid breastfeeding**

Evaluation

Positive therapeutic outcome
- Decreased cholesterol levels, serum triglyceride
- Improved ratio of HDLs

RARELY USED

plasma protein fraction (Rx)
(pler-ix′a-fore)
Plasmanate
Func. class.: Hematological agent
Chem. class.: Plasma volume expander
Pregnancy category C

Therapeutic outcome: Shift of fluid from extravascular into intravascular space

USES: Hypovolemic shock, hypoproteinemia, ARDS, preoperative cardiopulmonary bypass, acute liver failure, nephrotic syndrome, cardiogenic shock

CONTRAINDICATIONS
Hypersensitivity to this product or albumin, CHF, severe anemia, renal insufficiency, hyponatremia, cardiopulmonary bypass

DOSAGE AND ROUTES
Hypovolemia
Adult: **IV** INF 250-500 ml (12.5-25 g of protein), max 10 ml/min

Child: **IV** INF 10-30 ml/kg max 5-10 ml/min
Hypoproteinemia
Adult: **IV** INF 1000-1500 ml/day, max 8 ml/min

RARELY USED

plerixafor (Rx)
(pler-ix′a-fore)
Mozobil
Func. class.: Biological modifier
Chem. class.: Colony-stimulating factor
Pregnancy category D

Therapeutic outcome: Successful collection of stem cells

USES: For peripheral blood stem cell (PBSC) mobilization for collection and autologous transplant in non-Hodgkin's lymphoma, multiple myeloma; used with a granulocyte colony stimulating factor (G-CSF)

CONTRAINDICATIONS
Pregnancy **D**, hypersensitivity, breastfeeding

DOSAGE AND ROUTES
Adult: SUBCUT 0.24 mg/kg qd about 11 hr before initiating apheresis; give up to 4 consecutive days; give filgrastim 10 mcg/kg SUBCUT qd each AM beginning 4 days before the 1st evening dose of plerixafor and on each day of apheresis; give filgrastim before procedure

pomalidomide
(pom-a-lid′o-mide)
Pomalyst
Func. class.: TNF modifier
Chem. class.: Antineoplastic, biologic response modifier, hormone
Pregnancy category X

ACTION: Inhibits growth of tumor cells and induces apoptosis; can be used in those resistant to lenalidomide

Therapeutic outcome: Decreased growth of tumor cells

USES: Multiple myeloma in those who have received ≥2 treatments, including lenalidomide and bortezomib, and in whom disease has progressed within 60 days of completion of the treatment

CONTRAINDICATIONS
Breastfeeding, hypersensitivity

BLACK BOX WARNING: Pregnancy **(X)**

Precautions: Children, geriatric patients, accidental exposure, bone marrow suppression, uterine bleeding, dental disease, fungal/viral infections, smoking

> BLACK BOX WARNING: Thrombocytopenia

DOSAGE AND ROUTES
Adult: PO 4 mg on days 1-21

Hepatic/renal dose
Adult: PO bilirubin >2 mg/dl and AST/ALT >3× ULN or CCr >3 mg/dl, do not use

Available forms: Tabs 1, 2, 3, 4 mg

Implementation
• With or without dexamethasone; may use dexamethasone 40 mg on days 1, 8, 15, 22 of each cycle; if age >75 yr, decrease dexamethasone to 20 mg/dose

ADVERSE EFFECTS
CNS: Dizziness, fatigue, fever, headache, peripheral neuropathy
CV: Chest pain
GI: Constipation, diarrhea, nausea/vomiting
HEMA: Leukopenia, neutropenia, thrombocytopenia
META: Hypokalemia
MS: Arthralgia, back pain
RESP: Cough, dyspnea, pulmonary embolism, epistaxis
SYST: Secondary malignancy

Pharmacokinetics

Absorption	Unknown
Distribution	12%-44% protein binding
Metabolism	Unknown
Excretion	Unknown
Half-life	Unknown

Pharmacodynamics

Onset	Unknown
Peak	Unknown
Duration	Unknown

INTERACTIONS
Drug classifications
CYP3A4 inducers (rifampin, rifapentine, rifabutin, primadone, phenytoin, PHENobarbital, nevirapine, nafacillin, modafinil, griseofulvin, etraviral, efavirenz, barbituarates, bexarotene, bosentan, carBAMazepine, enzalutamide, dexamethasone): decreased pomalidomide effect; avoid concurrent use

CYP3A4 inhibitors (amprenavir, bocenavir, delavirdine, ketoconazole, indinavir, itraconazole, dalfopristin/quinupristin, ritonavir, tipranavir, fluconazole, isoniazid, miconazole); P-gb inhibitors: increased pomalidomide effect; avoid concurrent use

NURSING CONSIDERATIONS
Assessment

> BLACK BOX WARNING: Blood studies: monitor Hct, Hgb; thrombolytic disease may occur

> BLACK BOX WARNING: Monitor for pregnancy before treatment, pregnancy (**X**)

Patient/family education
• Instruct patient to avoid driving or hazardous activity during beginning of treatment

> BLACK BOX WARNING: Advise patient to use adequate contraception, pregnancy (**X**)

Evaluation

Positive therapeutic outcome
• Decreased growth of tumor cells

posaconazole (Rx)
(poe′sa-kon′a-zole)
Noxafil, Posanol ✦
Func. class.: Antifungal, systemic
Chem. class.: Triazole derivative
Pregnancy category C

ACTION: Inhibits a portion of cell wall synthesis; alters cell membranes and inhibits several fungal enzymes

Therapeutic outcome: Decreased fever, malaise, rash; negative C&S for infecting organism

USES: Prevention of aspergillus, candida infection, oropharyngeal candidiasis in the immunocompromised, chemotherapy-induced neutropenia, mucocutaneous candidiasis

CONTRAINDICATIONS
Hypersensitivity to this product or other systemic antifungal or azoles, fungal meningitis, onchomycosis or dermatomycosis in cardiac dysfunction, use with ergots, sirolimus, CYP3A4 substrates

Precautions: Pregnancy **C**, breastfeeding, children, hepatic/cardiac/renal disease

DOSAGE AND ROUTES
Adult/adolescent: PO 600 mg/day in 2-4 divided doses

Oropharyngeal candidiasis
Adult: PO 100 mg bid × 1 day, then 100 mg/day × 13 days

Oropharyngeal candidiasis resistant to fluconazole or itraconazole
Adult/Child ≥13 yr: PO 400 mg bid

Available forms: Oral susp 200 mg/5 ml

Implementation
PO route
• **Oral susp:** give after shaking well; use calibrated measuring device; take only with a full meal or liquid nutritional supplements such as Ensure; rinse measuring device after each use
• Store in a tight container in refrigerator; do not freeze

ADVERSE EFFECTS
CNS: *Headache, dizziness,* insomnia, fever, rigors, weakness, anxiety
CV: Hypo/hypertension, tachycardia, anemia, **QT prolongation, torsades de pointes**
GI: *Nausea, vomiting, anorexia, diarrhea,* cramps, abdominal pain, flatulence, **GI bleeding, hepatotoxicity**
GU: Gynecomastia, impotence, decreased libido
INTEG: *Pruritus,* fever, *rash,* **toxic epidermal necrolysis**
MISC: *Edema, fatigue,* malaise, hypokalemia, tinnitus, **rhabdomyolysis**

Pharmacokinetics

Absorption	Well absorbed, enhanced by food
Distribution	Protein binding 98%-99%
Metabolism	Liver
Excretion	Feces, 77% unchanged
Half-life	19-35 hr

Pharmacodynamics

Onset	Unknown
Peak	3-5 hr
Duration	Unknown

INTERACTIONS
Individual drugs
⚠ **Atorvastatin, lovastatin: do not use concurrently**
⚠ **BusPIRone, busulfan, clarithromycin, cycloSPORINE, diazepam, digoxin, felodipine, indinavir, isradipine, midazolam, niCARDipine, NIFEdipine, niMODipine, phenytoin, quiNIDine, ritonavir, saquinavir, tacrolimus, warfarin: increased levels, toxicity**
Haloperidol, chloroquine, droperidol, pentamidine; arsenic trioxide, levomethadyl: increased QT prolongation

Cimetidine, phenytoin: decreased posaconazole level
Didanosine, rifamycin: decreased posaconazole action
⚠ **Dofetilide, pimozide, quiNIDine, halofantrine: life-threatening reactions, increased QT prolongation**
Midazolam (oral), triazolam: increased sedation
QuiNIDine: increased tinnitus, hearing loss

Drug classifications
Antacids, H₂-receptor antagonists, rifamycins: decreased posaconazole action
Class IA/III antidysrhythmics, some phenothiazines, beta agonists, local anesthetics, tricyclics, CYP3A4 inhibitors (amiodarone, clarithromycin, erythromycin, telithromycin, troleandomycin), CYP3A4 substrates (methadone, pimozide, QUEtiapine, quiNIDine, risperiDONE, ziprasidone): increased QT prolongation
⚠ **Ergots: life-threatening reactions, increased QT prolongation**
Other hepatotoxic products: increased hepatotoxicity
Calcium channel blockers, HMG-CoA reductase inhibitors, vinca alkaloids: increased levels, toxicity
Oral hypoglycemics: increased severe hypoglycemia

Drug/food
Food: increased absorption

NURSING CONSIDERATIONS
Assessment
• **Rhabdomyolysis: assess for muscle pain, increased CPK, weakness, swelling of affected muscles; if these occur and if confirmed by CPK, product should be discontinued**
• **QT prolongation: monitor ECG for QT prolongation, ejection fraction; assess for chest pain, palpitations, dyspnea**
• Assess for type of infection; may begin treatment before obtaining results
• Assess for infection: temp, WBC, sputum, baseline, periodically, breakthrough infections may occur when used with fosamprenavir
• Monitor I&O ratio, potassium levels
• Monitor liver function tests (ALT, AST, bilirubin) if on long-term therapy
• Assess for allergic reaction: rash, photosensitivity, uricaria, dermatitis
⚠ **Assess for hepatotoxicity: nausea, vomiting, jaundice, clay-colored stools, fatigue**

Patient/family education
• Teach patient that long-term therapy may be needed to clear infection (1 wk-6 mo depending on infection)
• Advise patient to avoid hazardous activities if dizziness occurs
• Advise patient to take 2 hr before administration of other products that increase gastric pH (antacids, H₂-blockers, omeprazole, sucralfate, anticholinergics); to notify health care provider of all medications taken (many interactions)
• Teach the patient the importance of compliance with product regimen; to use alternative method of contraception
• **Teach patient to notify prescriber of GI symptoms, signs of hepatic dysfunction (fatigue, nausea, anorexia, vomiting, dark urine, pale stools)**
• Teach patient to take during meal or within 20 min of eating

Evaluation

Positive therapeutic outcome
• Decreased fever, malaise, rash, negative C&S for infecting organism

---

potassium acetate/ potassium bicarbonate (Rx, OTC)
K-Effervescent, Klor-Con EF, K-Vescent

potassium bicarbonate potassium chloride (Rx, OTC)
Neo-K ♦

potassium bicarbonate/ potassium citrate (Rx, OTC)

⚠ HIGH ALERT

potassium chloride (Rx, OTC)
Epiklor, Klor-Con, K-Tab, Micro-K, Odan K-20 ♦

potassium gluconate (Rx, OTC)
Kaon, Kaylixir, K-G Elixir, Potassium-Rougier ♦

Func. class.: Electrolyte, mineral replacement
Chem. class.: Potassium
Pregnancy category C

ACTION: Needed for adequate transmission of nerve impulses and cardiac contraction, renal function, intracellular ion maintenance

Therapeutic outcome: Potassium level 3.0-5.0 mg/dl

USES: Prevention and treatment of hypokalemia

CONTRAINDICATIONS
Renal disease (severe), severe hemolytic disease, Addison's disease, hyperkalemia, acute dehydration, extensive tissue breakdown

Precautions: Pregnancy **C**, cardiac disease, potassium-sparing diuretic therapy, systemic acidosis

DOSAGE AND ROUTES
Hypokalemia (prevention) (bicarbonate, chloride, gluconate)
Adult: PO 20 mEq/day in 1-2 divided doses
Child: PO 1-2 mEq/day in 1-2 divided doses

Hypokalemia, digoxin toxicity (acetate, chloride)
Adult: serum potassium conc > 2.5 mEq/L: **IV** max 10 mEq/l hr, with 24 hr dose max 200 mEq, initial dose of 20-40 mEq has been recommended; **PO** 40-100 mEq/day in 2-4 divided doses
Child: **IV** 0.25-0.5 mEq/g/dose, at 0.25-0.5 mEq/kg/hr; **PO** 2-5 mEq/day in divided doses

Available forms: Tabs for sol 6.5, 25 mEq; ext rel caps 8, 10 mEq; powder for sol 3.3, 5, 6.7, 10, 13.3 mEq/5 ml; tabs 2, 4, 5, 13.4 mEq; ext rel tabs 6.7, 8, 10 mEq; elix 6.7 mEq/5 ml; oral sol 2.375 mEq/5 ml; inj for prep of IV 1.5, 2, 2.4, 3, 3.2, 4.4, 4.7 mEq/ml

Implementation
PO route
• Do not break, crush, or chew ext rel tabs/caps or enteric-coated products
• Give with meal or after meal; take cap with full glass of liquid; dissolve effervescent tab, powder in 8 oz of cold water or juice; do not give IM, SUBCUT
• Store at room temperature

IV route
• Give through large-bore needle to decrease vein inflammation; check for extravasation; administer in large vein, avoiding scalp vein in child
• After diluting in large volume of **IV** sol give as an **IV** inf slowly to prevent toxicity; never give **IV** bol or IM

>> Potassium acetate
Additive compatibilities: Metoclopramide
• **Potassium chloride** must be diluted, concentrated potassium injections are fatal

---

Continuous IV infusion route
- Conc max 80 mEq/L for peripheral line, 120 mEq/L central line
- Dehydrated patients should receive 1 L of potassium-free hydration sol; then infuse 10 mEq/hr; in severe hypokalemia rate may be 40 mEq/hr

Y-site compatibilities: Acyclovir, aldesleukin, allopurinol, amifostine, aminophylline, amiodarone, ampicillin, atropine, aztreonam, betamethasone, calcium gluconate, cefmetazole, cephalothin, cephapirin, chlordiazePOXIDE, chlorproMAZINE, ciprofloxacin, cladribine, cyanocobalamin, dexamethasone, digoxin, diltiazem, diphenhydrAMINE, DOBUTamine, DOPamine, droperidol, edrophonium, enalaprilat, EPINEPHrine, esmolol, estrogens, ethacrynate, famotidine, fentaNYL, filgrastim, fludarabine, fluorouracil, furosemide, gallium, granisetron, heparin, hydrALAZINE, IDArubicin, indomethacin, inamrinone, regular insulin, isoproterenol, kanamycin, labetalol, lidocaine, LORazepam, magnesium sulfate, melphalan, meperidine, methicillin, methoxamine, methylergonovine, midazolam, minocycline, morphine, neostigmine, norepinephrine, ondansetron, oxacillin, oxytocin, PACLitaxel, penicillin G potassium, pentazocine, phytonadione, piperacillin/tazobactam, prednisoLONE, procainamide, prochlorperazine, propofol, propranolol, pyridostigmine, sargramostim, scopolamine, sodium bicarbonate, succinylcholine, tacrolimus, teniposide, theophylline, thiotepa, trimethaphan, trimethobenzamide, vinorelbine, zidovudine

>> Potassium chloride
Y-site compatibilities: Aldesleukin, amifostine, granisetron, LORazepam, midazolam, thiotepa

ADVERSE EFFECTS
CNS: Confusion
CV: Bradycardia, *cardiac depression*, dysrhythmias, arrest, peaking T waves, lowered R and depressed RST, prolonged P–R interval, widened QRS complex
GI: *Nausea, vomiting, cramps*, pain, *diarrhea*, ulceration of small bowel
GU: Oliguria
INTEG: Cold extremities, rash

Pharmacokinetics

Absorption	Unknown
Distribution	Unknown
Metabolism	Unknown
Excretion	Kidneys, feces
Half-life	Unknown

Pharmacodynamics

	PO	IV
Onset	30 min	Immediate
Peak	Unknown	Unknown
Duration	Unknown	Unknown

INTERACTIONS
Drug classifications
Angiotensin-converting enzyme inhibitors, calcium, diuretics (potassium-sparing), magnesium, potassium phosphate, **IV**, other potassium products: increased hyperkalemia

NURSING CONSIDERATIONS
Assessment
- Assess ECG for peaking T-waves, lowered R, depressed RST, prolonged PR interval, widening QRS complex, hyperkalemia; product should be reduced or discontinued
- Monitor potassium level during treatment (3.5-5.0 mg/dl is normal level)
- Monitor hydration status, I&O ratio; watch for decreased urinary output; notify prescriber immediately; check urinary pH in patients receiving the product as a urinary acidifier
- Assess cardiac status: rate, rhythm, CVP, PWP, PAWP if being monitored directly

Patient/family education
- Teach patient to eat foods rich in potassium after medication is discontinued
- Advise patient to avoid OTC products: antacids, salt substitutes, analgesics, vit preparations, unless specifically directed by prescriber; avoid licorice in large amounts, may cause hypokalemia, sodium retention
- Advise patient to report hyperkalemia symptoms or continued hypokalemia symptoms
- Tell patient to take cap with full glass of liquid; to dissolve powder or tab completely in at least 120 ml of water or juice; not to crush, chew caps or tabs
- Emphasize importance of regular follow-up and periodic potassium levels

Evaluation
Positive therapeutic outcome
- Absence of fatigue, muscle weakness, and decreased thirst and urinary output, cardiac changes
- Potassium level normal

pramipexole (Rx)

(pra-mi-pex′ol)

Mirapex, Mirapex ER

Func. class.: Antiparkinsonian agent

Chem. class.: Dopamine receptor agonist, nonergot

Pregnancy category C

ACTION: Selective agonist for D_2 receptors (presynaptic/postsynaptic sites); binding at D_3 receptor contributes to antiparkinson effects

Therapeutic outcome: Decreased symptoms of Parkinson's disease (involuntary movements)

USES: Idiopathic Parkinson's disease, restless leg syndrome

CONTRAINDICATIONS

Hypersensitivity

Precautions: Pregnancy **C**, renal/cardiac disease, MI with dysrhythmias, affective disorders, psychosis, preexisting dyskinesias, history of falling asleep during daily activities, rapid dose reduction

DOSAGE AND ROUTES

Initial treatment

Adult: PO from a starting dose of 0.375 mg/day given in 3 divided doses, increase gradually by 0.125 mg/dose at 5–7–day intervals until total daily dose of 4.5 mg is reached; ER 0.375 mg qd, may increase up to 0.75 mg/day, then increments of 0.75 mg/day ≤5-7 days, max 4.5 mg/day

Restless leg syndrome

Adult: PO 0.125 mg 2-3 hr before bedtime, increase gradually, max 0.5 mg/day

Renal dose

Adult: PO CCr 35-59 ml/min 0.125 mg bid, may increase q5-7day to 1.5 mg bid; CCr 15-34 ml/min 0.125 mg/day, may increase q5-7day to 1.5 mg/day

Available forms: Tabs 0.125, 0.25, 0.5, 1, 1.5 mg; cap ER 0.375, 0.75, 1.5, 3.0, 4.5 mg

Implementation

• Adjust dosage to patient's response
• Give with meals to decrease GI upset

ADVERSE EFFECTS

CNS: *Agitation, insomnia,* psychosis, hallucinations, depression, dizziness, headache, confusion, amnesia, dream disorder, asthenia, dyskinesia, hypersomnolence, sudden sleep onset, impulse-control disorders

CV: *Orthostatic hypotension,* edema, syncope, tachycardia, increased B/P, heart rate

EENT: Blurred vision

ENDO: Antidiuretic hormone secretion (SI-ADH)

GI: *Nausea, anorexia,* constipation, dysphagia, dry mouth

GU: Impotence, urinary frequency

HEMA: Hemolytic anemia, leukopenia, agranulocytosis

INTEG: Pruritus

Pharmacokinetics

Absorption	Well absorbed
Distribution	Widely distributed
Metabolism	Liver, minimally
Excretion	Kidneys, unchanged
Half-life	8 hr; 12 hr in geriatric

Pharmacodynamics

Onset	Unknown
Peak	2 hr
Duration	Unknown

INTERACTIONS

Individual drugs

Cimetidine, diltiazem, levodopa, quiNIDine, ranitidine, triamterine, verapamil: increased pramipexole levels

Metoclopramide: decreased pramipexole levels

Drug classifications

Butyrophenones, DOPamine agonists, phenothiazines: decreased pramipexole effect

NURSING CONSIDERATIONS

Assessment

• Monitor B/P, ECG, respiration during initial treatment; hypo/hypertension should be reported
• Assess mental status: affect, mood, behavioral changes, depression; complete suicide assessment
• Assess for involuntary movements in parkinsonism: akinesia, tremors, staggering gait, muscle rigidity, drooling; these symptoms should improve with therapy

⚠ **Assess for sleep attacks: may fall asleep during activities, without warning; may need to discontinue medication**

Patient/family education

• Advise patient that therapeutic effects may take several wk to a few mo
• Caution patient to change positions slowly to prevent orthostatic hypotension
• Instruct patient to use product exactly as prescribed; if product is discontinued abruptly, parkinsonian crisis may occur; if treatment is to be discontinued, taper over 1 wk; avoid alcohol, OTC sleeping products

Adverse effects: *italics* = common; **bold** = life-threatening

- Advise patient to notify prescriber if pregnancy is planned or suspected
- Teach patient to notify prescriber of impulse control disorders: shopping

Evaluation

Positive therapeutic outcome
- Decreased akathisia, other involuntary movements
- Improved mood

⚠ HIGH ALERT

pramlintide (Rx)
(pram′lin-tide)
Symlin
Func. class.: Antidiabetic
Chem. class.: Synthetic human amylin analog
Pregnancy category C

ACTION: Modulates and slows stomach emptying, prevents postprandial rise in plasma glucagon, decreases appetite, leads to decreased caloric intake and weight loss

Therapeutic outcome: Decreased polyuria, polydipsia, polyphagia; improved A1C

USES: As an adjunct to insulin therapy with uncontrolled type 1 or type 2 diabetes mellitus

CONTRAINDICATIONS
Hypersensitivity to this product or cresol, gastroparesis

> BLACK BOX WARNING: Hypoglycemia

Precautions: Pregnancy **C**, breastfeeding

DOSAGE AND ROUTES
Type 1 diabetes
Adult: SUBCUT prior to each meal (≥30 g carbohydrate), titrate up from 15 mcg to target dose of 60 mcg/dose, each dose titration should occur after no nausea for 3 days

Type 2 diabetes
Adult: SUBCUT 60 mcg prior to each meal (≥30 g CHO), titrate up to 120 mcg SUBCUT with each meal after no nausea for 3-7 days

Available forms: PEN 60, 120 (1000 mcg/ml sol for j-injection)

Implementation
- Pre-meal insulin should be decreased by 50% when starting and adjusted to therapeutic dose to prevent hypoglycemia

SUBCUT route
- Rotate inj sites, allow sol to warm to room temp before use
- Give immediately before mealtime or if 30 g of carbohydrates will be consumed
- Do not use if a meal is skipped
- Do not use if discolored; do not give in arm; absorption is variable
- Store at room temperature for up to 30 days; keep away from heat and sunlight; refrigerate all other supply

ADVERSE EFFECTS
CNS: *Headache,* fatigue, dizziness, confusion
EENT: Blurred vision
GI: *Nausea, vomiting, anorexia,* abdominal pain
INTEG: Inj site reactions, diaphoresis
META: Hypoglycemia
MS: Arthralgia
RESP: *Cough,* pharyngitis
SYST: *Systemic allergy*

Pharmacokinetics

Absorption	30%-40%
Distribution	Not bound to blood cells or albumin, 40% bound in plasma
Metabolism	Kidneys
Excretion	Unknown
Half-life	48 min

Pharmacodynamics

Onset	Unknown
Peak	20 min
Duration	3 hr

INTERACTIONS
Individual drugs
Acetaminophen: may increase effect of acetaminophen
Alcohol, disopyramide, insulin: increased hypoglycemia
Dextrothyroxine, niacin, triamterene: decreased hypoglycemia
Diphenoxylate, loperamide, octreotide: increased pramlintide action
Erythromycin, metoclopramide: do not use

Drug classifications
ACE inhibitors, anabolic steroids, androgens, corticosteroids, fibric acid derivatives: increased hypoglycemia
α-Glucosidase inhibitors, antimuscarinics, opiate agonist, tricyclics: increased pramlintide action
Estrogens, MAOIs, oral contraceptives, progestins, thiazide diuretics: decreased hypoglycemia
Phenothiazines: increased hyperglycemia

NURSING CONSIDERATIONS
Assessment
• Monitor fasting blood glucose, 2 hr post-prandial (80-150 mg/dl, normal fasting level; 70-130 mg/dl, normal 2 hr level); A1c may also be drawn to identify treatment effectiveness; also monitor weight, appetite
• **Assess for hypoglycemic reaction** (sweating, weakness, dizziness, chills, confusion, headache, nausea, rapid weak pulse, fatigue, tachycardia, memory lapses, slurred speech, staggering gait, anxiety, tremors, hunger)
• **Assess for hyperglycemia:** acetone breath, polyuria, fatigue, polydipsia, flushed, dry skin, lethargy

Patient/family education
• Advise patient that product does not cure diabetes but controls symptoms
• Advise patient to carry emergency ID as diabetic
• Teach patient to recognize hypoglycemia reaction: headache, fatigue, weakness, fast pulse
• Teach patient the dosage, route, mixing instructions, if any diet restrictions, disease process
• Advise patient to carry a glucose source (candy or lump sugar, glucose tabs) to treat hypoglycemia
• Teach patient symptoms of ketoacidosis: nausea, thirst, polyuria, dry mouth, decreased B/P, dry, flushed skin, acetone breath, drowsiness, Kussmaul respirations
• Advise patient that a plan is necessary for diet, exercise; all food on diet should be eaten; exercise routine should not vary
• Teach patient about blood glucose testing; make sure patient is able to determine glucose level
• Advise patient to avoid OTC products unless directed by prescriber, avoid alcohol
• Advise patient not to operate machinery or drive until effect is known
• Teach patient how to use pen

Evaluation

Positive therapeutic outcome
• Decrease in polyuria, polydipsia, polyphagia, clear sensorium; improved A1c, blood glucose; absence of dizziness; stable gait

TREATMENT OF OVERDOSE:
Glucose 25 g **IV**, via dextrose 50% sol, 50 ml or glucagon 1 mg SUBCUT

pramoxine topical
See Appendix B

---

prasugrel (Rx)
(pra′soo-grel)
Effient
Func. class.: Platelet aggregation inhibitor
Chem. class.: ADP receptor antagonist
Pregnancy category B

ACTION: Inhibits ADP-induced platelet aggregation

Therapeutic outcome: Absence of MI, stroke

USES: Reducing the risk of stroke, MI, vascular death, peripheral arterial disease in high-risk patients

CONTRAINDICATIONS
Hypersensitivity, stroke, TIA

> **BLACK BOX WARNING:** Active bleeding

Precautions: Pregnancy **B**, breastfeeding, children, hepatic disease, increased bleeding risk, neutropenia, agranulocytosis, renal disease, surgery, trauma, thrombotic thrombocytopenia purpura, Asian patients, weight <60 kg, CABG, geriatric, abrupt discontinuation

DOSAGE AND ROUTES
Adult/geriatric <75 yr and ≥60 kg: PO 60 mg loading dose, then 10 mg qd with aspirin (75-325 mg/day)
Adult/geriatric <75 yr and <60 kg: PO 60 mg loading dose, then 5 mg qd
Geriatric >75 yr: Not recommended

Available forms: Tabs 5, 10 mg

Implementation
• Give with food to decrease gastric symptoms
• Do not break tablets
• Do not discontinue therapy abruptly

ADVERSE EFFECTS
CNS: Headache, dizziness
CV: Edema, *atrial fibrillation*, bradycardia, chest pain, hyper/hypotension
GI: Nausea, vomiting, diarrhea
HEMA: Epistaxis, *leukopenia, thrombocytopenia, neutropenia, anaphylaxis, angioedema, anemia*
INTEG: Rash, hypercholesterolemia
MISC: Fatigue, *intracranial hemorrhage, secondary malignancy, angioedema*
MS: Back pain

Adverse effects: *italics* = common; **bold** = life-threatening

Pharmacokinetics

Absorption	Rapidly absorbed
Distribution	Unknown
Metabolism	Liver CYP3A4, CYP2B6
Excretion	Urine, feces
Half-life	7-8 hr

Pharmacodynamics

Onset	Unknown
Peak	30 min
Duration	Unknown

INTERACTIONS
Individual drugs
Abciximab, aspirin, eptifibatide, rifampin, tirofiban, ticlopidine, treprostinil: increased bleeding risk

Drug classifications
Anticoagulants, thrombolytics, NSAIDs, SSRIs: increased bleeding risk

NURSING CONSIDERATIONS
Assessment
⚠ **Assess for thrombotic/thrombocytic purpura: fever, thrombocytopenia, neurolytic anemia**
- Monitor hepatic studies: AST, ALT, bilirubin, creatinine (long-term therapy)
- Monitor blood studies: CBC, differential, Hct, Hgb, PT, cholesterol (long-term therapy)

> **BLACK BOX WARNING: Bleeding:** may be fatal, decreased B/P in those who have had CABG may be the first indication; bleeding should be controlled while continuing product; may use transfusion; do not use within 1 wk of CABG; may use lower doses in those <60 kg

Patient/family education
- Advise that blood work will be necessary during treatment
- Teach to report any unusual bruising, bleeding to prescriber; that it may take longer to stop bleeding
- Advise to take with food or just after eating to minimize GI discomfort
- Advise to report diarrhea, skin rashes, subcutaneous bleeding, chills, fever, sore throat
- Teach to tell all health care providers that prasugrel is used; may be withheld before surgery

Evaluation
Positive therapeutic outcome
- Absence of stroke, MI

pravastatin (Rx)
(pra′va-sta-tin)
Pravachol
Func. class.: Antilipidemic
Pregnancy category X

Do not confuse: Pravachol/Prevacid

ACTION: Inhibits biosynthesis of VLDL, LDL, which are responsible for cholesterol development, by inhibiting the enzyme HMG-CoA reductase

Therapeutic outcome: Decreasing cholesterol levels and LDL, increased HDL

USES: As an adjunct in primary hypercholesterolemia types IIa, IIb, III, IV, arthero-sclerosis; to reduce the risk of recurrent MI, primary/secondary CV events; reduce stroke, TIAs

CONTRAINDICATIONS
Pregnancy **X,** breastfeeding, hypersensitivity, active liver disease

Precautions: Past liver disease, alcoholism, severe acute infections, trauma, severe metabolic disorders, electrolyte imbalances, renal disease

DOSAGE AND ROUTES
Adult: PO 40-80 mg/day at bedtime (range 20-80 mg/day), start at 10 mg/day if also on immunosuppressants
Adolescent 14-18 yr: PO 40 mg/day
Child 8-13 yr: PO 20 mg/day
Geriatric: PO 10 mg/day, initially

Renal dose
Adult: PO 10-20 mg daily at bedtime, increase at 4-wk intervals

Available forms: Tabs 10, 20, 40, 80 mg

Implementation
- Give at bedtime only; give 1 hr before or 2 hr after bile acid sequestrants
- Store in cool environment in airtight, light-resistant container

ADVERSE EFFECTS
CNS: Headache, dizziness, fatigue, confusion
CV: Chest pain
EENT: Lens opacities
GI: Nausea, constipation, diarrhea, flatus, abdominal pain, heartburn, liver dysfunction, pancreatitis, hepatitis
GU: Renal failure (myoglobinuria)
INTEG: Rash, pruritus
MS: Muscle cramps, myalgia, myositis, rhabdomyolysis
RESP: Common cold, rhinitis, cough

Pharmacokinetics

Absorption	Poorly absorbed, erratic
Distribution	Protein binding 80%
Metabolism	Liver, extensively
Excretion	Feces (70%-75%); kidneys, unchanged (20%); breast milk (minimal)
Half-life	2 hr

Pharmacodynamics

Onset	Unknown
Peak	1-1½ hr
Duration	Unknown

INTERACTIONS
Individual drugs
Clarithromycin, clofibrate, cycloSPORINE, erythromycin, gemfibrozil, itraconazole, niacin: increased risk for myopathy

Drug classifications
Bile acid sequestrants: decreased pravastatin bioavailability
Protease inhibitors: increased risk of myopathy

Drug/herb
St. John's wort: decreased effect
Red yeast rice: increased adverse reactions
Eucalyptus: increased hepatotoxicity

Drug/lab test
Increased: CPK, liver function tests
Altered: thyroid function tests

NURSING CONSIDERATIONS
Assessment
• Assess nutrition: fat, protein, carbohydrates; nutritional analysis should be completed by dietitian before treatment
• Monitor triglycerides, esterol, cholesterol at baseline, throughout treatment; LDL and HDL should be watched closely; if increased, product should be discontinued
⚠ Rhabdomyolysis: assess for muscle tenderness, pain; obtain CPK; therapy should be discontinued
• Monitor ophth status yearly

Patient/family education
• Inform patient that compliance is needed for positive results to occur; not to double doses or skip doses
• Teach patient that risk factors should be decreased: high-fat diet, smoking, alcohol consumption, absence of exercise
• Advise patient to notify prescriber of weakness, tenderness, or limited mobility, blurred vision, severe GI symptoms, dizziness, headache, muscle pain, fever
⚠ Explain to patient that contraception is necessary, since product produces teratogenic effects, pregnancy X, not to breastfeed
• Advise patient to use sunscreen, protective clothing to prevent burns
⚠ Hepatic disease: Instruct patient to notify prescriber of lack of appetite, yellow sclera and skin, dark urine, abdominal pain, weakness

Evaluation
Positive therapeutic outcome
• Decreased cholesterol, serum triglyceride levels and improved ratio with HDL

prazosin (Rx)
(pra′zoe-sin)
Minipress
Func. class.: Antihypertensive
Chem. class.: α₁-Adrenergic blocker, peripheral
Pregnancy category C

ACTION: Blocks α-mediated vasoconstriction of adrenergic receptors, inducing peripheral vasodilatation

Therapeutic outcome: Decreased B/P in hypertension; decreased cardiac preload, afterload

USES: Hypertension

Unlabeled uses: Benign prostatic hypertrophy to decrease urine outflow obstruction, posttraumatic stress disorder (PTSD), scorpion venom poisoning

CONTRAINDICATIONS
Hypersensitivity

Precautions: Pregnancy C, breastfeeding, children, geriatric patients, prostate cancer, ocular surgery, orthostatic hypotension

DOSAGE AND ROUTES
Post-traumatic stress disorder (unlabeled)
Adult: PO up to 15 mg/day
Adolescents ≥ 15 yr: PO 1 mg at bedtime, then titrated to 1.5-4 mg at bedtime to relieve nightmares

Hypertension (unlabeled)
Adult: PO 1 mg bid or tid, increasing to 20 mg/day in divided doses if required, usual range 6-15 mg/day; max 1 mg initially, max 20-40 mg/day

Child: PO 5 mcg/kg q6hr; max 400 mcg/kg/day or 15 mg/day

Benign prostatic hyperplasia (unlabeled)

Adult: PO 2 mg bid

Available forms: Caps 1, 2, 5 mg

Implementation
• Severe hypotension may occur after first dose of this medication; hypotension may be prevented by reducing or discontinuing diuretic therapy 3 days before beginning prazosin therapy
• Give same time each day
• Store in airtight container at 86° F (30° C) or less
• Give without regard to meals
• Store at room temperature

ADVERSE EFFECTS

CNS: *Dizziness, headache, drowsiness,* anxiety, depression, vertigo, *weakness,* fatigue, syncope

CV: *Palpitations, orthostatic hypotension,* tachycardia, edema, rebound hypertension

EENT: Blurred vision, epistaxis, tinnitus, dry mouth, red sclera

GI: *Nausea,* vomiting, diarrhea, constipation, abdominal pain, pancreatitis

GU: Urinary frequency, incontinence, impotence, priapism, water and sodium retention

Pharmacokinetics

Absorption	60%
Distribution	Widely distributed
Metabolism	Liver, extensively; protein binding 97%
Excretion	Kidneys, unchanged (10%); bile (90%)
Half-life	2-3 hr

Pharmacodynamics

Onset	2 hr
Peak	1-3 hr
Duration	6-12 hr

INTERACTIONS

Individual drugs
Alcohol, nitroglycerin: increased hypotension
CloNIDine: decreased antihypertensive effect

Drug classifications
Antihypertensives, β-adrenergic blockers, phosphodiesterase inhibitors (vardenafil, tadalafil, sildenafil), diuretics, MAOIs: increased hypotension
NSAIDs: decreased antihypertensive effect

Drug/herb
Hawthorn: increased antihypertensive effect

Drug/lab test
Increased: urinary norepinephrine, VMA

NURSING CONSIDERATIONS

Assessment
• **Hypertension/CHF:** Monitor B/P, orthostatic hypotension, syncope; check for edema in feet, legs daily; monitor I&O, weight daily; notify prescriber of changes
• Assess for allergic reactions: rash, fever, pruritus, urticaria; product should be discontinued if antihistamines fail to help
• Assess for orthostatic hypotension; tell patient to rise slowly from sitting or lying position

Patient/family education
• Instruct patient not to discontinue product abruptly; stress the importance of complying with dosage schedule, even if feeling better; if dose is missed, take as soon as remembered; take at same time each day
• Advise patient not to use OTC products (cough, cold, allergy) unless directed by prescriber; also to avoid large amounts of caffeine, alcohol
• Emphasize the need to rise slowly to sitting or standing position to minimize orthostatic hypotension
• Teach patient to notify prescriber of mouth sores, sore throat, fever, swelling of hands or feet, irregular heartbeat, chest pain
• Caution patient to report excessive perspiration, dehydration, vomiting, diarrhea; may lead to fall in B/P
• Caution patient that product may cause dizziness, fainting, light-headedness; may occur during 1st few days of therapy; to avoid hazardous activities
• Teach patient how to take B/P and normal readings for age group; instruct to take B/P q7day

Evaluation

Positive therapeutic outcome
• Decreased B/P in hypertension

TREATMENT OF OVERDOSE:
Administer volume expanders or vasopressors, discontinue product, place patient in supine position

---

prednisoLONE (Rx)

(pred-niss'oh-lone)

Flo-Pred, Orapred, Prelone

Func. class.: Corticosteroid, synthetic

Chem. class.: Intermediate-acting gluco-corticoid

Pregnancy category C

Do not confuse: prednisoLONE/prednisONE

ACTION: Decreases inflammation by suppressing migration of polymorphonuclear leukocytes, fibroblasts; reversal to increase capillary permeability and lysosomal stabilization

Therapeutic outcome: Decreased inflammation, decreased adrenal insufficiency

USES: Severe inflammation, immunosuppression, neoplasms, asthma

CONTRAINDICATIONS

Hypersensitivity, fungal infections, varicella, viral infection

Precautions: Pregnancy **C**, breastfeeding, children, diabetes mellitus, glaucoma, osteoporosis, seizure disorders, ulcerative colitis, CHF, myasthenia gravis, thromboembolism, peptic ulcer disease, renal disease, Cushing syndrome, abrupt discontinuation, children, acute MI, GI ulcers, hypertension, hepatitis, psychosis

DOSAGE AND ROUTES

Primary (Addison's disease)/secondary adrenocortical insufficiency or for the treatment of congenital adrenal hyperplasia

Adult: PO 5-60 mg/day as a single dose or in divided doses

Adolescent/child/infant: PO 0.14-2 mg/kg or 4-60 mg/m²/day in 3-4 divided doses

Nonsuppurative thyroiditis

Adult: PO 5-60 mg/day as a single dose or in divided doses

Adolescent/child/infant: PO 0.14-2 mg/kg or 4-60 mg/m²/day in 3-4 divided doses

Management of symptomatic sarcoidosis; or treatment of hypercalcemia associated with sarcoidosis or with various cancers

Adult: PO 5-60 mg/day as a single dose or divided doses

Adolescent/child/infant: PO 0.14-2 mg/kg or 4-60 mg/m²/day in 3-4 divided doses

Adjunct in rheumatic disorders (ankylosing spondylitis, gout with gouty arthritis, juvenile rheumatoid arthritis (JRA)/juvenile idiopathic arthritis (JIA), post-traumatic osteoarthritis psoriatic arthritis, rheumatoid arthritis) or acute episodes or exacerbation of nonrheumatic inflammation (acute and subacute bursitis, epicondylitis, and acute nonspecific tenosynovitis)

Adult: PO 5-60 mg/day as a single dose or in divided doses

Adolescent/child/infant: PO 0.14-2 mg/kg or 4-60 mg/m²/day in 3-4 divided doses

Adjunct in carpal tunnel syndrome (unlabeled)

Adult: PO 20 mg/day × 2 wk, then 10 mg/day for an additional 2 wk relief

Maintenance therapy in selected cases of acute rheumatic carditis, systemic dermatomyositis (polymyositis), systemic lupus erythematosus (SLE); (unlabeled): temporal arteritis, Churg-Strauss syndrome, mixed connective tissue disease, polyarteritis nodosa, relapsing polychondritis, polymyalgia rheumatica, vasculitis, or Wegener's granulomatosis

Adult: PO 5-60 mg/day as a single dose or in divided doses

Adolescent/child/infant: PO 0.14-2 mg/kg or 4-60 mg/m²/day given in 3-4 divided doses

Corticosteroid-responsive respiratory disorders (airway-obstructing hemangioma in infant) (unlabeled), aspiration pneumonitis, berylliosis, chronic obstructive pulmonary disease (COPD), laryngotracheobronchitis (croup), Loeffler's syndrome, noncardiogenic pulmonary edema (unlabeled)

Adult: PO 5-60 mg/day as a single dose or in divided doses

Adolescent/child/infant: PO 0.14-2 mg/kg or 4-60 mg/m²/day in 3-4 divided doses

Asthma; bronchospasm prophylaxis (unlabeled)

Adult/adolescent: PO 40-80 mg/day in 1-2 divided doses until the peak expiratory flow (PEF) reaches 70% of predicted or personal best; total course of treatment is 3-10 days

---

Adverse effects: *italics* = common; **bold** = life-threatening

P

Child: PO 1 mg/kg/day (up to 60 mg) in 2 divided doses until PEF reaches 70% of predicted or personal best; if a patient is given systemic corticosteroids, continue PO corticosteroids for a total course of 3-10 days; tapering is not necessary for courses <1 wk

Acute asthma exacerbation on an outpatient basis

Adult/adolescent: PO 40-60 mg/day as a single dose or in 2 divided doses for 3-10 days
Child 5-12 yr: PO 1-2 mg/kg/day (up to 60 mg) in 2 divided doses for 3-10 days
Infant/child ≤4 yr: PO 1-2 mg/kg/day (up to 30 mg) in 2 divided doses for 3-10 days

Long-term prevention of symptoms in severe persistent asthma

Adult, adolescent, and child ≥12 yr: PO 7.5-60 mg once daily in the morning or every other day
Infant and child ≤11 yr: PO 0.25-2 mg/kg PO daily given as a single dose each morning or every other day

Hematologic disorders with thrombocytopenia (immune thrombocytopenia/idiopathic thrombocytopenic purpura (ITP), or secondary thrombocytopenia)

Adult: PO 5-60 mg/day as a single dose or in divided doses
Adolescent/child: PO 0.14-2 mg/kg or 4-60 mg/m²/day in 3-4 divided doses

Available forms: Tabs 5 mg; oral sol 5 mg/5 ml, 10 mg/5 ml, 15 mg/5 ml, 25 mg/5 ml; syrup 5 mg/5 ml; oral dissolving tab 10, 15, 30 mg

Implementation

- **Oral sol:** use calibrated measuring devices
- **Orally disintegrating tabs:** place on tongue, allow to dissolve, swallow; or swallow whole; do not cut, split

ADVERSE EFFECTS

CNS: *Depression,* flushing, sweating, headache, mood changes
CV: *Hypertension,* circulatory collapse, thrombophlebitis, embolism, tachycardia
EENT: Fungal infections, increased intraocular pressure, blurred vision
GI: *Diarrhea, nausea, abdominal distention,* GI hemorrhage, increased appetite, pancreatitis
INTEG: Acne, poor wound healing, ecchymosis, petechiae
MS: Fractures, osteoporosis, weakness, arthralgia, myopathy, tendon rupture

Pharmacokinetics

Absorption	Well absorbed (PO, IM), completely absorbed (**IV**)
Distribution	Widely distributed, crosses placenta
Metabolism	Liver, extensively
Excretion	Kidney, breast milk
Half-life	2-4 hr

Pharmacodynamics

	PO	IM (phosphate)	IV	IA/IL
Onset	1 hr	Rapid	Rapid	Slow
Peak	2 hr	1 hr	Unknown	Unknown
Duration	1½ days	Unknown	Unknown	Up to 1 mo

INTERACTIONS

Individual drugs

Alcohol, amphotericin B, cycloSPORINE, digitalis, indomethacin, NSAIDs: increased side effects
Ambenonium, isoniazid, neostigmine, somatrem: decreased effects of each specific product
Cholestyramine, colestipol, ePHEDrine, phenytoin, rifampin, theophylline: decreased action of prednisoLONE
Indomethacin, ketoconazole: increased action of prednisoLONE

Drug classifications

Antibiotics (macrolide), contraceptives (oral), estrogens, salicylates: increased action of prednisoLONE
Anticholinesterases, anticoagulants, anticonvulsants, antidiabetics, salicylates, toxoids, vaccines: decreased effects of each specific product
Azole antifungals, cycloSPORINE: increased toxicity
Barbiturates: decreased action of prednisoLONE
CYP3A4 inducers: decreased prednisoLONE effect
CYP3A4 inhibitors: increased prednisoLONE effect
Diuretics, salicylates: increased side effects
Quinolones: increased tendon rupture

Drug/lab test

Increased: cholesterol, sodium, blood glucose, uric acid, calcium, urine glucose
Decreased: calcium, potassium, T_4, T_3, thyroid
[131]I uptake test, urine 17-OHCS, 17-KS, PBI
False negative: skin allergy tests

NURSING CONSIDERATIONS
Assessment
• Monitor potassium, blood glucose, urine glucose while patient is on long-term therapy; hypokalemia and hyperglycemia may occur
• Monitor weight daily; notify prescriber of weekly gain >5 lb; monitor I&O ratio; be alert for decreasing urinary output and increasing edema
• Monitor B/P q4hr, pulse; notify prescriber if chest pain occurs
• Monitor plasma cortisol levels during long-term therapy (normal level 138-635 nmol/L [SI units] when measured at 8 AM)
• Assess adrenal function periodically for hypothalamic-pituitary-adrenal axis suppression
• **Assess infection:** increased temp, WBC even after withdrawal of medication; product masks infection symptoms
• **Assess for potassium depletion:** paresthesias, fatigue, nausea, vomiting, depression, polyuria, dysrhythmias, weakness, edema, hypertension, cardiac symptoms
• **Adrenal insufficiency: assess for nausea, vomiting, lethargy, restlessness, confusion**
• Assess mental status: affect, mood, behavioral changes, aggression
• Monitor temp; if fever develops, product should be discontinued
• Assess for systemic absorption: increased temp, inflammation, irritation (topical)

Patient/family education
• Advise patient to carry/wear emergency ID as steroid user
• Advise patient to notify prescriber if therapeutic response decreases; dosage adjustment may be needed
• Caution patient not to discontinue abruptly; adrenal crisis can result; take exactly as prescribed
• Caution patient to avoid OTC products: salicylates, cough products with alcohol, cold preparations unless directed by prescriber
• Teach patient all aspects of product usage including cushingoid symptoms
• **Teach patient symptoms of adrenal insufficiency: nausea, anorexia, fatigue, dizziness, dyspnea, weakness, joint pain**
• Advise patient that long-term therapy may be needed to clear infection (1-2 mo depending on type of infection)

Evaluation
Positive therapeutic outcome
• Decreased inflammation

prednisoLONE ophthalmic
See Appendix B

predniSONE (Rx)
(pred′ni-sone)
Rayos, Winpreo ✦
Func. class.: Corticosteroid
Chem. class.: Intermediate-acting glucocorticoid
Pregnancy category C

Do not confuse: predniSONE/methylPREDNISolone/prednisoLONE/PriLOSEC

ACTION: Decreases inflammation by increasing capillary permeability and lysosomal stabilization, minimal mineralocorticoid activity

Therapeutic outcome: Decreased inflammation, decreased adrenal insufficiency

USES: Severe inflammation, neoplasms, multiple sclerosis, collagen disorders, dermatologic disorders

CONTRAINDICATIONS
Hypersensitivity

Precautions: Pregnancy C, diabetes mellitus, glaucoma, osteoporosis, seizure disorders, ulcerative colitis, CHF, myasthenia gravis, renal disease, esophagitis, peptic ulcer, cataracts, coagulopathy, abrupt discontinuation, children, corticosteroid hypersensitivity, Cushing syndrome, thromboembolism, geriatrics, acute MI

DOSAGE AND ROUTES
Adult: PO 5-60 mg/day or divided bid-qid
Child: PO 0.05-2 mg/kg/day divided 1-4 ×/day

Nephrotic syndrome
Child: PO 2 mg/kg/day in divided doses until urine is protein-free for 3 consecutive days, then 1-1.5 mg/kg/day every other day × 4 wk

Multiple sclerosis
Adult: PO 200 mg/day × 1 wk, then 80 mg every other day × 1 mo

Asthma
Adult/adolescent: PO 40-80 mg/day in 1-2 divided doses until PEF is 70% of predicted or personal best
Child: PO 1 mg/kg (max 60 mg)/day in 2 divided doses until PEF is 70% of predicted or personal best

Adverse effects: *italics* = common; **bold** = life-threatening

Available forms: Tabs 1, 2.5, 5, 10, 20, 50 mg; oral sol 5 mg/5 ml; syr 5 mg/5 ml; del rel tab 1, 2, 5 mg

Implementation
• Give with food or milk to decrease GI symptoms; use measuring device for liquid route
• For long-term use, alternative product therapy is recommended, to decrease adverse reactions
• **Del rel tab:** swallow whole, do not break, crush, or chew; give once daily

ADVERSE EFFECTS
CNS: Depression, flushing, sweating, headache, mood changes
CV: Hypertension, thrombophlebitis, embolism, tachycardia, fluid retention
EENT: Fungal infections, increased intraocular pressure, blurred vision
GI: Diarrhea, nausea, abdominal distention, GI hemorrhage, increased appetite, pancreatitis
INTEG: Acne, poor wound healing, ecchymosis, petechiae
META: Hyperglycemia
MS: Fractures, osteoporosis, weakness

Pharmacokinetics

Absorption	Well absorbed
Distribution	Widely distributed, crosses placenta
Metabolism	Liver, extensively
Excretion	Kidney, breast milk
Half-life	3-4 hr

Pharmacodynamics

Onset	Unknown
Peak	1-2 hr; del rel 6-6½ hr
Duration	1½ days

INTERACTIONS
Individual drugs
Alcohol, amphotericin B, cycloSPORINE, digoxin: increased side effects
Ambenonium, isoniazid, neostigmine, sometrem: decreased effects of each specific product
Cholestyramine, colestipol, phenytoin, rifampin, theophylline: decreased action of predniSONE
Ketoconazole: increased action of predniSONE
NSAIDs: increased side effects, increased action of predniSONE

Drug classifications
Anticholinesterases, anticoagulants, anticonvulsants, antidiabetics, toxoids, vaccines: decreased effects of each specific product

Antiinfectives (macrolide), contraceptives (oral), estrogens: increased action of predniSONE
Barbiturates: decreased action of predniSONE
CYP3A4 inducers: decreased predniSONE effect
CYP3A4 inhibitors: increased predniSONE effect
Diuretics: increased side effects
Quinolones: increased tendon rupture
Salicylates: increased side effects, increased action of predniSONE, decreased effects of salicylates

Drug/herb
Ephedra (ma huang): decreased predniSONE effect

Drug/lab test
Increased: cholesterol, sodium, blood glucose, uric acid, calcium, urine glucose
Decreased: calcium, potassium, T_4, T_3, thyroid ^{131}I uptake test, urine 17-OHCS, 17-KS, PBI
False negative: skin allergy tests

NURSING CONSIDERATIONS
Assessment
• **Adrenal insufficiency: assess for nausea, vomiting, anorexia, confusion, hypotension, weight loss before and during treatment; HPA suppression may be precipitated by abrupt withdrawal**
• Monitor potassium, blood glucose, urine glucose while on long-term therapy; hypokalemia and hyperglycemia may occur
• Monitor weight daily; notify prescriber of weekly gain >5 lb; monitor I&O ratio; be alert for decreasing urinary output and increasing edema
• Monitor B/P, pulse; notify prescriber if chest pain occurs
• Monitor plasma cortisol levels during long-term therapy (normal level 138-635 nmol/L when measured at 8 AM)
• Assess adrenal function periodically for hypothalamic-pituitary-adrenal axis suppression
• Assess infection: increased temp, WBC even after withdrawal of medication; product masks infection symptoms
• **Assess for potassium depletion:** paresthesias, fatigue, nausea, vomiting, depression, polyuria, dysrhythmias, weakness, edema, hypertension, cardiac symptoms
• Assess mental status: affect, mood, behavioral changes, aggression
• Monitor temp; if fever develops, product should be discontinued

- Assess for systemic absorption: increased temp, inflammation, irritation (topical)

Patient/family education
- Advise patient that emergency ID as corticosteroid user should be carried or worn
- Advise patient to notify prescriber if therapeutic response decreases; dosage adjustment may be needed

⚠ Caution patient not to discontinue abruptly; adrenal crisis can result
- Caution patient to avoid OTC products: salicylates, cough products with alcohol, cold preparations unless directed by prescriber
- Teach patient all aspects of product use including cushingoid symptoms
- Teach patient symptoms of adrenal insufficiency: nausea, anorexia, fatigue, dizziness, dyspnea, weakness, joint pain
- Advise patient that long-term therapy may be needed to clear infection (1-2 mo depending on type of infection)

⚠ Teach patient to notify prescriber if pregnancy is planned or suspected; cleft palate, stillbirth, abortion reported

Evaluation

Positive therapeutic outcome
- Decreased inflammation

pregabalin (Rx)
(pre-gab'a-lin)
Lyrica
Func. class.: Anticonvulsant
Pregnancy category C
Controlled substance schedule V

ACTION: Binds to high-voltage–gated calcium channels in CNS tissues; this may lead to anticonvulsant action, similar to the inhibitory neurotransmitter GABA; anxiolytic, analgesic, and antiepileptic properties

Therapeutic outcome: Decreased seizure activity, decreased neuropathic pain

USES: Neuropathic pain associated with spinal cord injury, diabetic peripheral neuropathy, partial-onset seizures, postherpetic neuralgia, fibromyalgia

Unlabeled uses: Moderate pain, social anxiety disorder

CONTRAINDICATIONS
Hypersensitivity to this product or gabapentin, abrupt discontinuation

Precautions: Pregnancy C, breastfeeding, children <12 yr, geriatric, renal disease, PR interval prolongation, creatine kinase elevations, CHF (class III, IV), decreased platelets, drug abuse, dependence, glaucoma, myopathy, angioedema history, suicidal behavior

DOSAGE AND ROUTES
Diabetic peripheral neuropathic pain
Adult: PO/oral sol 50 mg tid, may increase to 300 mg/day (max) within 1 wk, adjust in renal disease

Partial onset seizures
Adult: PO/oral sol 75 mg bid or 50 mg tid; may increase to 600 mg/day (max)

Postherpetic neuralgia
Adult: PO/oral sol 150 mg/day in 2-3 doses, may increase to 300 mg/day in 2-3 divided doses, if higher dose is needed in 2-4 wk, may increase to 600 mg/day in 2-3 divided doses

Fibromyalgia, spinal cord injury/pain
Adult: PO/oral sol 75 mg bid, may increase to 150 mg bid within 1 wk and 225 mg bid after 1 wk

Renal dose
PO CCr 30-60 ml/min 75-300 mg/day in 2-3 divided doses; CCr 15-30 ml/min 25-150 mg/day in 1-2 divided doses, CCr <15 ml/min 25-75 mg/day in a single dose

Available forms: Caps 25, 50, 75, 100, 150, 200, 225, 300 mg; oral sol 20 mg/ml

Implementation
- Do not crush or chew caps; caps may be opened and contents put in applesauce or dissolved in juice
- Give without regard to meals
- Gradually withdraw over 7 days; abrupt withdrawal may precipitate seizures
- Store at room temperature away from heat and light
- Give hard candy, frequent rinsing of mouth, gum for dry mouth
- Provide assistance with ambulation during early part of treatment; dizziness occurs
- Provide seizure precautions: padded side rails; move objects that may harm patient
- Provide increased fluids, bulk in diet for constipation
- **Oral sol:** should be written in mg and calculated to mL

Adverse effects: *italics* = common; **bold** = life-threatening

ADVERSE EFFECTS

CNS: Dizziness, fatigue, confusion, euphoria, incoordination, nervousness, neuropathy, tremor, vertigo, somnolence, ataxia, amnesia, abnormal thinking

EENT: Dry mouth, blurred vision, nystagmus, amblyopia, sinusitis

GI: Constipation, flatulence, abdominal pain, weight gain, nausea, vomiting, increased appetite

GU: Gynecomastia

HEMA: Ecchymosis, thrombocytopenia

MS: Back pain, rhabdomyolysis, myopathy

MISC: Pruritus, orgasm/erectile dysfunction, peripheral edema, angioedema, suicidal ideation, drowsiness

RESP: Dyspnea

Pharmacokinetics

Absorption	Well absorbed
Distribution	Not bound to plasma proteins
Metabolism	Negligible
Excretion	90% unchanged, urine
Half-life	6 hr

Pharmacodynamics

Onset	Unknown
Peak	1.5 hr
Duration	Unknown

INTERACTIONS

Individual drugs

Alcohol: increased CNS depression

Drug classifications

Anxiolytics, barbiturates, general anesthetics, hypnotics, opiate agonists, phenothiazines, sedating H_1 blockers, sedatives, thiazolidinediones, tricyclics: increased CNS depression

Thiazolidinediones: increased weight gain/fluid retention; avoid use if possible

Drug/lab test

Increased: creatine kinase
Decreased: platelets

NURSING CONSIDERATIONS

Assessment

• Assess for seizures: aura, location, duration, activity at onset, use seizure precaution

• **Assess for pain:** location, duration, characteristics if using for diabetic neuropathy

• Monitor renal function tests: urinalysis, BUN, urine creatinine q3mo, creatine kinase; if markedly increased, discontinue

• Assess mental status: mood, sensorium, affect, behavioral changes, suicidal thoughts, behavior; if mental status changes, notify prescriber

⚠ Angioedema/hypersensitivity: monitor for blisters, hives, rash, dyspnea, wheezing; angioedema; if these occur discontinue: cross-hypersensitivity with this product and gabapentin may occur

⚠ Rhabdomyolysis and creatinine kinase elevations: monitor for muscle pain, tenderness, weakness accompanied by malaise or fever; product should be discontinued

• Hemolytic anemia may be severe in Asian, Mediterranean individuals

Patient/family education

• Advise patient to carry emergency ID stating patient's name, products taken, condition, prescriber's name and phone number

• Advise patient to avoid driving, other activities that require alertness: dizziness, drowsiness may occur

• Teach patient not to discontinue medication quickly after long-term use, taper over ≥1 wk; withdrawal-precipitated seizures may occur, not to double doses if dose is missed, take if 2 hr or more before next dose

• Teach patient to notify prescriber if pregnancy is planned or suspected; avoid breastfeeding

• Teach patient to report muscle pain, tenderness, weakness, when accompanied by fever, malaise

• Advise patient to avoid alcohol, live virus vaccines

Evaluation

Positive therapeutic outcome

• Decreased seizure activity; decrease in neuropathic pain

TREATMENT OF OVERDOSE:

Lavage, VS, hemodialysis

RARELY USED

primidone (Rx)

(pri'mi-done)
Mysoline, Sertan ✦
Func. class.: Anticonvulsant
Chem. class.: Barbiturate derivative
Pregnancy category D

Therapeutic outcome: Reduction in seizure activity

USES: Generalized tonic-clonic (grand mal), complex

CONTRAINDICATIONS

Pregnancy **D**, hypersensitivity to this product or barbiturates, porphyria, breastfeeding

DOSAGE AND ROUTES

Adult and child >8 yr: PO 125-250 mg at bedtime, increase by 125-250 mg/day q3-7day, usual dose 750-1500 mg/day in 3-4 divided doses, max 2 g/day in divided doses

Child <8 yr: PO 50-125 mg at bedtime, increase by 50-125 mg/day q3-7day, usual dose 10-25 mg/kg/day in 3-4 divided doses

Neonate: PO 12-20 mg/kg/day in 2-4 divided doses, start at lower dose and titrate

Renal dose
Adult: CCr 10-15 ml/min: increase interval between doses to 8-12 hr; CCr <10 ml/min: increase interval to 12-24 hr

---

⚠ HIGH ALERT

procainamide (Rx)
(proe′kane-ah-mide)
Func. class.: Antidysrhythmic (class IA)
Chem. class.: Procaine HCl amide analog
Pregnancy category C

ACTION: Depresses excitability of cardiac muscle to electrical stimulation and slows conduction velocity in atrium, bundle of His, ventricle; increases refractory period

Therapeutic outcome: Prevention of dysrhythmias

USES: Life-threatening ventricular dysrhythmias, paroxysmal atrial tachycardia, PSVT, Wolff-Parkinson-White (WPW) syndrome

CONTRAINDICATIONS

Hypersensitivity, severe heart block, torsades de pointes

BLACK BOX WARNING: Lupus erythromatosis

Precautions: Pregnancy **C**, breastfeeding, children, renal/hepatic disease, CHF, respiratory depression, cytopenia, dysrhythmia associated with digoxin toxicity, myasthenia gravis, digoxin toxicity

BLACK BOX WARNING: Bone marrow failure, cardiac arrhythmias

DOSAGE AND ROUTES
Ventricular tachycardia during CPR
Adult: IV loading dose 20 mg/min; either ventricular tachycardia resolves or patient becomes hypotensive; the QRS complex is widened by 50% of original width or total is 17 mg/kg (1.2 g for a 70 kg patient); may give up to 50 mg/min in urgent situations; maintenance 1-4 mg/min CONT IV INF; IM 50 mg/kg/day in divided doses q3-6hr
Child: IV PALS 15 mg/kg over 30-60 min

Renal dose
Adult: IV CCr 35-59 ml/min give 70% of maintenance dose; CCr 15-34 ml/min give 40%-60% maintenance dose; CCr <15 ml/min individualized

Available forms: inj 100, 500 mg/ml

Implementation
IM route
• IM inj in deltoid; aspirate to avoid intravascular administration, use only when unable to use IV

Direct IV route
• Dilute each 100 mg/10 ml of 0.9% NaCl, give at max 50 mg/min
Intermittent INF route
• Dilute 0.2-1 g/50-500 ml of D_5W (2-4 mg/ml) give over 30-60 min at max 25-50 mg/min, use inf pump

Y-site compatibilities: Alfentanil, amikacin, aminocaproic acid, aminophylline, amiodarone, amphotericin B lipid complex, amphotericin B liposome, anidulafungin, ascorbic acid, atenolol, atracurium, atropine, aztreonam, benztropine, bivalirudin, bleomycin, bumetanide, buprenorphine, butorphanol, calcium chloride/gluconate, caspofungin, ceFAZolin, cefmetazole, cefonicid, cefoperazone, cefotaxime, cefoTEtan, cefOXitin, cefTAZidime, cefTRIAXone, cefuroxime, cephalothin, chlorproMAZINE, cimetidine, cisatracurium, CISplatin, clindamycin, cyanocobalamin, cyclophosphamide, cycloSPORINE, cytarabine, DACTINomycin, DAPTOmycin, dexamethasone, digoxin, diphenhydrAMINE, DOBUTamine, DOCEtaxel, DOPamine, doxacurium, DOXOrubicin, doxycycline, enalaprilat, ePHEDrine, EPINEPHrine, epirubicin, epoetin alfa, eptifibatide, ertapenem, erythromycin, esmolol, etoposide, etoposide phosphate, famotidine, fenoldopam, fentaNYL, fluconazole, fludarabine, fluorouracil, folic acid, furosemide, gatifloxacin, gemcitabine, gentamicin, glycopyrrolate, granisetron, heparin, hydrocortisone, HYDROmorphone, IDArubicin, ifosfamide, indomethacin, insulin (regular), irinotecan, isoproterenol, ketorolac, labetalol, lidocaine, linezolid,

LORazepam, magnesium sulfate, mannitol, mechlorethamine, meperidine, metaraminol, methicillin, methotrexate, methoxamine, methyldopate, methylPREDNISolone, metoclopramide, metoprolol, mezlocillin, miconazole, midazolam, mitoXANtrone, morphine, moxalactam, multiple vitamins, mycophenolate, nafcillin, nalbuphine, naloxone, netilmicin, nitroglycerin, nitroprusside, norepinephrine, octreotide, ondansetron, oxacillin, oxaliplatin, oxytocin, PACLitaxel, palonosetron, pamidronate, pancuronium, pantoprazole, papaverine, PEMEtrexed, penicillin G potassium/sodium, pentamidine, pentazocine, PENTobarbital, PHENobarbital, phenylephrine, phytonadione, piperacillin, piperacillin-tazobactam, polymyxin B, potassium chloride, prochlorperazine, promethazine, propranolol, protamine, pyridoxine, quiNIDine, quinupristin-dalfopristin, ranitidine, remifentanil, ritodrine, rocuronium, sodium bicarbonate, succinylcholine, SUFentanil, tacrolimus, teniposide, theophylline, thiamine, thiotepa, ticarcillin, ticarcillin-clavulanate, tigecycline, tirofiban, tobramycin, tolazoline, trimetaphan, urokinase, vancomycin, vasopressin, vecuronium, verapamil, vinCRIStine, vinorelbine, vitamin B complex/C, voriconazole, zoledronic acid

Y-site incompatibilities: Milrinone

ADVERSE EFFECTS

CNS: *Headache, dizziness,* confusion, psychosis, restlessness, irritability, weakness, depression

CV: *Hypotension,* heart block, cardiovascular collapse, arrest, torsades de pointes

GI: Nausea, vomiting, anorexia, diarrhea, hepatomegaly, pain, bitter taste

HEMA: Systemic lupus erythematosus syndrome, agranulocytosis, thrombocytopenia, neutropenia, hemolytic anemia

INTEG: Rash, urticaria, edema, swelling (rare), pruritus, flushing, angioedema

SYST: SLE

Pharmacokinetics

Absorption	Well absorbed
Distribution	Rapidly distributed, protein binding 15%
Metabolism	Liver
Excretion	Kidneys, unchanged (50%-70%)
Half-life	2½-4½ hr; increased in renal disease

Pharmacodynamics

	IV
Onset	Rapid
Peak	½-1 hr
Duration	3-4 hr

INTERACTIONS
Individual drugs
Cimetidine, quiNIDine, ranitidine, trimethoprim: increased procainamide effect
Thioridazine: increased toxicity

Drug classifications
Antidysrhythmics, quinolones: increased toxicity
β-Adrenergic blockers: increased procainamide effects
Neuromuscular blockers: increased neuromuscular blocking effect

Drug/lab test
Increased: ALT, AST, alkaline phosphatase, LDH, bilirubin

NURSING CONSIDERATIONS
Assessment
• Assess for oxygenation or perfusion deficit: decreased B/P, chest pain, dizziness, loss of consciousness
• Assess respiratory status: auscultate lung fields for bibasilar crackles in patients with advanced CHF
• Monitor I&O ratio; electrolytes: potassium, sodium, chloride; watch for decreasing urinary output, possible retention
• Monitor liver function tests: AST, ALT, bilirubin, alkaline phosphatase

> **BLACK BOX WARNING: Cardiac dysrhythmias:** Monitor ECG continuously to determine product effectiveness; measure PR, QRS, QT intervals; check for PVCs, other dysrhythmias; check B/P continuously for hypo/hypertension; for rebound hypertension after 1-2 hr; prolonged PR/QT intervals, QRS complex; if QT or QRS increases by 50% or more, withhold next dose, notify prescriber

• Monitor ANA titer; during long-term treatment, watch for lupuslike symptoms
• Monitor for dehydration or hypovolemia
⚠ Monitor for CNS symptoms: confusion, seizures, psychosis, numbness, depression, involuntary movements; if these occur, product should be discontinued

> **BLACK BOX WARNING: Bone marrow suppression:** CBC q2wk × 3 mo; leukocyte, neutrophil, platelet counts may be decreased, treatment may need to be discontinued

- Monitor blood levels (therapeutic level 4-10 mcg/ml), ANA titer or *N*-acetylprocainamide levels 10-20 mcg/ml; notify prescriber of abnormal results; assess for toxicity: confusion, drowsiness, nausea, vomiting, tachydysrhythmias, oliguria
- Assess cardiac rate, respiration: rate, rhythm, character, chest pain, ventricular tachycardia, supraventricular tachycardia or fibrillation

Patient/family education
- Advise patient to report side effects immediately to prescriber; to take exactly as prescribed; if dose is missed take when remembered if within 3-4 hr of next dose, do not double doses
- Caution patient that dark glasses may be needed for photophobia; to use sunscreen or stay out of sun to prevent burns; avoid temperature extremes; impairment of heat-regulating mechanism can occur
- Advise patient to complete follow-up appointment with prescriber, including pulmonary function tests, chest x-ray
- Instruct patient that dry mouth may be relieved by frequent sips of water, hard candy, sugarless gum
- Caution patient to make position changes from lying to standing slowly to prevent orthostatic hypotension

> **BLACK BOX WARNING:** Advise prescriber immediately if lupuslike symptoms (joint pain, butterfly rash, fever, chills, dyspnea), leukopenia symptoms (sore mouth, gums, throat), or thrombocytopenia symptoms (bleeding, bruising) occur

- Teach patient how to take pulse and when to report to prescriber

Evaluation
Positive therapeutic outcome
- Decreased PVCs, ventricular tachycardia

TREATMENT OF OVERDOSE:
O_2, artificial ventilation, ECG, administer DOPamine for circulatory depression, diazepam or thiopental for seizures, isoproterenol

> **⚠ HIGH ALERT**

procarbazine (Rx)
(proe-kar′ba-zeen)
Matulane
Func. class.: Antineoplastic, alkylating agent
Chem. class.: Hydrazine derivative
Pregnancy category D

ACTION: Inhibits DNA, RNA, protein synthesis; has multiple sites of action; a nonvesicant

Therapeutic outcome: Prevention of rapidly growing malignant cells

USES: Lymphoma, Hodgkin's disease, cancers resistant to other therapy

Unlabeled uses: Brain, lung malignancies, other lymphomas, multiple myeloma, malignant melanoma, polycythemia vera

CONTRAINDICATIONS
Pregnancy **D**, breastfeeding, hypersensitivity, thrombocytopenia, bone marrow depression

Precautions: Cardiac/renal/hepatic disease, radiation therapy, seizure disorder, anemia, bipolar disorder, Parkinson's disease

> **BLACK BOX WARNING:** Requires a specialized care setting and an experienced clinician

DOSAGE AND ROUTES
Adult: PO 2-4 mg/kg/day for first wk; maintain dosage of 4-6 mg/kg/day until platelets and WBC fall; after recovery, 1-2 mg/kg/day
Child: PO 50 mg/m²/day for 7 days, then 100 mg/m² until desired response, leukopenia, or thrombocytopenia occurs; 50 mg/m²/day is maintenance after bone marrow recovery

Available forms: Caps 50 mg

Implementation
- Give with foods, fluids for GI upset; open cap and give with food/fluids for swallowing difficulty; administer as directed

ADVERSE EFFECTS
CNS: Headache, dizziness, seizures, insomnia, hallucinations, confusion, coma, pain, chills, fever, sweating, paresthesias, peripheral neuropathy
EENT: Retinal hemorrhage, nystagmus, photophobia, diplopia, dry eyes
GI: *Nausea, vomiting,* anorexia, diarrhea, constipation, dry mouth, stomatitis, elevated hepatic enzymes
GU: Azoospermia, cessation of menses
HEMA: Thrombocytopenia, anemia, leukopenia, myelosuppression, bleeding tendencies, purpura, petechiae, epistaxis, hemolysis
INTEG: *Rash,* pruritus, dermatitis, alopecia, herpes, hyperpigmentation
MS: Arthralgias, myalgias
RESP: Cough, pneumonitis, hemoptysis
SYST: Secondary malignancy

Pharmacokinetics

Absorption	Well absorbed
Distribution	Widely distributed, crosses blood-brain barrier
Metabolism	Liver
Excretion	Kidneys
Half-life	1 hr

Pharmacodynamics

Unknown

INTERACTIONS
Individual drugs
Alcohol: increased CNS depression

Caffeine, guanethidine, levodopa, methyldopa, reserpine: increased hypertension

Meperidine: hypotension; do not use together

Drug classifications
Anticoagulants, NSAIDs, platelet inhibitors, thrombolytics: increased bleeding risk

Antidepressants (tricyclics), MAOIs, SSRIs, SNRIs: confusion, seizures, hypertension

Antihistamines, barbiturates, hypotensive agents, opiates, phenothiazines: increased CNS depression

Sympathomimetics: disulfiram-like reaction, life-threatening hypertensive crisis

Drug/food
Tyramine-containing foods: increased disulfiram-like reaction, hypertensive crisis

NURSING CONSIDERATIONS
Assessment
⚠️ **Bone marrow suppression:** monitor CBC, differential, platelet count weekly; withhold product if WBC is <4000/mm³ or platelet count is <75,000/mm³; notify prescriber of results if WBC <20,000/mm³, platelets <150,000/mm³

• Monitor pulmonary function tests, chest x-ray films before, during therapy; chest film should be obtained q2wk during treatment; check for dyspnea, crackles, unproductive cough, chest pain, tachypnea

• **Hepatic/renal disease:** can cause accumulation of drug, increased toxicity; monitor renal function tests: BUN, serum uric acid, urine CCr before, during therapy; I&O ratio; report fall in urine output of 30 ml/hr; check for decreased hyperuricemia; monitor hepatic studies before, during therapy: bilirubin, AST, ALT, ALK phos, LDH, PRN or qmo

• Monitor for cold, fever, sore throat (may indicate beginning of infection); identify edema in feet, joint and stomach pain, shaking; prescriber should be notified

• **Assess for bleeding:** hematuria, guaiac, bruising or petechiae, mucosa or orifices; no rectal temp

• Assess for tyramine-containing foods in the diet; hypertensive crisis can occur

Patient/family education
• Teach patient to avoid use of products containing aspirin or NSAIDs, razors, commercial mouthwash, since bleeding may occur; to report symptoms of bleeding (hematuria, tarry stools)

• Caution patient to report signs of anemia (fatigue, headache, irritability, faintness, shortness of breath); CNS changes, diarrhea

• Advise patient to report any changes in breathing or coughing even several mo after treatment; to avoid crowds and persons with respiratory tract or other infections

• Inform patient hair loss is common; discuss the use of wigs or hairpieces

• Caution patient not to have any vaccinations without the advice of the prescriber; serious reactions can occur

• Advise patient that contraception is needed during treatment and for several mo after the completion of therapy; may cause infertility; avoid breastfeeding

• Teach patient to avoid sunlight, UV exposure; wear sunscreen or protective clothing

Evaluation
Positive therapeutic outcome
• Absence of swelling at night

• Increased appetite, increased weight

• Decreasing malignancy

---

prochlorperazine (Rx)
(proe-klor-pair′a-zeen)
Compro
Func. class.: Antiemetic/antipsychotic
Chem. class.: Phenothiazine, piperazine derivative
Pregnancy category C

Do not confuse: prochlorperazine/chlorproMAZINE

ACTION: Decreases DOPamine neurotransmission by increasing DOPamine turnover through blockade of the D_2 somatodendritic autoreceptor in the meso-limbic system

Therapeutic outcome: Decreased nausea, vomiting, decreased signs and symptoms of psychosis

USES: Nausea, vomiting, psychosis

CONTRAINDICATIONS
Hypersensitivity to phenothiazines, coma, infants/neonates/child <2 yr or <20 lb, surgery

Precautions: Pregnancy **C,** breastfeeding, geriatric, seizure, encephalopathy, glaucoma, hepatic disease, Parkinson's disease, BPH

> **BLACK BOX WARNING:** Increased mortality in elderly patients with dementia-related psychosis

DOSAGE AND ROUTES
Postoperative nausea/vomiting
Adult: IM 5-10 mg 1-2 hr before anesthesia; may repeat in 30 min; **IV** 5-10 mg 15-30 min before anesthesia; **IV INF** 20 mg/L D_5W or 0.9% NaCl 15-30 min before anesthesia, max 40 mg/day

Severe nausea/vomiting
Adult: PO 5-10 mg tid-qid; SUS REL 15 mg/day in AM or 10 mg q12hr; RECT 25 mg/bid; IM 5-10 mg; may repeat q3-4hr prn, max 40 mg/day
Child 18-39 kg: PO 2.5 mg tid or 5 mg bid; IM 0.132 mg/kg, q3-4hr prn, max 15 mg/day
Child 14-17 kg: PO/RECT 2.5 mg bid-tid; IM 0.132 mg/kg, q3-4hr prn, max 10 mg/day
Child 9-13 kg: PO/RECT 2.5 mg daily-bid; IM 0.132 mg/kg, q3-4hr prn, max 7.5 mg/day

Antipsychotic
Adult and child ≥12 yr: PO 5-10 mg tid-qid; may increase q2-3day, max 150 mg/day; IM 10-20 mg q2-4hr up to 4 doses, then 10-20 mg q4-6hr, max 200 mg/day; RECT 10 mg tid-qid, may increase by 5-10 mg q2-3day as needed
Child 2-12 yr: PO 2.5 mg bid-tid; IM 0.132 mg/kg, change to oral ASAP

Antianxiety
Adult and child ≥12 yr: PO 5 mg tid-qid, max 20 mg/day or >12 wk; IM 5-10 mg q3-4hr, max 40 mg/day; **IV** 2.5-10 mg; max 40 mg/day
Child 2-12 yr: IM 0.132 mg/kg, change to oral ASAP

Available forms: Syr 5 mg/ml; inj 5 mg/ml; tabs 5, 10, 25 mg; sus rel caps 10, 15 mg; supp 2.5, 5, 25 mg

Implementation
IM route
• Inject slowly in deep muscle mass; do not give SUBCUT; aspirate to avoid **IV** administration; do not administer sol with a precipitate; have patient lie down afterward for at least 30 min

Direct IV route
• No dilution needed, inject directly in a vein ≤5 mg/min, do not give as bolus
Intermittent IV infusion route
• May dilute 20 mg/L NaCl and give as inf 15-30 min prior to anesthesia induction

Y-site compatibilities: Amsacrine, calcium gluconate, CISplatin, cladribine, cyclophosphamide, cytarabine, DOXOrubicin, fluconazole, granisetron, heparin, hydrocortisone, melphalan, methotrexate, ondansetron, PACLitaxel, potassium chloride, propofol, sargramostim, SUFentanil, teniposide, thiotepa, vinorelbine, vit B/C

Y-site incompatibilities: Foscarnet

ADVERSE EFFECTS
CNS: Tardive dyskinesia, *euphoria, depression, EPS,* restlessness, tremor, dizziness, **neuroleptic malignant syndrome,** drowsiness, headache
CV: *Circulatory failure, tachycardia,* hypotension, ECG changes
EENT: Blurred vision
GI: Nausea, vomiting, anorexia, dry mouth, diarrhea, constipation, weight loss, metallic taste, cramps
HEMA: *Agranulocytosis*
MISC: Impotence
RESP: *Respiratory depression*

Pharmacokinetics

Absorption	Variably absorbed (PO); well absorbed (IM)
Distribution	Widely distributed, high concentration in CNS, crosses placenta
Metabolism	Liver, extensively; GI mucosa
Excretion	Kidneys, breast milk
Half-life	Unknown

Pharmacodynamics

	PO	PO-SUS REL	RECT	IM	IV
Onset	½ hr	Unkn	1 hr	10-20 min	4-5 min
Peak	Unkn	Unkn	Unkn	Unkn	Unkn
Duration	3-4 hr	10-12 hr	3-4 hr	4-6 hr; children: 12 hr	3-4 hr

Adverse effects: *italics* = common; **bold** = life-threatening

INTERACTIONS
Individual drugs
Lithium: decreased prochlorperazine effect

Drug classifications
Antacids, barbiturates: decreased prochlorperazine effect

Anticholinergics, antidepressants, antiparkinson products: increased anticholinergic effects

SSRIs, SNRIs: increased serotonin syndrome, increased neuroleptic malignant syndrome

CNS depressants: increased CNS depression

Drug/herb
Betel palm, kava: increased EPS

Dong quai: avoid use

Drug/lab test
Increased: liver function tests, cardiac enzymes, cholesterol, blood glucose, prolactin, bilirubin, PBI, ^{131}I, alkaline phosphatase, leukocytes, granulocytes, platelets

Decreased: hormones (blood and urine)

False positive: pregnancy tests, urine bilirubin

False negative: urinary steroids, 17-OHCS, pregnancy tests

NURSING CONSIDERATIONS
Assessment
• Assess mental status: orientation, mood, behavior, presence and type of hallucinations before initial administration and monthly; this product should significantly reduce psychotic behavior

• Check for swallowing of PO medication; check for hoarding or giving of medication to other patients

• Monitor I&O ratio; palpate bladder if low urinary output occurs, especially in geriatric; urinalysis recommended before, during prolonged therapy

⚠ Monitor bilirubin, CBC, liver function tests monthly; blood dyscrasias, hepatotoxicity may occur

• Assess affect, orientation, LOC, reflexes, gait, coordination, sleep pattern disturbances

• Monitor B/P with patient sitting, standing, and lying; take pulse and respirations q4hr during initial treatment; establish baseline before starting treatment; report drops of 30 mm Hg; obtain baseline ECG, Q-wave and T-wave changes

• Check for dizziness, faintness, palpitations, tachycardia on rising; severe orthostatic hypotension is common

⚠ Identify neuroleptic malignant syndrome: hyperpyrexia, muscle rigidity, increased CPK, altered mental status, seizures, fever, tachycardia, dyspnea, fatigue, loss of bladder control; notify prescriber

immediately; product should be discontinued

• Assess for EPS including akathisia (inability to sit still, no pattern to movements), tardive dyskinesia (bizarre movements of the jaw, mouth, tongue, extremities), pseudoparkinsonism (ragged tremors, pill rolling, shuffling gait); an antiparkinsonism product should be prescribed

• Assess for constipation, urinary retention daily; if these occur, increase bulk, water in diet

Patient/family education
• Teach patient to use good oral hygiene; frequent rinsing of mouth, sugarless gum for dry mouth since oral candidiasis may occur

• Caution patient to avoid hazardous activities until product response is determined; dizziness, blurred vision may occur

• Inform patient that orthostatic hypotension occurs often and to rise from sitting or lying position gradually; to remain lying down after IM inj for at least 30 min; tell patient to avoid hot tubs, hot showers, tub baths, since hypotension may occur; tell patient that in hot weather heat stroke may occur; take extra precautions to stay cool

• Advise patient to avoid abrupt withdrawal of this product, or EPS may result; product should be withdrawn slowly

• Teach patient to avoid OTC preparations (cough, hay fever, cold) unless approved by prescriber, since serious product interactions may occur; avoid use with alcohol, CNS depressants; increased drowsiness may occur; avoid activities requiring mental alertness

• Instruct patient to avoid sun or use sunscreen, sunglasses, and protective clothing to prevent burns

• Advise patient to take antacids 2 hr before or after taking this product

• Advise patient to report sore throat, malaise, fever, bleeding, mouth sores; if these occur, CBC should be done and product discontinued

• Teach patient not to double or skip doses

• Inform patient that urine may turn pink to reddish brown

• Instruct patient to report dark urine, clay-colored stools, bleeding, bruising, rash, blurred vision

• Advise patient that suppositories may contain coconut/palm oil

Evaluation
Positive therapeutic outcome
• Relief of nausea and vomiting

• Decrease in emotional excitement, hallucinations, delusions, paranoia

• Reorganization of patterns of thought, speech

TREATMENT OF OVERDOSE:
Lavage if orally ingested; provide airway; *do not induce vomiting or use EPINEPHrine*

progesterone (Rx)
(proe-jess'ter-one)
Crinone, Endometrin, Prochieve, Prometrium
Func. class.: Progestogen
Chem. class.: Progesterone derivative
Pregnancy category D

ACTION: Inhibits secretion of pituitary gonadotropins, which prevents follicular maturation, ovulation; stimulates growth of mammary tissue; antineoplastic action against endometrial cancer

Therapeutic outcome: Decreased abnormal uterine bleeding, absence of amenorrhea

USES: Contraception, amenorrhea, premenstrual syndrome, abnormal uterine bleeding, endometrial hyperplasia prevention, assisted reproductive technology (ART) gel

Unlabeled uses: Corpus luteum insufficiency

CONTRAINDICATIONS
Pregnancy **B**, thromboembolic disorders, reproductive cancer, genital bleeding (abnormal, undiagnosed), cerebral hemorrhage, ectopic pregnancy, PID, STDs, thrombophlebitis, hypersensitivity to this product, peanuts, or peanut oil

> **BLACK BOX WARNING:** Breast cancer

Precautions: Breastfeeding, hypertension, asthma, blood dyscrasias, gallbladder disease, CHF, diabetes mellitus, bone disease, depression, migraine headache, seizure disorders, renal/hepatic disease, family history of breast or reproductive tract cancer

> **BLACK BOX WARNING:** Cardiac disease, dementia

DOSAGE AND ROUTES
Infertility
Adult: Vag 90 mg/day (micronized gel); 100 mg 2-3 times/day, starting day after oocyte retrieval and up to 10 wk total

Amenorrhea/functional uterine bleeding
Adult: IM 5-10 mg/day × 6-8 doses

Endometrial hyperplasia prevention
Adult: PO 200 mg/day × 12 days

Assisted reproductive technology
Adult: GEL 90 mg (8%) vaginally daily, for supplementation; 90 mg (8%) vaginally bid for replacement; if pregnancy occurs, continue × 10-12 wk

Corpus luteum insufficiency (unlabeled)
Adult: VAG insert 90-100 mg bid-tid starting at oocyte retrieval and continuing up to 10-12 wk of gestation

Available forms: Caps 100, 200 mg; inj 50 mg/ml; powder micronized; vag gel 4%, 8%; vag insert 100 mg; supp 25, 100, 200, 500 mg, compounding kit 25, 50, 100, 200, 400 mg

Implementation
PO route
• Do not crush, break, chew caps, give one dose in AM
• With food or milk to decrease GI symptoms
• Start progesterone 14 days after estrogen dose, if given concomitantly
Vaginal route
• Wait at least 6 hr after any vaginal treatment before using vaginal gel
IM route
• Store in dark area
• Give titrated dose; use lowest effective dosage; give oil sol deep in large muscle mass; rotate sites; use after warming to dissolve crystals
• Check for particulate matter and discoloration prior to injecting

ADVERSE EFFECTS
CNS: *Dizziness, headache*, migraines, depression, *fatigue*, mood swings, dementia, drowsiness
CV: Hypotension, **thrombophlebitis**, edema, **thromboembolism, stroke, pulmonary embolism, MI**
EENT: Diplopia, retinal thrombosis
GI: *Nausea*, vomiting, anorexia, cramps, increased weight, **cholestatic jaundice**, *constipation*, abdominal pain
GU: Amenorrhea, cervical erosion, breakthrough bleeding, dysmenorrhea, vaginal candidiasis, nocturia, breast changes, *gynecomastia, testicular atrophy, impotence*, endometriosis, **spontaneous abortion**, breast pain, ectopic pregnancy
INTEG: Rash, urticaria, acne, hirsutism, alopecia, oily skin, seborrhea, purpura, melasma
META: Hyperglycemia
SYST: **Angioedema, anaphylaxis**

P

Pharmacokinetics

Absorption	Unknown
Distribution	Unknown
Metabolism	Unknown
Excretion	Breast milk
Half-life	Unknown

Pharmacodynamics

	IM	RECT	VAG
Onset	Unknown	Unknown	Unknown
Peak	Unknown	Unknown	Unknown
Duration	24 hr	24 hr	24 hr

INTERACTIONS
Drug classifications
Barbiturates, phenytoins: decreased progesterone effect

CYP3A4 inhibitors (cimetidine, clarithromycin, danazol, diltiazem, erythromycin, fluconazole, itraconazole, ketoconazole, troleandomycin, verapamil, voriconazole): increased progesterone effect

Drug/lab test
Increased: alkaline phosphatase, nitrogen (urine), pregnanediol, amino acids, factors VII, VIII, IX, X

Decreased: GTT, HDL

NURSING CONSIDERATIONS
Assessment
• Monitor B/P at beginning of treatment and periodically; check weight daily; notify prescriber of weekly weight gain >5 lb
• Monitor I&O ratio: be alert for decreasing urinary output, increasing edema, hypertension
• Assess liver function tests: ALT, AST, bilirubin periodically during long-term therapy
• Assess edema, hypertension, cardiac symptoms, jaundice
• Assess mental status: affect, mood, behavioral changes, depression
• Assess for hypercalcemia
• Assess cervical cytology
• Conduct breast exam

Patient/family education
• Teach patient to avoid activities requiring mental alertness until effects are realized; can cause dizziness
• Teach patient to report breast lumps, vaginal bleeding, edema, jaundice, dark urine, clay-colored stools, dyspnea, headache, blurred vision, abdominal pain, numbness or stiffness in legs, chest pain
• Teach patient to report suspected pregnancy
• Teach patient to avoid gel with other vaginal products; if to be used together, to separate by 6 hr; for vaginal route, teach patient proper insertion technique

Evaluation

Positive therapeutic outcome
• Decreased abnormal uterine bleeding
• Absence of amenorrhea
• Prevented pregnancy

⚠ HIGH ALERT

promethazine (Rx)
(proe-meth′a-zeen)
Promethagan
Func. class.: Antihistamine, H₁-receptor antagonist; antiemetic; sedative/hypnotic
Chem. class.: Phenothiazine derivative
Pregnancy category C

ACTION: Acts on blood vessels, GI, respiratory system by competing with histamine for H_1-receptor site; decreases allergic response by blocking histamine

Therapeutic outcome: Absence of allergy symptoms and rhinitis, absence of nausea/vomiting, sedation

USES: Motion sickness, rhinitis, allergy symptoms, sedation, nausea, preoperative and postoperative sedation

CONTRAINDICATIONS
Hypersensitivity to H_1-receptor antagonist, agranulocytosis, bone marrow suppression, breastfeeding, coma, jaundice, Reye's syndrome

> **BLACK BOX WARNING:** Infants, intraarterial/SUBCUT use, neonates, children, extravasation

Precautions: Pregnancy **C**, renal/cardiac/hepatic disease, asthma, seizure disorder, prostatic hypertrophy, bladder obstruction, glaucoma, COPD, GI obstruction, ileus, CNS depression, diabetes, sleep apnea, urinary retention

> **BLACK BOX WARNING: IV** use

DOSAGE AND ROUTES
Nausea/vomiting
Adult: PO/IM/**IV**/RECT 12.5-25 mg; q4-6hr prn
Child >2 yr: PO/IM/**IV**/RECT 0.25-0.5 mg/kg q4-6hr prn

Motion sickness
Adult: PO 25 mg bid; give 30-60 min before departure and q8-12hr prn
Child >2 yr: PO/IM/RECT 12.5-25 mg bid; give 30-60 min before departure and q8-12hr prn

---

Allergy/rhinitis (unlabeled)
Adult: PO 12.5 mg qid, or 25 mg at bedtime
Child ≥2 yr: PO 6.25-12.5 mg tid or 25 mg at bedtime

Sedation
Adult: PO/IM 25-50 mg at bedtime
Child ≥2 yr: PO/IM/RECT 12.5-25 mg at bedtime

Sedation (preoperative/postoperative)
Adult: PO/IM/IV 25-50 mg
Child ≥2 yr: PO/IM/IV 0.5-1.1 mg/kg

Available forms: Tabs 12.5, 25, 50 mg; supp 12.5, 25, 50 mg; inj 25, 50 mg/ml

Implementation
PO route
• With meals for GI symptoms; absorption may slightly decrease
• When used for motion sickness, 30 min-1 hr before travel

IM route
• IM inj in deep in large muscle; rotate site

Direct IV route

> **BLACK BOX WARNING:** Check for extravasation: burning, pain, swelling at **IV** site, can cause tissue necrosis

• Do not use if precipitate is present
• Rapid administration may cause transient decrease in B/P
• After diluting each 25-50 mg/9 ml of NaCl for inj; give 25 mg or less/2 min

Y-site compatibilities: Alfentanil, amifostine, amikacin, aminocaproic acid, amsacrine, anidulafungin, ascorbic acid, atenolol, atracurium, atropine, aztreonam, benztropine, bivalirudin, bleomycin, bumetanide, buprenorphine, butorphanol, calcium chloride/gluconate, CARBOplatin, caspofungin, chlorproMAZINE, cimetidine, ciprofloxacin, cisatracurium, CISplatin, cladribine, codeine, cyanocobalamin, cyclophosphamide, cycloSPORINE, cytarabine, DACTINomycin, DAPTOmycin, dexmedetomidine, digoxin, diltiazem, diphenhydrAMINE, DOBUTamine, DOCEtaxel, DOPamine, doxacurium, DOXOrubicin, doxycycline, enalaprilat, ePHEDrine, EPINEPHrine, epirubicin, epoetin, eptifibatide, erythromycin, esmolol, etoposide, famotidine, fenoldopam, fentaNYL, filgrastim, fluconazole, fludarabine, gemcitabine, gentamicin, glycopyrrolate, granisetron, HYDROmorphone, hydrOXYzine, IDArubicin, ifosfamide, insulin (regular), irinotecan, isoproterenol, labetalol, levofloxacin, lidocaine, linezolid, LORazepam, LR, magnesium sulfate, mannitol, mechlorethamine, melphalan, meperidine, metaraminol, methoxamine, methyldopate, metoclopramide, metoprolol, metroNIDAZOLE, miconazole, midazolam, milrinone, mitoXANtrone, morphine, mycophenolate, nalbuphine, naloxone, netilmicin, nitroglycerin, norepinephrine, octreotide, ondansetron, oxaliplatin, oxytocin, PACLitaxel, palonosetron, pamidronate, pancuronium, PEMEtrexed, pentamidine, pentazocine, phenylephrine, polymyxin B, procainamide, prochlorperazine, propranolol, protamine, pyridoxine, quiNIDine, quinupristin-dalfopristin, ranitidine, remifentanil, Ringer's, ritodrine, riTUXimab, rocuronium, sargramostim, sodium acetate, succinylcholine, SUFentanil, tacrolimus, teniposide, theophylline, thiamine, thiotepa, tigecycline, tirofiban, TNA, tobramycin, tolazoline, trastuzumab, trimetaphan, vancomycin, vasopressin, vecuronium, verapamil, vinCRIStine, vinorelbine, voriconazole

ADVERSE EFFECTS
CNS: *Dizziness, drowsiness,* poor coordination, fatigue, anxiety, euphoria, confusion, paresthesia, neuritis, EPS, **neuroleptic malignant syndrome**
CV: Hyper/hypotension, palpitations, tachycardia
EENT: Blurred vision, dilated pupils, tinnitus, nasal stuffiness, dry nose, throat, mouth, photosensitivity
GI: *Constipation,* dry mouth, nausea, vomiting, anorexia, diarrhea
GU: *Retention,* dysuria, frequency
HEMA: **Thrombocytopenia, agranulocytosis, hemolytic anemia**
INTEG: Rash, urticaria, photosensitivity
RESP: Increased thick secretions, wheezing, chest tightness, **apnea in pediatric patients**

Pharmacokinetics

Absorption	Well absorbed (PO, IM); erratically absorbed (RECT)
Distribution	Widely distributed; crosses the blood-brain barrier, placenta
Metabolism	Liver
Excretion	Kidneys, breast milk
Half-life	Unknown

Pharmacodynamics

	PO/IM/RECT	IV
Onset	20 min	3-5 min
Peak	Unknown	Unknown
Duration	4-12 hr	4-6 hr

Adverse effects: *italics* = common; **bold** = life-threatening

INTERACTIONS
Individual drugs
Alcohol: increased CNS depression
Heparin: decreased oral anticoagulants effect

Drug classifications
Antidepressants (tricyclics), barbiturates, CNS depressants, opiates, sedative/hypnotics: increased CNS depression
MAOIs: increased promethazine effect

Drug/lab test
False negative: skin allergy tests (discontinue antihistamines 3 days before testing)
False positive: urine pregnancy test
Interference: blood grouping (ABO), GTT

NURSING CONSIDERATIONS
Assessment

> **BLACK BOX WARNING:** Not to be used in children <2 yr: fatal respiratory depression may occur; use cautiously in children >2 yr: seizures, paradoxical CNS stimulation may occur

• **Neuroleptic malignant syndrome: assess for fever, confusion, diaphoresis, rigid muscles, elevated CPK, encephalopathy, discontinue product, notify prescriber**
• Assess respiratory status: rate, rhythm, increase in bronchial secretions, wheezing, chest tightness; provide fluids to 2 L/day to decrease secretion thickness
• Monitor I&O ratio: be alert for urinary retention, frequency, dysuria, especially geriatric; product should be discontinued if these occur
• **Monitor CBC during long-term therapy; blood dyscrasias may occur but are rare**
• Monitor cardiac status: VS, palpitations, increased pulse, hypo/hypertension

Patient/family education
• Inform patient that a false-negative result may occur with skin testing; these procedures should not be scheduled until 3 days after discontinuing use
• Advise patient to take 30 min before departure to prevent motion sickness
• Caution patient to avoid hazardous activities, activities requiring alertness, since dizziness may occur; instruct patient to request assistance with ambulation
• Advise patient to avoid alcohol, other depressants; serious CNS depression may occur
• Teach patient all aspects of product use; to notify prescriber if confusion, sedation, hypotension, jaundice, fever occur; to avoid driving and other hazardous activity if drowsiness occurs

• Advise patient to take 1 hr before or 2 hr after meals to facilitate absorption
• Caution patient not to exceed recommended dosage; dysrhythmias may occur
• Inform patient hard candy, gum, frequent rinsing of mouth may be used for dryness
• Advise that product may reduce sweating (heat stroke)

Evaluation
Positive therapeutic outcome
• Absence of motion sickness
• Absence of nausea, vomiting

> **⚠ HIGH ALERT**
>
> ## propafenone (Rx)
> (pro-paff′e-nown)
> **Rythmol, Rythmol SR**
> *Func. class.:* Antidysrhythmic (Class IC)
> **Pregnancy category C**

ACTION: Slows conduction velocity; reduces membrane responsiveness; inhibits automaticity; increases ratio of effective refractory period to action potential duration; β-blocking activity

Therapeutic outcome: Absence of arrhythmias

USES: Atrial fibrillation (single dose), sustained ventricular tachycardia, paroxysmal supraventricular tachycardia (PSVT) prophylaxis, supraventricular dysrhythmias

CONTRAINDICATIONS
2nd-, 3rd-degree AV block, right bundle branch block, cardiogenic shock, hypersensitivity, bradycardia, uncontrolled CHF, sick sinus syndrome, marked hypotension, bronchospastic disorders, electrolyte imbalance, Brugada syndrome

Precautions: Pregnancy **C**, breastfeeding, children, geriatric, CHF, hypo/hyperkalemia, nonallergic bronchospasm, renal/hepatic disease, hematologic disorders, myasthenia gravis, COPD

> **BLACK BOX WARNING:** Recent MI, cardiac arrhythmias, QT prolongation, torsades de pointes

DOSAGE AND ROUTES
PSVT
Adult: PO 150 mg q8hr; allow a 3-4 day interval before increasing dose, max 900 mg/day

---

Atrial fibrillation

Adult: PO 450 or 600 mg as a single dose; SR 225 mg q12hr, may increase to 325 mg q12hr, max 425 mg q12hr

Available forms: Tabs 150, 225, 300 mg, SR cap 225, 325, 425 mg

Implementation

- Begin treatment in hospital
- Remove other antiarrhythmics before starting propafenone
- Adjust dosage q3-4day, no sooner

ADVERSE EFFECTS

CNS: Headache, dizziness, abnormal dreams, syncope, confusion, **seizures**, insomnia, tremor, anxiety, fatigue

CV: **Supraventricular dysrhythmia, ventricular dysrhythmia, bradycardia,** prodysrhythmia, palpitations, AV block, intraventricular conduction delay, AV dissociation, hypotension, chest pain, asystole

EENT: Blurred vision, altered taste, tinnitus

GI: *Nausea, vomiting,* constipation, dyspepsia, cholestasis, abnormal hepatic studies, dry mouth, diarrhea, anorexia

HEMA: **Leukopenia, agranulocytosis, granulocytopenia, thrombocytopenia,** anemia, bruising

INTEG: Rash

RESP: Dyspnea

Pharmacokinetics

Absorption	Well absorbed
Distribution	Widely, crosses placenta
Metabolism	Rapid, liver, CYP1A2, CYP2D6, CYP3A4
Excretion	Kidneys
Half-life	2-32 hr, poor metabolizers 10-32 hr

Pharmacodynamics (antiarrhythmic)

Onset	Hours to several days
Peak	4-5 days
Duration	Several hr

INTERACTIONS

Individual products

Arsenic trioxide, chloroquine, clarithromycin, droperidol, erythromycin, haloperidol, levomethadyl, methadone, pentamidine, chlorproMAZINE, mesoridazine, thioridazine: increased QT prolongation

Cimetidine, quiNIDine, rifampin: decreased propafenone effect

CycloSPORINE, digoxin: increased serum levels

Metoprolol, propranolol: increased β-blocker effect

Warfarin: increased anticoagulation

Drug classifications

Local anesthetics: increased CNS effects

CYP1A2, CYP2D6, CYP3A4 inhibitors (protease inhibitors, quiNINE, PARoxetine, saquinavir, erythromycin, azole antifungals, sertraline, tricyclics): increased propafenone effects

Drug/food

Grapefruit juice: increased propafenone effect

Drug/herb

St. John's wort: decreased propafenone effect

Drug/lab test

Increased: CPK

NURSING CONSIDERATIONS

Assessment

- Monitor GI status: bowel pattern, number of stools

> **BLACK BOX WARNING:** Assess cardiac status: rate, rhythm, quality; ECG or Holter monitor prior to, during therapy; watch for PR, QT prolongation

- Monitor chest x-ray film, pulmonary function test during treatment
- Monitor I&O ratio; check for decreasing output; daily weight
- Monitor B/P for fluctuations

> **BLACK BOX WARNING:** Assess lung fields; bilateral crackles, dyspnea, peripheral edema, weight gain, jugular venous distention may occur in CHF patient

> **A** Assess toxicity: fine tremors, dizziness, hypotension, drowsiness, abnormal heart rate

Patient/family education

- Advise patient to avoid hazardous activities until response is known
- Advise patient to report fever, chills, sore throat, bleeding, shortness of breath, chest pain, palpitations, blurred vision
- Advise patient to take medication with food
- Advise patient to carry emergency ID identifying medication and prescriber
- Instruct patient not to use with grapefruit juice or St. John's wort

Evaluation

Positive therapeutic outcome

- Absence of dysrhythmias

TREATMENT OF OVERDOSE:

O_2, artificial ventilation, defibrillation ECG; administer DOPamine for circulatory depression, diazepam or thiopental for seizures, isoproterenol

P

proparacaine ophthalmic
See Appendix B

⚠ HIGH ALERT
propofol (Rx)
(pro′poh-fole)
Diprivan
Func. class.: Hypnotic
Pregnancy category B

ACTION: Produces dose-dependent CNS depression by activation of GABA receptor

Therapeutic outcome: Induction of anesthesia

USES: Induction or maintenance of anesthesia as part of balanced anesthetic technique; sedation in mechanically ventilated patients

CONTRAINDICATIONS
Hypersensitivity to product or soybean oil, egg, benzyl alcohol (some products)

Precautions: Pregnancy **B**, breastfeeding, children, geriatric, respiratory depression, severe respiratory disorders, cardiac dysrhythmias, labor and delivery, renal disease, hyperlipidemia

DOSAGE AND ROUTES
Anesthesia
Adult <55 yr and ASA I/II IV (Diprivan or generic): IV 40 mg q10sec until induction onset; maintenance: 100-200 mcg/kg/min or **IV BOL** 20-50 mg prn, allow 3-5 min between adjustments; Fresenius Propoven 1% **IV** 20-40 mg q10sec until induction then 3-6 mg/kg/hr
Child ≥3 yr or ASA I or II: IV Induction: 2.5-3.5 mg/kg over 20-30 sec when not premedicated or lightly premedicated
Child 2 mo-16 yr maintenance: IV 125-300 mcg/kg/min, lower dose for ASA III or IV

ICU sedation
Adult: IV 5 mcg/kg/min over 5 min; may increase by 5-10 mcg/kg/min over 5-10 min until desired response (Diprivan or generic): 0.3-4 mg/kg/hr, max 4 mg/kg/hr (Fresenius Propoven)

Available forms: Inj 10 mg/ml in 20 ml ampule, vials, syringes

Implementation
IV route
• Shake well before use; dilution is not necessary but if diluted, use only D₅W to ≥2 mg/ml; give over 3-5 min, titrate to needed level of sedation; use only glass containers when mixing, not stable in plastic; use aseptic technique when transferring from original container

• Only with resuscitative equipment available, only by qualified persons trained in anesthesia

Y-site compatibilities: Acyclovir, alfentanil, aminophylline, ampicillin, aztreonam, bumetanide, buprenorphine, butorphanol, calcium gluconate, CARBOplatin, ceFAZolin, cefoperazone, cefotaxime, cefoTEtan, cefOXitin, ceftizoxime, cefTRIAXone, cefuroxime, chlorproMAZINE, cimetidine, CISplatin, clindamycin, cyclophosphamide, cycloSPORINE, cytarabine, dexamethasone, diphenhydrAMINE, DOBUTamine, DOPamine, doxycycline, droperidol, enalaprilat, ePHEDrine, EPINEPHrine, esmolol, famotidine, fentaNYL, fluconazole, fluorouracil, furosemide, ganciclovir, glycopyrrolate, granisetron, haloperidol, heparin, hydrocortisone, HYDROmorphone, hydrOXYzine, ifosfamide, imipenem/cilastatin, inamrinone, regular insulin, isoproterenol, ketamine, labetalol, levorphanol, lidocaine, LORazepam, magnesium sulfate, mannitol, meperidine, mezlocillin, miconazole, morphine, nafcillin, nalbuphine, naloxone, nitroglycerin, norepinephrine, ofloxacin, PACLitaxel, PENTobarbital, PHENobarbital, piperacillin, potassium chloride, prochlorperazine, propranolol, ranitidine, scopolamine, sodium bicarbonate, sodium nitroprusside, succinylcholine, SUFentanil, thiopental, ticarcillin, ticarcillin/clavulanate, vecuronium, verapamil

Solution compatibilities: (If given together via Y-site) D₅W, D₅LR, LR, D₅/0.45% NaCl, D₅/0.2% NaCl

ADVERSE EFFECTS
CNS: Involuntary movement, headache, jerking, fever, dizziness, shivering, tremor, confusion, somnolence, paresthesia, agitation, abnormal dreams, euphoria, fatigue, increased ICP, impaired cerebral flow, seizures
CV: *Bradycardia, hypotension,* hypertension, PVC, PAC, tachycardia, abnormal ECG, ST segment depression, asystole, bradydysrhythmias
EENT: Blurred vision, tinnitus, eye pain, strange taste, diplopia
GI: *Nausea, vomiting, abdominal cramping,* dry mouth, swallowing, hypersalivation, pancreatitis
GU: Urine retention, green urine, cloudy urine, oliguria
INTEG: *Flushing, phlebitis, hives, burning/stinging at inj site,* rash, pain of extremities
MS: Myalgia
RESP: Apnea, *cough, hiccups,* dyspnea, hypoventilation, sneezing, wheezing, tachypnea, hypoxia, respiratory acidosis
SYST: Propofol infusion syndrome

Pharmacokinetics

Absorption	Completely absorbed
Distribution	Rapid
Metabolism	Liver, conjugation to active metabolites; 95%-99% protein binding
Excretion	Urine
Half-life	3-12 hr

Pharmacodynamics

Onset	15-30 sec
Peak	Unknown
Duration	Unknown

INTERACTIONS
Individual drugs
Alcohol: increased CNS depression

Drug classifications
Antipsychotics, CNS depressants (sedative-hypnotics, opioid analgesics), inhalational anesthetics, skeletal muscle relaxants: increased CNS depression
MAOIs: do not use within 10 days

Drug/herb
St. John's wort: increased propofol effect

NURSING CONSIDERATIONS
Assessment
• Assess inj site: phlebitis, burning, stinging
⚠ Monitor ECG for changes: PVC, PAC, ST segment changes; monitor VS
• Assess CNS changes: movement, jerking, tremors, dizziness, LOC, pupil reaction
• Assess allergic reactions: hives
⚠ Assess respiratory dysfunction: respiratory depression, character, rate, rhythm; notify prescriber if respirations are <10/min
⚠ Propofol infusion syndrome: assess for rhabdomyolysis, renal failure, hyperkalemia, metabolic acidosis, cardiac dysrhythmias, heart failure, usually between 35 and 93 hr after inf began, at >5 mg/kg/hr for >58 hr

Patient/family education
• Teach patient that this medication will cause dizziness, drowsiness, sedation; to avoid hazardous activities until drug effect wears off

Evaluation
Positive therapeutic outcome
• Induction of anesthesia

TREATMENT OF OVERDOSE:
Discontinue product; administer vasopressor agents or anticholinergics, artificial ventilation

---

⚠ HIGH ALERT

propranolol (Rx)
(proe-pran'oh-lole)
Inderal, Inderal LA, InnoPran XL
Func. class.: Antihypertensive, antianginal, antidysrhythmic (class III)
Chem. class.: β-Adrenergic blocker
Pregnancy category C

Do not confuse: Inderal/Toradol/Inderide/Adderall/Imuran, **propranolol**/Pravachol

ACTION: Nonselective β-blocker with negative inotropic, chronotropic, dromotropic properties

Therapeutic outcome: Decreased B/P, heart rate

USES: Chronic stable angina pectoris, hypertension, supraventricular dysrhythmias, migraine prophylaxis, pheochromocytoma, cyanotic spells related to hypertrophic subaortic stenosis, essential tremor, acute MI

Unlabeled uses: Prevention of variceal bleeding caused by portal hypertension, akathisia induced by antipsychotics, lithium-induced tremor

CONTRAINDICATIONS
Hypersensitivity to this product, cardiogenic shock, AV heart block, bronchospastic disease, sinus bradycardia, bronchospasm, asthma

Precautions: Pregnancy **C**, breastfeeding, children, diabetes mellitus, renal/hepatic disease, hyperthyroidism, COPD, myasthenia gravis, peripheral vascular disease, hypotension, cardiac failure, Raynaud's disease, sick sinus syndrome, vasospastic angina, smoking, Wolff-Parkinson-White syndrome, thyrotoxicosis

> BLACK BOX WARNING: Abrupt discontinuation

DOSAGE AND ROUTES
Dysrhythmias
Adult: PO 10-30 mg tid-qid; IV BOL 1-3 mg given 1 mg/min; may repeat in 2 min; may repeat q4hr thereafter
Child: PO 1 mg/kg/day divided in 2 doses, IV 0.01-0.1 mg/kg over 5 min

Hypertension
Adult: PO 40 mg bid or 80 mg/day (EXT REL) initially; usual dosage 120-240 mg/day bid-tid or 120-160 mg/day (EXT REL)
Child: PO 0.5-1 mg/kg/day divided q6-12hr

P

Adverse effects: *italics* = common; **bold** = life-threatening

Angina
Adult: PO 10-20 mg bid-qid, increase at 3-7 day intervals up to 160-320 mg/day, or 80 mg/day, increase at 3-7 day intervals up to 160-320 mg/day

MI prophylaxis
Adult: PO 180-240 mg/day tid-qid starting 5 days to 2 wk after MI

Pheochromocytoma
Adult: PO 60 mg/day × 3 days preoperatively in divided doses or 30 mg/day in divided doses (inoperable tumor)

Migraine
Adult: PO 80 mg/day (EXT REL) or in divided doses; may increase to 160-240 mg/day in divided doses
Child: PO 0.6-1.5 mg/kg/day divided q8hr
Child ≤35 kg (unlabeled): PO 10-20 mg tid

Essential tremor
Adult: PO 40 mg bid; usual dosage 120 mg/day

Available forms: Ext rel caps 60, 80, 120, 160 mg; tabs 10, 20, 40, 60, 80, 90 mg; inj 1 mg/ml; oral sol 4 mg, 8 mg/ml

Implementation
PO route
- Do not break, crush, chew, or open ext rel cap
- Do not use ext rel cap for essential tremor, MI, cardiac dysrhythmias; do not use InnoPran XL in hypertropic subaortic stenosis, migraine, angina pectoris
- Ext rel caps should be taken daily; InnoPran XL should be taken at bedtime
- May mix oral sol with liquid or semisolid food; rinse container to get entire dose
- Give with 8 oz water with food; food enhances bioavailability
- Do not give with aluminum-containing antacid; may decrease GI absorption

Direct IV route
- IV undiluted or diluted 10 ml D$_5$W for inj; give 1 mg or less/min

Intermittent IV infusion route
- May be diluted in 50 ml NaCl and run 1 mg over 10-15 min

Y-site compatibilities: Acyclovir, alfentanil, alteplase, amikacin, aminocaproic acid, aminophylline, anidulafungin, ascorbic acid, atracurium, atropine, azaTHIOprine, aztreonam, benztropine, bivalirudin, bleomycin, bumetanide, buprenorphine, butorphanol, calcium chloride/gluconate, CARBOplatin, caspofungin, cefamandole, ceFAZolin, cefmetazole, cefonicid, cefoperazone, cefotaxime, cefoTEtan, cefOXitin, cefTAZidime, ceftizoxime, cefTRIAXone, cefuroxime, cephalothin, cephapirin, chloramphenicol, chlorproMAZINE, cimetidine, CISplatin, clindamycin, cyanocobalamin, cyclophosphamide, cycloSPORINE, cytarabine, DACTINomycin, DAPTOmycin, dexamethasone, digoxin, diltiazem, diphenhydrAMINE, DOBUTamine, DOCEtaxel, DOPamine, doxacurium, DOXOrubicin, doxycycline, enalaprilat, ePHEDrine, EPINEPHrine, epirubicin, epoetin alfa, eptifibatide, ertapenem, erythromycin, esmolol, etoposide, etoposide phosphate, famotidine, fenoldopam, fentaNYL, fluconazole, fludarabine, fluorouracil, folic acid, furosemide, ganciclovir, gatifloxacin, gemcitabine, gemtuzumab, gentamicin, glycopyrrolate, granisetron, heparin, hydrocortisone, HYDROmorphone, hydrOXYzine, IDArubicin, ifosfamide, imipenem-cilastatin, inamrinone, irinotecan, isoproterenol, ketorolac, labetalol, levofloxacin, lidocaine, linezolid, LORazepam, magnesium, mannitol, mechlorethamine, meperidine, metaraminol, methicillin, methotrexate, methoxamine, methyldopate, methylPREDNISolone, metoclopramide, metoprolol, metroNIDAZOLE, mezlocillin, miconazole, midazolam, milrinone, minocycline, mitoXANtrone, morphine, moxalactam, multiple vitamins, mycophenolate, nafcillin, nalbuphine, naloxone, nesiritide, netilmicin, nitroglycerin, nitroprusside, norepinephrine, octreotide, ondansetron, oxacillin, oxaliplatin, oxytocin, palonosetron, pamidronate, pancuronium, papaverine, PEMEtrexed, penicillin G potassium/sodium, pentamidine, pentazocine, PENTobarbital, PHENobarbital, phenylephrine, phytonadione, piperacillin, polymyxin B, potassium chloride, procainamide, prochlorperazine, promethazine, propofol, protamine, pyridoxine, quiNIDine, quinupristin-dalfopristin, ranitidine, ritodrine, rocuronium, sodium acetate/bicarbonate, succinylcholine, SUFentanil, tacrolimus, teniposide, theophylline, thiamine, thiotepa, ticarcillin, ticarcillin-clavulanate, tigecycline, tirofiban, tobramycin, tolazoline, trimetaphan, urokinase, vancomycin, vasopressin, vecuronium, verapamil, vinCRIStine, vinorelbine, vitamin B complex/C, voriconazole, zoledronic acid

ADVERSE EFFECTS
CNS: Depression, hallucinations, *dizziness, fatigue,* lethargy, paresthesia, bizarre dreams, disorientation
CV: Bradycardia, *hypotension,* CHF, palpitations, AV block, peripheral vascular insufficiency, vasodilatation, pulmonary edema, dysrhythmias, cold extremities
EENT: Sore throat, laryngospasm, blurred vision, dry eyes

GI: Nausea, vomiting, diarrhea, colitis, constipation, cramps, dry mouth, hepatomegaly, gastric pain, **acute pancreatitis**
GU: Impotence, decreased libido, UTIs
HEMA: Agranulocytosis, thrombocytopenia
INTEG: Rash, pruritus, fever, **Stevens-Johnson syndrome, toxic epidermal necrolysis**
META: Hyperglycemia, hypoglycemia
MISC: Facial swelling, weight change, Raynaud's phenomenon
MS: Joint pain, arthralgia, muscle cramps, pain
RESP: Dyspnea, respiratory dysfunction, **bronchospasm,** cough

Pharmacokinetics

Absorption	Well absorbed (PO); slowly absorbed (ext rel); completely absorbed (**IV**)
Distribution	Widely distributed, crosses blood-brain barrier, protein binding 90%
Metabolism	Liver, extensively
Excretion	Kidneys
Half-life	3-8 hr; ext rel 8-11 hr

Pharmacodynamics

	PO	PO-EXT REL	IV
Onset	½ hr	Unknown	Rapid
Peak	1-1½ hr	6 hr	1 min
Duration	6-12 hr	24 hr	2-4 hr

INTERACTIONS
Individual drugs
Cimetidine: increased β-blocking effect
Disopyramide: increased negative inotropic effects
Haloperidol, prazosin, quiNIDine: increased hypotension
Propafenone: increased propranolol levels
Smoking: decreased propranolol levels

Drug classifications
Barbiturates: decreased β-blocking effect
Calcium channel blockers, neuromuscular blockers: increased effects
Phenothiazines: increased toxicity

Drug/herb
Hawthorn: increased antihypertensive effect
Avoid use with feverfew, ma huang: decreased antihypertensive effect

Drug/lab test
Increased: serum potassium, serum uric acid, AST, ALT, alkaline phosphatase, LDH
Decreased: blood glucose
Interference: glaucoma testing

NURSING CONSIDERATIONS
Assessment
• Monitor B/P during beginning treatment, periodically thereafter; pulse q4hr; note rate, rhythm, quality; check apical/radial pulse before administration; notify prescriber of any significant changes (pulse <50 bpm or systolic B/P <90 mm Hg)

> **BLACK BOX WARNING:** Abrupt withdrawal: taper over a few weeks; do not discontinue abruptly; dysrhythmias, angina, myocardial ischemia, or MI may occur; taper over at least a few weeks

⚠ **ECG continuously if using an antidysrhythmic IV, PCWP (pulmonary capillary wedge pressure), CVP (central venous pressure)**
• Check for baselines in renal, liver function tests before therapy begins and periodically thereafter
• Assess for edema in feet, legs daily; monitor I&O, weight daily; check for jugular vein distention, crackles bilaterally; dyspnea (CHF)
• Monitor skin turgor, dryness of mucous membranes for hydration status, especially geriatric
• Assess for headache, light-headedness, decreased B/P; may indicate need for decreased dose; may aggravate symptoms of arterial insufficiency

Patient/family education
⚠ **Teach patient not to discontinue product abruptly (life-threatening dysrhythmias, exacerbation of angina, MI); to take at same time of day either with or without food consistently; taper over at least a few wk**
• Teach patient not to use OTC products containing α-adrenergic stimulants (such as nasal decongestants, cold preparations); to avoid alcohol, smoking and to limit sodium intake as prescribed; blood glucose (diabetes mellitus)
• Teach patient how to take pulse and B/P at home; advise when to notify prescriber
• Instruct patient to comply with weight control, dietary adjustments, modified exercise program
• Instruct patient to carry/wear emergency ID to identify product being taken, allergies; tell patient product controls symptoms but does not cure
• Caution patient to avoid hazardous activities if dizziness, drowsiness are present
• **Teach patient to report symptoms of CHF:** difficulty breathing, especially on exertion or when lying down, night cough, swelling of

P

extremities or bradycardia, dizziness, confusion, depression, fever
- Advise patient that sensitivity to cold may occur
- Teach patient to monitor blood glucose; may mask symptoms of hypoglycemia
- Teach patient how to take pulse, B/P; withhold if <50 bpm or systolic B/P <90 mm Hg

Evaluation

Positive therapeutic outcome
- Decreased B/P in hypertension (after 1-2 wk)
- Decreased tremors
- Absence of dysrhythmias
- Decreased migraine headaches

TREATMENT OF OVERDOSE:
Lavage, **IV** atropine for bradycardia, **IV** theophylline for bronchospasm, digoxin, O_2, diuretic for cardiac failure, hemodialysis, **IV** glucose for hyperglycemia, **IV** diazepam (or phenytoin) for seizures

---

⚠ HIGH ALERT

propylthiouracil (Rx)
(proe-pill-thye-oh-yoor'a-sill)
Propyl-Thyracil ✤
Func. class.: Thyroid hormone antagonist (antithyroid)
Chem. class.: Thioamide
Pregnancy category D

ACTION: Blocks synthesis peripherally of T_3, T_4, inhibits organification of iodine

Therapeutic outcome: Decreased T_3, T_4 levels, hyperthyroid symptoms

USES: Preparation for thyroidectomy, thyrotoxic crisis, hyperthyroidism, thyroid storm

CONTRAINDICATIONS
Pregnancy **D**, breastfeeding, hypersensitivity, agranulocytosis, hepatitis, jaundice

Precautions: Infection, bone marrow depression, hepatic disease, fever

> BLACK BOX WARNING: Hepatic disease

DOSAGE AND ROUTES
Thyrotoxic crisis
Adult and child: PO 200-400 mg q4h for 1st 24 hr

Preparation for thyroidectomy
Adult: PO 600-1200 mg/day
Child: PO 10 mg/kg/day in divided doses

Hyperthyroidism
Adult: PO 100 mg tid increasing to 300 mg q8hr if condition is severe; continue to euthyroid state, then 100 mg daily-tid
Child >6 yr: PO 50 mg/day divided doses q8hr, titrate based on TSH/free T_4 levels
Neonate (unlabeled): PO 10 mg/kg/day in divided doses

Available forms: Tabs 50 mg

Implementation
- Give with meals to decrease GI upset
- Give at same time each day to maintain product level
- Give lowest dosage that relieves symptoms
- Store in light-resistant container
- Increase fluids to 3-4 L/day, unless contraindicated

ADVERSE EFFECTS
CNS: *Drowsiness, headache, vertigo, fever,* paresthesias, neuritis
GI: *Nausea, diarrhea, vomiting,* jaundice, hepatitis, loss of taste, liver failure, death
GU: Nephritis
HEMA: Agranulocytosis, leukopenia, thrombocytopenia, hypothrombinemia, lymphadenopathy, bleeding, vasculitis, periarteritis
INTEG: *Rash, urticaria, pruritus, alopecia, hyperpigmentation,* lupuslike syndrome
MS: Myalgia, arthralgia, nocturnal muscle cramps, osteoporosis

Pharmacokinetics
Absorption	Rapidly absorbed
Distribution	Crosses placenta, concentration in thyroid gland
Metabolism	Liver
Excretion	Urine, bile, breast milk
Half-life	1-2 hr

Pharmacodynamics
Onset	30-40 min
Peak	Unknown
Duration	2-4 hr

INTERACTIONS
Individual drugs
Heparin: decreased anticoagulant effect
Lithium: increased antithyroid effect
Potassium/sodium iodide: increased effects
Radiation: increased bone marrow depression

Drug classifications
Anticoagulants (oral): decreased anticoagulant effect
Antineoplastics: increased bone marrow depression
Phenothiazines: increased agranulocytosis

Drug/lab test
Increased: pro-time, AST, ALT, alkaline phosphatase

NURSING CONSIDERATIONS
Assessment
• Monitor pulse, B/P, temp; I&O ratio; check for edema (puffy hands, feet, periorbits); indicates hypothyroidism
• Check weight daily with same clothing, scale, time of day
• Hyperthyroidism: weight loss, nervousness, insomnia, fever, diaphoresis, tremors
• Hypothyroidism: constipation, dry skin, weakness, headache
• Monitor T_3, T_4, which are increased; check serum TSH, which is decreased; assess free thyroxine index, which is increased if dosage is too low; discontinue product 3-4 wk before radioactive iodine uptake test
⚠ **Blood dyscrasias: Monitor CBC with differential; leukopenia, thrombocytopenia, agranulocytosis**
⚠ **Overdose: Assess for peripheral edema, heat intolerance, diaphoresis, palpitations, dysrhythmias, severe tachycardia, increased temp, delirium, CNS irritability**
⚠ **Hypersensitivity: Assess for rash, enlarged cervical lymph nodes; product may have to be discontinued**
• **Hypoprothrombinemia:** assess for bleeding, petechiae, ecchymosis
• **Bone marrow depression:** assess for sore throat, fever, fatigue

> BLACK BOX WARNING: **Hepatotoxicity:**
> monitor LFTs before and during treatment; jaundice, nausea, vomiting, abdominal pain, anorexia, diarrhea, fatigue

• Monitor clinical response: after 3 wk should include increased weight, decreased pulse, decreased T_4

Patient/family education
• Advise patient to abstain from breastfeeding after delivery; product appears in breast milk
• Teach patient to take pulse daily and to keep graph of weight, pulse, mood
• **Advise patient to report redness, swelling, sore throat, mouth lesions, which indicate blood dyscrasias**
• Caution patient to avoid OTC products that contain iodine; that seafood, other iodine-containing foods may be restricted by prescriber
• Caution patient not to discontinue this medication abruptly; thyroid crisis may occur; stress patient compliance

• Teach patient that response may take several mo if thyroid is large
• **Teach patient symptoms/signs of overdose: periorbital edema, cold intolerance, mental depression; notify prescriber at once**
• Teach patient symptoms of inadequate dose: tachycardia, diarrhea, fever, irritability; prescriber should be notified to adjust dosage
• Teach patient to take medication exactly as prescribed, not to skip or double doses; missed doses should be taken when remembered up to 1 hr before next dose
• Instruct patient to carry/wear emergency identification indicating medication taken and condition being treated

Evaluation
Positive therapeutic outcome
• Weight gain
• Decreased pulse
• Decreased T_4
• Decreased B/P

---

protamine (Rx)
(proe´ta-meen)
Func. class.: Heparin antagonist
Chem. class.: Low-molecular-weight protein
Pregnancy category C

ACTION: Binds heparin, making it ineffective

Therapeutic outcome: Prevention of heparin overdose

USES: Heparin overdose; neutralizes heparin in procedures, hemorrhage

CONTRAINDICATION
Hypersensitivity

Precautions: Pregnancy **C,** breastfeeding, fish allergy, diabetes, previous exposure to protamine, insulins, heparin rebound or bleeding

DOSAGE AND ROUTES
Heparin overdose
Adult and child: IV 1 mg of protamine/100 units of heparin given; administer slowly over 1-3 min; max 50 mg/10 min

Enoxaparin overdose
Adult: IV 1 mg of protamine/1 mg enoxaparin

Dalteparin/tinzaparin overdose
Adult: IV 1 mg of protamine/100 anti-Xa unit

Available forms: Inj 10 mg/ml

Implementation

Direct IV route
• After reconstituting 50 mg/5 ml sterile bacteriostatic water for inj, shake; give 20 mg or less over 1-3 min

Y-site compatibilities: Alfentanil, amikacin, aminophylline, ascorbic acid, atracurium, atropine, azaTHIOprine, aztreonam, benztropine, bumetanide, buprenorphine, butorphanol, calcium chloride/gluconate, ceftazidime, chlorproMAZINE, cimetidine, clindamycin, cyanocobalamin, cycloSPORINE, digoxin, diphenhydrAMINE, DOBUTamine, DOPamine, doxycycline, enalaprilat, ePHEDrine, EPINEPHrine, epoetin alfa, erythromycin, esmolol, famotidine, fentaNYL, fluconazole, ganciclovir, gentamicin, glycopyrrolate, hydrOXYzine, imipenem-cilastatin, inamrinone, iohexol, iopamidol, iothalamate, isoproterenol, labetalol, lidocaine, magnesium, mannitol, meperidine, metaraminol, methoxamine, methyldopate, metoclopramide, metoprolol, miconazole, midazolam, minocycline, morphine, multiple vitamins, nalbuphine, naloxone, netilmicin, nitroglycerin, nitroprusside, norepinephrine, ondansetron, oxytocin, papaverine, pentazocine, phenylephrine, polymyxin B, potassium chloride, procainamide, prochlorperazine, promethazine, propranolol, pyridoxine, quiNIDine, ranitidine, Ringer's, ritodrine, sodium bicarbonate, succinylcholine, SUFentanil, theophylline, thiamine, tobramycin, tolazoline, trimetaphan, urokinase, vancomycin, vasopressin, verapamil

ADVERSE EFFECTS

CNS: Lassitude, flushing
CV: Hypotension, bradycardia, circulatory collapse, capillary leak
GI: Nausea, vomiting, anorexia
HEMA: Bleeding
INTEG: *Rash*, dermatitis, urticaria
RESP: Dyspnea, pulmonary edema, severe respiratory distress, bronchospasm
SYST: Anaphylaxis, angioedema

Pharmacokinetics

Absorption	Completely absorbed
Distribution	Unknown
Metabolism	Unknown
Excretion	Unknown
Half-life	Unknown

Pharmacodynamics

Onset	5 min
Peak	Unknown
Duration	2 hr

NURSING CONSIDERATIONS

Assessment
• Monitor blood studies (Hct, platelets, occult blood stools) q3mo
• Monitor coagulation tests (aPTT, ACT) 15 min after dose, then in several hr
• Monitor VS, B/P, pulse q30min, plus 3 hr after dose
⚠ Assess for hypersensitivity: skin rash, urticaria, dermatitis, cough, wheezing, have emergency equipment nearby; men who have had a vasectomy may be more prone to hypersensitivity
⚠ Assess for allergy to salmon; use with caution in these patients

Patient/family education
• Explain reason for medication and expected results; not to take if allergic to fish
• Caution patient to avoid contact activities that may result in bleeding

Evaluation

Positive therapeutic outcome
• Reversal of heparin overdose

pseudoephedrine (OTC)
(soo-doe-e-fed′rin)

ElixSure Cold, Eltor ✤, Nasofed, Sudafed, Sudafed 24 hour, Sudogest
Func. class.: Adrenergic
Chem. class.: Substituted phenylethylamine
Pregnancy category C

ACTION: Primary activity through α-adrenergic effects on respiratory mucosal membranes reducing congestion, hyperemia, edema; minimal bronchodilatation secondary to β-adrenergic effects

Therapeutic outcome: Decreased nasal congestion, swelling

USES: Nasal decongestant, otitis media adjunct, adjunct with antihistamines

CONTRAINDICATIONS
Hypersensitivity to sympathomimetics, closed-angle glaucoma

Precautions: Pregnancy C, breastfeeding, cardiac disorders, hyperthyroidism, diabetes mellitus, prostatic hypertrophy, hypertension

DOSAGE AND ROUTES
Adult and child >12 yr: PO 60 mg q6hr; EXT REL 120 mg q12hr or 240 mg q24hr
Geriatric: PO 30-60 mg q6hr prn
Child 6-12 yr: PO 30 mg q6hr, max 120 mg/day

Child 2-6 yr: PO 15 mg q6hr, max 60 mg/day

Available forms: Ext rel caps 120, 240 mg; oral sol 15 mg, 30 mg/5 ml; tabs 30, 60 mg; ext rel tabs 120, 240 mg

Implementation
• Swallow tab and ext rel cap whole; do not break, crush, or chew
• Avoid taking at or near bedtime if insomnia occurs
• Store at room temperature

ADVERSE EFFECTS
CNS: *Tremors, anxiety,* stimulation, insomnia, headache, dizziness, hallucinations, **seizures** (geriatric)
CV: Palpitations, tachycardia, hypertension, chest pain, **dysrhythmias, CV collapse**
EENT: Dry nose, irritation of nose and throat
GI: *Anorexia, nausea, vomiting,* dry mouth, ischemic colitis
GU: Dysuria

Pharmacokinetics
Absorption	Well absorbed
Distribution	Enters CSF, crosses placenta
Metabolism	Liver, partially
Excretion	Kidneys, unchanged (75%); breast milk
Half-life	7 hr

Pharmacodynamics
	PO	PO-EXT REL
Onset	15-30 min	1 hr
Peak	Unknown	Unknown
Duration	4-6 hr	12 hr

INTERACTIONS
Drug classifications
Antidepressants (tricyclics), MAOIs: hypertensive crisis, do not use together
Urinary acidifiers: decreased effect of pseudoephedrine
Urinary alkalizers, adrenergics, β-blockers, phenothiazines, tricyclics: increased effect of pseudoephedrine

NURSING CONSIDERATIONS
Assessment
• Assess for CNS side effects in the geriatric: excitation, seizures, hallucinations
• Monitor for nasal congestion; auscultate lung sounds; check for tenacious bronchial secretions; children with otitis media should be assessed for eustachian tube congestion
• Monitor B/P and pulse throughout treatment

Patient/family education
• Teach patient reason for product administration and expected results
• Instruct patient not to use continuously, or more than recommended dose; rebound congestion may occur
• Advise patient to check with prescriber before using other products, as product interactions may occur
• Advise patient to avoid taking near bedtime; stimulation can occur
• Caution patient not to use if stimulation, restlessness, tremors occur
• Notify parents of possible excessive agitation in children
⚠ Advise patient to notify prescriber of anxiety, slow or fast heart rate, dyspnea, seizures
• Ext rel: do not divide, crush, chew, or dissolve
• **Do not use within 14 days of MAOIs**

Evaluation
Positive therapeutic outcome
• Decreased nasal congestion

psyllium (OTC)
(sill'i-um)
Hydrocil, Leader Fiber Laxative, Metamucil, Natural Fiber, Natural Vegetable Fiber, Reguloid, Wal-Mucil
Func. class.: Laxative, bulk-forming
Chem. class.: Psyllium colloid
Pregnancy category C

ACTION: Bulk-forming laxative

Therapeutic outcome: Decreased constipation, decreased diarrhea in colitis

USES: Chronic constipation, ulcerative colitis, irritable bowel syndrome

CONTRAINDICATIONS
Hypersensitivity, intestinal obstruction, abdominal pain, nausea/vomiting, fecal impaction

Precautions: Pregnancy **C**

DOSAGE AND ROUTES
Adult: PO 1-2 tsp in 8 oz of water bid or tid, then 8 oz of water; or 1 premeasured packet in 8 oz of water bid or tid, then 8 oz of water
Child >6 yr: 1 tsp in 4 oz of water at bedtime

Available forms: Chew pieces 1.7, 3.4 g/piece; powder effervescent 3.4, 3.7 g/packet; powder 3.3, 3.4, 3.5, 4.94 g/tsp; wafers 3.4 g/wafer

Implementation
- Give alone for better absorption; give after mixing with water immediately before use; administer with 8 oz of water or juice followed by another 8 oz of fluid
- Administer in AM or PM (oral dose)
- Shake susp well

ADVERSE EFFECTS
GI: *Nausea, vomiting, anorexia, diarrhea,* cramps, intestinal/esophageal blockage

Pharmacokinetics
Absorption	None
Distribution	None
Metabolism	Unknown
Excretion	Feces
Half-life	Unknown

Pharmacodynamics
Onset	12-24 hr
Peak	2-4 days
Duration	Unknown

INTERACTIONS
Drug classifications
Cardiac glycosides, oral anticoagulants, salicylates: decreased absorption of each specific product

Drug/herb
Flax, senna: increased laxative

NURSING CONSIDERATIONS
Assessment
- Monitor blood, urine electrolytes if used often by patient; check I&O ratio to identify fluid loss
- Assess for cramping, rectal bleeding, nausea, vomiting; if these symptoms occur, product should be discontinued; identify cause of constipation; identify whether fluids, bulk, or exercise is missing from lifestyle
- Assess stool for color, consistency, amount, presence of flatulence

Patient/family education
- Discuss with patient that adequate fluid consumption is necessary
- Teach patient that normal bowel movements do not always occur daily
- Caution patient not to use in presence of abdominal pain, nausea, vomiting; tell patient to notify prescriber if constipation is unrelieved or if symptoms of electrolyte imbalance occur (muscle cramps, pain, weakness, dizziness, excessive thirst)
- Teach patient not to use laxatives for long-term therapy; bowel tone will be lost and will decrease
- Teach patient not to take at bedtime as a laxative; may interfere with sleep; also problems with lipid pneumonia
- Teach patient not to use with food or vitamin preparations; delays digestion and absorption of fat-soluble vitamins

Evaluation
Positive therapeutic outcome
- Decreased constipation in 12-24 hr

---

pyridostigmine (Rx)
(peer-id-oh-stig′meen)
Mestinon, Mestinon SR, Regonol
Func. class.: Cholinergic, anticholinesterase
Chem. class.: Tertiary amine carbamate
Pregnancy category C

ACTION: Inhibits destruction of acetylcholine, which increases concentration at sites where acetylcholine is released; this facilitates transmission of impulses across myoneural junction

Therapeutic outcome: Decreased action of nondepolarizing muscle relaxant; increased muscle strength in myasthenia gravis

USES: Nondepolarizing muscle relaxant antagonist, myasthenia gravis, pretreatment in nerve gas exposure (military only)

CONTRAINDICATIONS
Bradycardia, hypotension, obstruction of intestine, renal system, bromide, benzyl alcohol sensitivity, cholinesterase inhibitor toxicity

Precautions: Pregnancy C, seizure disorders, bronchial asthma, coronary occlusion, hyperthyroidism, dysrhythmias, peptic ulcer, megacolon, poor GI motility

DOSAGE AND ROUTES
Myasthenia gravis
Adult: PO 600 mg/day in 5-6 divided doses, max 1.5 g/day; IM/**IV** 2 mg or 1/30 of PO dose; SUS REL 180-540 mg/day or bid at intervals of at least 6 hr
Child: PO 7 mg/kg/day in 5-6 divided doses; IM/**IV** 0.05-0.15 mg/kg/dose

Nondepolarizing neuromuscular blocker antagonist
Adult: 0.6-1.2 mg IV atropine, then 0.1-0.25 mg/kg/dose
Child: IV 0.1-0.25 mg/kg/dose

Nerve gas exposure prophylaxis (military)
Adult: PO 30 mg q8hr if threat of exposure to Soman gas is anticipated, start several hours before exposure and discontinue upon exposure; after this product is discontinued, give antidotes (atropine, pralidoxime)

Available forms: Tabs 60 mg; ext rel tabs 180 mg; syr 60 mg/5 ml; inj 5 mg/ml

Implementation
• Only with atropine sulfate available for cholinergic crisis
• Only after all other cholinergics have been discontinued
• Increased doses for tolerance, as ordered
• Larger doses after exercise or fatigue, as ordered
• Do not break, crush, or chew sus rel tabs

PO route
• On empty stomach for better absorption

IV route
• Undiluted (5 mg/ml), give through Y-tube or 3-way stopcock, give 0.5 mg or less/min (myasthenia gravis); 5 mg/min (reversal of nondepolarizing neuromuscular blockers)

Y-site compatibilities: Heparin, hydrocortisone, potassium chloride, vit B/C
• Storage at room temperature

ADVERSE EFFECTS
CNS: Dizziness, headache, sweating, weakness, **seizures,** uncoordination, paralysis, drowsiness, LOC
CV: Tachycardia, dysrhythmias, bradycardia, AV block, hypotension, ECG changes, **cardiac arrest,** syncope
EENT: Miosis, blurred vision, lacrimation, vision changes
GI: *Nausea, diarrhea, vomiting, cramps, increased salivary and gastric secretions, peristalsis*
GU: Frequency, incontinence, urgency
INTEG: Rash, urticaria, flushing
RESP: **Respiratory depression, bronchospasm, constriction, laryngospasm, respiratory arrest**
SYST: Cholinergic crisis

Absorption	Poorly absorbed (PO)
Distribution	Widely distributed, crosses placenta
Metabolism	Liver, plasma cholinesterase
Excretion	Kidneys
Half-life	2 hr (**IV**); 4 hr (**PO**)

Pharmacodynamics

	PO	PO-EXT REL	IM/IV
Onset	20-30 min	½-1 hr	2-15 min
Peak	Unknown	Unknown	Unknown
Duration	3-6 hr	3-6 hr	2-4 hr

INTERACTIONS
Individual drugs
Atropine, gallamine, metocurine, pancuronium, tubocurarine: decreased action
Succinylcholine: increased action of pyridostigmine
Magnesium, mecamylamine, polymyxin, procainamide, quiNIDine: decreased action of pyridostigmine

Drug classifications
Aminoglycosides, anesthetics, antidysrhythmics, corticosteroids, quinolones: decreased action of pyridostigmine

NURSING CONSIDERATIONS
Assessment
• **Myasthenia gravis:** assess for fatigue, ptosis, diplopia, difficulty swallowing, SOB, hand/gait before and after product, improvement should be seen after 1 hr
• Monitor I&O ratio; check for urinary retention or incontinence
⚠ **Toxicity: assess for bradycardia, hypotension, bronchospasm, headache, dizziness, seizures, respiratory depression; product should be discontinued if toxicity occurs**
• Monitor VS, respiration; increased B/P during test and at baseline
• Monitor diabetic patient carefully, since this product lowers blood glucose

Patient/family education
• Advise patient to carry/wear emergency ID specifying myasthenia gravis, products taken
• Teach patient that product doesn't cure but relieves symptoms
• Teach patient to avoid driving, other hazardous activities until effect is known
• Advise patient not to drink alcohol
• Advise patient to take with food to decrease gastric side effects
• **Teach patient to report weakness (cholinergic crisis, or overdose), bradycardia**

Evaluation
Positive therapeutic outcome
• Increased muscle strength, hand grasp, improved gait, absence of labored breathing (if

P

severe); reversal of nondepolarizing neuromuscular blockers; prevention of nerve gas toxicity

TREATMENT OF OVERDOSE: Discontinue product, atropine 1-4 mg **IV**

---

pyridoxine (vitamin B₆) (OTC, Rx)
(peer-i-dox'een)
Equaline Vitamin B₆, Neuro-K, Walgreens Finest B-6, Walgreens Gold Seal Vitamin B₆
Func. class.: Vitamin B₆, water soluble
Pregnancy category A

ACTION: Needed for fat, protein, carbohydrate metabolism; enhances glycogen release from liver and muscle tissue; needed as coenzyme for metabolic transformations of a variety of amino acids

Therapeutic outcome: Absence of vit B₆ deficiency

USES: Vitamin B₆ deficiency associated with the following: inborn errors of metabolism, seizures, isoniazid therapy, oral contraceptives, alcoholism, polyneuritis

Unlabeled uses: Palmar-plantar erythrodysesthesia syndrome

CONTRAINDICATION
Hypersensitivity

Precautions: Pregnancy **A,** breastfeeding, children, Parkinson's disease, patients taking levodopa should avoid supplemental vitamins with >5 mg pyridoxine

DOSAGE AND ROUTES
RDA
Adult: PO (male) 1.7-2 mg; (female) 1.4-1.6 mg
Child 9-13 yr: PO 1 mg/day
Child 4-8 yr: PO 0.6 mg/day
Child 1-3 yr: PO 0.5 mg/day
Infant 7-12 mo: PO 0.3 mg/day

Vitamin B₆ deficiency
Adult: PO 5-25 mg/day × 3 wk
Child: PO 10 mg until desired response

Pyridoxine deficiency neuritis/ seizure (not drug induced)
Adult: PO without neuritis 2.5-10 mg/day, after corrected 2-5 mg/day; with neuritis 100-200 mg/day × 3 wk, then 2-5 mg/day
Child: PO without neuritis 5-25 mg/day × 3 wk, then 1.5-2.5 mg/day in a multivitamin; with neuritis 10-50 mg/day × 3 wk, then 1-2 mg/day
Neonate with seizures: IM/IV 50-100 mg as a single dose

Deficiency caused by isoniazid, cycloSERINE, hydrALAZINE, penicillamine
Adult: PO 100-300 mg/day
Child: PO 10-50 mg/day

Prevention of deficiency caused by isoniazid, cycloSERINE, hydrALAZINE, penicillamine
Adult: PO 25-100 mg/day
Child: PO 1.2 mg/kg/day

Palmar-plantar erythrodysesthesia syndrome (unlabeled)
Adult: PO 50-150 mg/day

Available forms: Tabs 10, 25, 50, 100 mg; ext rel tabs 100 mg; inj 100 mg/ml; ext rel caps 150 mg

Implementation
PO route
• Swallow ext rel cap and ext rel tabs whole; do not break, crush, or chew
IM route
• Rotate sites to avoid pain; burning or stinging at site may occur; give by Z-track to minimize pain
• Store in airtight, light-resistant container

IV route
• Give **IV** undiluted or added to most **IV** sol; give 50 mg or less/1 min if undiluted

Syringe compatibilities: Doxapram

Additive incompatibilities: Erythromycin, iron salts, kanamycin, riboflavin, streptomycin

ADVERSE EFFECTS
CNS: Paresthesia, flushing, warmth, lethargy (rare with normal renal function)
INTEG: Pain at inj site

Pharmacokinetics

Absorption	Well absorbed (PO)
Distribution	Stored in liver, muscle, brain; crosses placenta
Metabolism	Unknown
Excretion	Kidneys, unchanged (not used)
Half-life	Unknown

Pharmacodynamics

Unknown

INTERACTIONS
Individual drugs
Chloramphenicol, cycloSERINE, hydrALAZINE, isoniazid, penicillamine: decreased effects of pyridoxine
Levodopa: decreased effects of levodopa

Drug classifications

Contraceptives (oral), immunosuppressants: decreased effects of pyridoxine

NURSING CONSIDERATIONS
Assessment

• Monitor pyridoxine levels throughout treatment
• Assess nutritional status: yeast, liver, legumes, bananas, green vegetables, whole grains
• Assess for pyridoxine (B_6) deficiency: nausea, vomiting, dermatitis, cheilosis, seizures, irritability, dermatitis before, during treatment
• Assess neurological status: paresthesia, lethargy
• Monitor blood tests: Hct, Hgb

Patient/family education

• Teach patient to avoid other vitamin supplements unless directed by prescriber
• Advise patient to increase meat, bananas, potatoes, lima beans, whole grain cereals in diet which are high in vit B_6
• Caution patient not to increase dosage, since serious reactions may occur

Evaluation

Positive therapeutic outcome

• Absence of nausea, vomiting, anorexia, skin lesions, glossitis, stomatitis, edema, seizures, restlessness, paresthesia

pyrimethamine (Rx)

(peer-i-meth′a-meen)
Daraprim
Func. class.: Antimalarial, antiprotozoal
Chem. class.: Folic acid antagonist
Pregnancy category C

ACTION: Inhibits folic acid metabolism in parasite; prevents transmission by stopping growth of fertilized gametes

Therapeutic outcome: Prevention of malaria

USES: Malaria prophylaxis, antiprotozoal action against *Plasmodium vivax, Pneumocystis jiroveci*

CONTRAINDICATIONS

Hypersensitivity, chloroquine-resistant malaria, megaloblastic anemia caused by folate deficiency

Precautions: Pregnancy **C**, breastfeeding, geriatric patients, blood dyscrasias, seizure disorder, glucose-6-phosphate dehydrogenase (G6PD) disease, renal/hepatic disease

DOSAGE AND ROUTES
Prophylaxis of malaria

• Begin 2 wk before entering endemic area and continue for 6-10 wk after return
Adult and child >10 yr: PO 25 mg qwk
Child 4-10 yr: PO 12.5 mg qwk
Child <4 yr: PO 6.25 mg qwk

Malaria treatment

Adult/adolescent/child >10 yr: PO 25 mg/day × 2 days with sulfonamide
Child 4-10 yr: 25 mg/day × 2 days

Toxoplasmosis

Adult: PO 50-75 mg, then reduce by about 50% for 4-5 wk, with 1-4 g sulfADIAZINE × 1-3 wk, then reduce by 50% for 4-5 wk
Child: PO 1 mg/kg/day in 2 divided doses or 2 mg/kg/day × 3 days, then 1 mg/kg/day or divided twice daily × 4 wk, max 25 mg/day

Toxoplasmosis in AIDS patients

Adult: PO 100-200 mg/day × 1-2 days, then 50-100 mg/day × 3-6 wk, then 25-50 mg/day for life (given with clindamycin or sulfADIAZINE)

Available forms: Tabs 25 mg; combo tabs 500 mg sulfadoxine/25 mg pyrimethamine

Implementation
PO route

• Give leucovorin IM 3-9 mg/day × 3 days if folic acid deficiency occurs
• Give before or after meals at same time each day to maintain product level, decrease GI symptoms
• **Extemporaneous susp:** tabs may be crushed and mixed with 25 ml distilled water, sucrose-containing sol (1 mg/ml), shake well, stable for 5-7 days at room temp if mixed with sucrose-containing sol
• Store in tight, light-resistant container

ADVERSE EFFECTS

CNS: Stimulation, irritability, seizures, tremors, ataxia, fatigue, fever
CV: Dysrhythmias
GI: *Nausea, vomiting, cramps, anorexia,* diarrhea, atrophic glossitis, gastritis
HEMA: Thrombocytopenia, leukopenia, pancytopenia, megaloblastic anemia, decreased folic acid, agranulocytosis
INTEG: Skin eruptions, photosensitivity, Stevens-Johnson syndrome
RESP: Respiratory failure

P

Adverse effects: *italics* = common; **bold** = life-threatening

Pharmacokinetics

Absorption	Well absorbed
Distribution	Widely distributed; crosses placenta
Metabolism	Liver, extensively
Excretion	Kidneys, unchanged (30%); breast milk
Half-life	4 days

Pharmacodynamics

Onset	Unknown
Peak	2 hr
Duration	Unknown

INTERACTIONS
Individual drugs
Folic acid: increased synergistic action
Radiation: increased bone marrow suppression
Zidovudine: increased risk of megaloblastic anemia, agranulocytosis, thrombocytopenia

Drug classifications
Bone marrow depressants, folate antagonists: increased bone marrow suppression

NURSING CONSIDERATIONS
Assessment
• **Serious skin disorders: assess for Stevens-Johnson syndrome (swelling of face, lips, throat, fever)**

• **Monitor folic acid level; megaloblastic anemia occurs**
⚠ **Blood dyscrasias: assess blood studies, CBC, platelets; twice weekly if dosage is increased**
⚠ **Toxicity: assess for vomiting, anorexia, seizure, blood dyscrasia, glossitis; product should be discontinued immediately**

Patient/family education
• Instruct patient that compliance with dosage schedule, duration is necessary; that scheduled appointments must be kept or relapse may occur
• **Teach patient to report vision problems, fever, fatigue, bruising, bleeding, sore throat; may indicate blood dyscrasias**
• **Teach patient to report immediately skin rash; stop use**

Evaluation
Positive therapeutic outcome
• Decreased symptoms of toxoplasmosis
• Decreased symptoms of *Pneumocystis jiroveci* pneumonia
• Decreased symptoms of malaria

TREATMENT OF OVERDOSE:
Gastric lavage, short-acting barbiturate, leucovorin, respiratory support if needed

QUEtiapine (Rx)
(kwe-tie′a-peen)
SEROquel, Seroquel XR
Func. class.: Antipsychotic
Chem. class.: Dibenzodiazepine
Pregnancy category C

ACTION: Functions as an antagonist at multiple neurotransmitter receptors in the brain including $5\text{-}HT_{1A}$, $5\text{-}HT_2$, DOPamine D_1, D_2, H_1, adrenergic α_1, α_2 receptors

Therapeutic outcome: Decreased hallucinations and disorganized thought

USES: Bipolar disorder, bipolar I disorder, depression, mania, schizophrenia

CONTRAINDICATIONS
Hypersensitivity, breastfeeding

Precautions: Pregnancy **C**, geriatric, long-term use, seizures, hepatic disease, breast cancer, QT prolongation, CV disease, Parkinson's, brain tumor, hematological disease, torsades de pointes, cataracts, dehydration

> **BLACK BOX WARNING:** Children, suicide, dementia

DOSAGE AND ROUTES
Schizophrenia
Adult: PO (not at risk for hypotension) 25 mg bid on day 1, increase by 25-50 mg divided two to three times on day 2 and day 3 to a target of 300-400 mg/day in divided doses on day 4; make further dosage adjustments in 25-50 mg bid increments, max 800 mg/day
Adolescents 13-17 yr: PO 25 mg bid on day 1, 50 mg bid on day 2, 100 mg bid on day 3, 150 mg bid on day 4, 200 mg bid on day 5; ext rel 50 mg on day 1, then 100 mg on day 2 , 200 mg on day 3, 300 mg on day 4, 400 mg on day 5
Geriatric: PO ext rel 50 mg/day; may increase in 50 mg/day increments

Bipolar I disorder
Adult: PO (monotherapy or as adjunct to lithium or divalproex) 50 mg bid on day 1, 100 mg on day 2 in 2 divided doses as tolerated to 400 mg on day 4; range 400-800 mg/day; ext rel give in evening 300 mg qday day 1, then 600 mg qday day 2, then adjusted as tolerated

Psychotic disorders
Adult: PO 25 mg bid, titrate upward; XR: 300 mg/day in PM, range 400-800 mg/day

Depressive disorder (inadequate response to antidepressants alone)
Adult: PO EXT REL 50 mg/day in the PM on day 1, 2; on day 3 give 150 mg in the PM, max 600 mg/day
Geriatric: PO EXT REL 50 mg; may increase by 50 mg/day based on response; ext rel 50 mg in evening, max 800 mg/day

Available forms: Tabs 25, 50, 100, 200, 300, 400 mg; ext rel tab 50, 150, 200, 300, 400 mg
Implementation
- Give reduced dosage in geriatric patients
- Avoid use of CNS depressants
- Give **immediate release** without regard to meals
- Give **extended release** without food or with light meal, swallow whole, do not split, crush, chew
- Supervise ambulation until patient is stabilized on medication; do not involve in strenuous exercise program because fainting is possible; patient should not stand still for a long time
- Sips of water, sugarless candy, gum for dry mouth
- Store in airtight, light-resistant container

ADVERSE EFFECTS
CNS: EPS, pseudoparkinsonism, akathisia, dystonia, tardive dyskinesia, drowsiness, insomnia, agitation, anxiety, *headache*, **seizures, neuroleptic malignant syndrome,** dizziness, dystonia, restless legs syndrome
CV: Orthostatic hypotension, **tachycardia, QT prolongation,** CV disease, Parkinson's disease, **cardiomyopathy, myocarditis**
ENDO: SIADH, hyperglycemia
GI: Nausea, anorexia, constipation, abdominal pain, dry mouth
HEMA: **Leukopenia, agranulocytosis**
INTEG: Rash
META: Hyponatremia
MISC: Asthenia, back pain, fever, ear pain
MS: **Rhabdomyolysis**
RESP: Rhinitis
SYST: **Stevens-Johnson syndrome, anaphylaxis**

Pharmacokinetics

Absorption	Rapidly absorbed
Distribution	Widely distributed
Metabolism	Liver, extensively; inhibits P450 CYP3A4 enzyme system; 83% protein
Excretion	Excretion <1% unchanged urine
Half-life	≥6 hr

Adverse effects: *italics* = common; **bold** = life-threatening

Pharmacodynamics

Onset	Unknown
Peak	1.5 hr
Duration	Up to 12 hr

INTERACTIONS
Individual drugs

Alcohol: increased CNS depression

CarBAMazepine, phenytoin, rifampin, thioridazine: increased QUEtiapine clearance

**Chloroquine, clarithromycin, droperidol,
erythromycin, haloperidol, methadone,
pentamidine: increased QT prolongation**

Cimetidine: decreased QUEtiapine clearance

Erythromycin: increased effects of erythromycin

Fluconazole, itraconazole, ketoconazole: increased action of QUEtiapine

Levodopa: decreased effect of levodopa

Lithium: increased neurotoxicity

LORazepam: decreased effect of LORazepam

Drug classifications

Analgesics (opioid), antihistamines, sedatives-
hypnotics: increased CNS depression

Antihypertensives: increased hypotension

Barbiturates, glucocorticoids: increased
clearance of quetiapine, decreased
quetiapine effect

**β-agonists, class IA/III antidysrhythmics,
local anesthetics, phenothiazines (some),
tricyclics: increased QT prolongation**

DOPamine agonists: decreased effects of
DOPamine agonists

NURSING CONSIDERATIONS
Assessment

• Assess CV status: QT prolongation, tachycardia,
orthostatic B/P

> **BLACK BOX WARNING:** Mental status
> before initial administration, AIMS assess-
> ment; affect, orientation, LOC, reflexes, gait,
> coordination, sleep pattern disturbances;
> suicidal thoughts/behavior (child/young adult);
> dementia (geriatric patients)

> **BLACK BOX WARNING:** Not to be used in
> child <10 yr (immediate release) or <18 yr
> (extended release)

> **BLACK BOX WARNING: Suicide:** restrict
> amount of product given, usually suicidal
> thoughts, behavior occur early in treatment
> and in children/adolescents/young adults

• Check that patient swallows all PO medication; check for hoarding or giving of medication
to other patients

• Obtain baselines in blood glucose, liver
function tests, neurologic status, ophthalmologic
exam, weight, thyroid function tests, serum
electrolytes/creatinine/lipid profile/prolactin

• Monitor B/P with patient in sitting, standing,
and lying positions; take pulse and respirations
q4hr during initial treatment; establish baseline
before starting treatment; report drops of
30 mm Hg; obtain baseline ECG and monitor
Q- and T-wave changes

• Check for dizziness, faintness, palpitations,
tachycardia on rising; severe orthostatic
hypotension is common

⚠ **Identify for neuroleptic malignant
syndrome: hyperpyrexia, muscle rigidity,
increased CPK, altered mental status,
seizures, tachycardia, diaphoresis, hyper/
hypotension, fatigue; product should be
discontinued and prescriber notified
immediately**

• **Assess for EPS** including akathisia (inability
to sit still, no pattern to movements), tardive
dyskinesia (bizarre movements of the jaw,
mouth, tongue, extremities), pseudoparkinsonism (rigidity, tremors, pill rolling, shuffling
gait); an antiparkinson product should be
prescribed

Patient/family education

• Teach patient to use good oral hygiene;
frequent rinsing of mouth, sugarless gum for dry
mouth

• Caution patient to avoid hazardous activities
until product response is determined; dizziness,
blurred vision may occur

• Inform patient that orthostatic hypotension
occurs often; patient should rise from sitting
or lying position gradually; avoid hot tubs, hot
showers, and tub baths because hypotension
may occur; inform patient that heat stroke may
occur in hot weather, to take extra precautions
to stay cool, drink plenty of fluids

• Advise patient to avoid abrupt withdrawal of
this product or EPS may result; product should
be withdrawn slowly

• Teach patient to avoid OTC preparations
(cough, hayfever, cold) unless approved by
prescriber; serious product interactions may
occur; avoid use with alcohol, CNS depressants
because increased drowsiness may occur

• Advise patient to take medication only as
prescribed, not to use other products unless
approved by prescriber; not to stop abruptly

• Advise patient that follow-up is necessary
including LFTs, blood glucose, neurologic/
ophthalmic function, cholesterol profile, weight

• If drowsiness occurs, avoid hazardous
activities such as driving

• Advise patient to notify prescriber if pregnancy is planned, suspected; do not breastfeed
• **Advise patient to notify prescriber immediately of fever, difficulty breathing, fatigue, sore throat, rash, bleeding**

BLACK BOX WARNING: Suicide: thoughts, behavior, primarily in children/adolescents/young adults

Evaluation
Positive therapeutic outcome
• Decrease in emotional excitement, hallucinations, delusions, paranoia
• Reorganization of patterns of thought, speech

TREATMENT OF OVERDOSE:
Lavage, provide airway

quinapril (Rx)
(kwin'a-pril)
Accupril
Func. class.: Antihypertensive
Chem. class.: Angiotensin-converting enzyme (ACE) inhibitor
Pregnancy category D (2nd/3rd trimester)
Pregnancy category C (1st trimester)

Do not confuse: Accupril/Aciphex

ACTION: Selectively suppresses renin-angiotensin-aldosterone system; inhibits ACE, prevents conversion of angiotensin I to angiotensin II; results in dilatation of arterial, venous vessels

Therapeutic outcome: Decreased B/P in hypertension

USES: Hypertension, alone or in combination with thiazide diuretics, systolic CHF

CONTRAINDICATIONS
Children, hypersensitivity to ACE inhibitors, angioedema

BLACK BOX WARNING: Pregnancy D

Precautions: Breastfeeding, geriatric, impaired renal/liver function, dialysis patients, hypovolemia, blood dyscrasias, bilateral renal stenosis, cough, pregnancy **C** 1st trimester, hyperkalemia, aortic stenosis, African descent

DOSAGE AND ROUTES
Hypertension
Adult: PO 10-20 mg/day initially, then 20-80 mg/day divided bid or daily (monotherapy), start at 2.5 mg/day (with diuretics)
Geriatric: PO 10 mg/day, titrate to desired response (monotherapy), start at 2.5 mg/day (with diuretics), titrate ≥ 2 wk

Congestive heart failure
Adult: PO 5 mg bid, may increase qwk until 20-40 mg/day in 2 divided doses
Renal dose
Adult: PO CCr 61-89 ml/min start or 10 mg/day (hypertension), 5 mg bid (heart failure); CCr 30-60 ml/min 5 mg/day initially; CCr 10-29 ml/min 2.5 mg/day initially

Available forms: Tabs 5, 10, 20, 40 mg

Implementation
• Tabs may be crushed if necessary, without regard to food
• Store in airtight container at 86° F (30° C) or less
• Do not use with high-fat meal, decreases absorption
• Severe hypotension may occur after 1st dose of this medication; may be prevented by reducing or discontinuing diuretic therapy 3 days before beginning quinapril therapy

ADVERSE EFFECTS
CNS: Headache, dizziness, fatigue, somnolence, depression, malaise, nervousness, vertigo, syncope
CV: Hypotension, postural hypotension, syncope, palpitations, *angina pectoris*, **MI, tachycardia,** vasodilatation, chest pain
GI: Nausea, diarrhea, constipation, vomiting, gastritis, **GI hemorrhage,** dry mouth
GU: Increased BUN, creatinine, decreased libido, impotence
INTEG: **Angioedema,** rash, sweating, photosensitivity, pruritus
META: Hyperkalemia
MISC: Back pain, amblyopia
MS: Myalgia
RESP: Cough, pharyngitis, dyspnea

Pharmacokinetics
Absorption	≥60%
Distribution	Protein binding 97%, crosses placenta
Metabolism	Liver (active metabolites quinaprilat)
Excretion	Metabolites urine (60%), feces (37%)
Half-life	2 hr

Pharmacodynamics
Onset	½-1 hr
Peak	1-2 hr
Duration	24 hr

INTERACTIONS
Individual drugs
Aliskiren (diabetic patients): increased hyperkalemia
Alcohol: increased hypotension (large amounts)

Q

Adverse effects: *italics* = common; **bold** = life-threatening

Lithium: increased toxicity

HydrALAZINE, prazosin: use caution

Tetracycline: decreased absorption of tetracycline

Drug classifications

Adrenergic blockers, antihypertensives, diuretics, ganglionic blockers, nitrates, phenothiazines: increased hypotension

Diuretics (potassium sparing), potassium supplements, sympathomimetics, ACE/angiotensin II receptor antagonists, vasodilators: use caution

NSAIDs: decreased hypotensive effect of quinapril

Drug/herb

Cough: capsaicin

Decrease antihypertensive effect: ma huang

Drug/food

Hyperkalemia: do not use with potassium-containing salt substitutes; read label carefully

Drug/lab test

Increased: Potassium, creatinine, BUN, LFTs

NURSING CONSIDERATIONS
Assessment

• **Collagen vascular disease: monitor blood studies: neutrophils, decreased platelets; WBC with differential baseline, periodically q3mo; if neutrophils <1000/mm³ discontinue treatment**

• **Hypertension:** monitor B/P, check for orthostatic hypotension, syncope; if changes occur, dosage change may be required

• Monitor renal function tests (protein, BUN, creatinine) and periodically liver function tests, uric acid; glucose may be elevated; watch for increased levels that may indicate nephrotic syndrome and renal failure; monitor renal symptoms: polyuria, oliguria, frequency, dysuria

• Check potassium levels throughout treatment, although hyperkalemia rarely occurs

• **CHF:** check for edema in feet, legs daily, weight daily

BLACK BOX WARNING: Assess for pregnancy; pregnancy **D**; if pregnancy is suspected, discontinue product

Patient/family education

• Advise patient not to discontinue product abruptly; advise patient to tell all persons associated with care

• Teach patient not to use OTC products (cough, cold, allergy) unless directed by physician; serious side effects can occur; avoid high-fat meal at time of dose

• Inform patient that xanthines such as coffee, tea, chocolate, cola can prevent action of product

• Caution patient on the importance of complying with dosage schedule, even if feeling better; to continue with medical regimen to decrease B/P: exercise, cessation of smoking, decreasing stress, diet modifications

• Emphasize the need to rise slowly to sitting or standing position to minimize orthostatic hypotension; not to exercise in hot weather or increased hypotension can occur

• **Allergic reactions:** assess for allergic reactions: rash, fever, pruritus, urticaria; product should be discontinued if antihistamines fail to help

• Teach patient to notify prescriber of mouth sores, sore throat, fever, swelling of hands or feet, irregular heartbeat, chest pain, coughing, shortness of breath

• **Caution patient to report excessive perspiration, dehydration, vomiting, diarrhea; may lead to fall in B/P, maintain adequate hydration**

• Caution patient that product may cause dizziness, fainting, light-headedness; may occur during 1st few days of therapy; to avoid activities that may be hazardous

• Teach patient how to take B/P, and normal readings for age group

• Teach patient product may cause skin rash or impaired taste perception

BLACK BOX WARNING: Pregnancy **D**, to report if pregnancy is planned or suspected, do not breastfeed

Evaluation
Positive therapeutic outcome

• Decreased B/P in hypertension

TREATMENT OF OVERDOSE:
0.9% NaCl IV inf, hemodialysis

▲ HIGH ALERT

quiNIDine gluconate (Rx)
(kwin'i-deen)
quiNIDine sulfate (Rx)
Func. class.: Antidysrhythmic (class IA)
Chem. class.: QuiNINE dextro isomer
Pregnancy category C

Do not confuse: quiNIDine/quiNINE

ACTION: Prolongs action potential duration and effective refractory period, thus decreasing myocardial excitability; anticholinergic properties

Therapeutic outcome: Treatment of dysrhythmias

USES: Wolff-Parkinson-White syndrome, PVST, atrial fibrillation, flutter; paroxysmal atrial

---

tachycardia, ventricular tachycardia, malaria (**IV** quiNIDine gluconate)

Unlabeled uses: Singultus (hiccups)

CONTRAINDICATIONS

Hypersensitivity or idiosyncratic response, digoxin toxicity, blood dyscrasias, myasthenia gravis, AV block

Precautions: Pregnancy **C,** breastfeeding, children, geriatric, renal/hepatic disease, electrolyte imbalance, CHF, respiratory depression, bradycardia, hypotension, syncope

> **BLACK BOX WARNING:** Cardiac arrhythmias, MI

DOSAGE AND ROUTES
>> **QuiNIDine sulfate**
Atrial fibrillation/flutter/PVST/WPW
Adult: PO 200 mg q6-8hr × 5-8 doses; may increase daily until sinus rhythm is restored; max 4 g/day given only after digitalization; maintenance 200-300 mg tid-qid or 300-600 mg q8-12hr (EXT REL)

Hiccups (unlabeled)
Adult: PO 200 mg qid

>> **QuiNIDine gluconate**
Adult: PO 324-648 mg q8-12hr (EXT REL); IM 600 mg, then 400 mg q2hr; **IV** give 16 mg/min

Available forms: Gluconate: ext rel tabs 324, 330 mg; inj gluconate 80 mg/ml; **sulfate:** tabs 200, 300 mg; ext rel tabs 300 mg

Implementation
• Give AV node blocker (digoxin) before starting quiNIDine to avoid increased ventricular rate
PO route
• Do not break, crush, or chew ext rel tab
• Give on an empty stomach with a full glass of water; may be given with meals if GI irritation occurs, absorption will be decreased
• Ext rel forms not interchangeable
• Tab may be crushed and mixed with fluid or foods for patients with swallowing difficulties
IM route
• Give IM injection in deltoid, aspirate to avoid intravascular administration

> **Intermittent IV infusion route**
> • Give after diluting 800 mg/50 ml or more D$_5$W (16 mg/ml); give max 0.25 mg/kg/min, quiNIDine is absorbed by PVC tubing, minimize length; use inf pump

Y-site compatibilities: Alfentanil, amikacin, anidulafungin, argatroban, arsenic trioxide ascorbic acid, asparaginase, atenolol, atracurium, atropine, benztropine, bleomycin, bumetanide, buprenorphine, butorphanol, calcium gluconate, caspofungin, chlorproMAZINE,

cimetidine, CISplatin, cyanocobalamin, cycloSPORINE, DACTINomycin, digoxin, diltiazem, diphenhydrAMINE, DOBUTamine, DOCEtaxel, DOPamine, doxycycline, enalaprilat, ePHEDrine, EPINEPHrine, epoetin alfa, erythromycin, esmolol, etoposide, famotidine, fenoldopam, fentaNYL, fluconazole, fludarabine, gatifloxacin, gemcitabine, gentamicin, glycopyrrolate, granisetron, HYDROmorphone, IDArubicin, imipenem-cilastatin, irinotecan, isoproterenol, labetalol, lidocaine, linezolid, LORazepam, magnesium sulfate, mannitol, mechlorethamine, meperidine, metaraminol, methoxamine, methyldopate, metoclopramide, metoprolol, metroNIDAZOLE, miconazole, milrinone, mitoXANtrone, morphine, multiple vitamins, mycophenolate, nalbuphine, naloxone, nesiritide, netilmicin, nitroglycerin, norepinephrine, octreotide, ondansetron, oxaliplatin, PACLitaxel, palonosetron, pamidronate, pancuronium, papaverine, pentamidine, pentazocine, phenylephrine, phytonadione, polymyxin B, potassium chloride, procainamide, prochlorperazine, promethazine, propranolol, protamine, pyridoxine, ranitidine, ritodrine, succinylcholine, SUFentanil, tacrolimus, teniposide, theophylline, thiamine, thiotepa, tirofiban, tobramycin, tolazoline, trimetaphan, urokinase, vancomycin, vasopressin, verapamil, vinorelbine, voriconazole, zoledronic acid

ADVERSE EFFECTS
CNS: *Headache, dizziness,* involuntary movement, confusion, psychosis, restlessness, irritability, syncope, excitement, depression, ataxia
CV: **Hypotension,** *bradycardia, PVCs,* **heart block, cardiovascular collapse, arrest, torsades de pointes,** widening QRS complex, **ventricular tachycardia**
GI: Nausea, vomiting, anorexia, *diarrhea,* **hepatotoxicity,** abdominal pain
HEMA: **Thrombocytopenia, hemolytic anemia, agranulocytosis,** hypoprothrombinemia
INTEG: Rash, urticaria, **angioedema,** swelling, photosensitivity, flushing with severe pruritus
RESP: Dyspnea, **respiratory depression**

Pharmacokinetics
Absorption	Well absorbed (PO, IM), slowly absorbed (sus rel)
Distribution	Widely distributed, crosses placenta, protein binding 80%-90%
Metabolism	Liver
Excretion	Kidney unchanged, 10%-50% breast milk
Half-life	6-7 hr (prolonged in geriatrics, cirrhosis, CHF)

Pharmacodynamics

	PO (SULFATE)	(SULFATE ER)	(GLUCONATE PO)	IM	IV
Onset	½ hr			½ hr	5 min
Peak	1-6 hr	4 hr	3-4 hr	½-1½ hr	Unknown
Duration	6-8 hr	8-12 hr	6-8 hr	6-8 hr	6-8 hr

INTERACTIONS
Individual drugs
Amiodarone, cimetidine, NIFEdipine: increased quiNIDine level

Digoxin: increased digoxin level

NIFEdipine, sodium bicarbonate, verapamil: increased quiNIDine effect

Phenytoin, rifampin, sucralfate: decreased effects of quiNIDine

Propranolol: increased effect of propranolol

Reserpine: increased cardiac depression

Warfarin: increased levels of warfarin

Drug classifications
Antacids, carbonic anhydrase inhibitors, hydroxide suspensions: increased effects of quiNIDine

Anticholinergic blockers: increased vagolytic effects

Anticoagulants (oral): increased levels of anticoagulant

Antidepressants (tricyclics): increased effect of antidepressant

Antidysrhythmics: increased cardiac depression

Barbiturates, cholinergics: decreased effects of quiNIDine

Neuromuscular blockers: increased neuromuscular blocking

Phenothiazines: increased cardiac depression

Drug/herb
Hawthorn: increased quiNIDine effect, licorice

Drug/food
Grapefruit juice: decreased absorption, decreased metabolism

Drug/lab test
Increased: CPK

Interference: triamterene therapy interferes with quiNIDine test levels

Decrease: platelets, Hgb, granulocytes

NURSING CONSIDERATIONS
Assessment
• Monitor ECG continuously to determine product effectiveness, measure PR, QRS, QT intervals, check for PVCs, other dysrhythmias; monitor B/P continuously for hypo/hypertension; for rebound hypertension after 1-2 hr; check for dehydration or hypovolemia

• Monitor blood levels (therapeutic level 2-7 mcg/ml)

• Monitor I&O ratio, electrolytes (potassium, sodium, chloride); check weight daily; check for signs of CHF or pulmonary toxicity: dyspnea, fatigue, cough, fever, chest pain; if these occur, product should be discontinued

• Monitor liver function tests: AST, ALT, bilirubin, alkaline phosphatase

• Assess for CNS symptoms: confusion, psychosis, numbness, depression, involuntary movements; if these occur, product should be discontinued

• **Monitor cardiac rate, respiration: rate, rhythm, character, chest pain; watch for ventricular tachycardia, supraventricular tachycardia, or fibrillation that indicates toxicity**

Patient/family education
• Instruct patient to report adverse effects immediately to prescriber

• Instruct patient to complete follow-up appointments with health care provider including pulmonary function tests, chest x-ray, ophth and otoscopic exams

• Avoid grapefruit

Evaluation
Positive therapeutic outcome
• Resolution of dysrhythmias

RABEprazole (Rx)

(rab-ee-pray'zole)

Aciphex, Aciphex Sprinkle, Pariet ✦

Func. class.: Proton pump inhibitor

Chem. class.: Benzimidazole

Pregnancy category C

Do not confuse: Aciphex/Aricept/Accupril
RABEprazole/ARIPiprazole

ACTION: Suppresses gastric secretion by inhibiting hydrogen/potassium ATPase enzyme system in the gastric parietal cell; characterized as a gastric acid pump inhibitor, since it blocks the final step of acid production

Therapeutic outcome: Absence of duodenal ulcers; decreased gastroesophageal reflux

USES: Gastroesophageal reflux disease (GERD), severe erosive esophagitis, poorly responsive systemic GERD, pathologic hypersecretory conditions (Zollinger-Ellison syndrome, systemic mastocytosis, multiple endocrine adenomas); treatment of duodenal ulcers with or without antiinfectives for *Helicobacter pylori;* daytime, nighttime heartburn

CONTRAINDICATIONS

Hypersensitivity to this product or proton pump inhibitors (PPIs)

Precautions: Pregnancy **C**, breastfeeding, children, Asian patients, diarrhea, geriatric patients, gastric cancer, hepatic/GI disease, IBS, osteoporosis, pseudomembranous colitis, ulcerative colitis, vit B_{12} deficiency

DOSAGE AND ROUTES
Healing of duodenal ulcers
Adult: PO 20 mg/day × ≤4 wk, to be taken after breakfast

Erosive esophagitis/GERD
Adult: PO 20 mg/day × 4-8 wk; maintenance 20 mg qday

Adolescent and child ≥12 yr: PO 20 mg/day up to 8 wk, may use an additional course

Child 1-11 yr (≥ 15 kg): PO (sprinkle) 10 mg qday up to 12 wk; (<15 kg) 5 mg qday up to 12 wk; may increase to 10 mg qday if needed

H. pylori eradication
Adult: PO 20 mg bid × 7 days with amoxicillin 1 g bid × 7 days with clarithromycin 500 mg bid × 7 days

Pathologic hypersecretory conditions
Adult: PO 60 mg/day; may increase to 120 mg in 2 divided doses

Available forms: Del rel tabs 20 mg; delayed release caps 5, 10 mg

Implementation
PO route
- Do not break, crush, or chew del rel tab
- Give after breakfast daily with a full glass of water, without regard to food

ADVERSE EFFECTS

CNS: *Headache, dizziness, asthenia*

CV: Chest pain, angina, tachycardia, bradycardia, palpitations, peripheral edema

EENT: Tinnitus, taste perversion

GI: *Diarrhea, abdominal pain, vomiting, nausea, constipation, flatulence, acid regurgitation,* abdominal swelling, anorexia, irritable colon, esophageal candidiasis, dry mouth; **pseudomembranous colitis (rare)**

GU: UTI, frequency, increased creatinine, **proteinuria, hematuria,** testicular pain, glycosuria

HEMA: **Pancytopenia, thrombocytopenia, neutropenia, leukocytosis,** anemia

INTEG: Rash, dry skin, urticaria, pruritus, alopecia

META: Hypoglycemia, increased hepatic enzymes, weight gain

MISC: *Back pain,* fever, fatigue, malaise, **Stevens-Johnson syndrome**

RESP: *Upper respiratory tract infections, cough,* epistaxis, **pneumonia**

Pharmacokinetics

Absorption	Unknown
Distribution	Protein binding 96.3%
Metabolism	Liver, extensively by CYP2C19
Excretion	Kidneys, feces, metabolites
Half-life	1-2 hr

Pharmacodynamics

Unknown

INTERACTIONS
Individual drugs
Digoxin, nelfinavir/omeprazole: increased levels

Ketoconazole, itraconazole, iron salts, atazanavir/ritonavir, ampicillin: decreased levels

Calcium carbonate, sucralfate, vitamin B_{12}: decreased rabeprazole levels

Clarithromycin, phenytoin: increased levels of rabeprazole

Warfarin, clopidogrel: increased bleeding risk

Drug classifications
Benzodiazepines, antacids, other proton pump inhibitors, H_2 blockers: increased levels of rabeprazole

Drug/herb
St. John's wort: decreased levels of rabeprazole

R

Drug/lab test
Decreased: magnesium

NURSING CONSIDERATIONS
Assessment
• Assess GI system: bowel sounds q8hr, abdomen for pain and swelling, anorexia

⚠ **Pseudomembranous colitis: may occur with most antibiotic therapy; assess for watery diarrhea, abdominal pain, fever**

• **Vitamin B12 deficiency/cyanocobalamin/ hypomagnesemia:** may occur after 3-12 mo of treatment; use magnesium, vit B₁₂, cyanocobalamin supplement, if severe, discontinuing of product may be needed
• Monitor hepatic enzymes: AST, ALT, increased alkaline phosphatase during treatment
• **Serious skin reactions: assess for Stevens-Johnson syndrome**
• **Blood dyscrasias (rare): CBC with differential before and periodically during treatment**
• Obtain susceptibility testing if *H. pylori* treatment is ineffective; another antiinfective may be needed

Patient/family education
• Advise patient to report severe diarrhea; product may have to be discontinued
• Advise patient to notify prescriber if pregnancy is planned or suspected
• Teach patient to report diarrhea, black, tarry stools, product may need to be discontinued
• Inform diabetic patient that hypoglycemia can occur
• Caution patient to avoid driving and other hazardous activities until response to product is known, take delayed release tab whole, do not cut, break; that cap should be opened and sprinkled on food (applesauce)
• Caution patient to avoid alcohol, salicylates, NSAIDs; may cause GI irritation
• Advise patient to wear sunscreen, protective clothing to prevent burns

Evaluation
Positive therapeutic outcome
• Absence of epigastric pain, swelling, fullness; decreased symptoms of GERD after 4-8 wk

raloxifene (Rx)
(ral-ox′ih-feen)
Evista
Func. class.: Bone resorption inhibitor
Chem. class.: Hormone modifier, selective estrogen receptor modulator (SERM)
Pregnancy category X

ACTION: Tissue-selective estrogen agonist/ antagonist; agonist activity in bone and lipid metabolism, antagonistic activity on breast and uterus, reduces resorption of bone and decreases bone turnover

Therapeutic outcome: Absence or decrease of osteoporosis in postmenopausal women

USES: Prevention, treatment of osteoporosis in postmenopausal women, breast cancer prophylaxis in postmenopausal women with osteoporosis or in postmenopausal women at high risk for developing the disease

CONTRAINDICATIONS
Pregnancy **X**, breastfeeding, hypersensitivity

> **BLACK BOX WARNING:** Women with active or history of venous thromboembolic events

Precautions: Hepatic/CV disease, cervical/ uterine cancer, elevated triglycerides, pulmonary embolism

> **BLACK BOX WARNING:** Stroke

DOSAGE AND ROUTES
Hormone replacement
Postmenopausal women: PO 60 mg/day, max 60 mg/day

Available forms: Tabs 60 mg

Implementation
• Administer without regard to meals
• Add calcium supplement, vit D if lacking
• Do not use during prolonged bed rest

ADVERSE EFFECTS
CNS: Insomnia, depression, migraines
CV: Hot flashes, peripheral edema, **thromboembolism, stroke**
EENT: Retinal vein occlusion (rare)
GI: *Nausea,* vomiting, diarrhea, dyspepsia, abdominal pain
GU: Vaginitis, leukorrhea, *hot flashes,* cystitis, vaginal bleeding
INTEG: Rash, sweating
META: Weight gain, peripheral edema
MS: Arthralgia, myalgia, *leg cramps,* arthritis
RESP: Sinusitis, pharyngitis, increased cough, pneumonia, laryngitis, rhinitis, bronchitis, pulmonary embolism, flulike symptoms

Pharmacokinetics

Absorption	Unknown
Distribution	Highly protein bound
Metabolism	Unknown
Excretion	Feces, breast milk
Half-life	28-32 hr (elimination)

Pharmacodynamics

Onset	Unknown
Peak	Unknown
Duration	24 hr

INTERACTIONS
Individual drugs
Ampicillin, cholestyramine: decreased action of raloxifene

Desiccated thyroid, levothyroxine, liotrix: decreased action

Drug classifications
Anticoagulants: decreased action of anticoagulants

Highly protein-bound products, systemic estrogens: administer cautiously ibuprofen, diazepam, naprosen

Drug/food
Soy: decreased effect of raloxifene

Drug/lab test
Increased: apolipoprotein, corticosteroid-binding globulin, thyroxine-binding globulin (TBG)

Decreased: lipoprotein, LDL cholesterol, total cholesterol, calcium, total protein, albumin

NURSING CONSIDERATIONS
Assessment

> **BLACK BOX WARNING:** For history of stroke, TIA, thrombosis, atrial fibrillation, hypertension, smoking; venous thrombosis may occur; avoid prolonged sitting, discontinue 3 days before surgery or other immobilization

• Obtain bone density test baseline, periodically throughout treatment; bone-specific alkaline phosphatase; osteocalcin, collagen breakdown
• Monitor B/P q4hr, watch for increase caused by H_2O and sodium retention

Patient/family education

> **BLACK BOX WARNING:** Teach patients to discontinue product 72 hr before prolonged bedrest, to report possible blood clots immediately, usually during first few months of therapy

• Advise patient to avoid maintaining one position for long periods
• Advise patient to take calcium supplements, vit D if intake is inadequate
• Advise patient to increase exercise using weights
• Advise patient to stop smoking and to decrease alcohol consumption
• Inform patient that this product does not help control hot flashes
• Instruct patient to report fever, acute migraine, insomnia, emotional distress, UTI, or vaginal itching

• Provide product package insert and discuss with patient

> **BLACK BOX WARNING:** Teach patient to report swelling, warmth, or pain in calves

Evaluation
Positive therapeutic outcome
• Prevention, treatment of osteoporosis

raltegravir (Rx)
(ral-teg′ra-vir)
Isentress
Func. class.: Antiretroviral
Chem. class.: HIV integrase strand transfer inhibitor (ISTIs)
Pregnancy category C

ACTION: Inhibits catalytic activity of HIV integrase, which is an HIV-encoded enzyme needed for replication

Therapeutic outcome: Improvement in CD4, T-cell counts

USES: HIV in combination with other antiretrovirals

CONTRAINDICATIONS
Hypersensitivity, breastfeeding

Precautions: Pregnancy C, children, geriatric, hepatic disease, immune reconstitution syndrome, hepatitis, antimicrobial resistance, lactase deficiency

DOSAGE AND ROUTES
Adult and adolescent ≥16 yr: PO 400 mg bid, if using with rifampin give 800 mg bid

Available forms: Tabs 400 mg; chew tabs 25, 100 mg; granules for oral suspension 100 mg

Implementation
PO route
• Do not break, crush, or chew tabs
• May give without regard to meals, with 8 oz of water
• Store at room temperature
Oral suspension
• Open foil; use 5 ml of water in provided measuring cup; close, then swirl; don't turn upside down; use oral syringe to administer; use within 30 min; discard any remaining suspension

ADVERSE EFFECTS
CNS: *Fatigue,* fever, *dizziness, headache,* asthenia, **suicidal ideation**
CV: **MI**
GI: *Nausea,* vomiting, diarrhea, abdominal pain, gastritis, **hepatitis**

GU: Oliguria, proteinuria, hematuria, glomerulonephritis, acute renal failure, renal tubular necrosis
HEMA: Anemia, neutropenia
INTEG: Rash, urticaria, pruritus, pain or phlebitis at IV site, unusual sweating, alopecia
META: Hyperamylasia, hyperglycemia
MS: Myopathy, rhabdomyolysis
SYST: Immune reconstitution syndrome

Pharmacokinetics

Absorption	Max 3 hr if taken on empty stomach
Distribution	Unknown
Metabolism	Liver by uridine diphosphate glucuronosyltransferase (UGT A1A enzyme system)
Excretion	51% feces, 32% urine
Half-life	Terminal 9 hr

Pharmacodynamics

Unknown

INTERACTIONS
Individual drugs
Rifampin, efavirenz, tenofovir, tipranavir/ritonavir: decreased raltegravir levels

Drug classifications
Fibric acid derivatives, HMG-CoA reductase inhibitors: increased rhabdomyolysis, myopathy, elevated CPK
H_2 blockers, protein pump inhibitors, UGT1A1 inhibitors (atazanavir): increased raltegravir effect

Drug/lab test
Increased: total/HDL/LDL cholesterol

NURSING CONSIDERATIONS
Assessment
• **Rhabdomyolysis: Assess for calf pain, increased CPK; product should be discontinued**
• **HIV infection:** monitor CD4, T-cell count, plasma HIV RNA, viral load; resistance testing prior to therapy and at treatment failure
⚠ **Suicidal thoughts, behavior: monitor for depression, more common in those with mental illness**
⚠ **Immune reconstitution syndrome: usually during initial phase of treatment, may give antiinfective before starting**
• Monitor total HDL/LDL cholesterol baseline and periodically; all may be elevated
• Assess skin eruptions: rash, urticaria, itching

Patient/family education
• Teach patient to take as prescribed; if dose is missed, take as soon as remembered up to 1 hr

before next dose; do not double dose, do not share with others
• Teach patient that sexual partners need to be told that patient has HIV
• Advise patient that product does not cure infection, just controls symptoms, does not prevent infecting others
⚠ **Teach patient to report sore throat, fever, fatigue (may indicate superinfection)**
• Advise patient that product must be taken in equal intervals 2×/day to maintain blood levels for duration of therapy
• **Advise patient to notify prescriber immediately of suicidal thoughts, behavior**
• Advise patient to notify prescriber if pregnancy is planned or suspected, avoid breastfeeding

Evaluation
Positive therapeutic outcome
• Improvement in CD4, T-cell counts

⚠ HIGH ALERT
ramelteon (Rx)
(rah-mel′tee-on)
Rozerem
Func. class.: Sedative-hypnotic, anti-anxiety
Chem. class.: Melatonin receptor agonist
Pregnancy category C

ACTION: Binds selectively to melatonin receptors (MT_1, MT_2); thought to be involved in circadian rhythm and the normal sleep-wake cycle

Therapeutic outcome: Ability to fall asleep easily and decrease early-morning awakenings

USES: Insomnia (difficulty with sleep onset)

CONTRAINDICATIONS
Breastfeeding, infants, children, hypersensitivity

Precautions: Pregnancy C, hepatic disease, alcoholism, seizure disorder, sleep apnea, suicidal ideation, angioedema, depression, sleep-related behavior (sleepwalking), schizophrenia, bipolar disorder, alcohol intoxication, hepatic encephalopathy, aortic stenosis

DOSAGE AND ROUTES
Adult: PO 8 mg within 30 min of bedtime

Hepatic dose
Do not use in severe hepatic disease; use with caution in mild to moderate hepatic disease

Available forms: Tabs 8 mg

Implementation
- Give within 30 min of bedtime for sleepless-ness, give on empty stomach for fast onset
- Store in tight container in cool environment
- Do not break tabs, swallow whole

ADVERSE EFFECTS
CNS: *Dizziness, somnolence, fatigue, head-ache, insomnia, depression,* complex sleep-re-lated reactions: sleep driving, sleep eating, **sui-cidal thoughts/behavior,** syncope
GI: *Nausea, diarrhea,* dysgeusia, *vomiting*
MISC: Myalgia, arthralgia, decreased blood cortisol, influenza, upper respiratory tract infec-tion
SYST: **Severe allergic reactions, angio-edema**

Pharmacokinetics

Absorption	Rapidly absorbed
Distribution	Protein binding 82%
Metabolism	Rapid first-pass metabolism, liver
Excretion	84% urine, 4% feces
Half-life	2-5 hr metabolite

Pharmacodynamics

Onset	Unknown
Peak	½-1 ½ hr
Duration	Unknown

INTERACTIONS
Individual drugs
Alcohol, ciprofloxacin, fluconazole, fluvox-aMINE, ketoconazole: increased ramelteon effect, toxicity
Rifampin: decreased effect of ramelteon

Drug classifications
Antiretroviral protease inhibitors: possible toxicity
Anxiolytics, azole antifungals, barbiturates, CYP1A2 inhibitors, strong CYP2C9 inhibi-tors, strong CYP3A4 inhibitors hypnotics, sedatives: increased ramelteon effect, toxicity
Strong CYP inducers: decreased ramelteon effect
Potassium-sparing diuretics, potassium supple-ment, angiotensin II receptor agonists: in-creased hyperkalemia

Drug/food
High-fat/heavy meal: prolonged absorption, sleep onset reduced

Drug/lab test
Increased: protein level
Decreased: testosterone level

NURSING CONSIDERATIONS
Assessment
- **Sleep characteristics:** assess type of sleep problem: falling asleep, staying asleep; complex sleep disorders (sleep walking/driving/eating) after taking product
- Assess mental status: mood, sensorium, affect, memory (long, short), **suicidal thoughts/ behaviors**
- **Severe hypersensitivity reactions: Assess for angioedema (facial swelling); discon-tinue product; notify prescriber immediately**

Patient/family education
- Advise patient to avoid driving or other activities requiring alertness until product is stabilized; drowsiness may continue the next day
- Advise patient to avoid alcohol ingestion or CNS depressants
- Teach patient alternative measures to improve sleep: reading, exercise several hr before bed-time, warm bath, warm milk, TV, self-hypnosis, deep breathing
- Teach patient to report if pregnancy is planned or suspected (C), avoid breastfeeding
- Advise patient to take immediately before going to bed
- Advise patient not to ingest a high-fat/heavy meal before taking
- **Teach patient to report cessation of menses, galactorrhea (women), decreased libido, infertility, worsening of insomnia, behavioral changes, suicidal thoughts/ behavior**
- Med guide should be given to patient and reviewed

Evaluation
Positive therapeutic outcome
- Ability to sleep at night, decreased amount of early-morning awakening

ramipril (Rx)
(ra-mi′pril)
Altace
Func. class.: Antihypertensive
Chem. class.: Angiotensin-converting en-zyme (ACE) inhibitor
Pregnancy category D

Do not confuse: ramipril/enalapril, Altace/alteplase

ACTION: Selectively suppresses renin-an-giotensin-aldosterone system; inhibits ACE; pre-vents conversion of angiotensin I to angiotensin II; results in dilatation of arterial, venous vessels

Therapeutic outcome: Decreased B/P in hypertension

USES: Hypertension, alone or in combination with thiazide diuretics; CHF (after MI), reduction in risk of MI, stroke, death from CV disorders

CONTRAINDICATIONS
Breastfeeding, children, hypersensitivity to ACE inhibitors, history of ACE inhibitor–induced angioedema

> **BLACK BOX WARNING:** Pregnancy **D** (2nd/3rd trimesters)

Precautions: Impaired renal/liver function, dialysis patients, hypovolemia, blood dyscrasias, COPD, CHF, asthma, geriatric, renal artery stenosis, cough, African descent

DOSAGE AND ROUTES
Hypertension
Adult: PO 2.5 mg/day initially, then 2.5-20 mg/day divided bid or daily

CHF/Post MI
Adult: PO 1.25-2.5 mg bid, may increase to 5 mg bid

Reduction in risk of MI, stroke, death
Adult: PO 2.5 mg/day × 7 days, then 5 mg/day × 21 days, then may increase to 10 mg/day

Renal impairment
Adult: PO CCr <40 ml/min; reduce by 50%, titrate upward to max 5 mg/day

Available forms: Caps 1.25, 2.5, 5, 10 mg; tabs 1.25, 2.5, 5, 10 mg

Implementation
• Caps may be opened and added to food, mixture is stable for 24 hr at room temperature, 48 hr refrigerated
• Store in airtight container at 86° F (30° C) or less

ADVERSE EFFECTS
CNS: *Headache, dizziness,* anxiety, insomnia, paresthesia, fatigue, depression, malaise, vertigo
CV: *Hypotension,* chest pain, palpitations, angina, syncope, **dysrhythmia, heart failure, MI**
EENT: Hearing loss
GI: Nausea, constipation, vomiting, dyspepsia, dysphagia, anorexia, diarrhea, abdominal pain, **hepatitis, hepatic failure, pancreatitis, hepatic necrosis**
GU: Proteinuria, increased BUN, creatinine, impotence
HEMA: Decreased Hct, Hgb, **eosinophilia, leukopenia, pancytopenia, thrombocytopenia, agranulocytosis (rare)**
INTEG: Rash, sweating, photosensitivity, pruritus

META: *Hyperkalemia,* hyperglycemia
MISC: **Angioedema, toxic epidermal necrolysis, anaphylaxis, Stevens-Johnson syndrome**
MS: Arthralgia, arthritis, myalgia
RESP: Cough, dyspnea

Pharmacokinetics
Absorption	Well absorbed
Distribution	Not known, crosses placenta
Metabolism	Liver, extensively; protein binding 73%
Excretion	Urine
Half-life	Ramipril (5 hr), ramiprilat (13-17 hr)

Pharmacodynamics
Onset	½-1 hr
Peak	1-3 hr
Duration	24-72 hr

INTERACTIONS
Individual drugs
Do not use with aliskiren in moderate-severe renal disease
Alcohol: increased hypotension (large amounts)
Lithium: increased serum levels
HydrALAZINE, prazocin: increased toxicity
Indomethacin: decreased antihypertensive effect

Drug classifications
Adrenergic blockers, antihypertensives, diuretics, ganglionic blockers, nitrates: increased hypotension
Antacids: decreased absorption
Diuretics (potassium sparing), potassium supplements, sympathomimetics, vasodilators: increased toxicity
NSAIDs, salicylates: decreased antihypertensive effect

Drug/food
Potassium salt substitutes: increased hyperkalemia, avoid use

Drug/herb
Hawthorn: increased antihypertensive effect
Ephedra: decreased antihypertensive effect

Drug/lab test
Increased: LFTs, BUN, creatinine, glucose, potassium
Decreased: RBC, Hgb, platelets

NURSING CONSIDERATIONS
Assessment
• **Monitor blood tests: neutrophils, decreased platelets; WBC with differential baseline, periodically q3mo; if neutrophils are <1000/mm³, discontinue treatment**
• **Hypertension:** Monitor B/P baseline and regularly, check for orthostatic hypotension,

---

syncope; if changes occur, dosage may need to be changed

• **Renal disease: Monitor renal function tests: protein, BUN, creatinine, potassium, sodium; watch for increased levels that may indicate nephrotic syndrome and renal failure; monitor renal symptoms: polyuria, oliguria, frequency, dysuria; establish baselines in renal, liver function tests before therapy begins and monitor periodically; liver function tests, uric acid, and glucose may be increased**

• Check potassium levels throughout treatment, hyperkalemia occurs

• **CHF:** check for edema in feet, legs daily, weight daily

• **Allergic reactions: angioedema, Stevens-Johnson syndrome; rash, fever, pruritus, urticaria; product should be discontinued if antihistamines fail to help**

• Monitor electrolytes baseline and periodically, potassium may be increased

Patient/family education

• Caution patient not to discontinue product abruptly; advise patient to tell all persons associated with care

• Teach patient not to use OTC products (cough, cold, allergy) unless directed by physician; serious side effects can occur; xanthines such as coffee, tea, chocolate, cola can prevent action of product

• Instruct patient on the importance of complying with dosage schedule, even if feeling better; to continue with medical regimen to decrease B/P: exercise, cessation of smoking, decreasing stress, diet modifications

• Emphasize the need to rise slowly to sitting or standing position to minimize orthostatic hypotension; not to exercise in hot weather because increased hypotension can occur

• **Teach patient to notify prescriber of mouth sores, sore throat, fever, swelling of hands or feet, irregular heartbeat, chest pain, coughing, shortness of breath**

• Caution patient to report excessive perspiration, dehydration, vomiting, diarrhea; may lead to fall in B/P, maintain hydration

• Caution patient that product may cause dizziness, fainting, light-headedness; may occur during 1st few days of therapy; to avoid activities that may be hazardous

• Teach patient how to take B/P, and normal readings for age group

> **BLACK BOX WARNING:** Inform prescriber if pregnancy is planned or suspected, pregnancy **D,** do not breastfeed

Evaluation

Positive therapeutic outcome
• Decreased B/P in hypertension

TREATMENT OF OVERDOSE:
0.9% NaCl **IV** inf, hemodialysis

ranibizumab (Rx)
(ran-ih-biz′oo-mab)
Lucentis
Func. class.: Ophthalmic
Chem. class.: Selective vascular endothelial growth factor antagonist
Pregnancy category C

ACTION: Binds to receptor-binding site of active forms of vascular endothelial growth factor A (VEGF-A) that causes angiogenesis and cell proliferation

Therapeutic outcome: Prevention of increasing neovascular macular degeneration

USES: Macular degeneration (neovascular) (wet), macular edema after retinal vein occlusion (RVO)

CONTRAINDICATIONS
Hypersensitivity, ocular infections

Precautions: Pregnancy **C,** breastfeeding, children, retinal detachment, increased intraocular pressure

DOSAGE AND ROUTES
Adult: Intravitreal 0.3 mg (0.05 ml) of 10 mg/ml q28 days or 0.5 mg qmonth × 4 months, then 0.5 mg q3mo

Available forms: Sol for inj 6 mg/ml, 10 mg/ml

Implementation
• Given by ophthalmologist via intravitreal injection using adequate anesthesia; use 19-gauge filter
• Store in refrigerator; do not freeze
• Protect from light

ADVERSE EFFECTS
CNS: Dizziness, headache, peripheral neuropathy
EENT: Blepharitis, cataract, conjunctival hemorrhage/hyperemia, detachment of the retinal pigment epithelium, dryness/irritation/pain in the eye, visual impairment, vitreous floaters, ocular infection
GI: Constipation, nausea
MISC: Hypertension, UTI, **thromboembolism, non-ocular bleeding,** anemia, arthralgia
RESP: Bronchitis, cough, sinusitis, URI
INTEG: Impaired wound healing

R

Adverse effects: *italics* = common; **bold** = life-threatening

Pharmacokinetics

Absorption	Minimal
Distribution	None
Metabolism	None
Excretion	Elimination 9 days
Half-life	Unknown

Pharmacodynamics

Onset	Unknown
Peak	1 day
Duration	Unknown

INTERACTIONS
Individual drugs
Verteporfin photodynamic therapy (PDT): increased severe inflammation

NURSING CONSIDERATIONS
Assessment
• Assess for eye changes: redness, sensitivity to light, vision change, intraocular pressure change; report to ophthalmologist immediately, complete procedure with anesthesia and antibiotic prior to use, check perfusion of optic nerve after use

Patient/family education
• Teach patient that if eye becomes red, sensitive to light, or painful or if there is a change in vision, seek immediate care from ophthalmologist
• Teach patient reason for treatment, expected results
• **Hypersensitivity: monitor for inflammation**

Evaluation
Positive therapeutic outcome
• Prevention of increasing neovascular macular degeneration

---

ranitidine (Rx)
(ra-nit'i-deen)
Acid Reducer ❋, Nu-Ranit ❋, Zantac, Zantac-C ❋, Zantac EFFER-dose
Func. class.: H₂ histamine receptor antagonist
Pregnancy category B

Do not confuse: ranitidine/amantadine/rimantadine, **Zantac**/Xanax/Zofran/ZyrTEC

ACTION: Inhibits histamine at H_2 receptor site in the gastric parietal cells, which inhibits gastric acid secretion

Therapeutic outcome: Healing of duodenal ulcers or gastric ulcers; prevention of duodenal ulcers; decreased symptoms of gastroesophageal reflux disease (GERD), Zollinger-Ellison syndrome, or heartburn

USES: Short-term treatment of duodenal and gastric ulcers and maintenance; management of GERD, Zollinger-Ellison syndrome, active duodenal ulcers with *Helicobacter pylori* in combination with clarithromycin, hypersecretory conditions, stress ulcers, erosive esophagitis (maintenance), systemic mastocytosis, multiple endocrine adenoma syndrome, heartburn

Unlabeled uses: Prevention of aspiration pneumonitis, upper GI bleeding

CONTRAINDICATIONS
Hypersensitivity

Precautions: Pregnancy **B**, breastfeeding, child <12 yr, renal/hepatic disease

DOSAGE AND ROUTES
Erosive esophagitis
Adult: PO 150 mg qid for up to 12 wk
Child ≥1 mo: PO 5-10 mg/kg/day in 2-3 divided doses

Duodenal ulcer
Adult: PO 150 mg bid or 300 mg/day after PM meal or at bedtime, maintenance 150 mg at bedtime
Infant and child: PO 2-4 mg/kg bid, max 300 mg/day

Zollinger-Ellison syndrome
Adult: PO 150 mg bid, may increase if needed

Gastric ulcer
Adult: PO 150 mg bid × 6 wk, then 150 mg at bedtime
Infant/child: PO 2-4 mg/kg bid, max 300 mg/day

GERD
Adult: PO 150 mg bid

Renal dose
Adult: CCr <50 ml/min give 50% of dose or extend dosing interval

Available forms: Tab 75, 150, 300 mg; sol for inj 25 mg/ml; caps 150, 300 mg; syrup 15 mg/ml

Implementation
• Store at room temp
PO route
• May be given with or without meals
• Give antacids 1 hr before or 1 hr after this product
IM route
• No dilution needed; inject in large muscle mass, aspirate

IV direct route
- Dilute to max 2.5 mg/ml (50 mg/20 ml) using 0.9% NaCl (nonpreserved) or D$_5$W, give dose over ≥5 min (max 4 mg/ml)

Intermittent IV INF route
- Dilute to max 0.5 mg/ml with D$_5$W, 0.9% NaCl, give over 15-20 min (5-7 ml/min); premixed ready-to-use bags as 1 mg/ml (50 mg/50 ml), inf over 15-20 min

Continuous 24 hr IV INF route
- **Adult:** dilute 150 mg/250 ml of D$_5$W or 0.9% NaCl, run over 24 hr (6.25 mg/hr or as directed); use inf device and use within 48 hr; *Zollinger-Ellison:* dilute in D$_5$W or 0.9% NaCl, max concentration 2.5 mg/ml, use inf device

Y-site compatibilities: Acyclovir, aldesleukin, alemtuzumab, alfentanil, allopurinol, amifostine, amikacin, aminophylline, amphotericin B liposome, amsacrine, anikinra, anidulafungin, ascorbic acid, atracurium, atropine, aztreonam, bivalirudin, bumetanide, buprenorphine, butorphanol, calcium chloride/gluconate, CARBOplatin, ceFAZolin, cefepime, cefonicid, cefoperazone, cefotaxime, cefoTEtan, cefOXitin, cefTAZidime, ceftizoxime, cefTRIAXone, cefuroxime, chloramphenicol, chlorproMAZINE, cimetidine, ciprofloxacin, cisatracurium, CISplatin, clindamycin, cyanocobalamin, cyclophosphamide, cycloSPORINE, cytarabine, DACTINomycin, DAPTOmycin, dexamethasone, dexmedetomidine, digoxin, diltiazem, DOBUTamine, DOCEtaxel, DOPamine, doripenem, doxacurium, doxapram, DOXOrubicin, DOXOrubicin liposome, doxycycline, enalaprilat, ePHEDrine, EPINEPHrine, epirubicin, epoetin alfa, ertapenem, erythromycin, esmolol, etoposide, etoposide phosphate, famotidine, fenoldopam, fentaNYL, filgrastim, fluconazole, fludarabine, fluorouracil, folic acid, foscarnet, furosemide, ganciclovir, gemcitabine, gentamicin, glycopyrrolate, granisetron, heparin, hydrocortisone, HYDROmorphone, IDArubicin, ifosfamide, imipenem/cilastatin, inamrinone, indomethacin, isoproterenol, ketorolac, labetalol, levofloxacin, lidocaine, linezolid, LORazepam, magnesium sulfate, mannitol, mechlorethamine, melphalan, meperidine, metaraminol, methotrexate, methoxamine, methyldopate, methylPREDNISolone, metoclopramide, metoprolol, metroNIDAZOLE, midazolam, milrinone, mitoXANtrone, morphine, nalbuphine, naloxone, nesiritide, niCARdipine, nitroglycerin, nitroprusside, norepinephrine, octreotide, ondansetron, oxacillin, oxaliplatin, oxytocin, PACLitaxel, palonosetron, pancuronium, papaverine, PEMEtrexed, penicillin G, pentamidine, pentazocine, PENTobarbital, PHENobarbital, phentolamine, phenylephrine, phytonadione, piperacillin/tazobactam, potassium chloride, procainamide, prochlorperazine, promethazine, propofol, propranolol, protamine, pyridoxime, remifentanil, riTUXimab, rocuronium, sargramostim, sodium acetate/bicarbonate, succinylcholine, SUFentanil, tacrolimus, teniposide, theophylline, thiamine, thiopental, thiotepa, ticarcillin/clavulanate, tigecycline, tirofiban, tobramycin, tolazoline, trastuzumab, trimetaphan, urokinase, vancomycin, vecuronium, vinCRIStine, vinorelbine, warfarin, zidovudine, zoledronic acid

Y-site incompatibilities: Amphotericin B cholesteryl, caspofungin, diazepam, diazoxide, insulin, pantoprazole, phenytoin, quinupristin/dalfopristin, trimethoprim/sulfamethoxazole

ADVERSE EFFECTS

CNS: Headache, sleeplessness, dizziness, confusion, agitation, depression; hallucinations (geriatric)

CV: *Tachycardia, bradycardia,* premature ventricular contractions

EENT: Blurred vision, increased ocular pressure

GI: Constipation, abdominal pain, diarrhea, nausea, vomiting, *hepatotoxicity*

GU: Impotence, *acute interstitial nephritis (rare)*

INTEG: Urticaria, rash, fever

RESP: *Pneumonia*

SYST: *Anaphylaxis (rare)*

Pharmacokinetics

Absorption	Well absorbed (PO, IM), completely absorbed (**IV**)
Distribution	Widely distributed, crosses placenta
Metabolism	Liver (30%)
Excretion	Kidneys unchanged (70%)
Half-life	2-3 hr, increased renal disease

Pharmacodynamics

	PO	IM/IV
Onset	Unknown	Unknown
Peak	2-3 hr	15 min
Duration	8-12 hr	8-12 hr

INTERACTIONS
Individual drugs

Adefovir, pramipexole, procainamide, trospium, triazolam, memantine, saquinavir: increased effect of each product

Diazepam, metoclopramide: decreased absorption of ranitidine

Ketoconazole: decreased effect of ketoconazole

NIFEdipine, ext rel products: increased GI obstruction risk

Procainamide: increased absorption, toxicity

Drug classifications
Anticholinergics, antacids: decreased ranitidine absorption

Anticoagulants, sulfonylureas: increased absorption, toxicity

Benzodiazepines, calcium channel blockers: increased effect of each product

Cephalosporins: decreased effects of cephalosporins

Iron salts: decreased effects of iron salts

Drug/lab test
Increased: AST, creatinine, ALT

False positive: urine protein (multistix)

NURSING CONSIDERATIONS
Assessment
• **GI complaints:** assess patient with ulcers or suspected ulcers: epigastric or abdominal pain, hematemesis, occult blood in stools, blood in gastric aspirate before, throughout treatment

• Monitor I&O ratio, BUN, creatinine, CBC with differential monthly

Patient/family education
• Caution patient that gynecomastia, impotence may occur and are reversible after treatment is discontinued

• Advise patient to avoid driving, other hazardous activities until stabilized on this medication; drowsiness or dizziness may occur

• Inform patient that smoking decreases the effectiveness of the product; that smoking cessation should be considered

• Instruct patient that product must be continued for prescribed time to be effective and taken exactly as prescribed; doses should not be doubled; a missed dose should be taken when remembered up to 1 hr before next dose

• Advise patient to report bruising, fatigue, malaise; blood dyscrasias may occur

• Inform patient to report diarrhea, black tarry stools, sore throat, rash, dizziness, confusion, or delirium to prescriber immediately

• Teach patient to take once-daily dose before bedtime

Evaluation
Positive therapeutic outcome
• Decreased pain in abdomen, heartburn
• Healing of ulcers
• Absence of gastroesophageal reflux

ranolazine (Rx)
(ruh-no'luh-zeen)
Ranexa
Func. class.: Antianginal
Pregnancy category C

ACTION: Antianginal, antiischemic; unknown, may work by inhibiting portal fatty-acid oxidation

Therapeutic outcome: Decreased anginal pain and number of episodes

USES: Chronic stable angina pectoris; use in those that have not responded to other treatment options; should be used in combination with other antianginals such as amlodipine, β-blockers, or nitrates

CONTRAINDICATIONS
Preexisting QT prolongation, hepatic disease (Child-Pugh class A, B, C), hypersensitivity, hypokalemia, renal failure, torsades de pointes, ventricular dysrhythmia, ventricular tachycardia, hepatic cirrhosis

Precautions: Pregnancy **C**, breastfeeding, children, geriatric, renal disease, hypotension, females at risk for torsades de pointes

DOSAGE AND ROUTES
Adult: PO 500 mg bid and increased to 1000 mg bid based on response; max 1000 mg bid

Available forms: Ext rel tabs 500, 1000 mg

Implementation
• **Ext rel tabs:** Do not break, crush, or chew tabs; give products as prescribed; do not double or skip dose

• Give bid, without regard to meals
• Do not use with grapefruit juice

ADVERSE EFFECTS
CNS: *Headache, dizziness,* hallucinations
CV: Palpitations, **QT prolongation,** orthostatic hypotension
EENT: Tinnitus
GI: Nausea, vomiting, constipation, dry mouth
MISC: Peripheral edema
RESP: Dyspnea

Pharmacokinetics
Absorption	Varied absorption
Distribution	Protein binding 62%
Metabolism	Liver, extensively by CYP3A, CYP2D6 (lesser)
Excretion	Urine 75%, feces 25%
Half-life	7 hr

⚠ Nurse Alert　　　✸ Key NCLEX® Drug　　　>> Drug Specifics

Pharmacodynamics

Onset	Unknown
Peak	2-5 hr
Duration	Unknown

INTERACTIONS
Individual drugs
Haloperidol, chloroquine, droperidol, pentamidine, arsenic trioxide, levomethadyl; CYP3A4 substrates (methadone, pimozide, QUEtiapine, quiNIDine, risperiDONE, ziprasidone): increased QT prolongation

Digoxin, simvastatin: increased action of digoxin, simvastatin

Diltiazem, dofetilide, ketoconazole, PARoxetine, quiNIDine, sotalol, thioridazine, verapamil, ziprasidone: increased ranolazine action

Drug classifications
Anti-retroviral protease inhibitors: increased ranolazine absorption, toxicity

Class IA/III antidysrhythmics, some phenothiazines, β-agonists, local anesthetics, tricyclics; CYP3A4 inhibitors (amiodarone, clarithromycin, erythromycin, telithromycin, troleandomycin); CYP3A4 substrates (methadone, pimozide, QUEtiapine, quiNIDine, risperiDONE, ziprasidone): increased QT prolongation

Macrolide antibiotics, protease inhibitors: increased ranolazine action

Macrolides (clarithromycin, erythromycin, troleandomycin): increased QTc interval

Drug/food
Do not use with grapefruit or grapefruit juice

NURSING CONSIDERATIONS
Assessment
• Assess cardiac status: B/P, pulse, respiration, ECG; watch for prolongation of QT
• QT prolongation: ECG for QT prolongation, ejection fraction; assess for chest pain, palpitations, dyspnea
• Angina: characteristics of pain (intensity, location, duration, alleviating/precipitating factors)

Patient/family education
• Teach patient to avoid hazardous activities until stabilized on product, dizziness is no longer a problem
• Advise patient to avoid OTC drugs, grapefruit juice, drugs prolonging QTc (quiNIDine, dofetilide, sotalol, erythromycin, thioridazine, ziprasidone or protease inhibitors, diltiazem, ketoconazole, macrolide antibiotics, verapamil) unless directed by prescriber
• Advise patient to comply in all areas of medical regimen

• Teach patient to notify all health care providers of this product use
• Teach patient not to chew or crush, and to avoid grapefruit juice
• Advise patient to notify prescriber of palpitations, dizziness, fainting, edema, dyspnea
• For acute angina take other products prescribed; this product doesn't decrease acute attack

Evaluation
Positive therapeutic outcome
• Decreased anginal pain and number of episodes

---

rasagiline (Rx)
(ra-sa'ji-leen)
Azilect
Func. class.: Antiparkinson agent
Chem. class.: MAOI, type B
Pregnancy category C

ACTION: Inhibits MAO type B at recommended doses; may increase DOPamine levels

Therapeutic outcome: Improved symptoms in those with Parkinson's disease

USES: Idiopathic Parkinson's disease monotherapy or with levodopa

CONTRAINDICATIONS
Breastfeeding, hypersensitivity to this product or MAOIs, pheochromocytoma

Precautions: Pregnancy **C**, children, psychiatric disorders, severe hepatic disorders

DOSAGE AND ROUTES
Monotherapy
Adult: PO 1 mg/day

Adjunctive therapy
Adult: PO 0.5 mg/day, may be increased to 1 mg/day; change of levodopa dose in adjunct therapy; reduced levodopa dose may be needed

Hepatic dose
Adult: PO 0.5 mg in mild hepatic disease

Concomitant ciprofloxacin, other CYP1A2 inhibitors
Adult: PO 0.5 mg; plasma concentrations of rasagiline may double

Available forms: Tabs 0.5, 1 mg

Implementation
• Give with meals to prevent nausea; continuing therapy usually reduces or eliminates nausea; do not give with foods/liquids containing large amounts of tyramine
• Give reduced dose of carbidopa/levodopa cautiously

⚠ Renal failure: in dialysis, increase dose slowly

ADVERSE EFFECTS

CNS: Drowsiness, hallucinations, depression, headache, malaise, paresthesia, vertigo, syncope
CV: Angina, hypertensive crisis (ingestion of tyramine products), orthostatic hypotension
GI: *Nausea*, diarrhea, dry mouth, dyspepsia
GU: Impotence, decreased libido
HEMA: Leukopenia
INTEG: Alopecia, skin cancers
MISC: Conjunctivitis, fever, flu syndrome, neck pain, allergic reaction, alopecia
MS: Arthralgia, arthritis, dyskinesia, falls
RESP: Rhinitis

Pharmacokinetics

Absorption	Well absorbed
Distribution	Protein binding >88%-94%
Metabolism	Liver, CYP1A2
Excretion	Kidneys, half-life 3 hr
Half-life	Unknown

Pharmacodynamics

Unknown

INTERACTIONS
Individual drugs

Ciprofloxacin: increased levels of rasagiline up to twofold
⚠ Meperidine: do not give; serious reaction including coma and death may occur

Drug classifications

⚠ Analgesics, sympathomimetics: do not give; serious reaction including coma and death may occur
⚠ Antidepressants (tricyclics, SSRIs, SNRIs, mirtazapine, cyclobenzaprine): increased severe CNS toxicity
CYP1A2 inhibitors (atazanavir, mexiletine, taurine): increased levels of rasagiline up to twofold
⚠ MAOIs: increased hypertensive crisis

Drug/herb

⚠ St. John's wort, yohimbe: do not give

Drug/food

Do not use with food/liquids that contain large amounts of tyramine

Drug/lab test

Increased: LFTs
Decreased: WBCs

NURSING CONSIDERATIONS
Assessment

• **Assess for Parkinson's symptoms:** tremor, ataxia, muscle weakness and rigidity; baseline, periodically; assess for increased dyskinesia

and postural hypotension if used in combination with levodopa
• Assess mental status: hallucinations, confusion, notify prescriber
• **Assess for hypertensive crisis: severe headache, blurred vision, seizures, chest pain, difficulty thinking, nausea/vomiting, signs of stroke; any unexplained severe headache should be considered to be hypertensive crisis**
• Monitor arterial blood gases (ABGs), CBC with differential, LDH, serum bilirubin, creatinine, electrolytes, uric acid baseline and periodically
• **Assess for melanomas frequently, perform periodic skin exams by a dermatologist**
• Monitor cardiac status: B/P, ECG; periodically, orthostatic hypotension during first 2 months of treatment
• **Tyramine products: assess for foods, other medications, may lead to hypertensive crisis (tachycardia, bradycardia, chest pain, nausea, vomiting, sweating, dilated pupils)**

Patient/family education

• Advise patient to change position slowly to prevent orthostatic hypotension
• Instruct patient to avoid hazardous activities until stabilized; dizziness can occur
• Advise patient to rinse mouth frequently, use sugarless gum to alleviate dry mouth
• Teach patient to take as prescribed, not to miss dose or double doses; take missed dose as soon as remembered if several hours before next dose
• **Teach patient to prevent hypertensive crisis by avoiding tyramine foods >150 mg**
• **Teach patient to report signs of hypertensive crisis**
• Teach patient to avoid CNS depressants, alcohol
• If drowsiness, daytime sleepiness, or falling asleep occurs, product may need to be discontinued
• **Skin should be checked periodically for possible skin cancer**

Evaluation
Positive therapeutic outcome

• Improved symptoms in those with Parkinson's disease (decreasing tremors, ataxia, muscle weakness/rigidity)

rasburicase (Rx)

(rass-burr′i-case)
Elitek, Fasturtec ✤
Func. class.: Enzyme
Chem. class.: Recombinant urate-oxidase enzyme
Pregnancy category C

ACTION: Catalyzes enzymatic oxidation of uric acid into an inactive and a soluble metabolite (allantoin)

Therapeutic outcome: Decreased uric acid levels

USES: To reduce uric acid levels in children with leukemia, lymphoma, solid tumor malignancies who are receiving chemotherapy

CONTRAINDICATIONS

Hypersensitivity

> **BLACK BOX WARNING:** G6PD deficiency (Mediterranean, African descent), hemolytic reactions, or methemoglobinemia reactions to this product

Precautions: Pregnancy **C**, breastfeeding, children <2 yr, anemia

> **BLACK BOX WARNING:** Acute bronchospasm, angina, angioedema, patients of African or Mediterranean ancestry, hypotension, urticaria

DOSAGE AND ROUTES

Adult/adolescent/child/infant: IV INF 0.2 mg/kg as a single daily dose × 5 days

Available forms: Powder for inj 1.5, 7.5 mg/vial

Implementation

Intermittent IV INF route

• Reconstitute with diluent provided, add 1 ml of diluent/vial, swirl, withdraw amount needed and mix with 0.9% NaCl to final volume of 50 ml, use within 24 hr, give over 30 min, do not use filter, use different line, if not possible flush with ≥15 ml of NaCl before and after use
• Chemotherapy is started 4-24 hr after 1st dose

ADVERSE EFFECTS

CNS: *Headache,* fever
CV: Chest pain, hypotension
GI: *Nausea, vomiting, anorexia, diarrhea, abdominal pain, constipation, dyspepsia, mucositis*
HEMA: **Neutropenia with fever, hemolysis, methemoglobinemia**
INTEG: *Rash*
MISC: Edema
RESP: **Bronchospasm,** wheezing, dyspnea
SYST: **Anaphylaxis, hemolysis, methemoglobinemia, sepsis**

Pharmacokinetics

Absorption	Unknown
Distribution	Unknown
Metabolism	Unknown
Excretion	Unknown
Half-life	Elimination 16-21 hr

Pharmacodynamics

Unknown

INTERACTIONS
Individual drugs
Allopurinol: increased toxicity

NURSING CONSIDERATIONS
Assessment
• Monitor blood studies: BUN, serum uric acid, urine CCr, electrolytes, CBC with differential before, during therapy
• Monitor temp q4hr; fever may indicate beginning infection; no rectal temp
• **Assess for anaphylaxis (dyspnea, urticaria, flushing, wheezing, swelling of lips, tongue, throat); have emergency equipment nearby**
• **Assess for G6PD deficiency, hemolytic reactions, methemoglobinemia; these patients should not be given this agent, screen patients who are higher risk for these disorders**
• Assess GI symptoms: frequency of stools, cramping; if severe diarrhea occurs, fluid and electrolytes may need to be given

Patient/family education
• Advise of reason for therapy, expected results
• **Advise to report trouble breathing, jaundice, chest pain**

Evaluation
Positive therapeutic outcome
• Decreased uric acid levels in children when antineoplastics causing high uric acid levels are used

---

> **⚠ HIGH ALERT**   **R**
>
> ## regorafenib
> (re′goe-raf′e-nib)
> **Stivarga**
> *Func. class.:* Antineoplastic biologic response modifier; multikinase inhibitor
> *Chem. class.:* Signal transduction inhibitor (STI)
> **Pregnancy category D**

ACTION: Inhibits tyrosine kinase in patients with colorectal cancer

Therapeutic outcome: Decrease in spread or size of tumor

USES: Metastatic colorectal cancer in those who have received fluoropyrimidine, oxaliplatin, irinotecan-based chemotherapy, an anti-VEGF therapy; and an anti-EGFR therapy if *KRAS* wild type

CONTRAINDICATIONS
Pregnancy (D)

Adverse effects: *italics* = common; **bold** = life-threatening

Precautions: Breastfeeding, children, geriatric patients, cardiac/renal/hepatic/dental disease, fistula, GI bleeding or perforation, bone marrow suppression, infection, wound dehiscence, thrombocytopenia, neutropenia, immunosuppression

> **BLACK BOX WARNING:** Hepatic disease

DOSAGE AND ROUTES
Adult: PO 160 mg/day with a low-fat breakfast × 21 days of a 28-day cycle, cycles may be repeated

Available forms: Tabs 40 mg

Implementation
- Store at 77°F (25°C)
- Give at the same time each day with a low-fat breakfast that contains less than 30% fat such as 2 slices of white toast with 1 TBSP of low-fat margarine and 1 TBSP of jelly, and 8 oz of skim milk; or 1 cup of cereal, 8 oz of skim milk, 1 slice of toast with jam, apple juice, and 1 cup of coffee or tea
- Swallow tablets whole
- If a dose is missed, take as soon as possible that day; do not take 2 doses on the same day

Hand–foot skin reaction:
Reduce to 120 mg (grade 2 palmar–plantar erythrodysesthesia); hold if grade 2 toxicity does not improve in 7 days or recurs; hold for 7 days in grade 3 toxicity; reduce to 80 mg for recurrent grade 2 toxicity; discontinue if 80 mg is not tolerated
Hypertension:
Hold in grade 2 hypertension
Other severe toxicity (except hepatotoxicity)
Hold until toxicity resolves in grade 3 or 4 toxicity; consider the risk/benefits of continuing therapy in grade 4 toxicity, reduce dosage to 120 mg if grade 3 or 4 toxicity recurs, hold until toxicity resolves, then reduce to 80 mg; discontinue in those who do not tolerate 80-mg dose

Hepatic dose
Baseline mild (Child-Pugh class A) or moderate (Child-Pugh class B): No change; baseline severe hepatic impairment (Child-Pugh class C): use not recommended
AST/ALT elevations during therapy:
For grade 3 AST/AST level elevations, hold dose; if therapy is continued, reduce to 120 mg after levels recover; discontinue in those with AST/ALT > 20 × ULN; AST/ALT > 3 × ULN and bilirubin > 2 × ULN; recurrence of AST/ALT >5 × ULN despite a reduction to 120 mg

ADVERSE EFFECTS
CNS: Headache, tremor
CV: Hypertensive crisis, MI
EENT: Blurred vision, conjunctivitis
GI: Hepatotoxicity, GI hemorrhage, diarrhea, GI perforation, xerostomia
HEMA: Neutropenia, thrombocytopenia, bleeding
INTEG: Rash, alopecia
META: Hypokalemia
MISC: Fatigue, decreased weight, hand–foot syndrome, hypothyroidism

Pharmacokinetics
Absorption	Unknown
Distribution	Protein binding 99%
Metabolism	by CYP3A4, UGT1A0
Half-life	14–58 hr

Pharmacodynamics
Onset	Unknown
Peak	Unknown
Duration	Unknown

INTERACTIONS
Individual drugs
Simvastatin: Increased plasma concentrations of simvastatin
Warfarin: Increased plasma concentration of warfarin; avoid use; use low-molecular-weight anticoagulants instead

Drug classifications
CYP3A4 inhibitors (ketoconazole, itraconazole, erythromycin, clarithromycin): Increase: regorafenib concentrations
Calcium-channel blockers, ergots: Increased plasma concentrations of each product
CYP3A4 inducers (dexamethasone, phenytoin, carBAMazepine, rifampin, PHENobarbital): Decrease: regorafenib concentrations

Drug/food
Grapefruit juice; avoid use while taking product: Increased regorafenib effect

Drug/herb
St. John's wort: Decreased imatinib concentration

NURSING CONSIDERATIONS
Assessment

> **BLACK BOX WARNING:** Hepatic disease: fatal hepatotoxicity can occur; obtain LFTs baseline and at least every 2 wk × 2 mo, then monthly

⚠ **Fatal bleeding:** From GI, respiratory, GU tracts; permanently discontinue in those with severe bleeding

---

⚠ **Palmar–plantar erythrodysesthesia (hand–foot syndrome):** More common in those previously treated; reddening swelling, numbness, desquamation on palms, soles

⚠ **GI perforation/fistula:** Discontinue if this occurs, assess for pain in epigastric area, dyspepsia, flatulence, fever, chills

⚠ **Hypertension/hypertensive crisis:** Hypertension usually occurs in the first cycle in those with preexisting hypertension, do not start treatment until B/P is controlled; monitor B/P every wk × 6 wk, then at start of each cycle or more often if needed, temporarily or permanently discontinue for severe uncontrolled hypertension

Patient/family education
• Teach patient to report adverse reactions immediately: bleeding, rash
• Teach patient the reason for treatment, expected results
• Advise patient that effect on male fertility is unknown

Pregnancy (D): Teach patient to report if pregnancy is planned or suspected

Evaluation
Positive therapeutic outcome
• Decrease in spread or size of tumor

⚠ HIGH ALERT

remifentanil (Rx)
(re-me-fin′ta-nill)
Ultiva
Func. class.: Opiate agonist analgesic
Chem. class.: μ-Opioid agonist
Pregnancy category C
Controlled substance schedule II

ACTION: Inhibits ascending pain pathways in limbic system, thalamus, midbrain, hypothalamus

Therapeutic outcome: Maintenance of anesthesia

USES: In combination with other products in general anesthesia to provide analgesia

CONTRAINDICATIONS
Hypersensitivity

Precautions: Pregnancy **C**, breastfeeding, geriatric, increased ICP, acute MI, severe heart disease, GI/renal/hepatic disease, asthma, respiratory conditions, seizure disorders, bradyarrhythmias, child <12 yr

DOSAGE AND ROUTES
Adult: Induction IV 0.5-1 mcg/kg/min with a hypnotic or volatile agent; maintenance with isoflurane (0.4-1.5 MAC) or propofol (100-200 mcg/kg/min); CONT INF 0.25-0.4 mcg/kg/min
Child 1-12 yr: CONT IV INF 0.25 mcg/kg/min with isoflurane
Full-term neonate and infant up to 2 mo: CONT IV INF 0.4 mcg/kg/min with nitrous oxide

Available forms: Powder for inj, lyophilized 1, 2, 5 mg

Implementation
• Add 1 ml diluent/remifentanil
• Shake well; further dilute to a final concentration of 20, 25, 50 or 250 mcg/mg
• Interruption of inf results in rapid reversal (no residual opioid effect within 5-10 min)
• Store in light-resistant area at room temperature

Direct IV route
• Use only during maintenance of general anesthesia; inject into tubing close to venous cannula, give in nonintubated patients over 30-60 sec
CONT IV INF route
• Use infusion device, max 16 hr, do not use same tubing as blood, do not admix

Y-site compatibilities: Acyclovir, alfentanil, amikacin, aminophylline, ampicillin, ampicillin/sulbactam, aztreonam, bretylium, bumetanide, buprenorphine, butorphanol, calcium gluconate, ceFAZolin, cefepime, cefotaxime, cefoTEtan, cefOXitin, cefTAZidime, ceftizoxime, cefTRIAXone, cefuroxime, cimetidine, ciprofloxacin, cisatracurium, clindamycin, dexamethasone, digoxin, diltiazem, diphenhydrAMINE, DOBUTamine, DOPamine, doxacurium, doxycycline, droperidol, enalaprilat, EPINEPHrine, esmolol, famotidine, fentaNYL, fluconazole, furosemide, ganciclovir, gatifloxicin, gentamicin, haloperidol, heparin, hydrocortisone sodium succinate, HYDROmorphone, hydrOXYzine, imipenem/cilastatin, inamrinone, isoproterenol, ketorolac, lidocaine, LORazepam, magnesium sulfate, mannitol, meperidine, methylprednisoLONE sodium succinate, metoclopramide, metroNIDAZOLE, mezlocillin, midazolam, morphine, nalbuphine, nitroglycerin, norepinephrine, ondansetron, phenylephrine, pipericillin, potassium chloride, procainamide, prochlorperazine, promethazine, ranitidine, trimethroprim, SUFentanil, theophylline, thiopental, ticarcillin/clavulate, tobramycin, vancomycin, zidovudine

Solution compatibilities: D_5, 0.45% NaCl, LR, D_5LR, 0.9% NaCl

ADVERSE EFFECTS
CNS: Drowsiness, *dizziness,* confusion, *headache,* sedation, euphoria, delirium, agitation, anxiety
CV: Palpitations, **bradycardia**, change in B/P; facial flushing, syncope, **asystole**

EENT: Tinnitus, blurred vision, miosis, diplopia
GI: *Nausea, vomiting,* anorexia, constipation, cramps, dry mouth
GU: Urinary retention, dysuria
INTEG: Rash, urticaria, bruising, flushing, diaphoresis, pruritus
MS: Rigidity
RESP: Respiratory depression, apnea

Pharmacokinetics

Absorption	Complete
Distribution	70% protein binding
Metabolism	Unknown
Excretion	Urine
Half-life	Terminal 3-10 min

Pharmacodynamics

Onset	1-3 min
Peak	Unknown
Duration	Unknown

INTERACTIONS
Individual drugs
Alcohol: increased respiratory depression, hypotension, profound sedation

Drug classifications
Antihistamines, CNS depressants, phenothiazines, MAOIs, sedative/hypnotics: increased respiratory depression, hypotension, profound sedation

Drug/herb
Kava: increased CNS depression

NURSING CONSIDERATIONS
Assessment
• Monitor I&O ratio, check for decreasing output; may indicate urinary retention, especially in geriatric
• Assess CNS changes: dizziness, drowsiness, hallucinations, euphoria, LOC pupil reaction
• Assess allergic reactions: rash, urticaria
• **Assess respiratory dysfunction:** respiratory depression, character, rate, rhythm; notify prescriber if respirations are <12/min; CV status, bradycardia, syncope
• Monitor GI status: nausea, vomiting, anorexia, constipation
• Use pain scoring to determine pain perception

Patient/family education
• Advise patient to call for assistance when ambulating or smoking; drowsiness, dizziness may occur
• Advise patient to make position changes slowly to prevent orthostatic hypotension

Evaluation
Positive therapeutic outcome
• Maintenance of anesthesia

Do not confuse: Prandin/Avandia

ACTION: Causes functioning β-cells in pancreas to release insulin, leading to drop in blood glucose levels; closes ATP-dependent potassium channels in the β-cell membrane; this leads to opening of calcium channels; increased calcium influx induces insulin secretion

Therapeutic outcome: Blood glucose controlled

USES: Type 2 diabetes mellitus

CONTRAINDICATIONS
Hypersensitivity to meglitinides, diabetic ketoacidosis, type 1 diabetes

Precautions: Pregnancy **C**, breastfeeding, children, geriatric, cardiac disease, severe renal/hepatic disease, thyroid disease, severe hypoglycemic reactions

DOSAGE AND ROUTES
Adult: PO 0.5-4 mg with each meal, max 16 mg/day, adjust at weekly intervals; oral hypoglycemic-naïve patients or those with A1c <8% should start with 0.5 mg with each meal

Renal/hepatic dose
Adult: PO CCr 20-39 ml/min: 0.5 mg/day; titrate upward cautiously

Available forms: Tabs 0.5, 1, 2 mg

Implementation
• 15 min before meals: 2, 3, or 4 ×/day preprandially
• Skip dose if meal is skipped; add dose if meal is added
• Store in airtight container at room temperature

ADVERSE EFFECTS
CNS: *Headache, weakness,* paresthesia
CV: Angina
EENT: Sinusitis, tinnitus
ENDO: Hypoglycemia
GI: Nausea, vomiting, diarrhea, constipation, dyspepsia, **pancreatitis**
HEMA: Hemolytic anemia, leukopenia
INTEG: Rash, allergic reactions
MISC: Chest pain, UTI, allergy
MS: Back pains, arthralgia
RESP: URI, sinusitis, rhinitis, bronchitis

Pharmacokinetics

Absorption	Complete
Distribution	98% protein binding, crosses placenta
Metabolism	Liver by CYP3A4
Excretion	Urine/feces
Half-life	1 hr

Pharmacodynamics

Onset	30 min
Peak	1 hr
Duration	<4 hr

INTERACTIONS
Individual drugs

CarBAMazepine, rifampin: increased repaglinide metabolism

Chloramphenicol, deferasirox, fenofibrate, gemfibrozil, probenecid, simvastatin: increased effect of repaglinide

Erythromycin, ketoconazole, miconazole: decreased repaglinide metabolism

Gemfibrozil, isophane insulin (NPH): Do not use together

Isoniazid, phenobarbital, phenytoin, rifampin: decreased action of repaglinide

Levonorgestrel/ethinyl estradiol: increase in both

Drug classifications

Antifungals, CYP3A4 inhibitors, macrolides: decreased repaglinide metabolism

Barbiturates, CYP3A4 inducers: increased repaglinide metabolism

β-Adrenergic blockers, coumarins, MAOIs, NSAIDs, salicylates, sulfonamides: increased repaglinide effect

Calcium channel blockers, contraceptives (oral), corticosteroids, diuretics (thiazide), estrogens, phenothiazines, sympathomimetics, thyroid preparations: decreased repaglinide effect

CYP3A4, OATP1B1, CYP2C9 inhibitors: increased repaglinide effect

Drug/herb

Chromium, garlic, horse chestnut: increased antidiabetic effect

Drug/food

Decreased: repaglinide level; give before meals
Grapefruit juice: decreased repaglinide metabolism

Drug/lab test

Increased/decreased: glucose

NURSING CONSIDERATIONS
Assessment

• Assess for hypoglycemic or hyperglycemic reaction, which can occur soon after meals; dizziness, weakness, headache, tremor, anxiety, tachycardia, hunger, sweating, abdominal pain, monitor A1c, fasting, postprandial glucose during treatment

Patient/family education

• Teach patient technique of blood glucose monitoring using blood glucose meter
• Teach patient the symptoms of hypoglycemia and hyperglycemia, what to do about each
• Teach patient that product must be continued on daily basis; explain consequence of discontinuing product abruptly
• Advise patient to avoid OTC medications unless ordered by prescriber
• Advise patient that diabetes is a lifelong illness; product will not cure disease
• Advise patient to eat all food included in diet plan to prevent hypoglycemia; that if a meal is omitted, dose should be omitted; to have glucagon emergency kit available; to take repaglinide 15-30 min before meals 2, 3, or 4×/day
• Instruct patient to carry/wear emergency ID for emergency purposes

Evaluation
Positive therapeutic outcome

• Decrease in polyuria, polydipsia, polyphagia; clear sensorium; absence of dizziness; stable gait; blood glucose, A1c improvement

retapamulin topical
See Appendix B

retinoic acid
See tretinoin

Rh₀ (D) immune globulin, standard dose IM
HyperRHO SD, Rho Gam Ultra Filtered Plus
Rh₀ (D) immune globulin microdose IM
HyperRHO S/D mini-Dose, MICRhoGAM Ultra Filtered Plus, mini-Gamulin R
Rh₀ (D) immune globulin microdose (IM, IV)
Rhophylac
Rh₀ (D) immune globulin IV
Rhophylac, WinRho SDF
Func. class.: Immune globulins
Pregnancy category C

ACTION: Suppresses immune nonsensitized Rh₀ (D or Dᵘ)-negative patients who are exposed to Rh₀ (D or Dᵘ)-positive blood

Therapeutic outcome: Absence of Rh factor and transfusion error

USES: Prevention of isoimmunization in Rh-negative women exposed to Rh-positive blood given after abortions, miscarriages, amniocentesis, chronic idiopathic thrombocytopenic purpura (Rhophylac)

CONTRAINDICATIONS
Previous immunization with this product, Rh₀ (D)-positive/D^u-positive patient

> **BLACK BOX WARNING:** Hemolysis

Precautions: Pregnancy **C**

> **BLACK BOX WARNING:** Requires a specialized setting

DOSAGE AND ROUTES
To reduce risk of Rh isoimmunization antepartum/suppression of Rh isoimmunization postpartum following delivery of full-term infant
Adult and adolescent ≥16 yr: IM ([Hyper-RHO S/D] [full dose only]) 300 mcg (1500 international units) at 28 wk gestation, repeat within 72 hr of delivery of confirmed Rho(D)-positive infant; a dose is not needed after delivery, if delivery is within 3 wk of last dose and no fetal maternal hemorrhage of >15 ml of RBC; IM (RhoGam only) 300 mcg (1500 international units) at 26-28 wk gestation, repeat within 72 hr even if status of Rho is unknown or if 72 hr have passed; IM/IV (WinRho SDF only) 300 mcg (1500 international units) at 28 wk gestation; if given earlier in pregnancy, give at 12-wk intervals during pregnancy, a 120-mcg (600 international units) dose; IM/IV should be given as soon as possible and preferably within 72 hr of delivery of a confirmed Rho(D)-positive infant, and even if status is unknown give up to 28 days after delivery

Known or suspected massive feto-maternal hemorrhage (>15 ml of fetal RBC or >30 ml of fetal whole blood)
Adult and adolescent ≥16 yr: IM ([Hyper-RHO S/D] [full dose only]) 300 mcg (1500 international units) per every 15 ml of fetal blood cells or 30 ml of whole blood, multiple syringes may be injected IM at the same time in different sites, give within 72 hr of exposure, repeat dose within 72 hr of delivery; IM (RhoGAM only) 300 mcg (1500 international units) for every 15 ml of fetal blood cells or 30 ml of whole blood, give total dose within 72 hr of exposure; IM/IV (Win-Rho SDF only) if large fetomaternal hemorrhage

is suspected, give **IV** 9 mcg (45 international units) or IM 12 mcg (60 international units) for every ml of fetal whole blood, give **IV** 600 mcg (3000 international units) q8hr or IM 1200 mcg (6000 international units) q12hr until total dose is given, total dose should be given within 72 hr of exposure

Threatened abortion at any stage of pregnancy
Adult and adolescent ≥16 yr: IM ([Hyper-RHO S/D] [full dose only]) 300 mcg (1500 international units) as soon as possible; if given 13-18 wk gestation, give another 300 mcg (1500 international units) at 26-28 wk gestation; repeat dose within 72 hr of delivery; IM (RhoGam only) 300 mcg (1500 international units) as soon as possible and within 72 hr; IM/IV (Rhophylac only) 300 mcg (1500 international units) as soon as possible and within 72 hr; IM/IV (Win-Rho SDF only) 300 mcg (1500 international units) as soon as possible and within 72 hr, repeat dose at 12-wk intervals during pregnancy and 120 mcg (600 international units) as soon as possible after delivery and within 72 hr

Following spontaneous abortion, induced termination of pregnancy, or ectopic pregnancy that occurs ≤12 wk gestation
Adult and adolescent ≥16 yr: IM (Minidose, HyperRHO Minidose, MICRORhoGAM only) 50 mcg (250 international units) as soon as possible, give within 3 hr of spontaneous or surgical removal, if possible within 72 hr

Following spontaneous abortion, induced termination of pregnancy, or ruptured tubal pregnancy that occurs ≥13 wk
Adult and adolescent ≥16 yr: IM (full dose [HyperRHO S/D] RhoGAM only) 300 mcg (1500 international units) as soon as possible and within 72 hr of event

Following spontaneous abortion, induced termination of pregnancy, aminocentesis, chorionic villus sampling, abdominal trauma, ruptured tubal pregnancy, or percutaneous umbilical cord sampling up to 34 wk gestation
Adult and adolescent ≥16 wk: IM/IV (Win-Rho SDF only) 300 mcg (1500 international units) within 72 hr, repeat at 12-wk intervals during pregnancy, give 120 mcg (600 international units) as soon as possible and preferably within 72 hr of delivery

---

⚠ Nurse Alert   ✴ Key NCLEX® Drug   >> Drug Specifics

Available forms: Hyper RHO S/D solution for injection 1500 IU/prefilled syringe; MI-CRhoGAM Ultra Filtered Plus Solution for inj 50 mcg/ml; RhoGam Ultra Filtered Plus Solution for inj 50 mcg; Rhophylac Pre-Filled Syringes Solution for inj 300 mcg/2 ml; WinRho SDF Liquid for inj

Implementation

- BayRho-D is being changed to HyperRHO S/D
- HyperRHO S/D, MICRhoGAM, RhoGAM are given by IM only; do not give **IV**
- Rhophylac may be given IM or **IV**
- Inspect for particulate matter; do not use if particulate matter is present
- Reconstitution/dilution: no reconstitution or dilution is needed for BayRho-D (HyperRHO S/D), Rhophylac, MICRoGAM, RhoGAM, or the liquid formulation of WinRho SDF

IM route

- Use aseptic technique, observe for 20 min after administration
- Bring Rhophylac to room temperature before using
- Inject into the deltoid muscle of upper arm or anterolateral portion of the upper thigh; do not inject into gluteal muscle
- If dose calculated will need multiple vials or syringes, use different sites at the same time

IV route

- Use aseptic technique
- WinRhoSDF: remove entire contents of vial to obtain calculated dose; if partial vial contents are required for dosage calculation, withdraw the entire vial contents to ensure correct calculation; inf correct calculated dose over 3-5 min; do not inf with other fluids or products
- Rhophylac: bring to room temperature; inf by slow **IV**; observe for 20 min

ADVERSE EFFECTS

CNS: Lethargy
CV: Hypo/hypertension
INTEG: Irritation at inj site, fever
MISC: Infection, **ARDS**, anaphylaxis, pulmonary edema, **DIC**
MS: Myalgia

Pharmacokinetics

Absorption	Well absorbed
Distribution	Unknown
Metabolism	Unknown
Excretion	Unknown
Half-life	Unknown

Pharmacodynamics

Onset	Rapid
Peak	Unknown
Duration	Unknown

INTERACTIONS
Drug classifications

Live virus vaccines (measles, mumps, rubella): decreased antibody response to vaccine

NURSING CONSIDERATIONS
Assessment

- Assess for allergies, reactions to immunizations; previous immunization with this product
- Intravascular hemolysis: assess for back pain, chills, hemoglobinuria, renal insufficiency; usually when WinRho SDF is given in those with immune thrombocytopenia purpura
- Obtain type and cross-match of mother's blood and of neonate's cord blood; neonate must be $Rh_o(D)$-positive, mother must be $Rh_o(D)$-negative and (D^u)-negative, medication should be given if there is a doubt

Patient/family education

- Teach patient how product works; that product must be given after subsequent deliveries if subsequent babies are Rh-positive
- Intravascular hemolysis: Teach patient to report immediately: shaking, fever, chills, dark urine, swelling of hand or feet, back pain, SOB

Evaluation

Positive therapeutic outcome

- Prevention of $Rh_o(D)$ sensitization in transfusion error
- Prevention of erythroblastosis fetalis in subsequent $Rh_o(D)$-positive neonates

ribavirin (Rx)

(rye-ba-vye′rin)
Virazole
Func. class.: Synthetic antiviral
Chem. class.: Tricyclic amine
Pregnancy category X

ACTION: Prevents replication of DNA and RNA synthesis

Therapeutic outcome: Resolution of severe lower respiratory tract infections

Adverse effects: *italics* = common; **bold** = life-threatening

USES: Severe lower respiratory tract infections in infants and children

Unlabeled uses: Influenza A or B (early)

CONTRAINDICATIONS
Pregnancy **X,** breastfeeding, children <1 yr, hypersensitivity

Precautions: Epilepsy, renal/hepatic disease

DOSAGE AND ROUTES
Infant and young child: INH 20 mg/ml × 12-18 hr/day × 3-7 days

Available forms: Powder for reconstitution for aerosol 6 g/vial

Implementation
• Give by the Viratek small particle aerosol generator (SPAG-2), do not use other inhalation equipment
• May be given by an oxygen hood for infants, or a face mask may be attached to the SPAG-2
• Reconstitute 6 g of sterile water for inj or inh, place sol in the Erlenmeyer flask and dilute further to 20 mg/ml

ADVERSE EFFECTS
CNS: Dizziness, faintness
CV: Hypotension, cardiac arrest
EENT: Eye irritation, conjunctivitis, blurred vision, photosensitivity
INTEG: Rash

Pharmacokinetics

Absorption	Inhalation (systemic)
Distribution	To respiratory tract
Metabolism	Liver
Excretion	Respiratory tract
Half-life	9½ hr

Pharmacodynamics

Onset	Unknown
Peak	Inhalation's end
Duration	Unknown

INTERACTIONS
Individual products
Zidovudine: decreased antiviral action, increased toxicity

Drug classification
Cardiac glycosides: increased toxicity

NURSING CONSIDERATIONS
Assessment
• Assess allergies before initiation of treatment, reaction of each medication; list allergies on chart in bright red letters
• Monitor respiratory status: rate, character, wheezing, tightness in chest

• Obtain C&S test results before starting treatment

Patient/family education
• Teach patient and parents aspects of product therapy

Evaluation

Positive therapeutic outcome
• Absence of respiratory syncytial virus

riboflavin (vitamin B$_2$) (OTC)
(rye′bo-flay-vin)
Func. class.: Vitamin B$_2$, water soluble
Pregnancy category A

ACTION: Needed for respiratory reactions (catalyzes proteins) and for normal vision

Therapeutic outcome: Prevention or treatment of riboflavin deficiency

USES: Vitamin B$_2$ deficiency or polyneuritis; cheilosis adjunct with thiamine

Precautions: Pregnancy **A**

DOSAGE AND ROUTES
Deficiency
Adult: PO 5-30 mg/day
Child ≥12 yr: PO 3-10 mg/day, then 0.6 mg/1000 cal ingested

RDA
Adult: PO (Males) 1.3 mg; (females) 1.1 mg

Available forms: Tabs 5, 10, 25, 50, 100, 250 mg

Implementation
• Give with food for better absorption
• Store in airtight, light-resistant container

ADVERSE EFFECTS
GU: Yellow discoloration of urine (large doses)

Pharmacokinetics

Absorption	Well absorbed (by active transport)
Distribution	60% protein bound, widely distributed, crosses placenta
Metabolism	Unknown
Excretion	Kidneys (unchanged), excess amounts
Half-life	1-1½ hr

Pharmacodynamics

Unknown

INTERACTIONS
Individual drugs
Alcohol, probenecid: increased riboflavin need

Tetracycline: decreased action of tetracycline

Drug classifications
Antidepressants (tricyclics), phenothiazines: increased riboflavin need

Drug/lab test
False increase: urinary catecholamines

NURSING CONSIDERATIONS
Assessment
• Assess patient's nutritional status: liver, eggs, dairy products, yeast, whole grain, green vegetables

• Assess for vit B_2 deficiency: photophobia, cheilosis, stomatitis, ocular swelling

Patient/family education
• Inform patient that urine may turn bright yellow

• Instruct patient about needed addition of foods that are rich in riboflavin

Evaluation
Positive therapeutic outcome

• Absence of headache, GI problems, cheilosis, skin lesions, depression, burning itchy eyes, anemia

rifabutin (Rx)
(riff'a-byoo-tin)

Mycobutin

Func. class.: Antimycobacterial

Chem. class.: Rifamycin S derivative

Pregnancy category B

Do not confuse: rifabutin/rifampin/rifapentine

ACTION: Inhibits DNA-dependent RNA polymerase in susceptible strains

Therapeutic outcome: Antimycobacterial death of *Escherichia coli, Bacillus subtilis;* mechanism of action against *Mycobacterium avium* unknown

USES: Prevention of *M. avium* complex (MAC) in patients with advanced HIV infection

Unlabeled uses: *Helicobacter pylori* that has not responded to other treatment

CONTRAINDICATIONS
Hypersensitivity, active TB, WBC <1000/mm³, platelets <50,000/mm³

Precautions: Pregnancy **B**, breastfeeding, children, hepatic disease, blood dyscrasias

DOSAGE AND ROUTES
Adult: PO 300 mg/day (may take as 150 mg bid); max 600 mg/day

Renal dose

Adult: PO CCr <30 ml/min reduce dose by 50%

Available forms: Caps 150 mg

Implementation
• Give with meals to decrease GI symptoms; better to take on empty stomach 1 hr before or 2 hr after meal; high-fat food slows absorption, may take in 2 divided doses, may open capsule and mix with applesauce if unable to swallow whole

• Give antiemetic if vomiting occurs

ADVERSE EFFECTS
CNS: *Headache,* fatigue, anxiety, confusion, insomnia

GI: *Nausea, vomiting, anorexia, diarrhea,* heartburn, **hepatitis,** discolored saliva, **pseudomembranous colitis**

GU: Discolored urine

HEMA: Hemolytic anemia, eosinophilia, thrombocytopenia, leukopenia

INTEG: *Rash*

MISC: Flulike syndrome, shortness of breath, chest pressure

MS: Asthenia, arthralgia, myalgia

Pharmacokinetics

Absorption	Well absorbed
Distribution	Widely distributed
Metabolism	Liver
Excretion	Kidney
Half-life	45 hr

Pharmacodynamics

Onset	Unknown
Peak	2-3 hr
Duration	Unknown

INTERACTIONS
Individual drugs
Amprenavir, busPIRone, clofibrate, cycloSPORINE, dapsone, delavirdine, disopyramide, doxycycline, efavirenz, fluconazole, indinavir, ketoconazole, losartan, nelfinavir, nevirapine, phenytoin, quiNIDine, saquinavir, theophylline, zidovudine, zolpidem: decreased action of each specific product

Ritonavir: increased rifabutin level

R

Drug classifications

Anticoagulants, antidepressants (tricyclics), barbiturates, β-blockers, contraceptives (oral), corticosteroids, estrogens, sulfonylureas: decreased action of each specific product

Drug/food

High-fat foods: decreased absorption

Drug/lab test

Interference: folate level, vit B$_{12}$, BSP, gallbladder tests

NURSING CONSIDERATIONS
Assessment

- **Assess for active TB: chest x-ray, sputum culture, blood culture, biopsy of lymph nodes, obtain PPD test; product should be given only for MAC and never for TB**
- Monitor CBC for neutropenia, thrombocytopenia, eosinophilia
- **Pseudomembranous colitis: assess for diarrhea, abdominal pain, fever, fatigue, anorexia; possible anemia, elevated WBC and low serum albumin; stop product and usually give either vancomycin or IV metroNIDAZOLE**

Patient/family education

- Caution patient that compliance with dosage schedule and duration is necessary
- Instruct patient that scheduled appointments must be kept or relapse may occur
- **Instruct patient to notify prescriber if hepatitis, neutropenia, or thrombocytopenia occurs: sore throat, fever, bleeding, bruising, yellow sclera, anorexia, nausea, vomiting, fatigue, weakness; myositis: muscle or bone pain**
- Advise patient that urine, feces, saliva, sputum, sweat, tears may be colored red-orange; soft contact lenses may become permanently stained
- **Caution patients using oral contraceptives to use a nonhormonal method of birth control because rifabutin may decrease efficiency of oral contraceptives; to notify prescriber if pregnancy is planned or suspected**

Evaluation

Positive therapeutic outcome
- Decreased symptoms of *M. avium* in patients with HIV

rifampin (Rx)
(rif'am-pin)
Rifadin, Rofact ✦
Func. class.: Antitubercular
Chem. class.: Rifamycin B derivative
Pregnancy category C

Do not confuse: rifampin/rifabutin/rifaximin

ACTION: Inhibits DNA-dependent polymerase, decreases tubercle bacilli replication

Therapeutic outcome: Bactericidal against the following organisms: mycobacteria, *Staphylococcus aureus, Haemophilus influenzae, Neisseria meningitidis, Legionella pneumophila*

USES: Pulmonary TB, meningococcal carriers (prevention)

CONTRAINDICATIONS

Hypersensitivity to this product or rifamycins, active *Neisseria meningitidis* infection

Precautions: Pregnancy **C**, breastfeeding, children <5 yr, hepatic disease, blood dyscrasias

DOSAGE AND ROUTES
Tuberculosis

Adult: PO/**IV** max 600 mg/day as single dose 1 hr before or 2 hr after meals, or 10 mg/kg/day 5 days/wk or 2-3 ×/wk

Child >5 yr: PO/**IV** 10-20 mg/kg/day as single dose 1 hr before or 2 hr after meals, max 600 mg/day, with other antitubercular products

6-mo regimen: 2-mo treatment of isoniazid, rifampin, pyrazinamide, and possibly streptomycin or ethambutol; then rifampin and isoniazid × 4 mo

9-mo regimen: Rifampin and isoniazid supplemented with pyrazinamide or streptomycin or ethambutol

Meningococcal carriers

Adult: PO/**IV** 600 mg bid × 2 days, max 600 mg/dose

Child >5 yr: PO/**IV** 10-20 mg/kg bid × 2 days, max 600 mg/dose

Infant 3 mo-1 yr: PO 5 mg/kg bid for 2 days

Available forms: Caps 150, 300 mg; powder for inj 600 mg/vial

Implementation

- Do not give IM or SUBCUT
- **PO route**
- On empty stomach, 1 hr before or 2 hr after meals with a full glass of water; give with other products for TB

- Antiemetic if vomiting occurs
- Capsules may be opened and mixed with applesauce or gelatin

Intermittent IV INF route
- After diluting each 600 mg/10 ml of sterile water for inj (60 mg/ml), swirl, withdraw dose, and dilute in 100 ml or 500 ml of D₅W given as an inf over 3 hr, or if diluted in 100 ml, give over ½ hr; do not admix with other sol or medications

Y-site compatibilities: Amiodarone, bumetanide, midazolam, pantoprazole, vancomycin

ADVERSE EFFECTS

CNS: Headache, fatigue, anxiety, drowsiness, confusion
EENT: Visual disturbances
GI: *Nausea, vomiting, anorexia, diarrhea,* **pseudomembranous colitis,** *heartburn,* sore mouth and tongue, **pancreatitis,** elevated liver function tests
GU: **Hematuria, acute renal failure, hemoglobinuria**
HEMA: **Hemolytic anemia, eosinophilia, thrombocytopenia, leukopenia**
INTEG: Rash, pruritus, urticaria
MISC: Flulike syndrome, menstrual disturbances, edema, SOB, **Stevens-Johnson syndrome, toxic epidermal necrolysis, angioedema, anaphylaxis**
MS: Ataxia, weakness

Pharmacokinetics

Absorption	Well absorbed (PO), completely absorbed (**IV**)
Distribution	Widely distributed, crosses placenta
Metabolism	Liver—extensively
Excretion	Feces
Half-life	1-5 hr

Pharmacodynamics

	PO	IV
Onset	Rapid	Rapid
Peak	2-3 hr	Inf end
Duration	Unknown	Unknown

INTERACTIONS
Individual drugs
Acetaminophen, alcohol, chloramphenicol, clofibrate, cycloSPORINE, dapsone, digoxin, diltiazem, doxycycline, haloperidol, NIFEdipine, phenytoin, theophylline, verapamil, zidovudine: decreased effect of specific product
Isoniazid: increased hepatotoxicity

Drug classifications
Anticoagulants, antidiabetics, barbiturates, benzodiazepines, β-blockers, contraceptives (oral), glucocorticoids, hormones, imidazole antifungals: decreased effect of each product
Protease inhibitors: do not use together

Drug/lab test
Increased: alk phosphatase, ALT, AST, uric acid, bilirubin, eosinophils
Increased: LFTs
Decreased: Hgb
Interference: folate level, vit B₁₂

NURSING CONSIDERATIONS
Assessment
- Monitor liver function tests qmo: ALT, AST, bilirubin, decreased appetite, jaundice, dark urine, fatigue
- Monitor renal status: before, qmo: BUN, creatinine, output, specific gravity, urinalysis
- **Pseudomembranous colitis: assess for diarrhea, abdominal pain, fever, fatigue, anorexia; possible anemia, elevated WBC and low serum albumin; stop product and usually give either vancomycin or IV metro-NIDAZOLE**
- Monitor mental status often: affect, mood, behavioral changes; psychosis may occur
- **Infection:** assess sputum culture, lung sounds
- C&S should be performed before beginning treatment, during, and after therapy is completed
- **Serious skin reactions: assess for fever, sore throat, fatigue, ulcers, lesions in mouth, lips, rash; can be fatal**

Patient/family education
- Instruct patient that compliance with dosage schedule, duration is necessary
- Instruct patient that scheduled appointments must be kept or relapse may occur
- **Instruct patient to notify prescriber if hepatitis, neutropenia, or thrombocytopenia occurs: sore throat, fever, bleeding, bruising, yellow sclera, anorexia, nausea, vomiting, fatigue, weakness, diarrhea with pus, mucus, blood**
- Advise patient that urine, feces, saliva, sputum, sweat, tears may be colored red-orange; soft contact lenses may be permanently stained
- Caution patients using oral contraceptives to use a nonhormonal method of birth control because rifabutin may decrease the efficiency of oral contraceptives, to notify prescriber if pregnancy is planned or suspected

R

• Advise patient to avoid alcohol; hepato-toxicity may occur

Evaluation

Positive therapeutic outcome
• Decreased symptoms of TB

rifaximin (Rx)
(rif-ax′i-min)
Xifaxan
Func. class.: Misc. antiinfective
Chem. class.: Analog of rifampin
Pregnancy category C

Do not confuse: rifaximin/rifampin

ACTION: Binds to bacterial DNA dependent RNA polymerase, thereby inhibiting bacterial RNA synthesis

Therapeutic outcome: Bacterial action against *E. coli*

USES: Traveler's diarrhea in those ≥12 yr old, caused by *E. coli,* hepatic encephalopathy, irritable bowel syndrome

CONTRAINDICATIONS
Hypersensitivity to this product or rifamycins, diarrhea with fever, blood in stool

Precautions: Pregnancy **C**, breastfeeding, children, geriatric patients

DOSAGE AND ROUTES
Traveler's diarrhea
Adult and child ≥12 yr: PO 200 mg tid × 3 days without regard to meals

Hepatic encephalopathy
Adult: PO 550 mg bid

Available forms: Tabs 200, 550 mg

Implementation
• May be administered without regard to food

ADVERSE EFFECTS
CNS: Abnormal dreams, dizziness, insomnia, *headache,* fatigue, depression
CV: Hypotension, chest pain, peripheral edema, ascites
GI: *Abdominal pain, constipation, defecation urgency, flatulence, nausea, rectal tenesmus,* vomiting, ascites, **pseudomembranous colitis**
GU: Proteinuria, polyuria, increased urinary frequency
MISC: *Pyrexia,* motion sickness, tinnitus, rash, photosensitivity, **exfoliative dermatitis**
MS: Arthralgia, muscle pain, myalgia
RESP: Dyspnea, cough, pharyngitis

Pharmacokinetics

Absorption	Low, systemic
Distribution	Unknown
Metabolism	Induces CYP3A4
Excretion	Feces
Half-life	6 hr

Pharmacodynamics

Onset	Unknown
Peak	1-4 hr
Duration	Unknown

INTERACTIONS
Individual drugs
Afatinib: increased effect of afatinib

Drug/lab test
Increased: LFTs, potassium
Decreased: blood glucose, sodium

NURSING CONSIDERATIONS
Assessment
• Assess for GI symptoms: amount and character of diarrhea, abdominal pain, nausea, vomiting; do not use in those with blood in stool, increased temperature with diarrhea
⚠ Assess for overgrowth of infection and pseudomembranous colitis

Patient/family education
• Instruct patient to discontinue rifaximin and notify prescriber if diarrhea persists for more than 24-48 hr, if diarrhea worsens, or if blood is in stools and fever is present
• Advise patient to avoid hazardous activities if dizziness occurs
• Teach patient to take without regard to food
• Teach patient to take as directed, to consume all of the product prescribed

Evaluation
Positive therapeutic outcome
• Absence of infection

rilpivirine
(ril-pi-vir′ine)
Edurant
Func. class.: Antiretroviral
Chem. class.: Non-nucleoside transcriptase inhibitors (NNTIs)
Pregnancy category B

ACTION: Inhibits HIV-1 reverse transcriptase; unlike nucleoside reverse transcriptase inhibitors (NRTIs), it does not compete for binding nor does it require phosphorylation to be active.

Binds directly to a site on reverse transcriptase; causing disruption of the enzyme's active site thereby blocking RNA-dependent and DNA-dependent DNA polymerase activities

Uses: HIV in combination with other antiretrovirals

CONTRAINDICATIONS
Hypersensitivity

Precautions: Pregnancy category **B**, breastfeeding, immune reconstitution syndrome, antimicrobial resistance, pancreatitis, depression, suicidal ideation, neonates, infants, children, adolescents <18 yr, QT prolongation, torsades de pointes, hyperlipidemia, hypertriglyceridemia, hypercholesterolemia

DOSAGE AND ROUTES
Treatment of antiretroviral treatment-naive adults with human immunodeficiency virus (HIV) in combination with other antiretroviral agents
Adult: PO 25 mg/day with a meal; give with other antiretroviral agents. In antiretroviral-treatment–naive adults, rilpivirine is used as an alternative to efavirenz in NNRTI-based treatment regimens. Potential rilpivirine-based treatment regimens combine rilpivirine with either tenofovir plus emtricitabine or lamiVUDine, or abacavir plus emtricitabine or lamiVUDine, or zidovudine plus emtricitabine or lamiVUDine

Available forms: Tab 25 mg

Implementation
• Store at room temperature away from heat and moisture

ADVERSE EFFECTS
CNS: Depressed mood, dizziness, drowsiness, dysphoria, fatigue, headache, major depression, mood alteration, negative thoughts, suicide attempts
GI: Abdominal pain, cholecystitis, cholelithiasis, decreased appetite, diarrhea, elevated hepatic enzymes, hyperbilirubinemia, hypercholesterolemia, nausea, vomiting
GU: *Glomerulonephritis membranous/glomerulonephritis mesangioproliferative*

Pharmacokinetics

Absorption	Increased effect 40% (food), decreased effect 50% (high protein drink)
Distribution	Protein binding (99.7%) to albumin
Metabolism	Via oxidation CYP3A system
Excretion	Feces 25% excreted unchanged (85%); urine (6.1%)
Half-life	Terminal elimination 50 hr

Pharmacodynamics

Onset	Unknown
Peak	4-5 hr
Duration	Unknown

INTERACTIONS
Individual drugs
Aminoglutethimide, bexarotene, bosentan, efavirenz, flutamide, griseofulvin, metyrapone, modafinil, nafcillin, nevirapine, pioglitazone, primidone, ritonavir, topiramate: Decreased rilpivirine effect, treatment failure
Abarelix, alfuzosin, amiodarone, amoxapine, apomorphine, artemether, asenapine, chloroquine, ciprofloxacin, citalopram, cloZAPine, cyclobenzaprine, dasatinib, dolasetron, dronedarone, droperidol, eribulin, flecainide, fluconazole, gatifloxacin, gemifloxacin, haloperidol, iloperidone, lapatinib, levofloxacin, lopinavir, lumefantrine, maprotiline, mefloquinem, moxifloxacin, nilotinib, norfloxacin, octreotide, ofloxacin, OLANZapine, ondansetron, paliperidone, palonosetron, pentamidine, posconazole, QUEtiapine, ranolazine, saquinavir: Increased QT prolongation
Fluconazole, voriconazole: Increased rilpivirine adverse reactions, fungal infections

Drug classifications
CYP3A4 inducers (phenytoin, fosphenytoin, barbiturates, OXcarbazepine, carBAMazepine, rifabutin, rifampin, rifapentine, dexamethasone), proton pump inhibitors (PPIs): Decreased rilpivirine effect, treatment failure
H₂ receptor antagonists (cimetidine, famotidine, nizatidine, ranitidine): Decreased rilpivirine effect, treatment failure; give 12 hr before or 4 hr after rilpivirine
Antacids: Decreased rilpivirine effect; use 2 hr or more before, or 4 hr after rilpivirine
CYP3A4 inhibitors (aldesleukin, amiodarone, aprepitant, atazanavir, basiliximab, boceprevir, bromocriptine, chloramphenicol, clarithromycin, conivaptan, dalopristin, danazol, darunavir, dasatinib, delavirdine, diltiazem, dronedarone, efavirenz, erythromycin, ethinyl estradiol, fluconazole, FLUoxetine, fluvoxaMINE, fosamprenavir, fosaprepitant, IL-2, imatinib, indinavir, isoniazid, itraconazole, ketoconazole, lanreotide, lapatinib, miconazole, nefazodone, nelfinavir, niCARdipine, octreotide, posaconazole, quiNINE, ranolazine, rifaximin, tamoxifen, telaprevir,

R

Adverse effects: *italics* = common; **bold** = life-threatening

telithromycin, tipranavir, troleadomycin, verapamil, voriconazole, zafirlukast): Increased rilpivirine effect

Class IA/III antidysrhytmics, some phenothiazines, beta agonists, local anesthetics, tricyclics, CYP3A4 inhibitors (amiodarone, arsenic trioxide, clarithromycin, erythromycin, levomethadyl, telithromycin, troleandomycin); CYP3A4 substrates (methadone, pimozide, QUEtiapine, quiNIDine, risperiDONE, ziprasidone), halogenated anesthetics: Increased QT prolongation

Drug/food
Increased adverse reactions: grapefruit juice

NURSING CONSIDERATIONS
Assessment
• **HIV:** Assess symptoms of HIV, including opportunistic infections before and during treatment; some may be life-threatening; monitor plasma HIV RNA, CD4+, CD8+ cell counts, serum β-2 microglobulin, serum ICD+24 antigen levels; treatment failures occur more frequently in those with baseline HIV-1 RNA concs >100,000 copies/ml than in patients with concs <100,000 copies/ml; monitor serum cholesterol, lipid panel
• Antiretroviral drug resistance testing before initiation of therapy in antiretroviral treatment-naive patients
• For adults and adolescents, initiation of antiretroviral therapy is recommended in any patient with a history of an AIDS-defining infection; with a CD4 ≤500/mm³; who is pregnant; who has HIV-associated nephropathy; or who is being treated for hepatitis B (HBV) infection
⚠ **Suicidal thoughts/behaviors: Assess frequently for suicidal ideation; report any increase in depressive symptoms**
• **Hepatic disease:** monitor for elevated hepatic enzymes (>2.5 × ULN); grade 3 and 4 may be higher in patients co-infected with hepatitis B or C

Patient/family education
• Teach patient that product is not a cure but controls symptoms, that continuing use is required
• Teach patient that product must be taken in combination with other prescribed products
• Teach patient to advise prescriber of all products that are used
• Advise patient to report mood changes and depression immediately
• Teach patient to report if pregnancy is suspected immediately, do not breastfeed

Evaluation
Positive therapeutic outcome
• Control of HIV-related symptoms

RARELY USED

riluzole (Rx)
(ri-loo′zole)
Rilutek
Func. class.: Amyotropic lateral sclerosis (ALS) agent
Chem. class.: Benzathiazole
Pregnancy category C

Therapeutic outcome: Decreased symptoms of ALS

USES: ALS

CONTRAINDICATIONS
Hypersensitivity

DOSAGE AND ROUTES
Adult: PO 50 mg q12hr; take 1 hr before or 2 hr after meals

---

riociguat
(rye′oh-sig′ue-at)
Adempas
Func. class.: Antihypertensive/vasodilator
Chem. class.: Guanylate cyclase stimulator
Pregnancy category X

ACTION: Guanylate cyclase stimulator; also a vasoconstrictor

Therapeutic outcome: Decrease in B/P; decreased shortness of breath

USES: WHO Group I pulmonary arterial hypertension and WHO Group IV persistent/recurrent chronic thromboembolic pulmonary hypertension

CONTRAINDICATIONS
Breastfeeding, hypersensitivity

BLACK BOX WARNING: Pregnancy (X)

Precautions: Hypotension, hypovolemia, pulmonary edema, smoking

DOSAGE AND ROUTES
Adult: PO 1 mg tid, may start at 0.5 mg tid if needed; if systolic B/P remains >95 mm Hg, increase by 0.5 mg tid; increase no sooner than 2 wk, max 2.5 mg tid

---

Renal/hepatic dose
Adult: Not recommended in CCr <15ml/min or Child Pugh C

Available forms: Tabs 0.5, 1, 1.5, 2, 2.5 mg

Implementation
- Give tid without regard to food
- Do not discontinue abruptly
- If dose is missed, take at next scheduled dose; if stopped for ≥3 days, begin with initial dose

ADVERSE EFFECTS
CNS: Dizziness
CV: Hypotension, peripheral edema, palpitations
EENT: Sinusitis, rhinitis
GI: Constipation, gastritis, gastroesophageal reflux, nausea, vomiting
GU: Decreased sperm counts
HEMA: Anemia, bleeding, nosebleeds
RESP: Pulmonary edema

Pharmacokinetics

Absorption	Unknown
Distribution	95% protein binding
Metabolism	By P-gb, CYP1A1, CYP3A4, CYP#A, CYP2C8, CYP2J2
Excretion	Unknown
Half-life	Terminal 15 hr

Pharmacodynamics

Onset	Unknown
Peak	1.5 hr
Duration	Unknown

INTERACTIONS
Drug classifications
CYP3A4 inhibitors (amprenavir, aprepitant, atazanavir, clarithromycin, conivaptan, cycloSPORINE, dalfopristin, danazol, darunavir, erythromycin, estradiol, imatinib, itraconazole, ketoconazole, nefazodone, nelfinavir, propoxyphene, quinupristin, ritonavir, RU-486, saquinavir, tamoxifen, telithromycin, troleandomycin, zafirlukast): increased riociguat effect
Nitrates, nitric oxide donors, phosphodiesterase-5 inhibitors: do not use concurrently
Tobacco smoking: decreased riociguat effect

Drug/herbs
St. John's wort, ephedra (ma huang): require dosage change

NURSING CONSIDERATIONS
Assessment
- Pulmonary status: assess for improvement in breathing, ability to exercise; pulmonary edema may indicate venoocclusive disease

> **BLACK BOX WARNING:** Assess pregnancy status before giving this product; pregnancy category **X**

Patient/family education
- Teach patient the importance of complying with dosage schedule even if feeling better

> **BLACK BOX WARNING:** Teach patient to notify if pregnancy is planned or suspected (if pregnant, product will need to be discontinued, pregnancy test done monthly); to use 2 contraception methods while taking this product

- Instruct patient not to use OTC products including herbs, supplements, unless approved by prescriber

Evaluation
Positive therapeutic outcome
- Decrease in B/P; decreased shortness of breath

risedronate (Rx)
(rih-sed′roh-nate)
Actonel, Atelvia
Func. class.: Bone resorption inhibitor
Chem. class.: Bisphosphonate
Pregnancy category C

Do not confuse: Actonel/Actos

ACTION: Inhibits bone resorption; absorbs calcium phosphate crystal in bone and may directly block dissolution of hydroxyapatite crystals of bone

Therapeutic outcome: Increased bone mass, activity without fractures

USES: Paget's disease; prevention, treatment of osteoporosis in postmenopausal women; glucocorticoid-induced osteoporosis; osteoporosis in men

CONTRAINDICATIONS
Hypersensitivity to bisphosphonates, inability to stand or sit upright for ≥30 min, esophageal stricture, achalasia, hypocalcemia

Precautions: Pregnancy **C,** breastfeeding, children, renal disease, active upper GI disorders, dental disease, hyperparathyroidism, infection, vitamin D deficiency, coagulopathy, chemotherapy, asthma

DOSAGE AND ROUTES
Paget's disease
Adult: PO 30 mg/day × 2 mo; give calcium and vit D if dietary intake is lacking; if relapse occurs, retreatment is advised

R

Treatment/prevention of post-menopausal osteoporosis
Adult: PO 5 mg/day or 35 mg qwk or 75 mg/day × 2 consecutive days 2 × mo or 150 mg qmo

Glucocorticoid osteoporosis
Adult: PO 5 mg/day

Osteoporosis in men
Adult: PO 35 mg qwk

Renal dose
Adult: PO CCr <30 mg/min, avoid use

Available forms: Tabs 5, 30, 35, 75, 150 mg; tab, weekly 35 mg

Implementation
• Give PO for 2 mo to be effective in Paget's disease
• Give with a full glass of water; patient should be in upright position, give delayed release tablet in AM after breakfast, only use with food (delayed release)
• Administer supplemental calcium and vit D in Paget's disease
• Give daily ≥30 min before meals
• Store in cool environment out of direct sunlight

ADVERSE EFFECTS
CNS: Dizziness, headache, depression
CV: Chest pain, hypertension, atrial fibrillation
GI: *Abdominal pain,* diarrhea, *nausea,* constipation, esophagitis
MS: *Severe muscle/joint/bone pain,* osteonecrosis of the jaw, fractures
MISC: Rash, UTI, pharyngitis, hypocalcemia, hypophosphatemia, increased PTH
SYST: Angioedema

Pharmacokinetics

Absorption	Unknown
Distribution	To bones (50%)
Metabolism	Unknown
Excretion	Kidneys
Half-life	Terminal 23 hr

Pharmacodynamics
Unknown

INTERACTIONS
Drug classifications
Aluminum, antacids, calcium, iron, magnesium salts: decreased absorption of risedronate
NSAIDs, salicylates: increased GI irritation
H_2 antagonists, proton pump inhibitors: decreases absorption of delayed release risedronate; do not use together

Drug/food
Food: decreased bioavailability; take ½ hr before food or drinks other than water

Drug/lab test
Decreased: calcium, phosphorus

NURSING CONSIDERATIONS
Assessment
• **Paget's disease:** assess for headache, bone pain, increased head circumference
• **Osteoporosis:** in men or postmenopausal women; bone density study prior to and periodically during treatment
• **Hypocalcemia:** assess for paresthesia, twitching, laryngospasm, Chvostek's/Trousseau's signs
⚠ **Serious skin reactions: assess for angioedema**
⚠ **Assess for atrial fibrillation**
• Monitor phosphate, alkaline phosphatase, calcium; creatinine, BUN (renal disease)
• **Hypercalcemia:** assess for paresthesia, twitching, laryngospasm, Chvostek's/Trousseau's signs
⚠ **Assess dental health, cover with antiinfectives prior to dental extraction**

Patient/family education
• Advise patient to sit upright for ½ hr after dose to prevent irritation
• **Teach patient to notify prescriber immediately if difficulty swallowing, severe heartburn, or pain in chest**
• Instruct patient to comply with dietary restrictions, maintain good oral hygiene
• Advise patient to notify prescriber if pregnancy is planned or suspected

Evaluation
Positive therapeutic outcome
• Increased bone mass, absence of fractures

---

risperiDONE (Rx)
(res-pare'a-done)
RisperDAL, Risperdal Consta, Risperdal M-TAB
Func. class.: Antipsychotic
Chem. class.: Benzisoxazole derivative
Pregnancy category C

Do not confuse: RisperDAL/reserpine

ACTION: Unknown; may be mediated through both DOPamine type 2 (D_2) and serotonin type 2 (5-HT$_2$) antagonism

Therapeutic outcome: Decreased hallucinations and disorganized thought

---

USES: Irritability associated with autism, bipolar disorder, mania, schizophrenia

CONTRAINDICATIONS
Hypersensitivity, seizure

Precautions: Pregnancy **C**, children, geriatric, cardiac/renal/hepatic disease, breast cancer, Parkinson's disease, CNS depression, brain tumor, dehydration, diabetes, hematologic disease, seizure disorders, breastfeeding, abrupt discontinuation, suicidal ideation, phenylketonuria

> **BLACK BOX WARNING:** Increased mortality in elderly patients with dementia-related psychosis

DOSAGE AND ROUTES
Adult: PO 2 mg/day as a single dose or 2 divided doses, adjust dose at intervals of ≥24 hr and 1-2 mg/day as tolerated to 4-8 mg/day; IM establish dosing with PO prior to IM 25 mg q2wk, may increase to max 50 mg q2wk

Adolescent: PO 0.5 mg/day in AM or PM, adjust dose at intervals of ≥24 hr and 0.5-1 mg/day as tolerated to 3 mg/day

Geriatric: PO 0.5 mg daily-bid, increase by 1 mg qwk; IM 25 mg q2wk

Hepatic dose/renal dose
Adult: PO 0.5 mg, increase by 0.5 mg bid, then increase to 1.5 mg bid at intervals ≥1 wk

Available forms: Tabs 0.25, 0.5, 1, 2, 3, 4 mg; oral sol 1 mg/ml; orally disintegrating tabs 0.25, 0.5, 1, 2, 3, 4 mg; long-acting inj kit (Risperdal Consta) 12.5, 25, 37.5, 50 mg

Implementation
PO route
- Reduced dosage in geriatric patients
- Anticholinergic agent on order from prescriber, to be used for EPS
- Avoid use with CNS depressants
- Conventional tabs: give without regard to meals
- *Oral disintegrating tab* (Risperdal M-Tab): do not open blister pack until ready to use; tear 1 of the 4 units apart at perforation; bend corner where indicated; peel back foil; do not push tab through foil; remove from pack and place on tongue; tab disintegrates in seconds and can be swallowed with or without liquids, do not split or chew
- *Oral solution:* may dilute 3-4 oz of a beverage, measure dose using calibrated pipette, not compatible with tea, cola; compatible with water, coffee, orange juice, low-fat milk

IM route
- Only suspend in the diluent provided and with the supplied needle; prior to admixing, allow to come to room temperature for 30 minutes prior to reconstitution
- Remove colored cap from the vial without removing rubber stopper. Wipe top of the grey stopper with an alcohol wipe
- Peel back the blister pouch and remove the Vial Access Device by holding between the white luer cap and the skirt. Do not touch the spike tip at any time
- Place the vial on a hard surface and hold the base. Orient the Vial Access Device vertically over the vial so that the spike tip is at the center of the vial's rubber stopper
- With a straight downward push, press the spike tip of the Vial Access Device through the center of the vial's rubber stopper until the device securely snaps onto the vial top. Improper placement of the Vial Access Device on the vial could result in leakage of the diluent upon transfer
- Hold the base of the vial and swab the syringe connection point (blue circle) of the Vial Access Device with an alcohol wipe and allow to dry prior to attaching the syringe
- Avoid over-tightening, or syringe component parts may loosen from the syringe body
- While holding the white collar of the syringe, insert and press the syringe tip into the blue circle of the Vial Access Device and twist in a clockwise motion to secure the connection of the syringe to the Vial Access Device. Hold the skirt of the Vial Access Device during attachment to prevent it from spinning. Keep the syringe and the Vial Access Device aligned
- Inject the entire contents of the syringe containing the diluent into the vial
- Shake the vial vigorously for a minimum of 10 seconds while holding the plunger rod down with the thumb. Mixing is complete when the suspension appears uniform, thick, and milky colored, and all the powder is dispersed in liquid. The microspheres will be visible in liquid, but no dry microspheres remain
- Invert the vial completely and slowly withdraw the entire content of the suspension from the vial into the syringe. Tear the section of the vial label at the perforation and apply the detached label to the syringe for identification purposes
- While holding the white collar of the syringe, unscrew the syringe from the Vial Access Device, then discard both the vial and the Vial Access Device appropriately
- Select the appropriate color-coded needle provided with the kit. Two distinct needles are provided. The needle with the yellow colored hub and print is for injection into the gluteal muscle (2-inch needle) and the needle with the

R

Adverse effects: *italics* = common; **bold** = life-threatening

green colored hub and print is for deltoid muscles (1-inch needle). They are not interchangeable; do not use the needle intended for gluteal injection for deltoid injection, and vice versa

- Peel the blister pouch of the Needle-Pro safety device open halfway. Grasp the transparent needle sheath using the plastic peel pouch. To prevent contamination, do not touch the orange Needle-Pro safety device's luer connector. While holding the white collar of the syringe, attach the luer connection of the orange Needle-Pro safety device to the syringe with an easy clockwise twisting motion
- While holding the white collar of the syringe, grasp the transparent needle sheath and seat the needle firmly on the orange Needle-Pro safety device with a push and a clockwise twist. Seating the needle will secure the connection between the needle and the orange Needle-Pro safety device
- While holding the white collar of the syringe, pull the transparent needle sheath straight away from the needle. Do not twist the sheath since this may loosen the luer connection
- Re-suspension will be necessary prior to administration, since settling will occur after reconstitution. Re-suspend the microspheres in the syringe by shaking vigorously
- May refer to the Instructions for Use section of the product labeling for detailed visual aids that accompany the written instructions

Administration
- **Only for IM; do not give IV**
- Re-suspension will be necessary prior to administration, since settling will occur after reconstitution. Re-suspend the microspheres in the syringe by shaking vigorously
- Remove any air bubbles by tapping the syringe and slowly depressing the plunger with the needle in an upright position
- Inject the entire contents of the syringe into the upper outer quadrant of the gluteal area or the deltoid muscle of the arm; inject immediately after reconstitution to avoid settling. Gluteal injections should be alternated between the two buttocks
- After the injection is complete, press the needle into the orange Needle-Pro safety device by gently pressing the orange Needle-Pro safety device against a flat surface with one hand. As the orange Needle-Pro safety device is pressed, the needle will firmly engage into the orange Needle-Pro safety device
- Visually confirm full engagement of the needle into the Needle-Pro safety device, then appropriately discard both the used and unused needle provided in the dose pack

- Do not store the vial after reconstitution or the suspension may settle
- Do not combine 2 different dosage strengths of Risperdal Consta in a single administration
- The dose pack device is for single use only. Do not re-process for subsequent re-use because the integrity of the device may be compromised leading to a deterioration in performance
- *Stability after reconstitution:* Once in suspension, the product may remain at room temperature but must be used within 6 hr. Always re-suspend prior to administration if not used immediately
- When switching from oral to inj, give oral dose with first inj and continue for 3 wk, then discontinue

ADVERSE EFFECTS
CNS: *EPS (pseudoparkinsonism, akathisia, dystonia, tardive dyskinesia), drowsiness, insomnia, agitation, anxiety, headache,* neuroleptic malignant syndrome, dizziness, seizures, suicidal ideation, head titubation (shaking)
CV: Orthostatic hypotension, tachycardia, heart failure, sudden death (geriatric), AV block
EENT: Blurred vision, tinnitus
GI: *Nausea,* vomiting, *anorexia, constipation,* jaundice, weight gain
GU: Hyperprolactinemia, gynecomastia, dysuria
HEMA: Neutropenia, granulocytopenia
MS: Rhabdomyolysis
MISC: Renal artery disease; weight gain, hyperprolactinemia (child)
RESP: Rhinitis, sinusitis, upper respiratory infection, cough

Pharmacokinetics

Absorption	Unknown
Distribution	Unknown
Metabolism	Liver, extensively
Excretion	Urine 90%
Half-life	3-24 hr

Pharmacodynamics

Onset	Unknown
Peak	1-2 hr
Duration	Up to 12 hr

INTERACTIONS
Individual drugs
Alcohol: increased sedation
⚠ Chloroquine, clarithromycin, droperidol, erythromycin, haloperidol, methadone, pentamidine, thioridazine, ziprasidone: increased QT prolongation

---

CarBAMazepine: increased risperiDONE excretion

⚠ **Furosemide: increased risk of death in dementia-related psychosis**

Levodopa: decreased levodopa effect

⚠ **TraMADol: increased seizures**

⚠ **Valproic acid, verapamil: increased risperiDONE levels**

Drug classifications

Acetylcholinesterase inhibitors, CYP2D6 inhibitors, SSRIs: increased risperiDONE levels

Antipsychotics: increased EPS

⚠ **β-agonists, class IA/III antidysrhythmics, local anesthetics, some phenothiazines, tricyclics: increased QT prolongation**

CNS depressants: increased sedation

CYP2D6 inducers (carBAMazepine, barbiturates, phenytoin, rifampin): decreased risperiDONE action

CYP2D6 inhibitors (selective serotonin reuptake inhibitors): serotonin syndrome, neuroleptic malignant syndrome

Drug/herb

Echinacea: decreased risperiDONE effect

Drug/lab test

Increased: prolactin levels, blood glucose, lipids

NURSING CONSIDERATIONS
Assessment

• **Suicidal thoughts, behaviors often occur when depression is lessened; assess mental status: orientation, mood, behavior, presence and type of hallucinations before initial administration, monthly; this product should significantly reduce psychotic behavior**

• Monitor thyroid function test, blood glucose, serum electrolytes/prolactin/lipid profile, bilirubin, creatinine, weight, pregnancy test, CBC, LFTs, AIMS assessment, and weight baseline periodically

• Assess affect, orientation, LOC, reflexes, gait, coordination, sleep pattern disturbances

• **QT prolongation: Monitor B/P with patient in sitting, standing, and lying positions; take pulse and respirations q4hr during initial treatment; establish baseline before starting treatment; report drops of 30 mm Hg; obtain baseline ECG and monitor Q- and T-wave changes**

• Check for dizziness, faintness, palpitations, tachycardia on rising; severe orthostatic hypotension is common

⚠ **Assess for neuroleptic malignant syndrome: hyperpyrexia, muscle rigidity, increased CPK, altered mental status; product should be discontinued**

• EPS: Assess for akathisia (inability to sit still, no pattern to movements), tardive dyskinesia (bizarre movements of the jaw, mouth, tongue, extremities), pseudoparkinsonism (rigidity, tremors, pill rolling, shuffling gait); an antiparkinsonian product should be prescribed

• Assess for constipation, urinary retention daily; if these occur, increase bulk, water in diet

• Assess for weight gain, hyperglycemia, metabolic changes in diabetes, increased lipids

Patient/family education

• Teach patient to use good oral hygiene; frequent rinsing of mouth, sugarless gum for dry mouth

• Caution patient to avoid hazardous activities until product response is determined; dizziness, blurred vision may occur

• Inform patient that orthostatic hypotension occurs often; patient should rise from sitting or lying position gradually and remain lying down for at least 30 min after IM inj

• **Instruct patient to avoid hot tubs, hot showers, tub baths; hypotension may occur**

• Inform patient that heat stroke may occur in hot weather and to take extra precautions to stay cool

• Advise patient to avoid abrupt withdrawal of this product, or EPS may result; product should be withdrawn slowly

• Teach patient to avoid OTC preparations (cough, hay fever, cold) unless approved by prescriber; serious product interactions may occur; avoid use with alcohol, CNS depressants because increased drowsiness may occur

• Advise patient to use contraception, to inform prescriber if pregnancy is planned or suspected

⚠ **Teach patient to notify provider of suicidal thoughts/behaviors**

Evaluation
Positive therapeutic outcome

• Decrease in emotional excitement, hallucinations, delusions, paranoia

• Reorganization of patterns of thought, speech

TREATMENT OF OVERDOSE:
Lavage, provide airway

ritonavir (Rx)
(ri-toe′na-veer)
Norvir
Func. class.: Antiretroviral
Chem. class.: Protease inhibitor
Pregnancy category B

Do not confuse: ritonavir/retrovir

R

ACTION: Inhibits HIV-1 protease and prevents maturation of the infectious virus

Therapeutic outcome: Improvement of HIV-1 infection

USES: HIV-1 in combination with at least 2 other antiretrovirals

CONTRAINDICATIONS
Hypersensitivity

> **BLACK BOX WARNING:** Coadministration with other drugs

Precautions: Pregnancy **B,** breastfeeding, children, liver disease, pancreatitis, diabetes, hemophilia, AV block, hypercholesterolemia, immune reconstitution syndrome, neonates, cardiomyopathy, immune reconstitution syndrome

DOSAGE AND ROUTES
Adult/adolescent >16 yr: PO 600 mg bid; if nausea occurs, begin dose at ½ and gradually increase, max 1200 mg/day in divided doses
Adolescent ≤16 yr/child/infant: PO 400 mg/m² bid up to 1200 mg/day in divided doses; may start lower and escalate

Available forms: Caps 100 mg; oral sol 80 mg/ml, tab 100 mg

Implementation
• Oral sol: Shake oral sol well, use calibrated measuring device
• Store caps in refrigerator
• Mix liquid formulation with chocolate milk or liquid nutritional supplement to improve taste
• When switching from cap to tab, more GI symptoms may occur that will lessen over time
• Use dosage titration to minimize side effects
• Overdose: infants, children 43.2% alcohol, 26.57% propylene glycol oral solution, calculate total amount of alcohol, propylene glycol from all products given

ADVERSE EFFECTS
CNS: *Paresthesia*, headache, seizures, dizziness, insomnia, fever, asthenia, intracranial bleeding
CV: QT, PR interval prolongation
GI: *Diarrhea*, buccal mucosa ulceration, *abdominal pain, nausea, taste perversion*, dry mouth, *vomiting, anorexia*
INTEG: Rash
MISC: Asthenia, angioedema, anaphylaxis, Stevens-Johnson syndrome, increased lipids, lipodystrophy, toxic epidermal necrolysis
MS: Pain, rhabdomyolysis, myalgia

Pharmacokinetics
Absorption	Well
Distribution	Unknown
Metabolism	98% protein binding, liver
Excretion	Unknown
Half-life	3-5 hr

Pharmacodynamics
Onset	Unknown
Peak	2-4 hr
Duration	Unknown

INTERACTIONS
Individual drugs

> **BLACK BOX WARNING:** Amiodarone, astemizole, buPROPion, cisapride, cloZAPine, desipramine, encainide, ergotamine, flecainide, meperedine, midazolam, pimozide, piroxicam, propafenone, propoxyphene, quiNIDine, ranolazine, saquinavir, terfenadine, triazolam, zolpidem: toxicity, do not use together

Atovaquone, divalproex, ethinyl estradiol, lamoTRIgine, phenytoin, sulfamethoxazole, theophylline, voriconazole, zidovudine: decreased levels of each drug
Bosentan: increased levels of bosentan
Clarithromycin: increased level of both products
ddI: increased levels of both products
Fluconazole: increased ritonavir level

> **BLACK BOX WARNING:** Haloperidol, chloroquine, droperidol, pentamidine, arsenic trioxide, levomethadyl: increased QT prolongation

Nevirapine, phenytoin: decreased ritonavir levels

Drug classifications
Anticoagulants: decreased levels of anticoagulants
Azole antifungals, benzodiazepines, HMG-CoA reductase inhibitors, interleukins: toxicity, do not use together
Barbiturates, rifamycins: decreased ritonavir level

> **BLACK BOX WARNING:** Class IA/III antidysrhythmics, some phenothiazines, β-agonists, local anesthetics, tricyclics, CYP3A4 inhibitors (amiodarone, clarithromycin, erythromycin, telithromycin, troleandomycin), CYP3A4 substrates (dasatinib, methadone, pimozide, QUEtiapine, quiNIDine, risperiDONE, ziprasidone): increased QT prolongation

CYP2D6 inhibitors: toxicity, do not use together

Drug/herb
Red yeast rice: avoid use
St. John's wort: decreased ritonavir levels, avoid concurrent use

Drug/lab test
Increased: ALT, GGT, AST, CK, cholesterol, triglycerides, uric acid
Decreased: Hct, RBC, Hgb, neutrophils, WBC

NURSING CONSIDERATIONS
Assessment
• **QT prolongation: ECG for QT prolongation, ejection fraction; assess for chest pain, palpitations, dyspnea**
• **Rhabdomyolysis: muscle pain, increased CPK, weakness, swelling of affected muscles; if these occur and if confirmed by CPK, product should be discontinued**
⚠ **Immune reconstitution syndrome: may occur with combination therapy, may develop inflammatory response with opportunistic infection (MAC, Graves disease, Guillain-Barré syndrome, TB, PCP), may occur during initial treatment or months afterward**
• Assess signs of infection, anemia
• Monitor viral load and CD4, blood glucose, plasma HIV RNA, serum cholesterol, lipid profile baseline, throughout therapy
• Resistance testing prior to starting therapy and after treatment failure
• Assess liver function tests: ALT, AST; in those with hepatic disease, monitor q3mo
• Monitor C&S before product therapy; product may be taken as soon as culture is done; repeat C&S after treatment; determine the presence of other STDs
• Assess bowel pattern before, during treatment; if severe abdominal pain with bleeding occurs, product should be discontinued; monitor hydration
• **Serious skin disorders: Stevens-Johnson syndrome, angioedema; anaphylaxis, toxic epidermal necrolysis**

Patient/family education
• Teach patient to take as prescribed; if dose is missed, take as soon as remembered up to 1 hr before next dose; do not double dose
• Teach patient that product must be taken in equal intervals around the clock to maintain blood levels for duration of therapy
• Teach patient that product is not a cure for HIV; opportunistic infections may continue to be acquired, and others may continue to contract HIV from the patient
• Advise patient not to use St. John's wort, that it decreases this product's effect

• Inform that redistribution of body fat or accumulation of body fat may occur

Evaluation
Positive therapeutic outcome
• Decreasing symptoms of HIV
• Improving viral load and CD4 cell counts

⚠ HIGH ALERT

riTUXimab (Rx)
(rih-tuks'ih-mab)
Rituxan
Func. class.: Antineoplastic—miscellaneous; DMARD
Chem. class.: Murine/human monoclonal antibody
Pregnancy category C

ACTION: Directed against the CD20 antigen that is found on malignant B lymphocytes; CD20 regulates a portion of cell cycle initiation/differentiation

Therapeutic outcome: Decreased tumor size, prevention of spread of cancer

USES: Non-Hodgkin's lymphoma (CD20 positive, B-cell), bulky disease (tumors >10 cm), rheumatoid arthritis, Wegener's granulomatosis, microscopic polyangitis

CONTRAINDICATIONS
Hypersensitivity, murine proteins

Precautions: Pregnancy C, breastfeeding, children, geriatric, cardiac/renal/pulmonary conditions

> **BLACK BOX WARNING:** Exfoliative dermatitis, infusion-related reactions, progressive multifocal leukoencephalopathy

DOSAGE AND ROUTES
Relapsed or refractory low-grade or follicular, CD20 positive, B-cell non-Hodgkin's lymphoma (NHL)
Adult: IV 375 mg/m^2 qwk × 4 doses, may retreat with 4 more doses of 375 mg/m^2 qwk

First-line treatment of follicular, CD20-positive, B-cell non-Hodgkin's lymphoma (NHL), in combination with chemotherapy
Adult: IV 375 mg/m^2 on day 1 of each cycle for up to 8; may be given with cyclophosphamide IV 750 mg/m^2 on day 1, vinCRIStine IV 1.4 mg/m^2 (max of 2 mg) on day 1, and predniSONE 40 mg/m^2/day PO on days 1-5

Adverse effects: *italics* = common; **bold** = life-threatening

Single-agent maintenance therapy in patients with follicular, CD20-positive, B-cell non-Hodgkin's lymphoma (NHL) (complete or partial response following first-line treatment with riTUXimab in combination with chemotherapy)

Adult: IV 375 mg/m² IV q8wk × 12 doses as maintenance therapy starting 8 wk after the completion of induction chemotherapy with 8 doses of riTUXimab with 6-8 cycles of cyclophosphamide, vinCRIStine, and predniSONE 4-6 cycles of cyclophosphamide, DOXOrubicin, vinCRIStine, and predniSONE

As a component of the Zevalin (ibritumomab tiuxetan) regimen

Adult: IV; as a required component of the ibritumomab regimen; riTUXimab 250 mg/m² given within 4 hr prior to the administration of Yttrium-90 ibritumomab that may occur on day 7, 8, or 9

First-line treatment of diffuse large B-cell, CD20-positive non-Hodgkin's lymphoma (NHL), in combination with CHOP or other anthracycline-based chemotherapy regimen

Adult 18-59 yr: IV 375 mg/m² on day 1 of each cycle for up to 8 infusions

As single-agent maintenance therapy in patients with low-grade, CD20-positive, B-cell non-Hodgkin's lymphoma (NHL) with non-progressing disease (stable disease or better) following first-line treatment with cyclophosphamide, vinCRIStine, and predniSONE (CVP)

Adult: IV 375 mg/m² qwk × 4 wk repeated q6mo × 2 years (total of 16 doses) as maintenance therapy starting 4 wk after the completion of first-line chemotherapy with 6 to 8 cycles of cyclophosphamide, vinCRIStine, and predniSONE (CVP)

Available forms: Inj 10 mg/ml (100 mg/10 ml, 500 mg/50 ml)

Implementation

Intermittent IV infusion route
• Hold antihypertensive 2 hr before administration
• Administer after diluting to a final conc of 1-4 mg/ml; use 0.9% NaCl, D₅W, gently invert bag to mix; do not mix with other products
• Increase fluid intake to 2-3 L/day to prevent dehydration, unless contraindicated

• Store vials at 36° F-40° F; protect vials from direct sunlight; inf sol is stable at 36° F-46° F for 24 hr and at room temp for another 12 hr

Y-site compatibilities: Acyclovir, amifostine, amikacin, aminophylline, ampicillin, ampicillin/sulbactam, aztreonam, bleomycin, bumetanide, buprenorphine, busulfan, butorphanol, calcium gluconate, CARBOplatin, carmustine, ceFAZolin, cefoperazone, cefotaxime, cefoTEtan, cefOXitin, cefTAZidime, ceftizoxime, cefTRIAXone, cefuroxime, chlorproMAZINE, cimetidine, CISplatin, clindamycin, cyclophosphamide, cytarabine, DACTINomycin, DAUNOrubicin hydrochloride, dexamethasone, dexrazoxane, digoxin, diphenhydrAMINE, DOBUTamine, DOCEtaxel, DOPamine, DOXOrubicin liposome, doxycycline, droperidol, enalaprilat, etoposide phosphate, famotidine, fentaNYL, filgrastim, floxuridine, fluconazole, fludarabine, fluorouracil, ganciclovir, gemcitabine, gentamicin, granisetron, haloperidol, heparin, hydrocortisone, HYDROmorphone, IDArubicin, ifosfamide, imipenem/cilastatin, irinotecan, leucovorin, levorphanol, LORazepam, magnesium sulfate, mannitol, meperidine, mesna, methotrexate, methylPREDNISolone, metoclopramide, metroNIDAZOLE, mitoMYcin, mitoXANtrone, morphine, nalbuphine, netilmicin, PACLitaxel, pentamidine, piperacillin/tazobactam, plicamycin, potassium chloride, prochlorperazine, promethazine, ranitidine, sargramostim, streptozocin, teniposide, theophylline, thiotepa, ticarcillin/clavulanate, tobramycin, trimethoprim/sulfamethoxazole, trimethobenzamide, vinBLAStine, vinCRIStine, vinorelbine, zidovudine

Y-site incompatibilities: Aldesleukin, amphotericin B colloidal, ciprofloxacin, cycloSPORINE, DAUNOrubicin liposome, DOXOrubicin hydrochloride, furosemide, levofloxacin, minocycline, ondansetron, quinupristin/dalfopristin, sodium bicarbonate, topotecan, vancomycin

Additive incompatibilities: Do not admix with other products

ADVERSE EFFECTS

CNS: Life-threatening brain infection (progressive multifocal leukoencephalopathy)
CV: Cardiac dysrhythmias, heart failure, MI, superventricular tachycardia, hypertension, angina
GI: *Nausea, vomiting, anorexia,* GI obstruction/perforation
GU: Renal failure
HEMA: Leukopenia, neutropenia, thrombocytopenia, anemia
INTEG: *Irritation at inj site, rash,* fatal mucocutaneous infections (rare)

MISC: *Fever,* chills, asthenia, *headache,* angioedema, hypotension, myalgia, bronchospasm, ARDs

SYST: Stevens-Johnson syndrome, exfoliative dermatitis, toxic epidermal necrolysis, tumor lysis syndrome

Pharmacokinetics

Absorption	Unknown
Distribution	Binds to CD20 sites on lymphoma cells
Metabolism	Unknown
Excretion	Unknown
Half-life	Varies

Pharmacodynamics
Unknown

INTERACTIONS
Individual drugs
CISplatin: increased nephrotoxicity—avoid concurrent use; if used, monitor renal status

Drug classifications
Anticoagulants, NSAIDs: increased bleeding risk
Antihypertensives: increased hypotension, separate by 12 hr

NURSING CONSIDERATIONS
Assessment

> **BLACK BOX WARNING:** Assess for signs of fatal inf reaction: hypoxia, pulmonary infiltrates, ARDS, MI, ventricular fibrillation, cardiogenic shock; most fatal inf reactions occur with first inf, discontinue product

> **BLACK BOX WARNING:** Assess for signs of severe mucocutaneous reactions: Stevens-Johnson syndrome, lichenoid dermatitis, toxic epidermal lysis; signs occur 1-13 wk after product was given, discontinue treatment immediately

> **BLACK BOX WARNING:** Assess for tumor lysis syndrome: acute renal failure requiring hemodialysis, hyperkalemia, hypocalcemia, hyperuricemia, hyperphosphatasemia; allopurinol and adequate hydration may be needed

> **BLACK BOX WARNING: Multifocal leukoencephalopathy:** confusion, dizziness, lethargy, hemiparesis, monitor periodically

• Monitor CBC, differential, platelet count weekly; withhold product if WBC is <3500/mm³ or platelet count <100,000/mm³; notify prescriber of these results; product should be discontinued

• Monitor ECG, serum creatinine/BUN, electrolytes, uric acid
• Assess GI symptoms: frequency of stools, abdominal pain, perforation/obstruction may occur
⚠ Infection: assess for fever, increased temperature, flulike symptoms in those with WG and MPA, in those using DMARDs

Patient/family education
• Advise patient to report to prescriber possible infection (cough, fever, chills, sore throat), renal issues (painful urination, back/side pain), bleeding (gums, stools, bruising, urine, emesis, fatigue)
• Advise to avoid OTC products
⚠ Teach to use contraception during and up to 12 mo after therapy
• Avoid use with vaccines, toxoids

Evaluation

Positive therapeutic outcome
• Prevention of increasing cancer progression

⚠ HIGH ALERT

rivaroxaban
(ri-va-rox'a-ban)
Xarelto
Func. class.: Anticoagulant
Chem. class.: Factor Xa inhibitor
Pregnancy category C

ACTION: A novel, oral anticoagulant that selectively and potently inhibits coagulation factor Xa

Therapeutic outcome: Prevention of DVT, stroke, and systemic embolism

USES: For deep venous thrombosis (DVT) prophylaxis, pulmonary embolism (PE), in patients undergoing knee or hip replacement surgery; for stroke prophylaxis and systemic embolism prophylaxis in patients with nonvalvular atrial fibrillation

CONTRAINDICATIONS
Severe hypersensitivity

Precautions: Moderate or severe hepatic disease (Child-Pugh Class B or C), hepatic disease associated with coagulopathy, creatinine clearance <30 ml/min for use as DVT prophylaxis and <15 ml/min for stroke and systemic embolism prophylaxis in nonvalvular atrial fibrillation, dental procedures, neonates, infants, children, adolescents, pregnancy category C, aneurysm, diabetes retinopathy, breastfeeding, diverticulitis, endocarditis, geriatrics, GI bleeding, hypertension, obstetric delivery, peptic ulcer disease, stroke, surgery

DOSAGE AND ROUTES
Deep venous thrombosis (DVT) prophylaxis, which may lead to pulmonary embolism (PE) (knee or hip replacement surgery)
Administer the initial dose at least 6–10 hr after surgery once hemostasis has been established
Adult: PO 10 mg daily for 12 days after knee replacement surgery or for 35 days after hip replacement

Stroke prophylaxis and systemic embolism prophylaxis (nonvalvular atrial fibrillation)
Adult: PO 20 mg daily with the evening meal (CrCl > 50 ml/min); **converting from warfarin to rivaroxaban:** discontinue warfarin and start rivaroxaban when INR is <3; **converting from another anticoagulant other than warfarin to rivaroxaban:** start rivaroxaban 0-2 hr before the next scheduled evening administration of anticoagulant (omit that dose of anticoagulant); for continuous infusion of unfractionated heparin, stop the infusion and initiate rivaroxaban simultaneously; **converting from rivaroxaban to another anticoagulant with rapid onset (not warfarin):** Discontinue rivaroxaban and give the first dose of the other anticoagulant (oral or parenteral) at the time that the next dose of rivaroxaban would have been administered

Renal dose
Adult: PO (nonvalvular atrial fibrillation) CCr 15-50 ml/min, 15 mg/day; CCr <15 ml/min, avoid use; (treatment/prophylaxis of DVT/pulmonary embolism) CCr <30 ml/min, avoid use

Hepatic dose
Adult: PO Child-Pugh class B or C: avoid use

Available forms: Tab 10, 15, 20, 50 mg

Implementation
• For DVT prophylaxis: give daily without regard to food, give initial dose ≥6-10 hr after surgery when hemostasis has been established
• For stroke/systemic embolism prophylaxis: give daily with evening meal
• If dose is not given at correct time, give as soon as possible on the same day
• Unless pathological bleeding occurs, do not discontinue rivaroxaban in the absence of alternative

• Store at room temperature
• 15, 20 mg tablets should be taken with food, for those unable to swallow whole, 15 mg and 20 mg tablets may be crushed, mixed with applesauce, immediately following administration, instruct to eat, crushed tablets are stable in applesauce for up to 4 hr
• 10 mg tablet can be taken without regard to food

Nasogastric (NG) tube or gastric feeding tube
• Confirm gastric placement of tube
• Crush 15 mg or 20 mg tablet, suspend in 50 ml of water, and administer via NG or gastric feeding tube
• To minimize reduced absorption, avoid administration distal to the stomach
• Enteral feeding should immediately follow administration of a crushed dose
• Crushed tablets are stable in water for up to 4 hours

Missed doses
• Patients receiving 15 mg twice daily should take their missed dose immediately to ensure intake of 30 mg per day. Two 15-mg tablets may be taken at once followed by the regular 15 mg twice daily dose the next day
• For patients receiving once daily dosing, take the missed dose as soon as it is remembered

ADVERSE EFFECTS
GI: Cholestasis, cytolytic hepatitis, hyperbilirubinemia, increased hepatic enzymes, jaundice, nausea
HEMA: Adrenal bleeding, bleeding, cerebral hemorrhage, epidural hematoma, GI bleeding, hemiparesis, intracranial bleeding, retinal hemorrhage, retroperitoneal hemorrhage, subdural hematoma, thrombocytopenia
INTEG: Anaphylactic reaction, anaphylactic shock, blister, hypersensitivity, pruritus
SYST: Stevens-Johnson syndrome

> **BLACK BOX WARNING:** Active bleeding

> **BLACK BOX WARNING:** Abrupt discontinuation, epidermal/spinal anesthesia

Pharmacokinetics

Absorption	80%-100%
Distribution	Protein binding (92%-95%)
Metabolism	Oxidative degradation
Excretion	Urine (66%), feces (17%)
Half-life	5-9 hr; geriatric: 11-13 hr

Pharmacodynamics

Onset	Unknown
Peak	2-4 hrs
Duration	Unknown

INTERACTIONS
Individual drugs

Clarithromycin, conivaptan, erythromycin, itraconazole, ketoconazole, lopinavir/ritonavir, nicardipine: increased rivaroxaban effect, possible bleeding

CarBAMazepine, phenytoin, rifampin, ritonavir: decreased rivaroxaban effect

Amiodarone, azithromycin, darunavir, diltiazem, dronedarone, felodipine, fluconazole, lapatinib, mifepristone, nelfinavir, pantoprazole, posaconazole, quiNIDine, ranolazine, saquinavir, tamoxifen, telithromycin, verapamil: increased rivaroxaban effect in renal impairment

Drug classifications

NSAIDs, other anticoagulants, platelet inhibitors, salicylates, thrombolytics: increased rivaroxaban effect, possible bleeding

Drug/herb
St. John's wort: decreased rivaroxaban effect

Drug/food
Grapefruit juice: increased rivaroxaban effect in renal disease

Food: decreased rivaroxaban effect

NURSING CONSIDERATIONS
Assessment

> **BLACK BOX WARNING: Bleeding:** Monitor for bleeding, including bleeding during dental procedures, easy bruising, blood in urine, stools, emesis, sputum, epistaxis; there is no specific antidote

> **BLACK BOX WARNING: Abrupt discontinuation:** Avoid the abrupt discontinuation unless an alternative anticoagulant is used in those with atrial fibrillation; discontinuing puts patients at increased risk for thrombotic events; if this product must be discontinued for reasons other than pathological bleeding, consider administering another anticoagulant

• **Pregnancy/breastfeeding: pregnancy category C; identify if pregnancy is suspected or planned; pregnancy-related hemorrhage may occur, and anticoagulation cannot be monitored with standard laboratory testing; breastfeeding should be discontinued prior to use of this product**

> **BLACK BOX WARNING: Epidural/spinal anesthesia:** Epidural or spinal hematomas that may result in long-term/permanent paralysis may occur in patients who have received anticoagulants and are receiving neuraxial anesthesia or undergoing spinal puncture. The epidural catheter should not be removed <18 hr after the last dose of rivaroxaban; do not administer the next rivaroxaban dose <6 hr after the catheter removal; delay rivaroxaban administration for 24 hr if traumatic puncture occurs. Monitor for neuro changes

• **Hepatic/Renal disease: Increase in effect of this product in hepatic disease (Child-Pugh Class B or C), hepatic disease with coagulopathy; renal failure/severe renal impairment (creatinine clearance <30 ml/min in DVT prophylaxis and <15 ml/min for stroke/systemic embolism prophylaxis in nonvalvular atrial fibrillation); product should be discontinued in acute renal failure; reduce dose in those with atrial fibrillation and CrCl 15-50 ml/min; monitor renal function periodically (creatinine clearance, BUN)**

Patient/family education

• **Advise patient to report numbness of extremities, weakness, tingling, contact prescriber immediately (neuraxial anesthesia, spinal puncture)**

• Advise patient to report if pregnancy is planned or suspected, not to breastfeed

• Teach patient to report bleeding (bruising, blood in urine, stools, sputum, emesis, heavy menstrual flow) and to use soft toothbrush, electric shaver

• Advise patient to inform all health care providers of use; report to prescriber all products used, to take only as directed

• Advise patient to avoid abrupt discontinuation without another blood thinner

• Instruct patients, especially those with dental disease, in proper oral hygiene, including caution in use of regular toothbrushes, dental floss, and toothpicks.

Evaluation
Positive therapeutic outcome
• Prevention of DVT, stroke and systemic embolism

rivastigmine (Rx)
(riv-as-tig′mine)
Exelon, Exelon Patch
Func. class.: Anti-Alzheimer's agent
Chem. class.: Cholinesterase inhibitor
Pregnancy category B

ACTION: Potent selective inhibitor of brain acetylcholinesterase (AChE) and butycholinerase (BChE)

Therapeutic outcome: Decreased signs and symptoms of Alzheimer's dementia

USES: Mild to severe Alzheimer's dementia, mild to moderate Parkinson's disease dementia (PDD)

CONTRAINDICATIONS
Hypersensitivity to this product, other carbamates

Precautions: Pregnancy **B**, breastfeeding, children, renal/hepatic/respiratory disease, seizure disorder, asthma, urinary obstruction, peptic ulcer, increased intracranial pressure, surgery, GI bleeding, jaundice

DOSAGE AND ROUTES
Adult: PO 1.5 mg bid with food for 4 wk or more, may increase to 3 mg bid after 4 wk or more; may increase to 4.5 mg bid and thereafter 6 mg bid, max 12 mg/day; transdermal apply 4.6 mg/24 hr after 4 wk or more, may increase to 9.5 mg/24 hr; max 13.3 mg/24 hr; for those using 6-12 mg/day PO and switching to transdermal use one 9.5 mg/24 hr; for those using <6 mg/day PO and switching to transdermal use one 4.6 mg/24 hr

Available forms: Caps 1.5, 3, 4.5, 6 mg; transdermal patch 4.6, 9.5 mg/24 hr

Implementation
- Give with meals; take with AM and PM meal even though absorption may be decreased
- Provide assistance with ambulation during beginning therapy
- Discontinue treatment for several doses and restart at same or next lower dosage level if adverse reactions cause intolerance
- If treatment is interrupted for longer than several days treatment should be initiated with the lowest daily dose and titrated as indicated above

Transdermal route
- Apply to clean, hairless, dry skin; not in an area that clothing will rub; rotate sites daily; remove liner; apply firmly; may be used during water activities; avoid saunas, avoid excess sunlight or external heat, each 5 cm² patch contains 9 mg base, rate of 4.6 mg/24 hr, each 10 cm² patch is 18 mg base, rate of 9.5 mg/24 hr

ADVERSE EFFECTS
CNS: *Tremors, confusion, insomnia,* psychosis, hallucination, depression, dizziness, headache, anxiety, somnolence, fatigue, syncope, EPS, exacerbation of Parkinson's disease

CV: **QT prolongation, AV block, cardiac arrest, MI,** angina, palpitations

GI: *Nausea, vomiting, anorexia, abdominal distress, flatulence,* diarrhea, constipation, dyspepsia, colitis, eructation, fecal incontinence, GI bleeding/obstruction, GERD, gastritis, **pancreatitis**

MISC: UTI, asthenia, increased sweating, hypertension, flulike symptoms, weight change

Pharmacokinetics

Absorption	Rapidly, completely absorbed
Distribution	40% protein binding
Metabolism	To decarbamylated metabolite
Excretion	Kidney—metabolites, clearance lowered in geriatric, hepatic disease, increased nicotine use
Half-life	1½ hr

Pharmacodynamics

Onset	Unknown
Peak	1 hr
Duration	Unknown

INTERACTIONS
Individual drugs
Nicotine: increased metabolism, decreased blood level of rivastigmine

Drug classifications
Anticholinergics, phenothiazines, sedating H₁ blockers, tricyclics: decreased rivastigmine effect
Cholinergic agonists, other cholinesterase inhibitors: increased synergistic effect
NSAIDs: increased GI effects

NURSING CONSIDERATIONS
Assessment
- Monitor liver function tests: AST, ALT, alkaline phosphatase, LDH, bilirubin, CBC
- Assess for severe GI effects: nausea, vomiting, anorexia, weight loss, GI bleeding
- Monitor B/P, respiration during initial treatment; hypo/hypertension should be reported
- **Cognitive/mental status:** affect, mood, behavioral changes, depression; complete suicide assessment

Patient/family education
- Teach patient procedure for giving **oral sol**; use instruction sheet provided; teach application of **transdermal** product, to fold in half and discard, not to get in eyes, to wash hands after application, to not use heating pad, sauna, tanning bed
- Teach patient to notify prescriber of severe GI effects, do not discontinue abruptly

---

- Teach patient that product may cause dizziness, anorexia, weight loss

Evaluation

Positive therapeutic outcome

- Increased coherence, decreased symptoms of Alzheimer's disease, improved mood
- Teach patient to give with food in AM, PM
- Teach patient to report nausea, vomiting, diarrhea
- Advise to inform prescriber of all products taken

---

rizatriptan (Rx)

(rye-zah-trip′tan)
Maxalt, Maxalt-MLT
Func. class.: Migraine agent
Chem. class.: 5-HT$_1$-like receptor agonist
Pregnancy category C

ACTION: Binds selectively to the vascular 5-HT$_{1B/1D}$ receptor subtype, exerts antimigraine effect; causes vasoconstriction in cranial arteries

Therapeutic outcome: After treatment, relief of migraine

USES: Acute treatment of migraine

CONTRAINDICATIONS

Angina pectoris, history of MI, documented silent ischemia, Prinzmetal's angina, ischemic heart disease, concurrent ergotamine-containing preparations, uncontrolled hypertension, hypersensitivity, basilar or hemiplegic migraine

Precautions: Pregnancy C, breastfeeding, children, postmenopausal women, men >40 yr, geriatric, risk factors for CAD, hypercholesterolemia, obesity, diabetes, impaired renal/hepatic function

DOSAGE AND ROUTES

Adult: **PO** 5-10 mg single dose, redosing separate by 2 hr or more; max 30 mg/24 hr, use 5 mg in patient on propanolol; max 15 mg/24 hr

Available forms: Tabs (Maxalt) 5, 10 mg; orally disintegrating tabs (Maxalt-MLT) 5, 10 mg

Implementation

- Provide quiet, calm environment with decreased stimulation for noise, bright light, excessive talking
- Do not open blister pack until ready to use, put orally disintegrating tab on tongue to dissolve; swallow with saliva

ADVERSE EFFECTS

CNS: *Dizziness,* drowsiness, *headache, fatigue,* warm/cold sensation, flushing

CV: **MI, ventricular fibrillation, ventricular tachycardia, coronary artery vasospasm,** peripheral vascular ischemia, ECG changes
ENDO: Hot flashes, mild increase in growth hormone
GI: *Nausea,* dry mouth, diarrhea, abdominal pain, ischemic colitis
RESP: Chest tightness, pressure, dyspnea

Pharmacokinetics

Absorption	Unknown
Distribution	Unknown
Metabolism	Liver (metabolite)
Excretion	Urine/feces
Half-life	2-3 hr

Pharmacodynamics

Onset	10 min-2 hr
Peak	Unknown
Duration	Unknown

INTERACTIONS
Individual drugs

Cimetidine, isocarboxazide, pargyline, phenelzine, propranolol, trancyclomine: increased rizatriptan action
Ergot: increased vasospastic effects
Sibutramine: increased levels of sibutramine

Drug classifications

Contraceptives (oral), MAOIs, MAOIs (nonselective types A and B): increased rizatriptan action
Ergot derivatives, 5-HT$_1$ receptor agonists: increased vasospastic effects
Selective serotonin reuptake inhibitors: increased weakness, hyperreflexia, incoordination

Drug/herb
St. John's wort: serotonin syndrome

NURSING CONSIDERATIONS
Assessment

- Assess for stress level, activity, recreation, coping mechanisms
- Assess neurologic status: LOC, blurring vision, nausea, vomiting, tingling in extremities preceding headache
- **Ingestion of tyramine-containing foods:** Monitor for pickled products, beer, wine, aged cheese, food additives, preservatives, colorings, artificial sweeteners, chocolate, caffeine, which may precipitate these types of headaches

Patient/family education

- **Teach patient use of orally disintegrating tab:** instruct patient not to open blister until use, to peel blister open with dry hands, to place

R

tab on tongue, where it will dissolve, and to swallow with saliva (contains phenylalanine)
• Advise patient to report any side effects to prescriber
• Advise patient to use alternative contraception while taking product if oral contraceptives are being used
• Teach patient that product does not prevent or reduce number of migraines, main action is abortive, if first dose does not relieve pain, do not use more, notify prescriber

Evaluation

Positive therapeutic outcome
• Decrease in frequency, severity of headache

---

roflumilast
(roe-flue′mi-last)
Daliresp
Func. class.: Respiratory anti-inflammatory agent
Chem. class.: Phosphodiesterase-4 (PDE4) inhibitor
Pregnancy category C

ACTION: Roflumilast and the active metabolite (roflumilast N-oxide), selectively inhibit phosphodiesterase-4 (PDE4); not a bronchodilator; instead, inhibition of the PDE4 enzyme blocks the hydrolyses and inactivation of cyclic adenosine monophosphate (cAMP), resulting in intracellular cAMP accumulation; decreases inflammatory activity, PDE4 inhibition may affect migration and actions of pro-inflammatory cells (neutrophils, other leukocytes, T lymphocytes, monocytes, macrophages, fibroblasts)

Therapeutic outcome: Decreasing exacerbations in COPD

USES: For the prevention of COPD exacerbations in those with severe chronic obstructive pulmonary disease (COPD) associated with chronic bronchitis and a history of exacerbations

CONTRAINDICATIONS
Moderate to severe hepatic disease (Child-Pugh B or C)

Precautions: Pregnancy Category **C**, breastfeeding, neonates, infants, children, and adolescents, acute bronchospasm, anxiety, insomnia, depression, and/or suicidal ideation or behavior

DOSAGE AND ROUTES
Adult: **PO** 500 mcg/day

Available forms: Tab 500 mcg

Implementation
PO route
• Give without regard to meals
• Store at room temperature

ADVERSE EFFECTS
CNS: Anxiety, depression, dizziness, headache, insomnia, suicidal ideation, tremor
EENT: Rhinitis, sinusitis
GI: Abdominal pain, anorexia, diarrhea, dyspepsia, gastritis, nausea, vomiting, weight loss
GU: Urinary tract infection
MS: Back pain, muscle cramps/spasm
SYST: Infections, influenza

Pharmacokinetics

Absorption	80%
Distribution	Protein binding 99%
Metabolism	Exclusively by CYP3A4, CYP1A2
Excretion	Unknown
Half-life	17 hr (parent); 30 hr (metabolite)

Pharmacodynamics

Onset	Unknown
Peak	1 hr (parent drug); 8 hrs (metabolite)
Duration	Unknown

INTERACTIONS
Drug classifications
CYP3A4 inducers (alcohol, barbiturates, bexarotene, bosentan, carBAMazepine, dexamethasone, erythromycin, etravirine, fluvoxaMINE, ketoconazole, metyrapone, modafinil, nevirapine, OXcarbazepine, PHENobarbital, phenytoin, rifabutin, rifampin, ritonavir: decreased roflumilast effect
CYP3A4/CYP1A2 inhibitors (cimetidine, dalfopristin, delavirdine, enoxacin, indinavir, isoniazid, itraconazole, quinupristin, tipranavir): increased roflumilast effect
Oral contraceptives (gestodene and ethinyl estradiol): increased roflumilast effect
Fosamprenavir: altered effect

Drug/herb
St. John's wort: decreased roflumilast effect

NURSING CONSIDERATIONS
Assessment
• Monitor lung sounds and respiratory function baseline and periodically thereafter
• Assess behavioral changes including mood, depression and suicidal thoughts/behaviors

---

• Monitor liver function tests baseline and periodically thereafter; if increases in liver function studies occur, product should be discontinued
• Monitor weight baseline and periodically, as weight loss is common

Patient/family education
• Advise patient to take product as directed, do not skip or double doses, take missed doses as soon as remembered unless almost time for next dose
• Teach patient not to use OTC or other products without prescriber approval; not to discontinue other respiratory products unless approved by prescriber
• Advise patient not to be used for acute bronchospasm, but may be continued during acute asthma attacks
• **Suicidal thoughts/behaviors: Instruct patient to notify prescriber of worsening depression or suicidal thoughts/behaviors**

Evaluation

Positive therapeutic outcome
• Decreasing exacerbations in COPD

romiPLOStim (Rx)
(roe-mi-ploe′stim)
Nplate
Func. class.: Hematopoietin
Chem. class.: Thrombopoietin receptor agonist
Pregnancy category C

ACTION: A thrombopoietin-like fusion protein produced by DNA recombinant technology

Therapeutic outcome: Increase in platelet counts, absence of bleeding

USES: Chronic idiopathic thrombocytopenic purpura in patients who have had an insufficient response to corticosteroids, immunoglobulins, or splenectomy

CONTRAINDICATIONS
Hypersensitivity to this product or mannitol

Precautions: Pregnancy **C**, breastfeeding, malignancies, bleeding, bone marrow suppression, children

DOSAGE AND ROUTES
Thrombocytopenia in chronic idiopathic thrombocytopenic purpura (ITP) with insufficient response to corticosteroids, immunoglobulins, splenectomy
Adult: SUBCUT; initial dose is 1 mcg/kg SC qwk (based on actual body weight). Increase the

weekly dose by 1 mcg/kg until the patient achieves a platelet count ≥50,000/mm³; do not exceed a maximum weekly dose of 10 mcg/kg; use the lowest dose needed to achieve and maintain a platelet count ≥50,000/mm³; monitor CBC, including platelet counts, qwk until a stable platelet count is achieved; platelets ≥50,000/mm³ ≥4 wk without dose adjustment; then, monitor the CBC, including platelet counts, monthly. Once a stable dose is achieved, if the platelet count falls to <50,000/mm³, increase the dose by 1 mcg/kg/wk. If the platelet count increases to >200,000/mm³ for 2 consecutive wk, reduce dose by 1 mcg/kg; if the platelet count is >400,000/mm³, temporarily stop romiplostim, and continue to monitor the platelet count weekly; once the platelets are <200,000/mm³, restart, but reduce the previous dose by 1 mcg/kg/wk. RomiPLOStim may be administered concomitantly with other medical ITP therapies. If platelet counts exceed 50,000/mm³, other medical ITP therapies may be reduced or discontinued. Discontinue romiPLOStim if the platelet count does not increase to avoid important bleeding after 4 wk of therapy at max dose of 10 mcg/kg

Available forms: Inj vials 250, 500 mcg

Implementation
• Store vials in refrigerator, do not freeze; protect from light; diluted sol is stable refrigerated or at room temperature for 24 hrs
SUBCUT route
• Use 0.01 ml graduations syringe
• Discard any unused portion in vial; do not pool unused portions from vials
• Dilute 250 mcg/0.72 preservative-free sterile water for inj; 500 mcg/1.2 preservative-free sterile water for inj; final concentration 500 mcg/ml
• Gently swirl until dissolved; do not shake
• Do not use if discolored or if particulate matter is present
• Inj into outer aspect of upper arm or abdomen except for 2 inches around navel or front aspect of middle thigh; do not use areas that are bruised, scratched, or scarred
• Rotate inj sites

ADVERSE EFFECTS
CNS: *Dizziness, insomnia, headache,* fatigue
GI: Abdominal pain, dyspepsia, diarrhea
HEMA: **Thromboembolism, thrombosis,** bleeding, myelofibrosis, erythromelalgia
MS: Myalgia
SYST: **Secondary malignancy,** antibody formation

Pharmacokinetics

Absorption	Unknown
Distribution	Unknown
Metabolism	Unknown
Excretion	Unknown
Half-life	Terminal 1-34 days

Pharmacodynamics

Onset	Unknown
Peak	7-50 hr
Duration	Unknown

INTERACTIONS
Drug classifications
Anticoagulants, NSAIDs, platelet inhibitors, thrombolytics, salicylates: possible risk of bleeding

NURSING CONSIDERATIONS
Assessment
⚠ **Bone marrow suppression: If cytopenias occur, product should be discontinued; may use a bone marrow biopsy and straining for fibrosis**
• **Thromboembolic disease: Do not use to normalize patients, use only in those with thrombocytopenia in ITP, maintain platelets ≥50,000/mm³**
• Assess blood studies: CBC during treatment weekly and for 2 wks after discontinuing

Patient/family education
• Instruct patient to report bleeding, to avoid hazardous activities that may cause bleeding
• Inform the patient the reason for product and expected results
• Advise patient to report a missed dose to prescriber due to increased risk of bleeding
• Teach patient that lab tests will be done qwk and dose may be changed; if dose is not changed lab will be checked qmo; after drug is discontinued, labs will be checked qwk × 2 wk
• Teach patient to advise prescriber if spleen has been removed; bleeding or clotting problems
⚠ **Teach patient to notify prescriber if pregnancy is planned or suspected, pregnancy (C); if pregnancy occurs, call registry 877-675-2831**

Evaluation

Positive therapeutic outcome
• Increase in platelet counts, absence of bleeding

rOPINIRole (Rx)
(roe-pin'e-role)
Requip, Requip XL
Func. class.: Antiparkinsonian agent
Chem. class.: Dopamine-receptor agonist, nonergot
Pregnancy category C

Do not confuse: rOPINIRole/risperiDONE

ACTION: Selective agonist for DOPamine D₂ receptors (presynaptic/postsynaptic sites); binding at D₃ receptor contributes to antiparkinson effects

Therapeutic outcome: Decreased symptoms of Parkinson's disease (involuntary movements)

USES: Parkinsonism, restless legs syndrome

CONTRAINDICATIONS
Hypersensitivity

Precautions: Pregnancy **C**, cardiac/renal/hepatic disease, dysrhythmias, affective disorders, psychosis

DOSAGE AND ROUTES
Parkinson's disease
Adult: PO (regular release) Initially, 0.25 mg PO tid × first wk; gradually titrate at weekly intervals; wk 2: give 0.5 mg tid; wk 3: 0.75 mg tid; wk 4; titrate to 1 mg tid; after wk 4, may increase by 1.5 mg/day wk, max 9 mg/day total dose, and then by 3 mg/day qwk, max 24 mg/day; PO (ext rel) Initially, 2 mg/day × 1-2 wk, may increase by mg/day at intervals ≥1 wk based upon response; max 24 mg/day. If significant interruption of therapy occurs, retitration may be necessary

For conversion from immediate-release to ext rel tablets
Oral dosage (ext rel tablets):
Adults currently on 0.75-2.25 mg/day: Give 2 mg/day ext rel
Adults currently on 3-4.5 mg/day: Give 4 mg/day ext rel
Adults currently on 6 mg/day: Give 6 mg/day ext rel
Adults currently on 7.5-9 mg/day: Give 8 mg/day ext rel
Adults currently on 12 mg/day: Give 12 mg/day ext rel
Adults currently on 15-18 mg/day: Give 16 mg/day ext rel
Adults currently on 21 mg/day: Give 20 mg/day ext rel

Adults currently on 24 mg/day: Give 24 mg/day ext rel

For the treatment of restless legs syndrome (RLS)

Adult: PO (reg rel) Initially, 0.25 mg/day, give 1-3 hr before bedtime; days 3-7, may increase to 0.5 mg/day; at the beginning of wk 2 (day 8) the dose may be increased to 1 mg/day × 1 wk; weeks 3-6, dose may be titrated up by 0.5 mg/wk (from 1.5-3 mg over the 5-wk period), as needed to achieve desired effect; wk 7, may increase dose to 4 mg/day; dose is titrated based on clinical response; give all doses 1-3 hr before bedtime

Available forms: Tabs 0.25, 0.5, 1, 2, 3, 4, 5 mg; ext rel tab 2, 4, 6, 8, 12 mg

Implementation
- Give product until NPO before surgery
- Adjust dosage to patient's response
- Give with meals to decrease GI upset
- Test for diabetes mellitus, acromegaly if patient is receiving long-term therapy

ADVERSE EFFECTS
CNS: Dystonia, *agitation, insomnia,* dizziness, psychosis, hallucinations, depression, somnolence, **sleep attacks,** impulse-control disorders
CV: *Orthostatic hypotension,* hypotension, syncope, palpitations, **tachycardia,** hypertension
EENT: Blurred vision
GI: *Nausea, vomiting, anorexia, dry mouth,* constipation, dyspepsia, flatulence
GU: Impotence, urinary frequency
HEMA: **Hemolytic anemia, leukopenia, agranulocytosis**
INTEG: Rash, sweating
RESP: Pharyngitis, rhinitis, sinusitis, bronchitis, dyspnea

Pharmacokinetics
Absorption	Well absorbed
Distribution	Widely distributed
Metabolism	Liver, extensively by the liver by CYP450 CYP1A2 enzyme system
Excretion	Kidneys
Half-life	6 hr

Pharmacodynamics
Unknown

INTERACTIONS
Individual drugs
Cimetidine, ciprofloxacin, digoxin, diltiazem, enoxacin, erythromycin, fluvoxamine, levodopa, mexiletine, norfloxacin, tacrine, theophylline: increased effect of rOPINIRole
Metoclopramide: decreased rOPINIRole effect

Drug classifications
Butyrophenones, phenothiazines, thioxanthenes: decreased ropinirole effect

NURSING CONSIDERATIONS
Assessment
- Monitor B/P, respiration during initial treatment; hypotension or hypertension should be reported
- Assess mental status: affect, mood, behavioral changes, depression; complete suicide assessment
- **Parkinsonism:** assess for akinesia, tremors, staggering gait, muscle rigidity, drooling; these symptoms should improve with therapy
- ⚠ **Sleep attacks: assess for drowsiness, falling asleep without warning even during hazardous activities**

Patient/family education
- Teach patient to notify prescriber if pregnancy is planned or suspected, pregnancy (**C**), breastfeeding
- Teach patient to take with food to prevent nausea
- Teach patient to report hallucinations, confusion (usually in geriatrics)
- Advise patient that therapeutic effects may take several wk to a few mo
- Caution patient to change positions slowly to prevent orthostatic hypotension
- Instruct patient to use product exactly as prescribed; if product is discontinued abruptly, parkinsonian crisis may occur
- Teach patient that drowsiness, sleeping attacks may occur, to avoid driving or other hazardous activities until response is known
- Teach patient to avoid alcohol and CNS depressants (cough and cold products)
- Teach patient to notify prescriber of unusual urges

Evaluation
Positive therapeutic outcome
- Decreased akathisia, other involuntary movements
- Increased mood

ropivacaine (Rx)
(roe-pi′va-kane)
Naropin
Func. class.: Local anesthetic
Chem. class.: Amide
Pregnancy category B

ACTION: Competes with calcium for sites in nerve membrane that control sodium transport across cell membrane; decreases rise of depolarization phase of action potential

Therapeutic outcome: Maintenance of local anesthesia

USES: Peripheral nerve block, caudal anesthesia, central neural block, vaginal, epidural, spinal block

CONTRAINDICATIONS
Children <12 yr, geriatric, hypersensitivity to amide local anesthetics, severe liver disease, severe hypotension, complete heart block

Precautions: Pregnancy **B**, severe product allergies, hyperthyroidism, CV, hepatic/neurologic disease

DOSAGE AND ROUTES
Lumbar epidural block for C-section
Adult: 20-30 ml of 0.5% SOL, or 15-20 ml of 0.75% SOL

Thoracic epidural
Adult: 5-15 ml of 0.5%-0.75% SOL

Major nerve block
Adult: 35-50 ml of 0.5% SOL or 10-40 ml of 0.75% SOL

Labor pain epidural
Adult: 10-20 ml of 0.2% SOL, then 6-14 ml/hr

Postoperative (lumbar/thoracic epidural)
Adult: 6-14 ml/hr of 0.2% SOL

Infiltration/minor nerve block
Adult: 1-100 ml of 0.2% SOL or 1-40 ml of 0.5% SOL

Available forms: Inj 2, 5, 7.5 mg/ml

Implementation
• Give only with resuscitative equipment nearby
• Give only products without preservatives for epidural or caudal anesthesia
• Use new sol; discard unused portions

ADVERSE EFFECTS
CNS: Anxiety, restlessness, seizures, loss of consciousness, drowsiness, disorientation, tremors, shivering, paresthesia
CV: Myocardial depression, cardiac arrest, dysrhythmias, bradycardia, *hypo*/hypertension, fetal bradycardia
EENT: Blurred vision, tinnitus, pupil constriction
ENDO: Hypokalemia
GI: Nausea, vomiting
GU: Urinary retention
INTEG: Rash, urticaria, allergic reactions, edema, burning, skin discoloration at injection site, tissue necrosis

RESP: Status asthmaticus, respiratory arrest, anaphylaxis

Pharmacokinetics

Absorption	Complete
Distribution	Unknown
Metabolism	Liver
Excretion	Kidneys
Half-life	Unknown

Pharmacodynamics

Onset	2-8 min
Peak	Unknown
Duration	3 hr, varies with inj site

INTERACTIONS
Individual drugs
Amiodarone, cimetidine, ciprofloxacin, fluvoxaMINE, imipramine, theophylline: increased effect
Chloroprocaine: decreased action of ropivacaine
Enflurane, EPINEPHrine, halothane: increased dysrhythmias

Drug classifications
Antidepressants (tricyclics), MAOIs, phenothiazines: increased hypertension
Azole antifungals: increased effect

NURSING CONSIDERATIONS
Assessment
• Assess B/P, pulse, respiration during treatment
• Assess fetal heart tones during labor
• Assess allergic reactions: rash, urticaria, itching
• Assess cardiac status: ECG for dysrhythmias, pulse, B/P during anesthesia

Evaluation

Positive therapeutic outcome
• Anesthesia necessary for procedure

TREATMENT OF OVERDOSE:
Airway, O$_2$, vasopressor, **IV** fluids, anticonvulsants for seizures

> **⚠ HIGH ALERT**
>
> ## rosiglitazone (Rx)
> (rose-i-glye′ta-zone)
> **Avandia**
> *Func. class.:* Antidiabetic, oral
> *Chem. class.:* Thiazolidinedione
> **Pregnancy category C**

Do not confuse: rosiglitazone/pioglitazone, Avandia/Prandin

ACTION: Improves insulin resistance by hepatic glucose metabolism, insulin receptor kinase activity, insulin receptor phosphorylation

Therapeutic outcome: Decreased symptoms of diabetes mellitus

USES: Stable type 2 diabetes mellitus alone or in combination with sulfonylureas, metformin, or insulin

CONTRAINDICATIONS
Breastfeeding, children, hypersensitivity to thiazolidinediones, diabetic ketoacidosis, jaundice, type 1 diabetes

> **BLACK BOX WARNING:** NYHA III or IV acute heart failure, heart failure

Precautions: Pregnancy **C**, geriatric, thyroid/renal/hepatic disease, heart failure, NYHA class I, II

> **BLACK BOX WARNING:** MI

DOSAGE AND ROUTES
Adult: PO 4 mg/day or in 2 divided doses, may increase to 8 mg/day or in 2 divided doses after 12 wk; may be added to metformin, sulfonylureas at the adult dose

Available forms: Tabs 2, 4, 8 mg

Implementation
• Convert from other oral hypoglycemic agents if needed; change may be made without gradual dosage change; monitor blood glucose during conversion
• Give tabs crushed and mixed with meal or fluids for patients with difficulty swallowing
PO route
• Give once or in 2 divided doses without regard to food
• Store in airtight container in cool environment
• **Available only through the REMS Program 1-800-Avandia**

ADVERSE EFFECTS
CNS: Fatigue, *headache*
CV: CHF, MI, death (geriatric patients)
ENDO: Hyper/hypoglycemia
GI: Weight gain, hepatotoxicity, increased total cholesterol, LDL, HDL, decreased free fatty acids
MISC: Accidental injury, upper respiratory tract infection, sinusitis, anemia, back pain, diarrhea, edema, bone fractures (female), pulmonary/macular/peripheral edema
SYST: Anaphylaxis, Stevens-Johnson syndrome, lactic acidosis

Pharmacokinetics
Absorption	Unknown
Distribution	Protein binding 99.8%
Metabolism	Unknown
Excretion	Urine, feces, breast milk
Half-life	Elimination 3-4 hr

Pharmacodynamics
Onset	Unknown
Peak	6-12 wk
Duration	Unknown

INTERACTIONS
Individual drugs
FluvoxaMINE, gemfibrozil, ketoconazole: increased hypoglycemia; monitor glucose
Insulin: avoid concurrent use

Drug classifications
CYP2C5 inducers/inhibitors: may increase/decrease effect
Nitrates: avoid concurrent use

Drug/herb
Horse chestnut: increased antidiabetic effect

Drug/lab test
Increased: ALT, HDL, LDL, total cholesterol, blood glucose
Decreased: Hgb/Hct

NURSING CONSIDERATIONS
Assessment

> **BLACK BOX WARNING:** Use in NYHA III or IV acute heart failure is contraindicated; any deterioration in any cardiac status, discontinue product

> **BLACK BOX WARNING: CHF/MI:** assess for dyspnea, edema, weight gain ≥5 lb, jugular vein distention; may need to change or discontinue; do not use in acute coronary syndrome

• **Lactic acidosis: assess for dyspnea, abdominal pain, muscle pain; notify prescriber immediately**
• Assess for hypoglycemic reactions (sweating, weakness, dizziness, anxiety, tremors, hunger), hyperglycemic reactions soon after meals; monitor FBS, blood glucose glycosylated hemoglobin A1C (HbA1c)
• **Assess for systemic reactions: anaphylaxis, Stevens-Johnson syndrome**
• **Hepatotoxicity: check liver function tests periodically; AST, ALT (if ALT is >2.5 × ULN, do not use)**

• Monitor HbA2c, plasma lipids, lipoproteins, B/P, body weight baseline and
periodically during treatment

Patient/family education

• Teach patient that in order to use product,
provider/patient must be enrolled in the
Avandia-Rosiglitazone Access Program
• Teach patient to monitor capillary blood
glucose test, that periodic liver function tests are
mandatory; to report edema, weight gain
• Teach patient symptoms of hypo/hyperglyce-
mia, what to do about each
• Advise patient that product must be continued
on daily basis; explain consequence of discontinuing product abruptly
• Advise patient to avoid OTC medications,
nitrates, insulin, or herbal preparations unless
approved by prescriber
• Advise patient that diabetes is lifelong illness; that
this product is not a cure, only controls symptoms
• Advise patient that all food included in diet
plan must be eaten to prevent hypoglycemia
• Advise patient to carry/wear emergency ID
and glucagon emergency kit for emergencies
• Instruct patient to notify prescriber if oral
contraceptives are used
• Teach patient not to use if breastfeeding;
may be secreted in breast milk, may alter
blood glucose
• Hepatotoxicity: advise patient to report
nausea, vomiting, abdominal pain, fatigue, anorexia, dark urine, jaundice; to report macular
edema (change in vision) immediately
• Teach patient that 2 wk is needed to see a reduction in blood glucose, 2-3 mo to see full effect

Evaluation
Positive therapeutic outcome
• Decrease in polyuria, polydipsia, polyphagia;
clear sensorium; absence of dizziness; stable
gait; blood glucose, A1c improvement

rosuvastatin (Rx)
(roe-soo′va-sta-tin)
Crestor
Func. class.: Antilipemic
Chem. class.: HMG-CoA reductase
inhibitor
Pregnancy category X

ACTION: Inhibits HMG-CoA reductase,
which reduces cholesterol synthesis

Therapeutic outcome: Decreasing cholesterol levels

USES: As an adjunct in primary hypercholesterolemia (types IIa, IIb), mixed dyslipidemia
elevated serum triglycerides, homozygous/het-
erozygous familial hypercholesterolemia (FH),
slowing of atherosclerosis, CV disease prophylaxis, MI, stroke prophylaxis (normal LDL)

CONTRAINDICATIONS
Pregnancy **X**, breastfeeding, hypersensitivity, active liver disease

Precautions: Children <10 yr, geriatric,
past liver disease, alcoholism, severe acute infections, trauma, hypotension, uncontrolled seizure
disorders, severe metabolic disorders, electrolyte imbalances, severe renal impairment, hypothyroidism, Asian patients

DOSAGE AND ROUTES
Patient should first be placed on a cholesterol-
lowering diet

Hypercholesterolemia
Adult: PO 5-40 mg/day; initial dose 10 mg/day,
reanalyze lipid levels at 2-4 wk and adjust dosage
accordingly

Homozygous FH
Adult: PO 20 mg/day, max 40 mg; Asian patients
5 mg/day

Dose in patients taking cycloSPO-
RINE/gemfibrozil/lopinavir/ritona-
vir/atazanavir
Adult: 5 mg/day, max 10 mg/day

Heterozygous familial hypercho-
lesterolemia
**Females ≥1 yr post-menarche and ≥10 yr
and males ≥10 yr:** PO 5-20 mg/day individualized

Asian patients/predisposition for
myopathy
Adult: PO 5 mg/day

Atherosclerosis slowing
Adult: PO 10 mg/day (for those not taking cycloSPORINE or gemfibrozil)

Renal/hepatic dose
Adult: PO CCr <30 ml/min 5 mg daily; max
10 mg daily; avoid use in hepatic disease

Available forms: Tabs 5, 10, 20, 40 mg

Implementation
• May be taken at any time of day, with or
without food
• Store in cool environment in airtight, light-
resistant container

ADVERSE EFFECTS
CNS: *Headache, dizziness,* insomnia, paresthesia, confusion

GI: *Nausea, constipation, abdominal pain, flatus, diarrhea, dyspepsia, heartburn,* kidney failure, liver dysfunction, vomiting
HEMA: Thrombocytopenia, hemolytic anemia, leukopenia
INTEG: *Rash, pruritus*
MS: *Asthenia, muscle cramps, arthritis, arthralgia, myalgia,* myositis, rhabdomyolysis, leg, shoulder, or localized pain
RESP: Rhinitis, sinusitis, *pharyngitis,* increased cough

Pharmacokinetics

Absorption	Unknown
Distribution	88% protein bound, crosses placenta
Metabolism	Minimal liver metabolism (about 10%)
Excretion	Primarily in feces (90%)
Half-life	19 hr

Pharmacodynamics

Onset	Unknown
Peak	3-5 hr
Duration	Unknown

INTERACTIONS
Individual drugs
Alcohol: increased hepatotoxicity
Clofibrate, cycloSPORINE, gemfibrozil, niacin: increased myalgia, myositis
Warfarin: increased bleeding

Drug classifications
Antifungals (azole), antiretroviral protease inhibitors, fibric acid derivatives: increased myalgia, myositis
Bile acid sequestrants: increased effects

Drug/herb
St. John's wort: decreased rosuvastatin effect

Drug/lab test
Increased: CPK, liver function tests

NURSING CONSIDERATIONS
Assessment
• Assess diet: obtain diet history including fat, cholesterol in diet
• Monitor fasting cholesterol, LDL, HDL, triglycerides periodically during treatment
• Liver function: monitor liver function tests q1-2mo during the first 1½ yr of treatment; AST, ALT, liver function tests may increase
• Monitor renal function in patients with compromised renal system: BUN, creatinine, I&O ratio
• Obtain ophthalmic exam before, 1 mo after treatment begins, annually; lens opacities may occur

⚠ Rhabdomyolysis: Assess for muscle pain, tenderness, obtain CPK; if these occur, product may need to be discontinued; for Asian ancestry: increased blood levels, rhabdomyolysis

Patient/family education
• Advise to report suspected pregnancy, to use contraception while taking this product, pregnancy category X, not to breastfeed
• Advise that blood work and ophthalmic exam will be necessary during treatment
• Teach to report blurred vision, severe GI symptoms, dizziness, headache, muscle pain, weakness
• Teach that previously prescribed regimen will continue: low-cholesterol diet, exercise program, smoking cessation; liver injury (jaundice, anorexia, abdominal pain)

Evaluation
Positive therapeutic outcome
• Cholesterol at desired level after 8 wk

---

rufinamide (Rx)
(roo-fin′a-mide)
Banzel
Func. class.: Anticonvulsant
Chem. class.: Triazole derivative
Pregnancy category C

ACTION: May act through action at sodium channels; exact action is unknown

Therapeutic outcome: Decrease in severity of seizures

USES: Lennox-Gastaut syndrome

CONTRAINDICATIONS
Hypersensitivity, familial short QT syndrome

Precautions: Pregnancy **C**, breastfeeding, renal/hepatic disease, geriatric patients, child <16 yr, depression, dialysis, hazardous activities, suicidal ideation

DOSAGE AND ROUTES
Adult: PO 400-800 mg/day divided bid, increase by 400-800 mg/day q2day to 3200 mg/day
Child ≥4 yr: PO 10 mg/kg/day divided equally bid; increase by 10 mg/kg/day every other day to 45 mg/kg/day or 3200 mg/day, whichever is less

Available forms: Tabs 200, 400 mg; oral susp 40 mg/ml

Implementation
• **PO tabs:** Give with food, may give whole, crushed, or halved

---

• **Oral susp:** Shake well before use, use provided adapter and calibrated oral dosing syringe, insert adapter firmly in neck of bottle before use and keep in place for the duration of bottle use, insert dosing syringe into the adapter and withdraw dose from inverted bottle, replace cap after each use, use within 90 days of opening, give with food

ADVERSE EFFECTS

CNS: Dizziness, ataxia, drowsiness, fever, seizures, tremor, fatigue, headache, gait disturbance

EENT: Diplopia, blurred vision, nystagmus

GI: Nausea, hepatitis, vomiting

HEMA: Anemia, leukopenia, neutropenia, thrombocytopenia, lymphadenopathy

INTEG: Rash, urticaria, Stevens-Johnson syndrome

MISC: Edema, hematuria, influenzae, nephrolithiasis

Pharmacokinetics

Absorption	Unknown
Distribution	Unknown
Metabolism	Liver
Excretion	Kidneys
Half-life	Terminal 6-10 hr

Pharmacodynamics

Onset	Unknown
Peak	4-6 hr
Duration	Unknown

INTERACTIONS

Individual drugs

CarBAMazepine, PHENobarbital, phenytoin, primidone: decreased effect of rufinamide

Valproate: increased rufinamide effect

Drug classifications

Hormonal contraceptives: decreased effect

Drug/lab test

Increased: LFTs

NURSING CONSIDERATIONS

Assessment

• **Seizures:** Assess for duration, type, intensity precipitating factors

⚠ Assess mental status: mood, sensorium, affect, memory (long, short), increased suicidal thoughts/actions

Patient/family education

• Caution patient not to discontinue product abruptly; seizures may occur

• Advise patient to avoid hazardous activities until stabilized on product

• Instruct patient to carry emergency ID stating product use

• Instruct patient to notify prescriber if pregnancy is planned or suspected, to use alternative form of contraception; hormonal contraceptives may be decreased

• Inform patient to take adequate fluids

Evaluation

Positive therapeutic outcome

• Decrease in severity of seizures

salicylic acid topical
See Appendix B

salmeterol (Rx)
(sal-met'er-ole)
Serevent, Serevent Diskus
Func. class.: Adrenergic β₂ agonist, bronchodilator
Pregnancy category C

ACTION: Causes bronchodilatation by action on β₂ (pulmonary) receptors by increasing levels of cyclic AMP, which relaxes smooth muscle; with very little effect on heart rate, maintains improvement in FEV from 3 to 12 hr; prevents nocturnal asthma symptoms

Therapeutic outcome: Ease of breathing

USES: Prevention of exercise-induced asthma, bronchospasm, COPD

CONTRAINDICATIONS
Hypersensitivity to sympathomimetics, tachydysrhythmias, severe cardiac disease, monotherapy treatment of asthma

Precautions: Pregnancy **C**, breastfeeding, cardiac disorders, hyperthyroidism, diabetes mellitus, hypertension, prostatic hypertrophy, closed-angle glaucoma, seizures, acute asthma, as a substitute for corticosteroids, QT prolongation

> **BLACK BOX WARNING:** Asthma-related death, children <4 yr

DOSAGE AND ROUTES
Adult/child ≥4 yr: INH 50 mcg (one inhalation as dry powder); **exercise-induced bronchospasm:** 50 mcg (2 INH) ½-1 hr prior to exercise

Available forms: Inhalation powder 50 mcg/blister

Implementation
• Shake aerosol container, ask patient to exhale, then place mouthpiece in mouth, inhale slowly, hold breath, remove, exhale slowly; allow at least 1 min between inhalations
• Use this medication before other medications and allow at least 1 min between each
• Use spacing device for pediatric/geriatric patients
• Store in foil pouch; do not expose to temp >86° F (30° C); discard 6 wk after removal from foil pouch
• Use 1/2 hr prior to exercise for exercise-induced bronchospasm prevention
• Don't use spacer with this product

ADVERSE EFFECTS
CNS: *Tremors, anxiety,* insomnia, headache, dizziness, fever
CV: Palpitations, **tachycardia**, angina, hypo/hypertension, **dysrhythmias**
EENT: Dry nose, irritation of nose and throat
GI: Heartburn, nausea, vomiting, abdominal pain
MS: Muscle cramps
RESP: **Bronchospasm,** cough

Pharmacokinetics
Unknown

Pharmacodynamics
Onset	5-15 min
Peak	4 hr
Duration	12 hr

INTERACTIONS
Drug classifications
Antidepressants (tricyclics): increased salmeterol action
β-Adrenergic blockers: block therapeutic effect
Bronchodilators, aerosol: increased action of bronchodilator
CYP3A4 inhibitors (itraconazole, ketoconazole, nelfinavir, nefazodone, saquinavir): increased CV effects
MAOIs: increased action of salmeterol

Drug/herb
Betel palm, butterbur, coffee, cola nut, figwort, fumitory, guarana, hawthorn, lily of the valley, motherwort, plantain, tea (black, green), yerba maté: increased stimulation

NURSING CONSIDERATIONS
Assessment
• **Respiratory function:** assess vital capacity, FEV, ABGs, lung sounds, heart rate, rhythm (baseline)
• **Paradoxical bronchospasm: monitor for dyspnea, wheezing, chest tightness**

> **BLACK BOX WARNING:** Children should not use this product as monotherapy for asthma; use only with persistent asthma in those that are not well-controlled with a long-term asthma product

Patient/family education
• Caution patient not to use OTC medications because extra stimulation may occur
• Instruct patient to use this medication before other medications and to allow at least 1 min between each, to prevent overstimulation
• Teach patient how to use inhaler; to avoid getting aerosol in eyes; blurring may result; to wash

S

inhaler in warm water daily and dry; to avoid smoking, smoke-filled rooms, and persons with respiratory infections; review package insert with patient

• Instruct patient on administration of dose, not to use more than prescribed; serious side effects may occur

• Teach patient not to use for exercise-induced bronchospasm, never exhale into diskus, hold level, keep mouthpiece dry

• Teach patient not to use for treatment of acute exacerbation, a fast-acting β-blocker should be used instead

• Teach patient to report immediately dyspnea after use, if 1 canister or more is used in 2 mo time

• Teach patient to notify prescriber if >4 inhalations are needed, or if product is no longer working

• Advise patient not to get canister or mouthpiece wet, not to use spacer, not to exhale into mouthpiece

• Teach patient to take other products as prescribed

Evaluation

Positive therapeutic outcome
• Absence of dyspnea, wheezing
• Improved airway exchange
• Improved ABGs

TREATMENT OF OVERDOSE:
Administer a $β_2$-adrenergic blocker

⚠ HIGH ALERT

sargramostim (Rx)
(sar-gram'oh-stim)
Leukine, rhu GM-CSF
Func. class.: Biological modifier: cytokine
Chem. class.: Granulocyte-macrophage colony-stimulating factor (GM-CSF)
Pregnancy category C

Do not confuse: Leukine/leucovorin/ Leukeran

ACTION: Stimulates proliferation and differentiation of hematopoietic progenitor cells (granulocyte, macrophage)

Therapeutic outcome: WBC and differential recovery

USES: Acceleration of myeloid recovery in patients with non-Hodgkin's lymphoma, acute lymphoblastic leukemia, acute myelogenous leukemia, autologous bone marrow transplantation in Hodgkin's disease; bone marrow transplantation failure or engraftment delay; mobilization and transplant of peripheral blood progenitor cells (PBPCs)

Unlabeled uses: Aplastic anemia, Crohn's disease, ganciclovir- or zidovudine-induced neutropenia

CONTRAINDICATIONS
Hypersensitivity to GM-CSF, benzyl alcohol, yeast products; excessive leukemic myeloid blast in the bone marrow or peripheral blood, neonates

Precautions: Pregnancy **C**, breastfeeding, children, renal/hepatic/lung/cardiac disease, pleural/pericardial effusions, peripheral edema, leukocytosis, mannitol hypersensitivity, hepatic/renal disease

DOSAGE AND ROUTES
Myeloid recovery in Hodgkin's disease, non-Hodgkin's lymphoma, acute lymphocytic leukemia
Adult: IV 250 mcg/m²/day over a 2-hr period beginning 2-4 hr following infusion of bone marrow and not <24 hr after last dose of chemotherapy or radiotherapy
Child (unlabeled): SUBCUT/IV 250 mcg/m²/day beginning 2-4hr after infusion of bone marrow and not <24hr after last dose of chemotherapy

Acceleration of myeloid recovery
Adult: IV 250 mcg/m²/day × 14 days; give over 2 hr; may repeat in 7 days, may repeat 500 mcg/m²/day × 14 days after another 7 days if no improvement

Mobilization of PBPCs
Adult: IV/SUBCUT 250 mcg/m²/day during collection of PBPCs

After PBPC transplantation
Adult: IV/SUBCUT 250 mcg/m²/day until ANC >1500/mm³ × 3 days

Available forms: Powder for inj lyophilized 250 mcg; solution for injection 500 mcg/ml

Implementation
• Store in refrigerator; do not freeze
SUBCUT route
• No further dilution of reconstituted sol is needed; take care not to inject intradermally

Intermittent IV infusion route
• After reconstituting with 1 ml sterile water for inj without preservative; do not reenter vial; discard unused portion; direct reconstitution sol at side of vial; rotate contents, do not shake
• Dilute in 0.9% NaCl inj to prepare IV inf; if final concentration is <10 mcg/ml, add

---

human albumin to make a final concentration of 0.1% to NaCl before adding sargramostim to prevent adsorption; for a final concentration of 0.1% albumin, add 1 mg human albumin/1 ml 0.9% NaCl inj run over 2 hr **(bone marrow transplant or failure of graft)**; over 4 hr **(chemotherapy for AML)**; over 24 hr as cont inf **(PBPCs)**; give within 6 hr after reconstitution

Y-site compatibilities: Amikacin, aminophylline, aztreonam, bleomycin, butorphanol, calcium gluconate, CARBOplatin, carmustine, ceFAZolin, cefepime, cefotaxime, cefoTEtan, ceftizoxime, cefTRIAXone, cefuroxime, cimetidine, CISplatin, clindamycin, cyclophosphamide, cycloSPORINE, cytarabine, dacarbazine, DACTINomycin, dexamethasone, diphenhydrAMINE, DOPamine, DOXOrubicin, doxycycline, droperidol, etoposide, famotidine, fentaNYL, floxuridine, fluconazole, fluorouracil, furosemide, gentamicin, granisetron, heparin, IDArubicin, ifosfamide, immune globulin, magnesium sulfate, mannitol, mechlorethamine, meperidine, mesna, methotrexate, metoclopramide, metroNIDAZOLE, minocycline, mitoXANtrone, netilmicin, pentostatin, piperacillin/tazobactam, potassium chloride, prochlorperazine, promethazine, ranitidine, teniposide, ticarcillin, ticarcillin-clavulanate, trimethoprim-sulfamethoxazole, vinBLAStine, vinCRIStine, zidovudine

Y-site incompatibilities: Acyclovir, ampicillin, ampicillin/sulbactam, cefonicid, cefoperazine, cefTAZidime, chlorproMAZINE, ganciclovir, haloperidol, hydrocortisone, HYDROmorphone, hydrOXYzine, IDArubicin, imipenem/cilastatin, LORazepam, methylPREDNISolone sodium succinate, mitoMYcin, morphine, nalbuphine, ondansetron, piperacillin, sodium bicarbonate, tobramycin

ADVERSE EFFECTS

CNS: Fever, malaise, CNS disorder, weakness, chills, dizziness, syncope, headache
CV: *Transient supraventricular tachycardia*, peripheral edema, *pericardial effusion*, hypotension, tachycardia
GI: Nausea, vomiting, diarrhea, anorexia, *GI hemorrhage*, stomatitis, *liver damage*, hyperbilirubinemia
GU: Urinary tract disorder, abnormal kidney function
HEMA: *Blood dyscrasias, hemorrhage*
INTEG: Alopecia, rash, peripheral edema
MS: Bone pain, myalgia
RESP: Dyspnea

Pharmacokinetics

Absorption	Completely absorbed
Distribution	Unknown
Metabolism	Unknown
Excretion	Unknown
Half-life	Elimination **IV** 60 min; SUBCUT 2-3 hr

Pharmacodynamics

Onset	Rapid
Peak	2 hr
Duration	Unknown

INTERACTIONS
Individual drugs
Lithium: increased myeloproliferation

Drug classifications
Antineoplastics or radiation, separate by ≥24 hr
Corticosteroids: increased myeloproliferation

Drug/lab test
Increased: bilirubin, BUN, creatinine, eosinophils, LFTs, leukocytes

NURSING CONSIDERATIONS
Assessment
• **Monitor blood studies: CBC, differential count before treatment and twice weekly; leukocytosis may occur (WBC >50,000 cells/mm³, ANC >20,000 cells/mm³), platelets; if ANC >20,000/mm³ or 10,000/mm³ after nadir has occurred or platelets >500,000/mm³, reduce dose by ½ or discontinue; if blast cells occur, discontinue**
• Monitor renal/liver function tests before treatment: BUN, creatinine, urinalysis; AST, ALT, alkaline phosphatase; monitoring is needed twice a week in renal/hepatic disease
⚠ Gasping syndrome in neonates: assess for, due to benzyl alcohol hypersensitivity, do not use
• Assess for **hypersensitivity reactions**/rashes and local inj site reactions; usually transient
• Assess for increased fluid retention in cardiac disease, body weight, hydration status, pulmonary function
• Constitutional symptoms: asthenia, chills, fever, headache, malaise
• Assess for myalgia, arthralgia in legs, feet; use analgesics, antipyretics

Patient/family education
• Teach patient reason for medication and expected results
• Advise patient to notify nurse or prescriber of dyspnea
• Review all aspects of product use

Evaluation

Positive therapeutic outcome
- WBC and differential recovery
- Absence of infection

⚠ HIGH ALERT

saxagliptin (Rx)
(sax-a-glip′tin)
Onglyza
Func. class.: Antidiabetic, oral
Chem. class.: Dipeptidyl-peptidase-4
(DPP-4) inhibitor
Pregnancy category C

Do not confuse: saxagliptin/sitaGLIPtin

ACTION: Slows the inactivation of incretin hormones, improves glucose homeostasis, improves glucose-dependent insulin synthesis, lowers glucagon secretions and slows gastric emptying time

Therapeutic outcome: Decrease in polyuria, polydipsia, polyphagia; clear sensorium; absence of dizziness; stable gait; blood glucose at normal level

USES: Type 2 diabetes mellitus as monotherapy or in combination with other antidiabetic agents

CONTRAINDICATIONS
Hypersensitivity, angioedema

Precautions: Pregnancy **B,** geriatric, GI obstruction, thyroid disease, surgery, renal/hepatic disease, trauma, diabetic ketoacidosis (DKA), type 1 diabetes mellitus, heart failure

DOSAGE AND ROUTES
Adult: PO 2.5-5 mg; may use with other antidiabetic agents (metformin, pioglitazone, rosiglitazone), if used with insulin, a lower dose is needed; max 2.5 mg with strong 3A415 inhibitors

Renal dose
Adult: PO CCr ≤50 ml/min 2.5 mg/day

Available forms: Tabs 2.5; 5 mg

Implementation
PO route
- May be taken with or without food
- Conversion from other antidiabetic agents; change may be made with gradual dosage change
- Store in tight container at room temperature
- Do not break or cut tabs

ADVERSE EFFECTS
CNS: *Headache*
CV: Edema
EENT: Sinusitis
ENDO: Hypoglycemia (renal impairment)
GI: *Nausea, vomiting,* abdominal pain, **pancreatitis**
GU: UTI
INTEG: Urticaria, angioedema, anaphylaxis
META: Hypoglycemia
MISC: Lymphopenia, peripheral edema
RESP: Upper respiratory infection

Pharmacokinetics

Absorption	Rapidly
Distribution	Unknown
Metabolism	Unknown
Excretion	Kidneys 24% unchanged
Half-life	Terminal 2.5 hr, 3.1 hr metabolite

Pharmacodynamics

Onset	Unknown
Peak	1-4 hr
Duration	24 hr

INTERACTIONS
Individual drugs
Aripiprazole, cloZAPine, fosphenytoin, OLANZapine, phenytoin, QUEtiapine, risperiDONE, ziprasidone: decreased antidiabetic effect
Cimetidine, disopyramide: increased saxagliptin level
Cimetidine, FLUoxetine: increased hypoglycemia
Digoxin: increased levels of digoxin

Drug classifications
ACE inhibitors, estrogens, oral contraceptives, phenothiazines, progestins, protease inhibitors, sympathomimetics, thiazide diuretics: decreased antidiabetic effect
Androgens, β-blockers, corticosteroids, fibric acid derivatives, insulins, MAOIs, salicylates: increased hypoglycemia

Drug/herb
Garlic, horse chestnut: increased antidiabetic effect

Drug/lab test
Decreased: lymphocytes, glucose

NURSING CONSIDERATIONS
Assessment
- **Hypoglycemic reactions** (sweating, weakness, dizziness, anxiety, tremors, hunger); monitor blood glucose (BG) as needed
- Monitor CBC (baseline, q3mo) during treatment; check liver function tests periodically,

---

AST, LDH, renal studies: BUN, creatinine during treatment; glycosylated hemoglobin HbA1C
• **Heart failure:** history of risk factors for heart failure, use cautiously, in these patients
• **Pancreatitis: abdominal pain, nausea, vomiting; discontinue**

Patient/family education
• Teach patient to use regular self-monitoring of blood glucose using blood glucose meter
• Teach patient the symptoms of hypo/hyperglycemia; what to do about each
• Teach patient that product must be continued on daily basis; explain consequence of discontinuing product abruptly
• Advise patient to avoid OTC medications, alcohol, digoxin, exenatide, insulins, nateglinide, repaglinide, and other products that lower blood sugar, unless approved by prescriber
• Teach patient that diabetes is a lifelong illness; that this product is not a cure, only controls symptoms
• Teach patient that all food included in diet plan must be eaten to prevent hypo/hyperglycemia
• Teach patient to carry emergency ID
• Teach patient to take product without regard to food
• Teach patient to notify prescriber when surgery, trauma, or stress occurs, as dose may need to be adjusted

Evaluation
Positive therapeutic outcome
• Decrease in polyuria, polydipsia, polyphagia; clear sensorium; absence of dizziness; stable gait; blood glucose at normal level

---

RARELY USED

scopolamine (Rx)
(skoe-pol′a-meen)
Maldemar, Scopace, Transderm-Scop
Func. class.: Cholinergic blocker
Chem. class.: Belladonna alkaloid
Pregnancy category C

Therapeutic outcome: Absence of vomiting, secretions (preoperatively), involuntary movements

USES: Reduction of secretions before surgery, production of amnesia, prevention of motion sickness, Parkinson's symptoms

Unlabeled uses: Drooling (TD)

CONTRAINDICATIONS
Hypersensitivity, closed-angle glaucoma, myasthenia gravis, GI/GU obstruction, hypersensitivity to belladonna, barbiturates

DOSAGE AND ROUTES
Prevention of motion sickness
Adult: Transdermal 1 patch placed behind ear 4 hr before travel, reapply q3day

Parkinson's symptoms
Adult: PO 0.4-0.8 mg q8hr

Preoperatively
Adult: IM/IV/SUBCUT 0.32-0.65 mg; TD apply 1 patch PM before surgery or 1 hr before C-section

Nausea and vomiting
Adult: SUBCUT 0.6-1 mg
Child: SUBCUT 0.006 mg/kg; max 0.3 mg/dose

Drooling (unlabeled)
Adult: Transdermal 1.5 mg patch q3day

---

selegiline (Rx)
(se-le′ji-leen)
Eldepryl, Emsam, Zelapar
Func. class.: Antiparkinson agent
Chem. class.: MAOI, type B
Pregnancy category C

Do not confuse: Eldepryl/enalapril

ACTION: Increased dopaminergic activity by inhibition of MAO type B activity; not fully understood

Therapeutic outcome: Decreased symptoms of Parkinson's disease

USES: Adjunct management of Parkinson's disease in patients being treated with levodopa/carbidopa who have responded poorly to therapy, depression (transdermal)

Unlabeled use: Alzheimer's disease, depression

CONTRAINDICATIONS
Children/adolescents (suicide/hypertensive crisis), hypersensitivity, breastfeeding

Precautions: Pregnancy C

DOSAGE AND ROUTES
Adult: PO 10 mg/day in divided doses, 5 mg at breakfast and lunch with levodopa/carbidopa; after 2-3 days begin to reduce the dose of levodopa/carbidopa 10%-30%; **oral disintegrating tab** 1.25 mg (1 tab) initially, then 2.5 (2 tabs) dissolved on tongue daily before breakfast × 6 wk or more; max 2.5 mg/day; **transdermal** 6 mg/24 hr initially, increase by 3 mg/24 hr at ≥2 wk, up to 12 mg/24 hr if needed

S

Adverse effects: *italics* = common; **bold** = life-threatening

Alzheimer's disease (unlabeled)
Adult: PO 5 mg bid AM, PM

Available forms: Tabs 5 mg, caps 5 mg; oral disintegrating tabs 1.25 mg; transdermal 6 mg/24 hr (20 mg/20 cm²), 9 mg/24 hr (30 mg/30 cm²), 12 mg/24 hr (40 mg/40 cm²)

Implementation
- Do not use in children due to risk for hypertensive crisis
- Adjust dosage to patient's response
- Give with meals; limit protein taken with product
- Give at doses <10 mg/day because of risks associated with nonselective inhibition of MAO
- **Oral disintegrating tab:** peel back foil, place tab on tongue, allow to dissolve, swallow with saliva

Transdermal route
- Apply to dry, intact skin on upper torso/thigh or outer surface of upper arm q12hr

ADVERSE EFFECTS
CNS: Increased tremors, chorea, restlessness, blepharospasm, increased bradykinesia, grimacing, tardive dyskinesia, dystonic symptoms, involuntary movements, increased apraxia, hallucinations, dizziness, mood changes, nightmares, delusions, lethargy, apathy, overstimulation, sleep disturbances, headache, migraine, numbness, muscle cramps, confusion, anxiety, tiredness, vertigo, personality change, back/leg pain, suicide in children/ adolescents, suicidal ideation in adults

CV: Orthostatic hypotension, hypertension, dysrhythmia, palpitations; angina pectoris, hypotension, tachycardia, edema, sinus bradycardia, syncope, hypertensive crisis (children)

EENT: Diplopia, dry mouth, blurred vision, tinnitus

GI: *Nausea*, vomiting, constipation, weight loss, anorexia, diarrhea, heartburn, rectal bleeding, poor appetite, dysphagia, xerostomia

GU: Slow urination, nocturia, prostatic hypertrophy, hesitation, retention, frequency, sexual dysfunction

INTEG: Increased sweating, alopecia, hematoma, rash, photosensitivity, facial hair

RESP: Asthma, shortness of breath

Pharmacokinetics
Absorption	Well absorbed
Distribution	Widely distributed
Metabolism	Rapidly, liver
Excretion	Metabolites *N*-desmethyl-deprenyl, amphetamine, methamphetamine
Half-life	10 hr; oral disintegrating tab 1.3 hr

Pharmacodynamics
Onset	Unknown
Peak	½-2 hr
Duration	Unknown

INTERACTIONS
Individual drugs
Dextromethorphan: increased unusual behavior, psychosis

FLUoxetine, fluvoxaMINE, PARoxetine, sertraline: increased serotonin syndrome (confusion, seizures, fever, hypertension, agitation) discontinue 5 wk before selegiline

Levodopa/carbidopa: increased side effects

⚠ Meperidine: do not use, fatal reaction

Drug classifications
⚠ Antidepressants (tricyclics), opioids (especially meperidine): do not use, fatal reaction

Antihypertensives: increased hypotension

Drug/lab test
Decreased: VMA
False positive: urine ketones, urine glucose
False negative: urine glucose (glucose oxidase)
False increase: uric acid, urine protein

NURSING CONSIDERATIONS
Assessment
- Monitor cardiac status: tachycardia, bradycardia; B/P, respiration throughout treatment
- Assess mental status: affect, mood, behavioral changes, depression; perform suicide assessment, suicidal ideation may occur
- **Parkinson's symptoms:** assess for rigidity, unsteady gait, weakness, tremors; these should decrease in severity
- Assess opioids; if patient has received, do not give selegiline; fatal reactions have occurred

Patient/family education
- Caution patient to change positions slowly to prevent orthostatic hypotension
- ⚠ Hypertensive crisis: teach patient to report nausea, vomiting, sweating, agitation, change in mental status, headache, chest pain to prescriber immediately
- **Pregnancy:** teach patient to report if pregnancy is planned or suspected, pregnancy (**C**), avoid breastfeeding
- Teach patient to use during the day to prevent insomnia
- Caution patient to use product exactly as prescribed; if product is discontinued abruptly, parkinsonian crisis may occur
- Instruct patient to avoid foods high in tyramine: cheese, pickled products, wine, beer, large amounts of caffeine

• Instruct patient not to exceed recommended dose of 10 mg; might precipitate a hypertensive crisis; report severe headache or other unusual symptoms

⚠ Serotonin syndrome: teach patient to report twitching, sweating, shivering, diarrhea to prescriber immediately

• Teach patient to avoid heating pads, hot tubs when using transdermal products
• Teach patient to avoid hazardous activities until response is known

Evaluation

Positive therapeutic outcome
• Decreased symptoms of Parkinson's disease

TREATMENT OF OVERDOSE:
IV fluids for hypertension, **IV** dilute pressure agent for B/P titration

---

selenium topical
See Appendix B

---

sertraline (Rx)
(ser'tra-leen)
Apo-Sertraline ✦, Zoloft
Func. class.: Antidepressant
Chem. class.: Selective serotonin reuptake inhibitor (SSRI)
Pregnancy category C

Do not confuse: Zoloft/Zocor

ACTION: Inhibits serotonin reuptake in CNS, thus increasing action of serotonin; does not affect DOPamine, norepinephrine

Therapeutic outcome: Relief of depression, obsessive-compulsive disorder (OCD), posttraumatic stress disorder (PTSD), panic disorder

USES: Major depression, OCD, PTSD, social anxiety disorder, panic disorder, premenstrual dysphoric disorder (PMDD), separation anxiety disorder

CONTRAINDICATIONS
Hypersensitivity to this product or selective serotonin reuptake inhibitors

Precautions: Pregnancy **C**, breastfeeding, geriatric, renal/hepatic disease, epilepsy, recent MI, latex sensitivity (dropper of oral conc)

> BLACK BOX WARNING: Suicidal ideation, children

DOSAGE AND ROUTES
Adult/geriatric: PO 25-50 mg/day; may increase to a maximum of 200 mg/day, do not

change dose at intervals of <1 wk; administer daily in AM or PM
Child 6-12 yr: PO 25 mg/day, max 200 mg/day

Premenstrual disorders
Adult: PO 50-150 mg nightly

Hepatic dose
Adult: PO; use lower dose or less frequent dosing intervals

Available forms: Tabs 25, 50, 100 mg; oral sol 20 mg/ml

Implementation
• Administer dosage at bedtime if oversedation occurs during day; may take entire dose at bedtime; may crush
• Give with food, milk for GI symptoms
• Give crushed if patient is unable to swallow medication whole
• Use sugarless gum, hard candy; frequent sips of water for dry mouth
• **Oral concentration:** dilute before use with 4 oz (½ cup) of water, orange juice, ginger ale, or lemon/lime soda; do not mix with other liquids
• Store at room temperature; do not freeze
• Dropper contains latex

ADVERSE EFFECTS
CNS: *Insomnia, agitation, somnolence, dizziness, headache, tremor, fatigue,* paresthesia, twitching, confusion, ataxia, gait abnormality (geriatric), **seizures, neuroleptic malignant syndrome–like reactions, serotonin syndrome, suicidal ideation,** anxiety, drowsiness
CV: Palpitations, chest pain
EENT: Vision abnormalities, yawning, tinnitus, intraocular pressure
ENDO: Syndrome of inappropriate antidiuretic hormone (geriatric), diabetes mellitus
GI: *Diarrhea, nausea, constipation, anorexia, dry mouth,* dyspepsia, *vomiting, flatulence,* weight gain/loss, **hepatitis**
GU: *Male sexual dysfunction,* micturition disorder
INTEG: Increased sweating, rash, hot flashes
MISC: Hyponatremia, neonatal abstinence syndrome

Pharmacokinetics

Absorption	Well absorbed
Distribution	Unknown, steady state 1 wk
Metabolism	Liver, extensively
Excretion	Feces (14%)
Half-life	26 hr

S

Pharmacodynamics

Onset	Unknown
Peak	4.5-8.4 hr
Duration	Unknown

INTERACTIONS
Individual drugs
Cimetidine, warfarin: increased sertraline effect
CloZAPine: increased effects of cloZAPine
Diazepam: increased diazepam effect
Disulfiram: disulfiram reaction with oral conc
   due to alcohol content
Lithium: altered lithium levels
Phenytoin: increased effects of phenytoin
Pimozide: sertraline is contraindicated with
   pimozide, fatal reactions
Sibutramine, traZODone, busPIRone, linezolid,
   traMADol: increased serotonin syndrome, in-
   creased neuroleptic malignant syndrome
SUMAtriptan: increased SUMAtriptan effects
TOLBUTamide: increased effect of TOLBUTa-
   mide
Warfarin: increased warfarin effect

Drug classifications
Anticoagulants, NSAIDs, thrombolytics, platelet
   inhibitors, salicylates: increased bleeding risk
Antidepressants (tricyclics), benzodiazepines:
   increased effect
Highly protein-bound products: increased sertraline levels
SSRIs, SNRIs, serotonin-receptor agonists, tricyclics: increased serotonin syndrome, increased neuroleptic malignant syndrome
⚠ **MAOIs: fatal reactions**

Drug/herb
Kava, valerian: increased CNS effect
**SAM-e, St. John's wort, tryptophan: in-
creased effect of SSRIs, serotonin syndrome; do not use together**

Drug/lab test
Increased: AST, ALT
False positive: urine screen for benzodiazepines

NURSING CONSIDERATIONS
Assessment

> **BLACK BOX WARNING:** Assess mental status:
> mood, sensorium, affect, suicidal tendencies
> (child/young adult); increase in psychiatric
> symptoms: depression, panic attacks, OCD,
> PTSD, social anxiety disorder

• Identify alcohol consumption; if alcohol is
consumed, hold dose until AM
⚠ **Serotonin syndrome: assess for hyperthermia, hypertension, rigidity, delirium,
coma, myoclonus or neuroleptic**
malignant-like syndrome (muscle cramps,
fever, unstable B/P, agitation, tremors, mental changes)
⚠ **Bleeding (platelet serotonin depletion):
assess for GI bleeding, ecchymoses, epistaxis, hematomas, petechiae, hemorrhage)**
• LFTs, thyroid function test, growth rate, weight
baseline and periodically
• B/P (lying/standing), pulse q4hr; if systolic
B/P drops 20 mm Hg, hold product, notify
prescriber; VS q4hr in patients with CV disease
• Weight qwk; appetite may decrease with
product
• Urinary retention, constipation, especially in
geriatric patients

Patient/family education
• Teach patient that therapeutic effects may take
1 wk or longer
• Instruct patient to notify prescriber if
pregnant or planning to become pregnant or
breastfeed, pregnancy (**C**)
• Instruct patient to use caution in driving or
other activities requiring alertness because of
drowsiness, dizziness, blurred vision; to avoid
rising quickly from sitting to standing, especially
geriatric
• Advise patient to avoid alcohol ingestion,
other CNS depressants
⚠ **Teach patient not to discontinue medication quickly after long-term use: may
cause nausea, headache, malaise**
• Caution patient to wear sunscreen or large hat
because photosensitivity can occur
• Teach patient to increase fluids, bulk in diet if
constipation, urinary retention occur, especially
geriatric
• Instruct patient to take gum, hard sugarless
candy, or frequent sips of water for dry mouth
• Teach patient that medication may be taken
without regard to food
• **Serotonin syndrome: teach patient to
report agitation, nausea, vomiting, diarrhea,
twitching, sweating, shivering to prescriber
immediately**

> **BLACK BOX WARNING:** Teach patient that
> suicidal thoughts/behavior may occur (chil-
> dren/adolescents)

Evaluation
Positive therapeutic outcome
• Decrease in depression, OCD
• Absence of suicidal thoughts

TREATMENT OF OVERDOSE:
ECG monitoring, induce emesis, lavage, activated
charcoal, administer anticonvulsant

⚠ Nurse Alert   ✴ Key NCLEX® Drug   ≫ Drug Specifics

sildenafil (Rx)

(sil-den'a-fill)

Revatio, Viagra

Func. class.: Erectile agent; antihypertensive, peripheral vasodilator

Chem. class.: Selective inhibitor of cyclic GMP-PDE5

Pregnancy category B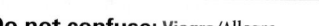

Do not confuse: Viagra/Allegra

ACTION: Enhances the effect of nitric oxide (NO) by inhibiting phosphodiesterase type 5 (PDE5), which is necessary for degrading cyclic GMP in the corpus cavernosum

Therapeutic outcome: Ability to achieve and maintain erection

USES: Treatment of erectile dysfunction, pulmonary hypertension; improvement in exercise ability

Unlabeled uses: Sexual dysfunction (women)

CONTRAINDICATIONS

Hypersensitivity to this product or nitrates

Precautions: Pregnancy **B**, anatomical penile deformities, sickle cell anemia, leukemia, multiple myeloma, retinitis pigmentosa, bleeding disorders, active peptic ulceration, CV/renal/hepatic disease, multidrug antihypertensive regimens, geriatric patients

DOSAGE AND ROUTES
Erectile dysfunction (Viagra only)

Adult male <65 yr: PO 50 mg 1 hr before sexual activity; may be increased to 100 mg or decreased to 25 mg; max frequency once/day

Adult ≥65 yr (male): PO 25 mg prn about 1 hr before sexual activity

Renal/hepatic dose

Adult: PO (Child-Pugh A, B) 25 mg, take 1 hr before sexual activity, do not use more than 1 ×/day; CCr <30 ml/min 25 mg starting dose

Pulmonary hypertension (Revatio only)

Adult: PO 20 mg tid, take 4-6 hr apart; **IV BOL** 10 mg tid

Available forms: Tabs 20, 25, 50, 100 mg, sol for inj 10 mg/12.5 ml

Implementation

• **Erectile dysfunction:** give approximately 1 hr before sexual activity, do not use more than once a day, give on empty stomach for better absorption

• Tab may be split

• **Pulmonary hypertension:** Give 3×/day, 4-6 hr apart

ADVERSE EFFECTS

CNS: *Headache, flushing, dizziness,* transient global amnesia, **seizures**

CV: **MI, sudden death, CV collapse,** TIAs, ventricular dysrhythmias, CV hemorrhage

MISC: *Dyspepsia, nasal congestion, UTI, abnormal vision, diarrhea, rash,* **NAION** (**nonarteritic ischemic optic neuropathy**), hearing loss, priapism, **sickle cell crisis**

Pharmacokinetics

Absorption	Rapidly, bioavailability (40%)
Distribution	Unknown
Metabolism	Liver (active metabolites)
Excretion	Feces, urine
Half-life	4 hr

Pharmacodynamics

Onset	Unknown
Peak	½-1½ hr
Duration	Unknown

INTERACTIONS
Individual drugs

Alcohol, amLODIPine: decreased B/P

Bosentan, rifampin, carBAMazepine, dexamethasone, phenytoin, nevirapine, rifabutin, troglitazone: decreased sildenafil levels

Cimetidine, erythromycin, itraconazole, ketoconazole, tacrolimus: increased sildenafil levels

Drug classifications

Antacids, barbiturates, CYP450 inducers: decreased sildenafil levels

Antiretroviral protease inhibitors: increased sildenafil levels

α-Blockers, angiotensin II receptor blockers: decreased B/P

A Nitrates: fatal fall in B/P; do not use together

Drug/food

Grapefruit: increased product effect

High-fat meal: decreased absorption

NURSING CONSIDERATIONS
Assessment

A Phosphodiesterase type 5 inhibitors with lopinavir/ritonavir (Kaletra): assess for hypotension, visual changes, prolonged erection, syncope; give only 25 mg q48hr and monitor for adverse reactions

S

Adverse effects: *italics* = common; **bold** = life-threatening

⚠ Identify organic nitrates that should not be used with this product
⚠ Assess for any severe loss of vision while taking this or any similar products; these products should not be used if vision loss has occurred
• Assess for MI, sudden death, CV collapse: Those with an MI within 6 mo, resting hypotension <90/50, resting hypertension >170/100, fluid depletion should use this product cautiously, may occur right after sexual activity to days afterward
• Sickle cell crisis (vasoocclusive crisis): when used for pulmonary hypertension, may require hospitalization

Patient/family education
• Teach patient that product does not protect against STDs, including HIV
• Teach patient that product absorption is reduced with a high-fat meal
• Teach patient that product should not be used with nitrates in any form
• Teach patient that tab may be split
• Teach patient to notify prescriber immediately and stop taking product if vision loss occurs
• Do not use more often than 100 mg in 24 hr
⚠ Teach patient to notify prescriber immediately and to stop taking product if vision/ hearing loss occurs or erection lasts >4 hr

Evaluation

Positive therapeutic outcome
• Ability to achieve and maintain an erection

---

silodosin (Rx)
(si-lo′do-seen)
Rapaflo
Func. class.: Selective α₁-adrenergic blocker, BPH agent
Chem. class.: Sulfamoylphenethylamine derivative
Pregnancy category B

ACTION: Binds preferentially to α_{1A}-adrenoceptor subtype located mainly in the prostate

Therapeutic outcome: Decreased symptoms of benign prostatic hyperplasia

USES: Symptoms of benign prostatic hyperplasia (BPH)

CONTRAINDICATIONS
Hypersensitivity, renal failure, hepatic disease

Precautions: Pregnancy **B**, breastfeeding, children, renal/hepatic disease, females, hypotension, ocular surgery, orthostatic hypotension, prostate cancer, syncope, geriatric patients

DOSAGE AND ROUTES
Adult: PO 8 mg/day with a meal; max 8 mg/day

Renal dose
Adult: PO CCr 30-49 ml/min 4 mg/day; CCr <30 ml/min not recommended

Available forms: Tabs 8 mg

Implementation
• Give with meal at same time of day
• Store at room temperature; protect from light and moisture

ADVERSE EFFECTS
CNS: *Dizziness, headache,* asthenia, insomnia, syncope
CV: Orthostatic hypotension
EENT: Nasal congestion, rhinorrhea, sinusitis
GI: Diarrhea, abdominal pain, jaundice
GU: Abnormal ejaculation, priapism, urinary incontinence
HEMA: Purpura

Pharmacokinetics

Absorption	Decreased with high-fat/high-calorie meal
Distribution	Extensive protein binding 97%
Metabolism	Liver
Excretion	Urine
Half-life	24 hr (metabolite)

Pharmacodynamics

Unknown

INTERACTIONS
Drug classifications
CYP3A4 inhibitors (clarithromycin, itraconazole, ritonavir, anti-retroviral protease inhibitors, aprepitant, chloramphenicol, conivaptan, dalfopristin, danazol, delavirdine, efavirenz, fosaprepitant, fluconazole, fluvoxaMINE, imatinib, isoniazid, mifepristone, nefazodone, tamoxifen, telithromycin, troleandomycin, voriconazole, zileuton, zafirlukast): increased silodosin effect

Drug/food
Grapefruit juice: increased silodosin effect

Drug/lab test
Increased: LFTs

NURSING CONSIDERATIONS
Assessment
• **Prostatic hyperplasia:** assess for change in urinary patterns, baseline and throughout treatment, testing for prostate cancer prior to administration is recommended

---

- Monitor BUN, uric acid, urodynamic studies (urinary flow rates, residual volume)
- Assess I&O ratios, weight daily, edema, report weight gain or edema
- B/P, monitor for orthostatic hypotension

Patient/family education
- Caution patient not to drive or operate machinery until effect is known
- Advise patient not to use with grapefruit juice
- Teach patient to take with same meal each day

Evaluation

Positive therapeutic outcome
- Decreased symptoms of benign prostatic hyperplasia

simeprevir
(sim-e′pre-vir)
Olysio
Func. class.: Antiviral, antihepatitis agent
Pregnancy category X

ACTION: Prevents formation of mature viral proteins by inhibiting hepatitis C viral (HCV) replication by blocking proteolytic activity of the hepatitis C virus NS3/4A protease

Therapeutic outcome: Decreased symptoms of chronic hepatitis C

USES: Chronic hepatitis C infection, hepatitis, (HCV, genotype 1) in adults with compensated liver disease

CONTRAINDICATIONS
Hypersensitivity, male-mediated teratogenicity, pregnancy (**X**) in combination

Precautions: Pregnancy **C** (alone), breastfeeding, Asian patients, liver transplant, UV exposure, hepatic disease, serious rash, children

DOSAGE AND ROUTES
Adult: **PO** 150 mg/day with food with peginterferon alfa and ribavirin × 12 wk

Available forms: Cap 150 mg

Implementation
- Give by mouth with food, swallow whole
- Do not use monotherapy; if peginterferon alfa or ribavirin is discontinued, discontinue simeprevir and do not restart
- Obtain NS3 Q80K polymorphism test before starting treatment
- Treatment-naïve/prior relapse: after initial 3-drug treatment, give another 12 wk with peginterferon alfa and ribavirin × another 12 wk; if HCV RNA concentrations ≥25 interstitial units/ml, discontinue all 3 drugs

- Prior nonresponders (partial/null): after initial 3-drug treatment give an additional 36 wk of peginterferon alfa and ribavirin; monitor HCV RNA at wk 4, 12, 24; if ≥25 interstitial units/ml, discontinue products

ADVERSE EFFECTS
EENT: Blurred vision, conjunctivitis
GI: Hyperbilirubinemia, nausea
INTEG: Exfoliative dermatitis, pruritus, photosensitivity, vasculitis
MISC: Rash, dyspnea

Pharmacokinetics
Absorption	Unknown
Distribution	99.9 % protein binding
Metabolism	Primarily by CYP3A4, also a mild inhibitor of intestinal CYP3A4 and CYP1A2
Excretion	91% feces
Half-life	40 hr

Pharmacodynamics
Onset	Unknown
Peak	Unknown
Duration	Unknown

INTERACTIONS
Individual drugs
Bromocriptine, chloramphenicol, cimetidine, dalfopristin/quinupristin, danazol, erythromycin, FLUoxetine, isoniazid, lanreotide, octreotide, zafirlukast: increased simeprevir effect

Drug classifications
CYP3A4 inhibitors: increased effects of these agents

NURSING CONSIDERATIONS
Assessment
- Allergic reaction: assess for rash, pruritus, exfoliative dermatitis
- **Asian patients: levels may be 3-fold to 4-fold higher**
- ⚠ **Pregnancy: if planned or suspected; if pregnant call the Pregnancy Registry 800-258-4263, pregnancy X in combination, obtain pregnancy test before using**
- Liver function tests; Monitor HCV, RNA concentrations at weeks 4, 12, and 24 and at end of treatment

Patient/family education
- Teach patient that optimal duration of treatment is unknown, that product is not a cure, that transmission may still occur
- Teach patient to avoid use with other medications unless approved by prescriber

S

- Teach patient to use protective clothing, sunscreen; photosensitivity may occur and can be severe
- Teach patient not to stop abruptly unless directed; worsening of hepatitis may occur
⚠ Teach patient to notify prescriber if pregnancy is planned or suspected, avoid breastfeeding; use 2 reliable forms of contraception, do not try to conceive for at least 6 mo after discontinuation of this drug combination
- Teach patient to use cautiously in sulfonamide allergy; do not take the drug as single agent; must use as combination therapy

Evaluation

Positive therapeutic outcome
- Decreased symptoms of chronic hepatitis C

silver nitrate 1% ophthalmic
See Appendix B

silver nitrate sulfacetamide sodium ophthalmic
See Appendix B

silver sulfADIAZINE topical
See Appendix B

simethicone (Rx, OTC)
(si-meth'i-kone)
Barriere ✦, Gas Relief ✦, Gas-Relief, Gas-X, Mylanta Gas, Mylanta Gas Relief, Mylicon, Ovol ✦, Phazyme
Func. class.: Antiflatulent
Pregnancy category C

Do not confuse: Mylicon/Mylanta Gas
Simethicone/Cimetidine

ACTION: Disperses, prevents gas pockets in GI system; lowers surface tension of gas bubbles

Therapeutic outcome: Belching or flatus

USES: Flatulence

Unlabeled uses: Dyspepsia

CONTRAINDICATIONS
Hypersensitivity, GI obstruction/perforation

Precautions: Pregnancy **C**, abdominal pain, fistula, hiatal hernia

DOSAGE AND ROUTES
Adult and child >12 yr: PO 40-125 mg after meals and at bedtime prn, max 500 mg/day

Child 2-12 yr: PO 40 mg after meals and at bedtime prn, max 240 mg/day
Child <2 yr: PO 20 mg qid prn

Available forms: Chew tabs 40, 150, 166 mg; tabs 60, 80, 95, 125 mg; drops 20 mg/0.3 ml; caps 95, 180 mg; caps, soft gel 125, 180 mg; oral dissolving film 62.5 mg

Implementation
- Give after meals and at bedtime
- Shake susp well before administering
- Chew tab should be chewed and not swallowed whole

ADVERSE EFFECTS
GI: Belching, rectal flatus, diarrhea

Pharmacokinetics
Absorption	None
Distribution	None
Metabolism	None
Excretion	None
Half-life	Unknown

Pharmacodynamics
Onset	Rapid
Peak	Unknown
Duration	3 hr

NURSING CONSIDERATIONS
Assessment
- Identify the reason for excess gas production: decreased bowel sounds, recent surgery, other GI conditions

Patient/family education
- Caution patient that tab must be chewed; to shake susp well before pouring

Evaluation

Positive therapeutic outcome
- Absence of flatulence

simvastatin (Rx)
(sim-va-stat'in)
Zocor
Func. class.: Antilipidemic
Chem. class.: HMG-CoA reductase inhibitor
Pregnancy category X

Do not confuse: Zocor/Cozaar/Zoloft

ACTION: Inhibits HMG-CoA reductase enzyme, which reduces cholesterol synthesis; this enzyme is needed for cholesterol production

Therapeutic outcome: Decreasing cholesterol levels and LDLs, increased HDLs

USES: As an adjunct in primary hypercholesterolemia (types IIa, IIb), isolated hypertriglyceridemia (Frederickson type IV) and type III hyperlipoproteinemia, CAD, heterozygous familial hypercholesterolemia; MI/stroke prophylaxis

CONTRAINDICATIONS
Pregnancy **X**, breastfeeding, hypersensitivity, active liver disease

Precautions: Past liver disease, alcoholism, severe acute infections, trauma, severe metabolic disorders, electrolyte imbalances, Chinese patients

DOSAGE AND ROUTES
Adult: PO 20-40 mg/day in PM initially, usual range 5-40 mg/day daily in PM max, 40 mg/day for most patients; max 80 mg/day (for patients taking 80 mg/day chronically without myopathy); dosage adjustments may be made at 4-wk intervals or more; those taking verapamil and amiodarone max 20 mg/day, max <80 mg for Chinese patients taking lipid-modifying niacin doses

With diltiazem/verapamil
Adult: PO 5-10 mg q PM, max 10 mg/day with amiodarone/amLODIPine/ranolazine
Adult: PO 5-20 mg q PM, max 20 mg/day
Child and adolescent ≥10 yr including girls ≥1 yr postmenarche: PO 10 mg q PM, range 10-40 mg/day

With amiodarone, amLODIPine, ranolazine
Adult: PO 5-20 mg/day in evening, max 20 mg/day

Heterozygous familial hypercholesterolemia
Adult: PO 40 mg qday in evening; make dosage adjustments q4wk

Available forms: Tabs 5, 10, 20, 40, 80 mg

Implementation
• Give 30 min before AM and PM meals
• Store in cool environment in tight container protected from light

ADVERSE EFFECTS
CNS: Headache, cognitive impairment
GI: Nausea, constipation, diarrhea, dyspepsia, flatus, abdominal pain, *liver dysfunction, pancreatitis,* hyperglycemia
INTEG: Rash, pruritus
MS: Muscle cramps, myalgia, *myositis, rhabdomyolysis,* myopathy
RESP: Upper respiratory tract infection

Pharmacokinetics
Absorption	85%
Distribution	Unknown
Metabolism	Liver—extensively
Excretion	70% feces, 20% kidneys
Half-life	3 hr

Pharmacodynamics
Unknown

INTERACTIONS
Individual drugs
Clarithromycin, clofibrate, cycloSPORINE, erythromycin, gemfibrozil, itraconazole, ketoconazole, niacin, danazol, delavirdine, nefazodone, verapamil, diltiazem, amiodarone, azole antifungals, telithromycin: increased myalgia, myositis, rhabdomyolysis
CycloSPORINE, gemfibrozil: do not use with simvastatin
Digoxin: increased digoxin levels
Warfarin: increased risk of bleeding

Drug classifications
Macrolide antiinfectives, protease inhibitors: increased myalgia, myositis, rhabdomyolysis
Increased: simvastatin effect ATP1B1 inhibitors

Drug/herb
Red yeast rice: increased simvastatin effect
St. John's wort: decreased effect

Drug/food
Increased: simvastatin level: grapefruit juice (large amounts)

Drug/lab test
Increased: CPK, liver function tests, HbA1C

NURSING CONSIDERATIONS
Assessment
• Assess nutrition: fat, protein, carbohydrates; nutritional analysis should be completed by dietitian before treatment is initiated
⚠ **Rhabdomyolysis: assess for muscle tenderness, increased CPK levels 10× ULN; therapy should be discontinued, more likely in those receiving >80 mg/day, first year of treatment, those ≥65 yr, females**
• Monitor bowel pattern daily; diarrhea may be a problem
• Monitor triglycerides, cholesterol baseline, throughout treatment; LDL, HDL, triglycerides and cholesterol should be watched closely at 6-8 wk and q6mo; if increased, product should be discontinued

Patient/family education
• Inform patient that compliance is needed for positive results to occur, not to double doses

- Advise patient to lower risk factors: high-fat diet, smoking, alcohol consumption, absence of exercise, smoking cessation
- **Advise patient to notify prescriber of planned or suspected pregnancy X**
- Teach patient to take in evening
- Teach patient to report muscle pain, weakness, abdominal pain, dark urine, yellowing of skin or eyes, memory loss

Evaluation

Positive therapeutic outcome
- Decreased cholesterol levels, serum triglycerides and improved ratio with HDLs

---

⚠ HIGH ALERT

sirolimus (Rx)
(seer-roe′li-mus)
Rapamune
Func. class.: Immunosuppressant
Chem. class.: Macrolide
Pregnancy category C

ACTION: Produces immunosuppression by inhibiting T-lymphocyte activation and proliferation

Therapeutic outcome: Prevention of rejection in organ transplant

USES: Organ transplants: to prevent rejection, recommended use is with cycloSPORINE and corticosteroids

CONTRAINDICATIONS
Breastfeeding, hypersensitivity to this product or to components of the product

Precautions: Pregnancy **C**, children <13 yr, severe cardiac/renal/hepatic disease, diabetes mellitus, hyperkalemia, hyperuricemia, hypertension, interstitial lung disease, hyperlipidemia, soy lecithin hypersensitivity

> BLACK BOX WARNING: Lymphomas, infection, other malignancies, liver transplant, requires a specialized setting, requires an experienced clinician

DOSAGE AND ROUTES
Adult/adolescent ≥40 kg: PO 2 mg daily with 6 mg loading dose
Child >13 yr <40 kg (88 lb): PO 1 mg/m²/day, 3 mg/m²/loading dose

Hepatic dose
Adult and child ≥13 yr <40 kg: PO reduce by 33% in maintenance dose (mild to moderate hepatic impairment); reduce by 50% in maintenance dose (severe hepatic impairment)

Available forms: Oral sol 1 mg/ml; tabs 0.5, 1, 2 mg

Implementation
- Administer prophylaxis for *Pneumocystis jiroveci* pneumonia for 1 yr after transplantation; prophylaxis for cytomegalovirus (CMV) is recommended for 90 days after transplantation in those at increased risk for CMV
- Use amber oral dose syringe and withdraw amount of oral sol needed from the bottle, empty correct dose into plastic/glass container holding 60 ml of water/orange juice, stir vigorously and have patient drink at once, refill container with additional 120 ml of water/orange juice, stir vigorously, and have patient drink at once; if using a pouch squeeze entire contents into container and follow preceding directions
- Give all medications PO if possible; avoid IM inj because bleeding may occur
- Give for 3 days before transplant surgery; patients should be placed in protective isolation, give at same time of day, give 4 hr after cycloSPORINE oral sol or caps, do not use with grapefruit juice
- Store protected from light; refrigerate; stable for 24 months

> BLACK BOX WARNING: Only those experienced in immunosuppressant therapy and transplant should use this drug; must use in a specialized care setting with adequate medical equipment

ADVERSE EFFECTS
CNS: *Tremors, headache, insomnia,* paresthesia, chills, fever
CV: Hypo/hypertension, atrial fibrillation, CHF, palpitations, tachycardia, peripheral edema, thrombosis
EENT: Blurred vision, photophobia
GI: Nausea, vomiting, diarrhea, constipation, hepatotoxicity
GU: UTI, albuminuria, hematuria, proteinuria, renal failure, nephrotic syndrome
HEMA: Anemia, thrombocytopenia purpura, leukopenia, pancytopenia
INTEG: *Rash, acne,* photosensitivity
META: Increased creatinine, edema, hypercholesterolemia, *hyperlipemia,* hypophosphatemia, weight gain, hyperglycemia, hypo/hyperkalemia, hyperuricemia, hypomagnesemia, hypertriglyceridemia
MS: Arthralgia

RESP: Pleural effusion, atelectasis, *dyspnea*, pneumonitis, pulmonary embolism/fibrosis
SYST: Lymphoma, exfoliative dermatitis

Pharmacokinetics

Absorption	Rapidly absorbed
Distribution	92% protein binding
Metabolism	Liver; extensively by CYP3A4 enzyme system
Excretion	Unknown
Half-life	57-63 hr

Pharmacodynamics

Onset	Unknown
Peak	1 hr single dose, 2 hr multiple dosing
Duration	Unknown

INTERACTIONS
Individual drugs
Bromocriptine, cimetidine, cycloSPORINE, danazol, erythromycin, metoclopramide: increased blood level
CarBAMazepine, PHENobarbital, phenytoin, rifamycin, rifapentine: decreased blood levels

Drug classifications
ACE inhibitors, angiotensin II receptor antagonists, cephalosporins, iodine-containing radiopaque contrast media, neuromuscular blockers, NSAIDs, penicillins, salicylates, thrombolytics: increased angioedema
Antifungal agents, calcium channel blockers, HIV protease inhibitors: increased blood levels
Live virus vaccines: decreased effect of vaccines

Drug/herb
St. John's wort: decreased sirolimus effect

Drug/food
Food: alters bioavailability, use consistently with or without food
Grapefruit juice: do not use with grapefruit juice

Drug/lab test
Increased: LFTs, alk phos, lipids, triglycerides, total cholesterol, BUN, creatinine, LDH, phosphate
Decreased: platelets, sodium
Increased or decreased: magnesium, glucose, calcium

NURSING CONSIDERATIONS
Assessment
⚠ **Wound dehiscence and anastomotic disruption:** assess wound, vascular, airway, ureteral, biliary, inhibition of growth factors; do not combine with corticosteroids, not recommended in lung or liver transplant

⚠ **Anaphylaxis, angioedema, exfoliative dermatitis:** assess for, more common when given with ACE inhibitors; do not use if a hypersensitivity reaction occurs
• **Bone marrow depression:** Hgb, WBC, platelets monthly during treatment; if leukocytes are <3000/mm³ or platelets <100,000/mm³, product should be discontinued or reduced; decreased Hgb level
• Monitor blood levels in those who may have altered metabolism, trough levels ≥15 ng/ml are associated with increased adverse reactions
• **Pulmonary fibrosis, pulmonary effusion, pneumonitis:** assess for dyspnea, cough, hypoxia; some fatal cases have occurred
• Monitor lipid profile: cholesterol, triglycerides; a lipid-lowering agent may be needed

> **BLACK BOX WARNING:** Creatinine/BUN, CBC, serum potassium

• Assess for infection and development of lymphoma
• Only those experienced in immunosuppressant therapy and organ transplantation should use this product; use only in renal transplant
• **High risk:** those with Banff grade 3 acute rejection or vascular rejection prior to cycloSPORINE withdrawal, dialysis dependent, creatinine >4.5 mg/dl, African descent, re-transplant, multiorgan transplant, high panel of reactive antibodies
• **Hepatotoxicity:** alk phos, AST, ALT, amylase, bilirubin: dark urine, jaundice, itching, light-colored stools; product should be discontinued

Patient/family education
• Instruct patient to report fever, rash, severe diarrhea, chills, sore throat, fatigue because serious infections may occur; clay-colored stools, cramping may indicate hepatotoxicity; fever, chills, sore throat (infection)
• Caution patient to avoid crowds or persons with known infections to reduce risk of infection
• Teach patient to use contraception before, during, and 12 wk after product has been discontinued, avoid breastfeeding
• Teach patient to use sunscreen, protective clothing to prevent burns
• Teach patient that lifelong use is required to prevent rejection
• Teach patient that continuing follow-up exams and blood work will be required
• Teach patient not to get on skin
• Teach patient how to use product
• Teach patient to take at same time, consistently, with or without regard to food
• Teach patient to take 4 hr after cycloSPORINE

S

Adverse effects: *italics* = common; **bold** = life-threatening

Evaluation

Positive therapeutic outcome

- Absence of graft rejection

⚠ HIGH ALERT

sitaGLIPtin (Rx)

(sit-a-glip′tin)

Januvia

Func. class.: Antidiabetic, oral

Chem. class.: Dipeptidyl-peptidase-4 inhibitor (DPP-4 inhibitor)

Pregnancy category B

ACTION: Slows the inactivation of incretin hormones; improves glucose homeostasis, improves glucose-dependent insulin secretion, lowers glucagon secretions and slows gastric emptying time

Therapeutic outcome: Decrease in polyuria, polydipsia, polyphagia; clear sensorium; absence of dizziness; stable gait; blood glucose at normal level

USES: Type 2 diabetes mellitus as monotherapy or in combination with other antidiabetic agents

CONTRAINDICATIONS

Angioedema, diabetic ketoacidosis (DKA)

Precautions: Pregnancy **B**, geriatric, hypersensitivity, GI obstruction, thyroid disease, surgery, renal/hepatic disease, trauma, breastfeeding, pancreatitis, hypercortisolism, hyperglycemia, hyperthyroidism, hypoglycemia, ileus, pituitary insufficiency, surgery, type 1 diabetes mellitus, adrenal insufficiency, burns, diabetic ketoacidosis

DOSAGE AND ROUTES

Adult: PO 100 mg/day; may use with other antidiabetic agents (metformin, pioglitazone, rosiglitazone) other than insulin

Renal dose

Adult: PO CCr 30-50 ml/min 50 mg qd; CCr <30 ml/min 25 mg qd

Available forms: Tabs 25, 50, 100 mg

Implementation

- May be taken with or without food
- Conversion from other antidiabetic agents; change may be made with gradual dosage change
- Store in tight container at room temperature
- Do not split, crush, chew, swallow whole

ADVERSE EFFECTS

CNS: *Headache*

ENDO: Hypoglycemia

GI: *Nausea, vomiting,* abdominal pain, diarrhea, pancreatitis, constipation

GU: Acute renal failure

MISC: Peripheral edema

SYST: Anaphylaxis, Stevens-Johnson syndrome, angioedema

Pharmacokinetics

Absorption	Rapidly
Distribution	Unknown
Metabolism	Unknown
Excretion	Kidneys, 79% unchanged
Half-life	Terminal 12.4 hr

Pharmacodynamics

Onset	Unknown
Peak	1-4 hr
Duration	Unknown

INTERACTIONS

Individual drugs

ARIPiprazole, cloZAPine, fosphenytoin, OLANZapine, phenytoin, QUEtiapine, risperiDONE, ziprasidone: decreased antidiabetic effect

Cimetidine, disopyramide: increased sitaGLIPtin level

Cimetidine, FLUoxetine: increased hypoglycemia

Digoxin: increased levels of digoxin

Drug classifications

ACE inhibitors, estrogens, oral contraceptives, progestins, phenothiazines, protease inhibitors, sympathomimetics, thiazide diuretics: decreased antidiabetic effect

Androgens, β-blockers, corticosteroids, fibric acid derivatives, insulins, MAOIs, salicylates, sulfonylureas: increased hypoglycemia

Drug/herb

Garlic, green tea, horse chestnut: increased antidiabetic effect

Drug/lab test

Increased: creatinine, LFTs

NURSING CONSIDERATIONS

Assessment

- **Hypoglycemic reactions:** assess for sweating, weakness, dizziness, anxiety, tremors, hunger, hyperglycemic reactions soon after meals
- Monitor CBC (baseline, q3mo) during treatment; check liver function tests periodically, AST, LDH, renal studies: BUN, creatinine during treatment; Hgb A1c
- Monitor blood glucose (BG) as needed
- **Serious skin reactions:** assess for swelling of face, mouth, lips, dyspnea, wheezing
- **Pancreatitis:** assess for severe abdominal pain, nausea, vomiting; discontinue product

---

• **Renal studies:** monitor BUN, creatinine during treatment, especially in geriatrics or those with renal disease
• Monitor hemoglobin A1C; monitor blood glucose as needed

Patient/family education
• Teach patient to use regular self-monitoring of blood glucose using blood glucose meter
• Teach patient the symptoms of hypo/hyperglycemia, what to do about each
• Teach patient that product must be continued on daily basis; explain consequence of discontinuing product abruptly
• Teach patient to notify prescriber if pregnancy is planned or suspected; to continue health regimen (diet, exercise)
• Advise patient to avoid OTC medications, alcohol, digoxin, exenatide, insulins, nateglinide, repaglinide, and other products that lower blood sugar, unless approved by prescriber
• Teach patient that diabetes is a lifelong illness; that this product is not a cure, only controls symptoms
• Teach patient that all food included in diet plan must be eaten to prevent hypo/hyperglycemia
• Teach patient to carry emergency ID
• Teach patient to notify prescriber immediately of hypersensitivity reactions (rash, swelling of face, trouble breathing)

Evaluation

Positive therapeutic outcome
• Decrease in polyuria, polydipsia, polyphagia; clear sensorium; absence of dizziness; stable gait, blood glucose, A1C improvement

---

sodium bicarbonate (Rx, OTC)
baking soda, Brosch-Neut, Citrocarbonate, Neut, Sellymin ✲
Func. class.: Alkalinizer; antacid
Chem. class.: NaHCO₃
Pregnancy category C

ACTION: Orally neutralizes gastric acid, which forms water, NaCl, CO_2; increases plasma bicarbonate, which buffers H^+ ion concentration; reverses acidosis **IV**

Therapeutic outcome: Correction of acidosis, gastric acid neutralization

USES: Acidosis (metabolic), cardiac arrest, alkalinization (systemic/urinary); antacid (PO); salicylate poisoning

CONTRAINDICATIONS
Respiratory/metabolic alkalosis, hypochloremia, hypocalcemia

Precautions: Pregnancy **C**, CHF, cirrhosis, toxemia, renal disease, hypertension, hypokalemia, breastfeeding, hypernatremia, Bartter's syndrome, Cushing's syndrome, hyperaldosteronism, children

DOSAGE AND ROUTES
Acidosis, metabolic (not associated with cardiac arrest)
Adult and child: IV INF 2-5 mEq/kg over 4-8 hr depending on CO_2, pH, ABGs

Cardiac arrest
Adult and child: IV BOL 1 mEq/kg of 7.5% or 8.4% SOL, then 0.5 mEq/kg q5-10min, then doses based on ABGs
Infant: IV 1 mEq/kg over several min (use only the 0.5 mEq/ml [4.2%] sol for inj)

Alkalinization of urine
Adult: PO 325 mg-2 g qid or 48 mEq/kg (4 g), then 12-24 mEq q4hr
Child: PO 84-840 mg/kg/day (1-10 mEq/kg), in divided doses q4-6hr

Antacid
Adult: PO 300 mg-2 g chewed, taken with water daily-qid

Available forms: Tabs 300, 325, 600, 650 mg; inj 4.2%, 5%, 7.5%, 8.4%

Implementation
PO route
• Antacid tab must be chewed and taken with 8 oz of water
• Dissolve effervescent tab in water
• May be used to neutralize gastric acid in peptic ulcer disease, given 1 and 3 hr after meals and at bedtime

Direct IV route
• Use in cardiac emergencies, use ampules or prefilled syringes only, give by rapid bolus dose, flush with 0.9% NaCl before and after use
Continuous IV infusion route
• Prepared sol or diluted in an equal amount of any dextrose/saline combination; administer 2-5 mEq/kg over 4-8 hr, max 50 mEq/hr; slower rate in children

Y-site compatibilities: Acyclovir, amifostine, asparaginase, aztreonam, bivalirudin, bumetanide, cefepime, cefmetazole, cefTRIAXone, chloramphenicol, cyclophosphamide, cytarabine, DAUNOrubicin, dexamethasone, DOXOrubicin, etoposide, famotidine, fentaNYL, filgrastim, fluconazole, fludarabine, furosemide,

S

Adverse effects: *italics* = common; **bold** = life-threatening

gallium nitrate, gemcitabine, gentamicin, granisetron, heparin, hydrocortisone sodium succinate, ifosfamide, indomethacin, insulin, ketorolac, labetalol, levofloxacin, lidocaine, linezolid, LORazepam, magnesium sulfate, melphalan, mesna, meperidine, methylPREDNISolone, metoclopramide, metoprolol, metroNIDAZOLE, milrinone, morphine, nafcillin, nitroglycerin, nitroprusside, PACLitaxel, palonosetron, pantoprazole, PEMEtrexed, penicillin G potassium, phenylephrine, phytonadione, piperacillin/tazobactam, potassium chloride, procainamide, propofol, propranolol, protamine, ranitidine, remifentanil, tacrolimus, teniposide, thiotepa, ticarcillin/clavulanate, tirofiban, tobramycin, tolazoline, vasopressin, vitamin B complex with C, voriconazole

Y-site incompatibilities: Allopurinol, amiodarone, amphotericin B, amphotericin B cholesteryl sulfate complex, ampicillin, anidulafungin, calcium chloride, calicum gluconate, caspofungin, cefotaxime, cefOXitin, cefuroxime, diazepam, diphenhydrAMINE, DOBUTamine, DOXOrubicin liposome, doxycycline, EPINEPHrine, fenoldopam, ganciclovir, haloperidol, hydrOXYzine, IDArubicin, imipenem/cilastatin, inamrinone, isoproterenol, lansoprazole, leucovorin, midazolam, nalbuphine, norepinephrine, ondansetron, phenytoin, prochlorperazine, promethazine, quinupristin/dalfopristin, sargramostim, trimethoprim/sulfamethoxazole, verapamil, vinCRIStine, vinorelbine

ADVERSE EFFECTS

CNS: Irritability, headache, confusion, stimulation, tremors, *twitching, hyperreflexia,* **tetany,** weakness, **seizures** caused by alkalosis
CV: Irregular pulse, **cardiac arrest,** water retention, edema, weight gain
GI: Flatulence, *belching, distention*
GU: Calculi
META: *Alkalosis*
MS: Muscular twitching, tetany, irritability

Pharmacokinetics

Absorption	Unknown
Distribution	Widely distributed—extracellular fluids
Metabolism	Unknown
Excretion	Kidneys
Half-life	Unknown

Pharmacodynamics

	PO	IV
Onset	2 min	Rapid
Peak	½ hr	Rapid
Duration	1-3 hr	Unknown

INTERACTIONS
Individual drugs
ChlorproPAMIDE, lithium: decreased effect of each specific product
Flecainide, mecamylamine, pseudoephedrine, quiNIDine, quiNINE: increased effects of each specific product

Drug classifications
Amphetamines, anorexiants, sympathomimetics: increased effects of each specific product
Barbiturates: decreased effects of barbiturates
Benzodiazepines: decreased effects of each specific product
Corticosteroids: increased sodium; decreased potassium, decreased effects of corticosteroids
Ketoconazoles: decreased effects of ketoconazoles
Salicylates: decreased effect of salicylates

Drug/herb
Oak bark: decreased action of sodium bicarbonate

Drug/lab test
Increased: sodium, lactate
Decreased: potassium

NURSING CONSIDERATIONS
Assessment
• Assess respiratory and pulse rate, rhythm, depth, lung sounds; notify prescriber of abnormalities
• Assess for CO_2 in GI tract; may lead to perforation if ulcer is severe
• **Fluid balance** (I&O ratio, weight daily, edema); notify prescriber of fluid overload, assess for edema, crackles, SOB
• Monitor electrolytes, blood pH, PO_2, HCO_3 during beginning treatment; ABGs frequently during emergencies
• Monitor extravasation with **IV** administration (tissue sloughing, ulceration, and necrosis)
• **Alkalosis:** irritability, confusion, twitching, hyperreflexia, stimulation, slow respirations, cyanosis, irregular pulse
• **Milk-alkali syndrome: confusion, headache, nausea, vomiting, anorexia, urinary stones, hypercalcemia**

Patient/family education
• Instruct patient to chew antacid tab and drink 8 oz of water; not to take antacid with milk because milk-alkali syndrome may result; not to use antacid for more than 2 wk
• **Advise patient to notify prescriber if indigestion is accompanied by chest pain; trouble breathing; diarrhea; dark, tarry stools; vomit that looks like coffee grounds; swelling of feet/ankles**

- Teach patient about sodium-restricted diet; to avoid use of baking soda for indigestion

Evaluation

Positive therapeutic outcome
- ABGs, electrolytes, blood pH, HCO_3 normal levels
- Decreased gastric pain

---

sodium biphosphate/ sodium phosphate (OTC)
Fleet Enema, Phospho-soda
Func. class.: Laxative, saline
Pregnancy category C

ACTION: Increases water absorption in the small intestine by osmotic action; laxative effect occurs by increased peristalsis and water retention

Therapeutic outcome: Absence of constipation

USES: Constipation, bowel or rectal preparation for surgery, examination

CONTRAINDICATIONS
Hypersensitivity, rectal fissures, abdominal pain, nausea/vomiting, appendicitis, acute surgical abdomen, ulcerated hemorrhoids, Na-restricted diets, renal failure, hyperphosphatemia, hypocalcemia, hypokalemia, hypernatremia, Addison's disease, CHF, ascites, bowel perforation, megacolon, imperforate anus

> **BLACK BOX WARNING:** GI obstruction, renal failure

Precautions: Pregnancy **C**

> **BLACK BOX WARNING:** Colitis, elderly, hypovolemia, renal disease

DOSAGE AND ROUTES
Adult: PO 20-30 ml (Phospho-soda)
Child: PO 5-15 ml (Phospho-soda)
Adult and child >12 yr: RECT enema (118 ml)
Child 2-12 yr: RECT ½ enema (59 ml)

Available forms: Enema 7 g/phosphate and 19 g/biphosphate/118 ml; oral sol 18 g phosphate/48 g biphosphate/100 ml

Implementation
PO route
- Give on empty stomach
- Mix oral sol in cold water
- Take alone for better absorption; do not take within 1 hr of other products

ADVERSE EFFECTS
CV: **Dysrhythmias, cardiac arrest,** hypotension, widening QRS complex
GI: *Nausea, cramps,* diarrhea
META: Electrolyte, fluid imbalances

Pharmacokinetics
Absorption	Up to 20% (rec)
Distribution	Unknown
Metabolism	Unknown
Excretion	Kidneys
Half-life	Unknown

Pharmacodynamics
	PO	Rect
Onset	½-3 hr	5 min
Peak	Unknown	Unknown
Duration	Unknown	Unknown

NURSING CONSIDERATIONS
Assessment
- Assess stools: color, amount, consistency
- Assess for bowel pattern, bowel sounds (frequency, intensity), flatulence, distention, increased temp, dietary patterns (fluid, bulk), exercise
- Assess for cramping, rectal bleeding, nausea, vomiting; if these symptoms occur, product should be discontinued

Patient/family education
- Advise patient not to use laxatives or enema for long-term therapy; bowel tone will be lost
- Teach patient that normal bowel movements do not always occur daily
- Caution patient not to use in presence of abdominal pain, nausea, vomiting
- Caution patient to notify prescriber if constipation is unrelieved or if symptoms of electrolyte imbalance occur: muscle cramps, pain, weakness, dizziness, excessive thirst
- Instruct patient to maintain adequate fluid consumption to help prevent constipation

Evaluation
Positive therapeutic outcome
- Decrease in constipation

S

Adverse effects: *italics* = common; **bold** = life-threatening

sodium polystyrene sulfonate (Rx)

(po-lee-stye′reen)

**Kalexate, Kayexalate, K-Exit ✖,
Kionex, SPS**

Func. class.: Potassium-removing resin
Chem. class.: Cation exchange resin

Pregnancy category C

ACTION: Removes potassium by exchanging sodium for potassium in body; occurs primarily in large intestine

Therapeutic outcome: Potassium levels within accepted range

USES: Hyperkalemia in conjunction with other measures

CONTRAINDICATIONS

Hypersensitivity to saccharin or parabens that may be in some products; GI obstruction, neonate (reduced gut motility)

Precautions: Pregnancy **C**, geriatric, renal failure, CHF, severe edema, severe hypertension, sodium restriction, constipation, GI bleeding, hypocalcemia

DOSAGE AND ROUTES

Adult: PO 15 g daily-qid; RECT enema 30-50 q1-2hr initially prn, then q6hr prn

Child (unlabeled): PO 1 g/kg q6hr prn; RECT 1 g/kg q2-6hr prn

Available forms: Powder for susp 453.6 g, 454 g; oral susp 15 g/60 ml

Implementation

PO route

• Powdered resin: Usually given orally as a suspension in water or in a syrup. Usually, the amount of fluid ranges 20-100 ml, depending on the dose, or 3-4 ml per g of resin. Suspensions should be freshly prepared and not stored for longer than 24 hr. The suspension may also be introduced into the stomach via a tube or the powdered resin may be mixed with the patient's food; the powder should not be mixed with foods or liquids that contain a large amount of potassium (bananas or orange juice)

Rectal route

• Precede retention enema with a cleansing enema; instruct patient to lie down on left side with lower leg extended and the upper leg flexed for support or place the patient in the knee-chest position. Gently insert a soft, large (French 28) rubber tube into the rectum for a distance of about 20 cm; the tip should be well into the

sigmoid colon. Tape the tube in place. Suspend the sodium polystyrene sulfonate powdered resin in 100 ml of an aqueous vehicle (water or sorbitol) which has been warmed to body temperature and introduce through the tube by gravity. The particles should be kept suspended by stirring the suspension during administration. Alternatively, 120-180 ml of a commercially available suspension may be administered as a retention enema after the suspension has been warmed to body temperature. Following administration, flush the tube with 50-100 ml of fluid and clamp the tube and leave in place. The suspension should be retained in the colon for at least 30-60 min or for several hours, if possible

• After several hours have passed, administer a cleansing enema using a nonsodium containing solution at body temperature. Up to 2 quarts of fluid may be necessary. Drain fluid through a Y-tube connection. Observe the drainage if sorbitol was used

ADVERSE EFFECTS

GI: *Constipation,* anorexia, nausea, vomiting, diarrhea (sorbitol), *fecal impaction,* gastric irritation

META: Hypocalcemia, hypokalemia, hypomagnesemia, sodium retention

Pharmacokinetics

Absorption	None
Distribution	None
Metabolism	None
Excretion	Feces
Half-life	Unknown

Pharmacodynamics

	PO	Rect
Onset	2-12 hr	2-12 hr
Peak	Unknown	Unknown
Duration	6-24 hr	4-6 hr

INTERACTIONS

Individual drugs

Sorbitol: increased colonic necrosis, do not use concurrently

Lithium: decreased effect of lithium

Drug classifications

Diuretics (loop), cardiac glycosides: increased hypokalemia

Magnesium/calcium antacids: increased metabolic acidosis

Thyroid hormones: decreased effect of thyroid hormones

NURSING CONSIDERATIONS
Assessment
• Assess bowel function daily: amount of stool, color, characteristics
• Assess for hypotension: confusion, irritability, muscular pain, weakness
• Hyperkalemia: assess for confusion, dyspnea, weakness, dysrhythmias
• Monitor electrolytes: potassium, sodium, calcium, magnesium; I&O ratio, weight daily
• **Monitor ECG for spiked T-waves, depressed ST segments, prolonged QT interval, and widening QRS complex**
• Monitor I&O ratio, weight daily; crackles, dyspnea, jugular vein distention, edema
• **Monitor for digoxin toxicity (nausea, vomiting, blurred vision, anorexia, dysrhythmia) in those receiving digoxin**

Patient/family education
• Explain reason for medication and expected results
• Teach patient to avoid laxatives, antacids, electrolyte-based products unless approved by prescriber
• Teach patient to use a low-potassium diet, provide sample diet

Evaluation
Positive therapeutic outcome
• Potassium level 3.5-5 mg/dl

sofosbuvir
(soe-fos'bue-vir)
Sovaldi
Func. class.: Antiviral, antihepatitis agent
Chem. class.: Adenosine monophosphate analog
Pregnancy category B

ACTION: Inhibits hepatitis C virus RNA polymerase by incorporating the polymerase into the viral RNA, also acts as a chain terminator

Therapeutic outcome: Decreased symptoms of chronic hepatitis C

USES: Chronic hepatitis C (genotypes 1, 2, 3, 4) with compensated liver disease

CONTRAINDICATIONS
Hypersensitivity, pregnancy (**X**) in combination; male-mediated teratogenicity

Precautions: Pregnancy (**B**), breastfeeding, children, hepatic/renal disease

DOSAGE AND ROUTES
Genotype 1, 4
Adult: PO 400 mg/day with peginterferon alfa and ribavirin × 12 wk; may consider use for genotype 1 with ribavirin × 24 wk

Genotype 2
Adult: PO 400 mg/day with ribavirin × 12 wk

Genotype 3
Adult: PO 400 mg/day with ribavirin or daclatasvir × 24 wk

Available forms: Tabs 400 mg

Implementation
• Give by mouth without regard to food
• Do not use as monotherapy

ADVERSE EFFECTS
CNS: Headache, chills, weakness, fatigue, fever, insomnia
GI: Diarrhea, hyperbilirubinemia
MISC: Rash, pruritus, neutropenia, anemia, myalgia

Pharmacokinetics
Absorption	Unknown
Distribution	61%-65% protein
Metabolism	Unknown
Excretion	By kidneys 80%
Half-life	0.4-27 hr

Pharmacodynamics
Onset	Unknown
Peak	½-2 hr
Duration	Unknown

INTERACTIONS
Individual drugs
OXcarbazepine, rifabutin, rifapentine, tipranavir: decreased sofosbuvir effect, avoid concurrent use

Drug classifications
P-glycoprotein (P-gp) inducers (carBAMazepine, PHENobarbital, phenytoin, rifampin): decreased sofosbuvir effect, avoid concurrent use

NURSING CONSIDERATIONS
Assessment
• Severe renal disease/eGFR <30 ml/min/1.73 m^2: monitor BUN, creatinine
• Monitor geriatric patients more carefully; may develop renal, cardiac symptoms more rapidly
⚠ **Pregnancy: if planned or suspected; if pregnant call the Pregnancy Registry 800-258-4263, obtain pregnancy test before starting treatment**

Adverse effects: *italics* = common; **bold** = life-threatening

Patient/family education
• Teach patient that optimal duration of treatment is unknown, that product is not a cure, that transmission may still occur
• Instruct patient to avoid use with other medications unless approved by prescriber
• Instruct patient not to stop abruptly unless directed, worsening of hepatitis may occur
🅰 Teach patient to notify prescriber if pregnancy is planned or suspected, use 2 forms of reliable contraception, avoid breastfeeding

Evaluation

Positive therapeutic outcome
• Therapeutic response: decreased symptoms of chronic hepatitis C

---

solifenacin (Rx)
(sol-i-fen'a-sin)
VESIcare
Func. class.: Urinary antispasmodic, anticholinergic
Chem. class.: Antimuscarinic receptor antagonist
Pregnancy category C

Do not confuse: Vesicare/Vesanoid

ACTION: Relaxes smooth muscles in urinary tract by inhibiting acetylcholine at postganglionic sites

Therapeutic outcome: Decreased dysuria, frequency, nocturia, incontinence

USES: Overactive bladder (urinary frequency, urgency, incontinence)

CONTRAINDICATIONS
Hypersensitivity, uncontrolled closed-angle glaucoma, urinary retention, gastric retention

Precautions: Pregnancy **C**, breastfeeding, children, geriatric patients, renal/hepatic disease, controlled closed-angle glaucoma, bladder outflow obstruction, GI obstruction, decreased GI motility, history of QT prolongation

DOSAGE AND ROUTES
Adult: PO 5 mg/day, max 10 mg/day

Renal/hepatic dose
Adult: PO CCr <30 ml/min 5 mg/day; Child-Pugh B max 5 mg/day

Available forms: Tabs 5, 10 mg

Implementation
PO route
• Without regard to meals
• Swallow product whole with water, liquid

ADVERSE EFFECTS
CNS: Anxiety, paresthesia, fatigue, *dizziness,* headache, confusion, delirium, depression, drowsiness, fatigue
CV: Chest pain, hypertension, QTc prolongation, peripheral edema, palpitations, sinus tachycardia
EENT: *Vision abnormalities, xerophthalmia,* nasal dryness
GI: *Nausea, vomiting, anorexia,* abdominal pain, *constipation,* dry mouth, dyspepsia
GU: Dysuria, urinary retention, frequency, UTI
INTEG: Rash, pruritus, angioedema, exfoliative dermatitis, erythema multiforme
MISC: Hyperthermia
RESP: Bronchitis, cough, pharyngitis, URI

Pharmacokinetics
Absorption	Rapid (90%)
Distribution	98% protein bound
Metabolism	Extensively metabolized by CYP3A4
Excretion	Excreted in urine (69%)/feces (22%)
Half-life	Terminal half-life 45-68 hr

Pharmacodynamics
Unknown

INTERACTIONS
Drug classifications
Azoles, macrolides, fluoroquinolones, class IA, III antidysrhythmics: increased QT prolongation
Benzodiazepines, hypnotics, opioids, sedatives: increased CNS depression
CYP3A4 inducers (carBAMazepine, nevirapine, phenobarbitol, phenytoin): decreased effects of solifenacin
CYP3A4 inhibitors (clarithromycin, diclofenac, doxycycline, erythromycin, isoniazid, ketoconazole, nefazodone, propofol, protease inhibitors, verapamil): increased action of solifenacin, max dose 5 mg

Drug/herb
St. John's wort: decreased effects

Drug/food
Grapefruit juice: increased effect

Drug/lab test
Increased: LFTs

NURSING CONSIDERATIONS
Assessment
• **Urinary patterns:** assess for distention, nocturia, frequency, urgency, incontinence
• **Allergic reactions:** assess for rash; if this occurs, product should be discontinued

---

- **Cardiac patients: monitor ECG for QT prolongation, avoid products that can increase QT prolongation**
- **Angioedema: assess for swelling of face, lips, tongue, larynx**

Patient/family education

- Caution patient to avoid hazardous activities; dizziness may occur
- Advise patient that constipation, blurred vision may occur, to notify prescriber if abdominal pain with constipation occurs
- Instruct patient to call prescriber if severe abdominal pain or constipation lasts for 3 or more days
- Advise patient that heat prostration may occur if used in a hot environment, sweating is decreased
- Teach patient to take without regard to food
- Teach patient to swallow tab whole, do not crush, chew

Evaluation

Positive therapeutic outcome

- Urinary status: decreased dysuria, frequency, nocturia, incontinence

---

somatropin (Rx)

(soe-ma-troe′pin)
Genotropin, Humatrope, Norditropin, Norditropin Flexpro, Nutropin, Nutropin AQ, Omnitrope, Saizen, Serostim, Tev-Tropin, Zorbtive
Func. class.: Pituitary hormone
Chem. class.: Growth hormone
Pregnancy category C

Do not confuse: somatropin/somatrem/ SUMAtriptan

ACTION: Stimulates growth; similar to natural growth hormone—both preparations are developed by recombinant DNA technique

Therapeutic outcome: Increase in height as a result of skeletal growth in pituitary growth hormone deficiency

USES: Pituitary growth hormone deficiency (hypopituitary dwarfism), children with human growth hormone deficiency, AIDS wasting syndrome, cachexia, adults with somatropin deficiency syndrome (SDS), short stature in Noonan syndrome, SHOX deficiencies; Turner's syndrome, Prader-Willi syndrome

CONTRAINDICATIONS

Hypersensitivity to benzyl alcohol, creosol, glycerin hypersensitivity (for medications that contain these products), closed epiphyses, acute respiratory failure, Prader-Willi syndrome with obesity, trauma

Precautions: Pregnancy **C**, breastfeeding, newborns, geriatric, diabetes mellitus, hypothyroidism, intracranial lesions, prolonged treatment in adults, scoliosis, sleep apnea, chemotherapy, respiratory disease

DOSAGE AND ROUTES

>> Genotropin

Child: SUBCUT 0.16-0.24 mg/kg/wk, divided into 6 or 7 daily inj, give in abdomen, thigh, buttocks
Adult: SUBCUT 0.4-0.8 mg/kg/wk divided in 6-7 daily doses

>> Humatrope

Child: SUBCUT/IM 0.006 mg/kg divided into equal doses either on 3 alternate days or 6 ×/wk, max 0.3 mg/kg/wk
Adult: IM 0.018 units/kg/day, max 0.0125 units/kg/day

Growth hormone deficiency

>> Nutropin/Nutropin AQ

Child: SUBCUT 0.3 mg/kg/wk

>> Serostim

Adult: SUBCUT at bedtime >55 kg 6 mg, 45-55 kg 5 mg, 35-45 kg 4 mg

>> Norditropin

Child: SUBCUT 0.024-0.034 mg/kg 6-7 ×/wk

Replacement of GH in GH deficiency

Adult: SUBCUT (Saizen) 0.005 mg/kg/day; may increase after 4 wk to max 0.01 mg/kg/day

Available forms: Powder for inj (lyophilized) 1.5 mg (4 international units/ml), 4 mg (12 international units/vial), 5 mg (13 international units/vial), 5 mg (15 international units/vial), rDNA origin, 5.8 mg (15 international units/ml), 6 mg (18 international units/ml), 8 mg (24 international units/vial), 10 mg (26 international units/vial), inj 10 mg (30 international units/vial); 5, 10, 15 mg/1.5 ml

Implementation

- Store in refrigerator for <1 mo; if reconstituted, <1 wk; do not use discolored or cloudy sol
- Give IM or subcut, do not use IV
- Discontinue therapy if final height is achieved or epiphyseal fusion occurs

S

Adverse effects: *italics* = common; **bold** = life-threatening

- Visually inspect parenteral products for particulate matter and discoloration

>> Genotropin

- Powder, filled in a two-chamber cartridge with the active substance in the front chamber and the diluent in the rear chamber. Available in a 5 mg cartridge (green tip) and a 12 mg cartridge (purple tip). The 5 and 12 mg cartridges can be used with the Genotropin Pen or the Genotropin Mixer. Also, in various doses ranging from 0.2 mg to 2 mg, in single use, auto-mix devices called Genotropin Miniquicks
- *Cartridges:* Store cartridges refrigerated prior to reconstitution, do not freeze; protect from light. A reconstitution device is supplied and is used to mix the powder and the diluent. After the powder and diluent are mixed, gently tip the cartridge upside down a few times until dissolved. DO NOT SHAKE. If the solution is cloudy, do not use. Following reconstitution, the 5 mg cartridge will contain a 5 mg/ml and the 12 mg cartridge will contain a 12 mg/ml solution; both the 5 mg and 12 mg cartridges contain overfill. The cartridges contain diluent with preservative (m-cresol) and may be stored refrigerated ≤28 days after reconstitution. Do not use the 5 mg and 12 mg cartridges in patients with m-cresol hypersensitivity
- *Genotropin Miniquicks:* After dispensing, but prior to reconstitution, store at or 77 degrees ≤3 mo. A reconstitution device is supplied and is used to mix the powder and diluent. Ten different strengths are available that each deliver a fixed volume of 0.25 ml. This product contains a diluent with no preservative, refrigerate after reconstitution and use within 24 hr. Use the reconstituted solution only once and discard any remaining

>> Humatrope

- Prior to reconstitution, store refrigerated
- *Vials:* Reconstitute each 5-mg vial with 1.5-5 ml of the diluent (contains m-cresol as a preservative) or Bacteriostatic Water for Injection (contains benzoyl alcohol as a preservative); sterile water for injection can be used with a hypersensitivity to both m-cresol and benzoyl alcohol. Direct the liquid against the glass vial wall. Swirl until contents are dissolved. Do not shake. If the solution is cloudy, do not use. Small, colorless particles may be present after refrigeration; this is not unusual for solutions containing proteins. Vials reconstituted with the diluent or bacteriostatic water are stable for 14 days when refrigerated; for vials reconstituted with sterile water, use the vial only once and

discard; if not used immediately, refrigerate and use within 24 hr; avoid freezing
- *Cartridges:* Reconstitute cartridges using ONLY the supplied diluent syringe; the cartridges are designed for use only with the Humatrope injection device. Once reconstituted, the cartridges are stable for up to 28 days when stored refrigerated. Store the injection device without the needle attached; avoid freezing reconstituted solutions

>> Norditropin

- Do not use reconstituted solution if cloudy or contains particulate matter
- Prior to use, store refrigerated
- Reconstitution of the cartridges is not required. The cartridge is intended for use only with the NordiPen injector; a prefilled, disposable pen, NordiFlex Pen injector, is also available. Each cartridge size (5 mg, 10 mg, or 15 mg per 1.5 ml cartridge) has a color-coded corresponding pen, which is graduated to deliver an appropriate dose based on the solution concentration; NordiPen and NordiFlex Pen allow for administration of a minimum 0.25-mg dose to a maximum 4.5-mg dose, depending on cartridge concentrations. Follow directions provided in Pen injector instruction booklet
- After a cartridge has been inserted into the NordiPen injector or once a NordiFlex pen is in use, the pen should be stored refrigerated and used within 4 wk. Alternatively, the 5-mg and 10-mg cartridges may be stored in the pen at room temperatures, no higher than 77° F, for up to 3 wk. NovoFine needles are recommended for administration. Wipe the stopper of the pen cartridge with rubbing alcohol

>> Nutropin

- Prior to reconstitution, store refrigerated
- Reconstitute each 5-mg vial with 1-5 ml bacteriostatic water for injection (benzyl alcohol preserved) and each 10-mg vial with 1-10 ml of bacteriostatic water for injection (benzyl alcohol preserved). If using for newborns, reconstitute with sterile water for injection. Direct the liquid against the glass vial wall. Swirl vial with a gentle rotary motion until contents are dissolved completely. Do not shake. If the solution is cloudy after reconstitution or refrigeration, do not use. Small, colorless particles may be present after refrigeration; this is not unusual for solutions containing proteins
- Solutions reconstituted with bacteriostatic water for injection are stable for 14 days refrigerated

---

- Solutions reconstituted with sterile water for injection should be used immediately and only once; discard any unused portions. Avoid freezing reconstituted solutions

Nutropin AQ

- Does not require reconstitution. Solution should be clear. Small, colorless particles may be present after refrigeration; this is not unusual for solutions containing proteins. Allow vial or pen cartridge to come to room temperature and gently swirl. If solution is cloudy, do not use
- *Vials:* Before needle insertion, wipe the vial septum with rubbing alcohol or antiseptic solution to prevent contamination by microorganisms that may be introduced by repeated needle insertions. Administer using sterile, disposable syringes and needles. Use syringes with small enough volume that the prescribed dose can be drawn from the vial with reasonable accuracy
- *Pen cartridge:* Two strengths are available: 10 mg and 20 mg; intended for use only with Nutropin AQ Pen. Each pen and cartridge are color coded to ensure accurate placement of the 10-mg or 20-mg cartridge into the appropriate pen. Do not use the 20-mg cartridge in the pen intended for the 10-mg cartridge, and vice versa. Wipe septum of pen cartridge with rubbing alcohol or antiseptic solution to prevent contamination by microorganisms that may be introduced by repeated needle insertions. Administer using sterile, disposable needles. Follow the directions provided in the Nutropin AQ Pen Instructions for Use. The Nutropin AQ 10 pen allows for administration of a minimum 0.1-mg dose to a maximum 4-mg dose, in 0.1-mg increments. The Nutropin AQ 20 pen allows for administration of a minimum 0.2-mg dose to a maximum 8-mg dose, in 0.2-mg increments
- *Prefilled device:* A prefilled multi-dose, dial-a-dose device is available in 3 strengths. Administer using disposable needles. Follow the directions provided in the Nutropin AQ NuSpin Instructions for Use. The Nutropin AQ Nuspin 5 allows for administration of a minimum dose of 0.05 mg to a maximum dose of 1.75 mg, in increments of 0.05 mg. The Nutropin AQ Nuspin 10 allows for administration of a minimum dose of 0.1 mg to a maximum dose of 3.5 mg, in increments of 0.1 mg. The Nutropin AQ Nuspin 20 allows for administration of a minimum dose of 0.2 mg to a maximum dose of 7 mg, in increments of 0.2 mg
- After initial use, vials, cartridges, and prefilled devices are stable for 28 days refrigerated; avoid freezing. Vials, cartridges, and prefilled devices are light sensitive; protect from light

Omnitrope

- Prior to reconstitution, store vials refrigerated. Store in the carton; Omnitrope is sensitive to light
- *Vials:* Reconstitute the vial with diluent provided using a sterile, disposable syringe. Swirl the vial gently, but do not shake. If the solution is cloudy after reconstitution, the contents must not be injected. After reconstitution, the 1.5-mg vial may be refrigerated ≤24 hr. The 1.5-mg vial does not contain a preservative and should only be used once; discard any remaining solution. The 5.8-mg vial diluent contains benzoyl alcohol as a preservative. After reconstitution, the contents must be used within 3 wk. After the first injection, store the 5.8-mg vial in the carton, to protect from light, in the refrigerator; avoid freezing
- *Omnitrope Pen 5 cartridge:* Each 5-mg cartridge must be inserted into the Omnitrope Pen 5 delivery system. Follow the directions provided in the Omnitrope Instructions for Use. The cartridge contains benzyl alcohol as a preservative. Once initially used, store refrigerated ≤28 days, protect from light, avoid freezing
- *Omnitrope Pen 10 cartridge:* Each 10-mg cartridge must be inserted into the Omnitrope Pen 10 delivery system. Follow the directions provided in the Omnitrope Instructions for Use. Once initially used, store refrigerated ≤28 days, protect from light, avoid freezing

Saizen

- Prior to reconstitution, store at room temperature
- *Vials:* Reconstitute each 5 mg vial with 1-3 ml bacteriostatic water for injection; reconstitute each 8.8-mg vial with 2-3 ml bacteriostatic water for injection (benzyl alcohol preserved). In patients with hypersensitivity to benzyl alcohol, the vials can be mixed with sterile water for injection. Direct the liquid against the glass vial wall. Swirl vial with a gentle rotary motion until contents are dissolved completely. Do not shake. The solution should be clear; if it is cloudy immediately after reconstitution or refrigeration, do not use. Small, colorless particles may be present after refrigeration; this is not unusual for solutions containing proteins. After reconstitution, store vials mixed with bacteriostatic water for injection refrigerated and use within 14 days. For vials mixed with sterile water for injection, the solution should be used immediately, and any unused portion should be discarded. Avoid freezing
- *Cartridges:* Available in 4-mg and 8.8-mg click.easy cartridges for use in a compatible injection device. A reconstitution device

supplied by the manufacturer is used to mix the Saizen with accompanying diluent containing metacresol. Cartridges reconstituted with the diluent containing metacresol are stable under refrigeration for up to 21 days. Avoid freezing

Serostim
• Prior to reconstitution, store vials and diluent at room temperature (15-30° C / 59-86° F).
• *Vials:* Reconstitute the 5-mg or 6-mg vials with 0.5-1 ml of supplied diluent (sterile water for injection). Reconstitute the 4-mg vial with 0.5-1 ml of bacteriostatic water for injection (benzyl alcohol preserved) and the 8.8-mg vial with 1-2 ml of bacteriostatic water for injection (benzyl alcohol preserved). Direct the liquid against the glass vial wall. Swirl vial with a gentle rotary motion until contents are dissolved completely. Do not shake. The solution should be clear; if it is cloudy immediately after reconstitution or refrigeration, do not use. Small, colorless particles may be present after refrigeration; this is not unusual for solutions containing proteins. If reconstituted with sterile water for injection, use within 24 hr. If reconstituted with bacteriostatic water for injection (benzyl alcohol preserved), the solution is stable for up to 14 days under refrigeration (2-8° C or 36-46° F). Avoid freezing
• *Cartridges:* Available in 8.8-mg click.easy cartridges for use in a compatible injection device. A reconstitution device is supplied by the manufacturer and is used to mix the Serostim with accompanying diluent containing metacresol. After reconstitution, cartridges are stable under refrigeration for up to 21 days. Avoid freezing

Serostim LQ
• Prior to use, store refrigerated
• Available in 6-mg single-use cartridges that do not require reconstitution. Administer using sterile, disposable syringes and needles
• Bring to room temperature prior to use. Discard single-use cartridge after use, even if some drug remains. Discard cartridges after the expiration date stated on the product. Do not freeze. Protect from light

Tev-Tropin
• Prior to reconstitution, store refrigerated
• Reconstitute each 5-mg vial with 1-5 ml bacteriostatic 0.9% sodium chloride (benzyl alcohol preserved) for injection. Direct the liquid against the glass vial wall. Swirl vial with a gentle rotary motion until contents are dissolved completely. Do not shake. The solution should be clear; if it is cloudy immediately after reconstitution, do not inject. Small, colorless particles may be present after refrigeration; this is not unusual for solutions containing proteins.

When administering to newborns, reconstitute with sterile normal saline for injection that is unpreserved
• Solution reconstituted with bacteriostatic 0.9% sodium chloride is stable for 14 days when stored refrigerated. Solution reconstituted with sterile normal saline should be used only once, with any remaining solution discarded. Avoid freezing

Valtropin
• Prior to dispensing, store vials and diluent refrigerated. After dispensing to patients, may be stored at or below 77° F for up to 3 months
• Reconstitute each 5-mg vial with the entire contents of the accompanying diluent, which contains metacresol as a preservative. If patients are allergic to metacresol, sterile water for injection can be used. Direct the liquid against the glass vial wall. Swirl vial with a gentle rotary motion until contents are dissolved completely. Do not shake. The solution should be clear; if it is cloudy or contains particulate matter immediately after reconstitution or after refrigeration, do not inject. The final concentration of the reconstituted solution is 3.33 mg/ml
• After reconstituted with the provided diluent, solutions can be stored refrigerated for up to 14 days. After reconstituted with sterile water for injection, use only one dose of Valtropin per vial and discard the unused portion if not used immediately

Zorbtive
• Unreconstituted vials of drug and diluent may be stored at room temperature until expiration date
• Reconstitute each vial of 4 mg, 5 mg, or 6 mg with 0.5-1 ml sterile water for injection, USP. Reconstitute each 8.8 mg with 1-2 ml bacteriostatic water for injection (0.9% benzyl alcohol preserved); in newborns or patients with a benzyl alcohol hypersensitivity, sterile water for injection can be used. Review manufacturer's labeling for expected concentrations. Direct the liquid against the glass vial wall. Swirl vial with a gentle rotary motion until contents are dissolved completely. Do not shake. The solution should be clear; if it is cloudy after reconstitution or refrigeration, do not use. Small, colorless particles may be present after refrigeration; this is not unusual for solutions containing proteins
• After reconstitution with sterile water for injection, use the solution immediately and discard any unused portion. When using bacteriostatic water for injection, reconstituted solutions are stable for up to 14 days refrigerated. Avoid freezing vials of drug or diluent, or reconstituted vials

IM route
- Inject deeply into a large muscle; aspirate prior to injection; rotate injection sites daily

Subcut route
- Volumes >1 ml of reconstituted solution is not recommended; do not inject intradermally
- Allow refrigerated solutions to come to room temperature prior to injection
- Subcutaneous injections may be given in the thigh, buttocks, or abdomen; rotate injection sites daily

ADVERSE EFFECTS

CNS: Headache, growth of intracranial tumor, fever, aggressive behavior
ENDO: *Hyperglycemia, ketosis, hypothyroidism*
GI: Nausea, vomiting
GU: *Hypercalciuria*
INTEG: Rash, urticaria, pain, inflammation at inj site; hematoma
MS: Tissue swelling, joint and muscle pain
SYST: Antibodies to growth hormone

Pharmacokinetics

Absorption	Well absorbed (SUBCUT/IM)
Distribution	Unknown
Metabolism	Unknown
Excretion	Unknown
Half-life	15-60 min

Pharmacodynamics

	IM/SUBCUT (growth)
Onset	Unknown
Peak	Unknown
Duration	7 days

INTERACTIONS
Drug classifications
Androgens, thyroid hormones: increased epiphyseal closure
Glucocorticosteroids: decreased growth
Insulins, antidiabetics: decreased antidiabetic effect, adjust dosage

Drug/lab test
Increased: glucose, urine glucose
Decreased: glucose thyroid hormones

NURSING CONSIDERATIONS
Assessment
- Assess for signs/symptoms of diabetes
- Identify growth hormone antibodies if patient fails to respond to therapy
- Monitor thyroid function tests: T_3, T_4, T_7, TSH to identify hypothyroidism, thyroid hormone replacement may be needed

- Assess for allergic reaction: rash, itching, fever, nausea, wheezing
- Assess for hypercalciuria: urinary stones; groin, flank pain; nausea, vomiting, frequency, hematuria, chills
- Monitor growth rate, bone age of child at intervals during treatment
- **Respiratory infection:** in those with Prader-Willi syndrome, may have sleep apnea, upper airway obstruction; discontinue if obstruction occurs
- Rapid growth: assess for slipped capital femoral epiphysis; may also occur in endocrine disorders
- Monitor ophthalmologic status baseline and periodically, intracranial hypertension may occur
- Identify creosol or benzyl alcohol hypersensitivity before use

Patient/family education
- Explain reason for medication and expected results; that treatment may continue for yr
- Advise patient that routine follow-up is needed to monitor growth rate
- Instruct parents on procedure for medication preparation and inj use; request demonstration, return demonstration; provide written instructions
- Teach patient to maintain growth record, report knee, hip pain or limping
- Advise patient treatment is very expensive

Evaluation

Positive therapeutic outcome
- Growth in children until epiphyseal plates close

S

sotalol (Rx)
(soe-ta'lole)
Betapace, Betapace AF, Rylosol ✦, Sorine
Func. class.: Antidysrhythmic, group III
Chem. class.: Nonselective β-blocker
Pregnancy category B

ACTION: Blockade of β_1- and β_2-receptors leads to antidysrhythmic effect, prolongs action potential in myocardial fibers without affecting conduction, prolongs QT interval, no effect on QRS duration

Therapeutic outcome: Decreased B/P, heart rate, AV conduction

USES: Life-threatening ventricular dysrhythmias; Betapace AF: to maintain sinus rhythm in symptomatic atrial fibrillation/flutter

CONTRAINDICATIONS

Hypersensitivity to β-blockers, cardiogenic shock, heart block (2nd or 3rd degree), sinus bradycardia, CHF, bronchial asthma, CCr <40 ml/min

> **BLACK BOX WARNING:** Congenital or acquired long QT syndrome, hypokalemia

Precautions: Pregnancy **B**, breastfeeding, major surgery, diabetes mellitus, renal/thyroid disease, COPD, well-compensated heart failure, CAD, nonallergic bronchospasm, electrolyte disturbances, bradycardia, peripheral vascular disease

> **BLACK BOX WARNING:** Cardiac dysrhythmias, torsades de pointes, ventricular dysrhythmias, ventricular fibrillation

DOSAGE AND ROUTES

Adult: PO initial 80 mg bid, may increase to total of 240-320 mg/day, each dosage increase is made after ≥3 days and QTc interval <550 msecs

Child >2 yr with normal renal function (un-labeled): PO 30 mg/m² tid, adjust dosage gradually after ≥36 hr to max 60 mg/m² tid

Renal dose
Adult: PO CCr 30-60 ml/min q24hr; CCr 10-29 ml/min q36-48hr; CCr <10 ml/min individualize dose

Life-threatening ventricular dysrhythmias
Adult: with CCr 40-60 ml/min **IV** 75 mg over 5 hr/day, monitor QTc at end of each infusion during initiation and titration; 80 mg PO = 75 mg **IV**; 120 mg PO = 112.5 mg **IV**; 160 mg PO = 150 mg **IV**

Betapace AF
Adult: PO initial 80 mg bid, titrate upward to 120 mg bid during initial hospitalization, monitor OTC interval for 2-4 hr after each dose

Renal dose (Betapace AF)
Adult: CCr >60 ml/min q12hr; CCr 40-60 ml/min q24hr; CCr <40 ml/min do not use

Available forms: Tabs 80, 120, 160, 240 mg; (Betapace AF) 80, 120, 160 mg; inj 150 mg/10 ml (15 mg/ml)

Implementation
PO route
• Given before meals, at bedtime, tab may be crushed or swallowed whole; give with food to prevent GI upset; reduce dosage in renal dysfunction

• **Betapace and Betapace AF are not interchangeable**
• Store in dry area at room temp; do not freeze

IV route
• Dilute to a volume of either 120 ml or 300 ml with D₅W, LR
• **75-mg dose:** withdraw 6 ml sotalol inj (90 mg), add 114 ml dilute to make 120 ml (0.75% mg/ml); or withdraw 6 ml sotalol inj (90 mg), add 294 ml, dilute to make 300 ml (0.3 mg/ml)
• **112.5-mg dose:** withdraw 9 ml sotalol inj, (135 ml), add 111 ml, dilute to 120 ml (1.125 mg/ml); or withdraw 9 ml sotalol (135 mg) and add 291 ml dilute to 300 ml (0.45 mg/ml)
• **150-mg dose:** withdraw 12 ml sotalol (180 mg), add 108 ml to 120 ml (1.5 mg/ml); or withdraw 12 ml of sotalol (180 mg), add 288 ml to 300 ml (0.6 mg/ml)
• Use inf pump and infuse 100 or 250 ml over 5 hr at a constant rate

ADVERSE EFFECTS

CNS: Dizziness, mental changes, drowsiness, fatigue, headache, catatonia, depression, anxiety, nightmares, paresthesia, lethargy, insomnia, decreased concentration
CV: Orthostatic hypotension, bradycardia, **CHF**, chest pain, **ventricular dysrhythmias, prolonged QT**, AV block, peripheral vascular insufficiency, palpitations, **prodysrhythmia, torsades de pointes;** Betapace AF: **life-threatening ventricular dysrhythmias**
EENT: Tinnitus, visual changes, sore throat, double vision, dry, burning eyes
GI: Nausea, vomiting, diarrhea, dry mouth, flatulence, constipation, anorexia, indigestion
GU: Impotence, dysuria, ejaculatory failure, urinary retention
HEMA: **Agranulocytosis, thrombocytopenic purpura (rare), thrombocytopenia, leukopenia**
INTEG: Rash, alopecia, urticaria, pruritus, fever, diaphoresis
MISC: Facial swelling, decreased exercise tolerance, weight change, Raynaud's disease
MS: Joint pain, arthralgia, muscle cramps, pain
RESP: **Bronchospasm**, dyspnea, wheezing, nasal stuffiness, pharyngitis

Pharmacokinetics

Absorption	Variable (30%)
Distribution	Crosses placenta, minimal penetration in CNS
Metabolism	Liver, protein binding 0%
Excretion	70% unchanged—kidneys
Half-life	10-24 hr, increased in renal disease

Pharmacodynamics

Onset	Several hr
Peak	Unknown
Duration	Unknown

INTERACTIONS
Individual drugs

> **BLACK BOX WARNING:** Haloperidol, chloroquine, droperidol, pentamidine; arsenic trioxide, levomethadyl: increased QT prolongation

Insulin: increased hypoglycemia
Lidocaine: increased effects of lidocaine
Nitroglycerin: increased hypotension
Theophylline: decreased bronchodilating effects of theophylline

Drug classifications

Antihypertensives, diuretics: increased hypotension
β₂-Agonists: decreased bronchodilating effects
Class IA/III antidysrhythmics, some phenothiazines, β-agonists, local anesthetics, tricyclics, CYP3A4 inhibitors (amiodarone, clarithromycin, erythromycin, telithromycin, troleandomycin), CYP3A4 substrates (methadone, pimozide, QUEtiapine, quiNIDine, risperiDONE, ziprasidone): increased QT prolongation
Sulfonylureas: decreased hypoglycemic effects
Sympathomimetics: decreased β-blocker effects

Drug/herb

Hawthorn: do not use concurrently

Drug/lab test

False: increased urinary catecholamines
Interference: glucose, insulin tolerance tests

NURSING CONSIDERATIONS
Assessment

> **BLACK BOX WARNING: QT syndrome:** Monitor B/P during beginning treatment, periodically thereafter; pulse q4hr; note rate, rhythm, quality; apical/radial pulse before administration; notify prescriber of any significant changes (pulse <50 bpm); monitor ECG continuously (Betapace AF); use QT interval to determine patient eligibility; baseline QT must be ≤450 msec, if ≥500 msec, frequency or dosage must be decreased or drug must be discontinued

> **BLACK BOX WARNING:** Requires a specialized care setting: for a minimum of at least 3 days on maintenance dose with continuous ECG monitoring, creatinine clearance, calculate before dosing

> **BLACK BOX WARNING:** Cardiogenic shock, acute pulmonary edema: do not use, as effect can further depress cardiac output

• Check for baselines in renal function tests, before therapy begins
• Assess for edema in feet, legs daily, monitor I&O ratio, daily weight; check for jugular vein distention, crackles, bilaterally, dyspnea (CHF)
⚠ **Abrupt discontinuation: do not discontinue abruptly; taper over 1-2 wk**
• Dose should be adjusted slowly, with at least 3 days between changes; monitor ECG for QT interval
• Monitor electrolytes (hypokalemia, hypomagnesemia); may increase dysrhythmias

Patient/family education

• Teach patient not to discontinue product abruptly, taper over 2 wk; may cause precipitate angina if stopped abruptly
• Teach patient not to use OTC products containing α-adrenergic stimulants (such as nasal decongestants, cold preparations); to avoid alcohol and smoking and to limit sodium intake as prescribed
• Teach patient how to take pulse and B/P at home, advise when to notify prescriber
• Instruct patient to comply with weight control, dietary adjustments, modified exercise program
• Caution patient to carry/wear emergency ID to identify product being taken, allergies
• Inform patient that product controls symptoms but does not cure
• Caution patient to avoid hazardous activities if dizziness, drowsiness are present
• Teach patient to report symptoms of **CHF:** difficulty breathing, especially on exertion or when lying down; night cough; swelling of extremities; bradycardia; dizziness; confusion; depression; fever
• Teach patient to take product as prescribed, not to double or skip doses; take any missed doses as soon as remembered if at least 4 hr until next dose
• Teach patient that hospitalization will be required for ≥3 days

Evaluation

Positive therapeutic outcome
• Absence of dysrhythmias

TREATMENT OF OVERDOSE:
Lavage; **IV** atropine for bradycardia; **IV** theophylline for bronchospasm; digoxin, O₂, diuretic for cardiac failure; hemodialysis; **IV** glucose for hyperglycemia; **IV** diazepam (or phenytoin) for seizures

spironolactone (Rx)

(speer′on-oh-lak′tone)

Aldactone, Novo-Spiroton ✦

Func. class.: Potassium-sparing diuretic
Chem. class.: Aldosterone antagonist

Pregnancy category D

Do not confuse: Aldactone/Aldactazide

ACTION: Competes with aldosterone at receptor sites in the distal tubule in the renal system, resulting in excretion of sodium chloride, water, retention of potassium, phosphate

Therapeutic outcome: Diuretic and antihypertensive effect while retaining potassium; lowered aldosterone levels

USES: Edema of CHF, hypertension, diuretic-induced hypokalemia, primary hyperaldosteronism (diagnosis, short-term treatment, long-term treatment), edema of nephrotic syndrome, cirrhosis of the liver with ascites

Unlabeled uses: CHF, hirsutism in women

CONTRAINDICATIONS

Pregnancy **D**, hypersensitivity, anuria, severe renal disease, hyperkalemia

Precautions: Breastfeeding, dehydration, renal/hepatic disease, electrolyte imbalances, metabolic acidosis, gynecomastia

> **BLACK BOX WARNING:** Secondary malignancy

DOSAGE AND ROUTES
Edema/hypertension
Adult: PO 25-200 mg/day in 1-2 divided doses

CHF
Adult: PO 12.5-25 mg/day, max 50 mg/day

Edema
Child: PO 1.5-3.3 mg/kg/day in single or divided doses

Hypertension
Child (unlabeled): PO 1.5-3.3 mg/kg in divided doses

Hypokalemia
Adult: PO 25-100 mg/day; if PO, potassium supplements must not be used

Primary hyperaldosteronism diagnosis
Adult: PO 400 mg/day × 4 days or 4 wk depending on the test, then 100-400 mg/day maintenance

Edema (nephrotic syndrome, CHF, hepatic disease)
Adult: PO 100 mg/day given as a single dose or in divided doses, titrate to response
Child: PO 1.5-3.3 mg/kg/day or 60 mg/m²/day given once daily or in 2-4 divided doses

Renal dose
Adult: PO CCr 10-50 ml/min; give dose q12-24hr; CCr <10 ml/min, avoid use

Polycystic ovary syndrome/ hirsutism in women (unlabeled)
Adult: PO 50-200 mg in 1-2 divided doses

Available forms: Tabs 25, 50, 100 mg

Implementation
• Give in AM to avoid interference with sleep
• Give with food if nausea occurs; absorption may be increased; take at same time each day
• Effect may take 2 wk

ADVERSE EFFECTS
CNS: Headache, confusion, drowsiness, lethargy, ataxia
ELECT: Hyperchloremic metabolic acidosis, hyperkalemia, hyponatremia
ENDO: Impotence, gynecomastia, irregular menses, amenorrhea, postmenopausal bleeding, hirsutism, deepening voice, breast pain
GI: Diarrhea, cramps, bleeding, gastritis, vomiting, anorexia, nausea, hepatocellular toxicity
HEMA: Agranulocytosis
INTEG: *Rash, pruritus,* urticaria

Pharmacokinetics

Absorption	GI tract; well absorbed
Distribution	Crosses placenta
Metabolism	Liver to canrenone (active metabolite)
Excretion	Renal; breast milk
Half-life	12-24 hr (canrenone)

Pharmacodynamics

Onset	24-48 hr
Peak	48-72 hr
Duration	Unknown

INTERACTIONS
Individual drugs
Aspirin: decreased action of spironolactone
Cholestyramine: increased hyperchloremic acidosis in cirrhosis
Digoxin: increased digoxin action
Lithium: increased action, toxicity

Drug classifications
ACE inhibitors, diuretics (potassium-sparing), potassium products, salt substitute: increased hyperkalemia

Anticoagulants: decreased effects of anticoagulants, monitor INR/PT
Antihypertensives: increased action
NSAIDs: decreased effect of spironolactone

Drug/food
Potassium-rich foods, potassium salt substitutes: increased hyperkalemia

Drug/herb
Ephedra: decreased antihypertensive effect
Hawthorn, horse chestnut: increased hypotension
St. John's wort: severe photosensitivity

Drug/lab test
Increased: BUN, potassium
Decreased: sodium, magnesium
Interference: 17-OHCS, 17-KS, radioimmunoassay, digoxin assay

NURSING CONSIDERATIONS
Assessment
• **Hypokalemia:** assess for polyuria, polydipsia, dysrhythmias including a U wave on ECG
• **Hyperkalemia:** assess for weakness, fatigue, dyspnea, dysrhythmias, confusion
• Assess fluid volume status: I&O ratios and record, count or weigh diapers as appropriate, weight, distended red veins, crackles in lung, color, quality, and specific gravity of urine, skin turgor, adequacy of pulses, moist mucous membranes, bilateral lung sounds, peripheral pitting edema; dehydration symptoms of decreasing output, thirst, hypotension, dry mouth and mucous membranes should be reported
• Monitor electrolytes: potassium, sodium, calcium, magnesium; also include BUN, ABGs, uric acid, CBC, blood glucose

> **BLACK BOX WARNING:** Secondary malignancy: assess periodically

Patient/family education
• Teach patient to take medication early in day to prevent nocturia
• Instruct patient to take with food or milk if GI symptoms of nausea and anorexia occur
• Teach patient to maintain a record of weight on a weekly basis and notify prescriber of weight loss of >5 lb
• Caution patient that this product causes an increase in potassium levels, that foods high in potassium should be avoided: oranges, bananas, salt substitutes, dried apricots, dates; avoid potassium salt substitutes; refer to dietitian for assistance planning
• Teach patient to take in AM, to prevent sleeplessness

• Teach patient to avoid hazardous activities until reaction is known
• Teach patient to notify prescriber if pregnancy is planned or suspected, pregnancy (**C**), do not breastfeed
• Teach patient not to use alcohol or any OTC medications without prescriber's approval; serious product reactions may occur
• Emphasize the need to contact prescriber immediately if muscle cramps, weakness, nausea, dizziness, or numbness occur
• Teach patient to take own B/P and pulse and record
• Teach patient to notify prescriber of cramps, diarrhea, lethargy, thirst, headache, skin rash, menstrual abnormalities, deepening voice, breast enlargement
• Advise patient that dizziness and confusion may occur; avoid driving or other hazardous activities if alertness is decreased
• Teach patient to continue taking medication even if feeling better; this product controls symptoms but does not cure the condition
• Advise patient with hypertension to continue other treatment (exercise, weight loss, relaxation techniques, cessation of smoking)

Evaluation

Positive therapeutic outcome
• Prevention of hypokalemia (diuretic use)
• Decreased edema
• Decreased B/P
• Decreased aldosterone levels
• Increased diuresis

TREATMENT OF OVERDOSE
• Lavage if taken orally, monitor electrolytes
• Administer sodium bicarbonate
• Monitor hydration, CV, renal status

stavudine d4t (Rx)
(sta′vu-deen)
Zerit
Func. class.: Antiretroviral
Chem. class.: Nucleoside reverse transcriptase inhibitor (NRTI)
Pregnancy category C

ACTION: Prevents replication of HIV-1 by inhibition of reverse transcriptase; causes DNA chain termination

Therapeutic outcome: Decreasing diarrhea, fatigue, night sweats; increased body weight

USES: Treatment of HIV-1; used in combination with other antiretrovirals

CONTRAINDICATIONS
Hypersensitivity to this product or zidovudine, didanosine, zalcitabine; severe peripheral neuropathy

> **BLACK BOX WARNING:** Lactic acidosis

Precautions: Breastfeeding, advanced HIV infections, bone marrow suppression, renal, peripheral neuropathy, osteoporosis, obesity

> **BLACK BOX WARNING:** Pregnancy **C**, hepatic disease, pancreatitis

DOSAGE AND ROUTES
Adult >60 kg: PO 40 mg q12hr
Adult <60 kg: PO 30 mg q12hr
Child <30 kg: PO 1 mg/kg q12hr
Child ≥30 kg ≤60 kg: PO 30 mg q12hr
Child >60 kg: PO 40 mg q12hr

Renal dose
Adult >60 kg: CCr 26-50 ml/min 20 mg q12hr; CCr 10-25 ml/min 20 mg q24hr
Adult <60 kg: CCr 26-50 ml/min 15 mg q12hr; CCr 10-25 ml/min 15 mg q24hr

Available forms: Caps 15, 20, 30, 40 mg; oral powder for sol 1 mg/ml

Implementation
• Give with or without meals; absorption does not appear to be lowered when taken with food
• Give product q4hr around the clock, even during night
• Shake susp well before using
• Use after hemodialysis

ADVERSE EFFECTS
CNS: *Peripheral neuropathy,* insomnia, anxiety, depression, dizziness, confusion, *headache,* chills/fever, malaise, neuropathy
CV: Chest pain, vasodilatation, hypertension
EENT: Conjunctivitis, abnormal vision
GI: Hepatotoxicity, *diarrhea, nausea, vomiting,* anorexia, dyspepsia, constipation, stomatitis, pancreatitis
HEMA: Bone marrow suppression, leukopenia, macrocytosis
INTEG: *Rash,* sweating, pruritus, benign neoplasms
MISC: Lactic acidosis, asthenia, lipodystrophy
MS: Myalgia, arthralgia
RESP: Dyspnea, pneumonia, asthma

Pharmacokinetics
Absorption	Rapidly absorbed, 82% bioavailability
Distribution	Cerebrospinal fluid
Metabolism	Unknown
Excretion	Kidneys, breast milk
Half-life	Elimination: 1-1.6 hr

Pharmacodynamics
Onset	Unknown
Peak	1 hr
Duration	Unknown

INTERACTIONS
Individual drugs
Chloramphenicol, dapsone, didanosine, ethambutol, hydrALAZINE, lithium, phenytoin, vinCRIStine, zalcitabine: increased peripheral neuropathy
Methadone, zidovudine: decreased stavudine effect
Probenecid: increased stavudine levels

Drug classifications
Myelosuppressants: increased myelosuppression

NURSING CONSIDERATIONS
Assessment

> **BLACK BOX WARNING:** Assess for lactic acidosis and severe hepatomegaly with steatosis; death may result; monitor LFTs

• Monitor viral load and CD4 counts, plasma HIV RNA baseline, throughout treatment
• Monitor for peripheral neuropathy: tingling, pain in extremities; if these occur, discontinue product, may not resolve after treatment is discontinued

> **BLACK BOX WARNING: Monitor for pancreatitis:** severe upper abdominal pain, weakness, fatigue, dyspnea, nausea, vomiting throughout treatment; if these occur, discontinue product

• Monitor blood tests: WBC, differential, RBC, Hct, Hgb, platelets, serum amylase, lipase, blood glucose, plasma hepatitis CRNA, pregnancy test, serum cholesterol, serum lipids, hepatitis serology, baseline and periodically
• Monitor renal function tests: urinalysis, protein, blood, serum creatinine
• Lipoatrophy/lipodystrophy during treatment
• Monitor bowel pattern before, during treatment
• Monitor fluid overload; product requires large volume to stay in sol

---

⚠ Nurse Alert   ✳ Key NCLEX® Drug   ≫ Drug Specifics

- Assess for weakness, tremors, confusion, dizziness, psychosis; if these occur, product may have to be decreased or discontinued

Patient/family education
- Teach patient signs of peripheral neuropathy: burning, weakness, pain, pricking feeling in the extremities
- Caution patient that this product should not be given with antineoplastics
- Inform patient that GI complaints and insomnia resolve after 3-4 wk of treatment
- Inform patient that product is not a cure for AIDS but controls symptoms
- Advise patient to call prescriber if sore throat, swollen lymph nodes, malaise, fever occur; may indicate presence of other infections
- Caution patient that even with product administration, virus is still infective and may be passed on to others
- Caution patient that follow-up visits must be continued because serious toxicity may occur; blood counts must be done q2wk
- Teach patient that product must be taken q4hr around the clock even during night
- Caution patient that serious product interactions with other medications may occur, check with prescriber first if taking chloramphenicol, dapsone, cisplatin, didanosine, ethambutol, lithium, antifungals

> **BLACK BOX WARNING:** Teach patient to notify prescriber if pregnancy is planned or suspected, fatal lactic acidosis may occur, pregnancy (**C**), avoid breastfeeding

- Inform patient that other products may be necessary to prevent other infections
- Inform patient that product may cause fainting or dizziness

Evaluation

Positive therapeutic outcome
- Decreased symptoms of HIV infection

⚠ HIGH ALERT

succinylcholine (Rx)
(suk-sin-ill-koe′leen)
Anectine, Quelicin
Func. class.: Neuromuscular blocker (depolarizing—ultra short)
Pregnancy category C

ACTION: Inhibits transmission of nerve impulses by binding with cholinergic receptor sites, antagonizing action of acetylcholine; causes release of histamine

Therapeutic outcome: Paralysis of skeletal muscles

USES: Facilitation of endotracheal intubation, skeletal muscle relaxation during orthopedic manipulations

CONTRAINDICATIONS
Hypersensitivity, malignant hyperthermia, trauma

Precautions: Pregnancy **C**, breastfeeding, geriatric or debilitated patients, severe burns, fractures (fasciculation may increase damage), electrolyte imbalances, dehydration, neuromuscular disease, respiratory disease, collagen diseases, glaucoma, eye surgery, renal/hepatic/cardiac disease

> **BLACK BOX WARNING:** Hyperkalemia, myopathy, rhabdomyolysis, children <2 yr

DOSAGE AND ROUTES
Adult: IV 0.3-1.1 mg/kg, max 150 mg, maintenance 0.04-0.07 mg/kg q5-10min as needed; CONT **IV** INF dilute to concentration of 1-2 mg/ml in D₅W or NS 10-100 mcg/kg/min
Child: IV initially 1-2 mg/kg; CONT **IV** INF not recommended

Available forms: Inj 20, 50, 100 mg/ml; powder for inj 100, 500 mg/vial, 1 g/vial

Implementation
- Store in refrigerator, powder at room temp; close tightly
- Give IV or IM; only experienced clinicians familiar with the use of neuromuscular blocking drugs should administer or supervise the use of this product
- Visually inspect parenteral products for particulate matter and discoloration prior to use
- Monitor heart rate and mechanical ventilator status during use

Rapid IV injection route
- Due to tachyphylaxis and prolonged apnea, this method is not recommended for prolonged procedures. Rapid IV injection of succinylcholine may result in profound bradycardia or asystole in pediatric patients; as with adults, the risk increases with repeated doses. Pretreatment with atropine may be needed
- No dilution of injection solution necessary
- Inject rapidly IV over 10-30 seconds

Continuous IV infusion route
- Not recommended for infants and children due to risk of malignant hyperthermia
- This route is preferred for long surgical procedures due to possible tachyphylaxis and prolonged apnea associated with administration of repeated fractional doses

---

• Dilute succinylcholine to a concentration of 1-2 mg/ml with D₅W, D₅NS, NS, or 1/6 M sodium lactate injection. One g of the powder for injection or 20 ml of a 50-mg/ml solution may be added to 1 L or 500 ml of diluent to give solutions containing 1 or 2 mg/ml, respectively. Alternatively, 500 mg of the powder for injection or 10 ml of a 50 mg/ml solution may be added to 500 ml or 250 ml of diluent to give solutions containing 1 or 2 mg/ml, respectively
• Infuse IV at a rate of 2.5 mg/min (range = 0.5-10 mg/min); adjust rate based on patient response and requirements

IM route
• Recommended for infants and other patients in whom a suitable vein is not accessible
• Inject into a large muscle, preferably high into the deltoid muscle. Aspirate prior to injection

Syringe compatibilities: Heparin

Y-site compatibilities: Etomidate, heparin, potassium chloride, propofol, vit B/C

Additive compatibilities: Amikacin, cephapirin, isoproterenol, meperidine, methyldopate, morphine, norepinephrine, scopolamine

Additive incompatibilities: Barbiturates, nafcillin, sodium bicarbonate

ADVERSE EFFECTS
CV: Bradycardia, tachycardia; increased, decreased B/P, **sinus arrest, dysrhythmias,** edema
EENT: Increased secretions, increased intraocular pressure
HEMA: Myoglobulinemia
INTEG: Rash, flushing, pruritus, urticaria
MS: Weakness, muscle pain, fasciculation, prolonged relaxation, myalgia, **rhabdomyolysis**
RESP: **Prolonged apnea, bronchospasm, cyanosis, respiratory depression,** wheezing, dyspnea
SYST: Anaphylaxis, angioedema

Pharmacokinetics

Absorption	Well absorbed (IM)
Distribution	Widely distributed, crosses placenta
Metabolism	Plasma (90%)
Excretion	Hydrolyzed in blood, excreted in urine (active/ inactive metabolites)
Half-life	Unknown

Pharmacodynamics

	IM	IV
Onset	2-3 min	1 min
Peak	Unknown	2-3 min
Duration	10-30 min	6-10 min

INTERACTIONS
Individual products
Clindamycin, enflurane, isoflurane, lincomycin, lithium, oxytocin, procainamide, quiNIDine: increased neuromuscular blockade
Theophylline: increased dysrhythmias

Drug classifications
Aminoglycosides, anesthetics (local), antibiotics (polymyxin), β-adrenergic blockers, cardiac glycosides, magnesium salts, opioids, thiazides: increased neuromuscular blockade

Drug/herb
Melatonin: blocks succinylcholine

NURSING CONSIDERATIONS
Assessment
• Assess for electrolyte imbalances (potassium, magnesium); may lead to increased action of this product
• Monitor VS (B/P, pulse, respirations, airway) until fully recovered; rate, depth, pattern of respirations, strength of hand grip
• Monitor I&O ratio; check for urinary retention, frequency, hesitancy
• **Recovery:** assess for decreased paralysis of face, diaphragm, leg, arm, rest of body
• **Allergic reactions:** assess for rash, fever, respiratory distress, pruritus; product should be discontinued if these occur

> **BLACK BOX WARNING: Myopathy, rhabdomyolysis:** in pediatric patients (rare)

Patient/family education
• Explain reason for medication and expected results
• Provide reassurance if communication is difficult during recovery from neuromuscular blockade; postoperative stiffness is normal, soon subsides

Evaluation
Positive therapeutic outcome
• Paralysis of jaw, eyelid, head, neck, rest of body

TREATMENT OF OVERDOSE:
Edrophonium or neostigmine, atropine, monitor VS; may require mechanical ventilation

---

sucralfate (Rx)

(soo-kral'fate)

Carafate, Sulcrate ✤

Func. class.: Protectant; antiulcer

Chem. class.: Aluminum hydroxide/
sulfated sucrose

Pregnancy category B

Do not confuse: Carafate/Cafergot

ACTION: Forms a complex that adheres to
ulcer site, adsorbs pepsin

Therapeutic outcome: Healing of ulcers

USES: Duodenal ulcer, oral mucositis, stomatitis after radiation of head and neck

Unlabeled uses: Gastric ulcers, gastroesophageal reflux

CONTRAINDICATIONS

Hypersensitivity

Precautions: Pregnancy **B**, breastfeeding,
children, renal failure, hypoglycemia (diabetics)

DOSAGE AND ROUTES

Duodenal ulcers

Adult: PO 1 g qid 1 hr before meals and at
bedtime

Child: PO 40-80 mg/kg/day divided

Available forms: Tabs 1 g; oral susp 1 g/10 ml

Implementation

• Do not break, crush, or chew tabs
• Give on empty stomach 1 hr before meals and
at bedtime
• Avoid antacids ½ hr before or 1 hr after tak-
ing this product
• Store at room temperature

ADVERSE EFFECTS

CNS: Drowsiness, dizziness

ENDO: Hyperglycemia (diabetes mellitus)

GI: *Dry mouth, constipation,* nausea, gastric
pain, vomiting, bezoar (critically ill patients)

INTEG: Urticaria, rash, pruritus

Pharmacokinetics

Absorption	Minimally absorbed
Distribution	Unknown
Metabolism	Not metabolized
Excretion	Feces (90%)
Half-life	6-20 hr

Pharmacodynamics

Onset	½ hr
Peak	Unknown
Duration	6 hr

INTERACTIONS

Individual drugs

Cimetidine, ranitidine: decreased absorption of
sucralfate

Digoxin, ketoconazole, phenytoin, tetracycline,
theophylline: decreased action of each specific product

Drug classifications

Antacids: decreased absorption of sucralfate

Fat-soluble vitamins: decreased action of fat-soluble vitamins

Fluoroquinolones: decreased absorption

NURSING CONSIDERATIONS

Assessment

• **GI symptoms:** assess for abdominal pain,
blood in stools
• **Hypoglycemia:** may occur in those with diabetes mellitus, monitor blood glucose carefully

Patient/family education

• Instruct patient to take medication on empty
stomach
• Caution patient to take full course of therapy,
not to use >8 wk, to avoid smoking
• Caution patient to avoid antacids within ½ hr
of product or 1 hr after this product
• Advise patient to increase fluids, bulk, exercise to lessen constipation

Evaluation

Positive therapeutic outcome

• Absence of pain or GI complaints

sulfamethoxazole/ trimethoprim (cotrimoxazole) (Rx)

(sul-fa-meth-ox'a-zole/trye-meth'oh-prim
[ko-trye-mox'a-zole])

**Bacter-Aid DS, Bactrim DS, Novo-
Trimel** ✤**, Nu-Cotrimox** ✤**, Septra,
Septra DS, SMZ/TMP, Sultrex**

Func. class.: Antiinfective

Chem. class.: Sulfonamide—
miscellaneous

Pregnancy category C

ACTION: Sulfamethoxazole (SMZ) interferes with bacterial biosynthesis of proteins by
competitive antagonism of PABA when adequate
levels are maintained; trimethoprim (TMP)

S

blocks synthesis of tetrahydrofolic acid; combination blocks two consecutive steps in bacterial synthesis of essential nucleic acids, protein

Therapeutic outcome: Absence of infection, based on C&S

USES: UTI, otitis media, acute and chronic prostatitis, shigellosis, chancroid, traveler's diarrhea, *Enterobacter, Escherichia coli, Haemophilus influenzae* (beta-lactamase negative), *Haemophilus influenzae* (beta-lactamase positive), *Klebsiella, Morganella morganii, Pneumocystis carinii, Pneumocystis jiroveci, Proteus mirabilis, Proteus, Shigella flexneri, Shigella sonnei, Streptococcus* pneumonia; **may also be effective for** *Acinetobacter baumannii, Actinomadura madurae, Actinomadura pelletieri, Bordetella pertussis, Burkholderia pseudomallei, Cyclospora cayetanensis, Haemophilus ducreyi, Isospora belli, Klebsiella granulomatis, Legionella micdadei, Legionella pneumophila, Listeria monocytogenes, Moraxella catarrhalis, Neisseria gonorrhoeae, Nocardia asteroides, Nocardia brasiliensis, Nocardia otitidiscaviarum, Pediculus capitis, Plasmodium falciparum, Providencia, Salmonella, Serratia, Shigella, Staphylococcus aureus* (MRSA), *Staphylococcus aureus* (MSSA), *Staphylococcus epidermidis, Stenotrophomonas maltophilia, Streptococcus pyogenes* (group A beta-hemolytic streptococci), *Streptomyces somaliensis, Toxoplasma gondii, Vibrio cholerae, Viridans* streptococci, *Yersinia enterocolitica*

CONTRAINDICATIONS
Pregnancy at term, breastfeeding, infants <2 mo, hypersensitivity to trimethoprim or sulfonamides, megaloblastic anemia, CCr <15 ml/min

Precautions: Pregnancy **C**, infants, geriatric, renal disease, G6PD deficiency, impaired renal/hepatic function, possible folate deficiency, severe allergy, bronchial asthma, UV exposure, porphyria, hyperkalemia, hypothyroidism

DOSAGE AND ROUTES
Based on TMP content

UTI
Adult: PO 160 mg TMP q12hr × 10-14 days
Child: PO 8 mg/kg TMP daily in 2 divided doses q12hr (treatment); 2 mg/kg/day (prophylaxis)

Otitis media
Child: PO 8 mg/kg TMP daily in 2 divided doses q12hr × 10 days

Chronic bronchitis
Adult: PO 160 mg TMP q12hr × 10-14 days

Pneumocystis jiroveci pneumonitis
Adult and child: PO 15-20 mg/kg TMP daily in 4 divided doses q6hr × 14-21 days; IV 15-20 mg/kg/day (based on TMP) in 3-4 divided doses for up to 14 days

Renal dose
Dosage reduction necessary in moderate to severe renal impairment (CCr <30 ml/min)

Available forms: Tabs 80 mg TMP/400 mg SMZ, 160 mg TMP/800 mg SMZ; susp 200 mg-40 mg/5 ml, 800 mg-160 mg/20 ml; IV 16 mg/80 mg/ml

Implementation
• Give with full glass of water to maintain adequate hydration; increase fluids to 2 L/day to decrease crystallization in kidneys
• Give medication after C&S; repeat C&S after full course of medication
• Store in airtight, light-resistant container at room temp
• Give without regard to meals

Intermittent IV infusion route
• Dilute 5 ml ampule/100-125 ml of D₅W, stable for 6 hr, give over ½ hr, do not refrigerate, if using Septra ADD-Vantage vials dilute each 10-ml vial in ADD-Vantage diluent containers containing 250 ml of D₅W, infuse over 60-90 min, change site q48-72hr

Y-site compatibilities: Acyclovir, aldesleukin, allopurinol, amifostine, atracurium, aztreonam, cefepime, cyclophosphamide, diltiazem, enalaprilat, esmolol, filgrastim, fludarabine, gallium, granisetron, HYDROmorphone, labetalol, LORazepam, magnesium sulfate, melphalan, meperidine, morphine, pancuronium, perphenazine, piperacillin/tazobactam, sargramostim, tacrolimus, teniposide, thiotepa, vecuronium, zidovudine

Y-site incompatibilities: Alfentanil, amikacin, aminophylline, amphotericin B colloidal, ampicillin, ampicillin/sulbactam, ascorbic acid, atropine, azaTHIOprine, benztropine, bumetanide, buprenorphine, butorphanol, calcium chloride/gluconate, caspofungin, ceFAZolin, cefotaxime, cefOXitin, cefTAZidime, cefTRIAXone, chloramphenicol, chlorproMAZINE, cimetidine, clindamycin, codeine, cyanocobalamin, cycloSPORINE, dantrolene, dexamethasone, diazepam, diazoxide, digoxin, diphenhydrAMINE, DOBUTamine, DOPamine, DOXOrubicin, doxycycline, ePHEDrine, EPINEPHrine, epirubicin, epoetin alfa, erythromycin, famotidine, fentaNYL, fluconazole, folic acid, furosemide, ganciclovir, gentamicin, glycopyrrolate, haloperidol, heparin, hydrALAZINE, hydrocortisone, hydrOXYzine,

IDArubicin, imipenem/cilastatin, inamrinone, indomethacin, insulin, isoproterenol, ketorolac, lidocaine, mannitol, mechlorethamine, metaraminol, methoxamine, methyldopate, methylPREDNISolone, metoclopramide, metoprolol, metroNIDAZOLE, midazolam, multi-vitamins, nafcillin, nalbuphine, naloxone, nitroglycerin, nitroprusside, norepinephrine, ondansetron, oxacillin, oxytocin, papaverine, penicillin G, pentamidine, pentazocine, PENTobarbital, PHENobarbital, phentolamine, phenylephrine, phenytoin, phytonadione, potassium chloride, procainamide, prochlorperazine, promethazine, propranolol, protamine, quinupristin/dalfopristin, ranitidine, sodium bicarbonate, succinylcholine, SUFentanil, thiamine, ticarcillin/clavulanate, tobramycin, tolazoline, trimetaphan, urokinase, vancomycin, verapamil, vinorelbine

ADVERSE EFFECTS

CNS: Headache, insomnia, hallucinations, depression, vertigo, fatigue, anxiety, seizures, product fever, chills, **aseptic meningitis**
CV: Allergic myocarditis
EENT: Tinnitus
GI: *Nausea, vomiting, abdominal pain,* stomatitis, **hepatitis,** glossitis, pancreatitis, diarrhea, **enterocolitis,** anorexia, **pseudomembranous colitis**
GU: **Renal failure, toxic nephrosis;** increased BUN, creatinine; crystalluria
HEMA: **Leukopenia, neutropenia, thrombocytopenia, agranulocytosis, hemolytic anemia, hypoprothrombinemia, Henoch-Schölein purpura, methemoglobinemia, eosinophilia I**
INTEG: Rash, dermatitis, urticaria, erythema, photosensitivity, pain, inflammation at injection site, **toxic epidermal necrolysis, erythema multiforme**
RESP: Cough, shortness of breath
SYST: **Anaphylaxis, systemic lupus erythematosus, Stevens-Johnson syndrome**

Pharmacokinetics

Absorption	Rapid
Distribution	Breast milk, crosses placenta, 68% protein bound
Metabolism	Liver
Excretion	Kidneys
Half-life	8-13 hr

Pharmacodynamics

Onset	Unknown
Peak	1-4 hr
Duration	Unknown

INTERACTIONS
Individual drugs
CycloSPORINE: decreased response
Dofetilide: increased levels of dofetilide
Methenamine: increased crystalluria
Methotrexate: increased bone marrow depression
Phenytoin: decreased hepatic clearance of phenytoin

Drug classifications
Anticoagulants (oral): increased anticoagulant effect
CYP2C9, CYP3A4 inducers: decreased hepatic clearance
Diuretics (potassium-sparing), potassium supplements: increased potassium levels
Diuretics (thiazide): increased thrombocytopenia
Sulfonylureas: increased hypoglycemic response

Drug/lab test
Increased: creatinine, bilirubin
Decreased: Hgb, platelets

NURSING CONSIDERATIONS
Assessment
• Monitor I&O ratio; note color, character, pH of urine if product administered for UTI; output should be 800 ml less than intake; if urine is highly acidic, alkalization may be needed
• Monitor renal function tests: BUN, creatinine, urinalysis (long-term therapy)
• Assess type of infection; obtain C&S before starting therapy
• Assess blood dyscrasias, skin rash, fever, sore throat, bruising, bleeding, fatigue, joint pain
• Assess allergic reaction: rash, dermatitis, urticaria, pruritus, dyspnea, bronchospasm, AIDS patients are more susceptible

Patient family education
• Teach patient to take each oral dose with full glass of water to prevent crystalluria; drink 8-10 glasses of water/day
• Teach patient to complete full course of treatment to prevent superinfection
• Teach patient to avoid sunlight or use sunscreen to prevent burns
• Teach patient to avoid OTC medications (aspirin, vit C) unless directed by prescriber
• If diabetic, teach patient to use Clinistix or Tes-Tape
• **Teach patient to use alternative contraceptive measures; decreased effectiveness of oral contraceptives may result**
• Teach patient to notify prescriber if skin rash, sore throat, fever, mouth sores, unusual bruising, bleeding occur

Evaluation

Positive therapeutic outcome
• Absence of pain, fever, C&S negative

---

sulfaSALAzine (Rx)
(sul-fa-sal′a-zeen)
**Azulfidine, Azulfidine EN-tabs,
Salazopyrin** ✤
Func. class.: GI Antiinflammatory, anti-rheumatic (DMARD)
Chem. class.: GI Sulfonamide
Pregnancy category B

Do not confuse: sulfaSALAzine/
sulfiSOXAZOLE

ACTION: Proproduct to deliver sulfapyridine and 5-aminosalicylic acid to colon; antinflammatory in connective tissue

Therapeutic outcome: Treatment of ulcerative colitis, rheumatoid arthritis

USES: Ulcerative colitis, rheumatoid arthritis, juvenile rheumatoid arthritis (Azulfidine EN-tabs)

Unlabeled uses: Crohn's disease

CONTRAINDICATIONS
Pregnancy at term, children <2 yr, hypersensitivity to sulfonamides or salicylates, intestinal, urinary obstruction, porphyria

Precautions: Pregnancy **B**, breastfeeding, impaired renal/hepatic function, severe allergy, bronchial asthma, megaloblastic anemia

DOSAGE AND ROUTES
Bowel disease
Adult: PO 3-4 g/day in divided doses; maintenance 2 g/day in divided doses q6hr
Child ≥6 yr: PO 40-60 mg/kg/day in 4-6 divided doses, then 30 mg/kg/day in 4 doses, max 2 g/day

Rheumatoid arthritis
Adult: PO 0.5-1 g/day, then increase daily dose by 500 mg qwk to 2 g/day in 2-3 divided doses

Juvenile rheumatoid arthritis
Child ≥6 yr: PO 30-50 mg/kg/24 hr, divided into 2 doses

Renal dose
Adult: PO CCr 10-30 ml/min give bid; CCr <10 ml/min give daily

Available forms: Tabs 500 mg; oral susp 250 mg/5 ml; del rel tabs 500 mg

Implementation
• Give with full glass of water to maintain adequate hydration; increase fluids to 2 L/day to decrease crystallization in kidneys; contact lenses, urine, skin may be yellow-orange
• Give total daily dose in evenly spaced doses and after meals to help minimize GI intolerance
• Give at bedtime
• Store in airtight, light-resistant container at room temperature

ADVERSE EFFECTS
CNS: Headache, confusion, insomnia, hallucinations, depression, vertigo, fatigue, anxiety, **seizures,** product fever, chills
CV: Allergic myocarditis
GI: *Nausea, vomiting, abdominal pain,* stomatitis, **hepatitis,** glossitis, **pancreatitis,** diarrhea
GU: Renal failure, toxic nephrosis, increased BUN, creatinine, crystalluria
HEMA: Leukopenia, neutropenia, thrombocytopenia, agranulocytosis, hemolytic anemia
INTEG: Rash, dermatitis, urticaria, **Stevens-Johnson syndrome,** erythema, photosensitivity
SYST: Anaphylaxis

Pharmacokinetics	
Absorption	Partially absorbed
Distribution	Crosses placenta
Metabolism	Liver
Excretion	Kidneys, breast milk
Half-life	6 hr

Pharmacodynamics	
Onset	1 hr
Peak	1½-6 hr
Duration	6-12 hr

INTERACTIONS
Individual drugs
AzaTHIOprine, mercaptopurine: increased leucopenia risk
CycloSPORINE: decreased effect of cycloSPORINE
Digoxin: decreased digoxin effect
Folic acid: decreased folic acid effect
Methotrexate: decreased renal excretion

Drug classifications
Anticoagulants (oral): increased anticoagulant effect
Hypoglycemics (oral): increased hypoglycemic response

Drug/food
Iron, folic acid will be poorly absorbed

Drug/lab test

False positive: urinary glucose test

NURSING CONSIDERATIONS

Assessment

• Monitor I&O ratio; note color, amount, character, pH of urine if product administered for UTIs; output should be 800 ml less than intake; if urine is highly acidic, alkalization may be needed

• Monitor kidney function tests: BUN, creatinine, urinalysis if on long-term therapy

⚠ **Blood dyscrasias: assess for rash, fever, sore throat, bruising, bleeding, fatigue, joint pain; monitor CBC before and q3mo**

⚠ **Allergic reaction: assess for rash, dermatitis, urticaria, pruritus, dyspnea, bronchospasm**

• **Ulcerative colitis, proctitis, other inflammatory bowel disease:** monitor character, amount, consistency of stools, abdominal pain, cramping, blood, mucus

• **Rheumatoid arthritis:** assess mobility, joint swelling, pain, activities of daily living

Patient/family education

• Advise patient to take each oral dose with full glass of water to prevent crystalluria

• Teach patient to avoid sunlight or to use sunscreen to prevent burns

• Teach patient to avoid OTC medication (aspirin, vit C) unless directed by prescriber

• Advise patient to notify prescriber if skin rash, sore throat, fever, mouth sores, unusual bruising, bleeding occur

• Advise patient to use rectal susp at bedtime and retain all night

Evaluation

Positive therapeutic outcome

• Absence of fever, mucus in stools or pain in joints

SUMAtriptan (Rx)

(soo-ma-trip′tan)

ALSUMA Auto-injector, Imitrex, Sumavel Dose Pro, Zecuity

Func. class.: Antimigraine agent
Chem. class.: 5-HT₁ receptor agonist
Pregnancy category C

Do not confuse: SUMAtriptan/somatropin

ACTION: Binds selectively to the vascular 5-HT₁ receptor subtype and exerts antimigraine effect; causes vasoconstriction in cranial arteries

Therapeutic outcome: Absence of migraines

USES: Acute treatment of migraine with or without aura and cluster headache

CONTRAINDICATIONS

Angina pectoris, history of MI, documented silent ischemia, Prinzmetal's angina, ischemic heart disease, **IV** use, concurrent ergotamine-containing preparations, uncontrolled hypertension, hypersensitivity, basilar or hemiplegic migraine

Precautions: Pregnancy **C**, breastfeeding, children <18 yr, postmenopausal women, men >40 yr, geriatric, risk factors for CAD, hypercholesterolemia, obesity, diabetes, impaired renal/hepatic function, overuse

DOSAGE AND ROUTES

Adult: SUBCUT 6 mg or less, may repeat in 1 hr, max 12 mg/24 hr; PO 25 mg with fluids if no relief in 2 hr, give another dose, max 200 mg/day; NASAL 1 dose of 5, 10, or 20 mg in one nostril, may repeat in 2 hr, max 40 mg/24 hr, 1 puff each nostril q2hr; TD 1 patch (6.5 mg/4 hr); after application push activation button

Hepatic dose
Adult: PO 25 mg, if no response after 2 hr, give up to 50 mg

Available forms: Inj 4, 6 mg/0.5 ml; tabs 25, 50, 100 mg; nasal spray 5 mg/100 mcl-units dose spray device 20 mg/100 mcl-units; transdermal patch 6.5 mg/4 hr

Implementation

PO route

• Swallow tab whole; do not break, crush, or chew

• Take with fluids as soon as symptoms appear; may take a second dose >4 hr, max 200 mg/24 hr

SUBCUT route

• Give by SUBCUT route only, avoid IM or **IV** administration, use only for actual migraine attack

• Give 1st dose supervised by medical staff in those with CAD or those at risk for CAD

Nasal route

• Spray once in 1 nostril, may repeat if headache returns, do not repeat if pain continues after 1st dose

Transdermal route

• Do not cut; apply to dry, intact skin of upper arm or thigh; do not use over scars, tattoos, cuts, scratches, burns, abrasions

• Apply another patch if headache is not relieved ≥2 hr after 1st patch; push activation button within 15 min of applying or patch will not work; do not bathe, shower, swim; may be taped with medical tape if needed

S

- Do not use with MRI
- Remove slowly, cleanse with soap and water, may cause redness
- Dispose of after folding in half

ADVERSE EFFECTS

CNS: *Tingling, hot sensation, burning, feeling of pressure, tightness, numbness, dizziness, sedation,* headache, anxiety, fatigue, cold sensation
CV: *Flushing,* MI, hypo/hypertension
EENT: Throat, mouth, nasal discomfort, vision changes
GI: Abdominal discomfort
INTEG: *Inj site reaction,* sweating
MS: *Weakness, neck stiffness,* myalgia
RESP: Chest tightness, pressure

Pharmacokinetics

Absorption	Well absorbed (SUBCUT)
Distribution	10%-20% plasma protein binding
Metabolism	Liver (metabolite)
Excretion	Urine, feces
Half-life	2 hr

Pharmacodynamics

	SUBCUT
Onset	10-20 min
Peak	10 min-2 hr
Duration	Up to 24 hr (pain relief)

INTERACTIONS
Individual drugs
Ergotamine: increased risk of vasospastic reaction

Drug classifications
Ergot derivatives: extended vasospastic effects
MAOIs, SSRIs, SNRIs, serotonin-receptor agonists: increased SUMAtriptan levels

Drug/herb
SAM-e, St. John's wort: serotonin syndrome

NURSING CONSIDERATIONS
Assessment
- **Serotonin syndrome: assess for delirium, coma, agitation, diaphoresis, hypertension, fever, tremors, may resemble neuroleptic malignant syndrome (in patients taking SSRIs, SNRIs)**
- Assess for tingling, hot sensation, burning, feeling of pressure, numbness, flushing, inj site reaction
- Assess B/P; signs/symptoms of coronary vasospasm
- Monitor stress level, activity, reaction, coping mechanisms of patient
- Assess neurologic status: LOC, blurring vision, nausea, vomiting, tingling in extremities preceding headache
- Assess for ingestion of tyramine-containing foods (pickled products, beer, wine, aged cheese), food additives, preservatives, colorings, artificial sweeteners, chocolate, caffeine, which may precipitate these types of headaches

Patient/family education
- Caution patient not to take more than 2 doses/day or 12 mg/day; allow at least 1 hr between doses
- Caution patient to avoid driving or hazardous activities if dizziness or drowsiness occurs
- Teach patient to report chest tightness, heat, flushing, drowsiness, dizziness, fatigue, sudden severe abdominal pain or any allergic reactions that occur to prescriber immediately
- Inform patient to report any side effects to prescriber
- Caution patient to use contraception when taking product, to notify prescriber if pregnancy is suspected or planned
- **Nasal spray:** one spray in one nostril, may repeat if headache returns, do not repeat if pain continues after 1st dose

Evaluation
Positive therapeutic outcome
- Decrease in frequency, severity of headache

⚠ HIGH ALERT

SUNItinib (Rx)
(soo-nit'in-ib)
Sutent
Func. class.: Antineoplastic—miscellaneous
Chem. class.: Protein-tyrosine kinase inhibitor
Pregnancy category D

ACTION: Inhibits multiple receptor tyrosine kinases (RTKs), some are responsible for tumor growth

Therapeutic outcome: Decrease in size of tumor

USES: Gastrointestinal stromal tumors (GIST) after disease progression or intolerance to imatinib; advanced renal carcinoma, pancreatic neuroendocrine tumors (pNET) in those with unresectable locally advanced/metastatic disease

CONTRAINDICATIONS
Pregnancy **D**, breastfeeding, hypersensitivity

Precautions: Children, geriatric, active infections, QT prolongation, torsades de pointes, stroke, heart failure

BLACK BOX WARNING: Hepatic disease

DOSAGE AND ROUTES
Gastrointestinal stromal tumors (GIST)/renal cell cancer
Adult: PO 50 mg/day × 4 wk, then 2 wk off; may increase or decrease dose by 12.5 mg; if administered with CYP3A4 inducers, give 87.5 mg/day; if given with CYP3A4 inhibitors give 37.5 mg/day

Pancreatic neuroendocrine (pNET)
Adult: PO 37.5 mg/day continuously, increase or decrease by 12.5 mg based on tolerance, avoid potent CYP3A4 inhibitors/inducers, if used with CYP3A4 inhibitor decrease SUNItinib dose to a minimum of 25 mg/day; if used with CYP3A4 inducer increase SUNItinib to a max of 62.5 mg/day

Available forms: Caps 12.5, 25, 50 mg

Implementation
• Give with meal and large glass of water to decrease GI symptoms
• Give nutritious diet with iron, vitamin supplement, low fiber, few dairy products
• Store at 25°C (77°F)

ADVERSE EFFECTS
CNS: **CNS hemorrhage**, headache, dizziness, insomnia, **seizures**, fatigue
CV: Hypertension, **left ventricular dysfunction; QT prolongation, cardiotoxicity, thrombotic microangiopathy, torsades de pointes**
ENDO: Hyper/hypothyroidism
GI: *Nausea*, **hepatotoxicity**, vomiting, dyspepsia, *anorexia, abdominal pain*, altered taste, *constipation*, stomatitis, mucositis, pancreatitis, diarrhea, **GI bleeding/perforation**
GU: **Nephrotic syndrome**
HEMA: **Neutropenia, thrombocytopenia, hemolytic anemia, leukopenia**
INTEG: *Rash, yellow skin discoloration*, depigmentation of hair or skin, alopecia
MS: Pain, arthralgia, myalgia, myopathy, **rhabdomyolysis**
RESP: Cough, dyspnea, **pulmonary embolism**
SYST: **Bleeding**, electrolyte abnormalities, hand-foot syndrome, **serious infection**

Pharmacokinetics

Absorption	Unknown
Distribution	Protein binding 95%
Metabolism	By CYP3A4
Excretion	Feces, small amount in urine
Half-life	Terminal 40-60 hr (SUNItinib); active metabolite 80-110 hr

Pharmacodynamics

Onset	Unknown
Peak	6-12 hr
Duration	Unknown

INTERACTIONS
Individual drugs
Acetaminophen: increased hepatotoxicity
Bevacizumab: microangiopathic hemolytic anemia; avoid concurrent use
Dexamethasone, carBAMazepine, PHENobarbital, phenytoin, rifampin: decreased SUNItinib concentrations
Haloperidol, chloroquine, droperidol, pentamidine, arsenic trioxide, levomethadyl: increased QT prolongation
Simvastatin: increased plasma concentrations
Warfarin: increased plasma concentration; avoid use with warfarin, use low-molecular-weight anticoagulants instead

Drug classifications
Calcium channel blockers: increased plasma concentrations
Class IA/III antidysrhythmics, some phenothiazines, β-agonists, local anesthetics, tricyclics, CYP3A4 inhibitors (amiodarone, clarithromycin, erythromycin, telithromycin, troleandomycin), CYP3A4 substrates (methadone, pimozide, QUEtiapine, quiNIDine, risperiDONE, ziprasidone): increased QT prolongation

Drug/herb
St. John's wort: decreased SUNItinib concentration

Drug/food
Grapefruit juice: increased plasma concentrations

NURSING CONSIDERATIONS
Assessment
• **Monitor ANC and platelets; if ANC <1 × 10⁹/L and/or platelets <50 × 10⁹/L, stop until ANC >1.5 × 10⁹/L and platelets >75 × 10⁹/L; if ANC <0.5 × 10⁹/L and/or platelets <10 × 10⁹/L, reduce dose by 200 mg; if cytopenia continues, reduce dose by another 100 mg; if cytopenia continues for 4 wk, stop product until ANC ≥1 × 10⁹/L**
• Assess CV status: hypertension, QT prolongation can occur; monitor left ventricular ejection fraction (LVEF) (MUGA) baseline periodically, ECG, B/P
• **Assess for renal toxicity: if bilirubin >3 × IULN, withhold SUNItinib until bilirubin levels return to <1.5 × IULN; electrolytes**

Adverse effects: *italics* = common; **bold** = life-threatening

> **BLACK BOX WARNING: Hepatotoxicity:**
> monitor liver function tests, before treatment
> and qmo; if liver transaminases >5 × IULN,
> withhold SUNItinib until transaminase levels
> return to <2.5 × IULN

• Assess for **CHF, adrenal insufficiency** in
those experiencing trauma
• Assess for bleeding: epistaxis rectal, gingival,
upper GI, genital, wound bleeding; tumor-
related hemorrhage may occur rapidly

Patient/family education
• Advise patient to report adverse reactions
immediately: shortness of breath, bleeding
• Teach patient reason for treatment, expected
result
• Teach patient that many adverse reactions may
occur: high B/P, bleeding, mouth swelling, taste
change, skin discoloration, depigmentation of
hair/skin
• Teach patient to avoid persons with known
upper respiratory infections; immunosuppression is common
• Teach to avoid grapefruit juice
• Teach patient to report if pregnancy is
planned or suspected, pregnancy D

Evaluation
Positive therapeutic outcome
• Decrease in size of tumor

---

suvorexant
(soo'voe-rex'ant)
Belsomra
Func. class.: Psychotropic—sedative/
hypnotic, anxiolytic
Chem. class.: Orexin receptor antagonist
Pregnancy category C

ACTION: Alters the signaling of neurotransmitters called orexins, which are responsible for
regulating the sleep–wake cycle

Therapeutic outcome: Normalized sleeping patterns

USES: The treatment of insomnia characterized by difficulties with sleep onset and/or sleep
maintenance

CONTRAINDICATIONS: Narcolepsy, hypersensitivity

Precautions: Preexisting respiratory disease,
COPD, breastfeeding, pregnancy **C**, labor, geriatrics, hepatic disease, sleep apnea, substance
abuse, alcohol use, suicidal ideation, mental
changes, depression

DOSAGE AND ROUTES
Adult: PO 10 mg every night within 30 min of
going to bed, and with ≥7 hr remaining before
the planned time of awakening, may increase to
maximum 20 mg every night

Available forms: Tabs 5, 10, 15, 20 mg

Implementation
• Give 30 min before bedtime
• Effect may be delayed if taken with food, take
on empty stomach for faster effect

ADVERSE EFFECTS
CNS: Amnesia, suicidal ideation, anxiety, dizziness, drowsiness, hallucinations, headache,
memory impairment
GI: Diarrhea

Pharmacokinetics

Absorption	Unknown
Distribution	High-protein binding
Metabolism	Unknown
Excretion	Feces (66%), urine (23%)
Half-life	Terminal half-life 12 hr

Pharmacodynamics

Onset	Unknown
Peak	2 hr
Duration	Unknown

INTERACTIONS
Drug classifications
CNS depressants: increased effects of both
    products
CYP3A inducers: decreased suvorexant effect
CYP3A inhibitors: avoid concurrent use

Drug/herb
Kava kava, melatonin, valerian: increased su-
    vorexant effect

NURSING CONSIDERATIONS
Assessment
• Sleeping patterns: waking in the night, inability to fall asleep, stay asleep, amnesia

Patient/family education
• Advise patient to use on an empty stomach for
faster effect
• Teach patient to report suicidal thoughts/
behaviors immediately
• Teach patient to avoid use with other products
unless approved by prescriber

Evaluation
Therapeutic response
• Normalized sleeping patterns

---

tacrolimus (PO, IV) (Rx)
(tak-row′lim-us)
Astagraf XL, Prograf
tacrolimus (topical) (Rx)
Protopic
Func. class.: Immunosuppressant
Chem. class.: Macrolide
Pregnancy category C

ACTION: Produces immunosuppression by inhibiting lymphocytes (T)

Therapeutic outcome: Prevention of rejection in organ transplant

USES: Organ transplants, to prevent rejection; **topical:** atopic dermatitis

Unlabeled uses: Severe recalcitrant psoriasis

CONTRAINDICATIONS
Hypersensitivity to this product or to some kinds of castor oil, long-term use (topical), child <2 yr (topical)

Precautions: Pregnancy **C**, breastfeeding, children <12 yr, severe renal/hepatic disease, diabetes mellitus, hyperkalemia, hyperuricemia, lymphomas, hypertension, acute bronchospasm, African descent, heart failure, seizures, QT prolongation

> **BLACK BOX WARNING:** Children <12 yr, lymphomas, infection, neoplastic disease, neonates, infants; requires a specialized setting and an experienced clinician; liver transplant (ext rel)

DOSAGE AND ROUTES
Kidney transplant rejection prophylaxis
Adult: IV 0.03-0.05 mg/kg/day as cont INF, give no sooner than 6 hr after transplantation

Liver transplant rejection prophylaxis
Adult: PO 0.1-0.15 mg/kg/day in 2 divided doses q12h, give no sooner than 6 hr after transplantation; **IV** 0.03-0.05 mg/kg/day as a cont INF, give no sooner than 6 hr after transplantation; ext rel caps 0.1 mg/kg qday preoperatively on empty stomach, 1st dose 12 hr prior to reperfusion and 0.2 mg/kg once daily postoperatively 1st dose within 12 hr of reperfusion but ≥ 4 hr after preoperative dose in combination with mycophenolate and corticosteroids

Heart transplant rejection prophylaxis
Adult: PO 0.075 mg/kg/day in 2 divided doses q12h, give no sooner than 6 hr after transplantation; **IV** 0.01 mg/kg/day as a cont INF, give no sooner than 6 hr after transplantation

Atopic dermatitis
Adult: TOP use 0.03% or 0.1% ointment, apply bid × 7 day after clearing of signs
Child 2-5 yr: TOP 0.03% ointment, apply bid × 7 day after clearing of signs

Available forms: Inj IV 5 mg/ml; caps 0.5, 1, 5 mg; ext rel cap 0.5, 1, 5 mg; ointment 0.03%, 0.1%

Implementation
PO route
• Give on empty stomach, food decreases absorption
• Give for several days before transplant surgery; patients should be placed in protective isolation
• Apply thin layers to affected skin only, rub in gently
• Use on small area of skin
• Extended release: Take in morning on empty stomach, 1 hr before or 2 hr after a meal
• Swallow whole; do not chew, divide, crush
• Do not use with alcohol
• If dose is missed up to 14 hr from scheduled dose, take dose, if >14 hr, skip
• Topical ointment has risk of developing cancer; use only when other options have failed

Continuous IV infusion route
• Give after diluting in 0.9% NaCl or D₅W to a concentration of 0.004-0.02 mg/ml as a cont inf

Y-site compatibilities: Alemtuzumab, alfentanil, amifostine, amikacin, aminophylline, amiodarone, amphotericin B colloidal, amphotericin B liposome, anidulafungin, atracurium, aztreonam, benztropine, bivalirudin, bleomycin, bumetanide, buprenorphine, busulfan, butorphanol, calcium acetate/chloride/gluconate, CARBOplatin, carmustine, caspofungin, ceFAZolin, cefoperazone, cefotaxime, cefoTEtan, cefOXitin, cefTAZidime, ceftizoxime, cefTRIAXone, cefuroxime, chloramphenicol, chlorproMAZINE, cimetidine, ciprofloxacin, cisatracurium, CISplatin, clindamycin, cyclophosphamide, cycloSPORINE, cytarabine, DACTINomycin, DAPTOmycin, dexamethasone, dexmedetomidine, dexrazoxane, digoxin, diltiazem, diphenhydrAMINE, DOBUTamine, DOCEtaxel, dolasetron, DOPamine, doripenem, doxacurium, DOXOrubicin hydrochloride, doxycycline, droperidol, enalaprilat, ePHEDrine, EPINEPHrine, epirubicin, ertapenem, erythromycin, esmolol, etoposide, etoposide phosphate, famotidine, fenoldopam, fentaNYL, fluconazole, fludarabine, foscarnet, fosphenytoin, gemcitabine, gentamicin, glycopyrrolate, granisetron, haloperidol, heparin, hydrALAZINE, hydrocortisone, HYDROmorphone, IDArubicin, ifosfamide, imipenem/cilastatin, inamrinone, insulin, isoproterenol, ketorolac, labetalol, leucovorin, levofloxacin, levorphanol, lidocaine, linezolid, LORazepam, magnesium sulfate, mannitol, mechlorethamine, meperidine, meropenem, mesna, metaraminol, methotrexate, methyldopate, methylPREDNISolone, metoclopramide, metoprolol, metroNIDAZOLE, micafungin, midazolam, milrinone, mitoMYcin, mitoXANtrone, mivacurium, morphine, multivitamins, nafcillin, nalbuphine, naloxone, nesiritide, niCARdipine, nitroglycerin, nitroprusside, norepinephrine, octreotide, ondansetron, oxacillin, oxaliplatin, oxytocin, PACLitaxel, palonosetron, pancuronium, PEMEtrexed, penicillin G, pentamidine, pentazocine, perphenazine, phentolamine, phenylephrine, piperacillin/tazobactam, potassium chloride/phosphates, procainamide, prochlorperazine, promethazine, propranolol, quinupristin/dalfopristin, ranitidine, remifentanil, rocuronium, sodium acetate/bicarbonate/phosphates, streptozocin, succinylcholine, SUFentanil, teniposide, theophylline, thiotepa, ticarcillin/clavulanate, tigecycline, tirofiban, tobramycin, tolazoline, trimethobenzamide, vancomycin, vasopressin, vecuronium, verapamil, vinCRIStine, vinorelbine, voriconazole, zidovudine, zoledronic acid

Y-site incompatibilities: Acyclovir, allopurinol, azaTHIOprine, cefepime, dantrolene, diazepam, diazoxide, espmeprazole, folic acid, ganciclovir, iron sucrose, levothyroxine, omeprazole, phenytoin, thiopental

ADVERSE EFFECTS
CNS: *Tremors, headache,* insomnia, paresthesia, chills, fever, seizures, posterior reversible encephalopathy syndrome, BK-virus-associated nephropathy, coma
CV: Hypertension, myocardial hypertrophy, prolonged QTc, cardiomyopathy
EENT: Blurred vision, photophobia
GI: Nausea, vomiting, diarrhea, constipation, GI bleeding
GU: Urinary tract infections, albuminuria, hematuria, proteinuria, renal failure, hemolytic uremic syndrome
HEMA: Anemia, leukocytosis, thrombocytopenia, purpura
INTEG: Rash, flushing, itching, alopecia
META: Hyperglycemia, hyperuricemia, hypokalemia, hyperkalemia

MS: Back pain, muscle spasms
RESP: Pleural effusion, atelectasis, dyspnea, interstitial lung disease
SYST: Anaphylaxis, infection, malignancy

Pharmacokinetics

Absorption	Erractically absorbed (PO), completely absorbed (**IV**)
Distribution	Crosses placenta, 75% protein binding
Metabolism	Liver to metabolite
Excretion	Kidney—minimal; breast milk, bile
Half-life	10 hr

Pharmacodynamics

	PO	IV
Onset	Unknown	Unknown
Peak	1-4 hr	Unknown
Duration	12 hr	12 hr

INTERACTIONS
Individual drugs
CarBAMazepine, PHENobarbital, phenytoin, rifamycin: decreased blood levels
Cimetidine, danazol, erythromycin, mycophenolate, mofetil: increased blood levels
CISplatin, cycloSPORINE: increased toxicity
Haloperidol, chloroquine, droperidol, pentamidine, arsenic trioxide, levomethadyl; CYP3A4 substrates (methadone, pimozide, QUEtiapine, quiNIDine, risperiDONE, ziprasidone): increased QT prolongation; do not use together
Ibuprofen: increased oliguria

Drug classifications
Aminoglycosides: increased toxicity
Antifungals, calcium channel blockers: increased blood levels
Class IA/III antidysrhythmics, some phenothiazines, β-agonists, local anesthetics, tricyclics, CYP3A4 inhibitors (amiodarone, clarithromycin, erythromycin, telithromycin, troleandomycin), CYP3A4 substrates (methadone, pimozide, QUEtiapine, quiNIDine, risperiDONE, ziprasidone): increased QT prolongation
Live virus vaccines: decreased effect of vaccines

Drug/herb
Astragalus, echinacea, melatonin: decreased immunosuppression, ginseng, St. John's wort

Drug/food
Decreased absorption of food
Grapefruit juice: increased effect of tacrolimus

Drug/lab test
Increased: glucose, BUN, creatinine
Decreased: magnesium, Hgb, platelets
Increased or decreased: LFTs, potassium

NURSING CONSIDERATIONS
Assessment
• **Monitor blood studies: Hgb, WBC, platelets during treatment monthly; if WBC is <3000/mm^3 or platelet count <100,000/mm^3, product should be discontinued or reduced; decreased Hgb level may indicate bone marrow suppression**
• **QT prolongation: ECG for QT prolongation, ejection fraction; assess for chest pain, palpitations, dyspnea**
• **Monitor liver function tests: alkaline phosphatase, AST, ALT, amylase, bilirubin, and for hepatotoxicity: dark urine, jaundice, itching, light-colored stools; product should be discontinued**
• Monitor serum creatinine/BUN, serum electrolytes, lipid profile, serum tacrolimus concentration
⚠ **Assess for anaphylaxis: rash, pruritus, wheezing, laryngeal edema; stop inf, initiate emergency procedures**

Patient/family education

BLACK BOX WARNING: Advise patient to report if pregnancy is planned or suspected

BLACK BOX WARNING: Advise patient to report symptoms of lymphoma

• **Instruct patient to report fever, rash, severe diarrhea, chills, sore throat, fatigue because serious infections may occur; clay-colored stools, cramping may indicate hepatotoxicity, signs of diabetes mellitus**
• Caution patient to avoid crowds or persons with known infections to reduce risk of infection, to avoid eating raw shellfish

BLACK BOX WARNING: Liver transplant: extended-release product should not be used due to increased female death rate

BLACK BOX WARNING: Specialized care setting, experienced clinician: this product should only be used when equipped and staffed with adequate supportive medical services and by those experienced in immunosuppressive therapy and organ transplantation

BLACK BOX WARNING: Children, infants, neonates: Not approved use of ointment in those <2 yr old, ext rel in those <16 yr not approved for pediatric kidney/heart transplant

Evaluation
Positive therapeutic outcome
• Absence of graft rejection
• Immunosuppression in autoimmune disorders

tadalafil (Rx)
(tah-dal′a-fil)
Adcirca, Cialis
Func. class.: Impotence agent
Chem. class.: Phosphodiesterase type 5 inhibitor
Pregnancy category B

ACTION: Inhibits phosphodiesterase type 5 (PDE5); enhances erectile function by increasing the amount of cyclic GMP, which causes smooth muscle relaxation and increased blood flow into the corpus cavernosum; improves erectile function for up to 36 hr

Therapeutic outcome: Erection

USES: Treatment of erectile dysfunction; pulmonary arterial hypertension (PAH) (Adcirca only), benign prostatic hyperplasia (BPH) with or without erectile dysfunction

CONTRAINDICATIONS
Newborns, women, children, hypersensitivity, patients taking organic nitrates regularly or intermittently, patients taking any α-adrenergic antagonist other than 0.4 mg once-daily tamsulosin

Precautions: Pregnancy **B**, although not indicated for women, anatomic penile deformities, sickle cell anemia, leukemia, multiple myeloma, CV/renal/hepatic disease, bleeding disorders, active peptic ulcer, prolonged erection

DOSAGE AND ROUTES
Erectile dysfunction
Adult: PO (Cialis) CCr 51-80 ml/min erectile dysfunction no adjustment; 20 mg/day initially, pulmonary hypertension; 10 mg, taken prior to sexual activity, dose may be reduced to 5 mg or increased to a max of 20 mg; usual max dosing frequency is once per day; once-daily dosing 2.5 mg/day at same time each day

BPH
Adult: PO 5 mg bid at the same time every day

Renal dose
Adult: PO CCr 31-50 ml/min 5 mg/day, max 10 mg q48hr; CCr <30 ml/min, max 5 mg q72hr

Hepatic dose
Adult: PO Child-Pugh class A, B, max 10 mg/day or 20 mg/day (pulmonary hypertension)

max 40 mg/day; Child-Pugh class C, not recommended

Concomitant medications
Ketoconazole, itraconazole, ritonavir, max 10 mg q72hr

Pulmonary hypertension
Adult: PO (**Adcirca only**) 40 mg qd; **Adult taking ritonavir:** PO 20 mg qd initially, then increase to 40 mg qd as tolerated

Available forms: Tabs 2.5, 5, 10, 20 mg; tab 20 mg (Adcirca)

Implementation
• **Sexual dysfunction:** give before sexual activity; do not use more than once a day
• **Pulmonary hypertension:** give Adcirca without regard to meals
• Product should not be used with nitrates in any form

ADVERSE EFFECTS
CNS: *Headache, flushing, dizziness,* seizures, transient global amnesia
CV: MI, hypotension, QT prolongation
INTEG: Stevens-Johnson syndrome, exfoliative dermatitis, urticaria
MISC: Back pain/myalgia, *dyspepsia, nasal congestion, UTI,* blurred vision, changes in color vision, *diarrhea,* pruritus, priapism, nonarteritic ischemic optic neuropathy (NAION), hearing loss

Pharmacokinetics

Absorption	Rapid; rate and extent of absorption of tadalafil are not influenced by food
Distribution	94% protein bound
Metabolism	Liver
Excretion	Excreted primarily as metabolites, feces, urine; plasma concentration 61% in feces, 36% in urine
Half-life	17.5 hr

Pharmacodynamics

Onset	Rapid
Peak	6 hr
Duration	Unknown

INTERACTIONS
Individual drugs
Alcohol, amlodipine, enalapril: decreased B/P
Bosentan: decreased effects of tadalafil

Itraconazole, ketoconazole, ritonavir: increased levels (although not studied, may also include other HIV protease inhibitors)

Drug classifications
⚠ Do not use with nitrates because of unsafe drop in B/P that could result in heart attack or stroke
α-blockers, angiotensin II receptor blockers: decreased B/P
Antacids: decreased effects of tadalafil

Drug/food
Grapefruit: increased tadalafil effect

NURSING CONSIDERATIONS
Assessment
• **Cialis:** assess for underlying cause of erectile dysfunction prior to treatment; organic nitrates that should not be used with this product; assess for severe loss of vision
• **Adcirca:** monitor hemodynamic parameters baseline and periodically

Patient/family education
• Teach patient to take 1 hr before sexual activity
• Teach patient not to drink large amounts of alcohol
• Advise that product does not protect against STDs, including HIV
• Instruct to tell physician if patient has a bleeding problem
• Advise that product should not be used with nitrates in any form
• Advise that product has no effect in the absence of sexual stimulation
• Instruct to seek medical help if an erection lasts more than 4 hr or if chest pain occurs
• Advise to notify physician of all medicines, vitamins, and herbs patient is taking, especially α-blockers, erythromycin, indinavir, itraconazole, ketoconazole, nitrates, ritonavir
• Advise that tadalafil is contraindicated for use with α-blockers except 0.4 mg/daily tamsulosin

Evaluation
Positive therapeutic outcome
• Sustainable erection
• Improvement in exercise ability (pulmonary hypertension)

⚠ HIGH ALERT

tamoxifen (Rx)
(ta-mox'i-fen)
Apo-Tamox ✦, **Soltamox, Tamofen** ✦,
Tamone ✦, **Tamoplex** ✦
Func. class.: Antineoplastic
Chem. class.: Antiestrogen
Pregnancy category D

ACTION: Inhibits cell division by binding to cytoplasmic estrogen receptors; resembles normal cell complex but inhibits DNA synthesis and estrogen response of target tissue

Therapeutic outcome: Prevention of rapidly growing malignant cells

USES: Advanced breast carcinoma that has not responded to other therapy in estrogen receptor–positive patients (usually postmenopausal), prevention of breast cancer, after breast surgery/radiation in ductal carcinoma in situ (DCIS)

Unlabeled uses: Mastalgia, pain/size of gynecomastia, ovulation stimulation, malignant carcinoid tumor, carcinoid syndrome, metaplastic melanoma, desmoid tumors, McCune-Albright syndrome (female pediatric patients)

CONTRAINDICATIONS
Pregnancy **D**, breastfeeding, hypersensitivity

> **BLACK BOX WARNING:** Thromboembolic disease

Precautions: Leukopenia, thrombocytopenia, cataracts, women of childbearing age

> **BLACK BOX WARNING:** Endometrial cancer, stroke

DOSAGE AND ROUTES
Breast cancer
Adult: PO 20-40 mg/day × 5 yr, doses >20 mg/day divide AM/PM

High risk for breast cancer
Adult: PO 20 mg/day × 5 yr

Ductal carcinoma in situ
Adult: PO 20 mg/day × 5 yr

McCune-Albright syndrome (unlabeled)
Child 2-10 yr (girls): PO 20 mg/day for up to 1 yr

Available forms: Tabs 10, 20 mg; oral solution 10 mg/5 ml

Implementation
• Do not break, crush, or chew tabs

• Give with food or fluids for GI upset; repeat dose may be needed if vomiting occurs
• Store in light-resistant container at room temperature
• Oral solution: use calibrated container; dose >20 mg/day should be divided morning and evening; may be used with food for gastric irritation

ADVERSE EFFECTS
CNS: *Hot flashes, headache, light-headedness,* depression, mood changes
CV: Chest pain, stroke, fluid retention, flushing
EENT: Ocular lesions, cataracts, retinopathy, corneal opacity, blurred vision (high doses)
GI: *Nausea, vomiting,* altered taste (anorexia)
GU: Vaginal bleeding, pruritus vulvae, uterine malignancies, *altered menses, amenorrhea*
HEMA: **Thrombocytopenia, leukopenia,** deep vein thrombosis
INTEG: *Rash,* alopecia
META: Hypercalcemia
RESP: **Pulmonary embolism**

Pharmacokinetics
Absorption	Adequately absorbed
Distribution	Unknown
Metabolism	Liver—extensively
Excretion	Feces—slowly, small amounts (kidneys)
Half-life	1 wk

Pharmacodynamics
Onset	Unknown
Peak	4-7 hr
Duration	Unknown

INTERACTIONS
Individual drugs
Aminoglutethimide, rifamycin: decreased tamoxifen levels
Bromocriptine: increased tamoxifen level
Letrozole: decreased levels of letrozole
PARoxetine: increased risk for death from breast cancer
Radiation: increased myelosuppression

Drug classifications
Anticoagulants: increased risk of bleeding
Cytotoxics: increased thromboembolic action
CYP2D6 inhibitors (antidepressants): decreased tamoxifen effect
CYP3A4 inducers (barbiturates, bosentan, carBAMazepine, efavirenz, phenytoin, nevirapine, rifabutin, rifampin): decreased tamoxifen effect
CYP3A4 inhibitors (aprepitant, antiretroviral protease inhibitors, clarithromycin, danazol, delavirdine, diltiazem, erythromycin,

T

Adverse effects: *italics* = common; **bold** = life-threatening

fluconazole, FLUoxetine, fluvoxaMINE, imatinib, ketoconazole, mibefradil, nefazodone, telithromycin, voriconazole): increased toxicity

Drug/herb
Black cohosh, dong quai, St. John's wort: avoid use

Drug/lab test
Increased: serum calcium, T_4, AST, ALT, cholesterol, triglycerides

NURSING CONSIDERATIONS
Assessment
• Monitor CBC, differential, platelet count weekly; withhold product if WBC is <4000/ mm^3 or platelet count is <75,000/mm^3; notify prescriber of results; monitor calcium levels (hypercalcemia is common); breast exam, mammogram, pregnancy test, bone mineral density, LFTs, serum calcium, serum lipid profile, periodic eye exams (cataracts, retinopathy)

⚠ **Assess for tumor flare: increase in bone, tumor pain during beginning treatment; give analgesics as ordered to decrease pain**

• **Assess for bleeding:** hematuria, guaiac, bruising or petechiae, mucosa or orifices q8hr, no rectal temp

> **BLACK BOX WARNING: Assess for uterine malignancies:** symptoms of stroke, PE that may occur in women with DCIS and women at high risk for breast cancer

Patient/family education
• **Teach patient to use nonhormonal contraception during treatment and for 2 months after discontinuing treatment**
• Teach patient to notify prescriber of stroke: blurred vision, headache, weakness on one side of the body; pulmonary embolism: chest pain, fainting sweating, difficulty breathing
• Instruct patient to report any complaints, side effects to prescriber; if dose is missed, do not double next dose; that use may be 5 yr
• Advise patient that vaginal bleeding, pruritus, hot flashes can occur and are reversible after discontinuing treatment
• **Instruct patient to report immediately decreased visual acuity, which may be irreversible; stress need for routine eye exams**
• Inform patient about who should be told about tamoxifen therapy
• Advise patient to report vaginal bleeding immediately; that tumor flare (increase in size or tumor, increased bone pain) may occur and will subside rapidly; may take analgesics for pain;

that premenopausal women must use mechanical birth control method because ovulation may be induced (teratogenic product)
• **Tumor flare: Advise patient that increase in size of tumor, increased bone pain may occur and will subside rapidly; may take analgesics for pain**
• Teach patient that hair loss may occur during treatment; a wig or hairpiece may make patient feel better; new hair may be different in color, texture
• Advise patient to increase fluids to 2 L/day unless contraindicated

Evaluation
Positive therapeutic outcome
• Decreased spread of malignant cells in breast cancer

---

tamsulosin (Rx)
(tam-sue-lo'sen)
Flomax
Func. class.: Selective α-adrenergic blocker, BPH agent
Chem. class.: Sulfamoyl phenethylamine derivative
Pregnancy category B

Do not confuse: Flomax/Fosamax/Volmax

ACTION: Binds preferentially to α IA-adrenoceptor subtype located mainly in the prostate

Therapeutic outcome: Decreased symptoms of benign prostatic hyperplasia (BPH)

USES: Symptoms of BPH

CONTRAINDICATIONS
Hypersensitivity

Precautions: Pregnancy **B,** breastfeeding, children, hepatic disease, CAD, severe renal disease, prostate cancer; cataract surgery (floppy iris syndrome)

DOSAGE AND ROUTES
Adult: PO 0.4 mg/day, increasing to 0.8 mg/day if required

Hepatic dose (moderate impairment)
Adult: PO reg rel 50 mg q8hr, titrate; ext rel 50 mg q24hr, titrate, max 100 mg q24hr; avoid use in severe impairment

Available forms: Caps 0.4 mg

Implementation
• Swallow caps whole; do not break, crush, or chew

- Store in airtight container at 86° F (30° C) or less
- Give without regard to food, but may be given with food to prevent GI symptoms; ½ hr after same meal each day
- If treatment is interrupted for several days, restart at lowest dose (0.4 mg/day)

ADVERSE EFFECTS

CNS: *Dizziness, headache,* asthenia, insomnia
CV: Chest pain, orthostatic hypotension
EENT: Amblyopia, floppy iris syndrome
GI: Nausea, diarrhea, dysgeusia
GU: Decreased libido, abnormal ejaculation, priapism
MS: Back pain
RESP: Rhinitis, pharyngitis, cough
SYST: Angioedema

Pharmacokinetics

Absorption	Well absorbed
Distribution	Not known; 98% plasma protein bound
Metabolism	Liver, extensively
Excretion	Kidneys
Half-life	9-15 hr

Pharmacodynamics

Unknown

INTERACTIONS
Individual drugs
Cimetidine: increased toxicity
Doxazosin, prazosin, terazosin, vardenafil: do not use together

Drug classifications
α-blockers: do not use together

Drug/food
Decreased: absorption with food

NURSING CONSIDERATIONS
Assessment
- Monitor CBC with differential and liver function tests; B/P and heart rate
- Monitor urodynamic studies/urinary flow rates, residual volume
- **Assess for BPH:** change in urinary patterns, baseline, throughout treatment; monitor I&O ratios, weight daily, edema, report weight gain or edema
- **Orthostatic hypotension:** monitor B/P standing, sitting

Patient/family education
- Teach patient not to discontinue product abruptly; emphasize the importance of complying with dosage schedule, even if feeling better;

if dose is missed take as soon as remembered; take at same time each day
- Teach patient not to use OTC products (cough, cold, allergy) unless directed by prescriber; also to avoid large amounts of caffeine
- Caution patient that product may cause dizziness, may occur during 1st few days of therapy; to avoid hazardous activities
- Teach patient to take ½ hr before same meal each day
- Teach patient about priapism (rare)
- Advise patient not to crush, break, chew caps

Evaluation

Positive therapeutic outcome
- Decreased symptoms of BPH

⚠ HIGH ALERT

tapentadol (Rx)
(ta-pen'ta-dol)
Nucynta, Nucynta ER
Func. class.: Analgesic, miscellaneous
Chem. class.: μ-Opioid receptor agonist
Pregnancy category C
Controlled substance schedule II

ACTION: Centrally acting synthetic analgesic; μ-opioid agonist activity is thought to result in analgesia; inhibits norepinephrine uptake

Therapeutic outcome: Relief of pain

USES: Moderate to severe pain

CONTRAINDICATIONS
Hypersensitivity, asthma, ileus

BLACK BOX WARNING: Respiratory depression

Precautions: Pregnancy **C**, breastfeeding, children <18 yr, increased intracranial pressure, MI (acute), severe heart disease, respiratory depression, renal/hepatic disease, GI obstruction, ulcerative colitis, sleep apnea, seizure disorder

BLACK BOX WARNING: Accidental exposure, avoid ethanol, substance abuse, neonatal opioid withdrawal/syndrome, potential for overdose, poisoning

DOSAGE AND ROUTES
Adult: PO 50-100 mg q4-6hr; may give second dose 1 hr or more after 1st dose; max 700 mg on day 1, 600 mg/day thereafter; ext rel 50 mg

q12hr (opioid-naive), titrate to 100-250 mg q12hr, max 250 mg q12hr

Hepatic disease
Adult: PO immediate rel/oral sol 50 mg q8hr; may titrate to response; ext rel 50 mg qday max 100 mg/day

Available forms: Tab 50, 75, 100 mg; tabs, ext rel 50, 100, 150, 200, 250 mg

Implementation
• Give with antiemetic if nausea, vomiting occur
• Give when pain is beginning to return; determine dosing interval by response
• Store in light-resistant area at room temperature
• Provide assistance with ambulation
• Provide safety measures: night-light, call bell within easy reach
• Not to crush, chew, break, or use with alcohol: ext rel product
• This is the preferred analgesic in those with altered cytochrome P450 or mild hepatic disease, mild to moderate renal disease

> **BLACK BOX WARNING:** These products have high potential for overdose, poisoning; may be fatal due to respiratory depression

ADVERSE EFFECTS
CNS: *Drowsiness, dizziness, confusion, headache, euphoria,* hallucinations, restlessness, syncope, anxiety, flushing, psychological dependence, insomnia, lethargy, tremor, **seizures**
CV: Palpitations, bradycardia, hypo/hypertension, orthostatic hypotension, sinus tachycardia
GI: *Nausea, vomiting, anorexia, constipation, cramps,* gastritis, dyspepsia, biliary spasms
GU: Urinary retention/frequency
INTEG: *Rash,* urticaria, diaphoresis, pruritus
RESP: Respiratory depression, cough
SYST: Anaphylaxis, infection, serotonin syndrome

Pharmacokinetics

Absorption	32%
Distribution	Protein binding 20%
Metabolism	Liver, extensively
Excretion	Urine 99%
Half-life	Terminal 4 hr

Pharmacodynamics

Onset	Unknown
Peak	Unknown
Duration	Unknown

INTERACTIONS
Individual drugs
Alcohol: increased effects with other CNS depressants

Drug classifications
Antipsychotics, opioids, sedatives/hypnotics, skeletal muscle relaxants: increased effects with other CNS depressants
MAOIs: increased toxicity
Serotonin-receptor agonists, SSRIs, SNRIs, tricyclics: increased serotonin syndrome

> **Black Box Warning:** Do not use with alcohol; fatal overdose may occur

Drug/herb
Kava, St. John's wort, valerian: increased sedative effect

NURSING CONSIDERATIONS
Assessment
• Monitor I&O ratio; check for decreasing output; may indicate urinary retention
• Assess CNS changes: dizziness, drowsiness, hallucinations, euphoria, LOC, pupil reaction
• Assess for allergic reactions: rash, urticaria, anaphylaxis
• **Serotonin syndrome:** Assess for increased heart rate, shivering, sweating, dilated pupils, tremors, high B/P, hyperthermia, headache, confusion; if these occur, stop product, administer a serotonin antagonist if needed

> **BLACK BOX WARNING:** Addiction risk, previous substance abuse before using extended-release product

> **BLACK BOX WARNING:** Identify if alcohol has been used before giving this product; may be fatal if used with tapentadol

> **BLACK BOX WARNING: Assess for respiratory dysfunction:** respiratory depression, character, rate, rhythm; notify prescriber if respirations are <10/min; also B/P, pulse

• **Assess for pain:** intensity, location, type, characteristics; need for pain medication by pain/sedation scoring; physical dependence

Patient/family education
• Teach patient to report any symptoms of CNS changes, allergic reactions
• Advise that physical dependency may result from extended use
• Inform that withdrawal symptoms may occur: nausea, vomiting, cramps, fever, faintness, anorexia

- Teach to avoid CNS depressants, alcohol
- Advise to avoid driving, operating machinery if drowsiness occurs

> **BLACK BOX WARNING:** Not to use with alcohol, may be fatal

Evaluation

Positive therapeutic outcome
- Decrease in pain

RARELY USED

tasimelteon
(tas'i-mel'tee-on)
Hetlioz
Func. class.: Anxiolytic/sedative/hypnotic
Pregnancy category C

USES: Sleep-wake disorder in the blind

CONTRAINDICATIONS: Hypersensitivity

DOSAGE AND ROUTES
Adult: **PO** 20 mg before bedtime at the same time every night; take without food

tavaborole topical
See Appendix B

tazobactam
See piperacillin/tazobactam

RARELY USED

tbo-filgrastim
(fil-gras'tim)
Neutrophil
Func. class.: Biologic modifier
Chem. class.: Short-acting granulocyte colony-stimulating factor (G-CSF)
Pregnancy category C

USES: Chemotherapy-induced neutropenia prophylaxis to reduce the duration of severe neutropenia in nonmyeloid malignancies

CONTRAINDICATIONS
Hypersensitivity

DOSAGE AND ROUTES
Adult: SUBCUT 5 mcg/kg/day

teduglutide
(te'due-gloo'tide)
Gattex
Func. class.: GI disorder agent
Chem. class.: Recombinant glucagonlike peptide-2 analog
Pregnancy category B

ACTION: Increases intestinal, portal blood flow, inhibits gastric acid secretion, decreases gastric motility

Therapeutic outcome: Increased absorption of nutrients

USES: Short bowel syndrome in patients who are dependent on parenteral support

Precautions: Pregnancy C, breastfeeding, diarrhea, pancreatitis, renal disease, electrolyte imbalances, GI obstruction, heart failure, neoplastic disease, bilary tract disease, cardiac disease, gastric cancer, GI disease

DOSAGE AND ROUTES
Adult: SUBCUT 0.05 mg/kg/day

Available forms: Powder for injection 5 mg

Implementation
SUBCUT route
- **Reconstitution:** Slowly inject the 0.5 ml of preservative-free sterile water for injection provided in the prefilled syringe into the vial; allow to stand for 30 sec and gently roll the vial between your palms for 15 sec; do not shake; allow to stand 2 min; if undissolved powder is present, roll the vial again until all material is dissolved; if the product remains undissolved after the second attempt, do not use; discard unused portion; use within 3 hr after reconstitution
SUBCUT injection
- Calculate dose, withdraw into a syringe, and give; do not use IV, IM; if a dose is missed, it should be given as soon as possible on the same day; two doses should not be given on the same day; alternate sites

ADVERSE EFFECTS
CNS: Headache, fatigue
GI: Nausea, abdominal pain, cholecystitis, cholestasis, **GI obstruction, pancreatitis,** vomiting

Pharmacokinetics

Absorption	Unknown
Distribution	Unknown
Metabolism	Unknown
Excretion	Unknown
Half-life	2 hr; 1.3 hr (short bowel syndrome)

Adverse effects: *italics* = common; **bold** = life-threatening

Pharmacodynamics

Onset	Unknown
Peak	Unknown
Duration	Unknown

INTERACTIONS
Individual drugs
Benzodiazepine, carBAMazepine, cycloSPORINE, digoxin, disopyramide, ethosuximide, flecainamide, lerothromixe, lithium, phenytoin, procainamide, quiNIDine, sirolimus, tacrolimus, theophylline, valproic acid, warfarin: increased absorption of each of these products

NURSING CONSIDERATIONS
Assessment
- GI symptoms: nausea, abdominal pain
- Monitor alk phos, amylase, bilirubin, serum electrolytes, lipase—baseline and q6mo

Patient/family education
- Instruct patient to notify prescriber of GI symptoms

Evaluation
Positive therapeutic outcome
- Increased absorption of nutrients

telaprevir
(tel-a′pre-vir)
Incivek
Func. class.: Antiviral, antihepatitis agent
Chem. class.: NS3/4A protease inhibitor
Pregnancy category B (alone); X (combination therapy)

ACTION: Prevents hepatitis C viral (HCV) replication by blocking the proteolytic activity of HCV NS3/4A serine protease; hepatitis C virus NS3/4A serine protease is an enzyme responsible for the conversion of HCV-encoded polyproteins to mature/functioning viral proteins. These proteins (NS4A, NS4B, NS5A, NS5B), are needed for viral replication.

Therapeutic outcome: Decreasing hepatitis C viral infection

USES: Chronic hepatitis C

CONTRAINDICATIONS
Pregnancy **X** in combination, male partners of women who are pregnant

Precautions: Breastfeeding, anemia, neutropenia, thrombocytopenia, HIV, hepatitis B, decompensated hepatic disease, in liver or other organ transplants, neonates, infants, children, adolescents <18 years of age

---

> **BLACK BOX WARNING:** Serious rash

DOSAGE AND ROUTES
For the treatment of chronic hepatitis C infection (genotype 1) in adults with compensated liver disease in patients without cirrhosis who are previously untreated or have relapsed after treatment with interferon and ribavirin therapy
Adult: PO 750 mg tid (q7-9hr) with peginterferon alfa and ribavirin; duration is determined by the patient's HCV RNA level at treatment wk 4, 12. If the HCV RNA is undetectable at wk 4, 12, give the three-drug regimen for 12 wk, then give an additional 12 wk of only peginterferon alfa and ribavirin (24 wk total); if the HCV RNA is detectable but ≤1000 international units/ml at wk 4, or 12, give the three-drug regimen for 12 wk, then an additional 36 wk of only peginterferon alfa and ribavirin (48 wk total)

Those without cirrhosis who are previously partial or null responders to interferon and ribavirin therapy/or those with cirrhosis
Adult: PO 750 mg tid (q7-9hr) with peginterferon alfa and ribavirin; give the three drug regimen for 12 wk, then another 36 wk (48 wk total) of only peginterferon alfa and ribavirin

Available forms: Tab 375 mg

Implementation
- Only use in combination with peginterferon alfa and ribavirin; never give as monotherapy
- Discontinue in hepatitis C virus (HCV) RNA concentrations ≥1000 international units/ml at wk 4 or 12 or a confirmed detectable HCV RNA concentration at wk 24
- Any contraindication to peginterferon alfa or ribavirin also applies to this product. See ribavirin monograph for additional information regarding contraindications and warnings associated with these products
- Give with food, not low-fat
- Store tabs at room temperature

ADVERSE EFFECTS
CNS: Fatigue
GI: Anorectal discomfort, diarrhea, dysgeusia, hemorrhoids, hyperbilirubinemia, nausea, pruritus ani, rectal burning, vomiting
HEMA: Anemia, decreased Hgb, leukopenia, lymphopenia, neutropenia, thrombocytopenia
INTEG: Drug reaction with eosinophilia and systemic symptoms (DRESS), pruritus, rash, Stevens-Johnson Syndrome (SJS); severe

---

⚠ Nurse Alert   ✴ Key NCLEX® Drug   >> Drug Specifics

rashes (bullous rash, skin ulcerations, and vesicular rash)
META: Increased uric acid

Pharmacokinetics

Absorption	Unknown
Distribution	59%-76% protein binding
Metabolism	Liver
Excretion	82% (feces)
Half-life	9-11 hr

Pharmacodynamics

Onset	Unknown
Peak	4-5 hrs
Duration	Unknown

INTERACTIONS
Individual drugs
Acetaminophen, alfentanil, aliskiren, almotriptan, alosetron, ALPRAZolam, aminophylline, amiodarone, amitriptyline, amLODIPine, ARIPiprazole, astemizole, atorvastatin, atorvastin, bepridil, boceprevir, bosentan, budesonide, bupivacaine, buprenorphine, busPIRone, carvedilol, cevimeline, chloroquine, cilostazol, cinacalcet, citalopram, clarithromycin, clomiPRAMINE, clonazePAM, clopidogrel, cloZAPine, colchicine, cyclobenzaprine, cycloSPORINE, dapsone, DAUNOrubicin, desipramine, desloratadine, dexamethasone, dexlansoprazole, dextromethorphan, diazepam, diclofenac, digoxin, diltiazem, disopyramide, disulfiram, DOCEtaxel, dolasetron, donepezil, DOXOrubicin, droperidol, dutasteride, ebastine, eletriptan, eplerenone, erlotinib, erythromycin, estazolam, eszopiclone, ethosuximide, etoposide, exemestane, felodipine, fentaNYL, fexofenadine, finasteride, flecainide, flunitrazepam, flurazepam, galantamine, gefitinib, glyburide, granisetron, halofantrine, haloperidol, HYDROcodone, ifosfamide, imipramine, indiplon, isradipine, irinotecan, itraconazole, ivermectin, ixabepilone, ketoconazole, lansoprazole, lidocaine, loperamide, loratadine, losartan, maraviroc, mefloquine, meloxicam, mirtazapine, mitoMYcin, montelukast, morphine, nateglinide, niCARdipine, NIFEdipine, nisoldipine, nortriptyline, omeprazole, ondansetron, oxybutynin, oxyCODONE, PACLitaxel, palonosetron, paricalcitol, plicamycin, posaconazole, prasugrel, praziquantel, propafenone, quazepam, QUEtiapine, quinacrine, quiNIDine, ramelteon, repaglinide, rifabutin, risperiDONE, ropivacaine, salmeterol, selegiline, sertraline, sibutramine, silodosin, sirolimus, sitaxsentan, solifenacin, SUFentanil, SUNItinib, tacrolimus, telithromycin, teniposide, terfenadine, testosterone, theophylline, tiagabine, tinidazole, tolterodine, tolvaptan, traMADol, traZODone, vardenafil, venlafaxine, verapamil, vinBLAStine, vinCRIStine, voriconazole, warfarin, and others: use cautiously; may need to reduce dose: increased effect, adverse reactions of each product

Alfuzosin, cisapride, ezetimibe, lovastatin, niacin with simvastatin and boceprevir, pimozide, simvastatin; oral midazolam, triazolam; sildenafil, tadalafil (pulmonary arterial hypertension): do not use concurrently; increased, life-threatening reactions of each product

Atazanavir, efavirenz, lopinavir with ritonavir, ritonavir: possible treatment failure

Drosperinone: increased hyperkalemia

Ethinyl estradiol: Decreased estrogen levels

Methadone: decreased effect of methadone

Drug classifications
CYP3A4 inhibitors (carBAMazepine, PHENobarbital, phenytoin, rifampin): decreased telaprevir effect

Ergots (dihydroergotamine, ergotamine, ergonovine, methylergonovine): do not use concurrently; increased, life-threatening reactions of each product

Phosphodiesterase type 5 (PDE5) inhibitors (for erectile dysfunction), systemic corticosteroids: use cautiously; may need to reduce dose: increased effect, adverse reactions of each product

Drug/herb
Do not use with St. John's wort

NURSING CONSIDERATIONS
Assessment
• **Pregnancy:** Pregnancy (X) combination therapy; obtain a pregnancy test prior to, monthly during, and for 6 months after treatment is completed; those who are not willing to practice strict contraception should not receive treatment with these products; report any cases of prenatal ribavirin exposure to the Ribavirin Pregnancy registry at (800) 593-2214
• **Anemia:** Monitor hemoglobin prior to, at treatment wks 4, 8, and 12, and as needed. If Hgb is less than 10 g/dl, decrease ribavirin dosage; if Hgb is less than 8.5 g/dl, discontinuation of therapy is recommended; telaprevir dosage should not be altered based on adverse reactions; Anemia may be managed through ribavirin dose modifications; never alter the dose of telaprevir. If anemia persists despite a reduction in ribavirin

dose, consider discontinuing telaprevir. If management of anemia requires permanent discontinuation of ribavirin, treatment with telaprevir must also be permanently discontinued. Once telaprevir has been discontinued, it must not be restarted; monitor CBC with differential at treatment wks 4, 8, 12, and at other treatment points as needed

> **BLACK BOX WARNING: Serious rash:**
> Assess for toxic epidermal necrolysis, Stevens-Johnson syndrome, eosinophilia, fever, mucosal skin erosion, mucosal ulceration, target lesions; if serious skin reaction occurs, immediately discontinue all components of the three-drug regimen and refer the patient for urgent medical care

• **Hepatitis C: Hepatitis C RNA baseline, wk 4 and 12**
• Thyroid function tests, LFTs, serum bilirubin/creatinine, BUN, bilirubin, serum electrolytes, serum uric acid, baseline and periodically during treatment

Patient/family education
• Teach patient that 3-drug regimen must be used, not to discontinue unless approved by prescriber
• Teach patient to take with food with fat for increased absorption
• Transmission of infection may still occur; use precautions
• Advise patient if dose is missed, take it within 6 hr of when dose should have been used; provide "Medication Guide"
• Teach patient to drink plenty of fluids to prevent dehydration
• Teach patient not to use other products (OTC, Rx, herbs, supplements) unless approved by prescriber
• **Instruct patient to use two forms of effective contraception (intrauterine devices and barrier methods) during treatment and for 6 months after treatment (pregnancy X), avoid breast feeding**

> **BLACK BOX WARNING:** If a serious skin reaction occurs, patients should be instructed to seek urgent medical care and all components of the triple-drug regimen must be discontinued immediately

Evaluation

Positive therapeutic outcome
• Decreasing hepatitis C viral infection, HCV-RNA level $\geq$ 1000 IU/ml at wk 4 and 12, confirm wk 24

telavancin (Rx)
(tel-a-van'sin)
Vibativ
Func. class.: Antiinfective—miscellaneous
Chem. class.: Lipoglycopeptide
Pregnancy category C

ACTION: Inhibits bacterial cell wall synthesis, disrupts cell membrane integrity, blocks glycopeptides

Therapeutic outcome: Negative culture

USES: Skin/skin structure infections caused by *Enterococcus faecalis*, *E. faecium*, *Staphylococcus aureus* (MSRA), *S. aureus* (MSSA), *S. epidermidis*, *S. haemolyticus*, *Streptococcus agalactiae* (group B), *S. dysgalactiae*, *S. pyogenes* (group A beta tremolytic), *S. anginosus*, *S. intermedius*, *S. constellates*, nosocomial pneumonia caused by susceptible gram-positive bacteria

CONTRAINDICATIONS
Hypersensitivity

Precautions: Breastfeeding, geriatric patients, renal disease, antimicrobial resistance, children, diabetes mellitus, diarrhea, GI disease, heart failure, hypertension, pseudomembranous colitis, QT prolongation, vancomycin hypersensitivity

> **BLACK BOX WARNING: Pregnancy C, females**

DOSAGE AND ROUTES
Complicated skin/skin structure infections
Adult: IV INF 10 mg/kg over 60 min q24hr × 7-14 days

Nosocomial pneumonia
Adult: IV INF 10 mg/kg q24hr × 7-21 days

Renal dose
Adult: IV CCr 30-50 ml/min 7.5 mg/kg q24hr; CCr 10-29 ml/min 10 mg/kg q48hr

Available forms: Lyophilized powder for inj 250, 750 mg

Implementation
• Use only for susceptible organisms to prevent drug-resistant bacteria
• Give antihistamine if red man syndrome occurs: decreased B/P, flushing of neck, face
• Store in refrigerator
• **Have EPINEPHrine, suction, tracheostomy set, endotracheal intubation equipment on unit; anaphylaxis may occur**

- Give adequate intake of fluids (2 L/day) to prevent nephrotoxicity
- Avoid IM, subcut use

Intermittent IV infusion route
- Administer after reconstituting with 15 ml D₅W sterile water for inj; 0.9% NaCl (15 mg/ml) 250 mg vial; add 45 ml to 750 mg vial (15 mg/ml) for dose of 150-800 mg; further dilute with 100-250 ml of compatible sol; for dose <150 mg or 800 mg, further dilute to a conc of 0.6-8 mg/ml with compatible sol; give over 60 min, **avoid rapid IV, may cause red man syndrome;** reconstituted or diluted solution is stable for 4 hr at room temperature, 7 hr refrigerated

Y-site compatibilities: Amphotericin B lipid complex (Abelcet), ampicillin-sulbactam, azithromycin, calcium gluconate, caspofungin, cefepime, cefTAZidime, cefTRIAXone, ciprofloxacin, dexamethasone, diltiazem, DOBUTamine, DOPamine, doripenem, doxycycline, ertapenem, famotidine, fluconazole, gentamicin, hydrocortisone, labetalol, magnesium sulfate, mannitol, meropenem, metoclopramide, milrinone, norepinephrine, ondansetron, pantoprazole, phenylephrine, piperacillin-tazobactam, potassium chloride/phosphates, ranitidine, sodium bicarbonate, sodium phosphates, tigecycline, tobramycin, vasopressin

ADVERSE EFFECTS
CNS: Anxiety, chills, flushing, headache, insomnia, dizziness
CV: QT prolongation, irregular heartbeat
EENT: Hearing loss
GI: Nausea, vomiting, pseudomembranous colitis, abdominal pain, constipation, diarrhea, metallic/soapy taste
GU: Nephrotoxicity, *increased BUN, creatinine,* renal failure, foamy urine
HEMA: Leukopenia, eosinophilia, anemia, thrombocytopenia
INTEG: Chills, fever, rash, thrombophlebitis at inj site, urticaria, pruritus, necrosis (red man syndrome)
SYST: Anaphylaxis, superinfection

Pharmacokinetics

Absorption	Unknown
Distribution	Unknown, protein binding 90%
Metabolism	Unknown, hepatic metabolism
Excretion	Urine 76%
Half-life	8-9 hr

Pharmacodynamics

Onset	Rapid
Peak	Unknown
Duration	Unknown

INTERACTIONS
Individual drugs
Adefovir, amphotericin B, bacitracin, cidofovir, CISplatin, colistin, cycloSPORINE, foscarnet, ganciclovir, IV pentamine acyclovir, pamidronate, polymyxin, streptozotocin, tacrolimus, zoledronic acid: increased toxicity, nephrotoxicity
Chloroquine, clarithromycin, dronedarone, droperidol, erythromycin, grepafloxacin, haloperidol, levomethadyl, methadone, pimozide, ziprasidone: increased QT prolongation

Drug classifications
Aminoglycosides, cephalosporins, nondepolarizing muscle relaxants: increased toxicity, nephrotoxicity
Class IA, III antidysrhythmics, some phenothiazines: increased QT prolongation

Drug/lab test
False increase: INR, PT, PTT

NURSING CONSIDERATIONS
Assessment
- Monitor I&O ratio; report hematuria, oliguria; nephrotoxicity may occur
- Monitor C&S throughout treatment
- Assess auditory function during, after treatment, hearing loss, ringing, roaring in ears; product should be discontinued
- **Pseudomembranous colitis: Monitor for diarrhea, fever, blood in stools, abdominal cramps; may be several weeks after therapy ends; report to prescriber immediately**

> **BLACK BOX WARNING:** Obtain a pregnancy test before use; if a woman has taken this product during pregnancy, the national registry should be notified at 866-658-4228

- **Anaphylaxis: Monitor for rash, itching, wheezing, laryngeal edema; discontinue and notify prescriber immediately; emergency equipment and EPINEPHrine should be nearby**
- Monitor B/P during administration; sudden drop may indicate red man syndrome; also flushing, pruritus, rash
- Assess respiratory status: rate, character, wheezing, tightness in chest

Patient/family education
• Teach all aspects of product therapy; culture may be taken after completed course of medication
• Advise patient to notify prescriber if infection continues
• That bitter taste, nausea, vomiting, headache may occur
• **Advise to report sore throat, fever, fatigue; could indicate superinfection; diarrhea (pseudomembranous colitis); hearing loss; rash, wheezing, tightness of chest, itching, tightening of throat (anaphylaxis)**
• **Teach patient to use contraception while taking this product; do not breastfeed; to notify prescriber if pregnancy is planned or suspected**

Evaluation

Positive therapeutic outcome
• Negative culture

---

telbivudine (Rx)
(tel-bi′vyoo-deen)
Sebivo ✦, Tyzeka
Func. class.: Antiretroviral
Chem. class.: Nucleoside reverse transcriptase inhibitor (NRTI)
Pregnancy category B

ACTION: Inhibits replication of HBV DNA polymerase, which inhibits HBV replication

Therapeutic outcome: Decreased hepatitis B serology

USES: Treatment of chronic hepatitis B

CONTRAINDICATIONS
Hypersensitivity, breastfeeding

Precautions: Pregnancy **B**, children, severe renal disease, anemia, organ transplant, dialysis, HIV, obesity, alcoholism; Hispanic or African descent (safety not established)

> **BLACK BOX WARNING:** Impaired hepatic function, lactic acidosis

DOSAGE AND ROUTES
Adult and adolescent >16 yr: PO 600 mg/day; max 600 mg/day

Renal dose
Adult: PO CCr 30-49 ml/min 600 mg tab q48hr or 400 mg oral sol/day; CCr <30 ml/min (not requiring dialysis) 600 mg tab q72hr or 200 mg oral sol/day

Available forms: Tabs 600 mg

Implementation
• Give with or without food with a full glass of water
• Store at room temperature

ADVERSE EFFECTS
CNS: *Fever, headache, malaise,* weakness, *dizziness, insomnia*
EENT: Taste change, hearing loss, photophobia
GI: *Nausea, vomiting, diarrhea, anorexia,* abdominal pain, hepatomegaly
INTEG: *Rash*
MISC: Lactic acidosis
MS: Myalgia, arthralgia, muscle cramps
RESP: Cough

Pharmacokinetics

Absorption	Unknown
Distribution	Steady state 5-7 days, protein binding 3.3%
Metabolism	Unknown
Excretion	Kidneys, unchanged
Half-life	Terminal 40-49 hr

Pharmacodynamics

Onset	Unknown
Peak	1-4 hr
Duration	Unknown

INTERACTIONS
Individual drugs
CycloSPORINE, erythromycin, hydrochloroquine, niacin, penicillamine, zidovudine, ZDV: increased myopathy risk
Do not use with pegylated interferon alfa-2a

Drug classifications
Any agent altering renal function: altered telbivudine levels
Azole antifungals, corticosteroids, fibric acid derivatives, HMG-CoA reductase inhibitors: increased myopathy risk

NURSING CONSIDERATIONS
Assessment

> **BLACK BOX WARNING:** Monitor liver function tests, hepatitis B serology, creatine kinase, periodically; monitor HBV DNA after 24 wk, if viral suppression is incomplete (≥300 copies/ml) start alternate therapy, monitor HBV DNA q6mo

---

Patient/family education

• Advise patient that GI complaints and insomnia may resolve after 3-4 wk of treatment
• Teach patient that product does not cure hepatitis B and does not stop the spread to others
• Teach patient that follow-up visits must be continued
• **Teach patient that serious product interactions may occur if OTC products are ingested; check with prescriber before taking**
• Advise patient that product may cause dizziness; avoid hazardous activities until response is known
• **Teach patient to report symptoms of cough, difficulty sleeping or excessive headache, muscle pain/weakness**
• **Teach patient to report progressive liver dysfunction: light-colored stools, dark urine, poor appetite, nausea, yellowing of skin, eyes**
• **Advise patient that product will not cure HBV, and precaution should be taken to protect others**

Evaluation

Positive therapeutic outcome
• Decreased hepatitis B serology

telmisartan (Rx)

(tel-mih-sar'tan)

Micardis

Func. class.: Antihypertensive
Chem. class.: Angiotensin II receptor (type AT$_1$)

Pregnancy category C (1st trimester) D (2nd/3rd trimesters)

ACTION: Blocks the vasoconstrictor and aldosterone-secreting effects of angiotensin II; selectively blocks the binding of angiotensin II to the AT$_1$ receptor found in tissues

Therapeutic outcome: Decreased B/P

USES: Hypertension, alone or in combination; stroke, MI prophylaxis (>55 yr) in those unable to take ACE inhibitors

Unlabeled uses: Heart failure, proteinuria in diabetic nephropathy

CONTRAINDICATIONS

Hypersensitivity

Precautions: Pregnancy **C** (1st trimester), breastfeeding, children, geriatric, hypersensitivity to angiotensin-converting enzyme (ACE) inhibitors, renal/hepatic disease, renal artery stenosis, dialysis, CHF, hyperkalemia, hypotension, hypovolemia, African descent

DOSAGE AND ROUTES

Adult: PO 40 mg/day; range 20-80 mg/day

Stroke, MI prophylaxis
Adult >55 yr: PO 80 mg/day

Available forms: Tabs 20, 40, 80 mg

Implementation

• Give without regard to meals
• Give increased dose to African American, Hispanic patients, B/P response may be reduced
• Do not remove from blister pack until ready to use

ADVERSE EFFECTS

CNS: Dizziness, insomnia, *anxiety,* headache, fatigue, syncope
GI: *Diarrhea,* dyspepsia, *anorexia, vomiting*
META: Hyperkalemia
MS: *Myalgia, pain*
RESP: *Cough, upper respiratory tract infection,* sinusitis, pharyngitis
SYST: **Angioedema**

Pharmacokinetics

Absorption	Unknown
Distribution	Highly protein bound
Metabolism	Liver, extensively
Excretion	Urine/feces
Half-life	Terminal 24 hr

Pharmacodynamics

Onset	3-hr
Peak	0.5-1 hr
Duration	Unknown

INTERACTIONS

Individual drugs
Digoxin: increased digoxin peak, trough concentrations

Drug classifications
ACE inhibitors, potassium-sparing diuretics, potassium salt substitutes: increased hyperkalemia
Antihypertensives, diuretics, NSAIDs: increased antihypertensive action

T

    Adverse effects: *italics* = common; **bold** = life-threatening

NSAIDs, salicylates: decreased antihypertensive effect

Drug/lab test
Increased: LFTs

NURSING CONSIDERATIONS
Assessment

BLACK BOX WARNING: Pregnancy test: if positive, stop treatment

• Monitor B/P, pulse q4hr; note rate, rhythm, quality; if severe hypotension occurs, place in supine position **IV** NS, usually occurs during first few weeks of treatment
• Monitor baselines in renal, electrolytes, liver function tests before therapy begins
• Assess edema in feet, legs daily
• Assess skin turgor, dryness of mucous membranes for hydration status
• **Overdose: dizziness, bradycardia or tachycardia**

Patient/family education
• Instruct patient to comply with dosage schedule, even if feeling better
• Advise patient to notify prescriber of mouth sores, fever, swelling of hands or feet, irregular heartbeat, chest pain
• Teach patient that excessive perspiration, dehydration, vomiting, diarrhea may lead to fall in blood pressure; consult prescriber if these occur
• Teach patient not to stop medication abruptly

BLACK BOX WARNING: Teach patient that product may cause dizziness, fainting; lightheadedness may occur; to avoid hazardous activities until response is known; to rise slowly from sitting to prevent drop in B/P

BLACK BOX WARNING: Advise patient to use contraception while taking this product, pregnancy category **D**, 2nd/3rd trimester

• Teach patient to notify prescriber of all prescriptions, OTC preparations, and supplements taken

Evaluation

Positive therapeutic outcome
• Decreased B/P

⚠ HIGH ALERT

temazepam (Rx)
(tem-az'a-pam)
Restoril
Func. class.: Sedative-hypnotic
Chem. class.: Benzodiazepine, short-intermediate acting
Pregnancy category X
Controlled substance schedule IV (USA), schedule F (Canada)

Do not confuse: Restoril/RisperDAL

ACTION: Produces CNS depression at limbic, thalamic, hypothalamic levels of the CNS; may be mediated by neurotransmitter γ-aminobutyric acid (GABA); results are sedation, hypnosis, skeletal muscle relaxation, anticonvulsant activity, anxiolytic action

Therapeutic outcome: Decreased insomnia

USES: Insomnia (short-term treatment, generally 7-10 days)

CONTRAINDICATIONS
Pregnancy **X,** breastfeeding, hypersensitivity to benzodiazepines

Precautions: Children <15 yr, geriatric, anemia, pulmonary/renal/hepatic disease, suicidal patients, product abuse, psychosis, acute closed-angle glaucoma, seizure disorders, angioedema, sleep-related behavior (sleep walking), COPD, dementia, myasthenia gravis, intermittent porphyria

DOSAGE AND ROUTES
Adult: PO 7.5-30 mg at bedtime
Geriatric: PO 7.5 mg at bedtime

Available forms: Caps 7.5, 15, 22.5, 30 mg

Implementation
• Without regard to food
• Give with food or milk to decrease GI symptoms; if patient is unable to swallow medication whole, tab may be crushed and mixed with foods or fluids
• Give sugarless gum, hard candy, frequent sips of water for dry mouth
• Store in tight container in cool environment
• 15-30 min before bedtime for sleeplessness

ADVERSE EFFECTS
CNS: *Lethargy, drowsiness, daytime sedation,* dizziness, confusion, light-headedness, headache, anxiety, irritability, complex sleep-related reactions (sleep driving, sleep eating), fatigue

---

CV: Chest pain, pulse changes, hypotension
EENT: Blurred vision
GI: Nausea, vomiting, diarrhea, heartburn, abdominal pain, constipation, anorexia
SYST: Severe allergic reactions

Pharmacokinetics

Absorption	Well absorbed
Distribution	Widely distributed, crosses placenta, crosses blood-brain barrier
Metabolism	Liver
Excretion	Kidneys, breast milk
Half-life	10-20 hr

Pharmacodynamics

Onset	½ hr
Peak	1-2 hr
Duration	6-8 hr

INTERACTIONS
Individual drugs
Alcohol: increased actions of both products
Cimetidine, disulfiram: increased effect of each specific product
Probenecid: increased effect of temazepam
Rifampin: decreased action of rifampin
Theophylline: decreased effects of theophylline

Drug classifications
Antacids: decreased effect of antacids
Contraceptives (oral): increased effect
CNS depressants: increased action of both products

Drug/herb
Chamomile, skullcap, valerian: increased CNS depression

Drug/food
Caffeine: decreased temazepam effect

Drug/lab test
Increased: AST/ALT
Decreased: radioactive iodine uptake
False increase: 17-OHCS

NURSING CONSIDERATIONS
Assessment
• Assess mental status: mood, sensorium, anxiety, affect, sleeping pattern (baseline, periodically), drowsiness, dizziness, especially geriatric; physical dependency, withdrawal symptoms: anxiety, panic attacks, agitation, orientation, headache, nausea, vomiting, muscle pain, weakness; indications of increasing tolerance and abuse

Patient/family education
• Inform patient that product may be taken with food, and that tab may be crushed or swallowed whole
• Advise patient not to use for everyday stress or longer than 3 mo unless directed by prescriber; not to take more than prescribed amount; may be habit forming; not to double or skip doses
• Caution patient to avoid OTC preparations unless approved by prescriber; alcohol and CNS depressants will increase CNS depression
• Advise patient to avoid driving, activities that require alertness, drowsiness may occur; to avoid alcohol ingestion or other psychotropic medications; to rise slowly or fainting may occur, especially in geriatric; that drowsiness may worsen at beginning of treatment
• Caution patient not to discontinue medication abruptly after long-term use; withdrawal symptoms include vomiting, cramping, tremors, seizures
• **Advise patient to use contraception while taking this product, to notify prescriber if pregnancy is planned or suspected, pregnancy X**
• Advise patient that complex sleep-related behavior may occur (sleep driving/eating)
• Teach patient to limit to 7-10 days continuous use

Evaluation
Positive therapeutic outcome
• Decreased anxiety, restlessness, sleeplessness (short-term treatment only)

TREATMENT OF OVERDOSE:
Lavage, VS, supportive care

⚠ HIGH ALERT

temozolomide (Rx)
(tem-oo-zole′oo-mide)
Temodar
Func. class.: Antineoplastic alkylating agents
Chem. class.: Imidazotetrazine derivative
Pregnancy category D

ACTION: A proproduct that undergoes conversion to 5-(3-methyl-1-triazeno) imidazole-4-carboxamide (MTIC); MTIC action prevents DNA transcription

Therapeutic outcome: Prevention of rapidly growing malignant cells

USES: Anaplastic astrocytoma with relapse, glioblastoma multiforme, malignant glioma

Adverse effects: *italics* = common; **bold** = life-threatening

Unlabeled uses: Metastatic melanoma

CONTRAINDICATIONS

Pregnancy **D**, breastfeeding, hypersensitivity to this product, carbazine, or gelatin

Precautions: Radiation therapy, renal/hepatic disease, bone marrow suppression, infection, geriatric, myelosuppression

DOSAGE AND ROUTES
Anaplastic astrocytoma
Adult: PO adjust dose based on nadir neutrophil and platelet counts 150 mg/m²/day × 5 days during 28-day cycle

Glioblastoma multiforme
Adult: PO/IV 75 mg/m²/day × 42 days with focal radiotherapy, then maintenance of 6 cycles

Malignant glioma
Adult: 150 mg/m²/day over 90 min day 1-5, q28day; may increase to 200 mg/m²/day on day 1-5, q28day if hematologic parameters permit

Available forms: Caps 5, 20, 100, 140, 180, 250 mg; powder for inj 100 mg

Implementation
PO route
• Give fluids IV or PO before chemotherapy to hydrate patient
• Give antiemetic 30-60 min before giving product to prevent vomiting, and prn; antibiotics for prophylaxis of infection
• **Capsules should not be opened; if accidentally damaged, do not allow contact with skin, or inhale; take caps one at a time with 8 oz of water at the same time of day; use cytotic handling procedure**
• Give on empty stomach at bedtime to prevent nausea/vomiting
• Store in light-resistant container in a dry area

IV route
• Bring vial to room temperature, discard if cloudy
• Inject 41 ml sterile water for inj into vial (2.5 mg/ml)
• Gently swirl, do not shake
Intermittent IV infusion route
• Withdraw up to 40 ml from each vial to make total dose and transfer to empty 250 ml PVC inf bag, flush before and after inf
• Run over 90 min
• Use reconstituted sol within 14 hr including inf time
• Do not admix

ADVERSE EFFECTS
CNS: Seizures, hemiparesis, dizziness, poor coordination, amnesia, insomnia, paresthesia, somnolence, paresis, ataxia, anxiety, dysphagia, depression, confusion
GI: Nausea, anorexia, vomiting, abdominal pain, constipation
GU: Urinary incontinence, UTI, frequency
HEMA: Thrombocytopenia, leukopenia, anemia, myelosuppression, neutropenia
INTEG: Rash, pruritus
MISC: Headache, fatigue, asthenia, fever, edema, back pain, weight increase, diplopia
RESP: Upper respiratory tract infection, pharyngitis, sinusitis, coughing
SYST: Anaphylaxis, secondary malignancy

Pharmacokinetics

Absorption	Rapid, complete
Distribution	Crosses blood-brain barrier
Metabolism	To MTIC and metabolite
Excretion	Urine, feces
Half-life	1.8 hr

Pharmacodynamics

Onset	Unknown
Peak	1 hr
Duration	Unknown

INTERACTIONS
Individual drugs
Digoxin: decreased action of digoxin
Radiation: increased toxicity, bone marrow suppression

Drug classifications
Anticoagulants, NSAIDs, platelet inhibitors, thrombolytics: increased bleeding risk
Antineoplastics: increased bone marrow suppression
Live virus vaccines, toxoids: increased adverse reactions, decreased antibody reaction

Drug/food
Decreased drug absorption

Drug/lab test
Decreased: Hgb, platelets, WBC, neutrophils

NURSING CONSIDERATIONS
Assessment
• Assess symptoms indicating severe allergic reaction: rash, pruritus, urticaria, purpuric skin lesions, itching, flushing; product should be discontinued
• Assess tumor response during treatment
• **Obtain CBC on day 22 (21 days after 1st dose), CBC weekly until recovery if ANC is <1.5 × 10⁹/L and platelets <100 × 10⁹/L, do not administer to patients that do not tolerate 100 mg/m²; myelosuppression usually occurs late in the treatment cycle**

• Assess for seizures, mental status throughout treatment
• Monitor renal function studies: BUN, creatinine, urine CCr before, during therapy; I&O ratio; report fall in urine output to <30 ml/hr
• Monitor temp q4hr (may indicate beginning of infection)
• **Monitor liver function tests before, during therapy (bilirubin, AST, ALT, LDH) as needed or monthly; note jaundice of skin or sclera, dark urine, clay-colored stools, itchy skin, abdominal pain, fever, diarrhea; hepatotoxicity can be serious and fatal**
• Assess for bleeding: hematuria, stool guaiac, bruising or petechiae, mucosa or orifices; check for inflammation of mucosa, breaks in skin

Patient/family education
• Teach patient to avoid use of products containing aspirin or NSAIDs, razors, commercial mouthwash, since bleeding may occur; to report symptoms of bleeding (hematuria, tarry stools)
• Instruct patient to report signs of anemia (fatigue, headache, irritability, faintness, shortness of breath)
• Caution patient not to have any vaccinations without the advice of prescriber; serious reactions can occur
• **Advise patient contraception is needed during treatment and for several months after completion of therapy; product has teratogenic properties, pregnancy D, not to breastfeed**

Evaluation

Positive therapeutic outcome
• Prevention of rapid division of malignant cells

RARELY USED

temsirolimus (Rx)
(tem-sir-oh′li-mus)
Torisel
Func. class.: Biological response modifier
Chem. class.: Kinase inhibitor, mTOR antagonist
Pregnancy category D

CONTRAINDICATIONS
Pregnancy **D**, breastfeeding, hypersensitivity to this product or to sirolimus, polysorbate 80

Precautions: Children <13 yr, females, severe pulmonary/renal/hepatic disease (bilirubin >1-1.5 × ULN or AST > ULN, but bilirubin ≤ULN), diabetes mellitus, hyperkalemia, hyperuricemia, hypertension, bone marrow suppression, hypertriglyceridemia/hyperlipidemia, surgery, brain tumor

DOSAGE AND ROUTES
Adult: IV 25 mg over 30-60 min qwk; treat until disease progression or severe toxicity occurs

Hepatic dose
Adult: IV (mild impairment) (bilirubin >1-1.5 × ULN or AST > ULN but bilirubin ≤ ULN)

⚠ HIGH ALERT

tenecteplase (TNK-tPA) (Rx)
(ten-ek′ta-place)
TNKase
Func. class.: Thrombolytic
Chem. class.: Tissue plasminogen activator
Pregnancy category C

ACTION: Activates conversion of plasminogen to plasmin (fibrinolysin): plasmin breaks down clots (fibrin), fibrinogen, factors V, VII; occlusion of venous access lines

Therapeutic outcome: Resolution of MI

USES: Acute MI, coronary artery thrombosis

CONTRAINDICATIONS
Hypersensitivity, arteriovenous malformation, aneurysm, active bleeding, intracranial, intraspinal surgery or trauma within 2 mo, CNS neoplasms, severe hypertension, severe renal disease, hepatic disease, history of CVA, increased ICP, stroke

Precautions: Pregnancy **C**, breastfeeding, children, geriatric, arterial emboli from left side of heart, hypocoagulation, subacute bacterial endocarditis, rheumatic valvular disease, cerebral embolism/thrombosis/hemorrhage, intraarterial diagnostic procedure or surgery (10 days), recent major surgery, dysrhythmias, hypertension

DOSAGE AND ROUTES
Total dose, max 50 mg, based on patient's weight
Adult <60 kg: IV BOL 30 mg, give over 5 sec
Adult 60-70 kg: IV BOL 35 mg, give over 5 sec
Adult 70-80 kg: IV BOL 40 mg, give over 5 sec
Adult 80-90 kg: IV BOL 45 mg, give over 5 sec
Adult ≥90 kg: IV BOL 50 mg, give over 5 sec, max 50 mg total dose

Available forms: Powder for inj, lyophilized 50 mg

Implementation

Intermittent IV infusion route
• Give as soon as thrombi are identified; not useful for thrombi >1 wk old

T

- Administer cryoprecipitate or fresh frozen plasma if bleeding occurs
- Give heparin after fibrinogen level >100 mg/dl; heparin inf to increase PTT to 1.5-2 × baseline for 3-7 days; **IV** heparin with loading dose is recommended
- Aseptically withdraw 10 ml of sterile water for inj from diluent vial, use red cannula syringe-filling device, inject all contents of syringe into product vial, direct into powder, swirl, withdraw correct dose, discard any unused sol; stand the shield with dose vertically on flat surface and passively recap the red cannula; remove entire shield assembly by twisting counterclockwise; give by **IV** bol
- **IV** therapy: use upper extremity vessel that is accessible to manual compression
- Provide bed rest during entire course of treatment
- Avoid venous or arterial puncture, inj, rectal temp, any invasive test
- Treat fever with acetaminophen or aspirin
- Apply pressure for 30 sec to minor bleeding sites; inform prescriber if this does not attain hemostasis; apply pressure dressing

ADVERSE EFFECTS

CV: Dysrhythmias, hypotension, pulmonary edema, **pulmonary embolism, cardiogenic shock, cardiac arrest, heart failure, myocardial reinfarction, myocardial rupture, tamponade, pericarditis, pericardial effusion, thrombosis, CVA**

HEMA: Decreased Hct, bleeding

INTEG: Rash, urticaria, phlebitis at **IV** inf site, itching, flushing

SYST: GI, GU, intracranial, retroperitoneal bleeding, surface bleeding, anaphylaxis

Pharmacokinetics

Absorption	Unknown
Distribution	Unknown
Metabolism	Liver
Excretion	Unknown
Half-life	20-24 min

Pharmacodynamics

Onset	Immediate
Peak	Unknown
Duration	Unknown

INTERACTIONS
Individual drugs

Aspirin, cefamandole, cefoperazone, cefoTEtan, clopidogrel, dipyridamole, indomethacin, phenylbutazone, ticlopidine: increased bleeding potential

Drug classifications

Anticoagulants, antithrombolytics, glycoprotein IIb, IIIa inhibitors, NSAIDs, SNRIs, SSRIs: increased bleeding

Drug/herb

Anise, basil, dong quai, fenugreek, feverfew, garlic, ginger, ginkgo, ginseng, green tea, horse chestnut: increased risk of bleeding

Drug/lab test

Increased: INR, PT, PTT

NURSING CONSIDERATIONS
Assessment

- **Assess for allergy:** fever, rash, itching, chills; mild reaction may be treated with antihistamines
- ⚠ **Assess for bleeding during 1st hr of treatment; hematuria, hematemesis, bleeding from mucous membranes, epistaxis, ecchymosis; may require transfusion (rare), continue to assess for bleeding for 24 hr**
- Monitor blood tests (Hct, platelets, PTT, protime, TT, aPTT) before starting therapy; protime or aPTT must be less than 2 × control before starting therapy; PTT or pro-time q3-4hr during treatment
- ⚠ **Cholesterol embolism: assess for blue-toe syndrome, renal failure, MI, cerebral/spinal cord/bowel/retinal infarction, hypertension; can be fatal**
- Assess for hypersensitive reactions: fever, rash, dyspnea; product should be discontinued
- Monitor VS, B/P, pulse, respirations, neurologic signs, temp at least q4hr; temp >104° F (40° C) indicates internal bleeding; systolic pressure increase >25 mm Hg should be reported to prescriber
- ⚠ **Assess for neurologic changes that may indicate intracranial bleeding**
- ⚠ **Assess for retroperitoneal bleeding: back pain, leg weakness, diminished pulses**

Patient/family education

- **Teach patient to notify prescriber immediately of severe headache**
- Advise patient to notify prescriber of bleeding, hypersensitivity, fast, slow, or uneven heart rate, feeling of fainting, blood in urine/stools, nose bleeds
- Teach patient about proper dental care to avoid bleeding

Evaluation

Positive therapeutic outcome

- Resolution of myocardial infarction

⚠ Nurse Alert   ✳ Key NCLEX® Drug   ≫ Drug Specifics

tenofovir (Rx)
(ten-oh-foh'veer)
Viread
Func. class.: Antiretroviral
Chem. class.: Nucleoside reverse transcriptase inhibitor (NRTI)
Pregnancy category B

ACTION: Inhibits replication of HIV-1 virus by competing with the natural substrate and then incorporating into cellular DNA by viral reverse transcriptase, thereby terminating cellular DNA chain

Therapeutic outcome: Improved symptoms of HIV-1 infection

USES: HIV-1 infection with at least 2 other antiretrovirals, hepatitis B

CONTRAINDICATIONS
Hypersensitivity

> **BLACK BOX WARNING:** Lactic acidosis

Precautions: Pregnancy **B**, breastfeeding, children, geriatric, renal disease, hepatic insufficiency, CCr <60 ml/min, osteoporosis, immune reconstitution syndrome

> **BLACK BOX WARNING:** Hepatic disease, hepatitis

DOSAGE AND ROUTES
Adult: PO 300 mg with meal; if used with didanosine, give tenofovir 2 hr before or 1 hr after didanosine

Renal dose
Adult: PO CCr 30-49 ml/min 300 mg q48hr; CCr 10-29 ml/min 300 mg q72-96hr; CCr <10 ml/min not recommended
Child ≥2 yr: PO 8 mg/kg/day approximate; ≥35 kg 300 mg/day; 28-34 kg 250 mg/day; 22-27 kg 200 mg/day; 17-21 kg 150 mg/day

Available forms: Tabs 150, 200, 250, 300 mg; oral powder 40 mg/scoop

Implementation
• Administer PO without regard to meals
• Store at 25° C (77° F)
• Give product 2 hr before or 1 hr after taking didanosine (if used)
• Oral powder: use scoop provided, mix powder into 2-4 oz (¼-½ cup) of applesauce or yogurt, do not mix with liquid, product will not mix; product is bitter; use immediately after mixing, clean scoop

ADVERSE EFFECTS
CNS: *Headache,* asthenia
GI: *Nausea, vomiting, diarrhea,* anorexia, *flatulence, abdominal pain,* **pancreatitis**
GU: **Renal failure, renal tubular acidosis/ necrosis, Fanconi syndrome**
HEMA: **Neutropenia, osteopenia**
INTEG: *Rash,* **angioedema**
META: **Lactic acidosis,** hypokalemia, hypophosphatemia
MS: *Myopathy,* **rhabdomyolysis**
SYST: Lipodystrophy

Pharmacokinetics
Absorption	Rapidly absorbed
Distribution	Extravascular space; bound to serum plasma <0.7%, to serum proteins <7.2%
Metabolism	Unknown
Excretion	Urine, unchanged (70%-80%)
Half-life	Terminal 17 hr

Pharmacodynamics
Onset	Unknown
Peak	1-2 hr
Duration	Unknown

INTERACTIONS
Individual drugs
Acyclovir, cidofovir, ganciclovir, valacyclovir, valganciclovir: increased level of tenofovir
Didanosine: increased level of didanosine when coadministered with tenofovir

Drug classifications
Increased: levels of tenofovir with any product that decreases renal function

NURSING CONSIDERATIONS
Assessment
• Monitor viral load, CD4+ T cell count, plasma HIV RNA, serum creatinine/BUN/phosphate

> **BLACK BOX WARNING: Hepatitis exacerbations:** Monitor resistance testing at start of therapy and at treatment failure

• Assess liver function tests: AST, ALT, bilirubin; amylase, lipase, triglycerides periodically during treatment
• Assess for bone, renal toxicity: if bone abnormalities are suspected, obtain tests: serum phosphorus, creatinine

T

Adverse effects: *italics* = common; **bold** = life-threatening

BLACK BOX WARNING: Lactic acidosis, severe hepatomegaly with steatosis: Obtain baseline LFTs, if elevated discontinue treatment; discontinue even if LFTs are normal but lactic acidosis, hepatomegaly are present, may be fatal

Patient/family education

• Instruct patient to take this product 2 hr before or 1 hr after taking didanosine (if used)
• Instruct patient to take product with meal
• Advise patients that GI complaints resolve after 3-4 wk of treatment
• **Caution patient not to breastfeed while taking this product**
• Inform patient that product must be taken daily even if patient feels better
• Advise patient to continue follow-up visits since serious toxicity may occur; blood counts must be done q2wk
• Inform patient that product controls symptoms but is not a cure for HIV; patient is still infectious, may pass HIV virus on to others
• Advise patient that other products may be necessary to prevent other infections
• Advise patient that changes in body fat distribution may occur

BLACK BOX WARNING: ⚠ Lactic acidosis: teach patient symptoms of lactic acidosis, to notify prescriber

Evaluation

Positive therapeutic outcome

• Decrease in signs/symptoms of HIV

terazosin (Rx)

(ter-ay'zoe-sin)
Func. class.: Antihypertensive
Chem. class.: α-Adrenergic blocker (peripherally acting)
Pregnancy category C

ACTION: Peripheral blood vessels are dilated, peripheral resistance is lowered; reduction in blood pressure results from α-adrenergic receptors being blocked

Therapeutic outcome: Decreased B/P in hypertension, decreased symptoms of benign prostatic hyperplasia (BPH)

USES: Hypertension, as a single agent or in combination with diuretics or β-blockers, BPH

CONTRAINDICATIONS

Hypersensitivity

Precautions: Pregnancy **C**, breastfeeding, children, prostate cancer, renal disease, syncope

DOSAGE AND ROUTES

Hypertension

Adult: PO 1 mg at bedtime, may increase dosage slowly to desired response; max 20 mg/day divided q12hr

Benign prostatic hyperplasia

Adult: PO 1 mg at bedtime, gradually increase up to 5-10 mg, max 20 mg divided q12hr

Available forms: Caps 1, 2, 5, 10 mg

Implementation

• May be used in combination with other antihypertensives
• Give at same time each day
• May be given with food to prevent GI symptoms
• Store in airtight container at 86° F (30° C) or less
• If treatment is interrupted for several days, restart with initial dose
• Give without regard to food
• Feeding tube: place cap in 60 ml of warm tap water, stir until liquid spills from ruptured shell (5 min), stir until cap dissolves, draw solution into oral syringe, give through feeding tube, flush with water

ADVERSE EFFECTS

CNS: *Dizziness, headache, drowsiness,* anxiety, depression, vertigo, weakness, fatigue, syncope
CV: *Palpitations, orthostatic hypotension,* tachycardia, *edema,* rebound hypertension
EENT: Blurred vision, epistaxis, tinnitus, dry mouth, red sclera, nasal congestion, sinusitis
GI: *Nausea,* vomiting, diarrhea, constipation, abdominal pain
GU: Urinary frequency, incontinence, impotence, priapism
RESP: Dyspnea, cough, pharyngitis

Pharmacokinetics

Absorption	Well absorbed
Distribution	Not known
Metabolism	Liver (50%)
Excretion	Kidneys unchanged (10%), feces unchanged (20%)
Half-life	9-12 hr

Pharmacodynamics

Onset	15 min
Peak	2-3 hr
Duration	24 hr

INTERACTIONS
Individual drugs
Alcohol, nitroglycerin, verapamil: increased hypotensive effects, not to drink alcohol

Drug classifications
Antihypertensives (other): increased hypotension
β-Blockers: increased hypotensive effects
Estrogens, NSAIDs, salicylates, sympathomimetics: decreased antihypertensive effect

Drug/herb
Hawthorn: increased antihypertensive effect
Ephedra: decreased antihypertensive effect

NURSING CONSIDERATIONS
Assessment
• **Hypertension:** monitor B/P, orthostatic hypotension, syncope; check for edema in feet, legs daily; I&O ratio; weight daily; notify prescriber of changes
• **Benign prostatic hyperplasia (BPH):** assess urinary patterns (hesitancy, frequency, change in stream, dribbling, dysuria, urgency)

Patient/family education
• Caution patient not to discontinue product abruptly; the importance of complying with dosage schedule, even if feeling better; if dose is missed take as soon as remembered; take medication at same time each day
• Teach patient not to use OTC products (cough, cold, allergy) unless directed by prescriber; to avoid large amounts of caffeine
• Emphasize the need to rise slowly to sitting or standing position to minimize orthostatic hypotension
• Teach patient to notify prescriber of mouth sores, sore throat, fever, swelling of hands or feet, irregular heartbeat, chest pain
• Caution patient to report excessive perspiration, dehydration, vomiting, diarrhea; may lead to fall in B/P
• Caution patient that product may cause dizziness, fainting, light-headedness; may occur during 1st few days of therapy; to avoid hazardous activities
• **Hypertension:** teach patient how to take B/P and normal readings for age group; to take B/P q7day; to continue with regimen including diet and exercise

Evaluation
Positive therapeutic outcome
• Decreased B/P in hypertension
• Decreased symptoms of BPH

TREATMENT OF OVERDOSE:
Administer volume expanders or vasopressors; discontinue product; place patient in supine position

---

terbinafine (Rx)
(ter-bin'a-feen)
LamISIL
Func. class.: Antifungal, systemic
Chem. class.: Synthetic allylamine derivative
Pregnancy category B

Do not confuse: LamISIL/LaMICtal/lamoTRIgine

ACTION: Interferes with cell membrane permeability in fungi such as *Trichophyton rubrum, Trichophyton mentagrophytes, Trichophyton tonsurans, Epidermophyton floccosum, Microsporum canis, Microsporum audouinii, Microsporum gypseum, Candida,* broad-spectrum antifungal

Therapeutic outcome: Resolution of fungal infection

USES: Onychomycosis of the toenail or fingernail due to dermatophytes, tinea capitis/corporis/cruris/pedis/versicolor

Unlabeled uses: Cutaneous candidiasis, tinea versicolor

CONTRAINDICATIONS
Hypersensitivity

Precautions: Pregnancy **B**, breastfeeding, children, chronic/active renal/hepatic disease GFR ≤50 mg/min, immunosuppression

DOSAGE AND ROUTES
Adult: PO 250 mg/day × 6 wk (fingernail); × 12 wk (toenail)

Available forms: Tabs 250 mg; oral granules 125, 187.5 mg

Implementation
• **PO:** give without regard to food
• **Granules:** take with food, sprinkle packet contents on pudding or non-acidic soft food, swallow without chewing, do not use fruit-based foods
• Store at 25° C (77° F), protect from light

ADVERSE EFFECTS
CNS: Depression
EENT: Tinnitus, hearing impairment
GI: Diarrhea, dyspepsia, abdominal pain, nausea, **hepatitis**
HEMA: Neutropenia

INTEG: Rash, pruritus, urticaria, Stevens-Johnson syndrome, photosensitivity
MISC: Headache, hepatic enzyme changes, taste, visual/olfactory disturbance

Pharmacokinetics

Absorption	80%
Distribution	Extensive, most to hair, scalp, nails; excreted in breast milk; protein binding 99%
Metabolism	Liver, extensively
Excretion	Unknown
Half-life	22 days or longer

Pharmacodynamics

Onset	Up to 1 wk
Peak	Several days-weeks
Duration	Several weeks

INTERACTIONS
Individual drugs
Atomoxetine: decreased metabolism of atomoxetine
Cimetidine: increased effect
CycloSPORINE: increased cycloSPORINE clearance
Dextromethorphan: increased levels
Rifampin: increased terbinafine clearance

Drug/herb
Cola nut, guarana, yerba maté, tea (black, green), coffee: side effects

Drug/lab test
Increased: LFTs

NURSING CONSIDERATIONS
Assessment
• Assess hepatic studies (ALT, AST) before beginning treatment; do not use in presence of hepatic disease
• Monitor CBC in treatment >6 wk
• Assess for continuing infection

Patient/family education
• Teach patient to notify prescriber of nausea, vomiting, fatigue, jaundice, dark urine, clay-colored stool, RUQ pain, that may indicate hepatic dysfunction
• Teach patient to avoid using OTC medication unless approved by prescriber
• Teach patient that treatment may take 10 wk (toenail), 4 wk (fingernail)

Evaluation

Positive therapeutic outcome
• Decrease in size, number of lesions

terbinafine topical
See Appendix B

terbutaline (Rx)
(ter-byoo'ta-leen)
Bricanyl ✤
Func. class.: Selective β$_2$-agonist; bronchodilator
Chem. class.: Catecholamine
Pregnancy category B

Do not confuse: terbutaline/TOLBUTamide/terbinafine

ACTION: Relaxes bronchial smooth muscle by direct action on β$_2$-adrenergic receptors through accumulation of cyclic AMP at β-adrenergic receptor sites; results are bronchodilatation, diuresis, and CNS and cardiac stimulation; relaxes uterine smooth muscle

Therapeutic outcome: Bronchodilatation with ease of breathing

USES: Bronchospasm

Unlabeled uses: Premature labor

CONTRAINDICATIONS
Hypersensitivity to sympathomimetics; closed-angle glaucoma, tachydysrhythmias

Precautions: Pregnancy **B**, breastfeeding, geriatric, cardiac disorders, hyperthyroidism, diabetes mellitus, prostatic hypertension, hypertension, seizure disorder

> **BLACK BOX WARNING:** Labor

DOSAGE AND ROUTES
Bronchospasm
Adult and child >12 yr: PO 2.5-5 mg q8hr; SUBCUT 0.25 mg q15-30min, max 0.5 mg in 4 hr
Adolescent ≤15 yr and child ≥12 yr: PO 2.5 mg tid, max 7.5 mg/day

Renal dose
Adult: PO CCr 10-50 ml/min 50% of dose; CCr <10 ml/min avoid use

Severe renal failure
Adult: PO avoid if GFR <10 ml/min

Tocolytic (preterm labor) (unlabeled)
Adult: SUBCUT 0.25 mg q20min to 6 hr, hold if pulse >120 bpm

Available forms: Tabs 2.5, 5 mg; inj 1 mg/ml

Implementation
• Use this medication before other medications and allow 5 min between each to prevent overstimulation

---

PO route
• Give PO with meals to decrease gastric irritation; tab may be crushed and mixed with food or fluid

SUBCUT route
• May give by SUBCUT route; do not give by IM route

Aerosol route
• Give after shaking; ask patient to exhale, place mouthpiece in mouth, then inhale slowly; hold breath, remove, exhale slowly; allow at least 1 min between inhalations
• Store in light-resistant container, do not expose to temperatures over 86° F (30° C)

IV route
• Give at 5 mcg q10min until contractions are stopped; use inf pump for correct dose; after ½-1 hr with no contraction decrease dose by 5 mcg; switch to PO dose when possible

Y-site compatibilities: Regular insulin

ADVERSE EFFECTS
CNS: Tremors, anxiety, insomnia, headache, dizziness, stimulation
CV: Palpitations, tachycardia, hypertension, dysrhythmias, **cardiac arrest, QT prolongation**
GI: Nausea, vomiting
META: Hypokalemia, hyperglycemia
RESP: Paradoxical bronchospasm, dyspnea

Pharmacokinetics

Absorption	Well absorbed (SUBCUT), partially absorbed (PO)
Distribution	Unknown
Metabolism	Liver, partially
Excretion	Unknown
Half-life	PO 3-4 hr, subcut 5-7 hr

Pharmacodynamics

	PO	INH	SUB-CUT	IV
Onset	½ hr	5-15 min	10-15 min	Rapid
Peak	1-2 hr	1-2 hr	½-1 hr	Unknown
Duration	4-8 hr	4-6 hr	1½-4 hr	Unknown

INTERACTIONS
Individual drugs
Arsenic trioxide, chloroquine, droperidol, haloperidol, levomethadyl, pentamidine: increased QT prolongation

Drug classifications
Beta agonists, class IA/III antidysrhythmics, CYP3A4 inhibitors (amiodarone, **clarithromycin, erythromycin, telithromycin, troleandomycin), CYP3A4 substrates (methadone, pimozide, QUEtiapine, quiNIDine, risperiDONE, ziprasidone), local anesthetics, some phenothiazines, tricyclics:** increased QT prolongation
β-Adrenergic blockers: do not use together, block therapeutic effect
MAOIs: increased chance of hypertensive crisis
Sympathomimetics: increased effects of both products

Drug/herb
Green tea (large amounts), guarana: increased effect

NURSING CONSIDERATIONS
Assessment
• Monitor respiratory function: vital capacity, FEV, ABGs, lung sounds, heart rate, rhythm (baseline)
• Determine that patient has not received theophylline therapy before giving dose; assess client's ability to self-medicate
• Monitor for evidence of allergic reactions; withhold dose and notify prescriber
• **Assess for paradoxical bronchospasm: dyspnea, wheezing; keep emergency resuscitative equipment nearby**

> **BLACK BOX WARNING:** Assess for labor: maternal heart rate, B/P, contractions, fetal heart rate; can inhibit uterine contractions, labor; monitor for hypoglycemia, do not use injectable product for prevention or treatment over 72 hr in preterm labor; do not use oral product for preterm labor

Patient/family education
• Advise patient not to use OTC medications; extra stimulation may occur; to use this medication before other medications and allow at least 5 min between each to prevent overstimulation
• Teach patient how to use inhaler; to avoid getting aerosol in eyes because blurring may result; to wash inhaler in warm water daily and dry; to avoid smoking, smoke-filled rooms, persons with respiratory infections; review package insert with patient
• **Teach patient that paradoxical bronchospasm may occur; to stop product immediately and notify prescriber; to limit caffeine products such as chocolate, coffee, tea, and colas**
• Instruct patient on administration of dose, not to use more than prescribed; serious side effects may occur; if taking PO regularly and dose is

T

missed, take when remembered; space other doses on new time schedule

Evaluation

Positive therapeutic outcome
- Absence of dyspnea, wheezing after 1 hr
- Improved airway exchange
- Improved ABGs

TREATMENT OF OVERDOSE:
Administer a β_2-adrenergic blocker

terconazole vaginal antifungal
See Appendix B

teriflunomide
(ter'i-floo'noe-mide)
Aubagio
Func. class.: Multiple sclerosis agent
Chem. class.: Pyrimidine synthesis inhibitor
Pregnancy category X

ACTION: Antiproliferative effects including peripheral T- and B-lymphocytes, might reduce inflammatory demyelination

Therapeutic outcome: Decreased symptoms of MS

USES: Reduction of the frequency of relapses or remitting MS

CONTRAINDICATIONS
Hypersensitivity

> BLACK BOX WARNING: Pregnancy: **X**

Precautions: Breastfeeding, alcoholism, diabetes mellitus, eosinophilic pneumonia, hepatitis, jaundice, male-mediated teratogenicity, pneumonitis, pulmonary disease/fibrosis, sarcoidosis, TB, vaccination

> BLACK BOX WARNING: Hepatic disease

DOSAGE AND ROUTES
Adult: PO 7 or 14 mg/day

Available forms: Tabs 7, 14 mg

Implementation
PO route
May be taken without regard to food

ADVERSE EFFECTS
CNS: Anxiety, headache
CV: Palpitations, hypertension, MI
EENT: Blurred vision, conjunctivitis, sinusitis

GI: Nausea, vomiting, diarrhea, cystitis
HEMA: Leukopenia, lymphopenia, neutropenia
INTEG: Acne vulgaris, alopecia, pruritus
META: Weight loss
MISC: Infection, cystitis

Pharmacokinetics

Absorption	Unknown
Distribution	Protein binding >99%
Metabolism	Unknown
Excretion	Unknown
Half-life	Median 18–19 days, peak 1–4 hr

INTERACTIONS
Individual drugs
Do not use with leflunomide

CycloSPORINE, eltrombopag, gefitinib: increased teriflunomide effect

Methotrexate: increased hepatotoxicity

Zidovudine: increased hematologic toxicity

Repaglinide, pioglitazone, rosiglitazone, PACLitaxel, naproxen, topotecan, bosentan, furosemide: increased effect of each agent

Warfarin, alosetron, DULoxetine, theophylline, tiZANidine, quiNINE, tamoxifen, bendamustine, rasagiline, rOPINIRole, selegiline, propafenone, mexiletine, lidocaine, anagrelide, cloZAPine, cinacalcet, caffeine: decreased effect of each agent, monitor closely

Cholestyramine, activated charcoal: decreased effect of teriflunomide

Drug classifications
Do not use with live virus vaccines

HMG-CoA reductase inhibitors: Increase: hepatotoxicity

Oral contraceptives: increased effect of oral contraceptives

NURSING CONSIDERATIONS
Assessment
- CNS symptoms: assess for anxiety, confusion, vertigo
- GI status: assess for diarrhea, vomiting, abdominal pain
- Cardiac status: assess for tachycardia, palpitations, vasodilation, chest pain

Patient/family education
- Teach patient that blurred vision can occur
- Advise patient to notify prescriber if pregnancy is planned or suspected
- Inform patient not to change dosing or stop taking without advice of prescriber

---

Evaluation

Positive therapeutic outcome
• Decreased symptoms of MS

teriparatide (Rx)
(tah-ree-par'ah-tide)
Forteo
Func. class.: Parathyroid hormone (rDNA)
Chem. class.: Teriparatide
Pregnancy category C

ACTION: Contains human recombinant parathyroid hormone, which stimulates new bone growth

Therapeutic outcome: Calcium levels at 9-10 mg/dl, decreased symptoms of hypocalcemia, hypoparathyroidism

USES: Postmenopausal women with osteoporosis, men with primary or hypogonadal osteoporosis who are at high risk for fracture, glucocorticoid-induced osteoporosis

CONTRAINDICATIONS
Hypersensitivity, increased baseline risk of osteosarcoma (Paget's disease, open epiphyses, previous bone radiation), bone metastases, history of skeletal malignancies, other metabolic bone diseases, preexisting hypercalcemia

Precautions: Pregnancy **C,** breastfeeding, children, urolithiasis, hypotension, use >2 yr

> **BLACK BOX WARNING:** Secondary malignancy

DOSAGE AND ROUTES
Adult: SUBCUT 20 mcg/day up to 2 yr (osteoporosis); use for years/lifetime is recommended (glucocorticoid-induced osteoporosis)

Available forms: Prefilled pen delivery device (delivers 20 mcg/day)

Implementation
• Store refrigerated; do not freeze
SUBCUT route
• Give by SUBCUT only, rotate inj sites
• Protect from freezing, light; refrigerate pen

ADVERSE EFFECTS
CNS: Dizziness, headache, insomnia, depression, vertigo
CV: Hypertension, angina, syncope
GI: Nausea, diarrhea, dyspepsia, vomiting, constipation
INTEG: Rash, sweating
MISC: Pain, asthenia, hyperuricemia
MS: Arthralgia, leg cramps, back/leg pain, weakness, **osteosarcoma (rare)**

RESP: Rhinitis, cough, pharyngitis, pneumonia, dyspnea

Pharmacokinetics
Absorption	Extensively, rapidly
Distribution	Unknown
Metabolism	Liver
Excretion	Kidneys
Half-life	Unknown

Pharmacodynamics
Onset	Rapid
Peak	½ hr
Duration	3 hr

INTERACTIONS
Individual drug
Digoxin: increased digoxin toxicity

Drug/lab test
Increased: calcium, uric acid, urinary calcium
Decreased: magnesium, phosphorus

NURSING CONSIDERATIONS
Assessment
• **Secondary malignancy: osteosarcoma depends on length of treatment, those at higher risk for osteosarcoma should not use this product**
• Monitor uric acid, chloride, magnesium, electrolytes, urine pH, vit D, phosphate for normal serum levels; serum calcium may be transiently increased after dosing (max at 4-6 hr after dose)
• Assess for bone pain, headache, fatigue, changes in LOC, leg cramps
• Monitor for signs of persistent hypercalcemia: nausea, vomiting, constipation, lethargy, muscle weakness
• Assess nutritional status: diet for sources of vit D (milk, some seafood), calcium (dairy products, dark green vegetables), phosphates (dairy products)

Patient/family education
• Advise patient of the symptoms of hypercalcemia
• Teach about foods rich in calcium
• Teach how to use delivery device, dispose of needles, not to share pen with others, use at same time of day
• Advise to sit or lie down if dizziness or fast heartbeat occurs after the first few doses
• Pen may be used for 28 days

Evaluation

Positive therapeutic outcome
• Increased bone mineral density

T

tesamorelin
(tes-a-moe-rel'in)
Egrifta
Func. class.: Pituitary hormone, growth hormone modifiers
Pregnancy category X

ACTION: Binds to growth hormone releasing factor receptors on the pituitary somatotroph cells; binding stimulates the production, release of endogenous growth hormone (GH)

Therapeutic outcome: Decreasing lipodystrophy in HIV patients

USES: Treatment of excess abdominal fat in HIV-infected patients with lipodystrophy

CONTRAINDICATIONS
Hypersensitivity to this product or mannitol, neoplastic disease, pregnancy **X**, disruption of the hypothalamic-pituitary axis (hypothalamic-pituitary-adrenal [HPA] suppression) resulting from hypophysectomy, hypopituitarism, pituitary tumor/surgery, radiation therapy of the head, head trauma, IV/IM administration

Precautions: Breastfeeding, CABG, diabetes, diabetic retinopathy, edema, geriatrics, children, infants, adolescents

DOSAGE AND ROUTES
Adult: SUBCUT 2 mg/day

Available forms: Powder for injection 1 mg

Implementation
SUBCUT route
• Visually inspect parenteral products for particulate matter and discoloration before use whenever solution and container permit
• To reconstitute use 2, 1 mg vials, inject 2.1 ml sterile water for injection into the first 1-mg vial; use the syringe with the needle already attached. To avoid foaming, push the plunger in slowly with the needle at a slight angle so the sterile water goes down the inside wall of the vial; with the needle and syringe attached to the vial, keep the vial upright and gently roll the vial for 30 sec until mixed; do not shake; remove all contents and put in next 1 mg vial, roll; withdraw 2.1 ml of the reconstituted solution
• Take the syringe out of the vial, place the needle cap on its side against a clean, flat surface; do not touch needle; hold syringe and slide the needle into cap; push the cap all the way or until it snaps shut; do not touch cap until it covers the needle completely
• Remove needle and insert a ½″ 27-G safety injection needle onto the syringe; use immediately;

throw away any unused product or used sterile water for injection
• Solution should be clear; do not use if discolored, cloudy, or has particles, but slight foaming is acceptable
• Inject subcut into abdomen; avoid scar tissues, bruises, or the navel; rotate injection sites in the abdomen; slowly push plunger down until all solution has been injected
• After removing the injection from the skin, flip back the needle shield until it snaps, covering the injection needle completely; keep pressing until you hear a click; that means the injection needle is protected
• Use a piece of sterile gauze to rub the injection site clean; if there is bleeding, apply pressure to the injection site with gauze for 30 seconds; if bleeding continues, apply a bandage to the site
• Properly dispose of used syringe, needles, vial, and sterile water for injection bottle in a sharps container

ADVERSE EFFECTS
CNS: Depression, flushing, headache, hypoesthesia, insomnia, night sweats, peripheral neuropathy paresthesias, spasms
CV: Chest pain, edema, hypertension, palpitations, peripheral edema
GI: Diarrhea, dyspepsia, nausea, upper abdominal pain, vomiting
INTEG: Flushing, injection site reactions, pruritus, rash, urticaria
MS: Arthralgia, carpal tunnel syndrome, joint swelling, myalgias, stiffness
RESP: *Upper respiratory tract infection*
SYST: Secondary malignancy

Pharmacokinetics

Absorption	Unknown
Distribution	Unknown
Metabolism	Unknown
Excretion	Unknown
Half-life	26 and 38 mins in healthy and HIV-infected patients, respectively, peak 0.15 hrs

Pharmacodynamics

Onset	Unknown
Peak	0.15 hrs
Duration	Unknown

INTERACTIONS
Individual drugs
Cortisone, predniSONE, simvastatin, ritonavir: decreased effect of each specific product

---

NURSING CONSIDERATIONS
Assessment
• **Lipsodystrophy:** Assess for sunken cheeks; thinning arms and legs; fat accumulation in the abdomen, jaws, and back of neck; after treatment these should lessen
• Monitor glycosylated hemoglobin A1C (HbA1C), serum IGF-1 concentrations, ophthalmologic exam

Patient/family education
• Explain reason for product and expected result
⚠ Teach patient to use contraception (pregnancy X)

Evaluation
Positive therapeutic outcome
• Decreasing lipodystrophy in HIV patients

---

testosterone (Rx)
(tess-toss′te-rone)
testosterone enanthate (Rx)
Delatestryl
testosterone cypionate (Rx)
Depo-Testosterone
testosterone pellets (Rx)
Testopel
testosterone transdermal (Rx)
Androderm
testosterone gel (Rx)
AndroGel Fortesta, Testim
testosterone buccal (Rx)
Striant
testosterone topical solution (Rx) gel
AndroGel, Axiron, Fortesta, Testim, Vogelxo
testosterone nasal gel (Rx)
Natesto
Func. class.: Androgenic anabolic steroid
Chem. class.: Halogenated testosterone derivative
Pregnancy category X
Controlled substance schedule III

ACTION: Increases weight by building body tissue; increases potassium, phosphorus, chloride, nitrogen levels; increases bone development; responsible for maintenance of secondary sex characteristics (male)

Therapeutic outcome: Increased hormone levels in eunuchoidism, decreased tumor growth in female breast cancer, onset of male puberty

USES: Female breast cancer, hypogonadism, eunuchoidism, male climacteric, oligospermia, impotence, vulvar dystrophies, low testosterone levels, delayed male puberty (inj)

CONTRAINDICATIONS
Pregnancy **X**, breastfeeding, severe renal/cardiac/hepatic disease, hypersensitivity, genital bleeding (rare), male breast/prostate cancer

Precautions: Diabetes mellitus, CV disease, MI, urinary tract disorders, prostate cancer, hypercalcemia

> **BLACK BOX WARNING:** Children, accidental exposure

DOSAGE AND ROUTES
Replacement
Adult: IM (enanthate or cypionate) 50-400 mg q2-4wk; transdermal (Testoderm) 4-6 mg applied q24hr; (Androderm, AndroGel) 5 mg applied q24hr; once daily (gel); topical sol (Axiron) 60 mg (2 pump activations) each AM; BUCCAL 1 buccal system (30 mg) to the gum region q12hr before meals/PM
Adult (male) and child: SUBCUT (pellets) 150-450 mg (2-6 pellets) inserted q3-6mo

Breast cancer
Adult: IM 50-100 mg 3 ×/wk (propionate) or 200-400 mg q2-4wk (cypionate or enanthate)

Delayed male puberty
Child >12 yr: IM up to 100 mg/mo for up to 6 mo

Available forms: Enanthate: inj 200 mg/ml; **cypionate:** inj 100, 200 mg/ml; pellets 75 mg; **transdermal** 2, 4 mg/24 hr; **gel** 1%, 1.62%, 10 mg/actuation; **buccal system** 30 mg; **topical solution** 30 mg/actuation

Implementation
• Administer diet with increased calories, protein; decreased sodium if edema occurs
• Administer supportive product if anemia occurs
• Give titrated dose; use lowest effective dose
• Give IM inj deep into upper outer quadrant of gluteal muscle; route can be painful
Transdermal route
• Apply Testoderm to skin of scrotum, Androderm to skin of back, upper arms, thighs, abdomen; area must be clean and dry, free of hair

　　Adverse effects: *italics* = common; **bold** = life-threatening

Gel route
- Products are not interchangeable, dosage and administration for AndroGel 1% differs from AndroGel 1.62%
- Apply daily to clean dry area on shoulders, upper arms, or abdomen; women, children should not touch gel or treated skin

Buccal system route
- Do not chew or swallow buccal system
- Rotate sites; place above incisor tooth on either side of mouth
- Open packet; place rounded side of surface against gum and hold firmly in place with finger over lip for 30 sec; if product falls off, replace with new system; discard in trash can away from children or pets

Topical solution
- Using the provided applicator, apply the solution to clean, dry, intact skin of the axilla, preferably at the same time each morning. Do not apply to any other part of the body. Allow the solution to dry completely before dressing. If an antiperspirant or deodorant is used, apply at least 2 min before applying the solution. The pump must be primed before the first use by fully depressing the pump mechanism 3 times and discarding any solution that is released during the priming. To dispense the solution, position the nozzle over the applicator cup and carefully depress the pump once fully; the cup should be filled with no more than 1 pump actuation (30 mg). With the applicator upright, place it up into the axilla and wipe steadily down and up into the axilla. Do not use fingers or hand to rub the solution. If multiple applications are necessary for the required dose, alternate application between the left and right axilla. When repeat application to the same axilla is necessary, allow the solution to dry completely before the next application. After use, rinse the applicator under running water and pat dry with tissue. Wash hands with soap and water
- Following application, allow the site to dry a few minutes before putting on clothing
- Direct contact of the medicated skin with the skin of another person can result in the transfer of residual testosterone and absorption by the other person. To reduce accidental transfer, the patient should cover the application site(s) with clothing (e.g., a T-shirt) after the solution has dried. The application site should be washed with soap and water prior to any skin-to-skin contact regardless of the length of time since application. In the case of direct contact, the other person should wash the area of contact with soap and water as soon as possible

- Patients should be advised that the topical solution is flammable; therefore, fire, flame, and smoking should be avoided during use
- Advise patients to avoid swimming or washing the application site until 2 hr following application of solution

ADVERSE EFFECTS
CNS: Dizziness, headache, fatigue, tremors, paresthesias, flushing, sweating, anxiety, lability, insomnia, carpal tunnel syndrome
CV: Increased B/P
EENT: Conjunctival edema, nasal congestion
ENDO: Abnormal GTT
GI: Nausea, vomiting, constipation, weight gain, cholestatic jaundice
GU: Hematuria, amenorrhea, vaginitis, decreased libido, decreased breast size, clitoral hypertrophy, testicular atrophy, gynecomastia, enlarged prostate
HEMA: Polycythemia
INTEG: Rash, acneiform lesions, oily hair and skin, flushing, sweating, acne vulgaris, alopecia, hirsutism
MS: Cramps, spasms

Pharmacokinetics

Absorption	Well but slowly absorbed
Distribution	Crosses placenta
Metabolism	Liver
Excretion	Kidneys, breast milk
Half-life	8 days (cypionate)
	10-100 min (base)

Pharmacodynamics

	IM (base)	IM (cypionate)	IM (enanthate)	IM (propionate)
Onset	Unknown	Unknown	Unknown	Unknown
Peak	Unknown	Unknown	Unknown	Unknown
Duration	1-3 days	2-4 wk	2-4 wk	1-3 days

INTERACTIONS
Individual drugs
ACTH, buPROPion: increased edema
Insulin: decreased glucose levels may alter need for insulin
Oxyphenbutazone: increased effects of oxyphenbutazone

Drug classifications
Adrenal steroids: increased edema
Anticoagulants: increased pro-time
Antidiabetics, oral: decreased need for oral antidiabetics

Drug/lab test

Increased: serum cholesterol, blood glucose, urine glucose

Decreased: serum Ca, serum K, T_4, T_3, thyroid ^{131}I uptake test, urine 17-OHCS, 17-KS, PBI

NURSING CONSIDERATIONS
Assessment
• Monitor patient's weight daily; notify prescriber if weekly weight gain is >5 lb; assess I&O ratio; be alert for decreasing urinary output, increasing edema
• Monitor B/P q4hr, Hgb/Hct
• Assess growth rate, bone age in adolescent because growth rate may be uneven (linear/bone growth) if used for extended periods
• Monitor electrolytes: potassium, sodium, chloride, calcium; cholesterol
• Monitor liver function tests: ALT, AST, bilirubin
• Assess edema, hypertension, cardiac symptoms, jaundice
• Assess mental status: affect, mood, behavioral changes, aggression
• **Assess signs of masculinization** in female: increased libido, deepening of voice, decreased breast tissue, enlarged clitoris, menstrual irregularities; male: gynecomastia, impotence, testicular atrophy
• **Assess hypercalcemia:** lethargy, polyuria, polydipsia, nausea, vomiting, constipation; product may have to be decreased
• **Assess hypoglycemia** in diabetics because oral antidiabetic action is increased

Patient/family education
• Inform patient that product needs to be combined with complete health plan: diet, rest, exercise
• Caution patient to notify prescriber if therapeutic response decreases; not to discontinue this medication abruptly
• Inform women patients to report menstrual irregularities; about changes in sex characteristics
• Discuss that 1-3 mo course is necessary for response in breast cancer
• Inform patient about application of transdermal patches: Testoderm to skin of scrotum, Androderm to skin of back, upper arms, thighs, abdomen; area must be dry and free of hair; may be reapplied after bathing, swimming
• Teach about changes in sex characteristics: priapism, gynecomastia, increased libido

Evaluation

Positive therapeutic outcome
• Decrease size of tumor in breast cancer
• Increased androgen levels

tetracaine ophthalmic
See Appendix B

tetracaine topical
See Appendix B

tetracycline (Rx)
(tet-ra-sye′kleen)
Func. class.: Antiinfective— broad-spectrum
Chem. class.: Tetracycline
Pregnancy category D

ACTION: Inhibits protein synthesis and phosphorylation in microorganisms; bacteriostatic

Therapeutic outcome: Bactericidal action against susceptible organisms: gram-positive pathogens *Bacillus anthracis, Clostridium perfringens, Clostridium tetani, Listeria monocytogenes, Nocardia, Propionibacterium acnes, Actinomyces israelii;* gram-negative pathogens *Haemophilus influenzae, Legionella pneumophila, Yersinia enterolitica, Yersinia pestis, Neisseria gonorrhoeae, Neisseria meningitidis*

USES: Syphilis, *Chlamydia trachomatis,* gonorrhea, lymphogranuloma venereum, uncommon gram-positive, gram-negative organisms, rickettsial infections

CONTRAINDICATIONS
Pregnancy **D**, breastfeeding, children <8 yr, hypersensitivity to tetracyclines

Precautions: Renal/hepatic disease, UV exposure

DOSAGE AND ROUTES
Susceptible gram-positive/gram-negative infections
Adult: PO 250-500 mg q6hr
Child >8 yr: PO 25-50 mg/kg/day in divided doses q6hr

Chlamydia trachomatis
Adult: PO 500 mg qid × 7 days

Syphilis
Adult and adolescent: PO 500 mg qid × 2 wk; if syphilis duration >1 yr, must treat 30 days

Brucellosis
Adult: PO 500 mg qid × 3 wk with 1 g of streptomycin IM 2 ×/day × 1 wk, and 1 ×/day the 2nd wk

Urethral, endocervical, rectal infections *(C. trachomatis)*
Adult: PO 500 mg qid × 7 days

Acne
Adult and adolescent: PO 250 mg q6hr, then 125-500 mg/day or every other day

Renal dose
Adult: PO CCr 51-90 ml/min give dose q8-12hr, CCr 10-50 ml/min give dose q12-24hr, CCr <10 ml/min give dose q24hr

Available forms: Caps 250, 500 mg

Implementation
PO route
- Give around the clock to maintain proper blood levels; give with food to increase absorption of product; do not give within 3 hr of other agents; product interactions may occur; take on an empty stomach (1 hr before or 2 hr after meals)
- Give with 8 oz of water
- Shake liquid preparation well before giving; use calibrated device for proper dosing
- Store in tight, light-resistant container at room temp

ADVERSE EFFECTS
CNS: Fever, headache, paresthesia
CV: Pericarditis
EENT: Dysphagia, glossitis, decreased calcification (permanent discoloration) of deciduous teeth, oral candidiasis, oral ulcers
GI: *Nausea,* abdominal pain, *vomiting, diarrhea,* anorexia, enterocolitis, hepatotoxicity, flatulence, abdominal cramps, epigastric burning, stomatitis, hepatitis, pseudomembranous colitis
GU: *Increased BUN,* azotemia, acute renal failure
HEMA: Eosinophilia, neutropenia, thrombocytopenia, leukocytosis, hemolytic anemia
INTEG: *Rash, urticaria, photosensitivity, increased pigmentation,* exfoliative dermatitis, pruritus, angioedema, Stevens-Johnson syndrome
MISC: Increased intracranial pressure, candidiasis

Pharmacokinetics
Absorption	60%-80% (PO), lower (IM)
Distribution	Widely distributed, some in CSF; crosses placenta
Metabolism	Not metabolized
Excretion	Unchanged—kidneys
Half-life	6-10 hr

Pharmacodynamics
Onset	1-2 hr
Peak	2-3 hr
Duration	Unknown

INTERACTIONS
Individual drugs
Cimetidine, NaHCO₃: decreased tetracycline effect
Digoxin: increased digoxin effect
Iron: forms chelates, decreased absorption
Methoxyflurane: fatal nephrotoxicity
Warfarin: increased warfarin effect

Drug classifications
Alkali products, antacids: decreased tetracycline effect
Penicillins: decreased penicillin effect

Drug/herb
Dong quai: increased photosensitivity

Drug/food
Decreased: absorption with dairy products; forms insoluble chelate

Drug/lab test
Increased: BUN, LFTs

NURSING CONSIDERATIONS
Assessment
⚠ Serious skin reactions: angioedema, Stevens-Johnson syndrome, exfoliative dermatitis, report immediately after stopping product
- Assess patient for previous sensitivity reaction
- Assess patient for signs and symptoms of infection including characteristics of wounds, sputum, urine, stool, WBC >10,000/mm³, temp; obtain baseline information before, during treatment
- Complete C&S testing before beginning product therapy to identify if correct treatment has been initiated
- Assess for allergic reactions: rash, urticaria, pruritus, chills, fever, joint pain; angioedema may occur a few days after therapy begins; EPINEPHrine, resuscitation equipment should be available for anaphylactic reaction
- Identify urine output; if decreasing, notify prescriber (may indicate nephrotoxicity); increased BUN, creatinine
- Pseudomembranous colitis: assess for diarrhea, abdominal pain, fever, fatigue, anorexia; possible anemia, elevated WBC and low serum albumin; stop product and usually give either vancomycin or IV metroNIDAZOLE

• **Assess for superinfection: perineal itching, fever, malaise, redness, pain, swelling, drainage, rash, diarrhea, change in cough, sputum if on prolonged therapy**

Patient/family education
• Teach patient to report sore throat, bruising, bleeding, joint pain; may indicate blood dyscrasias (rare)
• Advise patient to use sunscreen when outdoors to decrease photosensitivity reaction
• Advise patient to contact prescriber if vaginal itching, loose foul-smelling stools, furry tongue occur; may indicate superinfection; report itching, rash, pruritus, urticaria
• Teach patient to take 1 hr before bedtime to prevent esophageal ulceration
• Instruct patient to take all medication prescribed for the length of time ordered; product must be taken around the clock to maintain blood levels; do not give medication to others
• **Teach patient to notify prescriber immediately of diarrhea with pus, mucus, fever, abdominal pain**
• **Teach patient to notify prescriber if pregnancy is planned or suspected, pregnancy D**
⚠ **Teach patient not to use outdated products, as Fanconi syndrome (nephrotoxicity) may occur**

Evaluation
Positive therapeutic outcome
• Absence of signs/symptoms of infection (WBC <10,000/mm^3, temp WNL, absence of red, draining wounds)
• Reported improvement in symptoms of infection, resolution of infection, prevention of malaria

---

tetrahydrozoline nasal agent
See Appendix B

tetrahydrozoline ophthalmic
See Appendix B

---

theophylline (Rx)
(thee-off'i-lin)
Elixophyllin, Theo-24, Theochron, Uniphyl
Func. class.: Spasmolytic, bronchodilator
Chem. class.: Xanthine, ethylenediamine
Pregnancy category C

ACTION: Relaxes smooth muscle of respiratory system by blocking phosphodiesterase, which increases cyclic AMP, exact action unknown

Therapeutic outcome: Ability to breathe without difficulty

USES: Bronchial asthma, bronchospasm of COPD, chronic bronchitis, emphysema

CONTRAINDICATIONS
Hypersensitivity to xanthines, tachydysrhythmias

Precautions: Pregnancy **C**, children, geriatric, CHF, cor pulmonale, hepatic disease, active peptic ulcer disease, diabetes mellitus, hyperthyroidism, hypertension, seizure disorder

DOSAGE AND ROUTES
Acute exacerbations of reversible airway obstructions
Adult: PO/IV 5 mg/kg loading dose over 20-30 min

COPD, chronic bronchitis
Adult: IV 0.4 mg/kg/hr in nonsmokers or 0.7 mg/kg/hr in smokers
Adult, child >45 kg: Maintenance PO (regular release) 10 mg/kg/day, in divided doses q1-8hr; after 3 days increase dosage to 400 mg in divided doses q6-8hr; after 3 more days increase to 600 mg in divided doses q6-8hr; max 800 mg/day

Apnea of prematurity
Neonate: IV 4 mg/kg over 20-30 min, then maintenance IV/PO neonate ≥24 days 1.5 mg/kg q12h

Available forms: Cap, ext rel 100, 200, 300, 400 mg; tab ext rel 100, 200, 400, 450, 600 mg; elixir 80 mg/15 ml; sol for inj 250 mg/10 ml, 500 mg/20 ml

Implementation
PO route
• Do not crush or chew time release products
• Contents of bead-filled cap may be sprinkled over food for children's use
• Give PO with 8 oz water; to decrease GI symptoms; avoid food, absorption may be affected
• Store diluted sol for 24 hr if refrigerated

IV route
• Give loading dose over 20-30 min; max 20-25 mg/min; do not give by rapid IV; use only by cont inf

Y-site compatibilities: Acyclovir, ampicillin, aztreonam, ceFAZolin, cefoTEtan, cefTAZidime, cefTRIAXone, cimetidine, clindamycin, dexamethasone, diltiazem, DOBUTamine, DOPamine, doxycycline, erythromycin, famotidine, fluconazole, gentamicin, haloperidol, heparin, hydrocortisone, lidocaine, methyldopa, methylPREDNISolone, metroNIDAZOLE, midazolam, nafcillin, nitroglycerin, nitroprusside, penicillin G potassium, piperacillin, potassium chloride, ranitidine, ticarcillin, ticarcillin/clavulanate, tobramycin, vancomycin

ADVERSE EFFECTS

CNS: *Anxiety, restlessness, insomnia, dizziness, seizures,* headache, light-headedness, muscle twitching, tremors

CV: *Palpitations, sinus tachycardia,* hypotension, dysrhythmias, fluid retention with tachycardia

ENDO: Hyperglycemia

GI: *Nausea, vomiting, anorexia,* diarrhea, bitter taste, dyspepsia, gastric distress

INTEG: Flushing, urticaria

MISC: SIADH, urinary frequency

RESP: Increased rate, tachypnea

Pharmacokinetics

Absorption	Well absorbed (PO), slowly absorbed (ext rel)
Distribution	Crosses placenta, widely distributed
Metabolism	Liver
Excretion	Kidneys, breast milk
Half-life	6.5-10.5 hr; increased in liver disease, CHF, geriatric

Pharmacodynamics

	PO	PO–TIME REL	IV
Onset	Rapid	Slow	Immediate
Peak	1 hr	4-8 hr	Inf end
Duration	6 hr	12-24 hr	6-8 hr

INTERACTIONS

Individual drugs

CarBAMazepine: decreased theophylline level

Cimetidine, disulfiram, erythromycin, fluvoxaMINE, influenza vaccine, mexiletine, propranolol: increased theophylline action

Lithium: decreased effect of lithium

PHENobarbital, phenytoin, rifampin: decreased theophylline

Increased: dysrhythmias: halothane

Drug classifications

Anticoagulants: increased anticoagulant level

β-Adrenergic blockers: cardiotoxicity

Contraceptives (oral), corticosteroids, fluoroquinolones, interferons: increased theophylline action

Smoking: decreased theophylline level

Drug/herb

Coffee, cola nut, guarana, ma huang (ephedra), tea (black, green), yerba maté: increased toxicity

St. John's wort: decreased theophylline level

NURSING CONSIDERATIONS

Assessment

• Monitor theophylline blood levels (therapeutic level is 5-15 mcg/ml); toxicity may occur with small increase above 15 mcg/ml

• Monitor I&O; diuresis occurs; dehydration may result in children or geriatric

• Assess for signs of toxicity: irritability, insomnia, restlessness, tremors, nausea, vomiting

• Monitor respiratory rate, rhythm, depth; auscultate lung fields bilaterally; notify prescriber of abnormalities

• Assess for allergic reactions: rash, urticaria; if these occur, product should be discontinued

Patient/family education

• Advise patient to check OTC medications, current prescription medications for ePHEDrine, which increases stimulation, and to avoid alcohol, caffeine

• Caution patient to avoid hazardous activities; dizziness may occur

• Inform patient that if GI upset occurs, to take product with 8 oz of water; avoid food; absorption may be decreased

• Advise patient to notify prescriber of toxicity: nausea, vomiting, anxiety, insomnia, seizures

• Advise patient to notify prescriber of change in smoking habit; dosage may have to be changed

Evaluation

Positive therapeutic outcome
• Ability to breathe more easily

---

thiamine (vitamin B₁) (PO, OTC; IV, IM, Rx)

Betaxin ✣, Betalin S, Biamine, Revitonus, Thiamilate

Func. class.: Vitamin B₁
Chem. class.: Water soluble

Pregnancy category A

Do not confuse: thiamine/Tenormin

ACTION: Needed for pyruvate metabolism, carbohydrate metabolism

Therapeutic outcome: Prevention and treatment of thiamine deficiency

USES: Vit B₁ deficiency or polyneuritis, cheilosis adjunct with thiamine beriberi, Wernicke-Korsakoff syndrome, pellagra, metabolic disorders, alcoholism

---

⚠ Nurse Alert ✳ Key NCLEX® Drug ≫ Drug Specifics

CONTRAINDICATIONS
Hypersensitivity

Precautions: Pregnancy **A**

DOSAGE AND ROUTES
RDA
Adult: PO (Male) 1.2-1.5 mg; (female) 1.1 mg; (pregnancy) 1.4 mg; (breastfeeding) 1.4 mg
Child 9-13 yr: PO 0.9 mg
Child 4-8 yr: PO 0.6 mg
Child 1-3 yr: PO 0.5 mg
Infant 6 mo-1 yr: PO 0.3 mg
Neonate and infant to 6 mo: PO 0.3 mg

Beriberi
Adult: PO 5-30 mg qd or given in 3 divided doses × 1 month; IM/IV 5-30 mg qd or in 3 doses, then convert to PO
Child/infant: PO 10-50 mg qd × 2 wk, then 5-10 mg qd × 1 mo; IV/IM 10-25 mg/day × 2 wk, then 5-10 mg qd × 1 mo

Available forms: Tabs 50, 100, 250, 500 mg; inj 100 mg/ml; enteric-coated tabs 20 mg

Implementation
IM route
• Give by IM inj; rotate sites if pain and inflammation occur; do not mix with alkaline sol; Z-track to minimize pain
• Application of cold compress may decrease pain
• Store in airtight, light-resistant container

Direct IV route
• **IV** undiluted given over 5 min
Continuous IV infusion route
• Dilute in compatible **IV** sol

Syringe compatibilities: Doxapram

Y-site compatibilities: Famotidine

ADVERSE EFFECTS
CNS: Weakness, restlessness
CV: Collapse, pulmonary edema, hypotension
EENT: Tightness of throat
GI: Hemorrhage, *nausea, diarrhea*
INTEG: Angioneurotic edema, cyanosis, sweating, warmth
SYST: Anaphylaxis

Pharmacokinetics

Absorption	Well absorbed (PO, IM), completely absorbed (**IV**)
Distribution	Widely distributed
Metabolism	Liver
Excretion	Kidneys (unchanged—excess amounts)
Half-life	Unknown

Pharmacodynamics
Unknown

NURSING CONSIDERATIONS
Assessment
• **Anaphylaxis (IV only):** assess for swelling of face, eyes, lips, throat, wheezing
• **Thiamine deficiency:** assess for anorexia, weakness, pain, depression, confusion, blurred vision, tachycardia
• Assess nutritional status: yeast, beef, liver, whole or enriched grains, legumes

Patient/family education
• Teach patient necessary foods to be included in diet: yeast, beef, liver, legumes, whole grains

Evaluation
Positive therapeutic outcome
• Absence of nausea, vomiting, anorexia, insomnia, tachycardia, paresthesias, depression, muscle weakness

RARELY USED

thioridazine (Rx)
(thye-or-rid′a-zeen)
Func. class.: Antipsychotic (typical)
Chem. class.: Phenothiazine, piperidine
Pregnancy category C

Do not confuse: thioridazine/thiothixene/thorazine

ACTION: Depresses cerebral cortex, hypothalamus, limbic system, which control activity, aggression; blocks neurotransmission produced by dopamine at synapse; exhibits strong α-adrenergic, anticholinergic blocking action; mechanism for antipsychotic effects is unclear

Therapeutic outcome: Decreased signs and symptoms of psychosis

USES: Psychotic disorders, schizophrenia, behavioral problems in children, anxiety, major depressive disorders, organic brain syndrome

CONTRAINDICATIONS
Children <2 yr, hypersensitivity, coma, CNS depression

BLACK BOX WARNING: QT prolongation, cardiac dysrhythmias

Precautions: Pregnancy **C**, breastfeeding, seizure disorders, hypertension, hepatic/pulmonary disease, renal failure, BPH, glaucoma, phenothiazine hypersensitivity, suicidal ideation, smoking, Reye's syndrome, Parkinson's disease

Adverse effects: *italics* = common; **bold** = life-threatening

> **BLACK BOX WARNING:** Cardiac disease, dementia, AV block, bundle branch block, torsades de pointes

DOSAGE AND ROUTES
Psychosis
Adult: PO 25-100 mg tid, max dose 800 mg/day; dose is gradually increased to desired response, then reduced to minimum maintenance

Depression/behavioral problems/organic brain syndrome
Adult: PO 25 tid, range from 10 mg bid-qid to 50 mg tid-qid; max 800 mg/day for short period
Geriatric: PO 10-25 mg daily-bid, increase 4-7 days by 10-25 mg to desired dose, max 300 mg/day for short period
Child 2-12 yr: PO 0.5-3 mg/kg/day in divided doses, max 3 mg/kg/day

Available forms: Tabs 10, 25, 50, 100 mg

Implementation
• Decrease dosage in geriatric because metabolism is slowed
• Administer PO with full glass of water, milk; or give with food to decrease GI upset
• Give antacids 2 hr before or after this product
• Store in airtight, light-resistant container, oral sol in amber bottle

ADVERSE EFFECTS
CNS: *EPS (pseudoparkinsonism, akathisia, dystonia, tardive dyskinesia)*, **seizures, headache,** confusion, **neuroleptic malignant syndrome, dizziness,** drowsiness
CV: Orthostatic hypotension, **cardiac arrest,** ECG changes, **tachycardia, QT prolongation, torsades de pointes**
EENT: Blurred vision, glaucoma, dry eyes
GI: *Dry mouth, nausea, vomiting, anorexia, constipation,* diarrhea, jaundice, weight gain
GU: Urinary retention, urinary frequency, enuresis, impotence, amenorrhea, gynecomastia, ejaculation dysfunction, priapism
HEMA: Anemia, **leukopenia, leukocytosis, agranulocytosis**
INTEG: *Rash,* photosensitivity, dermatitis
RESP: **Laryngospasm,** dyspnea, **respiratory depression**

Pharmacokinetics

Absorption	Variably absorbed (tab)
Distribution	Widely distributed, high concentrations in CNS, crosses placenta, protein binding 91%-99%
Metabolism	Liver, extensively; GI mucosa
Excretion	Kidneys, breast milk
Half-life	26-36 hr

Pharmacodynamics

Onset	Erratic
Peak	2-4 hr
Duration	8-12 hr

INTERACTIONS
Individual drugs
Alcohol: oversedation
Aluminum hydroxide, magnesium hydroxide: decreased absorption

> **BLACK BOX WARNING:** Haloperidol, chloroquine, droperidol, pentamidine, arsenic trioxide, levomethadyl: increased QT prolongation

Lithium: decreased thioridazine levels

Drug classifications
Anesthetics (barbiturate), CNS depressants: oversedation
Antacids: decreased absorption
Anticholinergics: increased anticholinergic effects
Antiparkinson agents: decreased effect of these agents
Barbiturates: decreased thioridazine effect
Centrally acting antihypertensives: decreased antihypertensive effect

> **BLACK BOX WARNING:** Class IA/III antidysrhythmics, some phenothiazines, β-agonists, local anesthetics, tricyclics, CYP3A4 inhibitors (amiodarone, clarithromycin, erythromycin, telithromycin, troleandomycin); CYP3A4 substrates (methadone, pimozide, QUEtiapine, quiNIDine, risperiDONE, ziprasidone): increased QT prolongation; CYP2D6 inhibitors

Drug/lab test
Increased: liver function tests, prolactin, bilirubin, alk phos
Decreased: Hct/Hgb, platelets, granulocytes, leukocytes, neutrocytes, eosinophils

NURSING CONSIDERATIONS
Assessment
• Assess mental status: orientation, mood, behavior, presence of hallucinations, and type before initial administration and monthly; this product should significantly reduce psychotic behavior; assess affect, orientation, LOC, reflexes, gait, coordination, sleep pattern disturbances
• Check for swallowing of PO medication; check for hoarding or giving of medication to other patients
• Monitor I&O ratio; palpate bladder if low urinary output occurs, especially in geriatric; urinalysis recommended before, during prolonged therapy

• Monitor bilirubin, CBC, liver function tests monthly
• Monitor B/P sitting, standing, and lying, take pulse and respirations q4hr during initial treatment; establish baseline before starting treatment; report drops of 30 mm Hg; obtain baseline ECG, monitor Q- and T-wave changes
• Check for dizziness, faintness, palpitations, tachycardia on rising; severe orthostatic hypotension is common
• **QT prolongation: monitor ECG for QT prolongation, ejection fraction; assess for chest pain, palpitations, dyspnea**
⚠ Neuroleptic malignant syndrome: assess for hyperpyrexia, muscle rigidity, increased CPK, altered mental status, dyspnea, fatigue; product should be discontinued
• **EPS** including akathisia (inability to sit still, no pattern to movements), tardive dyskinesia (bizarre movements of the jaw, mouth, tongue, extremities), pseudoparkinsonism (ragged tremors, pill rolling, shuffling gate); an antiparkinsonian product should be prescribed
• Assess for constipation, urinary retention daily; if these occur, increase bulk, water in diet

Patient/family education
• Teach patient to use good oral hygiene; frequent rinsing of mouth, sugarless gum for dry mouth
• Advise patient to avoid hazardous activities until product response is determined; dizziness, blurred vision are common
• Inform patient that orthostatic hypotension occurs often and to rise from sitting or lying position gradually; to avoid hot tubs, hot showers, tub baths because hypotension may occur
• Instruct patient that in hot weather, heat stroke may occur; take extra precautions to stay cool
• Caution patient to avoid abrupt withdrawal of this product, or EPS may result; product should be withdrawn slowly
• Teach patient to avoid OTC preparations (cough, hay fever, cold) unless approved by prescriber; serious product interactions may occur; avoid use with alcohol, CNS depressants; increased drowsiness may occur
• Advise patient to use sunglasses and sunscreen to prevent burns
• Teach patient about EPS and necessity for meticulous oral hygiene because oral candidiasis may occur
• Advise patient to take antacids 2 hr before or after this product
• **Instruct patient to report sore throat, malaise, fever, bleeding, mouth sores; if these occur, CBC should be performed and**

product discontinued; may cause vision impairment, report to prescriber
• Advise patient that urine may be discolored

Evaluation

Positive therapeutic outcome
• Decrease in emotional excitement, hallucinations, delusions, paranoia
• Reorganization of patterns of thought, speech

TREATMENT OF OVERDOSE:
Lavage if orally ingested; provide airway; *do not induce vomiting or use EPINEPHrine*, CV monitoring, continuous ECG

RARELY USED

thyroid USP (desiccated) (Rx)
(thye′roid)
Armour Thyroid, Bio-Throid, Nature Thyroid, NP Thyroid
Func. class.: Thyroid hormone
Chem. class.: Active thyroid hormone in natural state and ratio
Pregnancy category A

ACTION: Increases metabolic rate; increases cardiac output, O_2 consumption, body temp, blood volume, growth, development at cellular level

Therapeutic outcome: Correction of lack of thyroid hormone

USES: Hypothyroidism, cretinism (juvenile hypothyroidism), myxedema

CONTRAINDICATIONS
Adrenal insufficiency, MI, thyrotoxicosis, porcine protein hypersensitivity

| BLACK BOX WARNING: Obesity treatment |

Precautions: Pregnancy **A**, breastfeeding, geriatric, angina pectoris, hypertension, ischemia, cardiac disease

DOSAGE AND ROUTES
Hypothyroidism
Adult: PO 60-65 mg/day, increased by 30 mg qmo until desired response; maintenance dose 65-120 mg/day
Geriatric: PO 7.5-15 mg/day, increase dose q6-8wk until desired response

Cretinism/juvenile hypothyroidism
Child: PO 15 mg/day, then 30 mg/day after 2 wk, then 60 mg/day after another 2 wk; maintenance dose 60-180 mg/day

T

Myxedema
Adult: PO 15 mg/day, double dose q2wk, maintenance 60-180 mg/day

Available forms: Tabs 16, 32, 60, 65, 98, 130, 195, 260, 325 mg; enteric-coated tabs 32, 65, 130 mg; sugar-coated tabs 32, 65, 130, 195 mg; caps 65, 130, 195, 325 mg

Implementation
• Give in AM if possible as a single dose to decrease sleeplessness; at same time each day to maintain product level
• Do not give with food because absorption will be decreased
• Give only for hormone imbalances; not to be used for obesity, male infertility, menstrual conditions, lethargy; give lowest dose that relieves symptoms; lower dosage in the geriatric and in cardiac diseases
• Store in airtight, light-resistant container
• Wean patient off medication 4 wk before RAIU test

ADVERSE EFFECTS
CNS: *Insomnia, tremors,* headache, **thyroid storm**
CV: *Tachycardia, palpitations, angina,* **dysrhythmias,** hypertension, **cardiac arrest**
GI: Nausea, diarrhea, increased or decreased appetite, cramps
MISC: Menstrual irregularities, weight loss, sweating, heat intolerance, fever

Pharmacokinetics

Absorption	Well absorbed
Distribution	Widely distributed, does not cross placenta
Metabolism	Liver, tissues
Excretion	Feces via bile, breast milk
Half-life	T_3, 2 days; T_4, 1 wk

Pharmacodynamics

Onset	1 hr
Peak	12-48 hr
Duration	Unknown

INTERACTIONS
Individual drugs
Aluminum, calcium, magnesium: decreased thyroid absorption

Drug classifications
Anticoagulants, oral: increased effects of anticoagulants
Antidepressants (tricyclic): increased antidepressant (tricyclics) effect
Bile acid sequestrants: decreased thyroid absorption
Catecholamines: increased effects of catecholamines
Estrogens: decreased thyroid hormone effect
Sympathomimetics: increased effects of sympathomimetics

NURSING CONSIDERATIONS
Assessment

> **BLACK BOX WARNING: Obesity treatment:** use can lead to serious or life-threatening toxicity

• Identify if the patient is taking anticoagulants, antidiabetic agents; document on chart
• Take B/P, pulse before each dose; monitor I&O ratio and weight every day in same clothing, using same scale, at same time of day
• Monitor height, weight, psychomotor development, growth rate if given to a child
• Monitor T_3, T_4, FTIs, which are decreased; radioimmunoassay of TSH, which is increased; radioactive iodine uptake (RAIU), which is increased if patient's dose of medication is too low
• Monitor pro-time; patient may require decreased dosage of anticoagulant; check for bleeding, bruising
• **Hyperthyroidism:** assess for increased nervousness, excitability, irritability, which may indicate that dose of medication is too high, usually after 1-3 wk of treatment
• **Hypothyroidism:** lethargy, cold intolerance, weight gain, constipation, muscle cramps, may indicate dosage is too low
• Assess cardiac status: angina, palpitation, chest pain, change in VS; the geriatric patient may have undetected cardiac problems; baseline ECG should be completed before treatment

Patient/family education
• Teach patient that product is not a cure but controls symptoms and that treatment is long-term, that strong odor is normal
• Instruct patient to report excitability, irritability, anxiety, sweating, heat intolerance, chest pain, palpitations, which indicate overdose
• Advise patient not to switch brands unless approved by prescriber; bioavailability may differ; do not take with food; absorption will be decreased
• Teach patient that product might be discontinued after giving birth; thyroid panel will be evaluated after 1-2 mo
• Teach patient that hyperthyroid child will show almost immediate behavior/personality change; that hair loss will occur in child and is temporary
• Caution patient that product is not to be taken to reduce weight

---

• Caution patient to avoid OTC preparations containing iodine; read labels; other medications should not be used unless approved by prescriber
• Teach patient to avoid iodine-containing food: iodized salt, soybeans, tofu, turnips, certain kinds of seafood and bread

Evaluation

Positive therapeutic outcome
• Absence of depression
• Weight loss, increased diuresis, pulse, appetite
• Absence of constipation, peripheral edema, cold intolerance, pale, cool dry skin, brittle nails, alopecia, coarse hair, menorrhagia, night blindness, paresthesias, syncope, stupor, coma, rosy cheeks
• Improved levels of T_3, T_4 by laboratory tests
• Child: Age-appropriate weight, height, and psychomotor development

TREATMENT OF OVERDOSE:
Withhold dose for up to 1 wk; acute overdose—gastric lavage or induce emesis, then activated charcoal; provide supportive treatment to control symptoms

RARELY USED
tiaGABine (Rx)
(tie-ah-ga′been)
Gabitril
Func. class.: Anticonvulsant
Pregnancy category C

Do not confuse: tiaGABine/tiZANidine

ACTION: Inhibits reuptake and metabolism of GABA; may increase seizure threshold, structurally similar to GABA; tiaGABine binding sites in neocortex, hippocampus

USES: Adjunct treatment of partial seizures in adults and children ≥12 yr

CONTRAINDICATIONS
Hypersensitivity

Precautions: Pregnancy C, breastfeeding, child <12 yr, geriatric, renal/hepatic disease, suicidal ideation/behavior, status epilepticus, mania, bipolar disorder, abrupt discontinuation, depression

DOSAGE AND ROUTES
When not given with a CYP3A4 enzyme, effect of tiaGABine is doubled; lower dosages are indicated
Adult: PO (those on an enzyme-inducing antiepileptic) 4 mg/day in divided doses, may increase by 4-8 mg qwk until desired response, max 56 mg/day
Child 12-18 yr: PO 4 mg/day, may increase by 4 mg at beginning of wk 2, may increase by 4-8 mg qwk until desired response, max 32 mg/day

Hepatic dose
Adult: PO reduce dose or increase dosing interval

Available forms: Tabs 2, 4, 12, 16 mg

Implementation
• Store at room temperature away from heat and light
• Provide assistance with ambulation during early part of treatment; dizziness occurs
• Provide seizure precautions: padded side rails; move objects that may harm patient
• Use with food

ADVERSE EFFECTS
CNS: *Dizziness, anxiety,* somnolence, ataxia, confusion, *asthenia,* unsteady gait, depression, suicidal ideation, seizures, tremor, hostility, EEG changes
CV: Vasodilatation, tachycardia, hypertension
ENDO: Goiter, hypothyroidism
GI: Nausea, diarrhea, vomiting, increased appetite
INTEG: Pruritus, rash, Stevens-Johnson syndrome, alopecia, hyperhidrosis
MS: Myalgia
RESP: Pharyngitis, coughing

Pharmacokinetics

Absorption	>95%
Distribution	Protein binding 96%
Metabolism	Liver
Excretion	Kidneys
Half-life	7-9 hr

Pharmacodynamics

Onset	Unknown
Peak	45 min
Duration	Unknown

INTERACTIONS
Individual drugs
CarBAMazepine, PHENobarbital, phenytoin, primidone: decreased effect of these products
Sevelamer: decreased tiagabine effect
Valproate: lower dose of tiaGABine may be required

Drug classifications
Alcohol, CNS depressants: increased CNS depression

Drug/food
High-fat meal: decreased rate of absorption

NURSING CONSIDERATIONS
Assessment
• Monitor renal function tests: urinalysis, BUN, urine creatinine q3mo
• Monitor liver function tests: ALT, AST, bilirubin
• **Assess description of seizures: location, duration, presence of aura; assess for weakness**
⚠ **Withdraw gradually to prevent seizures**
⚠ **May cause status epilepticus and unexplained death**
⚠ **Assess mental status: mood, sensorium, affect, behavioral changes, suicidal thoughts; if mental status changes, notify prescriber, increased affect and hypnomania may be present**

Patient/family education
• Advise patient to carry/wear emergency ID stating patient's name, products taken, condition, prescriber's name and phone number
• Advise patient to avoid driving, other activities that require alertness
• Teach patient not to discontinue medication quickly after long-term use
• Teach patient to notify prescriber if pregnancy is planned or suspected, avoid breastfeeding
⚠ **Teach patient to report suicidal thoughts, behaviors immediately**

Evaluation
Positive therapeutic outcome
• Decreased seizure activity; document on patient's chart

⚠ HIGH ALERT

ticagrelor
(tye-ka′gre-lor)
Brilinta
Func. class.: Platelet inhibitor
Chem. class.: ADP receptor antagonist
Pregnancy category C

ACTION: Reversibly binds to the platelet receptor, preventing platelet activation

Therapeutic outcome: Prevention of thromboembolism

USES: Arterial thromboembolism prophylaxis in acute coronary syndrome (ACS) (unstable angina, acute MI), including in patients undergoing percutaneous coronary intervention (PCI)

CONTRAINDICATIONS
Hypersensitivity, severe hepatic disease, bleeding

Precautions: Abrupt discontinuation, breastfeeding, children, infants, neonates, GI bleeding, hepatic disease, pregnancy C

DOSAGE AND ROUTES
Adult: **PO** Loading dose 180 mg with aspirin (usually 325 mg PO); then, give 90 mg bid with aspirin 75-100 mg/day, do not give maintenance doses of aspirin >100 mg/day

Available forms: Tab 90 mg

Implementation
PO route
• May be taken without regard to food
• Store at room temperature, in original container in dry place
• Discontinue 5-7 days before surgery
• Ensure entire dose is given by flushing mortar, syringe, NG tube with 2 additional 50 ml of water

ADVERSE EFFECTS
CNS: Dizziness, fatigue, headache
CV: Atrial fibrillation, bradyarrhythmias, chest pain, hypertension, hypotension, syncope, ventricular pauses
GI: Diarrhea, nausea
HEMA: Fatal bleeding
MISC: Back pain, gynecomastia, hyperuricemia
RESP: Cough, dyspnea

> **BLACK BOX WARNING:** Bleeding, intracranial bleeding

> **BLACK BOX WARNING:** Coronary artery bypass graft (CABG) surgery

Pharmacokinetics

Absorption	36%
Distribution	Protein binding >99%
Metabolism	By CYP3A4
Excretion	26% (urine)
Half-life	7 hr; 9 hr metabolite

Pharmacodynamics

Onset	Unknown
Peak	1.5 hr (product), 2.5 hr (metabolite)
Duration	≥8 hr

INTERACTIONS
Individual drugs
Simvastatin, lovastatin: increased effect
Digoxin: change in effect

Drug classifications

> **BLACK BOX WARNING:** Anticoagulants, NSAIDs, platelet inhibitors: increased bleeding risk

CYP3A4 inducers (carBAMazepine, dexamethasone, PHENobarbital, phenytoin, rifampin): decreased ticagrelor action

> **BLACK BOX WARNING:** CYP3A4 inhibitors (atazanavir, clarithromycin, dalfopristin, delavirdine, indinavir, isoniazid, itraconazole, ketoconazole, lopinavir, nefazodone, nelfinavir, quinupristin, ritonavir, saquinavir, telithromycin, tipranavir, voriconazole): increased bleeding risk

Drug/lab
Serum creatinine: increased

NURSING CONSIDERATIONS
Assessment
• Thromboembolism: Monitor CBC differential with platelet count baseline and periodically during treatment

> **BLACK BOX WARNING:** Assess for bleeding that may occur when aspirin is combined with this product, some bleeding can be fatal, usually aspirin doses >100 mg/day; watch for frank bleeding, hypotension

> **BLACK BOX WARNING:** CABG: Do not use in those undergoing CABG; discontinue ≥5 days before surgery

• **Abrupt discontinuation:** Do not discontinue abruptly, may increase risk for MI, stent thrombosis, death

Patient/family education
• Teach patient to take only as prescribed, do not skip or double doses, if a dose is missed, take next dose at scheduled time
• Advise patient to notify prescriber of chills, fever, bruising, bleeding; not to use aspirin ≥100 mg/day
• Teach patient not to use any Rx, OTC products, herbs without approval of prescriber; products with aspirin, NSAIDs may cause bleeding
• Instruct patient to notify all health care providers of product use
• Advise patient that product can be taken without regard to meals
• Teach patient it may take longer for bleeding to stop
• **Teach patient not to breastfeed**
• Advise patient to notify prescriber if pregnancy is planned or suspected

Evaluation
Positive therapeutic outcome
• Prevention of thromboembolism

ticarcillin/clavulanate (Rx)
(tye-kar-sill'in)
Timentin
Func. class.: Extended-spectrum penicillin, beta lactamase inhibitor
Chem. class.: Antiinfective— broad-spectrum
Pregnancy category B

ACTION: Interferes with cell wall replication of susceptible organisms; osmotically unstable cell wall swells, bursts from osmotic pressure; clavulanate inhibits β-lactamase and protects against enzymatic degradation of ticarcillin

Therapeutic outcome: Resolution of infection

USES: Respiratory, soft tissue, urinary tract infections; bacterial septicemia; effective for gram-positive cocci *(Staphylococcus aureus, Streptococcus faecalis, Streptococcus pneumoniae)*, gram-negative cocci *(Neisseria gonorrhoeae)*, gram-positive bacilli *(Clostridium perfringens, Clostridium tetani)*, gram-negative bacilli *(Bacteroides, Fusobacterium nucleatum, Escherichia coli, Proteus mirabilis, Salmonella, Morganella morganii, Proteus rettgeri, Enterobacter, Pseudomonas aeruginosa, Serratia, Peptococcus, Peptostreptococcus, Eubacterium)*

CONTRAINDICATIONS
Hypersensitivity to penicillins; neonates

Precautions: Pregnancy **B,** hypersensitivity to cephalosporins, renal disease

DOSAGE AND ROUTES
Systemic/urinary tract infections, moderate/severe infections
Adult ≥60 kg: IV INF 3.1 g q4-6hr
Adult <60 kg: IV INF 200-300 mg/kg/day q4-6hr
Child >60 kg: IV INF 3.1 g q4hr
Child <60 kg: IV INF 300 mg/kg/day q4hr
Full-term neonate/infant <3 mo (unlabeled): IV 50 mg/kg q4hr

Mild/moderate infections
Child ≥60 kg: IV INF 3.1 g q6hr
Child <60 kg: IV INF 200 mg/kg/day q6hr
Full-term neonate/infant <3 mo (unlabeled): IV 50 mg/kg q6hr

T

Renal dose
Adult: IV INF loading dose 3.1 g; CCr 60 ml/min 3.1 g q4hr; CCr 30-60 ml/min 2 g q4hr; CCr 10-30 ml/min 2 g q8hr; CCr <10 ml/min 2 g q12hr; CCr <10 ml/min with hepatic dysfunction 2 g q24hr

Available forms: Inj IM, **IV** 3 g ticarcillin and 0.1 g clavulanate; **IV** inf 3 g ticarcillin and 0.1 g clavulanate; powder for inj 3 g ticarcillin, 0.1 g clavulanate

Implementation
- Give product after C&S has been completed, give ≥q1hr before bactericidal antiinfectives, change IV site q48hr
- Have adrenalin, suction, tracheostomy set, endotracheal intubation equipment available
- Obtain scratch test results to assess allergy after securing order from prescriber; usually done when penicillin is only product of choice
- Store at room temperature, reconstituted sol for 12-24 hr or 3-7 days refrigerated

Intermittent IV infusion route
- Give **IV** after diluting 3.1 g or less/13 ml of sterile water or 0.9% NaCl (200 mg/ml), shake; may further dilute in 50-100 ml or more 0.9% NaCl, D₅W, or LR and run over ½ hr

Y-site compatibilities: Allopurinol, amifostine, amikacin, anidulafungin, atropine, aztreonam, bivalirudin, bumetanide, ceFAZolin, cefepime, cefotaxime, cefOXitin, cefTAZidime, ceftizoxime, cefTRIAXone, cefuroxime, chloramphenicol, cimetidine, clindamycin, cyclophosphamide, cycloSPORINE, dexamethasone, dexmedetomidine, digoxin, diltiazem, diphenhydrAMINE, DOCEtaxel, DOPamine, DOXOrubicin liposome, doxycycline, enalaprilat, EPINEPHrine, esmolol, etoposide phosphate, famotidine, fenoldopam, filgrastim, fluconazole, furosemide, gemcitabine, gentamicin, granisetron, heparin, hydrocortisone, HYDROmorphone, imipenem/cilastatin, insulin, isoproterenol, labetalol, levofloxacin, lidocaine, linezolid, LORazepam, melphalan, meperidine, methylPREDNISolone, metoclopramide, metoprolol, metroNIDAZOLE, milrinone, morphine, nitroglycerin, nitroprusside, norepinephrine, ondansetron, palonosetron, pantoprazole, PEMEtrexed, penicillin G potassium, perphenazine, phenylephrine, procainamide, propofol, propranolol, ranitidine, remifentanil, sargramostim, sodium bicarbonate, tacrolimus, teniposide, theophylline, thiotepa, tirofiban, tobramycin, vasopressin, verapamil, vinorelbine, voriconazole

Y-site incompatibilities: Acyclovir, amphotericin B cholesteryl sulfate, azithromycin, caspofungin, diazepam, DOBUTamine, drotrecogin, erythromycin, ganciclovir, haloperidol, hydrOXYzine, lansoprazole, phenytoin, promethazine, protamine, quinupristin/dalfopristin, trimethoprim/sulfamethoxazole

ADVERSE EFFECTS
CNS: Anxiety, coma, seizures, confusion, drowsiness
GI: *Nausea, vomiting, diarrhea,* increased AST, ALT, abdominal pain, glossitis, colitis, pseudomembranous colitis, hepatotoxicity
HEMA: Anemia, increased bleeding time, bone marrow depression, granulocytopenia
INTEG: Rash, urticaria, toxic epidermal necrolysis, pain at injection site
META: Hypokalemia, hypernatremia
SYST: Anaphylaxis, Stevens-Johnson syndrome, overgrowth of organisms

Pharmacokinetics
Absorption	Completely absorbed (**IV**)
Distribution	Widely distributed, crosses blood-brain barrier
Metabolism	Liver
Excretion	Kidneys
Half-life	64-68 min

Pharmacodynamics
	IV
Onset	Unknown
Peak	30-45 min
Duration	4 hr

INTERACTIONS
Individual drugs
Chloramphenicol: decreased antimicrobial effect of ticarcillin
Heparin: increased effect of heparin
Methotrexate: increased methotrexate level
Probenecid, sulfinpyrazone: increased ticarcillin concentration

Drug classifications
Aminoglycosides (**IV**): decreased antimicrobial effect of ticarcillin
Anticoagulants: increased bleeding
Contraceptives (oral): decreased effect of oral contraceptives
Erythromycins: decreased absorption
Macrolides, sulfonamides, tetracyclines: decreased ticarcillin effect

Drug/lab test
Increased: LFTs, sodium, eosinophils, INR, bleeding time, uric acid, bilirubin, BUN, creatinine, alk phos, LDH

Decreased: Hgb, potassium, platelets, WBC, granulocytes

False positive: urine glucose, urine protein, Coombs' test

NURSING CONSIDERATIONS
Assessment
- Infection: WBC, wound, temperature, sputum, urine, baseline and periodically
- **Pseudomembranous colitis: assess for diarrhea, abdominal pain, fever, fatigue, anorexia; possible anemia, elevated WBC, low serum albumin; stop product and usually give either vancomycin or IV metroNIDAZOLE**
- Monitor liver function tests: AST, ALT
- Monitor blood tests: WBC, RBC, Hgb, Hct, bleeding time, platelets, baseline and periodically
- Monitor renal function tests; sodium, potassium
- Assess skin eruptions after administration of penicillin to 1 wk after discontinuing product
- ⚠ **Assess for anaphylaxis: wheezing, rash, laryngeal edema; have emergency equipment nearby**
- **Serious skin reactions:** Stevens-Johnson syndrome, toxic epidermal necrolysis

Patient/family education
- Advise patient that C&S may be performed after completed course of medication
- Instruct patient to report sore throat, fever, fatigue (may indicate superinfection)
- Advise patient to carry/wear emergency ID if allergic to penicillins
- Advise patient to use alternative birth control methods instead of hormonal
- **Advise patient to report persistent diarrhea with blood, pus, mucus, or fever**

Evaluation

Positive therapeutic outcome
- Absence of fever, purulent drainage, redness, inflammation

TREATMENT OF OVERDOSE:
Withdraw product, maintain airway, administer EPINEPHrine, aminophylline, O$_2$, **IV** corticosteroids for anaphylaxis

ticlopidine (Rx)
(tye-cloe'pi-deen)
Func. class.: Platelet aggregation inhibitor
Chem. class.: Thienopyridine compound
Pregnancy category B

ACTION: Irreversible inhibition of platelet aggregation through antagonism of ADP

Therapeutic outcome: Decreased stroke by decreasing platelet aggregation

USES: Reducing the risk of stroke in high-risk patients

Unlabeled uses: Intermittent claudication, chronic arterial occlusion, subarachnoid hemorrhage, uremic patients with AV shunts/fistulas, open heart surgery, coronary artery bypass grafts, primary glomerulonephritis, diabetic neuropathy

CONTRAINDICATIONS
Hypersensitivity, severe liver disease, active bleeding, coagulopathy

> **BLACK BOX WARNING:** Agranulocytosis, neutropenia, thrombocytopenia, thrombotic thrombocytopenic purpura (TTP)

Precautions: Pregnancy **B**, breastfeeding, children, geriatric, past liver disease, renal disease, increased bleeding risk, peptic ulcer disease, surgery

> **BLACK BOX WARNING:** Anemia, hematological disease

DOSAGE AND ROUTES
Adult: PO 250 mg bid with food

Available forms: Tabs 250 mg

Implementation
- Give with food or after eating to decrease GI effects; may use methylPREDNISolone **IV** 20 mg to provide normal bleeding time in 2 hr

ADVERSE EFFECTS
CNS: Dizziness, headache, weakness
EENT: Tinnitus, epistaxis
GI: Nausea, vomiting, diarrhea, GI discomfort, **cholestatic jaundice, hepatitis,** increased cholesterol LDL, VLDL, triglycerides
GU: Hematuria
HEMA: **Bleeding (epistaxis, hematuria, conjunctival hemorrhage, GI bleeding), agranulocytosis, neutropenia, thrombocytopenia, thrombotic thrombocytopenic purpura**
INTEG: Rash, pruritus
META: Hypercholesterolemia, hypertriglyceridemia

T

Adverse effects: *italics* = common; **bold** = life-threatening

Pharmacokinetics

Absorption	Well absorbed
Distribution	Unknown
Metabolism	Liver, extensively; 98% protein binding
Excretion	Kidneys, unchanged product
Half-life	Increased with repeat dosing; 4-5 days (multiple doses)

Pharmacodynamics

Onset	Unknown
Peak	1-3 hr
Duration	Unknown

INTERACTIONS
Individual drugs

Abciximab, aspirin, eptifibatide, tirofiban: increased bleeding tendencies

Ambrisenten, fosphenytoin, phenytoin, theophylline: increased levels of each specific drug

Cimetidine: increased effects of ticlopidine

CycloSPORINE: decreased plasma levels of cycloSPORINE

Digoxin: decreased plasma levels of digoxin

Drug classifications

Antacids: decreased plasma levels of ticlopidine

Anticoagulants, NSAIDs, salicylates, SSRIs, thrombin inhibitors, thrombolytics: increased bleeding risk

CYP2C19, CYP2DC substrates: increased levels of each specific drug

Drug/herb

Ginger, ginkgo, garlic, feverfew, horse chestnut, green tea: increased bleeding risk

NURSING CONSIDERATIONS
Assessment

• Monitor liver function tests: AST, ALT, bilirubin, creatinine if patient is on long-term therapy (4 mo or more)

> **BLACK BOX WARNING:** Blood dyscrasias, bone marrow depression, do not use in those with a history of these conditions; monitor blood tests: CBC, Hct, Hgb, pro-time if patient is on long-term therapy; CBC q2wk × 3 mo therapy; thrombocytopenia, neutropenia may occur

> **BLACK BOX WARNING:** Monitor bleeding time baseline and throughout therapy, levels may be 2-5 × normal limit

Patient/family education

• Advise patient that blood studies are necessary during treatment

> **BLACK BOX WARNING:** Advise patient to report any unusual bleeding to prescriber

• Instruct patient to take with food or just after eating to minimize GI discomfort, not to double missed dose
• Caution patient to report side effects such as diarrhea, skin rashes, subcutaneous bleeding, signs of cholestasis (yellow skin and sclera, dark urine, light-colored stools)
• Advise patient that product should be discontinued 10-14 days before surgery
• Advise there are many drug and herb interactions; to avoid all OTC products unless approved by prescriber
• To take with food

Evaluation
Positive therapeutic outcome
• Absence of stroke

tigecycline (Rx)
(tye-ge-sye'kleen)
Tygacil
Func. class.: Broad-spectrum antiinfective
Chem. class.: Glycylcyclines
Pregnancy category D

ACTION: Inhibits protein synthesis and phosphorylation in microorganisms; bacteriostatic, structurally similar to the tetracyclines

Therapeutic outcome: Resolution of infection

USES: Complicated skin/skin structure infections: *Escherichia coli, Enterococcus faecalis* (vancomycin-susceptible only), *Staphylococcus aureus, Streptococcus agalactiae, S. anginosus* group, *S. pyogenes, Bacteroides fragilis*; complicated intraabdominal infections (*Citrobacter freundii*), *Enterobacter cloacae, Escherichia coli, Klebsiella oxytoca, K. pneumoniae, E. faecalis* (vancomycin-susceptible only), *S. aureus* (methicillin-susceptible only), *S. anginosus* group, *B. fragilis, Bacteroides thetaiotaomicron, B. uniformis, B. vulgatus, Clostridium perfringens, Peptostreptococcus micros*, community-acquired pneumonia

CONTRAINDICATIONS
Pregnancy **D**, breastfeeding, children <18 yr, hypersensitivity to tigecycline

Precautions: Renal/hepatic disease, hypersensitivity to tetracyclines, ventricular-associated hospital-acquired pneumonias

---

DOSAGE AND ROUTES

Adult: IV 100 mg, then 50 mg q12hr, **IV** INF is given over 30 min to 60 min q12hr; given for 5-14 days depending on infection

Hepatic dose (Child-Pugh C)
Adult: IV 100 mg, then 25 mg q12hr

Available forms: Powder for inj, lyophilized 50 mg

Implementation

• Tigecycline allergy test before using, obtain C&S, do not begin treatment before results

Intermittent IV infusion route

• Reconstitute each vial with 5.3 ml of 0.9% NaCl, or D₅W (10 mg/ml); swirl to dissolve; immediately withdraw 5 ml of the reconstituted sol and add to a 100-ml **IV** bag for inf (1 mg/ml); may be yellow or orange, if not, sol should be discarded; do not give if particulate matter is present, use a dedicated IV line or Y-site, flush with NS before and after use, give over ½ hr
• Store in tight, light-resistant container at room temperature, diluted sol at room temp for up to 24 hr, 6 hr in vial, and remaining time in IV bag, 48 hr refrigerated

Y-site compatibilities: Acyclovir, alfentanil, allopurinol, amifostine, amikacin, aminocaproic acid, aminophylline, amphotericin B liposome, ampicillin, ampicillin/sulbactam, argatroban, azithromycin, aztreonam, bivalirudin, bumetanide, buprenorphine, butorphanol, calcium chloride/gluconate, CARBOplatin, carmustine, caspofungin, ceFAZolin, cefepime, cefotaxime, cefoTEtan, cefOXitin, cefTAZidime, ceftizoxime, cefTRIAXone, cefuroxime, cimetidine, ciprofloxacin, cisatracurium, CISplatin, clindamycin, cyclophosphamide, cycloSPORINE, cytarabine, dacarbazine, DACTINomycin, DAPTOmycin, DAUNOrubicin hydrochloride, dexamethasone, dexmedetomidine, dexrazoxane, digoxin, diltiazem, diphenhydrAMINE, DOBUTamine, DOCEtaxel, dolasetron, DOPamine, doripenem, DOXOrubicin hydrochloride, DOXOrubicin liposome, droperidol, enalaprilat, EPINEPHrine, eptifibatide, ertapenem, erythromycin, esmolol, etoposide, etoposide phosphate, famotidine, fenoldopam, fentaNYL, fluconazole, fludarabine, fluorouracil, foscarnet, fosphenytoin, furosemide, ganciclovir, gemcitabine, gentamicin, glycopyrrolate, granisetron, haloperidol, heparin, hydrocortisone, HYDROmorphone, ifosfamide, imipenem/cilastatin, insulin, irinotecan, isoproterenol, ketorolac, labetalol, lansoprazole, lepirudin, leucovorin, levofloxacin, lidocaine, linezolid, LORazepam, magnesium sulfate, mannitol, mechlorethamine, melphalan, meperidine, meropenem, mesna, methohexital, methotrexate, methyldopa, metoclopramide, metoprolol, metroNIDAZOLE, midazolam, milrinone, mitoMYcin, mitoXANtrone, morphine, moxifloxacin, mycophenolate, nafcillin, nalbuphine, naloxone, nesiritide, nitroglycerin, nitroprusside, norepinephrine, octreotide, ondansetron, oxaliplatin, oxytocin, PACLitaxel, palonosetron, pamidronate, pancuronium, pantoprazole, PEMEtrexed, pentamidine, pentazocine, PENTObarbital, PHENobarbital, phenylephrine, piperacillin/tazobactam, potassium acetate/chloride/phosphate, procainamide, prochlorperazine, promethazine, propofol, propranolol, ranitidine, remifentanil, rocuronium, sodium acetate/bicarbonate/phosphate, streptozocin, succinylcholine, SUFentanil, tacrolimus, teniposide, theophylline, thiopental, thiotepa, ticarcillin/clavulanate, tirofiban, tobramycin, topotecan, trimethoprim/sulfamethoxazole, vancomycin, vasopressin, vecuronium, vinBLAStine, vinCRIStine, vinorelbine, zidovudine, zoledronic acid

Y-site incompatibilities: Amiodarone, amphotericin B colloidal, bleomycin, chloramphenicol, chlorproMAZINE, dantrolene, DAUNOrubicin liposome, diazepam, epirubicin, hydrALAZINE, IDArubicin, niCARdipine, phenytoin, quinapristin/dalfopristin, verapamil

ADVERSE EFFECTS

CNS: Headache, dizziness, insomnia
CV: Hypo/hypertension, phlebitis
EENT: Tooth discoloration
GI: *Nausea, vomiting, diarrhea,* anorexia, constipation, dyspepsia, **hepatotoxicity, hepatic failure, pseudomembranous colitis**
HEMA: **Anemia, leukocytosis, thrombocytopenia**
INTEG: *Rash,* pruritus, sweating, photosensitivity
META: Increased ALT, AST, BUN, lactic acid, alkaline phosphatase, amylase, hyperglycemia, hypokalemia, hypoproteinemia, bilirubinemia
MISC: Back pain, fever, abnormal healing, abdominal pain, abscess, asthenia, infection, pain, peripheral edema, local reactions
RESP: Cough, dyspnea
SYST: **Anaphylaxis**

Pharmacokinetics

Absorption	Unknown
Distribution	Protein binding 71%-89%
Metabolism	Not extensively
Excretion	22% unchanged, urine; primarily biliarily excreted
Half-life	Terminal 42 hr

T

Unknown

INTERACTIONS
Individual drugs
Warfarin: increased effect of tigecycline

Drug classifications
Oral contraceptives: decreased effect of tigecycline

Drug/lab test
Increased: amylase, LFTs, alk phos, BUN, creatinine, LDH, WBC, INR, PTT, PT
Decreased: potassium, calcium, sodium, Hgb/Hct, platelets

NURSING CONSIDERATIONS
Assessment

> **BLACK BOX WARNING:** Infection: Use only with confirmed or strongly suspected bacterial infection; do not use as a prophylactic

- **Pseudomembranous colitis: assess for diarrhea, abdominal pain, fever, fatigue, anorexia; possible anemia, elevated WBC, low serum albumin; stop product and usually give either vancomycin or IV metroNIDAZOLE**
- Assess for signs of anemia: Hct, Hgb, fatigue
- Monitor blood tests: PT, CBC, AST, ALT, BUN creatinine
- **Assess for allergic reactions:** rash, itching, pruritus, angioedema
- ⚠ Serious allergic skin reactions: assess for Stevens-Johnson syndrome, anaphylaxis
- Assess for nausea, vomiting, diarrhea; administer antiemetic, antacids as ordered
- **Assess for overgrowth of infection:** fever, malaise, redness, pain, swelling, drainage, perineal itching, diarrhea, changes in cough or sputum
- ⚠ **Toxicity: assess for pseudotumor cerebri, photosensitivity, anti-anabolic actions (azotemia, BUN, hypophosphatemia, metabolic acidosis): tigecycline is structurally similar to tetracycline**
- ⚠ **Assess for pancreatitis, hyperamylasemia: may be fatal; if these occur, discontinue; improvement usually occurs after product is discontinued**

Patient/family education
- Teach patient to avoid sun exposure; sunscreen does not seem to decrease photosensitivity
- Teach patient to avoid pregnancy while taking this product; fetal harm may occur; to avoid breastfeeding
- Teach patient to report burning, pain at inj site
- **Teach patient to report diarrhea, fatigue, abdominal pain**

Evaluation

Positive therapeutic outcome
- Decreased temp, absence of lesions, negative C&S

---

timolol (Rx)
(tye′moe-lole)
Apo-Timol ✦, Novo-Timol ✦
Func. class.: Antihypertensive; antiglaucoma
Chem. class.: Nonselective β-blocker
Pregnancy category C

ACTION: Competitively blocks stimulation of β-adrenergic receptor within vascular smooth muscle (decreases rate of SA node discharge, increases recovery time), slows conduction of AV node, decreases heart rate, which decreases O_2 consumption in myocardium; also decreases renin-aldosterone-angiotensin system; at high doses inhibits $β_2$ receptors in bronchial system

Therapeutic outcome: Decreased B/P, decreased arrhythmias, absence of death from MI, decreased aqueous humor in the eye, absence of migraine headaches

USES: Mild to moderate hypertension, migraine prophylaxis, to decrease mortality following MI

Unlabeled uses: Tremors, angina pectoris

CONTRAINDICATIONS
Hypersensitivity to β-blockers, cardiogenic shock, heart block (2nd or 3rd degree), sinus bradycardia, CHF, cardiac failure, severe COPD, asthma

Precautions: Pregnancy C, breastfeeding, major surgery, diabetes mellitus, thyroid/renal/hepatic disease, COPD, well-compensated heart failure, nonallergic bronchospasm, peripheral vascular disease

> **BLACK BOX WARNING:** Abrupt discontinuation

DOSAGE AND ROUTES
Hypertension
Adult: PO 10 mg bid, or 20 mg/day, may increase by 10 mg q7day, max 60 mg/day
Geriatric: PO Initiate dose cautiously

Myocardial infarction
Adult: 10 mg bid beginning 1-4 wk after MI for ≥2 yr

Glaucoma
Adult: Ophth 1 gtt daily or bid
Child: Ophth 1 gtt daily or bid (0.25% SOL only)

Migraine headache prevention
Adult: PO 10 mg bid, or 20 mg/day; may increase to 30 mg/day, 20 mg in AM, 10 mg in PM; discontinue if not effective after 8 wk

Available forms: Tabs 5, 10, 20 mg

Implementation
• Given before meals, at bedtime; tab may be crushed or swallowed whole; give with food to prevent GI upset; reduce dosage in renal dysfunction
• Store at room temp; do not freeze

ADVERSE EFFECTS
CNS: *Insomnia, dizziness,* hallucinations, anxiety, fatigue, depression, headache
CV: Hypotension, bradycardia, **CHF,** edema, chest pain, claudication, angina, AV block, ventricular dysrhythmias
EENT: *Vision changes,* sore throat, *double vision,* dry burning eyes
GI: *Nausea,* vomiting, **ischemic colitis,** diarrhea, *abdominal pain,* **mesenteric arterial thrombosis,** flatulence, constipation
GU: Impotence, urinary frequency
HEMA: **Agranulocytosis, thrombocytopenia, purpura**
INTEG: Rash, alopecia, pruritus, fever
META: Hypoglycemia
MUSC: *Joint pain, muscle pain*
RESP: **Bronchospasm,** dyspnea, cough, crackles, nasal stuffiness

Pharmacokinetics

Absorption	Well absorbed (PO), minimally absorbed (ophth)
Distribution	Protein binding <10%
Metabolism	Liver, extensively
Excretion	Breast milk
Half-life	3 hr

Pharmacodynamics

	PO
Onset	Unknown
Peak	2-4 hr
Duration	12-24 hr

INTERACTIONS
Individual drugs
Alcohol: increased hypotension, bradycardia (large amounts)
HydrALAZINE, methyldopa, prazosin, reserpine: increased hypotension, bradycardia
Insulin: decreased hypoglycemia
Thyroid hormones: decreased antihypertensive effect

Drug classifications
Anticholinergics, nitrates: increased hypotension, increased bradycardia
β₂-Adrenergic agonists: increased β-blocking effect
Calcium channel blockers: increased effects of calcium channel blockers
NSAIDs, salicylates, sympathomimetics: decreased antihypertensive effect
Sulfonylureas: decreased hypoglycemic effect
Theophyllines: decreased bronchodilatation

Drug/lab test
Increased: renal, liver function tests, uric acid
Interference: glucose, insulin tolerance test

NURSING CONSIDERATIONS
Assessment

> **BLACK BOX WARNING: Abrupt discontinuation:** may result in myocardial ischemia, MI, severe hypotension, ventricular dysrhythmias in those with preexisting cardiovascular disease

• Assess for headaches: location, severity, duration, frequency baseline, throughout treatment
• Monitor B/P during beginning treatment, periodically thereafter; pulse q4hr; note rate, rhythm, quality: apical/radial pulse before administration; notify prescriber of any significant changes (pulse <50 bpm)
• Check baselines in renal, liver function tests before therapy begins
• Assess for edema in feet, legs daily, monitor I&O ratio, daily weight; check for jugular vein distention, crackles bilaterally, dyspnea (CHF)
• Monitor skin turgor, dryness of mucous membranes for hydration status, especially geriatric

Patient/family education

> **BLACK BOX WARNING:** Teach patient not to discontinue product abruptly; taper over 2 wk; may cause precipitate angina if stopped abruptly

• Advise patient not to use OTC products containing α-adrenergic stimulants (nasal decongestants, cold preparations); to avoid alcohol, smoking; to limit sodium intake as prescribed

T

• Teach patient how to take pulse and B/P at home; advise patient when to notify prescriber
• Instruct patient to comply with weight control, dietary adjustments, modified exercise program
• Advise patient to carry/wear emergency ID to identify product being taken, any allergies; tell patient product controls symptoms but does not cure
• Caution patient to avoid hazardous activities if dizziness, drowsiness are present
• Teach patient to report symptoms of CHF; difficult breathing, especially on exertion or when lying down; night cough; swelling of extremities or bradycardia; dizziness; confusion; depression; fever
• Teach patient to take product as prescribed, not to double dose, skip doses; take any missed doses as soon as remembered if at least 4 hr until next dose
• Product masks hypoglycemia; monitor blood sugar

Evaluation

Positive therapeutic outcome
• Decreased B/P in hypertension (after 1-2 wk)
• Absence of dysrhythmias

TREATMENT OF OVERDOSE:
Lavage, **IV** atropine for bradycardia, **IV** theophylline for bronchospasm, digoxin, O_2, diuretic for cardiac failure, hemodialysis, **IV** glucose for hyperglycemia, **IV** diazepam (or phenytoin) for seizures

timolol ophthalmic
See Appendix B

🛆 HIGH ALERT

tinidazole (Rx)
(tye-ni´da-zole)
Tindamax
Func. class.: Antiprotozoal
Chem. class.: Nitroimidazole derivative
Pregnancy category C

ACTION: Interferes with DNA/RNA synthesis in protozoa

Therapeutic outcome: Decrease in infection

USES: Amebiasis, giardiasis, trichomoniasis

CONTRAINDICATIONS
Breastfeeding, hypersensitivity to this product or nitroimidazole derivative, pregnancy

Precautions: Pregnancy **C,** children, geriatric, hepatic disease, CNS depression, blood dyscrasias, candidiasis, seizures, viral infection, alcoholism

BLACK BOX WARNING: Secondary malignancy

DOSAGE AND ROUTES
Intestinal amebiasis
Adult: PO 2 g/day × 3 days
Adolescent/child ≥3 yr: PO 50 mg/kg/day × 3 days, max 2 g/day

Amebic involvement (liver)
Adult: PO 2 g/day × 3-5 days
Child ≥3 yr: PO 50 mg/kg/day × 3-5 days, max 2 g

Giardiasis
Adult: PO 2 g as a single dose
Child ≥3 yr: PO 50 mg/kg as a single dose, max 2 g

Trichomoniasis
Adult: PO 2 g as a single dose

Bacterial vaginosis
Adult (not pregnant): PO 2 g/day × 2 days with food or 1 g/day × 5 days with food

Available forms: Tabs 250, 500 mg

Implementation
• Administer to those >3 yr old
• Give with food; tabs can be crushed and mixed with artificial cherry syrup

ADVERSE EFFECTS
CNS: *Dizziness, headache, seizures, peripheral neuropathy,* malaise, fatigue
GI: *Nausea, vomiting,* anorexia, increased AST and ALT, constipation, abdominal pain, indigestion, altered taste
HEMA: Leukopenia, neutropenia
INTEG: Pruritus, urticaria, *rash,* oral candidiasis
SYST: Angioedema, cramping

Pharmacokinetics

Absorption	Unknown
Distribution	Crosses blood-brain barrier
Metabolism	Extensively in the liver
Excretion	Unchanged (20%-25%) in urine, (12%) feces
Half-life	12-14 hr

Pharmacodynamics

Unknown

INTERACTIONS
Individual drugs
Do not use within 2 wk of taking disulfiram

Cholestyramine, oxytetracycline: decreased action of tinidazole

CycloSPORINE, fluorouracil, lithium, tacrolimus: increased action

Drug classifications

Anticoagulants, hydantoins: increased action

CYP3A4 inducers (phenobarbital, phenytoin, rifampin): decreased action of tinidazole

CYP3A4 inhibitors (cimetidine, ketoconazole): increased action of tinidazole

Drug/herb

St. John's wort: increased or decreased tinidazole level

Drug/lab test

Increase: triglycerides, LDH, AST/ALT, glucose

Decrease: WBCs

NURSING CONSIDERATIONS
Assessment

• Giardiasis: obtain 3 stool samples several days apart beginning q3-4wk after treatment

• **Assess for amebic liver abscess:** monitor CBC, ESR, amebic gel diffusion test, ultrasound, total and differential leukocyte count

• Assess for signs of infection, anemia

• Assess bowel pattern before, during treatment

> BLACK BOX WARNING: **Secondary malignancy:** Avoid unnecessary use

Patient/family education

• Instruct patient to take with food to increase plasma concentrations, minimize epigastric distress and other GI effects; not to use alcoholic beverages during or for 3 days afterward

• Advise patient that in cases of trichomoniasis, both partners should be treated at the same time

• Teach patient to avoid alcohol, may cause disulfiram reaction

• Teach patient to avoid doing hazardous activities until reaction is known

• Teach patient that product causes taste change

• Teach patient not to use OTC, Rx or herbal products unless approved by prescriber

Evaluation

Positive therapeutic outcome

• Decrease in infection as evidenced by negative culture

tioconazole vaginal antifungal
See Appendix B

tiotropium (Rx)

(ty-oh′tro-pee-um)

HandiHaler, Spiriva, Spiriva Respimat

Func. class.: Anticholinergic, bronchodilator

Chem. class.: Synthetic quaternary ammonium compound

Pregnancy category C

Do not confuse: Spiriva/Inspra

ACTION: Inhibits interaction of acetylcholine at receptor sites on the bronchial smooth muscle, resulting in decreased cGMP and bronchodilatation

Therapeutic outcome: Improved breathing

USES: COPD, for long-term treatment, once daily maintenance of bronchospasm, associated with COPD including chronic bronchitis and emphysema

CONTRAINDICATIONS

Hypersensitivity to this product, atropine, or its derivatives

Precautions: Pregnancy **C**, breastfeeding, children, geriatric, closed-angle glaucoma, prostatic hypertrophy, bladder neck obstruction, renal disease

DOSAGE AND ROUTES

Adult: INH content of 1 cap/day (18 mcg) using HandiHaler inhalation device or 2 inh (spray) (2.5 mcg each) qday

Available forms: Powder for inhalation 18 mcg in blister packs containing 6 caps with inhaler; 30 caps with inhaler; spray inhaler (Respimat) 2.5 mcg/spray

Implementation
Inhalation route

• **Caps are for INH only; do not swallow**

• Immediately before administration, peel back foil until cap is visible (until "stop" line); open dust cap of HandiHaler by pulling upward, then open mouthpiece

• Place cap in center chamber; firmly close mouthpiece until it clicks, leaving dust cap open

• Hold HandiHaler with mouthpiece upward; press button in once, completely, and release; this allows medication to be released

• Breathe out completely; do not breathe into mouthpiece at any time

• Raise device to mouth and close lips tightly around mouthpiece

T

• With head upright, breathe in slowly/deeply, but allowing the cap to vibrate; breathe until lungs fill; hold breath and remove mouthpiece; resume normal breathing
• Repeat
• Remove used capsule and discard; close the mouthpiece and dust cap; store

Inhalation route (spray)
• Insert cartridge into inhaler; prime inhaler; must reprime once if not used for >3 days; if not used for >21 days, prime until aerosol is visible and 3 more times

ADVERSE EFFECTS
CNS: Depression, paresthesia
CV: Chest pain, increased heart rate
EENT: Dry mouth, blurred vision, glaucoma
GI: *Vomiting,* abdominal pain, constipation, dyspepsia
GU: Urinary difficulty, urinary retention, UTI
INTEG: Rash, **angioedema**
MISC: Candidiasis, flulike syndrome, herpes zoster, infections, angina pectoris
MS: Arthritis, myalgic leg/skeletal pain
RESP: *Cough, worsening of symptoms,* sinusitis, URI, epistaxis, pharyngitis

Pharmacokinetics

Absorption	Unknown
Distribution	Does not cross blood-brain barrier
Metabolism	Very little metabolized in the liver
Excretion	Excreted in urine, 72% protein binding
Half-life	5-6 days in animals

Pharmacodynamics
Unknown

INTERACTIONS
Drug classifications
Anticholinergics: avoid use with other anticholinergics

Drug/lab test
Increased: cholesterol, glucose

NURSING CONSIDERATIONS
Assessment
• For tolerance over long-term therapy; dose may have to be increased or changed
• **Respiratory status:** assess for dyspnea, rate, breath sounds before and during treatment; pulmonary function tests baseline and periodically; upper respiratory infection, cough, sinusitis

Patient/family education
• Teach patient how to use HandiHaler
• Teach patient signs of closed-angle glaucoma (eye pain, blurred vision, visual halos)
• Advise patient that product is used for long-term maintenance, not for immediate relief of breathing problems
• Caution patient to avoid getting the powder in the eyes; may cause blurred vision and pupil dilatation
• **Teach patient to report immediately blurred vision, eye pain, halos**
• Teach patient to keep caps in sealed blisters before use, store at room temperature

Evaluation
Positive therapeutic outcome
• Ability to breathe easier

---

tipranavir (Rx)
(ti-pran'a-veer)
Aptivus
Func. class.: Antiretroviral
Chem. class.: Protease inhibitor
Pregnancy category C

ACTION: Inhibits HIV protease; this prevents the maturation of virus

Therapeutic outcome: Prevention of worsening of HIV

USES: HIV in combination with other antiretrovirals

CONTRAINDICATIONS
Hypersensitivity

> **BLACK BOX WARNING:** Hepatic disease (Child-Pugh B to C)

Precautions: Pregnancy **C,** breastfeeding, children, renal disease, history of renal stones, sulfa allergy, hemophilia, diabetes mellitus, pancreatitis, alcoholism, immune reconstitution syndrome, surgery, trauma, infection

> **BLACK BOX WARNING:** Intracranial bleeding, hepatitis

DOSAGE AND ROUTES
Reduce dosage in mild or moderate hepatic impairment and ketoconazole coadministration
Adult: PO 500 mg coadministered with ritonavir 200 mg bid with food
Adolescent and child ≥2 yr: PO 14 mg/kg given with ritonavir 6 mg/kg bid or 375 mg/m^2 given with ritonavir 150 mg/m^2 bid; max 500 mg with ritonavir 200 mg bid

---

Available forms: Caps 250 mg; oral sol 100 mg/ml

Implementation
• Not to be used in those who are treatment naive
• Swallow cap whole; do not break, crush, or chew
• Store caps in refrigerator before use; after opening, store at room temp; use within 60 days
• Give after meals
• Give in equal intervals around the clock to maintain blood levels

ADVERSE EFFECTS
CNS: *Headache, insomnia,* dizziness, somnolence, fatigue, *fever,* **intracranial bleeding**
GI: *Diarrhea, abdominal pain, nausea, vomiting,* anorexia, dry mouth, **hepatitis B or C, fatalities when given with ritonavir, pancreatitis**
GU: Nephrolithiasis
INTEG: *Rash,* urticaria, lipodystrophy, serious rash
MS: Pain
OTHER: Asthenia, **insulin-resistant hyperglycemia,** *hyperlipidemia,* **ketoacidosis**

Pharmacokinetics

Absorption	Unknown
Distribution	Protein binding, 99.9%, steady state 7-10 days
Metabolism	CYP3A4
Excretion	80% feces
Half-life	Terminal 6 hr

Pharmacodynamics

Onset	Unknown
Peak	3 hr
Duration	Unknown

INTERACTIONS
Individual drugs
⚠ Amiodarone, astemizole, cisapride, flecainide, midazolam, pimozide, propafenone, quiNIDine, rifabutin, rifampin, terfenadine, triazolam: life-threatening dysrhythmias
Clarithromycin, zidovudine: increased levels of both products
Delavirdine, itraconazole, ketoconazole: increased tipranavir levels
Efavirenz, fluconazole, nevirapine: decreased tipranavir levels
Lovastatin, simvastatin: increased myopathy, rhabdomyolysis

Drug classifications
⚠ Ergots: life-threatening dysrhythmias
Oral contraceptives: increased levels of tipranavir
Rifamycins: decreased tipranavir levels

Drug/herb
St. John's wort: decreased tipranavir levels; avoid concurrent use

Drug/food
Grapefruit juice, high-fat, high-protein foods: decreased tipranavir absorption

Drug/lab test
Increased: AST, ALT, cholesterol, blood glucose, amylase, lipase, triglycerides

NURSING CONSIDERATIONS
Assessment
• Assess for signs of infection, anemia, the presence of other STDs

> **BLACK BOX WARNING:** Assess for hepatic studies: ALT, AST; total bilirubin, amylase, all may be elevated, discontinue in those with hepatic insufficiency or hepatitis or AST/ALT 10× upper limit or AST/ALT 5-10× ULN and total bilirubin 2.5× ULN; assess for anorexia, nausea, jaundice, hepatomegaly, clay-colored stools

• **HIV:** Monitor viral load, CD4, plasma HIV RNA, serum cholesterol/triglycerides during treatment
• Monitor bowel pattern before, during treatment; if severe abdominal pain with bleeding occurs, product should be discontinued; monitor hydration
• **Immune reconstitution syndrome: has been reported with combination antiretroviral therapy; patients may develop pain (MAC, CMV, PcP, TB) and autoimmune disease months after treatment**

> **BLACK BOX WARNING: Intracranial bleeding:** more common in those with trauma or surgery, or those taking antiplatelets or anticoagulants; assess for headache, nausea, vomiting, seizures, confusion, inability to speak; can be fatal

• Cushingoid symptoms: assess for buffalo hump, facial/peripheral wasting, breast enlargement, central obesity
• **Serious rash: if a serious rash occurs, product should be discontinued**
• Assess for allergies before treatment, reaction of each medication; place allergies on chart

Patient/family education
• Teach patient to take as prescribed; if dose is missed, take as soon as remembered up to 1 hr before next dose; do not double dose
• Teach patient that product must be taken in equal intervals around the clock to maintain blood levels for duration of therapy
⚠ Advise that hyperglycemia may occur; watch for increased thirst, weight loss, hunger, dry, itchy skin; notify prescriber
• Advise patient that product does not cure AIDS, only controls symptoms; not to donate blood
• Teach patient not to breastfeed
• Advise patient that redistribution of body fat may occur
• Teach patient not to use with other products unless approved by prescriber, many drug interactions
• Inform patient that product must be taken in combination with ritonavir
• Teach patient to stop product and notify prescriber if anorexia, nausea, vomiting, yellowing of skin or eyes, clay-colored stools, fatigue, pain in upper abdomen occur

Evaluation

Positive therapeutic outcome
• Prevention of viral replication

> **⚠ HIGH ALERT**
>
> ## tirofiban (Rx)
> (tie-roh-fee′ban)
> **Aggrastat**
> *Func. class.:* Antiplatelet
> *Chem. class.:* Glycoprotein IIb/IIIa inhibitor
> **Pregnancy category B**

ACTION: Antagonist of platelet glycoprotein (GP) IIb/IIIa receptor that leads to binding of fibrinogen and von Willebrand's factor, which inhibits platelet aggregation

Therapeutic outcome: Decreased platelet count

USES: Acute coronary syndrome in combination with heparin

CONTRAINDICATIONS
Hypersensitivity, active internal bleeding, stroke, major surgery, severe trauma within 30 days, intracranial neoplasm, aneurysm, hemorrhage, acute pericarditis, platelets <100,000/mm³, history of thrombocytopenia, coagulopathy, systolic B/P >180 mm Hg or diastolic B/P >110 mm Hg

Precautions: Pregnancy **B**, breastfeeding, children, geriatric, renal disease, bleeding tendencies, hypertension, platelets <150,000/mm³

DOSAGE AND ROUTES
Adult: IV 0.4 mcg/kg/min × 30 min, then 0.1 mcg/kg/min for 12-24 hr after angioplasty or atherectomy

Renal dose
Adult: IV CCr <30 ml/min 0.2 mcg/kg/min × 30 min, then 0.05 mcg/kg/min, during angiography and for up to 12-24 hr after angioplasty

Available forms: Inj 50 ml vials; inj premixed bag 50 mcg/ml in 100, 250 ml

Implementation
• Dilute inj: withdraw and discard 100 ml from a 500-ml bag of sterile 0.9% NaCl or D₅ and replace this vol with 100 ml of tirofiban inj from two vials
• Tirofiban inj for sol is premixed in containers of 500 ml 0.9% NaCl (50 mg/ml), give over 30 min
• Minimize other arterial/venous punctures, IM inj, catheter use, intubation to reduce bleeding risks
• Do not use if particulates are present
• Discard unused solution after 24 hr from start of infusion

Y-site compatibilities: Acyclovir, alfentanil, allopurinol, amifostine, amikacin, aminocaproic acid, aminophylline, amiodarone, ampicillin, ampicillin/sulbactam, anidulafungin, argatroban, arsenic trioxide, atracurium, atropine, azithromycin, aztreonam, bivalirudin, bleomycin, bumetanide, buprenorphine, butorphanol, calcium chloride/gluconate, capreomycin, CARBOplatin, carmustine, caspofungin, ceFAZolin, cefepime, cefotaxime, cefoTEtan, cefOXitin, cefTAZidime, ceftizoxime, cefTRIAXone, cefuroxime, chloramphenicol, chlorproMAZINE, cimetidine, ciprofloxacin, cisatracurium, CISplatin, clindamycin, cyclophosphamide, cycloSPORINE, cytarabine, DACTINomycin, DAPTOmycin, dexamethasone, dexmedetomidine, dexrazoxane, digoxin, diltiazem, diphenhydrAMINE, DOBUTamine, DOCEtaxel, dolasetron, DOPamine, doxacurium, DOXOrubicin, DOXOrubicin liposome, doxycycline, droperidol, enalaprilat, ePHEDrine, EPINEPHrine, epirubicin, eptifibatide, ertapenem, erythromycin, esmolol, etoposide, etoposide phosphate, famotidine, fenoldopam, fentaNYL, fluconazole, fludarabine, fluorouracil, foscarnet, fosphenytoin, furosemide, ganciclovir, gemcitabine, gentamicin, glycopyrrolate, granisetron, haloperidol, heparin, hydrALAZINE, hydrocortisone,

---

HYDROmorphone, IDArubicin, ifosfamide, imipenem/cilastatin, insulin, irinotecan, isoproterenol, ketorolac, labetalol, leucovorin, lidocaine, linezolid, LORazepam, magnesium sulfate, mannitol, mechlorethamine, melphalan, meperidine, meropenem, mesna, methylhexital, methotrexate, methyldopate, methylPREDNISolone, metoclopramide, metoprolol, metroNIDAZOLE, midazolam, milrinone, mitoXANtrone, morphine, mycophenolate, nafcillin, nalbuphine, naloxone, nesiritide, niCARdipine, nitroglycerin, nitroprusside, norepinephrine, octreotide, ondansetron, oxaliplatin, oxytocin, PACLitaxel, palonosetron, pamidronate, pancuronium, pantoprazole, PEMEtrexed, PENTobarbital, PHENobarbital, phentolamine, phenylephrine, piperacillin/tazobactam, potassium acetate/chloride/phosphates, procainamide, prochlorperazine, promethazine, propranolol, quinupristin/dalfopristin, ranitidine, remifentanil, rocuronium, sodium acetate/bicarbonate, streptozocin, succinylcholine, SUFentanil, tacrolimus, teniposide, theophylline, thiopental, thiotepa, ticarcillin/clavulanate, tigecycline, tobramycin, topotecan, vancomycin, vasopressin, vecuronium, verapamil, vinBLAStine, vinCRIStine, vinorelbine, voriconazole, zidovudine, zoledronic acid

Y-site incompatibilities: Amphotericin B colloidal, amphotericin B liposome, dantrolene, diazepam, phenytoin

ADVERSE EFFECTS
CNS: Dizziness, headache
CV: Bradycardia, hypotension
GI: Nausea, vomiting
HEMA: Bleeding, **thrombocytopenia**
INTEG: *Rash*
MISC: Dissection, edema, pain in legs/pelvis, sweating
SYST: *Anaphylaxis*

Pharmacokinetics

Absorption	Unknown
Distribution	Plasma clearance 20%-25%
Metabolism	Liver
Excretion	Urine/feces
Half-life	2 hr

Pharmacodynamics
Unknown

INTERACTIONS
Individual drugs
Abciximab, aspirin, cefamandole, cefoperazone, cefoTEtan, clopidogrel, dipyridamole, eptifibatide, heparin, ticlopidine, valproic acid: increased bleeding risk

Drug classifications
Heparins, NSAIDs, SNRIs, SSRIs, thrombin inhibitors: increased bleeding risk

NURSING CONSIDERATIONS
Assessment
• **Bleeding:** Monitor platelet counts, Hct, Hgb before treatment, within 6 hr of loading dose and at least daily thereafter; watch for bleeding from puncture sites, catheters, or in stools, urine
• **Multiple sclerosis, spinal cord injury:** assess muscle spasms, dizziness, drowsiness, difficulty moving, coordination, balance

Patient/family education
• Advise patient that it is necessary to quit smoking to prevent excessive vasoconstriction
• Teach signs/symptoms of bleeding, low platelets
• Advise that there are many drug and herb interactions, do not use unless approved by prescriber

Evaluation
Positive therapeutic outcome
• Treatment of acute coronary syndrome

tiZANidine (Rx)
(tye-za′na-deen)
Zanaflex
Func. class.: Skeletal muscle relaxant, central acting
Chem. class.: Imidazole
Pregnancy category C

Do not confuse: tiZANidine/tiaGABine

ACTION: Increases presynaptic inhibition of motor neurons and reduces spasticity by α_2-adrenergic agonism

Therapeutic outcome: Decreased pain/spasticity in multiple sclerosis

USES: Acute/intermittent management of increased muscle tone associated with spasticity, symptoms of MS

CONTRAINDICATIONS
Hypersensitivity

Precautions: Pregnancy **C**, breastfeeding, children, geriatric, renal/hepatic disease, hypotension

DOSAGE AND ROUTES
Adult: PO 8 mg q6-8hr; max 36 mg/24 hr

Renal dose
Adult: PO CCr <25 ml/min, start with lower dosage

Adverse effects: *italics* = common; **bold** = life-threatening

Available forms: Tabs 2, 4 mg; caps 2, 4, 6 mg

Implementation

- Give with meals for GI symptoms
- Store in airtight container at room temperature
- Give consistently either with or without food; food may affect absorption
- Titrate dose carefully

ADVERSE EFFECTS

CNS: *Dizziness,* somnolence, speech disorder, dyskinesia, nervousness, hallucination, psychosis
CV: Hypotension, bradycardia
GI: *Constipation, vomiting, dry mouth,* increased ALT, abnormal liver function tests
GU: Urinary frequency
OTHER: Blurred vision, pharyngitis, rhinitis, tremor, rash, muscle weakness

Pharmacokinetics

Absorption	Completely absorbed
Distribution	Widely distributed
Metabolism	Liver, extensively
Excretion	Kidneys, feces
Half-life	2½ hr

Pharmacodynamics

Onset	Unknown
Peak	1-2 hr
Duration	3-6 hr

INTERACTIONS
Individual drugs

Acyclovir, alcohol, amiodarone, ciprofloxacin, enoxacin, famotidine, fluvoxaMINE, norfloxacin, propafenone, tacrine, verapamil, zileuton: increased tizanidine levels; avoid concurrent use
Rasagiline: increased effect of rasagiline

Drug classifications

Antihypertensive: increased hypotension
CNS depressants: increased CNS depression

Drug/herb

Kava, St. John's wort: increased CNS depression

Drug/lab test

Increased: AST, alkaline phosphatase, ALT, serum glucose

NURSING CONSIDERATIONS
Assessment

- Assess for muscle spasticity baseline and throughout treatment
- Monitor B/P, heart rate
- Perform neurologic exam in spasticity: deep tendon reflexes, muscle tone, clonus, sensory function
- Monitor renal/liver function tests, electrolytes, CBC with differential during long-term treatment
- Assess for allergic reactions: rash, fever, respiratory distress; severe weakness, numbness in extremities
- Assess CNS depression: dizziness, drowsiness, psychiatric symptoms
- Check dosage, because individual titration is required

Patient/family education

- Advise patient not to discontinue medication quickly; spasticity will occur; product should be tapered off over 1-2 wk
- Advise patient not to take with alcohol, other CNS depressants; take as directed; if dose is missed, take as soon as remembered, unless it is almost time for next dose
- Caution patient to avoid altering activities while taking this product; to avoid hazardous activities if drowsiness or dizziness occurs; to rise from sitting or lying slowly to prevent fainting
- Teach patient to use gum, frequent sips of water for dry mouth
- Advise patient to avoid using OTC medications (cough preparations, antihistamines) unless directed by prescriber
- Notify prescriber if fainting, hallucinations, dark urine, stomach pain, yellowing of skin/eyes occurs
- Advise patient to rise slowly from lying or sitting to upright position to prevent orthostatic hypotension
- Teach patient to avoid hazardous activities until reaction is known
- Teach patient not to use other products unless approved by prescriber

Evaluation

Positive therapeutic outcome

- Decreased pain, spasticity

---

tobramycin (Rx)

(toe-bra-mye′sin)
TOBI, TOBI Podhaler
Func. class.: Antiinfective
Chem. class.: Aminoglycoside
Pregnancy category D

ACTION: Interferes with protein synthesis in bacterial cell by binding to ribosomal subunit, causing inaccurate peptide sequence to form in protein chain, causing bacterial death

Therapeutic outcome: Bactericidal effects for the following organisms: *Pseudomonas aeruginosa, Enterobacter, Escherichia coli, Providencia, Citrobacter, Staphylococcus, Proteus, Klebsiella, Serratia*

USES: Severe systemic infections of CNS, respiratory, GI, urinary tract, bone, skin, soft tissues, cystic fibrosis (nebulizer), *Acinetobacter calcoaceticus, Citrobacter, Enterobacter, Enterococcus, Escherichia coli, Haemophilus aegyptius, Haemophilus influenzae* (beta-lactamase negative), *Haemophilus influenzae* (beta-lactamase positive), *Klebsiella, Moraxella lacunata, Morganella morganii, Neisseria, Proteus mirabilis, Proteus vulgaris, Providencia, Pseudomonas aeruginosa, Serratia, Staphylococcus aureus* (MSSA), *Staphylococcus epidermidis, Staphylococcus, Streptococcus;* **may also be used for the following:** *Acinetobacter, Aeromonas, Bacillus anthracis, Salmonella, Shigella*

CONTRAINDICATIONS
Hypersensitivity to aminoglycosides

> **BLACK BOX WARNING:** Pregnancy **D**, severe renal disease

Precautions: Breastfeeding, geriatric, neonates, mild renal disease, myasthenia gravis, Parkinson's disease

> **BLACK BOX WARNING:** Hearing deficits, neuromuscular disease

DOSAGE AND ROUTES
Adult: IM/IV 3 mg/kg/day in divided doses q8hr; may give up to 6 mg/kg/day in divided doses q8-12hr; once-daily dosing (pulse dosing) (unlabeled) IV 5-7 mg/kg; dosing intervals are determined using a nomogram and are based on random levels drawn 8-12 hr after first dose
Child: IM/IV 6-7.5 mg/kg/day in 3-4 equal divided doses
Child ≥6 yr: NEB 300 mg bid in repeating cycles of 28 days on/28 days off; give inh over 10-15 min using a hand-held PARI LC PLUS reusable nebulizer with a DeVilbiss Pulmo-Aid compressor
Neonate <1 wk: IM/IV ≤4 mg/kg/day divided q12hr
Conventional dosing: Multiply the serum creatinine (mg/100 ml) by 6 to determine the dosing; to decrease the dose, divide the standard dose by the serum creatinine (mg/100 ml) to determine the lower recommended dose
Interval adjustment of extended-interval dosing of 5 or 7 mg/kg (unlabeled): Adjust doses based on serum concentrations and organism MIC; CCr 40-59 ml/min: 5 or 7 mg/kg IV q36hr; CCr 20-39 ml/min: 5 or 7 mg/kg IV q48hr; CCr <20 ml/min: 5 or 7 mg/kg IV once, then follow serial levels to determine time of next dose (serum concentration <1 mcg/ml)
Dose adjustment of extended dosing of 5 mg/kg (unlabeled): Adjust doses based on serum concentrations and organism MIC; CCr >80 ml/min: no dosage adjustment is needed; CCr 60-79 ml/min: 4 mg/kg IV q24hr; CCr 50 ml/min: 3.5 mg/kg IV q24hr CrCl 40 ml/min: 2.5 mg/kg IV q24hr; CrCl <30 ml/min: Use traditional dosing

Cystic fibrosis with *Pseudomonas aeruginosa*
Adult/adolescent/child: IV 2.5-3.3 mg/kg q8hr, neb 300 mg via inhalation bid × 28 days, then 28 days after

Available forms: Inj 10, 40 mg/ml; powder for inj 1.2 g; neb sol 300 mg/5 ml; powder for inh 28 mg

Implementation
IM route
- Give inj deeply in large muscle mass, aspirate
- Draw peak 1 hr after dose, trough right before next dose; absorption erratic

Nebulizer route
- The solution for nebulization is for inhalation only; use over 10-15 min

Inhalation route (TOBI Podhaler)
- Use with Podhaler device, do not swallow caps, use device for 7 days then discard
- Keep caps in blister pack until ready to use, administer other inhaled products or chest physiotherapy before
- While holding base of Podhaler device, unscrew lid, stand upright, unscrew mouthpiece; while holding body, tear blister card in half lengthwise along precut lines; peel back foil, place cap in chamber at top of device, reattach mouthpiece, and tighten; with mouthpiece pointed down, press blue button down with thumb, release; exhale completely, place mouth over mouthpiece, close lips, inhale with single breath, hold 5 sec, and exhale normally away from device; after a few normal breaths, repeat, unscrew mouthpiece, and remove cap: cap should be empty; repeat process 3 more times (total 4 caps); after use reattach mouthpiece and wipe with clean, dry cloth

Intermittent IV infusion route
- Visually inspect solution; do not use if discolored or if particulate is present

---

Adverse effects: *italics* = common; **bold** = life-threatening

- ADD-Vantage vials are for IV only and only for exactly 60 or 80 mg
- Give **IV** diluted in 50-100 ml of 0.9% NaCl, $D_{10}W$, D_5/0.9% NaCl, 0.9% NaCl, Ringer's, LR, D_5W (adult), inf over 20-60 min, volume for pediatric patients needs and should be sufficient to allow for 20-60 min infusion
- Flush after inf with D_5W, 0.9% NaCl
- Separate aminoglycosides and penicillins by $\geq$1 hr

Y-site compatibilities: Acyclovir, aldesleukin, alfentanil, alprostadil, amifostine, aminophylline, amiodarone, amsacrine, anidulafungin, ascorbic acid, atracurium, atropine, aztreonam, bivalirudin, bretylium, bumetanide, buprenorphine, butorphanol, calcium chloride/gluconate, CARBOplatin, caspofungin, chloramphenicol, cimetidine, ciprofloxacin, cisatracurium, CISplatin, clindamycin, cyanocobalamin, cyclophosphamide, cycloSPORINE, cytarabine, DACTINomycin, DAPTOmycin, dexmedetomidine, digoxin, diltiazem, diphenhydrAMINE, DOBUTamine, DOCEtaxel, DOPamine, doripenem, doxacurium, DOXOrubicin hydrochloride, DOXOrubicin liposome, doxycycline, enalaprilat, ePHEDrine, EPINEPHrine, epirubicin, epoetin alfa, ertapenem, esmolol, etoposide, etoposide phosphate, famotidine, fenoldopam, fentaNYL, filgrastim, fluconazole, fludarabine, fluorouracil, foscarnet, furosemide, gemcitabine, gentamicin, glycopyrrolate, granisetron, HYDROmorphone, ifosfamide, imipenem/cilastatin, isoproterenol, ketorolac, labetalol, levofloxacin, lidocaine, linezolid, LORazepam, magnesium sulfate, mannitol, mechlorethamine, melphalan, meperidine, metaraminol, methicillin, methotrexate, methoxamine, methyldopate, methylPREDNISolone, metoclopramide, metoprolol, metroNIDAZOLE, miconazole, midazolam, milrinone, minocycline, mitoXANtrone, morphine, moxalactam, multiple vitamins, nafcillin, nalbuphine, naloxone, niCARdipine, nitroglycerin, nitroprusside, norepinephrine, octreotide, ondansetron, oxaliplatin, oxytocin, PACLitaxel, palonosetron, pantoprazole, papaverine, penicillin G, pentazocine, perphenazine, PHENobarbital, phentolamine, phenylephrine, phytonadione, potassium chloride, procainamide, prochlorperazine, promethazine, propranolol, protamine, pyridoxime, quinupristin/dalfopristin, ranitidine, remifentanil, riTUXimab, rocuronium, sodium acetate/bicarbonate, succinylcholine, SUFentanil, tacrolimus, teniposide, theophylline, thiamine, thiotepa, ticarcillin/clavulanate, tigecycline, tirofiban, tolazoline, trastuzumab, trimetaphan, urokinase, vancomycin, vasopressin, vecuronium, verapamil, vinCRIStine, vinorelbine, voriconazole, zidovudine

Y-site incompatibilities: Allopurinol, amphotericin B cholesteryl, amphotericin B colloidal, amphotericin B liposome, azaTHIOprine, azithromycin, ceFAZolin, cefoperazone, cefoTEtan, cefTRIAXone, dantrolene, dexamethasone, diazepam, diazoxide, drotrecogin, folic acid, ganciclovir, heparin, indomethacin, oxacillin, PEMEtrexed, pentamidine, PENTobarbital, phenytoin, piperacillin/tazobactam, propofol, sargramostim, trimethoprim/sulfamethoxazole

ADVERSE EFFECTS

CNS: Confusion, depression, numbness, tremors, **seizures**, muscle twitching, **neurotoxicity**, dizziness, vertigo

CV: Hypo/hypertension, palpitations

EENT: *Ototoxicity*, deafness, visual disturbances, tinnitus

GI: *Nausea, vomiting, anorexia*, increased ALT, AST, bilirubin, hepatomegaly, **hepatic necrosis**, splenomegaly

GU: **Oliguria, hematuria, renal damage, azotemia, renal failure, nephrotoxicity**

HEMA: **Agranulocytosis, thrombocytopenia, leukopenia, eosinophilia**, anemia

INTEG: *Rash*, burning, urticaria, dermatitis, alopecia

Pharmacokinetics

Absorption	Well absorbed (IM), completely absorbed (**IV**)
Distribution	Widely distributed in extracellular fluids
Metabolism	Minimal liver
Excretion	Mostly unchanged (>90%) kidneys
Half-life	2-3 hr, increased in renal disease, neonates

Pharmacodynamics

	IM	IV	OPHTH
Onset	Rapid	Rapid	Rapid
Peak	1 hr	Inf end	Unknown
Duration	Unknown	Unknown	Unknown

INTERACTIONS

Individual drugs
Acyclovir, amphotericin B, bacitracin, cidofovir, CISplatin, ethacrynic acid, furosemide,

mannitol, methoxyflurane, polymyxin, vancomycin: increased ototoxicity, neurotoxicity, nephrotoxicity

Drug classifications

BLACK BOX WARNING: Aminoglycosides, cephalosporins, penicillins: increased ototoxicity, neurotoxicity, nephrotoxicity

NURSING CONSIDERATIONS
Assessment
• Assess patient for previous sensitivity reaction
Systemic route
• Assess patient for signs and symptoms of infection including characteristics of wounds, sputum, urine, stool, WBC >10,000/mm³, temp baseline, during treatment
• Complete C&S testing before beginning product therapy to identify if correct treatment has been initiated
• Assess for allergic reactions: rash, urticaria, pruritus, chills, fever, joint pain

BLACK BOX WARNING: Renal disease: Identify urine output; if decreasing, notify prescriber (may indicate nephrotoxicity); also, obtain BUN, creatinine, urine CCr (<80 ml/min) values; urinalysis daily for proteinuria, cells, casts; report sudden change in urine output

BLACK BOX WARNING: Pregnancy: identify if pregnancy is planned or suspected; pregnancy **(D)**

• Monitor blood studies: AST, ALT, CBC, Hct, bilirubin, LDH, alkaline phosphatase, Coombs' test monthly if patient is on long-term therapy
• Monitor electrolytes: potassium, sodium, chloride, magnesium monthly if patient is on long-term therapy
• Monitor for bleeding: ecchymosis, bleeding gums, hematuria, stool guaiac daily if patient is on long-term therapy
• **Assess for overgrowth of infection:** perineal itching, fever, malaise, redness, pain, swelling, drainage, rash, diarrhea, change in cough, sputum
• Obtain weight before treatment; calculation of dosage is usually based on ideal body weight but may be calculated on actual body weight
• Monitor VS during inf, watch for hypotension, change in pulse
• Assess IV site for thrombophlebitis including pain, redness, swelling q30min; change site if needed; apply warm compresses to discontinued site

BLACK BOX WARNING: Obtain serum peak, drawn at 30-60 min after **IV** inf or 60 min after IM inj, trough level drawn just before next dose; peak 4-12 mcg/ml, trough 1-2 mcg/ml, increased level may lead to serious toxicity

BLACK BOX WARNING: Monitor for deafness by audiometric testing, ringing, roaring in ears, vertigo; assess hearing before, during, after treatment, promptly

Patient/family education
• Teach patient to report sore throat, bruising, bleeding, joint pain; may indicate blood dyscrasias (rare)
• Advise patient to contact prescriber if vaginal itching, loose foul-smelling stools, furry tongue occur; may indicate superinfection

BLACK BOX WARNING: Advise patient to notify prescriber if pregnancy is planned or suspected, pregnancy **D**

• Advise patient to notify prescriber of diarrhea with blood or pus; may indicate pseudomembranous colitis
• Teach patient to avoid hazardous activities until response is known

Nebulizer route
• Advise patient to use multiple therapies first, then tobramycin, not to use if cloudy or contains particulates

Evaluation
Positive therapeutic outcome
• Absence of signs/symptoms of infection (WBC <10,000/mm³, temp WNL, absence of red, draining wounds)
• Reported improvement in symptoms of infection

TREATMENT OF OVERDOSE:
Withdraw product, hemodialysis, exchange transfusion in the newborn, monitor serum levels of product, may give ticarcillin or carbenicillin

tobramycin ophthalmic
See Appendix B

tocilizumab (Rx)
(toe′si-liz′oo-mab)
Actemra
Func. class.: DMARDs (Disease modifying anti-rheumatoid drugs)/tumor necrosis factor (TNF) modifier
Pregnancy category C

ACTION: Interleukin- 6 (IL-6) receptor inhibiting monoclonal antibody

Adverse effects: *italics* = common; **bold** = life-threatening

Therapeutic outcome: Ability to move more easily with less pain

USES: Rheumatoid arthritis, active systemic juvenile idiopathic arthritis

CONTRAINDICATIONS
Hypersensitivity

Precautions: Breastfeeding, pregnancy **C**, risk for GI perforation, active hepatic disease, severe neutropenia/thrombocytopenia, demyelinating disorders

> **BLACK BOX WARNING:** Invasive fungal infection, active TB

DOSAGE AND ROUTES
Monotherapy with or without methotrexate or other DMARDs, moderate-severe rheumatoid arthritis
Adult: **IV** 4 mg/kg over 1 hr q4wk, may increase to 8 mg/kg q4wk based on clinical response, max dose 800 mg/inf; do not initiate if ANC is >2000 and platelets are <100,000.

Juvenile idiopathic arthritis
Child ≥2 yr/adolescent ≥30 kg: **IV** 8 mg/kg over 1 hr q2wk
Child ≥2 yr/adolescent <30 kg: **IV** 12 mg/kg over 1 hr

Available forms: Sol for inj 80 mg/4 ml, 200 mg/10 ml, 400 mg/20 ml

Implementation

Intermittent IV route
• Visually inspect for particulate matter and discoloration before administration whenever solution and container permit, colorless to pale yellow liquid
• From a 100-ml infusion bag or bottle, withdraw a volume of 0.9% NaCl for inj equal to the volume of the tocilizumab solution required for the patient's dose
• Slowly add tocilizumab from each vial into the infusion bag or bottle. Gently invert the bag to avoid foaming. Fully diluted solutions are compatible with polypropylene, polyethylene, and polyvinyl chloride infusion bags and polypropylene, polyethylene, and glass infusion bottles
• The fully diluted sol for inf may be stored refrigerated or at room temp for up to 24 hours and should be protected from light. Do not use unused product remaining in vials; no preservatives
• Allow the fully diluted solution to reach room temp before infusing

• Give over 60 min with an infusion set. Do not administer as an **IV** push or bolus
• Do not infuse concomitantly in the same intravenous line with other drugs

ADVERSE EFFECTS
CNS: Headache, dizziness
CV: Hypertension
GI: Perforation, abdominal pain, gastritis, mouth ulcerations
HEMA: Neutropenia, thrombocytopenia
INTEG: Rash, infusion reactions
RESP: Upper respiratory infections, nasopharyngitis, bronchitis
SYST: Serious infections, anaphylaxis, infusion-related reactions, anti-tocilizumab antibody formation, secondary malignancy

Pharmacokinetics

Absorption	Unknown
Distribution	Unknown
Metabolism	Unknown
Excretion	Unknown
Half-life	~6 days with a single dose and ~11 days with multiple (steady state) doses

Pharmacodynamics
Unknown

INTERACTIONS
Individual drugs
CycloSPORINE, theophylline, warfarin: decreased product level

Drug classifications
CYP3A4 substrates (hormonal contraceptives, omeprazole, atorvastatin, simvastatin): decreased levels of these products
Live virus vaccines: Do not use together
TNF modifiers, DMARDs, immunosuppressives: avoid use due to increased risk of infection

NURSING CONSIDERATIONS
Assessment
• **Rheumatoid arthritis:** assess ROM, pain, stiffness baseline q1-2wk
• Monitor blood studies: CBC with differential, LFTs, platelet count, serum lipid profile, baseline and periodically

> **BLACK BOX WARNING:** Assess for infection before and periodically, obtain TB screening before beginning treatment

Patient/family education
• Teach patient that this treatment must continue unless safety or effectiveness is an issue; reason for use and expected result

---

BLACK BOX WARNING: Advise patient to avoid use of live vaccines, bring immunizations up to date before treatment

BLACK BOX WARNING: Instruct patient to report signs/symptoms of infection (including TB and Hepatitis B), invasive fungal infections, discontinue if infection occurs during administration; may use antituberculosis therapy prior to tocilizumab in past history of latent or active TB when adequate course of treatment cannot be confirmed and those with a negative TB with risk factors for infections, to avoid others with infections

• Teach patient to notify prescriber if pregnancy is planned or suspected, pregnancy (C); do not use if breastfeeding, consider using a nonhormonal contraceptive because contraception may be decreased
• Secondary malignancy: assess for malignancy periodically

Evaluation

Positive therapeutic outcome
• Ability to move more easily with less pain

tofacitinib

(toe′fa-sye′ti-nib)
Xeljanz
Func. class.: antirheumatic agent (disease modifying), immunomodulator/biologic DMARD
Chem. class.: Janus kinase inhibitor
Pregnancy category: C

ACTION: Affects the signaling pathway of Janus kinase

Therapeutic outcome: Decreased inflammation, pain in joints, decreased joint destruction

USES: Rheumatoid arthritis (moderately to severely active) in those who have taken methotrexate with inadequate response or intolerance

CONTRAINDICATIONS

Hypersensitivity

Precautions: Pregnancy (**C**), breastfeeding, neonates, infants, children, geriatric patients, neoplastic disease, ulcerative colitis, neutropenia, peptic ulcer disease, active infections, risk of lymphomas/leukemias, TB, posttransplant lymphoproliferative disorder (PTLD), kidney disease, diabetes mellitus, HIV, hypercholesterolemia, herpes virus infection reactivation, patients of Asian descent

BLACK BOX WARNING: Infection, secondary malignancy

DOSAGE AND ROUTES

Adult: PO 5 mg/day with or without methotrexate or other nonbiologic DMARDs

Available forms: Tabs 5 mg

Implementation
PO route
Give without regard to food

ADVERSE EFFECTS

CNS: Headache, paresthesias, insomnia, fatigue
CV: Hypertension
GI: Abdominal pain, nausea, **liver damage,** dyspepsia, vomiting, diarrhea, gastritis, **GI perforation, steatosis**
HEMA: Anemia, lymphocytosis, lymphopenia, neutropenia
INTEG: Rash, pruritus
MISC: Increased cancer risk, risk of infection (TB, invasive fungal infections, other opportunistic infections), may be fatal, posttransplant lymphoproliferative disorder (PTLD)

Pharmacokinetics

Absorption	Bioavailability 70%
Distribution	Protein binding 40% (albumin)
Metabolism	Mediated by CYP3A4
Excretion	Unknown
Half-life	3 hr

Pharmacodynamics

Onset	Unknown
Peak	0.5–1 hr
Duration	Unknown

INTERACTIONS
Drug classifications

BLACK BOX WARNING: Do not use with TNF modifiers, vaccines, potent immunosuppressants, other biologic DMARDS

CYP3A4 inhibitors (amprenavir, boceprevir, delavirdine, ketoconazole, indinavir, itraconazole, dalfopristin/quinupristin, ritonavir, tipranavir, fluconazole, isoniazid, miconazole): increased tofacinib effect

CYP3A4 inducers (rifampin, rifapentine, rifabutin, primidone, phenytoin, PHENobarbital, nevirapine, nafcillin, modafinil, griseofulvin, etravirine, efavirenz, barbiturates, bexarotene, bosentan, carBAMazepine, enzalutamide, dexamethasone): decreased tofacinib effect

Adverse effects: *italics* = common; **bold** = life-threatening

Drug/lab test
Increase: LFTs, cholesterol
Decrease: neutrophils, lymphocytes, Hct, Hgb

NURSING CONSIDERATIONS
Assessment
• Monitor lipid profile, Hct/Hgb WBC, LFTs
• RA: assess for pain, stiffness, ROM, swelling of joints before, during treatment

> **BLACK BOX WARNING:** Active infection, including localized infection: evaluate and test patients for active or active TB before use; treat with antimycobacterials before use of product; this product increases the risk of serious illness including fatal infections (pulmonary or extrapulmonary TB; invasive fungal infections; and bacterial, viral, and opportunistic infections); during and after use, monitor for infection including TB in those who tested negative for latent TB before use; if a serious infection develops, interrupt receipt until the infection is controlled, reactivation or viral infections is higher in those of Asian descent

> **BLACK BOX WARNING:** Secondary malignancy: lymphoma and other malignancies have been noted with product use

⚠ Epstein–Barr virus–associated post transplant lymphoproliferative disorder (PTLD): in kidney transplant patients when used with this product and immunosuppressives
• **Liver disease:** not recommended in severe liver disease, impairment; dose modification is needed with moderate liver impairment, monitor LFTs
⚠ GI perforation: assess in those with diverticulitis, peptic ulcer disease, or ulcerative colitis

> **BLACK BOX WARNING:** ⚠ Immunosuppression: obtain neutrophil and lymphocyte counts before use, do not start the product in lymphocyte count < 500 cells/mm³ or < ANC 1000 cells/mm³; for ANC >1000 cells/ mm³, monitor neutrophil counts after 4-8 wk and every 3 mo thereafter; lymphocyte count > 500 cells/ mm³, monitor lymphocyte counts every 3 mo

⚠ Anemia: determine Hgb, do not start in Hgb 9 g/dl; in Hgb 9 g/dl, monitor Hgb after 4-8 wk and every 3 mo thereafter
⚠ Pregnancy (C)/breastfeeding: use during pregnancy only if the potential benefit justifies the potential risk to the fetus; if pregnancy occurs, enrollment in the pregnancy registry is encouraged by calling 877–311–8972; discontinue product or breastfeeding, serious adverse reactions can occur in nursing infants

> **BLACK BOX WARNING:** Neoplastic disease (lymphomas/leukemias)

Patient/family education
• Teach patient not to have vaccines while taking this product
• Advise patient not to take any live virus vaccines during treatment
• Inform patient to report signs of infection, allergic reaction
⚠ Pregnancy C: teach patient to report if pregnancy is planned or suspected, do not breastfeed

Evaluation

Positive therapeutic outcome
• Decreased inflammation, pain in joints, decreased joint destruction

---

tolcapone (Rx)
(toll′cah-pone)
Tasmar
Func. class.: Antiparkinson agent
Chem. class.: Catecholamine inhibitor (COMT)
Pregnancy category C

ACTION: Selective, reversible inhibitor of catecholamine; used as adjunct to levodopa/carbidopa therapy

Therapeutic outcome: Increased ability to move and speak

USES: Parkinsonism

CONTRAINDICATIONS
Hypersensitivity, rhabdomyolysis

> **BLACK BOX WARNING:** Hepatic disease

Precautions: Pregnancy **C**, breastfeeding, cardiac/renal disease, hypertension, asthma, history of rhabdomyolysis

DOSAGE AND ROUTES
Adult: PO 100-200 mg tid, with levodopa/carbidopa therapy; max 600 mg/day; discontinue if no benefit in 3 wk

Available forms: Tabs 100, 200 mg

Implementation
• Administer tid with levodopa/carbidopa therapy

• Provide assistance with ambulation during beginning therapy
• Give without regard to food

ADVERSE EFFECTS

CNS: Dystonia, dyskinesia, dreaming, *fatigue, headache, confusion,* psychosis, hallucination, dizziness, sleep disorders
CV: *Orthostatic hypotension,* chest pain, hypotension
EENT: Cataract, eye inflammation
GI: *Nausea, vomiting, abdominal distress,* diarrhea, constipation, **fatal liver failure,** elevated liver function tests
GU: UTI, urine discoloration, uterine tumor, micturition disorder, hematuria
HEMA: **Hemolytic anemia, leukopenia, agranulocytosis**
INTEG: Sweating, alopecia
MS: **Rhabdomyolysis**

Pharmacokinetics

Absorption	Rapidly absorbed
Distribution	Protein binding 99%
Metabolism	Liver, extensively
Excretion	Urine (60%), feces (40%)
Half-life	2-3 hr

Pharmacodynamics

Onset	Unknown
Peak	2 hr
Duration	Unknown

INTERACTIONS
Individual drugs
Apomorphine, DOBUTamine, isoproterenol, α-methyldopa: may influence pharmacokinetics

Drug classifications
CNS depressants: increased CNS depression
MAOIs: decreased normal catecholamine metabolism; MAO-B inhibitor may be used

NURSING CONSIDERATIONS
Assessment
• **Hepatic disease:** monitor liver function tests: AST, ALT, alkaline phosphatase, LDH, bilirubin, CBC, if no improvement in 3 wk, discontinue
• Assess involuntary movements in parkinsonism: akinesia, tremors, staggering gait, muscle rigidity, drooling
• Monitor B/P, respiration during initial treatment; hypo/hypertension should be reported
• Monitor mental status: affect, mood, behavioral changes, avoid use in those with dystonia

Patient/family education
• Advise patient to change positions slowly to prevent orthostatic hypotension

• Advise patient that urine, sweat may change color
• Teach patient to notify prescriber if pregnancy is planned or suspected, pregnancy (**C**)
• Teach patient that CNS changes may occur, hallucinations, involuntary movement
• Teach patient to avoid hazardous activities until reaction is known, dizziness occurs
• Advise patient that nausea and diarrhea are common

> **BLACK BOX WARNING:** Advise patient to report signs of hepatic injury: clay-colored stools, jaundice, fatigue, appetite loss, lethargy, fatigue, itching, right upper abdominal pain

• Teach patient to report nausea, vomiting, anorexia
• May be taken without regard to food

Evaluation

Positive therapeutic outcome
• Decrease in akathisia, improved mood

tolnaftate topical
See Appendix B

tolterodine (Rx)
(tol-tehr′oh-deen)
Detrol, Detrol LA
Func. class.: Overactive bladder product
Chem. class.: Muscarinic receptor antagonist
Pregnancy category C

ACTION: Relaxes smooth muscles in urinary tract by inhibiting acetylcholine at postganglionic sites

Therapeutic outcome: Decreased symptoms of overactive bladder

USES: Overactive bladder (frequency, urgency), urinary incontinence

CONTRAINDICATIONS
Hypersensitivity, uncontrolled closed-angle glaucoma, urinary retention, gastric retention

Precautions: Pregnancy **C**, breastfeeding, children, renal/hepatic disease, controlled closed-angle glaucoma, bladder obstruction, QT prolongation, decreased GI motility

DOSAGE AND ROUTES
Adult and geriatric: PO 2 mg bid, may decrease to 1 mg bid; EXT REL 4 mg/day, may decrease to 2 mg if needed, max 4 mg/day

T

Hepatic disease
Adult: PO 1 mg bid (50% dose) or EXT REL 2 mg/day

Renal dose
Adult: PO CCr ≤30 ml/min reduce by 50%

Available forms: Tabs 1, 2 mg; ext rel caps 2, 4 mg

Implementation
• Swallow whole; give with liquids

ADVERSE EFFECTS

CNS: *Anxiety,* paresthesia, fatigue, *dizziness,* headache, increasing dementia, memory impairment
CV: Chest pain, hypertension, **QT prolongation**
EENT: Vision abnormalities, xerophthalmia
GI: *Nausea, vomiting, anorexia,* abdominal pain, constipation, dry mouth, dyspepsia
GU: Dysuria, retention, frequency, UTI
INTEG: Rash, pruritus
RESP: Bronchitis, cough, pharyngitis, upper respiratory tract infection
SYST: Angioedema, Stevens-Johnson syndrome

Pharmacokinetics

Absorption	Rapidly absorbed
Distribution	Highly protein bound
Metabolism	Liver, extensively by CYP2D6, a portion of the population may be poor metabolizers
Excretion	Urine/feces
Half-life	Unknown

Pharmacodynamics

Unknown

INTERACTIONS
Individual drugs
Chloroquine, clarithromycin, droperidol, erythromycin, grepafloxacin, halofantrine, haloperidol, methadone, pentamidine: increased QT prolongation
Festerodine: do not use in those with known hypersensitivity

Drug classifications
Antibiotics (macrolide), antifungal agents, antiretroviral protease inhibitors: increased action of tolterodine
Antimuscarinics: increased anticholinergic effect
β-agonists, class IA/III antidysrhythmics, local anesthetics, some phenothiazines, tricyclics: increased QT prolongation
Diuretics: increased urinary frequency

Drug/food
Increased: bioavailability of tolterodine

Drug/lab test
Increased: LFTs, bilirubin

NURSING CONSIDERATIONS
Assessment
• **Assess urinary patterns:** distention, nocturia, frequency, urgency, incontinence
• **Serious skin disorders: assess for angioedema, Stevens-Johnson syndrome; assess allergic reactions: rash; if this occurs, product should be discontinued**
• **QT prolongation: ECG for QT prolongation, ejection fraction; assess for chest pain, palpitations, dyspnea**

> **BLACK BOX WARNING:** Fatal hepatic injury: increased LFTs, bilirubin during first 18 mo of therapy in those with autosomal dominant polycystic kidney disease; assess for fatigue, anorexia, right upper abdominal pain, dark urine, jaundice; if these occur, discontinue product and do not restart if cause is liver injury

Patient/family education
• Advise patient to avoid hazardous activities; dizziness may occur, shortness of breath, urinary retention
• Advise patient not to drink liquids before bedtime, to swallow extended-release product whole
• Teach patient importance of bladder maintenance
• Teach patient to take with liquids; swallow whole

Evaluation

Positive therapeutic outcome
• Decreased urinary frequency, urgency

tolvaptan (Rx)
(tole-vap′tan)
Samsca
Func. class.: Antihypertensive
Chem. class.: Vasopressin receptor antagonist, V2
Pregnancy category C

ACTION: Arginine vasopressin (AVP) antagonist with affinity for V_2 receptors; level of circulating AVP in circulating blood is critical for regulation of water, electrolyte balance and is usually elevated in euvolemic/hypervolemic hyponatremia

Therapeutic outcome: Normal serum sodium level

USES: Hypervolemic/euvolemic hyponatremia in heart failure, cirrhosis, SIADH

CONTRAINDICATIONS
Hypersensitivity, hypovolemia, anuria

Precautions: Pregnancy **C**, breastfeeding, children, dehydration, geriatric patients, hyperkalemia, autosomal dominant PKD

> **BLACK BOX WARNING:** Alcoholism, malnutrition, hepatic disease

DOSAGE AND ROUTES
Adult: PO 15 mg qd; after 24 hr, may increase to 30 mg qd; max 60 mg/day for ≤30 days

Available forms: Tab 15, 30 mg

Implementation
- Give PO with or without food
- Avoid fluid restriction the first 24 hr
- Initiate in hospital setting

ADVERSE EFFECTS
CNS: Fever, dizziness
CV: Ventricular fibrillation, DIC, stroke, thrombosis
GI: *Nausea*, vomiting, *constipation*, colitis, hepatic injury
GU: Polyuria
HEMA: Bleeding
META: *Dehydration*, *hyperglycemia*, hyperkalemia, hypernatremia
MS: Rhabdomyolysis
RESP: Respiratory depression, pulmonary embolism

Pharmacokinetics

Absorption	Unknown
Distribution	Protein binding 99%
Metabolism	CYP3A4
Excretion	Unknown
Half-life	Terminal 12 hr

Pharmacodynamics

Onset	Unknown
Peak	2-4 hr
Duration	Unknown

INTERACTIONS
Drug classifications
CYP3A4 inducers (carBAMazepine, dexamethasone, etravirine, flutamide, griseofulvin, metyrapsone, modafinil, nafacillin, nevirapine, OXcarbazepine, phenytoin, rifampin, rifabutin, rifapendine, topiramate): decreased concentrations of tolvaptan

CYP3A4 inhibitors (efavirenz, fosamprenavir, quiNINE), P-gp inhibitors (azithromycin, cycloSPORINE, mefloquine, palperidone, propafenone, quiNIDine, testosterone): increased concentrations of tolvaptan

Drug/herb
St. John's wort: decreased tolvaptan effect

Drug/food
Grapefruit juice: do not use together

NURSING CONSIDERATIONS
Assessment
- Assess renal, hepatic function

> **BLACK BOX WARNING:** Monitor malnutrition, alcoholism, frequent sodium volume status; overly rapid correction of sodium concentration (>12 mEq/L per 24 hr) may result in osmotic demyelination syndrome; may occur in alcoholism, severe malnutrition, advanced liver disease, SIADH, correct sodium levels slowly

- Assess CV status: ventricular fibrillation, hypertension, monitor B/P, pulse
- Monitor electrolytes (sodium, potassium)

Patient/family education
- Teach patient to avoid pregnancy, breastfeeding while taking this product
- Advise of administration procedure and expected result
- Teach patient to report difficulty swallowing or speaking, seizures, dizziness, drowsiness: embolism may be the cause
- Teach patient to drink fluid in response to thirst
- Teach patient to not use grapefruit juice
- Teach patient to notify prescriber before using other products

Evaluation

Positive therapeutic outcome
- Correction of serum sodium levels

---

topiramate (Rx)
(toh-pire′a-mate)
Topamax, Topamax Sprinkle, Topiragen, Trokendi XR, Qudexy XR
Func. class.: Anticonvulsant—miscellaneous
Chem. class.: Monosaccharide derivative
Pregnancy category D

ACTION: Increased GABA activity; may prevent seizure spread as opposed to an elevation of seizure threshold

Therapeutic outcome: Absence of seizures

USES: Partial seizures in adults and children 2-16 yr old; tonic-clonic seizures; seizures in Lennox-Gastaut syndrome, migraine prophylaxis

Unlabeled uses: Infantile spasms, bulimia nervosa

CONTRAINDICATIONS
Hypersensitivity, metabolic acidosis, pregnancy **D**

Precautions: Breastfeeding, children, renal/hepatic disease, acute myopia, secondary closed-angle glaucoma, behavioral disorders, COPD, dialysis, encephalopathy, status asthmaticus, status epilepticus, surgery, paresthesias, maculopathy, nephrolithiasis

DOSAGE AND ROUTES
Adjunctive therapy
Adult/adolescent/child ≥10 yr: PO 25-50 mg/day initially, titrate by 25-50 mg/wk, up to 200-400 mg/day in 2 divided doses

Adult/adolescent/child ≥10 yr: PO (Qudexy XR, Trokendi XR) 50 mg qday; increase by 50 mg qwk during wk 2, 3, 4; increase by 100 mg qwk, wk 5, 6; final dose 400 mg qday

Child 2-9 yr: PO week 1 25 mg q PM, then 25 mg bid if tolerated (week 2), then increase by 25-50 mg/day each week as tolerated over 5-7 wk titration period, maintenance given in 2 divided doses; <11 kg minimum 150 mg/day, max 250 mg/day; 12-22 kg minimum 200 mg/day, max 300 mg/day; 23-31 kg minimum 200 mg, max 350 mg/day, 32-38 kg minimum 250 mg/kg, max 350 mg/day; >38 kg minimum 250 mg/day, max 400 mg/day; Qudexy XR 25 mg qday at night; may increase to 50 mg wk 2, if tolerated; increase by 25-50 mg each wk over 5-7 wk titration period; max dose based on weight

Migraine prophylaxis
Child ≤11 kg: PO Qudexy XR minimum 150 mg daily, max 250 mg daily; 12-22 kg minimum 200 mg daily, max 300 mg daily; 23-31 kg minimum 200 mg daily, max 350 mg daily; 32-38 kg minimum 250 mg daily, max 350 mg daily; >38 kg minimum 250 mg daily, max 400 mg daily

Adult: PO 25 mg/day initially, increase by 25 mg/day qwk up to 100 mg/day in 2 divided doses

Renal dose
Adult: PO CCr <70 ml/min ½ dose

Available forms: Tabs 25, 50, 100, 200 mg; sprinkle caps 15, 25 mg; ext rel caps 25, 50, 100, 200 mg; ext rel cap (sprinkles 24 hr) 25, 50, 100, 150, 200 mg

Implementation
- Do not break, crush, or chew tabs; very bitter
- May take without regard to meals
- Sprinkle cap can be given whole or opened and sprinkled on soft food; do not chew, drink water after sprinkle
- Store at room temp away from heat, light

Trokendi XR: swallow whole; do not sprinkle on food, crush, chew; not recommended for child <6 yr

Qudexy XR: may swallow whole or sprinkle on food (teaspoon); swallow immediately; do not crush, chew

ADVERSE EFFECTS
CNS: Dizziness, fatigue, cognitive disorder, *insomnia*, anxiety, depression, paresthesia, motor retardation, suicidal ideation, memory loss, tremor, poor balance, ataxia
CV: Flushing, chest pain
EENT: Diplopia, vision abnormality
GI: *Diarrhea, anorexia,* nausea, dyspepsia, abdominal pain, constipation, dry mouth, pancreatitis
GU: Breast pain, dysmenorrhea, menstrual disorder
INTEG: Rash, alopecia
MISC: Weight loss, leukopenia, metabolic acidosis, increased body temperature, unexplained death (epilepsy)
RESP: Upper respiratory tract infection, pharyngitis, sinusitis

Pharmacokinetics
Absorption	Well absorbed
Distribution	Crosses placenta, plasma protein binding (9%-17%), steady state 4 days
Metabolism	Unknown
Excretion	Kidneys unchanged 55%-97%
Half-life	19-25 hr

Pharmacodynamics
Onset	Unknown
Peak	2-4 hr
Duration	Unknown

INTERACTIONS
Individual drugs
Alcohol: increased CNS depression
Amitriptyline: increased effect of amitriptyline
CarBAMazepine, phenytoin, probenecid: decreased levels of topiramate
Digoxin: decreased levels of digoxin
Estrogen: decreased levels of estrogen

Hydrochlorothiazide, lamoTRIgine, metformin: increased topiramate levels

Lithium: decreased levels of lithium

RisperiDONE: decreased levels of risperidone

Valproic acid: decreased levels of both products

Drug classifications

Carbonic anhydrase inhibitors: increased kidney stone formation

CNS depressants: increased CNS depression

Oral contraceptives: decreased level of oral contraceptives

NURSING CONSIDERATIONS
Assessment

• **Bipolar disorder:** assess mood, behavior

⚠ **Assess mental status: mood, sensorium, affect, memory (long, short), especially in geriatric; suicidal thoughts/behavior**

• Assess for blood dyscrasias: fever, sore throat, bruising, rash, jaundice, epistaxis (long-term treatment only)

• **Assess seizure activity** including type, location, duration, and character; provide seizure precaution

• Monitor CBC during long-term therapy; serum bicarbonate

• Assess body weight and evidence of cognitive disorder

Patient/family education

• Teach patient to carry/wear emergency ID stating name, products taken, condition, prescriber's name and phone number

• Advise patient to avoid driving, other activities that require alertness, until response is known

• Teach patient not to discontinue medication abruptly after long-term use

• **Advise patient to use nonhormonal contraceptive; effect of oral contraceptives is decreased, pregnancy D**

• Teach patient to drink plenty of fluids to prevent kidney stones, vision loss may occur

• Teach patient that increased dietary intake might be necessary, weight loss may occur

• Teach patient to swallow extended-release product whole

Evaluation

Positive therapeutic outcome

• Decreased seizure activity

TREATMENT OF OVERDOSE:
Lavage, VS

⚠ HIGH ALERT

topotecan (Rx)
(to-poe′ti-kan)

Hycamtin

Func. class: Antineoplastic natural; topoisomerase inhibitor

Chem. class.: Camptothecin analog

Pregnancy category D

ACTION: Antitumor product with topoisomerase I–inhibitory activity; topoisomerase I relieves torsional strain in DNA by causing single-strand breaks; causes double-strand DNA damage

Therapeutic outcome: Decreased tumor size

USES: Metastatic ovarian cancer after failure of traditional chemotherapy, relapsed small cell lung cancer, cervical cancer

CONTRAINDICATIONS
Pregnancy **D**, breastfeeding, hypersensitivity, severe bone marrow depression

BLACK BOX WARNING: Neutropenia

Precautions: Children, renal disease, gelatin hypersensitivity

DOSAGE AND ROUTES
Metastatic carcinoma of the ovary after failure of first or subsequent chemotherapy; SCLC-sensitive disease after failure of first-line therapy

Adult: **IV** INF 1.5 mg/m² over 30 min/day × 5 days starting on day 1 of a 21-day course × 4 courses; may be reduced to 0.25 mg/m² for subsequent courses if severe neutropenia occurs

Relapsed small-cell lung cancer (SCLC) in those with a prior complete or partial response, 45 days from end of first-line treatment

Adult: PO 2.3 mg/m²/day on days 1-5 of a 21-day course

Renal dose

Adult: **IV** CCr 20-39 ml/min 0.75 mg/m²/day × 5 days on day 1 of a 21-day course

Available forms: Lyophilized powder for inj 4 mg; cap 0.25, 1 mg

Implementation

• Provide increased fluid intake to 2-3 L/day to prevent dehydration, unless contraindicated

---

Adverse effects: *italics* = common; **bold** = life-threatening

- Change **IV** site q48hr
- Store caps in refrigerator; IV INF unopened at room temperature; protect both from light

Intermittent IV infusion route
- Visually inspect for particulate matter and discoloration prior to use
- Reconstitute each 4-mg vial with 4 ml sterile water for injection; use immediately, no preservative
- Withdraw the appropriate volume of the reconstituted solution; dilute further in 0.9% NaCl or D_5W prior to administration
- The reconstituted solution is yellow or yellow-green
- Topotecan injection diluted for infusion is stable at room temperature with normal light for 24 hr
- Infuse over 30 min

ADVERSE EFFECTS
CNS: Arthralgia, *asthenia, headache,* myalgia, *pain,* weakness
GI: *Abdominal pain, constipation,* diarrhea, obstruction, *nausea,* stomatitis, *vomiting,* increased ALT, AST, anorexia
HEMA: Neutropenia, leukopenia, thrombocytopenia, anemia, sepsis
INTEG: *Total alopecia*
RESP: Dyspnea, cough, interstitial lung disease

Pharmacokinetics

Absorption	Rapidly, completely absorbed
Distribution	7%-35% protein binding
Metabolism	Liver
Excretion	Urine, feces to metabolites
Half-life	2.8 hr

Pharmacodynamics

Unknown

INTERACTIONS
Individual drugs
CISplatin: increased myelosuppression
Itraconazole, mefloquine, niCARdipine, quiNIDine, RU-486, tamoxifen, testosterone, verapamil: avoid giving together

Drug classifications
Anticoagulants, NSAIDs, platelet inhibitors, thrombolytics: increased bleeding risk
P-glycoprotein, breast cancer resistance protein inhibitors (amiodarone, clarithromycin, diltiazem, erythromycin, indinavir vaccines, toxoids: avoid using together

Drug/food
Grapefruit juice: avoid use

NURSING CONSIDERATIONS
Assessment
- Monitor liver function tests: AST, ALT, alkaline phosphatase, which may be elevated; creatinine, BUN

> **BLACK BOX WARNING:** Monitor CBC, differential, platelet count weekly; withhold product if WBC is <3500/mm^3 or platelet count is <100,000/mm^3; notify prescriber of these results; product should be discontinued

- Assess buccal cavity for dryness, sores or ulceration, white patches, oral pain, bleeding, dysphagia
⚠ **Interstitial lung disease (ILD): assess for fever, cough, dyspnea, hypoxia, may be fatal**

Patient/family education
- Advise patient to avoid foods with citric acid or hot flavor or rough texture if stomatitis is present; to drink adequate fluids
- Advise patient that total alopecia may occur; hair grows back but may be different in color and texture
- Advise patient to report stomatitis; any bleeding, white spots, ulcerations in mouth; tell patient to examine mouth daily; report symptoms

> **BLACK BOX WARNING:** Teach patient to report signs of anemia; fatigue, headache, faintness, shortness of breath, irritability

- Teach patient to rinse mouth tid-qid with water, club soda; brush teeth bid-tid with soft brush or cotton-tipped applicator for stomatitis; use unwaxed dental floss
⚠ **Teach patient to use effective contraception during treatment and up to 6 mo after, pregnancy (D), avoid breastfeeding**
- Advise patient to avoid OTC products without approval of prescriber
- Advise to avoid driving or other activities requiring alertness
- Advise to avoid vaccines, toxoids

Evaluation
Positive therapeutic outcome
- Decreased tumor size, spread of malignancy

RARELY USED

toremifene (Rx)

(tor-em'ih-feen)

Fareston

Func. class.: Antineoplastic

Chem. class.: Antiestrogen hormone

Pregnancy category D

Therapeutic outcome: Prevention of rapidly growing malignant cells

USES: Advanced breast carcinoma that has not responded to other therapy in estrogen-receptor-positive patients (usually postmenopausal)

CONTRAINDICATIONS

Pregnancy **D**, hypersensitivity, history of thromboembolism

BLACK BOX WARNING: QT prolongation

DOSAGE AND ROUTES

Adult: PO 60 mg/day

Available forms: Tabs 60 mg

traMADol (Rx)

(trah'mah-dol)

ConZip, Ultram, Ultram ER, Zytram ✦

Func. class.: Analgesic, miscellaneous

Pregnancy category C

Do not confuse: traMADol/Toradol

ACTION: Binds to μ-opioid receptors and inhibits reuptake of norepinephrine, serotonin

Therapeutic outcome: Relief of pain

USES: Management of moderate to severe pain, chronic pain, headache, osteoarthritis

CONTRAINDICATIONS

Hypersensitivity, acute intoxication with any CNS depressant, alcohol, asthma, respiratory depression

Precautions: Pregnancy **C**, breastfeeding, children, geriatric, seizure disorder, renal/hepatic disease, respiratory depression, head trauma, increased ICP, acute abdominal condition, product abuse, depression, suicidal ideation

DOSAGE AND ROUTES

Mild to moderate pain

Adult: PO 25 mg qd, titrate by 25 mg ≥3 days to 100 mg/day (25 mg qid), then may increase by 50 mg ≥3 days to 200 mg (50 mg qid), then 50-100 mg q4-6hr, max 400 mg/day; use caution in elderly

Geriatric >75 yr: PO <300 mg/day in divided dose

Hepatic dose

Adult: PO 50 mg q12hr

Renal dose

Adult (Child-Pugh C): PO CCr <30 ml/min q12hr, max 200 mg/day; do not use ext rel tabs

Moderate to severe chronic pain

Adult: PO-ER (Ultram ER) 100 mg daily, titrate upward q5day by 100 mg, max 300 mg/day; (Ryzolt) 100 mg, titrate upward q2-3day in 100-mg increments; max 300 mg/day; products are not interchangeable

Available forms: Tabs 50 mg; ext rel tab 100, 200, 300 mg; orally disintegrating tab 50 mg

Implementation

• Do not break, crush, or chew ext rel product

• Give with antiemetic for nausea, vomiting

• Administer when pain is beginning to return; determine dosage interval by patient response

• Store in cool environment, protect from sunlight

• Give with or without food; ext rel: always give with food, or always give on empty stomach

ADVERSE EFFECTS

CNS: Dizziness, CNS stimulation, somnolence, headache, anxiety, confusion, euphoria, *seizures*, hallucinations, sedation, **neuroleptic malignant syndrome–like reactions**

CV: Vasodilatation, orthostatic hypotension, tachycardia, hypertension, abnormal ECG

EENT: Visual disturbances

GI: Nausea, constipation, vomiting, dry mouth, diarrhea, abdominal pain, anorexia, flatulence, **GI bleeding**

GU: Urinary retention/frequency, menopausal symptoms, dysuria, menstrual disorder

INTEG: Pruritus, rash, urticaria, vesicles, flushing

SYST: **Anaphylaxis, Stevens-Johnson syndrome, toxic epidermal necrolysis, serotonin syndrome**

Pharmacokinetics

Absorption	Rapidly, almost completely absorbed
Distribution	Steady state 2 days
Metabolism	Extensively in liver, may cross blood-brain barrier
Excretion	Unchanged product 30% in urine, protein binding 20%
Half-life	Unknown

T

Pharmacodynamics

Unknown

INTERACTIONS
Individual drugs
Alcohol: increased CNS depression
CarBAMazepine: decreased tramadol level

Drug classifications
CYP3A4 inducers (barbiturates, bosentan, car-BAMazepine, efavirenz, nevirapine, phenytoin, rifabutin, rifampin): decreased tramadol effect

CYP3A4 inhibitors (aprepitant, antiretroviral protease inhibitors, clarithromycin, danazol, delavirdine, diltiazem, erythromycin, fluconazole, FLUoxetine, fluvoxaMINE, imatinib, ketoconazole, mibefradil, nefazodone, telithromycin, voriconazole): increased traMADol levels

MAOIs: inhibition of norepinephrine and serotonin reuptake; use together with caution

Opiates, sedative/hypnotics: increased CNS depression

SSRIs, SNRIs, serotonin-receptor agonists: increased serotonin syndrome

Drug/herb
Chamomile, hops, kava, skullcap, valerian: increased CNS depression

St. John's wort: avoid use

Drug/lab test
Increased: creatinine, liver enzymes
Decreased: Hgb

NURSING CONSIDERATIONS
Assessment
• **Pain:** assess location, type, character; give before pain becomes extreme
• Assess for increased side effects in renal/hepatic disease
• **Respiratory depression:** withhold if respirations <12/min
• Monitor I&O ratio: check for decreasing output; may indicate urinary retention
• Assess need for product
• Assess for constipation and bowel pattern; increase fluids, bulk in diet
⚠ **Hypersensitivity: usually after beginning treatment**
• Monitor CNS changes: dizziness, drowsiness, hallucinations, euphoria, LOC, pupil reaction
• Determine allergic reactions: rash, urticaria
• **Serotonin syndrome, neuroleptic malignant syndrome: assess for increased heart rate, shivering, sweating, dilated pupils, tremors, high B/P, hyperthermia, headache, confusion; if these occur, stop product, administer a serotonin antagonist if needed**

Patient/family education
• Teach patient to report any symptoms of CNS changes, allergic reactions
• Teach patient that drowsiness, dizziness, and confusion may occur; to call for assistance
• Instruct patient to make position changes slowly; orthostatic hypotension may occur
• Tell patient to avoid OTC medication and alcohol unless approved by prescriber
• Instruct patient not to discontinue abruptly, taper

Evaluation
Positive therapeutic outcome
• Decreased pain

⚠ HIGH ALERT

trametinib
(tra-me′ti-nib)
MeKinist
Func. class.: Antineoplastic biologic response modifier
Chem. class.: Signal transduction inhibitor (STI), tyrosine kinase inhibitor
Pregnancy category D

ACTION: Inhibits MEK-1, MEK-2 tyrosine kinase created in patients with malignant melanoma

Therapeutic outcome: Decrease in progression of disease

USES: Unresectable or metastatic BRAD V600E or BRAF V600K mutated malignant melanoma

CONTRAINDICATIONS
Pregnancy (**D**), hypersensitivity

Precautions: Breastfeeding, children, diarrhea, geriatric patients, hepatic disease, bone marrow suppression, infection, thrombocytopenia, neutropenia, immunosuppression

DOSAGE AND ROUTES
Adult: PO 2 mg/day, may be used in combination with dacarbazine or PACLitaxel in those with BRAF V600E

Management of treatment-related toxicity
Cutaneous toxicity
• **Grade 2 rash:** reduce dose by 0.5 mg (e.g., 2 mg/day to 1.5 mg/day) or discontinue in patients who are receiving trametinib 1 mg/day. In patients with an intolerable grade 2 rash that does not improve within 3 wk of a dosage reduction, withhold trametinib for up to 3 wk. If the rash is improved within 3 wk, resume therapy at a lower dose (reduce the previous

---

dose by 0.5 mg). If the rash does not improve within 3 wk, permanently discontinue.

• Grade 3 or 4 rash: withhold for up to 3 wk. If the rash is improved within 3 wk, resume at a lower dose (reduce the previous dose by 0.5 mg); discontinue in patients who are receiving trametinib 1 mg/day. If the rash does not improve within 3 wk, permanently discontinue.

Cardiac toxicity

• Asymptomatic cardiac toxicity and an absolute decrease in LVEF of ≥10% from baseline and below institutional lower limits of normal (LLN) from pretreatment value: withhold for up to 4 wk. If the LVEF is improved within 4 wk, resume at a lower dose (reduce the previous dose by 0.5 mg); discontinue in patients who are receiving 1 mg/day. If the LVEF does not improve to normal within 4 wk, permanently discontinue.

• Symptomatic CHF or an absolute decrease in LVEF of >20% from baseline and below institutional LLN: permanently discontinue

Ocular toxicity

• Grade 2 or 3 retinal pigment epithelial detachment (RPED): withhold for up to 3 wk. If the RPED improves to grade 1 or less within 3 wk, resume at a lower dose (reduce the previous dose by 0.5 mg); discontinue therapy in patients who are receiving 1 mg/day. If the RPED does not improve to at least grade 1 within 3 wk, permanently discontinue.

• Retinal vein occlusion: permanently discontinue therapy

Pulmonary toxicity

• Interstitial lung disease/pneumonitis: permanently discontinue

Other toxicity

• Grade 3 toxicity: withhold for up to 3 wk. If the toxicity improves to grade 1 or less within 3 wk, resume at a lower dose (reduce the previous dose by 0.5 mg); discontinue in patients who are receiving 1 mg/day. If the toxicity does not improve to at least grade 1 within 3 wk, permanently discontinue.

• Grade 4 toxicity: permanently discontinue

Available forms: Tabs 0.5, 2 mg

Implementation

• Give 1 hr before or 2 hr after a meal
• If dose is missed, take within 12 hr of missed dose; if >12 hr have passed, skip dose
• Follow cytotoxic handling procedures

ADVERSE EFFECTS

CNS: Dizziness
CV: Heart failure, hypertension, cardiomyopathy

EENT: Occular hemorrhage, retinal detachment, blurred vision
GI: Diarrhea, nausea, vomiting, abdominal pain, stomatitis
GU: Hematuria
INTEG: Rash, pruritus, acne, folliculitis, erythema
MISC: Elevated LFTs, hand-foot syndrome
MS: Rhabdomyolysis
RESP: Cough, dyspnea, pleural effusion, pneumonitis, edema

Pharmacokinetics

Absorption	Unknown
Distribution	Protein binding 97.4%
Metabolism	Unknown
Excretion	In feces
Half-life	Unknown

Pharmacodynamics

Onset	Unknown
Peak	1.5 hr
Duration	Unknown

INTERACTIONS
None known

NURSING CONSIDERATIONS
Assessment

• Monitor LFTs every mo × 3 mo, then as clinically indicated

Patient/family education

• Teach patient to report adverse reactions immediately, bleeding
• Teach patient about reason for treatment, expected results
• Teach patient to use effective contraception during treatment and up to 30 days after discontinuing treatment

Evaluation

Positive therapeutic outcome
• Decrease in progression of disease

trandolapril (Rx)
(tran-doe′la-prill)
Mavik
Func. class.: Antihypertensive
Chem. class.: Angiotensin-converting enzyme (ACE) inhibitor
Pregnancy category D (2nd/3rd trimester), C (1st trimester)

ACTION: Selectively suppresses renin-angiotensin-aldosterone system; inhibits ACE; prevents conversion of angiotensin I to angiotensin

Adverse effects: *italics* = common; **bold** = life-threatening

II, resulting in dilatation of arterial and venous vessels and lowered B/P

Therapeutic outcome: Decreased B/P in hypertension

USES: Hypertension alone or in combination, heart failure, after MI, LV dysfunction after MI

CONTRAINDICATIONS
Breastfeeding, hypersensitivity, history of angioedema

> **BLACK BOX WARNING:** Pregnancy **D**, pregnancy **C** (1st trimester)

Precautions: Geriatric, hyperkalemia, hepatic disease, bilateral renal stenosis, after kidney transplant, aortal/mitral valve stenosis, cirrhosis, severe renal disease, untreated CHF, autoimmune diseases, cough

DOSAGE AND ROUTES
Hypertension
Adult: PO 1 mg/day, 2 mg/day in African Americans, make dosage adjustment ≥1 wk; up to 8 mg/day

Heart failure (after MI/left ventricular dysfunction)
Adult: PO 1 mg/day, titrate upward to 4 mg/day if tolerated, 2-4 yr

Renal dose/hepatic dose
Adult: PO CCr <30 ml/min or hepatic disease 0.5 mg/day

Available forms: Tabs 1, 2, 4 mg

Implementation
• Store in airtight container at ≤77° F (≤25° C) or less
• Give without regard to food
• Space antacids by 2 hr after dose

ADVERSE EFFECTS
CNS: *Dizziness,* paresthesias, headache, *syncope,* fatigue, drowsiness, depression, sleep disturbances, anxiety, syncope
CV: *Hypotension,* **MI,** palpitations, angina, TIAs, **stroke,** bradycardia, dysrhythmias
GI: Nausea, vomiting, cramps, diarrhea, constipation, **pancreatitis,** *dyspepsia*
GU: Proteinuria, renal failure
HEMA: Agranulocytosis, neutropenia, leukopenia, anemia
INTEG: Rash, purpura, pruritus, **angioedema**
MISC: Hyperkalemia, hyponatremia, impotence, *myalgia, angioedema,* muscle cramps, asthenia, hypocalcemia, gout
RESP: Dyspnea, cough

Pharmacokinetics
Absorption	40%-60%
Distribution	Unknown
Metabolism	Liver
Excretion	Kidneys (33%), feces (66%)
Half-life	0.6-1.1 hr, 16-24 hr

Pharmacodynamics
Onset	½ hr
Peak	4-10 hr
Duration	>8 days

INTERACTIONS
Individual drugs
Levodopa, lithium, reserpine: increased effect of each specific product

Drug classifications
Antacids, NSAIDs, salicylates: decreased effect of trandolapril
Antihypertensives, diuretics: increased severe hypotension
Barbiturates, ergots, hypoglycemics, neuromuscular blocking agents: increased effects of each specific product
Diuretics (potassium-sparing): increased potassium levels
Phenothiazines: increased antihypertensive effects
Potassium supplements: increased potassium levels
Salt substitutes: increased potassium levels

Drug/lab test
Increased: potassium, LFTs, BUN, creatinine
Decreased: sodium, WBC

NURSING CONSIDERATIONS
Assessment
• Monitor blood tests: neutrophils, decreased platelets
• Monitor B/P, orthostatic hypotension, syncope; if changes occur dosage change may be required
• Monitor renal studies: protein, BUN, creatinine; increased levels may indicate nephrotic syndrome and renal failure
• Monitor renal symptoms: polyuria, oliguria, frequency, dysuria
• Establish baselines in renal, liver function tests before therapy begins
• Check potassium levels throughout treatment, although hyperkalemia rarely occurs
• Check for edema in feet, legs daily
• Assess for allergic reactions: rash, fever, pruritus, urticaria; product should be discontinued if antihistamines fail to help

BLACK BOX WARNING: Pregnancy: Identify if pregnancy is planned or suspected; pregnancy (**D**)

⚠ Hepatotoxicity (rare): assess for increased LFTs, jaundice, fulminating hepatic necrosis; if jaundice occurs, discontinue product
• Angioedema: of the face, edema of the extremities, mucus membranes, may need to discontinue
⚠ Hyperkalemia: monitor electrolytes, check potassium

Patient/family education
• Advise patient not to discontinue product abruptly; advise patient to tell all persons associated with health care
• Teach patient not to use OTC products (cough, cold, allergy) unless directed by physician; serious side effects can occur; xanthines, such as coffee, tea, chocolate, cola, can prevent action of product
• Instruct patient on the importance of complying with dosage schedule, even if feeling better; to continue with medical regimen to decrease B/P: exercise, cessation of smoking, decreasing stress, diet modifications
• Emphasize the need to rise slowly to sitting or standing position to minimize orthostatic hypotension; not to exercise in hot weather, which can cause increased hypotension
• Advise patient to notify prescriber of mouth sores, sore throat, fever, swelling of hands or feet, irregular heartbeat, chest pain, coughing, shortness of breath
• Caution patient to report excessive perspiration, dehydration, vomiting, diarrhea; may lead to fall in B/P
• Caution patient that product may cause dizziness, fainting, light-headedness; may occur during 1st few days of therapy; to avoid activities that may be hazardous
• Teach patient how to take B/P and normal readings for age group

BLACK BOX WARNING: Teach patient to notify prescriber if pregnancy is suspected or planned, pregnancy **D**

Evaluation

Positive therapeutic outcome
• Decreased B/P in hypertension

TREATMENT OF OVERDOSE:
Lavage, **IV** atropine for bradycardia, **IV** theophylline for bronchospasm, digoxin, O$_2$, diuretic for cardiac failure, hemodialysis

---

⚠ HIGH ALERT

trastuzumab (Rx)
(tras-tuz'uh-mab)
Herceptin
Func. class.: Antineoplastic—miscellaneous
Chem. class.: Humanized monoclonal antibody
Pregnancy category D

ACTION: DNA-derived monoclonal antibody selectively binds to extracellular portion of human epidermal growth factor receptor 2 (HER2); it inhibits proliferation of cancer cells

Therapeutic outcome: Decreasing symptoms of breast cancer

USES: Metastatic breast cancer with overexpression of HER2, early breast cancer (adjuvant, neoadjuvant), gastric cancer; previously untreated HER2 overexpressing metastatic gastric or gastroesophageal junction adenocarcinoma with CISplatin, 5-fluorouracil or capecitabine

CONTRAINDICATIONS
Pregnancy **D**, hypersensitivity to this product, Chinese hamster ovary cell protein

Precautions: Breastfeeding, children, geriatric, pulmonary disease, anemia, leukopenia

BLACK BOX WARNING: Cardiac disease, respiratory distress syndrome, respiratory insufficiency, infusion-related reactions, cardiomyopathy

DOSAGE AND ROUTES
Breast cancer
Several regimens may be used
Adult: IV 4 mg/kg given over 90 min, then maintenance 2 mg/kg given over 30 min; do not give as **IV** PUSH or BOL; may be given in combination with other antineoplastics

Gastric cancer
Adult: IV 8 mg/kg over 90 min on day 1, then 6 mg/kg over 30-90 min q21days from day 22, give with CISplatin 80 mg/m^2 on day 1 plus 5-fluorouracil 800 mg/m^2 CONT INF on days 1-5 or capecitabine 1000 mg/m^2 bid on days 1-14, repeat cycle q3wk

Available forms: Lyophilized powder 440 mg

Implementation
• Give acetaminophen as ordered to alleviate fever and headache
• Increase fluid intake to 2-3 L/day

T

Adverse effects: *italics* = common; **bold** = life-threatening

Intermittent IV infusion route
- Administer after reconstituting vial with 20 ml of bacteriostatic water for inj, 1.1% benzyl alcohol preserved (supplied) to yield 21 mg/ml, mark date on vial 28 days from reconstitution date; if patient is allergic to benzyl alcohol, reconstitute with sterile water for inj; use immediately; inf over 90 min; q3wk give 8 mg/kg loading dose over 90 min; subsequent doses 6 mg/kg may be given over 30-60 min
- Do not mix or dilute with other products or dextrose sol

ADVERSE EFFECTS

CNS: *Dizziness, numbness, paresthesias,* depression, *insomnia,* neuropathy, peripheral neuritis
CV: Tachycardia, CHF
GI: Nausea, vomiting, *anorexia, diarrhea,* abdominal pain, hepatotoxicity, dysgeusia
HEMA: *Anemia,* leukopenia
INTEG: *Rash,* acne, herpes simplex
META: Edema, peripheral edema
MISC: *Flulike symptoms; fever, headache, chills*
MS: Arthralgia, *bone pain*
RESP: *Cough, dyspnea, pharyngitis, rhinitis,* sinusitis, pneumonia, pulmonary edema/fibrosis, acute respiratory distress syndrome (ARDS)
SYST: Anaphylaxis, angioedema

Pharmacokinetics

Absorption	Unknown
Distribution	Unknown
Metabolism	Unknown
Excretion	Unknown
Half-life	1-32 days

Pharmacodynamics

Unknown

INTERACTIONS
Individual drugs
Cyclophosphamide: increased cardiomyopathy risk; avoid use
Warfarin: increased bleeding risk

Drug classifications
Anthracyclines: increased cardiomyopathy risk
Vaccines/toxoids: decreased immune response

NURSING CONSIDERATIONS
Assessment
- Monitor CBC, HER2 overexpression
- Assess for symptoms of infection; may be masked by product
- Assess CNS reaction: LOC, mental status, dizziness, confusion

> **BLACK BOX WARNING: CHF** and other cardiac symptoms: assess for dyspnea, coughing, gallop; obtain a full cardiac workup including ECG, echocardiogram, multigated angiogram

- Hypersensitivity reactions, anaphylaxis

> **BLACK BOX WARNING: Potentially fatal infusion reactions:** assess for fever, chills, nausea, vomiting, pain, headache, dizziness, hypotension; discontinue product

- **Pulmonary toxicity: assess for dyspnea, interstitial pneumonitis, pulmonary hypertension, ARDS; can occur after infusion reaction, those with lung disease may have more severe toxicity**

Patient/family education
- Advise patient to take acetaminophen for fever
- Teach patient to avoid hazardous tasks, since confusion, dizziness may occur
- Teach patient to report signs of infection: sore throat, fever, diarrhea, vomiting
- Inform patient that emotional lability is common; instruct patient to notify prescriber if severe or incapacitating
- **Advise patient to use contraception while taking this product, pregnancy D; avoid breastfeeding**

> **BLACK BOX WARNING:** Teach patient to report pain at infusion site

Evaluation
Positive therapeutic outcome
- Decrease in size of tumors

travoprost ophthalmic
See Appendix B

traZODone (Rx)
(tray'zoe-done)
Oleptro
Func. class.: Antidepressant—miscellaneous
Chem. class.: Triazolopyridine
Pregnancy category C

ACTION: Selectively inhibits serotonin, norepinephrine uptake by brain, potentiates behavioral changes

Therapeutic outcome: Decreased symptoms of depression after 2-3 wk

USES: Depression

CONTRAINDICATIONS
Hypersensitivity to tricyclics

Precautions: Pregnancy **C**, suicidal patients, severe depression, increased intraocular pressure, closed-angle glaucoma, urinary retention, cardiac/hepatic disease, hyperthyroidism, electroshock therapy, elective surgery, bleeding, abrupt discontinuation, bipolar disorder, breastfeeding, dehydration, hyponatremia, hypovolemia, recovery phase of MI, seizure disorders, prostatic hypertrophy, family history of long QT

> **BLACK BOX WARNING:** Suicidal ideation in children/adolescents

DOSAGE AND ROUTES
Depression
Adult: PO 150 mg/day in divided doses; may increase by 50 mg/day q3-4day, max 400 mg/day (outpatient), 600 mg/day (inpatient); EXT REL 150 mg/day in the evening, may increase gradually by 75 mg/day at 3 day intervals, max 375 mg/day

Geriatric: PO 25-50 at bedtime, increase by 25-50 mg q3-7day to desired dose, usual 75-150 mg/day

Child 6-18 yr (unlabeled): PO 1.5-2 mg/kg/day in divided doses, may increase q3-4day up to 6 mg/kg/day or 400 mg/day in divided doses, whichever is less

Available forms: Tabs 50, 100, 150, 300 mg; ext rel tabs 150, 300 mg

Implementation
• Give with food or milk for GI symptoms; crush if patient is unable to swallow medication whole
• Give dose at bedtime if oversedation occurs during day; may take entire dose at bedtime; geriatric may not tolerate once/day dosing
• Store in tight, light-resistant container at room temp; do not freeze

ADVERSE EFFECTS
CNS: *Dizziness, drowsiness,* confusion, headache, anxiety, tremors, stimulation, weakness, insomnia, nightmares, EPS (geriatric), increase in psychiatric symptoms, **suicide in children/adolescents**

CV: *Orthostatic hypotension, ECG changes, tachycardia,* **hypertension,** palpitations

EENT: *Blurred vision,* tinnitus, mydriasis

GI: *Diarrhea, dry mouth,* nausea, vomiting, **paralytic ileus,** increased appetite, cramps, epigastric distress, jaundice, **hepatitis,** stomatitis, constipation

GU: *Retention,* **acute renal failure, priapism**

HEMA: **Agranulocytosis, thrombocytopenia, eosinophilia, leukopenia**

INTEG: Rash, urticaria, sweating, pruritus, photosensitivity

Pharmacokinetics

Absorption	Well absorbed
Distribution	Widely distributed
Metabolism	Liver, extensively
Excretion	Kidneys, minimally unchanged
Half-life	4½-7½ hr

Pharmacodynamics

Onset	Unknown
Peak	1 hr without food, 2 hr with food
Duration	Unknown

INTERACTIONS
Individual drugs
Alcohol, carBAMazepine, digoxin, phenytoin: increased effect of each product

FLUoxetine, nefazodone: increased levels, increased toxicity, serotonin syndrome

Guanethidine, cloNIDine: decreased effects of each product

Warfarin: increased or decreased effects of warfarin

Drug classifications
Barbiturates, benzodiazepines, CNS depressants: increased effects

CYP3A4, 2D6 inhibitors (phenothiazenes, protease inhibitors, azole antifungals): increased effects of trazodone

MAOIs: increased hyperpyretic crisis, seizures, hypertensive episode, do not use within 14 days

SNRIs, SSRIs: increased toxicity, serotonin syndrome

Sympathomimetics (direct-acting): increased sympathomimetic effects

Sympathomimetics (indirect-acting): decreased effects

Drug/herb
Hops, kava, lavender, valerian: increased CNS depression

SAM-e, St. John's wort: increased serotonin syndrome

Drug/lab test
Increased: LFTs
Decreased: Hgb

NURSING CONSIDERATIONS
Assessment
• Monitor B/P (lying, standing), pulse q4hr; if systolic B/P drops 20 mm Hg hold product, notify prescriber; take vital signs q4hr in patients with CV disease
• Monitor blood tests: CBC, leukocytes, differential

- Monitor liver function tests: AST, ALT, bilirubin
- Check weight qwk; appetite may increase with product
- **Assess ECG for flattening of T wave, bundle branch block, AV block, dysrhythmias in cardiac patients**
- Assess for EPS primarily in geriatric: rigidity, dystonia, akathisia

> **BLACK BOX WARNING:** Assess mental status: mood, sensorium, affect, suicidal tendencies in children/adolescents; increase in psychiatric symptoms: depression, panic, not approved for children

- Monitor urinary retention, constipation; constipation is more likely to occur in children or geriatric
- **Withdrawal symptoms:** assess for headache, nausea, vomiting, muscle pain, weakness; do not usually occur unless product was discontinued abruptly
- Identify alcohol consumption; if alcohol is consumed, hold dose until AM
- **Serotonin syndrome, neuroleptic malignant syndrome: assess for increased heart rate, shivering, sweating, dilated pupils, tremors, high B/P, hyperthermia, headache, confusion; if these occur, stop product, administer a serotonin antagonist if needed**

Patient/family education
- Teach patient that therapeutic effects may take 2-3 wk
- Teach patient to use caution in driving or other activities requiring alertness because of drowsiness, dizziness, blurred vision; to avoid rising quickly from sitting to standing, especially geriatric
- Teach patient not to crush, chew ext rel product
- Caution patient to avoid alcohol ingestion, other CNS depressants
- Teach patient not to discontinue medication quickly after long-term use: may cause nausea, headache, malaise
- Advise patient to wear sunscreen or large hat because photosensitivity occurs
- Teach patient to increase fluids, bulk in diet if constipation, urinary retention occur, especially geriatric
- Advise patient to take gum, hard sugarless candy, or frequent sips of water for dry mouth
- Advise patient to rise slowly to prevent dizziness

> **BLACK BOX WARNING:** Teach family to watch for suicidal ideation or tendencies, usually in children/adolescents

- Teach patient to notify prescriber if pregnancy is planned or suspected, pregnancy (C), avoid breastfeeding

Evaluation

Positive therapeutic outcome
- Decrease in depression
- Absence of suicidal thoughts

TREATMENT OF OVERDOSE:
ECG monitoring, induce emesis, lavage, activated charcoal, administer anticonvulsant

treprostinil (Rx)
(treh-prah′stin-ill)
Remodulin, Tyvaso
Func. class.: Antihypertensive vasodilator
Chem. class.: Tricyclic benzidine prostacyclin analog
Pregnancy category B

ACTION: Direct vasodilatation of pulmonary, systemic arterial vascular beds, inhibition of platelet aggregation

Therapeutic outcome: Decreased pulmonary arterial hypertension (PAH)

USES: PAH, NYHA class II through IV

CONTRAINDICATIONS
Hypersensitivity to this product or other prostacyclin analogs

Precautions: Pregnancy **B**, breastfeeding, children, geriatric, past hepatic disease, renal/thromboembolic disease, abrupt discontinuation, **IV** administration

DOSAGE AND ROUTES
Pulmonary arterial hypertension (WHO group 1)
Adult: SUBCUT INF 1.25 ng/kg/min by cont INF, may reduce to 0.625 ng if not tolerated; may increase by 1.25 ng/kg/min qwk for first 4 wk, then 2.5 ng/kg/min qwk for remainder of INF; oral INH 3 breaths via Tyvaso INH system qid

Hepatic dose
Adult: SUBCUT INF 0.625 ng/kg ideal body weight/min and increase cautiously

Available forms: Inj 1, 2.5, 5, 10 mg/ml; neb sol 1.74 mg/2.9 ml

Implementation

SUBCUT INF route
- By continuous subcut infusion
- No dilution required

CONT IV INF route

- By surgically placed CV catheter using an ambulatory inf pump
- The IV pump, product, and patient education can be obtained from Priority Healthcare in the United States
- Must be diluted with sterile water for inj or 0.9% NaCl
- Calculate the concentration using this formula: diluted conc = [dose (ng/kg/min) × weight (kg) × 0.00006]/inf rate (ml/hr)
- Sudden decreased doses or abrupt withdrawal may worsen pulmonary atrial hypertension symptoms

Oral inhalation route

- Avoid skin or eyes, do not take orally; use Tyvaso Inhalation System only
- Patient should have a backup Optineb-ir device to avoid interruptions
- Follow instructions for use and cleaning
- Do not mix with other medications in Optineb-ir device
- Twist off cap and squeeze total contents into medicine cup, volume is sufficient for 4 treatments

ADVERSE EFFECTS

CNS: Dizziness, headache, syncope
CV: Vasodilatation, *hypotension, edema,* right ventricular heart failure
GI: Nausea, *diarrhea*
INTEG: *Rash,* pruritus
OTHER: Jaw pain, cough, throat irritation
SYST: Infusion site reactions, inf site pain, increased risk of infection

Pharmacokinetics

Absorption	Unknown
Distribution	Unknown
Metabolism	Liver, 90% protein binding
Excretion	Urine, feces
Half-life	2-4 hr, terminal

Pharmacodynamics

Unknown

INTERACTIONS
Individual drug
Aspirin: increased risk of bleeding

Drug classifications
Anticoagulants, NSAIDs, SSRIs, thrombin inhibitors: increased risk of bleeding
Antihypertensives, β-blockers, calcium channel blockers, diuretics, MAOIs, vasodilators: increased hypotension

NURSING CONSIDERATIONS
Assessment
- **Hypertension:** monitor B/P baseline and periodically
- Monitor liver function tests: AST, ALT, bilirubin, creatinine (long-term therapy)
- ⚠ Monitor blood tests: CBC; CBC q2wk × 3 mo, Hct, Hgb, pro-time (long-term therapy), ABGs
- ⚠ Monitor bleed time baseline and throughout; levels may be 2-5 × normal limit

Patient/family education
- Teach patient that blood work will be necessary during treatment
- Teach patient to report side effects such as diarrhea, skin rashes
- Teach patient that therapy will be needed for prolonged periods of time, sometimes years
- Advise patient that aseptic technique must be used in preparing and administering to prevent infection
- Teach that there are many drug and herb interactions
- Teach signs/symptoms of bleeding: blood in urine, stools
- Teach patient to avoid abrupt discontinuation
- Teach patient how to use inhaled solution and how to care for equipment

Evaluation

Positive therapeutic outcome
- Decreased pulmonary arterial hypertension

---

tretinoin (vitamin A acid, retinoic acid) (Rx)
(tret′i-noyn)
Avita, Renova, Retin-A, Retin-A Micro, Stieva-A ✦
Func. class.: Vitamin A acid/acne product, antineoplastic—miscellaneous
Chem. class.: Tretinoin derivative
Pregnancy category C (TOPICAL), D (PO)

ACTION: (Topical) Decreases cohesiveness of follicular epithelium, decreases microcomedone formation; (PO) induces maturation of acute promyelocytic leukemia, exact action is unknown

Therapeutic outcome: Decreased signs/symptoms of leukemia

USES: (Topical) Acne vulgaris (grades 1-3); (PO) acute promyelocytic leukemia, facial wrinkles, photoaging

CONTRAINDICATIONS

Hypersensitivity to retinoids or sensitivity to parabens

> **BLACK BOX WARNING:** Pregnancy **D** (PO)

Precautions: Pregnancy **C** (topical), breastfeeding, eczema, sunburn, sun exposure

> **BLACK BOX WARNING:** Rapid-evolving leukocytosis, respiratory compromise, acute promyelocytic leukemia differentiation syndrome, requires a specialized care setting, experienced clinician

DOSAGE AND ROUTES

Adult and child: TOP cleanse area, apply 0.025%-0.1% cream or 0.05% liquid at bedtime; cover lightly

Promyelocytic leukemia

Adult: PO 45 mg/m²/day given as 2 evenly divided doses until remission; discontinue treatment 30 days after remission or after 90 days of treatment, whichever is first

Available forms: Topical cream 0.01%, 0.02%, 0.025%, 0.05%, 0.1%; topical gel 0.025%, 0.04%, 0.05%, 0.1%; topical liquid 0.05%; caps 10 mg

Implementation
Topical route
• Apply using gloves or cotton, once daily before bedtime; cover area lightly using gauze
• Store at room temperature
• Wash hands after application
• Apply only to affected areas

ADVERSE EFFECTS

PO route
CNS: Headache, fever, sweating, fatigue
CV: Cardiac dysrhythmias, pericardial effusion
GI: Nausea, vomiting, **hemorrhage,** abdominal pain, diarrhea, constipation, dyspepsia, distention, **hepatitis**
META: Hypercholesterolemia, hypertriglyceridemia
RESP: Pneumonia, upper respiratory tract disease

Topical route
INTEG: Rash, stinging, warmth, redness, erythema, blistering, crusting, peeling, contact dermatitis, hypo/hyperpigmentation, dry skin, pruritus, scaly skin, retinoic acid syndrome (RAS)

Pharmacokinetics

Absorption	Small amounts
Distribution	Unknown
Metabolism	Unknown
Excretion	Kidneys
Half-life	Unknown

Pharmacodynamics

Unknown

INTERACTIONS

Individual drugs
Aminocaproic acid, aprotinin, tranexamic acid: increased thrombotic complications
Benzoyl peroxide, resorcinol, salicylic acid (topical), sulfur: increased peeling
Ketoconazole: increased plasma concentrations of tretinoin (oral)

Drug classifications
Alcohol, astringents, cleansers with drying effect, medicated, abrasive soaps: use with caution (topical)
Diuretics (thiazide), phenothiazines, quinolones, retinoids, sulfonamides, sulfonylureas: increased photosensitivity
Tetracyclines: increased ICP, risk of pseudotumor cerebri; do not use together

Drug/lab test
Increased: AST, ALT

NURSING CONSIDERATIONS

Assessment
Topical route
• Assess part of body involved, including time involved, what helps or aggravates condition, cysts, dryness, itching; lesions may become worse at beginning of treatment
PO route
• Monitor hepatic function, coagulation, hematologic parameters, also cholesterol, triglycerides

Patient/family education
Topical route
• Instruct patient to avoid application on normal skin, to avoid getting cream in eyes, nose, other mucous membranes
• Advise patient to avoid sunlight, sunlamps or to use protective clothing or sunscreen to prevent burns
• Advise patient that treatment may cause warmth, stinging; dryness, peeling will occur
• Inform patient that cosmetics may be used over product; not to use shaving lotions
• Inform patient that rash may occur during first 1-3 wk of therapy

---

- Caution patient that product does not cure condition, only relieves symptoms; that therapeutic results may be seen in 2-3 wk but may not be optimal until after 6 wk

PO route

> **BLACK BOX WARNING:** Advise patient to report to prescriber if pregnancy is planned or suspected, pregnancy **D** (PO)

Evaluation

Positive therapeutic outcome
- Decrease in size and number of lesions

tretinoin topical
See Appendix B

triamcinolone (Rx)
(trye-am-sin'oh-lone)
Aristospan, Kenalog-10, Kenalog-40, Tac-3, Tac-40, Triesence
Func. class.: Corticosteroid, synthetic; antiinflammatory
Chem. class.: Glucocorticoid, intermediate-acting
Pregnancy category C

ACTION: Decreases inflammation by suppressing migration of polymorphonuclear leukocytes, fibroblasts, reversal of increased capillary permeability and lysosomal stabilization

Therapeutic outcome: Decreased inflammation, normal immune response

USES: Severe inflammation, immunosuppression, neoplasms, asthma (steroid dependent), collagen, respiratory, dermatologic disorders, rheumatic disorders

CONTRAINDICATIONS
Hypersensitivity, neonatal prematurity, epidural/intrathecal administration (triamcinolone acetonide injections [Kenalog]), systemic fungal infections

Precautions: Pregnancy **C**, breastfeeding, diabetes mellitus, glaucoma, osteoporosis, seizure disorders, ulcerative colitis, CHF, myasthenia gravis, renal disease, esophagitis, peptic ulcer, acne, cataracts, coagulopathy, head trauma, children <2 yr, psychosis, idiopathic thrombocytopenia, acute glomerulonephritis, amebiasis, fungal infections, nonasthmatic bronchial disease, AIDS, TB, adrenal insufficiency, acute bronchospasm, acne rosacea, Cushing's syndrome, acute MI, thromboembolism

DOSAGE AND ROUTES
Adult: IM 40 mg qwk (acetonide), 5-48 mg into neoplasms (acetonide), 2-40 mg into joint or soft tissue (hexacetonide), 0.5 mg/sq in of affected intralesional skin (hexacetonide), 2-20 mg into joint or soft tissue (hexacetonide)

Severe/incapacitating allergic conditions such as asthma
Adult: IM (Trivaris) 60 mg, titrate; usual range 40-80 mg
Child: IM (Trivaris) 0.11-1.6 mg/kg/day (3.2-48 mg/m²/day) given in 3-4 divided doses

Available forms: Inj 3, 10, 40 mg/ml acetonide; inj 5, 20 mg/ml hexacetonide; inh 100 mcg/spray

Implementation
PO route
- Give with food or milk to decrease GI symptoms; tablet may be crushed

IM route
- Give IM inj deeply in large muscle mass; rotate sites; avoid deltoid; use 21-G needle
- Avoid SUBCUT administration, may damage tissue

Inhalation route
- Use spacer device for geriatric
- Give inh with water to decrease possibility of fungal infections; titrated dose, use lowest effective dose
- Give after cleaning aerosol top daily with warm water, dry thoroughly
- Store in cool environment; do not puncture or incinerate container

Topical route
- Apply only to affected areas; do not get in eyes
- Apply medication, then cover with occlusive dressing (only if prescribed), seal to normal skin, change q12hr; systemic absorption may occur
- Apply only to dermatoses; do not use on weeping, denuded, or infected areas
- Cleanse skin before applying product
- Continue treatment for a few days after area has cleared
- Store at room temperature

Nasal route
- Have patient clear nasal passages before administration; use decongestant if needed; shake inhaler, invert, tilt head backward, insert nozzle into nostril, away from septum; hold other nostril closed and depress activator, inhale through nose, exhale through mouth

ADVERSE EFFECTS
CNS: *Depression,* headache, mood changes
CV: *Hypertension,* **circulatory collapse, embolism,** tachycardia, edema

Adverse effects: *italics* = common; **bold** = life-threatening

EENT: Fungal infections, increased intraocular pressure, blurred vision

GI: *Diarrhea, nausea, abdominal distention,* **GI hemorrhage,** *increased appetite,* pancreatitis

HEMA: Thrombocytopenia

INTEG: Acne, poor wound healing, ecchymosis, petechiae

MS: Fractures, osteoporosis, weakness

Pharmacokinetics

Absorption	Well absorbed (PO, IM)
Distribution	Crosses placenta, widely distributed
Metabolism	Liver, extensively
Excretion	Kidney, breast milk
Half-life	2-5 hr, adrenal suppression 3-4 days

Pharmacodynamics

	PO	IM	TOPICAL	INH	INTRANA-SAL
Onset	Unknown	Unknown	Min to hr	1-2 wk	Unknown
Peak	1-2 hr	1-2 hr	Hr to days	Unknown	2-3 wk
Duration	3 days	Unknown	Hr to days	Unknown	Unknown

INTERACTIONS
Individual drugs

Alcohol, amphotericin B, cycloSPORINE, digoxin, indomethacin, quinolones: increased side effects

Ambenonium, isoniazid, neostigmine, somatrem: decreased effects of each specific product

Cholestyramine, colestipol, ePHEDrine, phenytoin, rifampin, theophylline: decreased action of triamcinolone

Indomethacin, ketoconazole: increased action of triamcinolone

Drug classifications

Anticholinesterases, anticoagulants, anticonvulsants, antidiabetics, salicylates: decreased effects of each specific product

Antidiabetic agents: increased need for antidiabetic agents

Antiinfectives (macrolide), carBAMazepine, contraceptives (oral), estrogens, salicylates: increased action of triamcinolone

Barbiturates: decreased action of triamcinolone

Diuretics, salicylates: increased side effects

Toxoids, vaccines: decreased effects of toxoids, vaccines

Drug/herb

Aloe, cascara sagrada, senna: increased hypokalemia

Drug/lab test

Increased: cholesterol, sodium, blood glucose, uric acid, calcium, urine glucose

Decreased: calcium, potassium, T_4, T_3, thyroid ^{131}I uptake test, urine 17-OHCS, 17-KS

False negative: skin allergy tests

NURSING CONSIDERATIONS
Assessment

• Monitor potassium, blood glucose, urine glucose while on long-term therapy; hypokalemia and hyperglycemia

• Monitor weight daily; notify prescriber of weekly gain >5 lb; I&O ratio; be alert for decreasing urinary output and increasing edema

• Monitor B/P q4hr, pulse; notify prescriber if chest pain occurs

• Monitor plasma cortisol levels during long-term therapy (normal level 138-635 nmol/L [SI units] when measured at 8 AM); adrenal function periodically for hypothalamic-pituitary-adrenal axis suppression

• Assess for infection: increased temp, WBC even after withdrawal of medication; product masks infection symptoms

• Assess for potassium depletion: paresthesias, fatigue, nausea, vomiting, depression, polyuria, dysrhythmias, weakness

• Assess mental status: affect, mood, behavioral changes, aggression

• Assess nasal passages during long-term treatment for changes in mucus (nasal)

• Monitor temp; if fever develops, product should be discontinued

• Assess for systemic absorption: increased temp, inflammation, irritation (topical)

Patient/family education

• Advise patient that emergency ID as corticosteroid user should be carried/worn; not to discontinue abruptly, taper dose

• Instruct patient to notify prescriber if therapeutic response decreases; dosage adjustment may be needed

---

- Caution patient to avoid OTC products: salicylates, alcohol in cough products, cold preparations unless directed by prescriber; to avoid live vaccines
- Advise patient on all aspects of product use including cushingoid symptoms
- Teach patient symptoms of adrenal insufficiency: nausea, anorexia, fatigue, dizziness, dyspnea, weakness, joint pain
- Teach patient that long-term therapy may be needed to clear infection (1-2 mo depending on type of infection)

Inhalation route
- Teach patient proper administration technique; to wash inhaler with warm water and dry after each use
- Teach patient all aspects of product use including cushingoid symptoms

Topical route
- Instruct patient to avoid sunlight on affected area; burns may occur

Nasal route
- Instruct patient to clear nasal passages if sneezing attack occurs, repeat dose
- Advise patient to continue using product even if mild nasal bleeding occurs; is usually transient
- Teach patient method of instillation after providing written instruction from manufacturer

Evaluation

Positive therapeutic outcome
- Decrease in runny nose (nasal)
- Decreased dyspnea, wheezing, dry crackles on auscultation (inh)
- Ease of respirations, decreased inflammation
- Absence of severe itching, patches on skin, flaking (topical)

triamcinolone nasal agent
See Appendix B

triamcinolone topical
See Appendix B

⚠ HIGH ALERT

triazolam (Rx)
(trye-az'oh-lam)
Apo-Triazo ✦, Gen-Triazolam ✦, Halcion
Func. class.: Sedative-hypnotic, antianxiety
Chem. class.: Benzodiazepine, short acting
Pregnancy category X
Controlled substance schedule IV (USA), targeted (CDSA IV) (Canada)

Do not confuse: Halcion/Haldol/halcinonide

ACTION: Produces CNS depression at limbic, thalamic, hypothalamic levels of CNS; may be mediated by neurotransmitter; γ-aminobutyric acid (GABA); results are sedation, hypnosis, skeletal muscle relaxation, anticonvulsant activity, anxiolytic action

Therapeutic outcome: Decreased anxiety, insomnia

USES: Insomnia (short-term), sedative/hypnotic

CONTRAINDICATIONS
Pregnancy **X,** breastfeeding, hypersensitivity to benzodiazepines

Precautions: Children <15 yr, geriatric, anemia, renal/hepatic disease, suicidal individuals, product abuse, psychosis, acute closed-angle glaucoma, seizure disorders, angioedema, respiratory disease, depression, sleep-related behaviors (sleep walking), intermittent porphyria, myasthenia gravis, Parkinson's disease

DOSAGE AND ROUTES
Adult: PO 0.125-0.5 mg at bedtime, max 0.5 mg/day
Geriatric: PO 0.0625-0.125 mg at bedtime, max 0.25 mg/day

Available forms: Tabs 0.125, 0.25 mg

Implementation
- Give with food or milk to decrease GI symptoms; if patient is unable to swallow medication whole, tab may be crushed and mixed with food or fluid
- Give sugarless gum, hard candy, frequent sips of water for dry mouth

ADVERSE EFFECTS
CNS: *Headache, lethargy, drowsiness, daytime sedation,* dizziness, confusion, light-headedness, anxiety, irritability, amnesia, poor coordination, complex sleep-related reactions (sleep driving, sleep eating)
CV: Chest pain, pulse changes, ECG changes
GI: Nausea, vomiting, diarrhea, heartburn, abdominal pain, constipation, **hepatic injury**
SYST: **Severe allergic reactions**

Pharmacokinetics

Absorption	Well absorbed
Distribution	Widely distributed, crosses placenta, crosses blood-brain barrier
Metabolism	Liver
Excretion	Kidneys, breast milk
Half-life	1.5-5.5 hr

T

Adverse effects: *italics* = common; **bold** = life-threatening

Pharmacodynamics

Onset	15-30 min
Peak	Unknown
Duration	6-8 hr

INTERACTIONS
Individual drugs
Alcohol: increased action of both products

Cimetidine, clarithromycin, disulfiram, erythromycin, isoniazid, probenecid: increased effects; do not use concurrently

Rifampin: decreased action of rifampin

Theophylline: decreased effects of theophylline

Drug classifications
Antacids: decreased effects of antacids

Antiinfectives (clarithromycin): increased effects

CNS depressants: increased effects of both products

Contraceptives (oral): increased effects; do not use concurrently

CYP3A4 inhibitors, protease inhibitors: increased triazolam levels

Smoking: decreased hypnotic effects

Drug/food
Grapefruit may increase action, avoid concurrent use

Drug/herb
Chamomile, hops, kava, lavender, valerian: increased CNS depression

Drug/lab test
Increased: AST, ALT, serum bilirubin

Decreased: radioactive iodine uptake

False increase: 17-OHCS

NURSING CONSIDERATIONS
Assessment
• Assess patient's mental status: mood, sensorium, anxiety, affect, sleeping pattern, drowsiness, dizziness, especially geriatric; physical dependency, withdrawal symptoms: anxiety, panic attacks, agitation, seizures, headache, nausea, vomiting, muscle pain, weakness; suicidal tendencies; for indications of increasing tolerance and abuse

• Monitor patient's B/P (lying, standing), pulse; if systolic B/P drops 20 mm Hg, hold product, notify prescriber

• Monitor blood tests: CBC during long-term therapy; blood dyscrasias have occurred rarely; decreased hematocrit, neutropenia may occur

• Monitor liver function tests: AST, ALT, bilirubin, creatinine LDH, alkaline phosphatase

• Monitor I&O ratio; indicate renal dysfunction

Patient/family education
• Advise patient that product may be taken with food or fluids, and tab may be crushed or swallowed whole

• Caution patient not to use for everyday stress or longer than 3 mo unless directed by prescriber; not to take more than prescribed amount; may be habit forming; not to double doses or skip doses

• Instruct patient to avoid OTC preparations unless approved by prescriber; alcohol and CNS depressants will increase CNS depression

• Caution patient to avoid driving, activities that require alertness because drowsiness may occur; to avoid alcohol ingestion or other psychotropic medications; to rise slowly or fainting may occur, especially geriatric; that drowsiness may worsen at beginning of treatment

• Teach patient to use reliable contraception, pregnancy X

• Teach patient that complex sleep-related behaviors (sleep eating/driving) may occur

• Advise patient not to discontinue medication abruptly after long-term use; withdrawal symptoms include vomiting, cramping, tremors, seizures; decrease dosage by 50% q2nights until 0.125 mg for 2 nights, then stop

Evaluation
Positive therapeutic outcome
• Decreased anxiety, restlessness, sleeplessness (short-term treatment only)

TREATMENT OF OVERDOSE:
Lavage, VS, supportive care

trifluridine ophthalmic
See Appendix B

trimethobenzamide (Rx)
(trye-meth-oh-ben′za-mide)
Tigan
Func. class.: Antiemetic, anticholinergic
Chem. class.: Ethanolamine derivative
Pregnancy category C

ACTION: Acts centrally by blocking chemoreceptor trigger zone, which in turn acts on vomiting center

Therapeutic outcome: Absence of nausea and vomiting

USES: Nausea, vomiting, prevention of postoperative vomiting

CONTRAINDICATIONS
Children (parenterally), hypersensitivity to opioids, shock

Precautions: Pregnancy **C**, children, geriatric, cardiac dysrhythmias, acute febrile illness, encephalitis, gastroenteritis, dehydration, electrolyte imbalances, Reye's syndrome

DOSAGE AND ROUTES
Postoperative vomiting
Adult: IM 200 mg followed by a second dose 1 hr later

Nausea/vomiting
Adult: PO 300 mg tid-qid; IM 200 mg tid-qid

Renal dose
Adult: IM CCr 15-30 ml/min give 50% of dose

Available forms: Caps 300 mg; inj 100 mg/ml

Implementation
PO route
• Cap may be swallowed whole or opened and mixed with food or fluids
IM route
• Administer IM inj in large muscle mass; aspirate to avoid **IV** administration
• Patient should remain lying down for 30 min after IM inj

Syringe compatibilities: Glycopyrrolate, HYDROmorphone, midazolam, nalbuphine

ADVERSE EFFECTS
CNS: *Drowsiness,* headache, dizziness, confusion, *vertigo,* EPS, disorientation, **coma, seizures,** depression
CV: Hyper/hypotension, palpitations, **cardiac dysrhythmias**
EENT: Dry mouth, blurred vision, photosensitivity
GI: Nausea, diarrhea, vomiting, difficulty swallowing
INTEG: Rash, urticaria, fever, chills, flushing, hyperpyrexia

Pharmacokinetics

Absorption	Unknown
Distribution	Unknown
Metabolism	Liver, extensively
Excretion	Kidneys
Half-life	Unknown

Pharmacodynamics

	PO	IM	RECT
Onset	20-40 min	15 min	10-40 min
Peak	Unknown	Unknown	Unknown
Duration	3-4 hr	2-3 hr	3-4 hr

INTERACTIONS
Individual drugs
Alcohol: increased effect

Drug classifications
CNS depressants: increased effect

NURSING CONSIDERATIONS
Assessment
• Monitor VS, B/P; check patients with cardiac disease more often
• Assess for signs of toxicity of other products or masking of symptoms of disease: brain tumor, intestinal obstructions
• Observe for drowsiness, dizziness
• Assess for nausea, vomiting before and after treatment

Patient/family education
• Teach patient to use good oral hygiene; frequent rinsing of mouth, sugarless gum for dry mouth
• Caution patient to avoid hazardous activities until product response is determined; drowsiness may occur
• Inform patient that orthostatic hypotension occurs often and to rise from sitting or lying position gradually; avoid hot tubs, hot showers, and tub baths because hypotension may occur
• Advise patient to remain lying down after IM inj for at least 30 min
• Inform patient that in hot weather, heat stroke may occur; take extra precautions to stay cool
• Teach patient to avoid OTC preparations (cough, hay fever, cold) unless approved by prescriber; serious product interactions may occur; avoid use with alcohol, CNS depressants, increased drowsiness may occur
• Teach patient about EPS
• Instruct patient to report sore throat, malaise, fever, bleeding, mouth sores; if these occur, CBC should be performed and product discontinued

Evaluation
Positive therapeutic outcome
• Decreased nausea, vomiting

triptorelin (Rx)
(trip-toe'rel-in)
Trelstar, Trelstar Depot, Trelstar LA
Func. class.: Gonadotropin-releasing hormone antagonist
Chem. class.: Synthetic decapeptide analog of LHRH
Pregnancy category X

ACTION: Inhibitor of pituitary gonadotropin secretion; initially increases LH and FSH, with increases in testosterone, reduction in sex steroid levels

Therapeutic outcome: Decreased signs/symptoms of advanced prostate cancer

USES: Advanced prostate cancer

CONTRAINDICATIONS
Pregnancy **X**, breastfeeding, hypersensitivity to this product or other LHRH agonists or LHRH

Precautions: Metastatic vertebral lesions, urinary tract obstruction, spinal cord compression, renal disease

DOSAGE AND ROUTES
Adult: IM 3.75 mg q4wk; 11.25 mg q12wk, 22.5 mg q24wk

Available forms: Microgranules, depot inj 3.75 mg, 11.25 mg

Implementation
• Give IM using implant, inserted by qualified person
• Use syringe with 20-G needle, withdraw 2 ml of sterile water for inj, inject into vial, shake well, withdraw vial contents, inject immediately

ADVERSE EFFECTS
CNS: Headache, insomnia, dizziness, lability, fatigue
CV: *Hypertension,* peripheral edema
ENDO: Gynecomastia, breast tenderness, hot flashes
GI: Nausea, vomiting, diarrhea
GU: Impotence, urinary retention, UTI
INTEG: Rash, pain on injection, pruritus, hypersensitivity
MISC: Anaphylaxis, angioedema
MS: Osteoneuralgia

Pharmacokinetics

Absorption	Unknown
Distribution	Unknown
Metabolism	CYP450
Excretion	Liver, kidneys
Half-life	3 hr

Pharmacodynamics

Unknown

INTERACTIONS
Drug/lab test
Increased: alk phos, estradiol, FSH, LH, testosterone levels
Decreased: testosterone levels, progesterone

NURSING CONSIDERATIONS
Assessment
• **Assess for severe hypersensitivity:** discontinue product and give antihistamines, have emergency equipment nearby
• Monitor I&O ratios; palpate bladder for distention in urinary obstruction
• Monitor for relief of bone pain (back pain)
• Assess levels of testosterone and PSA

Patient/family education
• Teach patient that gynecomastia may occur but will decrease after treatment is discontinued
• Advise patient to report allergic reaction immediately
• Teach patient that disease flare may occur at beginning of therapy
• Teach patient to use during pregnancy (X)

Evaluation
Positive therapeutic outcome
• More normal levels of PSA, acid phosphatase, alkaline phosphatase, testosterone level of <25 ng/dl, tumor response

trospium (Rx)
(trose′pee-um)
Sanctura, Sanctura XR
Func. class.: Anticholinergic, overactive bladder product, urinary antispasmodic
Chem. class.: Muscarinic receptor antagonist
Pregnancy category C

ACTION: Relaxes smooth muscles in bladder by inhibiting acetylcholine effect on muscarinic receptors

Therapeutic outcome: Absence of bladder distention, nocturia, frequency, urgency, incontinence

USES: Overactive bladder (urinary frequency, urgency)

CONTRAINDICATIONS
Hypersensitivity, uncontrolled closed-angle glaucoma, urinary retention, gastric retention, myasthenia gravis

Precautions: Pregnancy **C**, breastfeeding, children, renal/hepatic disease, controlled closed-angle glaucoma, ulcerative colitis, intestinal atony, bladder outflow obstruction

DOSAGE AND ROUTES
Adult: PO 20 mg bid, give 5 ml ≥1 hr prior to meals or on empty stomach ER 60 mg qAM

Renal dose
Adult: PO CCr < 30 ml/min 20 mg/day at bedtime
Geriatric ≥75 yr: PO titrate down to 20 mg/day based on response and tolerance

Available forms: Tabs 20 mg caps ER 60 mg

Implementation
• Take 1 hr before meals or on empty stomach

ADVERSE EFFECTS
CNS: Fatigue, dizziness, headache
CV: Tachycardia
EENT: Dry eyes, vision abnormalities
GI: Flatulence, abdominal pain, *constipation, dry mouth,* dyspepsia
GU: Urinary retention, UTI
INTEG: Dry skin, **angioedema**
MISC: **Heat stroke,** fever

Pharmacokinetics

Absorption	Rapidly absorbed (10%)
Distribution	Protein bound (50%-85%)
Metabolism	Not fully understood in humans; extensively metabolized
Excretion	Urine (6%), feces (85%); excreted in urine by active tubular secretion
Half-life	Unknown

Pharmacodynamics

Unknown

INTERACTIONS
Individual drugs
Alcohol: increased drowsiness
MetFORMIN, procainamide, quiNIDine, ranitidine, tenofovir, triamterene, vancomycin: increased or decreased action of trospium

Drug classifications
CNS depressants: increased drowsiness
Products excreted by active renal secretion (aMILoride, digoxin, morphine): increased or decreased action of trospium

Drug/food
High-fat meal: decreased absorption

NURSING CONSIDERATIONS
Assessment
• **Assess urinary patterns:** distention, nocturia, frequency, urgency, incontinence, voiding patterns

Patient/family education
• Advise patient to avoid hazardous activities; dizziness may occur
• Caution patient that alcohol may increase drowsiness
• Inform patient about anticholinergic effects that may occur
• Teach patient to avoid all other products unless approved by prescriber

Evaluation
Positive therapeutic outcome
• Correction of urinary status: absence of dysuria, frequency, nocturia, incontinence

T

Adverse effects: *italics* = common; **bold** = life-threatening

ulipristal (Rx)

(ue′li-pris′tal)
Ella
Func. class.: Progesterone agonist/antagonist-abortifacient
Pregnancy category X

ACTION: Binds to the progesterone receptor and prevents progesterone from occupying the receptor, postpones follicular rupture when taken immediately prior to ovulation

Therapeutic outcome: Absence of pregnancy

USES: Emergency contraception

CONTRAINDICATIONS

Pregnancy **X,** children/infants/neonates, postmenopausal females

Precautions: History of ectopic pregnancy, HIV

DOSAGE AND ROUTES

Adult/adolescent females: PO 30 mg (1 tab) as soon as possible within 120 hr (5 days) of unprotected intercourse or a known or suspected contraceptive failure

Available forms: Tab 30 mg

Implementation
• Administer without regard to food
• Store at room temperature, protect from light

ADVERSE EFFECTS

CNS: Dizziness, headache, fatigue
GI: Nausea, vomiting, abdominal pain
GU: Dysmenorrhea, breakthrough bleeding
INTEG: Acne vulgaris

Pharmacokinetics

Absorption	Unknown
Distribution	Protein binding >94%
Metabolism	Metabolized by CYP3A4
Excretion	Unknown
Half-life	Terminal half-life 27-38 hrs

Pharmacodynamics

Onset	Unknown
Peak	1 hr
Duration	Unknown

INTERACTIONS

Individual drugs
Bosentan, carBAMazepine, felbamate, griseofulvin, OXcarbazepine, phenytoin, rifampin, St. John's wort, topiramate, bexarotene, dexamethasone, etravirine, flutamide, metyrapone, modafinil, nafcillin, nevirapine, pioglitazone, rifabutin, itraconazole, ketoconazole: decreased effect of ulipristal

Aldesleukin, IL-2, amiodarone, atazanavir, basiliximab, chloramphenicol, cimetidine, clarithromycin, dalfopristin, danazol, darunavir, delavirdine, diltiazem, dronedarone, erythromycin, fluconazole, FLUoxetine, fluvoxaMINE, imatinib, isoniazid, lapatinib, nefazodone, nelfinavir, niCARdipine, octreotide, pantoprazole, quinupristin, ranolazine, saquinavir, tamoxifen, telithromycin, tipranavir, verapamil, voriconazole, zafirlukast: increased ulipristal effect and adverse reactions

Aprepitant, fosaprepitant, efavirenz, fosamprenavir, quiNINE, ritonavir: increased or decreased ulipristal effect

Drug classifications
Regular hormonal contraceptive methods: decreased contraceptive action
CYP3A4 inducers, barbiturates: decreased effect of ulipristal
CYP3A4 inhibitors: increased ulipristal effect and adverse reactions

Drug/herb
St. John's wort: decreased effect of ulipristal

NURSING CONSIDERATIONS
Assessment
• **Assess need for emergency contraception,** pregnancy planned or suspected, obtain pregnancy test before use (pregnancy **X**)
• Assess medications taken, many drug interactions may occur

Patient/family education
• Instruct patient that if vomiting occurs within 3 hours of taking the tablet, consider repeating the dose
• Advise patient to report to provider any side effects
• Explain reason for medication and expected results
• Advise patient to avoid use in breastfeeding

Evaluation

Positive therapeutic outcome
• Absence of pregnancy

undecylenic acid topical
See Appendix B

unoprostone ophthalmic
See Appendix B

valACYclovir (Rx)
(val-a-sye′kloh-vir)
Valtrex
Func. class.: Antiviral
Chem. class.: Synthetic acyclic purine nucleoside analog
Pregnancy category B

Do not confuse: valACYclovir/
valGANciclovir, **Valtrex**/Valcyte

ACTION: Interferes with DNA synthesis by conversion to acyclovir, causing decreased viral replication, time of lesional healing

Therapeutic outcome: Absence of itching, painful lesions; crusting and healing of lesions

USES: Treatment or suppression of herpes zoster (shingles), recurrent genital herpes, herpes labialis (cold sores), varicella, varicella-zoster

Unlabeled uses: Prevention of CMV infection in advanced HIV, posttransplant patients, Bell's palsy, herpes simplex virus prophylaxis

CONTRAINDICATIONS
Hypersensitivity to this product, acyclovir, valGANciclovir

Precautions: Pregnancy **B**, breastfeeding, geriatric, renal/hepatic disease, electrolyte imbalance, dehydration, hypersensitivity to penciclovir, famciclovir, ganciclovir, varicella

DOSAGE AND ROUTES
Genital herpes (suppressive initial)
Adult: PO 1 g bid × 10 days initially

Genital herpes (recurrent episodes)
Adult: PO 500 mg bid × 3 days

Genital herpes (suppressive therapy)
Adult: PO 1 g/day with normal immune function; 500 mg/day for those with ≤9 recurrences/yr; 500 mg bid in HIV-infected patients with CD4 ≥100

Reduction of transmission
Adult: PO 500 mg/day for source partner

Herpes zoster (shingles)
Adult: PO 1 g tid × 1 wk

Herpes labialis
Adult: PO 2 g bid × 1 day at first sign of lesions

Varicella (chickenpox) in immuno-competent patients
Adolescent and child ≥2 yr: PO 20 mg/kg/dose tid × 5 days, max 3 g/day; start at first sign, preferably within 24 hr of rash

Renal dose
Adult: PO CCr 30-49 ml/min 1g q12hr (herpes zoster); 1 g q12hr × 1 day (herpes labialis); CCr 10-29 ml/min 1 g q24hr (genital herpes/herpes zoster); 500 mg q24hr (recurrent genital herpes); CCr <10 ml/min 500 mg q24hr (genital herpes/herpes zoster), 500 mg q24hr (recurrent genital herpes)

Available forms: Tabs 500, 1000 mg

Implementation
• Give within 72 hr of outbreak (herpes zoster); as soon as possible (herpes labialis, genital herpes)
• Give orally before infection occurs
• Store at room temp; protect from light, moisture

ADVERSE EFFECTS
CNS: Tremors, lethargy, *dizziness, headache, weakness,* depression
ENDO: *Dysmenorrhea*
GI: *Nausea, vomiting, diarrhea, abdominal pain, constipation,* increased AST
HEMA: **Thrombocytopenic purpura, hemolytic uremic syndrome**
INTEG: *Rash*

Pharmacokinetics
Absorption	Unknown
Distribution	Crosses placenta, enters breast milk, protein binding 13.5%-17.9%
Metabolism	Converts to acyclovir
Excretion	Urine, as acyclovir
Half-life	2½-3½ hr

Pharmacodynamics
Unknown

INTERACTIONS
Individual drugs
Cimetidine, probenecid: increased blood levels of valACYclovir (only if renal disease is significant)

Drug/lab test
Increased: LFTs, creatinine
Decreased: WBC, platelets

NURSING CONSIDERATIONS
Assessment
- **Assess for signs of infection;** characteristics of lesions; therapy should be started at first sign of herpes and is most effective within 72 hr of outbreak
- Assess C&S before product therapy; product may be given as soon as culture is performed; repeat C&S after treatment; determine the presence of other STDs
- Assess bowel pattern before, during treatment
- Assess for skin eruptions: rash
- Assess allergies before treatment, reaction of each medication

⚠ **Assess for thrombocytopenic purpura, hemolytic uremic syndrome, may be fatal**

Patient/family education
- Advise patient to take as prescribed; if dose is missed, take as soon as remembered up to 2 hr before next dose; do not double dose, without regard to meals
- Instruct patient to take product orally before infection occurs; product should be taken when itching or pain occurs, usually before eruptions
- Inform patient that partners need to be told that patient has herpes; they can become infected; condoms must be worn to prevent reinfections
- Tell patient that product does not cure infection, just controls symptoms and does not prevent infection to others
- **Teach patient to report CNS changes (tremors, weakness, lethargy) immediately**

Evaluation
Positive therapeutic outcome
- Absence of itching, painful lesions; crusting and healed lesions

---

valGANciclovir (Rx)
(val-gan-sy′kloh-veer)
Valcyte
Func. class.: Antiviral
Chem. class.: Synthetic nucleoside
Pregnancy category C

Do not confuse: valGANciclovir/valACYclovir, **Valcyte**/Valtrex

ACTION: valGANciclovir is metabolized to ganciclovir; inhibits replication of human CMV in vivo and in vitro by selectively inhibiting viral DNA synthesis

Therapeutic outcome: Decreased proliferation of virus responsible for CMV retinitis

USES: Cytomegalovirus (CMV) retinitis in immunocompromised persons, including those with AIDS, after indirect ophthalmoscopy confirms diagnosis; prevention of CMV in transplantation; prevention of CMV in patients at risk going through transplant (kidney, heart, pancreas)

CONTRAINDICATIONS
Breastfeeding, hypersensitivity to ganciclovir or valACYclovir, absolute neutrophil count <500/mm³, platelet count <25,000/mm³, hemodialysis, liver transplant

Precautions: Children, geriatric, renal function impairment, hypersensitivity to acyclovir, penciclovir, famciclovir

> **BLACK BOX WARNING:** Preexisting cytopenias, secondary malignancy, infertility, anemia, pregnancy (**C**)

DOSAGE AND ROUTES
Treatment of CMV
Adult: PO induction 900 mg bid × 21 days with food; maintenance 900 mg/day with food

Transplant (CMV prophylaxis)
Adult/adolescent >16 yr: PO 900 mg/day with food starting within 10 days before transplantation until 100 days after transplantation
Infant ≥4 mo/child/adolescent ≤16 yr: PO give within 10 days of heart/kidney transplant; calculate dose as 7 × BSA × CCr and give a single daily dose

Renal dose
CCr ≥60 ml/min same dosage as above; CCr 40-59 ml/min 450 mg bid × 21 days, then 450 mg/day; CCr 25-39 ml/min 450 mg/day × 21 days, then 450 mg q2day; CCr 10-24 ml/min 450 mg q2day, then 450 mg 2 ×/week

Available forms: Tabs 450 mg; powder for oral sol 50 mg/ml

Implementation
PO tab
- Give with food for better absorption, avoid getting on skin, do not break tab
Oral SOL
- Measure 9 ml of purified water in graduated cylinder, shake bottle to loosen powder, add ½ liquid, shake well, add remaining water, shake, remove child-resistant cap and push bottle adapter into neck of bottle, close with cap, give using the dispenser provided
- Store liquid in refrigerator; do not freeze; throw away any unused portion after 49 days

---

ADVERSE EFFECTS

CNS: *Fever,* chills, **coma**, *confusion,* abnormal thoughts, dizziness, bizarre dreams, *headache,* psychosis, tremors, somnolence, *paresthesia,* **weakness**, **seizures**, insomnia

EENT: Retinal detachment in CMV retinitis

GI: *Abnormal liver function tests, nausea, vomiting, anorexia, diarrhea, abdominal pain,* **hemorrhage**

GU: **Hematuria**, increased creatinine, BUN

HEMA: **Granulocytopenia, thrombocytopenia, irreversible neutropenia, anemia, eosinophilia**

INTEG: *Rash,* alopecia, *pruritus,* urticaria, pain at inj site, phlebitis, **Stevens-Johnson syndrome**

MISC: Local and systemic infections and **sepsis**

Pharmacokinetics

Absorption	Well absorbed from GI tract
Distribution	Plasma protein binding unknown; crosses blood-brain barrier, CSF
Metabolism	Rapidly metabolized in intestinal wall and liver to ganciclovir
Excretion	Kidneys (ganciclovir)
Half-life	3-4½ hr

Pharmacodynamics

Onset	Unknown
Peak	1-3 hr
Duration	Unknown

INTERACTIONS

Individual drugs

Adriamycin, amphotericin B, cycloSPORINE, dapsone, DOXOrubicin, flucytosine, pentamidine, trimethoprim/sulfamethoxazole, vinBLAStine, vinCRIStine: increased toxicity

Didanosine: increased effect; monitor for adverse effects, toxicity

Imipenem/cilastatin: increased seizures

Mycophenolate: increased effect of both drugs

Probenecid: decreased renal clearance of valGANciclovir

Radiation, zidovudine: severe granulocytopenia; do not coadminister

Drug classifications

Antineoplastics, immunosuppressants: increased severe granulocytopenia; do not coadminister

Nucleoside analogs, other: increased toxicity

Drug/food

Absorption: increased with high-fat meal

Drug/lab test

Increased: creatinine

Decreased: RBC/WBC, Hct/Hgb

NURSING CONSIDERATIONS

Assessment

> **BLACK BOX WARNING: Assess for leukopenia/neutropenia/thrombocytopenia:** WBCs, platelets q2day during 2 ×/day dosing and then qwk

> **BLACK BOX WARNING: Malignancy:** monitor for malignancy; avoid accidental exposure of broken, crushed tabs, powder for solution; if these were in contact with skin, wash well with soap and water

> **BLACK BOX WARNING: Pregnancy:** considered potentially teratogenic; adequate contraception should be used

- Assess serum creatinine or CCr ≥q2wk
- Assess for CMV retinitis by ophthalmoscopy before beginning treatment and q2wk
- Obtain culture for CMV

Patient/family education

- Inform patient that product does not cure condition, that regular ophthalmologic and blood tests are necessary
- Caution patient that major toxicities may necessitate discontinuing product

> **BLACK BOX WARNING: ⚠ Caution patient to use contraception during treatment and that infertility may occur; men should use barrier contraception for 90 days after treatment**

- Instruct patient to take with food
- ⚠ Instruct patient to report seizures, dizziness; to avoid hazardous activities
- Caution patient to use sunscreen to prevent burns

Evaluation

Positive therapeutic outcome
- Decreased symptoms of CMV

TREATMENT OF OVERDOSE:

Maintain adequate hydration; dialysis may help reduce serum concentrations; consider use of hematopoietic growth factors

valproate (Rx)
(val-proh'ate)
Depacon
valproic acid (Rx)
Depakene, Stavzor
divalproex sodium (Rx)
Depakote, Depakote ER, Epival ✿
Func. class.: Anticonvulsant, vascular headache suppressant
Chem. class.: Carboxylic acid derivative
Pregnancy category D

ACTION: Increases levels of γ-aminobutyric acid (GABA) in the brain, which decreases seizure activity

Therapeutic outcome: Decreased symptoms of epilepsy, bipolar disorder

USES: Simple (petit mal), complex (petit mal), absence, mixed seizures, manic episode associated with bipolar disorder, prophylaxis of migraine, adjunct in schizophrenia, tardive dyskinesia, aggression in children with ADHD, organic brain syndrome, tonic-clonic (grand mal)/myoclonic seizures

Unlabeled uses: Rectal for seizures (valproic acid)

CONTRAINDICATIONS
Hypersensitivity, urea cycle disorders

> BLACK BOX WARNING: Pregnancy **D**, hepatic disease, pancreatitis

Precautions: Breastfeeding, geriatric

> BLACK BOX WARNING: Children <2 yr

DOSAGE AND ROUTES
Epilepsy
Adult and child: PO 10-15 mg/kg/day divided in 2-3 doses, may increase by 5-10 mg/kg/day qwk, max 60 mg/kg/day in 2-3 divided doses; **IV** ≤20 mg/min over 1 hr

Mania (divalproex sodium)
Adult: PO 750 mg/day in divided doses, max 60 mg/kg/day or 3000 mg/day

Mania (valproic acid: Stavzor)
Adult: DEL REL cap 750 mg/day in divided doses

Migraine (divalproex sodium)
Adult: PO 250 mg bid, may increase to 1000 mg/day; or 500 mg (Depakote ER) daily × 7 days, then 1000 mg/day

Available forms: Valproic acid: caps 250 mg; syr 250 mg/5 ml del rel cap (Stavzor) 125 mg; divalproex: del rel tabs 125, 250, 500 mg; ext rel tabs 250, 500 mg; sprinkle caps 125 mg; valproate: inj 100 mg/ml

Implementation
• Swallow tabs and caps whole; do not break, crush, or chew
• Sprinkle cap contents on food
• Give elixir alone; do not dilute with carbonated beverage; do not give syrup to patients on sodium restriction
• Give with food or milk to decrease GI symptoms

IV route
• Dilute dose with ≥50 ml D₅W, NS, LR
• Run over 60 min (20 mg/min)

ADVERSE EFFECTS
CNS: *Sedation, drowsiness,* dizziness, headache, incoordination, depression, hallucinations, behavioral changes, tremors, aggression, weakness, coma, suicidal ideation
CV: Hypotension/hypertension, chest pain, palpitations, peripheral edema
EENT: Visual disturbances, taste perversion
GI: *Nausea, vomiting, constipation, diarrhea, dyspepsia,* anorexia, cramps, hepatic failure, pancreatitis, toxic hepatitis, stomatitis, weight gain, dry mouth
GU: Enuresis, irregular menses
HEMA: Thrombocytopenia, leukopenia, lymphocytosis, increased pro-time, bruising, epistaxis, pancytopenia
INTEG: *Rash,* alopecia, photosensitivity, dry skin
META: Hyperammonemia, SIADH
RESP: Dyspnea

Pharmacokinetics
Absorption	Unknown
Distribution	Breast milk, crosses placenta, widely distributed, protein binding 90%
Metabolism	Liver
Excretion	Kidneys
Half-life	6-16 hr

Pharmacodynamics
Onset	15-30 min
Peak	1-4 hr
Duration	4-6 hr

INTERACTIONS
Individual drugs
Abciximab, cefoperazone, cefoTEtan, eptifibatide, heparin, tirofiban: increased bleeding risk

Alcohol: increased CNS depression

Cimetidine: decreased metabolism of valproic acid

ChlorproMAZINE, erythromycin, felbamate: increased valproic acid level

Phenytoin: increased action of phenytoin

Warfarin: increased bleeding

Drug classifications
Antidepressants (tricyclics), barbiturates: increased action

Antihistamines, barbiturates, MAOIs, opioids, sedative/hypnotics: increased CNS depression

Tricyclics: decreased seizure threshold

Drug/lab test
Increased: LFTs, bleeding time, ammonia

Decreased: sodium

False positive: ketones, urine

Interference: thyroid function tests

NURSING CONSIDERATIONS
Assessment
• Monitor blood tests: Hct, Hgb, RBC, serum folate, ammonia, platelets, pro-time, PTT, vit D if on long-term therapy

• Monitor liver function tests: AST, ALT, bilirubin, creatinine, failure; monitor for fever, anorexia, vomiting, lethargy, jaundice of skin, eyes that may occur during treatment, those with organic brain disorders, mental retardation, child <2 yr

• Monitor blood levels: therapeutic level 50-125 mcg/ml

• **Assess seizure disorder:** location, aura, activity, duration; seizure precautions should be in place

⚠ **Assess bipolar disorder: mood, activity, sleeping, eating, behavior; suicidal thoughts/behaviors**

⚠ **Hyperammonemic encephalopathy: can be fatal in those with urea cycle disorders (UCD); lethargy, confusion, coma, CV, respiratory changes; discontinue**

• **Assess migraines:** frequency, intensity

• Overdose symptoms: heart block, coma

> BLACK BOX WARNING: Assess for pancreatitis, may be fatal; may occur anytime during treatment or several months/years after discontinuing treatment

Patient/family education
• Teach patient that physical dependency may result from extended use

⚠ Instruct patient to report immediately suicidal thoughts/behaviors

• Instruct patient to avoid driving, other activities that require alertness

⚠ Advise patient not to discontinue medication quickly after long-term use; seizures may result

> BLACK BOX WARNING: ⚠ Advise patient to report visual disturbances, rash, diarrhea, light-colored stools, jaundice, protracted vomiting to prescriber

⚠ Advise patient to use contraception while taking this product, pregnancy D

• Instruct patient to drink plenty of fluids

Evaluation
Positive therapeutic outcome
• Decreased seizures

valsartan (Rx)
(val-zar'tan)
Diovan
Func. class.: Antihypertensive
Chem. class.: Angiotensin II receptor antagonist (type AT₁)
Pregnancy category D

Do not confuse: Diovan/Dioval

ACTION: Blocks the vasoconstrictor and aldosterone-secreting effects of angiotensin II; selectively blocks the binding of angiotensin II to the AT₁ receptor found in tissues

Therapeutic outcome: Decreased B/P

USES: Hypertension, alone or in combination, in patients >6 yr; CHF, after MI with left ventricular dysfunction/failure in stable patients

CONTRAINDICATIONS
Hypersensitivity, severe hepatic disease, bilateral renal artery stenosis

> BLACK BOX WARNING: Pregnancy D

Precautions: Breastfeeding, children, geriatric, CHF, hypertrophic cardiomyopathy, aortic/mitral valve stenosis, CAD, angioedema, renal/hepatic disease, hypersensitivity to ACE inhibitors, hyperkalemia, hypovolemia, African descent

DOSAGE AND ROUTES
Adult: PO 80 or 160 mg/day alone or in combination with other antihypertensives, may increase to 320 mg CHF

Geriatric: PO Adjust based on clinical response; may start with lower dose

Child/adolescent 6-16 yr: PO 1.3 mg/kg/day, max 40 mg/day

CHF
Adult: PO 40 mg bid, up to 60 mg bid

Post MI
Adult: PO 20 mg bid as early as 12 hr after MI, may be titrated within 7 days to 40 mg bid, then titrate to maintenance of 160 mg bid

Available forms: Tabs 80, 160, 320 mg

Implementation
• Administer without regard to meals

ADVERSE EFFECTS
CNS: *Dizziness, insomnia,* drowsiness, vertigo, headache, fatigue
CV: Angina pectoris, 2nd-degree AV block, cerebrovascular accident, hypotension, MI, dysrhythmias
EENT: Conjunctivitis
GI: Diarrhea, abdominal pain, nausea, hepatotoxicity
GU: Impotence, nephrotoxicity, renal failure
HEMA: *Anemia,* neutropenia
META: Hyperkalemia
MISC: Vasculitis, angioedema
MS: Cramps, myalgia, pain, stiffness
RESP: *Cough*

Pharmacokinetics
Absorption	Well absorbed
Distribution	Bound to plasma proteins
Metabolism	Extensive
Excretion	Feces, urine, breast milk
Half-life	9 hr

Pharmacodynamics
Onset	Up to 2 hr
Peak	2-4 hr
Duration	24 hr

INTERACTIONS
Individual drugs
Aliskiren: do not use concurrently
Gemfibrozil, rifampin, ritonavir, telithromycin: increased valsartan levels
Lithium: increased effects of lithium

Drug classifications
Diuretics (potassium-sparing, potassium supplements, ACE inhibitors): increased hyperkalemia

NSAIDs, salicylates: decreased antihypertensive effects

Drug/herb
Ephedra, ma huang: decreased antihypertensive effect
Hawthorn: increased antihypertensive effect

Drug/food
Decreased AUC by 40%
Salt substitutes with potassium: increased hyperkalemia

NURSING CONSIDERATIONS
Assessment
• Assess B/P (lying, sitting, standing), pulse q4hr; note rate, rhythm, quality periodically
• Monitor electrolytes: potassium, sodium, chloride; total CO_2
• Assess for angioedema: facial swelling, shortness of breath
• Obtain baselines in renal, liver function tests before therapy begins
• Assess blood tests: BUN, creatinine, before treatment
• Monitor for edema in feet, legs daily
• Assess for skin turgor, dryness of mucous membranes for hydration status; correct volume depletion before initiating therapy
• Overdose symptoms: bradycardia or tachycardia, circulatory collapse

Patient/family education
• Teach patient not to take this product if breastfeeding or pregnant, or have had an allergic reaction to this product
• If a dose is missed, instruct patient to take as soon as possible, unless it is within an hour before next dose
• Advise patient to comply with dosage schedule, even if feeling better
• Teach patient to notify prescriber of fever, swelling of hands or feet, irregular heartbeat, chest pain, persistent cough
• Advise patient excessive perspiration, dehydration, diarrhea may lead to fall in blood pressure; consult prescriber if these occur
• Inform patient that product may cause dizziness, fainting; light-headedness may occur, maintain hydration
• Instruct patient to avoid potassium supplements and foods, salt substitutes
• Caution patient to rise slowly to sitting or standing position to minimize orthostatic hypotension; how to take B/P

Evaluation

Positive therapeutic outcome
• Decreased B/P

vancomycin
(van-koe-mye′sin)
Vancocin
Func. class.: Antiinfective—miscellaneous
Chem. class.: Tricyclic glycopeptide
Pregnancy category B

ACTION: Inhibits bacterial cell wall synthesis, blocks glycopeptides

Therapeutic outcome: Bactericidal for the following organisms: staphylococci, streptococci, *Corynebacterium, Clostridium*

USES: *Actinomyces* sp., *Bacillus* sp., *Clostridium difficile, Clostridium* sp., *Enterococcus faecalis, Enterococcus faecium, Enterococcus* sp., *Lactobacillus* sp., *Listeria monocytogenes, Staphylococcus aureus* (MRSA), *Staphylococcus aureus* (MSSA), *Staphylococcus epidermidis, Staphylococcus* sp., *Streptococcus agalactiae* (group B streptococci), *Streptococcus bovis, Streptococcus pneumoniae, Streptococcus pyogenes* (group A beta-hemolytic streptococci), *Viridans streptococci;* may be effective against *Corynebacterium jeikeium, Corynebacterium* sp.; pseudomembranous colitis, staphylococcal enterocolitis, group A β-hemolytic streptococci, endocarditis prophylaxis for dental procedures, bacteremia, join/bone infections, osteomyelitis, pneumonia, septicemia

CONTRAINDICATIONS
Hypersensitivity, previous hearing loss

Precautions: Pregnancy **B** (PO); **C** (IV), breastfeeding, neonates, geriatric, renal disease

DOSAGE AND ROUTES
Serious staphylococcal infections
Adult: **IV** 500 mg (7.5 mg/kg) q6-8hr or 1 g (15 mg/kg) q12hr or 15-20 mg/kg q12hr
Child: **IV** 40-60 mg/kg/day divided q6-8hr
Neonate: **IV** 15 mg/kg initially followed by 10 mg/kg q8-24hr

Pseudomembranous/staphylococcal enterocolitis
Adult: PO 125 mg qid × 10-14 days
Child: PO (unlabeled) 40 mg/kg/day divided q6hr × 7-10 days, max 2 g/day

Endocarditis prophylaxis for dental procedure
Adult: **IV** 2 g divided
Child: **IV** 20 mg/kg over 1 hr; 1 hr before procedure

Renal dose
Adult: IV 15-20 mg/kg loading dose in seriously ill; individualize all other doses

Available forms: Cap 125, 250 mg; powder for inj **IV** 500, 750 mg; vials 1, 5, 10 g; dextrose sol for inj 500 mg/100 ml, 750 mg/150 ml, 1 g/200 ml

Implementation
• Give antihistamine if red man syndrome occurs: decreased B/P, flushing of neck, face; stop or slow infusion
• Give dose based on serum conc
• Give in equal intervals around the clock to maintain blood levels
• Store at room temp for up to 2 wk after reconstitution
• **Have adrenaline, suction, tracheostomy set, endotracheal intubation equipment on unit; anaphylaxis may occur**
• Provide adequate intake of fluids (2 L) to prevent nephrotoxicity
PO route
• Give without regard to food, swallow whole

Intermittent IV INF route
• Give after reconstitution with 10 ml of sterile water for inj (500 mg/10 ml); further dilution is needed for **IV**, 500 mg/100 ml of 0.9% NaCl, D₅W given as intermittent inf over 1 hr; decrease rate of inf if red man syndrome occurs
Continuous IV INF route (unlabeled)
• Reconstitute, then may inf 1-2 g in volume to give over 24 hr if intermittent **IV** route cannot be used

Y-site compatibilities: Acetylcysteine, acyclovir, alatrofloxacin, aldesleukin, alemtuzumab, alfentanil, allopurinol, alprostadil, amifostine, amikacin, amino acids injection, aminocaproic acid, amiodarone, amoxicillin-clavulanate, amsacrine, anidulafungin, argatroban, ascorbic acid injection, atenolol, atracurium, atropine, azithromycin, benztropine, bleomycin, bretylium, bumetanide, buprenorphine, butorphanol, calcium

V

chloride/gluconate, CARBOplatin, carmustine, caspofungin, cefpirome, chlorproMAZINE, cimetidine, ciprofloxacin, cisatracurium, CISplatin, clarithromycin, clindamycin, codeine, cyanocobalamin, cyclophosphamide, cycloSPORINE, cytarabine, DACTINomycin, DAUNOrubicin liposome, dexamethasone, dexmedetomidine, dexrazoxane, digoxin, diltiazem, diphenhydrAMINE, DOBUTamine, DOCEtaxel, dolasetron, DOPamine, doripenem, doxacurium, doxapram, DOXOrubicin, DOXOrubicin liposomal, doxycycline, enalaprilat, ePHEDrine, EPINEPHrine, epirubicin, eptifibatide, ertapenem, erythromycin, esmolol, etoposide, etoposide phosphate, famotidine, fenoldopam, fentaNYL, filgrastim, fluconazole, fludarabine, folic acid (as sodium salt), gallium, gemcitabine, gentamicin, glycopyrrolate, granisetron, HYDROmorphone, hydrOXYzine, ifosfamide, insulin, regular, irinotecan, isoproterenol, isosorbide, ketamine, labetalol, lactated Ringer's injection, lepirudin, levofloxacin, lidocaine, linezolid, LORazepam, magnesium sulfate, mannitol, mechlorethamine, melphalan, meperidine, meropenem, metaraminol, methyldopate, metoclopramide, metoprolol, metroNIDAZOLE, midazolam, milrinone, minocycline, mitoXANtrone, morphine, multiple vitamins injection, mycophenolate, nalbuphine, naloxone, nesiritide, netilmicin, niCARdipine, nitroglycerin, nitroprusside, norepinephrine, octreotide, ofloxacin, ondansetron, oxacillin, oxaliplatin, oxytocin, PACLitaxel (solvent/surfactant), palonosetron, pamidronate, pancuronium, papaverine, PEMEtrexed, penicillin G potassium/sodium, pentamidine, pentazocine, PENTobarbital, perphenazine, PHENobarbital, phentolamine, phenylephrine, phytonadione, piritramide, polymyxin B, potassium acetate/chloride, procainamide, prochlorperazine, promethazine, propranolol, protamine, pyridoxine, quiNIDine, ranitidine, remifentanil, rifampin, Ringer's injection, riTUXimab, sodium acetate/bicarbonate/citrate, succinylcholine, SUFentanil, tacrolimus, teniposide, thiamine, thiotepa, tigecycline, tirofiban, TNA (3-in-1), tobramycin, tolazoline, TPN (2-in-1), trastuzumab, urapidil, vasopressin, vecuronium, verapamil, vinBLAStine, vinCRIStine, vinorelbine, voriconazole, zidovudine, zoledronic acid

ADVERSE EFFECTS
CNS: Headache
CV: Cardiac arrest, vascular collapse (rare), hypotension, peripheral edema
EENT: *Ototoxicity, permanent deafness,* tinnitus, nystagmus

GI: Nausea, pseudomembranous colitis
GU: Nephrotoxicity: increased BUN, creatinine, albumin, fatal uremia
HEMA: Leukopenia, eosinophilia, neutropenia
INTEG: Chills, fever, rash, thrombophlebitis at inj site, urticaria, pruritus, necrosis (red man syndrome), skin/subcutaneous tissue disorders
MS: Back pain
RESP: Wheezing, dyspnea
SYST: Anaphylaxis, superinfection

Pharmacokinetics

Absorption	Poorly absorbed (PO), completely absorbed (**IV**)
Distribution	Widely distributed, crosses placenta
Metabolism	Liver
Excretion	PO, feces; **IV**, kidneys
Half-life	4-8 hr

Pharmacodynamics

	IV
Onset	Immediate
Peak	Inf end
Duration	Unknown

INTERACTIONS
Individual drugs
Acyclovir, adefovir, amphotericin B, capreomycin, CISplatin, colistin, cycloSPORINE, foscarnet, ganciclovir, methotrexate, pamidronate, IV pentamidine, polymyxin B, streptozocin, tacrolimus, zoledronic acid: increased ototoxicity or nephrotoxicity
Cholestyramine, colestipol, cidofovir: do not use concurrently
MetFORMIN: increased lactic acidosis

Drug classifications
Aminoglycosides, cephalosporins, NSAIDs: increased ototoxicity or nephrotoxicity
Nodepolarizing muscle relaxants: increased neuromuscular effects

Drug/lab test
Increased: BUN/creatinine, eosinophils
Decreased: WBC

NURSING CONSIDERATIONS
Assessment
• **Assess for infection:** WBC, urine, stools, sputum, wound characteristics, throughout treatment

---

• Monitor I&O ratio, BUN, creatinine; report hematuria, oliguria because nephrotoxicity may occur
• Monitor blood tests: WBC; serum levels; peak 1 hr after 1-hr inf 25-40 mg/L; trough before next dose 5-10 mg/L, especially in renal disease
• Obtain C&S before product therapy; product may be given as soon as culture is performed
• Assess auditory function during, after treatment; hearing loss, ringing, roaring in ears; product should be discontinued
• Monitor B/P during administration; sudden drop may indicate red man syndrome
• Assess for signs of infection
• **Red man syndrome: flushing of neck, face, upper body, arms, back; may lead to anaphylaxis, slow IV infusion to >1 hr**

Patient/family education
• Teach patient aspects of product therapy: need to complete entire course of medication to ensure organism death (7-10 days); culture may be performed after completed course of medication
• Advise patient to report sore throat, fever, fatigue; could indicate superinfection
• Instruct patient that product must be taken in equal intervals around the clock to maintain blood levels

Evaluation

Positive therapeutic outcome
• Absence of fever, sore throat
• Negative culture after treatment

vardenafil (Rx)
(var-den'a-fil)
Levitra, Staxyn
Func. class.: Impotence agent
Chem. class.: Phosphodiesterase type 5 inhibitor
Pregnancy category B

ACTION: Inhibits phosphodiesterase type 5 (PDE5); enhances erectile function by increasing the amount of cyclic GMP, which causes smooth muscle relaxation and increased blood flow into the corpus cavernosum

Therapeutic outcome: Erection

USES: Treatment of erectile dysfunction

CONTRAINDICATIONS
Hypersensitivity, coadministration of α-blockers or nitrates, renal failure, congenital or acquired QT prolongation

Precautions: Pregnancy **B**; not indicated for women, children, or newborns; hepatic impairment; retinitis pigmentosa; cardiovascular disease; anatomic penile deformities; sickle cell anemia; leukemia; multiple myeloma; bleeding disorders; active peptic ulceration; renal disease

DOSAGE AND ROUTES
Adult: PO 10 mg, taken 1 hr before sexual activity, dose may be reduced to 5 mg or increased to a max of 20 mg; max dosing frequency is once/day; orally disintegrating tab 10 mg 60 min before sexual activity; do not use with potent CYP3A4 inhibitors
Geriatric >65 yr: PO 5 mg initially, titrate as needed/tolerated

Hepatic dose (Child-Pugh B)
Adult: PO 5 mg, max 10 mg

Concomitant medications
Ritonavir, max 2.5 mg q72hr; for indinavir, ketoconazole 400 mg/day and itraconazole 400 mg/day, max 2.5 mg/day; for ketoconazole 200 mg/day, itraconazole 200 mg/day and erythromycin, max 5 mg/day

Available forms: Tabs 2.5, 5, 10, 20 mg; orally disintegrating tab 10 mg

Implementation
• Take approximately 1 hr before sexual activity; do not use more than once a day
• Orally disintegrating tabs are not interchangeable with film-coated tabs
• **Orally disintegrating tab:** place on tongue, allow to dissolve, do not use water

ADVERSE EFFECTS
CNS: *Headache, flushing, dizziness, insomnia,* seizures, transient global amnesia
CV: Hypertension, **MI, CV collapse,** chest pain
EENT: Conjunctivitis, tinnitus, photophobia, diminished vision, glaucoma, hearing loss
GU: Abnormal ejaculation; priapism
MISC: Rash, GERD, GGTP increased, **NAION (nonarteritic ischemic optic neuropathy),** dyspepsia
MS: Myalgia, arthralgia, neck pain
RESP: Rhinitis, sinusitis, dyspnea, pharyngitis, epistaxis

Pharmacokinetics	
Absorption	Rapid; reduced absorption with high-fat meal
Distribution	Bioavailability 15%; protein binding 95%
Metabolism	Liver
Excretion	Primarily in feces (91%-95%)
Half-life	4-5 hr

V

Adverse effects: *italics* = common; **bold** = life-threatening

Pharmacodynamics

Onset	20 min
Peak	½-1½ hr
Duration	<5 hr

INTERACTIONS
Individual drugs
Alcohol, amLODIPine, metoprolol, NIFEdipine: increased hypotension, do not use concurrently

Cimetidine, erythromycin, itraconazole, ketoconazole: increased levels

Clarithromycin, droperidol, procainamide, quiNIDine: serious dysrhythmias; do not use concurrently

Drug classifications
⚠ Do not use with nitrates because of unsafe decrease in B/P that could result in heart attack or stroke

α-Blockers, protease inhibitors: increased hypotension; do not use concurrently

Angiotensin II receptor blockers: increased hypotension; do not use concurrently

Antidysrhythmics class Ia, III, quinolones: serious dysrhythmias; do not use together

Antiretroviral protease inhibitors: increased vardenafil levels

Drug/food
High-fat meal: decreased absorption

Drug/lab test
Increase: CK

NURSING CONSIDERATIONS
Assessment
• **Assess for use of organic nitrates that should not be used with this product**
• **Assess for severe loss of vision while taking this or any similar products; these products should not be used if vision loss has occurred**

Patient/family education
• Advise that product does not protect against STDs, including HIV
• Teach that product absorption is reduced with a high-fat meal
⚠ **Instruct that product should not be used with nitrates in any form**
• Inform that product has no effect in the absence of sexual stimulation
• Teach that patient should seek immediate medical attention if erection lasts for more than 4 hr
• Advise to inform physician of all medications being taken
• **Teach patient to notify prescriber immediately and stop taking product if vision loss occurs**

Evaluation
Positive therapeutic outcome
• Sustainable erection

---

varenicline (Rx)
(var-e-ni′kleen)
Champix ✿, **Chantix**
Func. class.: Smoking cessation agent
Pregnancy category C

ACTION: Partial agonist for nicotine receptors; partially activates receptors to help curb cravings; occupies receptors to prevent nicotine binding

Therapeutic outcome: Smoking cessation

USES: Smoking deterrent

CONTRAINDICATIONS
Hypersensitivity, eating disorders

Precautions: Pregnancy **C**, breastfeeding, children <18 yr, geriatric, renal disease, recent MI, angioedema

> **BLACK BOX WARNING:** Bipolar disorder, depression, schizophrenia, suicidal ideation

DOSAGE AND ROUTES
Smoking cessation
Adult: PO therapy should begin 1 week prior to smoking stop date (i.e., take product plus tobacco for 7 days); titrate for 1 wk, days 1 through 3, 0.5 mg/day; days 4 through 7, 0.5 mg bid; day 8 through end of treatment 1 mg bid; treatment is 12 wk and may repeat for another 12 wk

Renal dose
Adult: PO CCr ≤50 ml/min, titrate to max 0.5 mg bid

Available forms: Tabs 0.5, 1 mg, Chantix continuing month PAK; Chantix starting month PAK

Implementation
• Do not break, crush, or chew tabs
• Give increased fluids, bulk in diet if constipation occurs
• Give with a full glass of water after eating
• Give sugarless gum, hard candy, or frequent sips of water for dry mouth

ADVERSE EFFECTS
CNS: Headache, agitation, dizziness, insomnia, abnormal dreams, fatigue, malaise, behavior changes, depression, suicidal ideation, suicide, amnesia, hallucinations, hostility, mania, psychosis, tremor

---

⚠ Nurse Alert   ✳ Key NCLEX® Drug   >> Drug Specifics

CV: Dysrhythmias, hypertension, palpitations, tachycardia, angina, hypotension, MI
EENT: *Blurred vision,* tinnitus
GI: *Nausea, vomiting,* anorexia, *dry mouth,* increased/decreased appetite, *constipation,* flatulence, GERD
GU: Erectile dysfunction, urinary frequency, menstrual irregularities
INTEG: Rash, pruritus, angioedema, Stevens-Johnson syndrome
MISC: Weight loss or gain
RESP: Dyspnea, rhinorrhea

Pharmacokinetics

Absorption	Unknown
Distribution	Steady state 4 days
Metabolism	Minimal
Excretion	Urine 92%, unchanged
Half-life	Elimination 24 hr

Pharmacodynamics

Onset	Unknown
Peak	3-4 hr
Duration	24 hr

NURSING CONSIDERATIONS
Assessment
• **Assess smoking history:** motivation for smoking cessation, years used, amount each day, assess for smoking cessation after 12 wk; if progress has not been made, product may be used for an additional 12 wk
• Assess for renal function in geriatric

BLACK BOX WARNING: Neuropsychiatric symptoms: assess for mood, sensorium, affect, behavioral changes, agitation, suicidal ideation; suicide has occurred; possible worsening of depression, schizophrenia, bipolar disorder

Patient/family education
• Teach patient that treatment for smoking cessation lasts 12 wk and another 12 wk may be required
• Teach patient to use caution in driving, other activities requiring alertness; blurred vision may occur
• Advise patient to set a date to quit smoking and initiate treatment 1 wk prior to that date
• Teach patient how to titrate product
• Advise patient not to use with nicotine patches unless directed by prescriber; may increase B/P
• Advise patient to notify prescriber if pregnancy is suspected or planned

• Teach patient common side effects to be expected

BLACK BOX WARNING: Instruct patient to notify prescriber immediately of change in thought/behavior (suicidal ideation, hostility, depression); stop product

Evaluation

Positive therapeutic outcome
• Smoking cessation

vasopressin (Rx)
(vay-soe-press′in)
Pressyn ✦
Func. class.: Pituitary hormone
Chem. class.: Lysine vasopressin
Pregnancy category C

ACTION: Promotes reabsorption of water by action on renal tubular epithelium; causes vasoconstriction on muscles in the GI system

Therapeutic outcome: Increased osmolality, decreased urine output in diabetes insipidus

USES: Diabetes insipidus (nonnephrogenic/nonpsychogenic), abdominal distention postoperatively, bleeding esophageal varices

CONTRAINDICATIONS
Hypersensitivity, chronic nephritis

Precautions: Pregnancy **C,** breastfeeding, CAD, asthma, renal/vascular disease, migraines, seizures

DOSAGE AND ROUTES
Diabetes insipidus
Adult: IM/SUBCUT 5-10 units bid-qid prn; CONT IV INF 0.0005 units/kg/hr, (0.05 milliunit/kg/hr), double dose q30min as needed
Child: IM/SUBCUT 2.5-10 units bid-qid prn; IM/SUBCUT 1.25-2.5 units q2-3day for chronic therapy

Abdominal distention
Adult: IM 5 units, then q3-4hr, increasing to 10 units if needed (aqueous)

Available forms: Sol for inj 20 units/ml

Implementation
IM/SUBCUT route
• May be given IM/SUBCUT for diagnosis of diabetes insipidus
• Give patient 16 oz water at administration to prevent nausea, vomiting, cramping

V

Adverse effects: *italics* = common; **bold** = life-threatening

ADVERSE EFFECTS

CNS: Drowsiness, headache, lethargy, flushing, vertigo
CV: Increased B/P, dysrhythmias, chest pain, cardiac arrest, shock, MI
EENT: Nasal irritation, congestion, rhinitis
GI: Nausea, heartburn, cramps, vomiting, flatus
GU: Vulval pain, uterine cramping
MISC: Tremor, sweating, vertigo, urticaria, bronchial constriction

Pharmacokinetics

Absorption	Erratically absorbed (IM)
Distribution	Widely distributed extracellular fluid
Metabolism	Liver, rapidly
Excretion	Kidneys, unchanged
Half-life	10-20 min

Pharmacodynamics

	IM	IV
Onset	1 hr	Unknown
Peak	Unknown	Unknown
Duration	3-8 hr	3-8 hr

INTERACTIONS
Individual drugs
CarBAMazepine, chlorproPAMIDE, clofibrate, fludrocortisone, urea: decreased antidiuretic effect
Demeclocycline, lithium: increased antidiuretic effect

Drug classifications
Tricyclics: increased antidiuretic effect

NURSING CONSIDERATIONS
Assessment
• Assess intranasal use: nausea, congestion, cramps, headache; usually decreased with decreased dose
• Monitor pulse, B/P when giving product **IV** or SUBCUT
• Monitor I&O ratio, weight daily, fluid/electrolyte balance; check for edema in extremities; if water retention is severe, diuretic may be prescribed; check for water intoxication: lethargy, behavioral changes, disorientation, neuromuscular excitability
• Small doses may precipitate coronary adverse effects; keep emergency equipment nearby

Patient/family education
• Teach patient technique for nasal instillation: to insert tube into nasal cavity to instill product

• Caution patient to avoid OTC products for cough, hay fever because these preparations may contain EPINEPHrine, decrease product response; do not use with alcohol
• Advise patient to carry/wear emergency ID specifying therapy, disease process (diabetes insipidus)
• Teach patient to measure/record I&O
• Teach patient to avoid alcohol, all OTC medications unless approved by prescriber

Evaluation
Positive therapeutic outcome
• Absence of severe thirst
• Decreased urine output, osmolality

vedolizumab
(ve′-doe-liz′ue-mab)
Entyvio
Func. class.: Immunosuppressive, biologic response modifier
Pregnancy category B

ACTION: A specific integrin receptor antagonist that inhibits the migration of specific memory T lymphocytes across the endothelium into inflamed gastrointestinal parenchymal tissue. The action reduces the chronic inflammatory process present in both ulcerative colitis and Crohn's disease

Therapeutic outcome: Lessening of ulcerative colitis and Crohn's disease

USES: For moderately to severely active ulcerative colitis/Crohn's disease; to reduce signs and symptoms, and to induce and maintain clinical remission in patients who have an inadequate response to conventional therapy

CONTRAINDICATIONS: Hypersensitivity

Precautions: Hepatic disease, infections, progressive multifocal leukoencephalopathy (PML), pregnancy **B,** breastfeeding

DOSAGE AND ROUTES
Adult: IV INF 300 mg; give over 30 min at weeks 0, 2, and 6 as induction therapy, then 300 mg q8wk

Available forms: Powder for injection 300 mg

Implementation
• Full response is usually observed by 6 wk; those who do not respond by week 14 are unlikely to respond
• Give as IV infusion only, do not use as an IV push or bolus

• Make sure all immunizations are up to date
• Reconstitute with 4.8 ml of sterile water for injection, using a syringe with a 21- to 25-gauge needle
• Insert the syringe needle into the vial and direct the stream of sterile water for injection to the glass wall of the vial; gently swirl the solution for 15 sec; do not shake
• Allow the solution to stand for up to 20 min at room temperature to allow for reconstitution and for any foam to settle
• Once dissolved, product should be clear or opalescent, colorless to light brownish yellow, and free of visible particulates. Discard if discolored or if foreign particles are present.
• Before withdrawing solution from vial, gently invert vial 3 times. Withdraw 5 ml (300 mg) of reconstructed product using a 21- to 25-gauge needle. Discard remaining product.
• Add the 5 ml (300 mg) of reconstituted product to 250 ml of sterile 0.9% sodium chloride and gently mix infusion bag. Do not mix with other medications. Administer solution as soon as possible; if necessary, solution may be stored for up to 4 hr refrigerated; do not freeze. Infuse over 30 min; after infusion, flush line with 30 ml of sterile 0.9% sodium chloride injection. Discard any unused infusion solution.

ADVERSE EFFECTS

CNS: Headache, fatigue, dizziness
GI: Nausea, vomiting
MISC: Rash, pruritus, infusion-related reactions
MS: Arthralgia, back pain
SYST: Anaphylaxis, progressive multifocal leukoencephalopathy (PML)

Pharmacokinetics

Absorption	Unknown
Distribution	Unknown
Metabolism	Unknown
Excretion	Unknown
Half-life	Unknown

Pharmacodynamics

Onset	Unknown
Peak	Unknown
Duration	Unknown

INTERACTIONS

Drug classifications
Antineoplastics, immunosuppressives: increased infection risk

Do not use with tumor necrosis factor (TNF) modifiers
Toxoids, vaccines: decreased immune response

NURSING CONSIDERATIONS
Assessment
• Ulcerative colitis/Crohn's disease: Monitor symptoms before and after treatment
• Liver dysfunction: Monitor for elevated hepatic enzymes, jaundice, malaise, nausea, vomiting, abdominal pain, and anorexia; these signs are predictive of severe liver injury that may be fatal or may require a liver transplant in some patients; if hepatic dysfunction is suspected, discontinue
• Tuberculosis (TB) latent/active: Obtain TB skin test both before and during treatment. Do not give in active infection such as influenza or sepsis.
• Progressive multifocal leukoencephalopathy (PML): Assess for increased weakness on one side of the body or clumsiness of limbs, visual disturbance, and changes in thinking, memory, and orientation leading to confusion and personality changes; severe disability or death can come over weeks or months

Patient/family education
• Teach patient about the symptoms of infection and to report to health care provider immediately
• Advise patient to report planned or suspected pregnancy, or if breastfeeding

Evaluation
Positive therapeutic response
• Lessening of ulcerative colitis and Crohn's disease

⚠ **HIGH ALERT**

vemurafenib
(vem-ue-raf′e-nib)
Zelboraf
Func. class.: Biologic response modifiers; signal transduction inhibitors (STIs)
Pregnancy category D

ACTION: Inhibitor of some mutated forms of BRAF serine threonine kinase, thereby blocking cellular proliferation in melanoma cells with the mutation. It also inhibits other kinases including CRAF, ARAF, wild-type BRAF, SRMA, ACK1, MAP4H5, and FGR. It is a potent adenosine triphosphate-competitive inhibitor of RAFs with a modest preference for mutant BRAF and CRAF as compared with wild-type BRAF.

Therapeutic outcome: Decreased spread of malignancy

USES: Unresectable or metastatic malignant melanoma with V600E mutation of the BRAF gene

CONTRAINDICATIONS
Hypersensitivity

Precautions: Pregnancy **D**, breastfeeding, children, infants, neonates, hepatic disease, QT prolongation, secondary malignancy, torsades de pointes, hypokalemia, hypomagnesium, sunlight exposure

DOSAGE AND ROUTES
Adult: PO 960 mg (4 tabs) bid about q12h

Dose adjustments for toxicity due to symptomatic adverse reactions or QTc prolongation for Grade 1 or tolerable Grade 2 adverse events: No dosage change

For intolerable Grade 2 or Grade 3 adverse events (1st episode): Interrupt treatment until toxicity resolves to grade ≤1; when resuming, reduce dosage to 720 mg-(3 tabs) bid

For intolerable Grade 2 or Grade 3 adverse events (2nd episode): Interrupt treatment until toxicity resolves to grade ≤1; when resuming, reduce dose to 480 mg (2 tabs) bid

For intolerable Grade 2 or Grade 3 adverse events (3rd episode) Discontinue treatment permanently

For Grade 4 adverse events (1st episode): Discontinue permanently or interrupt until toxicity resolves to grade ≤1; when resuming, reduce dose to 480 mg (2 tablets) bid

For Grade 4 adverse events (2nd episode): Discontinue permanently

Available forms: Tab 240 mg

Implementation
• Continue until disease progresses or unacceptable toxicity occurs
• Missed doses can be taken up to 4 hr before the next dose is due; take about 12 hr apart; take without regard to meals
• Swallow whole with a full glass of water; do not crush or chew
• Store at room temperature in original container

ADVERSE EFFECTS
CNS: Asthenia, fatigue, fever, dizziness, headache, muscle paralysis, peripheral neuropathy
CV: Atrial fibrillation, hypotension, peripheral edema, QT prolongation
EENT: Blurred vision, iritis, photophobia, uveitis
GI: Constipation, decreased appetite, diarrhea, dysgeusia, nausea, vomiting, weight loss
INTEG: Actinic keratosis, alopecia, hyperkeratosis, maculopapular rash, palmar-plantar erythrodysesthesia (hand and foot syndrome), papular rash, photosensitivity, pruritus, xerosis/dry skin
MS: Arthralgia, arthritis, back pain, extremity pain, musculoskeletal pain, myalgias
RESP: Cough
SYST: Anaphylaxis, secondary malignancy

Pharmacokinetics
Absorption	Unknown
Distribution	Protein binding 99%
Metabolism	Unknown
Excretion	94% feces
Half-life	30-120 hr

Pharmacodynamics
Onset	Unknown
Peak	Unknown
Duration	Unknown

INTERACTIONS
Individual drugs
Abarelix, alfuzosin, amoxapine, apomorphine, arsenic trioxide, asenapine, chloroquine, ciprofloxacin, citalopram, clarithromycin, cloZAPine, cyclobenzaprine, dasatinib, dolasetron, dronedarone, droperidol, eribulin, erythromycin, ezogabine, flecainide, fluconazole, gatifloxacin, gemifloxacin, grepafloxacin, halofantrine, haloperidol, iloperidone, indacaterol, lapatinib, levofloxacin, levomethadyl, lopinavir/ritonavir, magnesium sulfate, maprotiline, mefloquine, methadone, moxifloxacin, nilotinib, norfloxacin, octreotide, ofloxacin, OLANZapine, ondansetron, paliperidone, palonosetron, pentamidine, pimozide, posaconazole, potassium sulfate, probucol, propafenone, QUEtiapine, quiNIDine, ranolazine, rilpivirine, risperiDONE, saquinavir, sodium, sparfloxacin, SUNItinib, tacrolimus, telavancin, telithromycin, tetrabenazine, troleandomycin, vardenafil, vemurafenib, venlafaxine, vorinostat, ziprasidone: increased QT prolongation, torsades de pointes

Drug classifications
β-agonists, Class IA antiarrhythmics (disopyramide, procainamide, quiNIDine),
Class III antiarrhythmics (amiodarone,
dofetilide, ibutilide, sotalol), halogenated
anesthetics, local anesthetics, certain
phenothiazines (chlorproMAZINE, flu-
PHENAZine, mesoridazine, perphenazine,
prochlorperazine, thioridazine and trifluoperazine), tricyclic antidepressants:
increased QT prolongation, torsades de
pointes

CYP3A4 inducers (alcohol, barbiturates, bexarotene, carBAMazepine, erythromycin, etravirine, fluvoxaMINE, ketoconazole, metyrapone, modafinil, nevirapine, OXcarbazepine,
phenytoin, rifabutin, rifampin, ritonavir): decreased vemurafenib effect

CYP3A4/CYP1A2 inhibitors (cimetidine, dalfopristin, delavirdine, enoxacin, indinavir, isoniazid, itraconazole, quinupristin, tipranavir):
increased vemurafenib effect

Drug/lab test
Alkaline phosphatase, bilirubin, LFTs, serum
creatinine: increase

NURSING CONSIDERATIONS
Assessment
• **Hepatic disease:** Liver function test (LFT)
abnormalities, altered bilirubin levels, may
occur during treatment; monitor LFTs and
bilirubin levels prior to treatment, then monthly;
more frequent testing is needed in those
presenting with grade 2 or greater toxicities;
Laboratory alterations should be managed
with dose reduction, treatment interruption, or
discontinuation
• **QT prolongation:** has been reported with
the use of crizotinib; therefore, crizotinib
should be avoided in patients with QT
prolongation; Monitor ECG and electrolytes
in those with congestive heart failure,
bradycardia, electrolyte imbalance (hypokalemia, hypomagnesemia), or in those
who are taking concomitant medications
known to prolong the QT interval; treatment
interruption, dosage adjustment, treatment
discontinuation may be needed in those
who develop QT prolongation
• **Pregnancy/breastfeeding:** Identify if pregnancy is planned or suspected, pregnancy
category D, avoid breastfeeding
• Serum electrolytes

Patient/family education
• Teach patient/family that missed doses can be
taken up to 4 hr before the next dose is due to
maintain the twice-daily regimen

• Teach patient to use reliable contraception;
both women and men of childbearing age
should use adequate contraceptive methods
during therapy and for at least 90 days after
completing treatment, pregnancy (D)

Evaluation
Positive therapeutic outcome
• Decreased spread of malignancy

venlafaxine (Rx)
(ven-la-fax′een)
Effexor, Effexor XR
Func. class.: Second-generation SNRI
antidepressant—miscellaneous
Pregnancy category C

ACTION: Potent inhibitor of neuronal serotonin and norepinephrine uptake, weak inhibitor
of dopamine; no muscarinic, histaminergic, or
α-adrenergic receptors in vitro

Therapeutic outcome: Relief of depression

USES: Prevention/treatment of major depression, to treat depression at end of life; long-term
treatment of generalized anxiety disorder, panic
disorder, social anxiety disorder (Effexor XR only)

CONTRAINDICATIONS
Hypersensitivity

Precautions: Pregnancy **C,** breastfeeding,
geriatric, mania, recent MI, cardiac/renal/he-
patic disease, seizure disorder, hypertension,
eosinophilic pneumonia, desvenlafaxine hypersensitivity

> **BLACK BOX WARNING:** Children, suicidal ide-
> ation, bipolar disorder, interstitial lung disease

DOSAGE AND ROUTES
Depression
Adult: PO 75 mg/day in 2 or 3 divided doses;
taken with food, may be increased to 150 mg/
day; if needed may be further increased to 225
mg/day; increments of 75 mg/day should be
made at intervals of no less than 4 days; some
hospitalized patients may require up to 375 mg/
day in 3 divided doses; EXT REL 37.5-75 mg PO
daily, max 225 mg/day; give Effexor XR daily

Anxiety disorders
Adult: PO 75 mg/day or 37.5 mg/day × 4-7
days initially, max 225 mg/day

Hepatic dose
Adult: PO moderate impairment 50% of dose

Renal dose
Adult: PO CCr 10-70 ml/min reduce dose by
25%-50%; CCr <10 ml/min reduce by 50%

Hot flashes (unlabeled)
Adult (male, prostate cancer): PO 12.5 mg
bid × 4 wk
Adult female: PO 37.5-75 mg/day

Available forms: Tabs scored (Effexor) 25,
37.5, 50, 75, 100 mg; ext rel caps (Effexor XR)
37.5, 75, 150, 225 mg

Implementation
• Give with food or milk for GI symptoms
• Crush if patient is unable to swallow medica-
tion whole
• Store at room temperature; do not freeze

ADVERSE EFFECTS
CNS: *Emotional lability, dizziness, weakness,* apathy, ataxia, headache, tremors, hypertonia, euphoria, hallucinations, hostility, insomnia, anxiety, suicidal ideation in children/
adolescents, seizures, neuroleptic malignant syndrome–like reaction
CV: Angina pectoris, extrasystoles, postural hypotension, syncope, thrombophlebitis, hypertension, tachycardia, change in QTc interval,
increased cholesterol
EENT: *Abnormal vision,* taste, *ear pain*
GI: *Dysphagia, eructation,* colitis, gastritis,
gingivitis, *constipation,* stomatitis, stomach and
mouth ulceration, nausea, anorexia, dry mouth
GU: *Anorgasmia,* abnormal ejaculation, urinary frequency, decreased libido, impotence,
menstrual changes
HEMA: Thrombocytopenia, leukocytosis, leukopenia, abnormal bleeding
INTEG: Ecchymosis, acne, alopecia, brittle
nails, dry skin, photosensitivity, sweating, angio-
edema (ext rel), Stevens-Johnson syndrome
META: *Peripheral edema, weight loss,*
edema, glycosuria, hyperlipemia, hypokalemia
MS: Arthritis, bone pain, tenosynovitis, arthralgia
RESP: *Bronchitis, dyspnea,* cough
SYST: Neonatal abstinence syndrome

Pharmacokinetics

Absorption	Well absorbed
Distribution	Widely distributed, 27% protein binding
Metabolism	Liver, extensively
Excretion	Kidneys, 87%
Half-life	5 hr, 11 hr (active metabolite)

Pharmacodynamics

Unknown

INTERACTIONS
Individual drugs
Alcohol: increased CNS depression

Cimetidine: increased venlafaxine effect
CloZAPine, desipramine, haloperidol, warfarin:
increased levels of these products
Cyproheptadine: decreased venlafaxine effect
Indinavir: decreased effect of indinavir
Linezolid, methylene blue, sibutramine,
SUMAtriptan, traMADol, traZODone, tryp-
tophan: increased serotonin syndrome

Drug classifications
Antihistamines, opioids, sedative-hypnotics: increased CNS depression
MAOIs: hyperthermia, rigidity, rapid fluctuations of vital signs, mental status changes,
neuroleptic malignant syndrome
Salicylates, NSAIDs, platelet inhibitors, anticoagulants: increased bleeding risk
SSRIs, SNRIs, serotonin-receptor agonists:
increased serotonin syndrome

Drug/herb
Kava, valerian: increased CNS depression
St. John's wort: serotonin syndrome

Drug/lab test
Increased: alkaline phosphatase, bilirubin, AST, ALT,
BUN, creatinine, serum cholesterol, CPK, LDH
False positive: amphetamines, phencyclidine

NURSING CONSIDERATIONS
Assessment
• Monitor B/P (lying, standing), pulse q4hr; if
systolic B/P drops 20 mm Hg hold product, notify prescriber; take vital signs q4hr in patients
with CV disease
• Monitor blood tests: CBC, leukocytes, differential, cardiac enzymes if patient is receiving
long-term therapy
• Monitor liver function tests: AST, ALT, bilirubin
• Check weight qwk; weight loss or gain; appetite may increase, peripheral edema may occur

> **BLACK BOX WARNING:** Assess mental status:
> mood, sensorium, affect; increase in psychiat-
> ric symptoms: depression, panic; for suicidal
> ideation in children/adolescents, discuss with
> family members

• Monitor urinary retention, constipation;
constipation is more likely to occur in children
or geriatric
• **Assess for withdrawal symptoms:**
headache, nausea, vomiting, muscle pain, weakness; do not usually occur unless product was
discontinued abruptly, taper over 14 days
• Identify alcohol consumption; if alcohol is
consumed, hold dose
• Serotonin syndrome, neuroleptic malignant syndrome: assess for increased heart
rate, shivering, sweating, dilated pupils,

tremors, high B/P, hyperthermia, headache, confusion; if these occur, stop product, administer a serotonin antagonist if needed; usually worse if given with linezolid, methylene blue, tryptophan

Patient/family education
• Advise patient to notify prescriber of rash, hives, or allergic reactions
• Teach patient that therapeutic effects may take 2-3 wk
• Teach patient to use caution in driving or other activities requiring alertness because of drowsiness, dizziness, blurred vision; to avoid rising quickly from sitting to standing, especially geriatric
• Teach patient to avoid alcohol ingestion, other CNS depressants

Serotonin syndrome, neuroleptic malignant syndrome: advise patient to report immediately shivering, sweating, tremors, fever, dilated pupils

⚠ Advise patient to avoid pregnancy, breastfeeding while taking this product, birth defects have occurred when used in the 3rd trimester

⚠ Teach patient that worsening of symptoms, suicidal thoughts/behavior may occur in children, young adults

• Advise patient to take as prescribed, contents of capsule may be sprinkled on applesauce if unable to swallow whole

Evaluation

Positive therapeutic outcome
• Decreased depression, anxiety; sense of well-being
• Absence of suicidal thoughts

TREATMENT OF OVERDOSE:
ECG monitoring, induce emesis, lavage, activated charcoal, administer anticonvulsant

---

verapamil (Rx)
(ver-ap′a-mil)
Apo-Verap ✲, Calan, Calan SR, Chronovera ✲, Covera ✲, Isoptin, Isoptin SR, Novo-Veramil ✲, Tarka ✲, Veramil ✲, Verelan, Verelan PM
Func. class.: Calcium-channel blocker; antihypertensive; antianginal, antidysrhythmic (Class IV)
Chem. class.: Diphenylalkylamine
Pregnancy category C

ACTION: Inhibits calcium ion influx across cell membrane during cardiac depolarization; produces relaxation of coronary vascular smooth muscle; peripheral vascular smooth muscle; dilates coronary vascular arteries; decreases SA/AV node conduction; dilates peripheral arteries

Therapeutic outcome: Decreased angina pectoris, dysrhythmias, B/P

USES: Chronic stable vasospastic, unstable angina; dysrhythmias, hypertension, supraventricular tachycardia, atrial flutter or fibrillation

CONTRAINDICATIONS
Sick sinus syndrome, 2nd- or 3rd-degree heart block, hypotension <90 mm Hg systolic, cardiogenic shock, severe CHF, Lown-Ganong-Levine syndrome, Wolff-Parkinson-White syndrome

Precautions: Pregnancy C, breastfeeding, children, geriatric, CHF, hypotension, hepatic injury, renal disease, concomitant β-blocker therapy

DOSAGE AND ROUTES
Angina
Adult: PO 80-120 mg tid, increase qwk, max 480 mg/day

Dysrhythmias
Adult: PO 240-320 mg/day in 3-4 divided doses in digitalized patients
Adult: IV BOL 5-10 mg (0.075-0.15 mg/kg) over 2 min, may repeat 10 mg (0.15 mg/kg) ½ hr after first dose
Child 1-15 yr: IV BOL 0.1-0.3 mg/kg over >2 min, repeat in 30 min, max 5 mg in a single dose
Child 0-1 yr: IV BOL 0.1-0.2 mg/kg over ≥2 min, may repeat after 30 min

Hypertension
Adult: PO 80 mg tid, may titrate upward; EXT REL 120-240 mg/day as a single dose, may increase to 240-480 mg/day

Hepatic dose/geriatric/compromised ventricular function
Adult: PO 40 mg tid initially, increase as tolerated

Available forms: Tabs 40, 80, 120 mg; ext rel tabs 120, 180, 240 mg; inj 2.5 mg/ml in ampules, syringes, vials; ext rel caps 100, 200, 240, 300 mg

Implementation
PO route
• **Regular release:** give without regard to food
• **Extended release:** do not crush or chew ext rel products

V

- Cap may be opened and contents sprinkled on food; do not dissolve, chew cap
- Give once a day before meals at bedtime; sus rel give with food to decrease GI symptoms

Direct IV route
- Give by direct **IV** undiluted (Y-site, 3-way stopcock) over at least 2 min, or 3 min geriatric; discard unused sol; to prevent serious hypotension, patient should be recumbent for 1 hr or more, with continuous ECG and B/P monitoring
- **Do not use IV with IV β-blockers, may cause AV nodal blockade**

Y-site compatibilities: Alfentanil, amikacin, argatroban, ascorbic acid, atracurium, atropine, aztreonam, bivalirudin, bumetanide, buprenorphine, butorphanol, calcium chloride/gluconate, CARBOplatin, caspofungin, ceFAZolin, cefonicid, cefotaxime, cefoTEtan, cefOXitin, ceftizoxime, cefTRIAXone, cefuroxime, chlorproMAZINE, cimetidine, ciprofloxacin, clindamycin, cyanocobalamin, cyclophosphamide, cycloSPORINE, cytarabine, DACTINomycin, DAPTOmycin, dexamethasone, dexmedetomidine, digoxin, diltiazem, diphenhydrAMINE, DOBUTamine, DOCEtaxel, DOPamine, doxacurium, DOXOrubicin hydrochloride, doxycycline, enalaprilat, ePHEDrine, EPINEPHrine, epirubicin, epoetin alfa, eptifibatide, erythromycin, esmolol, etoposide, etoposide phosphate, famotidine, fenoldopam, fentaNYL, fluconazole, fludarabine, gemcitabine, gentamicin, glycopyrrolate, granisetron, heparin, hydrALAZINE, hydrocortisone, HYDROmorphone, ifosfamide, imipenem/cilastatin, inamrinone, insulin, isoproterenol, ketorolac, labetalol, levofloxacin, lidocaine, linezolid, LORazepam, magnesium sulfate, mannitol, mechlorethamine, meperidine, metaraminol, methotrexate, methoxamine, methyldopate, methylPREDNISolone, metoclopramide, metoprolol, metroNIDAZOLE, miconazole, midazolam, milrinone, mitoXANtrone, morphine, multivitamins, nalbuphine, naloxone, nesiritide, nitroglycerin, nitroprusside, norepinephrine, octreotide, ondansetron, oxaliplatin, oxytocin, PACLitaxel, palonosetron, papaverine, PEMEtrexed, penicillin G, pentamidine, pentazocine, phentolamine, phenylephrine, phytonadione, piperacillin/tazobactam, potassium chloride, procainamide, prochlorperazine, promethazine, propranolol, protamine, pyridoxime, quinupristin/dalfopristin, ranitidine, rocuronium, sodium acetate, succinylcholine, SUFentanil, tacrolimus, teniposide, theophylline, thiamine, ticarcillin/clavulanate, tirofiban, tobramycin, tolazoline, trimethaphan, urokinase, vancomycin, vasopressin, vecuronium, vinCRIStine, vinorelbine, voriconazole

Y-site incompatibilities: Acyclovir, albumin, aminophylline, amphotericin B cholesteryl, amphotericin B colloidal, amphotericin B liposome, ampicillin, ampicillin/sulbactam, azaTHIOprine, cefoperazone, cefTAZidime, chloramphenicol, dantrolene, diazepam, diazoxide, ertapenem, fluorouracil, folic acid, furosemide, ganciclovir, indomethacin, pantoprazole, PENTObarbital, PHENobarbital, phenytoin, piperacillin/tazobactam, propofol, sodium bicarbonate, thiotepa, tigecycline, trimethoprim/sulfamethoxazole

ADVERSE EFFECTS
CNS: *Headache, drowsiness,* dizziness, anxiety, depression, weakness, asthenia, fatigue, insomnia, confusion, light-headedness
CV: *Edema,* CHF, bradycardia, hypotension, palpitations, AV block, **dysrhythmias**
GI: *Nausea,* diarrhea, gastric upset, *constipation,* elevated liver function tests
GU: Impotence, nocturia, polyuria, gynecomastia
HEMA: Bruising, petechiae, bleeding
INTEG: Rash, bruising
MISC: Gingival hyperplasia
SYST: Stevens-Johnson syndrome

Pharmacokinetics

Absorption	Well absorbed (PO)
Distribution	Not known
Metabolism	Liver, extensively
Excretion	Kidneys (70%)
Half-life	Biphasic 4 min, 3-7 hr

Pharmacodynamics

	PO	PO-EXT REL	IV
Onset	1-2 hr	Unknown	1-5 min
Peak	½-1½ hr	5-7 hr	3-5 min
Duration	3-7 hr	24 hr	2 hr

INTERACTIONS
Individual drugs
CarBAMazepine, cycloSPORINE, digoxin, theophylline: increased levels of each specific product
Cimetidine, clarithromycin, erythromycin: increased effect of verapamil
FentaNYL, prazosin, quiNIDine: increased hypotension
Lithium: decreased lithium levels

Drug classifications
Antihypertensive, β-adrenergic blockers, nitrates: increased effects of verapamil, monitor for CV effects

---

Nondepolarizing muscle relaxants: increased effect

NSAIDs: decreased antihypertensive effect

Drug/herb
Ephedra (ma huang): increased hypertension
Ginseng, ginkgo: increased verapamil effect
St. John's wort: decreased verapamil effect

Drug/food
Grapefruit juice: increased hypotension

Drug/lab test
Increased: alkaline phosphatase, AST, ALT, BUN, creatinine, serum cholesterol

NURSING CONSIDERATIONS
Assessment
• CHF: Assess fluid volume status: I&O ratio and record; weight; distended red veins; crackles in lung; color; quality, specific gravity of urine; skin turgor; adequacy of pulses; moist mucous membranes; bilateral lung sounds; peripheral pitting edema; dehydration symptoms of decreasing output, thirst, hypotension, dry mouth, and mucous membranes should be reported
• Monitor B/P and pulse, pulmonary capillary wedge pressure (PCWP), central venous pressure, index, often during inf; notify prescriber if <50 bpm, systolic B/P <90 mm Hg
• Monitor ALT, AST, bilirubin daily; if these are elevated, hepatotoxicity is suspected
• Monitor platelets; if <150,000/mm³, product is usually discontinued and another product started
• Assess for extravasation; change site q48hr
• **Monitor cardiac status:** B/P, pulse, respiration, ECG
• Monitor renal/hepatic function tests during long-term treatment, serum potassium, periodically

Patient/family education
• Advise patient to increase fluids/fiber to counteract constipation
• Caution patient to avoid hazardous activities until stabilized on product and dizziness is no longer a problem
• Teach patient how to take pulse, B/P before taking product; to keep record or graph
• Instruct patient to limit caffeine consumption; to avoid alcohol, grapefruit, and OTC products unless directed by prescriber
• Advise patient to comply with medical regimen: diet, exercise, stress reduction, product therapy; to notify prescriber of irregular heartbeat, shortness of breath, swelling of feet and hands, pronounced dizziness, constipation, nausea, hypotension, **IV** calcium
• Teach patient to use as directed even if feeling better; may be taken with other CV products (nitrates, β-blockers)
• Caution patient not to discontinue abruptly; chest pain may occur
• **Advise to report chest pain, palpitations, irregular heartbeat, swelling of extremities, skin irritation, rash, tremors, weakness**
• **Instruct patient to notify prescriber if pregnancy is planned; may breastfeed (American Academy of Pediatrics)**

Evaluation
Positive therapeutic outcome
• Decreased anginal pain
• Decreased dysrhythmias
• Decreased B/P

TREATMENT OF OVERDOSE:
Defibrillation, atropine for AV block, vasopressor for hypotension, **IV** calcium

vigabatrin (Rx)
(vye-ga′ba-trin)
Sabril
Func. class.: Anticonvulsant
Chem. class.: GABA transaminase inhibitor
Pregnancy category C

ACTION: May inhibit reuptake and metabolism of GABA, may increase seizure threshold; structurally similar to GABA

Therapeutic outcome: Prevention of seizure activity

USES: Adjunct treatment of partial seizures in adults and children ≥12 yr, infantile spasm

CONTRAINDICATIONS
Hypersensitivity to this product

Precautions: Pregnancy **C**, breastfeeding, children <2 yr, geriatric patients, renal/hepatic disease, suicidal ideation/behavior, abrupt discontinuation

BLACK BOX WARNING: Visual disturbance

DOSAGE AND ROUTES
Partial seizures
Adult: PO 500 mg bid, titrate in 500-mg increments at weekly intervals, up to 1.5 g bid

V

Adverse effects: *italics* = common; **bold** = life-threatening

Infantile spasm
Infant >1 mo, child ≤2 yr: PO 50 mg/kg/day in 2 divided doses titrate in 25-50 mg/kg/day increments q3days, max 150 mg/kg/day

Renal dose
Adult: PO CCr 50-80 ml/min, reduce dosage by 25%; PO CCr 30-50 ml/min, reduce dosage by 50%; PO CCr 10-30 ml/min, reduce dosage by 75%

Available forms: Powder for oral sol 500 mg; tablet 500 mg

Implementation
PO route (tab)
- Give without regard to meals

PO route (oral solution)
- Reconstitute immediately before using
- Empty contents of appropriate number of packets into a clean cup
- For each packet, dissolve 10 ml of water, conc. 50 mg/ml; do not use other liquids
- Stir until dissolved; solution should be clear
- Use calibrated oral syringe to measure correct dosage
- Discard any unused solution

ADVERSE EFFECTS
CNS: Headache, memory impairment, *dizziness,* irritability, lethargy, malignant hyperthermia, insomnia, suicidal ideation
CV: Edema
EENT: Vision impairment
GI: Nausea, vomiting, diarrhea, increased appetite, abdominal pain, GI bleeding, hemorrhoids, weight gain, constipation
GU: Impotence, dysmenorrhea
HEMA: Anemia
INTEG: Pruritus, rash
RESP: Coughing, respiratory depression, pulmonary embolism

Pharmacokinetics

Absorption	>95%
Distribution	Widely; no protein binding
Metabolism	Not metabolized
Excretion	Urine 80% parent drug, slowed in renal disease
Half-life	7.5 hr

Pharmacodynamics

Onset	Unknown
Peak	2 hr
Duration	Unknown

INTERACTIONS
Individual drugs
AzaTHIOprine, chloroquine, deferoxamine, ethambutol, hydroxychloroquine, interferons, loxapine, mecasermin, rh-IGF-1, pentostatin, tamoxifen, thiothixene: increased serious ophthalmic effects (glaucoma, retinopathy); avoid concurrent use

Drug classifications
CNS depressants: increased CNS depression
Corticosteroids, phenothiazines, phosphodiesterase inhibitors: increased serious ophthalmic effects (glaucoma, retinopathy)

Drug/lab test
Decreased: ALT/AST

NURSING CONSIDERATIONS
Assessment

> BLACK BOX WARNING: ⚠ Visual impairment: prescribers must be registered with the SHARE program due to risk of permanent vision loss; if no clinical response in 2-4 wk in pediatric patients or 3 mo in adults, provide vision assessment; assess again after ≤4 wk, at least q3mo, and 3-6 mo after stopping product

- Monitor renal studies: urinalysis, BUN, urine creatinine q3mo in those with renal disease
- Monitor hepatic studies: ALT, AST, bilirubin
- Assess description of seizures: location, duration, presence of aura
- Assess mental status: mood, sensorium, affect, behavioral changes; if mental status changes, notify prescriber

Patient/family education
- Teach patient to carry emergency ID stating patient's name, products taken, condition, prescriber's name and phone number
- Advise patient to avoid driving, other activities that require alertness
- Inform patient not to discontinue medication quickly after long-term use
- Instruct patient to notify prescriber if pregnancy is planned or suspected
- ⚠ Instruct patient to report suicidal thoughts/behaviors immediately

---

⚠ Instruct patient to avoid alcohol; drowsiness, dizziness may occur

Evaluation

Positive therapeutic outcome
• Decreased seizure activity; document on patient's chart

---

vilazodone (Rx)
(vil-az'oh-done)
Viibryd
Func. class.: Antidepressant, miscellaneous

Pregnancy category C

ACTION: A novel antidepressant unrelated to other antidepressants, enhances serotoninergic action by a dual mechanism

Therapeutic outcome: Remission of depressive symptoms

USES: Major depression

CONTRAINDICATIONS
Concomitant use of MAOIs or within 14 days after discontinuing an MAOI or within 14 days after discontinuing vilazodone

Precautions: Abrupt discontinuation, bipolar disorder, bleeding, operating machinery, ECT, geriatrics, hepatic disease, hyponatremia, hypovolemia, infants, labor, pregnancy **C**, substance abuse, history of seizures, serotonin syndrome, neuroleptic malignant syndrome, use with serotonin precursors (e.g., tryptophan) or serotonergic drugs, suicidal ideation and worsening depression or behavior

> **BLACK BOX WARNING:** Child, suicidal ideation

DOSAGE AND ROUTES
Adult: PO 10 mg ×7 days, then 20 mg ×7 days, then 40 mg/day; if taking a potent CYP3A4 inhibitor, the max is 20 mg/day

Available forms: Tabs 10, 20, 40 mg

Implementation
• Administer with food to increase absorption
• Store at room temperature, away from moisture, heat
• Do not use within 2 wk of MAOIs

ADVERSE EFFECTS
CNS: Restlessness, dizziness, drowsiness, fatigue, mania, insomnia, migraine, **neuroleptic malignant-like syndrome**, paresthesias, **seizures, suicidal ideation**, tremor, night sweats, dream disorders

CV: Palpitations, ventricular extrasystole
EENT: Cataracts, blurred vision
GI: *Nausea*, vomiting, flatulence, *diarrhea, xerostomia*, altered taste, gastroenteritis, increased appetite
GU: Decreased libido, ejaculation disorder, increased frequency of urination, sexual dysfunction
HEMA: Bleeding, decreased platelets
INTEG: Sweating
MS: Arthralgia
SYST: **Neonatal abstinence syndrome, withdrawal, serotonin syndrome**

Pharmacokinetics

Absorption	Unknown
Distribution	Protein binding 96-99%
Metabolism	Metabolized by the liver by CYP 3A4 (major) and CYP2C19 and CYP2D (minor) and non-CYP pathways
Excretion	Unknown
Half-life	25 hr

Pharmacodynamics

Onset	Unknown
Peak	4-5 hr
Duration	Unknown

INTERACTIONS
Individual drugs
Selegline, busPIRone, dextromethorphan, fenfluramine, dexfluramine, lithium, meperidine, fentaNYL, methylphenidate, dexmethylphenidate, metoclopramide, mirtazapine, nefazodone, pentazocine, phenothiazines, haloperidol, loxapine, thiothixene, molidone: increased serotonin syndrome

Drug classifications
MAO inhibitors: do not use within 2 wk of SSRIs, SNRIs, serotonin receptor agonists, ergots, amphetamines: increased serotonin syndrome

Anticoagulants, NSAIDs, platelet inhibitors, salicylates, thrombolytics: increased bleeding
CYP3A4 inducers: decreased vilazodone effect
CYP3A4 inhibitors (clarithromycin, dronedarone, efavirenz, erythromycin, ketoconazole and others): increased vilazodone levels

Drug/herb
St. John's wort: increased serotonin syndrome

Drug/food
Grapefruit juice: avoid use

V

Adverse effects: *italics* = common; **bold** = life-threatening

Drug/lab test
Decreased: sodium

NURSING CONSIDERATIONS
Assessment
• Assess mental status: orientation, mood behavior initially and periodically.

> **BLACK BOX WARNING:** Initiate suicide precautions if indicated

• Assess for history of seizures, mania
• Monitor renal, hepatic status: hyponatremia
⚠ **Abrupt discontinuation:** do not discontinue abruptly; taper, monitor for symptoms of withdrawal; if intolerable, resume previous dose and decrease more slowly
⚠ **Serotonin syndrome/neuroleptic malignant syndrome:** nausea, vomiting, sedation, sweating, facial flushing, high B/P; discontinue product, notify prescriber

Patient/family education
• Teach patient to take as directed, with food, do not double doses, that follow-up will be needed
• Advise patient to avoid abrupt discontinuation unless approved by prescriber
• Instruct patient not to drive or operate machinery until effects are known
• Instruct patient not to use other products unless approved by prescriber, do not use alcohol
• Advise patient to contact prescriber if allergic reactions, personality changes (aggression, anxiety, anger, hostility), extreme sleepiness or drowsiness, confusion, nervousness, restlessness, clumsiness, numbness, tingling or burning pain in hands, arms, legs or feet, tremors, or having unusual behavior or thoughts about self-harm
• Instruct patient to notify prescriber if pregnancy is planned or suspected; avoid breastfeeding

> **BLACK BOX WARNING:** Suicidal thoughts/behaviors: discuss with family the possibility of suicidal thoughts/behaviors, to notify prescriber immediately if these occur

Evaluation
Positive therapeutic outcome
• Remission of depressive symptoms

⚠ HIGH ALERT

vinBLAStine (VLB) (Rx)
(vin-blast'een)
Velbe ✤
Func. class.: Antineoplastic
Chem. class.: Vinca rosea alkaloid
Pregnancy category D

Do not confuse: vinBLAStine/vinCRIStine/vinorelbine

ACTION: Inhibits mitotic activity, arrests cell cycle at metaphase; inhibits RNA synthesis, blocks cellular use of glutamic acid needed for purine synthesis; a vesicant

Therapeutic outcome: Prevention of rapid growth of malignant cells; immunosuppression

USES: Breast, testicular cancer; lymphomas; neuroblastoma; Hodgkin's, non-Hodgkin's lymphomas; mycosis fungoides; histiocytosis; Kaposi's sarcoma, Langerhan's cell histiocytosis

CONTRAINDICATIONS
Pregnancy **D**, breastfeeding, infants, hypersensitivity, leukopenia, granulocytopenia, bone marrow suppression, infection

> **BLACK BOX WARNING:** Intrathecal use

Precautions: Renal/hepatic disease, tumor lysis syndrome

> **BLACK BOX WARNING:** Extravasation

DOSAGE AND ROUTES
Breast cancer
Adult: IV 4.5 mg/m^2 on day 1 of every 21 days in combination with DOXOrubicin and thiotepa

Hodgkin's disease
Adult: IV 6 mg/m^2 on days 1 and 15 q28 days with DOXOrubicin (ABVD)
Child: IV 2.5-6 mg/m^2/day once q 1-2 wk × 3-6 wks; max weekly dose 12.5 mg/m^2

Available forms: Inj powder 10 mg for 10 ml **IV** inj; sol for inj 1 mg/ml

Implementation

IV inj route
• Administer **IV** after diluting 10 mg/10 ml NaCl; give through Y-tube or 3-way stopcock or directly over 1 min
Intermittent IV INF route
• Further dilute in 50-100 ml of NS, inf over 15-30 min

- Give by intermittent inf
- Sol should be prepared by qualified personnel only under controlled conditions
- Use Luer-Lok tubing to prevent leakage; do not let sol come in contact with skin; if contact occurs, wash well with soap and water

BLACK BOX WARNING: Give hyaluronidase 150 units/ml in 1 ml of NaCl, warm compress for extravasation for vesicant activity treatment

BLACK BOX WARNING: Do not administer intrathecally: fatal

Syringe compatibilities: Bleomycin, CISplatin, cyclophosphamide, droperidol, fluorouracil, leucovorin, methotrexate, metoclopramide, mitomycin, vinCRIStine

Y-site compatibilities: Allopurinol, amifostine, aztreonam, bleomycin, CISplatin, cyclophosphamide, DOXOrubicin, droperidol, filgrastim, fludarabine, fluorouracil, granisetron, heparin, leucovorin, melphalan, methotrexate, metoclopramide, mitomycin, ondansetron, PAClitaxel, piperacillin/tazobactam, sargramostim, teniposide, thiotepa, vinCRIStine, vinorelbine

Y-site incompatibilities: Furosemide

ADVERSE EFFECTS
CNS: Paresthesias, peripheral neuropathy, depression, headache, seizures, malaise
CV: Tachycardia, orthostatic hypotension, hypertension
GI: *Nausea, vomiting,* ileus, *anorexia, stomatitis, constipation,* abdominal pain, GI and rectal bleeding, hepatotoxicity, pharyngitis
GU: Urinary retention, renal failure, hyperuricemia
HEMA: Thrombocytopenia, leukopenia, myelosuppression, agranulocytosis, granulocytosis, aplastic anemia, neutropenia, pancytopenia
INTEG: *Rash, alopecia,* photosensitivity, extravasation, tissue necrosis
META: SIADH
SYST: Tumor lysis syndrome (TLS)
RESP: Fibrosis, pulmonary infiltrate, bronchospasm

Pharmacokinetics
Absorption	Complete bioavailability
Distribution	Crosses blood-brain barrier slightly
Metabolism	Liver—active antineoplastic
Excretion	Biliary, kidneys
Half-life	Triphasic <5 min, 50-155 min, 23-85 hr

Pharmacodynamics
Unknown

INTERACTIONS
Individual drugs
Bleomycin: increased synergism
Methotrexate: increased methotrexate action
MitoMYcin: increased bronchospasm
Phenytoin: decreased phenytoin level
Radiation: increased toxicity, bone marrow suppression; do not use together

Drug classifications
Anticoagulants, antiplatelets, NSAIDs, thrombolytics: increased bleeding risk
Antineoplastics: increased toxicity, bone marrow suppression
CYP3A4 inducers (barbiturates, bosentan, carBAMazepine, efavirenz, phenytoin, nevirapine, rifabutin, rifampin): decreased vinBLAStine effect
CYP3A4 inhibitors (aprepitant, antiretroviral protease inhibitors, clarithromycin, danazol, delavirdine, diltiazem, erythromycin, fluconazole, FLUoxetine, fluvoxaMINE, imatinib, ketoconazole, mebefradil, nefazodone, telithromycin, voriconazole): increased toxicity
Live virus vaccines: increased adverse reactions

Drug/herb
St. John's wort: avoid use

Drug/lab test
Increased: uric acid, bilirubin
Decreased: Hgb, platelets, WBC

NURSING CONSIDERATIONS
Assessment
- Monitor B/P (baseline and q15min) during administration
- Monitor CBC, differential, platelet count weekly; withhold product if WBC is <2000/mm³ or platelet count is <75,000/mm³; notify prescriber of results; recovery will take 3 wk; RBC, Hct, Hgb may be decreased; nadir occurs on days 4-10, and continues for another 1-2 wk

⚠ Tumor lysis syndrome: monitor for hyperkalemia, hyperphosphatemia, hyperuricemia; usually occurs with leukemia, lymphoma; alkalinization of the urine; allopurinol should be used to prevent urate nephropathy; monitor electrolytes and renal function (BUN, uric acid, urine CCR)
• Monitor renal function tests: BUN, serum uric acid, urine CCr before, during therapy; I&O ratio; report fall in urine output of 30 ml/hr; for decreased hyperuricemia
⚠ Bronchospasm: can be life threatening; usually occurs when giving mitoMYcin
• Monitor for cold, fever, sore throat (may indicate beginning of infection); notify prescriber if these occur
• Assess for bleeding: hematuria, guaiac, bruising or petechiae, mucosa or orifices q8hr, no rectal temp; avoid IM inj; use pressure to venipuncture sites
• Identify nutritional status: an antiemetic may need to be prescribed
• Assess for gout, joint pain, swelling, increased uric acid; allopurinol or other treatment may be used
• Assess for symptoms indicating severe allergic reactions: rash, pruritus, urticaria, itching, flushing, bronchospasm, hypotension; EPINEPHrine and resuscitative equipment should be nearby
• Hepatitis: transient hepatitis may occur with continuous IV

Patient/family education
• Teach patient to avoid use of products containing aspirin or NSAIDs, razors, commercial mouthwash because bleeding may occur; to report symptoms of bleeding (hematuria, tarry stools)
• Instruct patient to report signs of anemia, (fatigue, headache, irritability, faintness, shortness of breath)
• Caution patient to report any changes in breathing or coughing even several mo after treatment; avoid breastfeeding; may cause male infertility
• Advise patient that contraception will be necessary during treatment; teratogenesis may occur
• Advise patient to use sunscreen, wear protective clothing and sunglasses
• Inform patient that hair may be lost during treatment; a wig or hairpiece may make patient feel better; new hair will be different in color, texture
• Advise patient to avoid vaccinations during treatment; serious reactions may occur

• Teach patient to report signs/symptoms of infection: fever, chills, sore throat; patient should avoid crowds and persons with known infections
• Pregnancy: teach patient to notify prescriber if pregnancy is planned or suspected, pregnancy D, avoid breastfeeding, may cause male infertility
⚠ Instruct patient to avoid persons with known infections
⚠ Infection: instruct patient to report sore throat, flulike symptoms

Evaluation

Positive therapeutic outcome
• Decreased spread of malignant cells

⚠ HIGH ALERT

vinCRIStine (VCR) (Rx)
(vin-kris'teen)
Vincasar PFS
vinCRIStine liposomal
vin-kris'teen
Marqibo
Func. class.: Antineoplastic— miscellaneous
Chem. class.: Vinca alkaloid
Pregnancy category D

Do not confuse: vinCRIStine/vinBLAStine/ vinorelbine

ACTION: Inhibits mitotic activity, arrests cell cycle at metaphase; inhibits RNA synthesis, blocks cellular use of glutamic acid needed for purine synthesis; a vesicant

Therapeutic outcome: Prevention of rapid growth of malignant cells, immunosuppression

USES: Lymphomas, neuroblastomas, Hodgkin's disease, acute lymphoblastic and other leukemias, rhabdomyosarcoma, Wilms' tumor, non-Hodgkin's lymphoma, malignant glioma, soft-tissue sarcoma; **liposomal:** Philadelphia chromosome- negative ALL in second or greater relapse or that has progressed after 2 or more antileukemia therapies

CONTRAINDICATIONS
Pregnancy **D**, breastfeeding, infants, hypersensitivity, radiation therapy

BLACK BOX WARNING: Intrathecal use

Precautions: Renal/hepatic disease, hypertension, neuromuscular disease

BLACK BOX WARNING: Extravasation

DOSAGE AND ROUTES
Adult: IV 0.4-1.4 mg/m²/wk, max 2 mg
Child >10 kg: IV 1-2 mg/m²/wk, max 2 mg
Liposomal
Adult: IV 2.25 mg/m² over 1hr q7days

Available forms: Inj 1 mg/ml; liposomal 5 mg/31 ml injection kit

Implementation
IV route (vinCRIStine)

> **BLACK BOX WARNING:** Do not give intrathecally: fatal

- Administer **IV** after diluting with diluent provided or 1 mg/10 ml of sterile water or 0.9% NaCl; give through Y-tube or 3-way stopcock or directly over 1 min; do not use 5-mg vial for single doses

> **BLACK BOX WARNING:** Hyaluronidase 150 units/ml in 1 ml of NaCl; apply warm compress for extravasation

Y-site compatibilities: Acyclovir, alemtuzumab, alfentanil, allopurinol, amifostine, amikacin, aminocaproic acid, aminophylline, amiodarone, amphotericin B cholesteryl, amphotericin B lipid complex, amphotericin B liposome, ampicillin, ampicillin–sulbactam, anidulafungin, argatroban, arsenic trioxide, asparaginase, atenolol, atracurium, azithromycin, aztreonam, bivalirudin, bleomycin, bumetanide, buprenorphine, butorphanol, calcium chloride/gluconate, capreomycin, CARBOplatin, carmustine, caspofungin, ceFAZolin, cefoperazone, cefoTEtan, cefOXitin, cefTAZidime, ceftizoxime, cefTRIAXone, cefuroxime, chlorproMAZINE, cimetidine, ciprofloxacin, cisatracurium, CISplatin, cladribine, clindamycin, codeine, cyclophosphamide, cycloSPORINE, cytarabine, D₅W-dextrose 5%, dacarbazine, DACTINomycin, DAPTOmycin, DAUNOrubicin, DAUNOrubicin citrate liposome, dexamethasone, dexmedetomidine, dexrazoxane, digoxin, diltiazem, diphenhydrAMINE, DOBUTamine, DOCEtaxel, dolasetron, DOPamine, doxacurium, doxapram, DOXOrubicin, DOXOrubicin liposomal, doxycycline, droperidol, enalaprilat, ePHEDrine, EPINEPHrine, epirubicin, ertapenem, erythromycin, esmolol, etoposide, famotidine, fenoldopam, fentaNYL, filgrastim, fluconazole, fludarabine, fluorouracil, foscarnet, fosphenytoin, gallium, ganciclovir, garenoxacin, gatifloxacin, gemcitabine, gentamicin, granisetron, haloperidol, heparin, hydrocortisone sodium phosphate/succinate, HYDROmorphone, hydrOXYzine, ifosfamide, imipenem-cilastatin, inamrinone, insulin, regular, isoproterenol, ketorolac, labetalol, lepirudin, leucovorin, levofloxacin, levorphanol, lidocaine, linezolid, LORazepam, magnesium sulfate, mannitol, mechlorethamine, melphalan, meperidine, meropenem, mesna, methadone, methohexital, methotrexate, methylPREDNISolone, metoclopramide, metoprolol, metroNIDAZOLE, midazolam, milrinone, minocycline, mitoMYcin, mitoXANtrone, mivacurium, morphine, moxifloxacin, nalbuphine, naloxone, nesiritide, niCARdipine, nitroglycerin, nitroprusside, norepinephrine, octreotide, ondansetron, oxaliplatin, PACLitaxel (solvent/surfactant), palonosetron, pamidronate, pancuronium, PEMEtrexed, pentamidine, pentazocine, PENTobarbital, PHENobarbital, phenylephrine, piperacillin, piperacillin–tazobactam, potassium acetate/chloride/phosphates, procainamide, prochlorperazine, promethazine, propranolol, quinupristin-dalfopristin, ranitidine, remifentanil, riTUXimab, rocuronium, sargramostim, sodium acetate/phosphates, succinylcholine, SUFentanil, sulfamethoxazole-trimethoprim, tacrolimus, teniposide, theophylline, thiopental, thiotepa, ticarcillin, ticarcillin–clavulanate, tigecycline, tirofiban, tobramycin, topotecan, trastuzumab, trimethobenzamide, vancomycin, vasopressin, vecuronium, verapamil, vinBLAStine, vinorelbine, voriconazole, zidovudine, zoledronic acid

Y-site incompatibilities: Amphotericin B conventional colloidal, cefepime, diazepam, gemtuzumab, IDArubicin, lansoprazole, nafcillin, pantoprazole, phenytoin

IV route (vinCRIStine liposomal)
Supplied in single-use kit; inspect for particulates after preparation in pharmacy; give using separate line over 1 hr

ADVERSE EFFECTS
CNS: *Decreased reflexes, numbness, weakness, motor difficulties,* CNS depression, cranial nerve paralysis, **seizures,** peripheral neuropathy
CV: Orthostatic hypotension
EENT: *Diplopia*
GI: *Nausea, vomiting, anorexia, stomatitis,* **constipation, paralytic ileus, abdominal pain, hepatotoxicity**
GU: **Renal tubular obstruction**
HEMA: **Thrombocytopenia, leukopenia, myelosuppression, anemia**
INTEG: *Alopecia,* extravasation
SYST: **Tumor lysis syndrome (TLS)**

V

Pharmacokinetics

Absorption	Complete bioavailability
Distribution	Rapidly, widely distributed; crosses blood-brain barrier
Metabolism	Liver
Excretion	Biliary, in feces, crosses placenta
Half-life	Triphasic <5 min, 50-155 min, 23-85 hr

Pharmacodynamics

Onset	Unknown
Peak	Unknown
Duration	1 wk

INTERACTIONS
Individual drugs
Digoxin: decreased digoxin level

MitoMYcin-C: increased acute pulmonary reactions

Radiation: increased toxicity, bone marrow suppression; do not use together

Drug classifications
CYP3A4 inducers (barbiturates, bosentan, carBAMazepine, efavirenz, phenytoins, nevirapine, rifabutin, rifampin): decreased vinCRIStine effect

CYP3A4 inhibitors (aprepitant, antiretroviral protease inhibitors, clarithromycin, danazol, delavirdine, diltiazem, erythromycin, fluconazole, FLUoxetine, fluvoxaMINE, imatinib, ketoconazole, mibefradil, nefazodone, telithromycin, voriconazole): increased toxicity

Peripheral nervous system products: increased neurotoxicity

Vaccines/toxoids: decreased immune response

Drug/herb
St. John's wort: avoid use

Drug/lab test
Increased: uric acid

Decreased: Hgb, WBC, platelets, sodium

NURSING CONSIDERATIONS
Assessment
• Monitor CBC, differential, platelet count weekly; withhold product if WBC is <4000/mm³ or platelet count is <75,000/mm³; notify prescriber of results; platelets may increase or decrease

• Assess neurologic status: paresthesia, weakness, cranial nerve palsies, orthostatic hypotension, lethargy, agitation, psychosis; notify prescriber

• **Bronchospasm:** more common with mitoMYcin

• Identify for increased uric acid levels, joint pain in extremities; increase fluid intake to 2-3 L/day unless contraindicated

⚠ Tumor lysis syndrome: hyperkalemia, hyperphosphatemia, hyperuricemia, hypocalcemia; more common in leukemia, lymphoma, use alkalinization of urine with allopurinol, monitor electrolytes, renal function (BUN, urine, CCR, uric acid)

> **BLACK BOX WARNING:** Extravasation: Assess for pain, swelling, poor blood return; if extravasation occurs, local injection of hyaluronidase and moderate heat to area may help disperse product

Patient/family education
• Teach patient to avoid use of products containing aspirin or NSAIDs, razors, commercial mouthwash because bleeding may occur; to report symptoms of bleeding (hematuria, tarry stools)

• Instruct patient to report signs of anemia (fatigue, headache, irritability, faintness, shortness of breath)

• Caution patient to report any changes in breathing or coughing, even several mo after treatment

⚠ Pregnancy: instruct patient to notify prescriber if pregnancy is planned or suspected; advise patient that contraception will be necessary during and 2 mo after treatment; may be teratogenic, pregnancy D, avoid breastfeeding

• Inform patient that hair may be lost during treatment; a wig or hairpiece may make patient feel better; new hair will be different in color, texture

• Advise patient to avoid vaccinations during treatment; serious reactions may occur

• Teach patient to report signs/symptoms of infection: fever, chills, sore throat; patient should avoid crowds or persons with known infections

• Advise patient to increase fluids, bulk in diet, exercise to prevent constipation

⚠ Infection: instruct patient to report sore throat, fever, flulike symptoms; avoid persons with known infection

Evaluation
Positive therapeutic outcome
• Decreased spread of malignancies

⚠ HIGH ALERT

vinorelbine (Rx)

(vi-nor'el-bine)

Navelbine

Func. class.: Antineoplastic—
miscellaneous

Chem. class.: Semisynthetic vinca alkaloid

Pregnancy category D

ACTION: Inhibits mitotic spindle activity, arrests cell cycle at metaphase; inhibits RNA synthesis, blocks cellular use of glutamic acid needed for purine synthesis; a vesicant

Therapeutic outcome: Decreased spread of malignancy

USES: Unresectable, advanced non–small-cell lung cancer (NSCLC) stage IV; may be used alone or in combination with cisplatin for stage III or IV NSCLC

CONTRAINDICATIONS

Pregnancy **D**, breastfeeding, hypersensitivity, infants, granulocyte count <1000 cells/mm³ pretreatment

> **BLACK BOX WARNING:** Severe neutropenia, intrathecal use

Precautions: Children, geriatric, hepatic/pulmonary/neurologic/renal disease, bone marrow suppression

> **BLACK BOX WARNING:** Extravasation

DOSAGE AND ROUTES

Adult: **IV** 30 mg/m² qwk

ANC: 1000-1499, give 50% dose; <1000 hold dose; <1000 × 3 wk, discontinue

Hepatic dose

Adult: **IV** total bilirubin 2.1-3 mg/dl 15 mg/m² qwk; total bilirubin ≥3 mg/dl 7.5 mg/m²/day

Available forms: Inj 10 mg/ml

Implementation

> **BLACK BOX WARNING:** Do not give intrathecally: fatal

> **BLACK BOX WARNING:** Hyaluronidase 150 units/ml in 1 ml of 0.9% NaCl, warm compress for extravasation for vesicant activity treatment

• Antacid before oral agent; give product after evening meal before bedtime

Intermittent IV infusion route

• Dilute to 0.5-2 mg/ml with 0.9% NaCl, 0.45% NaCl, D₅W, D₅/0.45% NaCl, LR, Ringer's; give over 6-10 min into Y-site or central line; flush line

Continuous IV infusion route

• Give 40 mg/m² q3wk after **IV** bol of 8 mg/m²; may be given in combination with DOXOrubicin, fluorouracil, cisplatin

Y-site compatibilities: Amikacin, aztreonam, bleomycin, buprenorphine, butorphanol, calcium gluconate, CARBOplatin, cefotaxime, CISplatin, cimetidine, clindamycin, dexamethasone, enalaprilat, etoposide, famotidine, filgrastim, fluconazole, fludarabine, gentamicin, hydrocortisone, LORazepam, meperidine, morphine, netilmicin, ondansetron, plicamycin, streptozocin, teniposide, ticarcillin, tobramycin, vancomycin, vinBLAStine, vinCRIStine, zidovudine

ADVERSE EFFECTS

CNS: Paresthesias, peripheral neuropathy, depression, headache, **seizures**, weakness, jaw pain, asthenia

CV: Chest pain

GI: *Nausea, vomiting,* ileus, *anorexia, stomatitis,* constipation, abdominal pain, *diarrhea,* **hepatotoxicity, GI obstruction/perforation**

HEMA: **Neutropenia, anemia, thrombocytopenia, granulocytopenia**

INTEG: *Rash, alopecia,* photosensitivity, inj site reaction, necrosis

META: Syndrome of inappropriate diuretic hormone

MS: Myalgia

RESP: Shortness of breath, **dyspnea, pulmonary edema, acute bronchospasm, acute respiratory distress syndrome (ARDS)**

Pharmacokinetics

Absorption	Poor bioavailability (<50%)
Distribution	Highly bound to platelets, lymphocytes
Metabolism	Liver, to metabolite
Excretion	Bile
Half-life	43 hr

Pharmacodynamics

Onset	Unknown
Peak	1-2 hr
Duration	Unknown

INTERACTIONS

Drug classifications

NSAIDs, anticoagulants: increased bleeding risk

CYP3A4 inhibitors (antiretroviral protease inhibitors, aprepitant, clarithromycin,

Adverse effects: *italics* = common; **bold** = life-threatening

danazol, delavirdine, diltiazem, erythromycin, fluconazole, FLUoxetine, fluvoxaMINE, imatinib, ketoconazole, mibefradil, nefazodone, telithromycin, voriconazole): increased toxicity

CYP3A4 inducers (barbiturates, bosentan, carBAMazepine, efavirenz, phenytoins, nevirapine, rifabutin, rifampin): decreased vinorelbine effect

Drug/herb
St. John's wort: avoid use

Drug/lab test
Increased: LFTs, bilirubin
Decreased: Hgb, WBC, platelets

NURSING CONSIDERATIONS
Assessment
• Monitor B/P (baseline and q15min) during administration

> **BLACK BOX WARNING:** Monitor CBC, differential, platelet count before each dose; withhold product if WBC is <4000/mm³ or platelet count is <75,000/mm³; notify prescriber of results; recovery will take 3 wk; liver function tests: AST, ALT, bilirubin, LDH

⚠ **Bronchospasm:** more common with mitoMYcin; also dyspnea, wheezing; may be treated with oxygen, bronchodilators, corticosteroids, especially if there is underlying pulmonary disease

• Assess for dyspnea, crackles, unproductive cough, chest pain, tachypnea
• Monitor renal function tests: BUN, serum uric acid, urine CCr before, during therapy, I&O ratio; report fall in urine output of 30 ml/hr; for decreased hyperuricemia
• Monitor for cold, fever, sore throat (may indicate beginning **infection**); notify prescriber if these occur; effects of alopecia on body image
• **Assess for bleeding:** hematuria, guaiac, bruising or petechiae, mucosa or orifices q8hr: no rectal temp; avoid IM inj; use pressure on venipuncture sites
• **Assess for symptoms indicating severe allergic reactions: rash, pruritus, urticaria, itching, flushing, bronchospasm, hypotension; EPINEPHrine and resuscitative equipment should be nearby**
• Assess neurologic status: numbness, pain, tingling, loss of Achilles reflex, weakness, palsies

Patient/family education
• Teach patient to use liquid diet: cola, gelatin; dry toast or crackers may be added if patient is not nauseated or vomiting

• Advise patient to rinse mouth 3-4 ×/day with water and brush teeth 2-3 ×/day with soft brush or cotton-tipped applicators for stomatitis; use unwaxed dental floss
• Advise patient to avoid crowds, people with infections, vaccinations
• **Pregnancy: notify prescriber if pregnancy is planned or suspected; advise patient to use effective contraception during and for ≥2 mo after product is discontinued; pregnancy D, avoid breastfeeding**
• Teach patient hair may be lost but will grow back; new hair may be different texture, color
⚠ **Infection: report sore throat, fever, flulike symptoms**

Evaluation
Positive therapeutic outcome
• Decreased spread of malignant cells

> ⚠ **HIGH ALERT**

vismodegib
(vis′moe-deg′ib)
Erivedge
Func. class.: Antineoplastic biologic response modifier
Chem. class.: Signal transduction inhibitor (STI)
Pregnancy category: D

ACTION: A hedgehog (Hh) signaling pathway inhibitor

Therapeutic outcome: Decreased spread of tumor

USES: Patients who have metastatic basal cell carcinoma, locally advanced, that has recurred after surgery and who are not candidates for surgery/radiation

CONTRAINDICATIONS
Hypersensitivity, breastfeeding

> **BLACK BOX WARNING:** Intrauterine fetal death, male-mediated teratogenicity, pregnancy **(D)**

Precautions: Children, blood donation

DOSAGE AND ROUTES
Adult: PO 150 mg/day

Available forms: Cap 150 mg

Implementation
• Give without regard to food
• To be swallowed whole, do not open or crush caps

- If a dose is missed, do not take additional dose, take at usual time
- Store at 77°F (25°C)

ADVERSE EFFECTS

GI: Nausea, vomiting, dysgeusia
GU: Amenorrhea, azotemia
INTEG: Alopecia
META: Hyponatremia
MISC: Fatigue, decreased weight
MS: Arthralgia

Pharmacokinetics

Absorption	Unknown
Distribution	Protein binding >99%
Metabolism	Unknown
Excretion	Unknown
Half-life	Elimination 4 days

Pharmacodynamics

Onset	Unknown
Peak	Unknown
Duration	Unknown

INTERACTIONS

Drug classifications

Pgp inhibitors (amiodarone, clarithromycin, cycloSPORINE, diltiazem, erythromycin, indinavir, itraconazole, ketoconazole, nelfinavir, niCARdipine, propafenone, quiNIDine, ritonavir, saquinavir, tacrolimus, tamoxifen, verapamil); CYP2C19 substrates (amitriptyline, clomiPRAMINE, imipramine, citalopram, diazepam, phenytoin, PHENobarbital, lansoprazole, omeprazole, pantoprazole, RABEprazole, esomeprazole, clopidogrel, proguanil, propranolol, carisoprodol, chloramphenicol, cyclophosphamide, indomethacin, nelfinavir, nilutamide, progesterone, teniposide, warfarin): Increased effect of each product

NURSING CONSIDERATIONS

Assessment

> **BLACK BOX WARNING: Pregnancy D:** Verify pregnancy status of all women within 7 days before starting therapy; effective contraception is needed during and for 7 mo after treatment; men receiving this product should use condoms with spermicide (even after vasectomy) during sexual intercourse with female partners and for 2 mo after the last dose; report exposure during pregnancy to the Genentech Adverse Event Line

Patient/family education

> **BLACK BOX WARNING: Pregnancy D:** Teach patient to notify their provider immediately if pregnancy is suspected (or in a female partner for male patients); effective contraception is needed during and for 7 mo after treatment; men receiving this product should use condoms with spermicide (even after vasectomy) during sexual intercourse with female partners and for 2 mo after the last dose; if product is used during pregnancy or if the patient becomes pregnant during use, the woman (or female partner for male patients) should be apprised of the potential hazard to the fetus; encourage exposed women (either directly or through seminal fluid) to participate in the ERIVEDGE pregnancy pharmacovigilance program

- Teach patient about reason for treatment, expected results
- Teach patient if dose is missed, do not take, but resume scheduled doses; swallow whole
- Tell patient not to donate blood during therapy or for ≥7 months after conclusion of product

Evaluation

Positive therapeutic outcome
- Decreased spread of tumor

vitamin A (PO, OTC; IM, Rx)

Aquasol A, Del-Vi-A, Vitamin A
Func. class.: Vitamin, fat-soluble
Chem. class.: Retinol
Pregnancy category C (PO); X (parenteral)

ACTION: Needed for normal bone and tooth development, visual dark adaptation, skin disease, mucosa tissue repair; assists in production of adrenal steroids, cholesterol, RNA

Therapeutic outcome: Prevention, absence of vit A deficiency

USES: Vit A deficiency

CONTRAINDICATIONS

Pregnancy **X** (parenteral), hypersensitivity to vit A, malabsorption syndrome (PO), hypervitaminosis A, parenteral, **IV** administration

Precautions: Pregnancy **C** (PO), breastfeeding, impaired renal function, children, hepatic disease, infants, alcoholism, hepatitis

DOSAGE AND ROUTES
Adult and child >8 yr: PO 100,000-500,000 international units/day × 3 days, then 50,000 international units/day × 2 wk; dose based on severity of deficiency; maintenance 10,000-20,000 international units for 2 mo
Child 1-8 yr: IM 5000-15,000 international units/day × 10 days
Infant <1 yr: IM 5000-15,000 international units × 10 days

Maintenance
Child 4-8 yr: IM 15,000 international units/day × 2 mo
Child <4 yr: IM 10,000 international units/ day × 2 mo

Available forms: Caps 10,000, 25,000, 50,000 international units; drops 5000 international units; inj 50,000 international units/ml; tabs 10,000, 25,000, 50,000 international units

Implementation
PO route
• Give with food (PO) for better absorption; do not give **IV** because anaphylaxis may occur, IM only
• Oral preparations are not indicated for vit A deficiency in those with malabsorption syndrome
• Store in airtight, light-resistant container
IM route
• Give deep in large muscle mass; do not use deltoid muscle for administration of >1 ml

ADVERSE EFFECTS
CNS: Headache, increased ICP, intracranial hypertension, lethargy, malaise
EENT: Gingivitis, papilledema, exophthalmos, inflammation of tongue and lips
GI: Nausea, vomiting, anorexia, abdominal pain, *jaundice*
INTEG: Drying of skin, pruritus, increased pigmentation, night sweats, alopecia
META: Hypomenorrhea, hypercalcemia
MS: Arthralgia, retarded growth, hard areas on bone

Pharmacokinetics

Absorption	Rapidly absorbed
Distribution	Stored in liver, kidneys, lungs
Metabolism	Liver
Excretion	Breast milk
Half-life	Unknown

Pharmacodynamics

Unknown

INTERACTIONS
Individual drugs
Cholestyramine, colestipol, mineral oil: decreased absorption of vit A

Drug classifications
Contraceptives (oral), corticosteroids: increased levels of vit A

Drug/lab test
False increase: bilirubin, serum cholesterol

NURSING CONSIDERATIONS
Assessment
• Assess nutritional status: increase intake of yellow and dark green vegetables, yellow/orange fruits, vit A–fortified foods, liver, egg yolks
• Assess vit A deficiency: decreased growth; night blindness; dry, brittle nails; hair loss; urinary stones; increased infection; hyperkeratosis of skin; drying of cornea
• Identify vit A deficiency by plasma vit A, carotene level
• Assess for chronic vit A toxicity: increased calcium, BUN, glucose, cholesterol, triglyceride level

Patient/family education
• Instruct patient that if dose is missed, it should be omitted
• Inform patient that ophth exams may be required periodically throughout therapy
• Instruct patient not to use mineral oil while taking this product because absorption will be decreased
• Advise patient to notify prescriber of nausea, vomiting, lip cracking, loss of hair, headache
• Caution patient not to take more than the prescribed amount

Evaluation
Positive therapeutic outcome
• Increase in growth rate, weight
• Absence of dry skin and mucous membranes, night blindness

TREATMENT OF OVERDOSE:
Discontinue product

vitamin A acid
See tretinoin

vitamin B₁
See thiamine

vitamin B₁₂ (cyano-cobalamin) (PO, OTC; IM/SUBCUT, Rx)

(sye-an-oh-koe-bal′a-min)
Alphamin, Anacobin ✤, Bedoz ✤, Cobex, Cobolin-M Crystamine, Crysti-1000, Cyanabin ✤, Cyanoject, Cyomin, Ener-B, Hydrobexan, Hydro Cobex, Hydro-Crysti-12

Func. class.: Vitamin B₁₂, water-soluble vitamin

vitamin B₁₂a (hydroxocobalamin) (vit B₁₂) (Rx)

(hye-drox′o-ko-bal′a-min)
Hydro Cobex, Hydroxycobal, LA-12, Nascobal, Neuroforter, Rubesol-1000, Rubramin PC, Shovite, Vibral LA, Vibral, Vitamin B₁₂
Pregnancy category A

ACTION: Needed for adequate nerve functioning, protein and carbohydrate metabolism, normal growth, RBC development and cell reproduction

Therapeutic outcome: Prevention, correction of vit B₁₂ deficiency

USES: Vit B₁₂ deficiency; pernicious anemia; vit B₁₂ malabsorption syndrome; Schilling test; increased requirements with pregnancy, thyrotoxicosis, hemolytic anemia, hemorrhage, renal and hepatic disease

CONTRAINDICATIONS
Hypersensitivity, optic nerve atrophy

Precautions: Pregnancy **A**, breastfeeding, children

DOSAGE AND ROUTES
Cyanocobalamin
Adult: PO up to 1000 mcg/day; SUBCUT/IM 30-100 mcg/day × 1 wk, then 100-200 mcg/mo

Shilling test
Adult and child: IM 1000 mcg in 1 dose
Child: PO up to 1000 mcg/day; SUBCUT/IM 30-50 mcg/day × 2 wk, then 100 mcg/mo; NASAL 500 mcg qwk

Hydroxocobalamin
Adult: SUBCUT/IM 30-50 mcg/day × 5-10 days, then 100-200 mcg/mo
Child: SUBCUT/IM 30-50 mcg/day × 5-10 days, then 30-50 mcg/mo

Available forms: Cyanocobalamin: tabs 25, 50, 100, 250, 500, 1000, 5000 mcg; ext rel tabs 100, 200, 500, 1000 mcg; lozenges: 100, 250, 500 mcg; nasal gel 500 mcg/spray; inj 100, 1000 mcg/ml; hydroxocobalamin: inj 1000 mcg/ml

Implementation
PO route
• Give with fruit juice to disguise taste; administer immediately after mixing
• Give with meals if possible for better absorption; large doses should not be used because most is excreted

IM route
• Give by IM inj for pernicious anemia for life unless contraindicated

IV route
• May be mixed with TPN sol, but **IV** route is not recommended

Y-site compatibilities: Heparin, hydrocortisone sodium succinate, potassium chloride

Solution compatibilities: Dextrose/Ringer's or LR's combinations, dextrose/saline combinations, D₅W, D₁₀W, 0.45% NaCl, Ringer's or LR's sol, ascorbic acid

ADVERSE EFFECTS
CNS: Flushing, optic nerve atrophy
CV: **CHF**, peripheral vascular thrombosis, **pulmonary edema**
GI: *Diarrhea*
INTEG: Itching, rash, pain at inj site
META: Hypokalemia
SYST: **Anaphylactic shock**

Pharmacokinetics

Absorption	Well absorbed (IM, SUBCUT)
Distribution	Crosses placenta
Metabolism	Stored in liver, kidney, stomach
Excretion	50%-90% (urine), breast milk
Half-life	Unknown

Pharmacodynamics
Unknown

INTERACTIONS
Individual drugs
Aminosalicylic acid, chloramphenicol, cimetidine, colchicine: decreased absorption
PredniSONE: increased absorption

Drug classifications
Aminoglycosides, anticonvulsants, potassium products: decreased absorption

V

Drug/herb
Goldenseal: decreased vit B_{12} absorption

Drug/lab test
False positive: intrinsic factor

NURSING CONSIDERATIONS
Assessment
• Assess for deficiency: anorexia, dyspepsia on exertion, palpitations, paresthesias, psychosis, visual disturbances, pallor, red inflamed tongue, neuropathy, edema of legs
• Monitor potassium levels during beginning treatment in patients with megaloblastic anemia
• Monitor CBC for increase in reticulocyte count during 1st wk of therapy, then increase in RBC and hemoglobin; folic acid levels, vit B_{12} levels
• Assess nutritional status: egg yolks, fish, organ meats, dairy products, clams, oysters, which are good sources of vit B_{12}
• Monitor for pulmonary edema or worsening of CHF in cardiac patients

Patient/family education
• Instruct patient that treatment must continue for life if diagnosed as having pernicious anemia
• Advise patient to eat well-balanced diet from the food pyramid and comply with dietary recommendation
• Caution patient not to exceed the RDA of vit B_{12} because adverse reactions may occur

Evaluation
Positive therapeutic outcome
• Decreased anorexia, dyspnea on exertion, palpitations, paresthesias, psychosis, visual disturbances, edema of legs
• Prevention or correction of vit B_{12} deficiency

TREATMENT OF OVERDOSE:
Discontinue products

---

vitamin C (ascorbic acid) (OTC, Rx)
(as-kor'bic)
Acerca C, Apo-C ✽, Ascor L-500, Cenolate, Equaline Vitamin C, Walgreens Gold Seal, and many more
Func. class.: Vitamin C, water-soluble vitamin
Pregnancy category C

ACTION: Needed for wound healing, collagen synthesis, antioxidant, carbohydrate metabolism

Therapeutic outcome: Replacement and supplementation of vit C

USES: Vit C deficiency, scurvy, delayed wound and bone healing, chronic disease, before gastrectomy, dietary supplement

Unlabeled uses: Common cold prevention

CONTRAINDICATIONS
Tartrazine, sulfite sensitivity; G6PD deficiency

Precautions: Pregnancy **C**, gout, diabetes, renal calculi (large doses)

DOSAGE AND ROUTES
RDA
Neonate and up to 6 mo: PO 30 mg/day
Infant: PO 40-50 mg/day
Child 1-3 yr: PO 15 mg/day
Child 4-8 yr: PO 25 mg/day
Child 9-13 yr: PO 45 mg/day
Child 14-18 yr: PO 65 mg/day (females), 75 mg/day (males)
Adult: PO 50-500 mg/day

Scurvy
Adult: PO/SUBCUT/IM/**IV** 100 mg-250 mg daily × 2 wk, then 50 mg or more daily
Child: PO/SUBCUT/IM/**IV** 100-300 mg daily × 2 wk, then 35 mg or more daily

Wound healing/chronic disease/ fracture
May be given with zinc
Adult: SUBCUT/IM/**IV**/PO 200-500 mg daily for 1-2 mo
Child: SUBCUT/IM/**IV**/PO 100-200 mg added doses for 1-2 mo

Urine acidification
Adult: 4-12 g daily in divided doses
Child: 500 mg q6-8hr

Available forms: Tabs 25, 50, 100, 250, 500, 1000, 1500 mg; effervescent tabs 1000 mg; chewable tabs 100, 250, 500 mg; time-release tabs 500, 750, 1000, 1500 mg; time-release caps 500 mg; crystals 4 g/tsp; powder 4 g/tsp; liquid 35 mg/0.6 ml; sol 100 mg/ml; syr 20 mg/ml, 500 mg/5 ml; inj SUBCUT, IM, **IV** 100, 250, 500 mg/ml

Implementation
PO route
• Swallow time rel tabs or caps whole; do not break, crush, or chew
• Mix oral sol with foods or fluids
IM route
• Not to be diluted; give deep in large muscle mass

IV, direct route
• Give undiluted by *direct* **IV** 100 mg over at least 1 min, rapid inf may cause fainting

---

Intermittent IV infusion route
- Give by intermittent inf after diluting with D_5W, $D_{10}W$, 0.9% NaCl, 0.45% NaCl, LR, Ringer's sol, dextrose/saline, dextrose/Ringer's combinations; temp will increase pressure in ampules; wrap with gauze before breaking

Syringe compatibilities: Metoclopramide, aminophylline, theophylline

Syringe incompatibilities: CeFAZolin, doxapram

Y-site compatibilities: Warfarin

ADVERSE EFFECTS
CNS: Headache, insomnia, dizziness, fatigue, flushing
GI: Nausea, vomiting, diarrhea, anorexia, heartburn, cramps
GU: Polyuria, urine acidification, oxalate or urate renal stones, dysuria
HEMA: Hemolytic anemia in patients with G6PD
INTEG: Inflammation at inj site

Pharmacokinetics

Absorption	Readily absorbed (PO)
Distribution	Widely distributed; crosses placenta
Metabolism	Oxidation
Excretion	Kidneys, inactive; breast milk
Half-life	Unknown

Pharmacodynamics

Unknown

INTERACTIONS
Drug/lab test
False positive: negative in glucose tests (Clinitest, Tes-Tape)
False negative: occult blood (large dose), urine bilirubin, leukocyte determination

NURSING CONSIDERATIONS
Assessment
- Assess nutritional status for inclusion of foods high in vit C: citrus fruits, cantaloupe, tomatoes
- Assess for vit C deficiency before, during, and after treatment; scurvy (gingivitis, bleeding gums, loose teeth); poor bone development
- Monitor I&O ratio, polyuria; in patients receiving large doses, renal stones may occur; urine pH (acidification)
- Monitor ascorbic acid levels throughout treatment if continued deficiency is suspected
- Assess inj sites for inflammation, pain, redness, thrombophlebitis if in large doses

Patient/family education
- Teach patient necessary foods to be included in diet that are rich in vit C: citrus fruits, cantaloupe, tomatoes, chili peppers (red)
- Teach patient that smoking decreases vit C levels; not to exceed prescribed dose; increases will be excreted in urine, except time release
- Teach patient not to exceed RDA recommended dose, urinary stones may occur
- Teach patient using ascorbic acid for acidification of urine to test urine pH periodically

Evaluation
Positive therapeutic outcome
- Absence of anorexia, irritability, pallor, joint pain, hyperkeratosis, petechiae, poor wound healing
- Reversal of scurvy: bleeding gums, gingivitis, loose teeth

---

vitamin D (cholecalciferol, vitamin D₃ or ergocalciferol, vitamin D₂) (Rx, OTC)
Calciferol, Delta-D, Drisdol, Radiostol ✦, Radiostol Forte ✦, vitamin D, vitamin D₃
Func. class.: Vitamin D
Chem. class.: Fat-soluble vitamin
Pregnancy category C

Do not confuse: Calciferol/calcitriol

ACTION: Needed for regulation of calcium, phosphate levels; normal bone development; parathyroid activity; neuromuscular functioning

Therapeutic outcome: Prevention of rickets, osteomalacia, normal calcium/phosphate levels

USES: Vit D deficiency, rickets, renal osteodystrophy, hypoparathyroidism, hypophosphatemia, psoriasis, rheumatoid arthritis

CONTRAINDICATIONS
Hypersensitivity, hypercalcemia, renal dysfunction, hyperphosphatemia

Precautions: Pregnancy **C**, CV disease, renal calculi

DOSAGE AND ROUTES
Deficiency
Adult: PO/IM 12,000 international units/day, then increased to 500,000 international units/day
Child: PO/IM 1500-5000 international units/day × 2-4 wk, may repeat after 2 wk or 600,000 international units as single dose

Hypoparathyroidism

Adult and child: PO/IM 200,000 international units given with 4 g calcium tab

Available forms: Tabs 400, 1000, 50,000 international units; caps 25,000, 50,000 international units; oral sol 8000 international units/ml; inj 500,000 international units/ml, 500,000 international units/5 ml

Implementation

PO route

• PO may be increased q4wk depending on blood level
• Store in airtight, light-resistant container at room temperature

IM route

• Give inj deeply in large muscle mass, administer slowly, aspirate to avoid **IV** administration, rotate inj site

ADVERSE EFFECTS

CNS: Fatigue, weakness, drowsiness, **seizures,** headache, psychosis
CV: Hypertension, dysrhythmias
GI: Nausea, vomiting, anorexia, cramps, diarrhea, constipation, metallic taste, dry mouth
GU: Polyuria, nocturia, **hematuria, albuminuria, renal failure,** decreased libido
INTEG: Pruritus, photophobia
MS: Decreased bone growth, early joint pain, early muscle pain

Pharmacokinetics

Absorption	Well absorbed
Distribution	Stored in liver
Metabolism	Liver, sun
Excretion	Bile, kidney
Half-life	12-22 hr

Pharmacodynamics

	PO	IM
Onset	Unknown	Unknown
Peak	4 hr	Unknown
Duration	15-20 days	Unknown

INTERACTIONS

Individual drugs

Cholestyramine, colestipol, PHENobarbital, phenytoin: decreased effects of vit D
Verapamil: increased toxicity

Drug classifications

Antacids, diuretics (thiazide): increased toxicity

NURSING CONSIDERATIONS

Assessment

• Monitor BUN, urinary calcium, AST, ALT, cholesterol, creatinine, uric acid, chloride, magnesium, electrolytes, urine pH, phosphate—may increase; calcium should be kept at 9-10 mg/dl; vit D at 50-135 international units/dl, phosphate at 70 mg/dl; alkaline phosphatase may be decreased
• Monitor for increased blood level; toxic reactions may occur rapidly
• Assess for dry mouth, metallic taste, polyuria, bone pain, muscle weakness, headache, fatigue, tinnitus, change in LOC, irregular pulse, dysrhythmias, increased respirations, anorexia, nausea, vomiting, cramps, diarrhea, constipation; may indicate hypercalcemia
• Assess renal status: decreased urinary output (oliguria, anuria), edema in extremities, weight gain ≥5 lb, periorbital edema
• Assess nutritional status, diet for sources of vit D (milk, cod, halibut, salmon, sardines, egg yolk), calcium (dairy products, dark green vegetables), phosphates (dairy products)

Patient/family education

• Advise patient to omit dose if missed; to avoid vitamin supplements unless directed by prescriber
• Inform patient of necessary foods to be included in diet
• Advise patient to keep appointments for evaluation because therapeutic and toxic levels are narrow
• Instruct patient to report weakness, lethargy, headache, anorexia, loss of weight; to report nausea, vomiting, abdominal cramps, diarrhea, constipation, excessive thirst, polyuria, muscle and bone pain
• Caution patient to decrease intake of antacids and laxatives containing magnesium

Evaluation

Positive therapeutic outcome

• Calcium levels 9-10 ml/dl
• Decreasing symptoms of bone disease

vitamin E (OTC)

Aquasol E

Func. class.: Vitamin E
Chem. class.: Fat-soluble vitamin

Pregnancy category A

ACTION: Needed for digestion and metabolism of polyunsaturated fats, decreases platelet aggregation, decreases blood clot formation, promotes normal growth and development of muscle tissue, prostaglandin synthesis

Therapeutic outcome: Prevention and treatment of vit E deficiency

USES: Vit E deficiency, impaired fat absorption, hemolytic anemia in premature neonates, prevention of retrolental fibroplasia, sickle cell anemia, supplement in malabsorption syndrome

CONTRAINDICATIONS

IV use in infants

Precautions: Pregnancy **A**, anemia, breast-feeding, hypothrombinemia

DOSAGE AND ROUTES

Deficiency
Adult: PO 60-75 international units/day
Child: PO 1 international unit/kg (malabsorption)

Prevention of deficiency
Adult: PO 30 international units/day
Infant: PO 5 international units/day

Topical route
Adult and child: TOP apply to affected areas as needed

Available forms: Caps 100, 200, 400, 500, 600, 1000 international units; tabs 100, 200, 400 international units; drops 15 mg/0.3 ml; chew tabs 400 units; ointment, cream, lotion, oil

Implementation
PO route
• Chew chewable tabs well
• Sol may be dropped in mouth or mixed with food
• Store in airtight, light-resistant container
Topical route
• Apply topical to moisturize dry skin

ADVERSE EFFECTS

CNS: Headache, fatigue
CV: Increased risk of thrombophlebitis
EENT: Blurred vision
GI: Nausea, cramps, diarrhea
GU: Gonadal dysfunction
INTEG: Sterile abscess, contact dermatitis
META: Altered metabolism of hormones (thyroid, pituitary, adrenal), altered immunity
MS: Weakness

Pharmacokinetics

Absorption	20%-80% (PO)
Distribution	Widely distributed, stored in fat
Metabolism	Liver
Excretion	Bile
Half-life	Unknown

Pharmacodynamics

Unknown

INTERACTIONS

Individual drugs
Cholestyramine, colestipol, mineral oil, sucralfate: decreased absorption

Drug classification
Anticoagulants (oral): increased action of anticoagulants

NURSING CONSIDERATIONS

Assessment
• Assess nutritional status: intake of wheat germ, dark green leafy vegetables, nuts, eggs, liver, vegetable oils, dairy products, cereals
• Assess for vit E deficiency (usually in neonates): irritability, restlessness, hemolytic anemia

Patient/family education
• Inform patient necessary foods to be included in diet high in vit E
• Instruct patient to omit if dose is missed
• Instruct patient to avoid vit supplements unless directed by prescriber because overdose may occur

Evaluation

Positive therapeutic outcome
• Absence of hemolytic anemia
• Adequate vit E levels
• Improvement in skin lesions
• Decrease in edema

⚠ HIGH ALERT

vorapaxar
(vor′a-pax′ar)
Zontivity
Func. class.: Platelet inhibitor
Pregnancy category B

ACTION: Antagonizes the protease-activated receptor-1 (PAR-1) expressed on platelets

Therapeutic outcome: Absence of MI, stroke

USES: Secondary myocardial infarction prophylaxis or stroke prophylaxis or thrombosis prophylaxis for reduction of thrombotic cardiovascular events in patients with a history of myocardial infarction or with peripheral arterial disease

CONTRAINDICATIONS

BLACK BOX WARNING: Bleeding, intracranial bleeding, stroke

Precautions: Breastfeeding, coronary artery bypass graft surgery (CABG), geriatric patients, hepatic disease, labor, obstetric delivery, pregnancy **B**, renal impairment, surgery

DOSAGE AND ROUTES
Adult: PO 2.08 mg once daily with aspirin and/or clopidogrel

Available forms: Tab 2.08 mg

Implementation
• May be administered without regard to food

ADVERSE EFFECTS
CNS: Depression
EENT: Diplopia, retinopathy
HEMA: Anemia, bleeding
MISC: Rash

Pharmacokinetics

Absorption	Unknown
Distribution	Within 1 week of treatment reaches ≥80% inhibition of thrombin receptor; protein binding 99%
Metabolism	Unknown
Excretion	Primarily feces
Half-life	3-4 days, terminal approximately 8 days

Pharmacodynamics

Onset	Unknown
Peak	1 hr
Duration	Unknown

INTERACTIONS
Drug classifications
Beers Criteria
CYP3A inducers: decreased vorapaxar effect
Other platelet inhibitors, anticoagulants, calcium channel blockers, CYP3A inhibitors, estradiols, NSAIDs, rifampins, salicylates, SNRIs, SSRIs, thrombolytics: increased bleeding risk

NURSING CONSIDERATIONS
Assessment

> **BLACK BOX WARNING:** Assess for bleeding, including intracranial bleeding and stroke during treatment

• Bleeding should be suspected in any patient presenting with hypotension who has recently undergone surgery, coronary angiography, percutaneous coronary intervention (PCI), or CABG

Patient/family education
• Advise patient to report any unusual bruising, bleeding to prescriber; that it may take longer to stop bleeding
• Teach patient to take without regard to food

Evaluation
Positive therapeutic outcome
• Absence of MI, stroke

> **⚠ HIGH ALERT**
>
> ## voriconazole (Rx)
> (vohr-i-kahn′a-zol)
> **Vfend**
> *Func. class.:* Antifungal
> **Pregnancy category D**

Do not confuse: Vfend/Venofer

ACTION: Inhibits fungal CYP 450-mediation demethylation, needed for biosynthesis, causing leakage from cell membrane

Therapeutic outcome: Decreasing signs, symptoms of infection

USES: Invasive aspergillosis, serious fungal infections (*Candida* sp., *Scedosporium apiospermum*, *Fusarium* sp.), *Monosportum, Apiospermum*

CONTRAINDICATIONS
Pregnancy **D**, breastfeeding, children, hypersensitivity, severe bone marrow depression, severe hepatic disease

Precautions: Renal disease (**IV**); Asian/African descent, cardiomyopathy, cholestasis, chemotherapy, lactase deficiency, visual disturbances, renal failure, pancreatitis, QT prolongation, hypokalemia, ventricular dysrhythmias, torsades de pointes

DOSAGE AND ROUTES
Esophageal candidiasis
Adult/geriatric/child ≥12 yr: IV PO **≥40 kg** 200 mg q12hr; **<40 kg** 100 mg q12hr
Adult/geriatric/child ≥12 yr: IV loading dose 6 mg/kg q12hr × 2 dose, then 3-4 mg/kg q12hr; may switch to oral dosing

Candidemia of the skin, kidney, bladder wall, abdomen (non-neutropenic patients)
Adult/child ≥12 yr: IV loading dose 6 mg/kg q12hr × 24 hr, then 3-4 mg/kg q12hr × ≥14 days and ≥7 days after resolution of symptoms; PO after loading dose **>40 kg** 200 mg q12hr × ≥14 days and ≥7 days after resolution of symptoms; **<40 kg** 100 mg q12hr × ≥14 days and ≥7 days after resolution of symptoms

Invasive aspergillosis
Adult/adolescent: IV 6 mg/kg q12hr (loading dose) then 4 mg/kg q12hr, may reduce to 3 mg/kg q12hr if intolerable

---

Child ≥12 yr: IV 6 mg/kg q12hr, then 4 mg/kg q12hr

Renal dose
Adult: PO CCr <50 ml/min, use only orally

Hepatic dose
Adult: PO 6 mg/kg q12hr × 2 doses, then 2 mg/kg q12hr or 100 mg q12hr if ≥40 kg; 50 mg q12hr if <40 kg

Available forms: Tabs 50, 200 mg; powder for inj, lyophilized 200 mg, powder for oral susp 45 g (40 mg/ml after reconstitution)

Implementation
• Give 1 hr before or after meals
• Store at room temperature (powder, tabs)

Intermittent IV infusion route
• Give product only after C&S confirms organism, product needed to treat condition; make sure product is used in life-threatening infections
• Reconstitute powder with 19 ml water for inj to 10 mg/ml, shake until dissolved; infuse over 1-2 hr at a conc of 5 mg/ml or less; do not admix with other products, 4.2% sodium bicarbonate inf

Y-site compatibilities: Acyclovir, alfentanil, allopurinol, amifostine, amikacin, aminocaproic acid, aminophylline, amiodarone, amphotericin B liposome, ampicillin, ampicillin/sulbactam, anidulafungin, azithromycin, aztreonam, bivalirudin, bleomycin, bumetanide, buprenorphine, butorphanol, calcium acetate/chloride/gluconate, CARBOplatin, carmustine, caspofungin, ceFAZolin, cefotaxime, cefoTEtan, cefOXitin, cefTAZidime, ceftizoxime, cefTRIAXone, chloramphenicol, chlorproMAZINE, cimetidine, ciprofloxacin, cisatracurium, CISplatin, clindamycin, cyclophosphamide, cytarabine, dacarbazine, DACTINomycin, DAPTOmycin, DAUNOrubicin, dexamethasone, dexmedetomidine, dexrazoxane, digoxin, diltiazem, diphenhydrAMINE, DOBUTamine, DOCEtaxel, dolasetron, DOPamine, doripenem, doxacurium, doxycycline, droperidol, enalaprilat, ePHEDrine, EPINEPHrine, epirubicin, ertapenem, erythromycin, esmolol, etoposide, etoposide phosphate, famotidine, fenoldopam, fentaNYL, fluconazole, fludarabine, fluorouracil, foscarnet, fosphenytoin, furosemide, ganciclovir, gemcitabine, gentamicin, glycopyrrolate, granisetron, haloperidol, heparin, hydrALAZINE, hydrocortisone, ifosfamide, imipenem/cilastatin, inamrinone, insulin, irinotecan, isoproterenol, ketorolac, labetalol, leucovorin, levofloxacin, lidocaine, linezolid, LORazepam, magnesium sulfate, mannitol, mechlorethamine, melphalan, meperidine, meropenem, mesna, metaraminol, methohexital, methotrexate, methyldopate, methylPREDNISolone, metoclopramide, metoprolol, metroNIDAZOLE, midazolam, milrinone, mitoMYcin, morphine, nafcillin, nalbuphine, naloxone, niCARdipine, nitroglycerin, norepinephrine, octreotide, ondansetron, oxaliplatin, oxytocin, PACLitaxel, palonosetron, pancuronium, pentamidine, pentazocine, PENTobarbital, PHENobarbital, phentolamine, phenylephrine, piperacillin/tazobactam, potassium chloride/phosphates, procainamide, promethazine, propranolol, quinupristin/dalfopristin, remifentanil, rocuronium, sodium acetate/bicarbonate/phosphates, streptozocin, succinylcholine, SUFentanil, tacrolimus, teniposide, theophylline, thiotepa, ticarcillin/clavulanate, tirofiban, tobramycin, topotecan, trimethobenzamide, trimethoprim/sulfamethoxazole, vancomycin, vasopressin, vecuronium, verapamil, vinBLAStine, vinCRIStine, vinorelbine, zidovudine

Y-site incompatibilities: Amphotericin B colloidal, busulfan, cefepime, cyclopSPORINE, dantrolene, diazepam, DOXOrubicin, IDArubicin, mitoXANtrone, nitroprusside, pantoprazole, phenytoin, thiopental

ADVERSE EFFECTS
CNS: *Headache,* paresthesias, peripheral neuropathy, *hallucinations,* psychosis, EPS, depression, Guillain-Barré syndrome, insomnia, **suicidal ideation,** dizziness, fever
CV: **Tachycardia,** hyper/hypotension, vasodilatation, **atrial dysrhythmias, atrial fibrillation, AV block, bradycardia, CHF, MI, QT prolongation, torsades de pointes,** peripheral edema
EENT: Blurred vision, eye hemorrhage, *visual disturbances*
GI: *Nausea, vomiting, anorexia, diarrhea,* cramps, **hemorrhagic gastroenteritis, acute liver failure, hepatitis, intestinal perforation, pancreatitis**
GU: *Hypokalemia,* azotemia, **renal tubular necrosis, permanent renal impairment, anuria, oliguria**
HEMA: Anemia, **eosinophilia,** hypomagnesemia, **thrombocytopenia, leukopenia, pancytopenia**
INTEG: *Burning, irritation,* pain, necrosis at inj site with extravasation, dermatitis, *rash,* photosensitivity
MISC: Respiratory disorder
SYST: **Stevens-Johnson syndrome, toxic epidermal necrolysis, sepsis, melanoma (photosensitivity reaction)**

V

Adverse effects: *italics* = common; **bold** = life-threatening

Pharmacokinetics

Absorption	Unknown
Distribution	Unknown
Metabolism	CYP3A4/CYP2C9
Excretion	Via hepatic metabolism
Half-life	Elimination 6 hr (dose dependent)

Pharmacodynamics

Onset	Unknown
Peak	1-2 hr
Duration	Unknown

INTERACTIONS
Individual drugs

CISplatin, cycloSPORINE, polymyxin B, vancomycin: increased nephrotoxicity

CycloSPORINE, phenytoin, pimozide, predniso-LONE, quiNIDine, rifabutin, sirolimus, tacrolimus, warfarin: increased effects of each specific product

Digoxin: increased hypokalemia

Haloperidol, chloroquine, droperidol, pentamidine; arsenic trioxide, levomethadyl: increased QT prolongation

Drug classifications

Aminoglycosides: increased nephrotoxicity

Benzodiazepines, calcium channel blockers, ergots, HMG-CoA reductase inhibitors, non-nucleoside reverse transcriptase inhibitors, protease inhibitors, proton pump inhibitors, sulfonylureas, vinca alkaloids: increased effects of each specific product

Class IA/III antidysrhythmics, some phenothiazines, beta agonists, local anesthetics, tricyclics, CYP3A4 inhibitors (amiodarone, clarithromycin, erythromycin, telithromycin, troleandomycin); CYP3A4 substrates (methadone, pimozide, QUEtiapine, quiNIDine, risperiDONE, ziprasidone): increased QT prolongation

Corticosteroids, diuretics (thiazide), skeletal muscle relaxants: increased hypokalemia

Drug/herb

St. John's wort: do not use together

Drug/food

High-fat foods: avoid use with high-fat meals, take 1 hr before or after a meal

Drug/lab test

Increased: AST/ALT, alkaline phosphatase, creatinine, bilirubin

Decreased: Hgb/Hct, platelets, WBC

NURSING CONSIDERATIONS
Assessment

• Monitor VS q15-30min during first inf; note changes in pulse, B/P

• Monitor I&O ratio; watch for decreasing urinary output, change in specific gravity; discontinue product to prevent permanent damage to renal tubules

• Monitor blood tests: CBC, K, Na, Ca, Mg q2wk; BUN, creatinine weekly

• Monitor weight weekly; if weight increases >2 lb/wk, edema is present; renal damage should be considered

⚠ Assess for renal toxicity: increasing BUN, serum creatinine; if BUN is >40 mg/dl or if serum creatinine >3 mg/dl, product may be discontinued or dosage reduced

⚠ Assess for hepatotoxicity: increasing AST, ALT, alkaline phosphatase, bilirubin, baseline and periodically

• **Assess for allergic reaction:** dermatitis, rash; product should be discontinued, antihistamines (mild reaction) or EPINEPHrine (severe reaction) administered

• **Assess for hypokalemia:** anorexia, drowsiness, weakness, decreased reflexes, dizziness, increased urinary output, increased thirst, paresthesias

• **Assess for ototoxicity:** tinnitus (ringing, roaring in ears), vertigo, loss of hearing (rare)

• **QT prolongation: ECG for QT prolongation, ejection fraction; assess for chest pain, palpitations, dyspnea**

Patient/family education

• Teach that long-term therapy may be needed to clear infection (2 wk-3 mo depending on type of infection)

• Advise patient to notify prescriber of bleeding, bruising, or soft tissue swelling

• Teach to take 1 hr before or after meal (PO)

• Advise patient not to drive at night because of vision changes

• Advise to avoid strong, direct sunlight

• **Advise women of childbearing age to use effective contraceptive**

Evaluation

Positive therapeutic outcome

• Decreased fever, malaise, rash, negative C&S for infecting organism

vortioxetine

(vor'tye-ox'e-teen)

Brintellix

Func. class.: Antidepressant

Chem. class.: Serotonin modulator

Pregnancy category C

ACTION: Reuptake inhibition at the serotonin transporter and agonist, or antagonist effects at serotonin receptors

Therapeutic outcome: Decreased depression

USES: Major depressive disorder in adults

CONTRAINDICATIONS

Hypersensitivity, MAOI therapy

Precautions: Pregnancy **C**, breastfeeding, seizure disorder, bipolar disorder, hyponatremia, hypovolemia, children, suicidal ideation

DOSAGE AND ROUTES

Adult: PO 10 mg/day, may start with 5 mg/day initially, increase to 20 mg/day as tolerated, max 20 mg/day; poor metabolizers of CYP2D6 max 10 mg/day

Available forms: Tabs 5, 10, 20 mg

Implementation

• Give without regard to food

ADVERSE EFFECTS

CNS: Flushing, mania, vertigo, dizziness, suicidal attempts

GI: Nausea, diarrhea, dyspnea, constipation, vomiting, flatulence

GU: Impotence

INTEG: Pruritus

SYST: Serotonin syndrome, neonatal abstinence syndrome

Pharmacokinetics

Absorption	Unknown
Distribution	Protein binding 98%
Metabolism	Unknown
Excretion	Urine (59%), feces (26%)
Half-life	Unknown

Pharmacodynamics

Onset	Unknown
Peak	Unknown
Duration	Unknown

INTERACTIONS

Individual drugs

CarBAMazepine: decreased vortioxetine levels

Lithium, traMADol, traZODone: increased serotonin syndrome

Drug classifications

Anticoagulants, antiplatelets, NSAIDs, salicylates, thrombolytics: increased bleeding risk

Barbiturates, sedative/hypnotics, other CNS depressants: increased CNS effects

Serotonin receptor agonists, SSRIs, MAOIs, SNRIs (venlafaxine, DULoxetine): increased serotonin syndrome

Tricyclics: increased effect of tricyclics; use cautiously

Drug/herb

St. John's wort: increased serotonin syndrome

NURSING CONSIDERATIONS

Assessment

> **BLACK BOX WARNING:** Mental status: assess mood, sensorium, affect, suicidal tendencies, increase in psychiatric symptoms, depression, panic

• **Serotonin syndrome: monitor for increased heart rate, sweating, dilated pupils, tremors, twitching, hyperthermia, agitation**

• Alcohol consumption: if alcohol is consumed, hold dose until AM

• Sexual dysfunction: assess for impotence

Patient/family education

• Teach patient that therapeutic effect may take several wk

• Teach patient to use caution when driving, performing other activities that require alertness, because of drowsiness, dizziness, blurred vision; to report signs, symptoms, or bleeding

• Teach patient to avoid alcohol, other CNS depressants

> **BLACK BOX WARNING:** Teach patient that suicidal ideas, behaviors may occur in children or young adults

• Teach patient to notify prescriber if pregnant, planning to become pregnant, or breastfeeding, pregnancy **C**

> **BLACK BOX WARNING:** Teach patient about the effects of serotonin syndrome: nausea/vomiting, tremors; if symptoms occur, to discontinue immediately, notify prescriber

Evaluation

Positive therapeutic outcome

• Decreased depression

Adverse effects: *italics* = common; **bold** = life-threatening

> ⚠ **HIGH ALERT**
>
> ## warfarin (Rx)
> (war'far-in)
> **Coumadin, Jantoven**
> *Func. class.:* Anticoagulant
> **Pregnancy category X**

Do not confuse: Coumadin/Cardura/ Compazine

ACTION: Interferes with blood clotting by indirect means; depresses hepatic synthesis of vit K–dependent coagulation factors (II, VII, IX, X)

Therapeutic outcome: Prevention of clotting

USES: Antiphospholipid antibody syndrome, arterial thromboembolism prophylaxis, deep vein thrombosis, MI prophylaxis, post MI, stroke prophylaxis, thrombosis prophylaxis

CONTRAINDICATIONS

Pregnancy **X,** breastfeeding, hypersensitivity, hemophilia, leukemia with bleeding, peptic ulcer disease, thrombocytopenic purpura, hepatic disease (severe), malignant hypertension, subacute bacterial endocarditis, acute nephritis, blood dyscrasias, preeclampsia, eclampsia, hemorrhagic tendencies, surgery of CNS, eye, traumatic surgery with large open surface, bleeding tendencies of GI/GU/respiratory, stroke, aneurysms, pericardial effusion, spinal puncture, major regional/lumbar block anesthesia

> **BLACK BOX WARNING:** Bleeding

Precautions: Alcoholism, geriatric, CHF, debilitated patients, trauma, indwelling catheters, severe hypertension, active infections, protein C deficiency, polycythemia vera, vasculitis, severe diabetes, Asian patients (CYP2C9, protein C,S deficiency)

DOSAGE AND ROUTES

Adult: PO 2-10 mg/day × 3 days, then titrated to INR/pro-time

Adolescent/child/infant: PO 0.2 mg/kg/day titrated to INR

Available forms: Tabs 1, 2, 2.5, 3, 4, 5, 6, 7.5, 10 mg

Implementation
PO route

• Warfarin is usually given with **IV** heparin for 3 or more days, warfarin blood level may take several days

ADVERSE EFFECTS

CNS: *Fever,* dizziness, fatigue, headache, lethargy
CV: Angina, chest pain, edema, hypotension, syncope
GI: *Diarrhea,* nausea, vomiting, anorexia, stomatitis, cramps, **hepatitis,** cholestatic jaundice
GU: Hematuria
HEMA: Hemorrhage, agranulocytosis, leukopenia, eosinophilia, ecchymosis, anemia, petechiae
INTEG: *Rash,* dermatitis, urticaria, alopecia, pruritus
MISC: Epistaxis, hemoptysis, mouth ulcers, taste disturbances, priapism, dyspnea
MS: Bone fractures
SYST: Anaphylaxis, coma, cholesterol, microembolisms, **exfoliative dermatitis, purple toe syndrome**

Pharmacokinetics

Absorption	Well absorbed (PO), completely absorbed
Distribution	Crosses placenta, 99% plasma protein binding
Metabolism	Liver
Excretion	Kidney, feces (active, inactive metabolites)
Half-life	Effective ½-2½ days

Pharmacodynamics

	PO
Onset	12-24 hr
Peak	½-4 days
Duration	3-5 days

INTERACTIONS
Individual drugs

Allopurinol, amiodarone, chloral hydrate, chloramphenicol, cimetidine, clofibrate, clotrimoxazole, dextrothyroxine, diflunisal, disulfiram, erythromycin, furosemide, glucagon, heparin, indomethacin, isoniazid, mefenamic acid, metroNIDAZOLE, mifepristone, phenylbutazone, quiNIDine, RU-486, sulfinpyrazone, sulindac, thyroid: increased warfarin action

Aprepitant, azoTHIOprine, bosentan, carBAMazepine, dicloxicillin, ethchlorvynol, factor IX/ VIIa, griseofulvin, nafcillin, phenytoin, rifampin, sucralfate, sulfaSALAzine, thyroid, vitamin K: decreased warfarin action
Phenytoin: increased toxicity

Drug classifications

Antidepressants (tricyclic), ethacrynic acids, HMG-CoA reductase inhibitors, NSAIDs, oxyphenbutazones, COX-2 selective inhibitors, penicillins, quinolones, salicylates, selective serotonin reuptake inhibitors, steroids, sulfonamides, thrombolytics: increased warfarin action

Barbiturates, bile acid sequestrants, contraceptives (oral), estrogens: decreased warfarin action

Sulfonylureas (oral): increased toxicity

Drug/herb

Angelica, anise, basil, chamomile, chondroitin, dong quai, evening primrose, feverfew, garlic, ginger, ginkgo, ginseng, horse chestnut, kava, licorice, melatonin, red yeast rice, saw palmetto: increased risk of bleeding

Coenzyme Q10, St. John's wort: decreased anticoagulant effect

Drug/food

Vit K foods: decreased warfarin action

Drug/lab test

Increased: T_3 uptake, liver function tests
Decreased: uric acid

NURSING CONSIDERATIONS
Assessment

> **BLACK BOX WARNING:** Monitor blood studies (Hct, PT, platelets, occult blood in stools) q3mo; INR: in hospital daily after 2nd or 3rd dose; once in therapeutic range for 2 consecutive days, monitor 2-3× wk for 1-2 wk, then less frequently depending on stability of INR results; *Outpatient:* monitor every few days until stable dose, then periodically thereafter depending on stability of INR results, usually at least monthly

> **BLACK BOX WARNING:** Assess for bleeding gums, petechiae, ecchymosis, black tarry stools, hematuria; fatal hemorrhage can occur

- Monitor B/P, watch for increasing signs of hypertension
- Assess for fever, skin rash, urticaria
- Assess for needed dosage change q1-2wk

Patient/family education

- Caution patient to avoid OTC preparations unless directed by prescriber; may cause serious product interactions
- Advise patient that product may be withheld during active bleeding (menstruation), depending on condition
- Advise patient to use soft-bristle toothbrush to avoid bleeding gums, avoid contact sports, use electric razor, avoid IM inj
- Instruct patient to carry/wear emergency ID identifying product taken
- Advise patient to report any signs of bleeding: gums, under skin, urine, stools
- Teach patient to read food labels; limited intake of vit K foods (green leafy vegetables) is necessary to maintain consistent prothrombin levels

Evaluation

Positive therapeutic outcome
- Decrease of deep vein thrombosis
- Pro-time (1.3-2.0 × control)

Adverse effects: *italics* = common; **bold** = life-threatening

zafirlukast (Rx)

(za-feer'loo-cast)

Accolate

Func. class.: Bronchodilator

Chem. class.: Leukotriene receptor antagonist

Pregnancy category B

Do not confuse: Accolate/Accupril/Aclovate

ACTION: Antagonizes the contractile action of leukotrienes (LTC_4, LTD_4, LTE_4) in airway smooth muscle; inhibits bronchoconstriction caused by antigens

Therapeutic outcome: Ability to breathe more easily

USES: Prophylaxis and treatment of chronic asthma in adults/children >5 yr

CONTRAINDICATIONS

Hypersensitivity, hepatic encephalopathy

Precautions: Pregnancy **B**, breastfeeding, children, geriatric, hepatic disease, Churg-Strauss syndrome, acute bronchospasm

DOSAGE AND ROUTES

Adult and child ≥12 yr: PO 20 mg bid

Child 5-11 yr: PO 10 mg bid

Available forms: Tabs 10, 20 mg

Implementation

• Give PO 1 hr before or 2 hr after meals; absorption may be decreased if given with food

ADVERSE EFFECTS

CNS: Headache, dizziness, suicidal ideation, fever, insomnia

GI: Nausea, diarrhea, abdominal pain, vomiting, dyspepsia, hepatic failure, hepatitis

HEMA: Agranulocytosis

MISC: Infections, pain, asthenia, myalgia, fever, increased ALT, urticaria, rash, angioedema

Pharmacokinetics

Absorption	Rapidly absorbed
Distribution	Unknown
Metabolism	Extensively by CYP2C9, CYP3A4 enzyme systems, protein binding (99%)
Excretion	Feces
Half-life	10 hr

Pharmacodynamics

Onset	Unknown
Peak	3 hr
Duration	Unknown

INTERACTIONS

Individual drugs

Aspirin: increased plasma levels of zafirlukast

Erythromycin, theophylline: decreased plasma levels of zafirlukast

Warfarin: increased pro-time

Drug/food

Decreased: bioavailability of zafirlukast

NURSING CONSIDERATIONS

Assessment

• Assess respiratory rate, rhythm, depth; auscultate lung fields bilaterally; notify prescriber of abnormalities; not to be used for acute bronchospasm in acute asthma

• **Churg-Strauss syndrome (rare): assess adults carefully (eosinophilia, vasculitic rash, worsening pulmonary symptoms, cardiac complications, neuropathy), may be caused by reducing oral corticosteroids**

• **Hepatic disease:** Monitor liver function tests

• Assess for renal/pancreatic/visual function

Patient/family education

• Advise patient to check OTC medications, current prescription medications that may increase stimulation, do not stop other asthma medications unless instructed to do so

• Advise patient to avoid hazardous activities; dizziness may occur

• Advise patient that if GI upset occurs, to take product with 8 oz of water; avoid food if possible; absorption may be decreased

• Advise to take even if symptom-free

• **Advise patient to notify prescriber of nausea, vomiting, diarrhea, abdominal pain, fatigue, jaundice, anorexia, flulike symptoms (hepatic dysfunction)**

• Advise patient not to use for acute asthma episodes

• **Teach patient not to breastfeed**

Evaluation

Positive therapeutic outcome

• Ability to breathe more easily

⚠ HIGH ALERT

zaleplon (Rx)

(zal'eh-plon)

Sonata

Func. class.: Hypnotic, nonbarbiturate

Chem. class.: Pyrazolopyrimidine

Pregnancy category C

Controlled substance schedule IV

ACTION: Binds selectively to ω-1 receptor of the γ-aminobutyric acid type A ($GABA_A$)

---

receptor complex; results are sedation, hypnosis, skeletal muscle relaxation, anticonvulsant activity, anxiolytic action

Therapeutic outcome: Ability to sleep

USES: Insomnia (short-term treatment)

CONTRAINDICATIONS
Hypersensitivity, severe hepatic disease

Precautions: Pregnancy **C**, breastfeeding, children <15 yr, geriatric, renal/hepatic disease, psychosis, angioedema, respiratory disease, depression, sleep-related behavior (sleep walking), Asian descent, CNS depression

DOSAGE AND ROUTES
Adult: PO 10 mg at bedtime; may increase dosage to 20 mg at bedtime if needed; 5 mg may be used in low-weight persons
Geriatric: PO 5 mg at bedtime; may increase if needed

Available forms: Caps 5, 10 mg

Implementation
• Give ½-1 hr before bedtime for sleeplessness; give on empty stomach
• Store in tight container in cool environment

ADVERSE EFFECTS
CNS: *Drowsiness,* amnesia, depersonalization, hallucinations, hyperesthesia, paresthesia, somnolence, tremor, vertigo, dizziness, anxiety, *lethargy, daytime sedation,* confusion, **complex sleep-related reactions (sleep driving, sleep eating)**
CV: Chest pain, peripheral edema
EENT: Vision changes, ear/eye pain, hyperacusis, parosmia
GI: Nausea, anorexia, colitis, dyspepsia, dry mouth, constipation, abdominal pain
MISC: Asthenia, fever, headache, myalgia, dysmenorrhea
MS: Myalgia, back pain, arthritis
RESP: Bronchitis
SYST: **Severe allergic reactions**

Pharmacokinetics

Absorption	Rapidly absorbed
Distribution	Extravascular tissues, crosses blood-brain barrier; crosses placenta
Metabolism	Extensively, liver to inactive metabolites
Excretion	Kidneys
Half-life	1 hr

Pharmacodynamics

Onset	Rapid
Peak	1 hr
Duration	3-4 hr

INTERACTIONS
Individual drugs
Cimetidine: increased action of zaleplon

Drug classifications
CYP3A4 inhibitors/inducers: increased or decreased zaleplon levels

Drug/herb
Chamomile, hops, kava, valerian: increased CNS depression

Drug/food
High-fat/heavy meal: prolonged absorption, sleep onset reduced

NURSING CONSIDERATIONS
Assessment
• **Sleep disorders:** assess for type of sleep problem, falling asleep, staying asleep; monitor for complex sleep disorders
• Assess for previous product dependence or tolerance; if product dependent or tolerant, amount of medication should be restricted
• Monitor patient's mental status: mood, sensorium, affect, sleeping patterns, drowsiness, dizziness, suicidal tendencies, excessive sedation, impaired coordination

Patient/family education
• Inform patient that product is for short-term use only
• Teach patient to take immediately before going to bed
• **Advise patient that product may cause memory problems, dependence (if used for longer periods of time), changes in behavior/thinking, complex sleep-related behavior (sleep eating/driving)**
• Advise patient not to ingest a high-fat/heavy meal before taking
• Advise patient to avoid OTC preparations unless approved by a physician, to avoid alcohol ingestion or other psychotropic medications unless prescribed by a health care provider, that 1-2 wk of therapy may be required before therapeutic effects occur
• Caution patient to avoid driving, activities requiring alertness; drowsiness may occur; until medication response is known, tell patient that drowsiness may worsen at beginning of treatment
• Instruct patient not to discontinue medication abruptly after long-term use

Z

Evaluation
Positive therapeutic outcome
• Decreased sleeplessness

zanamivir (Rx)
(zan-a-mee′veer)
Relenza
Func. class.: Antiviral
Chem. class.: Neuramidase inhibitor
Pregnancy category C

ACTION: Inhibits neuramidase enzyme needed for influenza virus replication

Therapeutic outcome: Decreased symptoms of influenza types A and B for those who have been symptomatic for no more than 2 days

USES: Treatment of influenza types A and B for those who have been symptomatic for no more than 2 days

CONTRAINDICATIONS
Hypersensitivity

Precautions: Pregnancy **C,** breastfeeding, children <7 yr, geriatric, respiratory disease, angioedema, milk protein hypersensitivity, Reye's syndrome

DOSAGE AND ROUTES
Adult and child >7 yr: INH 2 inh (two 5-mg blisters) q12hr × 5 days, on the 1st day 2 doses should be taken with at least 2 hr between doses

Available forms: Blisters of powder for inhalation 5 mg

Implementation
• Give before exposure to influenza; continue for 5 days after contact
• Store in airtight, dry container

ADVERSE EFFECTS
CNS: *Headache, dizziness,* fatigue, seizures, self-injury, delirium (child)
EENT: Ear, nose, throat infections, throat discomfort
GI: *Nausea, vomiting, diarrhea*
RESP: Nasal symptoms, cough, sinusitis, bronchitis, bronchospasm
SYST: Angioedema

Pharmacokinetics

Absorption	4%-17% absorbed
Distribution	<10% protein binding
Metabolism	Not metabolized
Excretion	Kidneys unchanged
Half-life	2½-5 hr

Pharmacodynamics
Unknown

INTERACTIONS
Individual drugs
Intranasal influenza vaccine: decreased effect; separate by ≥48 hr, do not restart antiviral drugs for ≥2 wk

NURSING CONSIDERATIONS
Assessment
• Assess for symptoms of influenza A: increased temp, malaise, aches and pains
• Assess for skin eruptions, photosensitivity after administration of product
• Monitor respiratory status: rate, character, wheezing, tightness in chest
• Assess for allergies before initiation of treatment, reaction of each medication

Patient/family education
• Give patient "Patient's instructions for use" and review all points before using delivery system
• Teach patient to avoid hazardous activities if dizziness occurs
• Teach patient to use for the entire 5 days
• Inform patient that this product does not reduce transmission risk of influenza to others
• Advise patients with asthma or COPD to carry a fast-acting inhaled bronchodilator since bronchospasm may occur; to use scheduled inhaled bronchodilators before using this product

Evaluation

Positive therapeutic outcome
• Absence of fever, malaise, cough, dyspnea in influenza A

zidovudine (Rx)
(zye-doe′vue-deen)
Novo-AZT ✦, Retrovir
Func. class.: Antiretroviral
Chem. class.: Nucleoside reverse transcriptase inhibitor (NRTI)
Pregnancy category C

Do not confuse: Retrovir/ritonavir

ACTION: Inhibits replication of HIV-1 by incorporating into cellular DNA by viral reverse transcriptase, thereby terminating the cellular DNA chain

Therapeutic outcome: Decreased symptoms of HIV-1 infection

USES: Used in combination with at least 2 other antiretrovirals for HIV-1 infection

CONTRAINDICATIONS
Hypersensitivity

Precautions: Pregnancy **C**, breastfeeding, children, granulocyte count <1000/mm^3 or Hgb <9.5 g/dl, severe renal disease, obesity

> **BLACK BOX WARNING:** Impaired hepatic function, anemia, lactic acidosis, myopathy, neutropenia

DOSAGE AND ROUTES
HIV infections with other antiretrovirals
Adult: PO (tabs, caps, syrup) 600 mg/day in divided doses, either 200 mg tid or 300 mg bid in combination with other antiretrovirals; **IV** 1-mg/kg q4hr, initiate PO as soon as possible, up to 1000 mg

Adolescent/child ≥30 kg: PO (tabs/caps/syrup) 300 mg bid or 200 mg tid

Child 25 kg to <30 kg: PO (tabs/caps) 500 mg/day divided bid

Child 19 kg to <25 kg: PO (tabs/caps) 400 mg/day divided bid

Child/infant ≥4 wk and 13 kg to <19 kg: PO (tabs/caps) 300 mg/day divided bid

Child/infant ≥4 wk and 7 kg to <13 kg: PO (tabs/caps) 200 mg/day divided bid

Child/infant ≥4 wk and 5 kg to <7 kg: PO (tabs/caps) 150 mg/day divided bid

Infant ≥4 wk, child/adolescent ≥9 kg and <30 kg: PO (syrup) 18 mg/kg/day divided bid or tid

Infant ≥4 wk and 4 kg to <9 kg: PO (syrup) 24 mg/kg/day divided bid or tid

Perinatal transmission prophylaxis
Full-term neonate: PO (syrup) 2 mg/kg or **IV** 1.5 mg/kg q6hr starting 12 hr after birth; continue up to 6 wk of age

Prevention of maternal-fetal HIV transmission
Neonate ≥34 wk: PO 2 mg/kg/dose q6hr × 6 wk beginning 8-12 hr after birth; **IV** 1.5 mg/kg/dose over 30 min q6hr until able to take PO

Maternal (>14 wk gestation): PO 100 mg 5 ×/day until start of labor, then during labor/delivery **IV** 2 mg/kg over 1 hr followed by **IV** INF 1 mg/kg/hr until umbilical cord is clamped

Prevention of HIV after needlestick
Adult: PO 200 mg tid plus lamiVUDine 150 mg bid, plus a protease inhibitor for high-risk exposure; begin within 2 hr of exposure

Available forms: Caps 100 mg; tabs 300 mg; inj 10 mg/ml; oral syr 50 mg/5 ml

Implementation
PO route
- Give on empty stomach
- Do not take dapsone at same time as didanosine
- Store in cool environment; protect from light

Intermittent IV infusion route
- Give after diluting with D$_5$W; give over 1 hr (<4 mg/ml), do not give by direct **IV**
- Protect unopened product from light; use diluted solutions within 24 hr if stored at room temperature, 48 hr if refrigerated

Y-site compatibilities: Acyclovir, alemtuzumab, allopurinol, amikacin, amphotericin B, anidulafungin, argatroban, aztreonam, ceftazidime, cefTRIAXone, cimetidine, clindamycin, dexamethasone, DOBUTamine, DOPamine, erythromycin, fluconazole, fludarabine, gentamicin, heparin, imipenem/cilastatin, LORazepam, metoclopramide, morphine, nafcillin, ondansetron, oxacillin, pentamidine, phenylephrine, piperacillin, potassium chloride, ranitidine, sargramostim, tacrolimus, tobramycin, trimethoprim/sulfamethoxazole, vancomycin, zoledronic acid

Additive incompatibilities: Blood products or protein solutions

ADVERSE EFFECTS
CNS: *Fever, headache, malaise,* diaphoresis, *dizziness, insomnia,* paresthesia, somnolence, chills, tremor, twitching, anxiety, confusion, depression, lability, vertigo, loss of mental acuity, seizures, malaise

EENT: Taste change, hearing loss, photophobia

GI: *Nausea, vomiting, diarrhea,* anorexia, cramps, *dyspepsia, constipation,* dysphagia, *flatulence,* rectal bleeding, mouth ulcer, abdominal pain, hepatomegaly

GU: Dysuria, polyuria, frequency, hesitancy

HEMA: Granulocytopenia, anemia

INTEG: *Rash,* acne, pruritus, urticaria

MS: Myalgia, arthralgia, muscle spasm

RESP: Dyspnea, cough, wheezing

SYST: Lactic acidosis

Pharmacokinetics

Absorption	Well absorbed (PO), completely absorbed (**IV**)
Distribution	Widely distributed—crosses placenta, CSF, protein binding 38%
Metabolism	Liver, mostly
Excretion	Kidneys
Half-life	Terminal ½-3 hr

Z

Adverse effects: *italics* = common; **bold** = life-threatening

Pharmacodynamics

	PO	IV
Onset	Unknown	Rapid
Peak	½-1½ hr	Inf end
Duration	Unknown	Unknown

INTERACTIONS
Individual drugs
DOXOrubicin, ribavarin, staduvine: avoid concurrent use

Ganciclovir, radiation, SMZ/TMP, valganciclovir: increased bone marrow suppression

Methadone: increased zidovudine level

Drug classifications
Antineoplastics: increased bone marrow suppression

Interferons, NRTIs: decreased zidovudine levels

Drug/lab test
Increased: LFTs, granulocytes

Decreased: platelets, amylase, CPK

NURSING CONSIDERATIONS
Assessment
• **Assess for peripheral neuropathy:** tingling or pain in hands and feet, distal numbness; if these occur, product may be decreased or discontinued

• **Assess for pancreatitis: abdominal pain, nausea, vomiting, elevated liver enzymes; product should be discontinued because condition can be fatal**

• Assess children by dilated retinal examination q6mo to rule out retinal depigmentation

> **BLACK BOX WARNING:** Monitor blood counts q2wk; watch for decreasing granulocytes, Hgb; if low, therapy may have to be discontinued and restarted after hematologic recovery; blood transfusions may be required; monitor viral load, CD4 counts, LFTs, plasma HIV RNA, serum creatinine/BUN baseline and throughout treatment

> **BLACK BOX WARNING: Lactic acidosis, severe hepatomegaly with steatosis:** obtain baseline LFTs; if elevated, discontinue treatment; discontinue even if LFTs are normal but lactic acidosis, hepatomegaly are present: may be fatal

Patient/family education
• Caution patient to take on empty stomach; to use exactly as prescribed

• Advise patient to report signs of infection: increased temp, sore throat, flulike symptoms; to avoid crowds and those with known infections

• Instruct patient to report signs of anemia: fatigue, headache, faintness, shortness of breath, irritability

• Advise patient to report bleeding; avoid use of razors or commercial mouthwash

• Inform patient that hair may be lost during therapy (rare); a wig or hairpiece may make patient feel better

• Caution patient to avoid OTC products or other medications without approval of prescriber

• Caution patient not to have any sexual contact without use of a condom; needles should not be shared; blood from infected individual should not come in contact with another's mucous membranes, compliance with treatment is required

Evaluation
Positive therapeutic outcome
• Decreased infection; decreased symptoms of HIV infection, decreased viral load, increased CD4 counts

---

zinc (PO, OTC; IV, Rx)
(zink sul'fate)
Orazinc, PMS Egozinc ✦, Verazinc, Zinca-Pak, Zincate, Zinc 15, Zinc-220
Func. class.: Trace element; nutritional supplement
Pregnancy category C, parenteral

ACTION: Needed for adequate healing, bone and joint development, (23% zinc)

Therapeutic outcome: Replacement of zinc

USES: Prevention of zinc deficiency, adjunct to vit A therapy

Unlabeled uses: Wound healing

Precautions: Pregnancy C (parenteral), breastfeeding, hypocupremia, neonatal prematurity, neonates, renal disease

DOSAGE AND ROUTES
Dietary supplement (elemental zinc)
Adult/adolescent pregnant females: PO 11-13 mg/day

Nutritional supplement (IV)
Adult: IV 2.5-4 mg/day, may increase by 2 mg/day if needed

Child 1-5 yr: IV 50 mcg/kg/day

Adult and lactating female: PO 12-14 mg/day × 12 mo

Adult and adolescent male ≥14 yr: PO 11 mg/day
Adult female ≥19 yr: PO 8 mg/day
Adolescent female ≥14 yr: PO 9 mg/day
Child 9-13 yr: PO 8 mg/day
Child 4-8 yr: PO 5 mg/day
Child 1-3 yr: PO 3 mg/day
Infant 7-12 mo: PO 3 mg/day
Infant birth to 6 mo: PO 2 mg/day (adequate intake)

Wound healing (unlabeled)
Adult: PO 50 mg tid until healed (elemental iron)

Available forms: Tabs 66, 110 mg; caps 220 mg; inj 1, 5 mg/ml

Implementation
PO route
• Give with meals to decrease gastric upset; restrict dairy products, caffeine, which decrease absorption

IV route
• Part of TPN

ADVERSE EFFECTS
GI: Nausea, vomiting, cramps, heartburn, ulcer formation

Pharmacokinetivcs

Absorption	Poorly absorbed (**PO**), completely absorbed (**IV**)
Distribution	Widely distributed
Metabolism	Liver
Excretion	90% (feces), 10% (kidneys)
Half-life	Unknown

Pharmacodynamics

Unknown

INTERACTIONS
Drug classifications
Fluoroquinolones, tetracyclines: decreased absorption

Drug/food
Caffeine, dairy products: decreased absorption of PO zinc

NURSING CONSIDERATIONS
Assessment
• Zinc deficiency: poor wound healing, absence of taste, smell, slowing growth
• Alkaline phosphatase, HDL monthly in long-term therapy
• Monitor zinc levels during treatment

Patient/family education
• Inform patient that element must be taken for 3 mo to be effective
• Advise patient to report immediately nausea, diarrhea, rash, severe vomiting, restlessness, abdominal pain, tarry stools

Evaluation

Positive therapeutic outcome
• Absence of zinc deficiency
• Improved wound healing

OVERDOSE: Diarrhea, rash, dehydration, restlessness

ziprasidone (Rx)
(zi-praz'ih-dohn)
Geodon, Zeldox ✤
Func. class.: Antipsychotic/neuroleptic
Chem. class.: Benzisoxazole derivative
Pregnancy category C

ACTION: Unknown; may be mediated through both dopamine type 2 (D_2) and serotonin type 2 (5-HT_2) antagonism

Therapeutic outcome: Decreased signs/symptoms of psychosis

USES: Schizophrenia, acute agitation, acute psychosis, bipolar disorder, mania, psychotic depression, agitation

CONTRAINDICATIONS
Hypersensitivity, breastfeeding

Precautions: Pregnancy **C,** children, geriatric, renal/cardiac/hepatic disease, breast cancer, diabetes, AV block, CNS depression, seizure disorders, abrupt discontinuation, agranulocytosis, ambient temperature increase, suicidal ideation, torsades de pointes, strenuous exercise

> **BLACK BOX WARNING:** Increased mortality in elderly patients with dementia-related psychosis

DOSAGE AND ROUTES
Schizophrenia
Adult: PO 20 mg bid with food, adjust dosage every 2 days upward to max of 80 mg bid; IM 10-20 mg; may give 10 mg q2hr, doses of 20 mg may be given q4hr, max 40 mg/day (acute episodes); switch to PO as soon as possible

Bipolar disorder
Adult: PO 40 mg bid with food, on day 2 increase to 60 or 80 mg bid, then adjust to response; maintenance as adjunct to lithium/valproate 40-80 mg bid

Available forms: Tabs 20, 40, 60, 80 mg; inj 20 mg/ml single-dose vials

Z

Implementation

- Give reduced dosage in geriatric
- Give antiparkinsonian agent on order from prescriber, to be used for EPS
- Provide decreased stimulus by dimming lights, avoiding loud noises
- Store in tight, light-resistant container
- Provide supervised ambulation until patient is stabilized on medication; do not involve in strenuous exercise program because fainting is possible; patient should not stand still for a long time

PO route

- Take cap whole and with food, with plenty of fluid at same time of day
- Food increases absorption
- Store in airtight, light-resistant container

IM route

- Add 1.2 ml sterile water for inj to vial, shake vigorously until product is dissolved; give deeply in large muscle; do not mix with other products; do not use if particulates are present, keep patient recumbent for 30 min after injection
- Store injection at room temperature; protect from light; after reconstituting may be stored at room temperature × 24 hr, 7 days refrigerated

ADVERSE EFFECTS

CNS: *EPS (pseudoparkinsonism, akathisia, dystonia, tardive dyskinesia), drowsiness, insomnia, agitation, anxiety, headache,* **seizures, neuroleptic malignant syndrome,** dizziness, tremor, facial droop

CV: Orthostatic hypotension, **tachycardia, prolonged QT/QTc, sudden death, heart failure (geriatric), torsades de pointes**

EENT: Blurred vision, diplopia

ENDO: Metabolic changes, hyperprolactinemia (rare)

GI: *Nausea,* vomiting, *anorexia, constipation,* jaundice, weight gain, diarrhea, dry mouth, abdominal pain

GU: Enuresis, urinary incontinence, gynecomastia, impotence, priapism

MS: Decreased bone density

RESP: Rhinitis, dyspnea, infection, cough

INTEG: Rash, inj site pain, sweating

Pharmacokinetics

Absorption	Unknown
Distribution	Protein binding 99%
Metabolism	Liver, extensively to metabolite
Excretion	Unknown
Half-life	Terminal 7 hr

Pharmacodynamics

Onset	Unknown
Peak	PO 6-8 hr; IM 60 min
Duration	Unknown

INTERACTIONS

Individual drugs

Alcohol: increased sedation

Chloroquine, clarithromycin, droperidol, erythromycin, grepafloxacin, haloperidol, methadone, moxifloxacin, pentamidine: increased QT prolongation

CarBAMazepine, phenytoin, rifampin: increased excretion of ziprasidone

Ketoconazole: increased ziprasidone level

Lithium: increased EPS, possible neurotoxicity

Drug classifications

Antihypertensives: increased hypotension

Antipsychotics: increased EPS

β-agonists, class IA/III antidysrhythmics, local anesthetics, phenothiazines (some), tricyclics: increased QT prolongation

Barbiturates: increased excretion of ziprasidone

CNS depressants: increased sedation

SSRIs, SNRIs: increased serotonin syndrome, increased neuroleptic malignant syndrome

NURSING CONSIDERATIONS

Assessment

> **BLACK BOX WARNING:** Assess geriatric with dementia closely; heart failure, sudden death have occurred

- Assess mental status before initial administration, AIMS assessment
- Monitor bilirubin, CBC, liver function tests, fasting blood glucose, cholesterol profile; potassium, magnesium when taken with loop/thiazide diuretics qmo
- Monitor urinalysis before, during prolonged therapy
- Monitor B/P standing and lying; also pulse, respirations; take these q4hr during initial treatment; establish baseline before starting treatment; report drops of 30 mm Hg; watch for ECG changes; **QT prolongation may occur**
- Assess dizziness, faintness, palpitations, tachycardia on rising
- **Assess EPS,** including akathisia (inability to sit still, no pattern to movements), tardive dyskinesia (bizarre movements of the jaw, mouth, tongue, extremities), pseudoparkinsonism (rigidity, tremors, pill rolling, shuffling gait)
- ⚠ Assess for neuroleptic malignant syndrome: hyperthermia, increased CPK, altered mental status, muscle rigidity

---

• Assess constipation, urinary retention daily; if these occur, increase bulk and water in diet

Patient/family education
• Advise patient that orthostatic hypotension may occur and to rise from sitting or lying position gradually; avoid hot tubs, hot showers, tub baths because hypotension may occur
• Advise patient to avoid abrupt withdrawal of this product; EPS may result; product should be withdrawn slowly
• Advise patient to avoid OTC preparations (cough, hay fever, cold) unless approved by prescriber, since serious product interactions may occur; avoid use with alcohol, CNS depressants; increased drowsiness may occur
• Teach patient to avoid hazardous activities if drowsy or dizzy
• Advise patient to increase fluids to prevent constipation
• Teach patient to use sips of water, candy, gum for dry mouth
• Teach patient to report impaired vision, tremors, muscle twitching
• **Teach patient that in hot weather, heat stroke may occur; take extra precautions to stay cool**

Evaluation

Positive therapeutic outcome
• Decrease in emotional excitement, hallucinations, delusions, paranoia; reorganization of patterns of thought, speech

TREATMENT OF OVERDOSE:
Lavage if orally ingested; provide airway; *do not induce vomiting*

> ⚠ **HIGH ALERT**

ziv-aflibercept
(ziv-a-flih′ber-sept)

Zaltrap

Func. class.: Antineoplastic biologic response modifier

Chem. class.: Signal transduction inhibitor (STI)

Pregnancy category: C

ACTION: An angiogenesis inhibitor, a fusion protein that binds to vascular endothelial growth factors (VEGF-A, VEGF-B) and placental growth factor 1 and 2

Therapeutic outcome: Decrease in spread or size of tumor

USES: Metastatic colorectal cancer that is resistant or has progressed after an oxaliplatin-containing regimen in combination with 5-fluorouracil, leucovorin, irinotecan (FOLFIRI)

CONTRAINDICATIONS
Hypersensitivity

Precautions: Infertility, male-mediated teratogenicity, encephalopathy, hypertension, dental work, breastfeeding, children, neonates, geriatric patients, infection, neutropenia, pregnancy **(C)**

> **BLACK BOX WARNING:** Bleeding, GI bleeding/perforation, intracranial bleeding, surgery

DOSAGE AND ROUTES
Adult: IV 4 mg/kg over 1 hr on day 1 every 2 wk in combination with the FOLFIRI regimen (irinotecan 180 mg/m^2 over 90 min on day 1 with dl-racemic leucovorin 400 mg/m^2 over 2 hr) (infused at the same time, in same Y-line; then on day 1 by 5-fluorouracil 400 mg/m^2 as a bolus, then 2400 mg/m^2 as a 46-hr cont IV inf)

Available forms: Solution for injection 100 mg/4 ml; 200 mg/8 ml

Implementation
• Give before FOLFIRI chemotherapy; visually inspect for particulate matter and discoloration before use

Dilution and preparation
• Withdraw the calculated dose, add to 0.9% sodium chloride or dextrose 5% solution to 0.6–8 mg/mL; use polyvinyl chloride (PVC) infusion bags containing bis (2-ethylhexyl) phthalate (DHEP) or polyolefin infusion bags; do not re-enter the vial after first puncture; discard any unused portion; do not mix or combine with other drugs in the same infusion bag; the diluted solution may be stored refrigerated for ≤4 hr; discard any unused portion in the infusion bag

IV infusion
• Give diluted solution over 1 hr using a 0.2 micrometer polyethersulfone filter; do not use nylon or polyvinylidene fluoride (PVDF) filters; do not give IV push or bolus; do not mix or combine with other drugs in the same IV line; give using an infusion set made of one of the following: PVC containing DEHP, DEHP-free PVC containing trioctyl-trimellitate (TOTM), polypropylene, polyethylene-lined PVC, or polyurethane
Dosage adjustments for recurrent or severe hypertension
Hold until B/P is controlled and then permanently reduce dose to 2 mg/kg; discontinue in hypertensive crisis or hypertensive encephalopathy

---

Z

Adverse effects: *italics* = common; **bold** = life-threatening

Dosage adjustments for proteinuria
(2 g/24 hr)
Hold until proteinuria is <2 g/24 hr; if proteinuria recurs, hold therapy until proteinuria is <2 g/24 hr, then reduce to 2 mg/kg; discontinue in nephrotic syndrome or thrombotic microangiopathy

ADVERSE EFFECTS

CNS: Intracranial bleeding, headache, dizziness

CV: Hypertensive crisis, hypertension, stroke

GI: Nausea, hepatotoxicity, dyspepsia, GI hemorrhage, abdominal pain, GI perforation

GU: Proteinuria, hematuria

HEMA: Neutropenia, leukopenia

INTEG: Rash, pruritus, alopecia, hypersensitivity

MISC: Fatigue, epistaxis, night sweats, decreased weight, flulike symptoms, infection

RESP: Dyspnea, pulmonary embolism

Pharmacokinetics

Absorption	Unknown
Distribution	Unknown
Metabolism	Unknown
Excretion	Unknown
Half-life	Elimination 6 days

Pharmacodynamics

Onset	Unknown
Peak	Unknown
Duration	Unknown

NURSING CONSIDERATIONS
Assessment

BLACK BOX WARNING: ⚠ Severe bleeding: Assess for GI bleeding, intracranial bleeding, and pulmonary hemorrhage/hemoptysis; may be fatal; monitor patients for signs and symptoms of bleeding

BLACK BOX WARNING: ⚠ GI perforation: some cases are fatal; monitor patients for signs and symptoms of GI perforation; discontinue therapy if GI perforation develops

• **Poor wound healing:** hold ≥4 wk before elective surgery; after major surgery, do not restart for ≥4 wk and until the surgical wound is entirely healed

⚠ Severe hypertension/hypertensive crisis: usually occurs within the first 2 cycles (grade 3 or 4 hypertension); monitor B/P every 2 wk or more often if needed; treatment with antihypertensives may be needed; product may need to be discontinued

⚠ Severe proteinuria/nephrotic syndrome/thrombotic microangiopathy (TMA): monitor urine protein by dipstick analysis and urinary protein–to–creatinine ratio (UPCR); obtain a 24-hr urine collection for a UPCR >1; for proteinuria of <2 g/24 hr is temporarily hold doses until proteinuria is <2 g/24 hr; if proteinuria recurs, hold doses until proteinuria is <2 g/24 hr, then permanently reduce; discontinue in nephrotic syndrome or TMA

⚠ Febrile neutropenia, neutropenic infection/sepsis: monitor CBC with differential at baseline and before each cycle, hold FOLFIRI until the neutrophil count is ≥1.5 × 10⁹/L

⚠ Geriatric toxicity: assess for diarrhea, dizziness, asthenia, weight loss, and dehydration that can indicate toxicity

⚠ Pregnancy C/Breastfeeding: highly effective contraception during treatment and up to 3 mo after the last dose is needed for all patients of reproductive potential because infertility and male-mediated teratogenicity can occur; infertility can occur but is reversible within 18 wk after stopping product; do not breastfeed

Patient/family education

⚠ Pregnancy C/breastfeeding: teach that highly effective contraception should be used during treatment and up to 3 mo after the last dose in all patients of reproductive potential, infertility and male-mediated teratogenicity can occur; infertility is reversible within 18 wk after stopping product; do not breastfeed

• Teach patient about reason for treatment, expected results

BLACK BOX WARNING: ⚠ Notify prescriber immediately of bleeding, severe abdominal pain, poor wound healing

Evaluation

Positive therapeutic outcome
• Decrease in spread of size of tumor

zoledronic acid (Rx)
(zoh′leh-drah′nick ass′id)
Reclast, Zometa
Func. class.: Bone-resorption inhibitor
Chem. class.: Bisphosphonate
Pregnancy category D

ACTION: Inhibits normal and abnormal bone resorption; potent inhibitor of osteoclastic bone resorption; inhibits osteoclastic activity, reduces bone resorption and inhibits skeletal calcium release caused by stimulating factors released by tumors; reduction of abnormal bone resorption is responsible for therapeutic effect in hypercalcemia; may directly block dissolution of hydroxyapatite bone crystals

Therapeutic outcome: Serum calcium at normal level

USES: Moderate to severe hypercalcemia associated with malignancy; multiple myeloma; bone metastases from solid tumors (used with antineoplastics), active Paget's disease, osteoporosis, glucocorticoid-induced osteoporosis, osteoporosis prophylaxis in postmenopausal women

CONTRAINDICATIONS

Pregnancy **D**, breastfeeding, hypocalcemia, hypersensitivity to this product or bisphosphonates

Precautions: Children, geriatric, renal dysfunction, asthmatic patients, asthma, acute bronchospasm, anemia, chemotherapy, coagulopathy, dehydration, dental disease, diabetes mellitus, renal disease, electrolyte imbalance, hypertension, hypovolemia, phosphate hypersensitivity, infection, multiple myeloma

DOSAGE AND ROUTES
Hypercalcemia of malignancy
Adult: IV INF 4 mg, given as a single INF over ≥15 min, may re-treat with 4 mg if serum calcium does not return to normal within 1 wk

Multiple myeloma/metastatic bone lesions
Adult: IV INF 4 mg, given over 15 min q3-4wk

Osteoporosis
Adult: IV 5 mg over 15 min or more q12mo

Active Paget's disease
Adult: IV INF 5 mg over ≥15 min

Osteoporosis prophylaxis (Reclast), postmenopausal women
Adult: IV INF 5 mg every other yr

Osteoporosis prophylaxis (Reclast) taking systemic glucocorticoids
Adult: IV 5 mg qyr

Renal dose
Adult: IV INF CCr 50-60 ml/min 3.5 mg; CCr 40-49 ml/min 3.3 mg; CCR 30-39 ml/min 3 mg; CCr <30 ml/min don't use

Early breast cancer (unlabeled)
Adult: IV 4 mg q6mo with goserelin 3.6 mg subcut qmo and tamoxifen 20 mg/day or anastrozole 1 mg/day for 3 yr

Available forms: Sol for inj 4 mg/5 ml (Zometa); inj 5 mg/100 ml (Reclast)

Implementation
- Give acetaminophen before and for 72 hr after to decrease pain
- Sol reconstituted with sterile water may be stored under refrigeration for up to 24 hr **IV**
- Administer in separate IV line from all other products

Zometa
- Administer after reconstituting by adding 5 ml of sterile water for inj to each vial, then add up to ≥100 ml of sterile 0.9% NaCl, D₅W, run over ≥15 min

Reclast
- No further dilution required; inf over ≥15 min at constant rate; max 5 mg

ADVERSE EFFECTS
CNS: Dizziness, headache, anxiety, confusion, insomnia, agitation
CV: Hypotension, leg edema, *atrial fibrillation*, chest pain
GI: Abdominal pain, anorexia, constipation, nausea, diarrhea, vomiting, taste change
GU: UTI, possible reduced renal function, *renal damage*
META: Anemia, hypokalemia, hypomagnesemia, hypophosphatemia, hypocalcemia, increased serum creatinine
MISC: *Fever, chills, flulike symptoms*
MS: Severe bone pain, *arthralgias, myalgias*, osteonecrosis of the jaw

Pharmacokinetics

Absorption	Rapidly cleared from circulation
Distribution	Taken up mainly by bones; plasma protein binding ~22%
Metabolism	Not metabolized
Excretion	Kidneys (~50% eliminated in urine within 24 hr)
Half-life	Terminal 167 hr

Pharmacodynamics

Onset	Unknown
Peak	15 min
Duration	Max effect 7 days

INTERACTIONS
Individual drugs
Calcium, vitamin D: decreased zoledronic acid effect
Digoxin: hypomagnesemia, hypokalemia

Drug classifications

Aminoglycosides, NSAIDs, radiopaque contrast agents: increased neurotoxicity

Aminoglycosides, loop diuretics: decreased serum calcium

Infusion solutions (calcium-containing): do not mix with calcium-containing inf sol such as lactated Ringer's sol

Drug/lab test

Increased: creatinine

Decreased: calcium, phosphorus, magnesium, potassium, Hct/Hgb, RBC, platelets, WBC

NURSING CONSIDERATIONS
Assessment

• Assess renal function tests and calcium, phosphate, magnesium, potassium, creatinine; if creatinine is elevated hold treatment

• **Assess for hypocalcemia:** paresthesia, twitching, laryngospasm; Chvostek's/Trousseau's signs

• Assess dental status; cover with antiinfectives for dental extraction

• Assess for atrial fibrillation

Patient/family education

• Instruct patient to report hypercalcemic relapse: nausea, vomiting, bone pain, thirst

• Advise patient to continue with dietary recommendations including calcium and vit D; take a multiple vitamin daily, 500 mg of calcium, 400 international units vit D in multiple myeloma

• Teach patient if nausea/vomiting occur, eat small meals, use lozenges or chewing gum

• Advise patient if bone pain occurs, notify prescriber to obtain analgesic

• **Advise patient not to use during pregnancy**

• Instruct patient to continue good oral hygiene

Evaluation

Positive therapeutic outcome

• Calcium levels decreased to normal

TREATMENT OF OVERDOSE:

Correct clinically relevant reductions in serum calcium by administering **IV** calcium gluconate; in serum phosphorus, with potassium or sodium phosphate; in serum magnesium, with magnesium sulfate

ZOLMitriptan (Rx)

(zole-mih-trip′tan)

Zomig, Zomig-ZMT

Func. class.: Migraine agent, abortive

Chem. class.: $5HT_{1B}/5HT_{1D}$ receptor agonist (triptan)

Pregnancy category C

ACTION: Binds selectively to the vascular serotonin type 1 ($5HT_{1B}/5HT_{1D}$) receptor subtype, exerts antimigraine effect; causes vasoconstriction in cranial arteries

Therapeutic outcome: Decreased severity, frequency of headache

USES: Acute treatment of migraine with or without aura

CONTRAINDICATIONS

Angina pectoris, history of MI, documented silent ischemia, ischemic heart disease, uncontrolled hypertension, hypersensitivity, basilar or hemiplegic migraine, risk of CV events

Precautions: Pregnancy **C**, breastfeeding, children, postmenopausal women, men >40 yr, geriatric, risk factors for CAD, hypercholesterolemia, obesity, diabetes, impaired renal/hepatic function

DOSAGE AND ROUTES

Adult: PO start at 2.5 mg or lower (tab may be broken), may repeat after 2 hr, max 10 mg/24 hr; NASAL 1 spray in 1 nostril at onset of migraine, repeat in 2 hr if no relief

Available forms: Tabs 2.5, 5 mg; orally disintegrating tabs 2.5, 5 mg; nasal spray 2.5, 5 mg

Implementation

• Give with fluids as soon as symptoms of migraine occur

• Provide quiet, calm environment with decreased stimulation for noise, bright light, excessive talking

Orally disintegrating tablet

• Give orally disintegrating tablet after opening; do not crush or chew, allow to dissolve on tongue

ADVERSE EFFECTS

CNS: *Tingling, hot sensation, burning, feeling of pressure, tightness, numbness, dizziness, sedation*

CV: Palpitations, chest pain

GI: Abdominal discomfort, nausea, dry mouth, dyspepsia, dysphagia

MISC: Odd taste (spray)

MS: *Weakness, neck stiffness,* myalgia
RESP: Chest tightness, pressure

Pharmacokinetics

Absorption	Unknown
Distribution	25% plasma protein binding
Metabolism	Liver
Excretion	Urine, feces
Half-life	3-3½ hr

Pharmacodynamics

Onset	Unknown
Peak	Unknown
Duration	2-3½ hr

INTERACTIONS
Individual drugs
Cimetidine: increased half-life of ZOLMitriptan
Ergot: increased vasospastic effects
FLUoxetine, fluvoxaMINE, PARoxetine, sertraline: increased weakness, hyperreflexia, incoordination
Sibutramine: increased ZOLMitriptan levels

Drug classifications
Contraceptives (oral): increased half-life of ZOLMitriptan
Ergot derivatives: increased vasospastic effects
MAOIs: do not use within 2 wk
Selective serotonin reuptake inhibitors: increased weakness, hyperreflexia, incoordination

Drug/herb
SAM-e, St. John's wort: serotonin syndrome

Drug/lab test
Increased: alkaline phosphatase

NURSING CONSIDERATIONS
Assessment
• Assess for tingling, hot sensation, burning, feeling of pressure, numbness, flushing
• Assess neurologic status: LOC, blurring vision, nausea, vomiting, tingling in extremities preceding headache
• Monitor ingestion of tyramine foods (pickled products, beer, wine, aged cheese), food additives, preservatives, colorings, artifical sweeteners, chocolate, caffeine, which may precipitate these types of headaches
• Assess for serotonin syndrome if also taking an SSRI

Patient/family education
• Teach patient to report any side effects to prescriber
• Advise patient to use contraception while taking product

• Teach patient to report pain, rash, swelling of face
• Instruct patient not to double doses; if second dose is needed, wait at least 2 hr; disintegrating dosage form: do not split, break, alter

Evaluation

Positive therapeutic outcome
• Decrease in frequency, severity of headache

⚠ HIGH ALERT

zolpidem (Rx)
(zole-pi′dem)
Ambien, Ambien CR, Edluar, Zolpimist
Func. class.: Sedative-hypnotic
Chem. class.: Nonbenzodiazepine of imid-azopyridine class
Pregnancy category C
Controlled substance schedule IV

ACTION: Produces CNS depression at limbic, thalamic, hypothalamic levels of CNS; may be mediated by neurotransmitter γ-aminobutyric acid (GABA); results are sedation, hypnosis, skeletal muscle relaxation, anticonvulsant activity, anxiolytic action

Therapeutic outcome: Ability to sleep, sedation

USES: Insomnia, short-term treatment; insomnia with difficulty of sleep onset/maintenance (ext rel)

CONTRAINDICATIONS
Hypersensitivity to benzodiazepines

Precautions: Pregnancy C, breastfeeding, children <18 yr, geriatric, anemia, hepatic disease, suicidal individuals, product abuse, seizure disorders, angioedema, depression, respiratory disease, sleep apnea, sleep-related behavior (sleep walking), myasthenia gravis, pulmonary disease, next-morning impairments; females (lower dose needed)

DOSAGE AND ROUTES
Adult: PO 10 mg at bedtime × 7-10 days only; total dose max 10 mg; EXT REL 12.5 mg immediately before bedtime, may be useful for up to 24 wk in people 18-64 yr with primary insomnia; oral spray (Zolpimist) 10 mg (2 sprays) immediately before bedtime, max 10 mg/day; SL (Edluar) 10 mg just before bedtime
Geriatric: PO 5 mg at bedtime; EXT REL 6.25 mg

Available forms: Tabs 5, 10 mg; ext rel tabs 6.25, 12.5 mg; SL 1.75, 3.5, 5, 10 mg; oral spray 5 mg/spray

Z

Implementation
PO route
- Do not break, crush, or chew ext rel product or orally disintegrating tab
- Give ½-1 hr before bedtime for sleeplessness; give several hr before patient is to rise (to avoid hangover)
- Give with food or fluids; tab may be crushed or swallowed whole
- Do not use spray with or after a meal
- Store in airtight container in cool environment

ADVERSE EFFECTS
CNS: Headache, lethargy, drowsiness, daytime sedation, dizziness, confusion, light-headedness, anxiety, irritability, amnesia, poor coordination, complex sleep-related reactions (sleep driving, sleep eating), depression, somnolence, **suicidal ideation**, abnormal thinking/behavioral changes
CV: Chest pain, palpitation
GI: Nausea, vomiting, diarrhea, heartburn, abdominal pain, constipation
HEMA: Leukopenia, granulocytopenia (rare)
MISC: Myalgia
SYST: Severe allergic reactions, angioedema, anaphylaxis

Pharmacokinetics

Absorption	Rapidly absorbed
Distribution	Unknown
Metabolism	Liver—inactive metabolite
Excretion	Kidneys, breast milk
Half-life	2½ hr, increased in geriatric

Pharmacodynamics

Onset	PO up to 1.5 mg

INTERACTIONS
Individual drugs
Alcohol: increased action of both products

Drug classifications
CNS depressants: increased action of both products
CYP3A4 inhibitors/inducers: increased or decreased zolpidem levels

NURSING CONSIDERATIONS
Assessment
- Assess mental status: mood, sensorium, anxiety, affect, sleeping pattern, drowsiness, dizziness, especially geriatric; physical dependency, withdrawal symptoms: anxiety, panic attacks, agitation, seizures, headache, nausea, vomiting, muscle pain, weakness; **suicidal tendencies**; for indications of increasing tolerance and abuse

- Monitor B/P (lying, standing), pulse; if systolic B/P drops 20 mm Hg, hold product, notify prescriber
- Monitor I&O ratio for renal dysfunction

Patient/family education
- Advise patient that complex sleep-related behavior may occur (sleep driving/eating)
- Instruct patient that product may be taken with food or fluids, next-morning impairment may occur
- Caution patient not to use for everyday stress or longer than 3 mo unless directed by prescriber; not to take more than prescribed amount; may be habit forming; not to double or skip doses
- Caution patient to avoid OTC preparations unless approved by prescriber; alcohol and CNS depressants will increase CNS depression
- Advise patient to avoid driving, activities that require alertness, because drowsiness may occur; to avoid alcohol ingestion or other psychotropic medications; to rise slowly or fainting may occur, especially geriatric; that drowsiness may worsen at beginning of treatment
- Instruct patient not to discontinue medication abruptly after long-term use; withdrawal symptoms include vomiting, cramping, tremors, seizures
- Teach patient use of orally disintegrating tabs: place on tongue, allow to dissolve before swallowing
- Teach patient not to crush, chew, break ext rel tabs
- Teach patient to prime spray pump before using

Evaluation
Positive therapeutic outcome
- Ability to sleep at night
- Decreased amount of early-morning awakening if taking product for insomnia

TREATMENT OF OVERDOSE:
Lavage, VS, supportive care

---

zonisamide (Rx)
(zone-is′a-mide)
Zonegran
Func. class.: Anticonvulsant
Chem. class.: Sulfonamides
Pregnancy category C

ACTION: May act through sodium and calcium channels, but exact action is unknown; serotoninergic action

Therapeutic outcome: Decreased seizures

USES: Epilepsy, adjunctive therapy of partial seizures

CONTRAINDICATIONS

Hypersensitivity to this product or sulfonamides

Precautions: Pregnancy **C,** breastfeeding, children <16 yr, geriatric, allergies, renal/hepatic disease, psychiatric condition, hepatic failure, pulmonary disease, suicidal ideation

DOSAGE AND ROUTES

Adults and child >16 yr: PO 100 mg/day, may increase after 2 wk to 200 mg/day, may increase q2wk, max dose 600 mg/day

Available forms: Caps 25, 50, 100 mg

Implementation

• Give without regard to food, swallow whole

ADVERSE EFFECTS

CNS: Dizziness, insomnia, paresthesias, depression, fatigue, headache, confusion, somnolence, agitation, irritability, speech disturbance, **suicidal ideation, seizures, status epilepticus**
EENT: Diplopia, verbal difficulty, speech abnormalities, taste perversion, amblyopia, pharyngitis, rhinitis, tinnitus, nystagmus
GI: Nausea, constipation, anorexia, weight loss, diarrhea, dyspepsia, dry mouth, abdominal pain
GU: Kidney stones
HEMA: Aplastic anemia, granulocytopenia (rare), ecchymosis
INTEG: Rash
MISC: Flulike symptoms
SYST: Stevens-Johnson syndrome, metabolic acidosis

Pharmacokinetics

Absorption	Unknown
Distribution	Protein binding 40%
Metabolism	Liver
Excretion	Kidneys
Half-life	In RBCs 105 hr

Pharmacodynamics

Onset	Unknown
Peak	2-6 hr
Duration	Unknown

INTERACTIONS

Individual drugs

Alcohol: increased CNS depression

Drug classifications

CarBAMazepine, PHENobarbital, phenytoin: decreased half-life of zonisamide
CYP3A4 inducers, inhibitors: altered product levels

Drug/herb

St. John's wort: increased effect of zonisamide

Drug/food

Grapefruit: do not use together

Drug/lab test

Increased: BUN, creatinine

NURSING CONSIDERATIONS

Assessment

• Assess for seizures: duration, type, intensity, precipitating factors
• Renal function: albumin conc, BUN, urinalysis, creatinine; serum bicarbonate baseline, periodically
⚠ **Assess mental status: mood, sensorium, affect, memory (long, short); suicidal thoughts/behavior**
⚠ **Stevens-Johnson syndrome, aplastic anemia, fulminant hepatic necrosis; may cause death; monitor for rashes and hypersensitive reactions**
• Assess for rash, hypersensitivity reaction
• Obtain bicarbonate before treatment/periodically; metabolic acidosis may occur in child

Patient/family education

• Advise patient not to discontinue product abruptly; seizures may occur
• Advise patient to avoid hazardous activities until stabilized on product
• Advise patient to carry/wear emergency ID stating product use
• Teach patient not to use grapefruit juice
• Teach patient to notify prescriber of sore throat, fever, easy bruising
⚠ **Teach patient to notify prescriber of rash immediately; to notify prescriber of back pain, abdominal pain, blood in urine; to increase fluid intake to reduce risk of kidney stones**
⚠ **Teach patient to report suicidal thoughts, behaviors immediately**

Evaluation

Positive therapeutic outcome
• Decrease in severity of seizures

Adverse effects: *italics* = common; **bold** = life-threatening

Z

Alpha-adrenergic Blockers

ACTION: α-Adrenergic blockers bind to α-adrenergic receptors, causing dilatation of peripheral blood vessels and lower peripheral resistance resulting in decreased blood pressure.

USES: α-Adrenergic blockers are used for benign prostatic hyperplasia, pheochromocytoma, prevention of tissue necrosis, and sloughing associated with extravasation of IV vasopressors.

CONTRAINDICATIONS
Hypersensitive reactions may occur, and allergies should be identified before these products are given. Patients with myocardial infarction, coronary insufficiency, angina, or other evidence of coronary artery disease should not use these products.

IMPLEMENTATION
PO route
• Start with low dose, gradually increasing to prevent side effects
• Give with food or milk for GI symptoms

ADVERSE EFFECTS: The most common side effects are hypotension, tachycardia, nasal stuffiness, nausea, vomiting, and diarrhea.

PHARMACOKINETICS: Onset, peak, and duration vary among products.

INTERACTIONS: Vasoconstrictive and hypertensive effects of EPINEPHrine are antagonized by α-adrenergic blockers.

NURSING CONSIDERATIONS
Assessment
• Monitor electrolytes: potassium, sodium chloride, carbon dioxide
• Monitor weight daily, I&O
• Monitor B/P with patient lying, standing before starting treatment, q4hr thereafter
• Assess for nausea, vomiting, diarrhea
• Assess for skin turgor, dryness of mucous membranes for hydration status

Patient/family education
• Caution patient to avoid alcoholic beverages
• Advise patient to report dizziness, palpitations, fainting
• Instruct patient to change position slowly or fainting may occur
• Teach patient to take product exactly as prescribed; to avoid all OTC products (cough, cold, allergy) unless directed by prescriber

Evaluation
Positive therapeutic outcome
• Decreased B/P
• Increased peripheral pulses

Generic Names
α 1 blockers:
silodosin

Anesthetics—general/local

ACTION: Anesthetics (general) act on the CNS to produce tranquilization and sleep before invasive procedures. Anesthetics (local) inhibit conduction of nerve impulses from sensory nerves.

USES: General anesthetics are used to premedicate for surgery, and for induction and maintenance in general anesthesia. For local anesthetics, refer to individual product listing for indications.

CONTRAINDICATIONS
Persons with CVA, increased ICP, severe hypertension, and cardiac decompensation should not use these products since severe adverse reactions can occur.

Precautions: Anesthetics (general) should be used with caution in the geriatric, children <2 yr, and those with cardiovascular disease (hypotension, bradydysrhythmias), renal/hepatic disease, and Parkinson's disease. The precaution for anesthetics (local) is pregnancy.

IMPLEMENTATION
• Give anticholinergic preoperatively to decrease secretions
• Administer only with resuscitative equipment nearby
• Provide quiet environment for recovery to decrease psychotic symptoms

ADVERSE EFFECTS: The most common side effects are dystonia, akathisia, flexion of arms, fine tremors, drowsiness, restlessness, and hypotension. Also common are chills, respiratory depression, and laryngospasm.

PHARMACOKINETICS: Onset, peak, and duration vary widely among products. Most products are metabolized in the liver and excreted in urine.

INTERACTIONS: AOIs, tricyclics, and phenothiazines may cause severe hypo/hypertension when used with local anesthetics. CNS depressants will potentiate general and local anesthetics.

NURSING CONSIDERATIONS
Assessment
• Monitor VS q10min during **IV** administration, q30min after IM dose

Evaluation

Positive therapeutic outcome
• Maintenance of anesthesia
• Decreased pain

Generic Names

General anesthetics:
droperidol (high alert), **fentaNYL** (high alert), fentaNYL/droperidol, fentaNYL transdermal, fospropofol, midazolam, **propofol** (high alert)

Local anesthetics:
lidocaine, parenteral (high alert), penicillin G procaine, ropivacaine

Antacids

ACTION: Antacids are basic compounds that neutralize gastric acidity and decrease the rate of gastric emptying. Products are divided into those containing aluminum, magnesium, calcium, or a combination of these.

USES: Antacids decrease hyperacidity in conditions such as peptic ulcer disease, reflux esophagitis, gastritis, or hiatal hernia.

CONTRAINDICATIONS
Sensitivity to aluminum or magnesium products may cause hypersensitive reactions. Aluminum products should not be used by persons sensitive to aluminum. Magnesium products should not be used by persons sensitive to magnesium. Check for sensitivity before administering.

Precautions: Magnesium products should be given cautiously to patients with renal insufficiency, and during pregnancy and breastfeeding. Sodium content of antacids may be significant. Use with caution for patients with hypertension, or CHF or those on a low-sodium diet.

IMPLEMENTATION
• Advise patient not to take other products within 1-2 hr of antacid administration, since antacids may impair absorption of other products
• Give all products with an 8-oz glass of water to ensure absorption in the stomach
• Give another antacid if constipation occurs with aluminum products

ADVERSE EFFECTS: The most common side effect caused by aluminum-containing antacids is constipation, which may lead to fecal impaction and bowel obstruction. Diarrhea occurs often when magnesium products are given. Alkalosis may occur when systemic products are used. Constipation occurs more frequently than laxation with calcium carbonate. The release of CO_2 from carbonate-containing antacids causes belching, abdominal distention, and flatulence. Sodium bicarbonate may act as a systemic antacid and produce systemic electrolyte disturbances and alkalosis. Calcium carbonate and sodium bicarbonate may cause rebound hyperacidity and milk-alkali syndrome. Alkaluria may occur when products are used on a long-term basis, particularly in persons with abnormal renal function.

PHARMACOKINETICS: Duration is 20-40 min. If ingested 1 hr after meals, acidity is reduced for at least 3hr.

INTERACTIONS: Products whose effects may be increased by some antacids include quiNIDine, amphetamines, pseudoephedrine, levodopa, valproic acid, and dicumarol. Products whose effects may be decreased by some antacids include cimetidine, corticosteroids, ranitidine, iron salts, phenothiazines, phenytoin, digoxin, tetracyclines, ketoconazole, salicylates, and isoniazid.

NURSING CONSIDERATIONS
Assessment
• Assess for aggravating and alleviating factors of epigastric pain or hyperacidity; identify the location, duration, and characteristics of epigastric pain
• Assess GI symptoms, including constipation, diarrhea, abdominal pain; if severe abdominal pain with fever occurs, these products should not be given
• Assess renal symptoms, including increasing urinary pH, electrolytes

Evaluation

Positive therapeutic outcome
• Absence of epigastric pain
• Decreased acidity

Generic Names
aluminum hydroxide, bismuth subsalicylate, calcium carbonate, magaldrate, magnesium oxide, sodium bicarbonate

Anti-Alzheimer Agents

ACTION: Anti-Alzheimer agents improve cognitive functioning by increasing acetylcholine and inhibiting cholinesterase in the CNS. They do not cure the condition, but improve symptoms.

USES: Anti-Alzheimer agents are used for the treatment of Alzheimer's symptoms.

CONTRAINDICATIONS
Persons with hypersensitivity reactions should not use these products.

Precautions: Anti-Alzheimer agents should be used cautiously in pregnancy **(C)**, breastfeeding, sick sinus syndrome, GI bleeding, bladder obstruction, and seizures.

IMPLEMENTATION
• Give lowest possible dose for therapeutic result; adjust dose to response
• Provide assistance with ambulation during beginning therapy if dizziness, ataxia occur

ADVERSE EFFECTS: The most common side effects are nausea, vomiting, diarrhea, dry mouth, insomnia, dizziness, urinary frequency, incontinence, and rash. The most serious side effects are seizures and dysrhythmias.

PHARMACOKINETICS: Onset, peak, and duration vary widely among products. Most products are metabolized in the liver and excreted by the kidneys.

INTERACTIONS: Increased synergistic reactions may occur with succinylcholine, cholinesterase inhibitors, and cholingeric agonists. There may be a decrease in the action of anticholinergics, and there may be additive effects when used with cholinergic agents.

NURSING CONSIDERATIONS
Assessment
• B/P, hypo/hypertension
• Mental status: affect, mood, behavioral changes, depression, confusion
• GI status: nausea, vomiting, anorexia, diarrhea
• GU status: urinary frequency, incontinence

Patient/family education
• Instruct patient to report side effects, adverse reactions to healthcare provider
• Advise patient to use exactly as prescribed, at regular intervals
• Caution patient not to increase or abruptly decrease dose; serious consequences may result
• Inform patient that product is not a cure, but relieves symptoms

Evaluation

Positive therapeutic outcome
• Decrease in confusion
• Improved mood

Generic Names
donepezil, memantine, rivastigmine

Antianginals

ACTION: Antianginals are divided into the nitrates, calcium channel blockers, and β-adrenergic blockers. The nitrates dilate coronary arteries, causing decreased preload, and dilate systemic arteries, causing decreased afterload. Calcium channel blockers dilate coronary arteries and decrease SA/AV node conduction. β-adrenergic blockers decrease heart rate so that myocardial O_2 use is decreased. Dipyridamole selectively dilates coronary arteries to increase coronary blood flow.

USES: Antianginals are used in chronic stable angina pectoris, unstable angina, and vasospastic angina. Some (i.e., calcium channel blockers and β-blockers) may be used as dysrhythmics and in hypertension.

CONTRAINDICATIONS
Persons with known hypersensitivity, increased ICP, or cerebral hemorrhage should not use some of these products.

Precautions: Antianginals should be used with caution in pregnancy, breastfeeding, children, postural hypotension, renal disease, and hepatic injury.

IMPLEMENTATION
• Store protected from light, moisture; place in cool environment

ADVERSE EFFECTS: The most common side effects are postural hypotension, headache, flushing, dizziness, nausea, edema, and drowsiness. Also common are rash, dysrhythmias, and fatigue.

PHARMACOKINETICS: Onset, peak, and duration vary widely among coronary products. Most products are metabolized in the liver and excreted in urine.

INTERACTIONS: Interactions vary widely among products. Check individual monographs for specific information.

NURSING CONSIDERATIONS
Assessment
• Monitor orthostatic B/P, pulse
• Assess for pain: duration, time started, activity being performed, character
• Assess for tolerance if taken over long period
• Assess for headache, light-headedness, decreased B/P; may indicate a need for decreased dosage

---

Patient/family education
• Instruct patient to keep tabs in original container
• Instruct patient not to use OTC products unless directed by prescriber
• Advise patient to report bradycardia, dizziness, confusion, depression, fever
• Teach patient to take pulse at home; advise when to notify prescriber
• Advise patient to avoid alcohol, smoking, sodium intake
• Advise patient to comply with weight control, dietary adjustments, modified exercise program
• Teach patient to carry/wear emergency ID to identify product being taken, allergies
• Caution patient to make position changes slowly to prevent fainting

Evaluation

Positive therapeutic outcome
• Decrease, prevention of anginal pain

Generic Names
Nitrates:
isosorbide, nitroglycerin

β-adrenergic blockers:
atenolol, dipyridamole, metoprolol, nadolol, propranolol

Calcium channel blockers:
amLODIPine, **diltiazem** (high alert), niCARdipine, NIFEdipine, verapamil

Miscellaneous:
ranolazine

Antianxiety Agents

ACTION: Benzodiazepines potentiate the action of GABA, including any other inhibitory transmitters in the CNS, resulting in decreased anxiety. Most agents cause a decrease in CNS excitability.

USES: Anxiety is relieved in conditions such as generalized anxiety disorder and phobic disorders. Benzodiazepines are also used for acute alcohol withdrawal to prevent delirium tremens, and some products are used for relaxation before surgery.

CONTRAINDICATIONS
These products are contraindicated in hypersensitivity, acute closed-angle glaucoma, breastfeeding (diazepam), children <6 mo, and hepatic disease (clonazePAM).

Precautions: Antianxiety agents should be used cautiously in geriatric or debilitated patients. Usually smaller doses are needed since metabolism is slowed. Persons with renal/hepatic disease may show delayed excretion. ClonazePAM may increase the incidence of seizures.

IMPLEMENTATION
• Give with food or milk for GI symptoms; may give crushed if patient is unable to swallow whole (tabs only, no controlled or sustained-release products)

ADVERSE EFFECTS: The most common side effects are dizziness, drowsiness, blurred vision, and orthostatic hypotension. Most adverse reactions are mediated through the CNS. There is potential for abuse and physical dependence with some products.

PHARMACOKINETICS: Most of these agents are metabolized by the liver and excreted via the kidneys.

INTERACTIONS: Increased CNS depression may occur when given with other CNS depressants. These products should be used together cautiously. Alcohol should not be used, as fatal reactions have occurred. The serum concentration and toxicity may be increased when used with benzodiazepines.

NURSING CONSIDERATIONS
Assessment
• Assess B/P (lying and standing), pulse; if systolic B/P drops 20 mm Hg, hold product and notify prescriber; orthostatic hypotension can be severe
• Monitor renal/hepatic function tests: AST, ALT, bilirubin, creatinine, LDH, alkaline phosphatase
• Monitor physical dependency and withdrawal with some products, including headache, nausea, vomiting, muscle pain, and weakness after long-term use

Patient/family education
• Inform patient that product should not be used for everyday stress or long-term use; not to take more than prescribed amount since product is habit forming
• Caution patient to avoid driving and activities that require alertness since drowsiness and dizziness may occur
• Instruct patient to abstain from alcohol, other psychotropic medications unless directed by prescriber
• Caution patient not to discontinue abruptly; after extended periods, withdrawal symptoms may occur

Evaluation

Positive therapeutic outcome
• Decreased anxiety
• Increased relaxation

Generic Names

Benzodiazepines:
ALPRAZolam, chlordiazePOXIDE, clonazePAM, diazepam, LORazepam, midazolam, triazolam

Miscellaneous:
busPIRone, doxepin, hydrOXYzine, PARoxetine, venlafaxine

Antiasthmatics

ACTION: Bronchodilators are divided into anticholinergics, α/β-adrenergic agonists, β-adrenergic agonists, and phosphodiesterase inhibitors. Also included in antiasthmatic agents are corticosteroids, leukotriene antagonists, mast cell stabilizers, and monoclonal antibodies. Anticholinergics act by inhibiting interaction of acetylcholine at receptor sites on bronchial smooth muscle. α/β-adrenergic agonists act by relaxing bronchial smooth muscle and increasing diameter of nasal passages. β-adrenergic agonists act by action on β₂-receptors, which relaxes bronchial smooth muscle. Phosphodiesterase inhibitors act by blocking phosphodiesterase and increasing cAMP, which mediates smooth muscle relaxation in the respiratory system. Corticosteroids act by decreasing inflammation in the bronchial system. Leukotriene receptor antagonists decrease leukotrienes, and mast cell stabilizers decrease histamine; both act to decrease bronchospasm.

USES: Antiasthmatics are used for bronchial asthma; bronchospasm associated with bronchitis, emphysema, or other obstructive pulmonary diseases; Cheyne-Stokes respirations; and prevention of exercise-induced asthma. Some products are used for rhinitis and other allergic reactions.

CONTRAINDICATIONS

Persons with hypersensitivity, closed-angle glaucoma, tachydysrhythmias, and severe cardiac disease should not use some of these products.

Precautions: Antiasthmatics should be used with caution in pregnancy, breastfeeding, hyperthyroidism, hypertension, prostatic hypertrophy, and seizure disorders.

IMPLEMENTATION

• Give inhaled product after shaking; exhale, place mouthpiece in mouth, inhale slowly, hold breath, remove, exhale slowly
• Give PO product with meals to decrease gastric irritation

• Store inhaled product in light-resistant container; do not expose to temperatures >86° F (30° C)
• Give gum, small sips of water for dry mouth

ADVERSE EFFECTS: The most common side effects are tremors, anxiety, nausea, vomiting and irritation in the throat. The most serious adverse reactions are bronchospasm and dyspnea.

PHARMACOKINETICS: Onset, peak, and duration vary widely among products. Most products are metabolized by the liver and excreted in urine.

INTERACTIONS: Interactions vary widely among products. Check individual monographs for specific information.

NURSING CONSIDERATIONS
Assessment
• Monitor respiratory function: vital capacity, forced expiratory volume, ABGs, lung sounds, heart rate and rhythm, aggravating and alleviating factors

Patient/family education
• Caution patient to avoid hazardous activities; drowsiness or dizziness may occur with some products
• Instruct patient to obtain bloodwork as required; some products require blood levels to be drawn
• Advise patient to avoid all OTC medications unless approved by provider
• Instruct patient to report side effects, including insomnia, heart palpitations, light-headedness; these side effects may occur with some products

Evaluation

Positive therapeutic outcome
• Decreased severity and number of asthma attacks
• Absence of dyspnea, wheezing

Generic Names

Bronchodilators:
albuterol, arformoterol, **atropine** (high alert), formoterol, ipratropium, levalbuterol, terbutaline, theophylline, tiotropium

Adrenergics:
EPINEPHrine (high alert)

Corticosteroids:
beclomethasone, betamethasone, budesonide, cortisone, dexamethasone, flunisolide, fluticasone, hydrocortisone, methylPREDNISolone, predniSONE, triamcinolone

---

Leukotriene antagonists:
zafirlukast

Monoclonal antibodies:
omalizumab

Anticholinergics

ACTION: Anticholinergics inhibit the muscarinic actions of acetylcholine at receptor sites in the autonomic nervous system. Anticholinergics are also known as antimuscarinic products.

USES: Anticholinergics are used for a variety of conditions: decreasing involuntary movements in parkinsonism (benztropine, trihexyphenidyl); bradydysrhythmias (atropine); nausea and vomiting (scopolamine); and as cycloplegic mydriatics (atropine, hematropine, scopalamine, cyclopentolate, tropicamide). Gastrointestinal anticholinergics are used to decrease motility (smooth muscle tone) in the GI, biliary, and urinary tracts and for their ability to decrease gastric secretions (propantheline, glycopyrrolate).

CONTRAINDICATIONS
Persons with closed-angle glaucoma, myasthenia gravis, or GI/GU obstruction should not use some of these products.

Precautions: Anticholinergics should be used with caution in pregnant, breastfeeding, or geriatric patients, or in those with prostatic hypertrophy, CHF, or hypertension. Use with caution in the presence of high environmental temperature.

IMPLEMENTATION
PO route
• Give with or after meals to prevent GI upset; may give with fluids other than water
• Store at room temperature
• Give hard candy, frequent drinks, sugarless gum to relieve dry mouth

IM/IV route
• Give parenteral dose with patient recumbent to prevent postural hypotension
• Give parenteral dose slowly; keep in bed for at least 1 hr after dose; monitor VS
• Give after checking dose carefully; even slight overdose could lead to toxicity

ADVERSE EFFECTS: The most common side effects are dry mouth, constipation, urinary retention, urinary hesitancy, headache, and dizziness. Also common is paralytic ileus.

PHARMACOKINETICS: Onset, peak, and duration vary widely among products. Most products are metabolized in the liver and excreted in urine.

INTERACTIONS: Increased anticholinergic effects may occur when used with MAOIs, tricyclics, and amantadine. Anticholinergics may cause a decreased effect of phenothiazines and levodopa.

NURSING CONSIDERATIONS
Assessment
• Assess I&O ratio; retention commonly causes decreased urinary output
• Assess for urinary hesitancy, retention; palpate bladder if retention occurs
• Assess for constipation; increase fluids, bulk, exercise if this occurs
• Identify tolerance over long-term therapy; dosage may need to be increased or changed
• Assess mental status: affect, mood, CNS depression, worsening of mental symptoms during early therapy

Patient/family education
• Caution patient to avoid driving and other hazardous activities; drowsiness may occur
• Advise patient to avoid OTC medication: cough, cold preparations with alcohol, antihistamines unless directed by prescriber

Evaluation

Positive therapeutic outcome
• Decreased secretions
• Absence of nausea and vomiting

Generic Names
atropine (high alert), benztropine, glycopyrrolate, hyoscyamine, scopolamine (transdermal), solifenacin

Anticoagulants

ACTION: Anticoagulants interfere with blood clotting by preventing clot formation.

USES: Anticoagulants are used for DVT, pulmonary emboli, myocardial infarction, open heart surgery, disseminated intravascular clotting syndrome, atrial fibrillation with embolization, and in transfusion and dialysis.

CONTRAINDICATIONS
Persons with hemophilia and related disorders, leukemia with bleeding, peptic ulcer disease, thrombocytopenic purpura, blood dyscrasias, acute nephritis, and subacute bacterial endocarditis should not use these products.

Precautions: Anticoagulants should be used with caution in pregnancy, geriatric, and alcoholism.

IMPLEMENTATION
• Store in tight container (PO dose)

SUBCUT route
- Give at same time each day to maintain steady blood levels
- Do not massage area or aspirate when giving SUBCUT inj; give in abdomen between pelvic bones; rotate sites; do not pull back on plunger, leave in for 10 sec; apply gentle pressure for 1 min
- Do not change needles
- Avoid all IM inj that may cause bleeding

ADVERSE EFFECTS: The most serious adverse reactions are hemorrhage, agranulocytosis, leukopenia, eosinophilia, and thrombocytopenia, depending on the specific product. The most common side effects are diarrhea, rash, and fever.

PHARMACOKINETICS: Onset, peak, and duration vary widely among products. Most products are metabolized in the liver and excreted in urine.

INTERACTIONS: Salicylates, steroids, and nonsteroidal antiinflammatories will potentiate the action of anticoagulants. Anticoagulants may cause serious effects. Check individual monographs for specific information.

NURSING CONSIDERATIONS
Assessment
- Monitor blood tests (Hct, platelets, occult blood in stools) q3mo
- Monitor PTT, which should be 1½-2 × control, PPT; daily, APTT, ACT, INR
- Monitor B/P; watch for increasing signs of hypertension
- Monitor for bleeding gums, petechiae, ecchymosis, black tarry stools, hematuria
- Monitor for fever, skin rash, urticaria
- Monitor for needed dosage change q1-2wk

Patient/family education
- Advise patient to avoid OTC preparations that may cause serious product interactions unless directed by prescriber
- Inform patient that product may be held during active bleeding (menstruation), depending on condition
- Caution patient to use soft-bristle toothbrush to prevent bleeding gums; avoid contact sports; use electric razor
- Instruct patient to carry/wear emergency ID identifying product taken
- Instruct patient to report any signs of bleeding: gums, under skin, urine, stools

Evaluation

Positive therapeutic outcome
- Decrease of DVT

Generic Names
argatroban, dabigatran, **dalteparin** (high alert), **enoxaparin** (high alert), fondaparinux, **heparin** (high alert), **lepirudin** (high alert), **tinzaparin** (high alert), **warfarin** (high alert)

Anticonvulsants

ACTION: Anticonvulsants are divided into the barbiturates, benzodiazepines, hydantoins, succinimides, and miscellaneous products. Barbiturates and benzodiazepines are discussed in separate sections. Hydantoins act by inhibiting the spread of seizure activity in the motor cortex. Succinimides act by inhibiting spike and wave formation; they also decrease amplitude, frequency, duration, and spread of discharge in seizures.

USES: Hydantoins are used in generalized tonic-clonic seizures, status epilepticus, and psychomotor seizures. Succinimides are used for absence (or petit mal) seizures. Barbiturates are used in generalized tonic-clonic and cortical focal seizures.

CONTRAINDICATIONS
Hypersensitive reactions may occur, and allergies should be identified before these products are given.

Precautions: Persons with renal/hepatic disease should be watched closely.

IMPLEMENTATION
PO route
- Give with food, milk to decrease GI symptoms
- Provide good oral hygiene as it is important for patients taking hydantoins

ADVERSE EFFECTS: Bone marrow depression is the most life-threatening adverse reaction associated with hydantoins or succinimides. The most common side effects are GI symptoms. Other common side effects for hydantoins are gingival hyperplasia and CNS effects such as nystagmus, ataxia, slurred speech, and confusion.

PHARMACOKINETICS: Onset, peak, and duration vary widely among products. Most products are metabolized in the liver and excreted in urine, bile, and feces.

INTERACTIONS: Hydantoins cause decreased effects of estrogens, and oral contraceptives.

NURSING CONSIDERATIONS
Assessment
- Monitor renal function tests, including BUN, creatinine, serum uric acid, urine CCr before, during therapy

---

- Monitor blood tests: RBC, Hct, Hgb, reticulocyte counts weekly for 4 wk then monthly
- Monitor hepatic function tests: AST, ALT, bilirubin, creatinine
- Assess mental status, including mood, sensorium, affect, behavioral changes; if mental status changes, notify prescriber
- Assess for eye problems, including need for ophth examinations before, during, and after treatment (slit lamp, fundoscopy, tonometry)
- Assess for allergic reaction, including red, raised rash; if this occurs, product should be discontinued
- Assess for blood dyscrasias, including fever, sore throat, bruising, rash, jaundice
- Monitor toxicity, including bone marrow depression, nausea, vomiting, ataxia, diplopia, cardiovascular collapse, Stevens-Johnson syndrome

Patient/family education
- Advise patient to carry/wear emergency ID stating products taken, condition, prescriber's name, phone number
- Advise patient to avoid driving, other activities that require alertness

Evaluation
Positive therapeutic outcome
- Decreased seizure activity; document on patient's chart

Generic Names
Succinimides:
ethosuximide

Hydantoins:
fosphenytoin, phenytoin

Miscellaneous:
acetaZOLAMIDE, carBAMazepine, clonazePAM, diazepam, eslicarbazepine, ezogabine, gabapentin, lacosamide, lamoTRIgine, **magnesium sulfate** (high alert), rufinamide, tiaGABine, topiramate, valproate/valproic acid/divalproex sodium, vigabatrin, zonisamide

Barbiturates:
PHENobarbital (high alert), primidone, **thiopental** (high alert)

Antidepressants

ACTION: Antidepressants are divided into the tricyclics, MAOIs, and miscellaneous antidepressants (SSRIs). The tricyclics work by blocking reuptake of norepinephrine and serotonin into nerve endings and increasing action of norepinephrine and serotonin in nerve cells. MAOIs act by increasing concentrations of endogenous EPINEPHrine, norepinephrine, serotonin, and dopamine in storage sites in the CNS by inhibition of MAO; increased concentration reduces depression.

USES: Antidepressants are used for depression and, in some cases, enuresis in children.

CONTRAINDICATIONS
The contraindications for antidepressants are seizure disorders, prostatic hypertrophy, and severe renal/hepatic/cardiac disease depending on the type of medication.

Precautions: Antidepressants should be used cautiously in pregnant, geriatric, and suicidal patients; severe depression; schizophrenia; hyperactivity; and diabetes mellitus.

IMPLEMENTATION
PO route
- Give increased fluids, bulk in diet if constipation, urinary retention occur
- Give with food or milk for GI symptoms
- Give gum, hard candy, or frequent sips of water for dry mouth
- Store in airtight container at room temperature; do not refreeze
- Provide assistance with ambulation during beginning therapy since drowsiness/dizziness occurs

ADVERSE EFFECTS: The most serious adverse reactions are paralytic ileus, acute renal failure, hypertension, and hypertensive crisis, depending on the specific product. Common side effects are dizziness, drowsiness, diarrhea, dry mouth, urinary retention, and orthostatic hypotension.

PHARMACOKINETICS: Onset, peak, and duration vary widely among products. Most products are metabolized in the liver and excreted in urine.

INTERACTIONS: Interactions vary widely among products. Check individual monographs for specific information.

NURSING CONSIDERATIONS
Assessment
- Monitor B/P (lying, standing), pulse q4hr; if systolic B/P drops 20 mm Hg, hold product, notify prescriber; take VS q4hr in patients with CV disease
- Monitor blood tests: CBC, leukocytes, differential, cardiac enzymes if patient is receiving long-term therapy
- Monitor hepatic function tests: AST, ALT, bilirubin, creatinine
- Monitor weight weekly; appetite may increase with product

• Monitor for EPS primarily in geriatric: rigidity, dystonia, akathisia
• Assess mental status: mood, sensorium, affect, suicidal tendencies, increase in psychiatric symptoms (depression, panic)
• Check for urinary retention, constipation; constipation is more likely to occur in children, geriatric patients
• Assess for withdrawal symptoms: headache, nausea, vomiting, muscle pain, weakness; do not usually occur unless product was discontinued abruptly
• Identify alcohol consumption; if alcohol is consumed, hold dose until AM

Patient/family education
• Teach patient that therapeutic effects may take 2-3 wk
• Advise patient to use caution in driving or other activities requiring alertness because of drowsiness, dizziness, blurred vision
• Caution patient to avoid alcohol ingestion, other CNS depressants
• Instruct patient not to discontinue medication quickly after long-term use; may cause nausea, headache, malaise
• Instruct patient to wear sunscreen or large hat, since photosensitivity may occur

Evaluation

Positive therapeutic outcome
• Decreased depression

Generic Names

Tetracyclics:
mirtazapine

Tricyclics:
amitriptyline, clomiPRAMINE, desipramine, doxepin, imipramine, nortriptyline

Miscellaneous:
buPROPion, DULoxetine, levomilnacipran, traZODone, venlafaxine, vortioxetine

SSRIs:
citalopram, escitalopram, FLUoxetine, PARoxetine, sertraline

Antidiabetics

ACTION: Antidiabetics are divided into the insulins that decrease blood glucose, phosphate, and potassium and increase blood pyruvate and lactate and oral antidiabetics that cause functioning β-cells in the pancreas to release insulin and improve the effect of endogenous and exogenous insulin.

USES: Insulins are used for ketoacidosis and diabetes mellitus types 1 and 2; oral antidiabetics are used for diabetes mellitus type 2.

CONTRAINDICATIONS
Hypersensitive reactions may occur, and allergies should be identified before these products are given. Oral antidiabetics should not be used in juvenile or brittle diabetes, diabetic ketoacidosis, or severe renal/hepatic disease.

Precautions: Oral antidiabetics should be used with caution in pregnancy, breastfeeding, geriatric, cardiac disease, and in the presence of alcohol.

IMPLEMENTATION
PO route
• Give oral antidiabetic 30 min before meals
SUBCUT route
• Give insulin after warming to room temperature by rotating in palms to prevent lipodystrophy from injecting cold insulin
• Give human insulin to those allergic to beef or pork
• Rotate inj sites when giving insulin; use abdomen, upper back, thighs, upper arm, buttocks; keep a record of sites

ADVERSE EFFECTS: The most common side effect of insulin and oral antidiabetics is hypoglycemia. Other adverse reactions for oral antidiabetics include blood dyscrasias, hepatotoxicity, and, rarely, cholestatic jaundice. Adverse reactions for insulin products include allergic responses and, more rarely, anaphylaxis.

PHARMACOKINETICS: Onset, peak, and duration vary widely among products. Oral antidiabetics are metabolized in the liver, with metabolites excreted in urine, bile, and feces.

INTERACTIONS: Interactions vary widely among products. Check individual monographs for specific information.

NURSING CONSIDERATIONS
Assessment
• Monitor blood, urine glucose levels during treatment to determine diabetes control (oral products)
• Monitor fasting blood glucose, 2 hr PP (60-100 mg/dl normal fasting level) (70-130 mg/dl—normal 2-hr level)
• Assess for hypoglycemic reaction that can occur during peak time

Patient/family education
• Advise patient to avoid alcohol and salicylates except on advice of prescriber

---

- Teach patient symptoms of ketoacidosis: nausea, thirst, polyuria, dry mouth, decreased B/P, dry, flushed skin, acetone breath, drowsiness, Kussmaul respirations
- Teach patient symptoms of hypoglycemia: headache, tremors, fatigue, weakness; that candy or sugar should be carried to treat hypoglycemia
- Advise patient to test urine for glucose/ketones tid if this product is replacing insulin
- Advise patient to continue weight control, dietary restrictions, exercise, hygiene

Evaluation

Positive therapeutic outcome
- Decrease in polyuria, polydipsia, polyphagia
- Clear sensorium
- Absence of dizziness
- Stable gait

Generic Names

albiglutide, canagliflozin, dapagliflozin, **dulaglutide** (high alert), empagliflozin, glipiZIDE, glyBURIDE, **insulin aspart** (high alert), **insulin detemir** (high alert), **insulin glargine** (high alert), **insulin glulisine** (high alert), **insulin lispro** (high alert), **insulin, regular** (high alert), **insulin, regular concentrated** (high alert), insulin, zinc suspension (Lente), insulin, zinc suspension extended (Ultralente), liraglutide, linagliptin, metFORMIN, miglitol, pioglitazone, repaglinide, rosiglitazone, saxagliptin, sitaGLIPtin

Antidiarrheals

ACTION: Antidiarrheals work by various actions including direct action on intestinal muscles to decrease GI peristalsis or by inhibiting prostaglandin synthesis responsible for GI hypermotility, acting on mucosal receptors responsible for peristalsis, or decreasing water content of stools.

USES: Antidiarrheals are used for diarrhea of undetermined causes.

CONTRAINDICATIONS

The contraindications are persons with severe ulcerative colitis, and pseudomembranous colitis with some products.

Precautions: Antidiarrheals should be used with caution in pregnancy, breastfeeding, children, geriatric patients, dehydration.

IMPLEMENTATION
PO route
- Give for 48 hr only

ADVERSE EFFECTS: The most serious adverse reactions of some products are paralytic ileus, toxic megacolon, and angioneurotic edema. The most common side effects are constipation, nausea, dry mouth, and abdominal pain.

PHARMACOKINETICS: Onset, peak, and duration vary widely among products. Most products are metabolized in the liver and excreted in urine.

INTERACTIONS: Interactions vary widely among products. Check individual monographs for specific information.

NURSING CONSIDERATIONS
Assessment
- Monitor electrolytes (potassium, sodium, chloride) if on long-term therapy
- Monitor bowel pattern before; for rebound constipation after termination of medication
- Assess response after 48 hr; if no response, product should be discontinued
- Identify dehydration in children

Patient/family education
- Advise patient to avoid OTC products
- Caution patient not to exceed recommended dose

Evaluation

Positive therapeutic outcome
- Decreased diarrhea

Generic Names
bismuth subsalicylate, kaolin/pectin, loperamide

Antidysrhythmics

ACTION: Antidysrhythmics are divided into four classes and miscellaneous antidysrhythmics:
- Class I increases the duration of action potential and the effective refractory period and reduces disparity in the refractory period between a normal and infarcted myocardium; further subclasses include Ia, Ib, Ic
- Class II decreases the rate of SA node discharge, increases recovery time, slows conduction through the AV node, and decreases heart rate, which decreases O_2 consumption in the myocardium
- Class III increases the duration of action potential and the effective refractory period
- Class IV inhibits calcium ion influx across the cell membrane during cardiac depolarization; decreases SA node discharge, decreases conduction velocity through the AV node

Adverse effects: *italics* = common; **bold** = life-threatening

• Miscellaneous antidysrhythmics include those such as adenosine, which slows conduction through the AV node, and digoxin, which decreases conduction velocity and prolongs the effective refractory period in the AV node

USES: Antidysrhythmics are used for PVCs, tachycardia, hypertension, atrial fibrillation, and angina pectoris.

CONTRAINDICATIONS
Contraindications vary widely among products.

Precautions: Precautions vary widely among products.

ADVERSE EFFECTS: Side effects and
adverse reactions vary widely among products.

PHARMACOKINETICS: Onset, peak,
and duration vary widely among products.

INTERACTIONS: Interactions vary
widely among products. Check individual monographs for specific information.

NURSING CONSIDERATIONS
Assessment
• Monitor ECG continuously to determine product effectiveness, PVCs, or other dysrhythmias
• Assess for dehydration or hypovolemia
• Monitor B/P continuously for hypo/hypertension
• Monitor I&O ratio
• Monitor serum potassium
• Assess for edema in feet and legs daily

Patient/family education
• Advise patient to comply with dosage schedule, even if patient is feeling better
• Instruct patient to report bradycardia, dizziness, confusion, depression, fever

Evaluation
Positive therapeutic outcome
• Decrease in B/P in hypertension
• Decreased B/P, edema, moist crackles in CHF

Generic Names
Class Ia:
disopyramide, procainamide, quiNIDine

Class Ib:
lidocaine, parenteral (high alert), phenytoin

Class Ic:
flecainide, propafenone

Class II:
acebutolol, esmolol, propranolol, sotalol

Class III:
amiodarone (high alert), **dronedarone** (high alert), **ibutilide** (high alert)

Class IV:
verapamil

Miscellaneous:
adenosine (high alert), **atropine** (high alert), **digoxin** (high alert)

Antiemetics

ACTION: The antiemetics are divided into the 5-HT$_3$ receptor antagonists, the phenothiazines, and the miscellaneous products. The 5-HT$_3$ receptor antagonists work by blocking serotonin peripherally, centrally, and in the small intestine. The phenothiazines act by blocking the chemoreceptor trigger zone in the brain. The miscellaneous products work by either decreasing motion sickness or delaying gastric emptying.

USES: Antiemetics are used to prevent nausea and vomiting due to cancer chemotherapy, radiotherapy, and surgery (5-HT$_3$ receptor antagonists); some of the miscellaneous products (antihistamines) work by decreasing motion sickness. Most other products are used for many types of nausea and vomiting.

CONTRAINDICATIONS
Persons developing hypersensitive reactions should not use these products.

Precautions: Antiemetics should be used cautiously in pregnancy, breastfeeding, hepatic disease, and some GI disorders.

IMPLEMENTATION
• Give prophylactically, before nausea and vomiting occur, in cancer chemotherapy
• Store at room temperature vial/ampules, oral products

ADVERSE EFFECTS: The most common side effects are headache, dizziness, fatigue, and diarrhea.

PHARMACOKINETICS: Onset, peak,
and duration vary widely among products. Most products are metabolized by the liver and excreted by the kidneys.

INTERACTIONS: Interactions vary
widely among products. Check individual monographs for specific information. Other CNS depressants increase CNS depression.

NURSING CONSIDERATIONS
Assessment
• Assess reason for nausea, vomiting; absence of nausea and vomiting after giving product
• Monitor hypersensitivity reactions: rash, bronchospasm with some products

---

⚠ Nurse Alert   ✴ Key NCLEX® Drug   >> Drug Specifics

Patient/family education
• Caution patient to avoid hazardous activities if dizziness occurs; ask for assistance if hospitalized
• Instruct patient to rise slowly to prevent orthostatic hypotension
• Teach patient all aspects of product usage
• Teach patient conservative methods to control nausea and vomiting such as sips of water or other fluids and dry crackers

Evaluation

Positive therapeutic outcome
• Absence or decreasing nausea and vomiting after use

Generic Names
5-HT₃ antagonists:
dolasetron, granisetron, ondansetron, palonosetron

Phenothiazines:
chlorproMAZINE, prochlorperazine, promethazine

Miscellaneous:
aprepitant, meclizine, metoclopramide, scopolamine, trimethobenzamide

Antifungals (systemic)

ACTION: Antifungals act by increasing cell membrane permeability in susceptible organisms by binding sterols and decreasing potassium, sodium, and nutrients in the cell.

USES: Antifungals are used for infections of histoplasmosis, blastomycosis, coccidioidomycosis, cryptococcosis, aspergillosis, phycomycosis, candidiasis, sporotrichosis causing severe meningitis, septicemia, and skin infections.

CONTRAINDICATIONS
Persons with severe bone marrow depression or hypersensitivity should not use these products.

Precautions: Antifungals should be used with caution in renal/hepatic disease and pregnancy.

IMPLEMENTATION

IV route
• Give by **IV** using in-line filter (mean pore diameter >1 μm) using distal veins; check for extravasation, necrosis q8hr
• Give product only after C&S confirms organism, make sure product is used in life-threatening infections
• Provide protection from light during infusion; cover with foil
• Give symptomatic treatment as ordered for adverse reactions: aspirin, antihistamines, antiemetics, antispasmodics
• Store protected from moisture and light; diluted sol is stable for 24 hr

ADVERSE EFFECTS: The most serious adverse reactions include renal tubular acidosis, permanent renal impairment, anuria, oliguria, hemorrhagic gastroenteritis, acute liver failure, and blood dyscrasias. Some common side effects include hypokalemia, nausea, vomiting, anorexia, headache, fever, and chills.

PHARMACOKINETICS: Onset, peak, and duration vary widely among products. Most products are metabolized in the liver and excreted in urine.

INTERACTIONS: Interactions vary widely among products. Check individual monographs for specific information.

NURSING CONSIDERATIONS
Assessment
• Monitor VS q15-30min during first infusion; note changes in pulse, B/P
• Monitor I&O ratio; watch for decreasing urinary output, change in specific gravity; discontinue product to prevent permanent damage to renal tubules
• Monitor blood tests; CBC, potassium, sodium, calcium, magnesium q2wk
• Monitor weight weekly; if weight increases over 2 lb/wk, edema is present; renal damage should be considered
• Assess for renal toxicity: increasing BUN, if >40 mg/dl or if serum creatinine >3 mg/dl; product may be discontinued or dosage reduced
• Assess for hepatotoxicity: increasing AST, ALT, alkaline phosphatase, bilirubin
• Assess for allergic reaction: dermatitis, rash; product should be discontinued; antihistamines (mild reaction) or EPINEPHrine (severe reaction) administered
• Assess for hypokalemia: anorexia, drowsiness, weakness, decreased reflexes, dizziness, increased urinary output, increased thirst, paresthesias
• Assess for ototoxicity: tinnitus (ringing, roaring in ears), vertigo, loss of hearing (rare)

Patient/family education
• Teach patient that long-term therapy may be needed to clear infection (2 wk-3 mo depending on type of infection)

Evaluation
Positive therapeutic outcome
• Decreased fever, malaise, rash
• Negative C&S for infecting organism

Generic Names
amphotericin B, anidulafungin, fluconazole, isavuconazonium, itraconazole, ketoconazole, micafungin, nystatin, posaconazole, voriconazole

Antihistamines

ACTION: Antihistamines compete with histamines for H_1 receptor sites. They antagonize in varying degrees most of the pharmacologic effects of histamines.

USES: Antihistamines are used to control the symptoms of allergies, rhinitis, and pruritus.

CONTRAINDICATIONS
Hypersensitivity to H_1-receptor antagonists occurs rarely. Patients with acute asthma and lower respiratory tract disease should not use these products since thick secretions may result. Other contraindications include closed-angle glaucoma, bladder neck obstruction, stenosing peptic ulcer, symptomatic prostatic hypertrophy, breastfeeding, and in the newborn.

Precautions: Antihistamines must be used cautiously in conjunction with intraocular pressure since they increase intraocular pressure. Caution should also be used in pregnancy, breastfeeding, and geriatric patients and patients with renal/cardiac disease, hypertension, and seizure disorders.

ADVERSE EFFECTS: Most products cause drowsiness; however, loratadine and fexofenadine produce little, if any, drowsiness. Other common side effects are headache and thickening of bronchial secretions. Serious blood dyscrasias may occur, but are rare. Urinary retention, GI effects occur with many of these products.

PHARMACOKINETICS: Onset varies from 20-60 min, with duration lasting 4-24 hr. In general, pharmacokinetics vary widely among products.

INTERACTIONS: Barbiturates, opioids, hypnotics, tricyclics, and alcohol can increase CNS depression when taken with antihistamines.

NURSING CONSIDERATIONS
Assessment
- Check I&O ratio; be alert for urinary retention, frequency, dysuria; product should be discontinued if these occur
- Assess for blood dyscrasias: thrombocytopenia, agranulocytosis (rare)
- Assess for respiratory status, including rate, rhythm, increase in bronchial secretions, wheezing, chest tightness
- Assess for cardiac status, including palpitations, increased pulse, hypotension
- Assess CBC during long-term therapy, since hemolytic anemia, although rare, may occur

- Administer with food or milk to decrease GI symptoms; absorption may be decreased slightly
- Administer whole (sus rel tab)
- Provide hard candy, gum, frequent rinsing of mouth for dryness

Patient/family education
- Advise patient to notify prescriber if confusion, sedation, hypotension occur
- Caution patient to avoid driving and other hazardous activity if drowsiness occurs
- Instruct patient to avoid concurrent use of alcohol and other CNS depressants
- Inform patient to discontinue a few days before skin testing

Evaluation

Positive therapeutic outcome
- Absence of allergy symptoms, itching

Generic Names
brompheniramine, budesonide, cetirizine, chlorpheniramine, cyproheptadine, desloratadine, diphenhydrAMINE, fexofenadine, levocetirizine, loratadine, promethazine

Antihypertensives

ACTION: Antihypertensives are divided into angiotensin converting enzyme (ACE) inhibitors, β-adrenergic blockers, calcium channel blockers, centrally acting adrenergics, diuretics, peripherally acting antiadrenergics, and vasodilators. β-blockers, calcium channel blockers, and diuretics are discussed in separate sections. ACE inhibitors selectively suppress conversion of renin-angiotensin I to angiotensin II; dilatation of arterial and venous vessels occurs. Centrally acting adrenergics act by inhibiting the sympathetic vasomotor center in the CNS, which reduces impulses in the sympathetic nervous system; blood pressure, pulse rate, and cardiac output decrease. Peripherally acting antiadrenergics inhibit sympathetic vasoconstriction by inhibiting release of norepinephrine and/or depleting norepinephrine stores in adrenergic nerve endings. Vasodilators act on arteriolar smooth muscle by producing direct relaxation or vasodilatation; a reduction in blood pressure, with concomitant increases in heart rate and cardiac output, occurs.

USES: Antihypertensives are used for hypertension and for heart failure not responsive to conventional therapy. Some products are used in hypertensive crisis, angina, and for some cardiac dysrhythmias.

CONTRAINDICATIONS

Hypersensitive reactions may occur, and allergies should be identified before these products are given. Antihypertensives should not be used in children or in patients with heart block.

Precautions: Antihypertensives should be used with caution in geriatric and dialysis patients, and in the presence of hypovolemia, leukemia, and electrolyte imbalances.

IMPLEMENTATION
• Place patient in supine or Trendelenburg position for severe hypotension

ADVERSE EFFECTS: The most common side effects are marked hypotension, bradycardia, tachycardia, headache, nausea, and vomiting. Side effects and adverse reactions may vary widely between classes and specific products.

PHARMACOKINETICS: Onset, peak, and duration vary widely among products. Most products are metabolized in the liver, with metabolites excreted in urine, bile, and feces.

INTERACTIONS: Interactions vary widely among products. Check individual monographs for specific information.

NURSING CONSIDERATIONS
Assessment
• Monitor blood tests: neutrophil; decreased platelets occur with many of the products
• Monitor renal function tests: protein, BUN, creatinine; watch for increased levels, which may indicate nephrotic syndrome; obtain baselines in renal/hepatic function tests before beginning treatment
• Assess for edema in feet and legs daily
• Identify allergic reaction, including rash, fever, pruritus, urticaria: product should be discontinued if antihistamines fail to help
• Identify symptoms of CHF: edema, dyspnea, wet crackles, B/P
• Assess for renal symptoms: polyuria, oliguria, frequency

Patient/family education
• Instruct patient to comply with dosage schedule, even if feeling better
• Advise patient to rise slowly to sitting or standing position to minimize orthostatic hypotension

Evaluation
Positive therapeutic outcome
• Decrease in B/P in hypertension
• Decreased B/P, edema, moist crackles in CHF

Generic Names

Angiotensin-converting enzyme inhibitors:
benazepril, enalapril, fosinopril, lisinopril, quinapril, ramipril, trandolapril

Angiotensin II receptor blockers:
azilsartan, candesartan, eprosartan, irbesartan, losartan, olmesartan, telmisartan, valsartan

Centrally acting adrenergics:
cloNIDine, guanFACINE, methyldopa

Peripherally acting antiadrenergics:
doxazosin, prazosin, reserpine

Vasodilators:
ambrisentan, fenoldopam, hydrALAZINE, macitentan, minoxidil, **nitroprusside** (high alert)

Antiadrenergic: Combined α/β-blocker:
labetalol

Direct renin inhibitors:
aliskiren

Antiinfectives

ACTION: Antiinfectives are divided into several groups, which include but are not limited to penicillins, cephalosporins, aminoglycosides, sulfonamides, tetracyclines, monobactam, erythromycins, and quinolones. These products inhibit the growth and replication of susceptible bacterial organisms.

USES: Antiinfectives are used for infections of susceptible organisms. These products are effective against bacterial, rickettsial, and spirochete infections.

CONTRAINDICATIONS
Hypersensitive reactions may occur, and allergies should be identified before these products are given. Cross-sensitivity can occur between products of different classes (penicillins or cephalosporins). Often persons allergic to penicillins are also allergic to cephalosporins.

Precautions: Antiinfectives should be used with caution in persons with renal/hepatic disease.

IMPLEMENTATION
• Give for 10-14 days to ensure organism death, prevention of superinfection
• Give after C&S completed; product may be taken as soon as culture is obtained

ADVERSE EFFECTS: The most common side effects are nausea, vomiting, and diarrhea. Adverse reactions include bone marrow depression and anaphylaxis.

PHARMACOKINETICS: Onset, peak, and duration vary widely among products. Most products are metabolized in the liver. Metabolites are excreted in urine, bile, and feces.

INTERACTIONS: Interactions vary widely among products. Check individual monographs for specific information.

NURSING CONSIDERATIONS
Assessment
- Assess for nephrotoxicity: increased BUN, creatinine
- Monitor blood tests: AST, ALT, CBC, Hct, bilirubin; test monthly if patient is on long-term therapy
- Monitor bowel pattern daily; if severe diarrhea occurs, product should be discontinued
- Monitor urine output; if decreasing, notify prescriber; may indicate nephrotoxicity
- Assess for allergic reaction: rash, fever, pruritus, urticaria; product should be discontinued
- Assess for bleeding: ecchymosis, bleeding gums, hematuria, stool guaiac daily
- Assess for overgrowth of infection: perineal itching, fever, malaise, redness, pain, swelling, drainage, rash, diarrhea, change in cough, sputum

Patient/family education
- Teach patient to comply with dosage schedule, even if feeling better
- Advise patient to report sore throat, bruising, bleeding, joint pain; may indicate blood dyscrasias (rare)

Evaluation
Positive therapeutic outcome
- Absence of fever, fatigue, malaise, draining wounds

Generic Names
Aminoglycosides:
amikacin, azithromycin, clarithromycin, gentamicin, neomycin, streptomycin, tobramycin

Cephalosporins:
cefaclor, cefadroxil, ceFAZolin, cefdinir, cefditoren, cefepime, cefixime, cefotaxime, cefprozil, ceftibuten, cefuroxime, cephalexin, cephradine

Fluoroquinolones:
ciprofloxacin, gemifloxacin, levofloxacin, norfloxacin, ofloxacin

Ketolides:
telithromycin

Miscellaneous:
adefovir, dalbavancin, DAPTOmycin, doripenem, ertapenem, fidaxomicin, meropenem, oritavancin, peginterferon alfa-2a, telavancin, vancomycin

Penicillins:
amoxicillin/clavulanate, ampicillin/sulbactam, imipenem/cilastatin, nafcillin, penicillin G benzathine, penicillin G, penicillin G procaine, penicillin V, piperacillin/tazobactam, ticarcillin, ticarcillin/clavulanate

Sulfonamides:
sulfaSALAzine

Tetracyclines:
doxycycline, minocycline, tetracycline

Antilipidemics

ACTION: Antilipidemics are divided into three categories or subclassifications; HMG-CoA reductase inhibitors (statins), bile acid sequestrants, and miscellaneous products. The HMG-CoA reductase inhibitors work by reduction of an enzyme that is responsible for the beginning step in cholesterol production. Bile acid sequestrants work by binding cholesterol in the GI system. The miscellaneous products work by various actions.

USES: Primary hypercholesterolemia in individuals as an adjunct with other lifestyle changes.

CONTRAINDICATIONS
Persons breastfeeding (some products) or those with hypersensitivity to any product or severe hepatic disease should not take these products. Antilipidemics are identified as pregnancy category **X** on some products.

Precautions: Some products are identified as pregnancy category **C**.

IMPLEMENTATION
- Give as directed by health care provider; times will vary with medication used
- Provide protection from sunlight and heat

ADVERSE EFFECTS: The most common side effects are headache, dizziness, fatigue, insomnia, peripheral edema, dysrhythmias, sinusitis, pharyngitis, abdominal pain, diarrhea, constipation, flatulence, and back pain.

PHARMACOKINETICS: Pharmacokinetics and pharmacodynamics vary with each product.

INTERACTIONS: Interactions vary widely among products. Check individual monographs for specific information.

NURSING CONSIDERATIONS
Assessment
- Obtain a diet and lifestyle history, including exercise, smoking, alcohol, and stress-related activities

Patient/family education
- Teach patient all aspects of medication use
- Instruct patient to combine medication with lifestyle changes, including low-cholesterol diet, decreasing LDL in diet; avoid smoking, alcohol, and sedentary daily routine

Evaluation
Positive therapeutic outcome
- Decrease in triglycerides and LDL cholesterol levels

Generic Names

HMG-CoA reductase inhibitors:
atorvastatin, fluvastatin, lovastatin, pitavastatin, pravastatin, simvastatin

Bile acid sequestrants:
cholestyramine, colesevelam

Miscellaneous:
alirocumab, evolocumab, ezetimibe, fenofibrate, fenofibric acid, gemfibrozil, mipomersen, niacin, niacinamide

Antineoplastics

ACTION: Antineoplastics are divided into alkylating agents, antimetabolites, antibiotic agents, hormonal agents, and miscellaneous agents. Alkylating agents act by cross-linking strands of DNA. Antimetabolites act by inhibiting DNA synthesis. Antibiotic agents act by inhibiting RNA synthesis and by delaying or inhibiting mitosis. Hormones alter the effect of androgens, luteinizing hormone, follicle-stimulating hormone, or estrogen by changing the hormonal environment.

USES: Antineoplastics vary widely among products and classes of products. They are used to treat leukemia, Hodgkin's disease, lymphomas, and other tumors throughout the body.

CONTRAINDICATIONS
Hypersensitive reactions may occur, and allergies should be identified before these products are given. Also, persons with severe renal/hepatic disease should not use these products unless the benefits outweigh the risks.

Precautions: Persons with bleeding, severe bone marrow depression, or renal/hepatic disease should be watched closely.

IMPLEMENTATION
- Check **IV** site for irritation; phlebitis
- Have EPINEPHrine available for hypersensitivity reaction
- Give antibiotics for prophylaxis of infection
- Provide strict medical asepsis, protective isolation if WBC levels are low
- Provide comprehensive oral hygiene, using careful technique and soft-bristle brush

ADVERSE EFFECTS: Most products cause thrombocytopenia, leukopenia, and anemia. If these reactions occur, the product may need to be stopped until the problem is corrected. Other side effects include nausea, vomiting, glossitis, and hair loss. Some products also cause hepatotoxicity, nephrotoxicity, and cardiotoxicity.

PHARMACOKINETICS: Onset, peak, and duration vary widely among products. Most products cross the placenta and are excreted in breast milk and in urine.

INTERACTIONS: Toxicity may occur when used with other antineoplastics or radiation.

NURSING CONSIDERATIONS
Assessment
- Monitor CBC, differential, platelet count weekly; withhold product if WBC is <4000 or platelet count is <75,000; notify prescriber of results
- Monitor renal function tests: BUN, creatinine, serum uric acid, and urine creatinine clearance before, during therapy
- Monitor I&O ratio; report fall in urine output of 30 ml/hr
- Monitor temp q4hr (may indicate beginning infection)
- Monitor hepatic function tests before, during therapy (bilirubin, AST, ALT, LDH) monthly or as needed
- Assess for bleeding, including hematuria, guaiac, bruising or petechiae, mucosa, or orifices q8hr; obtain prescription for viscous lidocaine (Xylocaine)
- Identify jaundice of skin, sclera, dark urine, clay-colored stools, itchy skin, abdominal pain, fever, diarrhea
- Assess for edema in feet, joint pain, stomach pain, shaking
- Assess for inflammation of mucosa, breaks in skin

Patient/family education
- Advise patient to report signs of infection, including increased temp, sore throat, malaise

• Instruct patient to report signs of anemia, including fatigue, headache, faintness, shortness of breath, irritability

• Instruct patient to report bleeding and to avoid use of razors and commercial mouthwash

Evaluation

Positive therapeutic outcome
• Decreased tumor size

Generic Names

Alkylating agents:
bendamustine, **busulfan** (high alert), **CARBOplatin** (high alert), **carmustine** (high alert), chlorambucil, **CISplatin** (high alert), cyclophosphamide (high alert), **dacarbazine** (high alert), **melphalan** (high alert), oxaliplatin

Antimetabolites:
capecitabine, **cytarabine** (high alert), decitabine, **etoposide** (high alert), **fluorouracil** (high alert), mercaptopurine, **methotrexate** (high alert), PEMEtrexed

Antibiotic agents:
bleomycin (high alert), **DACTINomycin** (high alert), **DAUNOrubicin** (high alert), **DOXOrubicin** (high alert), **mitoMYcin** (high alert), **mitoXANtrone** (high alert)

Hormonal agents:
flutamide, fulvestrant, goserelin, **irinotecan** (high alert), **leuprolide** (high alert), megestrol, tamoxifen, **topotecan** (high alert)

Miscellaneous agents:
ado-trastuzumab, afatinib, alemtuzumab, anastrozole, azaCITIDine, belinostat, bortezomib, brentuximab, cabazitaxel, **ceritinib** (high alert), cetuximab, crizotinib, dabrafenib, dasatinib, eribulin, erlotinib, gemcitabine, ibritumomab, ibrutinib, idelalisib, imatinib, interferon alfa-2a, interferon alfa-2b, ipilimumab, irinotecan, ixabepilone, lapatinib, nilotinib, olaparib, palbociclib, panitumumab, pembrolizumab, pomalidomide, procarbazine, ranibizumab, riTUXimab, sipuleucel-T, sonidegib, trametinib, vemurafenib, **vinBLAStine** (high alert), **vinCRIStine** (high alert), **vinorelbine** (high alert)

Antiparkinsonian Agents

ACTION: Antiparkinsonian agents are divided into cholinergics, dopamine agonists, and monoamine oxidase type B inhibitors. Cholinergics work by blocking or competing at central acetylcholine receptors. Dopamine agonists work by decarboxylation to dopamine or by activation of dopamine receptors. Monoamine oxidase type B inhibitors increase dopamine activity by inhibiting MAO type B activity.

USES: Antiparkinson agents are used alone or in combination for patients with Parkinson's disease.

CONTRAINDICATIONS

Persons with hypersensitivity, closed-angle glaucoma, and undiagnosed skin lesions should not use these products.

Precautions: Antiparkinsonian agents should be used with caution in pregnancy, breastfeeding, children, renal/cardiac/hepatic disease, and affective disorder.

IMPLEMENTATION

• Give product up until NPO before surgery
• Adjust dosage depending on patient response
• Give with meals; limit protein taken with product
• Give only after MAOIs have been discontinued for 2 wk
• Assist with ambulation during beginning therapy if needed
• Test for diabetes mellitus and acromegaly if on long-term therapy

ADVERSE EFFECTS: Side effects and adverse reactions vary widely among products. The most common side effects include involuntary movements, headache, numbness, insomnia, nightmares, nausea, vomiting, dry mouth, and orthostatic hypotension.

PHARMACOKINETICS: Onset, peak, and duration vary widely among products. Most products are metabolized in the liver and excreted in urine.

INTERACTIONS: Interactions vary widely among products. Check individual monographs for specific information.

NURSING CONSIDERATIONS

Assessment
• Monitor B/P, respiration
• Assess mental status: affect, behavioral changes, depression, complete suicide assessment

Patient/family education
• Advise patient to change positions slowly to prevent orthostatic hypotension
• Instruct patient to report side effects: twitching, eye spasm; indicate overdose
• Advise patient to use product exactly as prescribed; if product is discontinued abruptly, parkinsonian crisis may occur

---

⚠ Nurse Alert   ✴ Key NCLEX® Drug   ≫ Drug Specifics

Evaluation

Positive therapeutic outcome
- Decrease in akathisia
- Improvement in mood

Generic Names
amantadine, benztropine, bromocriptine, carbidopa-levodopa, pramipexole, rasagiline, selegiline, tolcapone

Antiplatelets

ACTION: The antiplatelets are divided into the platelet aggregation inhibitors, platelet adhesion inhibitors, and the glycoprotein IIb, IIIa inhibitors. The platelet aggregation inhibitors work by action on thrombin; the platelet adhesion inhibitors work by inhibition of phosphodiesterase; and the glycoprotein IIb, IIIa inhibitors work by preventing fibrin from binding to glycoprotein IIb, IIIa receptors.

USES: Antiplatelets are used to prevent myocardial infarction and stroke; other products are used for coronary syndromes.

CONTRAINDICATIONS
Persons developing hypersensitive reactions should not use these products.

Precautions: Antiplatelets should be used cautiously in pregnancy, breastfeeding, and bleeding disorders.

IMPLEMENTATION
- Give with heparin or other aspirin (some products)
- Store at room temperature vial/ampules, oral products

ADVERSE EFFECTS: The most common side effects are headache, dizziness, bleeding, and diarrhea.

PHARMACOKINETICS: Onset, peak, and duration vary widely among products. Most products are metabolized by the liver and excreted by the kidneys.

INTERACTIONS: Interactions vary widely among products. Check individual monographs for specific information.

NURSING CONSIDERATIONS
Assessment
- Assess reason for use of these products
- Monitor hypersensitivity reactions with some products
- Monitor bleeding from orifices, stool urine
- Monitor blood tests: platelets, Hgb, Hct, PT/APTT, and INR

Patient/family education
- Caution patient to avoid hazardous activities if drowsiness, dizziness occurs; ask for assistance if hospitalized
- Teach patient all aspects of product usage

Evaluation

Positive therapeutic outcome
- Absence of MI, stroke, or other coronary syndromes

Generic Names
Platelet aggregation inhibitors:
cilostazol, clopidogrel, ticagrelor, ticlopidine

Platelet adhesion inhibitors:
dipyridamole

Glycoprotein IIb, IIIa inhibitors:
eptifibatide (high alert), **tirofiban** (high alert)

Antipsychotics

ACTION: Antipsychotics/neuroleptics are divided into several subgroups: phenothiazines, thioxanthenes, butyrophenones, dibenzoxazepines, dibenzodiazepines, and indolones and other heterocyclic compounds. Although chemically different, these subgroups share many pharmacologic and clinical properties. All antipsychotics work to block postsynaptic DOPamine receptors in the brain that are responsible for psychotic behavior, including hallucinations, delusions, and paranoia.

USES: Antipsychotic behavior is decreased in conditions such as schizophrenia, paranoia, and mania. These agents are also effective for severe anxiety, intractable hiccups, nausea, vomiting, behavioral problems in children, and for relaxation before surgery.

CONTRAINDICATIONS
Persons with liver damage, severe hypertension or coronary disease, cerebral arteriosclerosis, blood dyscrasias, bone marrow depression, parkinsonism, severe depression, or closed-angle glaucoma; children <12 yr; persons withdrawing from alcohol or barbiturates should not use antipsychotics until these conditions are corrected.

Precautions: Caution must be used when antipsychotics are given to geriatric patients, since metabolism is slowed and adverse reactions can occur rapidly. Renal/hepatic disease may cause poor metabolism and excretion of the product. Seizure threshold is decreased with these products; increases in the dose of anticonvulsants may be required. Persons with diabetes mellitus, prostatic hypertrophy, chronic respiratory disease, and peptic ulcer disease should be monitored closely.

IMPLEMENTATION
• Give antiparkinsonian agent if extrapyramidal symptoms occur
• Administer liquid conc mixed in glass of juice or cola since taste is unpleasant; avoid contact with skin when preparing liquid conc or parenteral medications
• Supervise ambulation until stabilized on medication; do not involve in strenuous exercise program, since fainting is possible; patient should not stand still for long periods
• Increase fluids to prevent constipation
• Give sips of water, candy, gum for dry mouth
• Patient should remain lying down for at least 30 min after IM inj

ADVERSE EFFECTS: The most common side effects include extrapyramidal symptoms such as pseudoparkinsonism, akathisia, dystonia, and tardive dyskinesia, which may be controlled by use of antiparkinsonian agents. Serious adverse reactions such as hypotension, agranulocytosis, cardiac arrest, and laryngospasm have occurred. Other common side effects include dry mouth and photosensitivity.

PHARMACOKINETICS: Onset, peak, and duration vary widely with different products and routes. Products are metabolized by the liver, are excreted in urine as metabolites, are highly bound to plasma proteins, cross the placenta, and enter breast milk. Half-life can be extended over 3 days.

INTERACTIONS: Because other CNS depressants can cause oversedation, these combinations should be used carefully. Anticholinergics may decrease the therapeutic actions of phenothiazines and also cause increased anticholinergic effects.

NURSING CONSIDERATIONS
Assessment
• Monitor bilirubin, CBC, hepatic function tests monthly, since these products are metabolized in the liver and excreted in urine
• Monitor I&O ratio: palpate bladder if low urinary output occurs, since urinary retention occurs with many of these products
• Assess affect, orientation, LOC, reflexes, gait, coordination, sleep pattern disturbances
• Assess dizziness, faintness, palpitations, tachycardia on rising
• Check B/P with patient lying and standing; wide fluctuations between lying and standing B/P

may require dosage or product change, since orthostatic hypotension is occurring
• Assess for EPS, including akathisia, tardive dyskinesia, pseudoparkinsonism

Patient/family education
• Advise patient to rise from sitting or lying position gradually, since fainting may occur
• Caution patient to avoid hot tubs, hot showers, or tub baths, since hypotension may occur
• Advise patient to wear sunscreen or protective clothing to prevent burns
• Advise patient to take extra precautions during hot weather to stay cool; heat stroke can occur
• Caution patient to avoid driving and other activities requiring alertness until response to medication is known
• Inform patient that drowsiness or impaired mental/motor activity is evident the first 2 wk, but tends to decrease over time

Evaluation
Positive therapeutic outcome
• Decrease in excitement, hallucinations, delusions, paranoia
• Reorganization of thought patterns, speech

Generic Names
Phenothiazines:
chlorproMAZINE, fluPHENAZine

Butyrophenone:
haloperidol

Miscellaneous:
ARIPiprazole, asenapine, iloperidone, loxapine, OLANZapine, paliperidone, QUEtiapine, risperiDONE, ziprasidone

Antipyretics

ACTION: The antipyretics act on the CNS to control fever and also inhibit prostaglandin production.

USES: Antipyretics are used to decrease fever.

CONTRAINDICATIONS
Persons developing hypersensitive reactions should not use these products.

Precautions: Antipyretics should be used cautiously in pregnancy, breastfeeding, geriatric patients, hepatic disease, and those with certain GI disorders.

IMPLEMENTATION
• Give around the clock to keep fever reduced
• Store at room temperature

⚠ Nurse Alert   ✳ Key NCLEX® Drug   >> Drug Specifics

ADVERSE EFFECTS: The most common side effects are nausea, vomiting, and rash.

PHARMACOKINETICS: Onset, peak, and duration vary widely among products. Most products are metabolized by the liver and excreted by the kidneys.

INTERACTIONS: Interactions vary widely among products. Check individual monographs for specific information.

NURSING CONSIDERATIONS
Assessment
• Monitor temp frequently
• Assess reason for use and expected outcome
• Monitor hypersensitivity reactions: rash, bronchospasm with some products

Patient/family education
• Teach patient all aspects of product usage

Evaluation

Positive therapeutic outcome
• Absence or decreasing fever after use

Generic Names
acetaminophen, aspirin, choline/magnesium salicylates, ibuprofen, ketoprofen, magnesium salicylate, naproxen, salsalate

Antiretrovirals

ACTION: Antiretrovirals act by blocking DNA synthesis.

USES: Antiretrovirals are used in HIV infections, chronic hepatitis C to slow the progression of the disease.

CONTRAINDICATIONS
Persons with hypersensitivity should not use these products.

Precautions: Antiretrovirals should be used cautiously in pregnancy, breastfeeding, and renal/hepatic disease. Protease inhibitors should be used cautiously in diabetes.

IMPLEMENTATION
• Give in equal intervals around the clock
• Store at room temperature

ADVERSE EFFECTS: The most common side effects are nausea, vomiting, anorexia, headache, and diarrhea. The most serious adverse reactions are nephrotoxicity and blood dyscrasias.

PHARMACOKINETICS: Onset, peak, and duration vary widely among products. Most products are metabolized by the liver and excreted by the kidneys.

INTERACTIONS: Interactions vary widely among products. Check individual monographs for specific information.

NURSING CONSIDERATIONS
Assessment
• Monitor for signs of HIV infection: increased CD4 counts, decreased viral load; signs of chronic hepatitis C
• Monitor patients with compromised renal system; since product is excreted slowly in poor renal system function, toxicity may occur rapidly

Patient/family education
• Instruct patient to report sore throat, fever, fatigue; may indicate superinfection
• Caution patient that product does not cure condition or prevent infecting others, but controls symptoms
• Instruct patient that product must be taken around the clock, in equal intervals to maintain blood levels for duration of therapy
• Instruct patient to notify prescriber of side effects such as bruising, bleeding, fatigue, malaise; may indicate blood dyscrasias

Evaluation

Positive therapeutic outcome
• Decreased viral load
• Increased CD4 count
• Improvement in the symptoms of HIV/AIDS

Generic Names
Nonnucleoside reverse transcriptase inhibitors:
delavirdine, efavirenz, etravirine, nevirapine, rilpivirine

Nucleoside reverse transcriptase inhibitors:
abacavir, didanosine, emtricitabine, lamiVUDine, stavudine d4t, tenofovir, zidovudine

Protease inhibitors:
atazanavir, **atazanavir/cobistat** (high alert), boceprevir, fosamprenavir, indinavir, nelfinavir, ritonavir, saquinavir, telaprevir, tipranavir

Fusion inhibitors:
enfuvirtide

Miscellaneous:
daclatasvir, dolutegravir, raltegravir

Antituberculars

ACTION: Antituberculars act by inhibiting RNA or DNA, or interfering with lipid and protein synthesis, thereby decreasing tubercle bacilli replication.

USES: Antituberculars are used for pulmonary tuberculosis.

CONTRAINDICATIONS

Persons with severe renal disease or hypersensitivity should not use these products.

Precautions: Antituberculars should be used with caution in pregnancy, breastfeeding, and hepatic disease.

IMPLEMENTATION

- Give some of these agents on empty stomach, 1 hr before meals (only for isoniazid and rifampin) or 2 hr after meals
- Give antiemetic if vomiting occurs
- Give after C&S is completed; monthly to detect resistance

ADVERSE EFFECTS: Adverse effects vary widely among products. Most products can cause nausea, vomiting, anorexia, and rash. Serious adverse reactions include renal failure, nephrotoxicity, ototoxicity, and hepatic necrosis.

PHARMACOKINETICS: Onset, peak, and duration vary widely among products. Most products are metabolized in the liver and excreted in urine.

INTERACTIONS: Interactions vary widely among products. Check individual monographs for specific information.

NURSING CONSIDERATIONS
Assessment

- Assess for signs of anemia: Hct, Hgb, fatigue
- Monitor hepatic function tests weekly: ALT, AST, bilirubin
- Monitor renal status before treatment and monthly thereafter: BUN, creatinine, output, specific gravity, urinalysis
- Monitor hepatic status: decreased appetite, jaundice, dark urine, fatigue

Patient/family education

- Teach patient that compliance with dosage schedule, duration is necessary
- Teach patient that scheduled appointments must be kept; relapse may occur
- Advise patient to avoid alcohol while taking product
- Advise patient to report flulike symptoms: excessive fatigue, anorexia, vomiting, sore throat; unusual bleeding, yellowish discoloration of skin/eyes

Evaluation

Positive therapeutic outcome
- Decreased symptoms of TB
- Negative culture

Generic Names
ethambutol, isoniazid, pyrazinamide, rifabutin, rifampin, streptomycin

Antitussives/Expectorants

ACTION: Antitussives suppress the cough reflex by direct action on the cough center in the medulla. Expectorants act by liquefying and reducing the viscosity of thick, tenacious secretions.

USES: Antitussives/expectorants are used to treat cough occurring in pneumonia, bronchitis, TB, cystic fibrosis, and emphysema; as an adjunct in atelectasis (expectorants); and for nonproductive cough (antitussives).

CONTRAINDICATIONS

Some products are contraindicated in pregnancy, breastfeeding, and hypothyroidism

Precautions: Some products should be used cautiously with asthma and in geriatric and debilitated patients.

IMPLEMENTATION

- Give decreased dosage to geriatric patients; their metabolism may be slowed
- Increase fluids to liquefy secretions
- Humidify patient's room

ADVERSE EFFECTS: The most common side effects are drowsiness, dizziness, and nausea.

PHARMACOKINETICS: Onset, peak, and duration vary widely among products. Some products are metabolized in the liver and excreted in urine.

INTERACTIONS: Interactions vary widely among products. Check individual monographs for specific information.

NURSING CONSIDERATIONS
Assessment

- Assess cough: type, frequency, character including sputum

Patient/family education

- Advise patient to avoid driving and other hazardous activities until stabilized on this medication
- Caution patient to avoid smoking, smoke-filled rooms, perfumes, dust, environmental pollutants, cleaners that increase cough

Evaluation

Positive therapeutic outcome
- Absence of cough

Generic Names
acetylcysteine, codeine, dextromethorphan, diphenhydrAMINE, guaiFENesin, HYDROcodone

Antivirals

ACTION: Antivirals act by interfering with DNA synthesis that is needed for viral replication.

USES: Antivirals are used for mucocutaneous herpes simplex virus, herpes genitalis (HSV-1, HSV-2), varicella infections, herpes zoster, and herpes simplex encephalitis.

CONTRAINDICATIONS
Persons with hypersensitivity or immunosuppressed individuals should not use these products.

Precautions: Antivirals should be used cautiously in pregnancy, breastfeeding, and renal/hepatic disease.

IMPLEMENTATION
• Give increased fluids to 3 L/day to decrease crystalluria when given **IV**
• Store at room temperature for up to 12 hr after reconstitution

ADVERSE EFFECTS: The most common side effects are nausea, vomiting, anorexia, headache, and diarrhea. The most serious adverse reactions are nephrotoxicity and blood dyscrasias.

PHARMACOKINETICS: Onset, peak, and duration vary widely among products. Most products are metabolized by the liver and excreted by the kidneys.

INTERACTIONS: Interactions vary widely among products. Check individual monographs for specific information.

NURSING CONSIDERATIONS
Assessment
• Monitor for signs of infection, anemia
• Monitor patients with a compromised renal system; since product is excreted slowly in poor renal system function, toxicity may occur rapidly
• Monitor renal function tests: urinalysis, BUN, serum creatinine or decreased CCr may indicate nephrotoxicity; I&O ratio; report hematuria, oliguria, fatigue, weakness; check for protein in the urine during treatment
• Assess C&S before treatment; agent may be given as soon as culture is taken; repeat C&S after treatment
• Monitor bowel pattern before, during treatment; if severe abdominal pain with bleeding occurs, agent should be discontinued

• Monitor skin reactions: rash, urticaria, itching
• Monitor hepatic function tests: AST, ALT
• Monitor blood tests: WBC, RBC, Hct, Hgb, bleeding time; blood dyscrasias

Patient/family education
• Instruct patient to report sore throat, fever, fatigue; may indicate superinfection
• Caution patient that product does not prevent infecting others or cure condition but controls symptoms
• Instruct patient that product must be taken around the clock in equal intervals to maintain blood levels for duration of therapy
• Instruct patient to notify prescriber of side effects such as bruising, bleeding, fatigue, malaise; may indicate blood dyscrasias

Evaluation
Positive therapeutic outcome
• Absence or control of infection

Generic Names
acyclovir, amantadine, cidofovir, daclatasvir, docosanol, entecavir, famciclovir, foscarnet, ganciclovir, lamiVUDine, maraviroc, oseltamivir, penciclovir, rapivab, ribavirin, simeprevir, sofosbuvir, valACYclovir, valGANciclovir, zanamivir

β-adrenergic Blockers

ACTION: β-blockers are divided into selective and nonselective blockers. Selective β-blockers competitively block stimulation of β_1-receptors in cardiac smooth muscle; these products produce chronotropic and inotropic effects. Nonselective blockers produce a fall in blood pressure without reflex tachycardia or reduction in heart rate through a mixture of β-blocking effects; elevated plasma renins are reduced.

USES: β-blockers are used for hypertension, ventricular dysrhythmias, and prophylaxis of angina pectoris.

CONTRAINDICATIONS
Hypersensitive reactions may occur, and allergies should be identified before these products are given. β-adrenergic blockers should not be used in heart block, CHF, or cardiogenic shock.

Precautions: β-blockers should be used with caution in pregnant and geriatric patients or in renal/thyroid disease, COPD, CAD, diabetes mellitus, and asthma.

IMPLEMENTATION
• Give PO before meals and at bedtime; tab may be crushed or swallowed whole
• Give reduced dosage in renal dysfunction

ADVERSE EFFECTS: The most common side effects are orthostatic hypotension, bradycardia, diarrhea, nausea, and vomiting. Serious adverse reactions include blood dyscrasias, bronchospasm, and CHF.

PHARMACOKINETICS: Onset, peak, and duration vary widely among products. Most products are metabolized in the liver, with metabolites excreted in urine, bile, and feces.

INTERACTIONS: Interactions vary widely among products. Check individual monographs for specific information.

NURSING CONSIDERATIONS
Assessment
• Monitor renal function tests: protein, BUN, creatinine; watch for increased levels that may indicate nephrotic syndrome; obtain baselines in renal/hepatic function tests before beginning treatment
• Monitor I&O ratio, weight daily
• Monitor B/P during beginning of treatment and periodically thereafter, pulse q4hr; note rate, rhythm, quality
• Monitor apical/radial pulse before administration; notify prescriber of significant changes
• Check for edema in feet and legs daily

Patient/family education
• Instruct patient to comply with dosage schedule, even if feeling better
• Caution patient to rise slowly to sitting or standing position to minimize orthostatic hypotension
• Advise patient to report bradycardia, dizziness, confusion, depression, fever
• Teach patient to take pulse at home; advise when to notify prescriber
• Instruct patient to comply with weight control, dietary adjustment, modified exercise program
• Advise patient to wear support hose to minimize effects of orthostatic hypotension
• Advise patient not to discontinue product abruptly; taper over 2 wk; may precipitate angina

Evaluation
Positive therapeutic outcome
• Decrease in B/P in hypertension
• Decreased B/P, edema, moist crackles in CHF

Generic Names
Selective β_1-receptor blockers:
acebutolol, atenolol, esmolol, metoprolol, nebibolol

β_2-receptor blocker:
indacaterol

Nonselective β_1 and β_2-blockers:
carteolol, nadolol, propranolol, timolol

Combined α_1, β_1, and β_2-receptor blocker:
labetalol

Bone Resorption Inhibitors

ACTION: Bone resorption inhibitors are divided into the biphosphonates and the selective estrogen receptor modulators. The biphosphonates act by absorbing calcium phosphate crystals in bone and may directly block dissolution of hydroxyapatite crystals of bone, inhibiting normal and abnormal bone resorption and mineralization. Selective estrogen receptor modulators act by reducing resorption of bone and decreasing bone turnover, mediated through estrogen receptor binding.

USES: Bone resorption inhibitors are used for prevention and treatment of osteoporosis in postmenopausal women, treatment of Paget's disease, and treatment of osteoporosis in men.

CONTRAINDICATIONS
Persons developing hypersensitive reactions or those with hypocalcemia should not use these products.

Precautions: Bone resorption inhibitors should be used cautiously in pregnancy, breastfeeding, the geriatric patient, renal/hepatic disease, and some GI disorders.

IMPLEMENTATION
• Give for 6 months or more in Paget's disease
• Store at room temperature

ADVERSE EFFECTS: The most common side effects are nausea, vomiting, headache, bone pain, and rash.

PHARMACOKINETICS: Onset, peak, and duration vary widely among products. Most products are taken up by the bones and excreted by the kidneys.

INTERACTIONS: Interactions vary widely among products. Check individual monographs for specific information.

NURSING CONSIDERATIONS
Assessment
• Assess reason for use and expected outcome
• Monitor bone density test; hormonal status (women) before starting treatment and thereafter
• Monitor hypercalcemia: paresthesia, twitching, laryngospasm; Chvostek's, Trousseau's signs

Patient/family education
- Instruct patient to remain upright for at least 30 min after taking to prevent esophageal irritation
- Teach patient all aspects of product usage
- Instruct patient to use weight-bearing exercise to increase bone density

Evaluation
Positive therapeutic outcome
- Increase in bone mass
- Absence of fractures

Generic Names
Bisphosphonates:
alendronate, etidronate, ibandronate, pamidronate, risedronate

Selective estrogen receptor modulator:
raloxifene

Monoclonal antibody:
denosumab

Calcium Channel Blockers

ACTION: Calcium channel blockers inhibit calcium ion influx across the cell membrane in cardiac and vascular smooth muscle. This action produces relaxation of coronary vascular smooth muscle, dilates coronary arteries, slows SA/AV node conduction, and dilates peripheral arteries.

USES: Calcium channel blockers are used for chronic stable angina pectoris, vasospastic angina, dysrhythmias, hypertension, and unstable angina.

CONTRAINDICATIONS
Persons with 2nd- or 3rd-degree heart block, sick sinus syndrome, hypotension of <90 mm Hg systolic, Wolff-Parkinson-White syndrome, or cardiogenic shock should not use these products, since worsening of those conditions may occur.

Precautions: CHF may worsen since edema may be increased. Hypotension may worsen, since B/P is decreased. Patients with renal/hepatic disease should use these products cautiously since they are metabolized in the liver and excreted by the kidneys.

IMPLEMENTATION
- Give PO before meals and at bedtime

ADVERSE EFFECTS: The most common side effects are dysrhythmias and edema. Also common are headache, fatigue, drowsiness, and flushing.

PHARMACOKINETICS: Onset, peak, and duration vary widely with route of administration. Products are metabolized by the liver and excreted in the urine primarily as metabolites.

INTERACTIONS: Increased levels of digoxin and theophylline may occur when used with these products. Increased effects of β-blockers and antihypertensives may occur with calcium channel blockers.

NURSING CONSIDERATIONS
Assessment
- Monitor cardiac system: B/P, pulse, respirations, ECG intervals (PR, QRS, QT)

Patient/family education
- Teach patient how to take pulse before taking product; patient should record or graph pulses to identify changes
- Advise patient to avoid hazardous activities until stabilized on this product since dizziness occurs frequently
- Inform patient of the need for compliance to all areas of medical regimen, including diet, exercise, stress reduction, and product therapy

Evaluation

Positive therapeutic outcome
- Decreased anginal pain
- Decreased B/P, dysrhythmias

Generic Names
amLODIPine, clevidipine, **diltiazem** (high alert), felodipine, isradipine, niCARdipine, NIFEdipine, verapamil

Cardiac Glycosides

ACTION: Cardiac glycosides act by inhibiting sodium and potassium ATPase and then making more calcium available to activate contracted proteins. Cardiac contractility and cardiac output are increased.

USES: Cardiac glycosides are used for CHF, atrial fibrillation, atrial flutter, atrial tachycardia, and rapid digitalization in these disorders.

CONTRAINDICATIONS
Hypersensitive reactions may occur, and allergies should be identified before these products are given. Also, persons with ventricular tachycardia, ventricular fibrillation, and carotid sinus syndrome should not use these products.

Precautions: Persons with acute MI and those who have or may develop serum potassium, calcium, or magnesium imbalances should use these products cautiously. Also, geriatric patients and those with AV block, severe respiratory disease, hypothyroidism, or renal/hepatic disease should exercise caution when these products are prescribed.

IMPLEMENTATION
• Give potassium supplements if ordered for potassium levels <3

ADVERSE EFFECTS: The most common side effects are cardiac disturbances, headache, hypotension, and GI symptoms. Also common are blurred vision and yellow-green halos.

PHARMACOKINETICS: Onset, peak, and duration vary widely with the route of administration. Digitoxin is inactivated by the liver, and inactive metabolites are excreted in urine. Digoxin is excreted in urine mainly as the parent product and metabolites.

INTERACTIONS: Toxicity may occur when used with diuretics, succinylcholine, quiNIDine, and thioamines. Increased blood levels may occur with propantheline bromide, spironolactone, quiNIDine, verapamil, aminoglycosides (PO), amiodarone, anticholinergics, and quiNINE. Diuretics may increase toxicity.

NURSING CONSIDERATIONS
Assessment
• Montior cardiac system: B/P, pulse, respirations, and increased urine output
• Monitor apical pulse for 1 min before giving product; if pulse <60, take again in 1 hr; if <60 notify prescriber
• Monitor electrolytes: potassium, sodium, chloride, calcium, magnesium; renal function tests, including BUN and creatinine; and blood tests, including AST, ALT, bilirubin
• Monitor I&O ratio, daily weights
• Monitor therapeutic product levels

Patient/family education
• Teach patient how to take pulse before taking product; patient should record or graph pulse to identify changes
• Advise patient to avoid hazardous activities until stabilized on this product since dizziness occurs frequently
• Inform patient of the need for compliance to all areas of medical regimen, including diet, exercise, stress reduction, product therapy

Evaluation
Positive therapeutic outcome
• Decreased weight, edema, pulse, respiration
• Increased urine output

Generic Names
digoxin (high alert)

Cholinergics

ACTION: Cholinergics act by preventing destruction of acetylcholine, which increases concentration at sites where acetylcholine is released. This exaggerates the effects of acetylcholine and facilitates transmission of impulses across the myoneural junction. Cholinergics may also act by stimulating receptors for acetylcholine.

USES: Cholinergics are used for myasthenia gravis, as antagonists of nondepolarizing neuromuscular blockade, postoperative bladder distention and urinary distention, postoperative ileus.

CONTRAINDICATIONS
Persons with obstruction of the intestine or renal system should not use these products.

Precautions: Caution should be used in patients with bradycardia, hypotension, seizure disorders, bronchial asthma, coronary occlusion, and hyperthyroidism, and in breastfeeding and children.

IMPLEMENTATION
• Give only with atropine sulfate available for cholinergic crisis
• Give only after all other cholinergics have been discontinued
• Give increased dosages if tolerance occurs
• Give larger doses after exercise or fatigue
• Give on empty stomach for better absorption
• Store at room temperature

ADVERSE EFFECTS: The most serious adverse reactions are respiratory depression, bronchospasm, constriction, laryngospasm, respiratory arrest, convulsions, and paralysis. The most common side effects are nausea, diarrhea, and vomiting.

PHARMACOKINETICS: Onset, peak, and duration vary widely among products. Most products are metabolized in the liver and excreted in urine.

INTERACTIONS: Interactions vary widely among products. Check individual monographs for specific information.

NURSING CONSIDERATIONS
Assessment
• Monitor VS, respiration q8hr
• Monitor I&O ratio; check for urinary retention or incontinence

---

• Assess for bradycardia, hypotension, bronchospasm, headache, dizziness, seizures, respiratory depression; product should be discontinued if toxicity occurs

Patient/family education
• Inform patient that product is not a cure; it only relieves symptoms (myasthenia gravis)
• Advise patient to carry/wear emergency ID specifying myasthenia gravis, products taken

Evaluation

Positive therapeutic outcome
• Increased muscle strength, hand grasp
• Improved muscle gait
• Absence of labored breathing (if severe)

Generic Names
bethanechol, physostigmine, pyridostigmine

Cholinergic Blockers

ACTION: Cholinergic blockers inhibit or block acetylcholine at receptor sites in the autonomic nervous system.

USES: Many cholinergic blockers are used to decrease secretions before surgery, to reverse neuromuscular blockade, and to decrease motility of the GI, biliary, and urinary tracts. Other products are used for parkinsonian symptoms, including dystonia associated with neuroleptic products.

CONTRAINDICATIONS
Hypersensitivity can occur, and allergies should be identified before administering these products. Persons with GI and GU obstruction should not use these products, since constipation and urinary retention may occur. They are also contraindicated in closed-angle glaucoma and myasthenia gravis.

Precautions: Caution must be used when these products are given to the geriatric patient, since metabolism is slowed. Also, persons with tachycardia or prostatic hypertrophy should use these products with caution.

IMPLEMENTATION
• Give with food or milk to decrease GI symptoms
• Give parenteral dose with patient recumbent to prevent postural hypotension; give dose slowly, monitoring VS
• Give hard candy, gum, frequent rinsing of mouth for dryness

ADVERSE EFFECTS: The most common side effects are dryness of the mouth and constipation, which can be prevented by frequent rinsing of the mouth and increasing water and bulk in the diet.

PHARMACOKINETICS: Onset, peak, and duration vary with route.

INTERACTIONS: Increase in anticholinergic effect occurs when used with opioids, barbiturates, antihistamines, MAOIs, phenothiazines, amantadine.

NURSING CONSIDERATIONS
Assessment
• Assess I&O ratio; be alert for urinary retention, frequency, dysuria; product should be discontinued if these occur
• Assess urinary hesitancy, retention; palpate bladder if retention occurs
• Assess constipation; increase fluids, bulk, exercise
• Assess for tolerance over long-term therapy; dosage may need to be changed
• Assess mental status: affect, mood, CNS depression, worsening of mental symptoms during early therapy

Patient/family education
• Caution patient to avoid driving and other hazardous activities if drowsiness occurs
• Advise patient to avoid concurrent use of cough, cold preparations with alcohol, antihistamines unless directed by prescriber
• Caution patient to use with caution in hot weather, since medication may increase susceptibility to heat stroke

Evaluation

Positive therapeutic outcome
• Absence of cramps
• Absence of EPS

Generic Names
atropine (high alert), benztropine, glycopyrrolate, scopolamine

Corticosteroids

ACTION: Corticosteroids are divided into glucocorticoids and mineralocorticoids. Glucocorticoids decrease inflammation by the suppression of migration of polymorphonuclear leukocytes, fibroblasts, increased capillary permeability, and lysosomal stabilization. They also have varied metabolic effects and modify the body's immune responses to many different stimuli. Mineralocorticoids act by increasing resorption of sodium by increasing hydrogen and potassium excretion in the distal tubule.

USES: Glucocorticoids are used to decrease inflammation and for immunosuppression. In addition, some products may be given for allergy, adrenal insufficiency, or cerebral edema. Mineralocorticoids are given for adrenal insufficiency or adrenogenital syndrome.

CONTRAINDICATIONS

Hypersensitivity may occur and should be identified before administering. Since these products mask infection, they should not be used in systemic fungal infections or amebiasis. Mothers taking pharmacologic doses of corticosteroids should not breastfeed.

Precautions: Caution must be used when these products are prescribed for diabetic patients since hyperglycemia may occur. Also, patients with glaucoma, seizure disorders, peptic ulcer, impaired renal function, CHF, hypertension, ulcerative colitis, or myasthenia gravis should be monitored closely if corticosteroids are given. Use with caution during pregnancy, in children, and in the geriatric patient.

IMPLEMENTATION

• Give with food or milk to decrease GI symptoms
• Give single daily or alternate-day doses in the morning before 9 AM (for replacement therapy)

ADVERSE EFFECTS: The most common side effects include change in behavior, including insomnia and euphoria; GI irritation, including peptic ulcer; metabolic reactions, including hypokalemia, hyperglycemia, and carbohydrate intolerance; and sodium and fluid retention. Most adverse reactions are dose dependent.

PHARMACOKINETICS: For oral preparations the onset of action occurs between 1-2 hr, and duration can be up to 2 days, with a half-life of 2-4 days. Pharmacokinetics vary widely among products. These products cross the placenta and appear in breast milk.

INTERACTIONS: Decreased corticosteroid effect may occur with barbiturates, rifampin, and phenytoin; corticosteroid dosage may need to be increased. There is a possibility of GI bleeding when used with salicylates and indomethacin. Steroids may reduce salicylate levels. When using with digoxin, glycosides, potassium-depleting diuretics, and amphotericin, serum potassium levels should be monitored.

NURSING CONSIDERATIONS
Assessment

• Monitor potassium, blood glucose, urine glucose while on long-term therapy; hypokalemia and hyperglycemia are common

• Monitor weight daily; notify prescriber if weekly gain of >5 lb since these products alter fluid and electrolyte balance
• Assess for potassium depletion: paresthesias, fatigue, nausea, vomiting, depression, polyuria, dysrhythmias, weakness
• Assess for mental status: affect, mood, behavioral changes, aggression; if severe personality changes occur, including depression, product may need to be tapered and then discontinued
• Monitor I&O ratio; be alert for decreasing urinary output and increasing edema
• Monitor plasma cortisol levels during long-term therapy (normal level is 138-635 nmol/L when drawn at 8 AM)
• Assess for infection: increased temp, WBC, even after withdrawal of medication; product masks symptoms of infection
• Assess for adrenal insufficiency: nausea, anorexia, fatigue, dizziness, dyspnea, weakness, joint pain

Patient/family education

• Advise patient that emergency ID as steroid user should be carried/worn
• Advise patient not to discontinue this medication abruptly; adrenal crisis can result
• Teach patient all aspects of product use, including cushingoid symptoms
• Instruct patient to take with meals or a snack
• Teach patient to avoid exposure to chickenpox or measles if taking immunosuppressives

Evaluation

Positive therapeutic outcome
• Decreased inflammation

Generic Names
Glucocorticoids:
beclomethasone, betamethasone, cortisone, dexamethasone, hydrocortisone, hydrocortisone sodium succinate, methylPREDNISolone, predniSOLONE, predniSONE, triamcinolone

Diuretics

ACTION: Diuretics are divided into subgroups: thiazides and thiazidelike diuretics, loop diuretics, carbonic anhydrase inhibitors, osmotic diuretics, and potassium-sparing diuretics. Each one of these subgroups differs in its mechanism of action. Thiazides and thiazide-like diuretics increase excretion of water and sodium by inhibiting resorption in the early distal tubule. Loop diuretics inhibit resorption of sodium and chloride in the thick ascending limb of the loop of Henle. Carbonic anhydrase inhibitors increase sodium excretion by decreasing sodium-hydrogen ion exchange throughout the renal tubule. Carbonic anhydrase inhibitors also decrease secretion of aqueous humor in the eye and thus decrease intraocular pressure. Osmotic diuretics increase the osmotic pressure of glomerular filtrate, thus decreasing net absorption of sodium. The potassium-sparing diuretics interfere with sodium resorption at the distal tubule, thus decreasing potassium excretion.

USES: Blood pressure is reduced in hypertension; edema is reduced in CHF; intraocular pressure is decreased in glaucoma.

CONTRAINDICATIONS
Persons with electrolyte imbalances (sodium, chloride, potassium), dehydration, or anuria should not be given these products until the problem is corrected.

Precautions: Caution must be used when diuretics are given to the geriatric patient, since electrolyte disturbances and dehydration can occur rapidly. Renal/hepatic disorders may cause poor metabolism and excretion of the product.

IMPLEMENTATION
- Give in AM to avoid interference with sleep if using product as a diuretic
- Give potassium replacement if potassium is less than 3 mg/dl

ADVERSE EFFECTS: Hypokalemia, hyperuricemia, and hyperglycemia occur most frequently with thiazide diuretics. Aplastic anemia, blood dyscrasias, volume depletion, and dehydration may occur when thiazide-like diuretics, loop diuretics, or carbonic anhydrase inhibitors are given. Side effects and adverse reactions vary widely for the miscellaneous products.

PHARMACOKINETICS: Onset, peak, and duration vary widely among the different subgroups of these products.

INTERACTIONS: Cholestyramine and colestipol decrease the absorption of thiazide diuretics. Concurrent use of thiazides with diazoxide may increase hyperuricemia, hyperglycemia, and antihypertensive effects of thiazides. Ototoxicity may occur when loop diuretics are used with aminoglycosides. Thiazide and loop diuretics may increase therapeutic and toxic effects of lithium.

NURSING CONSIDERATIONS
Assessment
- Monitor weight, I&O ratio daily to determine fluid loss; check skin turgor for dehydration
- Monitor electrolytes: potassium, sodium, chloride: include BUN, blood glucose, CBC, serum creatinine, blood pH, ABGs, uric acid, calcium; electrolyte imbalances may occur quickly
- Monitor B/P with patient lying, standing; postural hypotension may occur since fluid loss occurs from intravascular spaces first
- Assess for signs of metabolic alkalosis, including drowsiness and restlessness
- Assess for signs of hypokalemia with some products: postural hypotension, malaise, fatigue, tachycardia, leg cramps, weakness

Patient/family education
- Teach patient to take product early in the day (diuretic) to prevent nocturia

Evaluation
Positive therapeutic outcome
- Improvement in edema of feet, legs, sacral area daily if medication is being used in CHF
- Improvement in B/P if medication is being used as a diuretic
- Improvement in intraocular pressure if medication is being used to decrease aqueous humor in the eye

Generic Names
Thiazides:
chlorothiazide, hydrochlorothiazide

Thiazidelike:
chlorthalidone, indapamide, metolazone

Loop:
bumetanide, furosemide

Carbonic anhydrase inhibitors:
acetaZOLAMIDE

Potassium-sparing:
aMILoride, spironolactone

Osmotic:
mannitol, urea

Histamine H₂ Antagonists

ACTION: Histamine H₂ antagonists act by inhibiting histamine at H₂ receptor site in parietal cells, which inhibits gastric acid secretion.

USES: Histamine H₂ antagonists are used for short-term treatment of duodenal and gastric ulcers and maintenance therapy for duodenal ulcer and for gastroesophageal reflux disease.

CONTRAINDICATIONS
Persons with hypersensitivity should not use these products.

Precautions: Caution should be used in pregnancy, breastfeeding, children <16 yr,

Adverse effects: *italics* = common; **bold** = life-threatening

organic brain syndrome, and renal/hepatic disease.

IMPLEMENTATION

- Give with meals for prolonged product effect
- Give antacids 1 hr before or 1 hr after cimetidine
- Give **IV** slowly; bradycardia may occur; give over 30 min
- Store diluted sol at room temperature for up to 48 hr

ADVERSE EFFECTS: The most serious adverse reactions are agranulocytosis, thrombocytopenia, neutropenia, aplastic anemia, and exfoliative dermatitis. The most common side effects are confusion (not with ranitidine), headache, and diarrhea.

PHARMACOKINETICS: Onset, peak, and duration vary widely among products. Most products are metabolized in the liver and excreted in urine.

INTERACTIONS: Antacids interfere with absorption of histamine H_2 antagonists. Check individual monographs for specific information.

NURSING CONSIDERATIONS
Assessment
- Monitor gastric pH (>5 should be maintained)
- Monitor I&O ratio, BUN, creatinine

Patient/family education
- Advise patient that gynecomastia, impotence may occur but is reversible
- Caution patient to avoid driving and other hazardous activities until patient is stabilized on this medication
- Caution patient to avoid black pepper, caffeine, alcohol, harsh spices, extremes in temperature of food
- Caution patient to avoid OTC preparations: aspirin, cough, cold preparations
- Inform patient that product must be continued for prescribed time to be effective
- Advise patient to report bruising, fatigue, malaise; blood dyscrasias may occur

Evaluation

Positive therapeutic outcome
- Decreased pain in abdomen

Generic Names
cimetidine, famotidine, ranitidine

Immunosuppressants

ACTION: Immunosuppressants produce immunosuppression by inhibiting T lymphocytes.

USES: Most immunosuppressants are used for organ transplants to prevent rejection.

CONTRAINDICATIONS
Products are contraindicated in hypersensitivity.

Precautions: Caution should be used in pregnancy and severe renal/hepatic disease.

IMPLEMENTATION
- Give for several days before transplant surgery
- Give with meals for GI upset or place product in chocolate milk
- Give with oral antifungal for *Candida* infections

ADVERSE EFFECTS: The most serious adverse reactions are albuminuria, hematuria, proteinuria, renal failure, and hepatotoxicity. The most common side effects are oral *Candida* infection, gum hyperplasia, tremors, and headache. The most serious adverse reactions for azaTHIOprine are hematologic (leukopenia and thrombocytopenia) and GI (nausea and vomiting). There is a risk of secondary infection.

PHARMACOKINETICS: Onset, peak, and duration vary widely among products. Most products are metabolized in the liver and excreted in urine.

INTERACTIONS: Interactions vary widely among products. Check individual monographs for specific information.

NURSING CONSIDERATIONS
Assessment
- Monitor renal function tests: BUN, creatinine at least monthly during treatment, 3 mo after treatment
- Monitor hepatic function tests: alkaline phosphatase, AST, ALT, bilirubin
- Monitor product blood levels during treatment
- Assess for hepatotoxicity: dark urine, jaundice, itching, light-colored stools; product should be discontinued

Patient/family education
- Advise patient to report fever, chills, sore throat, fatigue since serious infections may occur
- Caution patient to use contraceptive measures during treatment and for 12 wk after ending therapy

Evaluation

Positive therapeutic outcome
- Absence of rejection

Generic Names

azaTHIOprine, **basiliximab** (high alert), cycloSPORINE, everolimus, muromonab-CD3, secukinumab, sirolimus, tacrolimus, vedolizumab

Laxatives

ACTION: Laxatives are divided into bulk products, lubricants, osmotics, saline laxative stimulants, and stool softeners. Bulks work by absorbing water and expanding to increase moisture content and bulk in the stool. Lubricants increase water retention in the stool, causing reabsorption of water in the bowel. Saline draws water into the intestinal lumen. Osmotics increase distention and promote peristalsis. Stimulants act by increasing peristalsis by direct effect on the intestine. Stool softeners reduce surface tension of liquid in the bowel.

USES: Laxatives are used as a preparation for bowel or rectal examination, for constipation, or as stool softeners.

CONTRAINDICATIONS

Persons with GI obstruction, perforation, gastric retention, toxic colitis, megacolon, abdominal pain, nausea, vomiting, and fecal impaction should not use these products.

Precautions: Caution should be used in rectal bleeding, large hemorrhoids, and anal excoriation.

IMPLEMENTATION

• Give alone only with water for better absorption; do not take within 1 hr of antacids, milk, or cimetidine
• Swallow tab whole; do not break, crush, or chew

ADVERSE EFFECTS: The most common side effects are nausea, abdominal cramps, and diarrhea.

PHARMACOKINETICS: Onset, peak, and duration vary among products.

INTERACTIONS: Interactions vary widely among products. Check individual monographs for specific information.

NURSING CONSIDERATIONS
Assessment

• Monitor blood, urine electrolytes if product is used often by patient
• Monitor I&O ratio to identify fluid loss
• Determine cause of constipation; identify whether fluids, bulk, or exercise is missing from lifestyle

• Assess for cramping, rectal bleeding, nausea, vomiting; if these symptoms occur, product should be discontinued

Patient/family education

• Caution patient not to use laxatives for long-term therapy; bowel tone will be lost; that normal bowel movements do not always occur daily
• Caution patient not to use in presence of abdominal pain, nausea, vomiting
• Advise patient to notify prescriber of abdominal pain, nausea, vomiting
• Advise patient to notify prescriber if constipation is unrelieved or if symptoms of electrolyte imbalance occur: muscle cramps, pain, weakness, dizziness

Evaluation

Positive therapeutic outcome
• Decrease in constipation

Generic Names

Bulk laxative:
psyllium

Osmotic agent:
lactulose

Saline laxatives:
magnesium salts, sodium biphosphate/sodium phosphate

Stimulants:
bisacodyl, senna

Stool softener:
docusate

Neuromuscular Blocking Agents

ACTION: Neuromuscular blocking agents are divided into depolarizing and nondepolarizing blockers. They act by inhibiting transmission of nerve impulses by binding with cholinergic receptor sites.

USES: Neuromuscular blocking agents are used to facilitate endotracheal intubation and skeletal muscle relaxation during mechanical ventilation, surgery, or general anesthesia.

CONTRAINDICATIONS

Persons who are hypersensitive should not be given this product.

Precautions: Caution should be used in pregnancy, breastfeeding, children <2 yr, thyroid disease, collagen disease, cardiac disease, electrolyte imbalances, dehydration, neuromuscular disease (myasthenia gravis), and respiratory disease.

IMPLEMENTATION
• Administer using nerve stimulator by anesthesiologist to determine neuromuscular blockade
• Administer anticholinesterase to reverse neuromuscular blockade
• Give **IV** undiluted over 1-2 min (only by qualified person, usually an anesthesiologist)
• Store in light-resistant, cool area
• Reassure patient if communication is difficult during recovery from neuromuscular blockade

ADVERSE EFFECTS: The most serious adverse reactions are prolonged apnea, bronchospasm, cyanosis, respiratory depression, and malignant hyperthermia. The most common side effects are bradycardia and decreased motility.

PHARMACOKINETICS: Onset, peak, and duration vary widely among products. Most products are metabolized in the liver and excreted in urine.

INTERACTIONS: Aminoglycosides potentiate neuromuscular blockade. Check individual monographs for specific information.

NURSING CONSIDERATIONS
Assessment
• Monitor for electrolyte imbalances (potassium, magnesium); may lead to increased action of this product
• Monitor VS (B/P, pulse, respirations, airway) q15min until fully recovered; rate, depth, pattern of respirations, strength of hand grip
• Monitor I&O ratio; check for urinary retention, frequency, hesitancy
• Assess for recovery: decreased paralysis of face, diaphragm, leg, arm, rest of body
• Assess for allergic reactions: rash, fever, respiratory distress, pruritus; product should be discontinued

Evaluation

Positive therapeutic outcome
• Paralysis of jaw, eyelid, head, neck, rest of body

Generic Names
pancuronium (high alert), **succinylcholine** (high alert), **vecuronium** (high alert)

Nonsteroidal Antiinflammatories

ACTION: Nonsteroidal antiinflammatories decrease prostaglandin synthesis by inhibiting an enzyme needed for biosynthesis.

USES: Nonsteroidal antiinflammatories are used to treat mild to moderate pain, osteoarthritis, rheumatoid arthritis, and dysmenorrhea.

CONTRAINDICATIONS
Persons with hypersensitivity, asthma, or severe renal/hepatic disease should not use these products.

Precautions: Caution should be used in pregnancy, breastfeeding, children, geriatric patients, bleeding/GI/cardiac disorders, and hypersensitivity to other antiinflammatory agents.

IMPLEMENTATION
• Give with food to decrease GI symptoms; however, best to take on empty stomach to facilitate absorption
• Store at room temperature

ADVERSE EFFECTS: The most serious adverse reactions are nephrotoxicity (dysuria, hematuria, oliguria, azotemia), blood dyscrasias, and cholestatic hepatitis. The most common side effects are nausea, abdominal pain, anorexia, dizziness, and drowsiness.

PHARMACOKINETICS: Onset, peak, and duration vary widely among products. Most products are metabolized in the liver and excreted in urine.

INTERACTIONS: Interactions vary widely among products. Check individual monographs for specific information.

NURSING CONSIDERATIONS
Assessment
• Monitor renal, hepatic, blood tests: BUN, creatinine, AST, ALT, Hgb, before treatment, periodically thereafter
• Monitor audiometric, ophth examination before, during, and after treatment.
• Check for eye, ear problems: blurred vision, tinnitus; may indicate toxicity

Patient/family education
• Advise patient to report blurred vision, ringing, roaring in ears; may indicate toxicity
• Caution patient to avoid driving, other hazardous activities if dizziness, drowsiness occurs, especially in geriatric patients
• Advise patient to report change in urine pattern, increased weight, edema, increased pain in

joints, fever, blood in urine; indicate nephrotoxicity

• Inform patient that therapeutic effects may take up to 1 mo to occur

Evaluation

Positive therapeutic outcome
• Decreased pain, stiffness in joints
• Decreased swelling in joints
• Ability to move more easily

Generic Names
celecoxib, diclofenac, etodolac, ibuprofen, indomethacin, ketoprofen, ketorolac, nabumetone, naproxen, piroxicam, sulindac

Opioid Analgesics

ACTION: These agents depress pain impulse transmission at the spinal cord level by interacting with opioid receptors. Products are divided into opiates and nonopiates.

USES: Most opioid analgesics are used to control moderate to severe pain and are used before and after surgery.

CONTRAINDICATIONS
Hypersensitive reactions occur frequently. Check for sensitivity before administering. These products should not be used if opioid addiction is suspected.

Precautions: Caution must be used when these products are given to persons with an addictive personality, since the possibility of addiction is so great. Also, persons with increased ICP may experience an even greater increase in ICP. Persons with severe heart disease, renal/hepatic disease, respiratory conditions, and seizure disorders should be monitored closely for worsening condition.

IMPLEMENTATION
• Give with antiemetic if nausea or vomiting occurs
• Give when pain is beginning to return; determine dosage interval by patient response
• Provide assistance with ambulation; patient should not be ambulating during product peak

ADVERSE EFFECTS: GI symptoms, including nausea, vomiting, anorexia, constipation, and cramps are the most common side effects. Other common side effects include lightheadedness, dizziness, and sedation. Serious adverse reactions such as respiratory depression, respiratory arrest, circulatory depression, and increased ICP may result but are less common and usually dose dependent.

PHARMACOKINETICS: Onset of action is immediate by **IV** route and rapid by IM and PO routes. Peak occurs from 1-2 hr, depending on route, with a duration of 2-8 hr. These agents cross the placenta and appear in breast milk.

INTERACTIONS: Barbiturates, other opioids, hypnotics, antipsychotics, or alcohol can increase CNS depression when taken with opioids.

NURSING CONSIDERATIONS
Assessment
• Monitor I&O ratio; be alert for urinary retention, frequency, dysuria; product should be discontinued if these occur
• Assess for respiratory dysfunction: respiratory depression, rate, rhythm, character; notify prescriber if respirations are <12/min
• Assess for CNS changes: dizziness, drowsiness, hallucinations, euphoria, LOC, pupil reaction
• Assess for allergic reactions: rash, urticaria
• Assess for need for pain medication, use pain scoring

Patient/family education
• Advise patient to report any symptoms of CNS changes, allergic reactions, or shortness of breath
• Caution patient that physical dependency may result when used for extended periods
• Teach patient that withdrawal symptoms may occur, including nausea, vomiting, cramps, fever, faintness, anorexia
• Advise patient to avoid alcohol and other CNS depressants

Evaluation
Positive therapeutic outcome
• Decrease in pain

Generic Names
buprenorphine, butorphanol, codeine, **fentaNYL** (high alert), fentaNYL transdermal, **HYDROmorphone** (high alert), **meperidine** (high alert), **methadone** (high alert), **morphine** (high alert), nalbuphine, **oxyCODONE** (high alert), **oxymorphone** (high alert), **pentazocine** (high alert), **remifentanil** (high alert)

Salicylates

ACTION: Salicylates have analgesic, antipyretic, and antiinflammatory effects. The analgesic and antiinflammatory activities may be mediated through the inhibition of prostaglandin synthesis. Antipyretic action results from inhibition of the hypothalamic heat-regulating center.

USES: The primary uses of salicylates are relief of mild to moderate pain and fever and in inflammatory conditions such as arthritis, thromboembolic disorders, and rheumatic fever.

CONTRAINDICATIONS
Hypersensitivity to salicylates is common. Check for sensitivity before administering. Persons with bleeding disorders, GI bleeding, and vit K deficiency should not use these products since salicylates increase pro-time. Children should not use these products since salicylates have been associated with Reye's syndrome.

Precautions: Caution is needed when salicylates are given to patients with anemia, renal/hepatic disease, and Hodgkin's disease. Caution should also be exercised in pregnancy and breastfeeding.

IMPLEMENTATION
• Give with food or milk to decrease gastric irritation; give 30 min before or 1 hr after meals with a full glass of water

ADVERSE EFFECTS: The most common side effects are GI symptoms and rash. Serious blood dyscrasias and hepatotoxicity may result when used for long periods at high doses. Tinnitus or impaired hearing may indicate that blood salicylate levels are reaching or exceeding the upper limit of the therapeutic range.

PHARMACOKINETICS: Onset of action occurs in 15-30 min, with a peak of 1-2 hr and a duration up to 6 hr. These products are metabolized by the liver and excreted by the kidneys.

INTERACTIONS: Increased effects of anticoagulants, insulin, methotrexate, heparin, valproic acid, and oral sulfonylureas may occur when used with salicylates. Aspirin may decrease serum concentrations of nonsteroidal antiinflammatory agents.

NURSING CONSIDERATIONS
Assessment
• Monitor renal/hepatic function tests: AST, ALT, bilirubin, creatinine, LDH, alkaline phosphatase, BUN if patient is on long-term therapy since these products are metabolized and excreted by the liver and kidney
• Monitor blood tests: CBC, Hct, Hgb, and pro-time if patient is on long-term therapy, since these products increase the possibility of bleeding and blood dyscrasias

• Assess for hepatotoxicity: dark urine, clay-colored stools, jaundiced skin and sclera, itching, abdominal pain, fever, diarrhea, which may occur with long-term use
• Assess for ototoxicity: tinnitus, ringing, roaring in ears; audiometric testing is needed before and after long-term therapy

Patient/family education
• Advise patient that blood sugar levels should be monitored closely if patient is diabetic
• Caution patient not to exceed recommended dosage; acute poisoning may result
• Inform patient that therapeutic response takes 2 wk in arthritis
• Caution patient to avoid use of alcohol since GI bleeding may result
• Advise patient to notify prescriber if ringing in the ears or persistent GI pain occurs
• Advise patient to take with full glass of water to reduce risk of lodging in esophagus

Evaluation
Positive therapeutic outcome
• Decreased pain, fever

Generic Names
aspirin, magnesium salicylate, salsalate

Sedatives/Hypnotics

ACTION: The sedatives/hypnotics depress the CNS; some products at the cerebral cortex, others inhibit transmitters in the CNS.

USES: Sedatives/hypnotics are used for the treatment of sleep disorders, seizures, muscle spasms, and alcohol withdrawal.

CONTRAINDICATIONS
Persons with hypersensitivity reactions should not use these products.

Precautions: Sedatives/hypnotics should be used cautiously in pregnancy **(C)** and breastfeeding.

IMPLEMENTATION
• Give lowest possible dose for therapeutic result; adjust dose to response
• Provide assistance with ambulation during beginning therapy if dizziness, ataxia occur

ADVERSE EFFECTS: The most common side effects are nausea and drowsiness. The most serious side effects are Stevens-Johnson syndrome, blood dyscrasias, and risk of dependency.

PHARMACOKINETICS: Onset, peak, and duration vary widely among products. Most products are metabolized in the liver and excreted by the kidneys.

INTERACTIONS: Increased CNS depression may occur with other CNS depressants such as alcohol, opiates, antipsychotics, and antidepressants.

NURSING CONSIDERATIONS
Assessment
• Monitor mental status: affect, mood, behavioral changes, depression, confusion; seizure activity

Patient/family education
• Inform patient that these products should only be used for short-term insomnia
• Caution patient not to drive or engage in other hazardous activities while taking these products
• Instruct patient to avoid breastfeeding while taking these products
• Instruct patient to avoid alcohol or other CNS depressants as drowsiness will increase
• Teach patient that some of the products take two nights to be effective
• Advise patient to report side effects, adverse reactions to health care provider
• Instruct patient to use exactly as prescribed, at regular intervals

Evaluation
Positive therapeutic outcome
• Ability to sleep throughout the night
• Absence or decreasing seizure activity

Generic Names
Barbiturates:
PHENobarbital (high alert)

Benzodiazepines:
chlordiazePOXIDE, clorazepate, diazepam, flurazepam, LORazepam, midazolam, oxazepam, temazepam, triazolam

Miscellaneous products:
chloral hydrate, dexmedetomidine, **droperidol** (high alert), eszopiclone, hydrOXYzine, promethazine, ramelteon, suvorexant, tasimelton, zaleplon, zolpidem

Skeletal Muscle Relaxants

ACTION: Most skeletal muscle relaxants inhibit synaptic responses in the CNS by stimulating receptors and decreasing neurotransmission, decreasing pain and spasticity.

USES: Skeletal muscle relaxants are used for musculoskeletal disorders with pain or spasticity related to spinal cord injuries.

CONTRAINDICATIONS
Persons with hypersensitivity should not use these products.

Precautions: Skeletal muscle relaxants should be used cautiously in pregnancy (**C**), breastfeeding, the geriatric patient, peptic ulcer, renal/hepatic disease, stroke, seizure disorder, and diabetes.

IMPLEMENTATION
• Give when pain is beginning to return, not after pain is severe
• Store in dry area, away from heat and sunlight

ADVERSE EFFECTS: The most common side effects are dizziness, weakness, fatigue, drowsiness, and headache. Some products can cause seizures, cardiovascular collapse, and severe CNS depression.

PHARMACOKINETICS: Pharmacokinetics vary widely among products. Check individual monographs for specific information.

INTERACTIONS: CNS depressants used with skeletal muscle relaxants may lead to increased CNS depression.

NURSING CONSIDERATIONS
Assessment
• Monitor pain: character, location, duration, alleviating/aggravating factors

Patient/family education
• Advise patient not to use with other CNS depressant unless prescriber approved
• Inform patient that many products require 1-2 mo of treatment for full effect
• Caution patient to avoid hazardous activities until response to medication is known
• Caution patient that most products should not be discontinued quickly, but tapered over 1-2 wk

Evaluation
Positive therapeutic outcome
• Decrease in pain or spasticity

Generic Names
Centrally acting:
baclofen, carisoprodol, cyclobenzaprine, diazepam, methocarbamol

Direct-acting:
dantrolene

Thrombolytics

ACTION: Thrombolytics activate conversion of plasminogen to plasmin (fibrinolysin). Plasmin is able to break down clots (fibrin).

USES: Thrombolytics are used to treat DVT, PE, arterial thrombosis, arterial embolism, arteriovenous cannula occlusion, lysis of coronary artery thrombi after MI, and acute evolving transmural MI.

CONTRAINDICATIONS

Persons with hypersensitivity, active bleeding, intraspinal surgery, neoplasms of the CNS, ulcerative colitis/enteritis, severe hypertension, renal/hepatic disease, hypocoagulation, COPD, subacute bacterial endocarditis, rheumatic valvular disease, cerebral embolism/thrombosis/hemorrhage, intra-arterial diagnostic procedure or surgery (10 days), and recent major surgery should not use these products.

Precautions: Caution should be used in arterial emboli from left side of heart and pregnancy.

IMPLEMENTATION

• Administer as soon as thrombi identified; not useful for thrombi over 1wk old
• Administer cryoprecipitate or fresh, frozen plasma if bleeding occurs
• Give loading dose at beginning of therapy; may require increased loading doses
• Give heparin after fibrinogen level is over 100 mg/dl; heparin INF to increase PTT to 1.5-2 × baseline for 3-7 days
• About 10% of patients have high streptococcal antibody titers requiring increased loading doses
• Give **IV** therapy using 0.8-μm filter
• Store reconstituted sol in refrigerator; discard after 24 hr
• Provide bed rest during entire course of treatment

ADVERSE EFFECTS: Serious adverse reactions include GI, GU, intracranial, and retroperitoneal bleeding and anaphylaxis. The most common side effects are decreased Hct, urticaria, headache, and nausea.

PHARMACOKINETICS: Onset, peak, and duration vary widely among products. Most products are metabolized in the liver and excreted in urine.

INTERACTIONS: Interactions vary widely among products. Check individual monographs for specific information.

NURSING CONSIDERATIONS
Assessment

• Monitor VS, B/P, pulse, respirations, neurologic signs, temp at least q4hr (increased temp is an indicator of internal bleeding), cardiac rhythm following intracoronary administration; systolic pressure increase of >25 mm Hg should be reported to prescriber

• Assess for neurologic changes that may indicate intracranial bleeding
• Assess retroperitoneal bleeding: back pain, leg weakness, diminished pulses
• Assess for allergy: fever, rash, itching, chills; mild reaction may be treated with antihistamines
• Assess for bleeding during 1st hr of treatment: hematuria, hematemesis, bleeding from mucous membranes, epistaxis, ecchymosis
• Monitor blood tests (Hct, platelets, PTT, PT, TT, APTT) before starting therapy; PT or APTT must be less than 2 times control before starting therapy; TT or PT q3-4hr during treatment

Patient/family education

• Teach patient to avoid venous or arterial puncture, injection, rectal temp
• Teach patient to treat fever with acetaminophen or aspirin
• Teach patient to apply pressure for 30 sec to minor bleeding sites; inform prescriber if this does not attain hemostasis; apply pressure dressing

Evaluation
Positive therapeutic outcome
• Resolution of thrombosis, embolism

Generic Names
alteplase (high alert), drotrecogin alfa, **tenecteplase** (high alert), **urokinase** (high alert)

Thyroid Hormones

ACTION: Thyroid hormones increase metabolic rates, resulting in increased cardiac output, O_2 consumption, body temp, blood volume, growth, development at cellular level, respiratory rate, and enzyme system activity.

USES: Thyroid hormones are used for thyroid replacement.

CONTRAINDICATIONS

Persons with adrenal insufficiency, myocardial infarction, or thyrotoxicosis should not use these products.

Precautions: Caution should be used in pregnancy (**A**) and breastfeeding. Geriatric patients and those with angina pectoris, hypertension, ischemia, cardiac disease, or diabetes mellitus or insipidus should be watched closely when using these products.

IMPLEMENTATION

• Give at same time each day to maintain product level
• Give only for hormone imbalances; not to be used for obesity, male infertility, menstrual conditions, lethargy
• Remove medication 4 wk before RAIU test

ADVERSE EFFECTS: The most common side effects include insomnia, tremors, tachycardia, palpitations, angina, dysrhythmias, weight loss, and changes in appetite. Serious adverse reactions include thyroid storm.

PHARMACOKINETICS: Pharmacokinetics vary widely among products. Check individual monographs for specific information.

INTERACTIONS
• Impaired absorption of thyroid products may occur when administered with cholestyramine, iron products (separate by 4-5 hr).
• Increased effects of anticoagulants, sympathomimetics, tricyclics, catecholamines may occur.
• Decreased effects of digoxin, glycosides, insulin, hypoglycemics may occur.
• Decreased effects of thyroid products may occur with estrogens.

NURSING CONSIDERATIONS
Assessment
• Monitor B/P, pulse before each dose
• Monitor I&O ratio
• Monitor weight daily in same clothing, using same scale, at same time of day
• Monitor height, growth rate if given to a child
• Monitor T_3, T_4, which are decreased; radioimmunoassay of TSH, which is increased; ratio uptake, which is decreased if patient is on too low a dosage of medication
• Assess for increased nervousness, excitability, irritability; may indicate too high a dosage of medication, usually after 1-3 wk of treatment
• Assess for cardiac status: angina, palpitation, chest pain, change in VS

Patient/family education
• Advise patient/family that hair loss will occur in children and is temporary
• Advise patient to report excitability, irritability, anxiety; indicates overdose
• Caution patient not to switch brands unless directed by prescriber
• Caution family that hypothyroid children will show almost immediate behavior/personality change
• Advise patient that treatment product is not to be taken to reduce weight
• Advise patient to avoid OTC preparations with iodine; read labels; to avoid iodine-containing foods: iodized salt, soybeans, tofu, turnips, some seafood, some bread

Evaluation

Positive therapeutic outcome
• Absence of depression

• Increased weight loss, diuresis, pulse, appetite
• Absence of constipation, peripheral edema, cold intolerance, pale, cool, dry skin, brittle nails, alopecia, coarse hair, menorrhagia, night blindness, paresthesias, syncope, stupor, coma, rosy cheeks

Generic Names
levothyroxine, liothyronine (T_3), liotrix, thyroid USP

Vasodilators

ACTION: Vasodilators act in various ways. Check individual monographs for specific action.

USES: Vasodilators are used to treat intermittent claudication, arteriosclerosis obliterans, vasospasm and muscular ischemia, ischemic cerebral vascular disease, hypertension, and angina.

CONTRAINDICATIONS
Some products are contraindicated in acute MI, paroxysmal tachycardia, and thyrotoxicosis.

Precautions: Caution should be used in uncompensated heart disease or peptic ulcer disease.

IMPLEMENTATION
• Give with meals to reduce GI symptoms
• Store in tight container at room temperature

ADVERSE EFFECTS: The most common side effects are headache, nausea, hypotension, hypertension, and ECG changes.

PHARMACOKINETICS: Onset, peak, and duration vary widely among products. Most products are metabolized in the liver and excreted in urine.

INTERACTIONS: Interactions vary widely among products. Check individual monographs for specific information.

NURSING CONSIDERATIONS
Assessment
• Assess bleeding time in individuals with bleeding disorders
• Assess cardiac status: B/P, pulse, rate, rhythm, character; watch for increasing pulse

Patient/family education
• Inform patient that medication is not cure, may need to be taken continuously
• Advise patient that it is necessary to quit smoking to prevent excessive vasoconstriction
• Advise patient that improvement may be sudden, but usually occurs gradually over several weeks

• Instruct patient to report headache, weakness, increased pulse, since product may need to be decreased or discontinued

• Instruct patient to avoid hazardous activities until stabilized on medication; dizziness may occur

Evaluation

Positive therapeutic outcome
• Ability to walk without pain
• Increased temp in extremities
• Increased pulse volume

Generic Names

amyl nitrite, bosentan, dipyridamole, hydrALA-ZINE, minoxidil, nesiritide

Vitamins

ACTION: The action of vitamins varies widely among products and classes. Check individual monographs for specific action.

USES: Vitamins are used to correct and prevent vitamin deficiencies.

CONTRAINDICATIONS

Hypersensitive reactions may occur, and allergies should be identified before these products are given.

IMPLEMENTATION

• Give PO with food for better absorption
• Store in tight, light-resistant container

ADVERSE EFFECTS: There is an absence of side effects or adverse reactions with the water-soluble vitamins (C, B). However, fat-soluble vitamins (A, D, E, K) may accumulate in the body and cause adverse reactions (refer to individual monographs).

PHARMACOKINETICS: Onset, peak, and duration vary widely among products. Check individual monographs for specific information.

NURSING CONSIDERATIONS
Patient/family education
• Advise patient not to take more than prescribed amount

Evaluation

Positive therapeutic outcome
• Absence of vitamin deficiency

Generic Names
Fat-soluble:
phytonadione (vitamin K_1), vitamin A, vitamin D, vitamin E

Water-soluble:
ascorbic acid (C), cyanocobalamin (B_{12}), pyridoxine (B_6), riboflavin (B_2), thiamine (B_1)

Miscellaneous:
multivitamins

Appendix A

Selected New Drugs

albiglutide
(al′-bi-gloo′-tide)
Tanzeum
Func. class.: Antidiabetic
Chem. class.: Incretin mimetic
Pregnancy category C

ACTION: Binds and activates known human GLP-1 receptor, mimics natural physiology for self-regulating glycemic control

USES: Type 2 diabetes mellitus; once-weekly dosing

Therapeutic outcome: Decreasing blood glucose level, A1C; decreasing polydipsia, polyphagia

CONTRAINDICATIONS
Hypersensitivity

> **BLACK BOX WARNING:** Medullary thyroid carcinoma, multiple endocrine neoplasia syndrome type 2 (MEN-2), thyroid cancer

Precautions: Pregnancy **C**, geriatric patients, severe renal/hepatic/GI disease, pancreatitis, vit D deficiency, breastfeeding, burns, children, colitis, diabetic ketoacidosis, infection, pseudomembranous colitis, surgery, thyroid disease, smoking, trauma, type 1 diabetes mellitus, vomiting

DOSAGE AND ROUTES
Adult: SUBCUT 30 mg q7days at any time of day; may increase to 50 mg q7days if needed

Available forms: Prefilled pen powder for inj 30, 50 mg

Implementation
• Store in refrigerator for unopened pen; may store at room temperature after opening for up to 30 days
SUBCUT route
• Give every 7 days (weekly); the dose can be given at any time of day without regard to meals
Reconstitution of the pen:
• The powder contained within the pen must be reconstituted before administration

• Twist the clear cartridge on the pen in the direction of the arrow until a "click" is heard. (You will also see a number "2" appear in the number window.) This action mixes the diluent with the powder
• Slowly and gently rock the pen side to side 5 times to mix. Do NOT shake the pen. Shaking the pen will cause foaming
• Patients using the product at home must wait 15 min for the 30-mg pen or 30 min for the 50-mg pen to ensure that the medicine is properly mixed and to avoid clogging the pen needle. In health care environments, a health care professional may have to wait up to 10 min after adding the diluent to see complete dissolution
• As long as the needle has not been attached, the pen can be used within 8 hr of reconstitution with the diluent
Preparing the pen for injection:
• Prime the pen before use
• Slowly rock the pen side to side 5 times. Do NOT shake; inspect for particulate matter; sol will be yellow in color and free of particles. A small amount of foam is normal
• Holding the pen upright, attach the supplied needle to the pen
• Tap the cartridge to bring bubbles to the top, remove bubbles by twisting until a number "3" appears in window. At the same time, the inj button will be automatically released from the bottom of the pen
• Once the needle is attached, the product must be administered immediately. The product can clog the needle if allowed to dry in the primed pen
SUBCUT administration using the pen:
• Inject SUBCUT into the thigh, abdomen, or upper arm. Once the needle is inserted, press the inj button until you hear a "click" and then hold the button for 5 additional sec to deliver the full dose.
• Inject SUBCUT into the thigh, abdomen, or upper arm, rotate sites to prevent lipodystrophy

ADVERSE EFFECTS

GI: Nausea, vomiting, diarrhea, dyspepsia, gastroesophageal reflux, **pancreatitis**

INTEG: Serious injection-site reactions

Adverse effects: *italics* = common; **bold** = life-threatening

Pharmacokinetics

Absorption	Unknown
Distribution	Steady state 4-5 wk
Metabolism	Unknown
Excretion	Unknown
Half-life	5 days

Pharmacodynamics

Onset	Unknown
Peak	3-5 days, increased in renal disease
Duration	Unknown

INTERACTIONS
Individual drugs
Digoxin: decreased action of digoxin

Niacin, dextrothyroxine, triamterene: decreased efficacy

Disopyramide, alcohol: increased hypoglycemia

Tacrolimus, cycloSPORINE: increased hyperglycemia

Drug classifications
ACE inhibitors, sulfonylureas, androgens, fibric acid derivatives: increased hypoglycemia

Phenothiazines, corticosteroids, anabolic steroids: increased hyperglycemia

Thiazide diuretics, estrogens, progestins, oral contraceptives, MAOIs: decreased efficacy

NURSING CONSIDERATIONS
Assessment
• Monitor blood glucose, A1C, during treatment to determine diabetes control

• Monitor CBC, renal studies (urinalysis, creatinine), baseline and periodically during treatment, report decreased blood counts, abnormal renal studies

> **BLACK BOX WARNING:** Medullary thyroid carcinoma, multiple endocrine neoplasia syndrome 2 (MEN-2), thyroid cancer: Monitor patient closely

• **Pancreatitis: Assess for severe abdominal pain, with or without vomiting, product should be discontinued**

• Assess for Hypo/hyperglycemic reaction that can occur soon after meals; for severe hypoglycemia, give **IV** D50W, then **IV** dextrose sol

• Monitor for nausea, vomiting, diarrhea, ability to tolerate product; may cause dehydration

Patient/family education
• Teach patient the symptoms of hypo/hyperglycemia and what to do about each; to have glucagon emergency kit available, carry sugar packets

• Advise patient that product must be continued on a weekly basis, explain consequences of discontinuing product abruptly; to take only as directed

• Direct patient to avoid OTC products unless approved by prescriber

• Teach patient that diabetes is a life-long illness; product will not cure diabetes

• Advise patient to carry emergency ID with prescriber, condition, and medications taken

• **Pancreatitis: If severe abdominal pain with or without vomiting occurs seek medical attention immediately**

• Advise patient to continue weight control, dietary restrictions, exercise, hygiene

• Teach patient that regular blood glucose monitoring and A1C testing is needed

• Teach patient to notify prescriber if pregnant or intending to become pregnant (**C**)

• Advise patient that it is important to read "Information for the Patient" and "Pen User Manual"; about self-injection

• Teach patient to review inj procedure before use, dispose of pen appropriately

Evaluation
Positive therapeutic outcome
• Improving blood glucose level, A1C; decreasing polydipsia, polyphagia, polyuria, clear sensorium, absence of dizziness

alirocumab (Rx)
(al′-i- rok′-ue-mab)
Praluent
Func. class.: Antilipemic
Pregnancy category C

ACTION: Binds to low-density lipoproteins, a human monoclonal antibody (IgG1)

Therapeutic outcome: Decreased cholesterol levels

USES: Heterozygous, familial hypercholesterolemia, atherosclerotic disease

CONTRAINDICATIONS
Hypersensitivity

Precautions: Pregnancy, breastfeeding

DOSAGE AND ROUTES
Adult: SUBCUT 75 mg q2wk, may increase to 150 mg q2wk if needed

Available forms: Prefilled pen 75 mg/1 ml, 150 mg/1 ml

Implementation
• If dose is missed give within 7 days of next dose; if over 7 days, wait until next scheduled dose

• Visually inspect for particulate matter and discoloration, solution is clear, colorless to pale yellow
• Warm to room temperature for 30-40 min before use. Use as soon as possible after warming
• Do NOT use the pre-filled pen or syringe if it has been at room temperature for ≥24 hr
• Give by SUBCUT inj into the thigh, abdomen, or upper arm. Rotate inj site with each inj.
• Do NOT inject into areas of active skin disease or injury (sunburn, rash, inflammation, skin infection)
• Do NOT administer with other injectable drugs at the same inj site

ADVERSE EFFECTS
CNS: Memory impairment, confusion
GI: Diarrhea
INTEG: Pruritus, injection-site reaction, erythema, ecchymosis
MISC: Edema
MS: Myalgia
RESP: Pharyngitis, sinusitis, cough
SYST: Infection, antibody formation

Pharmacokinetics

Absorption	Unknown
Distribution	Unknown
Metabolism	Unknown
Excretion	Unknown
Half-life	At steady state 17-20 days

Pharmacodynamics

Peak	3-7 days

INTERACTIONS
None known

Drug/lab test
Increased: LFTs

NURSING CONSIDERATIONS
Assessment
• **Hypercholesterolemia:** Obtain diet history: fat content, lipid levels (triglycerides, LDL, LDL-C 4-8 wk after start of titration, HDL, cholesterol); LFTs at baseline, periodically during treatment

Patient/family education
• Teach patient that compliance is needed
• Advise that risk factors should be decreased: high-fat diet, smoking, alcohol consumption, absence of exercise
• Advise patient to notify prescriber if pregnancy suspected, planned, or if breastfeeding
• Inform patient to report confusion, injection-site reactions

Evaluation
• Therapeutic response: decreased cholesterol, LDL; increased HDL

⚠ HIGH ALERT

atazanavir/cobicistat (Rx)
(at-a-za-na′veer/koe-bik′-i-stat)
Evotaz
Func. class.: Antiretroviral
Chem. class.: Protease inhibitor
Pregnancy category B

ACTION: Inhibits human immunodeficiency virus (HIV-1) protease, which prevents maturation of the infectious virus; it combines a protease inhibitor with an enhancer

Therapeutic outcome: Decreasing symptoms of HIV

USES: HIV-1 infection in combination with other antiretroviral agents

CONTRAINDICATIONS
Hypersensitivity, Child-Pugh Class C

Precautions: Pregnancy **B**, breastfeeding, children, geriatric, liver disease, alcoholism, antimicrobial resistance, AV block, diabetes, dialysis, elderly, women, hemophilia, hypercholesterolemia, immune reconstitution syndrome, lactic acidosis, pancreatitis, cholelithiasis, serious rash

DOSAGE AND ROUTES
Adults: PO 300 mg/150 mg qday in both treatment-naive and treatment-experienced patients
Adolescents (unlabeled): PO 300 mg/150 mg qday in combination with other antiretroviral agents as part of an alternative initial regimen (treatment-naïve)

Available forms: Tabs 300 mg/150 mg

Implementation
• Antiretroviral drug resistance testing (preferably genotypic testing) is recommended before initiation of therapy in antiretroviral treatment-naïve patients and before changing therapy for treatment failure
• Give with food

ADVERSE EFFECTS
CNS: Headache, depression, dizziness, insomnia, peripheral neuropathy
CV: Increased PR interval
EENT: Yellowing of sclera
GI: *Diarrhea, abdominal pain, nausea, vomiting,* **hepatotoxicity,** *cholelithiasis*
INTEG: *Rash,* **Stevens-Johnson syndrome,** *photosensitivity,* **DRESS**

MISC: Fatigue, fever, arthralgia, back pain, cough, lipodystrophy, pain, gynecomastia, nephrolithiasis, lactic acidosis, hyperbilirubinemia (pregnancy, females, obesity)

Pharmacokinetics

Absorption	Rapid, increased with food
Distribution	86% protein bound
Metabolism	Liver extensively by CYP3A4
Excretion	27% excreted unchanged in urine/feces (minimal)
Half-life	7 hr

Pharmacodynamics

Onset	Unknown
Peak	2 hr
Duration	Unknown

INTERACTIONS
Individual drugs

Clorazepate, clarithromycin, cycloSPO-RINE, diazepam, irinotecan, midazolam, pimozide, sildenafil, sirolimus, tacrolimus, triazolam, warfarin: increased levels resulting in toxicity

Didanosine, efavirenz, rifampin: decreased atazanavir levels

Indinavir: increased hyperbilirubinemia

Ritonavir, telaprevir: decreased telaprevir levels when used with atazanavir and ritonavir

Drug classifications

Antacids, H$_2$-receptor antagonists, proton pump inhibitors, CYP3A4 inducers: decreased atazanavir levels

Antidepressants (tricyclics), antidysrhythmics, ergots, calcium channel blockers, HMG-CoA reductase inhibitors, immunosuppressants, other protease inhibitors: increased levels resulting in increased toxicity

Contraceptives (oral), estrogens: increased effects (unboosted), decreased (boosted with ritonavir) CYP3A4 substrates, CYP3A4 inhibitors: increased atazanavir levels

Drug/herb

Red yeast rice: myopathy, rhabdomyolysis

St. John's wort: decreased atazanavir levels, avoid concurrent use

Drug/lab test

Increased: AST, ALT, total bilirubin, amylase, lipase, CK

Decreased: Hgb, neutrophils, platelets

Drug/food

Increased: drug bioavailability (to be taken with food)

NURSING CONSIDERATIONS
Assessment

• Assess for hepatic failure; hepatic studies: ALT, AST, bilirubin

• Assess for lactic acidosis, hyperbilirubinemia (females, pregnancy, obesity)

• Monitor PR interval in those taking calcium channel blockers, digoxin

• Assess for signs of infection, anemia, nephrolithiasis

• Monitor bowel pattern before, during treatment; if severe abdominal pain with bleeding occurs, product should be discontinued; monitor hydration

• Monitor viral load, CD4 count throughout treatment

• Serious rash (Stevens-Johnson syndrome, DRESS): most rashes last 1-4 wk; if serious, discontinue product

• Immune reconstitution syndrome: when given with combination antiretroviral therapy, time of onset is variable

Patient/family education

• Advise to take as prescribed with other antiretrovirals as prescribed; if dose is missed, take as soon as remembered up to 1 hr before next dose; do not double dose; do not share with others

• Teach that product must be taken daily to maintain blood levels for duration of therapy

• Advise patient to report yellowing of skin, sclera

• Instruct to notify prescriber if diarrhea, nausea, vomiting, rash occur; dizziness, lightheadedness; ECG may be altered

• Inform that product interacts with many products and St. John's wort; advise prescriber of all products, herbal products used

• Advise that redistribution of body fat may occur; the effect is not known

• Teach that product does not cure HIV-1 infection or prevent transmission to others, only controls symptoms

• Advise that if taking sildenafil or other phosphodiesterase type 5 inhibitors with atazanavir, there may be an increased risk of phosphodiesterase type 5 inhibitor-associated adverse events, including hypotension and prolonged penile erection; notify physician promptly of these symptoms

Evaluation
Positive therapeutic outcome

• Increasing CD4 counts; decreased viral load, resolution of symptoms of HIV-1 infection

> **⚠ HIGH ALERT**

ceritinib
(cerr-ah-tin'ib)
Zykadia
Func. class.: Antineoplastic—
Miscellaneous
Chem. class.: Protein-tyrosine kinase
inhibitor
Pregnancy category D

ACTION: A tyrosine kinase inhibitor targeting anaplastic lymphoma kinase (ALK); also targets insulinlike growth factors

Therapeutic outcome: Decreased progression of tumor

USES: Anaplastic lymphoma kinase (ALK)-positive metastatic non-small cell lung cancer (NSCLC) in patients who have progressed on or are intolerant to crizotinib

CONTRAINDICATIONS
Pregnancy (**D**), hypersensitivity

Precautions: Breastfeeding, children, geriatric patients, cardiac/hepatic disease, GI bleeding, bone marrow suppression, infection, diarrhea, hyperglycemia, diabetes mellitus, nausea/vomiting, pancreatitis, pneumonitis, QT prolongation, torsade de pointes, bradycardia, cardiac arrhythmias, electrolyte imbalances, corticosteroid therapy

DOSAGE AND ROUTES
Adults: PO 750 mg qday on an empty stomach until disease progression or unacceptable toxicity. Avoid the concomitant use of strong 3A4 inhibitors or inducers

Hepatic dose
Adult: PO ALT or AST >5 times above ULN and total bilirubin ≤ 2 times ULN: Hold product. When ALT/AST return to baseline or ≤ 3 times ULN, resume with a 150-mg dose reduction. Do not resume those unable to tolerate 300 mg qday

Available forms: Cap 150 mg

Implementation
Dosage adjustments due to treatment-related toxicity QTc prolongation: QTc >500 msec on at least 2 separate ECGs: Hold. When QTc returns to <481 msec (or baseline if >481 msec), resume with a 150-mg dose reduction. Do not resume in those unable to tolerate 300 mg qday.
• Any occurrence, QTc prolongation in combination with torsade de pointes or polymorphic ventricular tachycardia or signs/symptoms

of serious arrhythmia: Permanently discontinue
• Bradycardia: Symptomatic, but not life-threatening: Hold and evaluate other medications that may cause bradycardia. When asymptomatic or heart rate ≥60 bpm, resume with an adjusted dose, do not resume in those unable to tolerate 300 mg qday; life-threatening: discontinue product
• Lipase or amylase >2 times the upper limit of normal (ULN): Hold product and monitor serum lipase/amylase. When improved to <1.5 x ULN, resume with a 150-mg dose reduction. Do not resume in those unable to tolerate 300 mg qday
• Any grade interstitial lung disease (ILD) or pneumonitis: Permanently discontinue
• Severe or intolerable nausea, vomiting, or diarrhea despite appropriate medical therapy: Hold dose; when improved, resume with a 150-mg dose reduction. Do not resume in those unable to tolerate 300 mg qday
• Persistent hyperglycemia >250 mg/dL despite optimal antihyperglycemic therapy: Hold dose; when hyperglycemia is controlled, resume with a 150-mg dose reduction. Do not resume in those unable to tolerate 300 mg qday. If blood sugars cannot be controlled medically, discontinue
Dosage guidance in patients on strong CYP3A4 inducers/Inhibitors:
• Strong CYP3A4 inhibitors: Avoid concomitant use. If a strong CYP3A4 inhibitor is required, reduce the dose of ceritinib by approximately one-third, rounded to the nearest multiple of 150 mg; close monitoring of the QT interval is recommended. If the strong CYP3A4 inhibitor is discontinued, resume the previous dosage
• Strong CYP3A4 inducers: Avoid concomitant use
Take on an empty stomach. Do not give within 2 hr of a meal; swallow tablets whole; do not crush or dissolve; if a dose is missed, take as soon as remembered unless the next dose is due within 12 hr. Do not take 2 doses at the same time if missed; if vomiting occurs, do not give an additional dose. Take the next dose at the next scheduled time
Store at 77°F (25°C)

ADVERSE EFFECTS
CNS: Weakness, fatigue, paresthesias
CV: QT prolongation, torsade de pointes, bradycardia
EENT: Blurred vision
GI: *Nausea,* **hepatotoxicity,** vomiting, *anorexia,* **pancreatitis,** GERD, *abdominal pain,* diarrhea
INTEG: *Rash*

Adverse effects: *italics* = common; **bold** = life-threatening

META: Hyperglycemia, hyperphosphatemia, hyperamylasemia
MISC: Renal failure
RESP: Cough, dyspnea, pneumonitis

Pharmacokinetics

Absorption	Unknown
Distribution	Protein 97%
Metabolism	CYP3A4
Excretion	Unknown
Half-life	41 hr

Pharmacodynamics

Onset	Unknown
Peak	4-6 hr
Duration	Unknown

INTERACTIONS
Individual drugs
Acetaminophen: increased hepatotoxicity
Warfarin: increased plasma concentration of warfarin; avoid use with warfarin; use low molecular weight anticoagulants instead
Simvastatin: increased plasma concentrations of simvastatin

Drug classifications
CYP3A4 inhibitors (ketoconazole, itraconazole, erythromycin, clarithromycin): increased ceritinib concentrations
CYP3A4 inducers (dexamethasone, phenytoin, carBAMazepine, rifampin, PHENobarbital): decreased ceritinib concentrations

Drug/herb
Decreased: ceritinib concentration—St. John's wort

Drug/lab test
Increased: bilirubin, amylase, LFTs

NURSING CONSIDERATIONS
Assessment
• **Pregnancy: Assess for pregnancy before starting treatment, pregnancy category (D); effective contraception is needed during and for ≥ 2 wk after treatment**
• **QT prolongation: Assess for a history of cardiac arrhythmias, congestive heart failure, bradycardia, electrolyte imbalance, or congenital long QT syndrome. Correct electrolyte abnormalities before starting product**
• **Hyperglycemia:** Monitor for hyperglycemia, may be 6-8-fold in diabetic patients
• **Pancreatitis: Monitor for nausea, vomiting, severe abdominal pain**

Patient/family education
⚠ **Pregnancy (D): Teach patient to notify their provider immediately if pregnancy is** suspected; effective contraception is needed during and for ≥ 2wk after treatment; if product is used during pregnancy or if the patient becomes pregnant during use, the woman should be apprised of the potential hazard to the fetus
• Teach patient about reason for treatment, expected results
• Teach patient to report adverse reactions immediately: abdominal pain, nausea, vomiting, increased blood glucose in diabetics
• Advise patient to avoid OTC products unless approved by prescriber

Evaluation
Positive therapeutic outcome
• Decreased spread of tumor

daclatasvir
(dak-lat′-as-vir)
Daklinza
Func. class.: Antiviral, antihepatitis agent
Pregnancy category UK

ACTION: Active against chronic infections caused by genotype 3 hepatitis C virus (HCV); prevents viral RNA replication by impairing protein function

Therapeutic outcome: Decreased symptoms of chronic hepatitis C

USES: Chronic hepatitis C, genotype 3 with complicated liver disease

CONTRAINDICATIONS
Hypersensitivity

Precautions: Pregnancy (**UK**) breastfeeding, antimicrobial resistance, hepatic disease, hepatitis C with HIV coinfection, liver transplant

DOSAGE AND ROUTES
Adults: PO 60 mg qday with sofosbuvir 400 mg qday X 12 wk
Adults receiving strong CYP3A inhibitors: PO 30 mg qday with sofosbuvir 400 mg qday X 12 wk
Adults receiving moderate CYP3A inducers: PO 90 mg qday with sofosbuvir 400 mg qday X 12 wk

Available forms: Tabs 30, 60 mg

Implementation
• Give by mouth without regard to food
• Do not use as monotherapy, must be given with sofosbuvir

ADVERSE EFFECTS
CNS: Headache, fatigue
GI: Diarrhea, nausea

Pharmacokinetics

Absorption	Unknown
Distribution	99% protein binding
Metabolism	Liver, by CYP3A4, affected by P-glycoprotein (P-gp), organic anion transporting polypeptides (OATP1B1 and OATP1B3), breast cancer resistance protein (BCRP)
Excretion	Feces 88%
Half-life	Terminal half-life 12-15 hr

Pharmacodynamics

Onset	Unknown
Peak	2 hr
Duration	Unknown

INTERACTIONS
Drug classifications
Do not use with potent CYP3A4 inducers
P-glycoprotein(P-gp) substrates: increase of each product
Potent CYP3A4 inhibitors: Increased daclatasvir effect, reduce dose of daclatasvir
Moderate CYP3A4 inducers. Decreased daclatasvir effect, increase dose of daclatasvir

NURSING CONSIDERATIONS
Assessment
• **Liver transplant/cirrhosis:** May have lower sustained virologic response rates in cirrhosis and use in prior liver transplant is unknown
• **HIV/ hepatitis C coinfection:** All patients with HIV infection should be tested for hepatitis C, with continued annual screening advised for those persons considered high risk for acquiring hepatitis C. If hepatitis C and HIV coinfection is identified, consider treating both viral infections concurrently
• **Pregnancy/breastfeeding:** Unknown, give careful consideration for use in pregnancy and breastfeeding
• **Strong CYP3A4 inducers: Do not use concurrently, may lead to treatment failure, review patient's medication profile for potential drug interactions before starting treatment**
• **Hepatitis C:** Monitor plasma hepatitis C RNA and plasma HIV RNA baseline and during treatment

Patient/family education
• Teach patient that optimal duration of treatment is 12 wk; that product is not a cure; that transmission may still occur and must be taken with sofosbuvir
• Inform patient to avoid use with other medications, herbs, supplements unless approved by prescriber

• Teach patient not to stop abruptly unless directed; worsening of hepatitis may occur
• Advise patient to notify prescriber if pregnancy is planned or suspected or if breastfeeding

Evaluation
Positive therapeutic outcome
• Therapeutic response: decreased symptoms of chronic hepatitis C

⚠ HIGH ALERT
dulaglutide(Rx)
(doo-la-gloo'-tide)
Trulicity
Func. class.: Antidiabetic
Chem. class.: Incretin mimetic
Pregnancy category C

ACTION: Binds and activates known human glucagon-like peptide-1 (GLP-1) receptor agonist, mimics natural physiology for self-regulating glycemic control

Therapeutic outcome: Decreased polyuria, polydipsia, polyphagia; improved Hgb A1C

USES: Type 2 diabetes mellitus, once-weekly dosing

CONTRAINDICATIONS
Hypersensitivity

BLACK BOX WARNING: Medullary thyroid carcinoma, multiple endocrine neoplasia syndrome type 2 (men-2), thyroid cancer

Precautions: Pregnancy (C), breastfeeding, children, geriatric patients, severe renal/hepatic/GI disease, pancreatitis, vit D deficiency, burns, colitis, diarrhea, fever, GI bleeding/perforation/obstruction, ileus, infection, pseudomembranous colitis, thyroid disease, trauma, surgery, type 1 diabetes mellitus, tobacco smoking, vomiting

DOSAGE AND ROUTES
Adult: SUBCUT 0.75 mg qwk, may increase to 1.5 mg qwk

Available forms: Inj 0.75 mg/0.5 ml, 1.5 mg/0.5ml

Implementation
SUBCUT route
• Do not use as first-line therapy for those who have inadequate glycemic control on diet and exercise
• Administer the dose at any time of day, with or without meals

---

Adverse effects: *italics* = common; **bold** = life-threatening

- If a dose is missed, take as soon as remembered, take as soon as the next dose is due at least 3 days later, If it is more than 3 days after the missed dose, wait until the next regularly scheduled dose
- Give by **SUBCUT** only; do not give **IV** or **IM**; inject into the thigh, abdomen, or upper arm; rotate sites with each inj to prevent lipodystrophy
- Properly dispose of the pen or syringe
- Store in refrigerator for unopened pen; may store at room temperature after opening for up to 30 days, do not freeze
- When using concomitantly with insulin, give as separate injections. Never mix them together. The two injections may be injected in the same body region, but not adjacent to each other
- **Pre-filled pen administration:** Part of pen is glass; if dropped on a hard surface, do not use; uncap the pen after checking that it is locked; place base flat and firmly; unlock by turning the lock ring, press and hold green button, click will be heard; continue holding until another click is heard; inj is complete when the gray plunger is visible, remove the pen, dispose of used pen

ADVERSE EFFECTS

CNS: Fatigue
ENDO: Hypoglycemia
GI: Nausea, vomiting, diarrhea, anorexia, gastroesophageal reflux, pancreatitis, flatulence, abdominal pain, constipation
SYST: Secondary malignancy
INTEG: Injection-site reactions, rash, urticaria

Pharmacokinetics

Absorption	Unknown
Distribution	Unknown
Metabolism	Unknown
Excretion	Unknown
Half-life	5 days

Pharmacodynamics

Onset	Unknown
Peak	24-72 hr
Duration	Unknown

INTERACTIONS

Individual drugs

Alcohol, disopyramide: increased hypoglycemia
Dextrothyroxine, niacin, triamterene: decreased hypoglycemia efficacy

Drug classifications

ACE inhibitors, anabolic steroids, androgens, fibric acid derivatives, sulfonylureas: increased hypoglycemia

Corticosteroids, phenothiazines: increased hyperglycemia
Estrogens, MAOIs, oral contraceptives, progestins, thiazide diuretics: decreased hypoglycemia

NURSING CONSIDERATIONS

Assessment
- Monitor fasting blood glucose, A1C levels, postprandial glucose during treatment to determine diabetes control
- **Pancreatitis: severe abdominal pain, with/without vomiting; product should be discontinued**
- Assess for hypo/hyperglycemic reaction that can occur soon after meals; for severe hypoglycemia give **IV** D_5W, then **IV** dextrose solution
- Assess for nausea, diarrhea, vomiting, ability to tolerate product, may cause dehydration

Patient/family education
- Teach patient symptoms of hypo/hyperglycemia, what to do about each; to have glucagon emergency kit available; to carry a glucose source (candy, sugar cube) to treat hypoglycemia
- Advise patient that product must be continued on a weekly basis explain consequences of discontinuing product abruptly
- Teach patient that diabetes is a lifelong illness; product will not cure disease
- Advise patient to carry emergency ID
- Advise patient to continue weight control, dietary restrictions, exercise, hygiene
- Inform patient that regular blood glucose monitoring and A1C testing is needed
- Advise patient to notify prescriber if pregnant or intend to become pregnant
- **Pancreatitis: if severe abdominal pain with or without vomiting occurs, seek medical attention immediately**

Evaluation
Positive therapeutic outcome
- Decreased polyuria, polydipsia, polyphagia; improved Hgb A1C

---

evolocumab (Rx)

(e'-voe-lok'-ue-mab)
Repatha
Func. class.: Antilipemic
Pregnancy category unknown

ACTION: Binds to low-density lipoproteins, a human monoclonal antibody (IgG1)

USES: Heterozygous, familial hypercholesterolemia, atherosclerotic disease

---

CONTRAINDICATIONS
Hypersensitivity

Precautions: Pregnancy, breastfeeding, latex sensitivity

DOSAGE AND ROUTES
Heterozygous familial hypercholesterolemia or primary hyperlipidemia with established clinical atherosclerosis in patients who require additional lowering of LDL-C:

Adults: SUBCUT 140 mg q2wk or 420 mg qmo. If switching dosage regimens, administer the first dose of the new regimen on the next scheduled date of the previous regimen

Homozygous familial hypercholesterolemia in patients who require additional lowering of LDL-C:

Adults and adolescents: 420 mg qmo

Available forms: Auto injector 140 mg/ml, solutions for inj 140 mg/ml

Implementation
• Visually inspect for particulate matter and discoloration, solution is clear, colorless to pale yellow

SUBCUT route
• Prefilled syringe or SureClick autoinjector
• If stored in the refrigerator, warm to room temperature for ≥ 30 min before use. Do not shake
• Give into areas of the abdomen (except for a 2-in area around the umbilicus), thigh, or upper arm that are not tender, bruised, red, or indurated
• To use the 420-mg dose, give 3 injections consecutively within 30 min
• Rotate the site with each inj
• Do not administer with other injectable drugs at the same inj site

Prefilled syringe administration
• Do not pick up or pull the prefilled syringe by the plunger rod or gray needle cap. Hold the syringe by the barrel
• Pull the gray needle cap off. It is normal to see a drop of sol at the end of the needle. Do not remove any air bubbles in the syringe
• Pinch the skin inj site to create a firm surface approximately 2 in wide. Hold the pinch, and insert the needle into the skin using a 45- to 90-degree angle
• Push the plunger rod all the way down until the syringe is empty

• When done, release the plunger, and gently lift the syringe off skin

SureClick autoinjector administration
• Do not remove the orange cap until you are ready to inject
• Pull the orange cap off
• Stretch (thigh) or pinch (stomach or upper arm) the skin inj site to create a firm surface approximately 2 in wide. Hold the stretch or pinch, and place the autoinjector on the skin at 90 degrees
• Firmly push down onto the skin; when ready to inject, press the gray button. A click should be heard. Keep pushing on the skin and then lift the thumb. The inj could take about 15 sec. The window on the autoinjector will turn from clear to yellow when the inj is complete. A second click may be heard
• Remove the needle that will be automatically covered

ADVERSE EFFECTS
CNS: Memory impairment, confusion
GI: Diarrhea
MISC: Edema
MS: *Myalgia*
RESP: Pharyngitis, sinusitis, cough
SYST: Infection, antibody formation
INTEG: Pruritus, injection-site reaction, erythema, ecchymosis

Pharmacokinetics

Absorption	Unknown
Distribution	Unknown
Metabolism	Unknown
Excretion	Unknown
Half-life	At steady state 17-20 days

Pharmacodynamics

Onset	Unknown
Peak	3-7 days

INTERACTIONS
Drug/lab test
Increased: LFTs

NURSING CONSIDERATIONS
Assessment
• **Hypercholesterolemia:** obtain diet history; monitor fat content, lipid levels (triglycerides, LDL, HDL, total cholesterol), LFTs baseline and periodically during treatment

Patient/family education
• Teach patient that compliance is needed
• Advise that risk factors should be decreased: high-fat diet, smoking, alcohol consumption, absence of exercise

- Advise patient to notify prescriber if pregnancy suspected, planned, or if breastfeeding
- Teach patient to report confusion, injection-site reactions

Evaluation
- Positive therapeutic response: Decreased cholesterol, LDL; increased HDL

---

isavuconazonium (Rx)
(eye′ sa-vue-koe′ na-zoe′ nee-um)
Cresemba
Func. class.: Antifungal, systemic
Chem. class.: Triazole derivative
Pregnancy category C

ACTION: Exerts antifungal activity by inhibiting the synthesis of ergosterol, an essential component of the fungal cell membrane. The depletion of ergosterol within the fungal cell membrane results in increased cellular permeability causing leakage of cellular content

Therapeutic outcome: Decreasing signs, symptoms of infection

USES: *Aspergillus flavus, Aspergillus fumigatus, Aspergillus niger, Rhizopus oryzae,* Rucormycetes species; do NOT use for infections of *Candida, Blastomyces, Histoplasma* V

CONTRAINDICATIONS
Hypersensitivity, short QT syndrome

Precautions: Azole hypersensitivity, pregnancy **C**, breastfeeding, infusion-related reactions, hepatic disease

DOSAGE AND ROUTES
Invasive aspergillosis and invasive mucormycosis
Adults: **PO** loading dose of 2 caps (372 mg) q8hr X 6 doses. Then, 2 caps (372 mg) qday. Start maintenance dosing 12-24 hr after the last loading dose; **IV** loading dose of 372 mg q8hr X 6 doses, then 372 mg day; then 12-24 hr after the last loading dose give over 1 hr, use a 0.2- to 1.2-micron in-line filter and be administered over a minimum of 1 hr, an additional loading dose is not needed when switching to PO

Available forms: Caps 186 mg; powder for inj 382 mg

Implementation
PO route
- Swallow whole, do not chew, crush, dissolve, open the capsules; may be used without regard to food

IV route
- Visually inspect for particulate matter and discoloration. The diluted solution may contain translucent to white particulates which will be removed by the in-line filter

Reconstitution
- Reconstitute the dry powder with 5 mL sterile water for inj, gently shake until dissolved
- Storage: The reconstituted solution may be stored below 25 degrees C (77 degrees F) for a maximum of 1 hr before further dilution

Dilution
- Remove 5 mL of the reconstituted solution and add it to 250 mL of either 0.9% NaCI or D_5W (1.5 mg /mL)
- Gently mix the solution or roll the bag. DO NOT shake. Do not place in a pneumatic transport system
- Apply an in-line filter (0.2-1.2 micron), adhere an in-line filter reminder sticker to the infusion bag
- Give over ≤ 6 hr of dilution
- Storage: May be stored immediately after dilution at 2 to 8 degrees C (36 to 46 degrees F); administration MUST be completed within 24 hr of the time of dilution. Do NOT freeze
- Use product only after C&S confirms organism, product needed to treat condition; make sure product used in life-threatening infections
- Flush IV lines with 0.9% sodium chloride or 5% dextrose in water before and after administration of the infusion
- Must be administered through a 0.2-1.2 micron filter; give over ≥ 1 hr. Do not give by bolus. *Do not admix*

ADVERSE EFFECTS
CNS: *Headache,* paresthesias, peripheral neuropathy, *hallucinations,* depression, insomnia, dizziness, fever, vertigo, tremor, confusion
CV: tachypnea, supraventricular tachycardia, atrial fibrillation/flutter
EENT: Tinnitus
GI: *Nausea, vomiting, anorexia, diarrhea,* cramps, hepatitis, stomatitis
GU: *Hypokalemia,* renal failure
HEMA: Anemia, eosinophilia, hypomagnesemia, thrombocytopenia, leukopenia
INTEG: *Burning, irritation,* pain, necrosis at injection site with extravasation, rash
MISC: Cough

Pharmacokinetics

Absorption	Unknown
Distribution	Chinese patients (levels 40% lower), protein binding >99%
Metabolism	By CYP3A4, CYP3A5, UGT, P-gp, OCT2 enzymes
Excretion	Eliminated in urine/feces
Half-life	Unknown

Pharmacodynamics

Onset	Unknown
Peak	2 hrs (**PO**)
Duration	Unknown

INTERACTIONS
Individual drugs
CycloSPORINE, pimozide, quiNIDine, predniso-LONE, sirolimus, tacrolimus, warfarin, rifabutin, phenytoin: increased effects of each

Drug classifications
Benzodiazepines, calcium channel blockers, ergots, HMG-CoA reductase inhibitors, sulfonylureas, vinca alkaloids, proton pump inhibitors, NNRTIs, protease inhibitors: increased effects of each
CYP3A4 substrates: increased effect of these
CYP3A4 inhibitors: decreased effect of these

Drug/herb
• Do not use with St. John's wort

Drug/lab test
Increased: AST/ALT, alk phos, creatinine, bilirubin
Decreased: Hgb/Hct, platelets, WBC

NURSING CONSIDERATIONS
Assessment
• **Pregnancy: Test for pregnancy before starting treatment, pregnancy C, do not breastfeed**
• **Short QT syndrome: Do not use in this condition**
• Monitor VS q15-30min during first infusion; note changes in pulse, B/P
• Blood studies: Obtain CBC, potassium, sodium, calcium, magnesium, q2wk
• **Hepatotoxicity: Identify increasing AST, ALT, alk phos, bilirubin, baseline and periodically**
• **Allergic reaction:** Assess for dermatitis, rash; product should be discontinued, antihistamines (mild reaction) or epinephrine (severe reaction) administered
• **Hypokalemia:** Assess for anorexia, drowsiness, weakness, decreased reflexes, dizziness, increased urinary output, increased thirst, paresthesias
• **Ototoxicity:** Assess for tinnitus (ringing, roaring in ears), vertigo

Patient/family education
• Teach patient that long-term therapy may be needed to clear infection (2 wk-3 mo, depending on type of infection)
• Advise patient to notify prescriber of bleeding, bruising, soft-tissue swelling, dark urine, persistent nausea or diarrhea, headache, rash, yellow skin/eyes
• **Women of childbearing age should use effective contraceptive, pregnancy (C)**

Evaluation
• Therapeutic response: Resolution of fungal infection, negative C&S

RARELY USED

miltefosine
(mil′-te-foe′-seen)
Impavido
Func. class.: antiprotozoal/antileishmanial

USES: Treatment of visceral leishmaniasis caused by *L. donovani;* mucosal leishmaniasis caused by *L. braziliensis;* and cutaneous leishmaniasis caused by *L. braziliensis, L. guyanensis,* and *L. panamensis*

CONTRAINDICATIONS
Hypersensitivity, pregnancy (**D**)

DOSAGE AND ROUTES
Adult/adolescent/child ≥ 12 yr and ≥45 kg: PO 50 mg tid X 28 days
Adult/adolescent/child ≥ 12 yr and 30 to 44 kg: PO 50 mg bid X 28 days; HIV guidelines suggest 100 mg qday X 4 wk in adults and adolescents regardless of weight

secukinumab (Rx)
(sek′-ue-kin′-ue-mab)
Cosentyx
Func. class.: Immune response modifier
Pregnancy category B

ACTION: Interleukin (IL)-12, IL-23 antagonist

Therapeutic outcome: Decreasing plaque psoriasis

USES: Plaque psoriasis

CONTRAINDICATIONS
Hypersensitivity, active TB

Precautions: Pregnancy (**B**), breastfeeding, latex hypersensitivity, Crohn's disease, vaccination, infection

DOSAGE AND ROUTES
Adult: **SUBCUT** 300 mg at wk 0, 1, 2, 3, 4, and then q4wk thereafter

Adverse effects: *italics* = common; **bold** = life-threatening

Available forms: Sol for inj 150 mg/ml (pen, prefilled syringe) 2 packs, singles

Implementation
• Use by **SUBCUT** inj only
• Those with latex hypersensitivity should not handle cap of inj

SUBCUT Inj
• Patients may use the prefilled syringe or Sensoready pen after proper training; the lyophilized powder is for health care provider use only
• Each 300-mg dose is used as 2 **SUBCUT** inj of 150 mg
• Do not administer where skin is tender, bruised, erythematous, indurated, or affected by psoriasis.

Reconstitution of lyophilized powder:
• Allow to warm to room temperature for 15-30 min, use 1 ml sterile water for inj to reconstitute, rotate, do not shake or invert vial, allow to stand for 10 min, again rotate vial, allow to stand for another 5 min (150 mg/ml)
• Storage: Use immediately or refrigerate for up to 24 hr. Do not freeze. If refrigerated, allow reconstituted solution to reach room temperature (15-30 min) before administration

Preparation for use of prefilled syringe or Sensoready pen:
• Remove prefilled syringe or Sensoready pen from refrigerator and allow 15-30 min to reach room temperature
• Storage: The prefilled syringe or Sensoready pen should be used within 1 hr

ADVERSE EFFECTS
EENT: Ocular infections, sinusitis, oral ulceration, rhinitis, sinusitis
GI: Diarrhea
INTEG: Urticaria
SYST: Serious infections, anaphylaxis, antibody formation, candidiasis

Pharmacokinetics

Absorption	Unknown
Distribution	Interstitial fluid in lesional and non-lesional skin
Metabolism	Unknown
Excretion	Unknown
Half-life	22-31 days

Pharmacodynamics

Onset	Unknown
Peak	6 days
Duration	Unknown

INTERACTIONS
Drug classifications
Immunosupressives: avoid use with immunosuppressives

Vaccines: do not give concurrently with vaccines; immunizations should be brought up to date before treatment

Drug/lab test
Increased: LFTs

NURSING CONSIDERATIONS
ASSESSMENT
• **TB:** TB testing should be done before starting treatment
• Bring immunizations up to date before starting treatment
• **Infection: monitor for fever, sore throat, cough; do not use during active infections**
• **Malignancy: Skin cancer may occur especially in older patients who have used ultraviolet treatments with immunosuppressants**
• Assess for inj site pain, swelling

Patient/family education
• Advise patient that product must be continued for prescribed time to be effective, to use as prescribed
• Teach patient not to receive live vaccinations during treatment
• Teach patient to notify prescriber of possible infection (upper respiratory or other) or allergic reactions
• How to use pen and inj techniques and proper disposable

Evaluation
• Decreasing plaque psoriasis

⚠ HIGH ALERT

RARELY USED

sonidegib
(soe′-ni-deg′-ib)
Odomzo
Func. class.: Antineoplastic

Uses: Locally advanced basal cell carcinoma that has recurred following surgery or radiation therapy or in those who are not candidates for surgery or radiation therapy

CONTRAINDICATIONS
Hypersensitivity

Precautions:

> **BLACK BOX WARNING:** Pregnancy, intrauterine fetal death, contraceptive requirement

DOSAGE AND ROUTES
Adults: **PO** 200 mg qday until disease progression or unacceptable toxicity; take on an empty stomach $\geq$ 1 hr before or 2 hr after a meal. Avoid use with strong CYP3A inhibitors or strong and moderate CYP3A inducers.

Available forms: Cap 200 mg

Appendix B

Ophthalmic, Nasal, Topical, and Otic Products

OPHTHALMIC PRODUCTS

ANESTHETICS
lidocaine (Rx)
(lye'doe-kane)
Akten
proparacaine (Rx)
(proe-par'a-kane)
Alcaine, Diocaine ✚, Parcaine
tetracaine (Rx)
(tet'ra-kane)
Minims Tetracaine ✚, Tetracaine, TetraVisc

ANTIHISTAMINES
alcaftadine
(al-caf'tah-deen)
Lastacaft
azelastine (Rx)
(ay-zell'ah-steen)
emedastine (Rx)
(ee-med'a-steen)
Emadine
epinastine (Rx)
(ep-een-as'teen)
Elestat
ketotifen (Rx, OTC)
(kee-toh-tif'en)
Alaway, Claritin Eye, Zaditor, ZyrTEC Itchy Eye
levocabastine (Rx)
(lee-voh-cab'ah-steen)
Livostin
olopatadine (Rx)
(oh-loh-pat'ah-deen)
Pataday, Patanase, Pazeo

ANTIINFECTIVES
azithromycin (Rx)
(ay-zi-thro-my'sin)
AzaSite

besifloxacin (Rx)
(be'si-flox'a-sin)
Besivance
ciprofloxacin (Rx)
(sip-ro-floks'a-sin)
Ciloxan
erythromycin (Rx)
(er-ith-roe-mye'sin)
Ilotycin, Romycin
ganciclovir (Rx)
(gan-sye'kloe-vir)
Zirgan
gatifloxacin (Rx)
(gat-ih-floks'ah-sin)
Zymaxid
gentamicin (Rx)
(jen-ta-mye'sin)
Garamycin Ophthalmic, Gentak, Gentasol
levofloxacin (Rx)
(lee-voh-flock'sah-sin)
moxifloxacin (Rx)
(mox-i-flox'a-sin)
Moxeza, Vigamox
natamycin (Rx)
(nat-a-mye'sin)
Natacyn
ofloxacin (Rx)
(oh-floks'a-sin)
Ocuflox
silver nitrate 1% (Rx)
silver nitrate
sulfacetamide sodium (Rx)
(sul-fa-seet'a-mide)
Bleph-10
tobramycin (Rx)
(toe-bra-mye'sin)
Tobrasol, Tobrex
trifluridine (Rx)
(trye-floor'i-deen)
Viroptic

✚ Canada only

Adverse effects: *italics* = common; **bold** = life-threatening

β-ADRENERGIC BLOCKERS
betaxolol (Rx)
(beh-tax'oh-lole)
Betoptic
carteolol (Rx)
(kar-tee'oh-lole)
levobetaxolol (Rx)
(lee-voh-beh-tax'oh-lohl)
Betaxon
levobunolol (Rx)
(lee-voe-byoo'no-lole)
Betagen
metipranolol (Rx)
(met-ee-pran'oh-lole)
OptiPranolol
timolol (Rx)
(tym'moe-lole)
Betimol

CARBONIC ANHYDRASE INHIBITORS
brinzolamide (Rx)
(brin-zoh'la-mide)
Azopt
dorzolamide (Rx)
(dor-zol'a-mide)
Trusopt

CHOLINERGICS
(Direct-acting)
acetylcholine (Rx)
(ah-see-til-koe'leen)
Miochol-E
carbachol (Rx)
(kar'ba-kole)
Isopto Carbachol
pilocarpine (Rx)
(pye-loe-kar'peen)
Isopto Carpine

CHOLINESTERASE INHIBITORS
physostigmine (Rx)
(fi-zoe-stig'meen)

CORTICOSTEROIDS
dexamethasone (Rx)
(dex-a-meth'a-sone)
Maxidex
fluorometholone (Rx)
(flure-oh-meth'oh-lone)
Flarex, FML, FML Forte, FML S.O.P.

loteprednol (Rx)
(loe-tee-pred-nole)
Alrex, Lotemax
prednisoLONE (Rx)
(pred-niss'oh-lone)
Econopred Plus, Omnipred, Pred-Forte, Pred Mild
rimexolone (Rx)
(ri-mex'a-lone)
Vexol

MYDRIATICS
atropine (Rx)
(a'troe-peen)
cyclopentolate (Rx)
(sye-kloe-pen'toe-late)
Cyclogyl, Cylate
homatropine (Rx)
(home-a'troe-peen)
Isopto Homatropine
phenylephrine (OTC)
(fen-ill-ef'rin)
Neofrin

NONSTEROIDAL
ANTIINFLAMMATORIES
bromfenac (Rx)
(brome'fen-ak)
Prolensa
diclofenac (Rx)
(dye-kloe'fen-ak)
flurbiprofen (Rx)
(flure-bi'pro-fen)
Ocufen
ketorolac (Rx)
(kee-toe'role-ak)
Acular, Acuvail
nepafenac (Rx)
(ne-pa-fen'ak)
Ilevro, Nevanac

SYMPATHOMIMETICS
apraclonidine (Rx)
(a-pra-klon'i-deen)
Iopidine
brimonidine (Rx)
(brem-on'i-dine)
Alphagan P

OPHTHALMIC DECONGESTANTS/ VASOCONSTRICTORS

Iodoxamide
(loe-dox'ah-mide)
Alomide
naphazoline (Rx, OTC)
(naf-az'oh-leen)
AK-Con, All Clear AR Maximum Strength Ophthalmic Solution, All Clear Eye Drops, CVS Maximum Redness Relief Eye Drops, CVS Redness Relief Lubricant Eye Drops
oxymetazoline (Rx)
(ox-i-met-ah-zoh'leen)
Visine L.R.
tetrahydrozoline (OTC)
(tet-ra-hye-dro'zoe-leen)
Visine Original

MISCELLANEOUS OPHTHALMICS

bimatoprost (Rx)
(bih-mat'o-prost)
Latisse, Lumigan
latanoprost (Rx)
(la-tan'oh-prost)
Xalatan
travoprost (Rx)
(tra'voe-prost)
Travatan
unoprostone (Rx)
(yoo-noe-pros'tone)
Rescula

β-ADRENERGIC BLOCKERS

ACTION: Reduces production of aqueous humor by unknown mechanism

USES: Ocular hypertension, chronic open angle glaucoma

ANESTHETICS

ACTION: Decreases ion permeability by stabilizing neuronal membrane

USES: Cataract extraction, tonometry, gonioscopy, removal of foreign objects, corneal suture removal, glaucoma surgery (ophthalmic); pruritus, sunburn, toothache, sore throat, cold sores, oral pain, rectal pain and irritation, control of gagging (topical)

ANTIINFECTIVES

ACTION: Inhibits folic acid synthesis by preventing PABA use, which is necessary for bacterial growth

USES: Conjunctivitis, superficial eye infections, corneal ulcers, prophylaxis against infection after removal of foreign matter from the eye

ANTIINFLAMMATORIES

ACTION: Decreases inflammation, resulting in decreased pain, photophobia, hyperemia, cellular infiltration

USES: Inflammation of eye, eyelids, conjunctiva, cornea; uveitis, iridocyclitis, allergic conditions, burns, foreign bodies, postoperatively in cataract

CARBONIC ANHYDRASE INHIBITOR

ACTION: Converted to EPINEPHrine, which decreases aqueous production and increases outflow

USES: Open angle glaucoma, ocular hypertension

DIRECT-ACTING MIOTIC

ACTION: Acts directly on cholinergic receptor sites; induces miosis, spasm of accommodation, fall in intraocular pressure, caused by stimulation of ciliary, pupillary sphincter muscles, which leads to pulling away of iris from filtration angle, resulting in increased outflow of aqueous humor

USES: Primary glaucoma, early stages of wide angle glaucoma (less useful in advanced stages), chronic open angle glaucoma, acute closed angle glaucoma before emergency surgery; also neutralizes mydriatics used during eye exam; may be used alternately with mydriatics to break adhesions between iris and lens

CONTRAINDICATIONS
Hypersensitivity

Precautions: Pregnancy, breastfeeding, children, aphakia, hypersensitivity to carbonic anhydrase inhibitors, sulfonamides, thiazide diuretics, ocular inhibitors, renal/hepatic insufficiency

Implementation
• Storage at room temperature away from light

ADVERSE EFFECTS
CNS: Headache
CV: Hypertension, tachycardia, dysrhythmias
EENT: Burning, stinging
GI: Bitter taste

NURSING CONSIDERATIONS
Assessment
• Monitor ophthalmic exams and intraocular pressure readings
• Monitor blood counts; renal/hepatic function tests and serum electrolytes during long-term treatment

Patient/family education
• Teach how to instill drops
• Advise patient that product may cause burning, itching, blurring, dryness of eye area

Evaluation

Positive therapeutic outcome
• Absence of increased intraocular pressure

NASAL AGENTS

NASAL ANTIHISTAMINES
olopatadine (Rx)
(oh-low-pat′uh-deen)
Patanase

NASAL DECONGESTANTS
azelastine (Rx)
(ay-zell′ah-steen)
Astepro
EPINEPHrine (OTC)
(ep-i-neff′rin)
Adrenalin Nasal Solution
oxymetazoline (OTC)
(ox-i-met-az′oh-leen)
Afrin No Drip, Dristan 12-HR Nasal Spray, Mucinex Moisture, Mucinex Sinus-Max, Vicks Sinex, Vicks QlearQuil
phenylephrine (OTC)
(fen-ill-eff′rin)
4-Way Nasal Spray, Neo-Synephrine
tetrahydrozoline (OTC)
(tet-ra-hye-dro′zoe-leen)
Tyzine, Tyzine Pediatric

NASAL STEROIDS
beclomethasone (Rx)
(be-kloe-meth′a-sone)
Beconase AQ Nasal, Qnasl
budesonide (Rx)
(byoo-des′oh-nide)
Rhinocort Aqua
flunisolide (Rx)
(floo-niss′oh-lide)
fluticasone (Rx)
(floo-tic′a-son)
Veramyst
triamcinolone (Rx)
(trye-am-sin′oh-lone)
Allergy 24 HR Nasal Spray, Nasacort

NONSTEROIDAL ANTIINFLAMMATORY
ketorolac (Rx)
(kee′toe-role-ak)
Sprix

ACTION: Produces vasoconstriction (rapid, long acting) of arterioles, thereby decreasing fluid exudation, mucosal engorgement by stimulation of α-adrenergic receptors in vascular smooth muscle

Therapeutic outcome: Absence of nasal congestion

USES: Nasal congestion

CONTRAINDICATIONS
Hypersensitivity to sympathomimetic amines

Precautions: Pregnancy **C,** children <6 yr, geriatric, diabetes, CV disease, hypertension, hyperthyroidism, increased ICP, prostatic hypertrophy, glaucoma

DOSAGE AND ROUTES
Implementation
• Have patient tilt head back, squeeze bulb to create a vacuum, and draw correct amount of sol into dropper; insert 2 gtt of sol into nostril; repeat in other nostril
• Store in light-resistant container; do not expose to high temperature or let sol come into contact with aluminum
• Give for <4 consecutive days
• Provide environmental humidification to decrease nasal congestion, dryness

ADVERSE EFFECTS
CNS: Anxiety, restlessness, tremors, weakness, insomnia, dizziness, fever, headache
EENT: Irritation, burning, sneezing, stinging, dryness, rebound congestion
GI: Nausea, vomiting, anorexia
INTEG: Contact dermatitis

NURSING CONSIDERATIONS
Assessment
• Assess for redness, swelling, pain in nasal passages before, during treatment

---

- Assess for systemic absorption; hypertension, tachycardia; notify prescriber; systemic absorption occurs at high doses or after prolonged use

Patient/family education
- Advise patient that stinging may occur for several applications; drying of mucosa may be decreased by environmental humidification
- Caution patient to notify prescriber if irregular pulse, insomnia, dizziness, or tremors occur
- Teach patient proper administration to avoid systemic absorption
- Advise patient to rinse dropper with very hot water to prevent contamination

Evaluation
Positive therapeutic outcome
- Decreased nasal congestion

TOPICAL GLUCOCORTICOIDS

betamethasone (Rx)
(bay-ta-meth'a-sone)
Beben ♣, Betacort ♣, Betanate, Betnovate ♣, Celestoderm ♣, Del-Beta, Ectosone ♣, Metaderm ♣
betamethasone (augmented) (Rx)
(bay-ta-meth'a-sone)
Diprolene AF
clobetasol (Rx)
(kloe-bay'ta-sol)
Clobex, Cormax, Dermovate ♣, Olux Topical Foam, Temovate
desonide (Rx)
(dess'oh-nide)
Desonate, DesOwen, LoKara, Verdeso Foam
desoximetasone (Rx)
(dess-ox-i-met'a-sone)
Topicort
fluocinolone (Rx)
(floo-oh-sin'oh-lone)
Derma-Smoothe/FS oil, Lidemol ♣, Lyderm ♣, Synalar, Topsyn ♣
flurandrenolide (Rx)
(flure-an-dren'oh-lide)
Cordran, Denison 1/4 ♣, Denison Tape ♣
fluticasone (Rx)
(floo-tik'a-sone)
Cutivate

halcinonide (Rx)
(hal-sin'oh-nide)
Halog
hydrocortisone (Rx)
(hye-droe-kor'ti-sone)
Barriere-HC ♣, CaldeCORT Cortacet ♣, Cortalo, Cortate ♣, Cortef ♣, Corticreme ♣, Cortifoam, Cortoderm ♣, Hyderm ♣, Instacort, Neosporin Eczema Anti-Itch, Novo Hydrocort ♣, Nutracort , Nuzon, Sarna HC ♣, Unicort ♣
triamcinolone (Rx)
(trye-am-sin'oh-lone)
Dermasorb TA, Kenalog, Pediaderm TA, Trianide ♣, Triderm

ACTION: Antipruritic, antiinflammatory

Therapeutic outcome: Decreased itching, inflammation

USES: Psoriasis, eczema, contact dermatitis, pruritus; usually reserved for severe dermatoses that have not responded to less potent formulation

CONTRAINDICATIONS
Hypersensitivity, viral infections, fungal infections

Precautions: Pregnancy C

DOSAGE AND ROUTES
Adult and child: Apply to affected area

Implementation
- Apply only to affected areas; do not get in eyes
- Apply and leave site uncovered or lightly covered; occlusive dressing is not recommended—systemic absorption may occur
- Use only on dermatoses; do not use on weeping, denuded, or infected area
- Cleanse area before application of product
- Continue treatment for a few days after area has cleared
- Store at room temperature

ADVERSE EFFECTS
INTEG: *Acne, atrophy, epidermal thinning, purpura, striae*

NURSING CONSIDERATIONS
Assessment
- Monitor temp; if fever develops, product should be discontinued
- Monitor for systemic absorption, increased temp, inflammation, irritation

---

Patient/family education
- Teach patient to avoid sunlight on affected area; burns may occur
- Teach patient to limit treatment to 14 days

Evaluation
Positive therapeutic outcome
- Absence of severe itching, patches on skin, flaking

TOPICAL ANTIFUNGALS

clotrimazole (OTC)
(kloe-trye'ma-zole)
Canesten ✦, Clotrimaderm ✦, Cruex, Crux, Desenex, Lotrimin AF, Myclo ✦, Neo-Zol ✦

econazole (OTC)
(ee-kon'a-zole)
Ecoza

efinaconazole
(ef'in-a-kon'a-zole)
Jublia

ketoconazole (OTC)
(kee-toe-kon'a-zole)
Extina, Ketodan, Kuric, Xolegel

luliconazole
(loo'li-kon'a-zole)
Luzu

miconazole (OTC)
(mye-kon'a-zole)
Antifungal, Azolen, Baza, Cruex, Lotrimin AF, Micaderm, Novana, Triple Paste AF, Zeasorb-AF

nystatin (OTC)
(nye-stat'in)
Nodostine ✦, Nyamyc, Nyaderm ✦, Nystop, Pediaderm AF

selenium (OTC)
(see-leen'ee-um)

tavaborole
(ta'va-bor'ole)
Kerydin

terbinafine (OTC)
(ter-bin'a-feen)
LamISIL

tolnaftate (OTC)
(tole-naf'tate)
Absorbine Athlete's Foot Cream, Lamasil AF Topical Spray, Ting

undecylenic acid (OTC)
(un-deh-sih-len'ik)

ACTION: Interferes with fungal cell membrane permeability

Therapeutic outcome: Absence of itching and white patches of the skin

USES: Tinea cruris, tinea pedis, diaper rash, minor skin irritations; amphotericin B is used for *Candida* infections

CONTRAINDICATIONS
Hypersensitivity

Precautions: Pregnancy **B**, breastfeeding, children

DOSAGE AND ROUTES
Massage into affected area, surrounding area daily or bid, continue for 7-14 days, max 4 wk

Implementation
- Apply to affected area, surrounding area; do not cover with occlusive dressings
- Store below 30° C (86° F)

ADVERSE EFFECTS
INTEG: Burning, stinging, dryness, itching, local irritation

NURSING CONSIDERATIONS
Assessment
- Assess skin for fungal infections: peeling, dryness, itching before, throughout treatment
- Assess for continuing infection; increased size, number of lesions

Patient/family education
- Instruct to apply with glove to prevent further infection; not to cover with occlusive dressings
- Teach patient that long-term therapy may be needed to clear infection (2 wk-6 mo depending on organism); compliance is needed even after feeling better
- Teach patient proper hygiene: hand-washing technique, nail care, use of concomitant top agents if prescribed
- Caution patient to avoid use of OTC creams, ointments, lotions unless directed by prescriber
- Instruct patient to use medical asepsis (hand washing) before, after each application; to change socks and shoes once a day during treatment of tinea pedis
- Advise patient to report to health care prescriber if infection persists or recurs; if blisters, burning, oozing, swelling occur
- Caution patient to avoid alcohol because nausea, vomiting, hypertension may occur
- Caution patient to use sunscreen or avoid direct sunlight to prevent photosensitivity
- Advise patient to notify prescriber of sore throat, fever, skin rash, which may indicate overgrowth of organisms

---

Evaluation

Positive therapeutic outcome
- Decrease in size, number of lesions

TOPICAL ANTIINFECTIVES

azelaic acid (Rx)
(a-zuh-lay'ic)
Azelex, Finacea
bacitracin (OTC)
(bass-i-tray'sin)
Bacitin ✙
clindamycin (Rx)
(klin-da-my'sin)
Cleocin T, Clindacin ETZ, Clindacin PAC, Evocin
erythromycin (Rx, OTC)
(er-ith-roe-mye'sin)
Emgel, Emcin Clear, Ery, Erygel
gentamicin (Rx)
(jen-ta-mye'sin)
mafenide (Rx)
(ma'fe-nide)
Sulfamylon
metroNIDAZOLE (Rx)
(met-roh-nye'da-zole)
MetroGel, MetroCream, Noritate, Rosadan
mupirocin (Rx)
(myoo-peer'oh-sin)
Bactroban, Centany
retapamulin (Rx)
(re-tap'a-mue'lin)
Altabax
salicylic acid (Rx)
(sal'i-sil'ik)
Bensal HP, Demarest, Keralyt, Salacyn, Salvax, UltraSal-ER
silver sulfADIAZINE (Rx)
(sul-fa-dye'a-zeen)
Flamazine ✙**, Silvadene, SSD, Thermazene**
tretinoin (Rx)
(treh'tih-noyn)
Atralin, Avita, Refissa, Retin-A, Rrnova, Tretin-X

ACTION: Interferes with bacterial protein synthesis

Therapeutic outcome: Resolution of infection

USES: Skin infections, minor burns, wounds, skin grafts, primary pyodermas, otitis externa

CONTRAINDICATIONS
Hypersensitivity, large areas, burns, ulcerations

Precautions: Pregnancy **C**, breastfeeding, impaired renal function, external ear or perforated eardrum

Implementation
- Apply enough medication to cover lesions completely
- Apply after cleansing with soap, water before each application; dry well
- Apply to less than 20% of body surface area when patient has impaired renal function
- Store at room temperature in dry place

ADVERSE EFFECTS
INTEG: Rash, urticaria, scaling, redness

NURSING CONSIDERATIONS
Assessment
- Assess for allergic reaction: burning, stinging, swelling, redness
- Assess for signs of nephrotoxicity or ototoxicity

Evaluation

Positive therapeutic outcome
- Decrease in size, number of lesions

TOPICAL ANTIVIRALS

acyclovir (Rx)
(ay-sye'kloe-ver)
Zovirax Topical
penciclovir (Rx)
(pen-sye'kloe-ver)
Denavir

ACTION: Interferes with viral DNA replication

Therapeutic outcome: Resolution of infection

USES: Simple mucocutaneous herpes simplex, in immunocompromised clients with initial herpes genitalis

CONTRAINDICATIONS
Hypersensitivity

Precautions: Pregnancy **C**, breastfeeding

Implementation
- Apply with finger cot or rubber glove to prevent further infection

• Apply enough medication to cover lesions completely
• Apply after cleansing with soap, water before each application; dry well
• Store at room temperature in dry place

ADVERSE EFFECTS
INTEG: Rash, urticaria, stinging, burning, pruritus, vulvitis

NURSING CONSIDERATIONS
Assessment
• Assess for allergic reaction: burning, stinging, swelling, redness, rash, vulvitis, pruritus
• Assess for signs of nephrotoxicity or ototoxicity

Patient/family education
• Teach patient not to use in eyes or when there is no evidence of infection
• Advise patient to apply with glove to prevent further infection
• Advise patient to avoid use of OTC creams, ointments, lotions unless directed by prescriber
• Advise patient to use medical asepsis (hand washing) before, after each application and avoid contact with eyes
• Advise patient to adhere strictly to prescribed regimen to maximize successful treatment outcome
• Advise patient to begin using product when symptoms arise

Evaluation

Positive therapeutic outcome
• Decrease in size, number of lesions

TOPICAL ANESTHETICS

benzocaine (OTC)
(ben′zoe-kane)
Americaine Anesthetic, Anbesol Maximum Strength, Boil-Ease, Orajel
dibucaine (OTC)
(dye′byoo-kane)
Nupercainal
lidocaine (Rx, OTC)
(lye′doe-kane)
EnovaRx, Glydo, Lidomar, LidoRx, LTA, Solarcaine, Zilactin-L
pramoxine (OTC)
(pra-mox′een)
Prax, Proctofoam
tetracaine (OTC, Rx)
(tet′ra-cane)
Pontocaine, Viractin

ACTION: Inhibits conduction of nerve impulses from sensory nerves

Therapeutic outcome: Decreasing inflammation, itching, pain

USES: Oral irritation, sore throat, toothache, cold sore, canker sore, sunburn, minor cuts, insect bites, pain, itching

CONTRAINDICATIONS
Hypersensitivity, infants <1 yr, application to large areas

Precautions: Pregnancy **C**, children <6 yr, sepsis, denuded skin

DOSAGE AND ROUTES
Adult and child: TOP apply qid as needed; RECT insert tid and after each BM

Implementation
• Store in tight, light-resistant container; do not freeze, puncture, or incinerate aerosol container

ADVERSE EFFECTS
INTEG: Rash, irritation, sensitization

NURSING CONSIDERATIONS
Assessment
• Assess pain: location, duration, characteristics before, after administration
• Assess for infection: redness, drainage, inflammation; this product should not be used until infection is treated

Patient/family education
• Teach patient to avoid contact with eyes
• Teach patient not to use for prolonged periods: use for <1 wk; if condition remains, prescriber should be contacted

Evaluation

Positive therapeutic outcome
• Decreased redness, swelling, pain

TOPICAL MISCELLANEOUS

docosanol (OTC)
(doh-koh′sah-nohl)
Abreva
pimecrolimus (Rx)
(pim-eh-kroh-ly′mus)
Elidel

ACTION: Docosanol unknown; pimecrolimus may bind with macrophilin and inhibit calcium-dependent phosphatase

Therapeutic outcome: Decreased redness, swelling, pain

USES: Docosanol applied to fever blisters to promote more rapid healing; pimecrolimus used to treat mild to moderate atopic dermatitis in nonimmunocompromised patients ≥2 yr who are unresponsive to other treatment

CONTRAINDICATIONS
Hypersensitivity

Precautions: Pregnancy **C,** breastfeeding, dermal infections

DOSAGE AND ROUTES
Docosanol
Adult: TOP rub into blisters 5 ×/day until healing occurs

Pimecrolimus
Adult and child ≥2 yr: TOP apply thin layer 2 ×/day and rub in; use as long as needed

Implementation
• Apply to skin, rub in gently

ADVERSE EFFECTS
Docosanol
NONE known

Pimecrolimus
INTEG: Burning

NURSING CONSIDERATIONS
Assessment
• Assess skin condition (color, pain, inflammation) before, after administration
• Assess for signs and symptoms of skin infections (redness, draining lesions); if present, avoid use of product (pimecrolimus)

Patient/family education
• Advise patient to avoid contact between medication and eyes
• Instruct patient to discontinue use of product when condition clears

Evaluation

Positive therapeutic outcome
• Decreased inflammation, redness

VAGINAL ANTIFUNGALS

butoconazole (OTC)
(byoo-toh-kone′ah-zole)
Gynazol-1
clotrimazole (OTC)
(kloe-trye′ma-zole)
Canesten ✤, Gyne-Lotrimin 3, Gyne-Lotrimin 7, Myclo ✤

miconazole (OTC)
(mye-kon′a-zole)
Monistat 3, Monistat 7
terconazole (OTC)
(ter-kone′ah-zole)
Terazol 7, Tetrazol 3, Zazole
tioconazole (OTC)
(tye-oh-kone′ah-zole)
Gyne-Trosyd ✤, Monistat 1, Vagistat-1

ACTION: Interferes with fungal DNA replication; binds sterols in fungal cell membranes, which increases permeability, leaking of nutrients

Therapeutic outcome: Fungistatic/fungicidal against susceptible organisms: *Candida* only

USES: Vaginal, vulval, vulvovaginal candidiasis (moniliasis)

CONTRAINDICATIONS
Hypersensitivity

Precautions: Pregnancy, breastfeeding, children <2 yr

Implementation
Topical route
• Administer one full applicator every night high into the vagina
• Store at room temperature in dry place

ADVERSE EFFECTS
GU: Vulvovaginal burning, itching, pelvic cramps
INTEG: Rash, urticaria, stinging, burning
MISC: *Headache,* body pain

NURSING CONSIDERATIONS
Assessment
• Assess for allergic reaction: burning, stinging, itching, discharge, soreness

Patient/family education
• Instruct patient in asepsis (hand washing) before, after each application
• Teach patient to apply with applicator only; to avoid use of any other vaginal product unless directed by prescriber; sanitary napkin may prevent soiling of undergarments
• Instruct patient to abstain from sexual intercourse until treatment is completed; reinfection and irritation may occur
• Advise patient to notify prescriber if symptoms persist

Evaluation

Positive therapeutic outcome
• Decrease in itching or white discharge
(vaginal)

OTIC ANTIINFECTIVES

---

ciprofloxacin (Rx)
(sip′roe-flox′a-sin)
Cetraxal, Ofloxacin, Otiprio

ACTION: Inhibits protein synthesis in susceptible microorganisms

USES: Ear infection (external), short-term use

CONTRAINDICATIONS
Hypersensitivity, perforated eardrum

Precautions: Pregnancy **C**

Implementation
• After removing impacted cerumen by
irrigation
• After cleaning stopper with alcohol
• After restraining child if necessary
• After warming sol to body temp

ADVERSE EFFECTS
EENT: Itching, irritation in ear
INTEG: Rash, urticaria

NURSING CONSIDERATIONS
Assessment
• Assess for redness, swelling, fever, pain in ear,
which indicates superinfection

Patient/family education
• Teach patient correct method of instillation
using aseptic technique, including not touching
dropper to ear
• Inform patient that dizziness may occur after
instillation

Evaluation

Positive therapeutic outcome
• Decreased ear pain

Appendix C Vaccines and toxoids

GENERIC NAME	TRADE NAME	USES	DOSAGE AND ROUTES	CONTRAINDICATIONS
anthrax vaccine	BioThrax	Pre-/postexposure prophylaxis	**Preexposure** Adult: SUBCUT 0.5 ml at 0, 2, 4 wk, then 0.5 ml at 6, 12, 18 mo **Postexposure** Adult: SUBCUT 0.5 ml 0, 2, 4 wk, with antibiotics	Hypersensitivity
BCG vaccine	TICE BCG	TB exposure	Adult and child >1 mo: 0.2-0.3 ml Child <1 mo: Reduce dose by 50% using 2 ml of sterile water after reconstituting	Hypersensitivity, hypogamma-globulinemia, positive TB test, burns
diphtheria and tetanus toxoids, adsorbed	Tenivac	Induces antitoxins to provide immunity to diphtheria and tetanus	Adult and child ≥7 yr: IM (adult strength) 0.5 ml q4-8wk × 2 doses, then 3rd dose 6-12 mo after 2nd dose, booster IM 0.5 ml q10yr Child 1-6 yr: IM (pediatric strength) 0.5 ml q4wk × 2 doses, booster 6-12 mo after 2nd dose Infant 6 wk-1 yr: IM (pediatric strength) 0.5 ml q4wk × 3 doses, booster 6-12 mo after 3rd dose	Hypersensitivity to mercury, thimerosal; immunocompromised patients; radiation; corticosteroids; acute illness
diphtheria and tetanus toxoids and whole-cell pertussis vaccine (DPT, DTP)	DTwP, Tri-Immunol	Prevention of diphtheria, tetanus, pertussis	Doses vary Check product information	Hypersensitivity, active infection, poliomyelitis outbreak, immunosuppression, febrile illness
diphtheria and tetanus toxoids and acellular pertussis vaccine	Adacel, Boostrix, Daptacel, Infanrix			
diphtheria, tetanus, pertussis, haemophilus, polio IPV	Pentacel	Immunity to diphtheria, tetanus, pertussis, haemophilus, polio	Infant >6 wk and child ≤5 yr: IM 0.5 ml at 2, 4, 6, and 15-18 mo	Hypersensitivity, polio outbreak, acute infection, immunosuppression
diphtheria, tetanus, pertussis, polio vaccine IPV	Kinrix, Quadracel	Immunity to diphtheria, tetanus, pertussis, polio vaccine IPV	Child: IM 0.5 ml	Hypersensitivity, polio outbreak, acute infection, immunosuppression

Continued

Appendix C   Vaccines and toxoids—cont'd

GENERIC NAME	TRADE NAME	USES	DOSAGE AND ROUTES	CONTRAINDICATIONS
H1N1 influenza A (swine flu) virus vaccine	Influenza A (H1N1)	Immunity to H1N1	Adult <50 yr, adolescent, child ≥2 yr: Intranasal 1 dose (roughly 0.1 ml) into each nostril; child 2-9 yr repeat dose ≥4 wk later Adult, adolescent, child ≥3 yr: IM 0.5 ml as a single dose; child 3-9 yr repeat dose ≥4 wk later (Sanofi) (CSL); child 4-9 yr repeat dose ≥4 wk later (Novartis); infants ≥6 mo, child <36 mo: IM 0.25 ml, repeat in 4 wk (Sanofi) Adult: IM 0.5 ml as a single dose (GSK)	Hypersensitivity, febrile illness, active infection
haemophilus b conjugate vaccine, diphtheria CRM₁₉₇ protein conjugate (HbOC)	HibTITER	Polysaccharide immunization of children 2-6 yr against *H. influenzae* b, conjugate	**HibTITER (IM only)** Child: IM 0.5 ml Child 2-6 mo: 0.5 ml q2mo × 3 inj	
haemophilus b conjugate vaccine, meningococcal protein conjugate (PRP-OMP)	PedvaxHIB	Immunization of child 2, 4, 6 mo	Child 7-11 mo: Previously unvaccinated 0.5 ml q2mo inj Child 12-14 mo: Previously unvaccinated 0.5 ml × 1 inj **PedvaxHIB (IM only)** Child 2-14 mo: 0.5 ml × 2 inj at 2, 4 mo of age (6 mo dose not needed), then booster at 12-18 mo against invasive disease Child ≥15 mo: Previously unvaccinated 0.5 ml inj	
hepatitis A vaccine, inactivated	Havrix, VAQTA	Active immunization against hepatitis A virus	Adult: IM 1440 EL units (Havrix) or 50 units (VAQTA) as a single dose; booster dose is the same given at 6, 12 mo Child 2-18 yr: IM 720 EL units (Havrix) or 25 units (VAQTA) as a single dose, booster dose is the same given at 6, 12 mo	Hypersensitivity
hepatitis B vaccine, recombinant	Engerix-B, Recombivax HB	Immunization against all subtypes of hepatitis B virus	Varies widely	Hypersensitivity to this vaccine or yeast
human papillomavirus recombinant vaccine, quadrivalent	Gardasil	Prevention of HPV types 6, 11, 16, 18, cervical cancer, genital warts, precancerous dysplastic lesions, anal cancer/anal intraepithelial neoplasia	Adult up to 26 yr and child >9 yr to 26 yr: IM give as 3 separate doses; 1st dose as elected; 2nd dose 2 mo after 1st dose; 3rd dose 6 mo after 1st dose	Child <9 yr, pregnancy, breastfeeding, geriatric, active disease, hypersensitivity

influenza virus vaccine	Afluria, FluMist, Fluvirin, Fluzone	Prevention of seasonal influenza	Adult and child >12 yr: IM 0.5 ml in 1 dose Adult 18-64 yr: ID 0.1 ml as a single dose Child 3-12 yr: IM 0.5 ml, repeat in 1 mo (split) unless 1978-1985 vaccine was given; also given nasal Child 6 mo to 3 yr: IM 0.25 ml, repeat in 1 mo (split) unless 1978-1985 vaccine was given; also given nasal child ≤2 yr	Hypersensitivity; active infection, chicken egg allergy, Guillain-Barré syndrome, active neurologic disorders
Japanese encephalitis virus vaccine, inactivated	Ixiaro	Active immunity against Japanese encephalitis (JE)	Adult/child >3 yr: IM 0.5 ml (deltoid), then 0.5 ml 28 days later. Give the second dose ≥1 wk before potential exposure Child ≥2 mo to <3 yr: IM 0.25 ml (anterolateral aspect of the thigh or deltoid for children 1-2 yr with adequate muscle mass), then 0.25 ml 28 days later	Hypersensitivity to murine, thimerosal; allergic reactions to previous dose
measles, mumps, and rubella vaccine, live	M-M-R-II	Prevention of measles, mumps, rubella	Adult: SUBCUT 1 vial; 2 vials separated by 1 mo, in person born after 1957 Child >15 mo and adult: SUBCUT 0.5 ml	Hypersensitivity, blood dyscrasias, anemia, active infection, immunosuppression; egg, chicken allergy; pregnancy, febrile illness, neomycin allergy; neoplasms
measles, mumps, rubella, varicella	ProQuad	Immunity to measles, mumps, rubella, varicella	Child: SUBCUT 0.5 ml	Hypersensitivity to eggs, neomycin, cancer, radiation, corticosteroids, blood dyscrasias, active untreated TB
meningococcal polysaccharide vaccine	Menomune-A/C	Prophylaxis to meningococcal meningitis	Adult and child >2 yr: SUBCUT 0.5 ml	Hypersensitivity to thimerosal, pregnancy, acute illness
pneumococcal 7-valent conjugate vaccine	Prevnar	Immunity against *Streptococcus pneumoniae*	Child: IM 0.5 ml ×3 doses (7-11 mo); × 2 doses (12-23 mo); × 1 dose >2-9 yr	Hypersensitivity to diphtheria toxoid or this product
pneumococcal vaccine, polyvalent	Pneumovax 23	Pneumococcal immunization	Adult and child >2 yr: IM/SUBCUT 0.5 ml	Hypersensitivity, Hodgkin's disease, ARDS
poliovirus vaccine (IPV)	IPOL	Prevention of polio	Adult and child >2 yr: PO 0.5 ml, given q8wk × 2 doses, then 0.5 ml ½-1 yr after dose 2 Infant: PO 0.5 ml at 2, 4, 18 mo; booster at 4-6 yr; may also be given: IPV at 2, 4 mo, then TOPV at 12-18 mo, booster at 4-6 yr	Hypersensitivity, active infection, allergy to neomycin/streptomycin, immunosuppression, vomiting, diarrhea
rabies vaccine, human diploid cell (HDCV)	Imovax, RabAvert	Active immunity to rabies	**Preexposure** Adult and child: IM 1 ml day 0, 7, 21, or 28 (total 4 doses) **Postexposure** Adult and child: IM 1 ml on day 0, 3, 7, 14, 28 (total 5 doses)	No contraindications

Continued

Appendix C Vaccines and toxoids—cont'd

GENERIC NAME	TRADE NAME	USES	DOSAGE AND ROUTES	CONTRAINDICATIONS
rotovirus	RotaTeq, Rotarix	Prevents rotovirus	Infant: PO 3 doses given between 6 and 32 wk of age; 1st dose between 6-12 wk of age; 2nd and 3rd doses q4-10wk	Hypersensitivity to this product or latex, immunocompromised, blood products given within 6 wk, lymphatic disorders
tetanus toxoid, adsorbed	No trade name	Tetanus toxoid: Used for prophylactic treatment of wounds	Adult and child: IM 0.5 ml q4-6wk × 2 doses, then 0.5 ml 1 yr after dose 2 (adsorbed); SUBCUT/IM 0.5 ml q4-8wk × 3 doses, then 0.5 ml ½-1 yr after dose 3, booster dose 0.5 ml q10yr	Hypersensitivity; active infection, poliomyelitis outbreak, immunosuppression
typhoid vaccine, parenteral typhoid vaccine, oral	Typhim Vi Vivotif Berna Vaccine	Active immunity to typhoid fever	Adult: PO 1 cap 1 hr before meals × 4 doses, booster q5yr Adult and child >10 yr: SUBCUT 0.5 ml, repeat in 4 wk, booster q3yr Child 6 mo-10 yr: SUBCUT 0.25 ml, repeat in 4 wk, booster q3yr	Parenteral: Systemic or allergic reaction, acute respiratory or other acute infection, intensive physical exercise in high temperatures Oral: Hypersensitivity, acute febrile illness, suppressive or antibiotic products
typhoid Vi polysaccharide vaccine	Typhim Vi	Active immunity to typhoid fever	Adult and child ≥2 yr: IM 0.5 ml as a single dose, reimmunize q2yr 0.5 ml IM, if needed	Hypersensitivity, chronic typhoid carriers
Varicella-Zoster Virus Vaccine	Varivax, Zostavax	Prevention of varicella-zoster (chickenpox)	Adult and child ≥13 yr: SUBCUT 0.5 ml, 2nd dose SUBCUT 0.5 ml 4-8 wk later	Hypersensitivity to neomycin; blood dyscrasias, immunosuppression, active untreated TB, acute illness, pregnancy, diseases of lymphatic system
yellow fever vaccine	YF-Vax	Active immunity to yellow fever	Adult and child ≥9 mo: SUBCUT 0.5 ml deeply; booster q10yr Child 6-9 mo: same as above if exposed	Hypersensitivity to egg or chicken embryo protein, pregnancy, child <6 mo, immunodeficiency

Appendix D

Abbreviations and Pregnancy Categories

abd	abdomen		**GPC**	giant papillary conjunctivitis
ABG	arterial blood gas		**gr**	grain
ac	before meals		**GTT**	glucose tolerance test
ACE	angiotensin-converting enzyme		**gtt**	drops
ACT	activated clotting time		**GU**	genitourinary
ADA	American Diabetes Association		**GVHD**	graft-versus-host disease
ADH	antidiuretic hormone		**H$_2$**	histamine$_2$
ALT	alanine aminotransferase		**hCG**	human chorionic gonadotropin
ANA	antinuclear antibody		**Hct**	hematocrit
AP	anteroposterior		**HDCV**	human diploid cell rabies vaccine
APLA	antiphospholipid antibody syndrome		**Hgb**	hemoglobin
APTT	activated partial thromboplastin time		**H&H**	hematocrit and hemoglobin
ASA	acetylsalicylic acid, aspirin		**5-HIAA**	5-hydroxyindoleacetic acid
ASHD	arteriosclerotic heart disease		**HIV**	human immunodeficiency virus (AIDS)
AST	aspartate aminotransferase (SGOT)		**H$_2$O**	water
AV	atrioventricular		**HOB**	head of bed
bid	twice a day		**HR**	heart rate
BM	bowel movement		**hr**	hour
BMR	basal metabolic rate		**IBD**	inflammatory bowel disease
B/P	blood pressure		**IC**	intracardiac
BPH	benign prostatic hypertrophy		**ICP**	intracranial pressure
BPM	beats per minute		**ID**	intradermal
BS	blood sugar		**IgG**	immunoglobulin G
BUN	blood urea nitrogen		**IM**	intramuscular
C	Celsius (centigrade)		**inf**	infusion
CAD	coronary artery disease		**INH**	inhalation
cap	capsule		**inj**	injection
Cath	catheterization or catheterize		**I&O**	intake and output
CBC	complete blood cell count		**IPPB**	intermittent positive-pressure breathing
CHF	congestive heart failure		**IT**	intrathecal
CHo	carbohydrates		**ITP**	idiopathic thrombocytopenic purpura
cm	centimeter		**IUD**	intrauterine device
CNS	central nervous system		**IV**	intravenous
CO$_2$	carbon dioxide		**IVP**	intravenous pyelogram
cont	continuous		**K**	potassium
COPD	chronic obstructive pulmonary disease		**kg**	kilogram
CPAP	continuous positive airway pressure		**L**	liter
CPK	creatinine phosphokinase		**lb**	pound
CPR	cardiopulmonary resuscitation		**LDH**	lactic dehydrogenase
CCr	creatinine clearance		**LE**	lupus erythematosus
C&S	culture and sensitivity		**LH**	luteinizing hormone
C sect	cesarean section		**LLQ**	left lower quadrant
CSF	cerebrospinal fluid		**LMP**	last menstrual period
CTCL	cutaneous T-cell lymphoma		**LOC**	level of consciousness
CV	cardiovascular		**LR**	lactated Ringer's solution
CVA	cerebrovascular accident		**LUQ**	left upper quadrant
CVP	central venous pressure		**M**	meter
D&C	dilatation and curettage		**m**	minim
dir inf	direct infusion		**m^2**	square meter
dr	dram		**MAOI**	monoamine oxidase inhibitor
D$_5$W	5% glucose in distilled water		**mcg**	microgram
DVT	deep vein thrombosis		**mEq**	milliequivalent
ECG	electrocardiogram (EKG)		**mg**	milligram
EDTA	ethylenediamine tetraacetic acid		**MI**	myocardial infarction
EEG	electroencephalogram		**min**	minute
EENT	ear, eye, nose, and throat		**ml**	milliliter
EPS	extrapyramidal symptoms		**mm**	millimeter
ESR	erythrocyte sedimentation rate		**mo**	month
ext rel	extended release		**Na**	sodium
FBS	fasting blood sugar		**neg**	negative
FHT	fetal heart tones		**NGU**	nongonococcal urethritis
FSH	follicle-stimulating hormone		**NHL**	non-Hodgkin's lymphoma
g	gram		**NPO**	nothing by mouth (Lat. *nulla per os*)
GABA	γ-aminobutyric acid		**NS**	normal saline
GI	gastrointestinal		**O$_2$**	oxygen

OBS	organic brain syndrome		RUQ	right upper quadrant
OD	right eye		Rx	prescription
OR	operating room		SARS	severe acute respiratory syndrome
OS	left eye		SCr	serum creatinine
OTC	over-the-counter		SIMV	synchronous intermittent mandatory ventilation
OU	each eye		SL	sublingual
oz	ounce		SLE	systemic lupus erythematosus
p̄	after		SOB	shortness of breath
P56	Plasma-Lyte 56		sol	solution
PaCO$_2$	arterial carbon dioxide tension (pressure)		sp gr	specific gravity
PaO$_2$	arterial oxygen tension (pressure)		ss	one half
PAT	paroxysmal atrial tachycardia		STD	sexually transmitted disease
PBI	protein-bound iodine		SUBCUT	subcutaneous
pc	after meals		supp	suppository
PCI	percutaneous coronary intervention		sus rel	sustained release
PCWP	pulmonary capillary wedge pressure		syr	syrup
PEEP	positive end-expiratory pressure		T&A	tonsillectomy and adenoidectomy
PERRLA	pupils equal, round, react to light and accommodation		tab	tablet
			tbsp	tablespoon
pH	hydrogen ion concentration		TD	transdermal
PO	by mouth		temp	temperature
postop	postoperative		tid	three times daily
PP	postprandial		tinc	tincture
PPHN	persistent pulmonary hypertension of the newborn		TPN	total parenteral nutrition
preop	preoperative		TOP	topical
prn	as required		TSH	thyroid-stimulating hormone
PT	prothrombin time		tsp	teaspoon
PTT	partial thromboplastin time		TT	thrombin time
PVC	premature ventricular contraction		UA	urinalysis
q	every		UTI	urinary tract infection
q$_{AM}$	every morning		UV	ultraviolet
qhr	every hour		vag	vaginal
q2hr	every 2 hours		VMA	vanillylmandelic acid
q3hr	every 3 hours		vol	volume
q4hr	every 4 hours		VS	vital sign
q6hr	every 6 hours		WBC	white blood cell count
q12hr	every 12 hours		wk	week
qid	four times daily		wt	weight
qmo	every month		yr	year
q$_{PM}$	every night		>	greater than
qs	sufficient quantity		<	less than
qt	quart		=	equal
qwk	every week		°	degree
R	right		%	percent
RAIU	radioactive iodine uptake		α	alpha
RBC	red blood count or cell		γ	gamma
RLQ	right lower quadrant		β	beta
ROM	range of motion			

- For a list of the Institute for Safe Medicine Practices (ISMP) error-prone abbreviations, symbols, and dose designations, please see http://www.ismp.org/tools/errorproneabbreviations.pdf.
- For frequently asked questions regarding the 2010 National Patient Safety Goals, please visit The Joint Commission website at http://www.jointcommission.org/PatientSafety/NationalPatientSafetyGoals.

FDA Pregnancy Categories

A No risk demonstrated to the fetus in any trimester

B No adverse effects in animals, no human studies available

C Only given after risks to the fetus are considered; animal studies have shown adverse reactions, no human studies available

D Definite fetal risks, may be given despite risks if needed in life-threatening conditions

X Absolute fetal abnormalities; not to be used any time during pregnancy

Note: **UK** = Unknown fetal risk (used in this text but not an official FDA pregnancy category).

Appendix E

Immunization Schedules

Recommended Childhood and Adolescent Immunization Schedule—United States, 2010

Immunization Schedule for Persons Aged 0-6 Years

Vaccine ▼ / Age ►	Birth	1 month	2 months	4 months	6 months	12 months	15 months	18 months	19-23 months	2-3 years	4-6 years
Hepatitis B[*]	HepB	HepB				HepB					
Rotavirus[*]			Rota	Rota	Rota						
Diphtheria, Tetanus, Pertussis[*]			DTaP	DTaP	DTaP		DTaP	DTaP			DTaP
Haemophilus Influenzae Type b[b]			Hib	Hib	Hib[*]	Hib					
Pneumococcal[*]			PCV	PCV	PCV	PCV				PPSV	
Inactivated Poliovirus			IPV	IPV		IPV					IPV
Influenza[*]						Influenza (Yearly)					
Measles, Mumps, Rubella[*]						MMR	MMR				MMR
Varicella[*]						Varicella	Varicella				Varicella
Hepatitis A[*]						HepA (2 doses)				HepA Series	
Meningococcal[*]										MCV	MCV

Range of recommended ages

Certain high-risk groups

This schedule indicates the recommended ages for routine administration of currently licensed childhood vaccines, as of December 15, 2009, for children aged 0-6 years. Any dose not administered at the recommended age should be administered at any subsequent visit, when indicated and feasible. Additional vaccines may be licensed and recommended during the year. Licensed combination vaccines may be used whenever any components of the combination are indicated and other components of the vaccine are not contraindicated and if approved by the Food and Drug Administration for that dose of the series. **Providers should consult the respective Advisory Committee on Immunization Practices statement for detailed recommendations, including for high-risk conditions: http://www.cdc.gov/vaccines/pubs/ACIP-list.htm.** Clinically significant adverse events that follow immunization should be reported to the Vaccine Adverse Event Reporting System (VAERS). Guidance about how to obtain and complete a VAERS form is available at http://www.vaers.hhs.gov or by telephone, 800-822-7967.

[*]For complete information go to http://www.cdc.gov/vaccines/schedules/index

Immunization Schedule for Persons Aged 7-18 Years

Vaccine ▼ Age ▶	7-10 years	11-12 years	13-18 years
Tetanus, Diphtheria, Pertussis*		Tdap	Tdap
Human Papillomavirus*	*	HPV (3 doses)	HPV Series
Meningococcal*	MCV	MCV	MCV
Influenza*		Influenza (Yearly)	
Pneumococcal*		PPSV	
Hepatitis A*		HepA Series	
Hepatitis B*		HepB Series	
Inactivated Poliovirus*		IPV Series	
Measles, Mumps, Rubella*		MMR Series	
Varicella*		Varicella Series	

Range of recommended ages

Catch-up immunization

Certain high-risk groups

This schedule indicates the recommended ages for routine administration of currently licensed childhood vaccines, as of December 15, 2009, for children aged 7-18 years. Any dose not administered at the recommended age should be administered at any subsequent visit, when indicated and feasible. Additional vaccines may be licensed and recommended during the year. Licensed combination vaccines may be used whenever any components of the combination are indicated and other components of the vaccine are not contraindicated and if approved

by the Food and Drug Administration for that dose of the series. **Providers should consult the respective Advisory Committee on Immunization Practices statement for detailed recommendations, including for high-risk conditions: http://www.cdc.gov/vaccines/pubs/ACIP-list.htm.** Clinically significant adverse events that follow immunization should be reported to the Vaccine Adverse Event Reporting System (VAERS). Guidance about how to obtain and complete a VAERS form is available at http://www.vaers.hhs.gov or by telephone, 800-822-7967.

*For complete information go to http://www.cdc.gov/nip/recs/child-schedule.htm#printable.

Appendix F

Standard Precautions

The following precautions are used in the care of all patients regardless of their diagnosis or disease. They are also applied when handling or cleaning equipment or supplies that are potentially contaminated.

1. Wear gloves any time that you may contact blood, any moist body fluid (except sweat), secretions, excretions, nonintact skin, or mucous membranes.
2. Remove your gloves, wash your hands, and reapply clean gloves if your gloves become soiled with infective material.
3. Even if you are wearing gloves, remove them, wash your hands, and apply clean gloves *immediately before* contact with mucous membranes or nonintact skin.
4. Wear a protective cover gown of waterproof material if your clothing is likely to have substantial contact with infective material or if splashing of body fluids is likely.
5. Wear a face shield or goggles to protect your eyes if splashing of secretions is likely.
6. Any time a face shield or goggles are worn, wear a surgical mask to protect the mucous membranes of your nose and mouth. A surgical mask may be worn during certain sterile procedures without protective eyewear. However, protective eyewear is *never* worn without a surgical mask.
7. Handle needles, razors, broken glass, and other sharp objects with care. Needles should never be recapped. All sharps should be disposed of in a puncture-resistant sharps container.
8. Wash your hands before and after each patient contact.
9. Wash your hands before you apply and after you remove gloves. Do not assume that hand washing is unnecessary because gloves were worn. Do not wash your hands with gloves on them.
10. Gloves are used for the care of one patient only, then discarded.
11. Follow your facility policy for disposal of gloves and other contaminated items. These items are generally not disposed of in open trash containers. Facilities have designated disposal sites for these biohazardous waste materials.
12. Use resuscitation barrier devices as an alternative to mouth-to-mouth resuscitation.
13. Linen should be handled in a manner that prevents contamination of the outside of the container. Linen from isolation rooms was previously double bagged. Double bagging is no longer recommended since all linen is handled as potentially infectious. Double bag linen only if the outside of the bag becomes contaminated during the bagging process.

Appendix G

Illustrated Mechanisms and Sites of Action

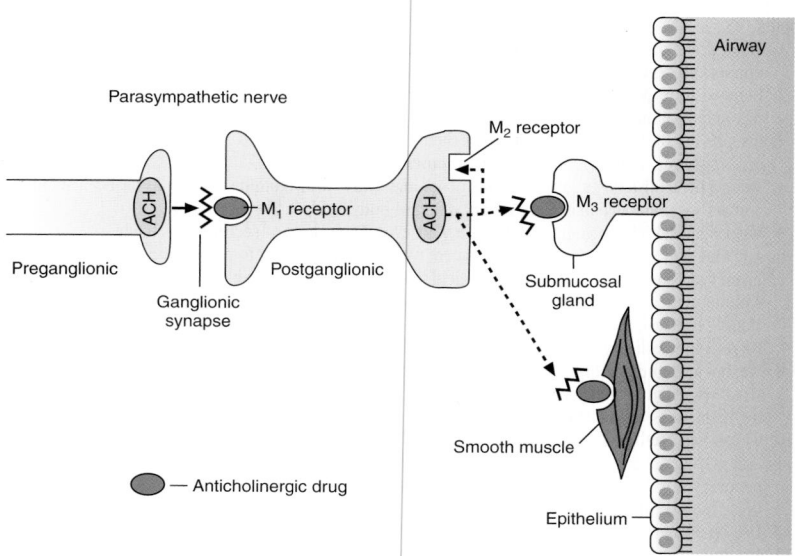

Fig. G-1 Sites and Mechanisms of Action: Anticholinergic Bronchodilators: Anticholinergic bronchodilators, such as ipratropium, work by blocking muscarinic-1 (M_1) receptors on postganglionic parasympathetic nerve endings and muscarinic-3 (M_3) receptors on the cell membranes of bronchial smooth muscles and submucosal glands. Normally, stimulation of the M_1 and M_3 receptors by acetylcholine (ACH) causes bronchoconstriction and mucus secretion from submucosal glands. Anticholinergic bronchodilators block these specific muscarinic receptors from the effects of acetylcholine, causing bronchial smooth muscle relaxation, bronchodilatation, and decreased mucus production. (From Gardenhire OS: *Rau's Respiratory Care Pharmacology,* ed 8, St. Louis, 2012, Mosby.)

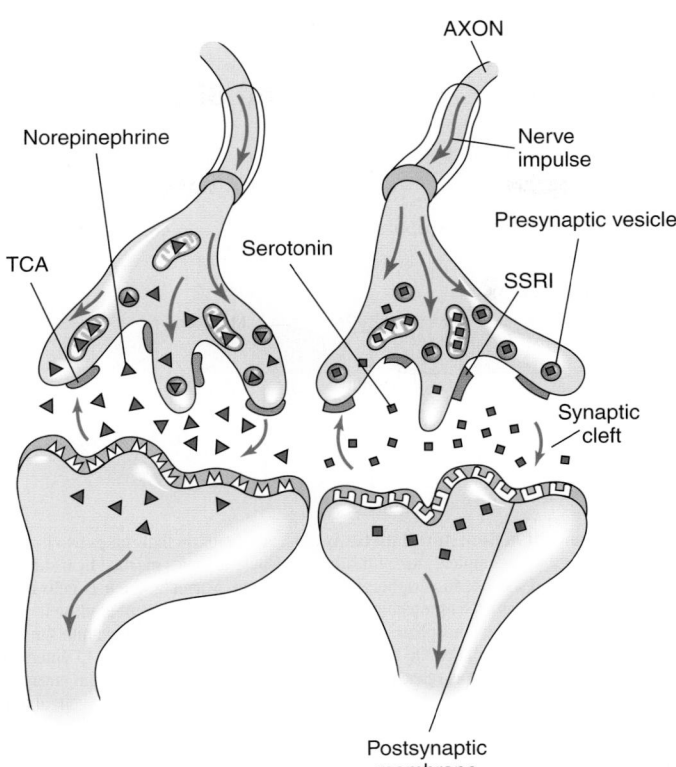

Fig. G-2 Mechanisms of Action: Antidepressants. Depression is thought to occur when levels of neurotransmitters, such as norepinephrine and serotonin, are reduced at postsynaptic receptor sites. These neurotransmitters affect a wide array of functions, including mood, obsessions, appetite, and anxiety. Antidepressants work by increasing the availability of these neurotransmitters at postsynaptic membranes and by enhancing and prolonging their effects. As a result, these agents improve mood, reduce anxiety, and minimize obsessions.

Antidepressants typically are classified as tricyclic antidepressants (TCAs), monoamine oxidase inhibitors (not shown), selective serotonin reuptake inhibitors (SSRIs), and atypical antidepressants (not shown). TCAs, such as amitriptyline and desipramine, primarily block norepinephrine reuptake at presynaptic membranes, thereby increasing the norepinephrine concentration at synapses and making more available at postsynaptic receptors.

SSRIs, such as FLUoxetine and PARoxetine, selectively inhibit serotonin uptake at presynaptic membranes. This action leads to increased serotonin availability at postsynaptic receptors. (From Gutierrez K: *Pharmacotherapeutics: Clinical Reasoning in Primary Care,* ed 2, Philadelphia, 2008, Saunders.)

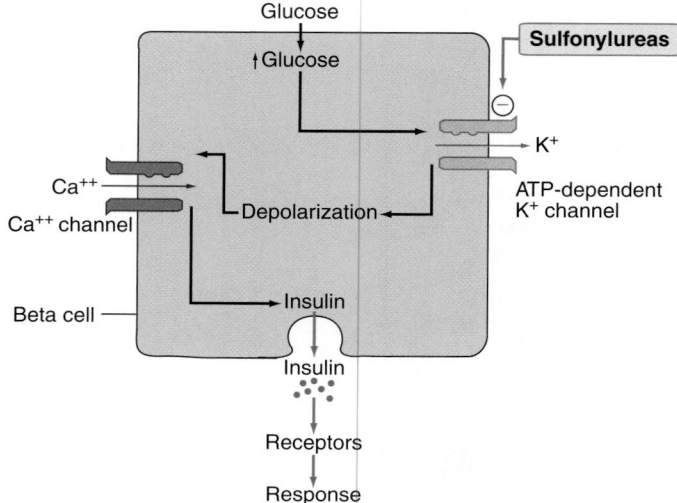

Fig. G-3 Mechanisms of Action: Antidiabetic Agents. Diabetes mellitus takes two forms: type 1 diabetes characterized by a complete lack of insulin and type 2 diabetes marked by insufficient insulin secretion, insulin resistance in peripheral tissues, or both. Normally, the beta cells in the pancreatic islets of Langerhans are responsible for secreting insulin. The rise of glucose levels in the beta cell triggers adenosine triphosphate (ATP)-dependent potassium (K^+) channels in the membranes of beta cells to close. Then the beta cells depolarize and calcium (Ca^{++}) enters the cell through Ca^{++} channel, and insulin is released from the cell. When circulating insulin engages with insulin receptors on cell membranes, it facilitates the movement of glucose into the cell, among other actions.

Type 1 diabetes is treated with the use of exogenous insulin, which mimics natural insulin in the body. Insulin takes many forms with varying degrees of onset, peak, and duration, including rapid, regular, intermediate, and long acting.

Type 2 diabetes is usually treated with oral agents. Sulfonylureas, such as glyBURIDE, block ATP-dependent K^+ channels in the cell membranes of beta cells, ultimately resulting in the release of insulin. (From Taylor: *Mosby's Crash Course Pharmacology,* St. Louis, 1998, Mosby.)

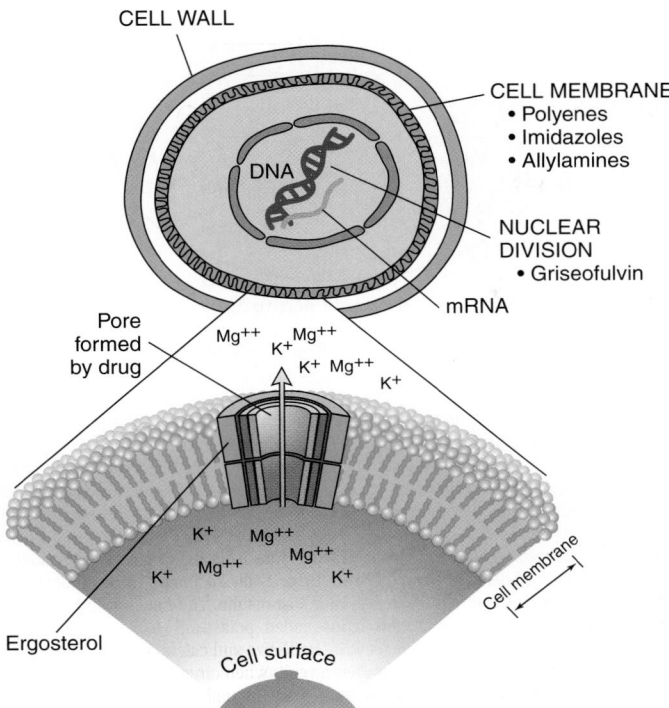

Fig. G-4 Sites and Mechanisms of Action: Antifungal Agents. Antifungal agents primarily affect fungi at one of two sites: the cell membrane or the cell nucleus. Most of these agents, such as polyene, imidazole, and allylamine antifungals, act on the fungal cell membrane. Polyene antifungals, such as amphotericin B, bind to ergosterol and increase cell membrane permeability. Imidazole antifungals, such as fluconazole and ketoconazole, interfere with ergosterol synthesis by inhibiting the cytochrome P_{450} enzyme system, altering the cell membrane, and inhibiting fungal growth. Allylamine antifungals, such as terbinafine, inhibit the enzyme squaline epoxidase, which disrupts ergosterol production—and cell membrane integrity. When cell membrane permeability increases, cellular components, including potassium (K^+) and magnesium (Mg^{++}), leak out. Loss of these cellular components leads to cell death.

Another antifungal agent, griseofulvin, directly affects the fungal nucleus, interfering with mitosis. By binding to structures in the mitotic spindle, it prevents cells from dividing, which eventually leads to their death. (From Gutierrez K: *Pharmacotherapeutics: Clinical Reasoning in Primary Care,* ed 2, Philadelphia, 2008, Saunders.)

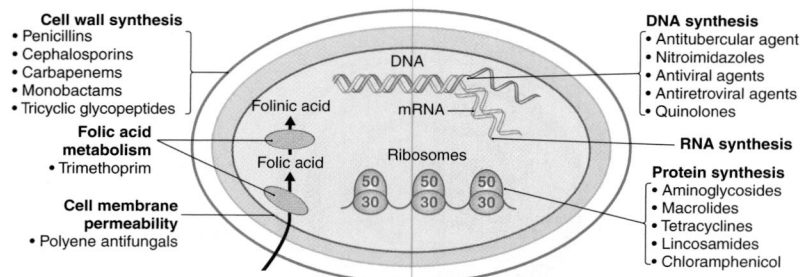

Fig. G-5 Sites and Mechanisms of Action: Antiinfective Agents. The goal of antiinfective therapy is to kill or inhibit the growth of microorganisms such as bacteria, viruses, and fungi. To achieve this goal, antiinfective agents must reach their targets, which usually occurs through absorption and distribution by the circulatory system. When the target is reached, a drug can kill or suppress microorganisms by:

• Inhibiting cell wall synthesis or activating enzymes that disrupt the cell wall, which leads to cellular weakening, lysis, and death. Penicillins (ampicillin), cephalosporins (ceFAZolin), carbapenems (imipenem), monobactams (aztreonam), and tricyclic glycopeptides (vancomycin) act in this way.

• Altering cell membrane permeability through direct action on the cell wall, which allows intracellular substances to leak out and destabilizes the cell. Polyene antifungals (amphotericin) work by this mechanism.

• Altering protein synthesis by binding to bacterial ribosomes (50/30) or affecting ribosomal function, which leads to cell death or slowed growth respectively. Aminoglycosides (gentamicin), macrolides (erythromycin), tetracyclines (doxycycline), lincosamides (clindamycin), and the miscellaneous antiinfective chloramphenicol use this action.

• Inhibiting DNA or RNA, including messenger RNA (mRNA), synthesis by binding to nucleic acids or interacting with enzymes required for their synthesis. Antitubercular agents (rifampin), nitroimidazoles (metroNIDAZOLE), antiviral agents (acyclovir), antiretroviral agents (stavudine), and quinolones (ciprofloxacin) act like this.

• Inhibiting the metabolism of folic acid and folinic acid or other cellular components that are essential for bacterial cell growth. The miscellaneous antiinfective trimethoprim employs this mechanism of action. (From Page C et al: *Integrated Pharmacology,* ed 3, St. Louis, 2006, Mosby.)

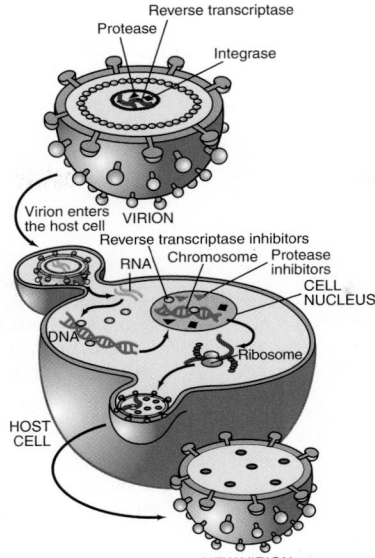

Fig. G-6 Mechanisms and Sites of Action: Antiretroviral Agents. When viruses reproduce, the infectious viral particle, or virion **(A)**, enters the host cell. The virion attaches to the cell's surface and then inserts itself into the host cell **(B)**. Once inside, the virion uncoats, and the enzyme reverse transcriptase makes two copies of the viral RNA: one copy is identical; the other is a mirror image. These two copies form double-stranded viral DNA that enters the host cell's nucleus, where it inserts itself into the host cell's DNA with the help of the enzyme integrase. Then viral DNA reprograms the host cell to produce additional viral RNA, which begins the process of forming new viruses. Specifically, messenger RNA (mRNA) instructs ribosomal RNA (rRNA) to produce a new chain of proteins and enzymes that are used to form new viruses. Protease cuts the chains, creating individual proteins. These combine with new RNA to create new virions, which bud and are released from the host cell **(C)**.

Antiretroviral agents target specific enzymes during viral reproduction. Nucleoside reverse transcriptase inhibitors, such as stavudine, interfere with the action of reverse transcriptase by mimicking naturally occurring nucleosides. Nucleotide reverse transcriptase inhibitors, such as tenofovir, block reverse transcriptase by competing with the natural substrate deoxyadenosine triphosphate and by causing DNA chain termination. Nonnucleoside reverse transcriptase inhibitors, such as delavirdine, work by directly binding to reverse transcriptase. As a result, no viral DNA is available to insert itself into the host cell's DNA. Protease inhibitors, such as indinavir, bind to and interfere with the action of protease; thus, the new chain of proteins formed by rRNA cannot be cut into individual proteins to make new viruses. (From Gutierrez K: *Pharmacotherapeutics: Clinical Reasoning in Primary Care,* ed 2, Philadelphia, 2008, Saunders.)

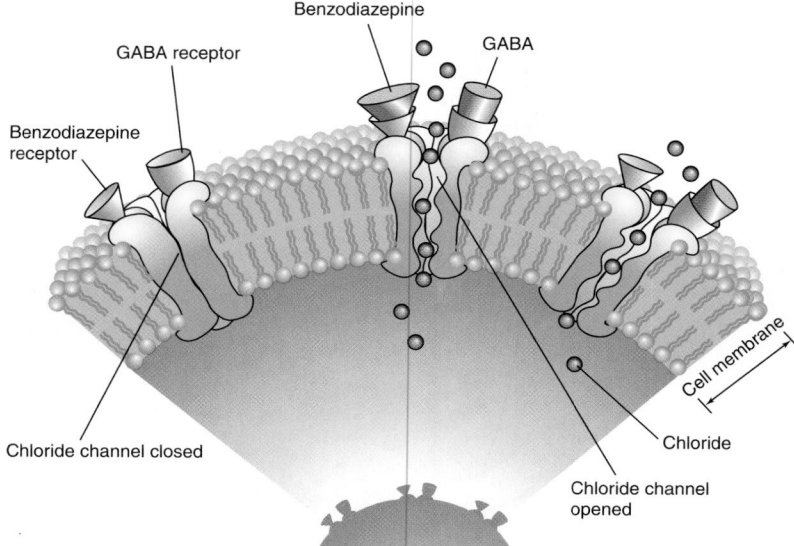

Fig. G-7 Mechanisms of Action: Benzodiazepines. Benzodiazepines reduce anxiety by stimulating the action of the inhibitory neurotransmitter, gamma-aminobutyric acid (GABA), in the limbic system. The limbic system plays an important role in the regulation of human behavior. Dysfunction of GABA neurotransmission in the limbic system may be linked to the development of certain anxiety disorders.

The limbic system contains a highly dense area of benzodiazepine receptors that may be linked to the antianxiety effects of benzodiazepines. These benzodiazepine receptors are located on the surface of neuronal cell membranes and are adjacent to GABA receptors. The binding of a benzodiazepine to its receptor enhances the affinity of a GABA receptor for GABA. In the absence of a benzodiazepine, the binding of GABA to its receptor causes the chloride channel in the cell membrane to open, which increases the influx of chloride into the cell. This influx of chloride results in hyperpolarization of the neuronal cell membrane and reduces the neuron's ability to fire, which is why GABA is considered an inhibitory neurotransmitter.

A benzodiazepine acts only in the presence of GABA. When it binds to a benzodiazepine receptor, it prolongs the time that the chloride channel remains open. This results in greater depression of neuronal function and a reduction in anxiety. (From Gutierrez K: *Pharmacotherapeutics: Clinical Reasoning in Primary Care,* ed 2, Philadelphia, 2008, Saunders.)

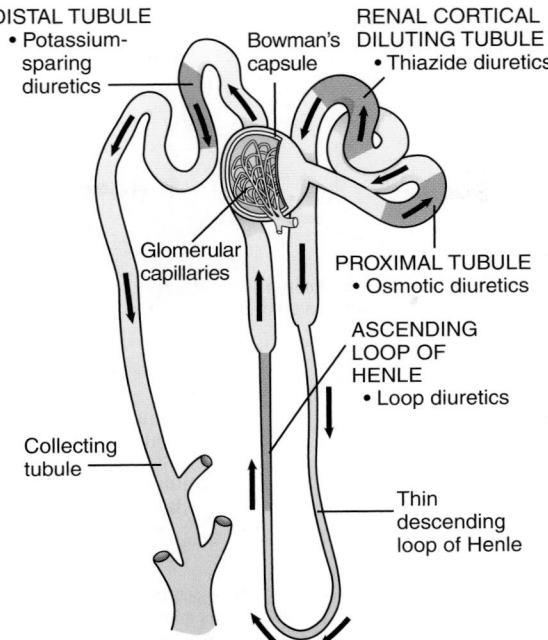

Fig. G-8 Sites of Action: Diuretics. Diuretics act primarily to increase water and sodium excretion by the kidneys, thereby increasing urine output. In the process, chloride, potassium, and other electrolytes may also be excreted. Most diuretics act by blocking sodium, water, and chloride reabsorption by peritubular capillaries in the nephrons. As a result, water and electrolytes remain in the convoluted tubules to be excreted as urine. The increased water and electrolyte excretion reduces blood volume—and ultimately blood pressure.

Diuretics belong to four major subclasses:

1. Thiazide diuretics, such as hydrochlorothiazide, act in the early portion of the distal convoluted tubule, called the cortical diluting segment. These drugs block sodium, chloride, and water reabsorption and promote their excretion along with potassium.

2. Loop diuretics, such as furosemide, act primarily in the thick ascending limb of the loop of Henle, blocking sodium, water, and chloride reabsorption. Then these substances are excreted along with potassium.

3. Potassium-sparing diuretics, such as spironolactone, act in the late portion of the distal convoluted tubule and collecting tubule. Here, they inhibit the action of aldosterone, leading to sodium excretion and potassium retention. Although triamterene and amiloride, two other potassium-sparing diuretics, act at the same site, they do not affect aldosterone. Instead, these drugs directly block the exchange of sodium and potassium, leading to decreased sodium reabsorption and decreased potassium excretion.

4. Osmotic diuretics, such as mannitol, work in the proximal convoluted tubule. As their name implies, these diuretics increase the osmotic pressure of the glomerular filtrate, inhibiting the passive reabsorption of water, sodium, and chloride. (From Gutierrez K: *Pharmacotherapeutics: Clinical Reasoning in Primary Care*, ed 2, Philadelphia, 2008, Saunders.)

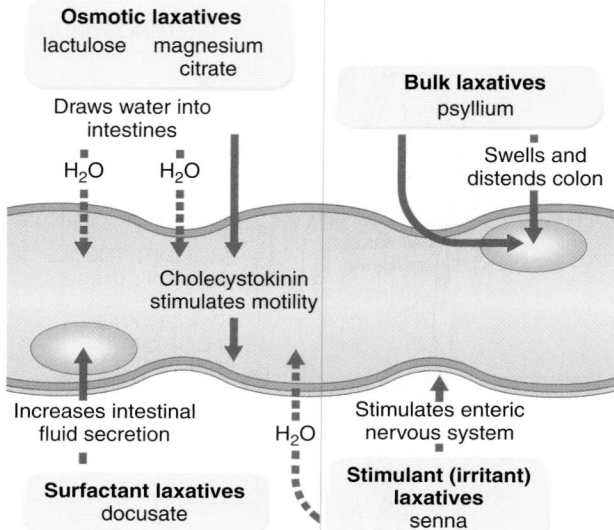

Fig. G-9 Mechanisms of Action: Laxatives. Laxatives ease or stimulate defecation. Typically, they are classified by their mechanism of action as bulk-forming, osmotic, stimulant, or surfactant laxatives.

Bulk-forming laxatives, such as psyllium, act in the small and large bowel. Because ingredients in these laxatives are undigestible, they remain within the stool and increase the fecal mass by drawing in water. These agents also enhance bacterial growth in the colon, further adding to the fecal mass.

Osmotic laxatives, such as lactulose, draw water into the intestinal lumen, causing the fecal mass to soften and swell. This osmotic action may be enhanced by the metabolism of colonic bacteria to lactate and other organic acids. These acids decrease colonic pH and increase colonic motility.

Stimulant (or irritant) laxatives, such as senna, act on the intestinal wall to increase water and electrolytes in the intestinal lumen. In addition, they directly irritate the colon, increasing motility.

Surfactant laxatives (or fecal softeners), such as docusate, reduce the surface tension of the stool, allowing water to enter it. These laxatives may also help to increase water and electrolyte excretion into the intestinal lumen, softening and increasing the fecal mass. (From Page C et al: *Integrated Pharmacology,* ed 3, St. Louis, 2006, Mosby.)

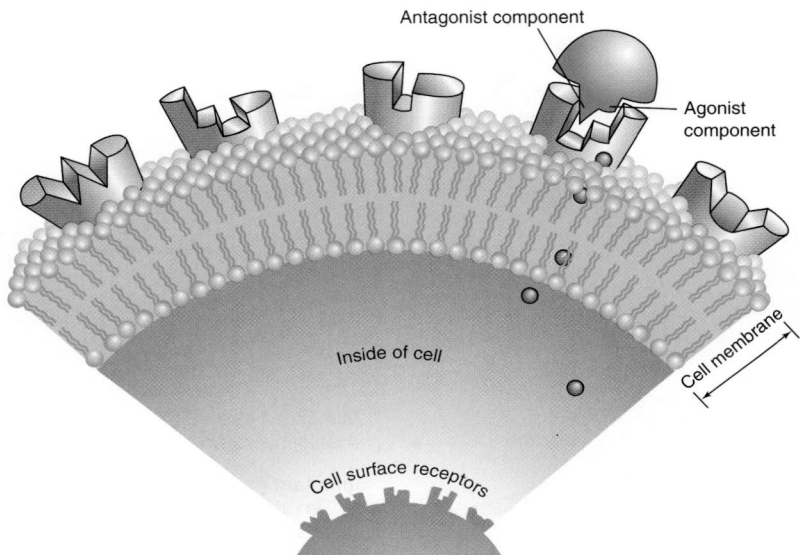

Fig. G-10 Mechanisms of Action: Narcotic Agonist-Antagonist Analgesics. Cell membranes have different types of opioid receptors, such as mu, kappa, and delta receptors. Opioid agonist-antagonists work by stimulating one type of receptor, while simultaneously blocking another type. As agonists, they work primarily by activating kappa receptors to produce analgesia and such other effects as CNS and respiratory depression, decreased GI motility, and euphoria. As antagonists, they compete with opioids at mu receptors, helping to reverse or block some of the other effects of agonists. (From Gutierrez K: *Pharmacotherapeutics: Clinical Reasoning in Primary Care,* ed 2, Philadelphia, 2008, Saunders.)

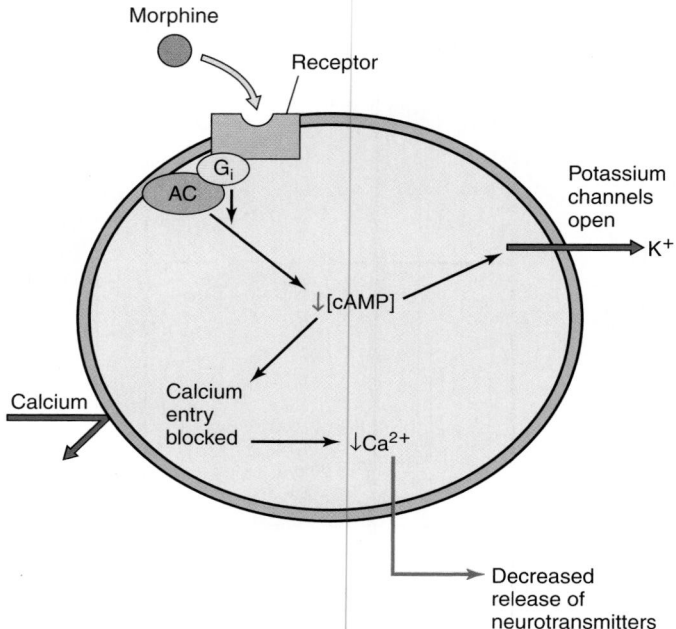

Fig. G-11 Mechanisms of Action: Narcotic Analgesics. Narcotic analgesics bind to three types of opioid receptors: mu, kappa, and delta receptors. They produce analgesia primarily by activating mu receptors. However, they also engage with and activate kappa and delta receptors, producing other effects, such as sedation and vasomotor stimulation.

When morphine or another narcotic analgesic binds to opioid receptors, activation occurs. The receptors send signals to the enzyme adenyl cyclase (AC) to slow activity by way of G proteins (G_i). Decreased adenyl cyclase activity causes reduced production of cyclic adenosine monophosphate (cAMP). A secondary messenger substance, cAMP is important for regulating cell membrane channels. A reduced cAMP level allows fewer potassium ions to leave the cell and blocks calcium ions from entering the cell. This ion imbalance—especially the reduced intracellular calcium level—ultimately decreases the release of neurotransmitters from the cell, thereby blocking or reducing pain impulse transmission. (From Minneman KP, Wecker L: *Brody's Human Pharmacology: Molecular to Clinical*, ed 4, St. Louis, 2005, Mosby.)

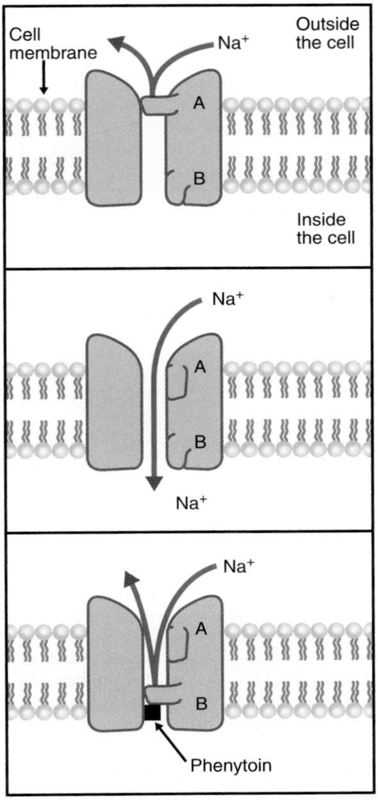

Fig. G-12 Mechanisms of Action: Phenytoin. Phenytoin, which is used to treat tonic-clonic seizures, acts in the motor cortex and brain stem, where the tonic phase of tonic-clonic seizures originates. By altering sodium transport across neuronal cell membranes, phenytoin stabilizes the cell membrane, reduces repetitive firing of the neurons, and halts or limits the spread of seizures. The first illustration shows a neuronal cell membrane in its resting state. The activation gate **(A)** of the sodium channel in the cell membrane is closed and blocks sodium (Na$^+$) from entering the cell. In the second illustration, a nerve impulse has caused depolarization and opening of the activation gate, allowing Na$^+$ to move into the cell. In the third illustration, depolarization continues and an inactivation gate **(B)** moves into the channel. This prevents Na$^+$ from moving into the cell. Phenytoin prolongs the inactivated state of the sodium channel by preventing reopening of the inactivation gate. By further preventing Na$^+$ from entering the cell, phenytoin slows impulse transmission, and thus slows the rate at which neurons fire. (From Minneman KP, Wecker L: *Brody's Human Pharmacology: Molecular to Clinical,* ed 4, St. Louis, 2005, Mosby.)

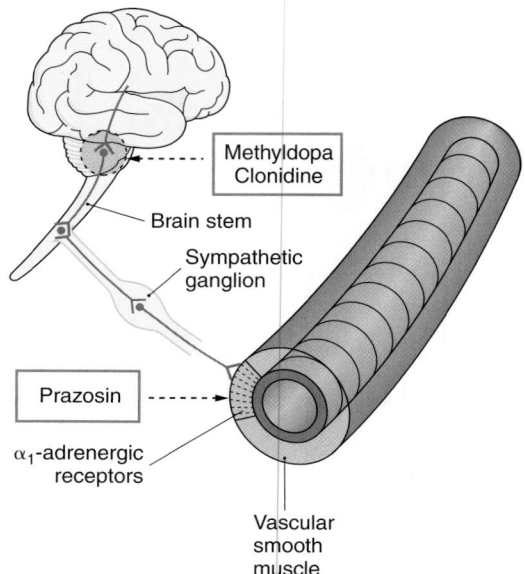

Fig. G-13 Sites of Action: Sympatholytics. Sympatholytics inhibit sympathetic nervous system (SNS) activity, which plays a major role in regulating B/P. Normally when the SNS is stimulated, nerve impulses travel from the cardiovascular center of the CNS to the sympathetic ganglia. From there, the impulses travel along postganglionic fibers to specific effector organs, such as the heart and blood vessels. SNS stimulation also triggers the release of norepinephrine, which acts primarily at alpha-adrenergic receptors.

Sympatholytics fall into two subclasses: central-acting α_2 agonists and peripheral-acting α_1-adrenergic antagonists. Central-acting α_2 agonists, such as methyldopa and cloNIDine, stimulate α_2-adrenergic receptors in the cardiovascular center of the CNS and reduce activity in the vasomotor center of the brain, interfering with sympathetic stimulation of the heart and blood vessels. This causes blood vessel dilatation and decreased cardiac output, which leads to reduced B/P.

Peripheral-acting α_1-adrenergic antagonists, such as prazosin, inhibit the stimulation of α_1-adrenergic receptors by norepinephrine in vascular smooth muscle, interfering with SNS-induced vasoconstriction. As a result, the blood vessels dilate, reducing peripheral vascular resistance and venous return to the heart. These effects, in turn, lead to decreased B/P. (From Prosser S, Worster B, Dewar K: *Applied Pharmacology for Nurses and Other Health Care Professionals,* St. Louis, 2000, Mosby.)

Appendix H

Photo Atlas of Drug Administration

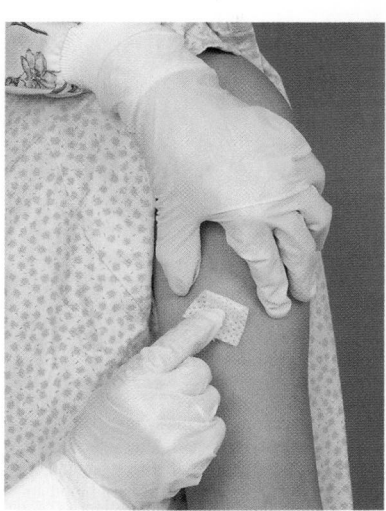

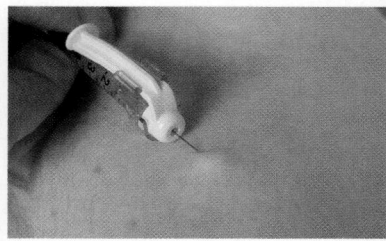

Fig. H-2 Intradermal Injection. For an intradermal injection, note formation of small bleb approximately 6 mm (¼ in) in diameter at injection site. (From Perry AG, Potter PA, and Elkin MK: *Nursing Interventions & Clinical Skills,* ed 5, St. Louis, 2012, Mosby.)

Fig. H-1 Administering an Injection. Cleanse site with antiseptic swab. Apply swab at center of site and rotate outward in circular direction for about 5 cm (2 in). (From Perry AG, Potter PA, and Elkin MK: *Nursing Interventions & Clinical Skills,* ed 5, St. Louis, 2012, Mosby.)

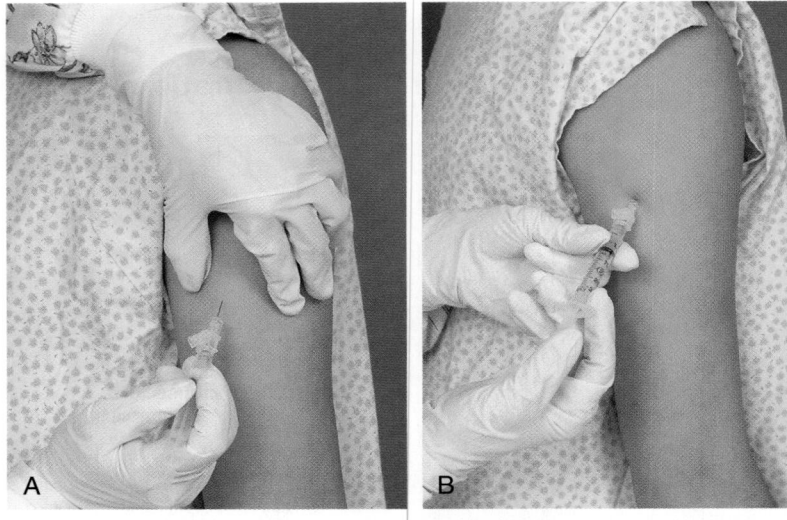

Fig. H-3 Subcutaneous Injection. **A,** For a subcutaneous injection, hold the syringe between the thumb and forefinger of the dominant hand as a dart, with the palm down. **B,** After injecting the needle at a 45- to 90-degree angle, grasp lower end of syringe barrel with nondominant hand to end of plunger. Avoid moving syringe while slowly pulling back on plunger to aspirate drug. If blood appears in syringe, remove needle, discard medication and syringe, and repeat procedure. *Exception:* Do not aspirate when giving heparin. (From Perry AG, Potter PA, and Elkin MK: *Nursing Interventions & Clinical Skills,* ed 5, St. Louis, 2012, Mosby.)

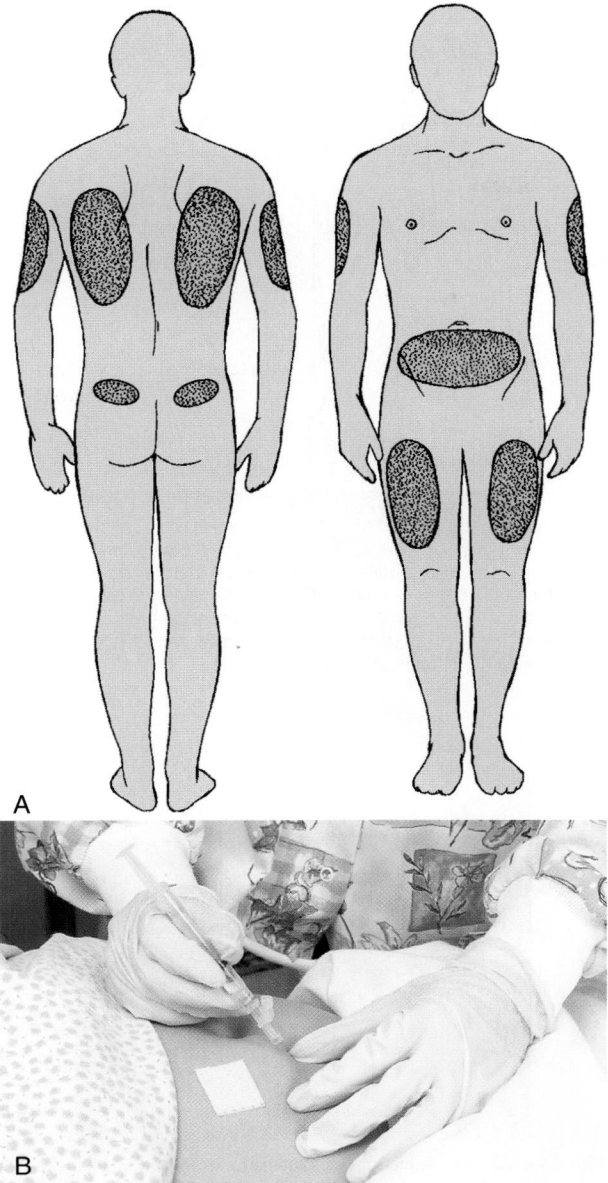

Fig. H-4 Subcutaneous Injection. A, Sites recommended for subcutaneous injections. **B,** Giving subcutaneous injection in the abdomen. (From Perry AG, Potter PA, and Elkin MK: *Nursing Interventions & Clinical Skills,* ed 5, St. Louis, 2012, Mosby.)

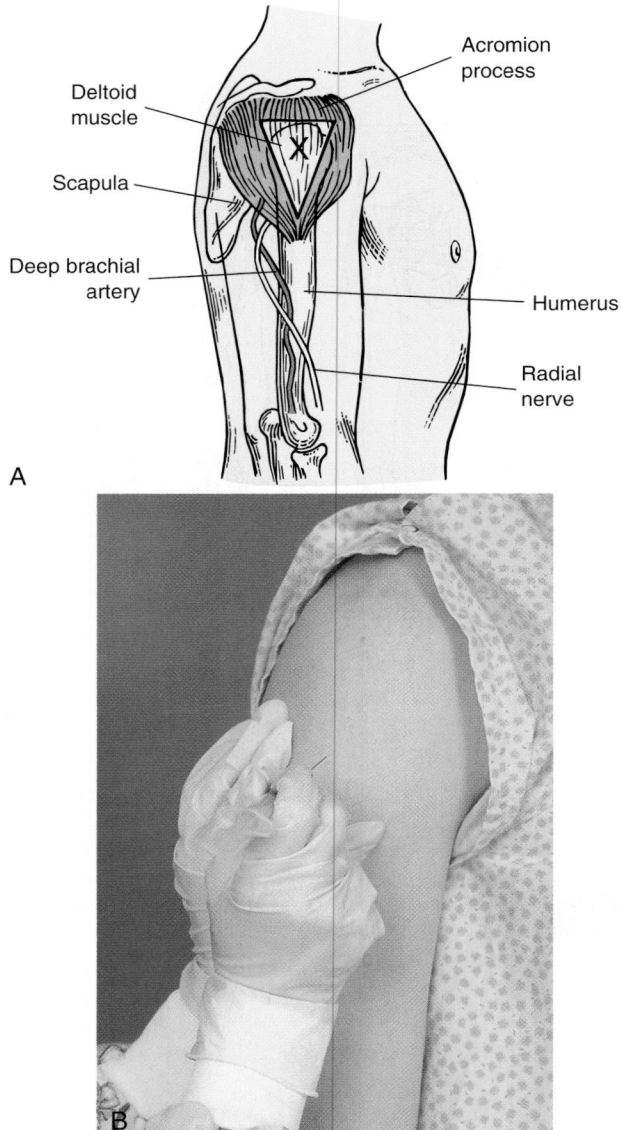

Fig. H-5 Deltoid Intradermal Injection. A, Landmarks for IM injection into the deltoid muscle. **B,** Giving IM injection in deltoid muscle. (From Perry AG, Potter PA, and Elkin MK: *Nursing Interventions & Clinical Skills,* ed 5, St. Louis, 2012, Mosby.)

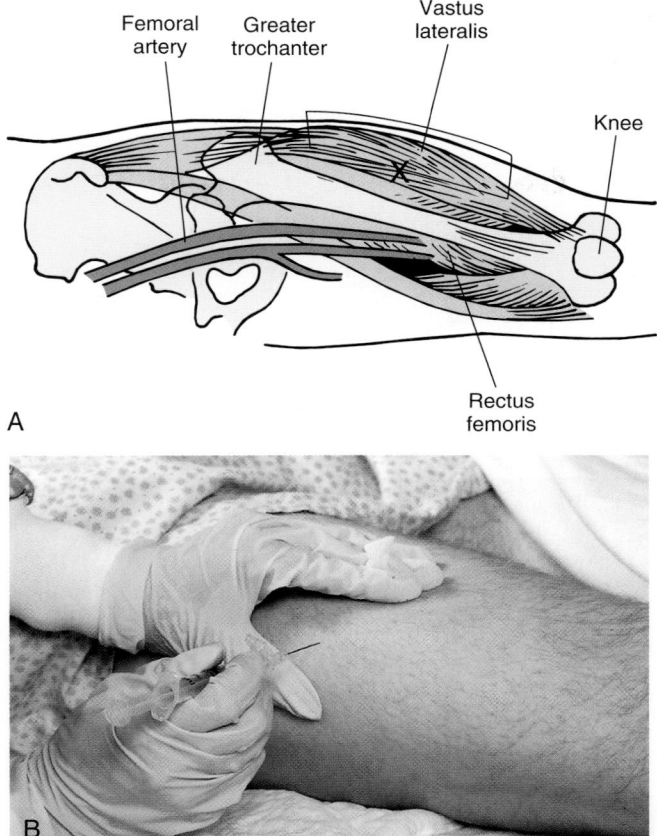

Fig. H-6 Vastus Lateralis Intramuscular Injection. A, Landmarks for IM injection in vastus lateralis. **B,** Giving IM injection in vastus lateralis site. (From Perry AG, Potter PA, and Elkin MK: *Nursing Interventions & Clinical Skills,* ed 5, St. Louis, 2012, Mosby.)

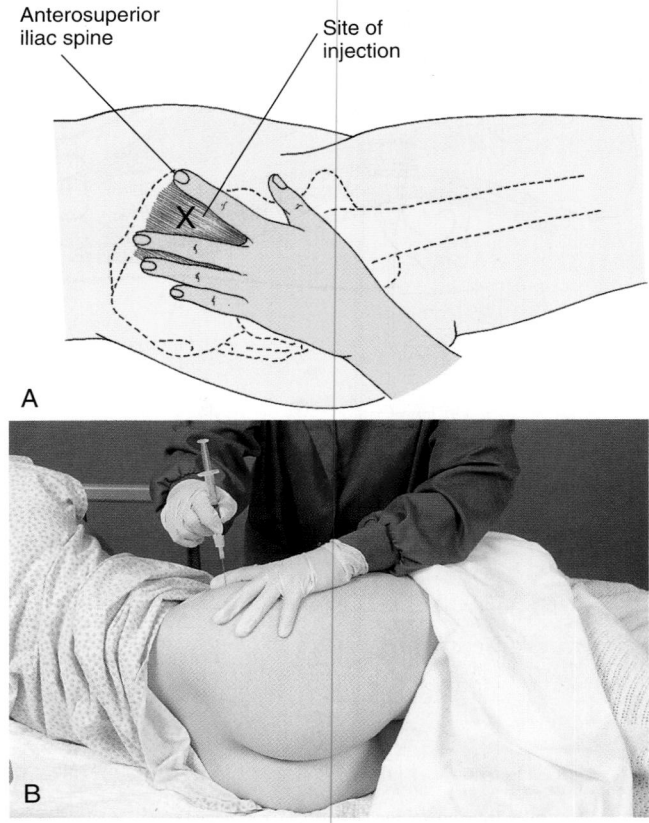

Fig. H-7 Ventrogluteal Intramuscular Injection. A, Anatomical view of ventrogluteal site. **B,** Giving IM injection into ventrogluteal muscle to avoid major nerves and blood vessels. (From Perry AG, Potter PA, and Elkin MK: *Nursing Interventions & Clinical Skills,* ed 5, St. Louis, 2012, Mosby.)

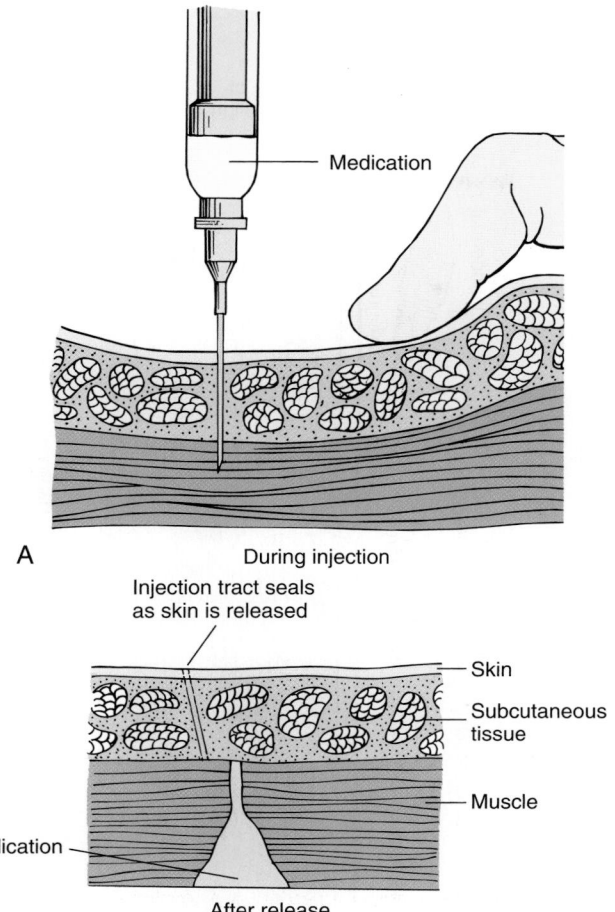

Fig. H-8 Z-Track Method of Injection. A, Pulling on overlying skin during IM injection moves tissues to prevent later tracking. **B,** The Z-track left after injection prevents the deposit of medication through sensitive tissue. (From Perry AG, Potter PA, and Elkin MK: *Nursing Interventions & Clinical Skills,* ed 5, St. Louis, 2012, Mosby.)

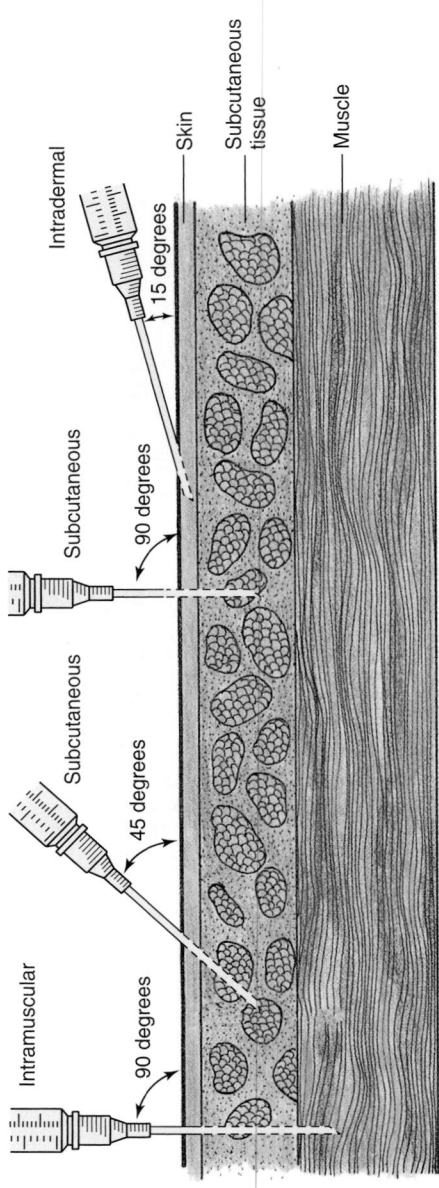

Fig. H-9 Comparison of Needle Angles. Comparison of angles of insertion for IM (90 degrees), SUBCUT (45 degrees and 90 degrees), and ID (15 degrees) injections. (From Potter PA, Perry AG: *Fundamentals of Nursing*, ed 7, St. Louis, 2009, Mosby.)

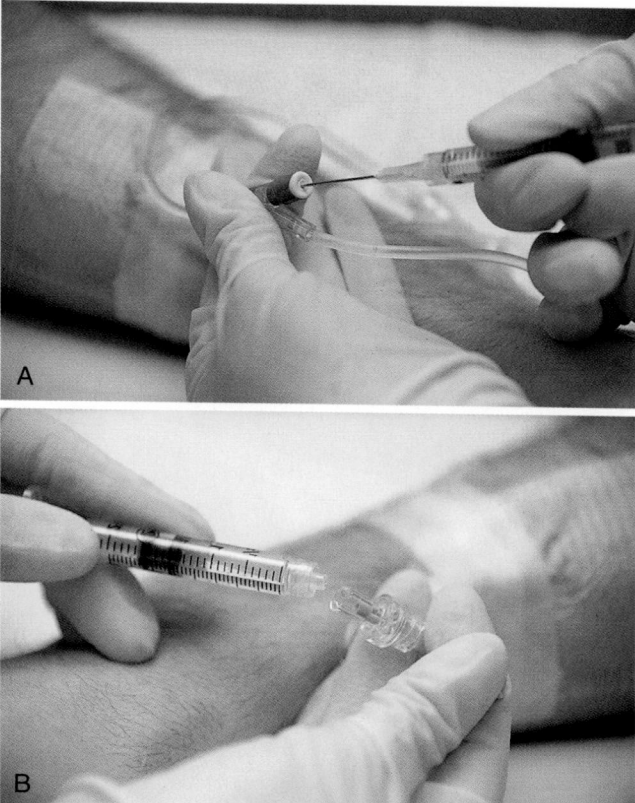

Fig. H-10 Administering Medication by IV Bolus (push). A, Needle system: Insert small-gauge needle of syringe containing prepared drug through center of injection port. **B,**Needleless system: Remove cap of needleless injection port. Connect tip of syringe directly. (From Potter PA, Perry AG: *Fundamentals of Nursing,* ed 6, St. Louis, 2005, Mosby.)

Continued

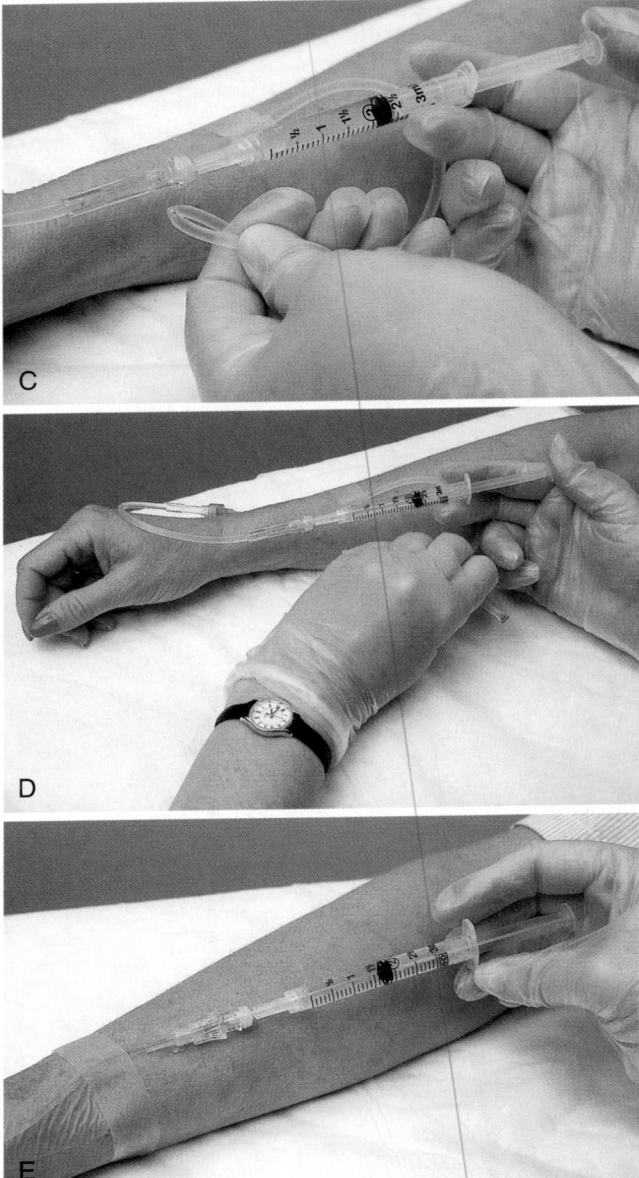

Fig. H-10, cont'd C, Occlude **IV** line by pinching tubing just above injection port. Pull back gently on syringe's plunger to aspirate blood return. **D,** After noting blood return, continue to occlude tubing and inject medication slowly over several minutes (read directions on drug package). Use watch to time administration. **E, IV** lock: Insert needle of syringe containing prepared drug through center of diaphragm. (From Potter PA, Perry AG: *Fundamentals of Nursing,* ed 6, St. Louis, 2005, Mosby.)

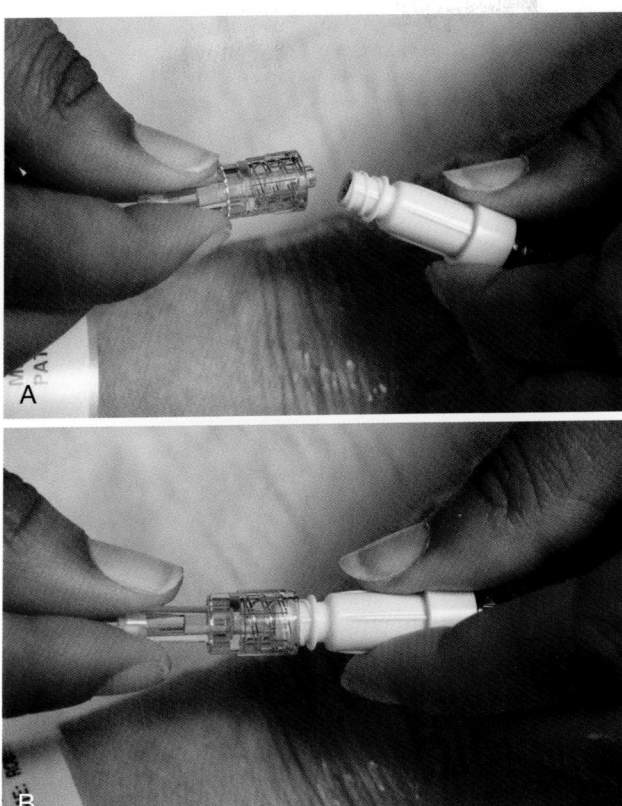

Fig. H-11 Administering IV Medication by Piggyback, Volume Administration Sets of Miniinfusors (Syringe Pump). Use needle-lock device to secure needle of secondary piggyback line through injection port of main line. (From Perry AG, Potter PA, and Elkin MK: *Nursing Interventions & Clinical Skills,* ed 5, St. Louis, 2012, Mosby.)

Index

Entries can be identified as follows: generic name, Trade Name, DRUG CATEGORY

Entries can be identified as follows: generic name, Trade Name, DRUG CATEGORY

Entries can be identified as follows: generic name, Trade Name, DRUG CATEGORY

Entries can be identified as follows: generic name, Trade Name, DRUG CATEGORY

Entries can be identified as follows: generic name, Trade Name, DRUG CATEGORY

- Does the patient have any allergies?
- Is the patient NPO?
- Is the patient taking any other medication and/or herbal supplements that may interact with this drug?
- Are there any vital signs that I need to check before administering the drug?
- Do I need to check any lab values (i.e., glucose)?
- Are there any other assessments that I need to make before giving this drug?

The 5 rights of medication administration

Always adhere to the 5 rights of medication administration when transcribing, preparing, administering, and documenting medications:

1. **Right patient:** Compare the patient's armband with the medication administration record. Compare the patient's name on the medication administration record (MAR) with that on the medication drawer or computerized equipment.
2. **Right drug:** Verify the correct medication by comparing the name on the label on the drug container with that written on the MAR.
3. **Right route:** Check the ordered route by reading the medication order, and verify the appropriateness of the route based on knowledge of the patient's condition.
4. **Right dose:** Always independently double-check dosages of medications with the pharmacy's calculations or with a second nurse. The nurse must also be aware of therapeutic dosages for each medication and question an order that is not within that range.
5. **Right time:** All medications should be administered within 30 minutes of the scheduled time. The medications must also be prepared to correlate appropriately with meal times and to avoid drug interactions.

Following appropriate drug administration, assess the patient for the expected therapeutic outcome and/or potential side effects.

Nomogram for Calculation of Body Surface Area

Place a straight edge from the patient's height in the left column to his or her weight in the right column. The point of intersection on the body surface area column indicates the body surface area (BSA). (Reproduced in Behrman RE, Kliegman RM, Jenson HB: *Nelson Textbook of Pediatrics*, ed 18, Philadelphia, 2007, WB Saunders; nomogram modified from data of E. Boyd by CD West.)

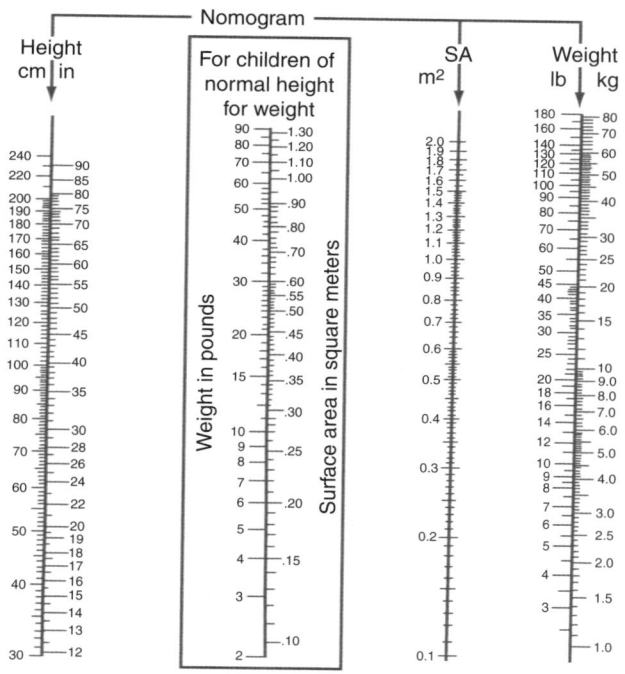

Alternative (Mosteller's formula):

$$\text{Surface area (m}^2\text{)} = \sqrt{\frac{\text{Height (cm)} \times \text{Weight (kg)}}{3600}}$$

Surface area rule:

$$\text{Child dose} = \frac{\text{Surface area (m}^2\text{)} \times \text{Adult dose}}{1.73 \text{ m}^2}$$

BMI formula:

$$\text{BMI} = \frac{\text{Weight (kg)}}{\text{Height (m}^2\text{)}}$$

Syringe Compatibility

	Atropine	Buprenorphine	Butorphanol	ChlorproMAZINE	Codeine	Diazepam	DimenhyDRINATE	DiphenhydrAMINE	Droperidol	Fentanyl	Glycopyrrolate	Heparin
Atropine			C	C		I	C	C	C	C	C	
Buprenorphine												
Butorphanol	C			C		I	I	C	C	C		
ChlorproMAZINE	C		C			I	I	C	C	C	C	C
Codeine						I						
Diazepam	I		I	I	I		I	I	I	I	I	
DimenhyDRINATE	C		I	I		I		C	C	C	I	
DiphenhydrAMINE	C		C	C		I	C		C	C	C	
Droperidol	C		C	C		I	C	C		C	C	I
Fentanyl	C		C	C		I	C	C	C		C	
Glycopyrrolate	C			C		I	I	C	C	C		
Heparin			I	C		I			I			
HydrOXYzine	C		C	C		I	I	C	C	C	C	
Meperidine	C		C	C		I	C	C	C	C	C	I
Metoclopramide	C		C	C		I	C	C	C	C		
Midazolam	C		C	C			I	C	C	C	C	
Morphine	C		C	C		I	C	C	C	C	C	I
Nalbuphine	C					I			C			
Pentazocine	C		C	C		I	C	C	C	C	I	I
Pentobarbital	C		I	I	I	I	I	I	I	I	I	
Perphenazine	C		C	C		I	C	C	C	C		
Prochlorperazine	C		C	C		I	I	C	C	C	C	
Promazine	C			C		I	I	C	C	C	C	
Promethazine	C		C	C		I	I	C	C	C	C	
Ranitidine	C			C			C	C		C	C	
Scopolamine Hbr	C		C	C		I	C	C	C	C	C	
Secobarbital	I		I	I	I	I	I	I	I	I	I	
Thiethylperazine			C			I						

Developed by Providence Memorial Hospital, El Paso, Texas.
NOTE: Give within 15 minutes of mixing.
C = compatible; I = incompatible; ☐ = no documented information.
* = compatibility depends on manufacturer, Wyeth and DuPont forms are incompatible.

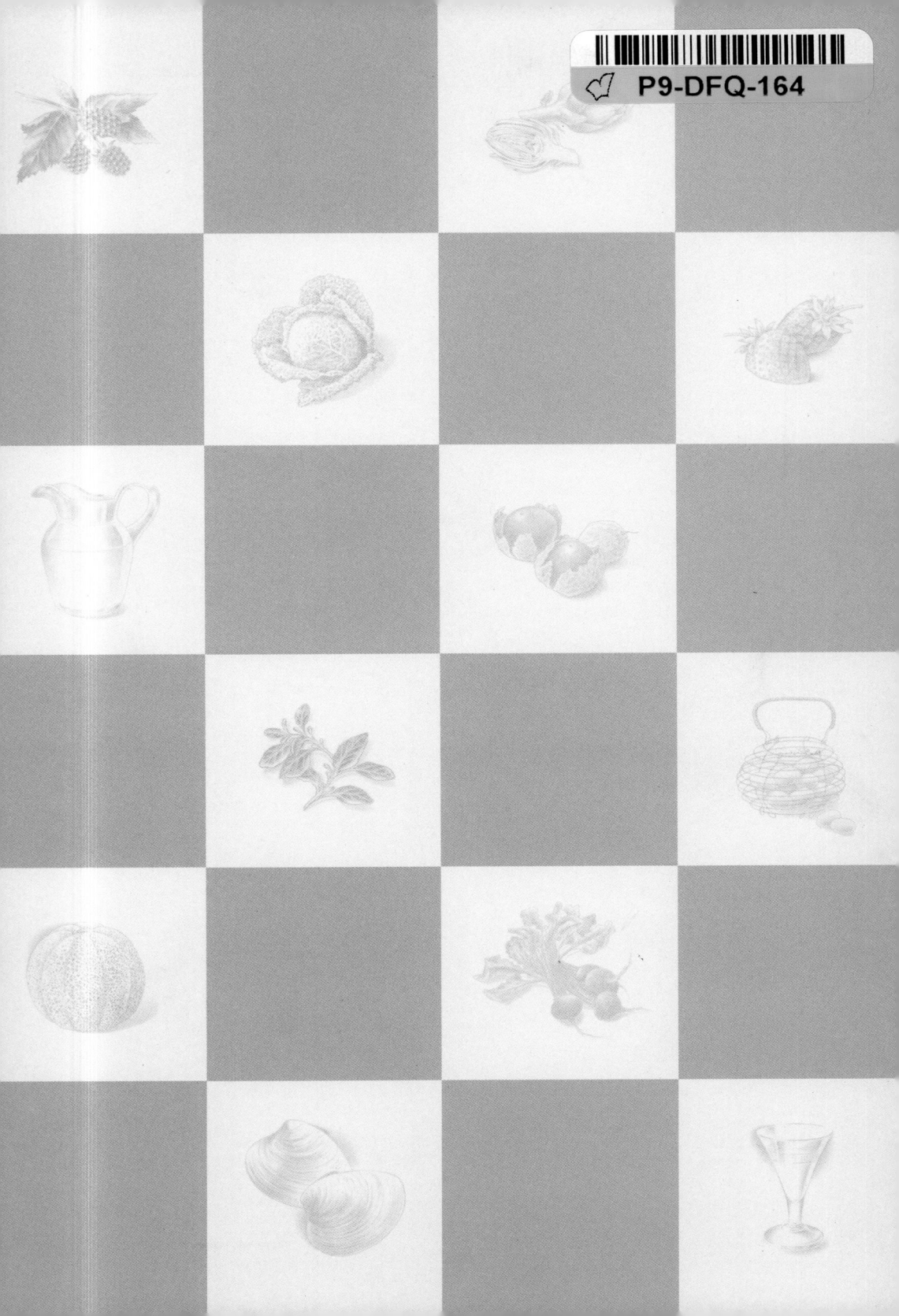

WILLIAMS-SONOMA

KITCHEN
COMPANION

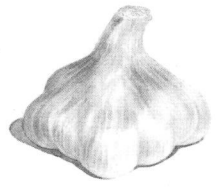

WILLIAMS-SONOMA

KITCHEN
COMPANION

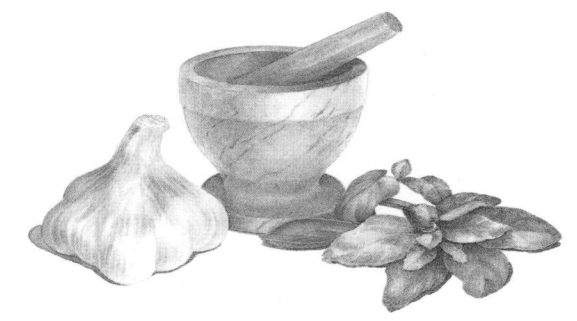

*the A to Z guide to everyday
cooking, equipment & ingredients*

GENERAL EDITOR
Chuck Williams

TEXT BY
Mary Goodbody,
Carolyn Miller & Thy Tran

ILLUSTRATIONS BY
Alice Harth

TIME
LIFE
BOOKS

Time-Life Books is a division of Time Life Inc.
Time-Life is a trademark of Time Warner Inc. and affiliated companies.

TIME LIFE INC.
CHAIRMAN AND CEO: Jim Nelson
PRESIDENT AND COO: Steven L. Janas

TIME-LIFE TRADE PUBLISHING
VICE PRESIDENT AND PUBLISHER: Neil Levin
SENIOR DIRECTOR OF ACQUISITIONS AND EDITORIAL RESOURCES: Jennifer L. Pearce
DIRECTOR OF NEW PRODUCT DEVELOPMENT: Carolyn Clark
DIRECTOR OF MARKETING: Inger Forland
DIRECTOR OF TRADE SALES: Dana Hobson
DIRECTOR OF CUSTOM PUBLISHING: John Lalor
DIRECTOR OF SPECIAL MARKETS: Robert Lombardi
DIRECTOR OF DESIGN: Kate L. McConnell
PROJECT MANAGER: Jennifer L. Ward

WILLIAMS-SONOMA
FOUNDER AND VICE-CHAIRMAN: Chuck Williams
BOOK BUYER: Cecilia Michaelis

WELDON OWEN INC.
CHIEF EXECUTIVE OFFICER: John Owen
PRESIDENT: Terry Newell
CHIEF OPERATING OFFICER: Larry Partington
VICE PRESIDENT, INTERNATIONAL SALES: Stuart Laurence
MANAGING EDITOR: Sarah Putman
COPY EDITOR: Sharon Silva
CONSULTING EDITOR: Norman Kolpas
EXPERT READERS: Pam Anderson, Molly Stevens, Susan Derecskey
ASSOCIATE EDITOR: Heather Belt
CREATIVE DIRECTOR: Gaye Allen
ART DIRECTOR: Jamie Leighton
DESIGN ASSISTANT: Sarah Gifford
BOOK DESIGN: Lori Barra and Andrew Faulkner, TonBo Designs
PRODUCTION DESIGNER: Jan Martí, Command Z
STUDIO MANAGER: Brynn Breuner
PRODUCTION ASSISTANTS: Linda Bouchard, Joan Olson
ILLUSTRATOR: Alice Harth
ILLUSTRATION EDITORS: Thy Tran, Judith Dunham
PRODUCTION DIRECTOR: Stephanie Sherman
PRODUCTION MANAGER: Chris Hemesath
PROOFREADERS: Desne Border, Ken DellaPenta, Carrie Bradley, Mu'frida Bell, Ellen Klages

Williams-Sonoma *Kitchen Companion* was conceived and produced by Weldon Owen Inc.,
814 Montgomery Street, San Francisco, California 94133, in collaboration with Williams-Sonoma,
3250 Van Ness Avenue, San Francisco, California 94109.

A Weldon Owen Production

First printed in 2000.
10 9 8 7 6 5 4 3 2 1

Printed in Hong Kong by Midas Printing Limited.

Library of Congress Cataloging-in-Publication Data:

Williams-Sonoma kitchen companion: the A to Z guide to everyday cooking,
equipment, and ingredients/Chuck Williams, general editor.
p. cm.
ISBN 0-7370-2051-2 (softcover)
1. Cookery—Encyclopedias. I. Williams, Chuck.
TX349.W47 2000
641.5'03—dc21
00-037386

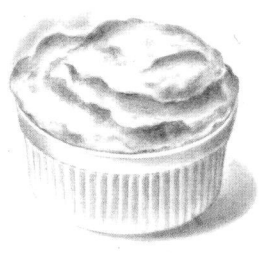

"Cooking is often
one disaster after another.
What you learn is the only thing
you can't fix is a soufflé."

—*Julia Child*

foreword

LIKE MANY GOOD IDEAS, THIS BOOK HAD ITS START IN AN UNEXPECTED WAY.

One morning, a letter arrived on my desk at Williams-Sonoma. It was from a frequent customer who had recently bought a muffin pan. "Chuck," she lamented, "no matter what I do, my muffins get very brown on top before they're cooked through. Please tell me how to keep the tops of my muffins from burning!"

The problem, I came to realize, is that nowadays fewer and fewer people have had a true understanding of cooking passed down to them. We once learned to cook by watching a parent or grandparent in the kitchen—seeing how they worked, discovering how they made adjustments to a recipe, and hearing their insights. Now, many people can only follow a recipe to the letter, unable to diverge from the stated steps and unable to compensate for gaps in the instructions or differing conditions in their own kitchens.

What if, I wondered, there was one compact book to which people could turn whenever they needed important everyday cooking information and needed it immediately? What if we could create the printed equivalent of having a knowledgeable companion standing by your side in the kitchen, one who could provide you with straightforward answers and commonsense advice at a glance?

This was the inspiration for Williams-Sonoma *Kitchen Companion*.

As our team of expert writers and editors went ahead with the project, we developed another goal for the book as well. We wanted to make it not just knowledgeable but also interesting and readable, a book you could pick up, dip into, and enjoy even when you weren't faced with a specific question or pressing problem. Consequently, we've done our best to make the entries intriguing and fun.

I hope you'll find this book a welcome addition to your own kitchen library, one to which you'll happily turn again and again.

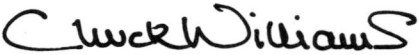

(If you're having problems with your own muffins, you'll find some possible solutions on page 297.)

How to Use This Book

WILLIAMS-SONOMA *KITCHEN COMPANION* is an everyday cooking reference for real-life cooks. It is meant to be used alongside a cookbook, cooking article, or recipe. It provides background information, clarifies unfamiliar terms, explains the whys behind recipe instructions, and helps the cook identify and avoid potential problems and pitfalls.

In order to achieve these goals, the book presents its information in a carefully structured format with the following key features used consistently throughout:

ALPHABETICAL ORGANIZATION For ease of reference, entries are presented in alphabetical order, from "Abalone" to "Zucchini."

INGREDIENT ENTRIES Basic ingredients receive their own entries and include general guidelines on selection, storage, and preparation. Broader entries such as "Fish" and "Spice" provide detailed glossaries of ingredients included in that category.

COOKWARE AND EQUIPMENT ENTRIES Important kitchen appliances receive separate alphabetical entries. Broader entries under such headings as "Bakeware," "Baking Tools," "Cooking Tools," and "Cookware" contain detailed subentries on a wide variety of items.

COOKING METHOD ENTRIES Key cooking methods such as "Frying" and "Roasting" are covered by extensive explanations.

TECHNIQUES AND TERMS ENTRIES Detailed entries explain cooking techniques and terms, from "Adjusting the Seasoning" to "Zesting."

CHARTS Throughout the book, charts provide easy, at-a-glance references to information such as cooking times and methods for various grains or acceptable substitutions for common ingredients.

STEP-BY-STEP "HOW TO'S" Many entries contain basic methods for preparing ingredients or for performing specific cooking techniques, all explained step by step.

ILLUSTRATIONS More than 800 line drawings illustrate ingredients, types of equipment, and step-by-step instructions.

CROSS-REFERENCES The book is extensively cross-referenced to help you quickly find the information you need however you might first try to look it up. Cross-references at the end of many entries also direct you to similar or related terms, ingredients, equipment, or techniques.

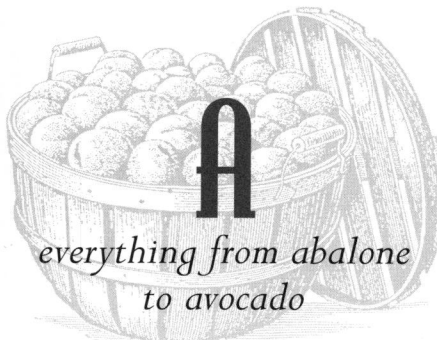

*everything from abalone
to avocado*

ABALONE With its sweet meat and beautiful shell lined with mother-of-pearl, this shellfish is native to the coasts of California and Alaska but is now rarely found fresh, and its harvesting is regulated. Most of us must settle for the canned version. If you come across live abalone in the fish market, snap it up, knowing you have a rare prize on your hands. Use it in recipes that call for squid, keeping in mind that, like squid, it overcooks easily and should be cooked for no longer than a minute or two.
Selecting Fresh abalone must be alive when you buy it. Check the meat inside the shell to make sure it moves when touched and that it looks plump and shiny. The shellfish should have a sweet smell, not an "off" odor. Canned and frozen abalone are available in Asian markets; frozen abalone is often pretenderized and can be very good.
Storing Live abalone should be kept refrigerated for no longer than 1 day. Canned abalone should be refrigerated after opening, covered with water, for not more than 4 days. Frozen will keep for 3 months.
Preparing Remove fresh abalone meat from its shell by running a knife under it to loosen it, and discard the innards, using only the large muscle. The meat of the abalone muscle is tough and must be

tenderized by pounding to make it palatable. Use a meat mallet or rolling pin to pound and flatten the muscle to a thickness of ¼ inch or less. Score the meat, cutting a series of shallow slashes across its surface, to keep it from curling as it cooks.

ACHIOTE Another name for annatto seed. See SPICE.

ACID The word *acid* may not sound appetizing, but the sour substances it names play important roles in food and cooking.

Vinegar, lemon juice, and wine are examples of acids used in cooking for flavor and astringency, contributing a tart, sour, or bitter note to a dish.

Like salt, an acid can preserve food, as in the case of the vinegar used for pickling.

An acid can react with an alkaline, or base, substance to form a gas, a critical step in baking. Baking powder, a mixture of acid and alkaline substances, releases carbon dioxide gas when exposed to moisture or heat, causing a baked good to rise.

Lemons.

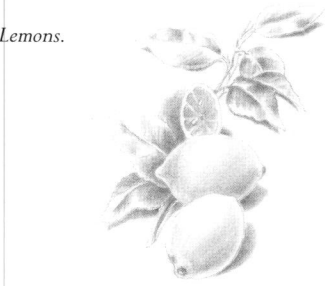

Acids break down proteins and are used to tenderize the surface of meats and fish. In the case of seviche, thin slices of fish or shellfish become firm and opaque when marinated in an acid, just as they would when cooked. On the other hand, acid added to vegetables and legumes will interfere with their cooking and softening.

Acids also act to prevent the discoloration of certain foods that occurs when they are cut and exposed to air. To slow the browning, lemon juice is commonly sprinkled or rubbed on the cut surfaces of fruits and vegetables.

See also BAKING POWDER & BAKING SODA; CREAM OF TARTAR; DISCOLORING; NONREACTIVE; VINEGAR.

ACIDULATED WATER See ACID; DISCOLORING.

ADJUSTING THE SEASONING
Many recipes instruct you to "adjust" or "correct" a given dish, usually near the end of the recipe. This means adding more salt, pepper, and any other appropriate herb or spice after tasting the cooked dish. Flavors meld and change as they cook, so it's important to gauge and adjust the seasoning to your liking just before serving. Take care to add seasonings in small amounts and to taste often when correcting. It is possible to add more but not to remove what you have already added. Also, do not taste a food until it has reached a stage at which you would consider it safe to eat. See also DONENESS; SEASONING; TASTING.

ADZUKI BEAN See BEAN, DRIED.

AGAR-AGAR See SEAWEED.

AIOLI (IY-o-lee) A pungent garlic-flavored mayonnaise that is highly popular in the south of France. The word derives from a combination of the Provençal words for garlic, *ail*, and oil, *oli*.

Quick Bite

In Provence, aioli is traditionally served with poached salt cod and boiled green beans, carrots, beets, and eggs for a festive summertime meal called *le grand aïoli*.

ALCOHOL Wine, beer, and spirits are fermented or distilled beverages, usually created from fruits or grains, that contain a percentage of ethyl alcohol, which can be intoxicating. They are added to both savory and sweet recipes for flavor. These versatile beverages can also add welcome color to a dish, as in the case of a ruby red wine sauce for poached fruit, or they can be used for basting meat to give it rich color and flavor. Wine is an especially popular ingredient in sauces and braising liquids. Through reducing, the flavor of the wine may be intensified and its consistency thickened, delivering a pleasing, fruity taste and rich body to the finished dish.

Alcohol adds more than just flavor and color to food. When spirits or wine are cooked, the alcohol in them does not completely evaporate. Between 5 and 85 percent of the alcohol may remain, depending on the cooking time, temperature, and type of beverage.

See also LIQUEUR; REDUCING; SPIRITS; WINE.

AL DENTE (AL DEN-tay) This Italian phrase, which literally means "to the tooth," indicates that pasta has been cooked until it is tender but still chewy, offering some resistance to the bite. The same term is also sometimes used as an indication of doneness for certain sturdy vegetables, such as green beans, carrots, and asparagus, and for risotto.

Removing pasta for testing.

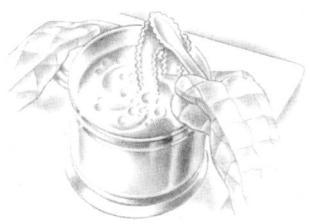

ALLSPICE See SPICE.

ALMOND See NUT.

ALUMINUM FOIL Found in virtually
every American home, aluminum foil is
one of the most versatile kitchen supplies.
It is useful for lining broiling and roasting
pans, for covering pans and baking dishes
that lack lids, for cooking food in a pocket
or pouch, and for wrapping cooked food
to keep it hot. Use it to tent turkeys and
chickens during the later stages of roasting
to prevent overbrowning, and to shield the
rims of pie crusts in the oven to keep them
from scorching. Many home cooks line the
bottom of the oven and the firebox of their
grill with heavy-duty aluminum foil to
deflect heat and ease cleanup.

When aluminum foil is used to line a
pan, an oven, or a firebox, its shiny side
should face outward. This deflects the heat
most effectively, promoting even cooking.

ANCHOVY This tiny fish makes a big impression, attracting or repelling people in
equal measure. Anchovies are indigenous to
the Mediterranean and the Atlantic coast-
lines of Spain and Portugal and are used
widely in the cuisines of those countries, as
well as in Italy and southern France. They
are an important ingredient in Caesar salad
and in tapenade, a boldly flavored paste
made from olives, capers, and anchovies.
When added to a dish during cooking, the
anchovy fillets will virtually dissolve,
leaving only a surprisingly subtle, nonfishy
dimension of flavor.
Selecting Anchovies are generally
boned, cured, packed in oil, and sold in
small cans. Rarely are they found fresh
in the United States. Look for them in the
canned fish section in 2-ounce jars or tins.
Although jarred are generally more expensive, they offer better flavor and texture.

In Italy, anchovies are also commonly
sold packed in salt, and many American
chefs and cooks prefer those. In delicatessens, salted anchovies are typically sold
by weight from a large opened can. They
must be boned and rinsed before using.

Anchovy fillets.

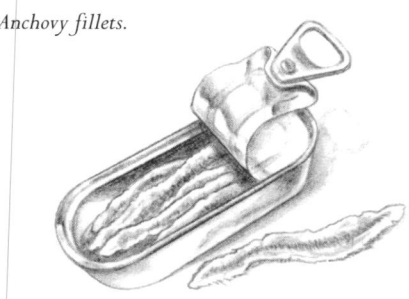

Storing Once a can of oil-packed fillets is
opened, transfer any leftover fillets and oil
to a small glass or plastic container, cover,
and refrigerate for up to 1 week. Add more
olive oil if needed to keep the fillets covered. Salted anchovies should be kept in a
tightly covered glass or other nonreactive
container (salt is corrosive) or a zippered
plastic bag in the refrigerator. They will
keep for several weeks. Once the seal is
broken on a tube of anchovy paste, the tube
should be refrigerated. Capped securely, it
will last for up to several months.
Preparing Lift oil-packed anchovies from
their oil and drain on paper towels before
using. Some cooks also rinse the oil-packed
fillets under cold running water.

To prepare salted anchovies for use,
rinse well under cold running water and
scrape off their skins with a small, sharp
knife. Split open along the backbone, cutting off the dorsal fins. Then pull out the
spines and rinse the fillets well. Pat dry
with paper towels, place in a glass or other
nonreactive bowl, pour in enough olive
oil to cover with a thin layer, cover tightly,
and refrigerate. Use within 2 weeks.

ANISEED See SPICE.

ANNATTO SEED See SPICE.

APPLE It should be easy to eat an apple a day, considering they are perhaps the most common tree fruit in the world. There are some 7,000 known apple varieties in the world today. Of course, far fewer are available to the average shopper. The most common varieties sold in the United States are Red Delicious, Golden Delicious, Granny Smith, Gala, and McIntosh. Keep an eye open, too, for recently revived heirloom apples, old-fashioned varieties that fell out of favor with big commercial growers because of difficulties in large-scale growing, storing, and shipping. Many kinds with excellent flavor and texture can now be found in farmers' or specialty markets.

Selecting Look for unbroken skin with good color and no soft brown spots. Whenever possible, buy newly harvested local apples. Most apples are picked in autumn or winter; a few summer varieties (Maiden Blush, Transparent, Gravenstein) exist. The Australian crop helps to fill American fruit bins in the summer.

Although some apple lovers may insist that the sweeter apples, such as the Fuji and the Gala, are good for eating out of hand, while tarter, firmer ones, such as the Granny Smith, are better suited for cooking and baking, such tart and sweet distinctions are completely subjective. See the Apple Glossary at right for a few pointers.

Storing Because apples continue to ripen at room temperature, refrigerate them in the cold back part of the refrigerator for 1 week or longer. If you plan to eat them soon after purchase, they can be held at room temperature for a few days.

Preparing A small, sharp knife is all you need for peeling and slicing apples, although a vegetable peeler may be easier for

Apple Glossary

Each apple variety has its own unique properties. Sample the range available in your local stores and farmers' markets to discover which ones you like. Following are some of the most popular varieties.

CORTLAND This red-skinned apple with snow-white flesh has a pleasing tartness and a firm texture. It is good for eating out of hand and for adding to fruit salads. Because it breaks down in cooking it is ideal for applesauce, although it is not as suitable for pies and the like.
EMPIRE Red- or green-skinned, this juicy apple with a tart-sweet flavor and creamy flesh is a cross between Red Delicious and McIntosh. It's good for applesauce and delicious eaten out of hand.
FUJI The Fuji, with its yellowish-green skin and juicy white flesh, has a sweet and slightly spicy flavor. This apple, developed in Japan in the 1960s, is particularly prized for eating out of hand.
GALA Native to New Zealand, the Gala is pleasantly sweet and crisp, with golden skin and a rosy overtone. It is best for eating raw, or for sautéing or slow baking.
GOLDEN DELICIOUS Sweet, juicy, and mild, this is probably the most widely available apple, good for eating raw, frying, and making pies. Its flesh does not darken as readily as that of other apples, and it holds its shape during baking. *continued*

Apple Glossary, continued

GRANNY SMITH Originally from Australia, this bright green apple boasts white, firm, juicy flesh that is sweet and tart at the same time. It is good for eating, sautéing, and baking.

HONEYCRISP This large apple, with its streaks of red and green, has a juicy, crisp flesh and mellow flavor. Good for eating raw or for a wide variety of cooking methods.

IDA RED A good-looking red apple with a hint of green, this mildly tart fruit is prized for baking and cooking.

JONAGOLD This cross between the Jonathan and the Golden Delicious has red-streaked yellow skin and firm, sweet, juicy white flesh. Use it for eating or cooking.

JONATHAN Most Jonathans are used for baking and cooking, although the golden apples with red stripes and juicy yellow flesh are good eaten raw, too.

MCINTOSH This is a fall favorite, with its red skin and crisp, white, juicy flesh. Macs, as they are affectionately known, have flesh that softens when cooked, making good applesauce.

NORTHERN SPY Red-blushed with green undertones, this juicy, sweet apple makes wonderful pies and sauces and holds its shape when baked. It is good for eating raw, too.

PIPPIN The term *pippin* turns up in a number of apple names, but the best known of them is the Newtown pippin, usually simply called pippin. This all-purpose apple, with its pale green or yellow skin 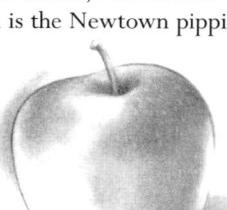 and creamy flesh, has a bright, tart, full flavor and firm texture that make it a favorite in pies.

RED DELICIOUS A popular eating apple that looks just how we all imagine an apple should. Unfortunately, due to overlong storage or supermarkets' selling the Red Delicious out of its natural season, many specimens have a mushy and tasteless flesh. Shop for your Red Delicious at a farmers' market so that you can buy in season and taste before you buy. This apple cooks down well into applesauce but is not recommended for baking or frying.

RHODE ISLAND GREENING A lovely green apple with crisp, tart, juicy, green-toned flesh that is excellent for pies and applesauce, as well as for eating out of hand.

ROME BEAUTY This large, red apple has sweet-tart, firm flesh and holds its shape when baked, which explains why it is among the most popular apples for filling with sweet or savory stuffings and baking whole.

WINESAP Sometimes called Stayman Winesap, this dark red apple has firm, crisp flesh and a sweet, winy flavor, characteristics that give it a loyal following among apple aficionados. It is not a good keeper, however, losing its crispness quickly. Its partisans recommend it for eating raw and for cooking.

YORK Mildly tart, this deep red apple with green stripes is a very good baking apple and makes fine applesauce.

the novice cook to use. Specially designed apple corers are available. Exposed apple flesh quickly discolors unless it is rubbed with lemon or other citrus juice. Since so many nutrients are in the skin of the apple, it is a good idea to leave it on when possible.

Quick Bite

Apples are grown widely, but those from colder northern climates are most prized. The Northeast and Pacific Northwest are the best-known apple-growing regions in the United States, with the largest crops coming from the states of Washington and New York.

See also CORING.

APRICOT Most apricots are canned, made into preserves, or dried, but once you experience a perfectly ripened fresh specimen, you will look forward to their brief season. Native to northern China, where they still grow wild, apricots are at their peak in July, but as they do not travel well, being easily bruised, they are not as widely available as peaches, nectarines, and other seasonal kin. They are small, too, less than half the size of a peach.

Selecting Look for fresh apricots with high golden color. When fully ripe, they will give slightly when gently pressed, similarly to a peach. Dark green unripe fruit will never ripen correctly. Light green unripe specimens may ripen satisfactorily.

Storing Eat ripe apricots as soon as possible. If you must store them, refrigerate them for up to 2 days. Those that are not fully ripe should be left at room temperature to ripen.

Preparing If a recipe requires peeled apricots, see BLANCHING.

See also DRIED FRUIT.

ARROWROOT See THICKENING.

ARTICHOKE Few vegetables look as forbidding as the artichoke. But for many cooks, this ungainly flower bud, harvested from a plant of the sizable thistle family, is a culinary treasure with a mild, nutty flavor to be savored. "Baby" artichokes are gaining in popularity and appearing on menus around the country, but most artichoke fanciers relish larger vegetables with more to them to enjoy. Baby artichokes are not immature artichokes, but simply small ones grown lower down on the plant. Whether large, medium, or small, all artichokes cultivated for commercial sale are Green Globe artichokes, which can be rounded or cone shaped.

Selecting The primary artichoke season is in early spring, followed by a second, smaller season in fall-winter. Buy artichokes that are heavy for their size. Look for tightly closed, olive green leaves and moist, healthy stems. A few purple streaks on the leaves are acceptable, but limp, brownish globes should be passed by. Some winter artichokes have black streaking, which indicates slight frost damage and is nothing to worry about. In fact, some artichoke lovers think these later vegetables are preferable to spring ones for their slightly nutty flavor. Baby artichokes should be olive green with tightly closed leaves.

If a recipe calls for artichoke hearts, use fresh ones or buy frozen or water-packed canned hearts, which are readily available in supermarkets. For cooked preparations, avoid small jars of marinated artichokes, as they add unwanted oil and flavorings to a recipe. They are, however, good in salads and as part of an antipasto spread.

Storing Sprinkle artichokes with a few drops of water and store in a perforated plastic bag in the coldest part of the refrigerator for up to 1 week. If cooking them on the day you buy them, leave them at cool room temperature. Once opened, marinated artichoke hearts will keep refrigerated for up to 2 weeks.

Quick Tip

Use only stainless-steel knives and cookware when preparing artichokes, since carbon steel, aluminum, and cast iron will discolor the vegetable within moments of cutting. No matter what you do, artichokes will darken somewhat, but fortunately this discoloration does not affect their flavor.

HOW TO *Trim an Artichoke*

1. Starting at the base, pull off and discard the tough outer leaves.

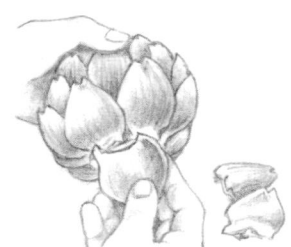

2. Cut the stem off flush with the bottom of the leaves and discard it.

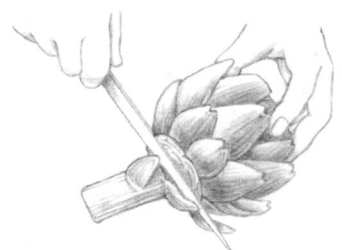

3. Using a serrated knife, slice off the top 1 to 2 inches of the remaining leaves to remove the thorns, or use kitchen shears to trim off each thorny leaf top. If you are not cooking the artichoke immediately, sprinkle all the cut surfaces with lemon juice to minimize discoloring.

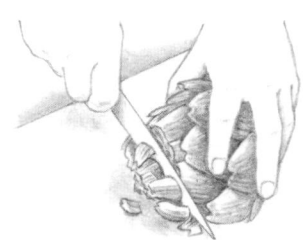

Removing the Choke Every large artichoke has an inedible fuzzy center, called a choke, that must be removed before eating. It is easiest to remove the choke after cooking since cooking softens the fibers, but some recipes direct you to remove the choke before cooking. Either way, there are several methods for removing the choke from an artichoke. You can halve the globes lengthwise and scrape the choke from either half with the edge of a spoon or with a small, sharp knife. You can also gently spread open the leaves from the top of a whole globe (this is easier after the top has been trimmed) and dig out the choke with a knife or spoon. This method is especially useful when making stuffed artichokes. After removing the choke this way, press the leaves back together to restore the artichoke's globe shape. If you want only the heart, you can remove all the leaves and then trim away the choke.

Artichoke hearts.

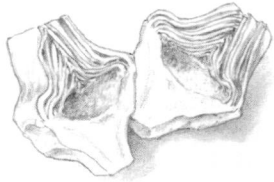

Or, you can serve a whole cooked artichoke with the choke intact and eat it as described in the section below entitled "Eating an Artichoke."

Baby artichokes can be as tiny as walnuts and do not have developed chokes, but you will still need to trim the stems, pull off the dark outer leaves, and cut away the spiny tops before cooking.

Artichokes are generally boiled or steamed, although they are also sometimes braised with other vegetables. They can be halved or quartered and roasted, as well. Baby artichokes are also delicious fried. If very young, they can be thinly sliced and eaten raw.

Quick Bite

Artichokes contain an acid called cynarin that causes most other foods or beverages you are consuming along with them to taste slightly sweet. This can make the crisp white wine with which you began your meal suddenly taste "off." To combat this effect, some cooks recommend serving Champagne or sparkling wine, rather than still wines, with artichokes.

Eating an Artichoke Eating an artichoke may sound like it takes a lot of effort, but the flavorful reward makes it well worth it. To eat large whole cooked artichokes, pull off the leaves one at a time, dip their thick, fleshy bases in melted butter, lemon juice, mayonnaise, vinaigrette, hollandaise sauce, or another dip, and then remove the sweet flesh from the bottom of each leaf by scraping it between your teeth. Discard the tough upper portion of the leaf. When you reach the last of the lighter-colored tender inner leaves, pull them out and discard them. If the fuzzy choke is not already removed, scrape it out with a spoon and eat the delicious heart.

See also BOILING; STEAMING.

ARUGULA Also known as rocket, this pleasantly peppery green has sword-shaped, deeply notched leaves usually no more than 2 or 3 inches long. Adding arugula to other milder salad greens results in a salad with a nicely sharp, spicy edge. It is much favored in Italy, where it is also used in pasta sauces and to top pizzas hot from the oven. Arugula can be added to soups and sauces, too.

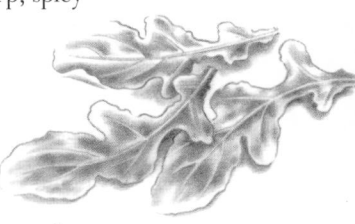

Selecting Arugula is generally sold in small bunches, often with the root ends standing in a shallow tub of water to maintain freshness. Occasionally it is sold as prewashed loose leaves. Look for fresh-looking bunches of long, slender, young leaves. Do not worry if they droop slightly. Mature arugula can be too sharply flavored for all but the most hard-core aficionado.

Storing Wrap the stems in damp paper towels and slip the bunch into a loosely sealed plastic bag, or wrap it loosely in a kitchen towel. Store loose leaves in a plastic bag. Store in the refrigerator crisper and use within 2 days.

Preparing Trim thick stalk ends and rinse the leaves thoroughly under cool water. Shake dry or spin in a salad spinner. Toss with other clean, dry greens.

See also GREENS, SALAD.

ASIAN PEAR See PEAR, ASIAN.

ASPARAGUS Among the produce market's tastiest harbingers of spring, asparagus is most delicious in its true season—but very good fresh asparagus is available all year long. These tall, crisp-tender spears can be pencil-thin or as thick as a man's thumb. Thin spears and thick each have their devoted followers. Steam or boil fresh spears vertically in an asparagus steamer or horizontally in a large frying pan (not a crowded saucepan) and serve hot, topped with melted butter and a squeeze of lemon juice, or cold, dressed with vinaigrette. Asparagus is heavenly when coated with olive oil and roasted in the oven or grilled. Slender spears are good sautéed in a bit of olive oil or but-ter and tossed with pasta; stockier spears are good additions to soups and stews. Canned and frozen are also available but are inferior to fresh.

Selecting Look for firm stalks and tight, dry, and often purple-tinged tips, avoiding those that are moist looking. The cut end should look freshly cut and not too dried out. If there is slight spreading at the top, the spears are still good. The length of the shoot should be all or mostly green. The white at the bottom should be discarded before cooking.

Most asparagus sold in the United States is green, but white asparagus, beloved in Europe, is becoming increasingly popular. It is the same vegetable, but given an exotic look and more delicate flavor by keeping the growing spears carefully covered with soil so only the tips emerge. This prevents sunlight from reaching the shoots and de-veloping their chlorophyll. There is also a purple variety, which turns green when cooked and tends to be a little sweeter than regular asparagus.

Storing Cook asparagus as soon as pos-sible after purchase. If you must store it, cut off an inch or so of the stalk at the base and set the bunch in a shallow pan of water for up to 4 days.

Preparing Bend the cut end of each spear until it breaks naturally. It will snap precisely where the fibrous, tough inedible portion begins.

Snapping off tough ends.

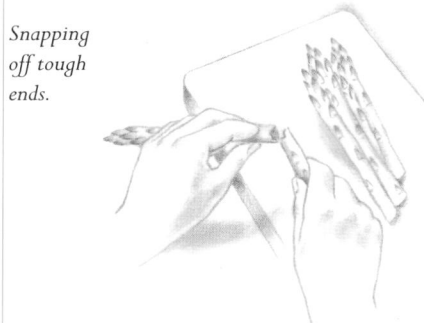

While the spears will be of unequal length, their flavor and texture will be uniformly glorious. If you favor a consistent length, trim snapped spears with a knife. If the spears have a thick or fibrous skin (check by taking a small bite), peel them to within about 1 inch of the tips.

Peeling asparagus.

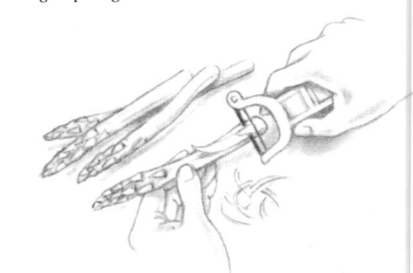

Quick Bite

Canned white asparagus from Spain, particu-larly from Navarre, is full flavored and tender, ideal for serving with a vinaigrette made from Spanish olive oil and sherry vinegar. In some people's opinion, these tinned Iberian spears rival the best fresh asparagus.

AVOCADO Buttery and rich, this tropical tree fruit is mistakenly regarded as a vegetable. The primary ingredient in guacamole, it is also wonderful in salads or sandwiches, and is frequently served halved, pitted, and filled with shrimp salad, chicken salad, or a thick mustard vinaigrette. Avocados are at their best when served raw or only slightly heated, as their silky texture and mildly nutty flavor do not hold up in cooking. Although high in fat—they contain about 30 percent unsaturated fat—avocados also boast a good amount of protein for a fruit.

Selecting Avocados are available year-round, with a large winter harvest filling market bins in January and February and a large summer harvest from June through August. Two major varieties are commonly available: the dark green, dimple-skinned Hass (or Haas) and the smoother, paler green Fuerte. The former has a far richer flavor and texture. Look for dark, rough skin when buying Hass and smooth, unblemished skin when buying Fuerte. Both varieties yield to gentle finger pressure when ripe. Avoid avocados that feel mushy or show signs of mold.

Storing Store ripe avocados at cool room temperature for up to 2 days, or in the refrigerator for up to 1 week. Keep unripe avocados in a warm, dark place. After a few days, they should pass the pressure test. When this occurs, you may cut and use the Fuerte avocado, but let the Hass ripen a day longer; too often, avocados are served before they are fully ripe, denying the eater the fruit's full, rich flavor. To speed the ripening process, put the avocado in a paper bag with an apple, a banana, or a tomato. Ethylene gases emitted by the other fruit will hasten ripening.

To store a cut avocado, wrap it in plastic wrap, smoothing the wrap right onto the fruit's cut surface to seal out air and prevent discoloring.

Preparing Since the flesh of an avocado quickly turns brown when exposed to air, cut the fruit just before serving. Sprinkling the cut flesh with a little lemon or lime juice will help slow the discoloring.

HOW TO *Halve an Avocado*

1. Using a small, sharp knife, cut the avocado in half lengthwise, cutting carefully around the large, round pit at the center.
2. Rotate the halves in opposite directions to separate them.

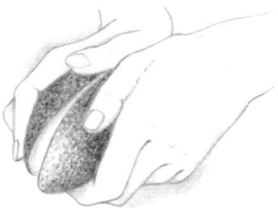

3. Scoop out the pit with the tip of a spoon and discard. Or, holding the avocado with a pot holder or kitchen towel to protect your hand, carefully strike the pit with the heel of a large, sharp knife so that the blade lodges in it, and draw out the pit.

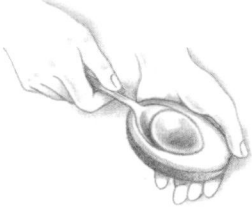

4. Ease a large spoon between the avocado flesh and the peel and gently scoop out the flesh, scraping as closely to the peel as possible. Alternatively, peel away the skin with the knife.

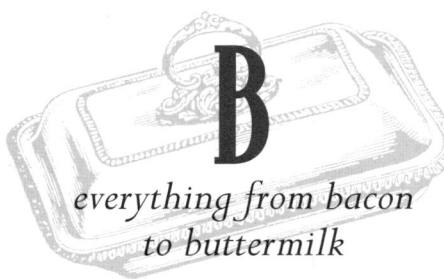

everything from bacon to buttermilk

b

BACK BACON See CANADIAN BACON.

BACON A little bit of bacon goes a long way—although it's easy to eat more than just a little! Cut from the belly (called the side) of the hog below the spareribs, it is cured and usually smoked, which contributes to its irresistible flavor. Bacon is delicious with eggs, crumbled over salads, used to top baked dishes, and in sandwiches: the BLT—bacon, lettuce, and tomato—is an American classic. In the South, bacon fat is traditionally used to cook mustard, collard, and other sturdy greens.

Generally, bacon is about 50 percent fat, although leaner versions can be as low as 33 percent fat. As bacon cooks, its fat becomes liquid and separates from the meat, a process known as rendering. If fat rendered from frying bacon is not used for the recipe at hand, it can be poured off into a tightly covered container, stored in the refrigerator or freezer, and used for sautéing or frying other foods. If you don't wish to use it for cooking, pour the fat off into a coffee can or similar container, keep the can in a cool, dark place, and add to it until the can is full. Then discard the fat sensibly (never down the sink!).

Selecting Most people buy bacon already cut into slices and packaged in clear plastic in the meat section of the market. Look for rosy pink meat and ivory fat. Buy thin-sliced, regular-sliced, or thick-sliced bacon, depending on your preference. Look for thick-sliced apple wood–smoked bacon for especially good flavor. Butchers also usually sell slab bacon, which is often of better quality than presliced. The slab is covered with rind, which you can ask the butcher to remove. You can also ask the butcher to slice the bacon, or you can slice it at home as needed. Whole slab bacon stays fresher longer than presliced and is often less expensive as well.

Storing All bacon should be refrigerated in its original packaging or carefully wrapped in plastic until ready to cook. It keeps for up to 2 weeks and can be frozen for up to 2 months.

Preparing Most bacon is fried, although it can be roasted, too, with very good results. Cooking bacon in the microwave requires a rack to help it cook evenly. Drain bacon on paper towels before serving.

Bacon Savvy

■ For perfect fried bacon, start with a dry pan. Heat the pan and bacon together over medium-low heat, tending it carefully and removing the slices when they are done to your liking—"soggy," crisp, or somewhere in between. If necessary, pour off the excess grease during cooking. Do not fall into the trap of cooking bacon over high heat. Cook it slowly.

■ You do not have to separate bacon slices before cooking them—this often results in tearing. They easily separate once they begin to cook.

■ To cook a large amount of bacon, place the strips in a roasting pan and roast in a 450°F oven until done to your liking. This can take 25 minutes. Separate the strips after 10 minutes and then turn them every 5 to 10 minutes, carefully pouring off the grease as needed.

See also CANADIAN BACON; PANCETTA; PORK.

BAGEL A roll-sized traditional Jewish yeast bread, round with a hole in the center, like a doughnut. Plain, or water, bagels have white interiors and a somewhat chewier texture than yellow egg-enriched bagels. Onions, garlic, salt, poppy seeds, sesame seeds, or raisins and cinnamon are common flavorings.

Traditionally, bagels are briefly boiled before they are baked, which leaves them chewy and shiny. Their dense texture and round shape make them tricky to slice, which has given rise to a small kitchen gadget called a bagel slicer: the bagel is held vertically in the tool and then sliced with a guillotine-like action. A long, serrated bread knife can be used as well, but watch your fingers.

Bagels are sold in Jewish delicatessens and bakeries, many food markets, and in specialized bagel shops, where an assortment of cream cheeses, or schmears, both plain and flavored (lox, chives, vegetables, honey), also is typically available.

BAIN-MARIE (BAN mah-REE) See WATER BATH.

BAKER'S PEEL See BAKING TOOLS.

BAKEWARE See page 24.

BAKING Put simply, "baking" refers to the method of cooking food in the dry heat of an oven. The term is sometimes applied to the process of cooking uniform pieces of meat, poultry, or seafood with a small amount of fat or liquid (or a combination of foods mixed with a sauce) in an open pan or dish in the hot, dry air of an oven.

When these foods are cooked alone in the oven, however, the process is usually called roasting—harkening back to the days when meats were roasted over an open flame. More generally, "baking" refers to the process of making baked goods such as breads, cakes, pastries, and pies, which are then cooked in an oven.

For centuries, home cooks baked nearly every day. If they hadn't, there would have been no bread on the table or cakes and cookies to sweeten daily life. Today, many home cooks are nervous about baking, believing it is too complicated to tackle. Undeniably, baking requires more precision than most other home cooking, but with just a few ingredients and the right equipment, anyone can produce towering cakes, crisp cookies, bubbling fruit pies, and golden loaves of bread. And, as with everything, baking gets easier with practice.

Before You Begin First, read the recipe all the way to the end. (This is good advice regardless of what you are cooking.) Read it again and make a shopping list of any ingredients and equipment you do not have. Once you have all the necessary ingredients, measure them carefully or otherwise prepare them according to the ingredient list (chop, grate, sift) and put them in small bowls or other containers. Assemble all necessary equipment and utensils ahead, too, and prepare the pans for baking. This may mean greasing and flouring them or lining them with waxed paper or parchment paper, according to the recipe. Experienced bakers always "prep" this way, never as they go along, to avoid needless delays or oversights.

Preparing Ingredients For many cake and cookie recipes, eggs and butter should be brought to room temperature. This helps to form a smooth batter. Room-temperature egg whites foam more quickly than cold whites, but cold eggs are easier to separate, so if a recipe calls for egg whites or yolks only, separate the eggs right out of the refrigerator and then let them come to room temperature before beating.

For pie and tart doughs, cold ingredients should be kept cold, especially the butter or shortening. If the fat is allowed to melt before the crust reaches the oven, the pastry will not be as flaky.

Quick Tip

If you forget to allow enough time for eggs and butter to reach room temperature, submerge cold eggs in a bowl of warm tap water (not hot, or you'll "cook" the eggs) for about 15 minutes. Soften butter in the microwave on a low setting, checking it every 20 to 30 seconds to make sure it is not melting.

Measuring Ingredients When measuring ingredients for baking, remember that accuracy is the key. Until you are an experienced baker, save your experimentation for stir-fries and pasta sauces. If you don't follow a cake or cookie recipe precisely, there's a good chance it won't turn out. Bread making is a bit more forgiving. See MEASURING for more detail.

Check Your Oven Whether you are baking a loaf of bread, a cake, or a batch of cookies, an accurate oven is important. Use an oven thermometer—available at kitchen shops, hardware stores, and food markets—to determine the oven's accuracy. Seek out a mercury type over the less sturdy, less reliable spring-style thermometer. Hang it from the rack in the middle of the oven, and then turn on the oven. Check the temperature after at least 20 minutes have passed. If it is off by 25° or 50°F, adjust for it when baking. For example, if you set the oven for 350°F and the oven thermometer reads 375°F, reduce the knob setting to 325°F during baking

to compensate. Or, depending on the type of oven you have, call your local electric or gas company; most will send a technician to your house to calibrate the oven, thus eliminating the need to make an adjustment each time you bake. Nevertheless, it is a good idea to leave the thermometer in the oven all the time to track its accuracy.

See also BLIND BAKING; BREAD; CAKE; COOKIE; CUSTARD; FLOUR; MEASURING; MOUSSE; PAN SIZES; PARCHMENT PAPER; PIE & TART; QUICK BREAD; YEAST.

BAKING DISH See BAKEWARE.

BAKING POWDER & BAKING SODA These everyday pantry items give a lift to cakes and cookies, muffins and quick breads. Baking powder and soda are chemical leaveners, unlike yeast, which is a living microorganism. Baking powder and soda work by reacting with both liquids and heat to release carbon dioxide gas, which in turn leavens the batter, causing it to rise as it cooks.

Baking Powder Baking powder is a mixture of an acid and an alkaline, or base, that is activated when it is exposed to moisture or heat and releases carbon dioxide. Cornstarch is a typical element of baking powder, serving to absorb moisture, keeping the powder dry, and preventing a reaction until liquid is added.

The principle of leavening baked goods this way was first discovered in the late 18th century, when carbonate-rich wood ash was used to give quick breads a rise.

Quick Tip

If in doubt about the viability of baking powder, drop a generous pinch into a little warm water. If it fizzes or bubbles, it is still good. If it sinks to the bottom of the cup, discard it.

Nearly all baking powder sold today is "double acting," which means that it contains two acids that react at two different times. The acids are typically cream of tartar and either sodium aluminum sulfate or anhydrous monocalcium phosphate. The first dissolves more quickly than the second, reacting with the base and releasing some gas as soon as it is mixed with the liquid in a recipe. The second dissolves more slowly and reacts later, when the batter is exposed to the heat of the oven. This second reaction makes double-acting baking powder a reliable leavener.

In days gone by, only single-acting baking powder was available. This powder reacted when first mixed with liquid, which meant the batter had to be baked immediately. If not, the gases responsible for leavening might escape before the batter was cooked. Although many recipes still recommend that batters made with baking powder be baked promptly, time is not as crucial as it used to be. Even so, do not leave the batter sitting for more than about 20 minutes before baking.

Baking Soda Also known as bicarbonate of soda or sodium bicarbonate, baking soda is an alkaline, or base, that releases carbon dioxide gas only when it comes into contact with an acidic ingredient, such as sour cream, yogurt, buttermilk, or citrus juice.

When a recipe calls for baking soda alone, rather than baking soda and baking powder, an acidic ingredient must also be present in the batter. Because baking soda is single, rather than double, acting, wet and dry ingredients for batters should be mixed separately. Then, as soon as the two mixtures are combined, the batter must go directly into its pan and straight into a preheated oven. Baking soda is useful for other household tasks, too, from deodorizing refrigerators to loosening burned bits of food on pan bottoms.

Selecting Commercially sold baking powders and sodas are generally excellent. Check the sell-by dates, particularly on baking powder, which will eventually lose its effectiveness. Some brands of double-acting baking powder include aluminum compounds. If you have any concerns about ingesting aluminum, look for aluminum-free brands in supermarkets and natural-food stores. The best-known example is Rumford, which comes in a red canister and performs as effectively as those with aluminum compounds. Sodium-free baking powders are available as well. They are less powerful, however, and so the amounts called for in recipes should be doubled. Single-acting baking powder is nearly impossible to find these days.

Quick Bite

If only baking soda is used in a recipe with an acidic ingredient, it reacts with and neutralizes the acidic ingredient. To help retain some of that pleasant acidity, as in a recipe for buttermilk biscuits, both baking powder and baking soda are used. Baking powder has a built-in acid, which gives the batter a lift without neutralizing all of the acidic ingredient.

Storing Keep baking powder and baking soda in a cool, dry place, although this is more important for baking powder. Both will last for at least 4 months, or for 6 months at most. Discard them after this point if you don't want a batch of leaden biscuits or a pitifully flat cake.

BAKING SHEET See BAKEWARE.

BAKING STONE See BAKING TOOLS.

BAKING TOOLS See page 28.

BALSAMIC VINEGAR See VINEGAR.

Bakeware

Have you ever bitten into a seemingly perfect cookie only to discover an unpleasant charred bottom? Had the cookie been baked on a sturdy cookie sheet, it would have been burn free.

The taste and texture of baked goods are affected by the surface on which they're cooked. Inexpensive pans and cookie sheets will warp with use, causing poor heat conduction and unevenly baked cakes, cookies, and breads. The best baking pans cook evenly, brown nicely, and resist sticking or burning. If you hope to enjoy your own baked treats, you owe it to yourself to invest in quality bakeware.

Bakeware Materials Pans are available in several different materials, each with its own advantages and disadvantages. Note that darker-colored materials may require lower heat and shorter baking time than lighter ones.

ALUMINUM A superb conductor of heat, aluminum heats evenly, so baked goods brown evenly. Once removed from the oven, it cools quickly. Select anodized aluminum, which has been treated with an electrolytic process to make it harder, denser, and more resistant to corrosion. Insulated aluminum is also a good choice, since it heats more slowly than regular aluminum, avoiding burnt bottoms.

CAST IRON Durable cast iron absorbs and releases heat more slowly than other metals, turning out delicate muffins with fine, thin crusts and moist interiors.

GLASS AND CERAMIC These materials, used mainly for baking dishes and pie dishes or plates, encourage browning because the radiant heat is conducted and retained well by them. Foods bake more quickly in glass and ceramic bakeware,

too, so you may need to reduce baking times and temperatures.

NONSTICK A nonstick coating ensures the easy release of baked goods and quick cleanup. Nonstick aluminum is a good heat conductor but is not always as sturdy as other materials, such as nonstick heavy-gauge steel. Look for a double-layer nonstick coating, and remember to use wooden or plastic utensils (such as a plastic spatula for removing cookies from a baking sheet) to avoid scratching the surface.

STEEL Heavy-gauge stainless steel is strong and easy to clean, a good choice for bakeware. Tinned steel is used in classic French baking; the shiny surface provided by the tin prevents overbrowning. Darkened steel pans, the choice of many professional bakers, are excellent absorbers and distributors of heat.

THE BASIC BAKER Following are the pans every home baker should have. While it is not necessary to buy every one of these pans at once, plan to stock your kitchen gradually with them over time. Note that

Quick Tip

Whatever the metal, a dark-colored pan absorbs heat more quickly than a light-colored one, and while this is desirable for some recipes, it can cause overbrowning of more delicate foods. Watch carefully and reduce oven temperature or shorten baking time.

the measurements given are taken on the inside of the pan.

BAKING DISH Used for everything from brownies to small roasts and lasagne, deep glass dishes (or metal pans) come in all shapes and sizes, but for the average home baker the most common are a 9-by-13-by-2-inch rectangular dish and an 8- or 9-inch square dish with 2-inch sides.

BAKING SHEET This rectangular metal pan with shallow, slightly sloping rims comes in several forms. The jelly-roll pan, so named because it is used to make sponge cakes that, after baking, are spread with a filling such as jelly and then rolled, is 10 by 15 inches with ½-inch rims. Half-sheet pans are 12 by 17 inches, half the size of large commercial baking sheets. Baking pans are handy for making rolls or croissants or may be used as roasting pans for small cuts of meat.

Quick Tip

A good baking sheet can play a strong supporting role for other bakeware. Placed beneath cake pans or under a soufflé dish, it will help retain more heat and conduct it into the cookware it accompanies, helping a cake or soufflé to rise higher than it otherwise would.

CAKE PAN Plan to buy at least two round cake pans in the sizes you are likely to use (check your recipes!): 1½ to 2 inches deep and 8 or 9 inches in diameter. American cake pans are not as deep as European ones. Choose good-quality, seamless, heavy metal pans. Square and rectangular pans also are often called for in some recipes—see Baking Dish, above, and Springform Pan, page 26.

COOKIE SHEET A flat metal pan, usually with a low rim on one or two ends, designed to allow for sliding cookies onto a cooling rack. Avoid very dark sheets, which will cause your baked goods to burn. Nonstick cookie sheets work well and are very easy to clean. Insulated cookie sheets, which have an interior air pocket between two layers of metal, guarantee that no cookie will ever have an overbrowned bottom. They do not, however, work well for thin, crisp cookies, which benefit from intense heat. You'll want two cookie sheets for big batches of cookies.

LOAF PAN Also called a bread pan, a standard loaf pan is 5 by 9 by 3 inches and may be metal or glass. A smaller pan, 4½ by 8½ by 2½ inches, is also useful. Metal loaf pans produce loaf cakes and quick breads with evenly browned crusts; glass dishes encourage fast browning, sometimes at the expense of the interior of the bread or cake. Can also be used for meat loaf.

MUFFIN PAN Standard muffin and cupcake pans have 6 or 12 cups, each capable of holding 6 to 7 tablespoons of batter. Muffin pans with jumbo cups or miniature, or gem, cups are also available. Muffin cups

continued

b

Bakeware, continued

can be lined with paper liners (although the crust is likely to come off with the paper) or greased before being filled.
Special muffin pans include those with wide, flat cups for making thin, crisp muffins; and pans with cups in such whimsical or holiday-theme shapes as hearts, stars, teddy bears, dinosaurs, flowers, cars, or Christmas trees. Although aluminum and steel are common materials, cast-iron pans with nonstick surfaces are ideal for making muffins.

PIE PAN Buy metal pie pans or glass or ceramic pie plates in 9- and 10-inch sizes. Glass pie plates let you see how the bottom crust is browning, although they are sometimes overzealous heat conductors that lead to a brown crust and an undercooked middle. Look for a wide rim to hold up the fluted edge of the crust.

Quick Tip

If you like to bake pies containing especially juicy fruit, look in specialty cookware stores for a pie pan with a juice-saver rim—an extra-wide rim that includes a shallow trough to capture juices that bubble from the crust, thus preventing them from dribbling and burning on the oven floor.

SPRINGFORM PAN This deep, round cake pan with sides secured by a clamp is especially useful for cheesecakes and other solid cakes. The sides expand when the clamp is released, making the cake easy to remove. A 9-inch diameter is the most commonly used size. Generally, springform pans should be used atop baking sheets to prevent batter from leaking onto the bottom of your oven.

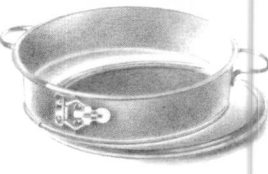

Quick Tip

If a recipe suggests placing a springform pan in a water bath, wrap the outside of the spring-form in a layer of aluminum foil, shiny side in (unless the recipe instructs otherwise), to prevent water seepage. See also WATER BATH.

TART PAN A tart pan has shallow, usually fluted sides and perhaps a removable bottom. An 11-inch metal tart pan with a removable bottom and a 10- or 11-inch solid tart pan are the most useful choices.

THE WELL-STOCKED BAKER As you experiment with baking and discover your own personal favorites you may decide to buy a few special pans.

BRIOCHE MOLD Also called a brioche pan, this circular mold with deeply fluted sides is used to bake the classic butter-and-egg-enriched French bread loaf of the same name. Made of darkened steel, stainless or tinned steel, porcelain, or glass.

CHARLOTTE MOLD Named for a classic baked French dessert in which buttery ladyfingers enclose a Bavarian cream filling. Made of tinned or stainless steel, and with slightly slanting sides that ease unmolding, the round mold can range in size from 6 ounces to 2 quarts.

MADELEINE PAN Unless you plan to bake the small French sponge cakes known as madeleines, you won't need this pan. But if you want to make the buttery sweets that Proust made famous, you cannot manage without it. Also called madeleine molds, the pans have shallow shell-shaped depressions, each about 3 inches long and 2 inches wide. Most pans make 8 to 12 cookies at a time.

PIZZA PAN These pans are usually 12 to 17 inches in diameter, with a very low, angled rim (about ½ inch high). Deep-dish pizza pans have 1½-inch sides and may be rectangular (about 12 by 8 inches or slightly larger) or round. They often have removable bottoms and may be equipped with a pan gripper that clamps onto the side of the pan to hold it steady while you cut the pizza into slices or squares. Round pans are available with perforated bottoms to encourage a crisp crust. Some pizza pans are insulated, similar to insulated baking sheets, to prevent the crust from burning or becoming overbrown.

POPOVER PAN Similar to a muffin pan, but specially designed to accommodate airier popovers as they rise. Muffin pans will work for popovers, too, but they are not the best choice, as the cups are closer together (popovers need room to crown). Cookware stores also offer individual popover molds made of black steel, although custard cups or individual soufflé dishes may be used in their place. Avoid aluminum, which trans-

mits the oven heat too quickly, overcooking the outside of the popover.

QUICHE DISH Similar to a tart pan, often made of steel with a removable bottom, with higher fluted sides to accommodate the deeper filling of a quiche. Quiche dishes made of ovenproof porcelain also double nicely as serving dishes.

SOUFFLÉ MOLD Designed with tall, straight sides so that the soufflé can rise straight and high, this dish is commonly circular, ranges in size from ½ to 2 quarts, and is porcelain. It is handsome enough to carry to the table. Smaller, individual-portion soufflé molds are available in some shops as well.

TUBE PAN Any pan with a central tube, a feature that helps the center of a cake to rise and bake evenly, is called a tube pan, but several different styles exist. Angel food cake pans sometimes have removable bottoms and small "feet" (or a tall central tube) extending above the rim, which permit the inverted pan to stand clear of the counter during cooling so no moisture is trapped. Fluted tube pans, called Bundt pans, and fluted and flared kugelhopf (also called kugelhupf or gugelhopf) pans have fixed bottoms and no feet. Tube pans hold from 1½ to 4 quarts of batter. For most uses, invest in one 10-inch tube pan.

Quick Tip

Tube pans can be used interchangeably with cake pans as long as they have the same capacity. But with more delicate recipes, such as for angel food cake, do not try to bake a tube pan recipe in a regular cake pan; the center of the cake may not cook properly.

See also PAN SIZES.

b

Baking Tools

Having the right tool for the job makes baking easier and more enjoyable. While you can roll out pastry dough with a wine bottle, or cut biscuits with an inverted water glass, these tasks go more smoothly with a rolling pin or a biscuit cutter.

If you buy good, sturdy tools, they will last for years and serve you well.

THE BASIC BAKER Every home baker should have the following tools. You don't need to buy every item listed here at once, but as time goes by, consider stocking your kitchen with most of them.

COOKIE AND BISCUIT CUTTERS Although some are made of plastic, the best cutters are made of metal, so that the cutting side holds its edge. Cookie cutters come in different shapes and sizes, from the basic round to holiday icons (jack-o'-lanterns, hearts, Christmas trees, Stars of David) and seasonal themes (leaves, flowers). Biscuit cutters are round and often fluted, and may come in nests of graduated sizes.

Quick Tip

A water glass will also work in a pinch for cutting cookies and biscuits. Thin crystal is best for slicing through dough.

COOLING RACK Because cakes, cookies, pies, and breads should be allowed to cool evenly, with air circulating on all sides, recipes call for cooling baked goods on wire racks. These come in squares, rectangles, or rounds and have small feet that raise them above the countertop. Most are made of chrome-plated metal, although some are made from stainless steel or nonstick aluminum. Buy sturdy racks that do not wobble on the counter. Have on hand two or three racks. You'll want enough to handle two cake layers or two sheets of cookies. Crisscrossing grids work well, leaving less of an indentation on your baked goods.

DOUGH SCRAPER Also called a bench scraper. This tool is used to lift dough (principally bread dough) as you work it, to scrape the remains of dough and flour from a board or countertop, and to divide pastry or bread dough into portions. Most dough scrapers have wooden or plastic handles and stainless-steel blades. Some have plastic blades, while others are constructed completely of stainless steel. All are rectangular, sometimes with rounded corners. Dough scrapers are also handy for scooping up and transferring chopped ingredients to a pan for sautéing, adding to a salad, or similar uses. Most such tasks executed by dough scrapers are relatively rugged work, so whatever type you decide on, look for a sturdy metal dough scraper that feels fairly hefty for its size. The little extra you might spend at the store will pay off in durability and efficiency at home.

FROSTING SPATULA Also called icing spatula or pastry spatula. This long, flat metal utensil with its slender, flexible, 6- to 12-inch-long blade resembles a round-tipped knife without a sharp edge. When the handle angles off the blade, the spatula is called an offset spatula. Both types will make frosting your cakes easier.

MEASURING SPOONS AND CUPS You will need a sturdy set of measuring spoons and two separate measures for dry and liquid ingredients. See MEASURING for more information.

MIXING BOWLS Stocking bowls in a range of materials, shapes, and sizes will help you tackle varied tasks more efficiently. For example, whipping egg whites and creaming butter call for deep bowls, while preparing and organizing ingredients for a cake call for a range of smaller bowls. See MIXING BOWL for more information.

MIXING SPOONS Wooden mixing spoons are favorites among cooks, although stainless-steel or sturdy plastic ones are also available. Wood does not conduct heat, so you won't burn your fingers, and wooden spoons are sturdy and inflexible, desirable qualities for most mixing tasks. They should be made of hardwoods such as beech or ash; softwoods can carry a resinous flavor. Segregate spoons used for baking from those used for savory preparations, as the latter may retain the taste of garlic and onions. Keep a mix of sizes for different tasks—small spoons for small quantities, large ones for mixing bowls of batter. See also SPOON.

PASTRY BLENDER Also known as a dough blender, this tool transforms fat and flour to a consistency suitable for pastry dough. It has a wooden or plastic handle anchoring a row of steel wires forming a U shape.

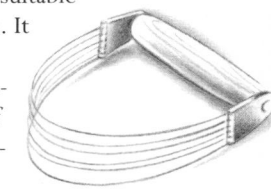

The wires act as cutters, reducing pieces of butter or other fat to the size of small peas or the consistency of meal. See CUTTING IN for more detail.

Quick Tip

If a pastry blender is unavailable, you can use a fork, 2 table knives, or a food processor to cut in butter or shortening.

PASTRY BRUSH This important tool is used to brush water, egg washes, melted butter, or glazes on pastry. The brushes are made with natural or nylon bristles, with the latter usually no more than $1\frac{1}{2}$ inches long and 1 to 2 inches wide. Goose-feather brushes are excellent for egg washes. Wash pastry brushes in hot, soapy water and keep them separate from brushes used for savory foods.

PREP BOWLS Baking is more relaxing when you precisely measure out, prepare, and line up all the ingredients before you start mixing. An assortment of small prep bowls helps you do just that. Look for glass or ceramic bowls, ranging from tiny vessels perfect for holding a single egg to larger sizes suitable for 2 cups of flour. Custard cups and ramekins also work.

continued

Baking Tools, continued

ROLLING PIN Rolling pins are available in different sizes and materials. For the most part, the type you choose is a matter of personal taste. Heavy, smooth wooden rolling pins are great for pie crusts and other types of dough. Some bakers prefer French-style pins without handles, either the straight dowel type or the kind with tapered ends, while others prefer pins with handles.

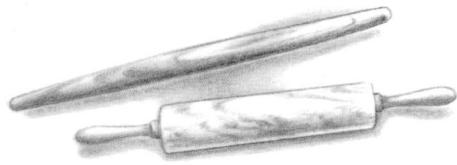

Professional models with good heft and ball bearings to keep the pin rolling smoothly are available. Marble or stainless-steel rolling pins are suggested for fine pastry work because they stay cool. Some rolling pins for pastry are even made with hollowed centers that can be packed with ice cubes, an elaboration that may go a bit too far. See also ROLLING OUT.

Quick Tip

If you're caught without a rolling pin, a clean wine bottle will work. Soak it in hot water, remove the label, dry it, and chill before using.

RUBBER SPATULA Also called a bowl scraper. This handy kitchen tool is used for getting every last bit of cake batter into pans, scraping down the sides of the mixing bowl when beating cookie dough, and scooping the last of the sour cream from its container. The best ones have blades made of silicone rubber, which won't melt or stick when used in a hot pan. Avoid plastic ones. The flexible blade is generally 2 inches wide by 3 inches long, although

smaller and larger ones are available. Some are slightly spoon shaped, which is great for stirring, folding, and scraping. Purchase a couple in different sizes for different tasks.

SIFTER Also known as a flour sifter or screen sifter. This is a metal or plastic canister fitted with two or three mesh screens and a handle that, when squeezed or turned, rotates an inside blade that forces

Quick Tip

If you don't have a sifter, a fine-mesh strainer with a handle is a good pinch hitter. Simply hold the strainer over a bowl and spoon in the flour or other ingredient. Then, gently tap the rim of the strainer with your hand to pass the contents through the mesh.

flour, lumpy cocoa powder or confectioners' sugar, or other dry ingredients through the screens to sift and aerate it. Sifters are sold in capacities ranging from 1 to 8 cups. A 2- or 3-cup capacity is most useful. See also SIFTING.

WHISK Wire whisks vary in length and diameter. The smallest are about 6 inches long, while the largest for the home baker are about 12 inches long. Three main types exist, each designed for a different task. Sauce whisks, which have somewhat elongated heads and relatively stiff wires, are used to mix ingredients thoroughly without adding excess air. Balloon whisks, which have rounded heads and more, thinner, lighter-gauge wires, are used to incorporate air into egg whites and cream. Flat whisks, sometimes called roux whisks, are used for whisking gravies and sauces. The flat shape allows you to get into the corners of a pan while also pressing out and smoothing lumps. As with rubber spatulas, you may need a couple of different sizes for different tasks. The best whisks have stainless-steel wires and sealed handles, so that no food can get into the handle. See also WHISKING.

b

THE WELL-STOCKED BAKER

Once you have the basic baking tools you need, you may want to add some specialty items that match your baking style.

BAKER'S PEEL Professional bread bakers use this wooden tool to slide loaves in and out of large ovens. Home cooks will find that a peel simplifies sliding a large loaf of bread dough or a fully loaded pizza onto a baking stone—and then retrieving it later.

BAKING STONE Also called a pizza stone, baking tile, or quarry tile. This is a flat rectangular, square, or round piece of unglazed stoneware used principally for baking breads and pizzas to produce crisp crusts. Appreciated for its efficient heat distribution, it is generally placed on the lowest rack or sometimes on the floor of the oven and preheated for at least 45 minutes or up to 1 hour before baking. The best ones are made of the same type of clay used to line kilns, as they are less apt to crack than ordinary clay baking stones. Wipe the cooled stones clean after use; do not use soap and water.

BREAD BOARD Any wooden board used mainly for kneading bread. Wood retains heat better than marble, tile, or granite, and yeast thrives in a warm environment, so home cooks whose kitchens have work surfaces in these materials often use a board for bread making.

CAKE ROUND Made of cardboard, this tool is used for both decorating and serving cakes. For easy frosting, a cake layer placed on a round can be balanced on the flat of your hand or on a decorating turntable. Each level on a tiered cake, such as a wedding cake, is supported by a cardboard round, which can be lifted off for serving. Buy cake rounds at cookware shops or bakeries or through catalogs, or cut rounds yourself from heavy, corrugated cardboard. See also FROSTING, ICING & GLAZE.

DECORATING COMB Also called a cake comb, an icing comb, or a comb scraper. These stainless-steel or plastic triangles with jagged teeth of varying size on each 3- to 4-inch edge are used to make decorative patterns in icings. Rectangular combs with a single serrated edge are also available.

DECORATING TURNTABLE Anyone who does a lot of cake decorating appreciates a turntable. Frosting and piping are much easier if you can turn the cake with a slight push and if it is raised above the work surface. An inexpensive "lazy Susan" works, but for the serious cake baker, a heavy metal turntable from a cookware shop or baking-supply house works best.

PASTRY BAG Also known as an icing bag, a decorating bag, a decorating tube, or a pastry tube. Pastry bags are made of plastic-lined canvas, plain canvas, polyester, nylon, or disposable plastic. Nylon and polyester are lightweight and easy to manipulate but can be slippery. The most useful bags are 8 to 12 inches long. Different pastry tips can be inserted into the narrow end of the conical bag, and frosting, whipped cream, or a similar mixture can be spooned into the wide end and piped out of the narrow end. If you plan to do much piping with a pastry bag, it is a good idea to have

continued

b

Baking Tools, continued

at least two bags, so that you can switch quickly back and forth between different colors of frosting without having to wash the bag. Pastry bags should be washed in warm, soapy water and turned inside out for drying. Be sure to keep bags used for savory preparations separate from those used for desserts. See also FROSTING, ICING & GLAZE; PIPING.

PASTRY BOARD Rolling out pastry calls for a smooth, hard, preferably cool surface. A pastry board may be made of hardwood or marble. Do not use it as a cutting board, or the surface will become rough (and marble will dull your knives). Marble boards stay cool, which is important for flaky pie dough. They can even be chilled in the refrigerator or on a cold back porch.

PASTRY CLOTH A piece of canvas cloth, measuring from 16 to 22 inches square, which facilitates rolling pastry by preventing it from sticking or sliding. Some are weighted or are fitted with clamps to hold them in place. Pastry cloths should be rubbed with flour before every use, and shaken and scraped clean afterward before storing. Wash them from time to time, since they may absorb fat and eventually become rancid. They are often sold accompanied by a rolling-pin sleeve made of the same fabric, which prevents the dough from sticking to the pin, a common problem for beginners. The sleeve must be rubbed with flour as well. See also PIE & TART; ROLLING OUT.

Quick Tip

In place of using a pastry cloth and sleeve, slip the dough between two sheets of waxed paper or parchment paper.

PASTRY CRIMPER Resembling large tweezers and sold in different patterns, pastry crimpers are used to seal together top and bottom crusts of pies and other filled pastries. The most common type is made of stainless steel and has serrated edges that can also be used to hull strawberries. See also CRIMPING; PIE & TART.

PASTRY WHEEL A tool used to cut out or trim rolled out pastry dough. Pastry wheels are circular straight or fluted blades attached to a handle that lets you roll them across the dough. They are useful for making strips or free-form shapes to top pies. Fluted pastry wheels are sometimes referred to as pastry jaggers for their jagged edges. Some manufacturers even produce double pastry wheels, with side-by-side blades that let you cut straight or fluted edges with a 180-degree turn of the handle.

PIE WEIGHTS Also known as pastry weights. These small aluminum or ceramic pellets are used to weight down pie dough when it is blind baked—that is, prebaked without a filling. A sheet of aluminum foil or parchment paper is fitted into the pastry-lined pan and then the weights are spread over the bottom to hold the pastry in place as it bakes. For more details, see BLIND BAKING.

Quick Tip

In a pinch, raw rice or dried beans work as pie weights. They should be discarded after a couple of bakings.

SCALE Choose a kitchen scale capable of weighing up to 10 pounds in no larger than ¼-ounce increments. The weighing bowl should be large enough to handle at least 2 cups of flour or an equivalent item. The best scales allow you to weigh ingredients in any bowl or container. Make sure that the scale weighs light items as accurately as it does heavy ones.

See also BREAD MACHINE; CROCKPOT; FOOD PROCESSOR; MIXER.

BAMBOO SHOOT A popular ingredient in the Asian pantry, bamboo shoots are ivory-colored, mild-flavored vegetables that provide refreshing, slightly crunchy texture. The shoots are harvested young and tender, when the bamboo plant, a grass related to edible grains such as wheat and oats, is green. Bamboo shoots are used in stir-fries and other typical Asian dishes.

Selecting Whole or sliced bamboo shoots canned in mild brine are more commonly available. Fresh ones are rarely encountered in markets outside Asia. Bamboo shoots also are found canned together with other vegetables such as water chestnuts and baby corn, usually labeled "stir-fry vegetables." Buy canned bamboo shoots in the ethnic-food aisle of the supermarket and in Asian markets.

Storing Once the can is opened, transfer the shoots to a plastic or glass container, cover with water, and refrigerate for up to 7 days. Changing the water once a day will keep them in good condition for up to another week.

Preparing Drain the canned shoots, slice them lengthwise if necessary, and use them in stir-fries or steamed dishes with beef, chicken, and/or vegetables.

BANANA Native to Asia, the banana is grown in most tropical regions of the world, with the largest and best crops coming from Latin America. The Cavendish is the familiar yellow variety found in most food stores, but other varieties are finding their way into markets with increasing frequency, particularly in areas where sizable Latin and Southeast Asian populations reside. These include lady's finger, apple, Canary, and Lakatan bananas. Most are small and plump, some are yellow, and others are rosy red. All taste, with varying degrees of sweetness, much like the Cavendish.

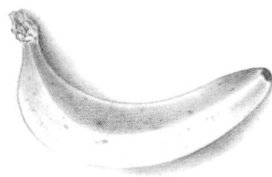

Cavendish banana.

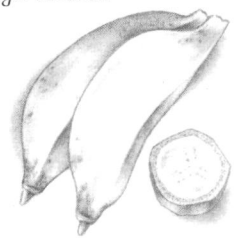

Lady's finger bananas.

Bananas ripen well off the tree, so they are picked nearly mature but still green, making them less vulnerable to bruising. During ripening, they emit ethylene gas, which in turn prompts the other bananas in a bunch to ripen. Put green bananas in a

Quick Tip

If you notice your bananas are darkening quickly but you aren't ready to eat them, freeze them now to use later for banana bread.

loosely closed paper bag with other underripe fruits (tomatoes, avocados, peaches), and they will speed the ripening of their companions. As bananas mature, the flesh softens and sweetens, and the skin turns from light green to light yellow to bright yellow and finally to yellow speckled with brown spots, at which point they are fully ripe, sweet, and tender.

Selecting For keeping around the house, buy bananas that are light green or light yellow with no, or very few, brown spots. Those with brown splotches are fully ripe and will quickly become overripe, unless you use them immediately. At this ripe stage, they don't travel well and may even bruise inside your shopping bag during the trip from market to home.

Quick Tip

Bananas can also be eaten as a frozen treat. Peel firm, ripe bananas and wrap them in plastic. They will keep for about 3 months. For an extra indulgence, dip the frozen bananas in melted chocolate.

Storing Bananas ripen nicely at normal room temperatures. If you choose less-ripe specimens, they will last for 5 to 7 days. If the fruit is ripe, refrigeration will not harm it, but the skin will turn black and the fruit may not last any longer than at room temperature. Peeled and wrapped in plastic, bananas freeze well for up to 3 months.

Preparing For slicing and mixing with other fruit, use firm, bright yellow bananas with only a few dark speckles. For banana bread and muffins, or for eating immediately out of hand, choose splotchier fruits, which will be softer and sweeter.

BAR See COOKIE.

BARBECUE SAUCE This tangy, thick sauce, an indispensable part of every pork or beef barbecue, varies from region to region—and from cook to cook. In many areas of the country, barbecue sauce is tomato based and slightly sweet and smoky. Other locales prefer a sharper-tasting vinegar- or mustard-based sauce. Trying different barbecue sauces is half the fun of eating barbecue. Most barbecue and grilling books have recipes for a basic barbecue sauce, made with ketchup, vinegar, brown sugar, onions, chiles, and other seasonings, but this is only the beginning.

Storing After opening, barbecue sauce should be refrigerated. It generally will keep for several months.

Preparing Barbecue sauce is often brushed on meat and poultry during the last several minutes of cooking for added flavor. The sugar present in most sauces will burn if the sauce is applied before the last 15 minutes or so, which is why most barbecue sauces should not be used as marinades. The sauces may be heated and served alongside the meat.

BARBECUING Although many people use this term interchangeably with grilling, the two are not the same. Barbecuing is cooking meat outdoors in a closed chamber by indirect heat. A low temperature is maintained for a long time, using fragrant, smoky wood or high-grade charcoal. This slow method results in meat so tender that it literally falls off the bone. Pork is the most traditional meat for barbecue, although beef is often barbecued, too, particularly in Texas. Chicken, turkey, and lamb are not strangers to this outdoor method either.

Quick Bite

In the old South, barbecuing was done in pits, with the cooks tending the fire and the meat (commonly a whole hog) for hours. This often meant staying up all night, sipping drinks, spinning yarns, and turning the cooking process into a social event.

The sauce that is served with barbecue is determined by region. Barbecued pork in Tennessee and western North Carolina is paired with a tomato-based sauce. In eastern North Carolina, the pork is treated to a vinegar-and-red-pepper sauce, while in South Carolina, a mustard-seasoned sauce is typical. Traditional Texas beef brisket barbecue is served without sauce, and Kansas City beef barbecue is served with a sweet, thick tomato sauce.

Barbecued meat is cooked at temperatures maintained between 185° and 250°F. Most red meat is cooked until its internal temperature reaches 180° to 185°F, although some, such as brisket, needs to reach slightly higher temperatures. Chicken is cooked to an internal temperature of 170° to 180°F. Traditionally, the heat source is hardwood or high-grade charcoal, not electricity or gas. Before cooking, the meat is usually rubbed with a spice mixture, called a dry rub, or marinated.

Home cooks rarely barbecue meat in the traditional way. But those who do are known to turn the activity into a passionate hobby, which often includes building a cooker. Enthusiasts also experiment endlessly with different rubs, marinades, and barbecue sauces. Barbecue contests are held throughout the United States but primarily in the South and Midwest. They can be small, informal gatherings or large, high-stake events. Among the latter perhaps the best known are two annual contests, Tennessee's Memphis in May and the American Royal in Kansas City, Missouri.

See also GRILLING; MARINATING; RUB.

BARDING Laying thin sheets of pork fat, called *bardes* by the French, or bacon slices over meat or poultry is called "barding." They may be secured with kitchen string if necessary. This traditional technique keeps lean cuts of meat and the lean breast meat of poultry, notably game birds, from drying out during roasting. After cooking, the fat is removed and discarded.

Layering the fat.

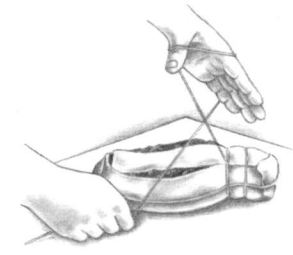

Securing with string.

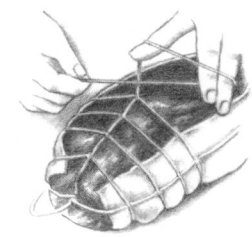

BARLEY See GRAIN.

BASIL See HERB.

BASTING When a recipe calls for basting, it means to pour, spoon, or brush liquid over food, most often meat or poultry, to give it good flavor and color during roasting. Basting is not just for turkeys. Indeed, any large item, from a standing rib roast to a pork loin to a whole chicken, also benefits from it. While the food is roasting, pull out the oven rack and brush or spoon accumulated pan juices or another liquid over the meat. Some cooks use a bulb baster, also called a turkey baster, to pour liquid over the meat. A metal baster is a better choice than a plastic one, which might be warped or melted by the hot fat.

Caution!

When cooking on an outdoor grill or under a broiler, many cooks like to baste food with the flavorful liquid in which it first marinated. Be advised, however, that marinades can harbor harmful bacteria from the meat, poultry, or seafood that they flavored. For this reason, stop basting with a marinade at least 5 minutes before the end of cooking, to allow sufficient time for the heat to kill off any bacteria. Or, bring the marinade to a boil for 5 minutes before basting with it.

While basting is a time-honored technique for adding moisture to meat, it doesn't actually achieve this goal. Quite simply, meat cannot absorb moisture during cooking. In fact, meat always loses moisture when it cooks, and no amount of basting can moisten dried-out meat or poultry. Basting does help prevent the food from drying out too quickly, but the best way to prevent meat from drying out is to avoid overcooking it. Larger cuts generally have enough fat in their connective tissues and, in the case of turkeys, skin, to keep the food moist. Small, lean pieces of meat, such as chicken breasts and pork tenderloins, can benefit from barding to keep them juicy. For more detail, see BARDING.

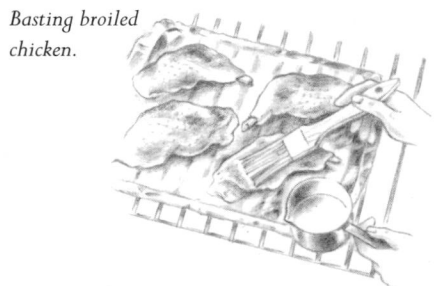

Basting broiled chicken.

Though it does not add moisture, basting does have its benefits. Basting liquids often are the accumulated pan juices, but they also can be melted butter, flavored or not, or various mixtures based on water, stock, wine, or beer. These all add flavor, and any that contain sugar or protein—in the form of butter, corn syrup, honey, preserves, stock or broth, wine, or beer—promote even browning. Too much sugar can cause scorching, however, so don't go overboard. Basting liquids also should include some fat, which is a flavor conductor.

BATTER Any smooth mixture that is thin enough to pour or spoon and that, when baked or fried, firms up to become a cake, bread, pancake, fritter, crisp coating, or similar item. Thinner batters are used to coat poultry, seafood, or vegetables, such as for batter-fried chicken or vegetable tempura. They rely 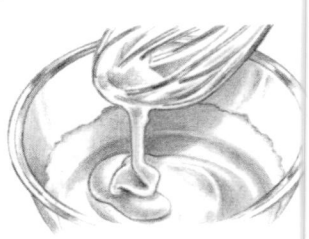 on properly heated deep oil to achieve the desired perfectly crisp, nongreasy results. So, too, do the slightly thicker batters that may be used to bind together diced or chopped ingredients cooked as fritters, from Indian *bhaji* to more familiar French and American-style croquettes. Most batters consist of flour, eggs, and a liquid such as milk or beer. Many also contain sugar and butter. Batters differ from doughs primarily in consistency. The former are thinner and must be contained, while the latter are thick.

See also FRYING.

BAY LEAF See HERB.

BEAN CURD See SOY FOODS.

Bean, Dried

Beans, peas, and lentils (known collectively as legumes) are among the most healthful of foods. They are low in fat and high in protein, fiber, carbohydrates, vitamins, and minerals.

Beans are a practical, economical food with a long shelf life, keeping well for a year when stored airtight in a cool, dry cupboard. Some beans have been sown by farmers since the Stone Age and were a pantry staple in ancient Rome and Athens. Today, from Boston baked beans and split pea soup to hummus and black beans with rice, dried legumes star regularly at tables around the world.

Nevertheless, some people avoid cooking dried legumes because of the relatively lengthy preparation. Hard as small pebbles, dried beans require rehydrating to soften them. This is generally done by soaking them before cooking. Depending on your schedule, you can, however, select a long- or quick-soak method, or no soaking plus longer cooking. Lentils and certain other dried legumes, such as split peas, do not require soaking and cook quickly in comparison to beans.

Selecting Dried legumes are sold prewashed in plastic bags and in bulk in some supermarkets and in health-food stores. Choose clean-looking beans and lentils that show no signs of shriveling and buy them from stores with good turnover.

Storing Store dried legumes in a cool, dry cupboard in their packaging or in a tightly lidded canister or jar. They will keep for up to 1 year. The older the dried legumes, the longer they will take to cook and the more water they will absorb. Once dried beans are cooked, they must be refrigerated to prevent spoilage.

Cooked beans or lentils freeze beautifully. When cooled, put them in a tightly lidded freezer-safe container or spoon them into a zippered plastic freezer bag and freeze for up to 1 year.

Preparing Most dried beans are soaked before cooking. Lentils and peas do not require soaking. Before soaking beans or cooking legumes, regardless of method, rinse them in a colander under cold running water, scooping them between your fingers to make sure any debris washes away. Dried beans and legumes used to be packaged somewhat carelessly. Today, they are generally clean, although you should still check them. Some recipes instruct you to "sort" or "pick over" the beans before rinsing them, which simply means to discard any misshapen beans or foreign matter (small stones and the like).

Picking over beans.

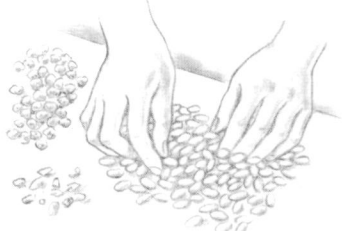

There are three methods for preparing beans: the long-soak method, the quick-soak method, and the no-soak method.

continued

Bean, Dried, continued

HOW TO *Soak Beans*

Your choice of which of the three soaking methods explained below for dried beans will depend entirely on your schedule: how soon ahead of time you decide to prepare a bean dish; whether you have the beans in your pantry or have to go out and buy them; and how much time you have available to do the actual cooking of the beans.

LONG-SOAK METHOD

1. Put the beans in a large pot or bowl and add cold water to cover by 3 inches or more.

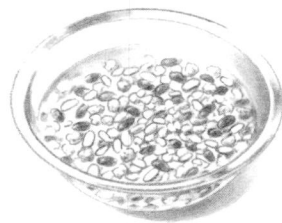

2. Soak at room temperature until visibly swelled and fully rehydrated, about 4 hours. Some recipes say to soak them overnight, but 4 hours is actually enough for any dried bean. If it suits your schedule, let the beans soak overnight or all day. Add additional water as necessary to keep them covered. Drain and proceed with the recipe.

QUICK-SOAK METHOD

1. Put the beans in a large pot and add cold water to cover by about 3 inches.
2. Bring the water to a rapid simmer over medium-high heat. Adjust the heat so the beans simmer vigorously for 2 minutes. Do not let the simmer turn into a full boil.
3. Remove the pot from the heat, cover, and let the beans cool in the liquid for at least 1 hour. Drain and proceed with the recipe.

NO-SOAK METHOD

Beans can be cooked without soaking. This is a satisfactory method, although soaking the beans will ensure even and thorough cooking. Omitting the step of soaking increases cooking times—but usually by no more than 30 to 40 minutes. To cook, drop the rinsed beans into boiling, lightly salted liquid and, when it returns to a boil, reduce the heat to very low, cover tightly, and cook until tender. Continue cooking as for soaked beans, adding more water as necessary to keep the beans covered. Test the beans for doneness every 10 to 15 minutes after the traditional cooking time is reached.

Quick Tip

Some cooks prefer cooking beans in a low (250°F) oven, rather than tending the pot simmering on top of the stove. Put the beans and cooking liquid in a covered casserole or Dutch oven and cook them for the same time as directed for stovetop cooking.

HOW TO *Cook Soaked Beans*

1. Put soaked and drained dried beans, or dried lentils or other legumes, in a pot and add cold water or stock to cover by several inches. Some recipes may say to add an onion, some garlic, herbs, or other flavorings at this point as well. Avoid acidic ingredients, such as tomatoes, which will toughen the beans and prevent them from softening.
2. Cooking beans with a bit of salt is not only acceptable, but preferable. Add about 1 teaspoon of salt to the cooking water for every 2 cups (about 1 pound) of dried beans. The old belief that salting will keep the beans from softening during cooking is based on the fact that an excessive amount of salt will interfere with their softening. A reasonable amount of salt will add good flavor and require only a slight adjustment at the end of cooking.
3. Bring to a boil over high heat, skim off the foam that rises to the top, and reduce the heat to low. Partially cover the pot and simmer the beans or lentils very gently. Slow cooking is essential; boiling the beans will cause their skins to split.

Cooking Times for Soaked Dried Beans

Legume	Cooking Time*
Adzuki beans	30 to 40 minutes
Appaloosa beans	1 to 1½ hours
Black beans	30 to 60 minutes
Black-eyed peas (no soaking required)	35 to 45 minutes
Cannellini	1 to 1½ hours
Chickpeas	1½ to 2 hours
Cranberry beans	1 to 1½ hours
Fava beans	2½ to 3 hours
Flageolets	1 hour
Great Northern beans	1 to 1½ hours
Kidney beans	1 to 1½ hours
Lentils, green or brown or Puy (no soaking required)	30 to 45 minutes
Lentils, red or yellow (no soaking required)	8 to 10 minutes
Lima beans	1 to 1½ hours
Mung beans	45 to 60 minutes
Navy beans	1½ to 2 hours
Pink beans	1 hour
Pinto beans	1 to 1½ hours
Soybeans	2½ to 3 hours
Split peas (no soaking required)	35 to 60 minutes

Cooking times in this chart are based on 1 cup dried beans or lentils, measured before soaking, which yields about 2½ to 3 cups when cooked. (If you are using the no-soak method, remember to increase these cooking times by 30 to 40 minutes.)

4. Check the liquid level every 30 or 40 minutes, adding more as necessary to keep the beans fully covered at all times. This helps them cook more evenly.

5. Test for doneness by mashing a cooled bean against the roof of your mouth with your tongue or pressing it between your thumb and forefinger. The bean should be soft but not mushy, retaining some shape. Cook the beans longer if you prefer them softer.

Quick Tip

Partially covering the bean-cooking pot helps the beans cook evenly and keeps the liquid from evaporating too quickly before the beans are done. It's always a good idea to check the water level of the beans occasionally.

continued

Bean, Dried, continued

Dried Legume Varieties Many of the following dried legumes may be substituted for one another in recipes. As a rule of thumb, feel free to use any other legume of similar size, color, or shape, letting common sense and your own tastes be your guides. Some of the most versatile and interchangeable of beans are those of the haricot family, which includes the various types of white, kidney, and pinto beans.

ADZUKI BEAN Small, reddish brown, sweet-tasting bean popular in Japanese and Chinese cooking. Also used to make the sweet bean paste used in some Asian desserts.

APPALOOSA BEAN A light beige bean with black to brown spots. Related to kidney beans and used similarly.

BLACK BEAN Also called turtle, Mexican, or Spanish black bean. Small and shiny black. Used widely in Latin American cooking for pot beans, soups, and dips.

BLACK-EYED PEA Also called cowpea or black-eyed bean. Cream colored and kidney shaped, with a characteristic black dot with a yellow center and a mild flavor. Native to India and Iran and widely consumed in Africa, these legumes require less soaking than most dried beans and are the centerpiece of hoppin' John, a classic Southern rice dish.

BORLOTTI BEAN See Cranberry Bean, below.

BROAD BEAN See Fava Bean, below.

BUTTER BEAN See Lima Bean, below.

CANNELLINI These ivory-colored beans go into traditional Italian minestrone soup. Great Northern beans may be substituted.

CECI BEAN See Chickpea, below.

CHICKPEA Also known as garbanzo bean or ceci bean. Rich, nutty-flavored, large beige bean with a firm texture. These are the main ingredient in hummus, the famed Middle Eastern spread.

COWPEA See Black-Eyed Pea, above.

CRANBERRY BEAN Also called Roman bean or borlotti bean. Mild-flavored, mottled reddish bean that loses its color during soaking and cooking. They can be substituted for dried lima beans and for kidney beans.

FAVA BEAN Also called broad bean, English bean, or horse bean. Large, light brown bean with a slightly bitter flavor and grainy texture. See also BEAN, FRESH.

FLAGEOLET Small, flavorful, pale green or white beans traditionally served with lamb dishes in French cooking.

GARBANZO BEAN See Chickpea, above.

GREAT NORTHERN BEAN Also called white bean. Small, oval-shaped white beans. Can be used in place of other small white beans such as navy and white kidney. They share these beans' mild flavor and creamy texture. Often used in Boston baked beans.

KIDNEY BEAN Large, dark red, pinkish, or white kidney-shaped beans. Sturdy and versatile. Color determines their most common usage, although they are interchangeable if color is not a concern. Red kidney beans are used in many Southwestern dishes. Pink kidney beans are called red beans in Louisiana and go into red beans and rice. White kidney beans, sometimes mistaken for cannellini, are used in Italian dishes and can be substituted for navy or Great Northern beans. Red kidney beans can be substituted for cranberry beans.

LENTIL Small and flat, lentils may be green, brown, yellow, red, pink, or mottled. Mild flavored and quick to cook, they are extremely versatile. Ocher-colored lentils are widely used in Indian cooking, where they are called dal. Puy lentils are small, dark green French lentils with a pleasantly mild flavor. They make good salads and soups and blend well with meats.

LIMA BEAN Also called butter bean. Large, flat, white to pale green, sweet-tasting bean. Lima beans are also sold frozen and are sometimes available fresh. Can be substituted for kidney and cranberry beans.

MUNG BEAN Also called mung pea. Small, round, gray-green bean used primarily in Asian cooking. When mung beans are split, they are called yellow mung beans or *moong dal*.

NAVY BEAN Small white bean with a mild flavor. Versatile and sturdy, navy beans can be used in place of white kidney or Great Northern beans.

PINK BEAN A smooth, kidney-shaped, pale red bean that turns reddish brown when cooked. The sweet-tasting, meaty bean is similar to kidney and pinto beans but longer in shape.

PINTO BEAN A pale brown bean with darker, sometimes pinkish streaks, which disappear during cooking. Used extensively in Southwestern cooking, where their full, earthy flavor is appreciated. These may be substituted for kidney beans or pink beans.

RED BEAN See Kidney Bean, above.

ROMAN BEAN See Cranberry Bean, above.

SOYBEAN Ivory, green, brown, or black rounded beans with mild flavor and a firm texture. These require long cooking. Although dried soybeans are available, most people instead consume soy in other forms: tofu, tempeh, miso, soy milk, soy sauce, and other soy products. Soy is considered extremely healthful. See also SOY FOODS.

SPLIT PEA Small, pale green or yellow dried legumes. Split peas cook quickly and are used as side dishes or, in their best-known role, as the basis for split-pea soup.

WHITE BEAN Rather than being a specific bean, this is a group of beans that includes Great Northern beans, navy beans, kidney beans, and cannellini. See also Great Northern Bean, above.

Quick Tip

Look in specialty-food stores and mail-order catalogs for the many different varieties of long-lost heirloom beans currently being recultivated by enterprising growers. Seek out such beautiful, flavorful, and evocatively named types as the Black Valentine, Pebble, Eye of Goat, Swedish Brown, Gigante, Tongue of Fire, Bisbee Red, Wren's Egg, and Zuni Shalako.

A Word on the Unmentionable

If beans, which are high in fiber, are not cooked thoroughly, they are hard to digest. And even when cooked properly, beans cause gas in many people because of the complex sugars that, paired with the fiber, also contribute to flatulence. Eating beans regularly is a good way to acquaint your system with them and reduce the problem significantly. Vinegar and commercial anti-gas products such as Beano, which can be sprinkled on the beans just before eating, help—but they are not magic remedies.

b

Bean, Fresh

Long a garden staple, fresh beans fall into two categories: pod beans and shell beans. Pod beans, such as green beans, are consumed whole, outer pod and inner seeds. Only the inner seeds of shell beans can be eaten, and the pod is discarded.

Some of the more popular varieties of fresh shell beans are lima beans and fava beans.

Fresh beans are harvested when young and tender—in most cases, the younger, the better. When shell beans are grown to full maturity, their fully developed inner seeds can be dried to become dried legumes (see BEAN, DRIED). While some shell beans, most notably fava beans and cranberry beans, are available in their fresh state early in the harvest season, most shell beans are sold dried.

Selecting Fresh beans should be firm with good bright color.

Green, wax, and lima beans are sold frozen and canned. If you cannot find them fresh and have a choice, choose frozen beans over canned, which tend to have a tinny taste and soft, mushy texture. All the fresh shell beans described here are available dried and canned.

Quick Bite

With the exception of haricots verts, romanos, and Chinese long beans, pod beans are rarely labeled anything other than "green beans."

Storing Put fresh beans into a perforated plastic bag and refrigerate for up to 5 days. They are best, however, when eaten within 2 days of purchase, as their "snap" diminishes with time. Once shelled, fresh shell beans should be used within 2 days.

Preparing Trim off brown-tipped ends and remove any strings along the length of pod beans. Split open shell beans along their seams to remove the beans, easing them out with your thumb as necessary.

Shelling beans.

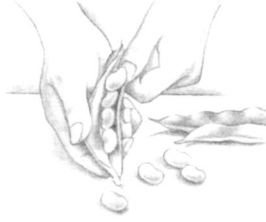

Fresh beans can be boiled, steamed, or added to soups and stews. Pod beans are often sautéed or stir-fried. Whatever recipe you choose, the important thing is not to overcook beans.

Fresh Bean Varieties

BORLOTTI BEAN See Cranberry Bean, below.

BROAD BEAN See Fava Bean, below.

BUTTER BEAN See Lima Bean, below.

CHINESE LONG BEAN Also called yard-long bean. Very long, rounded green pod bean used in Asian cooking and sold primarily in Asian markets, generally displayed bundled into loose skeins.

CRANBERRY BEAN Although usually eaten dried, the cranberry bean, a favorite of Italian American cooks, is available as a shell bean in some markets. The pod and inner seed should be the color of cream with a good representation of red speckles.

FAVA BEAN Also called broad bean, English bean, or horse bean. This shell bean is available fresh briefly in the spring in farmers' markets. Look for soft, pale green pods packed with pale green beans that resemble lima beans. They have a pleasingly bitter flavor.

Once removed from the pods, the beans should be peeled of their tough outer skin, which is slightly toxic, more so late in the season. To remove it, blanch the shelled beans for 1 minute in boiling water, let cool, then pinch the beans to remove the skin.

Skinning
fava beans.

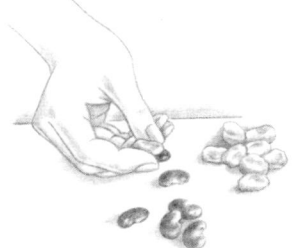

If the beans are young and fresh and no bigger than your thumbnail, skinning them may not be necessary, although some cooks find that even the skins of young beans impart too much bitterness. Fava beans are also sold dried.

FLAGEOLET Small, flavorful, pale green or white shell bean used in traditional French cooking. Flageolets are also sold canned and dried. The fresh beans can be difficult to find in the United States.

GREEN BEAN Also called snap bean, string bean, or runner bean. Green beans are eaten whole, pod and seeds, and taste mild and fresh with grassy overtones. The most familiar green bean is several inches long with a rounded pod. Buy evenly green ones that look as though they will snap decisively when broken. To prepare green beans, simply snap off the stem end and remove any strings along the length of the bean.

HARICOT VERT Also called French green bean or filet bean. Small, slender, dark green, young pod beans favored in France. Delicately flavored, they are more elegant, and commensurately expensive, than other green beans.

LIMA BEAN Also called a butter bean, the lima grows in wide, flat green inedible pods. Small beans are called baby limas. Look for green, velvety pods. The inner seed, the sweet-tasting edible portion, should be as green as possible. Avoid any with a white cast. Fresh lima beans may be difficult to find in some regional markets, while dried, canned, and especially frozen ones are commonly available.

ROMAN BEAN See Cranberry Bean, above.

ROMANO BEAN Also called Italian bean. A green pod bean, similar to green beans, but with slightly broader and more flattened pods and a somewhat more robust flavor and texture.

SNAP BEAN See Green Bean, above.

STRING BEAN See Green Bean, above.

WAX BEAN This is a green bean that is yellow rather than green. It has the same other characteristics as the green bean.

b

BEAN SPROUT See SPROUT.

BEATING Mixing vigorously until a single ingredient such as eggs or a mixture such as cake batter is smooth, well blended, and aerated. This is often accomplished with an electric mixer, although you can beat batters by hand with a spoon, whisk, manual egg beater, or fork. Eggs for scrambled eggs or French toast are commonly beaten by hand.

See also BATTER; DOUGH; EGG; FOLDING; MIXER; MIXING; WHIPPING; WHISKING.

BÉCHAMEL See SAUCE.

BEEF From the basic cheeseburger to the elegant standing rib roast, beef means eating well. Nothing satisfies a meat lover like a buttery beef tenderloin or a hearty beef stew, a sandwich piled high with corned beef or a juicy hamburger hot off the grill.

Beef Labeling Beef is graded by the United States Department of Agriculture (USDA) according to tenderness, flavor, and juiciness. All of these relate to the amount of white marbling, or intramuscular fat, the beef has. The best beef, with the most marbling and finest flavor, is graded "prime." Rarely is prime beef available anywhere but at premium butcher shops and steak houses. Most beef sold to consumers is "choice" or "select." It is generally leaner, although the leanness also depends on where on the animal the cut originated. Cuts from more active muscles, such as chuck and round, are naturally tougher and leaner than lightly used muscle sections, such as the rib and short loin. Though federal law mandates that all meat must be inspected, grading is voluntary. It is possible to find ungraded meat, but for assurance of quality, one should buy only prime, choice, or select grade beef.

In addition to the USDA grades, there is an increasing number of private labels or brands. For example, beef labeled "Certified Black Angus" is from the cattle of the same name, which is prized for its high-grade, top-quality beef. Although certified Angus beef may cost more than the meat of other breeds available at the market, it is preferred by many home cooks and restaurant chefs for its consistent quality.

Find a reliable butcher selling good meat at an independent shop or a supermarket, then develop a relationship with him or her. You will get good beef if you become a loyal and interested customer.

In recent years, with growing concerns for eating healthfully and light, beef was often dismissed as too high in saturated fat and cholesterol. Today, beef is bred to be more than 25 percent leaner than it was several decades ago, with less marbling and less outer fat in all grades. It is also generally sold in smaller cuts than it once was, with fewer roasts and more steaks, strips, and cubes, all of which are appropriate for lighter cooking methods such as grilling, broiling, and stir-frying. With these changes, cooks are starting to rediscover beef's healthful qualities, including its abundance of protein, iron, phosphorous, zinc, and B vitamins.

Selecting Look for bright red beef with light marbling (internal fat), fine texture, and nearly white outer fat but not much of it. The more marbling, the more tender and juicy the beef, and the best kind of marbling consists of many small deposits of intramuscular fat, rather than a few large globs. Vacuum-packed meat will appear purplish, but its color should brighten upon exposure to air. Be sure to press the meat (even through plastic) to make sure it feels firm. For ground beef, if you have a good butcher, ask him or her to grind it fresh for you. Otherwise, buy it already ground

ᕦᕤ Beef Glossary ᕦᕤ

Beef cuts.

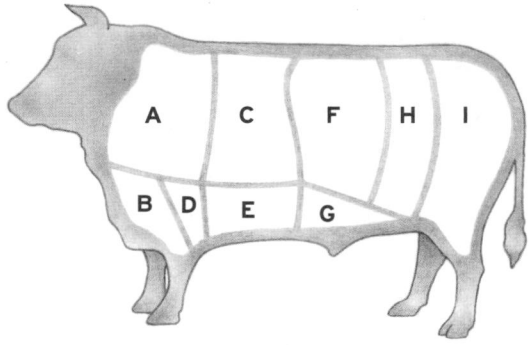

Cuts of meat are not labeled consistently from one region of the country to another—or even from one butcher shop to another. The following terms are based on the more universal primal cuts, large sections of beef that are then cut by the butcher into individual steaks and roasts. Understanding the nature of the primal cuts will help you decide what to buy for dinner and how to cook it. Never hesitate to ring the bell for the butcher at the supermarket and ask questions about a particular cut.

CHUCK (A) The muscular shoulder section, source of chuck steak, chuck roasts, and stewing beef, all tougher cuts best cooked by moist methods such as braising or stewing. Chuck roast makes the best pot roast. Ground chuck, a common type of ground beef, has a high proportion of fat, a robust flavor, and makes juicy hamburgers.

Chuck roast.

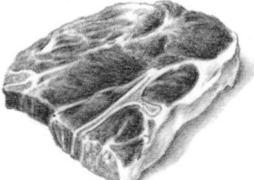

FORESHANK (B) Sold cubed or cut into bone-in slices, best suited for stewing, braising, or making stocks.

RIB (C) The meat nestled between the rib bones is flavorful, juicy, and tender. Rib cuts include flavorful rib-eye steaks for broiling or panfrying, short ribs for braising, and tender rib roasts and rib-eye roasts for oven roasting. A standing rib roast is a truly grand cut of beef, reserved for special occasions.

Standing rib roast.

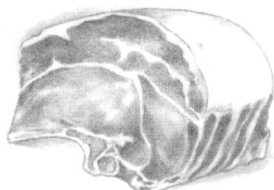

BRISKET (D) Cut into flat or pointed half briskets, which are often cured and simmered as corned beef. Briskets may also be braised.

Brisket.

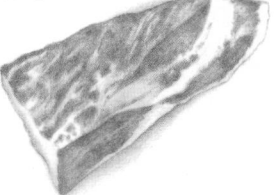

continued

⤙ Beef Glossary, continued ⤙

Quick Bite

When briskets are cured, they become corned beef. The "corn" in "corned beef" refers to corns, or grains, of salt used in the curing process.

PLATE (E) Source of short ribs and stew beef for braising and stewing, as well as ground beef. The inner muscle is sometimes sold as skirt steak, the traditional cut for fajitas. Good for braising, broiling, and grilling.

Short ribs.

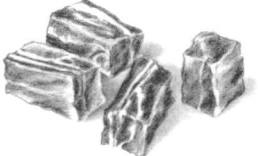

Skirt steak.

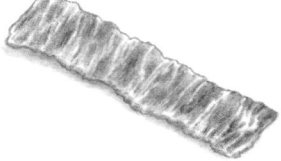

SHORT LOIN (F) Source of the finest steaks, T-bone, porterhouse, club, top loin, tenderloin (also known as filet mignon), fillet, and strip. Tenderloin cuts, from the bottom of the section, are considered the finest cuts of beef. Tenderloin roasts are wonderful for roasting or broiling.

T-bone steak.

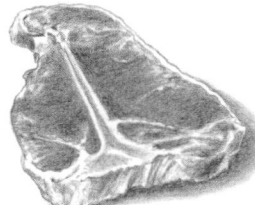

Fillet steaks.

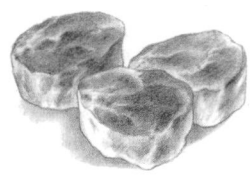

FLANK (G) Source of lean flank steak, for braising, grilling, and stir-frying, and ground beef.

Flank steak.

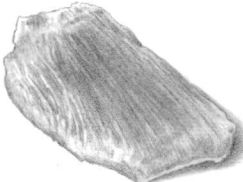

SIRLOIN (H) Source of sirloin steaks for broiling or roasting, as well as ground beef. Ground sirloin falls between ground chuck and ground round in terms of fat content and has a rich beef flavor.

Sirloin steak.

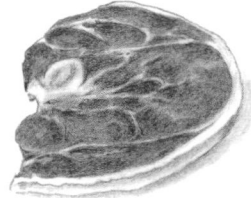

ROUND (I) Source of round (or rump) roasts for braising, broiling, or grilling, as well as ground beef. Ground round is extremely lean but a little tough. Top round is the most tender part of this beef section.

Boneless rump roast.

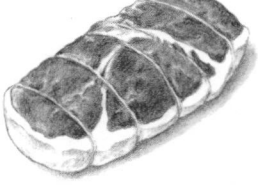

from a reliable vendor. Look for even red color and nice white fat throughout the meat. Avoid dark, brownish meat and grayish fat. Also pass up any beef that looks excessively moist or that has two-tone coloration.

Storing Leave meat in its wrapper and store it in the coldest part of the refrigerator, which is usually at the back of the bottom shelf, or in a meat drawer. (A refrigerator thermometer will tell you for sure.) If any juices are seeping from the store packaging, wrap the package in a layer of plastic wrap. Do not unwrap meat until just before cooking because unnecessary exposure to air adds to deterioration. Beef can be held for about 4 days in the refrigerator; in a cold meat drawer (with temperatures hovering around 30°F), it will keep for up to 5 days. Ground beef will keep for 2 days but is best if cooked on the day it is purchased. It also freezes well.

To freeze steaks, chops, and roasts, trim any excess fat, wrap the meat in freezer-weight plastic or put it into a zippered plastic freezer bag, and freeze for up to 10 months. Ground beef freezes best if divided into small amounts—patties, meatballs, or small meat loaves. Discard any beef that develops an "off" smell.

Preparing Beef cooks more evenly and stays juicier if it is allowed to come to room temperature first, but the time it takes to come to room temperature varies depending on the cut. Leave it on the counter for up to 2 hours, if possible, before cooking. This may not help a large roast, which will likely still be cold in the center after only 2 hours, but it will take the chill off a tenderloin. To be safe, however, don't leave any cuts of beef out for more than 2 hours, and don't leave ground beef out for more than 30 minutes.

Before cooking, trim excess fat from the outside of beef cuts, leaving a thin coating to protect the meat while it cooks. Cutting away all the fat contributes to dried-out meat. Meat that is not marinated should be trimmed just before cooking; meat that will be marinated should be trimmed before marinating.

Beef can be broiled, roasted, grilled, panfried, stewed, braised, and made into baked dishes and soups. As a general rule, the more tender cuts of beef—T-bone, sirloin, porterhouse, and strip steaks—benefit from quick, dry-heat methods of cooking, such as broiling, roasting, and grilling. The tougher, leaner cuts, including chuck, rump roast, and brisket, benefit from moist cooking, such as stewing, braising, and pot roasting. See the Beef Glossary at left for more details.

Beef that is roasted, grilled, or broiled (that is, cooked by a dry method) should be allowed to stand and "rest" for 5 to 25 minutes (depending on the size of the cut) before being carved. This gives the meat's juices, which rise to the surface during cooking, an opportunity to settle and redistribute themselves throughout the roast. The meat also firms up during the process and thus becomes easier to carve.

Doneness Temperatures for Beef	
Rare	120° to 130°F*
Medium-rare	130° to 140°F*
Medium	140° to 150°F*
Medium-well	150° to 160°F
Well-done	160° to 165°F

*Although these internal temperatures yield what many cooks feel are the optimum taste and texture, some are lower than those suggested by the U.S. Food Safety and Inspection Service guidelines; see Beef Safety, page 48, and DONENESS.

The best way to determine when beef is properly cooked is to gauge its internal temperature with an instant-read thermometer. When inserting the thermometer, make sure it does not touch bone, which can produce an inaccurate reading. Take the beef from the oven when the temperature reaches the lowest temperature in the range. The beef continues to cook from residual heat while standing.

Beef Safety In recent years there has been a good deal of media attention given to the need to cook meat properly in order to kill any potentially harmful bacteria. To make sense of these warnings, it is essential to understand the differences between whole cuts of beef, such as steaks and roasts, and ground beef. It is possible for the outside surface of beef cuts to become contaminated with bacteria during processing. These surface bacteria are rendered harmless by cooking, even if the interior is left rare or medium-rare. A problem arises, however, with ground beef, since during the grinding process any contamination on the surface can be mixed throughout the meat.

Ground beef should be cooked thoroughly, to 160°F in the center, to be perfectly safe. Steaks, roasts, and other whole cuts may safely be eaten rare if the surface of the beef has been cooked to 160°F, for example, if the surface is well seared, which would kill any bacteria.

Hands, utensils, and work surfaces that come into contact with raw beef must be washed in hot, soapy water to prevent bacteria spreading throughout the kitchen or to other foods.

See also CARVING; FOOD SAFETY; STOCK; individual cooking methods.

BEET Grandma might be surprised by the fuss being made over this hardy root vegetable. Beets were unglamorous kitchen staples for generations, but now they are showing up on every fashionable menu.

Also called beetroots, many boast a deep, rich red color combined with a sweet, earthy flavor and tender texture, making them a great favorite with chefs and home cooks alike.

Although beets will always be associated with their lovely deep red color, today it is not unusual to find pink, golden, white, and even striped beets in the market. These festive-looking vegetables have more or less the same flavor and texture as their red cousins, but provide unexpected color to dishes where the red beet is more commonly found.

Beets are served warm as a side dish, cold in salads, pickled, or made into the famous beet soup, borscht. Young, fresh-looking, bright green beet greens from small or medium-sized beets are delicious. Sauté or steam them as you would spinach.

Quick Tip

When working with red and pink beets, be prepared for beet-red stains on your hands and countertops. The color is difficult to remove from wood or plastic surfaces; you may want to work on waxed paper and wear gloves.

Selecting Beets are available all year, but are at their best in late summer and autumn. While most beets are about the size of small lemons, much smaller beets, about the size of large marbles, are in the markets now. Regardless of the size, look for firm, rounded vegetables with smooth skins and no noticeable bruising. Fresh beets, sold in bunches, should have the greens attached and 1 to 2 inches of root end, which looks like a tail. Do not buy beets with wilted, browning leaves—the leafy greens indicate the freshness of the beets. If the greens have been trimmed, look for bunches with at least 2 inches of stem still attached.

Storing Cut the greens from the root vegetable as soon as you get home, leaving 1 to 2 inches of stem attached. The beets will not spoil if left at cool room temperature for a few days, but they do best when refrigerated for up to 10 days. If they turn soft, discard them. Beet greens should be washed and cooked on the day they are bought. They do not keep well; if necessary, however, they may be put unwashed into a perforated plastic bag and refrigerated overnight. Canned and pickled beets should be refrigerated after opening. Canned beets will keep for 1 week after opening; pickled beets will keep for at least twice this period of time. Fully cooked and cooled whole beets can be frozen in zippered plastic freezer bags or rigid containers for up to 10 months.

Preparing Beets are best when cooked whole and unpeeled, then peeled and sliced, chopped, or mashed afterward. Roasting beets will help intensify their flavor and color, and you should wrap them in aluminum foil first, so you won't have to clean a pan. If boiling, leave about 1 inch of the stem and the root end intact to keep the beets from "bleeding" into the cooking water. Once they are fork-tender, let them cool and then slip off their skins.

For more information, see BOILING; ROASTING; STEAMING.

BELGIAN ENDIVE See CHICORY.

BELL PEPPER Also called sweet pepper. Bell peppers may be green, red, yellow, orange, brown, or purple. Some are blunt ended, while others are tapered, but the shape does not make any difference in the flavor.

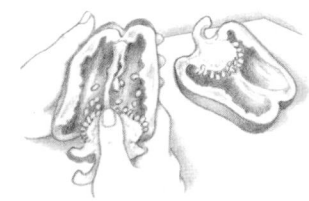

Bell peppers are available all year long. Green bell peppers are usually sharper flavored, more plentiful, and less expensive than peppers of other colors. They are immature and do not ripen once picked. Red bell peppers are simply a more mature (and sweeter) stage of green bell peppers. Other colors are separate varieties of pepper.

Use bell peppers raw in salads and for crudités. They often appear in sauces, stews, soups, relishes, and baked dishes. Large bells are excellent for stuffing and roasting, and any size pepper can be grilled. Bell peppers, particularly red ones, are delicious roasted and peeled, at which point they can be refrigerated in plastic bags or rigid containers—as is or covered with olive oil—for 3 to 4 days.

Selecting Buy firm, smooth, bright-colored peppers.

Storing Refrigerate the peppers as soon as you get them home, storing them loosely in a perforated plastic bag. Green peppers keep for at least 1 week, while red, yellow, orange, and purple peppers are best used within 5 or 6 days.

Preparing Cut the pepper in half at the equator or lengthwise. Remove a pepper's stem with your hands or a knife. Trim away the seeds and white membranes, or ribs, and cut to desired size and shape.

Stemming.

HOW TO *Roast and Peel Bell Peppers*

1. Using tongs or a large fork, hold the pepper over the flame of a gas burner, turning as needed, until the skin is blistered and charred black on all sides, 10 to 15 minutes. This may also be done in a broiler; watch the peppers carefully to prevent burning their flesh.

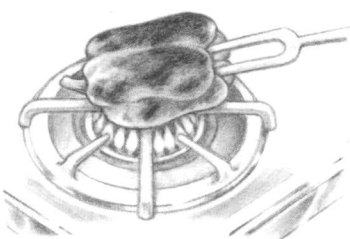

2. Once the skin is blackened and puffy, transfer the peppers to a paper bag and close loosely. This allows the peppers to steam as they cool and helps the skins to loosen.

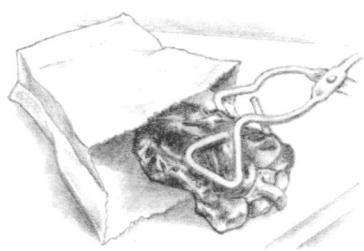

3. When cool, peel or rub away the charred skin. Do not worry if a little stays on the flesh. Don't rinse the peppers under running water, or you will wash away some flavor.

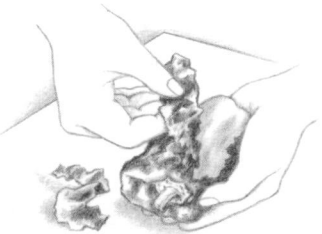

4. Lay the peppers on a cutting board. Using a small, sharp knife, slit each pepper lengthwise. Some liquid will run out, so have paper towels handy. Open the pepper and spread it on the cutting board. Cut around the stem end, then remove the stem, seeds, and membrane.

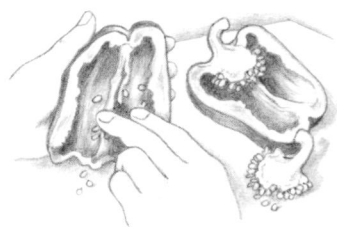

Quick Tip

When roasted whole, bell peppers accumulate sweet juices inside their cavities. If you like, peel and seed them over a bowl to catch those juices, then strain the juices to eliminate any seeds or bits of charred skin. If the roasted peppers will be used in a salad, add the juices to the dressing; or reserve them for adding extra flavor to a marinade or sauce.

HOW TO *Prepare Peppers for Stuffing*

Most recipes for stuffed bell peppers require parboiling the peppers first. Even if not specified, parboiling will make the peppers more tender.

1. Cut a slice ½ inch thick from the stem end of each pepper, leaving an opening like the top of a bowl. Remove the seeds and membrane.
2. Bring a large pot three-fourths full of water to a boil. Place a bowl of cold water nearby. Drop the peppers into the boiling water and cook until slightly softened, about 5 minutes.
3. Using tongs, transfer the peppers to the cold water to halt the cooking, then drain, cut side down, on paper towels.
4. When cool, stuff the peppers and cook according to individual recipes.

BERRY Berries are small, succulent fruits that grow on bushes, vines, or canes. They are available year-round, although they are more flavorful, plentiful, and affordable in the spring and summer months (except for

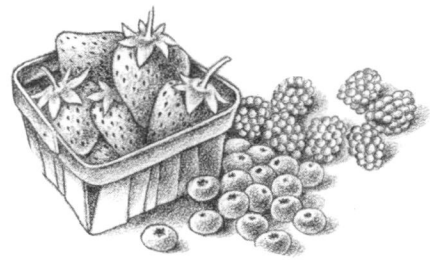

cranberries, which are in season in the autumn, and raspberries, which have a second harvest in fall).

Owing to their delicacy, many varieties must be hand-harvested, which contributes to their expense. Berries can be served raw or cooked into sauces, pies, relishes, and other sweet and savory preparations. They also make wonderful ice creams, sorbets, and preserves.

BLACKBERRY The blackberry is sweetest when completely black. When immature, blackberries are green or red. Blackberries are in season from late spring to early autumn and are best in high summer. Among the most fragile berries, blackberries should not be refrigerated for more than a day. Olallieberries are a kind of blackberry, and boysenberries and loganberries are blackberry hybrids. They may be freely substituted for one another or combined in recipes.

BLUEBERRY Blueberries are in season from late spring to late summer. They are dark blue and should have a powdery white bloom. When the bloom is gone, the berries are too old. Blueberries can be refrigerated for up to 1 week. Wild blueberries from Maine are legendary and, while they do not travel well, are increasingly available frozen. These wild berries (which are now domesticated as well) are smaller and darker than ordinary blueberries and usually very sweet.

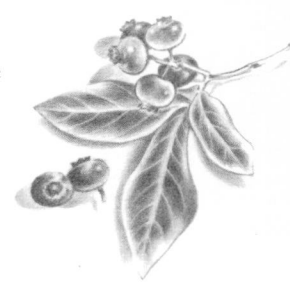

BOYSENBERRY This blackberry hybrid is a little larger and more purple to red hued than other cultivated blackberries. Boysenberries are preferred by some because of their sweet-tart flavor, juiciness, and large size.

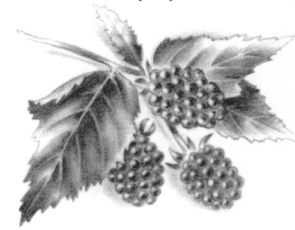

CRANBERRY Native to North America, the cranberry is an integral part of American cooking, from the cranberry relish served with the Thanksgiving turkey to the healthful glass of bottled cranberry juice. The berries are harvested throughout the fall, with most of the crop finding its way to commercial food processors for sauce and juice. Cranberries are too tart to eat raw on their own but lend themselves to savory and sweet preparations, marrying nicely with other fruits, such as apples and pears, and with nuts and grains. Fresh cranberries should be plump, firm, and dry and range from deep scarlet to light red. Both fresh and

b

frozen whole cranberries are usually packaged in plastic bags rather than sold loose. Refrigerate the berries for up to 1 month, or freeze them for up to 10 months.

CURRANT The red currant is grown in the United States, while both red and black currants are available in northern Europe, where they enjoy great popularity. Since they are both high in pectin, a natural jelling agent, most currants find their way into jams, preserves, jellies, and syrups. Although perfectly ripe currants are pleasing to anyone who likes slightly tart fruit, they are usually sweetened before they are eaten. Fresh currants are in season from early July through early August but are difficult to find in markets. If you locate them, buy small, firm berries and refrigerate them for no longer than 2 days. So-called dried currants are actually dried grapes, or raisins.

GOOSEBERRY This small berry, resembling a white-striped grape, is pale green and quite tart when underripe and gold, red, pink, white, or dark burgundy when ripe. Ripe gooseberries can be eaten straight from the plant, although they are sometimes very tart. Underripe berries are cooked and sweetened for making preserves, sauces, and pies. The berries are not readily available in markets in the United States but are popular in Europe. If you find them for sale, choose large, firm berries and refrigerate them for up to 3 days.

HUCKLEBERRY Close relatives of the blueberry, huckleberries, also called whortleberries, tend to be seedier and a little tarter and are not cultivated. One variety grows on the East Coast and another on the West Coast, with the latter being a true berry and the former a drupe, or a fruit with a center seed.

LOGANBERRY A blackberry hybrid developed in California and named after a Santa Cruz judge, James Logan. Loganberries are large and cone shaped, more purple than black, and decidedly juicy.

MARIONBERRY Another blackberry hybrid, often sold simply as "blackberries." Marionberries are sweet and firm enough to hold up in baking and in desserts.

MULBERRY These fragile berries with a sweet-sour flavor are rarely sold commercially. When ripe, they fall from the bush or tree and are gathered off the ground—mostly in home gardens. They look much like blackberries but come in white and red as well as black.

OLALLIEBERRY A large, fragrant blackberry hybrid that grows in California and is sweet and juicy. Because they are fragile and do not travel well, olallieberries are not usually available outside their region. They are most commonly found at farmers' markets, or at pick-your-own farms.

RASPBERRY For many people, this is the ultimate berry. Fragrant and subtly sweet-tart, raspberries, which grow on low, thorn-laden shrubs and have been cultivated for hundreds of years, can be red, black, or golden. All taste similar and all are extremely delicate, with hollow centers. Eat them as soon after purchase as possible. Raspberry season extends from June through October.

STRAWBERRY Bright red berries bursting with sweet flavor and blessed with a heady fragrance, strawberries are available all year, although they are best in the spring and early summer. Some large berries can taste good, but most giant supermarket berries do not. Shop for strawberries at farmers' markets, looking for smaller berries, preferably organic, with a rich, glossy red color and shiny green leaves. Avoid berries with white or green shoulders and brown or limp leaves. Tiny strawberries called wild or wood strawberries or *fraises des bois* are especially sweet. Hull strawberries before freezing them or using them for most preparations. To do so, use a small paring knife or a strawberry huller to carve out the white center core from the stem end of each berry.

Quick Tip

To bring out the flavor of lackluster berries, put them in a bowl (hull and slice strawberries first) and sprinkle with a little sugar, a tablespoon or two for every pint. Let them sit at room temperature for at least 15 minutes. The sugar draws moisture from the berries to make a sweet natural syrup.

Selecting Berries should be selected with care. Never buy them if they are moist, overly soft, pale colored, or show signs of mold. Do not buy berries if their cartons are leaking and wet, a sure sign that unseen fruits will be moldy. In fact, a quick check of the underside of the carton may very well let you see any mold that is growing on bruised fruit at the bottom; put that carton back. As a rule, berries are best in their natural season. Seek them out at large food stores, farmers' markets, and pick-your-own farms.

Frozen berries are often good. They are sold coated in sweet syrup or unsweetened. For recipes that call for fresh berries and require sugar to be added, use unsweetened frozen berries. If you plan to spoon the berries over ice cream, pound cake, or yogurt, sweetened berries are a fine choice, forming their own syrup as they thaw.

Storing Berries are fragile and should be handled with care. All require refrigeration, and they freeze well. Don't wash berries until just before you plan to eat them, as the moisture will encourage mold. If you don't plan to eat the berries within 1 to 2 days, rinse and dry them completely and then freeze them. Frozen berries will keep for 8 to 10 months.

HOW TO *Freeze Berries*

1. Put cranberries in the freezer in their original plastic bag packaging. Pack blueberries in rigid plastic containers and freeze. Spread more delicate raspberries, blackberries, and hulled strawberries in a single layer on a baking sheet and then freeze them. When firm, transfer to rigid plastic containers or zippered plastic freezer bags.

2. There is no need to thaw frozen berries for many recipes, including most sauces or ice creams. If a recipe calls for thawed berries, let them sit at room temperature for an hour or so. If necessary, transfer them to a colander to drain. You may capture the juice and use it for flavoring drinks or for other recipes.

Preparing While all fresh berries should be rinsed, they should not be soaked for any length of time, since they will absorb the water and turn mushy. For eating on their own, all berries—even the largest strawberries—should be left whole.

BEURRE BLANC See SAUCE.

BISCUIT Small, raised quick breads, biscuits are usually unsweetened and served piping hot. They are most readily associated with Southern cooking and generally are made from white flour, butter, a leavener, and milk or buttermilk. The most desirable qualities of a biscuit are tenderness, flakiness, and rich yet delicate flavor.

Add sugar to biscuit dough and it becomes shortcake, which can be split and topped with sweetened strawberries, peaches, or another fruit and sweetened whipped cream. Sweet biscuit dough is also used as a topping for fruit cobbler.

Biscuit cutters.

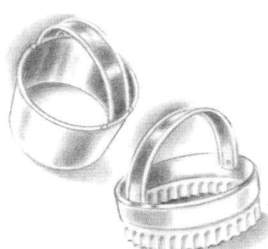

Like all quick bread batters, biscuit batter should be baked soon after mixing. As they bake, biscuits rise straight up, rather than spreading as many cookies do, and their tops turn golden brown. Once baked, they should be served hot from the oven, split and spread with butter, which will begin to melt immediately. They are also delicious with preserves or filled with ham or turkey. Biscuits spread with honey and served with fried chicken are old-fashioned comfort food.

Biscuit Savvy

■ When cutting the butter or other fat into the flour, work quickly so it does not melt too much before you put the dough in the oven. If the butter or fat becomes soft, it prevents the flakiness that characterizes good biscuits.

■ Biscuit dough can be mixed in a food processor. Take care not to overmix, using only on-off pulses. The fat should remain in discrete, flour-covered chunks the size of small peas.

■ When pouring the liquid (usually milk or buttermilk) into the flour-fat mixture, do it all at once. If it's added in small amounts and stirred after each addition, the dough will be overworked and the biscuits will not be flaky.

■ Do not overknead biscuit dough, or the biscuits will be tough. Gently knead just until the dough is smooth and cohesive but still soft and a little sticky.

■ Dip your biscuit cutter in flour to slice more easily through sticky dough.

■ When stamping out biscuits, do not twist the cutter. Lift straight up to prevent the sides of the dough from pinching together or twisting, which can inhibit rising or make misshapen or tough biscuits.

■ After cutting out as many biscuits as you can from the initial patting or rolling out, gather the dough remnants together, pat out, and cut out one more batch. Do not reroll scraps more than once, or your biscuits will be tough.

■ If you like a crisp crust, lightly brush the tops with water before baking. For soft biscuits, brush them with milk.

Quick Tip

If you don't have a biscuit cutter, use a cookie cutter or an inverted thin water glass. Another option is to pat the dough out into a square and cut out square-shaped biscuits with a chef's knife.

See also CUTTING IN.

BISCUIT CUTTER See BAKING TOOLS.

BLACK BEAN See BEAN, DRIED.

BLACKBERRY See BERRY.

BLACKENING A technique in which food, usually whole fish, fish fillets, or steak, is cooked in an extremely hot skillet, usually cast iron. The heat chars the exterior of the food so that it literally turns black. The quick cooking leaves the interior of the food tender and moist. Blackening is associated with Cajun cooking and was made popular by chef Paul Prudhomme of New Orleans. In traditional recipes for blackened food, the fish or meat is rubbed with a spice mixture before it is cooked. This forms a full-bodied blackened crispy crust that imparts extra aromatic flavor to the flesh beneath.

True blackening produces billows of smoke, so do not attempt this technique at home unless you have a well-ventilated kitchen. Most blackening is done in restaurant kitchens that are equipped with professional stoves capable of producing extremely high heat.

BLACK-EYED PEA See BEAN, DRIED; PEA, FRESH.

BLANCHING To submerge food—usually vegetables or fruits—in a generous amount of boiling water for a few seconds or for up to a minute or two before plunging it immediately into very cold water, preferably ice water, to stop the cooking process. The immersion in boiling water does not cook the food but just softens its texture. Plunging it into cold water sets a bright color as well. (This technique is also known as refreshing or shocking.) Blanching also makes some thin-skinned fruits, such as peaches or tomatoes, easier to peel, while leaving the inner flesh firm. Strong flavors—such as those of onions and garlic—may be mellowed by blanching, and sometimes cured meats—bacon, ham, salt pork—are blanched to reduce their saltiness.

Blanching is also necessary before freezing certain vegetables in order to disable the enzymes that would otherwise ruin their bright color and firm texture. Broccoli, Brussels sprouts, carrots, cauliflower, corn, green beans, okra, and English peas should all be blanched before they are frozen for this reason.

Tongs, large strainers with handles, pasta pots with perforated inserts, slotted spoons, and mesh skimmers may all be used for blanching. They allow you to move the food quickly from the hot water to the cold water so that it does not continue cooking longer than desired.

Foods may be blanched up to a day ahead of time and refrigerated until they are needed.

b

Quick Bite

The term *blanching* can also refer to cooking food partially in hot oil as a preparatory step in a recipe. French fries, for example, are often blanched in hot fat, drained, and then finished in fat at a higher temperature.

HOW TO *Blanch Vegetables for Freezing*

1. Plunge the vegetables into a large pot of boiling water for 20 seconds to 2 minutes. (Blanching time will depend on the recipe or on the size and hardness of the vegetables.) Begin counting from when the water starts to bubble again.

2. Using tongs, a strainer, or similar utensil, immediately transfer the vegetables to ice water. The water must be as cold as possible to ensure that they retain their bright color. Let the vegetables cool, but do not leave them soaking in the water.

HOW TO *Blanch Fruits for Peeling*

1. First cut out the stem and then score, or shallowly cut, an X in the blossom end of the fruit. This will help you remove the skin quickly.

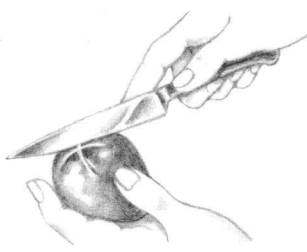

2. Plunge the fruit into a large pot of boiling water for 20 to 60 seconds. (Blanching time will depend on the recipe or on the size and hardness of the fruit.) Begin counting from when the water starts to bubble again. The fruit is ready when the skin begins to wrinkle. Remove it quickly—any longer and it may begin to cook.

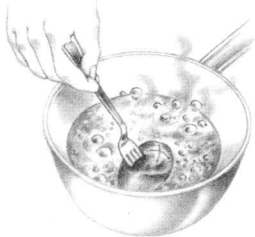

3. Using tongs, a strainer, a fork, or a similar utensil, transfer the fruit to very cold water, preferably ice water.
4. As soon as it is cool, remove the fruit from the water and peel away the skin, using your fingers or a small paring knife.

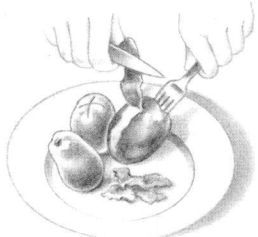

Quick Bite

In agriculture, blanching refers to covering a vegetable, such as asparagus, with straw or soil as it grows to prevent sunlight from activating its chlorophyll and turning it green.

BLENDER Also called liquefiers, blenders are excellent for puréeing soups and blending cold drinks such as milk shakes or fruit smoothies. Basic blenders can also be used to chop bread for fresh bread crumbs and to chop herbs. They can usually handle more liquid volume than food processors and are good complements to them. (Blenders do not aerate liquid well and they quickly overbeat delicate mixtures, so do not use them for whipping cream or beating egg whites.) When buying a blender, choose a sturdy, powerful model with a reliable motor that will last for years.

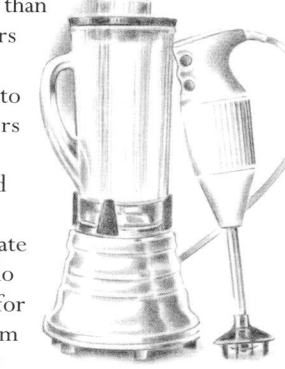

Standing Blenders These blenders have heavy metal or plastic bases that encase electric motors. A widemouthed, lidded canister, called a jar, is designed to fit on the base, permitting the motor to spin a small propeller-type blade inside the jar. Jars generally hold 5 to 8 cups, and most have lids fitted with removable center caps that double as 2-ounce measures. The removable cap also allows you to pour liquid into the blender while the motor is running without stopping to remove and replace the entire lid. Be sure to put the lid on while you're blending at higher speeds, and never stick a spoon or anything else into the jar while the blade is moving. Invest in a blender with a glass jar, as plastic retains odors. You don't want garlic-scented milk shakes or margaritas. Blenders can have as many as 16 or more speeds, although some, including many super-powered bar blenders, have only 2 speeds. Others have special ice-breaking capabilities. Don't try to break ice in your blender unless the instruction booklet assures you that your machine is up to the job.

Immersion Blenders Also called hand or handheld blenders, immersion blenders have an extended blade that is immersed in a food or mixture to blend or purée it. Immersion blenders are great for puréeing food in the container in which it is mixed or cooked. This means that they can blend larger amounts of food than will fit in the jar of a standing blender. Immersion blenders also tend to incorporate more air into a liquid and as such can be used to make frothy foam on creamed soups. These blenders usually have only 2 speeds, and the blade must be completely immersed in the food to prevent spattering. Many are designed to hang in a wall mount for easy storage. Some have whisk attachments or small containers for blending smaller amounts of food.

BLENDING To mix at least two ingredients so that they combine thoroughly and evenly. Chopped or minced vegetables and meat can be blended as well as liquid ingredients or dry ingredients. Blending differs from beating because its purpose is only to combine the ingredients, not to incorporate air into the mixture. It can be accomplished by spoon, fork, whisk, rubber spatula, electric mixer, food processor, blender, or your bare hands.

See also BEATING; BLENDER; CREAMING; MIXER; MIXING.

BLIND BAKING Also called prebaking, blind baking means partially or completely baking a pie or tart shell before filling it. Some very juicy pie fillings, such as berry and other fruit fillings, can make a bottom crust soggy, but partially baking a crust prevents the crust from absorbing too much liquid. Other pie and tart fillings, such as custard, are cooked separately from the crust or require no baking, and in these cases the crusts must be fully baked before they are filled. Follow the instructions given in your recipe.

HOW TO *Blind Bake*

1. After the dough is rolled out and fitted into the pans, carefully lay a sheet of aluminum foil or parchment paper over the dough and weight it down with a layer of raw rice, dried beans, or pie weights, small metal or ceramic balls designed specifically for this use. If using rice or beans, discard them after a couple of bakings.

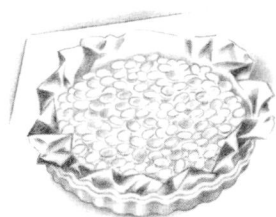

2. Bake according to the instructions in the recipe. If partially prebaking, this is usually until the sides of the crust are just set but still pale. If completely prebaking, it's until the crust is a deep golden brown. In either case, the recipe will instruct you to remove the weights and foil or paper after several minutes and continue cooking until the crust is ready. At this point, some recipes will instruct you to prick the crust with the tines of a fork to permit steam to escape before continuing.

3. If the filling is not baked in the crust, set the pan on a wire rack and let cool completely before filling, to prevent sogginess.

Blind baking generally takes from 25 to 40 minutes, depending on whether the shell is to be partially or fully baked, and on the ingredients, the size and thickness of the pastry, and the size of the pan.

Tiny tartlet shells, baked in individual tartlet molds, are nearly always blind baked. Because it is awkward to line small molds with foil, spray the outsides of same-shaped molds with cooking spray and set them inside the pastry-lined molds. Weight these with beans, rice, or pie weights and proceed as directed above.

See also BAKING; PIE & TART; ROLLING OUT.

BLUEBERRY See BERRY.

BOILING Heating liquid to its hottest point before it evaporates. At sea level, water boils at 212°F. (For boiling at high altitude, see HIGH-ALTITUDE COOKING.) When water, or any other liquid, boils, it moves rapidly and large air bubbles break through the surface in rapid succession. When this bubbling cannot be halted by stirring, cooks refer to it as a rapid, full, or rolling boil. When the bubbles are smaller and cling to the edges of the cooking pot so that the surface of the liquid gently undulates instead of rolls, the liquid is said to be simmering (about 185°F). A moderate boil is the state between these two: larger air bubbles rise to the surface than at a simmer, but at a slower pace than during a rolling boil. Simmering and moderately boiling liquids temporarily stop bubbling when stirred.

Boiling causes the liquid to convert to gas, which, in the case of water, takes the form of steam. (This steam can scald you just as boiling water can, so use caution!) Any liquid that is allowed to boil for a length of time will eventually disappear, with all the water in it converting to steam.

Solids, even those that have liquefied, will be left behind. When used deliberately in stock and sauce making, this process is called "reducing" or "cooking down" the liquid, allowing it to thicken and combine with the solids into a sauce or gravy.

Boiling is an intense method of cooking and should be used only for certain sturdy vegetables and dried pastas. Dried pasta is a particularly good candidate because a large pot of boiling water can disperse the starch that naturally comes off pasta as it cooks; as a result, the pasta will be neither gummy nor sticky. Even though the names of some meat dishes suggest that they are boiled, such as New England boiled dinner, the meat is actually gently simmered (called braising) or poached. Boiling any meat would in fact render it tough and tasteless.

Boiling Times for Various Foods

Food	Time
Artichoke, medium	30 to 40 minutes
Asparagus	
Thin spears	4 to 6 minutes
Thick spears	7 to 10 minutes
Beets	
Medium	30 to 35 minutes
Large	45 to 60 minutes
Broccoli	
Florets	3 to 5 minutes
Spears	7 minutes
Cauliflower	
Florets	3 to 5 minutes
Head	10 to 15 minutes
Corn on the cob	1 to 2 minutes
Pasta	
Strand pasta	6 to 8 minutes
Shaped pasta	8 to 12 minutes
Peas	3 to 5 minutes
Potatoes, cut into 1½- to 2-inch chunks	20 to 25 minutes

Use times only as a guideline when boiling food, relying on other tests to determine when the food is done. Taste the pasta and peas; pierce the potatoes and broccoli with a sharp knife to test for tenderness. Cooking times start when the water returns to a boil after the food is added.

Quick Tip

Boiling green vegetables in a lot of water helps retain their color but results in lost nutrients. Boiling them in smaller amounts of water retains nutrients but not as much color.

See also BLANCHING; HIGH-ALTITUDE COOKING; REDUCING; SIMMERING.

BOK CHOY Also called pak-choi, Chinese white cabbage, or white mustard cabbage, this common Asian vegetable is one of the best-known members of the extended Chinese cabbage family. Bok choy has long, white stalks with dark green leaves; a mild, chardlike flavor; and a crunchy texture. Baby bok choy is about half the size and more tender. Cut-up bok choy can be stir-fried, sautéed, or used raw in salads. Whole baby bok choy is good braised or steamed.

Selecting The stalks and leaves should be crisp, firm, and brightly colored. Avoid stalks with brown spots, bruising, or cracking or wilted leaves.

Storing Refrigerate bok choy in a plastic bag for up to 4 days.

Preparing Stalks and leaves may be used together or separately. Trim the stalks before using, removing the tough ends. If using leaves only, separate the leaves from the stalks and chop or shred as desired.

BONING Some recipes require removing the bones, sinews, and excess fat from meat or poultry. The terms *debone* and *fillet* also mean to bone. Many beginning cooks feel boning is too difficult to tackle, although with the right knife and a little practice it is an easy matter to bone a chicken breast or thigh. It is economical, too, because boneless cuts are pricier than bone-in cuts. Boning a tiny quail, a leg of lamb, or a whole fish, however, takes more skill, and you'll probably want to leave these tasks to the butcher or fishmonger.

Boned food cooks more quickly than bone-in food. It is well suited for poaching, sautéing, frying, and quick grilling.

A boning knife has a 6- or 7-inch-long, narrow blade that cuts through tendons and cartilage, slips easily between the flesh and bones of the meat or poultry, and is flexible enough to follow the contours of the bones.

b

HOW TO *Bone a Chicken Breast*
1. Skin the breast, if desired; pull off the skin and use a boning knife as needed to cut it free.
2. If starting with a whole breast, place the breast bone side up and slit down the center of the thin membrane covering the breastbone. Grasp the breast firmly at each end and flex it upward to pop out the breastbone. Pull out the bone, using a boning knife if needed. Cut through the center of the breast to split it in half, cutting away the tough sinews between the halves.

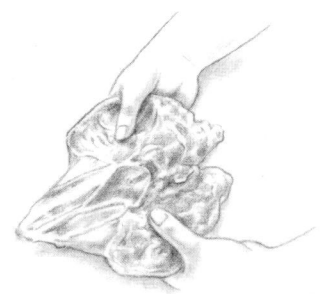

continued

3. To bone each breast half, starting along the rib side, insert a boning knife between the bones and meat. Following the curve of the bone with the knife and lifting the meat with your other hand, gradually cut the meat away from the bone. When you come to the wishbone, make a slit to remove the meat.

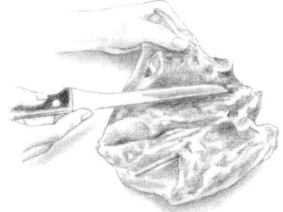

4. When the meat is free of the bone, trim away the tough membrane from the rib edge of the breast meat. Find the white tendon on the underside and remove it by scraping the meat away from it with your knife until it detaches from the breast. Trim the breast of any large bits of fat or skin.

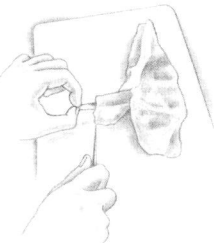

HOW TO *Bone a Chicken Thigh and Leg*

1. Skin the chicken, if desired; pull off the skin and use a boning knife as needed to cut it free.
2. Without separating the thigh and leg, cut along the thigh bone to expose it. Cut down the length of the leg to expose the leg bone.

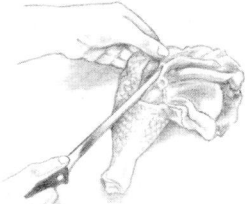

3. Using your fingers, push the meat away from the bones. Holding the thigh bone, let the thigh meat and the leg meat and bone hang from it.
4. Lay the meat on the cutting board, spreading it out as much as possible. Following the line where the meat is still attached, carefully cut the meat from the bones.

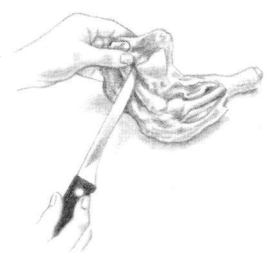

5. Carefully cut the leg meat from the thigh meat, if desired. For a more attractive presentation, trim away rough edges.

BORAGE See HERB.

BORLOTTI BEAN See BEAN, DRIED.

BOUILLON See BROTH.

BOUQUET GARNI (boo-KAY gahr-NEE) This French term refers to a bundle of herbs added at the start of cooking to a soup or stew to perfume it with flavor. A traditional bouquet garni includes parsley, thyme, and bay leaf and is most often tied in cheesecloth to make the herbs easier to retrieve and discard at the end of cooking. Other herbs and aromatics also may be added. Some rustic bouquets garnis are enclosed within pieces of celery or the dark-green leaves of a leek, the whole bundle securely tied with kitchen string.

BOWL See BAKING TOOLS; MIXING BOWL.

BOYSENBERRY See BERRY.

BRAISING To simmer food slowly in a moderate amount of liquid. Relatively tough cuts of meat, such as chuck roast and brisket, and fibrous vegetables, such as carrots, celery, and leeks, are excellent candidates for braising. Braising liquid can be water or more flavorful liquid such as broth, stock, wine, or beer. Onions, garlic, herbs, or other ingredients are often added to braising liquid for flavoring. Braising and stewing are closely related, although stews are made with more liquid and smaller pieces of food.

Meat to be braised is generally browned first in fat to give it color and add to its flavor. It is then cooked in a relatively small amount of liquid (usually only 1 to 2 inches deep) in a tightly closed pot or baking dish on the top of the stove over medium-low to medium heat or in a moderate (325° to 350°F) oven. The lid prevents liquid from evaporating, and the food is quickly surrounded by steam.

Quick Tip

In classic French-style braising, the vegetables that are cooked with the meat or poultry to impart their aromatic flavors are not necessarily served. Instead, fresh vegetables may be added toward the end of cooking for the benefit of their fresher color, texture, and flavor.

Braising results in tender, full-flavored dishes. Braised dishes are typically hearty, cold-weather fare. Some favorite braised dishes are pot roast, coq au vin, and lamb shanks. The braising times in the chart at right are based on braising in a tightly lidded pot in a 325°F oven or on top of the stove over medium heat, maintaining the liquid at a gentle simmer.

See also BROWNING.

BRAN See FLOUR.

BRAZIL NUT See NUT.

Braising Times for Various Foods	
Beef flank steak, 1¼ to 1¾ inches thick	1½ to 1¾ hours
Beef pot roast, 3 to 4 pounds	2 to 3 hours
Beef rump roast, 3 to 5 pounds	3½ to 4 hours
Beef short ribs	1½ to 2 hours
Belgian endive, halved lengthwise	40 to 45 minutes
Cabbage, shredded	20 to 25 minutes
Chicken, 3½ pounds or less	35 to 40 minutes
Chicken, 3¾ to 4 pounds	50 to 60 minutes
Chicken, 5 to 6 pounds	1¾ to 2 hours
Fennel bulb, quartered	20 to 25 minutes
Lamb shanks, 1 pound each	1½ to 2¼ hours
Lamb shoulder, 3 to 5 pounds	2 to 2½ hours
Lamb shoulder chops, ¾ to 1¼ inches thick	35 to 45 minutes
Pork chops, 1 to 1½ inches thick	35 to 50 minutes
Pork ribs, country style	1½ to 2¼ hours
Radicchio, cut into wedges	3 to 5 minutes
Veal shanks, 1 pound each	2 to 3 hours
Veal shoulder, 4 to 5 pounds	2 to 2½ hours

b

Bread

The most basic bread is made of flour, water, and a leavener, usually yeast. From this elemental triad come all breads, some of them made with specialty flours, others with sweeteners such as honey and molasses, and still others with fruits and nuts.

Breads can be formed into traditional or free-form loaves or into rolls or buns. Although most are leavened with yeast and thus dubbed yeast breads, others known as quick breads are raised with baking powder and baking soda or, in a few cases, eggs. See QUICK BREAD for more information.

Most people buy bread in the supermarket, where the selection is slowly but surely getting better. Today, large supermarkets may have in-store bakeries that sell fresh-baked European-style or rustic breads. These loaves tend to have a soft crumb (interior) and crisp 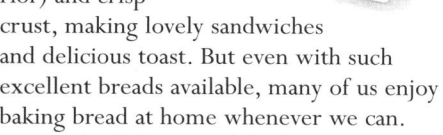 crust, making lovely sandwiches and delicious toast. But even with such excellent breads available, many of us enjoy baking bread at home whenever we can.

Nearly all flour used for bread baking is milled from wheat. Wheat flour contains glutenin, the protein in the bread that expands into elastic strands known as gluten to capture the gases released by the yeast during kneading, rising, and baking. Other flours, such as rye, corn, and rice, do not have glutenin, or they have such a tiny amount that it is not capable of raising bread. For this reason, recipes for breads made with other flours include wheat flour, too. Cake and pastry flours are rarely appropriate for breads because of their small amounts of glutenin.

Some recipes call for making a sponge, which is a very wet version of the bread dough and acts as a kind of head start for the yeast. The sponge, left at room temperature for an hour or longer (up to 36 hours), will swell as the yeast interacts with the flour and water. When it's time to make the bread, the sponge is mixed with more flour and other ingredients for a loaf with good texture and boosted flavor.

Water is the liquid used for most breads. Some recipes call for milk, which produces a very tender crumb. Except for the warm water used to activate the yeast, the water used in the recipe should be at room temperature. Tap water is generally fine, although some bakers think bottled or filtered water makes better-tasting bread. If your tap water tastes heavily of chemicals, you might want to consider buying water.

As a rule, breads contain very little fat, although some are rubbed with oil or softened butter before baking to encourage browning. A few recipes call for incorporat-

Quick Tip

To refresh a stale loaf of bread, sprinkle it with water, wrap it in aluminum foil, and bake it at 350°F until it is warm and soft. It will be good for one more use.

ing oil into the dough. Salt, on the other hand, is crucial to the taste of bread. A generous sprinkling brings out the flavor of the bread as nothing else will. Salt should be added to the dough with the bulk of the flour—never to the yeast and warm water mixture or to a sponge, as it inhibits the development of the yeast. See YEAST for further details.

Quick Tip

A little mold on a loaf of bread is not harmful. Cut it off and use the remaining bread. If numerous patches of mold are visible, however, discard the loaf.

In many bread recipes, a sprinkling of sugar or 1 teaspoon of honey is added to the yeast and water mixture to give the yeast a boost as it bubbles and swells. This small amount makes no significant contribution to the final flavor of the bread, and while the sweetener feeds the yeast, using it for proofing is not necessary. Of course, doughs for sweet breads, such as coffee cakes, dessert breads, muffins, cinnamon buns, and so on, are sweetened intentionally. Granulated and brown sugar, honey, and molasses are the most commonly used sweeteners, although some recipes call for maple syrup, barley malt, rice syrup, and organic cane sugar syrup.

Selecting Bread is a supermarket staple, and regular turnover is not usually a problem. Most stores stock fresh bread, but you should check the sell-by date to make sure it hasn't passed. Presliced soft-crusted loaves should feel relatively heavy and soft. Fresh-baked bread is generally better in quality than presliced, but it won't last as long. Crusty breads and rolls should feel firm but not rock solid.

Storing Store bread at room temperature, on a cupboard shelf or in a bread box or drawer. Fresh-baked bread may last only

1 or 2 days before going slightly stale (but perfect for fresh bread crumbs, stuffing, or French toast), while presliced bread should still be good 2 days after its sell-by date. Storing crusty bread in plastic bags will keep it fresh longer but will compromise the crust by making it soft.

Refrigeration can dry out bread, although pita bread and tortillas should be refrigerated. If you must refrigerate bread, put it in a zippered plastic bag to hold in moisture. Bread also freezes well enclosed in a zippered plastic freezer bag. Let frozen or refrigerated loaves come to room temperature in their packaging. Slices from a frozen loaf can be toasted without thawing, although they will defrost in a matter of minutes on the countertop.

b

Quick Tip

Don't be tempted to defrost bread in the microwave. Even a short stint in the microwave will dry it out. If you must defrost a muffin, roll, or slice of bread in the microwave, wrap it first in a paper towel to hold in moisture and microwave it for only a few seconds at a time.

Toasting Bread Breakfast fanciers almost always make toast part of their morning ritual. And while some eaters may opt for honey, others may reach for butter and cinnamon-sugar, and still others may insist on strawberry preserves. But the topping is not the only variable. Toasting may be a simple process, but the results vary greatly depending on the approach. Some people like to start with a slightly stale loaf, which produces more firm-textured toast, while fresh bread yields toast that is crisp on the outside while still tender within. Toasting at a higher heat has a similar effect. For more uniformly crisp toast, prepare the bread at a lower heat, which will dry it more before it turns golden.

continued

Bread, continued

Yeast Bread Savvy

- Yeast and gluten thrive in warmth, so bread benefits from a warm kitchen, warm hands, and a good, hot oven.
- After mixing the yeast and warm water together, stir in the minimum amount of flour called for in a recipe to achieve the right consistency. More can be added, but it can't be removed.
- When mixing the dough, use your hands and a sturdy spoon (many bread bakers like wooden spoons and earthenware bowls for mixing bread) until the dough holds together in a cohesive mass. It will not be smooth. This can be also done in a stand mixer fitted with the paddle attachment or a food processor fitted with a steel blade.

Mixing by hand.

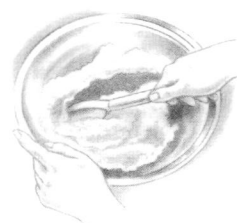

- For instructions on kneading, see KNEADING.
- A good test to determine if you have kneaded the bread long enough is to insert your fingertips into the dough. If the indentation springs back, the dough is well kneaded. The dough should also have a shiny look to its surface.
- Some heavy-duty stand mixers have dough hooks for kneading. Watch for the same indicators of properly kneaded dough as when kneading by hand.
- Kneaded dough is allowed to rise in an oiled or buttered bowl, after turning the dough to coat the surface. This coating prevents the dough from sticking to the bowl as it rises, allowing for a smooth and unimpeded leavening.

Placing in oiled bowl.

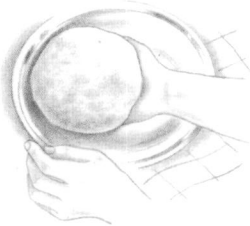

- Keep rising dough in a warm environment and allow ample time for the dough to rise. Most recipes call for dough to double in bulk.

Risen dough.

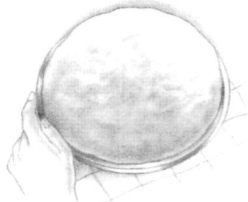

- Some breads benefit from second or even third risings, which help them develop finer texture and even more flavor. When repeated risings are called for, do not shape the dough into the desired loaf form until it has risen at least once.
- Bread will develop a finer texture and flavor if its rising is slowed by the cold of refrigeration. When time and your schedule allow, place the bowl of dough on a refrigerator shelf and leave it to rise slowly overnight.
- See PUNCHING DOWN and RELAXING for information on that step.
- Before baking, many bread recipes call for the top of a loaf to be slashed with a razor blade or sharp knife. These slashes enhance and increase crust area and promote more even rising in the oven.

- Most loaves are baked until they are well risen and lightly browned and sound hollow when tapped on the bottom. Take the bread from the oven, but do not turn the oven off. Turn the loaf from the pan into your hand (protected with an oven mitt) and literally knock on the bottom of the loaf with your bare knuckles. If it does not sound hollow, return it to the still-hot oven, checking it again after 5 to 7 minutes. If it does sound hollow, let it cool.
- Cool bread on wire racks to allow air to circulate. Allow the bread to cool completely before cutting—although it is tempting to cut it while warm and try a slice with butter melting on the hot crumb. However, the crumb will have the best flavor and texture if the bread is permitted to cool completely.

HOW TO *Shape Yeast Bread*

Following are simple instructions for shaping dough into the three basic loaf styles. In all cases, the dough should be allowed to rise after it has been shaped into a loaf, according to a recipe's instructions.

ROUND LOAF

The most basic of bread shapes, the round loaf nonetheless requires some technique to ensure an even, well-risen form.

1. After pressing the risen dough flat, form it into a ball. With both hands, stretch the sides of the dough downward and under, rotating the ball as you do so to form a tight, compact shape.

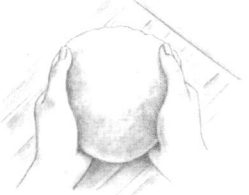

2. Pinch the seam closed to seal.

RECTANGULAR LOAF

All kinds of basic doughs may be baked in a loaf pan. Rolling up the dough and pinching its seams closed ensures a uniform, well-risen shape and even texture.

1. With a rolling pin, roll out a ball of dough into a flat, even rectangle of size specified. Starting at a short side, roll up the rectangle.

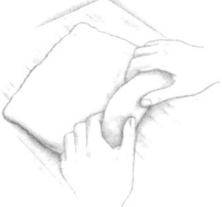

2. With your fingertips, pinch together the long seam and the spiral seams on both ends to seal them. Place the dough in a greased loaf pan with its long seam down.

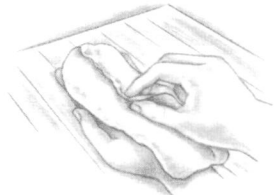

BRAIDED LOAF

Braiding, a traditional form for an egg loaf, is one of the easiest ways to prepare bread dough for a festive presentation.

1. Start with 3 ropes of dough of the length specified and braid them from the center to one end by alternately twisting the left- and right-hand ropes over the center rope. Pinch them together at one end. Braid from the center to the other end and pinch together to seal.

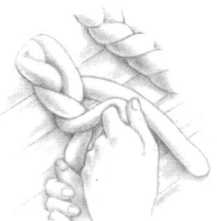

continued

Bread, continued

The Bread Basket Glossary

BAGEL A traditional, chewy Jewish bread made by forming dough into individually portioned doughnut shapes and then boiling them before baking. See BAGEL.

BAGUETTE A long, narrow loaf; also called French bread.

BOULE A rounded, free-form loaf with crisp crust.

BREADSTICKS Long, very narrow, crispy loaves of yeast bread, often coated with seeds. Also called *grissini*.

BRIOCHE Bread made from rich egg dough and traditionally baked in a mold so that it has a crowned top.

CHALLAH A high-rising, egg-rich yeast bread that is served at traditional Jewish holidays. The bread may be formed into elaborate loaves.

COUNTRY STYLE Any rustic, full-bodied, usually free-form yeast bread.

CROISSANT A flaky, buttery, half-moon-shaped bread made from a yeast dough similar to puff pastry. Croissants are often flavored with almond paste or filled with chocolate or cheese.

DANISH PASTRY A buttery pastry related to the croissant but sweeter and more breadlike.

FOCACCIA Yeast dough that is flattened, stretched, and dimpled before baking so that the finished loaf has a bumpy surface.

PITA A flat, round bread from the Middle East made with white or wheat flour and very little leavening. Known also as pocket bread or pita pockets, the bread forms a large hollow at the center as it bakes.

ROLL A wide variety of individual-portion breads, including the descriptively named clover-leaf and knot.

RYE A robust dark bread made from rye and wheat flour. See also FLOUR.

SODA BREAD In general, any bread leavened with baking soda, but more specifically, a traditional Irish loaf combining white and whole-wheat flours, buttermilk, baking soda, and salt.

SOURDOUGH Yeast bread with a tangy flavor, the result of a sourdough starter, or fermented mixture of flour, water, and yeast. Starters are kept for long periods of time, even passed from generation to generation. Atmospheric conditions contribute to the starter's flavor, which is why sourdoughs made from starters originating in a particular region (notably San Francisco) have a distinctive flavor.

STOLLEN Sweet yeast dough mixed with raisins, candied fruit, and citrus peel and juice and then folded into an oval shape before baking. Stollens are traditional holiday breads, particularly in Germany.

WHITE Refers specifically to those breads made from a dough of white-wheat flour.

WHOLE-GRAIN A general term applying to any bread that includes significant amounts of unrefined flour from any grain typically used in bread doughs.

See also BAGEL; BREAD CRUMBS; BREAD MACHINE; CORN BREAD; FLOUR; KNEADING; POPOVER; PUNCHING DOWN; QUICK BREAD; RISING; TORTILLA; UNMOLDING; YEAST.

BREAD BOARD See BAKING TOOLS.

BREAD CRUMBS Bread crumbs, fresh or dried, are the good cook's secret weapon, bestowing a crisp topping on casseroles and a crunchy coating on pan-fried meats. Dried bread crumbs, sold in canisters and cellophane packages, may be plain or seasoned and generally are finely ground. Seasoned dried crumbs, sometimes called Italian-style bread crumbs, often contain salt, herbs, and dried cheese and thus can interfere with other flavors in a dish. Be careful not to buy seasoned crumbs for a dessert preparation. Japanese-style dried bread crumbs, called *panko,* are sold in some supermarkets and in Asian food markets. They are delicate crystal-shaped crumbs that deliver an especially light, crisp texture to fried foods.

Fresh bread crumbs are almost always homemade (a few bakeries sell them), ground from slightly stale bread. About 2 ounces of bread, or 1 slice, makes about ½ cup bread crumbs. Making bread crumbs is a good way to use up the last few pieces of a loaf going stale.

Selecting When a recipe calls for bread crumbs, it usually means dried crumbs unless otherwise specified. Do not substitute one for the other, as fresh crumbs contain more moisture than dried and the two will behave differently in recipes.

Look for crumbs in a market with good turnover, checking their sell-by date before purchase. Even though packaged crumbs are dry, they will eventually become stale and contribute an "off" flavor to a dish. This is especially true of seasoned crumbs. If the crumbs are packed in clear cellophane, make sure they look fresh and dry.

Storing Store commercial dried bread crumbs in a cool, dry cupboard. They will keep for about 1 month after the sell-by date. Store homemade bread crumbs in a rigid plastic container or zippered plastic bag in the refrigerator for up to 1 month for dried and for 3 or 4 days for fresh. Freeze them for up to 1 year.

HOW TO *Make Bread Crumbs*

FRESH CRUMBS

1. Lay bread slices flat on the countertop and leave overnight to dry out, or "stale." Or use any bread a few days past its peak of freshness. Baguettes, whole-wheat breads, and egg breads make good crumbs.

2. Tear the bread into large pieces and process in a blender or food processor fitted with the metal blade to the texture you want.

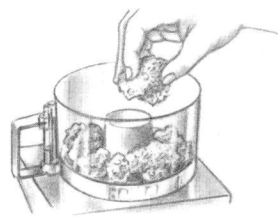

3. To season fresh crumbs, toss them with a teaspoon of olive oil for every cup, spread the crumbs on a baking sheet, and bake at 325°F, tossing once or twice, until crisp, 10 to 12 minutes. Add minced garlic, herbs, or spices to the olive oil for your flavor of choice.

DRIED CRUMBS

1. Let the bread dry out in a 200°F oven for about 1 hour. A hotter oven will brown the bread.

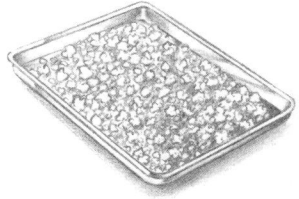

2. Break the bread into large pieces and then process in a blender or food processor into fine crumbs.

BREADING A crust or topping made primarily of bread crumbs, cracker crumbs, or another dry coating such as cornmeal. Breading is typically applied to foods that will be deep-fried or panfried. The crumbs, sometimes mixed with seasonings, grated cheese, or other ingredients, adhere to the food, such as a fritter, chicken breast, or fish fillet, and help it stay moist and tender during frying.

Breading is also the process by which these crumbs are applied to the food. Most often, the breading mixture is spread in a shallow dish, such as a pie dish, and the food is rolled in it, or the crumbs are patted on it. To help the crumbs stick, the food may first be dipped in beaten egg or another wet medium.

HOW TO *Bread Food*
Food should not be breaded until shortly before cooking. If allowed to sit too long with the coating, it will become gummy.
1. Dredge food in flour, turning to coat all sides and shaking off excess.
2. Dip food in beaten egg or another liquid, according to a recipe.
3. Place food in bread crumbs, patting in crumbs and again turning to coat all sides before shaking off excess.

BREAD MACHINE Bread dough is mixed, kneaded, raised, and baked in a bread machine. The process can be conveniently timed so that the bread is ready exactly when you want it—after work or first thing in the morning. Loaves baked in bread machines are shaped like the canister in which they are mixed and baked. Some people choose to mix, knead, and raise the dough in the machine but then shape it by hand and bake it in the oven.

See also BREAD.

BRIE See CHEESE.

BRINE A strong saltwater solution, a brine can be flavored with herbs, spices, or sugar, depending on its purpose. Brine is used to preserve or flavor food. Pickles are packed in brine; so is corned beef. The term "brining" means to immerse foods in brine or inject them with brine to preserve or flavor them, or both.

Caution!

Be sure to note that brine-cured meat is only partially cured and must still be cooked.

Soaking meat or poultry in brine to enhance its juiciness is an old-fashioned cooking technique that is now regaining popularity. Chefs and home cooks alike are discovering that a good brine bath adds flavor and juiciness to pork, chicken, turkey, even shrimp. Brining frozen shrimp for 15 to 20 minutes will refresh their texture after thawing. Depending on the food, brining can take from 30 minutes (for shrimp) to 2 days (for pork loin) to 2 weeks (for some pickles).

The brine must contain salt—for meat and poultry, use about a cup of kosher salt for every gallon of water—but other flavorings can be added, such as garlic, herbs, peppercorns, red pepper flakes, sugar, or honey. The brine can also include liquids other than water, such as cider, vinegar, beer, or wine. The salt should be kosher salt, which is free of additives. The liquid is brought to a boil to pick up the flavor of the herbs and spices, then thoroughly chilled before the food is added. The brine must cover the food completely. As the meat soaks, the salt will penetrate it, drawing in moisture and any other seasonings. The result is juicy, flavorful cooked meat and poultry that won't necessarily taste salty—just delicious.

See also CURING.

BROAD BEAN Another name for fava bean. See BEAN, DRIED; BEAN, FRESH.

BROCCOLI Broccoli is a cruciferous vegetable and is part of the cabbage family, as is cauliflower. In early stages of cultivation, these two vegetables resemble each other, and for hundreds of years, cooks made no distinction between them. Nowadays, we are perhaps more likely to cook broccoli than cauliflower. With its clusters of green florets topping thick stalks, broccoli is popular largely because it is readily available fresh all year long, is easy to cook, and is high in vitamins A and C and in iron.

Broccoli is at its best when briefly cooked. Although it can be eaten raw, too much of it can cause gastric distress. When cooked until soft, its flavor is strong and its texture unappealing. Consider steaming or stir-frying just until crisp-tender.

Selecting Buy heads with tightly clustered dark green or purplish florets and with no signs of yellowing or flowering. Stalks should be firm and fresh looking with healthy green leaves. Do not buy broccoli with tough or woody stems. The stalks of young, tender broccoli are slender, while those of older broccoli are thick and have hollow cores. Fresh broccoli, at its best from the fall through the spring, is available all year and usually is inexpensive.

Quick Bite

The small leaves on the broccoli stalk are higher in vitamin A than the florets, making them well worth eating.

Frozen broccoli is also readily available. Many markets sell only the florets, fresh or frozen, and these can be convenient for a quick weeknight dinner.

Storing Refrigerate broccoli as soon as you get it home. It will keep for 5 days in a perforated plastic bag. To freeze broccoli, trim the leaves and peel the stalks if they look a little woody. Cut the stalks and florets into small strips 1 to 3 inches long. Blanch the broccoli for about 5 minutes, plunge into cold water, drain, and freeze in freezer bags. Frozen broccoli keeps for about 1 year.

Preparing Trim the leaves on the broccoli stalk only if they appear discolored or unhealthy and cut away any tough portions on the bottoms of the stalks. If the stalk seems tough, peel it with a vegetable peeler or paring knife. Cut the broccoli lengthwise into manageable spears, usually about 3 inches long. Both the stalks and florets can be precooked by blanching or parboiling, particularly if you will be stir-frying or sautéing the vegetable. Florets cook more quickly than stalks, so split the stalks lengthwise only to the flower heads to cook them intact. Broccoli that is cooked until soft does not reheat well, but broccoli cooked until crisp-tender can be reheated.

Peeling broccoli stalks.

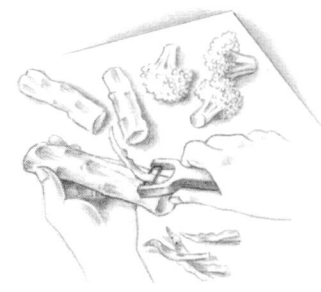

See also BLANCHING; BOILING; STEAMING.

BROCCOLI RABE Also called broccoli raab, rape, *rapini,* or Italian broccoli, broccoli rabe is a relative newcomer to the vegetable section of the average American market. The bright green vegetable, with its slender stalks and small florets, resembles a stunted head of broccoli, although it has many more leaves, which are small and jagged. Like broccoli, broccoli rabe is a cruciferous vegetable and is related to cabbage, turnips, and mustard. Chefs and home cooks alike appreciate its mild, pleasantly bitter taste with overtones of sweet mustard.

Broccoli rabe is popular in Italian cooking, where it may be sautéed in olive oil and garlic and served alongside meat or used as the basis of a pasta sauce. It can also be steamed, lightly braised, or blanched before sautéing, which reduces its bitterness. It is excellent cooked and chilled in salads or used to top pizzas.

Selecting Choose broccoli rabe with bright green florets and leaves and some open yellow flowers. Pass it up if the florets are yellowing. The stalks should be firm and can be slightly flexible. Some of the bottom leaves may appear slightly wilted, which is acceptable. Broccoli rabe is at its best during the autumn and winter.

Storing Refrigerate broccoli rabe in a perforated plastic bag for up to 3 days.

Preparing Trim any wilted leaves and any tough stem ends. As noted, some cooks blanch more mature broccoli rabe to reduce bitterness before sautéing it.

BROILING To cook relatively thin, tender cuts of meat, poultry, fish, or other food by placing them beneath and close to a high heat source. A broiler can be part of an oven or a separate unit. In general, foods are placed between 4 and 8 inches away from the broiler element. The best way to regulate the temperature is to move the food closer to or farther from the heat. Thicker cuts of meat and fish must be placed farther away from a broiler in order to cook properly. Otherwise, the outside will char before the inside cooks. During broiling, the food is set on a broiler pan, which has a perforated upper pan, or rack, that allows the fat to drip into the lower, deeper pan. To prevent sticking and for easy cleanup, spray the upper pan with nonstick cooking spray and line the lower pan with heavy-duty aluminum foil.

Broiler pan.

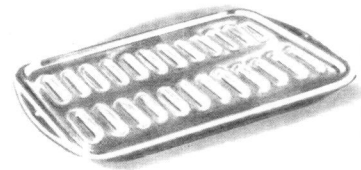

Broiling is a fast and efficient means of cooking foods without the addition of fat or liquids. The dry, radiant heat browns the surface of the food as it cooks it. Most meat or poultry should be turned at least once during broiling. Use tongs or a spatula, not a fork, to prevent juices from escaping. Fish, which is more delicate than meat and poultry, should not be turned during broiling unless it is very firm fleshed.

If using an electric broiler, let it preheat for about 5 minutes. Gas broilers do not require preheating—and as a rule do not reach the same high temperatures as electric broilers. When using an electric broiler, most manufacturers recommend keeping the oven or broiler door ajar to prevent the oven from overheating, which would cause the thermostat to turn off

Broiling Times for Various Foods

BEEF

Hamburger	1 inch thick	3 to 5 minutes for rare* 9 to 11 minutes for medium* 13 to 15 minutes for well done
Flank steak	1 inch thick	4 to 6 minutes for rare 7 to 9 minutes for medium
Club steak Porterhouse steak Sirloin steak T-bone steak	1 inch thick	4 to 6 minutes for rare 8 to 11 minutes for medium 12 to 16 minutes for well done
Filet mignon	1 inch thick	3 to 5 minutes for rare 6 to 8 minutes for medium

LAMB

Loin and rib chops	1 inch thick	5 to 7 minutes for rare 8 to 10 minutes for medium 12 to 14 minutes for well done

PORK

Loin and shoulder chops	1 inch thick	8 to 10 minutes for medium 12 to 15 minutes for well done
Tenderloin		10 to 12 minutes for medium 14 to 17 for well done

POULTRY

Small chicken (3 to 3½ pounds), split Bone-in chicken parts Turkey tenders or fillets		30 to 35 minutes 20 to 25 minutes 5 to 10 minutes

VEAL

Loin and rib chops	1 inch thick	8 to 10 minutes for rare 12 to 14 minutes for medium

FISH

Salmon	1 inch thick	5 to 6 minutes for medium-rare 7 to 10 minutes for medium
Tuna	1 inch thick	4 to 5 minutes for rare 6 to 7 minutes for medium-rare 7 to 10 minutes for medium

Although many cooks enjoy a touch of pink in their burgers, the U.S. Food Safety and Inspection Service recommends that ground beef be cooked to an internal temperature of 160°F to avoid all risk of bacterial contamination; see BEEF and DONENESS for more information.

the broiler. High-end gas stoves are often equipped with infrared broilers that heat very quickly to approximately 1500°F, about twice the temperature of other broilers. Food cooks nearly twice as quickly in these highly efficient units.

Most grilling recipes can be accomplished in a broiler instead. Broiling is also used to brown the top of casseroles, open-faced sandwiches, and gratins.

In the chart on page 71 are estimates of the total time it will take various foods to cook on a broiler pan positioned 4 to 6 inches from the heating element. Figure on turning meat or poultry once during cooking. Use these times as general guidelines. If you have an industrial stove, the broiler will be hotter than the broiler in a conventional home stove. Testing the temperature of the interior of the meat and poultry with a meat thermometer is the best gauge of doneness. Fish is done when it is opaque and the flesh is just beginning to flake when prodded with a fork.

About Pan Broiling Pan broiling is cooking rapidly in a skillet or sauté pan over high heat, without the addition of liquid or the use of a cover and very little or no fat. Similar to cooking on a grill or griddle, this dry-heat method develops flavor by browning the exterior of the food. Using a heavy pan and preheating it until very hot *before* adding the food are the two keys to successful pan broiling. This method works best for thin cuts of meat such as flattened boneless chicken breasts, veal scallops, or fish fillets that do not rely on long cooking or additional moisture for tenderness. One of the best-known variations of pan broiling is blackening.

BROTH Any commercially made and packaged stock made by cooking vegetables, chicken, beef, or fish in water is called a broth. These convenient products can be used as a base for soups, sauces, stews, braises, and pan gravies. Vegetable, chicken, beef, and fish broths are available in cans, in aseptic packaging, or frozen, or can be

Quick Bite

The term *broth* is sometimes also used to refer to a fortified homemade stock or soup, such as a Scotch broth.

made from bouillon cubes or powdered bouillon. Some commercial broths, like bouillon, are condensed and must be mixed with water. All of these products can be used in place of homemade stock, although they tend to be more salty, particularly bouillon cubes and powdered bouillon, and not as fresh tasting. Low-sodium and low-fat canned broths are available and allow more control in seasoning.

Selecting Choose a major brand, trying several until you find one you like best. Some cooks prefer the frozen or canned broths in health-food stores because they tend to be lower in sodium and additives.

Storing After opening, unused broth should be transferred to glass or plastic containers; do not store it in the can, or the broth will take on an unpleasant flavor. Refrigerate for up to 1 week. Store bouillon cubes and powdered bouillon at cool room temperature for up to 1 year. Broth in aseptic packaging can be held at cool room temperature for up to 1 year, but once opened should be refrigerated; it will keep for up to 1 week. Broth may be frozen for up to 3 months.

Preparing Use broth in any recipe calling for stock. Use it in place of water when cooking rice or beans for a flavor boost. Add it to stir-fries to reduce the amount of fat needed for cooking and to add flavor. But be careful with any recipe that calls for reducing or boiling down broth, since its sodium will become more concentrated as the liquid boils away. Use low-sodium broths for these dishes.

See also STOCK.

BROWNIE See COOKIE.

BROWNING When meat, poultry, or another food is cooked over high heat in an oiled or dry pan, the surface of the food quickly darkens and takes on an appealing brown color. It also gives the food a corresponding deeper flavor. For this reason, browning is often the first step in many braises and stews. It should be done quickly so as not to dry out the meat.

Quick Tip

Before browning, wipe meat or poultry dry with a paper towel and brown food in batches if necessary to prevent crowding in the pan. This keeps the food from steaming in the hot pan and results in a crisp, brown exterior.

Keeping the heat high and not overcrowding the pan are keys to successful browning. It also helps to understand that browning cannot occur in the presence of liquid or excessive moisture. This is why many recipes instruct you to dry meat or poultry before browning. Browning occurs at temperatures upward of 310°F, and, since water and other liquids cannot heat beyond 212°F, proper browning will never occur when water is present. Liquid fat, unlike water, can hold temperatures far above 310°F and is therefore an ideal medium for browning. And, since sugars and proteins brown readily, foods with a high amount of either will brown quickly.

Foods also brown in the oven during roasting. The skin of turkeys and chickens in particular will become brown, especially if you baste the birds with pan juices.

Cookies, cakes, and breads brown in the oven as their outer crusts cook.

See also BASTING; SEARING.

BROWN SUGAR See SUGAR.

BRUISING In its most familiar sense, this term refers to damaged spots or sections on fruits and vegetables. Once a fruit is bruised, a brownish discoloration starts to spread as cell walls break down, but this discoloration may be slowed down slightly by refrigerating the food.

Some foods are purposefully bruised so that their flavor is released. The aroma and flavor of herbs, spices, and garlic and onions are carried by their essential oils. When these foods are bruised, the oils are released and the flavor better infuses a dish. To bruise fresh or dried herbs, roll them between your fingers and thumb. To bruise hard spices, garlic, and onion, place them under the flat side of a chef's knife and carefully strike the flat side of the knife with the heel of your palm or your fist.

See also CRUSHING; SMASHING.

BRUSH See BAKING TOOLS; COOKING TOOLS.

BRUSSELS SPROUT Members of the cabbage family, Brussels sprouts grow on long, curving stalks as small, tightly closed heads that resemble tiny cabbages. The tops of the stalks have spreading leaves, making these impressive-looking plants when in the field. Brussels sprouts grow best in cool, coastal regions and are in season in the fall and winter. They may be boiled, braised, or steamed or parboiled and then sautéed.

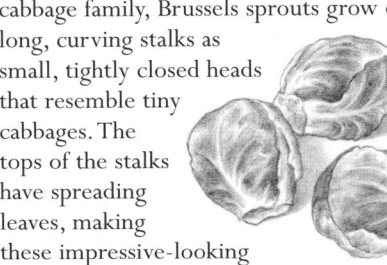

Selecting Buy fresh Brussels sprouts that are heavy for their size and bright green, with leaves clinging tightly to the heads. Avoid any with yellowing leaves, which indicate aging. They may be pale green at the base. Check that the stem ends are freshly cut. Also avoid soft heads with loose leaves. Small heads, about 1 inch in diameter, are usually preferable to large ones, which can be almost twice that size. If the large heads are dark green and firm, however, they should taste good. Fresh Brussels sprouts are sold loose or packed in pint baskets or small tubs, although at some farmers' markets you can buy them on the stalks. Brussels sprouts freeze well, so if fresh are not available, buy them frozen.

Storing Store in plastic bags or the original packaging in the refrigerator for up to 4 days, but try to eat them as soon as possible after purchase. To freeze, rinse and dry the heads, blanch for 4 to 5 minutes, depending on their size, refresh in cold water, drain, and freeze in sturdy freezer bags or rigid containers.

Preparing Rinse and dry the heads. Trim any brown outside leaves and trim away the stem ends. Cut a shallow X into the stem end before cooking so that the heads will cook quickly and evenly. Larger heads can be halved or quartered before cooking.

Quick Tip

If you are faced with loose-leafed Brussels sprouts, simply take apart the heads and separate and steam the individual leaves.

See also STEAMING.

BUCKWHEAT See GRAIN.

BUFFALO See GAME.

BULGUR See GRAIN.

BUNDT PAN See Tube Pan in BAKE-WARE.

BUTTER This essential dairy product is made by churning, or agitating, cream until the fats separate from the liquids, producing a semisolid fat. Butter is most often made from the 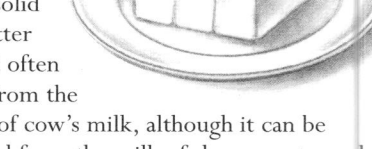 cream of cow's milk, although it can be churned from the milk of sheep, goats, and other mammals as well.

Butter is 80 to 85 percent milk fat. The rest is made up of milk solids (proteins) and water. Most commercially packaged butter has wrappers marked with tablespoon increments. Butter is sold in two

Quick Tip

When butter is heated, it will first melt, then begin to foam. When the foam is just beginning to subside, but before it begins to brown, the butter has reached the right temperature for cooking food.

basic styles. More familiar is salted butter, although many cooks favor unsalted butter, also called sweet butter, for two reasons. First, salt in the butter adds to the total amount of salt in a recipe, which can interfere with the taste. Second, unsalted butter is likely to be fresher, since it has no salt, which acts as a preservative and prolongs its shelf life. (If you're not planning to use it soon, you should freeze it.) If you have no choice when shopping, salted butter will work in most cooking recipes (you may want to taste and adjust other salt in the recipe), but it is not recommended as a substitute for unsalted butter in baking.

Storing Salted butter, if left wrapped and stored in a cold section of the refrigerator, will keep for about 2½ months, while wrapped unsalted butter will store well for about 1½ months. After that, the butter may begin to pick up refrigerator odors, thus losing its delicate flavor. Both types freeze well for up to 6 months in their original packaging. Once unwrapped, salted and unsalted butter should be eaten within 3 weeks. Even if wrapped, do not keep butter longer than 1 week beyond its sell-by date, unless you freeze it.

Buttering a Pan Buttering a pan means rubbing it with a thin film of softened butter. This can be done with a brush, your fingers, a wadded paper towel, or the wrapper from the butter. Or you can just grasp the stick of partially wrapped butter and use it to paint butter over the pan. In most cases, if a recipe instructs you to "grease" or "oil" the pan, you can use butter, margarine, or another fat. The layer of fat prevents food from sticking to the pan. Because butter burns at lower temperatures than refined vegetable oils, it is not recommended for greasing pans headed for very hot ovens.

As a general rule, when recipes call for buttering a pan, the relatively small amount of butter used is not listed but is in addition to any amount of butter called for among the actual ingredients.

Quick Tip

To soften butter in the microwave, put the butter in a microwave-safe glass dish and cover with waxed paper. Microwave on Defrost for 15 to 30 seconds. Check the butter and repeat if necessary. The larger the measurement, the longer the time in the microwave (1 cup, which is 16 tablespoons or 2 sticks, may take up to a minute to soften). Do not melt.

Butter Equivalents

1 cup	= 16 tablespoons = 8 ounces = 2 sticks	
¾ cup	= 12 tablespoons = 6 ounces = 1½ sticks	
½ cup	= 8 tablespoons = 4 ounces = 1 stick	
¼ cup	= 4 tablespoons = 2 ounces = ½ stick	

HOW TO *Clarify Butter*

Clarified butter keeps about three times as long as other butters because the milk solids, which can become rancid, have been removed. It is used for cooking but not as a spread, as it turns grainy when it cools and solidifies.

1. Melt at least 1 cup unsalted butter over low heat in a small pan or skillet.
2. Let the butter simmer undisturbed for 20 to 25 minutes. The water will evaporate and the white milk solids will collect at the bottom.
3. Skim any foam off the top of the butter.

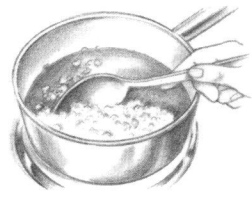

4. Remove the butter from the heat and carefully pour the clear, golden liquid through a fine sieve into a glass jar, leaving the white milk solids in the pan or sieve. Discard the solids.

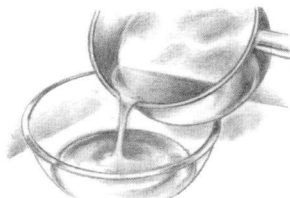

5. Cool the clarified butter completely, cover, and then refrigerate. It will keep for about 3 months.

BUTTER BEAN Another name for lima bean. See BEAN, DRIED; BEAN, FRESH.

BUTTERFLYING The technique of cutting a food nearly all the way through so that, instead of being split into two pieces, it can be opened up to lie relatively flat—like a book or, more poetically, a butterfly. Butterflying also allows fast, even cooking when the food is spread out flat and cooked, such as a boned leg of lamb on a charcoal grill. Butterflying also allows meat to be stuffed, rolled up, and tied before cooking. While most cooks think only of meat as a candidate for butterflying, the technique can also be applied to vegetables and fruits such as bell peppers and pears.

Butterflying a chicken breast.

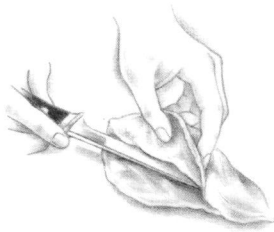

HOW TO *Butterfly Jumbo Shrimp*

1. After shelling and deveining (see SHRIMP), cut through the shrimp on the outside curve without slicing all the way through, so that the shrimp can be opened flat.

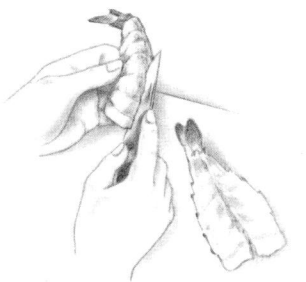

HOW TO *Butterfly and Stuff a Pork or Beef Tenderloin Roast*

1. Using a chef's knife, carefully cut a lengthwise slit along the center of the meat. As you cut, open the flaps of meat like a book, leaving them attached to each other and cutting to within about ½ inch of the opposite side.

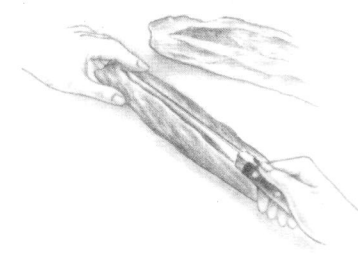

2. Place the slit tenderloin on a work surface with its cut side up and flaps opened flat. Using the smooth side of a meat pounder, pound the tenderloin evenly all over until it has the uniform thickness called for in the recipe.

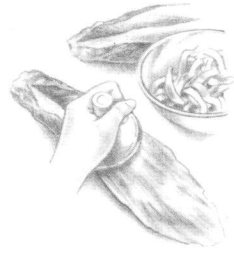

3. Evenly arrange the prepared stuffing lengthwise along the center of the butterflied tenderloin. Wrap both sides around the stuffing and, using lengths of kitchen string, securely tie the stuffed tenderloin at regular intervals.

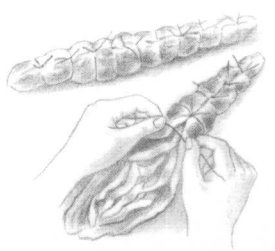

HOW TO *Butterfly a Whole Chicken*

1. Place the bird breast side down on a cutting board. Cut along one side of the backbone with kitchen shears or a large knife. Pull open the 2 halves of the bird and cut down the other side of the backbone to free it. Discard the backbone or save it for making stock.

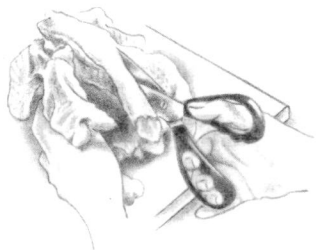

2. Turn the chicken breast side up, opening it as flat as possible. Cover it with plastic wrap and, using your hands, the smooth side of a meat mallet, or a rolling pin, press and pound it to break the breastbone and flatten the bird.

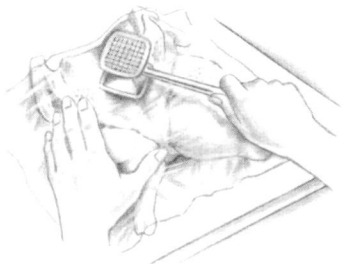

3. Make a small incision in the loose skin between thigh and breast, near the bottom of the breast, and push the ends of the drumsticks through the incisions to tuck them away neatly during cooking.

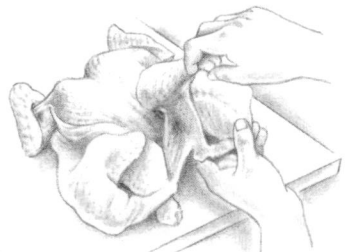

BUTTERMILK Traditionally, buttermilk is the liquid left behind when butter is churned from cream. Today, most buttermilk is a cultured product made by adding bacteria to skimmed milk (or sometimes whole milk) to convert the sugars to acids. Cultured buttermilk is thick—sometimes even bits of butter are added to give it more body and an old-fashioned appearance—and it tastes tangy. Your great-grandmother would never recognize it as the buttermilk she remembers from the days when she was a young girl.

Some people like to drink a tall glass of icy cold buttermilk. Perhaps more common, however, are buttermilk pancakes or waffles for weekend breakfasts. Buttermilk is also is used in various baking recipes, from cakes to scones, where it acts as a leavener when the acid in the buttermilk reacts with alkaline baking soda to create gas bubbles.

Storing Buttermilk will keep refrigerated for up to 10 days past its sell-by date. Use only what you need and return the carton to the refrigerator immediately. Do not let it sit out at room temperature, as buttermilk spoils easily.

Quick Tip

If a recipe calls for buttermilk and there's no time to go to the market, substitute sour milk. To make sour milk, add 1 tablespoon cider vinegar, distilled white vinegar, or lemon juice for every cup of whole, low-fat, or skim milk and let it sit at room temperature for about 10 minutes. The milk will curdle and is then ready to use. Likewise, buttermilk can be substituted for sour milk in a recipe.

See also BAKING POWDER & BAKING SODA; MILK.

b

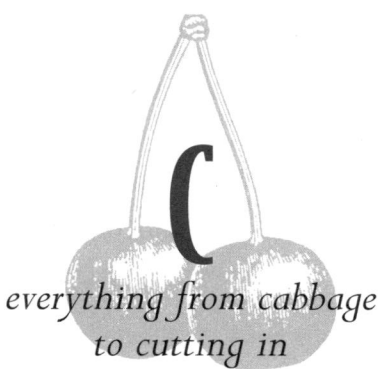

everything from cabbage to cutting in

CABBAGE Like broccoli and cauliflower, cabbage is a cruciferous vegetable, a group believed by some scientists to safeguard against certain forms of cancer. Fresh cabbage leaves may be pale green or red, with green cabbage (also called Dutch white) the most plentiful.

Green cabbage.

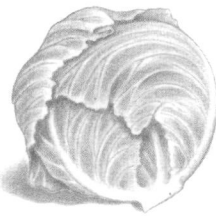

Red cabbage has thicker leaves, a faintly peppery taste, and a slightly higher price tag but is used in the same way. Another variety, savoy, has crinkled green leaves.

Savoy cabbage.

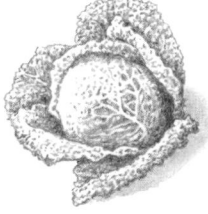

Chinese cabbage, also called napa or celery cabbage, is elongated and has wrinkly, light yellow-green leaves and a pearly white core. Cabbage is sold fresh all year long.

Cabbage is the primary ingredient in two popular preparations, coleslaw and sauerkraut. Whole leaves can be boiled or blanched until pliable and then stuffed and steamed. Whole cabbages can be stuffed as well, with a flavorful mixture tucked between the leaves. Chopped cabbage is added to soups and braises.

Chinese cabbage.

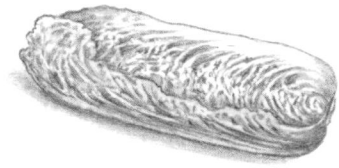

Selecting Buy firm, heavy heads of green, red, and savoy cabbage with closely furled leaves. An average head weighs about 2 pounds. Color is an indication of freshness. For example, green cabbages stored for too long lose pigment and look almost white. To ensure freshness, check the stem ends of cabbage heads to make sure the stem has not cracked around the base, which indicates undesirably lengthy storage. Chinese cabbage leaves should be crisp and unblemished and pale green with tinges of yellow and white.

Storing Refrigerate heads of green and red cabbage for up to 2 weeks, savoy and Chinese cabbage for 5 or 6 days. If you want to eat the cabbage raw, do so within

Quick Tip

Nothing combats the odor of cooking cabbage, despite old wives' tales about dropping a whole walnut or a chunk of bread into the cooking pot. Cooking it quickly helps, but a kitchen exhaust fan is the best defense.

3 or 4 days. Do not cut or shred cabbage until you are ready to use it. Store the unused portion intact, wrapped in plastic, and use within 2 days.

Preparing Pull off and discard any wilted outer leaves and cut the core from the head, either by cutting the head in half or quarters and slicing the core from the center, or by cutting around the core from the base.

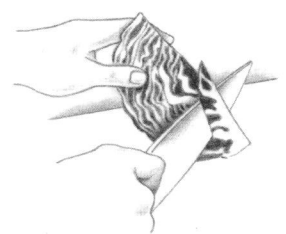

Coring cabbage.

Shred or slice cabbage for salads (a food processor makes quick work of the task).

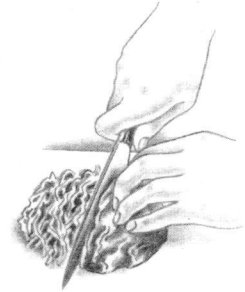

Cutting cabbage shreds.

See also BRAISING; SAUERKRAUT.

CAKE See page 80.

CAKE PAN See BAKEWARE.

CAKE ROUND See BAKING TOOLS.

CALAMARI See SQUID.

CALZONE The term *calzone,* Italian for "pantaloon," charmingly describes the shape of this pizza transformed into a turnover to be baked or deep-fried. Virtually any pizza can be made into a calzone. Essentially, pizza dough rounds are folded in half to conceal a filling. The technique is best suited to abundant fillings that will not sit well atop a pizza.

HOW TO *Shape a Calzone*

1. Prepare a pizza dough. Form the risen dough into individual-serving balls. On a lightly floured surface, roll each ball into a neat round about 10 inches in diameter or flatten and stretch the dough with your hands.

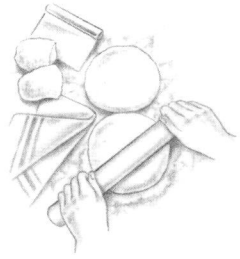

2. Prepare the filling. Mound it on the rolled-out dough, covering roughly half of it and leaving a generous rim.

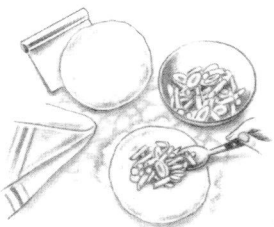

3. Using a brush dipped in water, lightly moisten the edges of the dough. Fold the uncovered portion over the filling, gently stretching it to cover the ingredients completely. Press and crimp the edges together to seal securely.

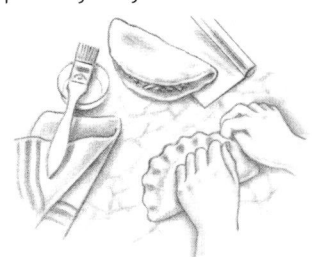

Cake

Most celebrations, whether large or small, planned or spontaneous, elegant or casual, call for a cake. Indeed, at weddings
and birthdays, a festively decorated cake is the culinary star. In
other instances, it transforms an ordinary meal into an occasion.

Cakes are usually made from batters composed of flour, milk (or another liquid),
sugar, eggs and often another leavener as
well, butter (or sometimes oil or shortening), and flavorings. The batter is baked
until its interior sets and becomes a crumb
and a firm exterior crust develops. As is the
case with all baked goods, the exact proportion of ingredients makes a significant
difference in the texture, flavor, and quality
of the finished cake. (The term *cake* also
may refer to any round, flat disk of food,
such as a crab cake, a pancake, or even a
yeast cake. In fact, the earliest cakes, which
date back at least as far as ancient Egypt,
were nothing more than sweet breads; cake
recipes featuring beaten eggs only began
to be popularized some time around the
17th century.)

Cakes are divided into two main types:
foam cakes and butter cakes. Foam cakes
have a high proportion of eggs, sugar, and
liquid to flour, and the air trapped in the
beaten eggs is the primary leavener. They
contain very little if any fat, such as butter
or oil, and so have a relatively dry and
spongy texture. Popular foam cakes include
angel food cake and sponge cake.

Butter cakes are richer and more velvety
and rely on the chemical leaveners, baking
powder and baking soda. They are made
with a comparatively high percentage of
butter. Typical butter cakes are American
layer cakes and pound cakes.

Some cakes, such as chiffon cake and the
classic French génoise, combine elements
of both types of cake.

Equipment Having the right equipment
makes cake baking easier, and for most
home baking needs, the basics are few.
Measuring cups and spoons, a mixing bowl
and spoon, a whisk for beating egg whites,
and a pair of round cake pans or a tube pan
are all you'll need for many recipes. Batters
can always be mixed by hand, but are more
easily whipped up with a handheld electric
mixer or in a stand mixer. For more details, see BAKEWARE; BAKING TOOLS.

Ingredients Begin with the freshest ingredients possible. When making cakes,
this pertains mainly to the butter, eggs, and
milk. If your baking powder or soda is
more than 6 months old, replace it to guarantee effectiveness. Be sure to use the right
kind of flour called for in a recipe, and
never use high-protein bread flour to make
a tender cake. For more detail, see FLOUR.

Preparing the Pans Properly prepared
pans are a crucial part of cake baking. A
poorly prepared pan can mean a cake will
stick to it and refuse to emerge without
tearing. Most recipes say to "grease (or butter) the pan," and some say to flour it as
well. Regardless of what the recipe says,
when a recipe requires greasing a pan, it is
always a good idea to line and flour the
pan as well. (Note that some cakes, such as
angel food cakes, are baked in dry pans.)

HOW TO *Prepare a Cake Pan*

1. Cut a waxed or parchment paper round or rectangle that will fit snugly in the bottom of the pan. Use the pan as a guide for tracing the right shape and size.
2. Rub the inside bottom and sides of the pan with butter, margarine, or vegetable shortening, or spray it lightly and evenly with un-flavored cooking spray.

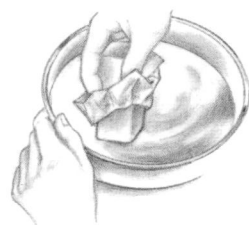

3. Lay the paper form in the pan and rub it with a little butter, margarine, or vegetable shortening, or spray it with a little cooking spray.

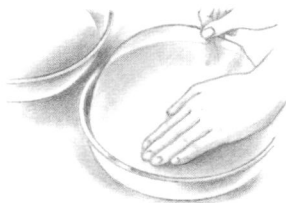

4. Sprinkle some flour on the paper form and on the sides of the pan. Holding the pan over the sink or work surface, turn and tilt the pan to distribute the flour evenly. Gently tap the excess flour from the pan and discard it. If you are baking a chocolate cake, use cocoa powder in place of flour, to avoid a contrasting white dusting on the brown cake.

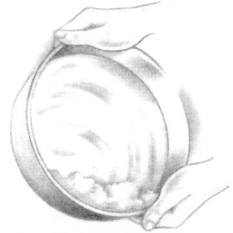

Mixing the Ingredients Every recipe is slightly different, but for most cakes the following techniques are recommended.

Before mixing, measure out and prepare all ingredients according to the ingredient list. Unless the recipe directs otherwise, the ingredients should be at room temperature. Start preheating the oven.

Quick Tip

Butter contributes good flavor but may burn if used for preparing cake pans for batters that bake at very high temperatures. Margarine and vegetable oil are better at high temperatures because they don't burn as readily. Unflavored cooking spray is convenient, too.

Stand mixers are valuable tools for making large quantities of cake batter or cakes that call for prolonged and vigorous beating to incorporate maximum air. If using a stand mixer, fit it with the paddle attachment to cream the butter (see CREAMING) and to mix the batter, and the whisk attachment for whisking egg whites or cream. If using a stand or handheld mixer, use a rubber spatula to scrape the flour up from the bottom of the bowl several times during mixing as well as from the sides.

Paddle and whip attachments.

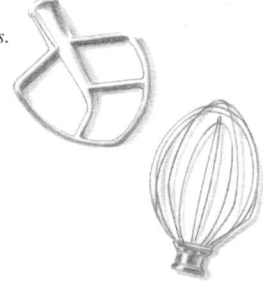

Do not overmix the batter. Mix it just until the flour is no longer visible or, if folding egg whites into batter, until only a few streaks of egg white remain.

continued

Cake, continued

Filling the Cake Pans When making layer cakes requiring two or more pans, pour equal amounts of batter into each, using a rubber spatula to smooth the surface. To ensure an equal amount of batter in each pan, use a kitchen scale. Weighing each filled pan and evening them out is the only way to end up with perfectly even layers. (Be sure also to account for any difference between the weight of the pans when empty.)

Once the pans are filled with batter, handle them gently. Though some cooks tap them once on the counter to release any large air bubbles, banging them roughly can release too much air from the batter and cause a cake to "fall," or sag in the center.

Baking the Cake Set the pans on the center rack in the preheated oven. Use an oven thermometer to check the accuracy of your oven, and adjust the temperature knob to compensate. If baking more layers than will fit on one oven rack, place the racks as close to the center of the oven as possible.

Do not open the oven door during baking until it's time to check for doneness. A considerable amount of heat escapes every time the oven door is opened. Also, banging an oven door shut can cause a cake to fall. Begin checking 8 to 10 minutes before the cake is supposed to be done.

Cooling the Cake Set the pan on a wire rack and let the cake cool for about 5 minutes. Place the wire rack on top of the cake and carefully invert the cake in its pan.

Inverting the cake pan.

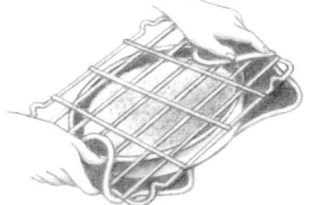

If the pan doesn't lift easily from the cake, give it a slight shake. The cake should fall from the pan.

Removing the pan.

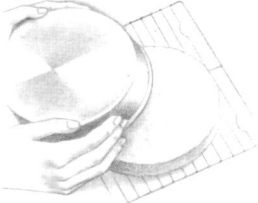

If necessary, before inverting the cake, loosen the sides of the cake with a table knife or tap the bottom of the pan, or both.

Loosening the cake.

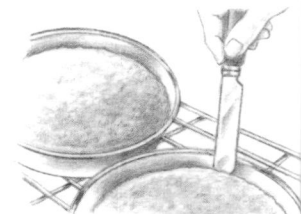

Peel the waxed or parchment paper from the bottom of the cake and discard. Let the cake cool completely before frosting and serving. See FROSTING, ICING & GLAZE for more information.

Storing and Freezing Cakes Wrap cooled, unfrosted cakes in plastic wrap, place in an airtight container or under an airtight cake dome, and store at room temperature for up to 2 days.

Store frosted cakes in the same manner as unfrosted cakes unless the frosting contains cream, in which case it should be refrigerated immediately; if it contains butter it should be left at room temperature for no more than 2 hours.

If a cake requires refrigeration, cover it loosely with plastic and refrigerate it for up to 3 days. Let most cakes come to room temperature before serving. To keep the plastic wrap from sitting directly on the frosting, insert evenly spaced toothpicks in the cake and rest the plastic on them.

To freeze cooled, unfrosted cakes, wrap them in freezer-weight plastic and freeze for up to 2 months for foam cakes and others with little fat. Butter cakes, which contain more fat, will keep for 6 months.

To freeze frosted cakes, put the frosted cakes in the freezer until the frosting hardens. Wrap them carefully in freezer-weight plastic and freeze for up to 1 month.

Let frozen cakes, still wrapped, defrost in the refrigerator or at room temperature. When they are partially defrosted, unwrap and let them come to room temperature.

Butter Cake Savvy

■ Start with room-temperature ingredients. Eggs should be large, unless otherwise specified.

■ When creaming the butter with sugar, start by thoroughly creaming the butter before adding any sugar. Then beat the butter and sugar together well. Be patient: it takes several minutes of beating for the butter and sugar mixture to become light and fluffy. See CREAMING for more details.

■ When mixing eggs into the batter, add them one at a time, incorporating each fully to create an emulsion.

■ Combine the dry ingredients (flour, salt, baking powder), whisking them 8 to 10 times, before they are mixed with the wet ingredients. This ensures that salt and leavening are evenly distributed in the batter.

■ Butter cakes are done baking when the top is lightly browned, the edges begin to pull away from the sides of the pans, and the surface springs back when you press the center with a fingertip. Another test: insert a toothpick, kitchen knife, or cake tester into the center. It should come out clean and dry, or, as some cakes require (check your recipe), with just a few crumbs clinging to the tester, showing that the center remains a bit more moist.

Foam Cake Savvy

■ Eggs separate more easily when cold but whip up better when room temperature. Separate the eggs as soon as you take them from the refrigerator, then let the whites sit out in a bowl for about 30 minutes to come to room temperature before beating them. See EGG for instructions on separating eggs.

■ If a recipe calls for whisking the eggs or egg whites over hot water, do not let the bottom of the bowl touch the water, or the eggs will cook.

■ Be sure to use a spotlessly clean bowl and beaters or whisk for beating egg whites. Any spot of grease or fat (including egg yolk) will prevent the whites from expanding to their full volume.

■ Lift the beaters or whisk from the whites and turn them upright to determine the state of their peaks. Soft peaks will gently fall over onto themselves, while stiff, dry peaks will stand straight up.

Soft peaks.

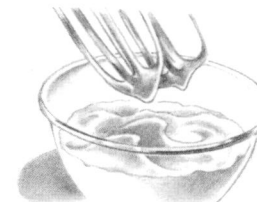

Stiff peaks.

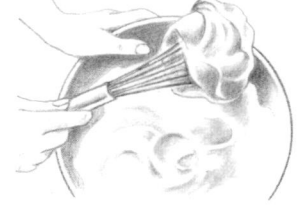

■ Overbeating eggs will cause them to clump and look somewhat chalky, and the cake will not rise as successfully.

■ Before baking, gently run a kitchen knife or small rubber spatula through the batter to deflate any large air bubbles.

continued

Cake, continued

- A foam cake is done when the top is golden and the cake springs back when gently pressed with a fingertip.
- For more about working with eggs, see EGG; FOLDING.

Cake Blues Got a problem with your cake? Find the explanation here.

BATTER CURDLES AND SEPARATES. Eggs were not added one at a time and beaten thoroughly after each addition; an electric mixer was set at too high a speed; and/or the eggs were too cold. Try adding 1 tablespoon of flour per egg and reducing the speed of the electric mixer.

CAKE DIDN'T RISE. Too much or not enough fat or liquid in the batter; batter was overbeaten; and/or oven temperature was too high.

CAKE IS TOUGH. Butter and sugar were underbeaten in the early stages of mixing; batter was overbeaten after the flour was added; not enough sugar; not enough baking powder; and/or not enough fat. Try brushing cake layers with sugar syrup or filling and frosting cake layers with a generous layer of moist frosting.

CAKE CRUMB IS STICKY. Too much sugar in the batter or sugar was too coarse.

TOP CRUST IS HARD. Oven temperature was too high; cake was overbaked; and/or cake was baked too close to the top of the oven. Try slicing off the top of the cake layer before frosting.

CAKE SINKS IN THE CENTER. Too much fat and/or sugar or leavening; batter was overbeaten; cake pan was too small; the filled cake pan was tapped too roughly on the countertop; the oven door was banged shut; or the oven temperature was too low. Try cutting out the fallen center and treating the cake like a tube cake; or, fill the depression with fruit or extra frosting.

CAKE PEAKS IN THE CENTER. Wrong type of flour was used (contained too much gluten); batter was overbeaten; too little fat and/or sugar in the batter; and/or oven temperature was too high. Try slicing the peaked center off the cake and frosting it.

TUNNELS RUN THROUGH THE CAKE. Not enough fat in the batter; batter was overbeaten; or wrong type of flour was used (contained too much gluten).

CRUST IS UNEVENLY COLORED. Too much leavener and/or sugar in the batter; not enough fat in the batter; oven temperature was too high or too low; oven heats unevenly. Try camouflaging with frosting.

CAKE ROSE UNEVENLY. Cake layers were crowded on the oven rack and heated unevenly. Bake each layer on its own rack. Trim the layers to even them out and camouflage with frosting.

Cake Styles There's a different type of cake to suit every taste. The following are some of the most popular choices:

AMERICAN LAYER CAKE A basic butter cake flavored with whatever suits the baker, from vanilla to coffee to strawberry, and usually frosted.

ANGEL FOOD CAKE Tall, single-layer, butterless white cake leavened with egg whites and baked in a tube pan. Seldom frosted.

CHIFFON CAKE This moist, light American classic falls somewhere between a foam cake (also contains lots of separated eggs) and a butter cake (although it uses oil rather than butter).

DEVIL'S FOOD CAKE Rich chocolate cake made from a mix of acidic and alkaline ingredients that produce a reddish hue.

GÉNOISE A delicate French sponge cake leavened by eggs only. Lends itself to layered and rolled cakes such as jelly rolls.

POUND CAKE Old-fashioned cake usually baked in a loaf pan and rarely frosted. Its name comes from the weight of each ingredient—butter, sugar, eggs, flour—traditionally needed to make one cake.

See also BAKING; BATTER; FLOUR; FROSTING, ICING & GLAZE; UNMOLDING.

CANADIAN BACON Cut from the loin of the hog, and cured but not always smoked, Canadian bacon, also called back bacon, is generally sliced thick. Many people appreciate its mild flavor and lean, meaty texture, which are closer to that of ham than bacon. It is used for eggs Benedict, the popular brunch dish that combines it with English muffins, eggs, and hollandaise sauce. Fully cooked, it can also be baked and fried.

Selecting Canadian bacon is widely sold in butcher shops and most food markets in both whole and presliced pieces.

Storing Canadian bacon should be refrigerated in its original packaging or carefully wrapped in plastic until ready to cook. Sliced Canadian bacon will keep for 3 to 4 days, while unsliced chunks will keep for up to 1 week. The bacon can also be frozen for up to 2 months.

Preparing Panfry Canadian bacon in a little fat over medium-high heat or broil it until lightly browned and fragrant. Drain on paper towels. Depending on the thickness of the slices, cooking can take as few as 3 minutes or as long as 10 minutes.

CANDY MAKING Most candy making involves working with sugar and a thermometer. With a little diligence and understanding, anyone can make toffee, caramel, fudge, and other candies.

The first step is often to make a sugar syrup by heating sugar and water together over high heat. The sugar dissolves easily, and the clear liquid goes through a number of stages as it rises in temperature and the water evaporates, increasing the syrup's concentration. The stages are defined progressively as thread, soft ball, firm ball,

hard ball, soft crack, hard crack, light caramel, and dark caramel (see chart, page 86). Those terms refer to the syrup's appearance and behavior, but they are best determined with an accurate candy thermometer, and candy recipes usually specify both the stage and the temperature, such as hard-ball stage and 265°F. The best kind of candy thermometer has a mercury bulb and column mounted on a protective metal casing fitted with a clip that attaches to the side of a pan.

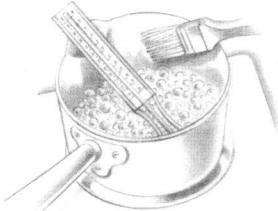

Using a candy thermometer.

While crystallization (the formation of very small crystals, not large ones) is desirable when making fudge or fondant, it should be avoided when making most other candies. In other words, the goal is usually to prevent crystals from forming. Otherwise, the resulting candy will be unpleasantly grainy. A little corn syrup or an acid such as cream of tartar or lemon juice added to the syrup impedes the development of crystals, but the best defense is to let the syrup boil undisturbed without jostling or stirring. Also, when first mixing the sugar and water, use a wooden rather

Caution!

Because the sugar gets very hot, burns can be severe. Always exercise extreme caution when cooking with sugar, protecting your hands and forearms with heavy oven mitts. And always keep a bowl of ice water next to the stove to cool down the bottom of a pan of sugar syrup quickly if it overheats.

than a metal spoon to prevent crystals. Sugar crystals do not adhere as readily to wood as they do to metal. Brushing down the sides of the pan with a pastry brush dipped in hot water as the sugar boils also prevents crystallization.

Sugar Syrup Savvy

- To test a thermometer for accuracy, bring water to a boil. Submerge the thermometer in the water for 1 or 2 minutes. If it does not register 212°F, adjust the temperature in the recipe accordingly.
- Before using a thermometer, put it in warm water to raise its temperature a little, particularly if the kitchen or storage drawer is cool.
- Cook sugar syrup on dry, cool days, if possible. If high humidity cannot be avoided, cook the syrup to the highest temperature for its stage—or even a few degrees higher. As the syrup cools, it will absorb humidity and may soften.
- Sifting lumpy granulated sugar after measuring will help it dissolve and prevent crystallization.
- Cooking the syrup in a heavy pan smaller than the burner lets the sides of the pan heat as well as the bottom.
- Once the sugar dissolves and the syrup boils, do not stir it.
- Use a clean brush dipped in hot water to brush sugar crystals down the sides of the pan into the syrup as it cooks.
- Soak pots and other utensils used for cooking sugar in hot tap water soon after use. The water will dissolve the sugar and facilitate washing. To loosen stubborn sugar, boil water in the pot.
- After removing a thermometer from hot syrup, submerge in hot water for easy cleaning. Cold water may crack it.

Sugar Syrup Stages

STAGE	TEMPERATURE	TEST
Thread	230° to 234°F	Syrup breaks into 1- or 2-inch threads when lifted from the pan and again when dropped into ice water. The threads do not form a ball.
Soft ball	234° to 240°F	When dropped into ice water and rolled between the fingers, the syrup forms a soft ball.
Firm ball	244° to 248°F	When dropped into ice water and rolled between the fingers, the syrup forms a ball that holds its shape.
Hard ball	250° to 265°F	When dropped into ice water and rolled between the fingers, the syrup forms a ball that holds its shape and also offers resistance when lightly squeezed.
Soft crack	270° to 290°F	When dropped into ice water, the syrup can be stretched into flexible strands.
Hard crack	300° to 310°F	When dropped into ice water, the syrup forms a mass that can be easily broken into two or three pieces.
Light caramel	320° to 338°F	When poured onto marble or a white dish, the syrup looks clear amber.
Dark caramel	350°F	The syrup turns dark brown or caramel color.

Checking the Stage Using a candy thermometer is the only foolproof way to determine when the syrup has reached a desired stage. However, the time-honored method used by many cooks is to drop a little of the syrup in ice water and then to try rolling it between the fingers to judge its stage by its appearance.

Caution!

Never touch hot syrup directly, as it will burn you badly!

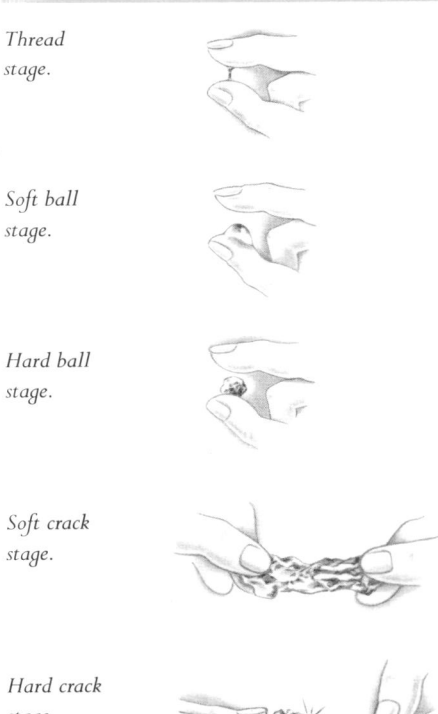

Thread stage.

Soft ball stage.

Hard ball stage.

Soft crack stage.

Hard crack stage.

Take care: a sugar syrup will continue cooking off the heat, and when cooked beyond the dark caramel stage, 350°F, it burns and will taste bitter.

See also CARAMELIZING; CHOCOLATE.

CANNELLINI See BEAN, DRIED.

CAN OPENER See COOKING TOOLS.

CANTALOUPE See MELON.

CAPER The small unopened flower buds of a shrub native to the Mediterranean, capers are unpleasantly bitter when raw. Once dried and packed in brine or salt, however, they add a pleasantly pungent flavor and a light crunch to meat, fish, and egg dishes and to various sauces. The smallest capers, called nonpareils, are from Provence, in southern France, and many culinary authorities consider them to be the finest capers. But how these edible flower buds are treated has more to do with their quality than does their size. If large pea-sized capers are packed in a mild brine or properly salted, they can add delicious flavor to any number of dishes.

Selecting Capers are usually sold in a vinegar brine and sealed in glass jars. Salted capers are harder to find, but they are usually carried in well-stocked Italian markets in bulk or in jars. Try a few brands before deciding which one you prefer.

Quick Bite

Caper berries are the fruit of the same shrub that produces capers. Popular throughout southern Europe, they are now finding their way into shops beyond the Continent. Olive shaped and with long stems, they are pickled or salted and, like capers, must be rinsed. They are especially delicious with firm, full-flavored cheeses.

Storing Unopened capers will keep for up to 1 year in a cool, dark cupboard. Once opened, they should be refrigerated, still covered with brine, and used within 9 months. Salted capers, packed in an airtight container, can be stored at room temperature for 6 months.

Preparing For capers in brine, drain them before using and gently blot dry with paper towels. For salted capers, thoroughly rinse and drain them. Blot them dry and taste them to be sure you have rinsed them enough to your taste. Do not soak them or they will lose flavor. Large capers may require chopping.

Quick Tip

Capers keep a long time, so if you spot a forgotten half-empty jar on your refrigerator shelf, consider pulling it out, taste-testing one, and using the capers to enliven sliced tomatoes, tuna salad, or stuffed eggs.

CARAMELIZING To heat sugar until it turns light to dark brown, or to cook other foods until natural sugars in them caramelize. Sugar becomes less purely sweet and develops a more complex flavor as it caramelizes. Sugar is considered caramelized when it registers between 320° and 350°F on a candy thermometer.

Caramelizing can be done in two ways: the sugar can be dissolved in water to make liquid syrup, or it can be sprinkled in a heavy pan and heated over a high flame. White or brown sugar, sprinkled over food and then heated under a broiler, is considered caramelized when it melts and darkens to form a crunchy, sweet crust, such as the topping on classic crème brûlée. (In restaurants, the sugar is caramelized with a standard-sized butane torch; home cooks can use miniature versions.) Caramelized sugar often lines serving dishes or custard cups for flan or crème caramel, too. Finally, when a mixture of sugar, corn syrup, and cream is caramelized to the soft-ball stage on a candy thermometer, and then butter and vanilla are added, you have cooked up a batch of chewy tan caramels.

Caution!

As with any sugar cooking, use great caution when caramelizing sugar, as any burns can be serious. Handle pans and utensils with heavy pot holders to avoid injury. Keep a bowl of ice water next to the stove to cool down the pan bottom quickly if the sugar syrup overheats.

HOW TO *Caramelize Sugar*

1. Put 2 parts granulated sugar to 1 part water in a heavy saucepan with a light-colored interior that lets you judge the color of the caramel. Enameled cast iron is a good choice.
2. Set the pan over medium-high heat and cook the mixture, shaking or tilting the pan in a circular motion, until the sugar dissolves.
3. Watching carefully and shaking or tilting the pan in a circle from time to time, bring the mixture to a boil and boil until the syrup begins to turn amber, about 3 minutes; the color will continue to darken slightly. Do not let it turn dark brown, or it will taste burned.
4. Immediately remove the pan from heat and use the caramel, as it thickens quickly. If necessary, remelt over low heat. Take care, as both caramel and pan will be very hot.

Other foods, such as onions, beets, and carrots, can be "caramelized" by cooking for a long time in a moderate oven or over medium-high to high heat so that their natural sugars, which caramelize during cooking, are accentuated. While this type of caramelizing is not precisely the same thing as caramelizing granulated cane sugar, it refers to a cooking method that emphasizes the sugar naturally occurring in many foods that are not ordinarily considered sweet. Although not always necessary, some cooks encourage caramelizing by sprinkling on a little extra sugar. This has become a popular way to prepare vegetables, particularly in recent years.

"Caramelized" is also used to refer to the darkened, flavorful drippings left on the bottom of a roasting pan after roasting meats and poultry.

See also CANDY MAKING; DEGLAZING; SUGAR.

CARAWAY SEED See SPICE.

CARDAMOM See SPICE.

CARROT Moms have long told kids that eating carrots guarantees good eyesight, so it is not surprising that nearly every kitchen has a few of these healthful root vegetables in the refrigerator bin. They turn up raw in lunch boxes and cooked in soups, stews, braises, salads, stir-fries, and vegetable side dishes. A favorite role is in moist carrot cake topped with cream cheese frosting. Another popular role—and one that is especially good for you—is bright orange carrot juice. Small carrots, already trimmed and peeled and packaged in 8- or 16-ounce plastic bags, have become popular as a quick and easy snack food.

> ## Quick Tip
>
> Carrots that have become slightly limp from overlong storage can be revived by a refreshing 30-minute soak in ice water.

Carrots, which are members of the parsley family, are among the least expensive of all vegetables. They are a good source of vitamin A, which actually accumulates during the months of storage after the carrots have been harvested. Their sweetness intensifies, too, during storage. Only beets have a higher sugar content among root vegetables.

> ## Quick Tip
>
> Carrot juice is deliciously sweet and refreshing and packs a wallop of vitamins and other nutrients. It attracts bacteria and so should never be stored for more than a day—unlike whole carrots. For the best taste and benefits, drink it immediately after juicing.

Selecting Look for smooth, firm, brightly colored carrots without cracks or any green, whitening, or sprouting around the stems. Larger carrots tend to have woody cores; baby carrots are tender but not especially sweet. Smaller, slender, mature carrots are the tastiest. Those with the feathery greens still attached, indicating freshness, generally are more expensive. They are not necessarily a better buy, however. The greens draw moisture and nutrients from the orange carrot roots and should be removed and discarded as soon as you get the carrots home (in many markets, the greengrocer will chop off the greens for you). Already trimmed carrots can be just as flavorful as those with their tops attached.

Storing Store carrots in plastic bags in the refrigerator for up to 2 weeks. They like both cool temperatures and high humidity. Do not store carrots near fruit such as bananas or apples, which emit ethylene gas and can give carrots a bitter flavor.

Preparing Trim off the root and stem ends. If the carrots are organic and on the

C

small side, simply scrub them under cold running water with a soft vegetable brush and use without peeling, since many nutrients will be lost if the peel is removed. If the carrots are not grown organically, peel them and trim at least an inch from the stem end, where pesticides concentrate. If the carrots have a woody core, remove it by halving the carrots lengthwise and cutting out the center with a small sharp knife.

See also STEAMING.

CARVING The art of removing meat or poultry from the bone and cutting it into attractive, serving-sized pieces. While some people are better at carving than others—and everyone improves with practice—performing this necessary task should not intimidate anyone. A good-quality sharp knife and a degree of confidence (as well as a healthy appetite!) facilitate carving as nothing else does.

A two-pronged carving fork to steady the roast is also very helpful.

Carving knife and fork.

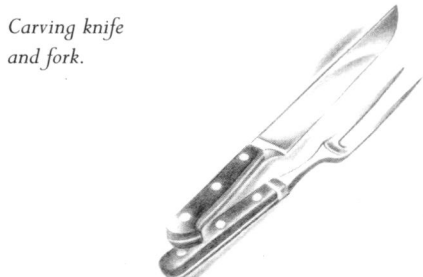

While an all-purpose slicing knife may be used for carving any type of roast, different knives are better suited to some roasts than to others. One with a long, flexible, but still sturdy blade is best for following the contours of a large turkey. A shorter, sturdier knife makes quick work of the smaller chicken. Long, straight blades with scalloped sides cut more readily through red meats. Whatever knife you use,

make sure it is well sharpened for easier, safer carving. A sturdy, slip-resistant carving board also facilitates the process by keeping the meat firmly in place.

Before carving roasted meat or poultry, let the roast rest, that is, sit at room temperature, for 10 to 25 minutes, depending on its size. This allows the juices time to settle and permits the internal temperature to stabilize. Some cooks suggest tenting a piece of aluminum foil over the meat to hold in the heat a bit, but this is generally ineffective unless the kitchen is very cold. It may also turn crispy poultry skin irretrievably soggy. Roasts are not meant to be served piping hot. Steaks, too, should be allowed to sit for 5 to 10 minutes before being sliced.

Carving board.

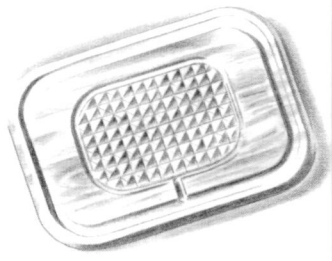

Meat should be carved across the grain. This produces a more handsome slice and avoids long strands of tough meat that can lodge in one's teeth. Also, the tougher the meat to be carved, the thinner the slice should be, again for ease of chewing. Finally, do not change the direction of the knife blade in midslice, or the pieces will be ragged and uneven.

Carve only the meat that will be consumed at the meal. The leftover meat will stay juicier if it remains uncarved. Once carved, the meat should be arranged attractively on a platter, usually in evenly overlapping slices, or placed directly on individual plates.

HOW TO *Carve a Turkey*

Generous in size, a turkey offers each diner an ample amount of dark leg meat and white breast meat. Carve only as much as you need to serve at one time, completing one side before starting the next.

1. With the turkey breast up, cut through the skin between leg and breast. Move the leg to locate the thigh joint, then cut through the joint to sever the leg. In the same way, remove the wing, cutting through the shoulder joint where it meets the breast.

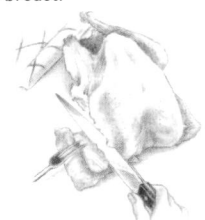

2. Cut through the joint to separate the drumstick and thigh. Carve both the drumstick and thigh, cutting thin slices parallel to the bone.

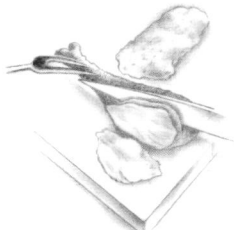

3. Just above the thigh and shoulder joints, carve a deep horizontal cut toward the bone, creating a base cut on one side of the breast. Starting near the breastbone, carve thin slices of breast meat vertically, cutting parallel to the rib cage and ending at the base cut.

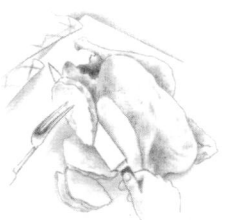

HOW TO *Carve a Chicken*

The basics of carving a chicken are similar to those for turkey. But because of the bird's smaller size, the drumstick and the thigh can be served whole and, depending on the number of mouths to feed, the entire chicken may be carved at once.

1. With the chicken breast up, cut through the skin between thigh and breast. Move the leg to locate the thigh joint, then cut through the joint to sever the leg. In the same way, remove the wing, cutting through the shoulder joint where it meets the breast.

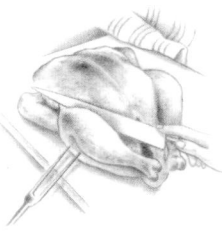

2. If the chicken is small, serve the whole leg as an individual portion. If it is larger, cut through the joint to separate the drumstick and thigh into 2 pieces. You may want to slice a large thigh into 2 pieces.

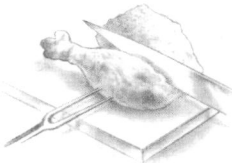

3. Starting at the breastbone, cut downward and parallel to the rib cage, cutting the meat into long, thin slices.

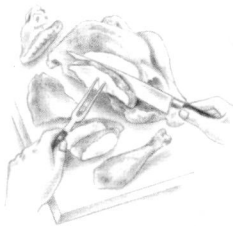

HOW TO *Carve a Bone-in Ham*

Whether you are carving a whole ham or a butt or shank end, the carving process is basically the same: cutting parallel slices perpendicular to the bone, which are then freed by cutting along the bone.

1. Starting at the widest end of the ham, cut a vertical slice about ¼ inch thick and perpendicular to the bone. The slice will remain attached to the ham.

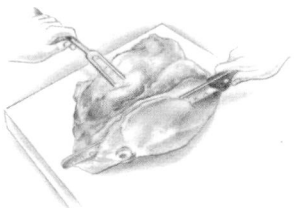

2. Continue making cuts of the same width and parallel to the first, cutting as many slices as you wish to serve.

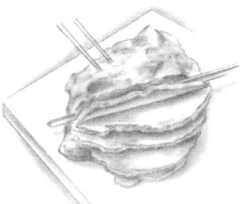

3. Free the slices from the bone: cut horizontally through the base of the slices, with the knife blade parallel to the bone. When all the meat has been removed from the first side, turn the ham over and repeat on the second side.

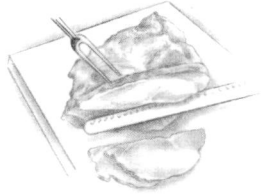

HOW TO *Carve a Boneless Roast or Ham*

1. Set the roast on end, leaving the twine in place to hold the roast together. Remove the twine as you reach it.
2. Hold the roast steady by inserting the fork below where you are slicing. Cut horizontal slices ¼ to ½ inch thick; arrange on a platter.
3. For a smaller roast, set the roast on its side and make vertical slices.

HOW TO *Carve a Prime Rib of Beef*

A prime rib of beef is fairly simple to carve, provided you have a long, sharp knife and a sturdy fork to steady the roast. You may wish to leave some slices attached to the ribs, for anyone who likes gnawing the meat on the bone.

1. Place the roast bone side down and steady it by inserting a carving fork. Using a long, sharp, sturdy blade, cut a vertical slice across the grain from one end of the roast down to the rib bone, much like slicing a loaf of bread. Then, holding the knife parallel with the rib bones, cut along the bone to free the slice.

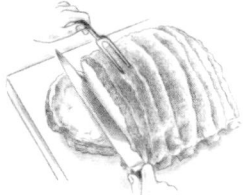

2. Cutting parallel to the first slice, continue to carve ¼- to ¾-inch-thick slices. As individual rib bones are exposed, cut between them and the meat to remove them, or leave them attached to meat slices if preferred.

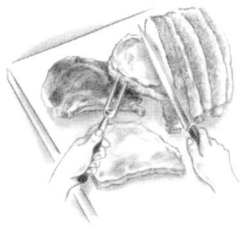

HOW TO *Carve a Leg of Lamb*

Shaped like an irregular, elongated pear, a leg of lamb presents a challenge. The keys to successful carving lie in cutting parallel to the bone and providing guests with slices from both sides of the leg.

Before cooking a bone-in leg of lamb, be sure to ask the butcher to remove the hip bone, to save you work.

1. Firmly grasp the protruding end of the shank bone with a kitchen towel and tilt it slightly upward. Using a long, sharp knife, carve a first slice from the rounded, meaty side of the leg at its widest point, cutting away from you and roughly parallel to the bone.

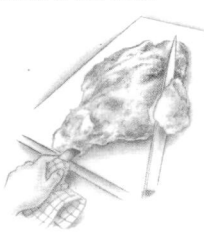

2. Cutting parallel to the first slice, continue carving the meat in thin slices until you have as many slices as you need.

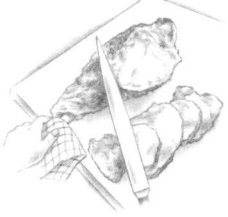

3. Grasping the bone, rotate the leg of lamb to expose its other, flatter side—the inner side of the leg, which is slightly more tender. Still cutting parallel to the bone, carve slices.

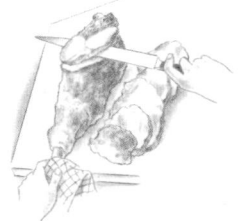

CASHEW See NUT.

CASSEROLE The casserole, a savory baked dish that mixes two or more ingredients and can be eaten with a fork alone, is an American culinary standard—a preparation that gained popularity with busy cooks in the 1950s and has never lost its appeal. The same term is used for the deep oven-proof dish in which the food is cooked. Such dishes often have lids and may be round, oval, rectangular, or square. They can be made from any number of materials, ranging from tempered glass to earthenware to porcelain to stoneware to enameled cast iron. A popular material for casserole dishes is the familiar heat-resistant glass that is often referred to by its trademarked name: Pyrex.

Quick Tip

Casseroles are soft and often creamy and therefore may be complemented well by a crunchy topping. A mixture of buttered bread crumbs and grated Parmesan cheese sprinkled over the top and allowed to brown during the final minutes of baking adds texture.

Noodles and rice are common casserole ingredients and are often combined with a creamy, thick sauce. Classic casseroles include tuna noodle and macaroni and cheese. Lasagne is also a casserole. These and many other dishes are baked in casserole dishes that can go directly from the oven to the table for serving.

Casseroles are great favorites with cooks who like or need to plan ahead, since many freeze well. They should be cooked thoroughly, allowed to cool just to room temperature, covered with foil or the casserole lid, and frozen. Most can be reheated directly from the freezer in a moderate (350°F) oven for about an hour, or until bubbling hot. If you want to brown the top, uncover the dish during the final 10 to 15 minutes of cooking.

Many baking dishes can be used for cooking casseroles. Most casserole dishes are relatively deep and have handles or lips and a noticeable heft to them. The most popular sizes hold from 2½ to 5 quarts, although some dishes hold as little as 1½ quarts, while others hold up to 7 quarts.

All casserole dishes are oven safe, but not all are meant to be used on top of the stove. Make sure you know which are flame resistant, either by reading the tags when you buy them or by using common sense: pottery casseroles usually are not meant for stove-top cooking, while shock- and heat-resistant glass ones, such as Pyrex, are. Many casserole dishes, particularly those made by large commercial companies, can go directly from the refrigerator or freezer into a hot oven without cracking. These are usually dishwasher safe, too. Those made by artisan potters tend to be more fragile.

See also COOKWARE.

CAULIFLOWER Mark Twain once described cauliflower as "cabbage with a college education." A member of the cabbage family, cauliflower is akin to broccoli, which it closely resembles.

Firm, compact, creamy white florets form a head, which is the primary edible portion of the cauliflower. The inner leaves are edible, too, and taste somewhat like collard greens. Unfortunately, they are rarely sold with the cauliflower, and even the green leaves near the stem end are usually removed. If you grow cauliflower, don't discard the leaves.

Cauliflower has a mild flavor that marries nicely with cheese and with vegetables such as green beans and carrots. It can be cooked and then puréed for soup. The florets are also good raw or blanched in salads or served on a crudité platter.

Quick Tip

Adding a few drops of lemon juice or a little milk to the cooking water helps cauliflower retain its creamy white color. As with cabbage, there is no way to prevent an odor's emanating from the cauliflower during cooking. Cut cauliflower into small florets, cook them quickly, and turn on exhaust fans and open windows to disperse any odor.

Selecting Cauliflower is in season in the fall, although it is available throughout most of the winter. Look for firm, tight heads without bruises or brown spots, with evenly colored ivory or cream florets. A few varieties of cauliflower have a green or purple tinge, which is natural and does not change the taste. If any leaves remain, they should be green and fresh looking. Avoid cauliflower with loosely packed or spreading florets. It is acceptable if a few green shoots are showing among the florets, or if the florets look a little grainy or bristly.

Storing Store cauliflower in a loose, perforated plastic bag in the refrigerator for up to 1 week. If you do not use the entire head, plan to eat the remaining florets within a day. Or, you may freeze them, first blanching them in lightly salted water for about 3 minutes, draining, and then putting them in rigid containers or plastic bags in the freezer for up to 1 year. Once cooked, cauliflower keeps for only 1 or 2 days in the refrigerator.

Preparing Remove any leaves from the stem end of the head, separate the head into florets, and rinse under cold running water. Trim off any brown spots. Cauliflower can be cooked whole as well and the florets separated after cooking. Steam or boil cauliflower until tender and toss with a little butter or lemon juice, or other vegetables, before serving.

See also BOILING; STEAMING.

CAVIAR Nearly synonymous with elegance, fresh, icy-cold caviar is one of history's most enduring luxuries. It is the roe (eggs) of various members of the sturgeon family, and although the roe of other fish such as salmon, whitefish, trout, and lumpfish also are sold under the name, they are not "true" caviar.

The best and most expensive caviar is from the three types of sturgeon that swim in the Caspian Sea and its tributaries: beluga, osetra, and sevruga. American sturgeon, most of which are farmed in California, also produce good caviar. Another good-quality caviar, called kaluga, is exported from China.

Beluga, considered the finest, has the largest grains, ranging from light gray to inky black. The grains have a firm, crisp texture and a clean, fresh, pleasingly salty

Quick Tip

Although some people who indulge in caviar may have been born with silver spoons in their mouths, silver and caviar do not mix. The silver interacts with the caviar grains, giving them a metallic taste. Serve this delicacy with mother-of-pearl or bone caviar paddles, antique ivory spoons, or gold spoons. Small plastic spoons are fine, too.

flavor. Some caviar lovers prefer osetra. It has a bolder, nuttier flavor, and the grains, which may be quite small, can be inky or very pale. The grains of sevruga caviar are

Quick Bite

The "caviar" sold at room temperature in vacuum-packed jars is not true caviar but rather less-desirable lumpfish roe that has been dyed black, gray, or red. Many people use it for hors d'oeuvres.

smaller and saltier than those of beluga or osetra. Many prefer sevruga's more pronounced flavor, and of the three classic caviars, it is the least costly.

Selecting Buy caviar from a reputable merchant in a shop with good turnover. It should be fresh packed in jars or tins that are stored at temperatures between 28° and 31°F. The eggs should be plump and whole and covered with a sheen of oil but not drenched in it. They should be light to dark gray (almost black), depending on the variety. Ideally, these grains pop when pressed against the roof of your mouth with your tongue, releasing their light, intoxicating flavor. Choose caviar labeled *malossol,* Russian for "lightly salted." When the tin or jar is opened, the grains should smell only slightly fishy or of the sea. Some manufacturers pasteurize the caviar to extend its shelf life, although aficionados avoid this, dismissing the resulting slightly softer texture and diminished flavor.

Storing A good caviar merchant will pack your purchase in an insulated bag for transportation home. Even so, do not make any stops. Store the caviar in the coldest part of the refrigerator, which is usually at the back of the bottom shelf or in a meat drawer. If it is already opened, serve the caviar within 24 hours. If not, it will keep in the refrigerator for up to 2 weeks.

Preparing The traditional way to serve caviar is ice cold, scooped straight from the tin or jar into a bowl on a bed of shaved ice. Many caviar lovers like it simple—no adornments—but others pair it with such accompaniments as thin toast points, chopped hard-boiled eggs, crème fraîche, sour cream, lemon slices, and chopped onions. Caviar also marries well with potatoes, blinis, and eggs. Chilled Champagne or vodka is a good partner.

CAYENNE PEPPER See SPICE.

CECI BEAN See BEAN, DRIED.

CELERIAC See CELERY ROOT.

CELERY This bland yet satisfyingly crunchy vegetable is so commonplace, we seldom think of it when pondering the vegetable kingdom. Yet nearly every refrigerator contains a head, and countless recipes list celery as an ingredient. Everyday celery is Pascal celery. A northern European variety of white celery (also called golden celery) is sometimes grown under cover to keep it from turning green. It is far rarer than Pascal celery.

A head of celery consists of several pale or darker green leafy ribs attached at a lighter-colored base. The inner section of this base is the celery heart, the tender, light-colored ribs in the center of the head, prized as an ingredient in some salads and braised dishes. These ribs are smaller than the outer ribs, but they are not always significantly smaller.

Celery is frequently matched with onions and carrots as the base for soups, stews, casseroles, and other savory dishes. Its mild flavor easily blends with others and its crispness disappears during cooking. The ribs can be served raw, either plain or filled with soft cheese or peanut butter, or chopped and added to tuna or chicken salads.

Celery hearts.

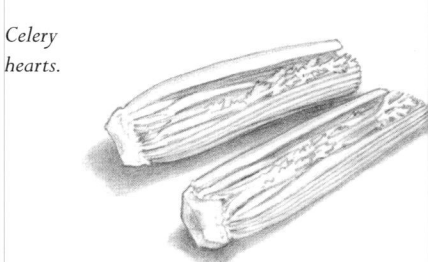

Selecting Buy firm, crisp heads with few blemishes and healthy-looking green leaves. Pass on any heads with ribs that do not look as though they will snap decisively when broken. Some heads are trimmed of leaves and bagged in plastic; these may be called "celery hearts," although they also include a good portion of the ribs.

Storing Refrigerate whole heads of celery in a perforated plastic bag in the vegetable crisper for up to 2 weeks.

Preparing Separate the ribs from the head only as needed. Wash them thoroughly under cold running water and trim off both ends. With few exceptions, new celery varieties have eliminated the need for

Quick Bite

Mirepoix, a classic French mixture of diced onions, carrots, and celery, flavors stocks, stews, and sauces and serves as a bed for roasting meat. Once they have given up all their flavor, the vegetables are generally strained from the stock or sauce.

removing strings from the ribs. Refresh slightly tired celery ribs with a 30-minute soak in ice water.

CELERY ROOT If you have ever ordered *céleri-rave rémoulade* in a Paris bistro, you will have tried this tough-looking vegetable in one of its most sophisticated guises: julienned raw and tossed with mustard mayonnaise. Also called celeriac, celery knob, or turnip-rooted celery, celery root is the root of a celery plant (not the same variety that produces the familiar supermarket celery bunches) grown specifically for its root, although both the leaves and stalks are edible. The gnarled, knobby brown root bulb may look impenetrable, but once the outside is peeled, the tender ivory flesh is delicious either raw (usually shredded in salads) or cooked. Celery root tastes similar to common celery but has a more pronounced nutty, earthy flavor and a softer, denser texture. Boil it as you would a potato, then mash; add it to stews or soups; or chop or shred it raw and add it to salads.

Selecting Buy firm, medium-sized roots, about the size of small grapefruits, that feel heavy for their size and are free of bruising and soft spots. Tangled root ends are acceptable, as are any green stalks growing from the top. Celery root is available from early fall through early spring.

Storing Trim any greenery and root ends from the celery root and store the unwashed roots in a perforated plastic bag in the vegetable crisper of the refrigerator for 3 to 5 days.

Preparing Scrub the celery root with a stiff bristle brush under cold running water. Trim the root further if it appears tough or particularly fibrous and then use a vegetable peeler or small, sharp knife to peel the brown skin. Immediately sprinkle the root with lemon juice to prevent discoloring. For cooking, cut, chop, or shred the root using a knife, food processor, or shredder.

CELERY SEED See SPICE.

CHANTERELLE See MUSHROOM.

CHARBROIL To broil meat or poultry over charcoal to the point where its surface begins to turn black and char.

CHAYOTE (chy-OH-tee) Also called vegetable pear, mirliton, or christophine. A soft-skinned, large, pear-shaped squash with light green or white skin and pronounced ridges running from top to stem end. The skin is not edible, and while many preparations suggest discarding the large, flat seed, it is perfectly edible in smaller, younger chayotes and can be cooked along with the chayote and eaten as a snack. The chayote has a somewhat mild flavor, not unlike zucchini, and is popular in Mexico and Central America, where it is indigenous. The flesh is cut into pieces and steamed, boiled, baked, or braised. Chayotes can also be split and cooked like a squash, or the flesh can be eaten raw in salads.

Selecting Buy firm, heavy-feeling chayotes with healthy-looking skin. Avoid those with soft spots or wrinkling, which indicate age. They should also look clean, with no trace of soil. Soft bristles on the skin are acceptable.

Storing Store in a perforated plastic bag in the refrigerator for up to 2 weeks.

Preparing Wash the chayote under cold running water. Like a potato's, a chayote's skin can be cut away before cooking or slipped off the vegetable after cooking, depending on what makes the most sense for a recipe. If a slimy substance escaping from the skin of the uncooked vegetable irritates your skin, peel the chayote under running water. (This is a common irritant, not harmful, and it disappears during cooking.) Discard the skin and single seed, unless you decide to cook it. You can also cut the flesh into pieces and steam, boil, bake, or braise it as you would zucchini or summer squash.

CHEDDAR See CHEESE.

CHEESE See page 100.

CHEESECAKE Most home bakers appreciate cheesecake for two reasons: it lends itself to advance preparation, and it generally gets rave reviews. This classic indulgence is irresistible to nearly everyone, even the most dedicated dieter.

American-style cheesecakes, commonly made with cream cheese, are so satiny smooth they melt in your mouth. Italian-style cheesecakes, made from lightly grained cheese (usually ricotta) mixed with flour, have drier textures but make equally impressive desserts.

Fillings Cheesecakes can be either sweet or savory. While they traditionally are made with cream cheese or ricotta, they can also include cottage cheese, Cheddar cheese, Swiss cheese, and farmer cheese. The cheese is blended with eggs, sugar or another sweetener (for sweet cheesecakes), and flavorings, poured into a pan, and baked. Flour and cornstarch are common thickeners, although too much cornstarch, in particular, will toughen the cake. Cream, sour cream, or yogurt adds smoothness and lightens the texture while adding richness. Chocolate is a popular flavor addition, but other crowd pleasers are ginger, citrus zest, espresso powder, chopped nuts, nutmeg, cinnamon, raisins, extracts, and candied fruit. Fruit and chocolate glazes are favorite toppings.

Unbaked cheesecakes generally rely on gelatin to stabilize them. Follow the recipe carefully and never use more than is called for, or the cake will be rubbery.

Crusts Cheesecake crusts typically are crumb crusts made with graham crackers, crumbled chocolate wafers, gingersnaps, or soda crackers. Other ingredients such as nuts, coconut, or citrus zest may be added to the crumbs to enhance the taste or texture. Cheesecakes also may be baked in traditional pastry crusts or shortcake crusts, or they can be baked without a crust in a buttered pan.

HOW TO *Form a Crumb Crust*
1. Put the crust ingredients in a food processor fitted with the metal blade. Process until the mixture forms fine crumbs that begin to stick together.
2. Drape plastic wrap over your hand to form a glove and press the crumb mixture firmly and evenly into a springform pan or other pan as directed in the recipe.

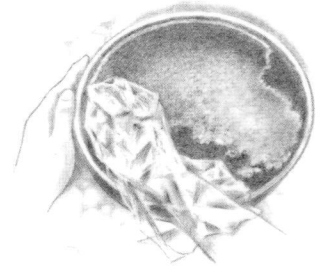

3. If directed, bake the crust for about 10 minutes to firm it up. Let the crust cool before filling it.

Cheesecake Savvy

- Beginning with all ingredients at room temperature ensures the creamiest, most easily blended batter.
- Before you start to mix the ingredients, beat the cream cheese by itself until it is completely free of lumps, light, and smooth. Trying to rid the batter of lumps later won't be successful.
- For perfect creaminess, never overbake a cheesecake. Baking the cheesecake in a water bath will help. (See WATER BATH.) If using a springform pan, wrap it in aluminum foil before placing it in the water, to avoid seepage.
- Take the cheesecake from the oven when the center still quivers; it will continue to cook outside the oven and will firm up. Overbaked cheesecakes will crack as they cool.
- To unmold a crustless cheesecake baked in a solid pan, run a flexible knife around the inside edge of the pan when the cake is taken from the oven, and then let the cake cool completely. Unmold the cake by putting a flat platter or plate over the pan and inverting it. Shake very gently or tap the bottom of the pan to release the cheesecake. If it is still reluctant to unmold, put the pan over a low flame or in a heated cast-iron frying pan for a few seconds and try again. To avoid this problem, bake cheesecakes in a springform pan. (See BAKEWARE.)
- To freeze a cheesecake, let cool completely in the pan, chill in the refrigerator for several hours, then carefully wrap the cheesecake, still in the pan, with freezer-weight plastic and freeze for up to 3 months. Thaw in the refrigerator and, when it is still very cold, release the sides of the pan or unmold the cake. Bring the cheesecake to room temperature before serving.

Quick Tip

While most cheesecakes are eaten cold, Italian-style cheesecakes based on ricotta are also delicious warm. Let them cool for about 20 minutes before slicing and serving; briefly reheat leftover slices in a low oven.

CHEESECLOTH Also called butter muslin, cheesecloth is lightweight, 100 percent cotton gauze, free of dyes and finishes. It is primarily used for straining and filtering, as it does not fall apart when wet or submerged in boiling water and never imparts any flavor to the food.

Cheesecloth is perhaps best known as the material used to hold the herbs for a bouquet garni or any bundle of herbs or spices. It is useful for holding a whole fish, such as salmon, during poaching. Cheesecloth is also employed for straining stocks, sauces, and jellies and for draining the whey from curds in fresh cheeses (hence its name) and the excess liquid from yogurt. Some cooks soak cheesecloth in melted butter or oil and drape it over turkey or chicken during roasting to add fat and flavor and promote browning.

Fine-mesh cheesecloth, preferred for jelly making and other fine straining needs, is generally found in kitchenware shops. Standard coarse-mesh cheesecloth is sold with other kitchen equipment in supermarkets, general houseware stores, and hardware stores, and while it is suitable for making bundles of herbs and poaching fish, it may be too coarse for straining fine liquids such as consommé or fruit jelly. Many sauce recipes recommend using a double layer of coarse-mesh cheesecloth to imitate a finer mesh. Handy cheesecloth bags for herbs are sold in many specialty-food stores, too, although making your own from hand-cut squares is less costly.

C

Cheese

Hundreds of cheeses with unique tastes and textures are enjoyed throughout the world, but they are all created from the same basic ingredients and by the same basic process.

The fresh or pasteurized milk of cows, sheep, or goats is first treated with enzymes, such as rennet, to separate it into creamy curds and watery whey, and then the curds are concentrated by various methods. The nuances of each unique cheese develop from the most minute variations in what the animals eat, the time of year the cheese is made, the method used to make the cheese, and how and where the cheese makers store and age the cheese.

Jack, mozzarella, and Swiss cheeses.

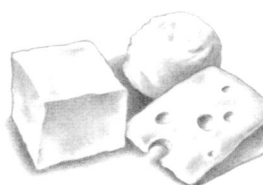

Cheeses can be divided into two basic categories: fresh and ripened (aged). Most fresh cheeses are simply curds separated from and drained of their watery whey, while ripened cheeses undergo aging to develop an infinite variety of textures and complex flavors. The longer a cheese ages, the drier and more flavorful it becomes. The same cheese may be eaten when young and soft or later after it is transformed by aging and drying. Fresh and ripened are, however, only the two most basic categories. Cheeses are grouped by a number of distinctive qualities, and these categories overlap in many cases.

Fresh Cheeses Very mild and soft, unripened fresh cheeses are used often in desserts and in some main-course recipes, breakfast dishes, and sandwiches. Some have a slightly acidic taste.

COTTAGE CHEESE A mild-flavored fresh cheese characterized by large or small curds mixed with a little milk or cream. Also called pot cheese. Unlike creamed, or regular, cottage cheese, dry-curd cottage cheese is not mixed with milk or cream.

CREAM CHEESE A mild, tangy fresh cheese made from whole milk and extra cream. Most commercial brands contain stabilizers and other additives. Cream cheese blends deliciously with other ingredients, such as herbs, chutneys, jellies, chocolate, and fruit. It is the primary ingredient in many cheesecakes and various hors d'oeuvres dips, and bagels are hardly bagels without a generous smear of cream cheese.

Quick Tip

Many baking recipes have been developed using full-fat, block cream cheese such as Philadelphia brand. Do not substitute light, whipped, or natural cream cheese for block cream cheese, and never use fat-free cream cheese in these recipes.

CRÈME FRAÎCHE Not everyone agrees that this cultured cream product is a fresh cheese, although many cheese makers say it is. Its silken texture and pleasing sour, mildly nutty flavor make it similar to sour cream, but sweeter and even more indulgent. See CRÈME FRAÎCHE.

C

FARMER CHEESE Similar in flavor to cottage cheese but with no curds. Instead, it is pressed into a block that can be sliced.

FROMAGE BLANC A mild fresh cheese made from skim or whole milk, with or without cream added. It is eaten flavored with sugar as a simple dessert and also used in cooking.

MASCARPONE A very soft, rich, smooth fresh Italian cheese made from cream, with a texture reminiscent of sour cream. Sold in plastic tubs.

NEUFCHÂTEL A mild, creamy, spreadable yellow cheese made in Normandy, France. In the United States, low-fat cream cheese is often called Neufchâtel and is used in recipes that attempt to cut calories and fat.

PROVOLONE Most commonly made from cow's milk, provolone is sold when young and mild and as a sharper, tangier aged cheese. Also available smoked.

QUESO FRESCO A Mexican cow's milk cheese made from fresh curds pressed into round molds. The result is a soft, crumbly, slightly grainy cheese similar in taste to ricotta or farmer cheese.

RICOTTA A whey-based cheese made by heating the whey left over from making sheep's, goat's, or cow's milk cheeses. Most Italian ricotta is made from sheep's milk. It takes no solid form but is sold in plastic containers. Fresh Italian ricotta is superb. See also Ricotta Salata, page 102.

Stretch-Curd Cheeses The mild Italian cheeses in this category, known in Italy as *pasta filata,* are made by immersing the curds in hot water and then kneading and stretching (or "stringing") them. In general, the cheeses melt smoothly over bread, pasta, vegetables, or poultry and also are good for slicing and using in sandwiches.

MOZZARELLA Mild, creamy cheese made from cow's or water buffalo's milk curd formed into balls. It may be salted or not.

If possible, seek out fresh mozzarella, which is sold surrounded by a little of the whey, rather than the rubbery products made in large factories.

STRING CHEESE A popular snack food, particularly with children, string cheese is mozzarella cheese that has been pulled into strings, or strands, and then packaged in plastic so that it is shaped like short, fat sticks. It is also called Armenian-style string cheese, rope, or braided cheese. String cheese is rarely, if ever, used in cooking.

Soft-Ripened Cheeses Uncooked and unpressed (that is, the curds are left to firm naturally), these cheeses are aged for a very short time after being transferred to molds. Their texture is usually soft enough to spread, and they have an edible rind that is powdery white or orange in color. Some of the rinds of the stronger-flavored cheeses have been washed in brine, brandy, or even beer to add flavor during aging. Since the flavors of these cheeses are easily lost when heated, they are rarely used in cooking (except for Brie, which is sometimes baked in a pastry or almond crust).

BOURSAULT A rich, nutty French cheese with a creamy texture. Made from pasteurized or unpasteurized cow's milk. Most aficionados prefer the unpasteurized cheese, but it is rare outside Europe.

BRIE A sublimely smooth, ivory cheese with an edible rind, made from cow's milk, pasteurized or unpasteurized (again, rare outside Europe). Brie should be served only when ripe and so soft it is almost—but not quite—runny. It is sold in flat rounds of various sizes.

CAMEMBERT This cow's milk cheese, similar to Brie, has a yellow interior and edible rind. Camembert should be as soft as bread dough when ripe and ready to eat.

continued

Cheese, continued

LIMBURGER A soft, slightly salty, full-flavored cow's milk product with a powerful aroma that dissuades some from trying the tasty cheese. The rind is washed in brine during ripening, which contributes to the development of the cheese's smell.

PONT L'ÉVÊQUE A full-flavored French cow's milk cheese similar to Brie and Camembert but with a stronger flavor. The cheese, with its light brown crust and pale yellow interior, is packed in square wooden boxes.

RICOTTA SALATA A mild, pure white, rindless sheep's milk cheese with a smooth texture and pleasantly sweet flavor. Ricotta salata is most readily associated with Sicily, Sardinia, and the southern part of Italy. The cheese is aged for at least 3 months, although in Sicily it may be aged far longer, until firm and appropriate for grating. It is served in much the same way as feta cheese (rather than as fresh ricotta cheese) or used to top pasta.

TELEME Resembling a tangy Brie and aged for about 3 weeks, this cheese of northern California is made from extra-rich milk.

Semisoft Cheeses Cooked but not pressed, these cheeses are soft but can be sliced. They are ideal for melting on sandwiches and on baked dishes.

HAVARTI An extremely mild cow's milk cheese sold in blocks and without rind, peppered with small indentations. It is as mild as Monterey jack and just as adaptable for sandwiches and melting. Originally from Denmark but now made in the United States and elsewhere.

MONTEREY JACK A soft, white, mild cow's milk cheese that originated in California, either with tiny "eyes" or smooth, depending on where it is made. Jack is often sold infused with hot red chiles and called "pepper jack." A dry version is also made, which was used by West Coast Italian Americans to replace Parmesan when it was in short supply during World War II.

MUENSTER When made in America, this cheese is very mild and smooth with great melting properties. French Muenster is fuller flavored with an odiferous rind and nutty overtones. German and Danish Muensters (or Münsters) fall between the two in terms of flavor and are formed into rounds, rather than rectangles.

PORT-SALUT A mild French cow's milk cheese with a creamy, yellow interior.

TALEGGIO An aromatic Italian cow's milk cheese with a pale brown rind and ivory interior and a bold, nutty, fruity flavor.

Semifirm (or Semihard) Cheeses These uncooked, pressed, and aged cheeses are dense in texture and ivory to pale yellow in color. They are popular for eating with bread and fruit, for sandwiches, and for cooking, as they melt nicely.

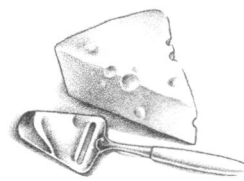

Semifirm cheese with plane.

ASIAGO An Italian cow's milk cheese sold in wheels and, when semifirm, pleasantly sharp tasting and covered with an inedible rind. Also available fresh (mild) and aged (sharper). American Asiago is very mild.

CHEDDAR This cow's milk cheese is appreciated for its sharp, salty flavor, which ranges from mild to sharp. Farmhouse Cheddars are stronger tasting than other American Cheddars.

EDAM Mildly tangy cow's milk cheese with a smooth interior covered with red wax, traditionally produced in the Netherlands in a town of the same name.

EMMENTHALER A cow's milk cheese produced in the mountains of Europe, most notably Switzerland, and distinguished by its random holes, which range in size from small to quite large. Ivory colored and mildly nutty in flavor.

FONTINA A mild, fruity Italian cow's milk cheese with a pleasing firmness and light but heady aroma.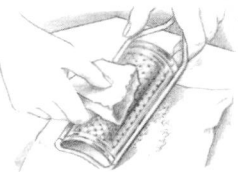

GOUDA A mild cow's milk cheese encased in red wax that is similar to Edam, above, although less tangy. Also made from goat's milk.

GRUYÈRE This smooth, creamy cow's milk cheese is produced in Switzerland and France and revered for its nutty yet mild flavor.

JARLSBERG A cow's milk cheese made from partially skimmed milk and characterized by its hole-filled interior and mild, slightly nutty flavor.

MANCHEGO A Spanish sheep's milk cheese with a mild, pale yellow interior dotted with holes and tasting mild and a little salty.

RACLETTE A sweet, fruity cheese with an inedible rind and pale beige interior. This cheese, produced in Switzerland and France, melts beautifully and is used for the classic Swiss melted cheese and potato dish of the same name.

REBLOCHON Very smooth, sweet, fruity French cheese sold formed into disks and sandwiched between two paper-thin wooden rounds. Reblochon is made with pasteurized or unpasteurized milk, the latter difficult to find outside of France.

SWISS A generic term for a variety of cheeses typified by Switzerland's Emmenthaler, above. Swiss cheeses are noted for their mild, nutlike flavor, semifirm texture, and network of holes or "eyes."

Firm (or Hard) Cheeses These cheeses are cooked, pressed, and aged for a firm, compact texture. Perfect for grating, some have a granular texture and a hard rind. Fine examples of these same cheeses are sometimes enjoyed as part of a cheese course at the end of a meal.

Grating cheese.

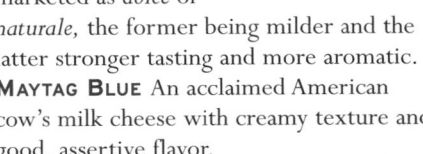

PARMESAN A wonderful grating cheese, Parmesan is an ivory-colored cow's milk cheese with a distinctive, salty flavor. See also PARMESAN.

PECORINO ROMANO A pleasantly salty Italian sheep's milk cheese with a grainy texture. Primarily used for grating.

Blue-Veined Cheeses These cheeses are inoculated with the spores of special molds to develop a fine network of blue veins for a strong, sharp, peppery flavor and a crumbly texture. Most blue cheeses can be crumbled, diced, spread, and sliced. Depending on the cheeses' moisture content, however, some hold their shape when sliced better than do others.

DANISH BLUE A cow's milk cheese with bold, straightforward flavor and smooth, creamy, moist texture.

GORGONZOLA An exceptional cow's milk cheese from Italy with a moist, creamy texture and complex flavor. May be marketed as *dolce* or *naturale,* the former being milder and the latter stronger tasting and more aromatic.

MAYTAG BLUE An acclaimed American cow's milk cheese with creamy texture and good, assertive flavor.

ROQUEFORT A sheep's milk cheese from France with a moist, crumbly interior and true, clean, strong flavor. Some Roqueforts are rather salty.

STILTON A cow's milk cheese from England with firm texture and an assertive flavor.

continued

Cheese, continued

Goat's Milk Cheeses Made from pure goat's milk or a blend of goat's and cow's milk. Mild, creamy, and only slightly tangy when fresh, goat cheeses become distinctly sharp in flavor as they age and harden. They are molded in a variety of shapes, such as logs and wheels, and may be coated with dried herbs, leaves, or ash. The French term for goat cheese is *fromage de chèvre,* which is often shortened to "chèvre" (SHEV).

BANON A soft, flavorful, somewhat spicy French goat cheese formed into disks and traditionally wrapped in chestnut leaves. Banons may sometimes be sprinkled with herbs or spices instead.

BÛCHERON Aged French goat's milk cheese sold in logs.

CROTTIN French goat's milk cheese shaped into thick rounds or short logs. Most have soft, mild, pure white interiors of young goat cheese; others are made from stronger, aged goat cheese.

FETA Sometimes made from goat's milk, but more generally from sheep's. See Sheep's Milk Cheeses, below.

MONTRACHET Mild, young French goat's milk cheese sold in logs with bright white interiors and spreadable texture. The term has become a generic designation for any young, fresh goat's milk cheese.

Sheep's Milk Cheeses

FETA A young cheese, traditionally made in Greece, Bulgaria, and Corsica (France) of sheep's milk. It usually has a crumbly texture that, in some cases, may be creamy as well. The pleasant, salty flavor of the white cheese is accentuated by the brine in which the cheese is pickled. American, Australian, Danish, and German feta cheeses are often made from cow's milk but taste very like sheep's milk feta. The cheese may also be made from goat's milk.

Double- and Triple-Cream Cheeses Cow's milk cheeses with cream added to increase the fat content for an extremely soft, smooth texture and a rich, slightly sweet flavor. By law, double-cream cheeses must have at least 60 percent milk fat, while triple-cream cheeses must have 75 percent or more. They can be either fresh or ripened.

BOURSAULT See Soft-Ripened Cheeses, page 101.

BOURSIN A creamy cheese flavored with herbs or garlic, or both.

BRILLAT-SAVARIN A buttery, very rich and creamy French cheese sent to market while still young and light.

EXPLORATEUR A full-flavored, creamy French cheese with a pale ivory interior and a bloomy edible rind.

PETIT-SUISSE A bright white, fresh French cheese sold in small logs with a very soft texture and sweet-tart flavor. Sometimes sold mixed with fruit.

Selecting A specialized cheese dealer with a rapid turnover will offer the best-quality cheeses. Look for cheeses with uniform color and veining, avoiding any with cracks or color changes near the rind. Although they may smell strong, cheeses should not have a sour or ammoniated odor. Wedges freshly cut from a larger wheel will retain more flavor. Before buying, ask for a small piece to sample. Because cheese stales quickly after grating, buy grating cheese in a single piece and grate it at home. When substituting another cheese for one specified in a recipe, try to use a cheese from the same general category for similar results.

Storing Because of their high moisture content, soft and fresh cheeses do not keep as long as aged firm and semifirm cheeses. Refrigerated, softer cheeses will keep for 1 week to 10 days, while harder ones can be stored for 2 to 4 weeks. Some very hard ones, like Parmesan, will keep for up to 10 months. Wrap cheese first in waxed paper to hold in the moisture and then double wrap it with a tight seal of plastic wrap or aluminum foil.

Preparing Cheese meant to be enjoyed as an appetizer, as a first course, or at the end of a meal is at its best served at room temperature. Remove the cheese from the refrigerator about an hour before serving.

In order to keep it moist and flavorful, grate or shred cheese just before serving or using in a recipe. Perforated metal cheese graters come in a variety of shapes and sizes, from the familiar box grater to the rotary grater. For more details, see GRATING; SHREDDING.

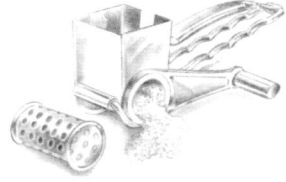

Rotary cheese grater/shredder.

The most popular devices for cutting cheese (other than a knife) are the cheese slicer, fitted with a taut wire that glides through a block of cheese, and the cheese plane or shaver. The plane, with its rounded or triangular blade, has a slot near the handle that has a sharp edge capable of shaving cheese as it is pulled across its surface. This device works well for semifirm cheeses, but should not be used for soft cheeses.

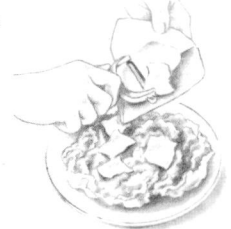

Cheese slicer.

Small cheese cleavers resemble larger butcher cleavers and are good for cutting cheese—and not much more.

The Cheese Course An array of quality cheeses may be served as an elegant alternative to dessert. To highlight a good selection of cheeses, present them simply on a tray, platter, or small marble or wooden cutting board, lining the surface with grape leaves (if you like). Make it easy for guests to help themselves by including appropriate cutting instruments, such as a sharp, broad-bladed knife for hard cheeses, a sharp knife with a pronged tip for semihard cheeses, a blunt-bladed knife for cutting and spreading soft cheese, and a cheese plane for shaving slices from blocks. Provide bread or crackers, fresh fruit (apples, pears, grapes) or dried fruits (apricots, nectarines, dates), and/or nuts, and wine.

Three or four cheeses is adequate. More will confuse the palate. When composing the tray, pick cheeses with contrasting textures and flavors. For example, try pairing Stilton, a mild goat cheese, and Fontina; or serve a wedge of Cheddar, Explorateur, and Gruyère with fresh fruit, slices from a baguette, and some walnuts or pecans. Some classic combinations are Cheddar with apples and Burgundy; Port-Salut with grapes and sweet Riesling; Stilton with pears, walnuts, and Port; and fresh goat cheese with dates. Remember, too, even a single delightful cheese can make a memorable impression.

Quick Bite

Dry natural cheese rinds occur as the cheese air-dries; they are generally not eaten. Soft white rinds, such as that on Brie, are a bloom of white mold; these are edible. Yellow to dark red washed rinds result from the cheese's being washed with one of a variety of liquids; these are not usually eaten. Artificial rinds may be produced from wax, ashes, or leaves and are not eaten.

C

CHERIMOYA Also known as the custard apple. This large tropical fruit has pale green skin and is slightly flattened and heart shaped. But the most distinctive visual clues to its identity are the overlapping leaf imprints that make the fruit look like an upside-down artichoke. The interior is white and creamy and studded with black seeds. Its texture is like firm custard, and while some say its flavor is a combination of bananas and mangoes, with a hint of strawberries, others declare it reminds them of pineapple. Cherimoyas are ripe when their leathery skin turns a brownish green and they give slightly when gently pressed, much like a peach or an avocado.

Selecting These fruits transport well and usually arrive at the market unripe. Buy firm, heavy cherimoyas with even-colored green skin. Avoid fruit with brown spots, although one or two are acceptable. Cherimoyas are sold in some supermarkets as well as Asian and Latin markets. Their season runs from November through April.

Storing If not yet ripe, let cherimoyas ripen at cool room temperature out of direct sunlight. If ripe, eat the fruit or wrap it in plastic and refrigerate for up to 3 days.

Preparing Cherimoya is best eaten chilled with a spoon. Cut the fruit in half and scoop out the flesh. Discard the seeds. Unless eating immediately, sprinkle a little lemon or lime juice on the flesh to prevent browning. Serve with citrus fruits or heavy cream, or cube and add to fruit salads. Cherimoyas are never cooked. But their tender, fragrant, and flavorful flesh is sometimes puréed for use in refreshing tropical punches or fruit sauces or as an ingredient in frozen desserts.

CHERRY Even if life isn't always just a bowl of cherries, a bowl of cherries can make anybody's life a little sweeter. Perfectly ripe cherries are a nearly unrivaled treat. Their short season is anticipated by all but the most jaded eaters.

Cherries are related to other one-seeded stone fruits, called drupes, most closely to plums, but also to peaches and nectarines. Two primary types exist: sweet and sour (or tart). Sweet cherry varieties include the deep red, plump Bing, the bright red, late-blooming Lambert, and the light-colored Royal Ann. 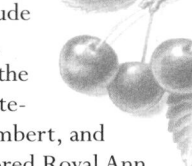 Sour cherries need to be cooked and are usually processed for canned pie filling, preserves, and juice.

Selecting Cherries are harvested when ripe; they do not ripen significantly off the tree. Their season runs from late May to very early August, peaking in June and early July. When buying sweet cherries, make sure they are large, plump, smooth, and dark colored for their variety (golden cherries such as Royal Anns are meant to be pale) and have firm stems. The darker the cherry, the sweeter its flavor. Avoid any that are pale colored (again, for their variety) and rock hard, which indicates immature fruit, or those that are wet, sticky,

Quick Tip

Cherry pits, which should not be eaten, have the flavor of almonds, which explains the fruit's affinity for dishes that include almonds and other nuts. A drop of almond extract added to cherry pie or cobbler filling or to cherry sauce enhances the cherry flavor.

bruised, excessively soft, or have shriveled stems, all signs of age. Cherries with the stems attached are desirable; once the stem is removed, the cherries spoil more rapidly.

Sour cherries are rarely sold fresh. If they are available, however, buy them following the same guidelines as for sweet cherries. Most taste too tart for pleasant eating out of hand, but they are good when sweetened for pies or preserves and other baking or cooking uses. Morello and Montmorency are two well-known varieties.

Quick Bite

Maraschino cherries are made from light-colored or white cherries such as Royal Anns or Rainiers, which are pitted and macerated in sugar syrup to preserve them. The cherries are then dyed red or green (unlike in the past, dyes used nowadays are considered safe) and packed in syrup. They are used as a garnish—the cherry on top of the ice cream sundae or in cocktails such as whiskey sours and old-fashioneds. Maraschino cherries are so named because they once were soaked in maraschino liqueur, a now-rare practice.

Both sweet and sour cherries are available pitted and canned, packed in water or syrup, or frozen. The latter generally have a better texture and taste than canned. Whenever you can, substitute fresh sweet or sour cherries for canned. A pound of fresh cherries can replace a 1-pound can of sour cherries. Once they have been pitted, the fresh cherries will yield the same 2 cups the can holds.

Storing Put fresh cherries in a plastic bag and refrigerate immediately. Eat them within 3 days. Canned cherries will keep for 1 year unopened in a cool, dark cupboard. Once opened, transfer the cherries to a covered glass, plastic, or ceramic container and refrigerate for up to 1 week.

Preparing If using fresh cherries in pies or the like, pit the fruit with a cherry pitter or small, sharp knife.

Pitting with a cherry pitter.

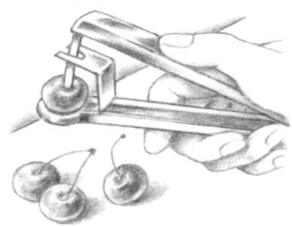

If the recipe calls for canned sour cherries and you wish to use fresh sweet cherries, reduce the amount of sugar and add a little lemon juice to taste. This works very well for cherry pie, cherry sauce for ice cream, or cherry topping for cheesecake.

CHERVIL See HERB.

CHESTNUT See NUT.

CHÈVRE Goat's milk cheese; see CHEESE for information.

CHICKEN Long gone are the days when Sunday dinner meant roast chicken. Everyone still loves a good roasted chicken, but modern cooks are just as likely to skin it, bone it, or cut it into parts, then bake, broil, braise, stir-fry, or grill it.

Chicken forms the perfect canvas for both sweet and spicy flavorings, marrying as successfully with apples, onions, or orange marmalade as with chiles and ginger or tomatoes, garlic, and wine. Its bones make a flavorful stock that can be used as a base for soups, sauces, and gravies.

Chicken Labeling Poultry can be labeled as "fresh" only if it has never been held at temperatures below 26°F. If chicken has been frozen and then thawed for sale, the label will say "previously frozen." Buy fresh chicken when possible. If given a choice between frozen and previously frozen, pick frozen, as chicken deteriorates quickly after thawing.

The terms *natural, free-range,* and *organic* are used to indicate a higher-quality chicken that also costs more in most cases. These terms have specific and different Food and Drug Administration (FDA) definitions and are not synonymous.

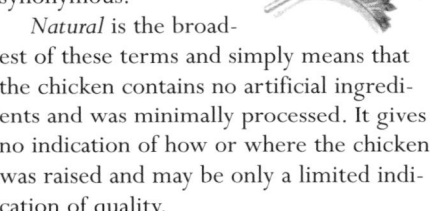

Natural is the broadest of these terms and simply means that the chicken contains no artificial ingredients and was minimally processed. It gives no indication of how or where the chicken was raised and may be only a limited indication of quality.

Free-range refers to a chicken that was allowed access to the outside. While this label is designed to invoke the image of a bird that has spent its time pecking and scratching in fresh air and developing meaty, leaner muscles, this is not always the case. Some free-range poultry is decidedly better quality than others, but it is important to judge for yourself rather than just following the label.

The final and most stringent category is *organic*. This means that the chicken producer has undergone a lengthy certification process to prove that the chickens have been raised in free-range conditions, without hormones or antibiotics, and on exclusively organic feed.

Before deciding to spend money for natural, free-range, or organic chicken, talk with the butcher or, if possible, a local chicken farmer at the farmers' market. Ask how the chicken was raised and what it was fed. This kind of knowledge is the best defense against buying mass-produced chicken that is misleadingly sold under the "free-range" or "natural" label.

Selecting Buy Grade A chicken, which is the grade most readily available to consumers. The bird should have even coloring, whether pale yellow or ivory. The color reflects the type of food the chicken was fed. Look for plump birds with well-defined breasts and legs. Press gently on the meat (through the plastic); it should be firm and resilient. Any visible fat should be white to light yellow. The skin should be unbroken, clean, and dry looking. Be sure to buy chicken before the sell-by date, which is a week after the bird was processed. If a chicken smells "off," you probably will be able to detect it even through plastic wrap. If you don't notice anything wrong at the store and the chicken smells bad when you open the package at home, return the poultry to the place where you bought it. If in doubt, do not eat it.

Storing Chicken is highly perishable and a potential haven for salmonella bacteria. Refrigerate raw chicken as soon as possible after purchase. Plan to cook chicken no more than 2 days after purchase, or else freeze it as soon as you get it home.

If you're planning to cook them soon, store chicken parts in the original packaging in the coldest part of the refrigerator, which is usually at the back of the bottom shelf or in a meat drawer. (A refrigerator thermometer will tell you for sure.) If the chicken is leaking, wrap the package in another layer of plastic, slip it into a plastic bag, or place it in a bowl or on a plate.

Chicken freezes well. Unwrap it from its original packaging and rinse the chicken under cool water. Remove any giblets and use within 24 hours. Pat the chicken dry and wrap in freezer-weight plastic or a zippered plastic freezer bag. Freeze for up to 6 months. Thaw the chicken in the refrigerator, which is the safest and surest way to do it. If time is a consideration, thaw plastic-wrapped chicken (or chicken parts) in a bowl of cool water, but tend it carefully and cook it as soon as it is thawed. Leaving thawed chicken at room temperature for any length of time is dangerous. You can also defrost chicken parts in the microwave on a low setting. Watch these carefully, however, to prevent them from cooking on the surface before they are completely thawed, and cook them immediately upon defrosting.

Preparing Trim the chicken or chicken parts of excess fat, skin (if desired), and tough gristle, if any. Wash it (inside the cavity as well, if preparing whole chicken) with cold running water and pat dry. Be sure to wash hands, utensils, and working surfaces in hot, soapy water after working with chicken.

Cutting up a whole chicken or boning a breast or thigh is not as difficult as you might think; see BONING and DISJOINTING. Reserve the bones and trimmings for making stock.

Many recipes call for browning the chicken as the first step. This gives the bird an appealing color, especially if it is going to be braised in liquid afterward. Chicken can also be sautéed, stir-fried, broiled, roasted, grilled, and used in stews, casseroles, and soups and to make stock.

Regardless of how you prepare chicken, be sure to cook it thoroughly. There are a few old-fashioned tests for determining when it is done: cook until the meat is no longer pink at the bone, the juices run clear when a thigh is pierced with a knife, or the breast meat is opaque throughout. The best way to determine doneness, however, is to insert an instant-read thermometer into the thickest part of the thigh, making sure it doesn't touch the bone.

Doneness Temperatures for Chicken	
Thigh	165° to 175°F
Breast	150° to 160°F*

Although these temperatures yield what many cooks feel are the optimum taste and texture for breast meat, a temperature of less than 160°F is lower than that suggested by the U.S. Food Safety and Inspection Service guidelines; see Chicken Safety, below, and DONENESS.

Chicken Safety It's important to handle chicken—and all poultry—safely. Raw chicken may harbor bacteria such as salmonella that can make a healthy adult very ill and may kill small children, elderly people, or anyone with a compromised immune system. Safe handling means:

- When preparing raw chicken, use a cutting board reserved only for flesh foods.
- Make sure no raw chicken or chicken juice comes in contact with other food. Wash the countertop, cutting board, knives and other utensils, and your hands with hot, soapy water immediately after working with chicken. Try to prepare the chicken before or after preparing other ingredients or dishes to avoid cross-contamination. See also FOOD SAFETY.
- Never serve marinade that was used for raw chicken without first bringing it to a boil and cooking it for at least 5 minutes to kill any bacteria.
- For more information about the doneness temperatures suggested by the U.S. Food Safety and Inspection Service, see DONENESS.
- Don't let raw or cooked birds sit at room temperature for more than 1 hour—or ½ hour in hot weather.
- Stuff whole birds right before cooking. After cooking, test the stuffing with a

C

thermometer; it should reach a temperature of 165°F. If it does not, transfer it to a baking dish and return it to the oven until the temperature is reached.

■ After the meal, remove the stuffing from the bird and store it separately in a tightly covered container in the refrigerator for no more than 2 days.

See also BONING; BUTTERFLYING; CARVING; CORNISH GAME HEN; DISJOINTING; GIBLETS; STOCK; TRUSSING; individual cooking methods.

Quick Tip

Whether it has been roasted, broiled, grilled, braised, stewed, or poached, chicken is one of the most versatile of leftovers. Use large slices of cooked chicken for sandwiches. Smaller scraps from a whole bird are ideal for tossing together with mayonnaise, thinly sliced celery, fresh herbs, and other embellishments such as nuts or raisins to make a chicken salad.

∼ Chicken Glossary ∼

Most chickens in the market weigh between 3 and 4 pounds. They are classified as broiler-fryers, a combination of what used to specify two different sizes of bird. These all-purpose birds can be broiled, fried, grilled, roasted, or, when on the large side, braised or stewed. While you can find the other chicken types listed here, they are not as readily available in supermarkets as they once were. If you want a specific size, you may need to ask a butcher for help. Weight and size are determined by age and are therefore an indication of tenderness—the smaller the bird, the more tender the meat.

POUSSIN The youngest chicken, weighing about 1 pound and also known as spring chicken. These tiny birds are tender and sweet tasting. They can be broiled, grilled, roasted, or sautéed. Substitute Cornish game hens.

BROILER Very young chicken weighing between 1 and 2¾ pounds. Broilers have fine-textured meat and delicate flavor. Excellent for broiling, grilling, roasting, or sautéing. Unfortunately, most chickens this size are sold to restaurants and are hard to find in the supermarket.

FRYER Very young chicken weighing from 1½ to 2¾ pounds. The parts from a fryer are small enough to cook all the way through during deep-frying before the skin becomes too crisp. Chickens are rarely sold as plain fryers anymore; instead they are sold as broiler-fryers and weigh up to 4 pounds.

BROILER-FRYER Young chicken weighing between 2¾ and 4 pounds. Its flavorful meat with good texture is recommended for broiling, frying, grilling, roasting, braising, and even stewing.

BROILER HEN Also called stewing chicken or fowl, this older bird weighs between 4 and 6 pounds and is recommended for stewing, braising, or making stock. The meat is full flavored but dry and benefits from these moist cooking methods.

ROASTER Chicken weighing between 3 and 5 pounds and with more meat than a broiler, which makes this tender bird ideal for roasting, although it can also be braised or stewed.

CAPON A plump chicken created by castrating a male bird, capons weigh between 5 and 8 pounds and are sweet, juicy, and great for roasting.

CHICKPEA See BEAN, DRIED.

CHICORY Members of this family of pleasantly bitter greens have a range of uses, from salads to braises to grilled side dishes. One is even made into a beverage. There is a good deal of name confusion, however, which includes Belgian endive, curly endive, escarole, frisée, and radicchio.
BELGIAN ENDIVE This chicory is grown in two steps. First, it is planted in a field and harvested, and the tops are cut off and thrown away.
The roots are then placed in a dark room for a few weeks, where they sprout and are care-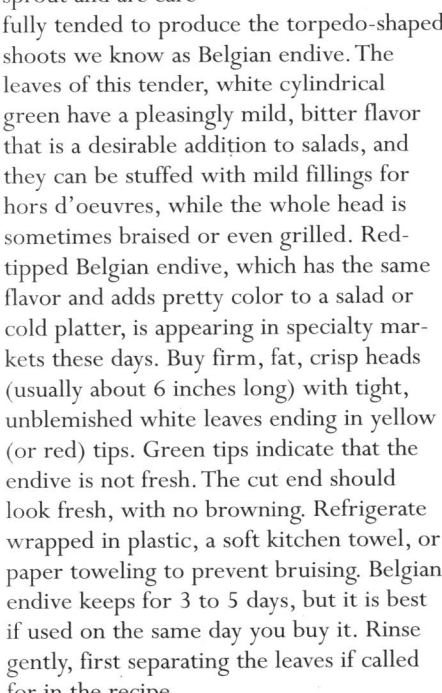fully tended to produce the torpedo-shaped shoots we know as Belgian endive. The leaves of this tender, white cylindrical green have a pleasingly mild, bitter flavor that is a desirable addition to salads, and they can be stuffed with mild fillings for hors d'oeuvres, while the whole head is sometimes braised or even grilled. Red-tipped Belgian endive, which has the same flavor and adds pretty color to a salad or cold platter, is appearing in specialty markets these days. Buy firm, fat, crisp heads (usually about 6 inches long) with tight, unblemished white leaves ending in yellow (or red) tips. Green tips indicate that the endive is not fresh. The cut end should look fresh, with no browning. Refrigerate wrapped in plastic, a soft kitchen towel, or paper toweling to prevent bruising. Belgian endive keeps for 3 to 5 days, but it is best if used on the same day you buy it. Rinse gently, first separating the leaves if called for in the recipe.
CURLY ENDIVE A close cousin of escarole (see below), this frilly, somewhat bitter

green is also known as chicory or curly chicory. It has narrow, spiky, finely curled leaves and a creamy white heart. It is used primarily in salads, tossed with olive oil and lemon juice. Available year-round; 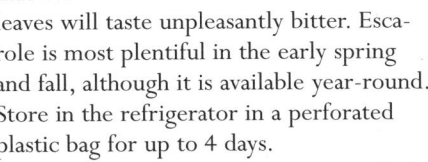select crisp heads with good color. Slip into a perforated plastic bag and refrigerate for up to 4 days.
ESCAROLE Also known as common chicory, broad chicory, or Batavian endive, escarole has loose, broad, green, tangy outer leaves, wide white stalks, and a yellow-green heart. The leaves can be chopped and mixed with other salad greens, cooked as a green, or added to soups or pasta sauces. Buy crisp, green heads with no browning. If too many of the leaves look thick or tough, pass on that head—those leaves will taste unpleasantly bitter. Escarole is most plentiful in the early spring and fall, although it is available year-round. Store in the refrigerator in a perforated plastic bag for up to 4 days.

Quick Bite

Since the late 18th century, certain types of chicory have been cultivated specifically for their large tap roots, which, when roasted, ground, and steeped in water, produce a dark brown, bitter beverage resembling coffee. Chicory is traditionally added to coffee in New Orleans to produce the familiar local brew.

FRISÉE French cooks have long used this flavorful green in salads—it is especially nice with pears and walnuts or as a bed for grilled chicken or fish. It is basically slightly immature curly endive, with smaller heads and a more delicate and tender leaf. Select and store in the same way. It is available year-round.

RADICCHIO A variety of chicory native to Italy and characterized by its variegated purplish red leaves and bitter taste. The sturdy raw leaves hold up

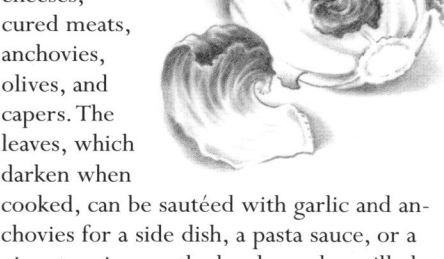

well in a salad, and their assertive flavor is nicely matched with cheeses, cured meats, anchovies, olives, and capers. The leaves, which darken when cooked, can be sautéed with garlic and anchovies for a side dish, a pasta sauce, or a pizza topping, or the heads can be grilled. Winter through early spring is the peak season for radicchio, although it is available most of the year in many locales. Look for

---

Quick Tip

Salads are rarely made with chicories alone. They would taste far too bitter, unless wilted with a warm dressing. Try mixing the bitter greens with milder butterhead varieties, such as Bibb or Boston, or oakleaf. Chicories are also good in salads containing nuts and fruits.

---

a head with a white core that is firm and has no holes or blemishes. Avoid those with moist leaves. Store in the refrigerator in a perforated plastic bag for up to 1 week.

See also GREENS, SALAD.

CHILE See page 114.

CHILE OIL Used extensively in Asian cooking and now finding its way into Western kitchens, chile oil is a red-hued vegetable oil whose color and heat are derived from steeping hot red chiles in oil. Drizzle a small amount in stir-fries and sautés to add a bit of fire.

Selecting Buy chile oil in small quantities from a store with good turnover. Asian markets and specialty-food stores are the best sources.

Storing Store at room temperature in a cool, dry cupboard for up to 4 months. Chile oil will keep for up to 8 months in the refrigerator, but like all oils, it will turn cloudy when chilled.

CHILE PASTE A very hot condiment made of chopped or ground chiles and (usually) vinegar and salt, used extensively throughout Southeast Asia, China, and Korea. Depending on the place of origin, different seasonings, such as garlic, ginger, soybeans, sesame oil, and even sugar, are added. Use it with caution. There are numerous brands and types for sale in Asian markets, which may be labeled "chile paste" or "chile sauce." (These should not be confused with the relatively benign commercial American product called chile sauce, a tomato-based sauce that is only slightly spicier than ketchup and is commonly used to make cocktail sauce to serve with shrimp and other seafood.)

Selecting Look for chile paste in Asian markets and specialty-food shops. Try several kinds to find what you like best. Those labeled chile-garlic sauce, a condiment with roots in Vietnam, are usually the hottest. Other pastes, which may include soy oil, are usually a little milder.

Storing Once opened, chile paste should be stored in the refrigerator, where it will keep for up to 1 year.

CHILI A thick, robust stew native to the American Southwest and also beloved elsewhere, seasoned with fresh or dried chiles, dried chile powder, or the spice blend known as chili powder. Traditional chilis may feature simply chiles and small pieces of pork or beef; other popular embellishments include tomatoes, herbs, pinto beans or black beans, and a little cornmeal as a thickener. Chili cook-offs are widespread, with devotees developing secret recipes based on rare chile types or blends and a wide range of other seasonings, meats, poultry, or game.

See also CHILE; CHILI POWDER.

CHILI POWDER A commercial spice blend that usually combines dried chiles, cumin, oregano, garlic, cloves, and coriander. It is used to season chili, as well as any other dishes that benefit from its distinctive, slightly spicy flavor, such as eggs, cheese dishes, and even tuna salad.

Some cooks prefer to season their pots of chili with pure ancho chile powder, claiming it provides excellent flavor and a good level of heat.

Selecting Most supermarkets will carry one or two standard brands of chili powder in jars or packets in the seasonings section. Look in specialty-food stores for chili seasoning mixes from smaller, regional labels, which may offer the more authentic flavor some chili aficionados are seeking.

Storing Store both types of powder in tightly capped containers in a cool, dry cupboard for up to 6 months.

CHILLING The cooling of food to below room temperature but above freezing is known as chilling. Recipes often instruct the cook to chill such items as custards, salads, gelatin-based dishes, fruit soups and desserts, and pâtés and terrines before serving.

Because food is most vulnerable to bacteria growth between the temperatures of 40°F and 140°F, chilling food to below 40°F keeps it safer. While it's a good idea to let food cool down before you put it in the refrigerator (otherwise it will heat up the entire refrigerator), don't let it sit at room temperature for more than 2 hours at most. Thick stews and soups, particularly dishes like chili, are the most difficult to cool down since they hold heat so effectively. Stirring foods as they cool redistributes the heat and makes them cool faster. Some recipes—in particular those for meat stocks—instruct you to set the pot in ice water, lowering the temperature of the food quickly before refrigerating.

C

Quick Tip

Divide large pots of food into smaller, shallower containers to expedite chilling.

HOW TO *Chill Food*

1. Let hot food cool slightly on the kitchen counter or carefully plunge the pot or saucepan into an ice-water bath. For the bath, put a stopper in the sink drain and fill the sink with cold water and ice cubes. Be careful not to swamp the food with water. Stir the food occasionally to expedite cooling.

2. As soon as it is no longer hot—but not completely cool, either—transfer the food to the coolest section of the refrigerator, usually the back of the bottom shelf. Do not cover.

3. When it is cold, cover it, and keep it refrigerated until ready to use.

See also COOLING.

Chile

From Sumatran saté to Sichuan stir-fry, Kashmiri red korma to Angolan *piri-piri* sauce, Mexican chiles rellenos to Jamaican jerk seasoning, chiles deliver heat, add color, and deepen the flavor of dishes around the globe.

Familiar sights to travelers from Luong Prabang to Lima, Biarritz to Bangkok are strings of bright red chiles drying in the summer sun.

Over centuries of domestication, hundreds of chile varieties have been developed. Requiring hot summers, they grow well in tropical areas. Diverse and versatile, chiles can be large or tiny, mild or fiery, sprinkled as a seasoning or cooked as a vegetable. They are left whole for stuffing, sliced for pickling, diced into salsa, puréed into sauces, dried and roasted for smoky flavor, and ground finely for seasoning. Hot sauces and salsas have helped to make chiles immensely popular.

Chile Varieties Many chile varieties, both fresh and dried, are widely available. Among the most popular are the following:

ANAHEIM A mild fresh green chile measuring 6 to 10 inches long. Anaheims are classically used for chiles rellenos. Anaheims have a tough skin and are often roasted or charred to remove the skin before using. They also are the chiles you find cooked and chopped in cans labeled "green chiles." Use them in place of poblanos. When dried, Anaheims, which turn a deep burgundy, are typically called California chiles.

ANCHO A mild, dark reddish brown or brick red, squat-looking dried poblano chile. About 4 inches long, anchos can pack a bit of heat along with their natural sweetness. Ancho chile powder is available in Latin markets and is generally considered to make the best pure ground chili powder. Use California chiles (see Anaheim, above) or mulato chiles when anchos are not available.

ÁRBOL About 3 inches long, narrow, and very hot. These chiles are bright orange when fresh and red to orange when dried.

BANANA Long yellow fresh chile, 5 to 6 inches, with a mild flavor. When allowed to mature, these turn red.

CASCABEL Globe-shaped, deep red, medium-hot dried chile usually no more than $1\frac{1}{2}$ inches in diameter. Its toasted flavor is appreciated in sauces and soups.

CAYENNE A tapered, bright red chile, about 3 inches long, pleasingly hot and smoky tasting. Most of the cayenne chile crop is ground into the familiar red powder.

CHIPOTLE A dried and smoked jalapeño chile, with lots of flavor and lots of heat. These dark brown chiles are about 3 inches long and may be bought either dried or in cans or jars, packed in an oniony tomato mixture called adobo sauce.

C

FRESNO A mild-to-hot fresh chile about 3 inches long. Usually red, but sometimes a less ripe one may be yellow or green. The red ones are sometimes mistaken for jalapeños.

GUAJILLO Narrow, dark red dried chile with a lot of heat and bold flavor. The guajillo is 5 to 6 inches long and resembles the New Mexico chile. When fresh, it is called the *mirasol* and is difficult to find outside of Mexico. The guajillo is interchangeable with the dried árbol.

HABANERO Some consider this small (1½ to 2 inches long) fresh chile the hottest—and certainly its heat exceeds those of virtually all those commercially available—but it also has a lovely citrusy bouquet and flavor. Closely related to Scotch bonnets, they are most often green, but can also be red or orange.

HUNGARIAN CHERRY PEPPER A small, sweet, bright red, round chile measuring about 2 inches or less in diameter. This pleasant-tasting chile does not pack much punch and often is pickled.

JALAPEÑO Ranging from mildly hot to fiery, the fleshy jalapeño is usually green but can also be red. Jalapeños measure from 2 to 4 inches long and are widely cultivated and available in most of the world. Jalapeños are also sold canned, whole or sliced, and pickled. Use in place of any hot chile—serranos or Thai in particular. Substitute 2 or 3 jalapeños for 1 habanero or Scotch bonnet.

MULATO Sweet mild-to-hot dried chile that is so dark it almost looks black; it is 5 to 6 inches long. Similar in taste and heat to the ancho but with sweet undertones.

NEW MEXICO Large red or green fresh chile (6 to 8 inches long) with moderate-to-hot bite. Also available dried. New Mexicos can be substituted for guajillos and are at their best when roasted.

PASILLA Also called *chile negro*. Dark, narrow, and wrinkled, this 6-inch-long dried chile is sweet and hot. A good substitute for ancho.

PEQUÍN A very small, very hot fresh or dried chile, measuring no more than ½ inch across, which may be round or tapered. This is not a variety of chile but instead a term for any tiny, hot chile and may be any one of a number of different kinds.

POBLANO Large and fairly mild, the dark green fresh poblano is about 5 inches long and has broad shoulders. Poblanos have a nutty flavor and are often stuffed for chiles rellenos. They usually should be roasted and peeled. Substitute Anaheims for poblanos if necessary. When dried, these are called ancho chiles.

SCOTCH BONNET Smaller than the habanero, only 1 to 1½ inches long, the Scotch bonnet is extremely hot. The little round fresh chiles are green, yellow, orange, or red. Use Scotch bonnets interchangeably with habaneros or 3 or 4 jalapeños.

SERRANO Similar to jalapeños in heat intensity, the serrano is sleeker and tends to have more consistent heat. About 2 inches long, serranos may be green or red and can be used in place

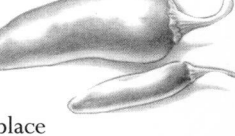

continued

Chile, continued

of jalapeños in any recipe. Although they are most often available fresh, occasionally you may find dried serrano chiles, which are called *serranos secos*. They are hot.

THAI Small, thin green or red chiles, usually only about 1 inch long. Also known as bird chiles. Thai chiles are very hot.

Selecting It is not always necessary to use the exact chile called for in a recipe. In fact, many recipes simply use phrases such as "small hot chiles" or "hot red chiles," rather than identify a specific type. Choose

Quick Tip

To impart just a little of a chile's warmth to a dish, sauté a fresh or dried pepper in the cooking oil and then remove it before adding other ingredients.

a chile based on how it is described in a recipe, what's available in your local market or on hand in your pantry, and your own taste buds.

When buying fresh chiles, select firm, bright chiles that are free of blemishes, moldy stems, soft spots, or wrinkling. In general, the smaller and more pointed the chile, the hotter it is. If you want heat, select small, green, pointed chiles, such as serranos or jalapeños. Small red chiles pack a punch, too, so don't go by color alone. Larger or rounder chiles, such as Anaheim or poblano, tend to be milder. But don't take this as gospel: although habaneros and Scotch bonnets are both relatively broad-shouldered chiles with blunt tips, they are considered among the hottest varieties known to humankind.

In the Southwest, some of the chile harvest is also frozen. Check in markets of the region, in mail-order catalogs of regional foods, or on the Internet. They make excellent replacements for fresh chiles.

When buying dried chiles, look for flexible pods rather than brittle ones. They will be wrinkled and perhaps a little twisted, but should have good, uniform color. Dried chiles may be sold loose or packaged in plastic or cellophane. They also may be woven into colorful, attractive wreaths and sprays. These are wonderful while fresh, but beware of letting them stay too long on the kitchen wall, as the heat of the room will dry them out and they will collect dust and possibly harbor insects.

Chiles are at their peak in late summer to early fall. Visit Asian and Latin American markets for specialty chiles, and look for whole dried chiles and canned chiles in sauce at Mexican markets and in the ethnic-foods aisle in major grocery stores. Ground cayenne and chile flakes, also known as red pepper flakes, appear in the spice section of supermarkets, while pickled peppers and hot sauces are in the condiment aisle.

Storing If you plan to use fresh chiles within 2 days of purchase, you can keep them at room temperature. For storage of up to 1 week, refrigerate them in perforated plastic bags to prevent molding. Alternatively, wrap the chiles first in a paper bag or paper towel to absorb excess moisture, then place them in a plastic bag. Refrigerate for 1 week or freeze for 6 months. Although dried chiles can be hung in the corner of your kitchen, they will fare better if stored in an airtight container away from light and moisture. Keep ground chiles in a cool, dry place for no longer than 6 months.

Quick Tip

If you are not sure about a chile's heat level, add a little at a time; you can always add more. If preparing a dish in advance, remember that the heat chiles impart to a dish increases with time.

Preparing The compound that gives chiles their heat, known as capsaicin, is concentrated in the white membranes, or ribs, inside the chile. The heat is transferred from these membranes to the attached seeds. To lessen the heat of a chile, trim off the membrane and scrape away the seeds.

Caution!

Wear gloves when working with hot chiles to prevent burns to your fingers. The heat of chiles can linger for hours on your skin, so thoroughly wash your hands, the cutting board, and the knife with hot, soapy water as soon as you have finished working with them. Avoid touching your face, especially your eyes and lips, or other sensitive areas before you complete this thorough washing process.

HOW TO *Toast Dried Chiles*

Dried chiles are toasted in Mexican and other cuisines to make them flexible and intensify their flavor. This step is especially necessary if the chiles are dried out and brittle. Toasted chiles are either ground dry or soaked and ground.

1. Place the chiles on a griddle or in a heavy cast-iron frying pan over medium heat.
2. Turn the chiles frequently with tongs until they are fragrant and lightly toasted.
3. Transfer to a plate to cool.

HOW TO *Roast and Peel Fresh Chiles*

1. Preheat the broiler.
2. Lay whole chiles on an aluminum foil—lined broiler pan and broil about 6 inches from the heat, turning as needed, until the skin is blistered and charred black on all sides, 10 to 15 minutes. Watch the chiles carefully to avoid burning their flesh.
3. Once the skin is blackened and puffy, transfer the chiles to a paper bag and close loosely. This allows the chiles to steam as they cool and helps the skins to loosen.

4. When cool, peel or rub away the charred skin. Do not worry if a little stays on the flesh. Don't rinse the chiles under running water, or you will wash away flavor.

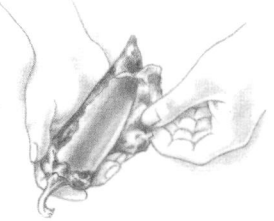

5. Lay the chiles on a cutting board. Using a small, sharp knife, slit each pepper lengthwise.

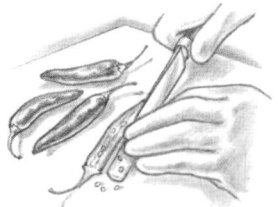

Some liquid will run out at this stage, so have paper towels handy. Open the chile and spread it on the cutting board.

6. Cut around the stem end, then remove the stem, seeds, and membrane.

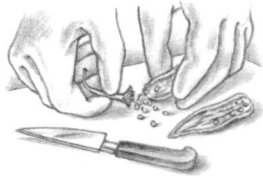

Quick Tip

If your mouth is aflame from eating chiles, drink milk or eat a slice of bread or a mouthful of cooked rice. Dairy products and starches will help neutralize the burning sensation.

See also BELL PEPPER; PIMIENTO.

CHINESE LONG BEAN See BEAN, FRESH.

CHINESE PARSLEY Another name for cilantro; see HERB.

CHINESE WHITE CABBAGE See BOK CHOY.

CHINOIS See STRAINER.

CHIPOTLE See CHILE.

CHIVE See HERB.

CHOCOLATE For many, it is the ultimate indulgence of choice. Never mind Champagne and caviar; bring on the rich, elegant Belgian chocolate or, in a pinch, the mass-produced chocolate bar.

We all know how wonderful it is, but defining chocolate is elusive. Chocolate is an ingredient, a flavor, a candy. It begins with cocoa beans, originally harvested in Central America but now cultivated in equatorial regions around the world. The beans are fermented, roasted, shelled, and crushed into bits called nibs. The nibs, which are more than 50 percent cocoa butter, the fat of chocolate, are ground and compressed into a mass called chocolate liquor—which with only a little further refining becomes unsweetened chocolate. Or, depending on the amount of sugar added, the chocolate liquor becomes bittersweet, semisweet, or sweet chocolate, all called dark chocolate. The addition of milk solids results in milk chocolate. When about three-fourths of the cocoa butter is removed and the remaining chocolate liquor is pulverized into powder, it becomes cocoa powder.

Much like coffee, chocolate manufacturing starts with beans or blends of beans. How the beans are harvested and fermented, how they are roasted, and then how the chocolate liquor is processed and how much extra cocoa butter is added (for smoothness and richness) all contribute to the end product. This explains why some chocolates are quite inexpensive, while others are remarkably pricey.

From unsweetened to the finest bittersweet, all chocolate has culinary uses. Because sugar and fat content vary from one variety to another, it is unadvisable to substitute one type of chocolate for another in a recipe. Take the time to find the right chocolate to suit your needs.

Selecting Buy chocolate from a store with good turnover. The packaging should be clean and neat. Avoid any that looks old, shopworn, or dusty. Acceptable baking and cooking chocolate is sold in supermarkets, while specialty shops sell better, more expensive, often imported brands. Better chocolate often produces a better baked good or candy. But for many chocolate aficionados, "better" is a matter of personal taste and experimentation. Most of all, buy the kind you like. Just make sure it's the right type of chocolate (unsweetened, bittersweet, cocoa powder, and so on).

Storing Store chocolate, well wrapped in aluminum foil and plastic wrap, at cool room temperature. Do not keep chocolate, especially milk and white chocolates, near foods with strong odors or flavors. If you refrigerate or freeze chocolate, wrap it very carefully in a double layer of plastic (freezer weight for the freezer) and allow it to come to room temperature before unwrapping it. When properly stored, dark chocolate keeps for up to 1 year; milk and white chocolates keep for up to 8 months.

Preparing Chocolate is nearly always melted for cooking and baking purposes. While this can be done over direct heat, you'll risk burning the chocolate. Better to do it in a double boiler or a microwave.

Chop the chocolate coarsely before melting it to speed the process. Do this carefully on a cutting board, using a large knife.

Chopping chocolate.

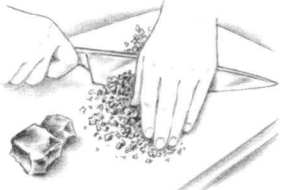

HOW TO *Melt Chocolate on the Stove Top*

1. Chop the chocolate into large chunks and transfer it to the top pan of a double boiler.
2. Set the top pan of the double boiler over barely simmering water in the bottom pan. Make sure the water does not touch the bottom of the pan holding the chocolate. Do not let the water boil. Any moisture or steam that comes in contact with the chocolate could cause it to seize, or stiffen.
3. As it melts, stir the chocolate every now and then with a wooden spoon. When the chocolate is liquefied, remove the top of the double boiler from the bottom and set aside to cool slightly, unless otherwise instructed in a recipe. Do not cover the chocolate as it cools.

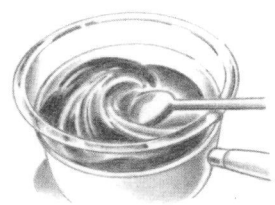

HOW TO *Melt Chocolate in a Microwave Oven*

1. Chop the chocolate into large chunks and transfer it to a microwave-safe dish.
2. Heat the chocolate on Medium (50 percent power) and check it after the first minute.
3. Keep checking it every 30 or 40 seconds to prevent scorching.
4. When the chocolate looks shiny and softened, remove it from the microwave. It will not melt completely in the microwave but will become smooth and liquid upon stirring.

HOW TO *Make Chocolate Curls*

1. Slightly soften a 3- to 4-inch chunk of chocolate in the microwave oven on Medium (50 percent power). Use a vegetable peeler to pare pretty, delicate curls from the softened chocolate. Refrigerate the curls until ready to use.

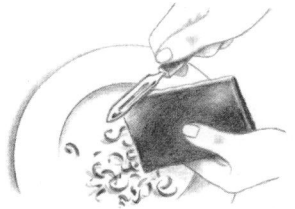

HOW TO *Make Chocolate Shavings*

1. Use a vegetable peeler or knife to shave flat, thin shavings from a room-temperature block of chocolate.

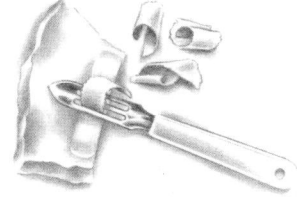

What Is Tempering? When cocoa butter crystals in chocolate harden into a stable crystalline pattern, the chocolate is said to be in temper. All chocolate leaves the manufacturer in temper, but when

C

stored incorrectly, it may go out of temper. When melted, it goes out of temper, too. A process called tempering restabilizes the crystals, so that when the chocolate cools and rehardens, it is smooth and glossy and breaks with a satisfying snap. When untempered chocolate cools, it is dull, grainy, and may even remain soft or sticky.

Tempering is done by heating and cooling the chocolate to particular temperatures. Different chocolates require different temperatures. Chocolate that is to be used in cakes, cookies, brownies, and mousses does not need to be tempered. Candy makers, however, must temper chocolate for dipping or enrobing.

Quick Tip

To use chocolate for dipping without tempering it, melt the chocolate with 2 teaspoons of vegetable shortening for every 8 ounces of chocolate. The shortening will keep the chocolate looking shiny and smooth after it cools.

Chocolate Blues Got a problem with your chocolate? You can find the simple explanation here.

CHOCOLATE LOOKS PALE, POWDERY, AND BLOTCHY. The appearance, called bloom, is the result of storage at too warm a temperature or in too humid an environment. The chocolate can still be used; the flavor and texture are only slightly altered.

MELTED CHOCOLATE IS HARD, STIFF, AND LUMPY. Chocolate has seized, or come into contact with a bit of moisture during melting and stiffened up. To salvage it, remove from the heat and work in a bit of water, a tablespoon at a time. This restored chocolate will be smooth and shiny and fine for use in icings and fillings, but will not work in recipes where the chocolate must set up, such as for candies. See SEIZING for more information.

Chocolate Glossary

many kinds of chocolate are created by adding ingredients such as sugar or milk to chocolate liquor. Some general variations and additions are described below.

BAKING CHOCOLATE See Unsweetened Chocolate, below.

BITTER CHOCOLATE See Unsweetened Chocolate, below.

BITTERSWEET CHOCOLATE Made from chocolate liquor sweetened with sugar and blended with additional cocoa butter. This chocolate is at least 35 percent chocolate liquor, with sugar making up about 40 percent of its weight. In general, European dark chocolates are called bittersweet, while American dark chocolates are called semisweet. For everything but the most specialized confectionery, the two can be used interchangeably in baked goods, frostings, sauces, and candies. Bittersweet chocolate also has devoted fans who eat it right out of the wrapper.

CHOCOLATE CHIPS These small droplets of semisweet, milk, or white chocolate let you incorporate the confection evenly into batters or doughs, of which a favorite example is chocolate chip cookies. Although their slightly lower cocoa butter content helps them keep their shape when baked, chocolate chips also melt easily and evenly, eliminating the need to chop blocks or bars of chocolate for melting.

Chocolate Glossary, continued

COCOA POWDER Made by removing nearly all the cocoa butter from chocolate liquor and then grinding it to an unsweetened powder. While less fatty than other chocolate, it still contains about 22 percent cocoa butter. Do not confuse this unsweetened powder with sweetened cocoa drink mixes.

Alkalized, or Dutch-processed, cocoa powder is treated with an alkali to make it milder and more soluble than nonalkalized cocoa powder. Nonalkalized or natural cocoa powder is lighter in color but bolder in flavor than the alkalized powder. Both types of cocoa powder have their roles in baking and cooking, and one is not better than the other. Nonalkalized cocoa powder is always used for devil's food cake, because when the mildly acidic cocoa powder reacts with the baking soda in the recipe it gives the cake crumb its characteristic reddish hue. Use the kind of cocoa powder specified in the recipe. If none is specified, use either.

COUVERTURE CHOCOLATE High-quality dark chocolate used for specialty candy making. Because of its relatively high percentage of cocoa butter, it melts smoothly, making it easier for enrobing, dipping, and molding chocolate. When properly tempered and cooled, it forms a thin, glossy shell. You will find couverture chocolate in some specialty-food shops and in mail-order catalogs.

DARK CHOCOLATE A term to describe any sweetened chocolate without milk solids, usually referring to bittersweet and semisweet chocolates.

MILK CHOCOLATE This familiar chocolate contains milk solids, cocoa butter, and sugar. Milk chocolate is most often eaten out of hand in the form of a candy bar, although it appears in recipes from time to time. It should not be substituted for bittersweet or semisweet chocolate, except in the form of chips for chocolate chip cookies.

PLAIN CHOCOLATE In the United States, the term *plain chocolate* refers to unsweetened chocolate, while in Great Britain the term commonly refers to bittersweet chocolate. See Unsweetened Chocolate, below.

SEMISWEET CHOCOLATE This dark chocolate is at least 35 percent chocolate liquor. Semisweet chocolate is what Europeans call bittersweet; the terms are interchangeable.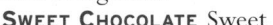

SWEET CHOCOLATE Sweet chocolate is dark chocolate that is sweeter than semisweet but is not milk chocolate. It is an ingredient rarely called for in recipes, except for German chocolate cake, named for the chocolate's inventor.

UNSWEETENED CHOCOLATE Chocolate liquor that is refined but not sweetened. Also called baking, plain, or bitter chocolate. This product is used only for baking and cooking—never for eating out of hand.

WHITE CHOCOLATE A mixture of cocoa butter, sugar, and milk solids but no chocolate liquor. Some manufacturers market a product called confectionery coating, which is like white chocolate but contains vegetable fat instead of cocoa butter and is less expensive.

C

CHOPPING Cutting food into irregular pieces that are small enough that they require no further cutting at the table, or are easy to mix or otherwise work with. *Chopping* is a general term; some more specific ways of cutting include dicing, cubing, julienning, and mincing. See the Chopping Glossary, below.

HOW TO *Chop*

Chopping is a common kitchen chore. For many chopping tasks, a knife is used in a specific way for efficiency.

1. Make sure that any large pieces are roughly cut into manageable pieces and that herbs—thick stems removed and discarded—are piled into a neat, fairly compact mass.
2. Grip the knife handle close to the blade, extending your thumb along the side of the blade if you wish, and rest the fingertips of your other hand on top of the knife's tip to keep it in contact with the cutting board.
3. Move the knife heel up and down rhythmically, trying not to lift the tip from the board.

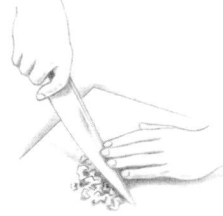

4. Use a graceful, rolling motion, pushing the knife down and forward, rather than jerking the knife straight up and down.

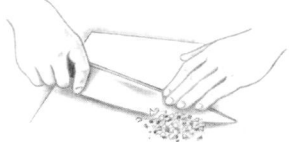

5. As the mass of food is chopped smaller, use the knife occasionally to gather the food again into tight, mounded piles. Try not to chop too much at a time, or it will spill off the board.

To chop carrots, peppers, onions, or other larger vegetables coarsely, grip the knife handle as described above and with the other hand hold the item being chopped. While keeping the tip of the knife on the board, lift the heel of the knife and cut down through the food in a smooth, even stroke. Adjust the position of the food as you cut, sliding it closer to the blade of the knife, while being careful to keep your fingertips well away from the cutting edge.

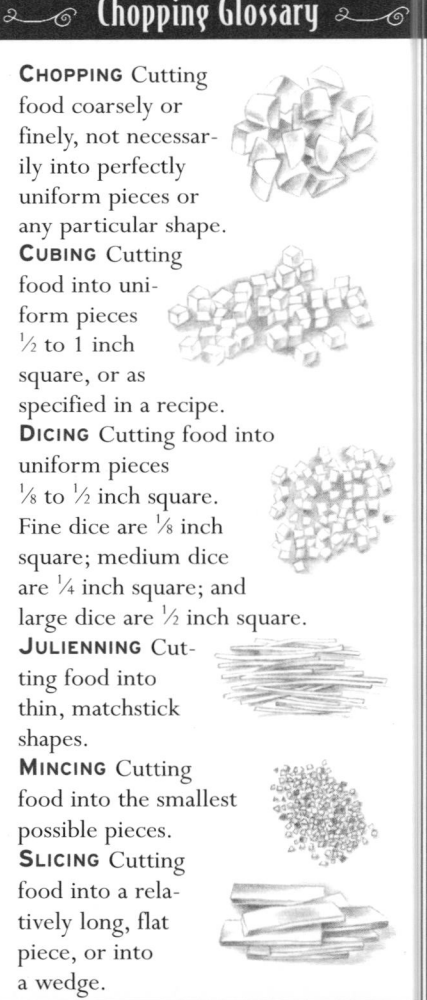

Chopping Glossary

CHOPPING Cutting food coarsely or finely, not necessarily into perfectly uniform pieces or any particular shape.

CUBING Cutting food into uniform pieces ½ to 1 inch square, or as specified in a recipe.

DICING Cutting food into uniform pieces ⅛ to ½ inch square. Fine dice are ⅛ inch square; medium dice are ¼ inch square; and large dice are ½ inch square.

JULIENNING Cutting food into thin, matchstick shapes.

MINCING Cutting food into the smallest possible pieces.

SLICING Cutting food into a relatively long, flat piece, or into a wedge.

Heavy knives and cleavers are the most common tools for chopping. Although the food processor makes quick work of sizable amounts of ingredients, it generally does not offer the kind of precision required when certain recipes call for food to be cut into uniform cubes or dice. In such cases, a chef's knife usually works best.

Cutting boards and sharp knives facilitate chopping. Cutting boards provide traction so that food will not slip away as you work. Dull knives are actually more dangerous than sharp ones, as you have to work harder, pressing the knife into the food, and there is more chance it will slip. The Italian mezzaluna (a curved blade with a wooden handle at each end) can also make quick work of chopping tasks.

See also CUBING; CUTTING BOARD; DICING; KNIFE; MINCING; SLICING.

CHOPSTICKS Arguably the most indispensable tool in both the Asian kitchen and dining room, chopsticks make perfect sense when eating dishes such as stir-fries in which the food is cut into bite-sized pieces before cooking. Chopsticks are held in one hand, between the thumb and forefinger. The bottom stick is held stationary, while the top one is moved up and down by the forefinger to grasp the food in a pincerlike grip. Chopsticks are also used for scooping rice and noodles into the mouth from a bowl held close to the face. Long chopsticks, useful in the kitchen for stir-frying and deep-frying and at the table for serving, are available in Asian markets.

Using chopsticks.

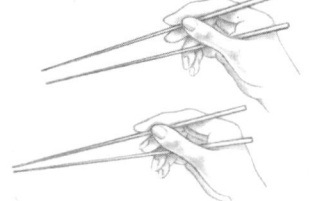

CHRISTOPHINE See CHAYOTE.

CHUTNEY A condiment that originated in India but is now made in a number of countries, chutney comes in countless styles, offering taste sensations ranging from sweet, hot, and tart to bitter. Most commonly served alongside curries and other savory dishes, chutneys may be raw or cooked mixtures of fruits or herbs, and usually also include vinegar, sugar, chiles, and spices. They may be used to cool the mouth when eating spicy foods or to add punch to milder ones. Some are thin enough to serve as dips, while others are chunky and thick and can be spread on bread or crackers or spooned onto a plate. Chutney can also be stirred into tuna or chicken salad for a flavor boost.

Selecting Most supermarkets carry the classic mango chutney called Major Grey's and may have some others, too. For a wider variety, look for bottled chutneys at Indian or Pakistani markets or specialty shops. Some of these markets may sell their own freshly prepared chutneys as well.

Storing Bottled chutneys, like jams and similar preserves, will keep unopened for up to 1 year in a cool, dark cupboard. Once opened, they will last 3 months or longer in the refrigerator. Fresh chutneys containing sugar will keep for up to 1 week in the refrigerator. Most others will keep for up to 2 days in the refrigerator.

Quick Bite

The name *chutney* derives from the Sanskrit word *chatni,* "for licking."

CILANTRO See HERB.

CINNAMON See SPICE.

CITRUS See individual fruits; ZESTING.

CLAM The clam is one of the most versatile members of the shellfish family. While clams are most often steamed, tender hard-shelled clams can be eaten raw, like oysters, with a squeeze of lemon juice and perhaps a dab of cocktail sauce. Clams are also terrific tossed with pasta in cream or tomato sauce, stuffed, and in the classic rice-based dish from Spain called paella. They also turn up in seafood stews, dips, and other dishes that benefit from their fresh, clean, sweet flavor. Clam chowder, whether white (milk or cream based) or red (tomato based), is a classic soup along the Atlantic coast. Deep-fried clams are another Eastern seaboard classic.

In addition to belonging to the broad category of shellfish, clams are classified as mollusks, along with abalone, scallops, mussels, and oysters. They are also bivalves, which is a general term referring to any creature with a soft body enclosed between two hinged shells.

Clams are either hard shelled or soft shelled, and different varieties are found in the Atlantic and the Pacific. Atlantic hard-shelled clams are called quahogs and come in various sizes, from small little-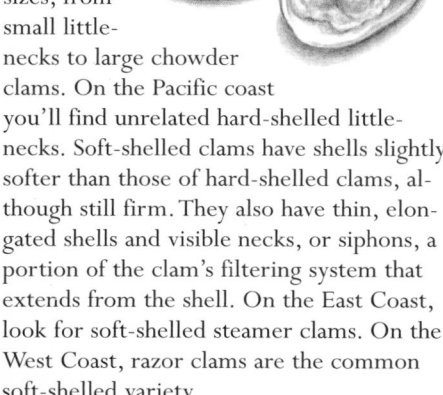necks to large chowder clams. On the Pacific coast you'll find unrelated hard-shelled littlenecks. Soft-shelled clams have shells slightly softer than those of hard-shelled clams, although still firm. They also have thin, elongated shells and visible necks, or siphons, a portion of the clam's filtering system that extends from the shell. On the East Coast, look for soft-shelled steamer clams. On the West Coast, razor clams are the common soft-shelled variety.

Selecting Buy the freshest clams you can find from a reputable fish merchant. They are sold live in the shell or freshly shucked and packed in pint and quart containers that usually contain clam liquor (or liquid), too. Hard-shelled quahog clams should have firm, finely textured gray shells with no yellowing; other hard-shelled clams should have even-colored, firm shells. The clams

Quick Bite

Soft-shelled clams are known as steamers on the East Coast, due to a simple and favorite way of preparing them. The clams are steamed open, and the steaming liquid is served with the clams, along with melted butter.

should not be open—if one gapes a little, prod it gently. If it does not close immediately, do not buy it. An open shell is the sign of a dead clam. Shucked hard-shelled clams should be plump and moist with clear liquor and a fresh and briny aroma.

Soft-shelled clams should be oval and evenly colored, with a neck, or siphon, protruding from the shell. To check for freshness, tap the neck. It should pull back toward the shell. The shells will not close as tightly as those of hard-shelled clams.

If you cannot find good fresh clams, you may be able to substitute frozen or canned ones. They will provide good flavor in pasta sauces, clam dips, and seafood broths but will not be as plump and juicy, so don't try them in paella or fried clams. Quick-frozen clams, available in some fish markets, are your best bet after fresh clams. Bottled clam juice, usually shelved near the canned seafood in supermarkets, can be substituted for fish stock or broth in recipes.

Storing Fresh clams in the shell should not be suffocated by being enclosed in a plastic bag or submerged in water. Instead, lay them on a flat tray or in a shallow bowl, cover them with a damp cloth, and refrigerate. Or put them in a mesh bag in a large bowl and refrigerate. Serve them the same day you buy them for the best flavor and texture, and certainly within 2 days.

Ready-shucked clams will also keep in the refrigerator for up to 2 days, although they are best eaten as soon after purchase as possible. Keep them in a tightly lidded container and push them to the back of the refrigerator where it is coldest.

Store canned clams in a cool, dark cupboard for up to 1 year and use them as soon as they are opened. If you can't use them immediately, transfer them to a plastic or glass container with a lid and refrigerate for no more than 2 days. Keep frozen clams in the freezer until ready to use, and use within 1 month of purchase.

Preparing Check over clams for any open shells. If their shells do not quickly shut tight after prodding, discard them.

Scrub clam shells well under running water with a soft-bristled brush to get rid of sand and grit. Soft-shelled clams, because of their slightly gaping shells, tend to be sandier than hard-shelled.

Scrubbing clams.

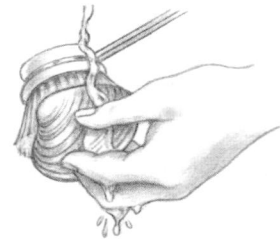

Clams may be cooked in the shell, which will open as they cook, or a recipe may require you first to shuck them, removing them from their shells. Opening hard-shelled clams calls for some dexterity, but the meat is easy to free from the open shell by scooping the knife around the perimeter. Briefly steaming clams to open them is easier than shucking them before cooking.

HOW TO *Purge Clams*

The traditional method of cleaning clams includes the step of soaking them in salt water to encourage them to purge any sand caught in their shells. This is not necessary unless you have very sandy soft-shelled clams. If the clams look clean and tightly closed, simply scrub them under cold running water before shucking or steaming them open. If you find sand in the clam liquor from the shell or steaming liquid, you can strain it through a coffee filter or doubled fine-mesh cheesecloth before using it. Alternatively, let the sand sink to the bottom and don't pour off the last few drops of sandy liquid.

1. Place the clams in a large bowl or pot and cover with fresh seawater, if available. If not, mix up a batch of cold, salted water. To create an approximation of the salinity of the ocean, dissolve 5 to 6 tablespoons of salt per gallon of tap water.
2. Discard any clams that do not sink to the bottom. Let the other clams soak for 3 or 4 hours.
3. Drain and rinse with cool water.

Caution!

Clams and other bivalves filter the shallow coastal waters in which they live through their shells. If the water is contaminated, eating the clams can result in illness. Most clams sold in stores and restaurants are purchased from wholesalers who vouch for the safety of the waters in which the clams were harvested. Other outlets, such as small roadside stands or pickup trucks parked near the beach, are not as reliable. If you gather clams yourself, ascertain that the waters have been tested and deemed safe for harvesting. Pay close attention to any posted signs. If there is any question, contact local officials or the state's department of agriculture, the agency that monitors local offshore waters.

Clam Glossary

BUTTER Small, sweet Pacific clam, also called moneyshell. Can be eaten raw when small—2 to 3 inches in diameter—but toughens as it grows and is then best cooked.

CHERRYSTONE A small hard-shelled Atlantic clam, measuring up to a maximum of 3 inches in diameter. Cherrystones are delicious raw or cooked.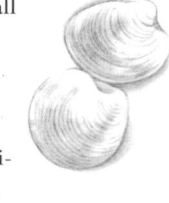

GEODUCK Pronounced "gooeyduck," this large clam (weighing as much as 3 pounds) calls the Pacific home, where it is best gathered during very low spring tides. These strange-looking soft-shelled clams have a long neck that can measure up to 3 feet and are delicious eaten raw or lightly cooked once their tough outer skin is removed. The interior meat is good in soups and stews.

LITTLENECK There are two kinds. The smallest of the hard-shelled clams, Atlantic littlenecks measure from 1½ to 2¼ inches in diameter. These are particularly sweet and delicious raw or very gently cooked. Pacific littlenecks are not related. Because they are a little tough, they should be steamed.

MAHOGANY A hard-shelled clam from Atlantic waters with a dark, reddish brown shell and pinkish meat. Also called ocean quahog, it has a flavor similar to that of large quahogs.

MANILA Also called Japanese clam. A small, sweet clam farmed off the Pacific coast of the United States, although it is not native. Most are harvested when they are barely 1 inch in diameter. Great favorites among chefs, they can be served raw or very lightly steamed.

PISMO A hard-shelled Pacific clam, quite rare and prized, is now most abundant in Baja California. Pismo clams are harvested when about 5 inches in diameter. Their tender, sweet adductor muscle is eaten raw, while the body meat is added to chowder or deep-fried.

QUAHOG Pronounced "coe-hog." A large hard-shelled clam from the Atlantic, measuring more than 3 inches in diameter. The flavor is sweet, but not quite as sweet and salty as smaller hard-shelled clams.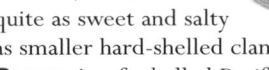

RAZOR A soft-shelled Pacific clam with a neck extending from its dark, narrow sharp shell. This clam is shaped like an old-fashioned straight razor, which explains its name and also explains its fairly sharp edges. Handle these clams with care. Razor clams require relatively long cooking and are good simmered in soups, stews, or sauces. They are found in both the Atlantic and the Pacific.

STEAMER A soft-shelled clam from the Atlantic Ocean. Also known as long-neck, fryer, or maninose clam. Its 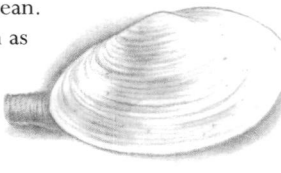 thin, oval shell measures 3 to 4 inches long. The meat is sweet and mild.

SURF This large hard-shelled Atlantic clam represents a big harvest along the Eastern seaboard. Also known as the skimmer, sea, or bar clam, it is good added to sauces and soups.

HOW TO *Shuck Clams by Hand*

A clam knife, with a squat, wide blade and thick handle for easy gripping, will make the job of prying open clam shells a much easier task.

1. For protection from a slip of the knife, use a folded cloth or oven mitt to hold the clam in one hand. (Hold the clam over a bowl to catch any clam liquor that might escape, and if it is sandy, strain the accumulated liquor through a coffee filter before using.)

2. Slide the clam knife sideways into the crack between the shells. When the knife penetrates the clam shell, sever the muscle at the hinge end of the shell and pry the shell open.

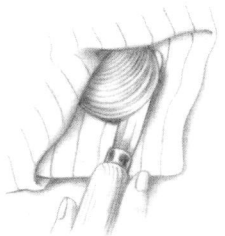

3. Run the knife around the clam meat to free it and then remove it. If serving the clam on the half shell, remove and discard the top shell.

HOW TO *Shuck Clams by Steaming*

Another, easier method of extracting clams from their shells is to steam them for a brief period of time. If using the clams in a recipe, make sure you pull them out of the pot just as soon as they open, and be careful not to overcook them.

1. Using a steamer rack in a large pot, steam clams over simmering water just until their shells barely open, not more than 5 minutes.

2. Run a knife around the clam meat to free it and then remove it.

Canned clams lend themselves to various preparations. Because they are already cooked, they require only gentle heating or no cooking at all. Frozen clams should thaw completely in the refrigerator and then be treated as fresh clams (they are not already cooked). Use them as soon as they defrost; do not refreeze them, or their texture will be destroyed.

CLARIFYING See BUTTER; STOCK.

CLAY POT Clay has been a material used to fashion cooking pots since ancient times. Today, most cookware is made from metal alloys or treated ceramic, but many loyal cooking enthusiasts still praise unglazed clay pots. The porous properties of these pots promote slow, moist, even cooking. And when the food is done, it can be served in the handsome clay pot. These pots are also known as terra-cotta bakers, Römertopfs, or Roman pots.

The most popular food for cooking in a clay pot is chicken. The pots, usually oval in shape with a domed lid, are designed to hold a whole chicken along with accompanying vegetables and, usually, broth. As it bakes, the food simultaneously steams and braises for deliciously succulent meat. Other meats, fish, and vegetables are cooked in unglazed clay pots, too.

Clay pots are meant for oven cooking, not stove top. Most are microwave safe. They should be soaked in cold water before every use to trap water in the porous clay, which forms steam during cooking. As a rule they are not dishwasher safe and should be cleaned carefully after each use. Be sure to follow the manufacturer's instructions for overall care.

See also COOKWARE.

CLOUD EAR See MUSHROOM.

CLOVE See SPICE.

COCOA See CHOCOLATE.

COCONUT Growing on palm trees in tropical climates, the coconut is the world's largest nut. Its nutmeat is firm, creamy, and snowy white, while its hollow center is filled with a sweet but watery liquid called coconut water or, erroneously, milk.

Coconut is a rich and generous nut, giving us not only coconut meat, but also coconut sugar and oil and the makings for coconut milk and cream. Coconut is a favorite ingredient for sweet baked goods, such as cakes, pies, and cookies, and for savory dishes, such as curries, often added in the form of coconut milk.

Selecting Hard, green outer shells are removed from coconuts before they are sent to market. The smaller, rounder brown shell, covered with hairy fibers, is left intact. Choose heavy coconuts filled with liquid. Shake the coconut near your ear, listening for the liquid inside. The more water sloshing around inside the nut, the fresher it is. Coconuts are available all year around but are more plentiful in the fall and winter months.

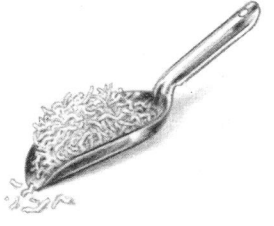

Shredded coconut.

Bags or cans of grated, shredded, and flaked dried coconut are sold in the baking-supply aisles of supermarkets and smaller grocery stores. This processed coconut is nearly always sweetened, although it is possible to buy unsweetened coconut in some supermarkets, in health-food stores, and in specialty-food stores. The bags contain dry coconut flakes or shreds, while canned flakes usually are moister. Check your recipe to be sure you buy the correct type.

The coconut "milk" you drain from the nut is more correctly called coconut water. It is different from the coconut milk often used in curries or sweetened coconut cream, which is mostly used to make tropical drinks such as the piña colada. For more detail, see COCONUT MILK.

HOW TO *Crack a Coconut*

1. Drive a long nail, ice pick, or other sharp spike through one of the three smooth "eyes" at one end of the coconut.
2. Drain the liquid and drink it immediately or refrigerate it for up to a few hours.
3. Put the nut on a hard surface—the floor or porch—and hit it with a hammer until it cracks.
4. Break the shell apart using your hands, the hammer, or another sturdy tool.

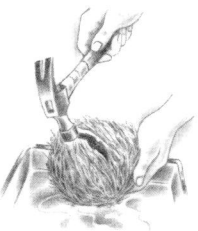

5. Very carefully cut the white meat from the shell with a knife. Peel the brown skin from the coconut meat.

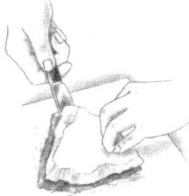

6. Grate or chop the meat using a box grater, rotary grater, food processor, or small, sharp knife, depending on how you will be using it.

Storing Store the unopened nut in the refrigerator for up to a month. Once the water is drained, drink it within a few hours. The coconut meat will keep, wrapped in plastic and refrigerated, for 5 days. Dried or canned coconut will keep in the refrigerator, covered with plastic wrap, for up to 1 month.

Quick Tip

Coconut shells can be easier to crack if they are heated or frozen first. These steps make the shell brittle, making it easier to crack. After draining the liquid, bake the coconut in a 375°F oven for about 15 minutes. Hit it with a hammer as soon as it is removed from the oven. Alternatively, put the coconut in the freezer for 2 or 3 hours beforehand. Both methods also work for removing meat once the coconut is open. Heating or freezing the broken shell makes it easier to pry the meat from it.

See also COCONUT MILK.

COCONUT CREAM See COCONUT MILK.

COCONUT MILK With its rich and nutty flavor, coconut milk, made by soaking grated coconut in water, is an essential ingredient throughout the tropics. It thickens sauces, turns rice dishes creamy, flavors desserts, smoothes out soups, and is a perfect foil for the heat of chiles. Coconut milk should not be confused with canned sweetened coconut cream, sometimes labeled "cream of coconut," which is used primarily for desserts and tropical drinks.
Selecting Good-quality coconut milk is available in cans or frozen in Asian and Latin markets.
Storing Store opened coconut milk in a lidded glass or plastic container for up to

Quick Tip

When using coconut milk for a Thai curry, avoid shaking the can. Instead, skim off the thick coconut cream that has settled on top, and heat it in place of oil for cooking the curry paste and aromatics. Later, stir in the remaining coconut milk to make the sauce.

3 days in the refrigerator. Unopened canned coconut milk can be kept for up to 1 year.
Preparing The solids in coconut milk separate and rise as cream does in cow's milk. For coconut cream, spoon the cream from the top of the opened can and reserve the remaining milk for another use. For recipes calling for coconut milk, shake the can vigorously before opening. If need be, whisk to remove the more stubborn lumps.

HOW TO *Make Your Own Coconut Milk*
1. Soak freshly grated coconut or dried, unsweetened coconut flakes in an equal amount of hot water (that is, 1 cup flakes to 1 cup water) until the coconut has softened.
2. Process briefly in a blender or food processor just until barely smooth.
3. Pour the mixture onto a large double layer of cheesecloth or a linen dishtowel draped over a bowl.
4. Gather the cloth around the coconut mixture and squeeze tightly to extract as much of the fluid as you can.
5. Repeat steps 1–4 up to two times, if desired. The subsequent pressings will yield thinner coconut milk. Use the batches separately, or mix them for uniform flavor and consistency.

CODDLING An exceedingly gentle form of cooking. Coddled eggs have been cooked just so that they are no longer raw but still extremely soft. They are sometimes cooked in a lidded porcelain dish called an egg coddler. The eggs are cracked into the coddler, covered, and then lowered into a pan of simmering water. Note that coddling does not raise the temperature of an egg above 160°F, which is necessary to kill salmonella bacteria. See also EGG.

COFFEE For many of us, a day without coffee (and its caffeine boost) is a day when we are 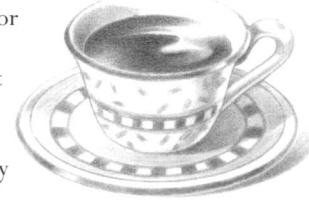 destined to feel sluggish and dull. Luckily, coffee is a ready staple in most kitchens, and specialized coffeehouses have proliferated in recent years, so that cappuccino, latte, and espresso are ours for the asking, any time of the day or night.

Coffee is brewed from beans harvested from trees that grow in tropical regions. After processing to remove the pulp and skins that enclose them, the beans are roasted and mixed to produce various blends—some so distinctive they practically announce themselves, and others quite ordinary but still unmistakably coffee. Coffee is also a favorite flavoring, starring in ice cream, cream pies, cakes, and candies, and often costarring with chocolate. Coffee-flavored liqueurs such as Kahlúa are delightful, too, as an ingredient in dessert recipes and on their own.

Most ordinary coffee is made from robusta beans, which grow at lower altitudes and are widely cultivated, primarily in Brazil and Indonesia. Coffee of distinction is more likely to be brewed from arabica beans, which thrive at high altitudes. Some of the best-tasting arabica beans are grown in Kenya, in Africa, and Sumatra and Sulawesi (formerly Celebes), in Indonesia. Beans from Costa Rica, Guatemala, and Colombia also can be exceptional. The famous Jamaican Blue Mountain beans produce remarkable coffee, but the harvest is small. Although Hawaiian coffee makes up only a small percentage of the world's crop, it is of high quality.

Origin alone does not determine the quality of the coffee. Coffee beans must be roasted to bring out their rich, heady flavor and, depending on the producer, this process differs. There is good reason coffee is often referred to by its roast, since this is perhaps the single most important process in coffee production. After roasting, the beans may or may not be combined for blends.

Essentially, various roasts produce darker or lighter cups of coffee. Standard American roast is a medium-light roast. It also is called breakfast roast and produces coffee that is neither particularly strong nor dark. This is the brewed coffee most often sold at convenience stores, diners, fast-food outlets, and many restaurants. Medium-dark roasted beans produce darker, richer coffee. A good example is Viennese roast, but the brewed coffee, while full flavored, does not have the full body of darker roasts. Dark-roasted coffee beans, usually dubbed French or Italian roast, produce a black, full-bodied cup of coffee and are used for making espresso.

Quick Bite

A good rule of thumb: "tropical" names—Sumatra, Jamaica, Kenya—refer to the source of beans, while European names—French, Italian, Viennese—describe the roast.

All coffee contains some amount of the stimulating compound known as caffeine. Caffeine, as much as flavor, is what attracts many of us to coffee. It perks us up in the morning and increases mental acuity. It also prevents some of us from falling asleep at night, and its sudden absence from our daily diet can bring on headaches and crabbiness. Some people are minimally affected by caffeine; others feel better overall when they drink only decaffeinated brew. Caffeine is removed by two methods, the water process and the solvent process, with the former resulting in a better-tasting cup. Decaffeinated coffee is approximately 97 percent caffeine-free.

Quick Tip

Different coffeemakers call for different grinds. French presses, for example, need coarse grounds. Consult your owner's manual or a good coffee merchant.

Selecting Buy coffee beans from a reputable merchant with good turnover. There are many roasts and blends, so experiment until you find those you prefer.

A coffee merchant will grind beans for you. While coffee beans do start to lose flavor once they are ground, if you drink a lot of coffee and can replenish your supply regularly, this is not a bad option.

Home bakers rely on instant coffee and espresso for flavoring. Instant coffee is sold as powder, freeze-dried crystals, or dehydrated granules. Instant espresso is commonly dehydrated granules and produces a slightly darker cup than instant coffee.

Storing Store the coffee beans you use every day in a cool cupboard, sealed in an airtight container, for up to 2 weeks. Beans can also be refrigerated for up to 1 month if you don't think you will use them up in a couple weeks' time. Well wrapped in plastic, coffee beans freeze for up to 3 months, which is useful if you like to buy your beans in bulk or like to store them in a weekend house. If you buy preground coffee, store it in an airtight container in a cool, dark place for up to 2 weeks.

Preparing Coffee tastes best when brewed from freshly ground beans. As soon as they are ground, coffee beans begin to lose essential oils and flavor. Check your local kitchenware or coffee stores for a small, efficient coffee grinder. Grind only as many beans as you need at the time. All coffee must be brewed with hot water. The optimum water temperature for brewing is 200°F (not quite boiling). When making coffee manually, bring the water to a boil and then let it cool briefly before brewing.

Coffee-Making Methods Most people make drip coffee, the method in which hot water passes through the ground coffee and then drips through a filter into a waiting pot. Electric drip coffeemakers are convenient, but a pot of well-made manual drip coffee probably tastes better. The latter allows you to heat the water to just the right temperature and also to moisten and stir the grounds as you begin to brew, which releases the flavor more evenly.

Drip pot.

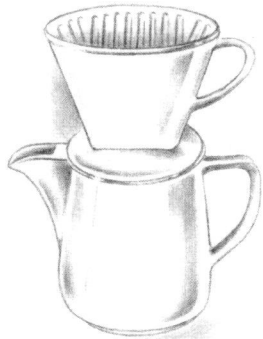

Quick Tip

Keeping coffee warm in an electric coffeemaker or on the stove will soon result in a burnt flavor. Pouring freshly made coffee into a thermos (or making drip coffee directly into a thermos) will keep coffee flavorful for hours.

French press or plunger coffeemakers, in which a plunger fitted with a screen is pushed through a mixture of grounds and water, are another option. This method is easy and quick, but the coffee often contains sediment and cools quickly.

Plunger pot.

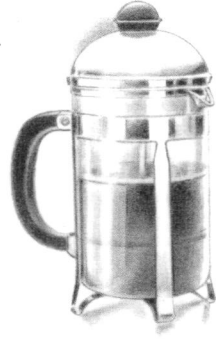

The percolator, in which boiling water passes through the grounds over and over during brewing, does not result in a good-tasting cup. When coffee is brewed for too long—more than a few minutes— more bitter-tasting elements of the beans are extracted and affect the coffee's flavor.

Whichever method you use, coffee should be served promptly after brewing for the best-tasting cup.

Coffee Savvy

- Begin with freshly ground beans, and grind only as much coffee as you need for a pot.
- For best results, use a manual drip pot fitted with a paper filter. Make sure the pot is scrupulously clean and free of soapy residue.
- Measure 2 level tablespoons (one coffee measure) of ground coffee for every 6 fluid ounces (¼ cup) of water.

Quick Tip

Coffee does not reheat well. Discard cold, left-over coffee or use it to make iced coffee.

- Start with cold tap water. Often, hot tap water has been sitting in a water heater and may taste stale or slightly metallic. If the water tastes of chemicals or is otherwise unpleasant, use bottled water.
- Bring the water to a boil, remove from the heat, and let cool slightly. The water should be 200°F, just below boiling, when it blends with the coffee.
- Before pouring the water into the grounds, moisten them with a little of the hot water and stir to distribute it.
- Once the coffee is brewed, serve it immediately. Pour the remaining coffee into a thermos to keep it warm.
- Do not let coffee boil. Boiling destroys its flavor.

COLANDER See STRAINER.

COLLARD See GREENS, DARK.

CONDENSED MILK See MILK.

CONFECTIONERS' SUGAR See SUGAR.

CONFIT When meat or poultry is cooked slowly in a large amount of its own fat until very tender and then stored in a pot or other container and completely covered with fat, it is called confit. This French method was developed originally as a way to preserve salt-cured meat and fowl, most notably pork and goose. Today, duck or goose confit is found on menus of upscale restaurants. Both are key ingredients in classic cassoulet. The poultry or meat for confit no longer is cured, although it usually is well seasoned. Some chefs cook vegetables such as green onions, yellow onions, and garlic slowly in oil and call the preparation a confit.

CONVERSION See MEASURING.

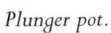

COOKIE See page 134.

COOKIE CUTTER See BAKING TOOLS.

COOKIE SHEET See BAKEWARE.

COOKING Home-cooked meals are more than simple sustenance: just as they nourish our bodies, so do they nourish our spirits. Nearly miraculous transformations in flavor, aroma, texture, and appearance take place when heat is applied to ingredients. Basic strategies will make the task of cooking easy and pleasurable, regardless of your level of expertise.

- Read through the recipe twice to make sure you have the ingredients, equipment, and time required. Make a shopping list based on the recipe, first checking the cupboard and refrigerator.
- Determine substitutions for any hard-to-find ingredients. See SUBSTITUTIONS & EQUIVALENTS.
- Decide which dishes or recipe steps can be prepared ahead of time.
- Allow sufficient time for foods to defrost or reach room temperature.
- Prepare the ingredients according to the ingredient list before you move on to the method of a recipe. This may involve chopping, dicing, slicing, or measuring ingredients; separating eggs; or letting ingredients soften at room temperature.
- Use the correct size pot, pan, or skillet. Good recipes will specify or will simply presume a medium-sized pan.
- Cook at the suggested temperatures. Use an oven thermometer to make sure your oven is accurate, adjusting the temperature dial accordingly.
- Use all your senses in the kitchen. Well-written recipes will give you visual, tactile, taste, and aromatic cues, as well as timing instructions.

- Taste dishes as you cook, adding such ingredients as herbs, spices, wine, vinegar, citrus juice and zest, chiles, sugar, and salt and pepper as needed. Long cooking, such as stewing and braising, alters the flavors of foods more so than stir-frying and sautéing do. Add seasonings with a measured hand, keeping in mind that you can always use more, but it's difficult to disguise an overused herb or spice. Always taste just before serving and adjust the seasoning accordingly.
- Clean up as you go. Put jars and bottles away as you finish with them. Wash bowls and utensils when you have a spare minute or soak them in the sink.
- When you run out of an ingredient, make a note of it. Don't trust your memory to kick in a few days later.

As much as many of us would like a large, spacious, well-designed kitchen with yards of shelving, few of us have one. Instead, we have to make adjustments and use space carefully. Following are some common-sense approaches to organizing your kitchen to make cooking more efficient.

- Plan your cupboard contents so that the foods you use often (oil, sugar, spices) are easy to reach. Store infrequently used items on higher or lower shelves.
- Put more perishable foods, such as chocolate and dried herbs, in cupboards distant from heat and light.
- Arrange the refrigerator so that frequently used foods, such as butter, milk, and juice, are easy to reach.
- Keep countertops clutter free. You'll be less eager to cook if you have to clear a space before you can begin.
- Make use of space-saving devices such as racks hung inside cupboard doors, below-cabinet shelving, pot racks, drawer organizers, and stacking bins.

See also HIGH-ALTITUDE COOKING; LOW-FAT COOKING.

Cookie

Chocolate chip. Gingersnap. Spice. Peanut butter. Cookies come in just about every flavor you can imagine. They are wonderful tucked into lunch boxes for a midday lift or dipped into milk while you watch the 11 o'clock news.

Cookies can be made from dough that is dropped onto baking sheets; rolled and cut out, and then placed on sheets; piped with a pastry bag; pushed through a cookie press; or molded by hand; and then baked. Some cookie doughs must be refrigerated to firm them up before baking. Others, such as those for bar cookies like brownies, are made from soft batter that is smoothed into a square or rectangular pan and cut into squares or bars after baking and cooling. Even no-bake versions of both cookies and bars exist, too.

*Using a
cookie cutter.*

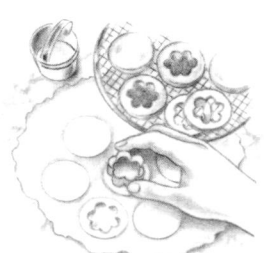

Equipment Cookies and bars are simple to make with the equipment most home bakers have. A mixing bowl, wooden spoon, and two baking sheets (or a pan for bars) will suffice in many cases. Recipes can be mixed by hand but are more easily assembled with a handheld electric mixer or in a stand mixer. The rapid beating also incorporates more air and lightens the batter. See also BAKEWARE; BAKING TOOLS.

Ingredients Cookies and bars rarely require expensive or hard-to-find ingredients. Most are simple mixtures of flour, butter, sugar, eggs, and flavorings. Nearly all recipes call for all-purpose flour, unsalted butter, granulated sugar, and large eggs. The flour may require sifting before measuring; the butter usually is softened or melted; and the eggs should be at room temperature. Most cookies and bars are leavened with small amounts of baking powder or baking soda.

General simplicity aside, a home cook setting out to make a batch of cookies should also bear in mind that they are a form of pastry. As in pastry making and other forms of baking, precise measuring of ingredients and following of recipe instructions will help ensure success.

HOW TO *Make Drop Cookies*
1. With a tablespoon, scoop up a spoonful of batter and use a second spoon to push it off onto a baking sheet, spacing the cookies at least 2 inches apart on all sides.

HOW TO *Roll Dough for Refrigerator Cookies*
1. Spoon the dough down the center of a sheet of waxed paper. Roll the dough up inside the paper, forming a log of whatever shape you desire—cylinder or rectangular block.
2. Refrigerate until firm. Unwrap, slice, and bake as directed in the recipe.

HOW TO *Use a Cookie Press*

Cookie presses work best with fairly firm, pliable dough. For opening the tube and pressing the cookies, consult your owner's manual, as models vary.

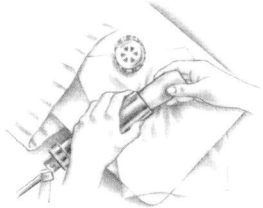

1. Roll the dough into a log with a diameter slightly smaller than that of the cookie press cylinder and about the same length. See How to Roll Dough for Refrigerator Cookies, above, step 1.

2. Unwrap the dough (no chilling is necessary) and slip it into the cookie press.

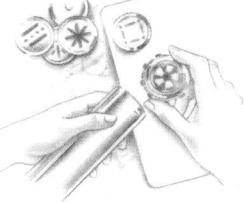

3. Select a design plate. Fit the plate into its holder and screw it securely onto the press.

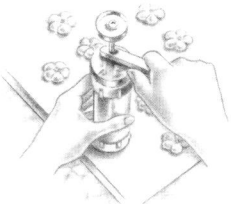

4. Hold the press upright, securely grasp the handle, and, applying even pressure, press out the dough to form cookies.

Cookie Savvy Recipes vary, but for most cookie baking, the following techniques are useful:

- If a recipe simply says to grease the baking sheet or pan, use softened butter or margarine, vegetable oil, or unflavored cooking spray. Butter, which burns at lower temperatures than oil, is not recommended for cookies that bake at high temperatures. Alternatively, line the baking sheets with parchment paper or nonstick liners, available in cookware shops. This eliminates some cleanup.

- Stir cookie batter just until the flour disappears, or your cookies may be tough.

- When rolling out cookie dough, work on a lightly floured surface, start at the center of the dough disk, and use gentle strokes. See also ROLLING OUT.

- If using a cookie cutter, dust it lightly with flour to avoid sticking. Press the cookie cutter straight into the dough and then lift it without twisting.

- After cutting out as many cookies as you can from the initial rolling out, gather the remnants of dough together, pat out, and cut out one more batch of cookies. Do not reroll scraps more than once unless you're working with a very rich and buttery dough; if you do, your subsequent cookies may be tough.

- If cookie dough softens too much during rolling and becomes limp and sticky, refrigerate it for 10 or 15 minutes, until firm enough to roll and cut.

- Be sure to leave ample room for spreading between dropped cookies. Don't try to crowd too many cookies on a sheet for each batch.

- Set the timer for the least amount of time if a range is given in a recipe. Use an oven thermometer to gauge the accuracy of your oven.

- If baking more than one sheet of cookies at a time, switch the baking sheets from

continued

C

Cookie, continued

the upper to lower rack and rotate them halfway through the baking time to ensure even cooking.

- Let baking sheets cool completely between batches, or, to save time, get each new batch ready on a piece of parchment paper, then slide it onto the sheet and move them directly into the oven. If you drop dough onto baking sheets still hot from baking the last batch of cookies, the dough will begin to cook, softening and spreading, before you've dropped all the cookies.
- For bar cookies, line the baking pan with aluminum foil for easy removal of the bars after baking.

Lining the baking pan.

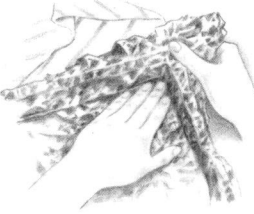

Removing from the pan.

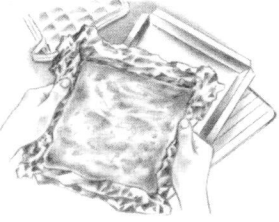

- If you can't bake all the cookies at once, refrigerate the dough for up to 24 hours, even if it is not called refrigerator dough. Cover the bowl with plastic wrap or aluminum foil before refrigerating. There is no need to bring the dough to room temperature before continuing with baking. The exception is bar cookies, which nearly always should be baked immediately after mixing. Their batter will deflate if left to sit for any length of time.

Storing Many cookie doughs can be frozen, particularly those designed for rolling into logs and slicing. Other good candidates include stiff, buttery doughs. See FREEZING for more details.

Most baked cookies and bars can be stored at room temperature for up to 3 days. Soft cookies with lots of fat, such as chocolate chip, will not keep as long as crispier ones, such as biscotti. When fully cooled, cookies or cut bars should be transferred to an airtight container, such as a cookie tin or rigid plastic container. Bars that have not been cut and removed from the pan can be covered with foil and set aside at room temperature for up to a day. For longer storage, the bars should be transferred to an airtight container.

Most cookies and bars can be frozen for long storage. Let them cool completely and then wrap them individually or in small stacks in plastic wrap. Pack the wrapped cookies snugly in rigid plastic containers, or in zippered plastic freezer bags, pressing out as much air as possible. Label the packages with their contents and date. Most can be frozen for up to 3 months.

Defrost frozen cookies, still wrapped, at room temperature or in the refrigerator. The choice depends on when you want to serve them. It also depends on whether the cookies or bars are to be served cold (in which case, defrost them in the refrigerator) or at room temperature. Most cookies will defrost within 2 hours, although some very thin, crisp cookies will defrost in 30 minutes or less. Serve cookies as soon as possible after they are defrosted. They are not as moist as fresh baked and therefore tend to go stale faster.

Do not store crisp and cakey cookies together. The crisp cookies will absorb moisture from the others and soften. Store frosted or topped cookies in single layers, separated by waxed or parchment paper to prevent them from sticking together.

Cookie Blues Got a problem with your cookies? Find the simple explanation here.

DOUGH RIPS AND TEARS WHEN ROLLED OUT. Hot, humid weather makes rolling tricky. Bake on cool, dry days, or chill the dough before rolling and be sure to rub the rolling pin and work surface with ample flour. If the dough softens so that it rips and tears, refrigerate it for about 20 minutes and rub the rolling pin with a little more flour.

SOME COOKIES BROWN TOO QUICKLY. Sugar-rich doughs brown more than do other types of dough. Use insulated baking sheets (see BAKEWARE) or line the sheets with foil. Check your oven temperature with a thermometer and lower the heat if necessary. Also, note that dark-colored sheets promote more rapid baking and may require lowering the heat by 20° to 25°F.

COOKIES SPREAD TOO MUCH IN THE OVEN. Dough was placed on a hot baking sheet; allow sheet to cool or prepare each batch on parchment paper, transfer it to the sheet, and place sheet directly in the oven.

COOKIES ON ONE BAKING SHEET BURN AND THOSE ON THE OTHER DON'T. One sheet may be too close to the bottom of the oven, so the cookies are baking more quickly. Bake the cookies a sheet at a time on a rack in the top third of the oven, or switch and rotate the sheets as the cookies bake.

COOKIES STICK TO THE BAKING SHEET. You may have left the cookies on the baking sheet too long. Lift them off with a spatula 2 to 3 minutes after they are removed from the oven and transfer them to wire racks to let them cool completely.

Quick Tip

For most home baking, two baking sheets and two or three large cooling racks are adequate. If you often bake large batches of cookies, however, consider stocking more of both for the most efficient use of time.

The Cookie Jar Cookies come in nearly every shape, size, and flavor.

BISCOTTI In Italy, all cookies are *biscotti*. Here, the term refers to Italian cookies that are baked twice—first in loaf form, then sliced and baked a second time.

BROWNIE The quintessential bar cookie, made from chocolate and sometimes containing nuts. Some brownies are fudgy and dense, while others are more cakelike.

GINGERBREAD MAN Children love this spice cookie made from a molasses-rich dough easily cut into figures, baked, and decorated with piped icing.

MACAROON A light cookie made from almonds pounded to a moist paste, then mixed with beaten egg whites and sugar and baked until the edges are golden.

MADELEINE Traditionally baked in distinctive shell-shaped molds, this delicate French cookie has a consistency reminiscent of sponge cake.

OATMEAL A chewy drop cookie made from a dough of rolled oats, flour, sugar, eggs, and butter. Raisins and nuts are often added.

SHORTBREAD A crumbly, rich bar cookie made from dough composed of flour, sugar, and a generous measure of butter.

SPRITZ A buttery German cookie made by pressing a rich dough through a cookie press fitted with any one of a variety of plates, from rosettes to ribbons to ropes.

TOLL HOUSE The ultimate American cookie. Created by a Massachusetts innkeeper in 1939, who discovered that small pieces of chocolate mixed into dough stay firm when baked.

TUILE A thin, fragile cookie made from an egg white–rich batter that is piped or dropped onto baking sheets. While still hot from the oven, the cookies are gently shaped over a rolling pin to recall Mediterranean roof tiles. The same batter is used to make cornets, "cigarettes," and cups.

See also BAKEWARE; BAKING; BAKING TOOLS; MEASURING; ROLLING OUT.

COOKING METHODS A good cook will learn to master all the varied methods by which foods are cooked, namely, baking, braising, grilling, roasting, sautéing, steaming, stewing, and stir-frying. More important still, a good cook will develop a sound knowledge of which cooking methods work best for particular types of foods.

In general, tender and small food items such as shrimp and scallops or thin slices of boneless poultry must be cooked quickly to keep them from toughening or drying out. Foods with a chewy, dense texture, such as stew meats, need long, slow cooking with moisture to achieve tenderness. Some foods, such as squid and flank steak, are tender only if cooked either very briefly or for a long time.

Foods intended to be quickly sautéed or stir-fried should be inherently tender or should be cut up into pieces that will cook quickly. Some vegetables also benefit from blanching to soften them slightly before they are sautéed. Meat destined for roasting should be a tender cut with some marbling or interior fat, or it can be barded (see BARDING). Tougher or very lean cuts, such as veal and pork, are often braised rather than roasted.

Dry vs. Moist Cooking Methods

DRY METHODS	MOIST METHODS
Baking	Boiling
Frying	Braising
Grilling	Poaching
Roasting	Steaming
Sautéing	Stewing
Stir-frying	

See also individual cooking methods; individual foods; TECHNIQUES.

COOKING SPRAY Also called vegetable oil spray, baking oil spray, canola oil spray, or olive oil spray, cooking spray is canned oil packed under pressure, dispersed by a propellant, and used to grease pots and pans. Cooking spray also is handy for lubricating the racks on charcoal and gas grills. Food, too, can be sprayed to prevent sticking during cooking, although the sprays are not recommended as substitutions for liquid oils in recipes. Using cooking spray is healthful as well as convenient because in general you use less oil than if you were pouring or brushing it over a surface.

Caution!

Never aim cooking spray toward an open flame, and use caution with it when grilling or cooking on a gas burner. The flame can travel back up the stream of spray and seriously burn you or cause an explosion.

Selecting Most cooking sprays are mixtures of soybean or canola oil, lecithin, water, and a propellant. Select the contents best suited for the type of cooking you do. Some contain flour as well, which is convenient for use on cake pans but undesirable for coating a sauté pan; others contain olive oil, which, because it burns at lower temperatures than soybean and canola oils

Quick Tip

Look for refillable spray bottles that use a pumping mechanism to build enough pressure to propel oil with about the same intensity as a can of commercial cooking spray. These devices allow you to spray high-quality olive oil or your favorite balsamic vinegar over salad greens, or to use peanut or canola oil from your own bottles to grease pans.

and because it imparts a distinct flavor, is not recommended for baking. Olive oil spray does add a little nice flavor when cooking onions, garlic, peppers, and other savory foods.

Storing Store the cans at cool room temperature in a dark cupboard. Do not refrigerate and do not let the cans reach temperatures exceeding 120°F, or they may explode. Manufacturers suggest using the sprays at temperatures between 68° and 75°F and not keeping them for more than 6 months after purchase.

Preparing Aim the spray nozzle at the pan or food and press it quickly several times, moving the stream across the surface of the pan or grill. In a short time the surface will be covered with a thin, even coating. If cooking on top of the stove, let the coated pan get hot before adding food.

Quick Bite

Approximately eight 1-second spritzes of oil from a can of commercial cooking spray equal ½ teaspoon oil.

COOKING TOOLS See page 140.

COOKWARE See page 146.

COOLING A loose term that can mean anything from allowing a pan to cool until you can comfortably hold it to letting food cool to room temperature. Cakes and other baked goods are set on racks to cool so that air can circulate around them, while soup and coffee are allowed to cool only until they don't burn the tongue. Many recipes call for cooling cooked foods "just until cool enough to handle"—that is, until you can just comfortably hold them—before peeling or slicing.

There's no trick to cooling. Simply remove the food from the heat source and let

it sit. Once cool, any moist, protein-based food should be served or chilled. Leaving food at room temperature too long invites bacterial growth. Never let perishable protein-based food (meats, poultry, soups, stocks, casseroles, custards, and the like) sit out for more than 2 hours at most.

See also CHILLING.

COOLING RACK See BAKING TOOLS.

CORIANDER When fresh, another name for cilantro; see HERB. For dried, see SPICE.

CORING To remove the central core of a fruit or vegetable. Heads of cabbage and lettuce usually require coring, as do apples, pears, and quince. Tomatoes, zucchini, and pineapples frequently are cored, too. Unless a recipe calls for the food to be kept whole, as for stuffing, you can simply cut it into halves or quarters and cut out the core from each piece.

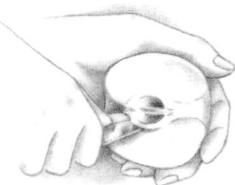

Coring apple half with knife.

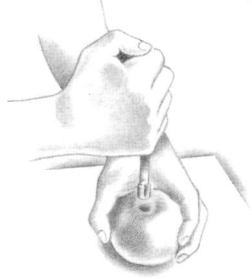

Coring whole apple with corer.

If you core a lot of fruit and vegetables, consider buying specialty corers. If the task comes up only now and then, you might want to save drawer space for other tools.

Cooking Tools

Stocking a kitchen with a selection of useful cooking tools is a lifelong process—and one you cannot begin too soon. Some gadgets may quickly lose their initial appeal, while others will wear out, get lost, or break; but if you invest in high-quality cooking tools they will last for decades. Good knives, sturdy bowls, and well-made pots and pans will never let you down.

THE BASIC COOK Following are the tools every home kitchen should have.

BRUSHES Natural-bristle brushes suitable for brushing foods with marinades, sauces, glazes, and other liquids should be firmly rooted in the handle. Handles can be made of wood or heavy-duty plastic and must be easy to grasp and long enough to allow dexterity. Wash the brushes after each use in hot, soapy water, flick them to remove excess water, and then air dry. Keep brushes used for savory foods separate from those used for dessert making.

Other useful brushes include soft- to medium-bristle vegetable brushes, good for cleaning potatoes, carrots, and other firm vegetables, and soft brushes appropriate for cleaning mushrooms.

CAN OPENER It can be frustrating to use a can opener that doesn't work well, so choose a high-quality one. The most popular can openers are manual geared ones. Variations on this style include those that remove tops from cans without producing sharp edges and those that mount on the wall. Electric can openers can stand on the countertop or be mounted.

COLANDER A bowl-shaped metal device perforated with small holes. Ideal for draining boiled foods such as pasta or vegetables. See also STRAINER.

CORKSCREW A simple metal spiral or other device designed to pull corks from wine bottles. See also CORKSCREW.

CUTTING BOARD A portable work surface. Cutting boards of various sizes and materials are used for knife work in the preparation or serving of food. See also CUTTING BOARD.

EGG BEATER Precursor of the handheld electric mixer, this convenient old-fashioned device quickly turns two bladed beaters by means of a hand-cranked ratchet wheel, easily whipping up egg whites, cream, or batters.

FORK Not just for eating at table, forks are used while cooking or serving to pierce, pick up, or steady foods. Large two-pronged carving forks steady roasts during carving; smaller ones turn steaks on the grill, or, smaller still, spear pickles from a jar. Large forks with 3 or more tines may be used for picking up and serving foods as varied as bacon, spaghetti, or sauerkraut. Even ordinary table forks may be used for many of the above-mentioned tasks.

GRATER A device used to grate food into fine particles with the aid of sharp, pointy rasps arrayed on a flat surface. (The same term is also sometimes used erroneously to refer to a shredder, since a box grater, a common kitchen tool, includes both shredding sides and a rasp-surfaced grating side containing sharp-edged holes.) See GRATING for details.

KNIFE Good, sharp knives in a few basic styles are kitchen essentials. See KNIFE for more information.

LADLE At least one ladle is essential in every kitchen. The bowl should be made of stainless steel or rigid, heat-resistant plastic and large enough to scoop up a good measure of soup, stew, or chili. The handle should be heat resistant as well and long enough for easy use. Small ladles are useful for saucing foods and skimming stocks.

MEASURING SPOONS AND CUPS Measuring spoons, sized from ⅛ teaspoon to 1 table-spoon, are fashioned from metal or plastic and usually bundled together. Liquid measures are made from clear tempered glass or plastic and generally measure up to 1 or 2 cups. This allows the cook to set the cup on the counter and view the liquid amount at eye level to get an accurate reading. Dry measures generally range from ¼ to 1 cup, are made of metal or rigid plastic, and are sold in nesting sets. See MEASURING for details on using measuring cups correctly.

MIXING BOWL Every kitchen should have an assortment of bowls in a range of sizes. Larger bowls contain mixtures as you stir and toss, while smaller-sized bowls are good for holding ingredients that have been prepared for a recipe. Bowls come in a range of sizes and materials; see MIXING BOWL for more information.

PEPPER MILL So many recipes nowadays call for pepper freshly ground from whole dried peppercorns that a pepper mill is an essential for even basic kitchens. Look for a sturdy model made from either wood or plastic, with a hardened-steel grinder that adjusts by the turn of the screw at the top of the mill to provide ground pepper of varying degrees of coarseness or fineness.

POTATO MASHER A handheld tool with a handle attached to a perforated or bent

wire grid, used to mash cooked potatoes by pressing down on them repeatedly. Choose a sturdy masher made of stainless steel. Some ingenious models include two parallel grids, the lower one of which is attached to a spring in the handle, making the mashing action more efficient. See also Potato Ricer, page 145, and MASHING.

POT HOLDERS AND OVEN MITTS Essential for taking pots from the stove and pans from the oven, pot holders and oven mitts should be thickly padded and large enough to perform their designated tasks with safety. Do not skimp on these. Square pot-holders should be generous in size, and glovelike oven mitts should reach above the wrist and be well insulated. Mitts designed to reach nearly to the elbow are especially useful for taking large pans from the oven and for working over a hot grill.

Oven mitt.

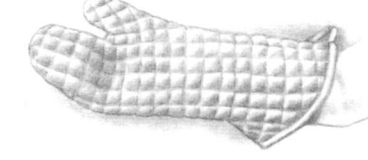

SCISSORS AND SHEARS Every kitchen should have at least one pair of scissors in the drawer to cut parchment paper, kitchen string, cheesecloth, fresh herbs, fruits, and even pickles. Basic kitchen scissors should have stainless-steel blades and one serrated edge. Heavier and longer poultry shears are useful for cutting chicken pieces and trimming fat and skin. Specialized scissors—shellfish shears, grape shears, pizza shears—can be acquired as the need arises.

Poultry shears.

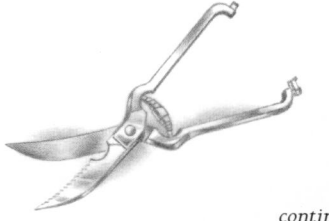

continued

Cooking Tools, continued

SPATULA Most people think of metal spatulas, hamburger or pancake turners, when they think of spatulas. These measure from 2 to 4 inches wide, have thin edges for slipping under food, and may have short or long handles. Flexible rubber spatulas, excellent for blending ingredients and scraping bowls, can have blades of varying sizes, heatproof or not. Wooden spatulas are good for lengthy stirring and for sautéing, as they won't heat up and burn your hands. Use heatproof silicone rubber and wooden spatulas on nonstick surfaces to avoid scratches; metal spatulas are fine for grills and heavy-duty frying pans. Long, narrow frosting (or icing) spatulas make quick work of frosting cakes.

Frosting spatula (top) and rubber spatula (bottom).

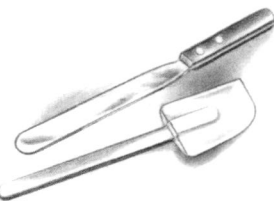

SPOON An assortment of wooden, plastic, and metal spoons, both solid and slotted, is useful. See SPOON for more details.

Slotted spoon.

STEAMER BASKET Also known as vegetable steamer or folding steamer. Steamer baskets are collapsible contraptions made of perforated metal with fanned sides that allow them to adjust to fit into a number of different-sized pans. They sit on small feet so they hold food above the boiling or simmering water, ensuring that the steam will circulate around the food to yield the best results. See also STEAMING.

STRAINER Also called a sieve. Strainers are used to separate out lumps or larger particles from ingredients, drain off liquid from solids, or purée soft foods. Made of fine or coarse wire mesh, they come in a variety of sizes. See STRAINER for details.

STRING Kitchen string, also called kitchen twine, is used for trussing chicken and tying roasts, as well as numerous other tasks. The string should be soft and pliable, and preferably linen—which won't burn.

THERMOMETER Every kitchen should have a meat thermometer. There are two kinds: a probe type, which is inserted into the meat at the beginning of cooking and left there until the proper temperature is reached, and an instant-read type, which is inserted toward the end of the cooking period to test for doneness. Most cooks prefer instant-read thermometers. They are more accurate and make a smaller hole in the meat, thus releasing fewer juices.

Instant-read thermometer.

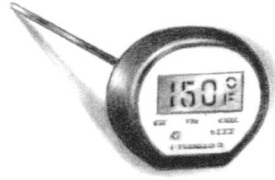

You can also use an instant-read thermometer to test different sections of the same piece of food, as well as more than one piece of food, and they are more convenient for grilled and panfried foods. Insert a meat thermometer in the center of a piece of meat or a roast, or on the inside of the thickest part of the thigh of a bird; make sure the thermometer is not touching bone. See BAKEWARE for information on oven thermometers and SAFETY for information on refrigerator thermometers. See also CANDY MAKING; DONENESS; and individual meats.

TIMER This invaluable little gadget is your best friend if you're cooking several dishes at once, are cooking in the midst of company, or are doing other tasks at the same time as cooking. Timers range in complexity from the simple spring-activated ones to digital timers that can time three different recipes at once. Most new stoves now have built-in oven timers. A clip-on timer that attaches to your apron is helpful when grilling outdoors.

Quick Tip

Always use a portable timer when you've put anything on a burner or in the oven but you are not staying in the kitchen. Take the timer with you so you'll hear it, and you'll save yourself the heartache of a burned pot.

TONGS These scissorlike tools, with their blunt ends capable of grasping food, are extremely useful. Some are fitted with finger loops, similar to scissors; others have a V-shaped holding end, which allows a bit more control. Most are 10 to 12 inches long; longer tongs are available for grilling. Tongs are useful for handling hot food, picking up pieces of meat without piercing them (and losing juices), tossing salads, checking pasta for doneness, and arranging food on plates. Many longer tongs are outfitted with a locking device

that keeps them closed during storage—a real space saver for a crowded utensil drawer.
VEGETABLE PEELER Sharp-edged blades and easy-to-hold handles define good vegetable peelers. Swivel-bladed peelers are more maneuverable, hugging the curves of vegetables and lessening your work. They will dull after several years of use and usually are replaced, not sharpened.
WHISK With a head of looped thin metal wires, a whisk is used to rapidly beat or whip ingredients. Also known as whips, whisks are made in various sizes and shapes for various uses. Elongated sauce whisks are the basic model, used to mix ingredients thoroughly without adding excess air. See also WHISKING.

THE WELL-STOCKED COOK

Specialty tools make particular tasks easier and cooking more pleasant. Once you have stocked the basics, you may want to add a few extras.
BULB BASTER Also called a turkey baster, this plastic, glass, or metal tube with a squeezable bulb at one end resembles a giant eyedropper. It is used to baste turkeys and other meats. See also BASTING.
CHERRY PITTER A tool that speeds the process of pitting cherries. The pitter has a hollowed-out cradle in which a single cherry is placed, and then a rod is pushed through it, forcing out the pit and leaving the fruit whole. This simple device doubles as an olive pitter. See CHERRY.
CHINOIS A fine cone-shaped strainer used for making stock, jellies, or purées. See also STRAINER.

continued

Cooking Tools, continued

EGG SLICER This tool is used to achieve uniform slices of hard-boiled eggs for salads, hors d'oeuvre platters, and other uses. The egg is placed on a rounded, slotted base attached to a frame composed of about 10 fine wires. The frame is pushed down through the egg, slicing it perfectly.

FUNNEL Metal and rigid plastic are the most common materials for funnels. Make sure they are not too large for your storage space and that the working ends fit easily in bottles and jars.

GARLIC PRESS Tool capable of mincing a peeled clove of garlic, so that it can be mixed more easily with other ingredients. The hinged tool is fitted with a perforated hopper and a plunger that squeezes the garlic through the perfora- tions. Some have a third arm accessory with small teeth that fit through the perfora- tions to push out the garlic waste. Others have plastic tubes for storing pressed garlic. The most useful are the simplest, made of metal rather than plastic. If you like garlic and use it a lot, look in specialty cookware shops or catalogs for oversized garlic presses capable of holding and pressing several cloves at a time.

HEAT DIFFUSER A disk that sits directly on a stove burner to shield fragile pots or delicate contents—hollandaise sauce, chocolate—from direct heat by diffusing it through two sheets of perforated metal with an air space between them. A second type of diffuser is a thick steel disk that stands about ¾ inch above the burner, the air space between the two modifying the intensity of the heat. The most popular brand of the latter type is the Flame-Tamer, a name that has become nearly synonymous with the tool itself.

ICE CREAM SCOOP Two styles of scoop are popular for spooning frozen ice cream and sherbet from containers: the dipper scoop and the half-sphere scoop. The dipper has a thick handle and a rounded, shallow bowl. The handle is hollow and transmits heat from your hand to the dipper. The half- sphere scoop has a full, deep bowl and a trigger-released metal wire that pushes the ice cream from the scoop. Some specialty shops and catalogs also carry electrically heated scoops that cut through ice cream more easily.

MEAT MALLET A mallet is useful for pounding boneless meat and poultry pieces until thin for quick and even cooking. Also called a meat pounder, although pounders tend to have one smooth side for flattening only, while mallets often have two sides, one with blunt teeth that help break down fibers in the meat, thus tenderizing it.

MELON BALLER Also known as a vegetable scoop, potato baller, or melon-ball scoop, this hand tool has a small bowl about 1 inch in diameter at one end used for making decorative balls from melon or other semi- firm foods. It is useful for coring some foods, such as pears, or preparing them for stuffing. Some scoops have a second, slightly smaller bowl at the opposite end of the handle.

MORTAR AND PESTLE This primitive pair of tools used for pounding and grinding in- gredients consists of a sturdy bowl-shaped mortar and a heavy, cylindrical pounder or pestle. While their work is often replaced nowadays by such mechanized tools as spice mills and food processors, the duo remains an excellent way to grind up spices or nuts, or to pound garlic together with fresh basil and pine nuts for pesto sauce at its most rustic. The best material for a mortar is marble, which is heavy, sturdy, and will not absorb food odors; heavy-duty ceramic models are also good. Pestles may be made from wood, metal, marble, or ceramic.

PIZZA WHEEL Although pizzas and open tarts can be cut with serrated knives, using a rotating pizza wheel, or pizza cutter, is more efficient. The sharp-edged wheels are from 2 to 4 inches in diameter; the metal or wooden handles are short and sturdy and are fitted with a protective thumb guard. Buy the sturdiest pizza wheel you can find, making sure it has a strong handle and a large thumb guard.

POTATO RICER A useful device for making smooth mashed potatoes and similar dishes. A plunger pushes potatoes through a perforated basket, reducing them to the consistency of grains of rice that are then stirred into a fluffy mass. See also RICING.

REAMER A handheld or freestanding tool designed to squeeze the juice from lemons, usually by means of a mound-shaped ridged surface pressed and twisted against and into a cut lemon half to help squeeze out the juice. See also JUICING.

SALAD SPINNER Also called a salad washer, this plastic device allows you to dry greens quickly and efficiently. Most salad spinners are 3-piece plastic contraptions with a perforated inner basket that is spun so that the water is removed from the washed greens by centrifugal force.

SALT GRINDER With the growing popularity of various types of coarse salt and sea salt, this handheld mill makes it possible to use them at table, reducing the flavorful salts to finer particles for seasoning individual portions of food. Unlike pepper mills, whose steel mechanisms would corrode with prolonged exposure to salt, these feature hardwood or heavy-duty plastic grinding mechanisms that crush the salt with the turn of a key, dispensing it from below.

SKEWERS Also called kabob or brochette skewers. Made of metal, wood, or bamboo, skewers have sharp points for pushing them through food. Metal skewers sometimes have looped handles to prevent food from sliding off. See also GRILLING.

SKIMMER Designed to skim frothy scum or foam from the tops of simmering stocks and other liquids, with a long handle and a large, shallow bowl of wire mesh or perforated metal. May also be used to remove pieces of food from hot fat when deep-frying. See also STRAINER.

STRAWBERRY HULLER Tweezerlike tinned steel tool with broad blades used to pluck the green stem from a strawberry without bruising the fruit. Also handy for picking out small bones that often remain in fish fillets.

ZESTER The citrus zester's metal blade at the end of a short handle is fitted with a row of 4 to 6 sharp-edged holes that allow for the removal of thin strips of the colorful outermost part of the peel while leaving behind the bitter white pith. See also ZESTING.

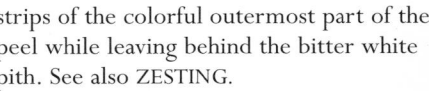

See also BAKEWARE; BAKING TOOLS; COOKWARE; GRILLING; KNIFE.

C

Cookware

The most important long-term investment the home cook makes is in cookware. Some would argue that it is more crucial to successful cooking than stove tops or ovens, as the kind and quality of cookware greatly affects the final outcome of a dish.

Peek into the cupboards of the best cooks you know and you likely will find an eclectic assortment of pots and pans of varying sizes, shapes, materials, and hefts.

Many beginning cooks, or those setting up a new kitchen, want to buy a complete set of pots and pans, all made by the same manufacturer and with the same design. While this is a convenient idea—and surely the matching pots and pans look handsome hanging from a pot rack—this is not the ideal way to buy cookware. Instead, select a few pieces at a time, building your stock over time as you learn more about cooking in general and your own cooking style in particular. As with all kitchen equipment, look for solid equipment that will last a lifetime. Lower-quality pots and pans tend to warp and dent easily, often do not hold heat well, and will probably end up needing to be replaced.

COOKWARE MATERIALS Different metals and alloys and different gauges (thicknesses) work most effectively for different cooking tasks.

ALUMINUM Heats rapidly and evenly, is durable and relatively inexpensive, but reacts with acidic foods and can impart a metallic taste. It also tends to warp if not of sufficient gauge. Select anodized aluminum, which has been treated with an electrolytic process to make it harder, denser, and resistant to corrosion.

CAST IRON Heats more slowly than some other materials but holds the heat extremely well and uniformly, even at high temperatures, making it good for frying and searing. It reacts with acidic foods and can impart a metallic taste. By the same token, it imparts a little iron into the food, which is beneficial. Regular cast iron is heavy and should always be dried after washing to prevent rusting. Enameled cast iron holds heat extremely well and is good for long, slow cooking but is prone to chipping and staining. See also SEASONING.

COPPER Heats and cools rapidly and evenly. Many cooks feel copper is the preferred metal for cookware. Copper cookware must be lined to avoid reactions with foods. Copper pans with stainless steel interiors and alloyed-aluminum and aluminum cores, which are durable and handsome, are a good compromise. They have good heft and heat quickly and evenly.

ENAMELED STEEL A good choice. Today's enameled steel is heavy and durable. It will not react with acidic foods.

GLASS Tempered to withstand both stovetop cooking and baking. It holds heat well and is noncorrosive, but heat conduction is not as uniform as with metal and there is the danger of breaking and cracking if glass cookware is mishandled.

NONSTICK SURFACES These popular coatings have steadily improved over the years. Unlike in the past, coatings today do not affect the metal's ability to conduct heat. In addition, they are durable and very easy to clean. Keep in mind that although nonstick is helpful for making omelets, oatmeal, and rice, it will interfere with browning meat.

STAINLESS STEEL Does not react with acidic ingredients and will not corrode, but it is a poor absorber of heat. Cladded stainless steel, that is, stainless steel exterior with a carbon core, boasts rapid and uniform heat conduction. Stainless steel with a layered alloyed-aluminum and aluminum core or an aluminum disk bottom also heats quickly and evenly, does not corrode, and is durable.

THE BASIC COOK Following are the pots and pans every kitchen should have.

BAKING DISH A shallow, rectangular dish made of tempered glass, porcelain, earthenware, or a pan made of metal, this all-purpose item works well for roasting meat or vegetables and baking brownies, gratins, or bread pudding.

BROILER PAN Also called a broiler tray, this rectangular pan is made to fit under a broiler's heat elements. Standard size is 9 by 12 inches and 1½ to 2 inches deep. Broiler pans come with a removable slotted tray to hold the food and allow drippings to fall into the bottom of the pan. Many oven manufacturers supply a broiler pan with their ovens.

CASSEROLE Deeper than your average baking dish, a casserole may be made of metal, porcelain, or stoneware, and usually comes with a fitted lid.

DUTCH OVEN Large, round or oval pots with tight-fitting lids and two loop handles used for slow cooking on top of the stove or in the oven. Most are made of enameled cast iron, although some are

made of regular cast iron or other uncoated metals. They range from 4 to 12 quarts; 8 or 9 quarts is recommended for most home kitchens. Also called heavy casseroles and stew pots.

FRYING PAN See Skillet, page 148.

ROASTING PAN AND RACK A large rectangular pan with handles that is sometimes fitted with a removable rack to hold the meat or turkey above the bottom of the pan. Roasting pans should be made from metal heavy enough to prevent them from warping or denting.

SAUCEPAN A simple round pan with either straight or sloping sides. In general, saucepans range in size from 1 to 5 quarts. Most useful is the 2-quart size. Traditional saucepans are twice as wide as they are high. This facilitates rapid evaporation, so that a sauce thickens and cooks efficiently. Straight-sided saucepans with high sides are ideal for longer cooking, since the liquid will not boil away so quickly. Slant-sided saucepans, commonly called chef's pans, with outwardly flaring sides, promote rapid evaporation, making them excellent for sauce making. The best materials for saucepans are anodized aluminum or aluminized steel.

SAUTÉ PAN Also known as a straight-sided frying pan. Sauté pans have a high, angled handle and relatively high sides so that the food can be flipped inside the pan and won't bounce out. The sides are 2½ to 4 inches high, with 3 inches being the height preferred by many cooks. Sauté pans are also very nice for braised dishes or any stove-top recipe that uses a lot of liquid. They may measure from 6 to 14¼ inches in diameter, and volume capacities generally

continued

Cookware, continued

range from one 1 to 7 quarts, with 2½ to 4 quarts being the most useful for the home cook. Sauté pans often have lids.

Sauté pan (top) and skillet (bottom).

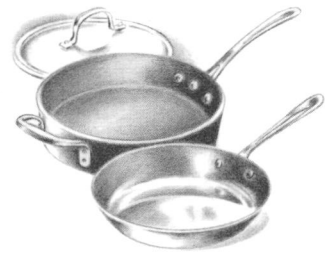

SKILLET Also called a frying pan, this broad pan is often confused with a sauté pan, but traditionally differs in that it has sides that flare outward, making it useful for cooking foods that must be stirred or turned out of the pan. Most kitchens should have both a smaller one, 9 or 10 inches across the bottom, and a larger one, 12 or 14 inches. Skillets do not have lids. The best materials are anodized aluminum or cast iron; if you buy two, make one of them nonstick.

STOCKPOT Also known as a spaghetti pot or soup pot, a stockpot is a high, narrow pot designed for minimal evaporation during long cooking. Stockpots are fitted with two looped handles for easy lifting and tight-fitting lids. They should be made of heavy-gauge metal with good heft. The smallest stockpots have an 8-quart capacity. Most home cooks find stockpots with 10- to 12-quart capacities to be the most useful.

THE WELL-STOCKED COOK You may eventually want to acquire these more specialized pots and pans, depending on the types of cooking you do.

CLAY POT Also known as clay cooker, terracotta baker, clay chicken pot, Römertopf, or Roman pot. Unglazed clay pots are meant for oven cooking, not stove top. Most are microwave safe. Because they are porous and because they are saturated with water before every use, they promote especially moist, succulent food. Chicken and other poultry are the most popular foods to cook in the pots, which are handsome enough to carry to the table for serving. See also CLAY POT.

CREPE PAN A small, shallow pan with flared sides that permit crepe batter to cook quickly and evenly. Its relatively long, flat handle is shaped so that the pan can be rotated easily during cooking. See also CREPE.

DEEP AND DOUBLE ROASTER This extra-deep roasting pan effectively creates a smaller oven within the environment of your kitchen's oven, speeding cooking time and promoting browning by holding in heat all around a roast. Most double roasters come with lids that transform them into large-sized dutch ovens. Some lids are mirror images of the bottom pans and offer the added convenience of effectively providing you with an additional roasting pan.

DOUBLE BOILER A set of two pans, one nesting atop the other, outfitted with one lid that fits both pans. A small amount of water is barely simmered in the lower pan, while ingredients are placed in the top pan to heat them gently, keep them warm, or melt them. See also DOUBLE BOILER.

FISH POACHER Specifically designed to fit whole fish (and can be used for large fillets), this deep, lidded poaching pan comes in a range of shapes and sizes. The most classic of these is a long, rectangular pan that fits across two burners, perfect for holding a side of salmon or even a whole salmon; a perforated rack fits inside, on which the fish may be easily lowered into or lifted from the poaching liquid. Smaller, oval poachers are ideal for whole flatfish such as sole, while a traditional rectangular French pot called a *turbotière* is made expressly for the cooking of whole turbot.

GRATIN DISH Shallow baking dish designed to maximize surface area for the formation of a well-browned, crisp crust. Gratin dishes of varying sizes may be made from metal, enameled metal, porcelain, or earthenware. See GRATIN.

GRIDDLE Flat rectangles or rounds of cast iron or cast aluminum, often with a non-stick finish, griddles sit flat on the stove top and are designed to be heated over one or two burners. They are used to

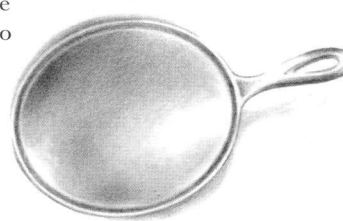

cook pancakes, eggs, bacon, thin steaks, cheese sandwiches, and more. Most have depressed rims to catch grease.

GRILL PAN A cast-iron skillet with ridges across the bottom for "grilling" meat or fish indoors. Some grill pans are designed for use in the broiler, others on top of the stove, fitting over one or two burners. Made of cast iron or anodized aluminum.

KETTLE In the old days, a kettle was any large pot used to boil water. Today, the word more specifically refers to teakettles designed to boil water quickly and to pour

Quick Tip

Not all pots and pans are made to sit on a burner, just as many are not made to go in the oven. Some can go from burner to oven, but not all. Be sure to read the instructions carefully that come with your pots and pans to determine if they are flameproof, ovenproof, or both. Flameproof means the pot or pan can go on a burner, whether it heats with gas flames, electric coils, or thermal induction. Ovenproof means the pot or pan can go into the oven.

it safely from an angled spout. Teakettles hold from 2 to 5 quarts and should have a removable lid for filling and cleaning and a stay-cool handle. A stockpot is often referred to as a soup kettle.

MULTIPURPOSE POT This tall pot with a tight-fitting lid is fitted with a perforated insert that cooks up to 2 pounds of pasta, which can be lifted from the pot for easy draining, as well as a steamer insert. Multipurpose pots usually have 6- or 8-quart capacities. They are useful for blanching.

OMELET PAN A shallow pan with rounded sloping sides, a long handle, and, preferably, a nonstick surface, for easy cooking and folding of omelets.

PASTA POT See Multipurpose Pot, above.

WOK This ingenious Chinese pan is a versatile cooking device ideal for stir-frying, deep-frying, and steaming. Traditionally made of plain steel, a good retainer of heat, the wok has a rounded bottom that allows small pieces of food to be rapidly tossed and stirred, while the gradually sloping sides help to keep the food inside the pan.

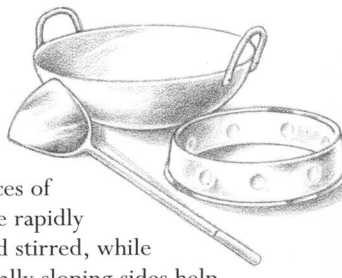

CORKSCREW Designing the perfect corkscrew is as challenging as designing the perfect mousetrap, but this has not stopped equipment designers from trying. Numerous devices for getting the cork out of a wine bottle are on the market, and in most cases which one you choose is a matter of personal preference. Most work well after a bit of practice, although a few are better than others. It is always a good idea to try out a new corkscrew on a bottle of inexpensive wine.

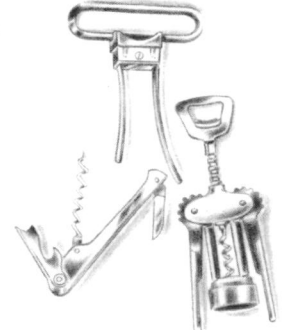

Corkscrews.

Corkscrews are no longer simply hefty screws topped with a perpendicular wooden handle. The twin-bladed cork puller consists of two slim metal shafts designed to grab the cork on either side while you pull it from the bottle. This style is especially useful for brittle older corks. Some find it tricky to use, but after a bit of practice, you'll be glad never to shred another cork. The double-screw corkscrew relies on two screws, one to invade the cork, the other to pull it from the bottle. When the screw on the double-wing corkscrew is twisted into the cork, two side handles are forced up; when they are pushed down, the cork rises from the bottle. Once you get the hang of the waiter's knife, tucked into the pocket of nearly every good waiter, it works beautifully. The tool has a handle that hooks onto the side of the bottle while the screw enters the cork. The cork is then levered from the bottle—and can be levered back into the bottle, too. Professional vintners and serious hobbyists often use a professional lever corkscrew, which effortlessly pulls corks from the bottles and just as effortlessly pushes them back. The tools are large and expensive. Finally, a device called a Screwpull is popular with many wine lovers. The specially engineered screw easily enters the cork as a levered handle is turned in one direction, and then, when the handle is turned in the other direction, the cork is pulled from the bottle.

CORN One of the joys of summer in temperate climates is eating freshly picked sweet corn. The briefly cooked kernels are sweet and crisp and usually need no more than a sprinkling of salt and pepper, or perhaps a pat of butter. The season for this golden grain, which many people erroneously consider a vegetable, is fleeting, and corn lovers anticipate it just as happily as they do the tomato crop, frequently pairing the two at meals. But corn plays an important role in our culinary universe year-round, not just during its short season.

Corn, whose true name is maize, is one of the world's most important crops. It is used to make oil, corn syrup, cornstarch, cornmeal, breakfast cereal, bread, and tortillas. In addition, field corn is fed to cattle and hogs, which is perhaps its most expansive role. Not all corn is yellow. Some types are white or a mixture of white and yellow kernels. Blue corn, grown in the

Southwest and Mexico, is used mainly for chips, cornmeal, and flour. Popcorn, a sizable crop, is used for only one thing.

See also BOILING; CORN BREAD; CORNMEAL; POLENTA.

Selecting Sweet corn is sold fresh, canned, and frozen. When fresh, it is sold on the cob, usually still in its outer green husk. It is at its best when just picked, with the freshest ears usually found at farmers' markets. Choose ears with green husks with no signs of browning or drying. They should feel cool, never noticeably warm. The silk, or tassels, should be pale yellow and moist, showing no signs of drying or rot. Whether the kernels are yellow or white, or a combination of the two, they should be tightly packed in even rows and look plump and juicy. Freshness is more crucial than the color of the kernel. If shopping in a supermarket, buy corn only if it is displayed in a refrigerated section. The ear may be partially husked and wrapped in plastic, revealing the kernels.

Quick Bite

When you tear back the husk to view the corn in the market, you are shortening its shelf life. Once the husk is removed, the corn begins to lose moisture and freshness more quickly.

Corn kernels are sold frozen, and you can sometimes find frozen corn on the cob. Frozen corn retains much of its good flavor and texture and can be used in place of fresh corn in many recipes.

Storing Fresh sweet corn should be kept wrapped in its husks in a cool place—a cooler or the refrigerator—until you are ready to cook it, preferably for no longer than a day. The natural sugar in corn begins to turn to starch the minute the ear is picked, so corn should be consumed as soon as possible after harvest. But this time-

Corn Glossary

CORN HUSKS, DRIED Dried corn husks (outer leaves) used to wrap tamales, sold packaged in specialty and Mexican stores. Corn husks are not meant to be eaten, but they give the tamales a deeper corn flavor.

CORNMEAL Any meal ground from dried corn, whether made from yellow, white, or blue corn; fine, medium, or coarse in texture; ground by millstones or steel rollers; and with or without the corn's husk and germ included. See CORNMEAL; POLENTA.

GRITS A ground meal of yellow or white hominy, cooked like cornmeal to a thick porridge. See also GRAIN.

HOMINY Mildly sweet-tasting, firm-textured kernels of dried white or yellow corn that have been soaked in a lye solution to slough off their hulls. See also GRAIN.

POLENTA Italian-style cornmeal, cooked in either water or stock until it becomes thick and porridgelike. See GRAIN; POLENTA.

POPCORN A type of corn that, because of its composition and ratio of protein to starch, "pops" through its outer skin and expands when heated.

SAMP Dried hominy that has been broken into large pieces or pounded into coarse meal, less refined than grits. Grits can be used in place of samp in most recipes.

honored admonishment about corn is not as true as it once was. Growers have developed new supersweet and sugar-enhanced varieties that make longer storage (and, consequently, long-distance shipping) possible. This means that some fresh in-season corn will keep for more than a day, and that out-of-season corn on the cob now may be quite delicious, although traditional summertime feasts of golden fried chicken and butter-slathered ears of corn seldom taste as good on a blustery fall day.

Preparing Strip the husks and silk from the ears, snapping the leaves off the bottom along with any remaining stem (unless you want to keep it as a handle for eating). Stubbornly clinging strands of corn silk can be removed by scrubbing the corn under cold running water with a vegetable brush.

To cut kernels from the cob, uncooked or cooked, break the cob in half and hold each cob half upright, flat end down. Using a sharp knife, slice straight down between the kernels and the cob, but not too deeply, to avoid the kernels' fibrous bases. If you want the corn milk for a recipe, place the cob's flat end in a shallow bowl as you cut. Run the back of the knife blade along the length of the ear after removing the kernels to squeeze every drop into the bowl.

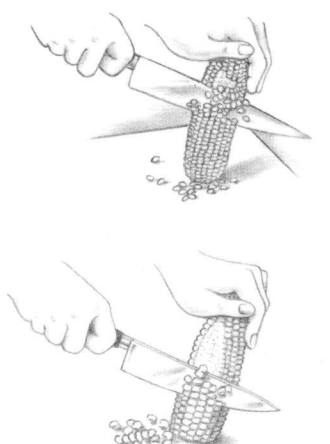

To get creamed corn or just the corn pulp and not the kernels, first score the individual rows of kernels by running the tip of your knife down each row. Then, stand-ing the ear on one end, run a spoon or the back of a knife blade along the kernels with enough pressure to express the milk and pulp but leave the skin behind.

You can drop fresh corn into boiling water and cook it quickly, or grill it or roast it in the oven or on a barbecue, usually brushed first with oil or butter and wrapped in foil. Four or five ears may be cooked successfully in the microwave. The kernels can be cut from the cob and sautéed, steamed, boiled, or added to soups, fritters, puddings, stews, casseroles, salads, and fresh relishes.

See also BOILING.

CORN BREAD An American favorite, corn bread is a quick bread made with cornmeal. Because of the inclusion of flour and sugar, corn bread in the North tends to be cakier and sweeter than Southern corn bread, made with just cornmeal, liquid, salt, leavener, and a little fat. Corn bread can be made with any type of cornmeal. Stone-ground cornmeal gives the bread fuller flavor and better texture, but corn bread is still good made with ordinary steel-cut cornmeal. Commercial mixes yield acceptable breads, although they tend to be sweet. Like all quick breads, corn bread should be baked immediately after the batter is mixed.

Corn bread usually is baked in a square or rectangular pan or, more traditionally, a cast-iron skillet, and sometimes in a loaf pan, muffin cups, or corn-stick pans, for bread shaped like ears of corn. While most modern recipes call for baking the bread in the oven, skillet corn bread can be "baked" on top of a stove, over a campfire, or nestled in the hot ashes of a fireplace. Many recipes, particularly those from the South, call for melting butter or bacon fat in the pan and then pouring the batter into the hot pan, resulting in a crisp, tender crust.

A lightly sweetened corn bread, split and spread with an aromatic honey, is good for breakfast, while a more savory version is wonderful with stews, soups, and chili. In recent years, making corn bread with roasted peppers or hot chiles such as jalapeños, and sometimes with Cheddar cheese as well, has become popular, especially as an accompaniment to chili.

See also CORNMEAL; QUICK BREAD.

CORNED BEEF See BEEF.

CORNISH GAME HEN Also known as a rock Cornish game hen or Cornish hen. This diminutive bird is a hybrid of two kinds of poultry, the Cornish game cock and the white Plymouth Rock hen. The Cornish game hen weighs from 1 to 1¼ pounds and is large enough to serve one or two people. Sold frozen in almost every supermarket, Cornish hens are available fresh, or fresh hens may be ordered. They may be substituted for poussins, chicken, and squabs and are usually roasted or grilled, either halved or whole. They may also be braised. Because of their delicate flavor, these birds pair well with mild marinades and sauces.

Selecting Choose fresh hens when possible; they should smell fresh and have no discoloration. The flesh should be firm and resilient. Packaged birds should not have accumulated liquid in the package. Frozen birds should not have pink-tinged ice.

Storing Store in the refrigerator in the original packaging, adding a layer of plastic to birds wrapped only in butcher paper. Use within 2 days of purchase.

Preparing One Cornish hen will feed one or two people. Prepare as for any poultry: remove the innards, wash and pat dry, and pluck any remaining feathers with a pair of tweezers or needle-nosed pliers.

See also CHICKEN; SQUAB.

CORNMEAL Made from yellow, white, or blue corn, cornmeal can be ground fine, medium, or coarse, and any one of these grinds can be used in recipes requiring cornmeal, unless otherwise specified. There is no difference between yellow and white cornmeal in terms of taste and usage, although yellow cornmeal has more vitamin A. Blue cornmeal is considered a specialty food and produces pleasingly nutty, full-flavored baked goods.

Stone-ground cornmeal is preferred by many home cooks because it contains the germ of the corn, giving it a fuller, slightly nutty flavor and more nutrients. It is literally ground between stones, often powered by water (for water-ground cornmeal), rather than steel-cut by more modern, industrialized equipment. Stone-ground cornmeal is softer, moister, and more perishable than steel-cut. Other cornmeal, labeled "enriched degerminated," contains only the starchy endosperm and has a longer shelf life. Cornmeal is used to make cornbread, polenta, corn pudding, spoon bread, Johnnycakes, and batter bread. It is also sprinkled on baking stones to keep pizza and focaccia doughs from sticking.

Selecting Buy stone-ground cornmeal if possible. Health-food stores and farmers' markets often sell cornmeal ground by small mills. These meals tend to be tastier than others, so try them if you can. Otherwise, buy the cornmeal available at the market, checking the sell-by date, particularly if the cornmeal is one of the more perishable stone-ground varieties.

Storing Stone-ground cornmeal will become rancid and stale with age. It must be stored in the refrigerator, where it will keep for up to 4 months. Degerminated cornmeal in an airtight container can be stored at cool room temperature for up to 1 year.

See also CORN; CORN BREAD; POLENTA.

CORNSTARCH A highly refined, silky powder made from the endosperm of the corn kernel and used to thicken sauces, puddings, fruit fillings and glazes, and stews. Sauces and glazes thickened with cornstarch have a glossy sheen, unlike those thickened with flour, which are opaque. Cornstarch has nearly twice the thickening power of flour.

Selecting Buy any commercial brand of cornstarch in the size of box suited to your cooking needs.

Storing Store cornstarch in a cool, dry cupboard for up to 1 year after its sell-by date. In humid climates, enclose the box in a plastic bag.

Preparing Cornstarch should be whisked with a small amount of cold water (1 part cornstarch to 3 parts liquid) to make what is called a slurry before it is added to a dish. It is then cooked gently for a minute or so to eliminate any starchy taste. Take care not to let the liquids boil once the cornstarch has been added, or the sauce will thin out.

See also THICKENING.

CORN SYRUP This syrup, made from cornstarch, is used to sweeten everything from commercial candies and jams to snack cakes and cookies. It also is used in home cooking and baking. Available in dark and light versions, corn syrup does not crystallize when heated, which makes it desirable for candy making. It also adds moisture and chewiness to cakes and cookies. Dark corn syrup has more flavor than light syrup. Imitation pancake syrups are made by adding maple flavoring to corn syrup.

Selecting Corn syrup is sold in glass bottles. Buy either dark or light, depending on your cooking needs or recipe.

Storing Store unopened corn syrup in a cool, dark cupboard for up to 6 months after the sell-by date. Once opened, it should be stored in the same cupboard for up to 6 months. To discourage spoiling, keep the syrup tightly capped and wipe any spillage from the outside of the bottle.

Preparing Use as directed in individual recipes. Light corn syrup can be used in place of dark, although it's generally best to use what a recipe directs. The reverse is not always true because dark corn syrup might add too much flavor to some dishes. Dark or light corn syrup can be used in place of honey in recipes, although you should expect it to be sweeter than honey, with a less interesting flavor. Light corn syrup can be substituted in equal measure for granulated sugar in many instances, although not in baking. Dark corn syrup can be substituted for molasses, although it is not as sweet.

CORRECTING THE SEASONING See ADJUSTING THE SEASONING.

COTTAGE CHEESE See CHEESE.

COURT-BOUILLON (KOOR bwee-YAWN) A stock requiring only short cooking (*court* means "short" in French) and used most often to cook fish, seafood, and vegetables. Court-bouillon may be used as a poaching or braising liquid and then discarded, or can become the base for a sauce. It is made from water and aromatic vegetables such as onions, celery, and carrots, along with a bouquet garni.

Court-bouillon also contains an acidic ingredient, such as vinegar, lemon juice, or wine, useful for keeping fish firm during poaching. Vegetable stock can be used in place of court-bouillon, although if using it to cook fish, add a dash of lemon juice.

See also BOUQUET GARNI.

COUSCOUS Couscous is a pasta made from semolina flour, which is coarsely ground from the hulled berries of durum wheat. The semolina is mixed with water and salt, formed into tiny, round pellets, and then steamed and dried. Some couscous also contains plain whole-wheat flour, or it also may be made from ground millet, corn, or barley.

Like other pastas, couscous does not have much flavor on its own but takes well to combining with other, stronger-flavored foods. Couscous is a staple throughout North Africa, where it is cooked in a double-tiered pot called a *couscousière*. For the hearty, traditional dish, also known as couscous, lamb or chicken, vegetables, and spices cook in the lower tier while the small grains of couscous steam in the perforated top tier, where they are flavored by the aromatic vapor produced below.

Selecting Buy regular or instant (quick-cooking) couscous, regular or large-grained, depending on the recipe and your needs. Regular couscous takes a little longer to cook than instant and is a little lighter and fluffier. Most recipes can be made with either, however, and instant couscous is often easier to find in the market. Couscous is available in most supermarkets and health-food stores and also in Middle Eastern markets and specialty stores. It usually is sold in packages but is sometimes available in bulk.

Storing Once its package is open, couscous should be stored in a cool, dry cupboard and will keep very well for at least 3 months and far longer in the refrigerator. A sealed package keeps indefinitely in a cool, dry place.

Preparing When cooking couscous, the goal is to let the grains absorb moisture and swell as much as possible. Many cooks feel regular couscous, not instant, does a better job of this, and steaming is the best way to cook it. Steam regular couscous in a perforated basket or sieve above boiling water for 20 to 30 minutes, or cook it in boiling liquid for about 10 minutes and then let it stand for 15 to 20 minutes until softened and swelled. Stir instant couscous into boiling water, remove from the heat, and let it sit for 5 to 10 minutes to soften and expand. Using a fork, be sure to fluff the couscous to separate the grains before serving.

COWPEA See BEAN, DRIED.

CRAB Crabs, like lobsters and shrimp, are crustaceans. Hundreds of varieties of crabs live in the world's waters. In the United States, a crab's popularity is determined by its local availability: along the Atlantic and Gulf coasts, blue crabs are eaten most often; in southern Florida, stone crabs are considered delicacies; along the Pacific coast from southern California to Washington, the Dungeness is the crab of choice; and in Alaska, king crab and snow crab reign supreme.

Like lobsters, crabs must be kept alive until cooking, after which their shells turn bright red. They are a little more tricky to eat than lobster, although in crab-eating regions such as Charleston and Maryland's eastern shore, folks think nothing of the messy task. In other parts of the country, many people prefer buying the sweet, velvety crabmeat out of the shell and already cooked, although you'll have better flavor if you extract the meat yourself. On the West Coast, Dungeness crab is usually sold cooked but still in the shell, although it is possible to buy the giant shellfish live for cooking at home. Alaskan king crab and snow crab are nearly always sold cooked and frozen except in Alaska, where they can be bought fresh.

Selecting Live hard-shelled crabs should move their claws with some vigor when poked. Live soft-shelled crabs should look moist and soft, with no hint of hardening shell. When you lift a crab, if its claws drop, reject it. Ideally, buy them immedi-

ately before you plan to cook them, and go directly home from the market. The only exception is if a fishmonger will pack the crabs in seaweed and then in special boxes for transport.

Cooked crabmeat usually is pasteurized and sold in cans or vacuum-packed plastic bags. It is commonly served cold, in salads or with cocktail sauces, as heating diminishes its flavor, although it is also used to

Crab Glossary

The following entries describe the characteristics and uses of the six types of crab most widely available in North America. Thousands of other edible crab species exist, however, leading to the possible availability of other local types in coastal areas. Feel free to substitute any variety of crabmeat that appeals to you for another in a recipe.

ALASKAN KING CRAB The best meat found in this type of crab is located in the long, spindly legs. The legs are cooked and frozen before being shipped.

BLUE CRAB Plentiful and popular on the Atlantic and Gulf coasts, these pleasant, mild-flavored crabs have dark green to black shells. They are used for much of the pasteurized crabmeat sold across the country, although they are also served whole. See also Soft-Shelled Crab, below.

DUNGENESS CRAB Large and delicious, the Dungeness is usually sold cooked in markets on the West Coast—and with increasing frequency elsewhere across the country.

SNOW CRAB A type of spider crab found in Alaskan waters with skinny legs and flavorful meat. The claws are available frozen, already cracked for easy eating, but most of the catch is used for crabmeat.

SOFT-SHELLED CRAB Before they reach their full maturity, blue crabs shed their hard shells several times. When they do, they are known as soft-shelled crabs during the days before they grow new, larger hard shells. Available from the spring to early autumn, they are meant to be eaten whole, soft shell and all.

STONE CRAB The only part of the stone crab that is eaten is the claws. When a crab is caught, a claw is pulled off the live crab. The crab is then returned to the sea where it will eventually grow a new one. The claws are usually sold cooked and eaten cold—except in southern Florida, where they are cooked and served hot.

make crab cakes. Some fishmongers sell crab meat freshly cooked and unpasteurized, packed in plastic tubs. This is usually meat from blue crabs. Lump crabmeat, also called backfin or jumbo, is the most desirable, as it is white meat taken from the center of the body and is in the largest pieces. Flake crabmeat is light and dark meat from the center and legs and is in smaller pieces; it's still tasty. If possible, avoid cooked crabmeat that has been frozen.

Storing Although it is always best to cook live crabs on the day you purchase them, properly packed live crabs can be refrigerated for up to 2 days. Lay them in a shallow bowl and nestle the bowl in a larger one containing ice. Cover the crabs with a damp kitchen towel or with wet seaweed, if it came with the crabs. Replace the ice as needed. Properly stored, the crabs should still be alive after a day or so. Discard any that are no longer living.

Freshly cooked crabmeat will keep in the refrigerator for 2 days; if the crabmeat has been frozen and thawed, eat it on the day you buy it. Pasteurized crabmeat packed in vacuum-sealed bags will keep in the refrigerator for 3 to 4 weeks. Frozen crab will keep in the freezer for 4 months; thaw in the refrigerator.

HOW TO *Clean Hard-Shelled Crabs*

Blue crabs can be cleaned while still alive or after they are cooked. For eating whole, they are cleaned after cooking; for soups and stews, they are cleaned first.

1. Rinse the crab under cold running water and scrub it with a small brush to remove any sand and grit.
2. Plunge the crab into boiling water for about 30 seconds and then rinse it under cold water to halt the cooking. (If it is already cooked, ignore this step.)
3. Using your hands, twist off the crab's legs and claws and set them aside.

4. Turn the crab upside down, and use your thumb to peel back and twist the apron off the body. The apron is the small triangular shell flap on the underside of the crab.

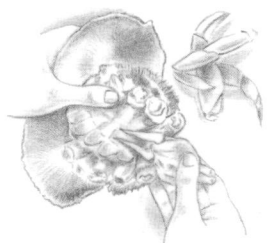

5. Insert your thumbs into the small crevice between the underside of the crab's body and its top shell. Pull them apart, lifting the top shell off the body and keeping the body intact.

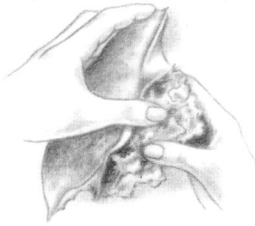

6. Pull or scrape out the liver and dark gray intestines from the center of the body, along with any roe you might find (the roe is dark before cooking and orange afterward). Scrape and rinse out the top shell if it is to be used in serving the crab. When the shell of Dungeness crab is removed for eating, underneath are its edible organs and fat called "crab butter" or "crab mustard." This yellow mass should be saved and eaten with the crab.

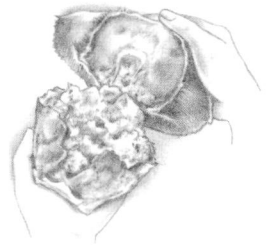

continued

7. Using a spoon or your fingers, scrape or pull off the spongy, feather-shaped white gills, known as "dead man's fingers," from either side of the body.

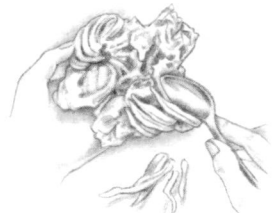

8. In blue crabs, remove the sand sac in the head behind the eyes. For Dungeness crabs, lift out the white intestine that runs along the back and remove the small mouth section as well.

9. If the crab is uncooked, cut the center section of the body in half or quarters using a sharp knife. Use the crab in soup or stock. If it is already cooked, break the crab's body in half to reveal the meat. Using your fingers, a knife, or a lobster pick, remove the meat from all the body cavities.

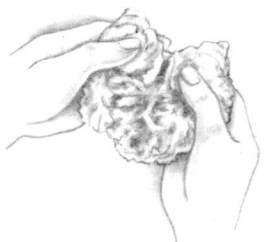

10. Using a mallet or lobster cracker, crack the shells of the claws in several places, as well as any legs large enough to contain a good amount of meat. Break away the shell pieces and remove the meat with your fingers or a lobster pick.

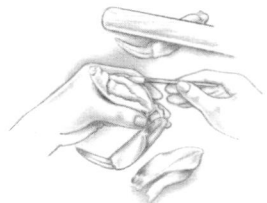

HOW TO *Clean Soft-Shelled Crabs*

1. Rinse quickly under cold water.

2. Turn the crab over and pull off and discard the apron, the small triangular shell flap on the underside of the crab.

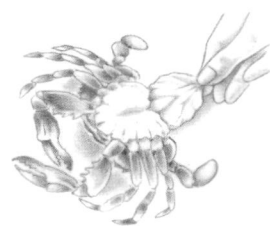

3. With a small knife or sharp scissors, cut off the crab's eyes—but not the entire head—by making a straight cut about ¼ inch behind the mouth and eyes.

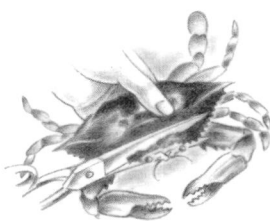

4. Squeeze the body gently and use the point of a knife to pull out the small bubblelike sand sac that hides behind the mouth.

5. Fold back the points of the top shell on either side of the crab to expose the spongy, feather-shaped white gills and pull off the gills from either side of the body.

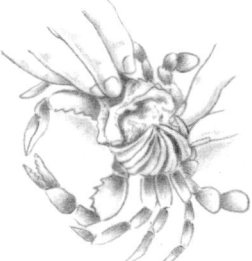

6. Cook immediately.

CRANBERRY See BERRY.

CRANBERRY BEAN See BEAN, DRIED; BEAN, FRESH.

CRAYFISH A small freshwater crustacean, which abounds in the South (where it is called crawfish). Crayfish resemble tiny lobsters. They are prized for their sweet, succulent tail meat. Usually cooked by steaming or boiling, they are eaten hot or cold on their own or shelled in gumbos or other Cajun and Creole dishes.
Selecting Crayfish should be bought alive or frozen.
Storing Store live crayfish in the refrigerator covered with a damp kitchen towel for no more than 1 or 2 days. Keep frozen crayfish for up to 3 months. Once defrosted, they should not be refrozen, or their texture will deteriorate. Cooked crayfish may be refrigerated for up to 3 days.
Preparing Before cooking, discard any dead crayfish. Like lobster and crab, crayfish will turn red when they are cooked, usually within 5 minutes. Take care not to overcook them.

CREAM People of a certain age may remember the days when the milkman left glass bottles of milk on the back stoop every morning. The unhomogenized milk naturally separated, with the cream rising to the top, hence the vernacular expressions that compare cream and excellence. These days, nearly all commercial milk is homogenized, a process that uniformly disperses the fat throughout the milk, so that the cream cannot separate from it.

Fresh milk contains fat, and it is this fat that makes cream sublime. Cream is sold according to the amount of milk fat it contains, with heavy cream containing the most and half-and-half the least. In between are light whipping cream and light cream. Cream is also used to make sour cream, cream cheese, and ice cream.

Nearly all cream sold by large dairies today is ultrapasteurized, which involves heating the cream to 300°F to kill certain microorganisms and extend shelf life, but which gives it a mildly cooked taste and makes it a little harder to whip.

Selecting Buy the kind of cream called for in a recipe. To make whipped cream, buy heavy cream (whipping cream) or light whipping cream. Light cream and half-and-half will not whip. Some specialty stores and farmers' markets sell minimally processed cream that has not been put through the ultrapasteurization process. This cream whips better but is more perishable. For most sauce-making purposes, buy heavy cream.

Storing Cream should be kept in the coldest part of the refrigerator, usually the back of the bottom shelf. Unopened ultra-pasteurized cream will keep for about a month, or 3 or 4 days past the sell-by date. Once opened, it will keep for up to 4 days. Other cream will keep for 2 or 3 days after its sell-by date. Heavy cream can be frozen for up to 4 months and used for baking, frostings, and sauces, but once frozen and defrosted, it will not whip. When using cream, pour just the amount of cream you need from the carton and return the carton to the refrigerator as quickly as possible. Do not pour room-temperature cream back into the carton; instead, store it separately in a lidded glass jar.

Quick Tip

Cream that is reaching the end of its life will form flecks in hot coffee, a result of its interacting with the acid in the beverage. It is still fine to use at this point, but it also is time to put cream on your shopping list. When cream is spoiled you will know it by a single whiff.

Preparing Whip chilled heavy or light whipping cream in a metal bowl with a whisk, an egg beater, a handheld mixer, or in a stand mixer fitted with a whisk. For the best results, put the bowl and whisk or beaters in the refrigerator for an hour or more to chill them. Blenders are not recommended, as they don't aerate the cream properly and are apt to whip it into butter, but large amounts of cream can be whipped in a food processor fitted with a specially designed whipping attachment. The cream will not, however, ever reach the same billowing heights it will in a bowl. Process the cream just until it rises in the bowl and thickens. Still, beware of overbeating, which can happen quickly in a food processor. For most uses, whip cream just until it forms soft peaks. When the whisk is lifted from the cream, the cream should form a peak that gently falls to one side. For piping, cream should be whipped to

ᴖ‿ᴗ Cream Glossary ᴖ‿ᴗ

HEAVY CREAM This cream has the most milk fat, containing between 36 and 40 percent but averaging about 36 percent. Whips up to a very dense and stable whipped cream, less voluminous than light cream, which can be useful for piped cake decorations. Also can be labeled heavy whipping cream or just whipping cream.

LIGHT WHIPPING CREAM Contains only slightly less milk fat than heavy cream, from 30 to 36 percent. Whips up to a softer, slightly more voluminous whipped cream than heavy cream does.

LIGHT CREAM Similar to half-and-half, this product is also known as coffee cream or table cream and contains 15 to 20 percent milk fat. It cannot be whipped.

HALF-AND-HALF A mixture of milk and cream, containing from 10 to 18 percent milk fat. It is used for coffee, to pour over cereal and berries, and in many creamed soup recipes. You can make your own, in a pinch, by combining equal parts milk and heavy cream. It cannot be whipped.

stiff peaks, which hold their shape and stand upright when the whisk is lifted.

Whipped cream, soft peaks.

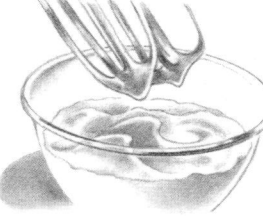

Whipped cream, stiff peaks.

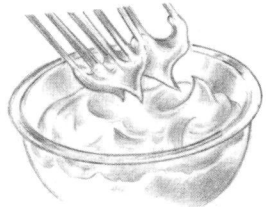

See also MILK; SOUR CREAM.

CREAM CHEESE See CHEESE.

CREAMING A recipe for cake batter or cookie dough typically starts with instructions to "cream the butter" or "cream the butter with the sugar."

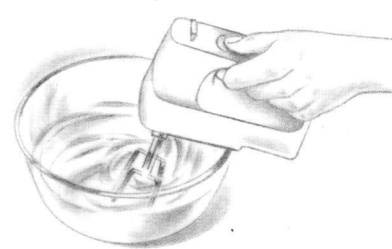

Creaming means beating fat, or fat plus another ingredient, until it becomes soft and smooth. You should first whip or beat softened (not melted) butter alone until it expands, lightens in color, and is as soft and smooth as possible. This can be done using an electric mixer or by hand with a wooden spoon or wire whisk. Give the

butter a little time to cream—it may take 3 or 4 minutes with an electric mixer, or longer by hand, to reach the desired stage. Do not rush this step; thorough creaming aerates the butter and contributes to the lightness of the final product.

Once the butter is creamed, add the sugar, again beating until the mixture is fluffy and light. At this point, the mixture may be referred to as batter. Creamed batter is often described as soft, smooth, and pale yellow or ivory. The grains of sugar should be fully incorporated into the butter. If you rub a little creamed batter between your fingertips, it should not feel gritty. Besides sweetening the batter, the sharp, crystalline edges of the sugar actually cut into the butter and create many tiny air bubbles. In fact, the creamed mixture has almost twice the original volume of its two components when sufficient time has been taken to do it correctly.

When adding other ingredients such as flour and eggs to creamed batter, be sure not to overwork it, or you may destroy the air bubbles and the resultant lightening effect of creaming.

CREAM OF TARTAR This powdery white substance, found in every supermarket and most kitchens, is potassium tartrate, a by-product of wine making. Once a common leavening agent for breads made without yeast, today cooks use it to stabilize egg whites so that they whip up well. (The common ratio is ⅛ teaspoon cream of tartar for each egg white.) Also used in candy making, cream of tartar inhibits sugar from crystallizing. Some cake recipes, such as angel food cake, include cream of tartar for whiter, finer crumbs and greater loft. It also contributes to the creaminess of frostings. Cream of tartar, an acid, is mixed with baking soda, an alkaline, to make commercial baking powder.

Selecting Buy any reliable brand of cream of tartar, which usually is packaged in a jar or can with a tight-fitting lid.
Storing Store it in a cool, dry cupboard for up to 1 year.

CRÈME BRÛLÉE (KREM broo-LAY)

A rich, satiny egg custard topped with a thin caramel crust. This dessert is a standard on restaurant menus, and a growing number of home cooks are attempting it in their own kitchens. The juxtaposition of textures—creamy custard and brittle caramel—has sent this indulgence to the top of many dessert lovers' lists of all-time favorites.

In restaurants today, the caramel topping usually is made by scattering granulated white or brown sugar over cold custard and passing a very hot butane torch over the sugar to melt and caramelize it. Such devices are now being made in miniature size for the home cook, but most nonprofessionals rely on hot broilers to melt the sugar.

Alternatively, one can pour hot, liquid caramel over cold custards and allow it to harden to a shiny crust. The advantage of this latter method is that the dessert can be assembled 10 to 12 hours ahead of time; the disadvantage is that the caramel crust will soften as the dessert sits. The ultimate crème brûlée has a still-warm, brittle, dark caramel crust on top of a cool, creamy custard.

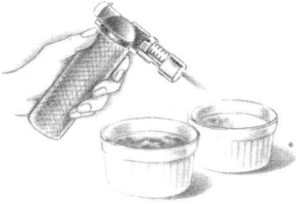

Caramelizing the sugar.

Crème Brûlée Savvy

■ If using an electric broiler, preheat it for at least 5 minutes so that it is very hot (gas broilers require no preheating). Position the broiler pan 2 to 3 inches from the heat to cook the sugar quickly without heating the custard.

■ Do not take the custard-filled ramekins from the refrigerator until the last minute. The interaction of the cold custard and hot sugar is crucial to forming a good crisp topping.

■ If using brown sugar, sift it to remove any lumps before sprinkling it evenly over the custards. Or use granulated brown (or white) sugar, which requires no sifting.

■ Place the custards in a water bath to keep them from heating up. For more details, see WATER BATH.

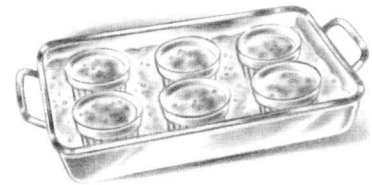

■ Turn the ramekins during broiling if necessary to help the sugar melt and caramelize as evenly as possible.

■ For the best effect, serve crème brûlée immediately after preparing it.

See also CARAMELIZING; CUSTARD; WATER BATH.

CRÈME FRAÎCHE (KREM FRESH)

A soured, cultured cream product, originally from France, crème fraîche is similar to sour cream. The silken, thick cream is tangy and sweet, with a hint of nuttiness, and adds incomparable flavor when used as a topping for berries and pastry desserts. It is also delicious paired with smoked salmon and trout, and lends a velvety smoothness and rich flavor to soups and sauces. Crème fraîche, which is 30 percent fat, is not always easy to find, and many home cooks make their own (see below).

Selecting Crème fraîche is sold in some supermarkets as an ultrapasteurized cream product. It is far more expensive than cream or sour cream. Because it loses flavor as it sits on the refrigerator shelf, buy it as fresh as possible. It is also sold in gourmet markets and cheese shops, often made by the purveyor or a local supplier. No two are exactly the same.

Storing Refrigerate for up to 2 weeks. Homemade crème fraîche will keep in a covered container for 1 week.

HOW TO *Make Crème Fraîche*

1. To make 1 cup crème fraîche, combine 1 cup heavy cream and 1 tablespoon buttermilk in a small saucepan over medium-low heat. Heat to lukewarm. Do not allow it to simmer.
2. Remove from the heat, cover, and allow to thicken at warm room temperature, which can take from 8 to 48 hours, depending on your taste and recipe needs.
3. Once it is as thick and flavorful as you want it, refrigerate to chill well before using.

CREMINO See MUSHROOM.

CREPE (KREP or KRAPE) A very thin pancake made from a pourable batter. Anyone who has stopped at a sidewalk crepe stand in France wants to try to duplicate that experience back home. Crepes are filled or sauced with creamy, savory mixtures and served for brunch or light suppers or with sweet mixtures for dessert. Crepes can be folded around a filling into halves, quarters, or envelopes.

Filled and folded crepes.

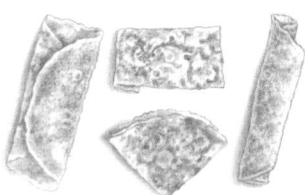

They can also be rolled into open-ended rolls, or stacked with filling between the layers and cut into wedges like a cake. The term *crepe* applies both to the pancakes and to the final dish. The pancakes can be made well ahead of time, stacked, and refrigerated and then filled and reheated. They also freeze well. Unlike other pancakes, crepes are not leavened, so they do not puff up when cooked.

Crepe batter must be made ahead of time, since it needs to chill for at least an hour (and will keep as long as 12 hours). During chilling, the flour expands and absorbs the liquid, a step that is essential for tender crepes. Crepes destined for dessert are often made from a slightly sweetened batter, while those for savory fillings are made with an unsweetened batter.

Crepes should be cooked in a small skillet or in a crepe pan, which is a small, shallow pan with flared sides and a long, flat handle, just large enough to cook one crepe at a time. Its configuration makes it easy to rotate the pan, first to spread the melted butter over its surface, and then the batter. The shape also makes it easy to flip the crepe during cooking.

Crepe pan.

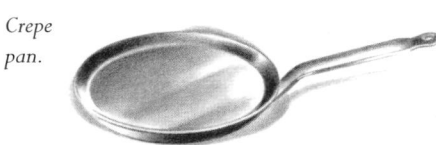

Crepe Savvy

- Crepe batter should be very smooth and free of lumps. Whip the batter in a blender or food processor, or use a whisk if mixing by hand. Beat the eggs into the batter one at a time and add the milk gradually while stirring to ensure a smooth batter. Some cooks recommend straining the whisked batter to eliminate even the tiniest clumps of flour.

- Before adding melted butter to the batter, let it cool down for 1 to 2 minutes to avoid curdling the eggs.
- When putting butter in the heated crepe pan, use only enough to film the bottom. Brush on the fat as you need it before starting a new crepe. It averages out to about ½ teaspoon butter per crepe. If using a nonstick pan, it is not necessary to grease it, although the butter also adds good flavor.
- Ladle in only enough batter to spread in a thin layer as you tilt the pan. This is usually 3 to 4 tablespoons batter for a 7-inch crepe.

Swirling batter.

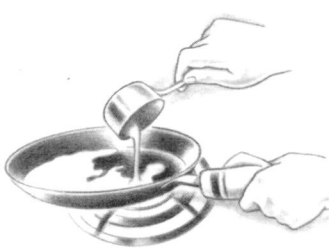

- If needed, run a knife around the edge of the crepe after it has set a bit to keep it from sticking.
- If you cannot flip the crepe by shaking the pan, slip a small knife or spatula under the pancake and turn it, using the tool or your fingers.

Flipping a crepe.

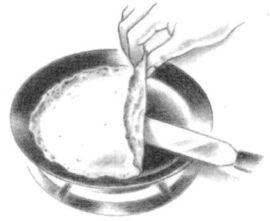

- Placing a square of waxed paper atop each crepe as you stack them will prevent them from sticking together.

CREPE PAN See COOKWARE.

CRIMPING To seal together the edges of two pieces of pastry dough by pressing the dough with the tines of a kitchen fork, the side of a knife, or a pastry crimper. Crimping differs from fluting in that you press down the dough with a tool in order to seal it, while fluting means to make a decorative shape with your fingers. Crimping is a good way to seal together securely the uncooked crusts of a double-crust pie, which may then be fluted if desired. See also BAKING TOOLS; PIE & TART.

CROCKPOT Ranging in size from 1 to 6 quarts, these handy covered electric pots slowly cook moist dishes such as stews, soups, and braises, allowing safe, unattended slow cooking. Sometimes known as slow cookers, they can be filled in the morning with soup or stew ingredients and left for the day. While generally favored for their convenience, some older models may cook foods unevenly. Newer appliances have resolved this problem and work extremely well. When using, follow instructions carefully to avoid overcooking and to ensure that food is cooked at the correct temperatures for safety.

CRUDITÉ (krew-dee-TAY) Crudités are trimmed whole or sliced vegetables served raw or lightly blanched or steamed and accompanied with a dip. A crudité platter is a colorful and healthful addition to a buffet table or cocktail party menu. For a festive touch, scoop out a large bell pepper or small pumpkin and serve the dip in it.

CRUMBLING To break food into small bits between your fingertips. Semisoft cheeses such as feta and Roquefort frequently are crumbled, as are dried herbs to bring out their flavor.

CRUSHING To turn a larger piece of food into many small particles, using your fingers, a rolling pin, a mortar and pestle, a mallet, or a tool specifically designed for the job. A garlic press crushes whole cloves of garlic; a rolling pin crushes crackers enclosed in a plastic bag. See also BRUISING; SMASHING.

CRUST See CHEESECAKE; PIE & TART.

CRYSTALLIZING Forming sugar crystals during cooking, which turns a syrup or other preparation gritty. Crystallizing is desirable in some instances, as with fudge, but unacceptable for most other candies. See also CANDY MAKING.

Fruits and edible flowers may be crystallized, or dipped or cooked in sugar syrup. This makes them into an elegant decoration. Also called candied or iced fruits or flowers, they can be found in specialty stores and mail-order catalogs.

CUBING To cut food, often meat and poultry, into small, uniformly sized pieces ½ to 1 inch square. This helps them cook evenly, and the bite-sized configuration makes them ready for use in stir-fries, soups, and stews. Smaller cubes, ⅛ to ½ inch square, are generally called dice. See also CHOPPING; DICING.

CUCUMBER This watery, mild-flavored, crunchy green vegetable shows up in green salads, on crudité platters, and as a garnish on cold plates. Chilled cucumber soup is a summer delight, and a cucumber sandwich is the darling of the afternoon tea lover. While fresh cucumbers can be steamed or lightly sautéed, they are most often consumed raw. Perhaps the best thing to happen to cucumbers is pickling. This versatile vegetable takes famously to long soaks in flavorful brines.

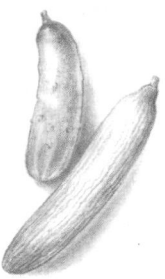

Slicing cucumbers.

Although numerous varieties of cucumbers are grown in home gardens, most supermarkets, greengrocers, and farmers' markets carry only two basic types: slicing varieties and pickling varieties. Slicing cucumbers are further divided into outdoor and hothouse, or English, varieties. Nearly all of the small, finger-length gherkin cucumbers, used to make little pickles called cornichons, are sold directly to food companies. Occasionally, however, they show up at farmers' markets and specialty greengrocers, and pickle makers snap them up. They are easy to grow, too, and many backyard gardeners harvest bumper crops.

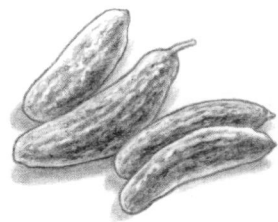

Pickling cucumbers.

Selecting When choosing slicing cucumbers—the type used in salads and other cold preparations—look for slender, dark green vegetables without yellowing or shriveling. Outdoor varieties should be 8 to 10 inches long and 1 to 1½ inches in diameter at the center. Many are coated with wax, which makes them shiny and helps preserve them. Avoid these if you can, as waxed skin must be peeled, and with the skin goes the vitamin A. Hothouse

Quick Tip

For pretty cucumber garnishes, use a vegetable peeler to create alternating stripes of dark green peel and light green flesh, and then slice the cucumber into thin disks.

cucumbers, usually sold wrapped in plastic, should be 12 to 16 inches long and have thin, smooth skin.

Storing Store cucumbers in a perforated plastic bag in the refrigerator for 5 days. Do not put cucumbers in the coldest part of the refrigerator; they prefer temperatures just above 40°F (the temperature of most refrigerators). Sliced cucumber will keep refrigerated in a covered container for 2 days.

Preparing Unless the skin is waxed, there is no need to peel cucumbers. Check for wax by scraping the cucumber with a fingernail. Pickling cucumbers should be scrubbed with a vegetable brush under cold running water to remove loose spines.

Cucumbers may be seeded for stuffing or before slicing crosswise for a salad.

HOW TO *Seed a Cucumber*

1. Slice the cucumber in half lengthwise.
2. Use a melon baller or spoon to scoop out the seeds and the surrounding pulpy matter.

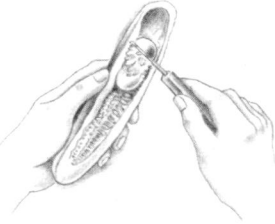

3. Proceed with stuffing or place the cucumber flat side down on a cutting board and slice crosswise.

CUMIN See SPICE.

CURDLING When eggs get too hot, their proteins react and they clump and expel moisture, a condition called curdling. When hollandaise sauce "breaks" or when custard separates, it is curdled and considered spoiled, or at least in need of salvage. On the other hand, when cream mixed with an acid such as buttermilk thickens and lumps, it becomes crème fraîche, a happy situation indeed but curdling nonetheless. Scrambled eggs are curdled eggs and are, of course, delicious. Cheese is made with milk and cream that have been allowed to curdle as one of the early steps in the cheese-making process.

Scrambled eggs.

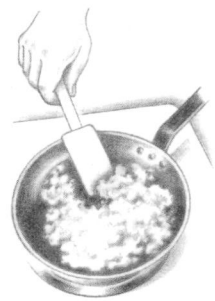

As desirable as curdling may be in some instances, for the home cook it usually spells disaster. The best way to avoid curdling is to monitor the heat. When cooking mixtures containing eggs, heat them gently and slowly, just to the point of thickening. Eggs to be added to hot liquids should be "tempered" first, by mixing a little of the hot liquid into them to warm them up. Then they can be stirred into the larger amount of hot liquid without curdling. See EGG for more detail.

Fat also prevents curdling, so when making recipes involving milk or cream plus an acidic ingredient, be wary of substituting a lower-fat version of the milk or cream called for in the recipe. It may cause curdling, whereas the full-fat version would have worked beautifully.

CURING Any process that preserves fresh food, usually meat or fish, by salting, brining, or smoking. Salting, which usually involves mixing the salt with sugar and/or herbs and spices, is used for gravlax (cured salmon) and other fish and for some hams such as prosciutto, which is salted and then left to cure in the open air. Brining, which is curing in a salt solution, is used for corned beef, pickles, and sauerkraut, among other foods. Smoking is used for everything from fish to whole chicken to cheese to nuts. Some, but not all, smoked foods are cured by dry salting or brining before smoking. There are two kinds of smoking: cold smoking, used for foods to be eaten raw (salmon) or later cooked (bacon); and hot smoking, used for foods that require no further cooking (chicken, certain sausages).

See also BRINE; SMOKING.

CURLY CHICORY See CHICORY.

CURLY ENDIVE See CHICORY.

CURRANT See BERRY; DRIED FRUIT.

CURRY Curry is a distinct flavor, immediately recognizable, but made from a mixture of seasonings and not dependent on any one ingredient. It is also a stewlike dish flavored with curry powder or curry paste. Curry is most readily associated with Indian cooking, although bold and pungent curries are made in Southeast Asia, most

---

Quick Tip

In most recipes, curry powder is cooked in a little oil to release its flavors. Curry paste, too, is cooked with a little fat, such as oil or coconut milk or cream, in a hot wok as the first step for many Southeast Asian dishes.

---

notably in Thailand; in Jamaica and other parts of the Caribbean; and in Mozambique and other countries in Africa. Curry leaves, which resemble small lemon leaves, smell of curry and are used in a number of Southeast Asian and Indian recipes and, not surprisingly, are components of many commercial curry powders.

Quick Bite

The best curry powders and pastes are made with whole spices that are first roasted and then ground. Cooks select the individual spices depending on the kind of curry they plan to cook, then grind the spices by hand in a mortar to ensure they are not overground.

In many Indian and Pakistani home kitchens, curry powder is made fresh daily or at least every few days. In other countries, it generally is sold already mixed and may be mild or spicy. Although numerous spices are ground together to make the powder, and the mixtures vary from region to region, and house to house, among the most common ingredients are cumin, curry leaves, cardamom, coriander seeds, fennel seeds, mustard seeds, mace, fenugreek, red and black peppers, and turmeric.

Curry paste, made throughout Southeast Asia, usually includes fresh ingredients such as lemongrass, galangal, garlic, onions, green or red chiles, and cilantro. Curry pastes are often classified as green, red, or yellow, depending on their ingredients. (Indian and Pakistani cooks also make curry paste, but curry powder is more widely used in Indian cooking.)

Selecting Curry powder is sold in supermarkets. The flavor of the widely distributed commercial brands may pale in comparison to those sold in specialty stores and from mail-order catalogs specializing in spices. Try a few different curry powders before selecting a brand you like. Curry paste is sold in Southeast Asian and Indian markets and in some specialty-food markets. Some are far hotter than others, so choose with discretion. Look for it in plastic tubs, jars, and cans. Curry leaves are available fresh and dried in Indian markets. They are 1 to 2 inches long and about ½ inch wide.

Quick Tip

Madras curry powder, a blend popular in southern India, is the most common type of curry powder sold commercially in countries where curry powders are not made at home. When a recipe calls for generic curry powder, it is acceptable to use Madras curry powder.

Storing Curry powder loses flavor after 2 months of storage in a cool, dry cupboard. Curry paste will keep in the cupboard for 6 months and once opened should be refrigerated, where it will keep for 2 or 3 months. Fresh curry leaves, often sold on the stalk, can be stored in the refrigerator for several days and freeze well for up to 6 weeks. Dried leaves will keep for 2 or 3 months, although their flavor dissipates as they age.

CUSTARD Custard is a mixture of eggs and milk or cream cooked just until the proteins in the ingredients thicken to form a soft, smooth, satiny dish that slides smoothly over the tongue. Both sweet and savory custards are among the world's most enduring comfort foods.

Sweet baked custards can be as simple as a *pot de crème* (vanilla cup custard) and as elegant as a crème brûlée or crème caramel. Spain's national dessert, flan, is made with sweetened condensed milk for richness. Savory baked custards are made following the same basic principles as those for sweet custards.

Custards are served in their ramekins, spooned from larger molds, or unmolded and plated. Those to be unmolded, such as crème caramel, contain whole eggs and a higher ratio of egg to milk or cream. This produces a firmer custard. Sleek, softer custards served in molds tend to be less stable. These may be made with egg yolks alone, as the proteins in egg whites are not needed to add stability.

Custard sauces, or stirred custards, are made from milk or cream, eggs, and sugar. They are cooked on the stove top, resulting in a different consistency: they are pourable. Perhaps the best-known custard sauce is English custard, or crème anglaise. This is the most basic of custard sauces and greatly appreciated by chefs and home cooks alike. From this basic sauce, you can make chocolate-, coffee-, mocha-, or almond-flavored custard sauces. Many ice creams are simply frozen English custard.

Pastry cream, or crème pâtissière, is yet another type of custard. Cornstarch and flour are added to the eggs, milk, and sugar for a firmer mixture and more stable custard. It is used to fill cream puffs, eclairs, fruit tarts, and cakes. Pastry cream can be flavored with chocolate, fruit, coffee, or crushed nuts.

Some home cooks fear making custards, concerned that they will curdle and clump or that they will toughen up and "weep," exuding water. The way to guarantee success is to control the heat, cooking the custard slowly and evenly, and to avoid overcooking it. This is necessary both during initial cooking on top of the stove and baking in the oven.

Baked Custard Savvy

■ Because milk may develop a skin when it has boiled, it should not boil or even simmer. Cook the milk or cream and sugar only until the sugar dissolves and the liquid is hot.

- Before eggs are added to hot milk or cream, "temper" them by whisking in just a little of the hot liquid to warm them up. This heats them up gradually to prevent curdling. The mixture can be returned to the pan and whisked into the hot liquid.
- Many custard recipes call for cooking the mixture until it is thick enough to "coat the back of a spoon." To test if the density is correct, carefully run your finger along the custard coating the spoon. If the path it makes stays in place and does not flow back onto itself, the custard is ready to be removed from the heat. To avoid overcooking custard, cook it just until it reaches this stage.

Testing the thickness.

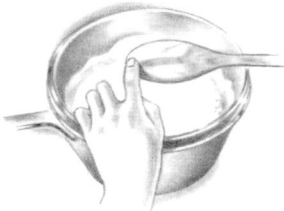

- Strain the custard into its baking container(s). Straining dissipates air bubbles and any lumps, producing a smooth consistency.
- Bake the custard in a water bath for gentle, even cooking. See WATER BATH.
- Don't let the custard's center set fully in the oven. It should still wiggle slightly, or a knife inserted in the center should come out moist. Carefully remove the custard from the oven and let cool, still in its water bath. Since the custard continues to cook for a few minutes outside the oven, taking it out just before it is firm prevents overcooking and tough, weeping custard. When the water bath is lukewarm, remove the custard and let it cool to room temperature.
- If the custard's center cooks through in the oven and an inserted knife comes

out completely clean and dry, remove the custard dish from the water bath and carefully submerge it halfway in a shallow pan or sink filled with cold water and ice cubes. This will quickly arrest the cooking.

Custard Sauce Savvy

- Cook the custard ingredients in a heavy saucepan, keeping the heat very low. The custard should hover between 160° and 170°F. As an extra precaution, use a heat diffuser; see COOKING TOOLS.
- Use a wooden spoon or silicone rubber spatula to stir custard. Both are more efficient at scraping the bottom of the pan than metal spoons.
- Stir the custard very carefully and gently. Hard, fast stirring can break the sauce and make it runny.
- Be patient. The custard sauce will thicken slowly, and slow cooking is the best safeguard against curdling. Don't raise the heat to hurry it up.
- To test for correct thickness, allow the custard to coat the spoon or spatula and carefully run your finger across the tool. A trail should remain that does not immediately run together.
- When custard sauce settles (any bubbles have dissipated), looks glossy, and feels noticeably thicker as you stir it, it's ready to remove from the heat.
- Once it is off the heat, continue to stir the sauce for a few minutes until completely thickened.
- Even if the sauce does not come out perfectly smooth, it will still taste good. Strain it to rid it of lumps.

Storing To chill custard, let it cool on the countertop and then place in the refrigerator until cold. Once it is cold, lay a piece of parchment or waxed paper directly on the surface of the custard to prevent a skin from forming and refrigerate. Custard will keep for 2 days.

Reheat custard sauce by setting it in a container in a larger saucepan of hot, but not simmering or boiling, water. Stir the custard until warm.

See also CRÈME BRÛLÉE; CURDLING; PUDDING; TEMPERING.

CUTTING BOARD Among the most indispensable pieces of kitchen equipment, a cutting board is frequently a built-in feature of contemporary kitchens. But even the simplest kitchen should have at least one portable cutting board.

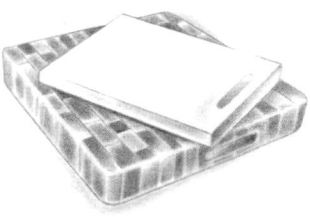

Wood and polyethylene boards.

Portable cutting boards are most commonly made of wood or polyethylene, a soft but rigid plastic. Marble and tempered glass boards, less familiar in many kitchens, are not recommended for cutting, as they will dull your knives, but they are appreciated by pie and pastry cooks for rolling out dough because they stay cool. Cutting boards made of very hard rubber, which once were reserved for chefs, are now available in limited supply to everyday home cooks.

Portable cutting boards may measure only 6 by 10 inches, although larger ones are more useful. For most kitchen work, boards should measure at least 12 by 18 inches and be ¾ to 1½ inches thick.

Cutting boards are used to chop meat, vegetables, herbs, and fruit; to knead bread; and to roll pastry. Using one protects the countertop and also is easier on knives. The sharp blade holds its edge longer when used on a cutting board.

Whether to buy wooden or polyethylene cutting boards is mainly a question of personal preference. In past years, controversy raged over which material was better in terms of safety. Polyethylene was believed to harbor fewer microorganisms and so was touted as being more sanitary than wood. More recently, wood was found to be safer, although these findings did not declare polyethylene unsafe. Whichever material you choose, it is a good idea to keep one cutting board for meat and chicken only and another for vegetables and other uses. This will limit the possibility of cross-contamination, or transferring flesh-borne bacteria to other foods in the kitchen. See also FOOD SAFETY.

The best wooden cutting boards are made of maple, oak, cherry, birch, and walnut and are all hardwoods with a long life. Cutting boards are traditionally made by laminating end-grain or edge-grain pieces of the wood, which naturally have some give. A wooden carving board with depressed grooves around the perimeter and a shallow well is preferred for slicing cooked meats and poultry, as escaping cooking juices are captured in the grooves. This board may be smooth on the reverse side and so is doubly useful.

As a rule, polyethylene cutting boards are lighter in weight than wooden boards. Most have rough, pebbly surfaces, which prevent food from slipping. Some have small feet on the underside; others are designed to be used on both sides.

Caring for Cutting Boards Carefully clean all cutting boards after each use and store away from heat, which can cause even heavy wood to warp and split. Every month or two, rinse both wooden and polyethylene boards with a mild solution of bleach and warm water, 4 cups of water to 1 teaspoon of bleach, to sanitize them. After bleaching them, rinse well with hot water.

Wooden Board Savvy

- Before using a new wooden board, rub it with tasteless, odorless mineral oil to season it. Use a wadded-up paper towel or small brush to spread a thin layer of oil over the wood. Rub it with fine steel wool and then let the oil soak in for 5 or 10 minutes. Wipe it dry with a soft cloth or paper towel and store. Repeat this seasoning process once a month for 10 to 12 months. After this time, oil the board periodically, particularly if the wood appears dry.
- After each use, wash the board with dishwashing liquid and a soft brush. Rinse well with hot water and dry completely before storing.
- For caked-on food, use a dough scraper to remove it and then wash the board. See BAKING TOOLS.
- If a board absorbs odors, clean it with lemon juice or salt, or a mixture of the two. Rinse well and dry before storing.
- Never let a wooden board soak in a sink of water or put it in the dishwasher. It will absorb water and warp.

Polyethylene Board Savvy

- After each use, wash the board with dishwashing liquid and a soft brush. Rinse well with hot water and dry before storing.
- Many of these boards are dishwasher safe. The heat of the dishwasher sanitizes them, although it may also warp some boards over time.
- These boards can be soaked in a sink of water, but it is rarely necessary and best avoided, as they could warp slightly.

CUTTING IN The technique of combining flour and fat for flaky pastry. Cutting in is accomplished by systematically working the flour and fat with a pastry blender, two table knives, or a fork until it resembles coarse crumbs. A food processor also is an effective and fast way of accomplishing the same thing. Cutting in differs from rubbing in only in that you do not use your fingertips exclusively. Using utensils instead of warm hands keeps the mixture cooler and is preferred for flaky pastry.

HOW TO *Cut Fat into Flour*

1. Measure out and whisk together the flour and other dry ingredients in a large bowl, then chop up the chilled fat called for in a recipe—usually butter, vegetable shortening, or a combination—before putting it into the flour. Toss the chunks of fat in the flour until they are coated.

2. Using a pastry blender or fork, preferably chilled, repeatedly slice through the fat as you turn the bowl quarter turns with your other hand. To use two knives, hold a knife in each hand and draw the knife blades across each other in a scissoring motion. (You can also use your fingertips to break down the fat to smaller pieces, but try not to handle it too much or you risk warming and melting the fat.) If using a food processor, fit it with the metal blade.

Using a pastry blender.

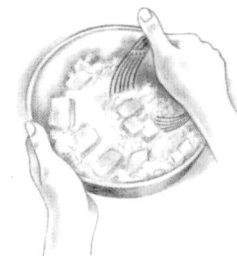

3. Keep tossing the fat in the flour as you slice, and wipe the fat off the blade occasionally to keep from mashing it. Continue slicing until the fat resembles small peas or coarse crumbs.

For flaky pie crust, take care that the flour and fat do not become too finely mixed or pasty. Small chunks of flour-coated fat result in light, flaky pastry; pieces that are too small or partially melted ones result in dense, crumbly pastry. See also BISCUIT; PIE & TART; RUBBING IN.

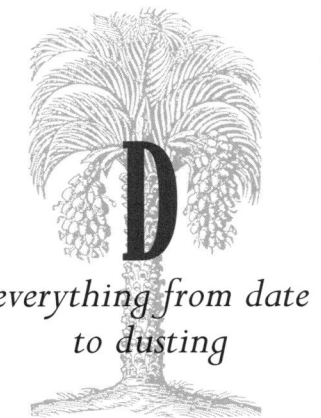

everything from date to dusting

DAIKON See RADISH.

DANDELION GREENS See GREENS, DARK.

DASH See MEASURING.

DATE Sweet, sticky, splendid dates grow in heavy profusion on towering date palm trees that flourish in the desert climates of North Africa and the Middle East. They are also grown domestically, mainly in California's arid Coachella Valley. Nearly all dates are sold fresh, although because of dates' naturally tacky consistency, many date lovers believe they are eating dried fruit. Another reason for this misconception is the dates' high sugar content and concentrated flavors, which, in terms of taste, make them more akin to dried fruits. Dates are also dried (see also DRIED FRUIT).

Dates are classified as being soft, semi-dry, or dry. Soft dates have a high moisture content and soft texture. They must be harvested by hand because of their fragility and then refrigerated to prevent deterioration. Medjool, Khadrawy, and Halawy are common varieties of soft dates. Semidry dates have a lower moisture content and firmer texture. They can be mechanically harvested and are packed in moisture-proof packages that are stocked on shelves rather than refrigerated. Deglet Noor (the most popular date sold in the United States) and Zahidy are the best-known semidry dates. Finally, dry dates, known also as bread dates, have an extremely high sugar content and low moisture content. Theory is the most common variety. Home cooks frequently pit dates, stuff the cavities with savory or sweet fillings, and serve them as hors d'oeuvres or after-dinner sweets. Dates are also tossed into stuffings for pork and duck and baked into cookies, breads, and cakes.

Selecting Dates are available year-round, although their peak season is from October through January, making them favorite holiday treats. Look for dates in the produce section of markets, usually in moisture-proof packages. Choose plump, shiny dates, and avoid any that are excessively sticky or covered with crystallized sugar. The exception is Medjool, which may have a dusting of natural sugar. Some dates are sold pitted.

Quick Tip

To prevent dates for baked goods from sticking to the knife as you chop them, dust the knife blade with flour.

Storing Tightly wrap soft and semidry dates in plastic and refrigerate for up to 3 weeks. Dry dates, well packaged, will keep refrigerated for 10 to 12 months.

Preparing All dates have pits, which must be removed before using the fruits in cooking or eating out of hand.

DEBEARDING Removing a mussel's beard, which looks like a little tuft of stringy dark hair extending from some shells, as part of the cleaning process. See MUSSEL.

DEBONING See BONING.

DECANTING Pouring wine from its original bottle into a glass container called a decanter. Before the advent of modern wine-making practices, wines were decanted as a matter of course to separate the liquid from the sediment that naturally collected in the bottles. Today, unless one is serving an older red wine or vintage Port, it rarely is necessary to decant wine for this or any other reason, as wines now are generally quite clear and can be served from the bottle with no danger of the wine drinker's imbibing bitter sediment. A very young or tannic wine may be decanted and allowed to "breathe" and soften for up to several hours before serving. This period of breathing is not recommended for older wines, as their bouquet fades rather quickly after pouring.

See also WINE.

DECORATING COMB See BAKING TOOLS.

DECORATING TURNTABLE See BAKING TOOLS.

DEEP-FRYING See FRYING.

DEFROSTING See FOOD SAFETY; FREEZING; THAWING.

DEGLAZING Using liquid to dislodge and dissolve the browned bits of meat, poultry, or other sautéed or fried food that become stuck to the pan bottom as a result of cooking. The liquid, usually wine, stock, or water, is added to the pan after the food has been removed. The liquid is heated over medium-high or high heat, and the cook stirs it with a wooden spoon or spatula and scrapes the pan bottom at the same time to free the browned bits. Before long, the flavorful liquid is reduced, meaning it partially cooks away or evaporates. The resulting sauce is often called a reduction sauce or pan sauce. See also REDUCING; SAUTÉING.

DEGREASING As stocks and pan drippings simmer and as they cool, the fat in them rises to the top. Degreasing means removing this fat for a clearer soup or sauce.

During stock making, the liquid should be kept at a gentle simmer so that the fat extracted from the meat and bones rises to the surface rather than becoming an integral part of the stock, which would happen if it was boiled. When the fat rises to the surface, the simmering stock can be degreased by skimming off the fat with a spoon or mesh skimmer (see COOKING TOOLS). Then, as the stock cools, any remaining fat separates from the liquid and also rises to the top. As the fat gathers, you can blot it up gently with a wadded paper towel.

If the liquid is chilled, the fat solidifies in a layer on top, which easily can be lifted off the surface with a large spoon or spatula.

Degreasing chilled stock.

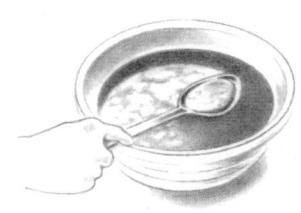

This same technique can be applied to the fat left in a roasting pan with the drippings. Use a spoon or mesh skimmer to remove excess fat from the surface of the drippings before making gravy.

See also GRAVY; SAUCE; SKIMMING; STOCK.

DEVEINING To remove the dark intestinal vein in a shrimp or lobster, which can be bitter, gritty, and unsightly. Once it is cooked, the intestinal vein is harmless—its removal is simply a matter of aesthetics. See LOBSTER; SHRIMP.

DICING Cutting food, often vegetables or fruit, into small, uniform cubes, usually ⅛ to ¼ inch square, which ensures that they will cook evenly and makes them easy to eat. Food cut into larger uniform pieces is considered cubed.

Cutting dice.

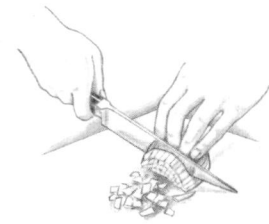

See also CHOPPING; CUBING.

DILL See HERB.

DIRECT HEAT See GRILLING.

DISCOLORING When some fruits and vegetables are peeled and exposed to the air, oxygenation causes them to darken, or turn brown, which is referred to as discoloring. This happens most commonly in low-acid fruits (such as apples and bananas) and vegetables (such as artichokes and eggplants). While the browning does not cause any harm, it does cause the food to lose some of its visual appeal.

A little acid, usually lemon juice or vinegar, slows the discoloring. It may be sprinkled over or rubbed on the cut apples, avocados, or bananas. Or, to avoid adding an acidic bite, the food may be submerged in acidulated water, which is water that has been mixed with a little lemon juice, vinegar, or another acid. The proportion of acid to water is fairly low—about 1 tablespoon per quart of water—so the flavor of the acid is not imparted to the food. Exact

> ## Quick Tip
>
> Fruits and vegetables that discolor when cut and exposed to air: apple, artichoke, avocado, banana, cauliflower, celery root, cherry, eggplant, fig, Jerusalem artichoke, lotus root, mushroom, nectarine, parsnip, peach, pear, potato, rutabaga, yam.

measurements generally are not important, however, except in the case of recipes that call for cooking vegetables and fruits in properly acidulated water. But remember, acid does not *prevent* discoloration; it simply slows it down. Over time, the cut surface will brown.

On the other hand, acid actually causes browning of some green vegetables. Acidic dressings and sauces will darken or discolor broccoli, green beans, and asparagus if the vegetables are allowed to stand in the liquid. For this reason, most recipes suggest tossing cold vegetable salads just before serving. Also, cooking green vegetables with acidic ingredients such as tomatoes or corn will cause them to turn a drab green.

See also ACID.

DISJOINTING The availability of precut chicken pieces has made disjointing—cutting up a whole, uncooked chicken—an endangered art. Yet, it is a simple process, and a whole chicken not only will cost you less than an equivalent weight of already-cut pieces, but also will yield backbones and other trimmings for the stockpot.

HOW TO *Disjoint a Chicken*

1. Place the chicken, breast up and drumsticks toward you, on a cutting board. With a sharp, heavy knife, cut through the skin between the thigh and body. Locate the joint by moving the leg, then cut through the joint to remove the leg. Repeat on the other side.

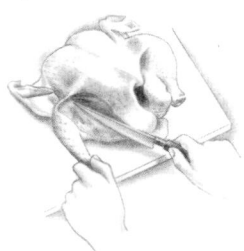

2. Move the drumstick to locate the joint connecting it to the thigh. Cut through the joint to separate the 2 pieces. Repeat with the other leg.

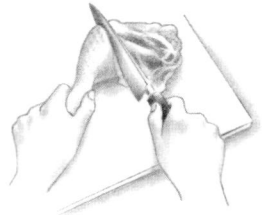

3. Move a wing to locate its joint with the body. Cut through the joint to remove the wing. Repeat with the other wing.

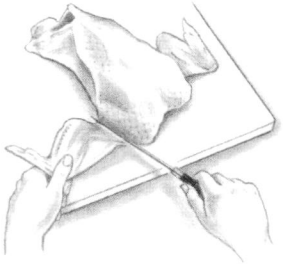

4. Starting at the neck opening, cut along both sides of the chicken, separating the breast section from the remainder of the bird.

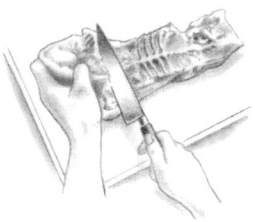

5. Holding the breast skin side down, slit the thin membrane covering the breastbone along its center. Grasp the breast firmly at each end and flex it upward to pop out the breastbone. Pull out the bone, using the knife if necessary to help cut it free.

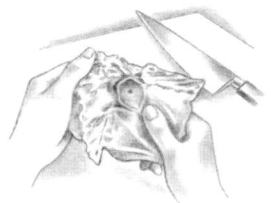

6. Place the breast skin side down on the cutting board. Cut along the center of the breast to split it in half.

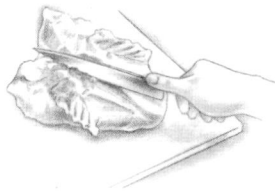

Disjointed and neatly trimmed, a whole chicken yields 8 serving-sized pieces ready for cooking: 2 each of thighs, legs, breasts, and wings. Before cooking, be sure to rinse the pieces with cold water and pat dry with paper towels.

d

DOLLOP A generous spoonful of a substance, usually a smooth, soft one such as whipped cream or sour cream. A dollop is not a precise measurement but generally signifies the amount of topping spooned atop a bowl of soup or a dessert, such as the swirl of sour cream that floats on a serving of borscht or the whipped cream that crowns strawberry shortcake.

DONENESS The degree to which food is cooked or baked so that it is ready to eat. Do not rely on a recipe's cooking time alone to judge a dish's doneness, a common pitfall for inexperienced cooks. Good recipes provide tests in addition to time for doneness. For example, you might be instructed to sauté onions "until translucent," toast spices "until browned and fragrant," or bake a cake "until a toothpick inserted into the center comes out clean." Pay attention to these cues as you follow a recipe; in time, you may rely more on your senses than on stated cooking times.

However, you should note that because of safety issues, internal temperature is the best way to judge when meat or poultry is done. Use an accurate meat thermometer and insert it into the meatiest part of the roast or bird, such as the thigh of a chicken or the heart of a pork loin, making sure it does not touch bone. (Bone conducts heat, skewing the reading.) See individual foods, or the guidelines below.

U.S. Government Doneness Guidelines The U.S. Food Safety and Inspection Service suggests temperatures for cooked meat and poultry to ensure the maximum degree of safety for consumers. A minimum temperature of 160°F is needed to destroy bacteria. Many people choose to cook food to a lower temperature for juicier flesh and fuller flavor. If you are pregnant or older, are cooking for young children or older people, have a compromised immune system, or want to limit your exposure to bacterial risk as much as possible, you may want to observe these guidelines:

Safe Doneness Temperatures	
Whole beef cuts (roasts, steaks)	160°F
(For rare meat, 145°F in the center is safe, except for rolled roasts or mechanically tenderized cuts.)	
Whole pork cuts (roasts, chops)	160°F*
Whole poultry	160°F*
Ground meat or poultry	160°F
Poultry stuffing	165°F
Casseroles with meat or egg	165°F

Some pork and poultry cuts will still have traces of pink at this temperature and can be cooked longer for a more appealing appearance of doneness.

See also FOOD SAFETY.

DOTTING Topping fruit pie fillings, gratins, or other foods with small slices or dabs of butter before baking. The butter should be scattered evenly over the food, so that it will seep consistently throughout the food as it melts during baking. Dotted butter provides richness and moisture and assists in browning.

DOUBLE BOILER A double boiler is a set of two pans, one nested atop the other with room for water to simmer in the pan below. Delicate foods such as chocolate, custards, mousses, and cream sauces are placed in the top pan to heat them gently, or to melt them in the case of chocolate. Double boilers are also good places to keep foods warm without cooking them further, or at least not too quickly. The top pan should not touch the water beneath it, and the water is not meant to boil. A tight fit between the pans ensures that no water or steam mixes with the ingredients, which can cause melting chocolate to stiffen, or seize.

You can easily create your own double boiler by placing a heat-resistant mixing bowl or slightly smaller saucepan over a larger one, although it may not be as steady or the fit as tight.

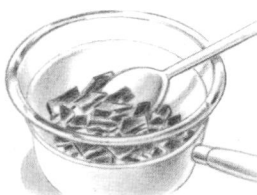

Melting chocolate in a makeshift double boiler.

DOUGH An unbaked, pliable mixture of flour and liquid, which may also include eggs, fat (such as butter), sugar, salt, and leaveners. Doughs, which are thicker and firmer than batters, do not require containment in a bowl. Bread and biscuit doughs, for example, are scraped from the bowl and worked, or kneaded, on a work surface. They are softer than cookie and pastry doughs, which have a higher ratio of flour to liquid and are rolled (with a rolling pin) or patted (with fingertips) into smooth, thin rounds or rectangles. See also BAKING; BATTER; BISCUIT; BREAD; COOKIE; PIE & TART; QUICK BREAD.

DOUGH BLENDER Another term for pastry blender; see BAKING TOOLS.

DOUGH SCRAPER See BAKING TOOLS.

DRAINING Foods cooked in water or other liquid until tender and edible may be drained before they are served. Pasta, potatoes, vegetables, and other foods are drained in colanders. Foods soaked in liquids, such as raisins that are plumped

or clams left in salt water to purge sand, are also drained before cooking. Foods with a high moisture content, such as yogurt or ricotta cheese, may be drained in a strainer or through cheesecloth, thus thickening as the liquid seeps from them. Watery vegetables, such as eggplant and cucumbers, benefit from being cut, salted, and left to drain in a colander or on paper towels.

Draining differs from straining in that you reserve the liquid when you strain, and usually discard it when you drain.

DREDGING To coat with flour or another dry ingredient, such as cornmeal or bread crumbs, often seasoned. Food is sprinkled with the dry ingredient, dragged through it, or shaken with it.

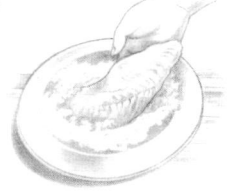

Dredging in flour.

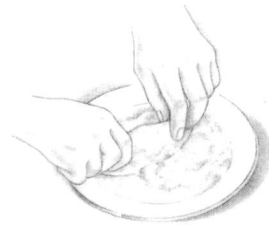

Turning to coat.

Alternatively, the food and coating may be placed in a plastic bag and shaken together.

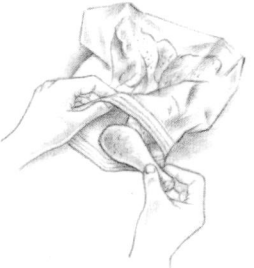

Dredging in a plastic bag.

After dredging, the food should be shaken to remove excess coating. Do not dredge food too far in advance of cooking, or the coating will absorb moisture from the food and become gummy. Laying dredged food on a wire rack also helps avoid gumminess.

Dredged food is usually sautéed, fried or deep-fried, or baked. The coating helps it brown nicely and retain moisture, and adds a nice crispiness.

DRESSING A light sauce used to moisten and flavor salad greens and other raw vegetables. Classic salad dressings are variations of vinaigrettes—mixtures of oil, vinegar, and seasonings such as salt, pepper, fresh herbs, garlic, and mustard. Other dressings are mayonnaise based.

When tossing a salad with dressing, use a light hand. Mix the greens or other vegetables with a relatively small amount of dressing, distributing it with numerous tossings. Do not drench the greens, and dress salad greens just before serving to keep them crisp.

Dressing can also refer to the bread-based mixture used to accompany turkey, chicken, and other poultry. Practically speaking, the terms dressing and stuffing are interchangeable, but with regional preferences. In the East and the South, dressing may be cooked in or out of the bird, while elsewhere, stuffing is cooked inside the bird and dressing is baked in a separate buttered casserole alongside it.

See also GREENS, SALAD; STUFFING; VINAIGRETTE.

Quick Tip

Mix a salad dressing in the bottom of the serving bowl up to an hour or so before dinner. Lightly pile greens on top, cover, and refrigerate, then toss just before serving.

DRIED FRUIT Using sunshine or the heat of kilns, many fruits are dried for prolonged storage and to give them an intense flavor and chewy texture. Some fruits, such as sticks of papaya or disks of cored pineapple, are candied to help preserve them and enhance their flavor.

Selecting Look for more recently dried and packaged fruits, which have a softer texture than older dried fruits. Health-food stores and farmers' markets, which often have more rapid turnovers of stock, are good places to shop.

Storing Store dried fruits in airtight containers at room temperature for up to 1 month or refrigerated for up to 6 months.

Preparing Depending on the recipe, dried fruits may be used whole or cut up, and are sometimes soaked in hot water, liqueur, or another liquid for about 20 minutes to "plump" or reconstitute them.

See also LIQUEUR; PLUMPING.

DRIPPINGS The liquid that collects in the roasting pan when large cuts of meat or poultry are roasted or fried is called drippings or pan drippings. Once degreased (the fat skimmed from the surface), the flavorful drippings are used to make gravy or sauces. The term *drippings* also applies to bacon drippings, namely, the melted fat rendered from bacon during cooking, which is used to cook other foods in turn. This fat could clog drains, and should be collected in an empty can and then discarded with the trash if not used for cooking purposes. See DEGLAZING; DEGREASING; GRAVY.

Dried Fruit Glossary

APPLE Typically sold in thin rings, dried apples may be sweet or tart, depending on the variety.

APRICOT Pitted whole or halved fruit, sweet and slightly tangy.

CHERRY Dried sour cherries have lovely sweet flavor and are increasingly available. Pitted before drying, they resemble raisins in shape and may be used in the same way.

CURRANT While fresh currants are berrylike fruits grown and used widely in Europe, dried currants are actually Zante grapes, tiny raisins with a distinctively tart-sweet flavor. If they are unavailable, substitute raisins.

DATE The sugars of this desert-grown fruit become even more concentrated when dried, though they are generally eaten fresh.

FIG The dried form of this compact and succulent black, green, or golden fruit is distinguished by the slightly crunchy texture of its many tiny seeds.

PEACH Halved or quartered, pitted, and flattened fruit; sweet and slightly tangy.

PEAR Halved, seeded, and flattened fruit, retaining the fresh pear's distinctive profile.

PRUNE Variety of dried plum, with a rich, dark, fairly moist flesh.

RAISIN Variety of dried grapes, popular as a snack on their own. For baking, use seedless dark raisins or golden raisins.

DRIZZLING To dribble a liquid, such as olive oil, melted butter, or chocolate sauce, lightly and irregularly over food. Sliced tomatoes are drizzled with olive oil, corn on the cob is drizzled with melted butter, and sliced strawberries are drizzled with chocolate sauce. For extra sweetness and a pretty pattern, drizzle melted white chocolate over a cake or other baked good.

To drizzle, put the liquid in a small ladle or cup and gently swirl it over the surface of the food. Or, dip a fork in the liquid and drizzle the liquid from the ends of the tines. Drizzle olive oil by placing your thumb over the mouth of the bottle, leaving just a tiny gap, and shaking it back and forth over the food. Specialized spouts that allow drizzling are also available for olive oil and other bottles. A plastic squeeze bottle can be used to drizzle mustard over a hot dog or caramel sauce over a bowl of ice cream.

DRY INGREDIENTS Flour, sugar, salt, baking powder, baking soda, cocoa, and cornmeal are all examples of dry ingredients. They are mixed with fats and wet ingredients—butter, eggs, water, milk, cream—to make batters and doughs. Many baking recipes suggest mixing the dry ingredients together before combining them with the wet ingredients. Depending on the recipe, this may be done by whisking or sifting them together. Not all recipes require sifting, but it is never a bad idea to spoon the dry ingredients into a shallow bowl and mix them with a large wire whisk, using 8 or 9 strokes. This aerates the dry ingredients, which helps with rising, and also distributes salt or leavening evenly throughout the mixture.

See also BAKING; MEASURING; SIFTING; WET INGREDIENTS; WHISKING.

DRY RUB See RUB.

DUCK Similar in size (but not shape) to a chicken, a duck is a treat many people order only in restaurants, rarely thinking to cook it at home. This is a shame because duck is rich and full flavored and no more difficult to cook than other poultry.

Duck is hunted recreationally during the fall. None of this game can be sold commercially. Only farm-raised duck is

Quick Bite

Although traditionally a wild duck, the mallard is now sometimes farm raised. It has pleasantly gamy meat.

available to the consumer, and most of this reaches the market frozen. If you can find fresh duck, buy it, as it is tastier than frozen. Duck is marketed when only months old and is often labeled as duckling.

With its mild, tender, lean meat, White Pekin is the most commonly available type of duck. Over the years, Long Island, New York, has become the leader in the breeding and raising of this delicious bird, and so today White Pekin is often referred to as Long Island duckling. A Muscovy reaches market slightly older than other ducks (nearly 3 months old), which results in mature, especially flavorful breast meat. The prized breasts may be marketed as *magrets*. The Muscovy is raised for excellent foie gras, too.

Quick Bite

Moulards are a cross between a male Muscovy and a female White Pekin duck. Most of them are raised for foie gras.

Selecting Most likely the duck you buy at the supermarket or from a butcher will be frozen; it should be solidly frozen with no signs of thawing. If it is fresh, look for smooth skin without discoloration. Duck breast is considered the finest part of the duck and often is sold separately.

Storing Store fresh duck in the cold rear section of the refrigerator in its original packaging and cook it within 2 days. Store duck tightly wrapped in the freezer for up to 6 months.

Preparing Let frozen duck defrost in the refrigerator for a day. To avoid the growth of harmful bacteria, do not let it defrost on the countertop. If time is an issue, it can be defrosted in cool water. Submerge the duck, still in its plastic packaging, in cool water for 2 to 3 hours, changing the water every 30 minutes or so to keep it cold. Once thawed, the duck can be kept in the refrigerator for another day but should not be refrozen. Bring to room temperature before cooking, then cook it promptly.

Remove any lumps of duck fat from the cavity before cooking a whole duck, or strain the rendered fat left in the pan after cooking and use it to cook potatoes or eggs.

See also FOIE GRAS; GAME.

DUMPLING WRAPPER See NOODLE.

DUSTING To sprinkle food with a light layer of a powdery ingredient such as confectioners' sugar or cocoa, usually for decorative purposes. To dust food (or to garnish plates), use a small, fine-mesh strainer. Put the sugar in the strainer and gently tap the side of it as you move it over the food, leaving a fine, even coating.

Cake pans may be dusted with flour or cocoa after being greased, which helps to prevent the batter from sticking.

See also BAKING.

DUTCH OVEN See COOKWARE.

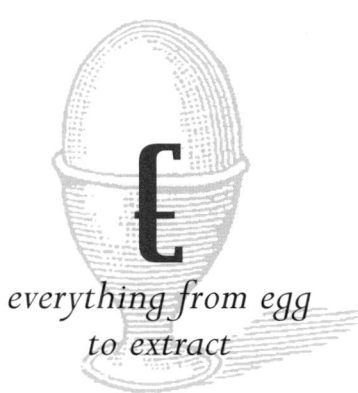

everything from egg to extract

EGG See page 183.

EGG NOODLE See NOODLE; PASTA.

EGGPLANT Native to Africa and Asia, eggplants are commonly associated with the cooking of the Mediterranean, as illustrated by the many Italian and French dishes that feature them, such as eggplant parmigiana, caponata, and ratatouille. But eggplant turns up with equal, if not more, frequency in Chinese, Indian, Southeast Asian, and Middle Eastern cuisines.

The most familiar eggplant, called a globe eggplant, is usually large, egg or pear shaped, with a thin, shiny, deep purple skin that looks almost black.

Globe eggplant.

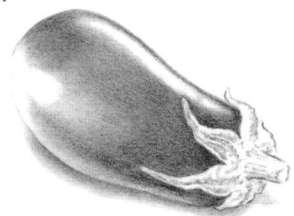

Asian eggplants, also purple skinned—some lavender, some deep purple—are smaller, longer, and narrower.

Other varieties may be slightly smaller and have white, rose, green, or variegated skin. The color of the skin does not determine the flavor of the vegetable.

Asian eggplants.

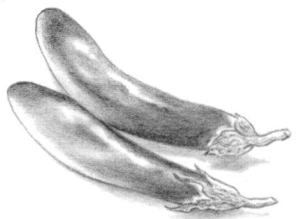

Mild, meaty eggplant flesh lends itself to countless simple, everyday preparations. In many countries, it is served in place of meat (which is saved for special occasions).
Selecting Eggplants are available year-round but are at their best from July through September. Choose smooth, firm, glossy-skinned eggplants with green caps and stems. Avoid any that are torn, bruised, or scarred, or that have brown, dried caps. Smaller eggplants are generally sweeter than large ones, and the vegetables should feel heavy for their size.
Storing Refrigerate eggplants in perforated plastic bags in the vegetable crisper for 4 or 5 days. They are best if cooked sooner rather than later, and if cooking on the day of purchase, let the vegetable sit at room temperature until ready to cook.
Preparing Large eggplants can be bitter, which explains why so many recipes suggest salting the cut-up vegetable, a step that draws out the bitterness. Salting also extracts excess moisture, which may interfere with the success of some recipes. As eggplants have become more commonplace in supermarkets, growers have been offering smaller, sweeter vegetables, which rarely

need salting. If the eggplant is large or old, or if the flesh looks dark and watery, however, you'll want to salt it after slicing. If frying eggplant, it's always a good idea to salt it, or at least press it gently to remove excess moisture. If the vegetables appear firm and quite dry, you can skip this step. Simply rinse the whole vegetable under cold running water and proceed with a recipe. Peeling is needed only if the skin seems thick and tough.

HOW TO *Salt Eggplant*

Salt an eggplant to remove bitterness or excess moisture that can interfere with the finished dish.

1. Cut the eggplant as directed in a recipe, and sprinkle pieces with coarse salt on all sides.
2. Put the pieces in a stainless steel or plastic colander set in the sink or over a plate and let drain for about 30 minutes.
3. Spread the eggplant on a double thickness of paper towels and, using a clean kitchen towel or more paper towels, gently press to squeeze out excess moisture.
4. Wipe with paper towels to remove excess salt. Do not rinse under running water, as the eggplant will absorb the water.

The flesh of an eggplant will discolor when exposed to the air for any length of time. To prevent this, sprinkle with a little lemon juice. Do not submerge in acidulated water, as the eggplant will absorb the water and turn soggy.

Quick Tip

A chemical reaction is produced when eggplant is cooked in aluminum, resulting in a metallic taste.

When sautéing or panfrying eggplant, be careful not to use more oil than needed. The eggplant will absorb nearly any amount of oil you pour into the pan. To combat this tendency, quickly cook the vegetable in a little oil over high heat.

Quick Bite

In Europe, an eggplant is called an aubergine, a word that also is used to describe its distinctive purple color.

EGG WASH Beaten whole eggs, yolks, or whites mixed with water, milk, or cream and used as a glaze on baked goods.

EMULSION An emulsion is a stabilized mixture that contains two or more liquids that would ordinarily not combine, such as oil and vinegar. While some emulsions are temporary, such as vinaigrette, others are more stable, such as mayonnaise. All emulsions require vigorous blending, such as shaking or whisking. When you shake a bottle of vinaigrette dressing and the ingredients mix together, you've created a temporary emulsion.

Whisking together an emulsion.

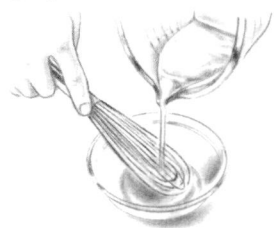

A stable emulsion also requires an agent known as an emulsifier to help hold the other ingredients together. Egg yolks are popular emulsifiers in the kitchen for recipes such as mayonnaise, hollandaise sauce, and Caesar dressing. Other emulsifying agents include mustard (which helps explain its presence in many vinaigrettes) and cream.

See also MAYONNAISE; VINAIGRETTE.

Egg

A common kitchen ingredient, the egg is as much a staple as sugar, flour, salt, and milk. But eggs are small miracles. They can be eaten by themselves—fried, boiled, scrambled, poached, baked—or added to numerous other dishes, both sweet and savory, to provide flavor, color, and consistency.

Cookies, cakes, soufflés, omelets, custards, and quiches cannot be made without breaking a few eggs.

Eggs are nutritional powerhouses, supplying protein; vitamins A, D, and E; and minerals such as phosphorus, manganese, iron, calcium, and zinc. Egg whites, also known as albumen, are among the most healthful of foods, being low in fat and high in protein. The yolks, on the other hand, contain the fat and cholesterol—and the most flavor.

Selecting Chicken eggs, by far the most commonly marketed and eaten eggs, are graded according to quality and size. Quality refers to freshness rather than nutrition. The highest-quality eggs, determined at time of packing, are AA, which have thick whites and firm, plump yolks. Grade A eggs fall only shortly behind in terms of quality. (Grade B eggs are low quality and rarely make it to the retail market.) In terms of size, eggs are labeled jumbo, extra-large, large, medium, small, and peewee. Most recipes are developed for large eggs, and while other sizes may

be substituted, you may have to adjust the recipe. For more details, see SUBSTITUTIONS & EQUIVALENTS. Fertile eggs from hens that have mated are considered a delicacy in some cultures, but these eggs offer no difference in nutritional value and do not keep as well.

Buy large AA eggs if possible. Look for those without cracks and with clean shells. All eggs destined for the commercial market have been carefully washed and coated with a natural mineral oil to prevent the introduction of bacteria.

Check the sell-by date, which should be as distant as possible.

Storing Store eggs in a cold area of the refrigerator where the temperature is below 40°F. Do not leave eggs at room temperature: a day on a countertop ages them as much as a week in the refrigerator.

Store eggs in their cartons. Don't transfer them to the egg racks found in some refrigerators. They may not stay cold enough, as the door exposes them to changing temperatures as it opens and closes. The carton helps keep them cold and less likely to pick up refrigerator odors. Additionally, eggs should be stored with the broad ends up, which is how they are packed. This keeps the yolk centered.

Unbroken eggs refrigerated in their carton will keep for 5 weeks past their sell-by

continued

Egg, continued

date. As they age, the whites will thin and become more transparent and the yolks will flatten, but the nutritional value of the eggs will not diminish. Use older eggs for baking, reserving the fresher ones for other cooking. Older egg whites are easier to whip up into voluminous meringue than absolutely fresh eggs, while fresh eggs are best for emulsified sauces such as hollandaise and mayonnaise.

Recipes will sometimes call for egg whites or egg yolks only, leaving you with leftover parts of eggs. Refrigerate uncooked egg whites in a tightly lidded glass or plastic container for up to 5 days. Refrigerate uncooked egg yolks in a glass or plastic container covered with a little water and tightly lidded for up to 2 days. Uncooked whole eggs removed from the shell can be stored in the same way and for the same length of time as egg yolks, but without the layer of water floated on top.

Quick Tip

If you find yourself with an excess of egg whites because a recipe used yolks alone, use them to make meringue, angel food cake, or egg-white omelets, or add them to whole eggs for more healthful scrambled eggs. If, on the other hand, you have an excess of egg yolks, get ready to make ice cream, mayonnaise, or chocolate mousse.

Freezing Eggs Remove whole eggs from their shells and place in a rigid container. (Never freeze eggs in the shell.) Stir lightly to break the yolks; do not stir briskly, or air bubbles may be incorporated. Cover, leaving only ½ inch of headroom, and freeze for up to 9 months. To freeze egg whites only, combine them in a rigid container, cover, and freeze for up to 1 year. To freeze egg yolks only, combine

them, as with whole eggs, add a pinch of salt or sugar, seal, and freeze for up to 9 months. When thawed to room temperature, frozen egg whites will whip up more easily than fresh whites. Use thawed, frozen whole eggs and egg yolks as you would fresh, for baking or omelets.

Preparing The best way to crack an egg is to tap it sharply against a flat surface such as a countertop—not a bowl rim. Holding the egg lengthwise over a container, break it in half, letting the white and yolk plop into it. If any shell gets into the bowl, use another piece of egg shell, a spoon, or a fork to remove it. (See also Egg Safety, below.)

HOW TO *Separate an Egg*

Cold eggs separate more easily than room-temperature eggs. If possible, take the eggs from the refrigerator immediately before separating them.

1. Position 2 small bowls side by side: 1 for the whites, the other for the yolks.
2. Crack the egg sharply on its equator, making a clean break.

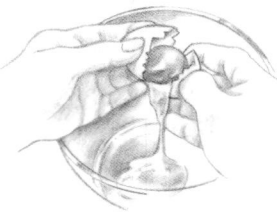

3. Pour the yolk and whites into your clean cupped hand, letting the whites run through your fingers into one of the bowls, or use an egg separator in place of your hand. Slide the remaining yolk into the other bowl. (An egg separator is a small, bowl-shaped device with a center depression made to hold the yolk while the egg white slides through slots on the side into a waiting bowl.) Or, pass the egg yolk back and forth from one shell half to the other, letting the whites slip into the bowl. (See also Egg Safety, below.)

Egg separator.

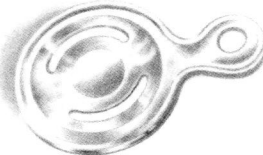

4. If any yolk gets into the whites, they will not beat properly. Whites in the yolks will make no difference to the recipe. If separating more than 1 egg, you may want to use 3 bowls to avoid any risk of yolks getting into egg whites. Crack each egg over an empty bowl and transfer the whites to the egg white bowl, the yolks to the yolk bowl.

Egg Whites Savvy

- When beating egg whites, start with a spotlessly clean bowl and whisk. Any spot of grease or fat (including egg yolk) will prevent egg whites from expanding to their full volume. A ceramic or glass bowl with slippery sides is not the best choice, and plastic tends to be a bit oily; stainless steel works better. The best choice is copper, which chemically interacts with the eggs whites to make them more stable and beautifully satiny. If using a copper bowl, cream of tartar may be omitted from a recipe.
- Egg whites may be beaten with a hand-held electric mixer or stand mixer, fitted with the whisk attachment, or by hand with a whisk. (Some cooks think hand-beating incorporates the most air, yielding a very stable foam.) Food processors and blenders do not aerate well.
- Beat egg whites thoroughly, according to the directions given in a particular recipe, in order to incorporate plenty of air. Once the whites foam, they will begin to increase in volume and will become opaque white rather than translucent. Lift the whisk or beaters from the whites to determine the state of their peaks. When the eggs are beaten to soft

peaks, they will gently fall over to one side, while eggs beaten to stiff, dry peaks will stand upright.

Soft peaks.

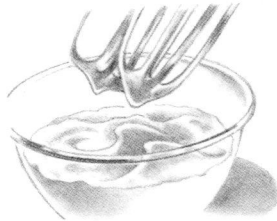

Stiff peaks.

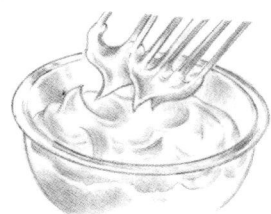

- Do not overbeat egg whites, or they will become clumpy and grainy and act less effectively in delicate baked goods.
- Fold beaten egg whites into a batter gently to avoid deflating them. See also FOLDING.

Egg Safety In recent years, raw eggs have been at the center of a controversy over their safety, namely, the incidence of salmonella bacteria present in some eggs. Recipes using raw eggs disappeared from the pages of newspapers, magazines, and cookbooks for years, but some are gradually reappearing in print now that the risk is better understood.

Salmonella bacteria can be found in a number of organisms, including poultry, meat, fish, and eggs. According to the American Egg Board, the incidence of salmonella in eggs is low, about 1 chance out of 20,000 overall. If an infected egg is properly stored so that the bacteria cannot

continued

Egg, continued

multiply, a healthy person probably will not get sick from eating it. Risk increases when a number of eggs are mixed together and

---

Quick Bite

The color of an egg's shell has nothing to do with the flavor or nutrition of the egg. The breed of chicken that laid the egg determines the shell's color.

---

a single contaminated egg infects the entire batch, as could happen in restaurant kitchens. If you are pregnant or older, are cooking for young children or for pregnant or older people, have a compromised immune system, or want to limit your exposure to bacterial risk as much as possible, you may want to observe these guidelines:

- Buy eggs only from refrigerated cases.
- Keep all eggs refrigerated, whether they are in the shell or out.
- Do not leave eggs at room temperature for longer than 30 minutes.
- Make sure your hands, work surfaces, and utensils are clean.
- Refrigerate leftovers containing eggs as soon as possible. Put them in shallow containers so that they cool quickly.
- Use only clean, unbroken eggs. Discard cracked eggs.
- To be especially cautious, do not let the shell come into contact with the egg after it is broken, either by passing the yolk back and forth between the shell halves as

---

Quick Tip

Room-temperature eggs blend better with sugar and fat than cold eggs. To take the chill off refrigerated eggs, put them in a bowl of cool water for about 30 minutes before adding them to cookie doughs and cake batters.

---

you separate the egg or by scooping other broken shell out of the egg.

- Cook eggs so that they are held at 140°F for at least 3½ minutes or reach a temperature of 160°F. Soft-boiled, poached, and coddled eggs do not reach 160°F.
- Avoid foods made with raw eggs, such as hollandaise sauce, béarnaise sauce, mayonnaise, and Caesar dressing.

A Basket of Breakfast Eggs

FRIED Cooked in butter or other fat, fried eggs can be finished "sunny-side up," that is, never flipped and with the yolk a bright yellow; or "over easy," that is, flipped and cooked briefly to set the yolk further.

OMELET Beaten eggs are cooked in a shallow pan, producing a firm exterior and soft interior, then typically folded over or rolled around a savory filling.

Quick Tip

When it comes to eggs, the fresher the better. If you have access to a farm stand that sells fresh eggs, buy them and use them for making soft-boiled, fried, scrambled, or poached eggs.

POACHED A classic topping for corned beef hash, poached eggs are cooked in simmering water or other liquid until the whites are set and opaque.

SCRAMBLED Whole eggs beaten, preferably with a little water, and then cooked slowly and stirred gently until thickened but still soft and moist.

SOFT-BOILED Eggs cooked in the shell until the whites are opaque and the yolks are hot and runny. Traditionally eaten directly from the shell in an eggcup.

Egg Substitute Made mainly of egg whites and thus lacking rich flavor, egg substitute is recommended for anyone avoiding the fat and cholesterol in egg yolks. Use in some baking, such as brownies and cookies, for scrambling, or in sauces.

See also CURDLING; FOOD SAFETY.

ENDIVE Also known as Belgian endive or witloof, this member of the chicory family is widely grown in Belgium, the principal source of the endive sold in North American markets. It relies on a painstaking, nonmechanized cultivation method (the reason for its high price) that calls for forcing chicory roots to sprout in a darkened, humid room, to yield small, white (or sometimes red-tipped), tightly furled, bullet-shaped heads. These carefully tended vegetables are fragile, and, while they travel well to foreign markets, they should be handled carefully at every step, including once you get them home. See also CHICORY.

ENOKI See MUSHROOM.

EPAZOTE See HERB.

ESCAROLE The robust, slightly curled leaves of this chicory relative are, like all chicory varieties, slightly bitter, but pleasingly so. The ruffled-leafed heads are particular favorites of Italian cooks, who add the leaves to a light broth for a simple soup or sauté the leaves quickly in olive oil with garlic and red pepper flakes and then toss them with pasta. See also CHICORY.

EVAPORATED MILK See MILK.

EVAPORATING A liquid heated to a certain temperature will boil, and agitating molecules will escape into the air, or evaporate. When water evaporates, it escapes in the form of a vapor called steam. The steam remains at a constant temperature just above the boiling point (212°F or 100°C for water at sea level). For this reason, steaming is a gentle, stable way to cook food and keep it moist.

Boiled long enough, a liquid will be reduced to only dry solids or trace residue.

Cooks take advantage of this process of evaporation to concentrate flavors and thicken sauces. In candy making, the water in boiling sugar syrup gradually evaporates, changing the temperature, density, and color of the syrup. See also BOILING; CANDY MAKING; DEGLAZING; HIGH-ALTITUDE COOKING; REDUCING; SAUCE.

EXTRACT Concentrated flavorings made from plants such as vanilla beans or almonds. Extracts, which are commonly used to flavor sweet dishes, are created by evaporating or distilling the plant's essential

Quick Tip

Because fats hold essential oils particularly well, add extracts while creaming the butter and sugar in a cake or cookie recipe to get the best flavor dispersion. As a general rule, use 1 teaspoon extract to flavor each 2 cups of food.

oils, which give it its distinctive flavor, and then suspending these oils in alcohol. In the United States, an extract labeled "pure" must contain only essential oils distilled from natural plants. Imitation flavorings, such as imitation vanilla extract, try to replicate the flavor of natural foods, sometimes using synthetic compounds. Artificial flavorings mimic foods that do not exist naturally, such as root beer or butterscotch. **Selecting** Use pure extracts whenever possible. They may cost more, but they have stronger, more complex flavors than either imitation or artificial products. **Storing** Store in a cool, dark cupboard. Extracts will keep for up to 1 year.

Quick Bite

In Britain and Australia, extracts are referred to as *essences*.

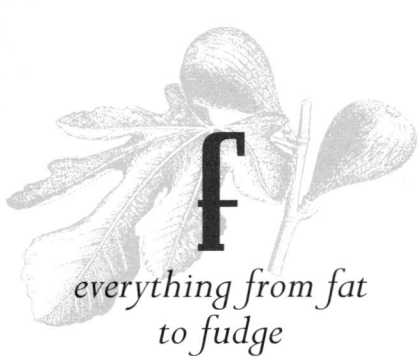

f

*everything from fat
to fudge*

f

FAT & OIL Too often demonized nowadays, fats and oils (the latter being fats that are liquid at room temperature) play an essential role in the kitchen. In sautéing, stir-frying, and panfrying, they lubricate food and cooking vessel alike, preventing sticking, and they transfer heat efficiently, promoting browning. In deep-frying, they become the cooking medium itself. In baking, they are used to grease pans, preventing batters and doughs from sticking. As part of those same batters and doughs, they give tenderness to the crumbs of breads and cakes and flakiness to pastries of all kinds. In dressings and sauces, and as spreads for bread, they add a smooth consistency. Particular fats and oils also contribute their distinctive and satisfying flavors to any recipe in which they appear.

Fats and Health With 9 calories per gram, fat is a concentrated calorie source, yielding two and a quarter times the energy by weight that a protein or carbohydrate offers. As a result, eating a high-fat diet without getting enough exercise can lead to weight gain and illnesses associated with obesity.

All fats from animal sources contain some cholesterol. This substance plays important roles in our bodies, helping to build cell membranes, nerve fibers, and hormones, for example. But because our livers actually manufacture all the cholesterol we need, diets high in animal fats introduce excess cholesterol, which can be deposited on arterial walls and lead to high blood pressure, heart disease, or stroke.

Different types of fat in food affect our bodies in different ways. Saturated fats, namely, those from animal sources, coconut and palm oils, and cocoa butter, bring excess levels of cholesterol to the blood. Another saturated fat is the trans fat that results when vegetable oil is hydrogenated to form margarine or solid shortenings. By contrast, the polyunsaturated fats found in most ordinary vegetable oils tend to lower blood cholesterol levels. But they are prone to oxidation, which can increase the buildup of plaque on arterial walls. Monounsaturated fats, such as olive and canola oils, not only lower blood cholesterol but also resist oxidation and are considered the healthiest choices of all.

Medical researchers generally recommend that we get no more than 30 percent of our daily calories from fat. No more than one-third of those should come from saturated fat, and as much as possible should come from monounsaturated fats.

Selecting Apart from the health-related issues already discussed, your choice of fat or oil for cooking will depend on three factors. One is whether a solid fat or liquid oil is required. Some baking recipes, for example, rely for their consistency on the ability to cut solid cubes of butter into little pieces covered in flour, or on the ability of solid fat to "cream" to a smooth, fluffy consistency when mixed with sugar. Another factor is whether or not the particular flavor of a fat or an oil is desired, an especially important question with flavorful olive oil. Finally, the temperature to which an oil or

Oil Glossary

I n most markets, the shelves devoted to cooking oils display a wide range of choices, from vegetable oils to nut oils to seed oils. The following, including notes on their uses, are the most common.

CANOLA OIL Bland oil pressed from rapeseed, a relative of the mustard plant. High in monounsaturated fat. Good for general cooking and baking, but can smell unpleasant at high frying temperatures.

COCONUT OIL Popular as a deep-frying oil in Indian and Malaysian kitchens, imparting rich flavor. High in saturated fat.

CORN OIL Deep golden, relatively flavorless all-purpose oil largely used for general cooking and deep-frying.

GRAPESEED OIL Pressed from grape seeds and mild in flavor. Heats to very high temperatures and is suitable for frying. Also popular in salad dressings and marinades.

HAZELNUT OIL Highly flavorful oil, usually imported from France, pressed from toasted hazelnuts and used sparingly to enrich dressings and to flavor savory and sweet dishes. With its low smoke point, it is not used for cooking.

OLIVE OIL Prized oil produced in Mediterranean countries, California, and Australia from the fruit of the olive tree. Extra-virgin olive oil, a term applied to products pressed without the use of heat or chemicals, has a clear green or brownish hue and a fine, fruity, sometimes slightly peppery flavor, and is low in acidity. Use it in dressings or as a seasoning or condiment. Those olive oils labeled "mild," "light," "pure," or simply "olive oil" will have less fragrance and color than extra-virgin and are better suited to light cooking such as sautéing. All olive oils, and especially extra-virgin oils, are high in healthful monounsaturated fat.

PEANUT OIL Pressed from peanuts, which give it a hint of rich, nutty flavor, unless it is a refined version. Popular in Chinese cooking for stir-frying or deep-frying, it also may be used in salad dressings and dipping sauces.

SAFFLOWER OIL Widely available, flavorless oil pressed from safflower seeds, with a high smoke point. High in polyunsaturated fat.

SESAME OIL Deep amber–colored oil pressed from toasted sesame seeds and used as a seasoning in Chinese and Japanese kitchens. A pale golden, fairly flavorless cold-pressed sesame oil, sold in health-food stores, may be used for sautéing but is not a suitable substitute in recipes that call for Asian oil.

SOYBEAN OIL Bland oil pressed from soybeans, with a high smoke point suitable for deep-frying.

SUNFLOWER SEED OIL Pale, light, flavorless oil high in poly- and monounsaturated fats. Good all-purpose oil, used for everything from deep-frying to sautéing to salad dressings.

VEGETABLE OIL Commercial term applied to general-purpose oils that may be composed of corn, safflower, canola, or other oils, blended and filtered to have a pale color, neutral flavor, and high smoke point.

WALNUT OIL Rich-tasting, deep brown nut oil imported from France or Italy and used as a seasoning on its own or blended into dressings or sauces. Walnut oil is not good for frying because of its low smoke point.

f

Fat Glossary

The well-stocked kitchen always has a good range of solid cooking fats on hand for sautéing, frying, and baking.

BUTTER Imparts the rich, creamy flavor of cow's milk. Used for brief, lower-heat sautéing (it tends to burn) or to enrich sauces or baked goods. See also BUTTER.

LARD Pure pork fat rendered from back and kidney fat, very rich in flavor and with the finest known as leaf lard. Favored by some bakers for the flaky texture and rich taste it gives to pastry. Has a high smoke point, making it suitable for deep-frying.

MARGARINE Butter substitute made from hydrogenated vegetable oil. With the exception of reduced-fat margarine, may be used for baking or frying. See also MARGARINE.

SCHMALTZ A rich, flavorful ingredient used in traditional Jewish cooking, schmaltz is rendered chicken fat, sold in Jewish delis and some well-stocked food stores. Used for brief sautéing and to enrich savory dishes such as matzo balls.

SHORTENING This term applies in general to any solid fat used in baking. More specifically refers to vegetable shortening, a type of hydrogenated solid vegetable fat manufactured for use in baking or deep-frying. See also SHORTENING; VEGETABLE SHORTENING.

SUET Pure beef fat rendered from solid white fat from the kidney and loin, particularly prized in Europe for the rich taste it gives to pastries and deep-fried dishes.

a fat can be heated before it begins to break down and smoke, called its smoke point, will determine the use to which it can be put, from no-heat use in dressings to high-temperature deep-frying. See the Oil Glossary on page 189 for a few tips.

With some oils, you'll have a choice of refined and unrefined. Asian sesame oil is a good example of an unrefined oil, which contains some flavorful solids in suspension. Peanut and corn oils also are found in both forms. Unrefined oils are generally not best for cooking, as their smoke points are fairly low, but they are full of flavor and good for dressings. Refined oils are better for cooking but are largely flavorless.

Storing The enemies of fat are light, water, and heat. Exposure to any of these will promote rancidity. Store solid animal fats such as butter or lard in the refrigerator in their original packaging or, after

Quick Tip

When oil being heated becomes fragrant and shimmers, it is hot and ready to cook with.

opening, in a covered container. Unopened packages also may be frozen for up to 6 months. You can keep shortening still sealed in its original packaging in a cool, dry place indefinitely. Once opened, it will keep for up to 1 year. Store oils in airtight containers away from light and heat. Flavorful nut oils, which go rancid more quickly, should be bought in small quantities and kept refrigerated, which will likely turn them solid. Bring to room temperature before use.

See also BUTTER; COOKING SPRAY; FRYING; LOW-FAT COOKING; MARGARINE; SMOKE POINT; VEGETABLE SHORTENING.

FAVA BEAN See BEAN, DRIED; BEAN, FRESH.

FENNEL Also known as sweet fennel or finocchio. The fennel plant's leaves, seeds, and stems all have a sweet, faintly aniselike flavor. The stems of fennel swell and overlap at the base of the plant to form a bulb with white to pale green ribbed layers that are similar to celery in appearance and texture. The pretty green leaves are light and feathery and slightly resemble fresh dill. Use them as a bed for steaming fish or in small amounts as a garnish. Originating in the Mediterranean, the fennel bulb appears often in Italian and Scandinavian cuisines. It can be eaten raw or grilled, baked, braised, or sautéed.

Selecting Choose fresh fennel bulbs that are smooth and tightly layered with no cracks or bruises. Fat, rounded bulbs with white and pale green color will tend to be more succulent than thin or yellow ones. Avoid any with wilted leaves or dried layers. Now available year-round, fennel is at its peak from late fall through winter. Grocers sometimes incorrectly label fennel as "sweet anise."

Storing Keep fennel bulbs in a perforated plastic bag in the refrigerator for up to 5 days. If kept too long, they will lose their flavor and toughen.

HOW TO *Trim and Cut Fennel*
1. Remove the green stems and leaves, saving them to flavor or garnish other dishes such as soups or fish.
2. Discard the outer layer of the bulb if it is tough and cut away any discolored areas.
3. Cut the bulb in half lengthwise and remove the base of the core if it is thick and solid.
4. Gently separate the layers with your hands and rinse well to remove any grit between them.
5. Slice or cut as directed in a recipe.

Quick Tip
While grilling, toss a handful of dried or fresh fennel stems onto the charcoal to infuse meat or fish with a light anise flavor.

See also BRAISING; SPICE.

FENUGREEK See SPICE.

FERMENTATION Some of the most important and most flavorful foods in the world, from bread, buttermilk, yogurt, cheese, and chocolate to beer and wine, depend on fermentation. Complex flavors emerge and textures change as yeast and bacteria are allowed to multiply in the food and break down large sugar or starch chains into smaller molecules, creating carbon dioxide and alcohol in the process. In some cases the gas produced during fermentation is trapped, making bread dough rise and Champagne bubbly. In other cases, it is released, as with still wine and cheese.

FETA See CHEESE.

FIG Among the world's oldest known foods, the fig was immortalized by the ancient poets, offered to early Olympic athletes during training, and long ago used in place of expensive or nonexistent sugar. The trees flourish in warm climates, where they can live for over a century and grow to a height of more than 100 feet. The soft, pear-shaped "fruit" is, in fact, a flower 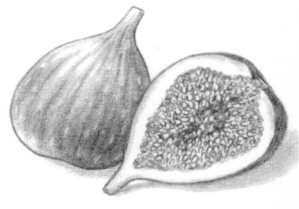 swollen and turned in on itself, while the many tiny "seeds" are the actual fruit of the tree.

There are more than 150 varieties of figs, with skin that can be purple, green, yellow, brown, or white and flesh that ranges from pale gold to deep, rich red. Among the best-known varieties are green-skinned, white-fleshed Adriatic; the small, dark purple, sweet-tasting Mission (also known as Black Mission and California Black); the gold-skinned Calimyrna; the yellow-green, virtually seedless Kadota; and the nutty, amber-hued Smyrna. When dried, figs become delightfully chewy and even sweeter.

Fresh figs are delicious when poached or baked in tarts or paired with poultry or game. Use dried figs like raisins, chopping them and adding them to muffins, quick breads, cookies, couscous, or rice pilafs.

Selecting Fresh figs are available twice a year. The first crop, which is the smaller of the two, arrives in the market in June and lasts through July, but the fruits themselves are larger and more flavorful than the harvest from the second crop. The second crop begins in early September and runs through mid-October. Because they do not ripen off the tree, figs must be picked ripe and are quite fragile. They must be handled exceedingly carefully, which accounts for their usually high price tag.

Choose figs that are soft to the touch but not wrinkled, mushy, or bruised. Look for plump figs with firm stems and good color free of gray or tan spots. Figs with a webbing of delicate fissures, stretch marks revealing particularly moist and sweet fruit, are highly prized—a classic farmers' market treat. A sour aroma indicates an over-ripe fig that has begun to ferment.

Figs are widely available dried. Often sold in blocks or rounds, they lose their shape if packed too tightly. For better quality, buy dried figs in bulk at specialty markets or health-food stores. Dried figs should still be slightly soft.

Storing Fresh figs are highly perishable and should be eaten as soon after purchase as possible. If need be, they can be refrigerated for 1 to 2 days, arranged in a single layer on a tray lined with paper towels. They do not ripen if left at room temperature, but if they are just a little too firm to enjoy right away, they will soften enough to eat in a day or so.

Dried figs will keep in a cool, dry place for 1 or 2 months or in the refrigerator or in an airtight container or plastic bag for up to 6 months.

Preparing Rinse fresh figs and pat dry gently just before serving. Some recipes call for peeling them, a step that is purely aesthetic and generally unnecessary, since the entire fruit is edible. Overhandling will bruise the delicate fruit.

Quick Tip

Slit whole dried figs, stuff them with walnuts, and serve with a glass of tawny Port for an elegant after-dinner nibble.

FILBERT Another name for hazelnut; see NUT.

FILLET (fil-LAY) As a noun, the term *fillet* (sometimes spelled *filet,* especially when the subject is beef) signifies a piece of boneless fish, meat, or poultry. As a verb, "to fillet" means to remove the bones from fish, meat, or poultry, thus producing a fillet. With a little practice and a good narrow-bladed, rigid, sharp boning knife, home cooks can bone fish, chicken, or meat, but most people leave the job to the fishmonger or butcher. See also BONING.

FILO (FEE-loh) Also spelled "phyllo." These large, paper-thin sheets of dough create the flaky layers of many Middle Eastern and Greek sweet and savory pastries.

Honey-sweet baklava, cinnamon-infused *bisteeya,* and rich *spanakopita* all depend on filo for their delicate crusts. Filo also replaces more time-consuming puff pastry and tart doughs in recipes that highlight convenience and light texture.

Selecting Traditionally stretched into expansive nearly transparent sheets by master bakers, commercially produced filo is now widely available. The machine-rolled and frozen filo in major grocery stores is a good alternative to the fresh sheets sold at Middle Eastern markets. A 1-pound box will generally have 20 to 24 sheets, each measuring about 12 inches wide and 18 inches long. Try to buy them from a source with a high turnover. Long-frozen filo sheets will tend to stick together in clumps and break easily once thawed. Fresh sheets may be slightly smaller than frozen ones.

Storing Well-wrapped filo can be frozen for up to 6 months. Once thawed, an unopened box will keep in the refrigerator for up to 3 weeks. Defrosted filo should not be frozen again. You can wrap unused sheets in several layers of plastic wrap and return them to the refrigerator for up to 1 week; however, they may lose some of their pliability. Seal fresh filo in plastic wrap and refrigerate for up to 3 days.

Preparing For pliable sheets that do not stick or tear, thaw frozen filo in the refrigerator for 24 hours. Before beginning to layer or shape the sheets, be sure your work surface is clean and dry, your filling is cool, and all your ingredients and equipment are ready at hand. Although more fat between the layers means richer flavor and flakier texture, you can use as little as 1 teaspoon melted butter or olive oil for each layer. Clarified butter (see BUTTER) results in the crispiest pastry, but simple melted butter or a healthier butter-oil mix will work as well.

Quick Tip

With moist fillings, keep the filo layers dry and crisp by sprinkling a teaspoon of bread or cookie crumbs on each sheet after spreading the butter or oil. Sprinkle additional crumbs on the layer just beneath the filling.

Carefully unwrap the filo sheets from their packaging and spread them flat on a large tray or baking sheet. Cover the stack with plastic wrap or waxed paper, and then drape the whole tray with a damp cloth. Working with filo is not nearly as difficult as many believe. The most important points to remember are to bring the filo to room temperature, to work quickly, and to keep the sheets covered to prevent them from drying out. Filo layers can be used in place of homemade strudel dough or as a variation for pie or tart pastry.

HOW TO *Butter and Layer Filo*

1. Lightly coat a pan or baking sheet with melted butter or olive oil.
2. Remove only 1 sheet of filo at a time, using both hands to lift it up straight by 2 corners. Lay the sheet of filo down in the pan.
3. Dot the filo with the butter or oil, and then brush outward to the filo's edges to spread the fat evenly.

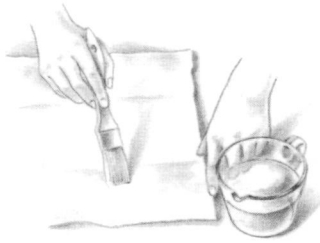

4. Repeat with the desired number of layers.
5. Coat the outside surfaces of the completed pastry with fat to encourage a golden brown color. Bake as directed.

fish

As the old saying goes, "There are a lot of fish in the sea." And that's not to mention the fish found in oceans, gulfs, lakes, rivers, reservoirs, streams, ponds, and bayous.

With the growing awareness of the benefits to be derived from eating this generally low-fat source of protein, more and more kinds of fish are turning up on menus and in markets, to be enjoyed as appetizers or main courses, on their own or in a wide range of salads, soups, sandwiches, pastas, and other preparations.

Selecting Use your eyes and nose to help you discern quality and freshness. All fish should look moist and bright and have a fresh, clean scent. Steer clear of products with discoloration, dryness, or even the slightest hint of an "off" aroma. Whole fish, in general, should look almost alive, with clear eyes; bright, intact scales and skin; and red, moist gills.

To find the best-quality fish, start with a reliable fishmonger or the seafood department of a well-stocked food store with frequent turnover. The staff should be readily able to tell you the origin of a fish and whether it is fresh or defrosted frozen. They should also willingly clean, scale, skin, fillet, or otherwise prepare the fish to your specifications.

Because fish tend to spoil more quickly than other animal proteins at normal refrigeration temperatures, all products at a fishmonger or seafood department should be displayed on crushed ice or in refrigerated cases with thermometers that clearly display a temperature of 33°F or lower.

Frozen fish also can be excellent if they were frozen on board the ship, soon after being caught. Avoid any that look dry, indicating freezer burn, or that come in packages containing liquid that has frozen, a sign of defrosting and refreezing—and of damage to the fish's texture.

Several popular kinds of fish are also commonly sold in other forms, including smoked, canned, pickled, and salted.

Storing Refrigerate fresh fish the moment you get it home and, ideally, cook it the day you buy it. To keep it in optimum condition for use on the following day, refrigerate the wrapped package in a baking pan—or any container large enough to hold it—and cover it with ice. Do not let the flesh of fish come in contact with ice, or it will cause freezer burn and leach out flavor. Always protect the flesh with plastic or some kind of barrier. Whole fish may sit directly in ice with no deterioration.

Frozen fish will keep well for 1 to 2 months in a freezer with a maximum temperature of 0°F. To defrost frozen fish, leave it on a tray or plate in the refrigerator for 24 hours, then store in a pan or tray of ice until ready to cook.

Preparing Hundreds of different types of fish, each with its own unique characteristics, are caught and eaten around the world. Most fish, however, can be classified in several simple ways that provide guidance on how to prepare, cook, and eat them.

LEAN FISH VS. OILY FISH Many fish, such as cod, sea bass, sole, and snapper, have mild-tasting, very lean flesh that calls for cooking with liquid or some fat to keep it moist. They are best when cooked by

f

moist-heat methods, such as braising, poaching, or steaming, or when cooked in fat, as in frying or sautéing. When cooked by grilling, broiling, or roasting, they need to be either diligently basted or wrapped up to contain their juices. By contrast, more distinctively flavored, oily-fleshed fish, such as salmon, tuna, mackerel, and eel, do well when cooked by nearly all dry-heat methods—sautéing, frying, grilling, roasting, baking—virtually basting themselves, although they also can be good when cooked by moist-heat methods. See also COOKING METHODS.

FIRM FISH VS. DELICATE FISH Some fish, such as cod, snapper, sole, and trout, have fairly delicate flesh that requires careful cooking. Their fillets, for example, may fall apart during grilling, so the fish should only be grilled whole. Other varieties, such as swordfish or tuna, have a meaty texture, almost akin to steak, that can stand up to almost any cooking method.

FLATFISH VS. ROUND FISH Fish that are flat and narrow, such as sole or flounder, cook quickly, whether they are left whole or boned to yield 4 thin fillets. They do well with rapid methods, such as sautéing, but can disintegrate or dry out if cooked too long. Large fish with a rounded body, such as salmon, swordfish, or tuna, yield a wider variety of cuts—including large fillets, boneless medallions, and cross-sectional bone-in steaks—that adapt well to a wide range of cooking methods.

Testing for Doneness Common kitchen wisdom holds that, whatever cooking method is used, any piece of fish should be cooked for a total of 10 minutes for each inch of thickness at its widest point. As the moistness and texture of fish vary widely from species to species, however, it is wise to start checking for doneness after 8 minutes have elapsed.

To test for doneness, use the tip of a small, sharp knife to separate the flakes of the fish or otherwise cut into it at its thickest point. Unless you are deliberately cooking to medium or medium-rare, as some contemporary recipes for salmon and tuna indicate, the fish should be just opaque but still moist at its center and easy to flake. If it is already flaking without being prodded, it is likely overdone.

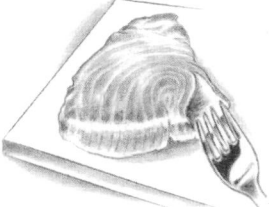

Testing fish for doneness.

A School of Fish

ANCHOVY This small, strong-tasting, oily saltwater fish is generally sold as fillets, either packed in salt or canned in oil. See also ANCHOVY.

BLUEFISH A rich-tasting, oily-fleshed saltwater fish found in Atlantic waters that is best cooked by a dry-heat method such as broiling or grilling.

CARP The mild taste and moist, meaty texture of this pale-fleshed, slightly oily freshwater fish is best highlighted by moist cooking such as braising or frying.

CATFISH This fairly firm-textured, white-fleshed freshwater fish can be cooked any way you like: fried, grilled, broiled, steamed, sautéed, or braised. Farm-raised specimens will have the mildest flavor.

COD Mild tasting, delicate, and lean, this white-fleshed saltwater fish takes well to any method but grilling.

EEL Found in both fresh- and saltwater, this long, slithery fish has rich-tasting, meaty, oily flesh that is good when broiled, grilled, braised, or stewed. Smoked eel, occasionally found in specialty-food stores, is especially delicious.

FLOUNDER A family of lean, delicate flatfish requiring quick cooking by any method.

continued

f

Fish, continued

HADDOCK Lean, mild, delicate saltwater fish similar to cod that may be cooked by any method.

HALIBUT Mild-flavored, lean, fairly firm-fleshed saltwater fish that may be cooked by any method.

HERRING Oily, flavorful, tender saltwater fish that is usually pickled, although fresh herring may be grilled or broiled.

MACKEREL Oily, flavorful, tender saltwater fish similar to herring that is likewise usually pickled, although the fresh fish may be grilled, broiled, or braised.

MONKFISH A white-fleshed saltwater fish, sometimes called the "poor man's lobster" for its meaty texture and mild, sweet flavor. May be cooked by any method.

PERCH Lean, mild, firm-fleshed freshwater fish that may be cooked by any method.

PIKE Mild-tasting and sweet, very lean, firm-fleshed freshwater fish that takes well to any cooking method.

ROCKFISH Delicate, mild-flavored, lean saltwater fish that takes well to any cooking method except grilling.

SABLE Rich, oily saltwater fish that is suitable for cooking by any method.

SALMON A firm, meaty, oily fish that may be poached, baked, roasted, panfried, steamed, broiled, or grilled. See SALMON.

SARDINE Small, slender, oily saltwater fish usually sold in cans. Fresh sardines are excellent cooked by dry heat. They are also good for pickling.

SEA BASS Lean, tender but meaty, white-fleshed saltwater fish suitable for cooking by any method.

SHAD Oily freshwater fish with a mild, sweet taste and tender texture best complemented by dry-heat cooking or sautéing. Shad roe, the delicate egg sac, is a springtime specialty, cooked by brief sautéing.

SHARK A family of lean, meaty-textured saltwater fish, of which some of the most commonly eaten varieties are the shortfin mako, the black tip, and the spiny dogfish. Shark may be cooked by any method.

SMELT Small, slender, oily saltwater fish with tender texture and mild, sweet flavor. Best quickly cooked by dry heat. Also known as whitebait in its smallest form, which is fried and eaten whole.

SNAPPER A family of tender but firm, lean, mild saltwater fish, of which red snapper and yellowtail snapper are the most popular varieties. Snapper may be cooked by any method.

SOLE A family of lean, delicate ocean flatfish, among which common varieties are Dover, lemon, petrale, and rex. May be cooked by any method, but only briefly.

STURGEON Very firm-textured, oily, rich-tasting salt- or freshwater fish, may be cooked by any method.

SWORDFISH Firm-textured, somewhat oily, rich-tasting white-fleshed ocean fish that may be cooked by any method.

TROUT Delicate, somewhat oily freshwater fish that may be cooked by dry heat. Excellent when smoked.

TUNA Meaty, flavorful, oily saltwater fish that is good cooked by any method and is excellent raw as sashimi or sushi. Also commonly available canned. See TUNA.

TURBOT Mild, tender white-fleshed saltwater flatfish that can be cooked by dry- or moist-heat methods.

WHITEFISH Oily, tender, flavorful freshwater fish that can be cooked by any method and is a favorite smoked fish.

See also CAVIAR; FILLET; FLAKING; individual cooking methods.

Quick Bite

Oily-fleshed fish, especially herring, anchovy, salmon, tuna, sardine, mackerel, and swordfish, are rich in a type of healthful polyunsaturated fat called omega-3 fatty acids.

FISH SAUCE Southeast Asians use fish sauce in much the same way Westerners use salt, both as a cooking seasoning and at the table. It is a clear liquid, ranging from amber to dark brown, and famous (or infamous) for its pungent aroma and strong, salty flavor.

The best-quality fish sauce is pressed from small fish, commonly anchovies, that have been salted, packed in barrels, and fermented for several months under the steady heat of the tropical sun. Fish sauce is called *nam pla* in Thailand, *nuoc mam* in Vietnam, *tuk trey* in Cambodia, and *patis* in the Philippines. In the Southeast Asian kitchen, these add depth to almost every savory dish, and at the table, fish sauce is mixed with various seasonings, such as lime juice, rice vinegar, sugar, black pepper, and chiles, and then used as a dipping sauce. Not surprisingly, the sauce is also high in protein.

Selecting The first pressing of the salted and fermented fish produces liquid with the clearest color and the most balanced flavor. A lighter color indicates a more subtle flavor, best as a table condiment and in dipping sauces. The darker fish sauces, which are used more often in cooking, tend to taste stronger and saltier.

Storing Fish sauce will keep indefinitely if stored in a cool, dark place.

FLAGEOLET See BEAN, DRIED; BEAN, FRESH.

FLAKING To separate food, especially cooked or canned fish, into its natural layers. Typically a fork is used to ease the layers apart. Sometimes the purpose of flaking is to break up the food sufficiently for easy mixing; other times larger flakes are desired for an attractive appearance, such as for a composed salad. Flaking can also be a test for when fish is done cooking: if a fork inserted vertically into a piece of fish separates the layers easily and reveals the flesh to be opaque throughout, the fish is done.

FLAMBÉING To pour warmed liquor over food and ignite its fumes. Flambéing, or flaming, is often used to prepare sauces and desserts at tableside for a dramatic presentation, but it also has a culinary purpose. Liquor is often used to flavor dishes, and burning off the alcohol tempers its harshness and accentuates the flavor. Not all the alcohol actually burns off; anywhere from 5 to 85 percent may remain in the dish, an important consideration for anyone avoiding alcohol. Flambéed dishes are not as popular as they once were, but flambéing is an essential element in coq au vin, bananas Foster, crêpes Suzette, cherries jubilee, baked Alaska, and the traditional English plum pudding served at Christmastime.

Restaurant chefs usually tilt their pans slightly over a gas burner to ignite the fumes. Don't try this professional technique at home; it is easier and safer to use a long kitchen or fireplace match. If you have a chafing dish or a portable burner, you can flambé at the table.

Caution!

- Brandy or an 80-proof liquor is best for flambéing. Higher-proof alcohol is too volatile, and anything lower in proof won't flame as effectively.
- When using a gas stove, always pour alcohol from a bottle into a pan that is well away from the heat. The flame from a gas burner can follow the alcohol into the bottle and cause it to burst.
- Be careful not to let long hair or loose sleeves catch fire, and don't lean your face too close to the pan as you ignite the alcohol fumes.

f

HOW TO *Flambé*

1. Have the dish with its sauce gently simmering over very low heat.
2. Warm the liquor in a small pan just until it is hot but not boiling. It can also be warmed in a microwave, allowing 15 to 20 seconds for every ¼ cup of liquor. The liquor must be warmed first in order to flambé successfully.
3. Remove the pan holding the food to be flamed from the burner, or turn the burner off. Pour the warmed liquor evenly over the food.
4. Without stirring, return the pan to the heat or turn the burner back on. Light a long match and hold it 1 to 2 inches above the food to light the fumes. Do not touch the match to the food or the liquor itself.
5. Wait for the flames to subside completely, or shake the pan gently or cover it with a lid if necessary to smother them. The longer you let the flames burn, the more alcohol you will burn off. Alcohol carries flavor, some of which you may wish to retain in the dish.

Quick Tip

To garnish with flames: Just before serving a dish, soak sugar cubes with liquor, arrange them decoratively on or around the food, and then ignite the fumes rising from the cubes.

FLAME-TAMER A brand-name heat diffuser; see COOKING TOOLS.

FLATTENING See POUNDING.

FLOUR The product that results from grinding grains, dried vegetables, or nuts into a fine powder. Flours provide the body and substance of breads, noodles, cakes, and cookies. They also thicken sauces and serve as coatings for fried meat and vegetables. One of the oldest and most

important foods in the human diet, the first flour was ground over 14,000 years ago.

In common usage, the term *flour* generally refers to ground wheat grain. Stone-ground flour retains more nutrients and flavor than flour milled with steel rollers, which heat the grain, changing its flavor. The first milling breaks the wheat grain and separates its three components. The outer hull, or bran, is rich in nutrients; the wheat germ contains the seed's embryo that will later sprout; and the endosperm, which makes up most of the grain and provides most of its starch, will become white flour. Since bran and germ contain oils that spoil quickly, they are removed to extend the shelf life of white flour, which is then fortified with vitamins and minerals to replace the lost nutrients. It will lighten naturally as it ages, but much of the flour sold is bleached chemically. Although not as white as chemically bleached flour, unbleached flour has a better flavor.

Storing Try to buy flour in amounts that you can use in 4 to 6 months. It will keep longer but is best used fresh. Transfer flour to an airtight container and keep it in a cool, dry place away from light. Because the bran and germ contain oils, whole-wheat flour will go rancid quickly if stored at room temperature. Wrap it tightly and keep it in the refrigerator for up to 6 months or in the freezer for up to 1 year.

About Sifting Passing flour through a fine mesh filters out lumps and creates a lighter, smoother texture. Although many flours come presifted, it is still a good idea to sift flour before you use it for cakes, cookies, and other tender baked goods. Read a recipe closely to see if it asks you to sift before or after measuring.

About Wheat Flour There are two general types of wheat grown. Soft wheat, found in milder climates, has less protein and more starch. Hard wheat generally grows in colder areas and is ground into bread and pasta flour. These natural variations in wheat, plus different kinds of processing, make for several different styles of wheat flour. For a baker, the most important difference to understand is the protein content, which can range from 5 to 15 percent. The varying levels of protein help determine the difference between tender cupcakes and chewy bread. A higher protein content in the flour used in bread baking allows a dough to form a strong, elastic network of interlocking strands, called gluten, to capture the gases needed to raise the bread. If low-protein cake flour is used in a bread recipe, the gluten structure will not be strong enough and the bread will not rise properly or attain a chewy texture. If high-protein bread flour is used in a cake recipe, it will have a tough, sturdy texture that no one wants in a cake. The following types of flour are arranged by protein content, from highest to lowest, to help you choose the right one for a particular use.

HIGH-GLUTEN FLOUR High-protein flour, milled from hard wheat and treated to remove a relatively high percentage of its starch. It is commonly mixed with flours that are very low in protein, such as rye.

BREAD FLOUR An unbleached, hard-wheat flour. Its high protein content creates an elastic dough for higher rise and more structure in breads, pizza crusts, and pastas. Some bread flours include malted barley flour to feed the yeast.

ALL-PURPOSE FLOUR A mixture of soft and hard wheats, with the bran and germ removed. This is the popular general-use flour that is good for a wide range of foods, from sauces to cookies to quick breads to pancakes to fritter batters.

WHOLE-WHEAT FLOUR Milled from whole grains of wheat. Since it still contains the bran and germ, whole-wheat flour has

Quick Tip

For best flavor and texture, do not replace all the all-purpose flour in a recipe with whole-wheat flour. Substitute one-fourth to three-fourths of the white flour, depending on taste. Add liquids gradually, as you may need to use less than you would if using only all-purpose flour.

more flavor, higher nutritional value, and darker color than white flour. It also absorbs more liquid, is denser after baking, and contains more fat. Because it contains more parts of the whole grains, whole-wheat flour has a lower protein content than all-purpose flour.

SELF-RISING FLOUR A relatively soft, or lower-protein, all-purpose flour mixed with baking powder and salt, intended as a convenience when making biscuits, quick breads, and cookies. Its leavening power decreases gradually after 2 or 3 months, which is one reason that many bakers prefer to use all-purpose flour and add rising agents themselves for consistent results.

PASTRY FLOUR With slightly more protein than cake flour, pastry flour offers the additional structure needed for puffed and layered pastry dough but is still more tender than all-purpose flour.

CAKE FLOUR Milled from soft wheat and containing cornstarch, cake flour is low in protein and high in starch. It gives cakes a light crumb. Cake flour has also undergone a bleaching process that increases its ability to hold water and sugar, so cakes made with cake flour are less likely to fall.

Quick Bite

Flour contains starch, which acts as a thickener in sauces and gravies. See THICKENING.

f

About Specialty Flours Flour is generally understood to be basic wheat flour, but there are other grains, vegetables, and nuts that can be ground into flour as well. The term *meal* refers to other coarsely ground grains.

BUCKWHEAT FLOUR A dark flour with a nutty, slightly sweet flavor and firm texture. Used to make soba noodles in Japan, crepes in Brittany, and pancakes and blini throughout Eastern Europe and Russia.

CHESTNUT FLOUR A flavorful, extremely fine flour ground from dried chestnuts. Used in desserts in Italy and Hungary.

CHICKPEA FLOUR Called *farinata* in Italy and *besan* in India. Ground from dried chickpeas, a rich flour used to make flat breads, dumplings, and fritters.

CORN FLOUR Finely ground white or yellow cornmeal. In Great Britain, the term *cornflour* refers to cornstarch.

MASA HARINA Literally "dough flour" in Spanish, a form of cornmeal used in Mexico to make tortillas and tamales. Whole corn kernels are cooked in a caustic mineral lime solution to remove their hulls, then dried and ground into flour.

OAT FLOUR Sweet, earthy flour made from finely ground groats. It makes particularly soft and moist baked goods.

Quick Tip

Gluten-forming proteins are plentiful in wheat but appear in much smaller amounts in rye and oats. Gluten-free grains include buckwheat, corn, and rice. Flours ground from vegetables or nuts such as chickpea and chestnut also do not form gluten, so these flours are traditionally used to make unleavened, or flat, breads. Replace no more than one-third of a recipe's wheat flour with oat or rye flour. You may substitute up to one-fourth of the wheat flour with gluten-free or nongrain flours.

POTATO FLOUR Ground from steamed and dried potatoes. Used to thicken delicate sauces and to make tender cakes and cookies. Also called potato starch.

RICE FLOUR Ground from white rice. Long-grain rice flour is used as a wheat substitute in baked goods and to obtain a light, crispy texture in crackers and cookies. Short-grain, or glutinous, rice flour gives Asian sweets their soft, chewy texture. In Japan, the flour is ground from cooked rice and then mixed with water and cooked to make the familiar sticky national sweet known as *mochi*. Neither should be confused with rice powder, which is exceedingly fine. Flour ground from brown rice has a nutty flavor and darker color.

Quick Tip

Both fat and acid will inhibit the development of gluten strands, which is good for pastry (and bad for bread). Less gluten will help make a dough easier to roll out and more tender after baking. When making pastry, for every cup of flour, add 1 teaspoon of lemon juice or 2 tablespoons of oil to the wet ingredients called for in a recipe.

RYE FLOUR A slightly bitter and tangy flour, second only to wheat flour in the world of bread baking, that makes a dense, heavy bread. Dark rye flour retains more of the bran than medium rye.

SEMOLINA FLOUR Ground from a particular variety of wheat, called durum wheat, that is especially hard (that is, high in protein) and used primarily for making dried pasta. High-quality pasta will be made from 100 percent durum semolina. Semolina flour is also used to make desserts such as cake and pudding.

See also BREAD; KNEADING; MEASURING; QUICK BREAD; SIFTING; SUBSTITUTIONS & EQUIVALENTS; THICKENING.

FLUFFING To make a mixture or dish light and airy, usually by gently stirring and lifting with a fork. Grains of rice, for example, are compact after cooking, but fluffing will separate them and lighten the overall texture of the rice.

FLUTING Decorative shaping of the edge of a pie crust. The edge of a single-crust pie can simply be pressed into gentle curves with fingertips or pinched into a ropelike pattern. The edges of double-crust pie are generally crimped with a fork both to seal the top and bottom crusts together and to make a decorative pattern. See also CRIMPING; PIE & TART.

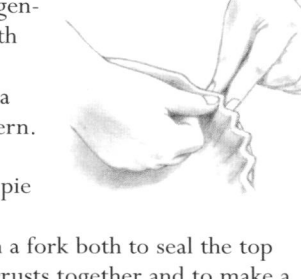

FOCACCIA A moist, rustic flat bread from northern Italy, traditionally made from a soft yeast dough that is spread into a pan, dimpled deeply with fingertips, and then generously drizzled with olive oil and sprinkled with sea salt before baking. Contemporary focaccia may also be sprinkled with other ingredients, such as fresh rosemary, shredded basil, olives, grated cheese, paper-thin tomato slices, or caramelized onions.

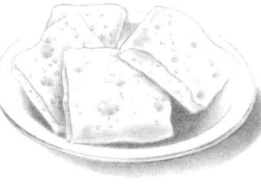

Selecting Look for rounds or rectangular sheets in the bakery sections of grocery stores or in Italian bakeries or delis.
Storing Best eaten as soon after baking as possible. To keep focaccia longer, wrap well with plastic and foil and freeze for up to 1 month.

FOIE GRAS (FWAH GRAH) specialty of the Gascony, Alsace, and Périgord regions of France, foie gras is a luxurious delicacy. Literally "fat liver" in French, foie gras is the greatly enlarged liver of a goose or duck that has been force-fed a special diet, usually of corn. Foie gras is silky in texture, creamy beige to light yellow with tinges of pink, and buttery rich in flavor, lacking the assertive flavors usually associated with liver. Good-quality foie gras is produced in countries other than France, including Israel, Poland, Hungary, Canada, and the United States, although supplies everywhere are limited.

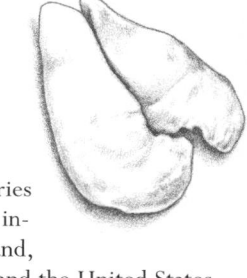

Selecting Foie gras from geese has a mellow flavor and rich texture. Livers from ducks will have a more intense, almost winy flavor. Color is not a good indicator of quality, but the highest grade of livers will be large and firm—never spongy. Buy foie gras from gourmet markets or specialty meat shops. It is available year-round. Cooked whole foie gras, foie gras mousse, and purée are available in cans.

❧ Foie Gras Grades ❧

FOIE GRAS GRADE A Weighs no less than 14 ounces and has no imperfections. Smooth and buttery, it is ideal for sautéing.
FOIE GRAS GRADE B Softer than Grade A and with slight imperfections. Weighs 11 to 13 ounces. Can be sautéed or baked.
FOIE GRAS GRADE C Meaty though small. Weighs 7 to 10 ounces. Rarely available to the consumer.

---

f

Storing Since fresh foie gras is highly perishable, use it as soon as possible after purchase. If necessary, wrap well in plastic and refrigerate for up to 2 days. Whole uncooked livers packaged in heavy plastic Cryovac can be kept refrigerated for 3 to 4 weeks. A whole foie gras can be frozen for up to 2 months, but its texture may suffer. Store canned foie gras in a cool, dry place for up to 1 year.

Preparing Whole, fresh foie gras has two lobes that must be carefully trimmed of all traces of green bile and white fat. Let the liver come to room temperature before preparing. Separate the lobes and pull out all veins.

Duck foie gras is often simply sautéed quickly only until still pink. (Cooked for a long time or at temperatures higher than 195°F, it will melt into a pool of fat.) Goose foie gras, which is fattier and even more likely to melt, is better chopped or ground into pâté, which is slowly cooked in a dish called a terrine. When pâté is served in a terrine, it is called a terrine; when it is unmolded, it is called pâté.

Quick Bite

What happens to the rest of the bird? These meaty specimens are used to make confit and other rich poultry dishes. Duck breasts, called *magrets,* are particularly large and tasty.

FOLDING This mixing technique is used to combine two ingredients or mixtures with different densities. Light, airy mixtures, such as beaten egg whites or whipped cream, will lose their loft if incorrectly folded into heavier batters, and your cake or soufflé won't rise properly. It is a simple but crucial technique. Use a firm but light hand when folding, and don't overdo it: stop folding once the mixtures are just blended.

HOW TO *Fold*

1. Spoon one-fourth of the lighter mixture, such as beaten egg whites, atop the heavier mixture, such as batter.
2. With a long-handled rubber spatula, slice down through both mixtures and sweep the spatula along the bottom of the bowl. Bring the spatula with a gentle circular motion up and over the contents. The goal is to lift up some of the heavier batter from the bottom of the bowl and gently "fold" it over the top of the lighter mixture without deflating the lighter mixture.

Folding in egg whites.

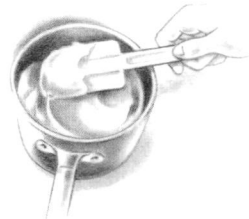

3. Rotate the pan or bowl a quarter turn and repeat the down-across-up-over motion. Continue in this manner, rotating the bowl each time, until the lighter mixture is incorporated. This initial folding of just one-fourth of the lighter mixture allows the rest of it to be folded in more easily.
4. Add the remaining lighter mixture. Fold as explained above, quickly but gently, just until the mixtures are evenly incorporated. A little streaking is fine. Overmixing will deflate the lighter mixture.

FONTINA See CHEESE.

FOOD GUIDE PYRAMID In 1992, the United States Department of Agriculture (USDA) and the Department of Health and Human Services unveiled the official Food Guide Pyramid. Studies had linked high-fat and high-salt diets to heart problems, high blood pressure, and cancer and other degenerative diseases, and the pyramid was designed to illustrate which foods in which quantities were considered most beneficial to overall good health.

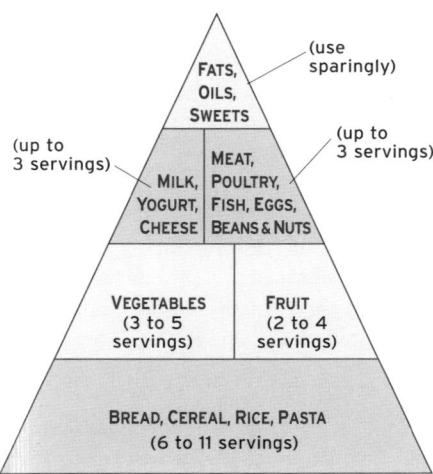

A refinement of the old-fashioned "four basic food groups," the pyramid's shape reflects current nutritional recommendations. Grains and cereals are the pyramid's wide foundation. Fats, oils, and sweets should be eaten "sparingly," illustrated by their placement in the narrow tip.

The recommended number of servings each day may seem high. Keep in mind, though, that the USDA's definition of 1 serving is less than what the average person might eat at one sitting. For example, a single serving in the bread group is just 1 slice of bread or ½ cup pasta. In the meat group, a serving might be 3 ounces of lean beef, 1 tablespoon of peanut butter, or 1 egg, while the average person might eat at least twice that in a sitting.

FOOD MILL Used to purée cooked or very soft foods, usually fruits or vegetables, a food mill looks like a stainless-steel or sturdy plastic saucepan with a perforated bottom and an interior crank-shaped handle. It also may have arms that extend for fitting it securely over a bowl. At the bottom of the mill is a circular, paddle-shaped blade that rotates against a disk perforated with small holes. As you turn the handle, the blade forces food through the holes and into a bowl or other receptacle, trapping any seeds, peels, or fibers in the mill. Some mills have interchangeable disks with holes of varying sizes for creating purées of various consistencies, while others have a single fixed disk. Food mills treat food more gently than food processors and produce more even-textured purées.

FOOD PROCESSOR Efficient, powerful, and capable of performing a wide variety of functions in the kitchen, food processors have become so popular in the past quarter century or so that recipe writers often assume they are as readily available as blenders and electric mixers.

Most models consist of a straight-sided work bowl that sits on a motorized base. Various disks and blades fit on a rotating shaft at the center of the bowl. The all-purpose, S-shaped metal blade chops, blends, mixes, and purées. Other attachments include disks for shredding, grating, or slicing; a plastic blade for kneading dough; and a disk for julienning. (See page 204.) A feed tube allows you to add ingredients while the food processor is running.

Despite their popularity, food processors are not capable of performing every kitchen task. Their powerful motors can easily overwork foods, sometimes making a mush if you are not careful. They are not recommended for mashing potatoes (it makes them gummy), nor can they normally be used for beating egg whites or whipping cream. Sometimes a whip attachment is available, but generally the machine is incapable of aerating these ingredients sufficiently for good loft. If you plan to mix very dense dough, make sure your processor motor is powerful enough, or the motor may dangerously overheat.

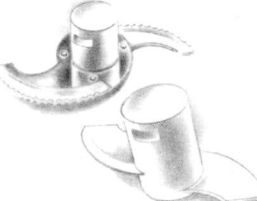

Metal blade and dough blade.

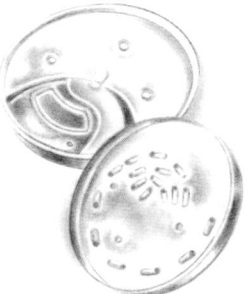

Slicing and shredding disks.

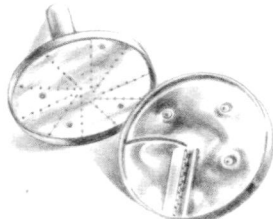

Grating and julienne disks.

Food Processor Savvy

■ To avoid having to wash the bowl when chopping several ingredients in succession, start with the driest and mildest ones and finish with the stronger, moister ingredients, such as onions. If needed, wipe out the work bowl with a dry paper towel between ingredients.
■ For easier cleanup after processing sticky foods, lightly coat the blades, disks, and work bowl with flavorless vegetable oil before use.
■ If the work bowl leaks between the blade and the shaft or under the lid, it is probably holding too much liquid. Process smaller batches, or strain the liquid out first and purée the solids separately.
■ Chopping large amounts of chocolate or stale bread will dull the blade. Crushing ice cubes may damage it.
■ Because the blade crushes ingredients as it chops, some cooks avoid using the food processor with ingredients that are easily bruised, such as onions, garlic, or fresh basil.
■ When scraping foods out of the work bowl, prevent the blade from falling into the bowl or pan with the food. Hold the bowl with your thumb inserted in the blade port on the bottom, pressing against the blade to keep it in place, with your fingers resting on the side.

FOOD SAFETY A few simple precautions and smart cooking habits will help safeguard you from the possibility of illness caused by the small amounts of bacteria naturally present in food.

Safe Shopping

■ Always check sell-by dates printed on food packaging.
■ When buying fresh meat or poultry, make sure that the package is not leaking. If there is any moisture, slip the package into a plastic bag so that it does not drip onto other fresh foods.
■ Buy eggs, meat, poultry, and fish only from refrigerated cases and only in good

condition. Avoid those with "off" odors or discoloration.

- Put perishables into your shopping cart last, and put them away first as soon as you get home.
- Avoid packaged foods in cans or jars with dents or bulges.

Safe Storage

- Check and follow use-by dates printed on food packaging.
- See food safety and general storage guidelines given in the individual ingredient entries of this book as well as under DONENESS.
- Use your physical senses, along with common sense, in judging whether any ingredients are in good condition. If you have any doubt, throw it out.
- In the refrigerator, place any packaged raw or defrosting frozen meat, seafood, or poultry on a dish or rimmed tray to catch any juices that might leak out.
- When recipes state to store food in the coldest part of the refrigerator, this usually means the back of the bottom shelf or in a meat drawer. (A refrigerator thermometer will tell you for sure.)
- Large quantities of hot food should be allowed to cool to room temperature before refrigerating; otherwise, the heat of the food can lower the internal temperature of the refrigerator, compromising the safety of the other food stored there. Spoon it into several small, shallow containers, stir it occasionally, and don't cover it. This will speed the cooling process. Refrigerate within 2 hours.
- Don't keep your refrigerator jammed full of food. Air needs to be able to circulate around the stored food to keep it at the correct temperature. At the same time, an empty refrigerator (or freezer compartment) is not as efficient as one with a good amount of food. The cold food helps maintain the temperature.

- Buy a refrigerator thermometer to make sure your food is refrigerated safely. The thermometer should be placed on the top shelf close to the door. Leave it overnight, then check to make sure the temperature is no more than 40°F.

Safe Food Preparation

- Before and after you handle any ingredients, especially raw seafood, poultry, and meat, wash your hands thoroughly with lots of warm water and soap.
- After preparing any foods, thoroughly wash all the kitchen tools, cutting surfaces, and dishware that touched them with lots of warm water and soap.
- Before cooking poultry, use cold running water to rinse off the bird, outside and inside the cavity.
- Before you cook fruits and vegetables or eat them raw, rinse them thoroughly with cold running water, scrubbing them as needed. Some fruits and vegetables are waxed to enhance appearance and lengthen storage. These commercial waxes are not toxic, but they can trap pesticide residues, so scrub them off thoroughly before eating.
- Rinse lettuce, spinach, and other greens thoroughly, even those bought in sealed plastic packages.
- Always use separate cutting boards for animal products and for produce. Thoroughly wash the boards after each use. Periodically sterilize polyethylene boards in the dishwasher at its hottest setting, or wash wooden or polyethylene boards with a solution of 4 cups warm water and 1 teaspoon household bleach.
- In preparation for cooking, do not leave perishable food out of the refrigerator for more than 2 hours. In warm weather, reduce this time to no more than 1 hour. As soon as possible, and no more than 2 hours after serving, refrigerate or freeze leftovers.

f

Caution!

If you are pregnant or older, are cooking for young children or older people, have a compromised immune system, or want to limit your exposure to bacterial risk as much as possible, you may want to observe even stricter guidelines for leaving out any perishable food, limiting it to 30 minutes.

Safe Cleanup

- Wipe up spilled foods quickly and thoroughly from counters and floors to avoid the growth of bacteria.
- Use fresh, clean kitchen towels, replacing them frequently, especially if they get soiled or damp.
- Run sponges, scrubbing pads, and brushes through the dishwasher every week or so to sterilize them. Alternatively, boil or microwave them for 2 minutes.

See also BEEF; CHICKEN; DONENESS; PORK; SAFETY.

FREEZING Freezing is one of the easiest and most nutritious ways to preserve food. Meats, fish, fruits, vegetables, breads, and many finished dishes all freeze well if certain guidelines are followed.

Understanding what happens in the freezer will help make sense of the rules. When food is frozen, the water in the food freezes, thus stopping (or slowing) the normal cell activity that would otherwise cause deterioration and spoilage. When foods are frozen quickly at extremely low temperatures (as is the case in commercial food manufacture), the ice crystals in the frozen water are tiny and do very little to disrupt the food's cell structure. When food is frozen at higher temperatures (for example, the temperature of a home freezer), it freezes more slowly and larger ice crystals

form. These larger crystals are actually sharp enough to puncture the food's cell walls. When the food thaws, there will be far greater deterioration than is the case with commercially frozen food.

In the interest of keeping cell damage and water loss to a minimum, try to freeze food as quickly as you can. Fluctuations in temperatures that allow partial thawing and then refreezing lead to extensive damage and textural degradation.

Food that is not well protected from the dry, cold air of the freezer will suffer freezer burn, extreme drying that ruins both texture and flavor. Freezer burns appear as dried, white, or darkened areas on the surface of the food. When preparing foods for freezing, wrap them carefully and expel excess air from their packaging to limit their exposure to air.

The most common form of freezer spoilage after freezer burn is rancidity. Fats can eventually turn rancid in the freezer, and the freezer life of frozen foods is directly correlated to their fat content. Exposure to air promotes rancidity, so again careful wrapping before freezing helps slow the process.

Freezer Savvy

- Maintain the freezer temperature as close to 0°F as possible.
- Cool all foods completely before transferring to containers and freezing.
- If possible, remove excess air from containers: fold down bags to squeeze out all the air you can.
- Divide large batches into the smaller quantities that you would be using at one time, such as portions of pesto in ice-cube trays, tomato sauce in pint containers, chicken breasts in pairs.
- Be sure to mark the date and contents on packages with a permanent marker, and mark containers the same way using tape or another removable label. It may

seem obvious to you at the moment, but 3 months from now you'll be hard-pressed to remember what is in that well-wrapped package at the back of the freezer.

- Don't try to freeze too much food at once, as this may lower the freezer temperature. When putting unfrozen food into the freezer, leave plenty of space between the packages or containers. Once completely frozen, the food can be closely stacked.
- Once the food is frozen, a full freezer is the most efficient freezer.
- When buying frozen food at the grocery store from open freezer cases, be sure that the entire package of food is sitting well below the indicated freeze line, marked on the side of the case, and that the contents are completely frozen. Return home as quickly as possible to prevent any thawing before transferring the food to your own freezer.

About Freezer Materials and Containers

ALUMINUM FOIL Aluminum foil is not the best material for cold storage. It creates mysterious little bundles in the refrigerator, unless you take the time to label. It also turns brittle under freezing temperatures and does not form the most secure seal. If you want to wrap food for the freezer in foil, wrap it first in waxed paper or plastic wrap. Use only heavy-duty freezer foil, not the lightweight version that can tear easily and disintegrates quickly. And do not use foil for highly acidic foods, since they may react and create "off" flavors and dark colors.

FREEZER PAPER Laminated with foil, glassine, cellophane, or rubber latex to provide protection against freezer burn. Be sure to seal completely with freezer tape. Freezer paper can be used over cardboard, plastic, or foil for additional protection.

PLASTIC

- Bags: Look for zippered bags made of heavy-duty plastic that are specially made to withstand freezing temperatures. Place the bag in a container to keep it upright and open for easy filling. Once full, eliminate excess air (to help prevent freezer burn and rancidity), seal closed, and then freeze it on a flat surface. When the contents are hard, stack the bags for efficient storage.
- Wrap: Heavy-duty plastic wrap is a good alternative. It seals out more air than bags do and does not waste space in the freezer. Wrap foods with at least two layers for the best protection.
- Containers: In addition to liquid foods such as soups and stews, fragile foods such as berries are best frozen in plastic containers to prevent bruising or squashing. Do not use a container larger than 2 quarts, or the food will take too long to freeze. The best containers are airtight, resist water and grease, and are made of materials that will not crack at low temperatures. Fairly rigid containers made of heavy plastic are ideal. Clean milk cartons can be cut down to fit specific foods, then tightly sealed in freezer bags. Leave ½ inch of headroom for dry foods and 1 inch for liquids, to allow for expansion during freezing. Square containers stack easily and use freezer space most efficiently. If using glass, look for dual-purpose glass jars specifically treated to withstand the cold temperatures of the freezer. A wide mouth allows easier removal of frozen food. Cardboard will eventually allow flavors to enter and moisture to escape. Check that lids in every case seal tightly.
- Vacuum-sealed: Vacuum-sealed plastic requires a machine or a special valve to suck out as much air as possible before sealing food in heavy-duty plastic.

f

TRAY FREEZING This method is ideal for berries, shrimp, ravioli, individual pastries, or other small foods that you want to keep distinct. Spread foods in a single layer, preferably not touching, on a baking sheet or tray. Freeze until the individual pieces are firm, transfer to a plastic bag (or a rigid plastic container if the food is particularly fragile), and return to the freezer.

About Freezing Foods

VEGETABLES Certain enzymes that break down vegetables, changing their color, flavor, texture, and nutrient content and shortening their shelf life, continue to work in the freezer. Blanching destroys these enzymes and helps to halt deterioration. Unblanched freezing is acceptable for onions, peppers, and herbs.

Frozen vegetables will have better texture and flavor if they are cooked without thawing. (An exception is corn on the cob, which should be partially thawed before cooking.) Steaming is the ideal method for cooking frozen vegetables.

FRUITS Select only fully ripe, but slightly firm, fruits for the freezer. Those with more delicate textures, such as papayas, mangoes, pears, watermelons, and avocados, do not generally freeze well. Although not usually blanched, most fruits, especially sliced ones, benefit from a light coating with granulated sugar or mixing with a light sugar syrup before they are frozen, to keep them firm, improve their flavor, and prevent oxidation. Berries and other small fruits are best kept whole, but larger ones should be peeled and cut as you would to the point of cooking. Sprinkle lemon juice over fruits that tend to brown when cut. See also DISCOLORING.

The higher the water content, the mushier the fruit will be upon thawing. Berries are a good example. Thaw fruits only partially and serve them while still slightly firm. Once thawed, frozen fruit tends to have more juice than an equal measure of fresh fruit. Cut back on the liquid called for in recipes. Adjust also for any sugar added before freezing.

MEATS, POULTRY, AND FISH Fresh meat and poultry freeze well, and fish freezes less well. Remember that fat can turn rancid in the freezer, so lean cuts freeze better and last longer than fatty ones. Also, unsaturated fats (in fish, chicken, and pork) turn rancid more quickly than saturated fats (in beef). Finally, ground meat and poultry have the shortest shelf life of all, because grinding increases the meat's exposure to oxygen, which promotes rancidity. Cured meats, such as bacon, ham, and sausage, fare less well, lasting no more than 1 to 2 months. The salt and other additives used in curing promote deterioration.

Reduce the amount of air in contact with the meat to prevent rancidity and freezer burn. Rancid meat will have an "off" odor and flavor, and freezer-burned meat will have a tough texture and "off" flavor.

Meats lose water as they thaw, making them drier when cooked. Those thawed too quickly will lose more liquid. Thaw meat in the refrigerator for the best quality and for safety. Immerse plastic-wrapped meat in cool water for faster thawing. Cook thawed meat or fish promptly.

BREADS Yeast breads and quick breads (banana bread, muffins, biscuits) freeze well, both before and after they are baked. Cooked batter breads like waffles also freeze well.

For unbaked breads, freeze wet batters in their containers and firm doughs on a baking sheet or in their pans until hard. Remove and wrap well. When ready to bake, return the bread, unthawed, to its pan and proceed with baking, allowing 15 to 20 minutes extra cooking time.

For baked breads, wrap and freeze as soon as they have cooled completely. To reheat, unwrap them, sprinkle lightly with water for a crispier crust, and heat, un-thawed, at 325°F until warmed through.

CAKES For unfrosted baked layers, cool cakes completely. Return them to their pans to give support while freezing. Once firm, remove the layers from the pans and wrap them well with freezer-weight plastic wrap. Thaw in the refrigerator, keeping them well wrapped. For frosted layers, freeze the entire cake unwrapped, then wrap and return to the freezer.

COOKIES For unbaked dough, form even logs of dough, then wrap in freezer-weight plastic and freeze. Slice the logs as instructed in a recipe and bake while still frozen. For drop cookies, form them on a baking sheet, freeze them on the sheet, and then transfer drops to a plastic bag. To bake, arrange them on the baking sheet again and bake as directed. Allow about 5 minutes extra cooking time in both cases. For baked cookies, use a plastic container or wrap the cookies in short stacks. Thaw at room temperature or in the microwave.

COOKED DISHES Stews, casseroles, sauces, and filled breads and pastries usually freeze well. (The exceptions are wheat flour–thickened sauces and stews that contain pasta or potatoes.) For best texture, do not overcook dishes that you plan to freeze, and do not thaw before reheating. If you freeze them in an ovenproof container, thawing is simple. For stews and casseroles, cover and reheat in a 350°F oven. Filled pastries and pies should be reheated at 375° to 400°F.

For soups, use less liquid, stop cooking 10 minutes before the soup is finished, and omit any potatoes for freezing. Add cooked potatoes or raw pasta and additional liquid while reheating over very low heat until completely thawed. For soups containing milk, cream, or egg yolks, it is best to whisk after thawing to prevent curdling. Reheat cream soups in a double boiler.

FRIED FOODS Some hardier fried foods, especially yeast breads and battered or breaded food, can be frozen. Those with a denser, sturdier structure fare better.

- Freezing before cooking: Once the food is breaded or battered, arrange it on a parchment-lined baking sheet and freeze until firm. Transfer to plastic freezer bags and freeze for up to 3 months.
- Freezing already-fried food: Once the food is completely cooled, spread it in a single layer on a rack-lined baking sheet and place it in the freezer until firm. Transfer to heavy plastic freezer bags and freeze for up to 3 months.
- To reheat: Arrange the food, without the pieces touching, on a rack-lined baking sheet. Bake at 325°F just until crisp and hot. Serve immediately. Once the food is rewarmed, do not refreeze it.

FOODS THAT DO NOT FREEZE WELL
- Cream sauces, custards, and creamy fillings thickened with wheat flour.
- Cooked rice, unless incorporated into a casserole.
- Meringue, cooked egg whites, or icings made from egg whites.
- Cheese.
- Cooked potatoes (the exception being half-cooked french fries).
- Delicate fried foods such as fritters.
- Salad greens, celery, cabbage, cucumbers (unless already brined and pickled).
- Emulsified sauces, like mayonnaise.

See also THAWING; individual foods.

FRISÉE See CHICORY; GREENS, SALAD.

FRITTATA This Italian dish resembles a crustless quiche, a mixture of eggs, cheese, and other ingredients cooked slowly in a skillet until firm. Its preparation differs from a French omelet in that ingredients are mixed into the uncooked egg, rather than used as a filling.

f
—

Frosting, Icing & Glaze

For every great cake, there is a sweet, rich, silky coating that complements it perfectly. Although just about anything spread on the outside of a cake goes by the name frosting, it is actually only one of three ways to cover a cake: frosting, icing, or glaze.

Thick, fluffy, and sweet, frostings hold their shape, lending themselves to dramatic swirls and high peaks. Popular frostings include buttercream, seven-minute, white mountain, and simple whipped cream.

A fine line divides frostings and icings. In general, icings are slightly shinier and thinner than frostings. The two terms are frequently interchanged. Royal icing is the most common icing.

Thinner than either frostings or icings, glazes are poured, drizzled, or brushed on cakes, tarts, and pastries. As they cool and dry, they become smooth and shiny. Glazes can be as simple as confectioners' sugar mixed with lemon juice, or apricot jelly melted with liqueur. Ganache and poured fondant are also glazes.

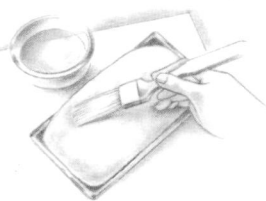

Glazing a bread loaf.

Ingredients Bring all the ingredients to room temperature and always sift the sugar first to get rid of lumps. Sugar is the base of virtually all frostings, icings, and glazes. Eggs, butter, milk, and cream add necessary richness and body.

Equipment For frosting or icing a cake, have on hand the following equipment:

waxed paper, a straight or offset stainless-steel frosting spatula to spread frosting quickly and smoothly, a cake round or a decorating turntable to rotate the cake, toothpicks, a serrated knife, and a decorating comb or pastry bag (if desired).

HOW TO *Cut a Cake Round*
Professional bakers use cardboard cake rounds to carry, arrange, and frost cake layers without any cracking or breaking. They are also excellent for supporting the layers in the freezer. Cake rounds are available at baking supply stores, but you can make them easily yourself.

1. Trace the bottom of the cake pans on heavy, corrugated cardboard.
2. Cut out the rounds. Making them the same size as the pan is easiest for decorating. A round can be slightly larger if it will be used under the bottom layer for serving the cake.
3. If you plan to reuse them, cover the rounds with aluminum foil.
4. Transfer cooled cake layers onto the rounds to frost them.

Preparing the Cake Layers Gently curved tops on the cake layers are fine. If you need to even out sharply peaked layers, hold a large serrated knife flat against the top, with the blade parallel to the work surface, and gently saw off the dome. Frosting will spread more easily and cleanly if you place any trimmed layers cut side down.

f

Cake layers can be cut in half for thinner, more elegant layers. Mark the halfway point on the side of a layer with toothpicks, sticking them in partway. Hold a long, serrated knife parallel to the work surface and cut from the outside edge of the cake toward its center, using the toothpicks to guide the knife. Turn the cake as you cut. Use a cardboard round or a plate to lift away the top layer. If the crust seems tough or if it is darker than both the interior of the cake and the frosting, you can trim it away with a serrated knife. The cut surfaces will shed crumbs readily, however, interfering as you frost. To help seal in crumbs, brush the cake surface with melted jelly or simple syrup and let set.

*Cutting
cake layers.*

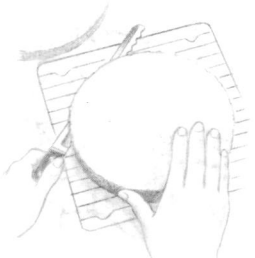

HOW TO *Frost a Layer Cake*

A cake must be completely cool before you begin frosting. If it is still even slightly warm, the frosting or glaze will melt and not adhere. A decorating turntable will make the job easier.

1. To keep the cake plate clean while frosting, arrange 4-inch-wide strips of waxed paper in a square to cover the edges of the plate. Center the cake on the plate, making sure the strips are under the edge of the cake. After you finish, pull the strips away.
2. Lightly brush away all the loose crumbs from the surface of the cake. If your cake layers are just slightly domed on top, to ensure a well-balanced cake, place the first layer with its top side down.

3. Spread ½ to ¾ cup frosting on the top of the first layer. If you are using a filling different from the outer frosting, leave a ½-inch unfrosted border around the edge, to allow for its spreading from the weight of the next layer.
4. Place the second layer over the first layer, checking that the edges of the layers are even with each other. Tap the top of the cake gently to set the second layer. (If the second layer is not the top layer, place it domed side down. If it is the top layer, it may be set either way.)

Quick Bite

The top of a cake can be rounded or flat, depending on how the layers are placed. Facing the flat sides of two layers together will reveal a straight line of filling when the cake is sliced.

5. Apply the crumb layer, a very thin layer of frosting on the top and sides of the cake. This will trap crumbs and keep them from appearing on the finished surface of the cake. If you find the frosting too stiff to spread easily, thin it with a tiny amount of milk or water.

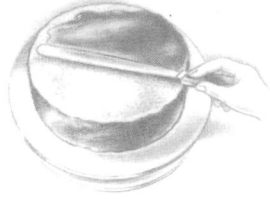

6. Frost the sides, sweeping up and creating a rim above the edge of the cake. It should be ¼ to ½ inch thick. Do not apply too much frosting. Keep in mind the richness of the frosting and the relative amount of cake.

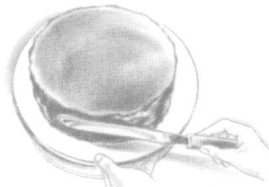

continued

f

Frosting, Icing & Glaze, continued

7. Drop the rest of the frosting at 3 or 4 points on the top layer of the cake. Using a frosting spatula, spread the frosting, sweeping out from the center and meeting the rim of frosting at a clean right angle. Use gentle pressure and smooth back-and-forth strokes.

8. Smooth the top and any excess frosting that may have fallen down the sides.

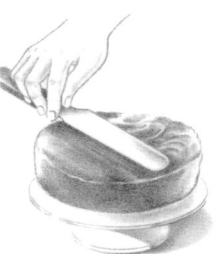

9. If desired, use a decorating comb or pastry bag to decorate the cake. For information on using a pastry bag to decorate a cake, see PIPING.

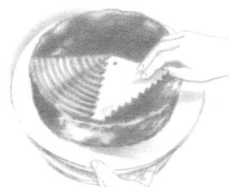

How Much Frosting Will I Need?

For thinner frostings, you will need the lesser amounts. When filling and covering a cake with light, fluffy frosting, plan on using the larger amounts.

Frosting Amounts	
8- or 9-inch cake, 2 layers	2½ to 3 cups
8- or 9-inch cake, 3 layers	3 to 3½ cups
10-inch tube cake	3 to 3½ cups
13 x 9-inch sheet cake	3½ to 4 cups
12 large cupcakes	1½ to 2 cups

You can fill layers with the same frosting, or use another mixture with contrasting flavor, texture, and color. Lemon curd, custard, chopped nuts, fresh fruit, and fruit purées make excellent fillings.

HOW TO *Glaze a Cake*

You must work quickly with warm glaze, so have everything at hand.

1. Set the cake or filled and stacked cake layers on a rack placed over a baking sheet.

2. Pour the glaze over the cake all at once, aiming at its center and letting the glaze flow down the sides. For a tube cake, pour in a steady stream as you circle the top of the cake.

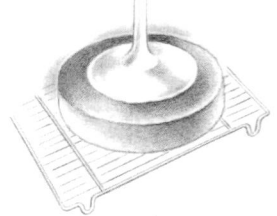

3. Immediately spread the glaze over still-exposed areas with a spatula. Work quickly. Ease the glaze gently, but do not swirl or press with the spatula. Let the glaze cool until set.

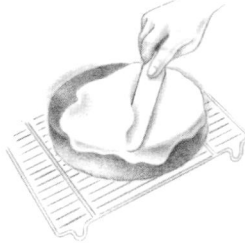

4. Resist the temptation to fix spots or smears. If needed, however, you can moisten the spatula and carefully smooth out imperfections.

See also BAKING TOOLS; GANACHE; PIPING.

FRUIT, DRIED See DRIED FRUIT.

FRUIT, FRESH See RIPENING; individual fruits.

FRYING French fries, fish and chips, crispy chicken, clam strips, spring rolls, tempura, doughnuts, and beignets—frying undeniably produces some of the world's most delectable foods. Grilling and sautéing may be the focus of more modern recipes, but frying, especially deep-frying, gives food a light, crisp texture and deep golden color difficult to achieve with any other method.

Ordinary frying, also called panfrying, means to cook food in a pan with a moderate amount of fat or oil over medium heat. Panfrying is similar to sautéing, but generally requires more fat, more time, and less heat. It is a good method for larger pieces of meat, such as thick pork chops, bone-in chicken parts, and hefty hamburgers. Firmer vegetables, such as pearl onions or potatoes, may also be panfried. (Very soft, juicy foods, such as ripe tomatoes, are not suitable for frying since they tend to liquefy at high temperatures.) In deep-frying, the food is immersed in a greater amount of fat and cooks for a shorter amount of time than in panfrying.

Stir-frying, a frying technique developed in Asia, uses a special bowl-shaped pan, small cuts of food, and very little oil. See STIR-FRYING.

Coatings for Frying Although some sturdy foods, such as potatoes or doughnuts, do not need coatings to protect them from the heat, most benefit from a coating that provides a crisp crust and a buffer from the hot fat. Food is sometimes dredged with flour first to help the coating adhere. Coat delicate or particularly moist foods, including fish, shellfish, chicken, zucchini, onions, and cheese.

BATTER Since batters are thin, they are best suited to foods that will keep their shape and are easily dunked, such as crisp vegetables, dry fruits, and firm fish. Different ingredients in batters have different effects. Eggs and flour provide protection from the hot oil. Milk encourages deep browning, sugar in a batter causes quick browning, and water or club soda makes light batters. Beer gives batter sweet flavor and airiness. Yeast adds additional lightness, and butter adds richness.

CRUMB COATING Crumb coating helps hold together flaky mixtures and provides a crisp crust for such foods as soft cheeses, delicate fish, and crab cakes. Coatings include cracker crumbs, bread crumbs, cornmeal, rice flakes, and ground nuts.

WRAPPER In Asia, thin wrappers enclose whole shrimp, small pieces of meat, or mixed fillings. Spring rolls and fried wontons are examples of these fried tidbits.

Fat and Oil for Frying Use refined fats and oils with high smoke points. Peanut, soybean, corn, safflower, and grapeseed oil, as well as vegetable shortening, will easily withstand the high heat of frying. Clarified butter and coconut and palm oils give crisp texture and incomparable flavor but are less used now because of their high amounts of saturated fat. Also less used today by home cooks are animal-rendered fats such as lard, beef fat, or duck fat, but they do contribute wonderful flavor. Extra-virgin olive oil and toasted sesame oil will quickly smoke and burn, while canola oil can give off an unpleasant odor. See also FAT & OIL.

f

Quick Tip

The secret to Japanese tempura is using thinly sliced foods, cold batter, and a light hand in stirring the batter.

Deep-frying Accessories and Equipment Glossary

BIRD'S NEST BASKETS A nesting pair of small, round, scoop-shaped baskets with long handles. Smaller potato nest baskets are used to form potato slices into basket shapes, while larger tools are made for shaping tortillas and wonton skins.

DEEP FRYER Also known as a deep-fat fryer. Stove-top deep fryers are fitted with a fry basket that fits comfortably in a heavy bottom pan. Both basket and pan have long handles. When frying in stove-top fryers, use an accurate thermometer. Electric deep fryers are cased in metal and stay-cool plastic and are fitted with a control panel and built-in thermometer, making them easier to use. Although fryers with capacities of 2½ quarts are available, a 4- to 5-quart fryer is more practical, and many home cooks prefer an even larger one.

FRYING PAN A large pan with straight or slightly flared sides, preferably made of a heavy material such as cast iron, to retain heat and prevent temperature fluctuations. For deep-frying, it must be deep enough for the sides to extend several inches above the surface of the oil, while for panfrying, 4 inches is the minimum height.

MESH SKIMMER Used to skim off bits of batter and food in oil to prevent burning and a bitter flavor from forming.

PAPER TOWEL Used to absorb grease when draining fried foods.

RACK Draining fried foods on a sturdy wire rack set on a baking sheet produces crispier, less soggy results than paper towels. Also used to keep fried foods warm in the oven.

SLOTTED SPOON A spoon with perforations that allow fat to drain away when lifting out food. A second slotted spoon may be used to transfer food from batter to oil.

SPATTER GUARD Also called a splatter screen. A large, round, flat mesh lid with a long handle that is placed over frying food to prevent oil spatters.

SPIDER Small, wire-netted, basketlike skimmer used for removing foods from hot oil and draining them.

THERMOMETER Large, high-temperature thermometer that clips to the side of the pan. Be sure the tip does not touch the bottom of the pan.

TONGS For adding, turning, and removing food from hot oil quickly and easily.

WIRE BASKET LINER Wire basket with a long handle that nests inside a pan of oil, placed there before the food is added. Lift the basket gently to remove a whole batch of food at once.

WOK The wok is a good choice for deep-frying, as it will hold a large amount of oil and is responsive to rapid changes in temperature.

Quick Tip

For a subtle flavor, season the oil for panfrying with spices and aromatics such as cumin, dried chiles, or garlic cloves as it is heating. Use a large mesh ball for easy removal, or scoop out the flavorings with a skimmer. In either case, remove the flavorings before the oil becomes hot enough to scorch them.

About Deep-frying Although deep-frying has received a bad health rap in recent years, proper frying actually results in minimal oil absorption. Food is immersed in oil at 350° to 375°F, which causes the water in a food to evaporate instantly, converting it to steam that will push out any oil trying to seep into the food. If the temperature of the oil is too low, there will be no outward push of steam and the food will absorb the oil instead, becoming greasy. The key to deep-frying is maintaining the oil at the proper temperature.

Taking Precautions Hot fat or oil is dangerous. If allowed to get too hot (400°F or beyond, where most will reach their smoke points), it can burst into flame. A few commonsense precautions will help avoid any accidents:

■ Use thick oven mitts that reach well beyond your wrists when frying to avoid spatter burns.

Caution!

If hot fat or oil catches fire, *do not* attempt to douse it with water. Extinguish the fire by smothering it with the pot's lid or baking soda or with a class ABC fire extinguisher. Always have one of these means for putting out the flames on hand before starting to deep-fry. If unable to control the fire, leave the house and call the fire department.

■ Make sure the pot's handle is turned away from the front of the stove.

■ Use a deep-frying thermometer when frying, and do not let the fat heat to 400°F or beyond.

■ Gently lower the food into the oil with tongs or a slotted spoon. Do not drop it into the oil and allow it to splash.

■ Clean any oil drips on the outside of the pan, which could catch fire.

■ Hold the fried food above the oil for a few seconds to let any excess drip back into the pot, rather than onto the burner.

Frying Savvy

■ In panfrying, the oil should reach no more than halfway up the sides of the food; the depth will depend on what type of food is being cooked. For deep-frying, use oil at a depth of at least 2 inches, and use enough oil to cover the food by at least ¾ inch. Use a large, deep pan, however, and never fill it more than one-third full of oil.

■ For deep-frying, use a deep-frying thermometer. Adjust the heat to maintain the oil at the temperature specified in the recipe (350° to 375°F), keeping its temperature as constant as possible. Adding food in small batches will prevent large drops in temperature as well as ensuring even immersion in the oil.

■ Having foods at room temperature prevents a drop in oil temperature. (Exceptions are recipes that call for chilling to keep a delicate dough or soft food firm.)

■ Remove excess moisture from the surface of food before cooking, and keep liquids away from the hot oil. Liquids can cause spatters and explosions when they come in contact with hot oil.

■ Use a slotted spoon to lower food into hot fat. If you drop it in, the fat may spatter and burn you.

■ Fry a small amount of food at a time. Overcrowding the pan will quickly

f

lower the temperature, causing the food to absorb the oil, to stick together, and to cook unevenly.

- Fry more mildly flavored foods first, then cook successively stronger-flavored foods, as the oil will carry the flavors of the foods. Fry vegetables before meat, and meat before fish.
- Use a fine-mesh skimmer to remove small bits of batter or food from the fat during frying and between batches. This will keep the oil from obtaining a bitter, scorched flavor.
- When deep-frying in batches, let the oil regain its correct frying temperature between each batch of food.
- Drain fried foods on a rack set on a baking sheet. If no rack is available, drain food on several layers of paper towels or a clean brown paper bag.
- Salt just before serving. If salted too far in advance, the food will become tough and soggy.
- Always try to serve food as soon after frying as possible. If it must be held, arrange the food on a rack on a baking sheet and place it in a 225°F oven for up to 30 minutes.

Quick Tip

When the surface of the oil shows expanding circles and small bubbles, it is very hot, or almost smoking.

Serving Fried Foods To help soak up any excess oil, fold a cloth or heavy paper napkin on the serving plate before arranging the food on it.

Serve savory fried food with lemon wedges, fruity vinegars, spicy dips, or other tart, fresh sauces that will temper the richness.

Reusing Oil If oil is used to deep-fry a small amount of food and the food was not

Quick Tip

Foods containing relatively high amounts of sugar, such as beets, sweet potatoes, dough-nuts, and fritters, require a slightly lower deep-frying temperature (350°F). Otherwise the sugar in them will burn before the food cooks thoroughly.

strongly flavored and none of it burned, you can reuse the oil after straining it carefully. Let it cool completely, strain it through a coffee filter, and store it in an airtight container in the refrigerator for up to 3 months. Add at least one-fourth of its volume in fresh oil the next time that you use it. Do not fry with the same oil more than three times. Every time you heat oil, it deteriorates a bit and its smoke point is lowered. Eventually, the oil will no longer be able to hold temperatures sufficient to fry food properly. If needed, you can fry thick slices of fresh potatoes in the oil to clarify it before cooking. Oil should not have any "off" or rancid smell.

See also BATTER; BREADING; DREDGING; FAT & OIL; SMOKE POINT; STIR-FRYING.

FRYING PAN Also known as a skillet; see COOKWARE.

FUDGE An old-fashioned, rich, smooth confection made from chocolate or cocoa, butter, sugar, corn syrup, and other ingredients such as milk, half-and-half, and cream. This traditional American candy, a favorite of New England cooks, usually contains walnuts and vanilla extract, and sometimes citrus zest, dried fruits, or marshmallow is added.

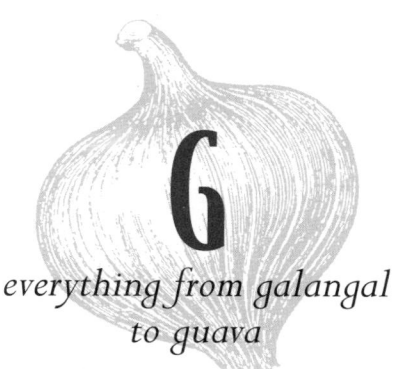

6

*everything from galangal
to guava*

GALANGAL (GAH-leng-gall) An aromatic seasoning with a hot, peppery, somewhat resinous flavor, galangal looks like a root but is actually an underground stem called a rhizome. Used throughout Southeast Asia, it resembles its relative ginger and is sometimes called Thai ginger. It has pink shoots, cream-colored fibrous flesh, and pale yellow skin with thin, dark stripes circling the rhizome. In Thailand, galangal is crushed with lemongrass, garlic, and chiles in the mortar as the base for curries. Thin slices of the rhizome infuse soups throughout Southeast Asia, while in Indonesia it replaces common ginger. If galangal is unavailable, some cooks recommend substituting ginger and black pepper with a bit of bay leaf to mimic the flavor.

Selecting Dried slices and sometimes the fresh or frozen rhizome can be found in Southeast Asian markets. When buying it fresh, look for firm specimens with smooth skins. Also sold are dried slices packaged in plastic and a less flavorful powder available in bottles.

Storing Keep fresh galangal in the refrigerator, wrapped in a paper towel inside a plastic bag, for up to 2 weeks. Store dried and powdered galangal away from air, light, and heat for up to 6 months.

Preparing Soak dried slices in warm water for 10 minutes before using.

If fresh galangal is used in chunks or slices and is not eaten, no peeling is necessary. If it will be consumed, peel and cut as directed before adding to a recipe.

GAME Our definition of game has changed considerably in recent times. Not so long ago, the term applied specifically to the meat of animals hunted in the wild, from birds such as wild turkey and duck, pheasant, and quail to animals such as deer, antelope, moose, and elk. All such meats are characterized by their robust flavor and relatively dark flesh, the result of their varying diets and active lives. Today, while such game still has its devotees and is available not only to hunters but also through specialty mail-order catalogs and websites, many more people are enjoying farm-raised game that is processed to uniform standards and has a milder flavor than its wild counterparts. Among the most popular types, available in well-stocked food stores and butcher shops, are buffalo, the meat of the American bison, leaner and slightly stronger tasting than beef; quail, small, flavorful birds with dark meat; squab, a type of pigeon, with dark, meaty breasts; and venison, the lean meat of deer, with dark red color, fine-grained dense texture, and a robust flavor.

GANACHE A smooth mixture of melted chocolate and cream. While still barely warm, it is poured over cakes and tortes to form a smooth glaze. Once cooled, it is whipped to become the filling for chocolate truffles and various pastries.

GARBANZO BEAN Also known as chickpea; see BEAN, DRIED.

GARLIC An edible bulb, garlic is a pungent member of the *Allium* genus, along with the onion. Each bulb, or head, of garlic is a cluster of 12 to 16 cloves, individually covered and collectively wrapped with papery, white to purplish red skin. Garlic is fundamental to cuisines around the world. Few kitchen staples arouse as much interest as humble garlic—revered for its therapeutic properties, endowed with both divine and devilish power, and reviled for its persistent odor. Shortsighted rulers in ancient Rome stayed clear of it, while suggesting that the peasant class should consume it for strength and good health.

Selecting Choose plump heads with smooth, firm cloves. Pass up those with soft, withered spots or green sprouts. The largest crop of garlic is harvested in midsummer, but garlic is widely available year-round. The strongly flavored, white-skinned American variety peaks in the middle of summer; milder, purplish red Mexican or Italian garlic comes to market in spring. Commercially prepared garlic paste, chopped garlic in oil, and peeled whole cloves are available as well, as are minced, flaked, and powdered forms.

Storing Keep whole garlic heads in an open container in a cool, dark, well-ventilated place for up to 2 months. To help prevent the heads from drying out, leave the papery skin on and break off individual cloves only as needed. Once separated, unpeeled cloves will keep for up to 1 week. Chop only as much garlic as you will use right away. Although chopped garlic can be refrigerated, sealed in an airtight container to prevent the transfer of odor and flavor to other foods, the volatile oils in garlic that give it its flavor begin to break down as soon as it is crushed or chopped. It will discolor, and the flavor will take on unpleasant tones. Commercial garlic paste and commercial chopped garlic will keep in the refrigerator for up to 3 months.

Garlic Glossary

ELEPHANT GARLIC With heads as large as a small orange, elephant garlic is not a variety of garlic, but instead a close relative to the leek. The flavor of its enormous cloves is much milder than that of ordinary garlic.

GARLIC SHOOTS Resembling chives, garlic shoots are the tender stems and flowers of an immature garlic plant, with a hint of garlic's flavor. Sprinkle raw over green salads, fold inside omelets, or add to light pasta dishes.

GREEN GARLIC Harvested just before the garlic plant begins to form cloves and available in the spring at farmers' markets, green garlic resembles large green onions with a tinge of pink at the bulb. Grill to accompany meat or fish.

Quick Tip

Sprinkle garlic cloves with a little salt to prevent them from sticking to the knife blade as you chop. Just be sure to allow for the salt when seasoning the dish.

Preparing Some recipes call for whole garlic cloves, while others specify sliced, chopped, minced, or crushed garlic. Garlic added to long-cooking recipes can be left in larger pieces so its flavors can be coaxed out over time, imbuing the dish with a mellow garlic flavor. Minced garlic has a hotter, more volatile flavor that will disperse quickly but is good for uncooked or quickly cooked foods where you want a pronounced garlic flavor. Crushing garlic will release much more of its aromatic oils than simply slicing or chopping it. Garlic presses make short work of mincing garlic, although some cooks believe their pressure creates bitterness. Some presses do not require you to peel the garlic cloves first.

Many cooks believe that even the beginnings of a green shoot spoil the sweet flavor of garlic. If you spy a green shoot starting to emerge, halve the clove and cut out the shoot.

Garlic is often sautéed as a first step in a recipe. Sauté garlic just until it is golden. If it scorches, it becomes unpleasantly bitter. To prevent burning, cook garlic over low heat, or add it to a pan after onions have been cooked slightly, in order to cook it for a shorter period of time. You can also cook crushed cloves briefly in hot oil to flavor it and then discard them before adding other ingredients.

HOW TO *Peel Garlic*
When you're faced with a heap of garlic cloves to peel, any one of the following will help loosen the skins:
- Crush cloves gently with the flat side of a knife blade.

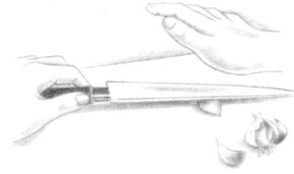

- Heat separated cloves in a dry skillet over medium-low heat for 30 seconds to 1 minute.
- Microwave a whole head of garlic for 1 minute and individual cloves for 5 seconds. Let cool slightly before peeling.

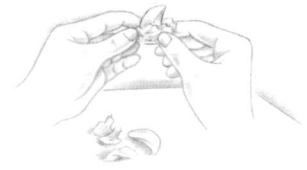

- Blanch in boiling water for 1 minute and drain.
- Roll the cloves 1 or 2 at a time in a flat sheet of rubber such as a jar-lid gripper. Kitchenware stores sell special rubber tubes specifically designed for this task.

HOW TO *Roast Garlic*

Roasted garlic purée is excellent spread on warm bread, whisked into sauces and soups, or mashed into potatoes.

1. Peel away the loose, papery outer layers of a whole head of garlic, leaving just enough skin to hold the cloves together. Cut off just enough of the top to expose the garlic cloves.
2. Center the head of garlic on a square of aluminum foil. Drizzle with olive oil or water. If desired, sprinkle with dried thyme or oregano. Wrap the foil tightly around the garlic.
3. Roast at 425°F degrees until soft, for about 30 minutes. Let the cloves cool slightly before unwrapping them.
4. Squeeze the head of garlic from base to top, like a tube of toothpaste, to extract the purée. Or, serve it whole at the table and let each diner squeeze his or her own cloves.

GARNISHING A slim slice of melon or a delicately fanned strawberry can add appealing color and freshness to an otherwise plain plate of food. Asian chefs train for years to learn the art of carving intricate flowers and animals to adorn dishes and platters. More casual American cuisine may call for only a sprig of flowering thyme on the rim of a dinner plate or a few vegetables propped against a roast. More and more chefs believe that garnishes should be edible and complement the flavor and appearance of the serving platter or composed plate. Remember, simpler is better. You don't want to detract from what should be the main focus of the dish—the food itself.

GELATIN Refrigerate homemade stock, and you will see the effect of natural gelatin: the stock will thicken and turn into a loose jelly. Gelatin is an odorless, colorless, tasteless thickener derived from collagen, a protein extracted from the bones, cartilage, and tendons of animals. Without gela-

tin, many fillings, mousses, puddings, and molded desserts, as well as marshmallows and jellied candies, would lose their shape. Although many cooks may not use it from one season to the next, gelatin is a common kitchen staple.

Quick Tip

Raw pineapple, papaya, fig, guava, kiwifruit, and fresh ginger contain enzymes that inhibit the setting of gelatin. Cook these foods first or use canned versions when adding them to any gelatin mixture.

Selecting Look for powdered unflavored gelatin packaged in small paper envelopes in the baking section of grocery stores. Clear, paper-thin sheets of unflavored leaf gelatin are available at gourmet and specialty baking stores. Leaf gelatin is not as convenient to use, but many bakers prefer it to the powdered form because it results in a smoother and clearer consistency. Although powdered and leaf gelatin can be used interchangeably in any recipe, their thickening powers may vary slightly.

Fruit-flavored gelatins are sold in small boxes in supermarkets. Do not confuse flavored gelatins with desserts such as Jell-O.

Storing Unflavored gelatin will keep for up to 3 years if sealed in an airtight container and stored in a cool, dry place. Flavored gelatin will keep for 1 year.

Quick Tip

Do not put a hot gelatin mixture into the freezer, as it can turn chewy and the surface will crack.

Preparing One envelope or 4 sheets of unflavored gelatin will jell 2 cups of liquid. Each ¼-ounce envelope of unflavored gelatin contains 1 scant tablespoon powder.

Softening gelatin first in a small amount of cold liquid will help it dissolve evenly when combined with the rest of the ingredients in a recipe. Once softened, gelatin then must be warmed with liquid to activate the protein. Finally, it must be allowed to cool and jell. Once this process is begun and the gelatin is softened, it should be used immediately. Do not boil gelatin, or it will lose its setting power. Although you should not stir gelatin while it soaks to avoid forming strings, be sure to stir it thoroughly into other mixtures.

Gelatin can set almost any liquid, from stock or tomato juice to Champagne or cream. Flavored gelatins are easy to use and generally require nothing more complicated than being stirred into very hot water; follow the package directions.

Keep homemade jelled foods cold to retain their shape. Prepared foods containing gelatin, such as marshmallow or jellied candies, do not require refrigeration.

HOW TO *Use Unflavored Powdered Gelatin*

1. Sprinkle 1 envelope (1 tablespoon) powdered gelatin over ¼ cup cold liquid and let it soften for about 5 minutes. Do not stir. It will swell slightly and develop a spongy consistency.
2. Stir the softened gelatin mixture directly into about 1¾ cups hot liquid.
3. Before stirring it into cold liquid in a recipe, heat the softened gelatin in a double boiler over hot water, swirling the pan until the gelatin is completely dissolved.
4. Proceed as directed in the recipe.

Quick Bite

Agar-agar, a tasteless, dried seaweed extract used in Asian kitchens, is prized by vegetarians as a replacement for animal-based gelatin. See also SEAWEED.

HOW TO *Use Unflavored Leaf Gelatin*

1. Soak the sheets in cold water for 15 to 20 minutes. They will resemble wet plastic wrap.
2. Transfer the sheets to a small saucepan, leaving behind the soaking liquid. Heat gently over very low heat until liquefied completely. Shake or swirl the pan, but do not stir.
3. Stir the melted gelatin into about 2 cups of hot liquid and proceed as directed in the recipe.

GIBLETS The small paper package tucked inside the cavity of most purchased whole birds, such as chickens and turkeys, contains the giblets, a term usually referring to the heart, gizzard, and liver of the poultry. Except for the liver, these parts can be used to make gravy, stock, or soup. The liver can be cooked separately and is often considered a delicacy. Giblets also make a nice addition to bread stuffings.

What Do I Do with Giblets?

1. Rinse the giblets well.
2. Simmer them (minus the liver, which would cloud the stock and may be cooked separately) in water with herbs and chopped aromatics such as garlic or onion for about 30 minutes, or until cooked through completely, to make a little stock for a sauce.
3. Finely dice the cooked giblets and stir into gravy or stuffing. Gravy made this way is called giblet gravy.

GIN See SPIRITS.

GINGER The brown, gnarled, knobby appearance of fresh ginger belies its refreshing and slightly sweet flavor. It also packs a fair amount of spiciness. Although mistakenly called a root, ginger is actually a rhizome, or underground stem. A kitchen staple throughout Asia, ginger is an essential aromatic in countless dishes. It adds a fresh note to rich dishes.

The cream- and pink-colored shoots of the rhizome, known as young ginger, are available during the summer in Asian grocery stores. They are more delicate in texture and flavor than mature ginger, the more fibrous, 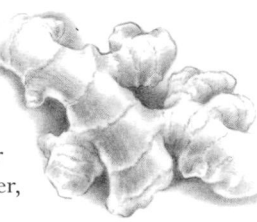 commonly found ginger with the papery brown skin. Crystallized ginger, candied in sugar syrup and then coated with granulated sugar, adds sweet-spicy flavor to dessert fruit fillings, cake batters, ice cream, or fruit salad. Familiar to anyone who loves sushi, pickled ginger is used in Japan as a palate cleanser. Ground dried ginger adds a delightful fragrance and flavor to many breads, cookies, and cakes.

Selecting Look for ginger that is hard and heavy, with an unbroken peel that is thin, light colored, smooth, and shiny. As ginger ages, it becomes darker and more flavorful but also drier and more fibrous. Avoid wrinkled ginger or pieces that give to moderate finger pressure. Young ginger should be a creamy pink color and have smooth, paper-thin skin. Fresh ginger is sold all year long in supermarkets and green grocers. Choose or break off the size piece that best accommodates your needs. Look for crystallized ginger sold in bulk at health-food stores or in small jars in specialty-food stores or grocery stores. Pickled ginger is available in Asian markets.

Storing Store ginger in a cool, dry place for up to 3 days or in the refrigerator for up to 3 weeks. To keep ginger from developing mold in the refrigerator, wrap it first in a paper towel or small paper bag and then in a plastic bag. Ginger freezes relatively well. Cut off slices as needed from the still-frozen rhizome. Store powdered ginger, often called ground ginger, in an airtight container in a cool, dark cupboard and replace every 6 months.

Preparing When a recipe calls for gingerroot, it simply means fresh ginger. If the ginger will be eaten (rather than just used to flavor a dish), peel it with a vegetable peeler or paring knife before using. Like garlic, ginger will have a more intense flavor when crushed or grated rather than simply sliced or chopped. Crush ginger slices with the flat side of a knife blade. To "mince" ginger quickly, crush a small, peeled chunk in a garlic press.

Quick Tip

When a recipe calls for a knob of ginger, it means a chunk of ginger usually about an inch long. Remove before serving the dish.

A ginger grater is a small, flat ceramic tool with tiny, very sharp teeth covering its surface. A knob of peeled ginger rubbed across the notches will fall away in tiny bits, leaving the fibers behind.

Ginger grater.

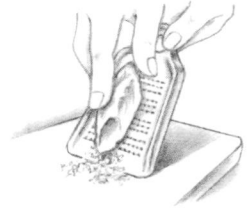

GLAZE See FROSTING, ICING & GLAZE.

GLUTEN See BREAD; FLOUR.

GOOSEBERRY See BERRY.

GORGONZOLA See CHEESE.

GOUDA See CHEESE.

GRAIN See page 224.

GRANITA See SORBET.

GRAPE Grapes come in many sizes and colors, from tiny ones that look like peppercorns to giants that could be mistaken for plums, from sparkling silver-green to deep purple-black. They reflect the specific local conditions of soil and climate in which they were cultivated, developing what the French call *goût terroir,* or "the taste of the land."

Nearly 90 percent of the grapes grown for wine and table belong to the European species *Vitis vinifera.* This includes seedless table grapes like red Emperor, crunchy Flame, and the oblong green Thompson, as well as famous wine varietals such as Chardonnay, Merlot, and Cabernet Sauvignon.

Native to North America, *Vitus labrusca,* or slip-skin grapes, have easily removable peels that make them ideal for jams, jellies, and juice. The Concord grape, starring in such childhood favorites as peanut butter and jelly sandwiches, is the best-known example of this type of grape species.

Whatever their species, grapes find themselves more popularly divided into two broad color categories, red or green, although some countries see things differently and classify grapes as black or white. Grape eaters, and thus grape growers, also further define their fruits by whether they have seeds or are seedless.

Grape leaves, primarily used as wrappers (for appetizers such as rice-stuffed dolmas, or for encasing cheeses or meats for grilling), are also edible. Use young, fresh leaves (blanch to soften), or purchase jars of brined leaves (rinse before using).

Selecting Choose grape bunches with plump, firm fruits, passing over those with fruits that are soft, withered, bruised, or easily brushed from their stems. Green grapes with a hint of yellow or amber are the ripest and sweetest. Red grapes should have no tinge of green in their skin. Darker grapes tend to have tougher skins than the lighter varieties. Bloom is a naturally occurring white powdery substance that covers freshly harvested grapes. Each of the many varieties of grapes peaks during different months, but most come to market between May and September, with a few arriving later into February. Grapes do not become sweeter once harvested.

Storing Remove and discard any bruised or spoiled grapes. Keep grape bunches in a perforated plastic bag in the refrigerator for up to 1 week. To freeze whole grapes, spread small clusters or individual fruits on a baking sheet. Freeze completely and then transfer them to an airtight container and keep in the freezer for up to 6 months.

Preparing Since they are highly susceptible to pests and molds, most grapes have been treated with chemicals, so be sure to rinse well. Let drain on paper towels to dry. Since they are most flavorful at room temperature, remove grapes from the refrigerator at least 30 minutes before serving.

HOW TO *Seed Grapes*

1. Grapes are more easily seeded if halved first, but if you need to keep them whole, use a clean bobby pin to remove the seeds. Holding the two prongs of the pin, insert the crook into the stem end of the grape, hook the seeds, and pull them out.

Quick Tip

Freeze a cluster of grapes and eat them on a hot day to cool off.

Grain

Quite literally, a world of grain awaits the adventurous cook eager to journey beyond such tried-and-true staples as rice and oats. In all their various forms, these edible seeds of cultivated grasses or other plants are outstanding sources of carbohydrate, fiber, protein, and other nutrients.

Grains may be used in virtually every course of the meal and at any time of day: as breakfast cereals or savory side dishes; to add both flavor and texture to salads, soups, stews, casseroles, and stuffings; and as the foundation of or embellishment to a wide array of desserts and baked goods. In addition, of course, many grains are finely ground to make flours.

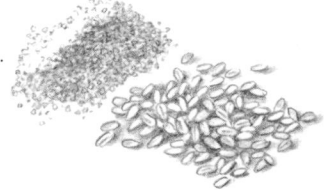

Bulgur and wheat berries.

Selecting Most well-stocked food stores carry a wide assortment of grains. Look in their specialty or ethnic-foods sections for less common types. For the widest selection, go to a large health-food store, where you will most likely find such unusual varieties as quinoa and triticale.

Storing Any whole grains, or cracked grains made from whole grains, will still contain their germ, which is rich in oil. For this reason, they are prone to turning rancid relatively quickly. Buy in small quantities, no more than you will use in a few months. Store in an airtight container in the refrigerator for up to 6 months. By contrast, polished grains—that is, those that have been hulled and de-germed—generally keep well in an airtight container at cool room temperature for up to 1 year.

A Cornucopia of Grains

BARLEY This ancient grain was probably the first one cultivated. Despite a long history of sustaining humankind, its primary uses now are in soups and to make Scotch whisky. It should not be forgotten by the home cook, since its nutty flavor and chewy texture lend themselves to delicious preparations. Barley can be cooked as a risotto-style dish, added to stews, and used cooked cold in salads. It can be bought whole and hulled, flaked, and pearled. Most recipes call for it in the common pearled form, meaning hulled and polished to a pearl-like shape and sheen.

BUCKWHEAT A grain probably native to Mongolia or Siberia. Kasha, the tan-colored, pyramid-shaped seeds of buckwheat, has a pleasantly sour, nutlike taste and robust texture. A popular choice for side dishes in eastern Europe and Russia, the grains are usually pan-toasted before being cooked to tenderness in boiling water.

BULGUR Made from wheat that has been steamed, dried, and cracked, nutty-tasting bulgur is most commonly found in Middle Eastern and Balkan cooking, used much as other cuisines use rice. Tabbouleh, a salad with parsley, onion, tomatoes, and lemon juice, is a well-known dish based on bulgur. Cracked wheat is sometimes mistaken for bulgur. See Wheat, page 227.

CORNMEAL Finely or coarsely ground, dried, whole or polished kernels of yellow or white corn. See also CORNMEAL.

COUSCOUS Not a grain but a pasta. See also COUSCOUS.

GRITS Also known as hominy grits, this is a ground meal of yellow or white hominy. Cooked to a thick porridge, grits, a favorite throughout the American South, is served as a side dish at breakfast, lunch, or dinner. The grain is available in three forms: regular coarsely ground, slow-cooking grits; finer quick-cooking grits; and precooked and dried instant grits, which reconstitute with the addition of boiling water.

HOMINY Dried corn kernels that have been soaked in an alkali such as lime or lye, washed to remove the outer skin, and boiled for several hours. In the end, the kernels resemble soft, white, rather puffed-up kernels of corn. Hominy is sold as either whole kernels or cracked into coarse bits that are cooked in boiling liquid. Whole-kerneled hominy is called samp. Served with butter or cream as a side dish.

KAMUT (ka-MOOT) Kamut is an ancient Egyptian grain. It is an unhybridized relative of durum wheat, similarly high in protein, with a sweet almost buttery taste.

KASHA See Buckwheat, above.

MILLET A common ingredient in birdseed mixtures, these pale yellow, spherical, bland-tasting grains are also cooked in liquid, swelling considerably to make a side dish or breakfast cereal popular in southern Europe, northern Africa, and Asia.

OATS Rich, robust, and flavorful, this favorite grain of northern Europe, Scotland, and Ireland is enjoyed in many forms: whole hulled oats; rolled or old-fashioned oats; quick-cooking rolled oats; and quick-cooking instant oats. Whatever their form, oats are most commonly eaten as a breakfast cereal or used in baking.

POLENTA The Italian name for cornmeal and the Italian dish made from it. See also POLENTA.

QUINOA (KEEN-wah) An ancient staple of the Incas of Peru, these highly nutritious grains look like spherical sesame seeds. When steamed, quinoa has a mild taste and light texture that lends itself well to pilafs, casseroles, salads, or breakfast dishes. Quinoa must be rinsed before cooking because the grain has a natural residue that is very bitter tasting.

RICE Many different types of this most widespread of cereal grains are sold for use in a broad variety of different preparations. See also RICE.

RYE Soft-textured, slightly sour grain native to eastern Europe. Rye is sold either as whole berries, the round seeds seen in rye bread, which can be cooked in soups, stews, casseroles, or stuffings; as cracked unpolished kernels, excellent in pilafs or as a morning cereal; as rolled flakes, to be cooked for breakfast; or as a fine flour for baking. See also FLOUR.

TRITICALE (trih-tih-KAY-lee) A hybrid of wheat and rye first cultivated in Scotland in the late 19th century, triticale has a full, nutty flavor. Like both its parent grains, the berries may be cooked whole and used in a wide ranges of dishes. Low in gluten, triticale flour may be used as a supplement to wheat flour in baking.

continued

g

Grain, continued

Grain-Cooking Timetable

This chart provides basic cooking directions for 1 cup grain. Add ½ to 1 teaspoon salt if desired.

TYPE	LIQUID	METHOD	YIELD
Barley, pearl	4 cups	Add to boiling liquid. Simmer 45 minutes. Drain.	3 to 3½ cups
Bulgur	2 cups	Add to cold water. Bring to a boil, then simmer, covered, 10 to 12 minutes.	2½ to 3 cups
Cornmeal (polenta)	3 to 4 cups, depending on desired consistency (thick or thin)	Add to cold liquid, amount to vary with desired consistency. Bring to a boil, then simmer, stirring frequently, 20 to 45 minutes.	3 to 4 cups
Grits, regular	See Cornmeal, above.		
Hominy	See Cornmeal, above.		
Kamut	3 cups	Add to boiling liquid. Bring to a boil for 2 to 3 minutes, then simmer, covered, for 1½ to 2 hours. Drain if necessary.	3 cups
Kasha	1½ cups	Add to cold liquid. Bring to a boil, then simmer, covered, 10 to 12 minutes.	2 cups
Millet	2 cups	Add to boiling liquid; simmer, uncovered, 15 minutes. Remove from heat, cover, and let stand 10 minutes.	3 cups
Oats, quick-cooking	2 cups	Add to boiling liquid; simmer, covered, 1 minute. Remove from heat and let stand, covered, 3 minutes.	2 cups
Oats, rolled	2 cups	Add to boiling liquid; simmer, uncovered, 5 to 8 minutes.	1¾ cups
Oats, steel-cut	2½ cups	Add to boiling liquid; simmer, covered, 20 to 25 minutes.	3 cups
Quinoa	2 cups	Rinse thoroughly. Add to boiling liquid; simmer, covered, 12 to 15 minutes.	3 cups
Rye berries	3 cups	Add to boiling liquid; simmer, covered, until tender, about 1 hour, adding more liquid as needed. Drain if necessary.	3 cups
Triticale	See Rye berries, above.		
Wheat berries	See Rye berries, above.		
Wheat, cracked	2 cups	Add to cold liquid. Bring to a boil, then simmer, covered, 30 to 45 minutes, depending on coarseness of grain.	3 cups

Wheat Source of the flour we use for
most of our baked goods and pasta,
wheat also may be enjoyed like other
grains. Dark brown, chewy, and rich-
tasting whole wheat berries are boiled
in water for use as a breakfast cereal, a
side dish, or an enhancement for stuffings or baked goods. So, too, are particles of coarse to finely ground cracked
wheat. Cracked wheat may look like
bulgur, but it has not been steamed, so
it requires boiling to soften fully. See
also Bulgur, page 224, and FLOUR.

Preparing The chart at left provides
basic cooking directions for 1 cup of
any listed grain. Please note that specific recipes may call for other cooking
techniques or times.

Grain Terminology The following
terms apply to the structure and processing of grains:

Berries Plump individual whole
grains, particularly of wheat and rye.

Endosperm The soft inner portion
of a grain, loaded with nutrients; often
the only part of it that is eaten.

Flake Flat pieces of grain formed
either by pressing between high-
pressured rollers or by fine slicing.

Germ The embryo contained within
every whole grain, which would grow
if the grain were planted and watered.
The oil-rich germ is often removed
during milling to prevent flour from
going rancid. It is nutritious, however,
and is often sold separately.

Hull The tough outer husk of some
grains such as barley, oats, and rice.

Pearl A term for polishing grains,
like barley, to remove their tough hulls.

Rolled Applies particularly to oats
that are hulled and then steamed and
flattened between rollers into quick-
cooking flakes.

See also CORN; CORNMEAL;
COUSCOUS; FLOUR; POLENTA; RICE.

GRAPEFRUIT The grapefruit is a relative newcomer in culinary history. It didn't
come on the scene until the 18th century,
when it was bred from a cross between oranges and pomelos. It is the second largest
citrus fruit, after the pomelo, and is grown
primarily in the United States. It has a tart,
refreshing flavor and a wealth of juice.
Depending on the variety, the pulp ranges
in color from white to pale pink to ruby
red. The peel is always yellow, although
some varieties sport a pinkish blush. Many
seedless varieties are available.

Selecting Choose grapefruits that are
firm and heavy for their size. Avoid fruits
that have soft spots or a puffy appearance.
Small blemishes on the peel are generally
not indicative of a poor interior.

Storing Grapefruits can be left out at
room temperature for 1 week or kept in
the refrigerator for up to 3 weeks. They
will be juicier and sweeter if brought back
to room temperature before serving.

Grapefruit spoons.

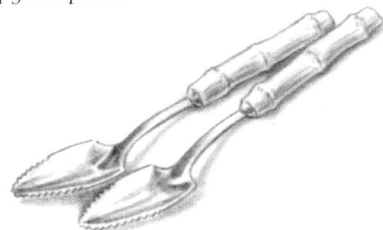

Preparing Cut grapefruits in half along
their equators. Specially designed grapefruit spoons and angled grapefruit knives,
both with serrated edges, permit the
drowsy morning grapefruit eater to free
the juicy sections easily from the tough
membranes. There are even grapefruit
bowls armed with sharp points to hold the
grapefruit in place. Lacking any of these
accoutrements, use a small, sharp knife to
cut all the way around the circumference
of the halved grapefruit, loosening the

g

segments from the peel, and then cut along either side of each section to separate it from the membrane.

Cutting grapefruit segments.

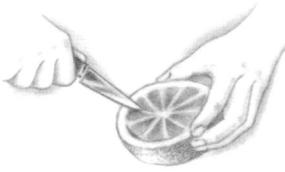

GRATIN Any recipe with the term *gratin, gratinée,* or *au gratin* in its name refers to a dish covered with a browned and crisp crust, usually of bread crumbs (sometimes mixed with bits of butter), cracker crumbs, finely ground nuts, grated or shredded cheese, or similar topping. The dish, usually some form of seafood, meat, poultry, or vegetable bound with a white sauce, is slipped into an oven or under a broiler to brown the crust. Specially designed shallow, usually oval heavy gratin dishes allow for a particularly large surface area, which increases each diner's share of the desirable crispy crust.

Gratin dish.

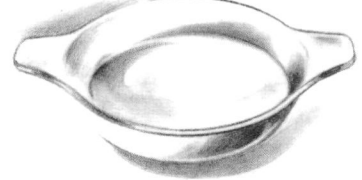

GRATING This term turns up in a wide variety of recipes. It calls for transforming a food into tiny particles, usually by rubbing it over sharp, pointy rasps on a flat grater surface.

Among likely candidates for grating are Parmesan cheese for pasta, lemon zest for cookie dough, bread crumbs for a meat loaf, or nutmeg for a pumpkin pie. The objective of grating is often to make foods cook, melt, dissolve, or blend more quickly and easily.

Grating and shredding cheese.

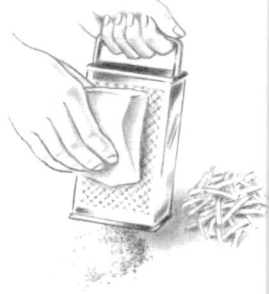

Different types of graters are available. The box grater, a common kitchen tool, includes both a rasp-surfaced grating side and

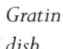

one or more shredding sides (medium or large holes with one raised edge).

Rotary graters, in which food is fed through a small hopper and grated by a rotating drum or disk, speed the job; they include handheld types and hand-turned countertop models.

Rotary cheese grater.

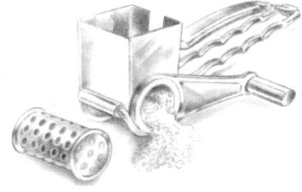

Food processors also come with grating disks among their other attachments.

Fine-rasped nutmeg graters are designed for freshly grating whole nutmegs and include a small compartment for storing the spice. Although most graters are made of stainless steel, small porcelain ginger graters, a standard tool in Asia, easily grate the fibrous rhizome—and can also be used for citrus zest.

Quick Tip

Use a pastry or vegetable brush to clean between the holes of graters.

See also CHEESE; GINGER; NUTMEG; SHREDDING.

GRAVY A sauce that accompanies roasted or panfried meat and is prepared with the meat's own drippings and juices. Traditional gravies call for briefly cooking flour in the drippings to make a light roux. Some cooks, however, use cornstarch or the reduction method as a thickener instead. Gravy can be enriched and flavored with stock, milk, cream, wine, bacon fat, butter, herbs, or tiny pieces of meat or giblets.

HOW TO *Make Gravy*

1. While the roast rests before carving, carefully pick up the roasting pan and pour off all but 3 to 5 tablespoons of the fat.

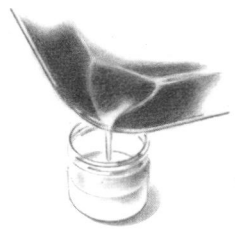

2. Place the roasting pan over medium heat. Sprinkle in 1 to 3 tablespoons all-purpose flour, stirring rapidly to incorporate it with the fat and pan juices and to break up any lumps. Cook briefly, stirring, until lightly browned.

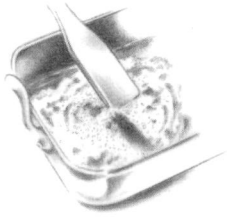

3. Raise the heat to high and, stirring vigorously, pour in hot stock or water and bring to a boil. Reduce the heat to medium and simmer, stirring often, for 5 minutes. Stir in more stock if necessary to achieve a saucelike consistency.

4. Season the gravy to taste with salt and pepper. Pour through a fine-mesh sieve into a warmed gravy boat, stir in a tablespoon of minced fresh herb (if desired), and serve hot.

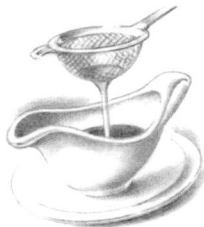

See also DEGLAZING; GIBLETS; REDUCING; SAUCE; THICKENING.

GREAT NORTHERN BEAN See BEAN, DRIED.

GREEN BEAN See BEAN, FRESH.

GREEN ONION Also known as a scallion; see ONION.

GREENS, DARK Hearty in flavor and high in nutrients, dark greens, also known as cooking greens, are no longer limited to the braising pot. Young, tender leaves can replace lettuce on sandwiches or be added to the salad bowl. Represented by several different vegetable families, they range in flavor from lemony sorrel to peppery turnip greens. See also CABBAGE; GREENS, SALAD.

Selecting Look for fresh, crisp leaves free of blemishes, yellowed spots, or tiny insect holes. Do not buy greens if they are wilted or dried out. Small, young leaves will have a milder flavor, and more and more greens are now available as tender "baby" leaves. Look for greens tied in bunches or washed, chopped, and sealed in plastic bags. (Even though the latter are prewashed, they should be rinsed well again before using.) Baby greens are sold in bulk or in plastic bags. Greens are available year-round in large markets, but most are at their peak from late winter to early spring. Exceptions are turnip greens, in late fall; spinach, spring and fall; beet greens, during the summer and early fall; and Swiss chard, arriving in early spring and lingering through the fall.

A Guide to Dark Greens

BEET GREENS Closely related to chard, beet greens have smooth, thin leaves and an earthy flavor. See also BEET.

BROCCOLI RABE Long, slender, sometimes tough stems with dark green, rippled leaves. Bright yellow broccoli rabe flowers are also edible. See also BROCCOLI RABE.

COLLARD GREENS Large, thick, dark green leaves, each branching from a thick central stem. The flavor is mild, but the tough texture calls for long cooking. A favorite in the American South.

DANDELION GREENS Although unwelcome on most lawns, the pale green, sharply sawtoothed leaves of the dandelion have a pleasantly bitter flavor. The larger and older the leaves, the stronger and tougher they will be. Dandelion cultivated specifically for eating grows longer leaves and is more tender than its wild cousin. (Do not pick greens from lawns that have been treated with chemicals or from busy roadsides.)

ESCAROLE A slightly bitter member of the chicory family with broad, ruffled leaves. Eaten cooked or raw. See also CHICORY.

KALE A member of the cabbage family, with firm, tightly crinkled leaves on long stems. Sturdy kale is dark green in color, has an earthy flavor similar to cabbage, and holds its texture well in cooking.

MUSTARD GREENS Light green, with hints of yellow. Different varieties range in size, shape, and sharpness. Large-leafed mustards tend to be sweeter than those loosely formed into heads, which have a pungent bite. Small, curled mustards have the hottest, spiciest flavor.

SORREL Delicate, triangular leaves with a strongly tart flavor similar to that of rhubarb. The paler the leaves, the more delicate the flavor. Sorrel discolors with cooking, but it lends a bright, pleasantly sour flavor when puréed into soups and sauces.

SPINACH Dark green leaves and earthy, faintly bitter flavor. There are several varieties of spinach: some have thick, crinkled leaves, while others are smooth and flat. Small, immature leaves, marketed as baby spinach, are sold in bulk in many markets and are an excellent salad green.

SWISS CHARD Also known as chard. Large, crinkled leaves on fleshy, ribbed stems. There are two varieties: one with red stems and another with pearly white stems. Red chard, also marketed as rhubarb or ruby chard, has a slightly earthier flavor, while chard with white stems tends to be sweeter.

TURNIP GREENS Among the most assertive of the dark greens. Rarely eaten raw, turnip greens have rich flavor when slowly braised. Often mixed with collard and mustard greens. See also TURNIP.

Storing Since greens will continue to draw nutrients and moisture from their roots after harvesting, trim off the greens and store them separately if you plan to eat the roots as well. Wrap unwashed greens in a clean, damp kitchen towel or damp paper towels, then cover them loosely with a plastic bag. They will keep in the refrigerator for 3 to 5 days. Generally, the sturdier greens will keep for a longer period of time than the delicate ones, although their flavor may become stronger—and perhaps unpleasant—with age.

Preparing The textured leaves of greens often trap large amounts of dirt and sand, especially the leaves of darker varieties. Wash well just before using: Fill the sink or a large bowl with cool water, immerse the greens, then lift them out, letting the grit settle at the bottom. Repeat a few times until no grit is left behind.

Washing spinach.

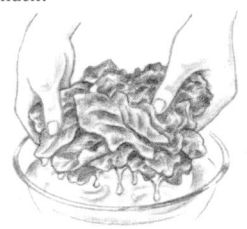

HOW TO *Remove Stems*

When stems are fibrous and leaves are tender, you'll want to remove the stems before cooking. Use a paring knife to cut away the wide, thick stems of tougher greens such as chard or mustard. For thin stems of tender greens:

1. Gently fold a leaf in half lengthwise along the stem with the vein side out.
2. Holding the folded leaf in one hand, quickly tear the stem away along with the tough center vein.

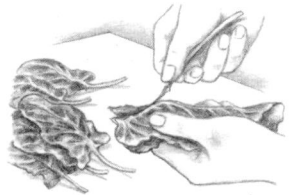

Most tender greens, such as spinach and broccoli rabe, can be simply sautéed. Tougher greens, such as kale and chard, may need a quick blanch to tenderize them and remove some of their bitterness.

GREENS, SALAD Once upon a time, a wedge of iceberg drizzled with thick dressing qualified as the ultimate in salads. But a quick glance today down any produce aisle will reveal that greens have come a long way. From pale romaine hearts to tender baby spinach, from frilly tufts of frisée to elegantly tapered heads of Belgian endive, there is an endless variety of color, flavors, and textures that you can toss in your salad bowl. Mesclun, a mix of baby greens, is now a staple in markets and restaurants, while imports from Europe and Asia have added zip and flair to the salad course. The French believe that anything added to greens beyond a sprinkle of fresh herbs spoils a salad, but Americans love to combine vegetables, greens, and other ingredients in explosions of color and texture. Europeans traditionally follow the main course with refreshing, palate-cleansing greens, while Americans serve salads as an opening course to stimulate the palate. Whatever your preferences (and iceberg lettuce has even made a comeback!), explore the steadily expanding world of greens and make salads a delicious part of every meal.

Selecting Choose heads that are densely packed and heavy for their size. Avoid any wilted or browned greens. If you are buying greens sealed in cellophane bags, check their freshness date and look closely, especially at the bottom of the bag, for any leaves that are discolored or wet. Baby greens are available in bulk and packaged in cellophane bags. Grocery stores stock lettuce greens year-round, but during the cool months of spring and fall, look for locally grown young greens, especially at the farmers' market.

Select greens from the different groups and don't hesitate to experiment with colors, textures, and flavors to make a salad that suits your taste.

A Salad Bowl of Greens

DELICATE LEAVES WITH SWEET FLAVOR:
BIBB LETTUCE Also called limestone. Very tender, pale green leaves loosely gathered in a small, rosettelike head.
BUTTER LETTUCE Also called Boston lettuce. Loose head with soft, "buttery"-textured, light green leaves. Similar to Bibb, but larger.
GREEN-LEAF OR RED-LEAF LETTUCE Large, ruffled leaves gathered at their stems to form an open, loose head. Mild and delicate in flavor, it is a popular all-purpose salad green. Red-leaf variety has a deep red blush on the leaf edges.
MÂCHE Also called field salad, corn salad, or lamb's lettuce, for it appears in early spring with the lambs. Very delicate and mild, with oval leaves that grow in small, loose bunches.
MESCLUN A varied mixture of young, tender greens. Mesclun, which is a Provençal word for "mix," is traditionally a salad consisting of the first greens and herbs of spring, hence its other name, spring mix. The mixes vary greatly but usually include a wide range of color and textures.
OAKLEAF LETTUCE 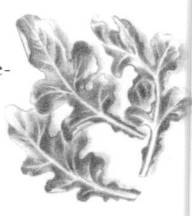 Tender, mild lettuce with notched leaves resembling those of the oak tree, sometimes fringed in red. Also sometimes applies to red-leaf lettuces.

CRISP LEAVES WITH MILD FLAVOR:
ICEBERG LETTUCE Also known as crisp-head lettuce. Bland, crisp, thick leaves are good for adding crunch to salad mixes and sandwiches. Very pale green, blending nearly to pale yellow or ivory at the center. The sturdy leaves from the tightly layered, round heads can serve as cups to hold minced salads or other appetizers.
ROMAINE An elongated head of crisp, sturdy leaves that are juicy and sweet. The traditional lettuce for Caesar salad, it can hold up well to strongly flavored dressings and firm garnishes. The pale and crunchy inner leaves of romaine hearts are sometimes sold separately.
SPINACH Slightly bitter-tasting dark green leaves. For use raw in salads, it is best to select small baby spinach leaves, often sold already washed and prepackaged; they have the mildest flavor and best texture.
LEAVES WITH NUTTY AND SWEET FLAVOR:
MIZUNA Originally from Japan, now grown domestically. Long and feathery leaves with a sweet, mild cabbage flavor.
SALAD SAVOY An ornamental variety of kale, tasting faintly of cauliflower. Has small ruffled leaves with stems and leaves streaked in pinkish purple or creamy white.
LEAVES WITH BITTER OR PEPPERY FLAVOR:
ARUGULA Also called rocket. Its dark green, deeply notched leaves resemble small, elongated oak leaves. Nutty, tangy, and slightly peppery in flavor. Larger leaves are more pungent. See also ARUGULA.

BELGIAN ENDIVE Crisp leaves in a small, cylindrical head. See CHICORY; ENDIVE.
CURLY ENDIVE Also known as curly chicory. Loose, bushy head of narrow, frilly leaves with long stems. Pale yellow center leaves have a milder taste. See also CHICORY.
ESCAROLE A green with broad, ruffled leaves and a slightly bitter flavor, similar to curly and Belgian endive. Popular green for wilted salads. See also CHICORY.
FRISÉE Young curly endive. Lacy leaves gathered loosely, with tender, pale green outer leaves and a pale yellow to white heart. See also CHICORY.
WATERCRESS Small, round, dark green leaves on short, delicate stems. Its refreshing, peppery flavor can turn bitter with age. See also WATERCRESS.
CRISP AND BRIGHTLY COLORED LEAVES:
RADICCHIO Grows in round or elongated heads. Complements other greens with its deep ruby red color and pleasantly bitter flavor. See also CHICORY.
RED CABBAGE Thinly sliced into strips and tossed into salads for color and texture. See also CABBAGE.
RED ENDIVE A reddish purple variety of Belgian endive. See also CHICORY; ENDIVE.
Storing Store greens unwashed in plastic bags. Although best if eaten the day of purchase, soft-leaved greens will keep for up to 4 days in a plastic bag in the crisper of the refrigerator. Firmer lettuces such as romaine will keep for up to 10 days.

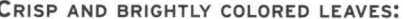

Preparing Immerse greens in a large bowl or sink filled with cool water. Discard any wilted or yellowed leaves. Lift out the greens gently, and repeat the washing until the water is clear. A salad spinner is ideal for drying greens, but shaking them gently in a clean kitchen towel will also absorb excess moisture. Be sure to dry the greens as much as possible, for excess water will dilute the dressing and prevent it from coating the leaves. If you have time, put the washed greens in the refrigerator to crisp.

To prevent discoloration and bruising, tear leaves instead of cutting them. (Romaine leaves, however, are traditionally cut.) Do not dress salad greens until just before serving them; acid and salt in the dressing will quickly wilt the leaves. The lighter and softer the leaf, the more quickly it will wilt. Milder greens are best in simple salads with few ingredients and less acidic vinaigrettes. More strongly flavored greens, such as the chicories, can stand up to other ingredients, including thinly sliced fruit and vegetables, citrus segments, cheese, and toasted nuts.

HOW TO *Wash Greens in Advance*

Washed lettuce can stay crisp in the refrigerator for up to a day. This is also a convenient way to transport lettuce for a picnic or a potluck.

1. Rinse the greens well, then shake off most but not all of the water.
2. Spread a clean kitchen towel flat and arrange the leaves in a single layer on the towel.
3. Gently roll up the towel with the leaves, jelly-roll fashion, being careful not to crush the leaves. Loosely cover the roll with a large plastic bag or plastic wrap.
4. When ready, unwrap and unroll the lettuce and continue as needed.

See also DRESSING; GREENS, DARK; SALAD; VINAIGRETTE.

GRIDDLE See COOKWARE.

GRILLING Nothing defines summer like grilling in the backyard. Cooking food on a grid placed over a fire, from fanning the charcoal to relishing the burnt ends, is a favorite pastime on leisurely August weekends. And now, with the steadily growing manufacture of sophisticated gas grills for the outdoors and simple grill pans for the indoors, grilling has become a way to cook in every season, for every occasion.

Direct vs. Indirect Heat Cooking food directly over smoldering coals or gas flame is called direct-heat grilling. It is an intense, high-heat method ideal for thin cuts of meat, fish, and vegetables that require less than 25 minutes to cook. On a gas grill, direct heat can be achieved by turning all the burners beneath the food to medium-high or high.

On the other hand, some recipes call for cooking by indirect heat. For charcoal grills, this means piling up charcoal opposite where the food will be placed, allowing for slower cooking. Gas grills simply need to be turned to very low or completely off beneath the food. This method works well with whole poultry, roasts, and other large cuts that would not cook all the way through over direct heat before their surfaces burned. Indirect-heat cooking, which is similar to roasting, also eliminates the flare-ups caused by fat dripping directly onto hot coals or flame, which can scorch food.

Indirect-heat grilling.

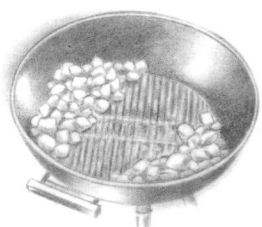

If you will be cooking only by indirect heat, you can arrange the coals on either side of the grill and cook the food at the center. If you will be using both methods or direct heat only, pile the charcoal on one side of the grill.

Before placing food on the grill, nestle a drip pan in the area of low heat, to catch juices and to reflect heat toward the food.

Types of Grills Despite the wide variety of grill styles, only three basic different kinds of grills exist, classed according to their source of heat. In charcoal grills, charcoal is burned until heated through, then spread into a single layer for flavorfully smoky heat. With charcoal, the heat level can be difficult to control.

A gas grill, commonly fueled by propane, emits gas flames that in turn heat ceramic briquettes or lava rocks. Once hot, the rocks cook the food. With gas burners and knob controls like a stove, the heat of gas grills can be adjusted. (Even set to high, a gas grill can never achieve the high temperatures of hardwood and charcoal, and purists claim that the food never acquires the flavor delivered by a good charcoal fire. Nonetheless, for most backyard cooks, the convenience of the gas grill more than makes up for any difference.)

Lastly, for indoor use, there are various models of electric grills. Some can cook enough food for up to six people. Powered by electricity, these tabletop appliances rarely reach the high temperatures of outdoor gas or charcoal grills. Open tabletop grills are shaped like hibachis; closed tabletop grills resemble large waffle makers with plates that may be grooved or smooth. The two sides close, sandwiching and cooking food that is placed between them. When using an electric grill, be sure to cook near an open window or exhaust fan.

One of the most common designs for an outdoor grill is the kettle grill, a spherical, covered design intended for promoting good heat circulation. A kettle grill has a domed lid that efficiently directs heat back down to the food and may be high enough to accommodate a whole turkey. Most kettle grills use charcoal, but gas models are also available.

Kettle grill.

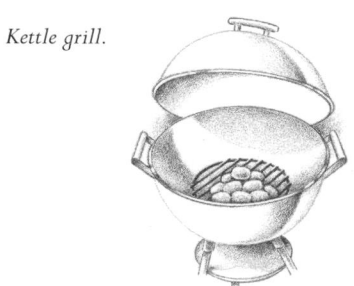

Hibachis are small, inexpensive uncovered square-cornered grills. Although good for picnics and grilling in tight spaces, they can hold only a few servings at a time. They are available as portable charcoal grills or electric tabletop appliances.

Double hibachi.

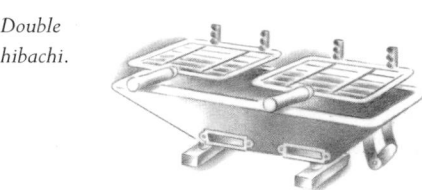

Range-top grills are sometimes an option, too. Some stoves include a dedicated grill section, while others offer a grate as an accessory to replace two of the burners. Range-top grills require powerful exhaust fans to avoid filling a room with smoke.

Fuel An array of fuels offers varying levels of flavor, convenience, and cost. The basic fuel for gas grills is liquid propane, which is sold in large, metal tanks. Be sure to keep track of the propane level so that you don't run out midway through cooking steaks at your next party. Color-coded magnetic patches attached to the side of the tank will clearly display the fuel's level.

With charcoal grills, you can use briquettes or natural hardwood charcoal. Briquettes are charcoal and sawdust pressed together in small, square-shaped coals. They are more widely available and less expensive than hardwood charcoal, but additives can impart unwanted flavors. Avoid briquettes that contain petroleum, nitrates, sand, or clay as fillers. Some contain starter for instant lighting and bits of wood for hints of hardwood flavor. Natural hardwood charcoal—mesquite, hickory, oak—is well worth its higher price. Virtually all carbon, these hardwood chunks light quickly, burn cleanly and slowly, and produce higher heat than either briquettes or gas.

Fuel choices.

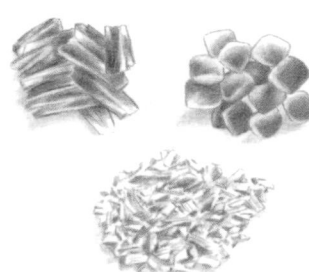

Wood chips add excellent flavor to grilled foods. Fruit woods such as apple, cherry, almond, grape, or olive have subtle aromas, while stronger woods such as mesquite or hickory give off more assertive smoke. For the best flavor, use them during slow cooking. You can use the chips dry for strong, smoky flavors, or soak them in water, beer, or wine for steamy, moist heat.

FOUR WAYS TO USE WOOD CHIPS

- Fill a drip pan with chips.
- Seal chips in a sheet of heavy-duty aluminum, forming a flat envelope. Poke holes in the package and place on coals.
- Scatter chips directly on the coals. For a subtler flavor, soak the chips in water

for at least 30 minutes before throwing them on the coals.
- Use them in the smoker box of a gas grill. Follow manufacturer's instructions.

Quick Tip

To infuse food quickly with fragrant smoke, soak a handful of woody herbs such as rosemary or thyme, spices such as cinnamon sticks or star anise, fresh fennel fronds, or grapevine cuttings in water for at least 15 minutes (to prevent burning), then drain and toss onto hot coals.

Starters The challenge of starting and maintaining a fire lends outdoor grilling much of its mystique. Gas grills were designed to bypass the difficulties and, for some, the fun. You need simply open the fuel valve of the propane tank, light the flames as directed by the manual, and then turn the knobs to adjust the heat level. Allow 15 to 20 minutes for a gas grill to heat completely.

Charcoal
chimney starter.

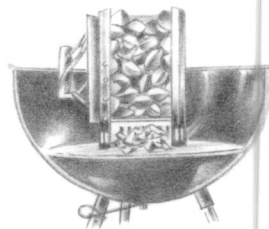

Charcoal grills, on the other hand, call for more finesse. If you grill frequently, consider purchasing a charcoal chimney. Resembling a large coffee can with a handle and holes circling the bottom, it lights coals quickly without the use of lighter fluid. Place crumpled newspaper in the bottom section, center the chimney in the grill, pour charcoal into the top compartment, and light the paper below. The flames burning upward inside the chimney will heat the charcoal. When they are ready, pour the coals from the chimney into the grill. If you need to add more preheated coals for extended cooking, add them to the grill on top of the burning coals as needed to continue grilling. Always let fresh coals burn down a bit before grilling food over them.

If you do not have a chimney, pile charcoal in a neat heap at the center of the grill. Soak the coals with lighter fluid and then light them. Although inexpensive and popular, lighter fluid gives off chemical flavors, especially if too much is used. Allow it to burn off completely before beginning to cook. Nontoxic solid cubes of odorless and smokeless paraffin lighter (or paraffin-soaked corn cobs), tucked into a pile of charcoal, can replace newspapers or liquid starter. An electric starter, basically an iron coil attached to a handle, requires an outlet, but it will heat your charcoal quickly and easily. Keep it away from high-traffic areas, however, since the combination of a cord and a bare element is a potential hazard.

Grilling Accessories and Equipment

Buy utensils with extra-long wooden handles to keep your fingers away from the heat.

BASTING BRUSH Use a wide natural bristle brush, and avoid plastic bristles, as they will melt.

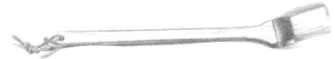

DRIP PAN Use a small, shallow metal pan to place under the meat during indirect cooking. You can also fill it with water for slow-cooking ribs or with wood chips for smoking.

HINGED BASKET Folding, two-part rectangular or oval baskets that enclose whole fish, hamburgers, or mixed vegetables.

MITTS Look for thick, flame-retardant materials and extra-long cuffs.

SKEWERS Invest in sturdy, stainless steel skewers if you grill brochettes frequently. Bamboo skewers are simple and inexpensive, but they tend to burn even with presoaking. Wide, flat skewers and double-pronged ones provide additional support for turning food. Long rosemary sprigs, stripped of their lower leaves and soaked for an hour, make beautiful and aromatic skewers.

SPECIALTY GRIDS Variously shaped mesh sheets and baskets to hold small, odd shaped, or delicate foods on top of the grill's standard grid or grill rack.

THERMOMETER For long cooking with lower heat, insert an instant-read thermometer in the vent opening to monitor the temperature inside the grill without opening the lid. See also COOKING TOOLS.

TONGS Extra-long tongs make turning and removing foods quick and easy without piercing them and losing juices.

WIRE BRUSH Stiff wire bristles scrape residue off the grill rack.

When Is the Charcoal Ready?

- After the flames die down, wait until a fine layer of white ash covers all of the charcoal pieces before spreading them. When using briquettes, wait until all traces of red are gone before cooking, to ensure that the food does not take on chemical or coal flavors.
- For a low-tech way to gauge the heat level of coals, hold your hand about 4 inches above the fire, or at the point where the food will be cooking. Keep your hand there as long as you comfortably can and count: 1 to 2 seconds is a hot fire, 3 to 4 seconds is a medium-hot fire, and 5 seconds or more is considered a low fire.

Grill Savvy

- If the grill rack is not clean when you're ready to cook, let the residue burn off while the charcoal is burning down to the point at which it is covered with white ash. Then scrape the rack clean before placing food on it.
- Be sure to preheat the grill rack, which helps keep food from sticking to it. Oiling it will also help. See FAT & OIL for more details. When grilling delicate foods such as fish, cut a large potato into thick slices and rub it on the grill rack before grilling. Its starch will coat the metal and help prevent sticking.
- For cooking most foods, place the rack 4 to 6 inches from the charcoal.
- Cover the grill to increase the heat level and the intensity of the smoky flavor. For a crispier char, leave the lid off.
- Adjust the vents as needed to keep the desired heat level. Opened wide, they will allow more air in for a hotter fire. Closed slightly, they will dampen the heat. Do not close them all the way unless you want to put out the fire.
- To keep a charcoal fire hot for extended cooking times, scatter 10 to 15 unlit, chemically untreated charcoal pieces at 30-minute intervals, or add a large number that have been lit separately in a chimney placed in a heatproof container, such as an old roasting pan or disposable aluminum pan.
- To prevent burning, brush on glazes or sauces, especially those containing sugar, toward the end of cooking.

Cleaning Up

- After cooking, cover the grill and allow the heat of the dying coals or gas flames to burn off the residue.
- Clean the cooled grill rack with a stiff wire brush or scrubbing pad.
- Clean the grill after every use, so the food does not dry on the rack.
- If your grill doesn't have an ash collector or a way for ashes to drop into a pan below, wait until the ash is completely cool, scoop it out, and discard it in a nonflammable container.
- Make sure all the vents are clear.
- To clean lava rocks, let cool completely, place in a heavy paper bag, and shake to knock off any bits of food. Do not wash the rocks with detergent.

Caution!

- Never spray liquid starter on already-lit charcoal.
- Do not leave a grill unattended, especially if children or pets are present.
- Do not grill indoors (except with an indoor grill pan).
- Place the grill away from foliage, dry grass, or other highly flammable material.
- Keep a water hose ready in case of fire.
- Store starter in a safe, secure place away from the grill.

See also BARBECUING; MARINATING; RUB.

GRILL PAN See COOKWARE.

GRINDING To crush foods such as grains, spices, nuts, seeds, or coffee to a fine texture. Various kinds of equipment are employed to grind ingredients, from large mill stones and industrial steel rollers to countertop electric appliances and old-fashioned mortars and pestles. Because they are not subjected to the heat of steel rollers, stone-ground products retain more flavor and tend to have more distinctive textures. Although grinding your own spices or coffee at home just before using them takes time, they will boast fuller flavors than already-ground ones, as their aromatic components will not already have dissipated upon exposure to air.

See also COFFEE; NUT; SPICE.

GRITS See GRAIN.

GRUYÈRE See CHEESE.

GUAVA Long enjoyed in Central and South America, the delicious and sweet-smelling guava is popular in tropical countries around the world. Vaguely pear shaped, guavas can be as small as a walnut or as large as an apple, depending on the variety. Their skin may be pale yellow or light green, while their flesh may be white, pink, yellow, or red. The flavor of the flesh can bring to mind strawberries, bananas, pineapple, or all three. Some varieties are seedless, but others have numerous small edible seeds, especially toward the center. The best varieties have a creamy texture and a soft rind that can be eaten as well.

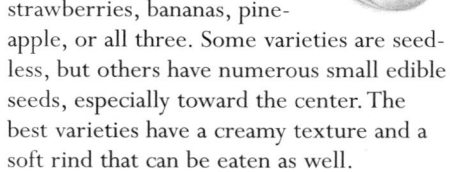

Enjoy ripe guavas out of hand, peeling and seeding them if needed. Slice them and toss gently with starfruit and kiwifruit for a colorful tropical salad. Puréed and strained guavas can thicken a fruity sauce for poultry or pork or flavor mousses, ice cream bases, whipped cream, or custards for desserts. They won't hold up to long cooking but can be gently simmered or poached briefly in sugar syrup.

Selecting Like avocados, guavas should yield to gentle pressure. Although small scuffs and scars are natural, avoid any fruit with discolored, soft spots. Sniff the fruit and choose one with an especially floral bouquet. When unripe, they may have a slight musky fragrance but should emit hints of sweetness. Since they do not survive shipping well, most guavas found in markets are grown domestically and are available from September to February.

Latino markets and some specialty supermarkets sell guava paste in firm, dark red blocks. In Latin America, it is typically sliced and served paired with a mild white cheese as a dessert, or is sometimes eaten alone, much like a candy bar. Check supermarkets for guava jelly, jam, nectar, and frozen purée, as well as cans of the whole fruit. In general, these products lack the fresh fruit's delicate, distinctive flavor but are convenient to use.

Storing Unripe guavas have an astringent bite, but they ripen quickly if stored at room temperature, especially in a paper bag. Once guavas are fully ripe, keep them in a plastic bag in the refrigerator for no more than 3 to 4 days.

Guava paste can be stored indefinitely in a sealed container at room temperature. Store guava purée in the freezer and the jellied or canned fruit in a cool, dark place for up to 1 year.

Preparing Peel and seed guavas if desired or called for in a recipe.

GUGELHOPF PAN See BAKEWARE.

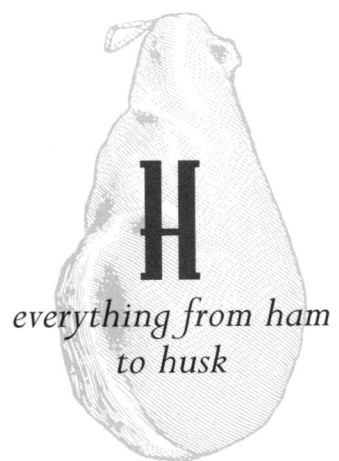

*everything from ham
to husk*

h

HABANERO See CHILE.

HALF-AND-HALF See CREAM.

HAM Ham is a portion of the lean hind leg of a pig that has been cured, or preserved, and flavored, often by smoking. The curing is done by various methods, depending on the style of ham. Traditional European hams, like Italian prosciutto and Spanish serrano, are dry-cured in salt and air-dried. In the United States, the hind leg of the pig is traditionally dry-cured or cured in brine (which is known as pickle curing), then smoked and aged for months to become country ham, the best-known version of which is the Smithfield ham of Virginia. Some country hams are sugar-cured, which means that the brine used for curing includes sugar, and other variations exist in other regions of the United States. American country hams must be soaked, simmered, and then baked before eating. Most European dry-cured hams and American country hams are highly flavored and fairly salty and are usually eaten in thin slices. European dry-cured hams may be used as an ingredient in cooked dishes but are not otherwise cooked before eating.

Aside from traditional ham, there is mass-produced ham. Most such hams are cured by injection, which takes considerably less time. A solution of brine is introduced into the pork through a needle. These hams may be smoked at this point (or given another injection, this time with liquid smoke) and then partially or fully cooked. Mass-produced hams are usually given only a "light cure," using a less-salty brine than country hams; they are also generally only lightly smoked or not smoked at all. The result is a milder tasting ham that is juicier and more tender than country ham, but with less distinctive flavor and texture. It is the type of ham with which many Americans are best acquainted.

Selecting Mass-produced hams are sold either fully or partially cooked. Fully cooked are labeled "ready to serve" or "heat and serve" and may be baked again before serving, but only to heat them through. Partially cooked require additional cooking. They are available with or without the bone, although bone-in hams are generally more flavorful. Sometimes the hams are sold spiral sliced for convenience.

Avoid hams labeled "with natural juices," "water added," or "ham and water product," which means that they have retained some of the water used in the brine-injected curing process. Instead, reach for those marked "no water added" or simply "ham." These latter hams are aged longer—for

Quick Bite

Picnic hams are made from the picnic shoulder, or front leg, of the pig; they are fattier and less expensive than hams from the hind leg.

at least a year—to create a more complex flavor and denser meat than their water-logged counterparts. However, some people prefer the moister, milder meat of shorter-aged hams.

Storing Whole or half hams will keep for no longer than 1 week in the refrigerator. Ham, because of its high salt content, is not a good candidate for long-term freezing; the flavor suffers.

HOW TO *Bake a Fully Cooked Ham*
1. If there is a rind, cut it off and trim away all but about ½ inch of the outer layer of fat.
2. For a ham to be presented whole at the table, score the remaining coat of fat diagonally in two directions to make diamond shapes; stud the center of each diamond with a whole clove.
3. Bake in a preheated 325°F oven until a meat thermometer registers 140°F at the center of its thickest part, which, depending on the size of the ham, will take 1 to 1½ hours. If desired, glaze with marmalade; a mixture of brown sugar, mustard, and honey; or melted cranberry sauce during the last 30 minutes of cooking.

HOW TO *Bake a Partially Cooked Ham*
1. Trim and score the ham as directed above.
2. Bake in a 350°F oven until a meat thermometer registers 155°F at the center of its thickest part, allowing 10 to 12 minutes per pound. If desired, glaze the ham during the last 30 minutes of cooking, using one of the glazes suggested for a fully cooked ham, above.

See also CARVING; PORK; PROSCIUTTO.

HAMBURGER Although the term sometimes refers to ground or chopped beef, it usually evokes the American favorite, a beef patty slipped into a bun. The hamburger's ancestral namesake is the pounded beefsteak served in 19th-century Hamburg, Germany, but it was in the United States that countless diners and fast-food chains immortalized this humble meal. The standard burger comes on a round bun, topped with some favorite combination of cheese, mayonnaise,

> ## Quick Tip
> Ground chuck, 80 to 85 percent lean, is ideal for juicy, tender, and flavorful burgers. You can use ground round or sirloin, but the leaner meat will have less flavor.

ketchup, mustard, onion, pickle, tomato, and lettuce. In recent years, however, a new class of gourmet burgers has introduced such up-to-date adornments as arugula and blue cheese, and burgers of tofu, poultry, grains, or vegetables now appear as menu options alongside their meaty cousins on many restaurant menus.

HARICOT VERT See BEAN, FRESH.

HAZELNUT See NUT.

HEAPING Describes a measure that is slightly more full than level, such as "1 heaping tablespoon." See also MEASURING.

HEART OF PALM The tender, edible core of a young cabbage palm tree is a delicacy in tropical countries. Hearts of palm are slender and white, with many thin, concentric layers, like a leek. They resemble thick stalks of white asparagus, have a taste reminiscent of artichokes, and are tossed with vinaigrette and served as part of a salad, or are included in lightly cooked dishes.

Selecting Fresh hearts of palm are rarely seen in markets outside of tropical regions,

h

but they are commonly available canned in water in well-stocked food stores. If you do come across fresh ones, buy stalks that are not dried, split, or separated in layers.

Storing Since they are highly perishable, store fresh hearts in a perforated plastic bag in the refrigerator and use them within 2 days. Once opened, canned hearts should be transferred to a glass, plastic, or ceramic container, covered with water, and refrigerated for up to 1 week.

Preparing Blanch fresh hearts for 30 seconds to remove bitterness. To remove any tinny taste from canned hearts, soak them in water and a little lemon juice for 10 minutes before using.

HEAT DIFFUSER See COOKING TOOLS.

HERB See page 244.

HIGH-ALTITUDE COOKING At high altitudes, cooks must adjust cooking times and temperatures. Due to the decrease in air density and air pressure, water molecules turn to steam more readily, thus boiling at lower temperatures than at sea level. Foods require longer cooking to compensate for this heat loss. The higher the altitude, the greater the difference.

Small adjustments will correct most of the effects of low pressure. Trial and error will determine exact changes for each dish. For best results, however, follow recipes written specifically for high altitudes.

Adjusting Time and Temperature
Cook food at higher heat or for a longer amount of time.

- Increase oven temperature by 25°F.
- Expect to boil or simmer food for a few minutes more.
- Starting at 4,000 feet, expect to simmer stews 1 hour more for every additional 1,000 feet.

- When deep-frying, decrease the oil temperature 3°F for every 1,000 feet above sea level, to prevent food from overbrowning on the outside while undercooking inside.

Adjusting Liquid Since liquids evaporate more rapidly at higher elevations, ingredients will become drier. The higher the elevation, the greater the loss of liquid.

- Increase the amount of liquid in recipes, adding 2 to 4 tablespoons to every 1 cup of liquid.
- Add several cups more liquid for boiling pasta and legumes.
- Double-wrap already baked breads and cakes to prevent drying out.

Boiling Point at High Altitudes

ELEVATION	FAHRENHEIT	CELSIUS
Sea level	212°	100°
2,000 feet	208°	98°
5,000 feet	203°	95°
7,500 feet	198°	92°
10,000 feet	195°	90°
15,000 feet	185°	85°

Adjusting Ingredients

LEAVENING At 3,000 feet above sea level, bread baking takes on new dimensions—literally. Baking powder, baking soda, and even yeast produce gas more quickly at high altitudes. And with less air pressure for baked goods to rise against, they can tower to greater heights. Unfortunately, they collapse more quickly, too, because they lack the time necessary to develop the structure to support themselves.

- Decrease leavening by one-fourth the amount required at sea level.
- Watch yeast dough carefully as it rises. Punch it down and let rise a second time

until doubled. With recipes that call for two risings, add a third rising.

OTHER INGREDIENTS

- Reduce every 1 cup of sugar by 1 to 2 tablespoons.
- Do not beat egg whites beyond soft peaks for meringues or cake batters. They will dry out too much, collapse easily, and add too much unstable air.
- Add an additional whole egg to delicate, airy batters (popovers, sponge cakes) to provide additional leavening.

HOISIN SAUCE A thick, sweet, reddish brown sauce made from soybeans, sugar, garlic, Chinese five-spice powder or star anise, and a hint of chile. It can be thick and creamy or thin enough to pour. Used throughout China, hoisin sauce is rubbed on meat and poultry before roasting to give them a sweet flavor and red color. It sometimes appears as a condiment but should be added with caution, as its strong flavor can easily overpower most foods.

Selecting Hoisin sauce is available in large cans, but smaller jars are more practical and are usually of better quality. Look for it in Asian markets or the ethnic-food aisle of major grocery stores.

Storing The sauce keeps indefinitely in the refrigerator. Once opened, transfer canned hoisin sauce to a glass jar or an airtight plastic container.

HOMINY See GRAIN.

HONEY The old adage "busy as a bee" has its basis in reality. A hive of bees must fly over 55,000 miles and visit 2 million flowers to produce a single pound of honey, the sweet, syrupy liquid that bees make from flower nectar to feed their hive, and that children, tea drinkers, and bakers love.

Honey arrives at market in three basic forms. Most common is liquid honey,

extracted from the honeycomb by centrifugal force, gravity, or straining. Liquid honey is usually pasteurized and filtered. Sold in a crystallized state, spun honey, also called granulated or crème honey, can be spread like butter at room temperature. Comb honey comes just as the bees produced it—still in its wax comb, which is edible as well. Cut comb honey, a variation, contains small chunks of the honeycomb.

Selecting Depending on the source of the nectar, honey ranges from almost white to deep, rich brown. The flavor changes according to the plants that surround any given hive. In general, the lighter the honey's color, the more delicate its flavor.

LIGHT AND MILD HONEYS Acacia, alfalfa, clover, lavender, orange blossom, rosemary.

DARK AND STRONG HONEYS Basswood (pale color but assertive flavor), buckwheat, chestnut, eucalyptus, tupelo, wildflower.

Caution!

Do not feed honey to children younger than 1 year old. The honey may contain bacterial spores that can cause infant botulism.

Storing Liquid and spun honey will keep for 1 year or more if stored in an airtight container at room temperature. Liquid honey may crystallize at colder temperatures; this is harmless. Comb honey will keep in a cool, dark cupboard for 6 months.

To reliquefy honey that has crystallized, remove the lid and set the jar in a pan of very hot water for 10 to 20 minutes, or microwave it in 30-second intervals, stirring after each one, until clear.

h

Herb

An Italian roast lacking rosemary, a Thai salad in need of cilantro, Scandinavian gravlax missing dill, Lebanese tabbouleh minus mint—without fresh and fragrant herbs, cuisines around the world would lose their heart and soul.

As immigrants share their traditional dishes and as travelers explore the tables of distant countries, cooks everywhere are discovering the power of herbs. Grocery stores now offer an ever-expanding selection of fresh herbs: alongside curly parsley appear bouquetlike bunches of delicate chervil, heady oregano, velvety sage, and perhaps three different varieties of thyme. Whether simmered in a simple broth, stirred into a sauce, or sprinkled over a fruit tart, fresh herbs enliven dishes with their perfume and infuse them with their distinct flavors. Although leafy and delicate herbs may lose significant flavor when dried, many other herbs, such as rosemary, dill, and thyme, dry well. Convenient to use and handy for last-minute inspirations, quality dried herbs are an important part of any kitchen's basic pantry. Since dried herbs have more concentrated flavors, use about one-fourth the amount of the dried form in place of fresh.

Herb or Spice? Although the two are used for similar purposes, herbs and spices actually refer to distinct categories of seasonings. Herbs are the fragrant leaves and tender stems of green plants, having an almost floral bouquet and more delicate flavors. Spices, on the other hand, generally come from woody plants, many of them native to the world's tropical regions. Most familiar in their dried forms, spices can be taken from the rhizomes, stems, buds, seeds, or bark of the plants, where concentrated amounts of their complex aromatic components result in significantly stronger flavors. Cinnamon, nutmeg, ginger, and clove all display the intense aromatic qualities of spices.

Selecting Choose fresh herbs that look bright, fragrant, and healthy. Avoid those that have wilted, yellowed, or blackened leaves or moldy stems. Herbs may be packaged in plastic bags or thin plastic containers, or simply gathered with rubber bands. Young, tender hothouse herbs make delicate garnishes but have less flavor than larger, hardier field-grown herbs. Although herbs with blossoms make attractive edible garnishes, leaves picked from plants without buds or flowers will have more flavor. When buying dried herbs, buy small amounts from a reputable specialty market that sells them in bulk with a high turnover or choose small glass jars containing large bright green flakes. A higher-priced brand usually ensures higher quality.

A Bouquet of Herbs

BASIL Traditionally used in kitchens throughout the Mediterranean and in Southeast Asia, basil is one of the world's best-loved herbs. Although related to mint, basil tastes faintly of anise and cloves. Italians use it in pesto, often pair it with tomatoes, and consider it essential to a classic minestrone. In Thailand and Vietnam, basil is often combined with fresh mint for seasoning stir-fries, curries, and, in the case of Vietnam, salads.

Quick Bite

More than 60 varieties of basil exist. Familiar green basil, also called sweet basil, has a mild anise flavor. Purple basil, also known as opal basil, has smaller leaves and tastes a little spicier than sweet basil. Lemon basil has a mild and pleasing citrus flavor.

BAY Elongated gray-green leaves used to flavor sauces, soups, stews, and braises, imparting a slightly sweet, citrusy, nutty flavor. Usually sold dried, bay leaves should be re-moved from a dish before serving, as they are leathery and can have sharp edges.

Quick Tip

Use fresh bay leaves as you would dried leaves, but add them with a light hand and ex-pect more flavor in the finished dish. Milder French bay (called laurel in Europe) can be used in greater quantities than California bay.

BORAGE Fresh or dried leaves that, when finely chopped, impart a light flavor remi-niscent of cucumber to vegetables, salads, soups, stews, and other dishes. Purple borage flowers may be used as a garnish.

CHERVIL A spring-time herb with a taste reminiscent of parsley and anise. It goes particularly well with poultry and seafood, with carrots, and in salads.

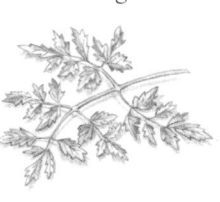

CHIVE These slender, bright green stems are used to give an onionlike flavor without the bite. The slender, hollow, grasslike leaves can be snipped with a pair of kitchen scissors to any length and scattered over scrambled eggs, stews, salads, soups, tomatoes, or any dish that would benefit from a boost of mild oniony flavor. Chives do not take well to long cooking—they lose flavor and crispness and turn a dull grayish green.

CILANTRO Also called fresh coriander and Chinese parsley, cilantro is a distinctly flavored herb with legions of loyal followers—and some emphatic detractors. Used extensively in the cuisines of Mexico, the Caribbean, India, Egypt, Thailand, Vietnam, and China, as well as in numerous others, cilantro asserts itself with a flavor that can't be missed. Some describe its taste as being citrusy or minty; others find hints of sage and parsley; others describe it as soapy. It is used fresh, as it loses flavor when dried. The herb is best added at the end of cook-ing; its flavor disappears during long expo-sure to heat.

Quick Tip

Cilantro and flat-leaf (Italian) parsley look somewhat similar and can be mistaken for each other. Check each bunch carefully. If in doubt, give it a sniff or taste a leaf.

DILL Fine, feathery leaves with a distinct aromatic flavor. Often used in savory pas-tries, baked vegetables, and, of course, in the making of pickles.

continued

h

Herb, continued

EPAZOTE A pungent herb, possibly indigenous to Mexico, that has no substitute for its unusual flavor. Although seldom available commercially outside Mexico or India, it is easily grown from seed and is self-sowing. It can be used dried, after the twigs are discarded, but its flavor is greatly diminished.

LAVENDER Highly perfumed blossoms, leaves, and stalks of a flowering plant that grows wild in southern France, where it is a signature seasoning. Use sparingly to season lamb or poultry, or infuse syrups for use in dessert making.

Quick Bite

Lavender is a signature ingredient in *herbes de Provence,* a traditional French herb blend that often also contains marjoram, rosemary, sage, and summer savory.

LEMON BALM A sweet, lemon-scented herb used with fresh fruit and in egg dishes, soups, and salads.

LEMON VERBENA A strongly lemon-scented herb, native to South America. Use sparingly, fresh or dried, to flavor fruit or custard desserts or herbal teas.

MARJORAM This Mediterranean herb, which has a milder flavor than its close relative oregano, is best used fresh. Pair it with tomatoes, eggplant, beans, poultry, and seafood.

MINT Refreshing herb available in many varieties, with spearmint the most common. Used fresh to flavor a broad range of savory preparations, including spring lamb, poultry, and vegetables, or to garnish desserts.

OREGANO Aromatic, pungent, and spicy herb, also known as wild marjoram, used fresh or dried as a seasoning for all kinds of savory dishes. Especially compatible with tomatoes and other vegetables.

PARSLEY Adds vibrant color and pleasing flavor to almost any savory dish. The two most popular varieties are curly-leaf parsley and flat-leaf, or Italian, parsley. Both have a refreshing and faintly peppery flavor, but flat-leaf parsley's flavor is stronger and more complex and is preferred in cooking. The hardier curly-leaf parsley garnishes many a dinner plate, and although not as flavorful, it can be substituted for the flat-leaf variety.

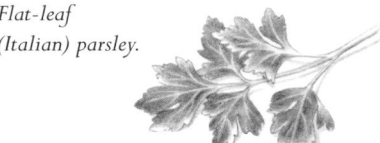

Flat-leaf (Italian) parsley.

ROSEMARY Used fresh or dried, this Mediterranean herb has a strong, fragrant flavor well suited to meats, poultry, seafood, and vegetables. It is a particularly good complement to chicken and lamb.

SAGE Soft, gray-green sage leaves are sweet and aromatic. Used fresh or dried, they pair well with poultry, vegetables, or fresh or cured pork.

SORREL Delicate, triangular leaves with a highly tart flavor. Lends bright, pleasantly sour flavor when puréed into soups and sauces.

SUMMER SAVORY More delicate than its cousin winter savory, summer savory has a scent reminiscent of thyme and a faintly bitter, almost minty flavor. Add in small amounts to stews, beans, and meat dishes or use to infuse vinegar.

TARRAGON With its distinctively sweet flavor that recalls anise, tarragon is used to season salads, egg and vegetable dishes, and fish and chicken dishes.

THYME One of the most important culinary herbs of Europe, thyme delivers a floral, earthy flavor to all types of food, including vegetables (especially roots and tubers) and poultry. One variety, lemon thyme, adds a subtle citrus note.

WINTER SAVORY This shrublike Mediterranean evergreen herb has a strong, spicy flavor that some cooks liken to thyme. It complements dried beans and lentils, meats, poultry, and tomatoes.

Storing Wrap in damp paper towels, then wrap in a plastic bag and refrigerate for 3 to 5 days. Take care with fragile herbs, such as chives and basil, for they bruise and discolor easily. To keep long-stemmed herbs, such as parsley, basil, and cilantro, for up to 10 days, trim off the ends of their stems, remove any yellowed leaves, and place the bunch in a container of water, like a bouquet of flowers. Drape a bag loosely upside down over the leaves, secure with a rubber band around the mouth of the jar, and refrigerate. Remove sprigs as needed. To prepare a large amount of herbs in advance with little loss of flavor, chop them up to 24 hours ahead. Then, place them in an airtight container, cover them with a damp paper towel, seal the lid, and store in the refrigerator.

Quick Tip

At many farmers' markets you can find herbs with roots still attached. Immersed in a glass of water, they will keep fresh for weeks.

Store dried herbs in airtight containers away from both light and heat. Buy in small amounts, replacing them after 4 to 6 months, as they fade in color, fragrance, and flavor. Although cork tops and prominently displayed racks add decorative touches to your kitchen, they only allow herbs to lose their flavor more quickly.

Quick Tip

Forgot about that bunch of thyme at the bottom of the vegetable bin? Herbs that are a little weary can be redeemed by a soaking in vinegar. Crush the herbs gently in a nonreactive container, pour in just enough warm vinegar to cover, and refrigerate overnight. Use in a flavorful vinaigrette or a cooked sauce.

continued

Herb, continued

Preparing Since fresh herbs can be sandy, rinse them well under cold running water, or dunk them gently in a bowl filled with water. Do not wash them until needed, however, to preserve their flavor and lengthen their storage life. To release their aromatic oils, crush dried herb flakes before using. Before searing or roasting meats, try to remove any herbs clinging to the surface of the meat, to prevent them from scorching.

As a general rule, fresh herbs are best added toward the end of cooking, for the better appreciation of their lighter flavors, which can dissipate rapidly. Dried herbs, more concentrated in flavor, are usually added earlier in the preparation of a dish, so that their aromas may permeate it and mingle with other ingredients. For more complex flavor, add herbs at two different points in cooking: dried at the beginning to intermingle with the other ingredients, and then fresh at the end of cooking to deliver a bright burst of flavor.

About Crushing Dried Herbs

Recipes using dried herbs often call for them to be crushed before adding to a dish. Crushing reduces the herbs to finer particles and helps release their aromatic oils, increasing the flavor they impart. To crush a small amount of herbs, place them in the palm of one hand and press down with the thumb of the other, twisting your thumb as you do so. Large quantities of herbs may also be crushed using a mortar and pestle.

Crushing dried herbs.

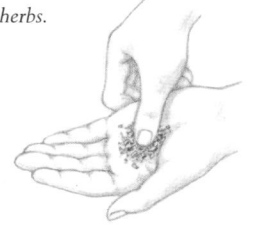

About Mincing Fresh Herbs

Begin with dry herbs; otherwise, they will stick to the knife. Rinse them far enough ahead of time for them to dry fully, or use a paper towel to pat them dry. Remove the leaves and discard the thick stems (or reserve for adding to the stockpot). Then, keeping fingers safely clear, chop the leaves with a good-sized chef's knife, holding down the knife tip with one hand so that it never leaves the cutting board and moving your chopping wrist and hand rhythmically. Gather the herb repeatedly into smaller and tighter clumps and chop until it is as fine as you want it. As a rule, herbs are finely chopped. A pair of scissors or a mezzaluna also comes in handy for mincing.

Chopping parsley tops.

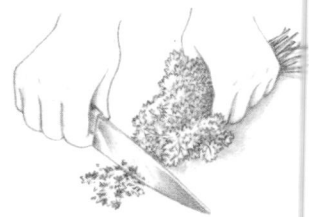

Mincing parsley.

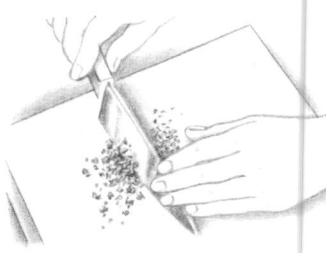

Quick Tip

A food processor minces large amounts of herbs quickly, but it also crushes and bruises them. Mince fresh herbs by hand if you have the time. See also MINCING.

See also BOUQUET GARNI.

HONEYDEW See MELON.

HORSERADISH A thick, gnarled root of a plant in the cabbage family that is native to Europe and Asia. The root has a refreshing, spicy bite that perks up everything from beef brisket to boiled beets. It is blended into sour cream to accompany smoked fish, into whipped cream to partner a rib roast, or into cocktail sauces to eat along with shellfish. It is available fresh but is more commonly used already grated, mixed with vinegar or beet juice, and packed in glass bottles labeled as prepared or commercial horseradish. It is also dried and sold as powder. Getting into the habit of using fresh horseradish pays off, for the flavor is purer and cleaner.

Selecting Fresh horseradish appears in markets from late fall to early spring. Look for firm roots free of wrinkles, soft spots, and mold. Prepared horseradish is available bottled in jars with white vinegar, but since some brands can be quite vinegary, a better

---

Quick Tip

Do not cook horseradish. While strong and biting when raw, the root is easily tamed by heat.

---

alternative is to reconstitute dried horseradish powder with water just before using—or at least try several brands and decide which you prefer. The horseradish packed in white vinegar is called white horseradish, while the horseradish packed in beet juice is called red horseradish.

Storing Keep the fresh root wrapped first in a paper bag or paper towels, then in a plastic bag. Store in the refrigerator for up to 3 weeks. The root freezes well and will grate easily into small flakes while frozen. Once opened, bottled horseradish should be refrigerated; it will keep for up to 4 months. Longer storage will not cause the horseradish to spoil, but it will lose its punch. Powdered horseradish may be stored in a cool place for up to 1 year.

Preparing Wash fresh horseradish roots, then peel. Trim away any green areas, for they will be unpleasantly bitter. Like parsnip, a large horseradish root will have a tough, fibrous core that should be removed and discarded. Horseradish quickly turns brown once cut. Prepare it just before serving, sprinkle it with a little lemon juice or vinegar to prevent discoloring, and use nonreactive containers.

HOT PEPPER See CHILE.

HUCKLEBERRY See BERRY.

HULL The dry outer covering of a fruit, seed, or nut. The term also refers to the leafy base where a stem connects to a fruit, as in a strawberry. Generally, both types of hulls are removed from food, either during processing or by the cook.

HUSK The dry papery sheath found on certain vegetables and fruits, the best known example of which is the corn husk. In Mexico—and wherever Mexican food is served—dried corn husks are used as wrappers for the ubiquitous tamale. Another common husk-covered market item is the tomatillo, a sour, green tomato-like vegetable that is a popular base for salsas.

h

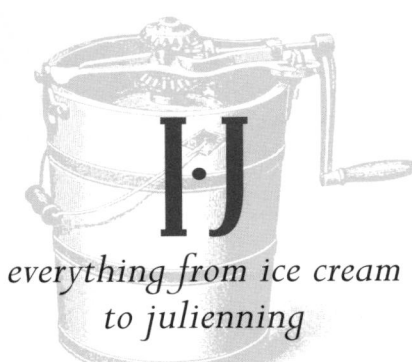

I·J

everything from ice cream to julienning

i·j

ICE See SORBET.

ICE CREAM See page 252.

ICED TEA See TEA.

ICING See FROSTING, ICING & GLAZE.

INDIRECT HEAT See GRILLING.

ITALIAN BEAN Another name for romano bean; see BEAN, FRESH.

ITALIAN BROCCOLI See BROCCOLI RABE.

JALAPEÑO See CHILE.

JAM & JELLY Most of us use these two terms interchangeably, and if pressed to explain the difference between them, we are likely to struggle. In truth, the distinction is quite simple. While both are sweet preserves (so called because added sugar slows spoilage), usually of fruit but sometimes of vegetable-fruits such as chiles or herbs such as mint, jams contain the edible portion of the fruit in its entirety and are therefore chunky, while jellies have been

strained to achieve a perfectly smooth consistency and often a crystalline clarity. In certain recipes, your choice can make a significant difference. Jams, for example, may serve as a simple filling for tartlets, having sufficient body to partner a crisp pastry shell. Jellies, by contrast, are sometimes employed as a glaze for sweets such as pastries or even for cooked meats: they are melted (sometimes with a little liqueur) and then spooned over the food.

JARLSBERG See CHEESE.

JELL To become firm or gelatinous, especially from a mostly liquid state. Jelling is usually a controlled process, using ingredients such as gelatin, pectin, or sugar to thicken food or to form it into specific shapes. It can also refer to protein-rich stocks or sauces that naturally jell as they cool. See also GELATIN; PECTIN.

JELLY See JAM & JELLY.

JELLY-ROLL PAN See BAKEWARE.

JERUSALEM ARTICHOKE Not from Jerusalem and not an artichoke, this delicate vegetable owes its name to the Italian word for sunflower, *girasole*—although admittedly it is a leap from there to *Jerusalem artichoke*. Also known as sunchokes, these are the small tubers of a sunflower plant native to North America. Knobby and beige skinned, they resemble fresh ginger in appearance. Their crisp, ivory flesh has a sweet, slightly nutty flavor that is delicious raw, thinly sliced in salads, as well as steamed, sautéed, or baked.

Selecting Look for Jerusalem artichokes that are small and firm, with smooth, unblemished skin. As with potatoes, do not buy them if they have sprouts or a green tinge. They are in season from midautumn through early spring and are at their best when harvested a few weeks after a frost.

Storing Jerusalem artichokes will keep at room temperature for 4 days. Or wrap first in a paper bag or paper towels, then in a plastic bag, and store in the vegetable bin of the refrigerator for up to 2 weeks.

Quick Tip

To prevent discoloring, avoid cooking Jerusalem artichokes in reactive pans made of aluminum or cast iron.

Preparing Wash Jerusalem artichokes well, scrubbing gently to remove dirt and grit. They will darken when cut and exposed to air. Sprinkle pieces with lemon juice to prevent discoloring. The tubers also bruise easily, so handle them with care. They do not need to be peeled, but their thin skin peels off easily after cooking.

JICAMA (HICK-uh-muh) A large, round tuber shaped like a turnip with golden beige skin and crisp, juicy, sweet white flesh. Jicama is also known as yam bean, and for good reason: like beans, it is a member of the legume family. It is eaten both fresh and cooked in Mexico, the American Southwest, and throughout Asia. Jicama is at its best raw or very briefly cooked, but you can also steam, fry, roast, or boil and purée it much like potatoes. It pairs especially well with citrus fruits and chiles. Peel a jicama's thick skin before using. Cut it into thin, wedge-shaped slices and toss with olive oil, fresh lime juice, and a pinch of chili powder for a healthy snack or a refreshing accompaniment to Mexican

dishes. Because it does not discolor, jicama is perfect for crudité platters, coleslaws, hors d'oeuvres, and both green and fruit salads. Its crunchy texture makes it a convenient substitute for water chestnuts in stir-fries.

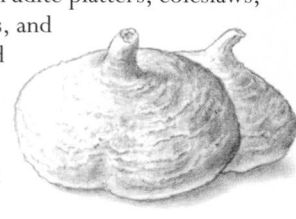

Selecting Choose a jicama that is firm and heavy for its size. Jicamas arrive at market in a range of sizes, from a convenient ½ pound to a rather unwieldy 5 or 6 pounds. Buy the size you need; girth does not indicate toughness or starchiness, although the thickness of the skin does. The skin should be thin and smooth, with no cracks or soft spots. Scratch the skin to check that it is thin and the flesh is juicy. The tuber is widely available year-round but is at its best from late fall to late spring.

Storing You can leave an uncut jicama at room temperature for 2 to 3 days. It will keep for up to 3 weeks in the refrigerator if stored unwrapped in the vegetable bin. Once cut, wrap the unused portion with plastic wrap and refrigerate for up to 1 week longer. To keep peeled, cut pieces fresh, cover them with water and refrigerate for no longer than 4 days.

HOW TO *Peel Jicama*

Cut a large jicama in half if you do not plan to use all of it.

1. If needed, cut it into manageable wedges.
2. With a sharp paring knife, trim both the stem and root ends.
3. Cut and lift up a small piece of the peel near the stem end, then tear a wide strip of the peel down. Repeat in segments with the remaining peel. The skin is too tenacious to be removed with a vegetable peeler.
4. If the jicama has another tough layer beneath the peel, repeat step 3 to remove it as well.

i·j

Ice Cream

Ancient Romans carried snow down from the Alps to fashion some of the earliest ice creams, and the Chinese reportedly were serving flavored ices as early as 1100 B.C.

The Turks were busy, too, whipping up fruit ices and fruit drinks, concoctions that some historians believe are the forerunners of today's sherbet. Italians invented the first machine-made ices, however, and perfected commercial freezing. Once enjoyed only by the wealthy, who could afford the pricey transport of ice and snow, ice cream is now enjoyed by all, young and old alike, in winter and summer.

Ingredients Ice cream has several essential ingredients or components, and each plays a carefully balanced role. Fat from cream and milk imparts richness, smoothness, and flavor. Too much fat, however, will cause the mixture to curdle and form small lumps.

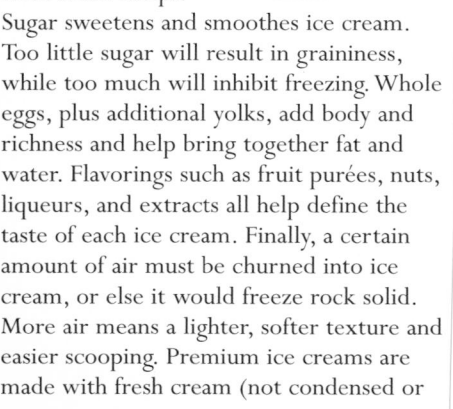

Sugar sweetens and smoothes ice cream. Too little sugar will result in graininess, while too much will inhibit freezing. Whole eggs, plus additional yolks, add body and richness and help bring together fat and water. Flavorings such as fruit purées, nuts, liqueurs, and extracts all help define the taste of each ice cream. Finally, a certain amount of air must be churned into ice cream, or else it would freeze rock solid. More air means a lighter, softer texture and easier scooping. Premium ice creams are made with fresh cream (not condensed or powdered milk), real eggs, and natural flavorings. They have very little air added.

Other Frozen Treats

FROZEN YOGURT Made from either low-fat or nonfat yogurt, along with skim milk or a mixture of milk and cream. Although the amount of fat in frozen yogurt can vary widely, in general it tends to have lower amounts than ice cream. Stabilizers take the place of most of the fat.

GELATO Contains only a minimal amount of air that is incorporated naturally in the mixing process. Gelato (and some premium ice cream) is so dense that it requires a slightly lower serving temperature, a perfect point at which the scoop is firm but not hard, yet not so soft that it melts immediately. Recipes usually include more egg yolks, more milk, and less cream than regular ice cream. In the end, gelato actually has less fat than its more conventional kin. Its low percentage of air, however, makes for an extremely creamy treat.

GRANITA A grainy-textured ice made by continued scraping and refrigerating of the mixture. See SORBET.

ICE Similar to a sorbet. A frozen mixture of ice and liquid, typically coffee, fruit juice, wine, or an herbal infusion. See SORBET.

ICE MILK With less fat than ice cream, ice milk tends to have a lighter texture.

SHERBET Made with fruit or fruit juice and (in some places) a small amount of milk. Sherbets tend to be coarser in texture than ice cream, with a slightly tarter flavor. See SORBET.

SORBET Contains no milk, cream, or eggs, only ice, sweeteners, and flavoring such as fresh fruit. See SORBET.

Equipment There are two basic kinds of ice-cream makers. A hand-operated maker consists of a hand-cranked bucket with a smaller canister inside and a dasher, or stirrer. A combination of ice and rock salt fills the gap between the bucket and the canister to chill down the ice-cream base. A popular variation involves a canister filled with liquid coolant that does not require ice; the liquid-gel canister simply needs to prefreeze for at least 1 day. Electric ice cream makers all have motors but range from wooden buckets that still require ice to large, imported gelato churners with self-contained refrigeration that make rich gelato with the touch of a button.

Homemade Ice Cream Savvy For best results when making homemade ice cream, follow these guidelines:

- If making a custard-based ice cream, cook the base gently in a double boiler to prevent scorching. Straining will remove all lumps.
- Be sure to refrigerate the base overnight, or for at least 4 hours. This helps bring together the flavors and prevents ice crystals from forming as the ice cream is churned, improving the final texture. Also, if you're using a machine that requires ice, less ice will be required later to cool the base and thus churning time will be reduced.
- Expect the base to taste sweeter than you would like the finished ice cream to. Food tastes less sweet when it is cold.
- Do not use only heavy cream if you want fine texture. The ice cream will be quite dense. Add condensed milk or half-and-half to lighten the consistency.
- If using a machine that requires ice, crushing ice increases its surface area. The cold will transfer more efficiently to the ice cream base.

- If using a machine that requires salted ice, use coarse salt, not table salt, since it dissolves more slowly.
- Continuous stirring, especially once the base begins to thicken, will decrease the size the of ice crystals that form and result in a smoother ice cream.
- Ice cream can be served immediately from the ice cream freezer while still somewhat soft, not unlike a frozen custard or fast-food soft-serve products. Or it can be transferred to your refrigerator freezer to set and harden for at least 3 hours before serving for a more familiar thick, solid consistency.
- Add fruit after freezing but before hardening. Or stir it in just before serving the ice cream.
- Berries can be used raw, but fruits such as peaches, pears, and plums should be poached in syrup for better flavor and texture. Poaching fruits such as kiwifruit and pineapple will also deactivate enzymes in them that would break down the ice cream.
- Be careful when adding alcohol to ice cream, since it lowers the freezing point. Too much alcohol will prevent ice cream from setting properly.
- Rinse salt well from all parts of the ice cream maker to prevent corrosion.

Ice Cream Blues Got a problem with your homemade ice cream? Find the simple explanation here.

MY HOMEMADE ICE CREAM IS LUMPY. The base was not strained, the egg coagulated; the base was not stirred evenly; or the paddle didn't scrape the sides of the canister enough to incorporate all the ingredients.

MY HOMEMADE ICE CREAM IS GRAINY. Too much water or alcohol in the base; not enough fat or sugar in the base; the cream curdled from too high of a fat content or from the base's being too acidic; the base churned too slowly; or the container was overfilled.

JUICING Various gadgets have been designed for juicing, from a handheld wooden reamer for squeezing out some lemon juice to large machines for extracting a drink from the hardest beet. The simple, classic citrus juicer resembles a shallow bowl with a deeply fluted, inverted cone that fits into a citrus half and a spout for pouring freshly squeezed orange or grapefruit juice into breakfast glasses. Fancier versions may include a mechanized cone or a perforated base for catching seeds and pulp.

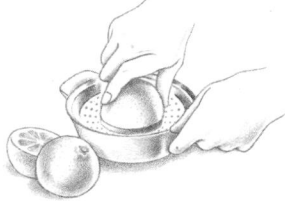

Juicing citrus with a reamer.

Tall, mechanical presses have a small, domed compartment for holding citrus halves. Press down on the lever, and juice drains into a cup set below. If you're ready to move on to carrot juice, then you'll need a big, heavy juice extractor. These machines grind and then separate the juice from the pulp, seeds, and peels of denser fruits and vegetables.

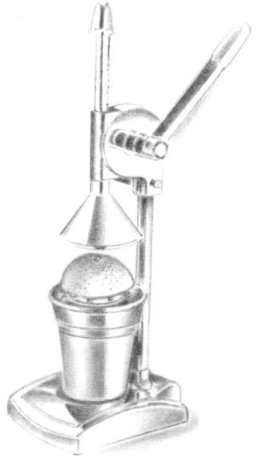

Mechanical citrus press.

JULIENNING Refers to cutting food into long, thin strips, which in turn are called a "julienne." Vegetables are most commonly julienned, although meats and cheeses may be prepared this way, too.

HOW TO *Julienne*

1. Cut the vegetable, here a carrot, into pieces the length of the desired julienne strips.

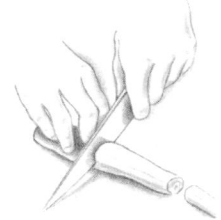

2. Cut each piece lengthwise into slices as thick as the desired julienne.

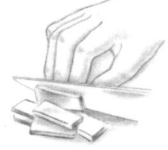

3. Stack the slices and cut them lengthwise into the julienne.

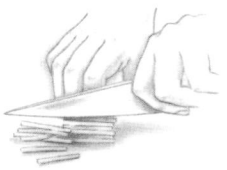

Alternatively, you can use a mandoline or the julienne-cutting disk of a food processor, especially for large quantities.

Quick Tip

To julienne basil or other leaves, stack several together, roll up lengthwise into a compact bundle, and thinly slice crosswise. These thin ribbons are also called a chiffonade.

JUNIPER BERRY See SPICE.

K

*everything from kabob
to kumquat*

Quick Tip

Thread shrimp to be grilled on 2 parallel soaked wooden skewers to keep the shrimp from twisting.

KABOB The term *kabob* comes from the Turkish *siskebabi,* or "spit-roasted meat." On streets throughout the Middle East, vendors sit by narrow metal braziers, fanning charcoal and tending to a multitude of skewers. In recipes that date back to ancient Greece, chunks of lamb absorb flavor from a mixture of olive oil, lemon juice, and herbs such as oregano, cumin, or rosemary. The marinated meat is threaded onto skewers, grilled, and then tucked into warm pita bread along with salad and pickles to make tasty sandwiches. At a Middle Eastern kabob house, the meat might be drizzled

Quick Tip

When grilling lamb kabobs, consider using twigs or branches of rosemary as fragrant skewers. Select sturdy, straight twigs at least 6 inches long. Strip off all leaves except for a tuft at one end. Use a kitchen knife to trim the other end into a point that can pierce the lamb cubes.

with paprika oil and served over broken pita with tomato and yogurt sauces.

While lamb is the traditional kabob meat, beef, veal, fish, chicken, vegetables,

and even tofu also appear on skewers. If you prepare kabobs at home, remember always to leave a little space between the pieces to allow for flavorful browning. If packed together too tightly, the pieces will steam and cook unevenly. Flat, metal skewers hold chunks of food more securely in place and also conduct heat to aid in quick and even cooking. Some cooks like to serve kabobs that combine meat and vegetables. This can be done one of two ways: by either threading them together on the same skewer or slipping them onto separate skewers. The former method creates a wonderful exchange of flavors and textures, while the latter better allows for different cooking times and guarantees that the meat browns well. See also GRILLING.

Chicken and mushroom kabobs.

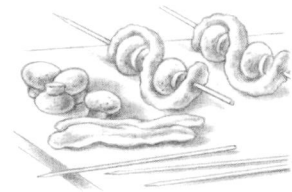

KAFFIR LIME A large, slightly pear-shaped citrus fruit grown throughout Southeast Asia, with a thick, bumpy, yellow-green peel and distinctive double leaves attached in pairs, end to end. The lime's juice is rarely used in the kitchen, but its highly aromatic peel and leaves add a fresh, tart flavor and flowery perfume to soups, curries, and grilled fish. The kaffir lime is traditionally used in the cuisines of cooks in Indonesia and Thailand.

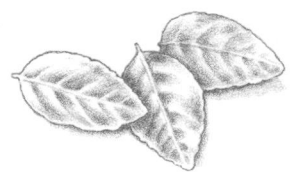

*Kaffir
lime leaves.*

Selecting You may find the fresh fruits
or their leaves in a Southeast Asian market,
but more common are frozen leaves and
dried or powdered peel. Look in the freezer
section for the leaves, packaged in small
plastic bags. They are also available dried,
like bay leaves. Dried peel, sold in small
bags, offers more flavor than powdered.
Storing Keep the frozen leaves wrapped
tightly in freezer-weight plastic in the
freezer for up to 1 year and use as needed.
The dried peel will keep for 3 to 4 years
and the dried leaves for up to 1 year if
sealed in an airtight container and kept
away from heat and light.
Preparing When adding the leaves to
a curry, sauce, or soup, partially tear the
fresh and frozen leaves lengthwise to release more of their flavor. Or cut a fresh or
frozen leaf crosswise into very thin strips
to sprinkle over stir-fries, salads, or grilled
fish or chicken. If using dried peel, soak it
briefly in warm water first and then mash
it before using.

KALE See GREENS, DARK.

KAMUT See GRAIN.

KASHA See GRAIN.

KETTLE See COOKWARE.

KIDNEY BEAN See BEAN, DRIED.

KIWIFRUIT A relatively recent import
from New Zealand, kiwifruit was once
called the Chinese gooseberry. The small,
egg-shaped fruit has a distinctive fuzzy
brown peel and lime green flesh with a
sunburst pattern of tiny black seeds. Early
on, kiwifruit's bright color, unique sweet-
tart flavor, and exotic pedigree
made it the darling
of restaurant
chefs. After
appearing for
years as garnishes
on dramatic nouvelle
cuisine plates, kiwifruits have now joined
apples, bananas, and oranges as standard
fare in fruit bowls and salads. They can also
be puréed and used as a sauce for desserts
or frozen in a sorbet.
Selecting Choose fruits heavy for their
size and free of bruises. Like peaches, kiwifruits are ready for eating when they give
to gentle pressure. Handle them with care,
for they bruise easily. They are widely available year-round. California's crop peaks
from winter to spring, while the New
Zealand fruits appear in our markets in
summer and fall.

Quick Tip

Kiwifruit contains the same powerful tenderizing enzymes as papaya. Rub or marinate
meats with kiwifruit before grilling or roasting.

Storing Leave kiwifruits at room temperature until they soften. Accelerate the
ripening by enclosing the fruits in a paper
bag with an apple or a banana. Once ripe,
keep kiwifruits in a plastic bag in the refrigerator for up to 1 week.
Preparing Peel off the fuzzy skin with a
vegetable peeler, using a gentle sawing motion. Or, if the fruit is soft and ripe, simply
cut it in half and scoop out the flesh in one
piece with a spoon. Slice a kiwifruit crosswise to highlight the pattern of its seeds.

k

KNEADING Folding and pressing dough repeatedly, to develop the structure of bread and other baked goods. During kneading, the gluten in flour interlocks to create an elastic network that captures gases and stretches as the bread rises. The rhythmic, tactile nature of kneading accounts for much of the meditative mystique of bread baking.

HOW TO *Knead by Hand*

A bread dough may require 5 to 20 minutes of kneading, with most taking about 10 minutes. (Scones and biscuits should be kneaded only 5 to 10 turns.)

1. Gather the dough in a ball and place it on a hard, stationary work surface that has been lightly dusted with flour.
2. Flour your hands to prevent sticking. Push firmly into the center of the dough with the heel of your hand.

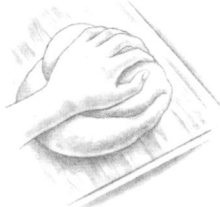

3. With your other hand, fold the dough in half toward you, and then rotate it a quarter turn.

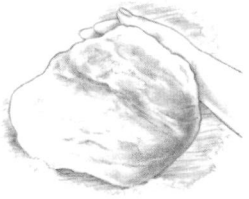

4. Repeat, adding more flour as necessary to keep it from sticking and working it into the dough as you knead. Do not add more flour than necessary, using any measurements in the recipe as a guide. Continue until the dough is smooth and elastic, or as directed in the recipe.

Kneading Savvy

- Many bakers prefer kneading on a wood surface; it holds in warmth and creates a hospitable environment for the yeast.
- Use a dough scraper to gather and turn a particularly soft, moist dough.
- Some doughs such as brioche or rye breads are slightly sticky. To knead these, lightly coat your hands or the machine kneading attachments with oil.
- If you end up adding too much flour during kneading, sprinkle the dough lightly with warm water and continue kneading until the dough is soft again.
- Scrape off and discard any dried bits of flour that stick to your palm. If incorporated back into the dough, they will bake into hard, pebblelike lumps.
- Some recipes call for adding more flour during the kneading process. If a recipe calls for a range of flour amounts, mix the dough first with the smaller measure and then slowly incorporate more while you continue to knead. The dough should remain soft enough to work but not be wet or too sticky.
- A good test to determine if you have kneaded long enough is to push your fingertips into the dough. If the indentation springs back, the dough has been kneaded sufficiently. The dough should also have a satiny surface.
- To take a break, cover the dough and leave it for 5 to 10 minutes.

Many bakers are happy to let a machine knead the dough. Food processors come with a plastic kneading blade, and heavy-duty stand mixers have dough hooks. When using either, keep an eye on the dough. While it is almost impossible to overknead a bread dough by hand, it can happen easily in a machine. An overkneaded dough will suddenly turn gooey and inelastic.

See also BREAD; FLOUR.

k

KNIFE No good cook can accomplish much without this most fundamental and versatile of tools. With a well-made, keenly sharpened kitchen blade of the right size and shape, you can easily and efficiently do everything from paring a few small fruits for a salad or garnish to cutting enough for a big batch of jam, from removing bones from a single chicken breast to carving and serving a large holiday roast for a dozen family members.

Basic kitchen knives.

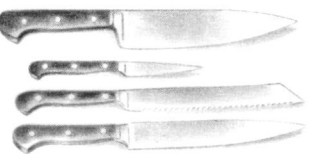

Knife Materials The sharpness of the knife is the secret to efficient, safe cutting. A dull blade cuts reluctantly, leading to excessive force, possible slippage, and a threat of injury. Knives with blades made of carbon steel, which could be honed to razor sharpness, were once the sharpest available; harder stainless steel simply could not hold an edge as well. That, however, is no longer the case, as today's best knives are made of carbon–stainless steel alloys that combine the best of both metals. They sharpen well and are easy to maintain, yet offer stainless steel's resistance to rusting or pitting from humidity or acidic ingredients.

For secure, durable construction and good balance, look for knives with full tangs—that is, those in which the metal of the blade visibly extends through the entire length of the handle. Most knife handles are made of wood, resin-impregnated wood, plastic, or rubber. Whatever the material, they should be securely attached to the tang, usually with visible metal rivets. In addition, the entire knife should feel well balanced in your hand.

Knives are sold in a wide variety of shapes and sizes, both individually and in sets that might include a sharpening steel and a knife block as well.

HOW TO *Use a Knife*

1. The knife handle should feel comfortable and secure in your grip.

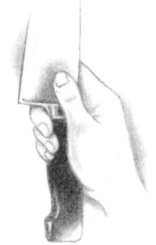

2. Hold the food to be cut with your fingertips curled away from the knife blade.

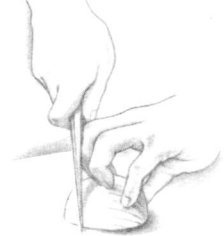

Knife Storage and Maintenance Knives should never be stored loose in kitchen drawers or in receptacles with other utensils. Such practices can result in injuries or a dull or nicked blade. Always store your knives in a knife block, rack, or

Quick Tip

Some experienced cooks say that all they need in their kitchens are a chef's knife and a paring knife. Start with the best-quality examples of those you can find that fit your budget and feel good to you. Add others from the list as dictated by your cooking habits and by the kinds of foods you like to prepare.

special drawer insert containing slots for blades, or on a magnetic bar mounted somewhere safely away from casual reach.

To safeguard the edges of your blades, always work on a resilient surface made of wood or soft plastic, avoiding hard or slick surfaces. Never use the blade for scraping.

Wash knives individually and carefully by hand with hot, soapy water, drying them immediately. Never immerse them in a sinkful of water. Prolonged soaking can loosen handles, and the knives could also accidentally be picked up by their sharp blades. Do not clean them in dishwashers, which can dull the blade.

Before you put a knife away after use, it's a good idea to sharpen it briefly. The best home tool to use is a sharpening steel, available wherever good-quality knives are sold. Swipe each side of the cutting edge a few times across and along the length of the steel, alternating sides and holding the blade at about a 15-degree angle to the long metal rod. This process will realign the sharp cutting edge.

When your knives seem to be cutting at anything less than their best, and your sharpening efforts no longer seem to have an effect, check with the shop where you bought them or with a local butcher shop or food-store meat department. The personnel should be able to hone the blades to keen new edges or recommend a professional who can do it at a reasonable cost.

⌁⟋ Basic Knife Styles ⟋⌁

CHEF'S KNIFE A larger, evenly proportioned, tapered blade, of which the most useful usually averages 8 inches long. Most often used for chopping as well as for slicing, dicing, julienning, or mincing of ingredients.

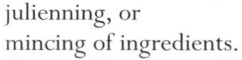

PARING KNIFE A small, evenly proportioned, tapered blade usually 3 to 4 inches long. Used for paring and slicing fruits and vegetables and for chopping small quantities.

BREAD KNIFE A straight, serrated blade at least 8 inches long. The serrated edge cuts easily through the tough crusts of breads or through the delicate skins of tomatoes that might otherwise be crushed by an ordinary knife.

CARVING KNIFE A long, sturdy blade for slicing through and serving roasted meats such as beef or ham.

SLICING KNIFE A long, slender, fairly flexible blade, well adapted to carving roast poultry and whole fish.

UTILITY KNIFE Similar to a paring knife but slightly larger, with a blade 6 to 8 inches long. Used for peeling and slicing or for carving small cuts of meat.

BONING KNIFE About the length of a utility knife, this tool has a very narrow, curve-edged blade that maneuvers more easily around the bones of raw poultry or meat.

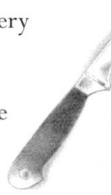

KOSHER Derived from *kashruth,* Hebrew for "proper" or "fit," *kosher* refers to food that accords with the strict dietary laws of Judaism. The laws originate from the Bible but have been expounded and refined by rabbinic legislation into a complex code on preparing and eating food.

Diverse Jewish communities have creatively adapted their local cuisines to the dietary laws, but the same basic tenets are followed throughout the world. Most of the guidelines concern meat, fish, and dairy, since all fruits, vegetables, and grains in their natural state are pareve, or neutral.

An Overview of Kosher Laws

MEAT An animal used for meat must both chew its cud and have split hooves. Beef, veal, lamb, and goat are kosher, but pork is not. Wild game is not kosher. Animals must be slaughtered quickly and painlessly. In kosher slaughtering, a specially trained butcher uses a sharp knife to kill the animal in a single stroke without stunning or maiming it. Afterward, the meat must be drained of all blood by salting. Because nerves and lobes of fat are also forbidden, large cuts of beef, veal, and lamb require the complete removal of these tissues.

NO MEAT WITH DAIRY The Bible's prohibition against boiling a calf in its mother's milk, out of respect for life and death, led to an absolute division between meat and dairy ingredients. The two cannot be mixed together in the same dish or even served within the same meal. The utensils, equipment, and dishware used to prepare and serve meat and dairy dishes must also be kept completely separate from each other. In addition, cheese cannot contain the coagulating agent rennet, an enzyme derived from an animal's stomach.

POULTRY Wild game birds, such as pheasants, are forbidden. Like meat, poultry must be slaughtered and prepared according to kosher law. It cannot mix with dairy.

FISH Only fish with fins and scales are allowed. Thus all shellfish such as shrimp, lobster, and squid are not kosher. Fish does not require special preparation, and some followers consider it neutral, meaning it can be served with meat or dairy.

WINE Because of their importance in the Sabbath meal, all wines, including brandies and other grape products, require strict rabbinic supervision during preparation.

KUGELHOPF PAN See BAKEWARE.

KUMQUAT

No other member of the citrus fruit family may be popped into the mouth whole and chewed up, peel, seeds, and all. Resembling a miniature orange and measuring little more than 1½ inches long, this Asian native takes its name from the Chinese *kam kwat,* meaning "gold-orange." Two main species exist: the oval kumquat (*Fortunella margarita*) and the round kumquat (*F. japonica*). The tender peel is sweet and contrasts pleasantly with the slightly tart, juicy pulp within.

Selecting Choose kumquats that are firm and free of blemishes. Avoid fruit with wrinkled or dull skin. Available from November to June, kumquats are at their peak during the winter months.

Preparing In addition to being eaten whole (be sure to remove any stems first), kumquats are canned, candied, preserved in brandy, cooked in syrup, and used in jams, marmalades, and pickles. Try dipping fresh kumquats in chocolate, or slice them crosswise as a decoration for cakes, pastries, or other desserts.

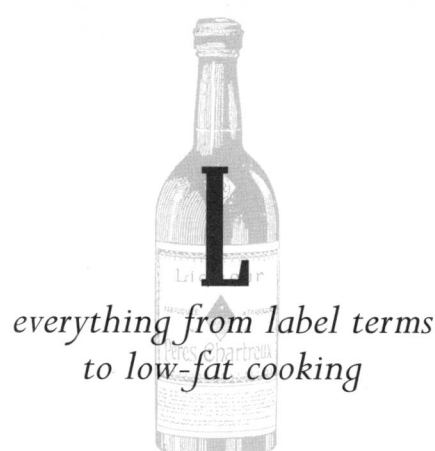

everything from label terms to low-fat cooking

LABEL TERMS Mouthwatering photographs, colorful logos, and catchy names help push foods off grocery-store shelves and into our shopping carts. A stroll down any aisle will also uncover those food-company phrases designed to seduce increasingly health-conscious shoppers: "low fat," "fat free," "low sodium," "low cholesterol." To protect consumers and to standardize labels, the Food and Drug Administration (FDA) has strictly defined an entire vocabulary of health claims. The FDA has also staked out precious space on food packaging to provide accurate, easy-to-read information on the nutritional content of processed foods.

Nutrition Labeling Since the Nutrition Labeling and Education Act of 1990, most processed and prepackaged foods in the United States must display nutrient information. The Nutrition Facts panel, in a standard format, is now a familiar sight on the back of most bags, boxes, bottles, and cans in a grocery store.

All foods that have more than one ingredient must declare a complete list of ingredients, presented in descending order of their amount in the food. In addition to using consistent serving sizes, package labels must clearly state the amount of total calories, calories from fat, total fat, saturated fat, cholesterol, sodium, total carbohydrates, dietary fiber, sugars, protein, vitamin A, vitamin C, calcium, and iron. A second column of numbers, the Percent Daily Values, shows how the food's nutritional content compares to the National Academy of Science's recommended daily allowances (RDA). These guidelines suggest minimum quantities of certain nutrients that are necessary to good health, such as vitamins and minerals. It also suggests maximum amounts of nutrients that may be detrimental to one's health in large quantities, such as fat, cholesterol, and sodium.

What's in a Word? The FDA has strict definitions of certain descriptions that are commonly used on food labels.

FREE Used in conjunction with fat, saturated fat, cholesterol, sodium, sugars, or calories, indicates that the food contains none at all or only a "physiologically inconsequential" amount of the component.

LOW Regulated, along with "little," "few," and "low source of." Foods labeled "low" in any particular component can contain, per serving, no more than a designated amount of that component.

    Low Fat: 3 g fat
    Low Saturated Fat: 1 g saturated fat
    Low Sodium: 140 mg sodium
    Very Low Sodium: 35 mg sodium
    Low Cholesterol: 20 mg fat, with 2 g
      of saturated fat
    Low Calorie: 40 calories

LEAN Indicates meat, poultry, and seafood with less than 10 g fat, 4.5 g saturated fat, and 95 mg cholesterol per serving.

EXTRA LEAN Indicates meat, poultry, and seafood with less than 5 g fat, 2 g saturated fat, and 95 mg cholesterol per serving.

LIGHT Designates a food that contains two-thirds of the calories or half of the fat contained in the regular version of the

1

food. However, it can also describe the color or texture of a food, not just its caloric or fat content.

FRESH Used for preservative-free foods that have never been heated or frozen.

Freshness Dating Milk and other dairy products have long been date-stamped, but now cereal, soda, beer, even batteries and film boast freshness dates. The sell-by date on food packaging indicates when the food is past its prime. Stores will pull a product from its shelves by the sell-by date. This does not mean the food has spoiled, but since there are no standards for freshness coding, the exact number of days the food can still be eaten varies. Milk tends to last no longer than 5 days after the sell-by date, while eggs can be good a month later. "Best if used by" recommends the last day for preparing or serving the food; it does not refer to selling or safety. In general, avoid buying food on or near its freshness date if you will not be using all of it immediately.

Some egg packers in the United States stamp cartons with a "Julian date," so-called for the Roman name of the calendar we all use, on the day they are packed. These dates begin with number 1 on January 1 and end with 365 on December 31. The eggs can be stored for up to 5 weeks beyond this date. It may take a little calculating to decipher the Julian date, but it's worth examining the carton for it.

LADLE See COOKING TOOLS.

LAMB Mild and tender lamb, the meat of a young sheep, is a far cry from the tough, gamy flesh of adult sheep, or mutton. Today, nothing helps define an upscale restaurant menu like a rack of lamb; and as kabobs, *tagine,* and *korma* enter our national lexicon, lamb is finding a new following in places far from the rugged terrain trod by the shepherds who originally dined on such dishes.

The lamb sold in supermarkets and at butcher shops is graded "prime" or "choice," United States Department of Agriculture (USDA) grades indicating quality and tenderness. For special occasions, splurge for the superior marbling (intermuscular fat that gives meat delicious flavor, tenderness, and juiciness) of prime meat. Spring lamb, sometimes called genuine lamb or simply lamb, specifies, by USDA regulation, a lamb less than a year old. The term once referred to the much-anticipated young, tender meat of the early season, but year-round production has largely diluted the term's significance. Most of the lamb that comes to market now is between 5 and 7 months old, thereby falling into the category of spring lamb. Baby lamb is 6 to 10 weeks old, and milk-fed or hothouse lambs drink a strict diet of milk only. Both have delicate flesh that cooks to a nearly white color. Lamb raised in the United States tends to be larger, meatier, and milder in flavor than lamb from Australia and New Zealand.

One-year-old, or yearling, lamb has darker, gamier flesh. Two-year-old mutton has an especially assertive flavor. Although many Europeans prefer the older, more flavorful mutton, it is nearly impossible to find in the United States and is increasingly difficult to locate even in Europe.

Selecting Fresh, young lamb will have rosy, fine-grained flesh and firm, white fat. Avoid cuts with yellowed fat. When buying trimmed racks, look for slender, pale bones.

Storing Store fresh lamb in the refrigerator for 2 to 3 days. Use ground lamb within 1 day of purchase. If sealed in heavy-duty plastic or placed in a zippered plastic freezer bag, lamb will keep in the freezer for 4 to 6 months. Do not freeze ground lamb or cooked lamb dishes for more than 3 months. Thaw frozen meat and cooked dishes slowly in the refrigerator.

~ Lamb Glossary ~

Lamb cuts.

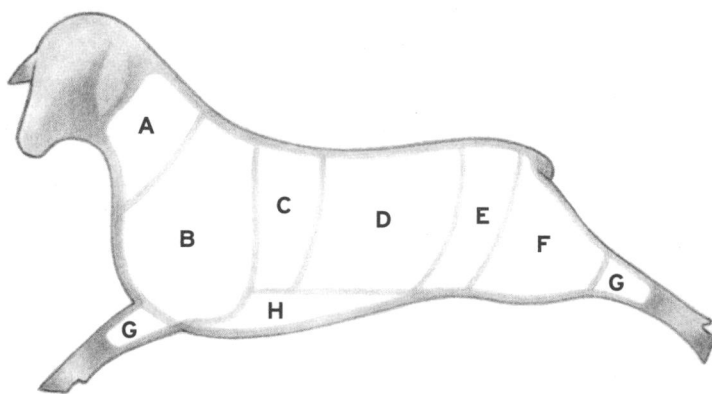

L amb destined for the market is divided into large primal, or wholesale, cuts that butchers divide into smaller cuts, individual portions for cooking and serving. Understanding the recommended cooking techniques for primal cuts will help you decide what to buy for dinner.

NECK (A) Meat from the neck section, rich in flavor but tough, is most commonly sold as ground lamb for lamb burgers and casseroles.

SHOULDER (B) This large cut contains firm, flavorful meat streaked with a moderate amount of fat. It yields shoulder chops for grilling or broiling; cubes of stewing meat for braising and kabob meat for grilling; ground lamb; and convenient rolled boned roasts for roasting or braising.

RIB (C) With its tender, rich meat, the rib section is one of the better sections of the lamb. It yields rib chops for sautéing, broiling, or grilling, as well as the whole roast composed of the chops left intact, known as rack of lamb or, when formed into a circle, a crown roast. For

the best flavor, use high heat to roast, broil, or grill racks of lamb just until they are done medium-rare or medium.

Rib chop.

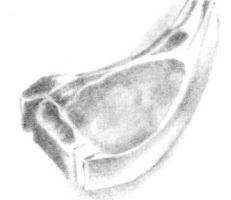

Rack of lamb.

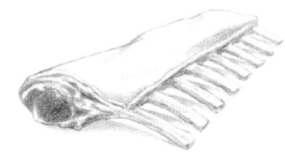

LOIN AND FLANK (D) Little-used muscles in the loin make for some of the most tender cuts of lamb. The loin is the source of compact tenderloin and loin chops, best broiled, grilled, or sautéed, as well as whole loin roasts, often boned and tied. Tough but flavorful flank meat is most often sold ground.

continued

⁓ Lamb Glossary, continued ⁓

SADDLE (E) The lamb's saddle portion contains the tender, well-marbled sirloin, which may be roasted whole or cut into sirloin chops and steaks for grilling, broiling, and sautéing. For grilled kabobs, chunks of boneless sirloin are ideal.

LEG (F) The firm, flavorful leg meat may be roasted whole or cut into cubes for kabobs or stew. If buying a bone-in leg, look for a French-style or three-quarter leg of lamb, with its upper pelvic bones removed, allowing for easier carving. Boned, butterflied, and marinated, a small leg is succulent when grilled or broiled. See boning and butterflying instructions at right.

SHANKS (G) This is the lower, shin section of the leg. Hearty, economical, and full flavored, the tough shank meat requires long, gentle braising. A few hours of gentle simmering will result in rich, moist, spoon-tender meat. The small, lean foreshank is usually braised as an individual-serving cut. The hind shank may be cut into thick, crosswise slices, or it may be boned and cut into stew meat for slow braising.

BREAST (H) This thin cut runs along the belly. The fatty, flavorful meat, with its many tiny rib bones, may be boned and cooked whole by braising, which results in tender meat, or it may be cut up and braised or grilled as lamb riblets. The breast is also sold ground for making grilled lamb burgers.

HOW TO *Bone and Butterfly a Leg of Lamb*

1. If possible, start with a leg that is still cold from the refrigerator and thus firm. Gripping the surrounding white skin with a cloth or paper towel, tear away the outer membrane. With a thin, sharp boning knife, trim away tough skin and excess external fat.

2. The large, rounded hipbone at the broad end of the leg and the S-shaped aitchbone attached to it form the pelvic bone. Making short, shallow cuts with the tip of the knife, outline the pelvic bone.

3. Slowly cut deeper and scrape away the meat, uncovering the bone down to where it meets the leg's ball-and-socket joint. Cut the tendons attached to the pelvic bone and remove it.

4. Holding the shank bone at the narrow, pointed end of the leg, sever the tendons connecting the meat to the base of the bone. (At this point, the leg can be trussed and roasted as a French-style leg of lamb.) Keeping the knife angled close to the bone, cut the meat away from the shank bone down to its joint. Sever the tendons and remove the shank bone.

5. Cutting into the muscle, trace the leg bone with the tip of the knife. Ease the leg bone out, carefully scraping and cutting away the meat under it as well as the tendons at both ends. Remove the leg bone.

6. To butterfly the boned leg, holding the knife blade parallel to the work surface, cut into the thickest part of the leg meat from the center outward toward the edge to open it out in a flap. Take care not to cut completely through the meat. The result should be a large, flat piece of meat of relatively uniform thickness.

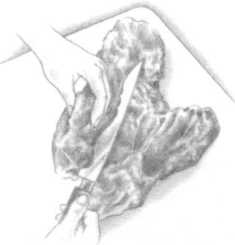

Preparing For the most succulent, tender meat, serve grilled, broiled, roasted, or panfried lamb slightly pink in color. If cooked to well done, the meat will be tough and dry, and it will take on a gamy flavor.

Quick Tip

Lamb fat has an assertive, unpleasant flavor. On roasts, leave no more than a ¼-inch-thick layer. Take care not to remove the thin, translucent membrane, which serves to hold the meat together.

Check the internal temperature of the meat with an instant-read thermometer. Since meat continues to cook and rise in temperature as it rests, remove the lamb when it registers 5° to 10°F less than the desired finished temperature.

Internal Temperatures for Lamb

Rare	125°F*
Medium-rare	130°F*
Medium	140°F*
Ground lamb	140°F*

Although these temperatures yield what many cooks feel are the optimum taste and texture for these foods, they are lower than those suggested by the U.S. Food Safety and Inspection Service guidelines; see DONENESS.

See also CARVING; ROASTING.

LARD See FAT & OIL.

LARDING To insert strips of fat into a lean cut of meat to add flavor and moisture during dry-heat cooking, such as roasting. The strips are inserted using a special tool called a larding needle. For a simpler technique with similar effect, see BARDING.

LEAVENING The formation of gas bubbles in batters or doughs that will expand during cooking, to lighten baked goods and give them an airy texture. Chemical substances such as baking powder and baking soda react with liquids and heat to create carbon dioxide. Yeast also gives off carbon dioxide, a natural by-product created as the microorganisms digest sugar and starches. When whipped, the proteins of eggs, especially the whites, create a foamy network of tiny air bubbles. The gases created by all these leaveners will expand when heated, causing foods to rise. By the time the gases dissipate, the structure provided by the starches and proteins of other ingredients, such as flour and sugar, will have set into a solid that is stable enough to hold itself. For more details, see BAKING POWDER & BAKING SODA; YEAST.

LEEK Resembling a giant green onion, with its bright white stalk and its long, overlapping green leaves, the leek is the mildest member of the onion family. Native to the Mediterranean region and essential to classic French cuisine, leeks bring a hint of both garlic and onion to the dishes they flavor. They can serve as a component of *mirepoix,* a classic French seasoning mixture; meld with other ingredients such as potatoes in standard preparations like vichyssoise; or star in a gratin or quiche. Raw leeks can also be sliced and added to salads.

Selecting Choose smaller leeks with dark green leaves that are crisp, firm, and free of blemishes. Check to make sure that the roots are light in color and still pliable. Avoid darkened, dried roots and wrinkled, wilted leaves.

Storing Keep leeks in a plastic bag in the refrigerator for up to 5 days.

Preparing Because leeks grow partly underground, grit is often lodged between the layers of their leaves. Wash them thoroughly before cooking.

HOW TO *Clean Leeks*

1. Trim off the roots and the tough, dark green tops of the leaves. If the outer layer is wilted or discolored, peel it away and discard.
2. Quarter or halve the stalk lengthwise. If using the leek whole, leave the root end intact.

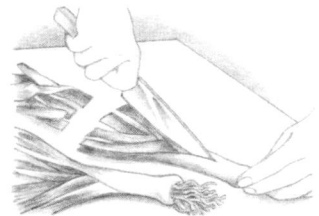

3. Rinse well under cold running water, separating the layers and rubbing the leaves to remove any silt between them.

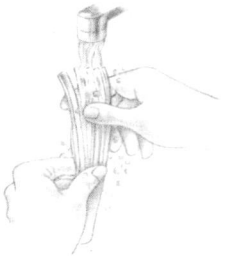

4. If a recipe calls for sliced leeks, slice the white and lighter green parts crosswise.

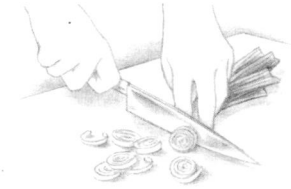

LEGUME See BEAN, DRIED; BEAN, FRESH; PEA, FRESH.

LEMON Although too sour to eat alone, lemons are an important seasoning in the kitchen and appear at the table in an endless parade of dishes. This small but versatile fruit was cultivated in tropical regions of Asia and India for centuries before the Moors introduced it to Europe. In refreshing dishes such as Latin America's seviche and Southeast Asia's lemon beef, the acidity in the juice turns seafood and thinly sliced meat opaque and firm, much as cooking does. Lemon is also a popular flavoring for pastries, cakes, and other baked goods.

Many dishes benefit from a grating of fragrant lemon peel or a squeeze of its tart juice. Lemon serves as a healthful substitute for salt in low-sodium diets, and its juice is used in place of vinegar to add fruity zing to almost any dressing.

Quick Tip

Add lemon juice or oil at the end of cooking for the freshest flavor.

Selecting Choose lemons heavy for their size and free of blemishes or soft spots. Lemons with smooth, glossy rinds offer the most juice, but buy lemons with thick, bumpy skin only when you need their zest. Although available year-round, lemons peak during the winter months.

Fresh lemons are so widely available that it shouldn't be difficult to avoid commercially packaged lemon juices, whether in glass bottles or in faux lemons fashioned out of squeezable plastic. The fresh will always supply a better flavor. In an emergency, frozen pure lemon juice is a good substitute. Look for it in the freezer section next to juice concentrates, thaw it, and store it in the refrigerator for up to a month. Natural lemon oil is another way to add lemon flavor to recipes. To preserve its flavor, store the oil in the refrigerator for up to 2 years.

Quick Bite

The Meyer lemon, a hybrid, was discovered by a man named Frank Meyer in 1908. Although the exact derivation of the Meyer lemon is disputed, many believe it is a cross between a lemon and a mandarin orange, as hinted at by its rounder shape, yellow-orange color, sweeter flavor, and flowery fragrance. Its peak season is November to May.

Storing Lemons can stay at room temperature for around 1 week. For longer storage, up to 1 month, keep them in plastic bags in the refrigerator.

Putting the Squeeze on Lemons

Like most citrus fruits, lemons release their juice more readily if you try the following:

- Store them at room temperature. If a lemon is still cold from the refrigerator, microwave it on High for 20 seconds.
- Roll them firmly against a hard, flat surface or between your palms to crush some of their inner membranes.
- Use a reamer. Its fluted ribs will extract every last drop. Take care not to rub too hard, though, or you will crush the pith and infuse the juice with some of its bitterness. A fork inserted into the cut surface of the lemon then rotated back and forth will work almost as well as a reamer.

If you have extra lemons, squeeze their juice and freeze it in an ice cube tray. Once hardened, transfer the lemon juice cubes to a plastic bag and add as needed during cooking.

See also ACID; DISCOLORING; JUICING; ZESTING.

LEMONGRASS An aromatic herb used throughout Southeast Asia, lemongrass flavors soups, curries, and grilled dishes from Myanmar to Malaysia. Resembling a green onion in shape, lemongrass has long, thin, graygreen leaves that meet and overlap along a woody, ivory-colored stem with bits of pale pink coloration.

Selecting Once found only in Asian markets, fresh lemongrass is now widely available in supermarkets. Look for firm stalks with no sign of fading or drying. In Asian stores, you can find small containers of finely minced lemongrass in the refrigerator or freezer sections. The herb is also available as dried shreds or a powder; avoid both forms, as they have none of the herb's fresh, lemony aroma. Lemongrass is traditionally paired in Asia with chicken, pork, seafood, tofu, tomatoes, and chiles, and is used in preparations ranging from soups to stir-fries to stews. The leaves make a refreshing infused tea.

Quick Tip

Simmer finely chopped lemongrass in equal parts sugar and water to make a fragrant syrup with an appealing lemony flavor. Store in an airtight container in the refrigerator. Uses include sweetening iced tea, drizzling over orange slices, glazing grilled chicken, and poaching fruit.

Storing Trim away the green leaves and refrigerate lemongrass in a plastic bag for up to 2 weeks. For convenient use, shred lemongrass stalks in a food processor or blender, and then freeze in a zippered plastic freezer bag for up to 6 months.

Preparing Only the pale bottom part of the stalk is used in cooking. Crush the stalk with a pestle or the side of a knife blade before chopping. Since its fibers are tough, lemongrass needs to be minced finely or removed from a dish before serving, much like a bay leaf. To infuse stock, slice lemongrass thinly on a sharp diagonal or cut it into 2-inch lengths and pound lightly. Both methods will help release more of the herb's flavor, while the latter allows a more easy removal of the pieces later.

LEMON VERBENA See HERB.

LENTIL See BEAN, DRIED.

LETTUCE See GREENS, SALAD.

LICHEE Or lichi. See LITCHI.

LILY BUD Also called golden needle or, mistakenly, tiger lily bud, lily bud is the dried, unopened blossom of the Chinese lily. Long, thin, golden, and earthy in flavor, lily buds measure 2 to 3 inches in length and appear frequently in Chinese vegetarian dishes. They also turn up in hot-and-sour soup, mu shu pork, and other dishes.
Selecting Lily buds should be a rich burnished gold and still soft and pliable. Pass up any that are dark and brittle. Look for lily buds in Asian markets, packaged in 4- or 8-ounce plastic bags.
Storing Transfer the buds to an airtight, glass jar and store in a cool, dark place for up to 6 months.
Preparing Before cooking, soak the dried lily buds in warm water for about 20 minutes until softened. Do not leave

them longer, or they may lose flavor. Drain and then trim off the hard stems. Knot the buds at their centers, individually or in small bundles, to keep them intact in stir-fries and braises. For delicate soups, tear the buds lengthwise into 3 or 4 shreds. This will also release more of their flavor.

LIMA BEAN See BEAN, DRIED; BEAN, FRESH.

LIME Smaller and more delicate than lemons, their yellow-skinned cousins, limes are tart with a hint of sweetness. They are an essential ingredient in the cuisines of Southeast Asia, Latin America, Africa, the West Indies, and the Pacific Islands. Lime can be used in place of lemon in nearly any recipe. Twist a bit of the zest into cocktails or add thin slices to a summery punch. In tropical countries, fresh lime juice deepens the flavor of sweet, musky fruits like papaya and guava. Lime pickles accompany Indian curries, fresh lime juice infuses Cuban chicken soup, and lime wedges accompany Mexican beer.

Familiar grocery store limes are Persian limes. Smaller, rounder Key limes grow in southern Florida. With thin, leathery skin and an abundance of seeds, highly tart Key limes lend their name to the famous pie. They appear fresh only occasionally in specialty produce markets, but look for good-quality bottled Key lime juice in gourmet shops. They are also known as the Mexican or West Indian lime.

Key lime.

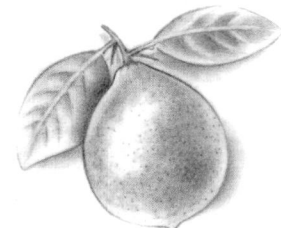

Selecting Buy smooth, glossy limes that are plump and heavy for their size. Avoid any with dull skin or soft spots. Pick Persian limes with dark green rind. Fully ripe Key limes have a yellowish rind and green flesh. Although available year-round, fresh limes peak from May to October.

Storing Limes can be stored at room temperature for 3 to 5 days. More perishable than lemons, limes fare better in a plastic bag in the refrigerator. Exposure to light and air will rapidly diminish the amount and tartness of their juice. Store lime oil in the refrigerator.

Preparing See LEMON for basic information on juicing citrus fruits.

See also JUICING; KAFFIR LIME; LEMON; ZESTING.

LIQUEUR See page 270.

LIQUID INGREDIENTS See MEASURING; WET INGREDIENTS.

LITCHI Also spelled lichi, lichee, and lychee. With pearly white, translucent flesh encased in a roughly textured, bright red shell, this fragrant tropical fruit is a luxury even in its native land of southern China. In Western countries, litchis are most commonly found packed in syrup. When dried, the fruit shrivels and looks and tastes similar to a raisin. Pour canned litchis over a shallow dish of cracked ice for a refreshing, simple dessert, or over vanilla or coconut ice cream.

Selecting Fresh litchis appear in Asian markets in late spring to early summer.

Fresh litchis.

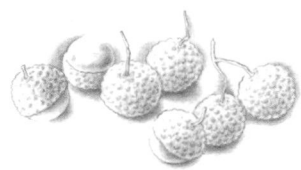

Look for fresh fruit with shells that are still rosy red or pink. Hardened, brownish fruits are old, dry, and flavorless. Litchis are also available canned in syrup, dried and packaged in plastic bags, or candied.

Canned litchis.

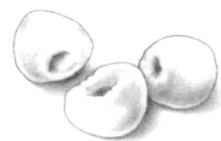

Look for them in Asian markets and well-stocked supermarkets.

Storing Fresh, whole litchis will keep in a plastic bag in the refrigerator for up to 2 weeks. Store canned or dried litchis in a cool, dark place for up to 2 years.

Preparing If you are lucky enough to find fresh litchis, enjoy them as a dessert on their own. With a paring knife, split open the thin shell. You can scoop out the flesh with a small spoon, pinching or cutting away the smooth seed at the center.

l

Liqueur

Often called crèmes, liqueurs are spirits flavored by natural extracts, essential oils, pure fruit syrups, sugar syrups, or, in the case of liqueurs of lesser quality, chemical extracts.

The flavors can come from fruits, nuts, spices, herbs, coffee, or chocolate.

A liqueur may be sipped in small quantity as an after-dinner drink or used to flavor desserts and sauces. Sometimes a fruit brandy, or eau-de-vie, may be served as a liqueur; see SPIRITS.

Cooking with Liqueurs Take care not to add too much liqueur to a dish, for the concentrated sweet flavor can easily

Liqueur Flavors

FLAVOR	LIQUEUR
Almond	amaretto; crème d'amandes; crème de noyaux; Noyau de Poissy
Anise	anisette; ouzo; pastis; Pernod; sambuca
Apricot	crème d'abricot; Abricotine; Apry
Banana	crème de banane
Cherry	crème de cerise; maraschino (sweet); Cherry Rocher; Peter Heering; Wishniac
Chocolate	crème de cacao; Chocolat Suisse; Chéri-Suisse (chocolate-cherry); Vandermint (chocolate-mint); Sabra (chocolate-orange)
Coffee	Kahlúa; Kona; Pasha; Tía Maria
Currant, black	crème de cassis
Hazelnut	Frangelico
Herbs & Flowers	Chartreuse (herbs); Chartreuse verte (herbs); Bénédictine (herbs); Liquore Galliano (herbs); crème de rose (rose); crème de violette (violet)
Melon	Midori
Orange	Cointreau; Curaçao; Grand Marnier; mandarine; Triple Sec
Pear	Birnengeist
Peppermint	crème de menthe; peppermint schnapps
Pineapple	crème d'ananas
Plum	prunelle; sloe gin
Vanilla	crème de vanille
Walnut	nocello; nocino

become cloying. The alcohol level of liqueurs tends to be relatively high, most fall between 50 and 100 proof, and their flavors are intense. As a general guideline, add no more than 2 tablespoons of liqueur to every 1 cup of sauce or batter. Remove a pan from the heat before stirring in a liqueur, and avoid letting the mixture sit too long before serving, since the flavors of liqueurs dissipate quickly when exposed to heat and air.

Pair liqueurs with dishes to accentuate the same flavor, such as adding almond-flavored amaretto to whipped cream that you plan to serve with an almond-crust tart; or to provide a pleasing complement to another ingredient, such as tart orange-flavored Grand Marnier with sweet strawberries. Food that combines well with a certain fruit will also match a liqueur derived from that same fruit, such as duck and cherries with kirsch. When soaking dried fruit for a recipe, try replacing the water or fruit juice with a related or contrasting liqueur, such as cherries in maraschino or dried cranberries in orange-flavored Cointreau. Liqueurs are also a nice touch in cream fillings, soufflés, ice creams, fruit compotes, and dessert sauces. Pour a little into hot drinks like hot chocolate or coffee.

Quick Bite

Bénédictine, which was developed in 1510 by Dom Bernardo Vincelli, a monk resident in the French Abbey of Fécamp, is believed to be the world's oldest liqueur. He reportedly poured his "elixir" for the resident monks, who sipped it as a cure for fatigue.

See also SPIRITS.

LOAF PAN See BAKEWARE.

LOBSTER On a candlelit table or in a clambake on the beach, a bright orange lobster is one of the undisputed icons of special occasions. Although once so plentiful that American colonists dismissed it as food for the poor, lobster now demands royal treatment in upscale restaurants and commands equally majestic prices.

Lobsters can be divided into two broad categories: clawed lobsters and spiny lobsters. Clawed lobsters are what most of us think of when we think "lobster." This includes orange and black American lobsters, also called Maine lobsters, which live in

American lobster.

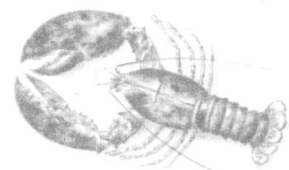

the cold waters off Newfoundland and New England. (Orange lobsters are blue-black when uncooked, turning orange when cooked.) They appear at market from July through November. Although similar to the American lobster, blue-black European lobsters are now scarce and extremely expensive. Some believe European lobsters have more delicate flavor and texture, but others can detect no significant difference.

Spiny lobsters, also known as rock lobsters or *langoustes,* lack large claws but are easily recognized by their extra-long antennae and the thin spines covering their hard shell. Cold-water spiny lobsters found near South Africa and Australia boast better quality meat than the warm-water species from Florida and the Caribbean. California spiny lobsters are rarely found beyond the markets of southern California and western Mexico. Actually sea-dwelling crayfish, live spiny lobsters arrive only at local markets from August to March. Their tails, however, with flesh slightly tougher and not as sweet as that of the American lobster, are widely available frozen.

Although New England purists insist that only drawn butter and corn should appear next to lobster on the dinner table, the sweet, rich flavor of this popular crustacean pairs well with a wide range of flavors, from dill, tarragon, basil, parsley, and saffron to mustard, lemongrass, and lime. Avocado, cucumber, citrus fruits, white wine, brandy, cream, coconut milk, chiles, and eggs are just a handful of the ingredients that are often matched with lobster.

Selecting When buying a live lobster, choose one that proves especially feisty. Hold a lobster up, grasping its sides safely behind its claws, to check that it quickly snaps its tail tightly under its body. Any that are sluggish and apathetic have been in the tank too long. Captured lobsters are not fed, so their meat will shrink away with time. Likewise, when purchasing a whole cooked lobster, make sure that its tail curls, an indication that it was still alive when it was dropped into the cooking pot.

A lively debate rages between those who prefer the firmer flesh of male clawed lobsters and those who like the sweet flesh of females. Also hotly contested are the merits of succulent 1-pound "chicken" lobsters versus fleshy 3-pound "jumbos." Those who have braved 10-pounders swear that the giants are just as sweet and tender. Most lobsters sold at markets fall between 1¼ and 2 pounds.

Quick Tip

How to subdue live lobsters: Place them in the freezer for 5 to 10 minutes before cooking.

He or She?

- Male lobsters have somewhat larger claws, and female lobsters grow slightly wider tails.
- Females have thin, soft, feathery swimmerets on the underside of their tails; these will later hold their eggs. Male lobsters have long, hard, spiky swimmerets.
- The red roe inside a female lobster may be a delicacy, but strict laws require that all females with eggs on their swimmerets be returned to the water.

Although missing one or both claws, less expensive "culls" taste just as good in soups, stews, or salads. If you lack a reliable local source for live lobsters, numerous companies can ship them to you overnight. Frozen lobster tails, usually from spiny lobsters, and already cooked whole lobsters can give you a head start on recipes.

Quick Tip

Lobster tails will curl during cooking. For a straight tail, stretch a live lobster flat and tie it firmly to a wooden spoon, ruler, or stick before boiling or steaming. If cooking the tail only, insert a skewer just beneath the shell.

Storing If not cooking them immediately, cover live lobsters with a damp cloth or wet newspaper, place them in a small cardboard box or large, heavy paper bag, and refrigerate. Although best if prepared as soon as possible after purchase, you can keep them in the refrigerator for up to 2 days, if needed. Expect the quality of the meat to diminish significantly with each day. Leave the rubber bands on in order to prevent mishaps with snapping claws. Do not immerse lobsters in tap water, for they will quickly die. Uncooked tails can be kept in the freezer in a zippered plastic freezer bag for 3 to 4 months, but cooked lobster will turn mushy and flavorless if frozen.

HOW TO *Halve and Clean Lobster*

These steps can be followed to prepare an uncooked lobster for grilling, roasting, or broiling.

1. If you have purchased a live lobster, plunge it into boiling water for about 30 seconds and then rinse it under cold water to halt the cooking. (If it is already cooked, ignore this step.) Alternatively, set the lobster on a firm surface and securely hold the lobster's tail with a folded cloth to prevent slipping. Insert the tip of a large chef's knife straight down through the back of the lobster to the board, piercing the cross mark in the area between the first and second pairs of thin legs.

2. Cut the lobster's head in half lengthwise. If desired, hold an uncooked lobster over a bowl to catch the juices.

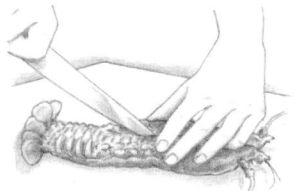

3. Turn the lobster around, hold its head, and cut the rest of the lobster sharply in half.

4. Lift away and discard the sand sac near the head. Using the tip of the knife, carefully remove the gray intestinal vein that runs along the lobster's back.

5. With a small spoon, scoop out the liver, known as the tomalley, which will be black if uncooked and green if cooked, and any coral, or eggs, which will be black if uncooked and bright red if cooked. Reserve both for sauce as needed.

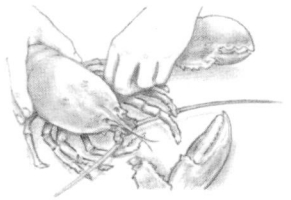

6. For a neater look, cut away the legs and claws. Crack claws in a few places with a lobster cracker or mallet, so diners can easily reach the meat inside.

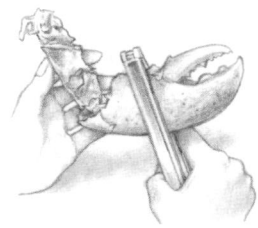

7. Before serving cooked lobsters, remove the pale, feathery gills along the sides of the lobster's body. If desired, loosen the cooked tail meat from its shell for easier eating. If you have them, provide lobster picks, small two-pronged forks designed specifically for the purpose.

HOW TO *Boil Lobster*

Serve boiled lobster with a dipping sauce such as melted butter, tarragon mayonnaise, chile-lime sauce, extra-virgin olive oil and lemon juice, or melted butter flavored with a touch of vanilla.

1. Bring a large pot of water to a full boil. To ensure quick cooking, use 1 gallon for 1 lobster; add 1 quart for each additional lobster.

2. Drop a live lobster in headfirst, taking care to avoid any splashing from its tail. Once the water returns to a boil, reduce the heat to maintain a gentle simmer.

3. Cook a lobster 8 minutes for the first pound plus 2 minutes for each additional ¼ pound. Remove with tongs and let the lobster cool slightly before serving.

Quick Tip

Traditionally, lobsters are boiled, but they can be steamed over 1 to 2 inches of water.

HOW TO *Remove Meat from Cooked Lobsters*

1. Drain any residual water from boiled or steamed lobsters by making a small cut between the eyes on the lobster head. Hold the lobster by its tail over a sink to drain the excess cooking liquid from underneath the shell.

2. Firmly twist off the claws from the body. With a lobster cracker or mallet, break the hard shell of each claw in several places. Pull away the shell pieces, taking care not to damage the claw meat if a recipe calls for it to be left whole.

3. Insert the tip of a large, sharp, sturdy knife into the point where the tail and body sections meet, and carefully cut lengthwise through the tail. Turn the lobster around and continue to cut from the center through the head, cutting the lobster into 2 equal halves.

4. Pull out and discard the black vein that runs the length of the body meat, as well as the small sand sac at the base of the head. Remove the white meat from the shell. If you like, reserve the green tomalley, or liver, and any bright red roe, which can be added to lobster dishes for extra flavor.

5. Firmly grasp the fins of a tail half with one hand. With the other, firmly pull out the tail meat in a single piece, using a fork to pry it loose if needed. Repeat with the other tail half.

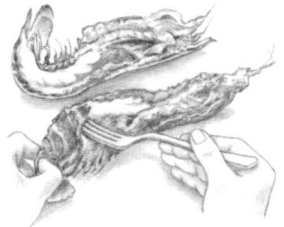

What to Do with All Those Shells

■ Simmer them with aromatics and herbs to make a rich lobster stock.

■ Crush the shells and heat gently with butter for 15 minutes. Ladle through a fine-mesh strainer, pressing down to extract as much flavor as possible. Add small amounts of the intensely flavored butter to sauces, spread on sandwiches, or use to top fish. Store covered in the refrigerator for up to 1 month or freeze for up to 1 year.

LOGANBERRY See BERRY.

LOTUS While its spectacular blossoms appear in water gardens from India to Japan, other parts of the lotus plant play flavorful roles in the kitchen.

Lotus leaf.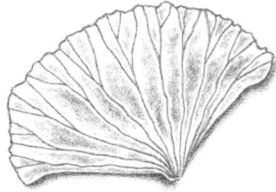

Dried and used as wrappers, the large leaves lend their subtle fragrance and flavor to small bundles of savory and sweet fillings to be steamed. The ivory-colored roots have a crisp texture and sweet flavor. Thin slices are excellent stir-fried or deep-fried as tempura, while thick ones are good braised with other vegetables. Lotus seeds are one of the celebrated "eight treasures" of Chinese dishes, adding their nutty flavor to many festive preparations.

Selecting Look for lotus in Asian markets or in the specialty produce section of major supermarkets. When selecting lotus roots, look for smooth, unblemished specimens and check at the trimmed ends for flesh that is still pale and moist. They may also be found cut in slices and vacuum packed in heavy plastic bags. Both the leaves and the pale, round seeds are available dried and packaged. Lotus seeds are also available canned or in bulk.

Storing Keep whole roots in the vegetable bin of the refrigerator for no longer than 1 week. Once cut or peeled, the unused portion should be immersed in lightly acidulated water to prevent darkening (see DISCOLORING) and returned to the refrigerator for up to 2 days. The dried leaves and seeds will keep indefinitely in an airtight container in a cool, dark place. Drain the canned seeds, transfer them to a container, add fresh water to immerse them completely, cover, and refrigerate them for up to 5 days.

Preparing Snap off whole sections of lotus root as needed. Peel the streaked, buff-colored skin with a vegetable peeler. Cut the roots crosswise into thick or thin slices according to a recipe, keeping them in acidulated water to prevent browning. Soften the dried leaves in boiling water. To prepare the seeds for cooking, drain them, remove the bitter green bud at their center, and boil until softened.

LOW-FAT COOKING In recent years, low-fat cooking has become enormously popular. Cookbooks and magazines promoting ways to cut fat and calories abound; supermarket shelves bulge with reduced-fat and fat-free products; an ever-growing list of restaurants are putting heart-safe or low-fat dishes on their menus; and even fast-food chains, long-standing bastions of high-fat foods, have cut the fat by offering such healthful alternatives as grilled chicken sandwiches and salad bars.

Quick Tip

Nonfat or reduced-fat products such as sour cream, cream cheese, cottage cheese, and mayonnaise don't always work in a recipe the way their regular counterparts do. Rather than simply substituting, seek out recipes specifically created for these products.

Low-fat cooking experts often disagree on how much protein and total fat to consume daily, and self-proclaimed gurus promising rapid weight loss if you follow a certain diet are everywhere. But a few commonsense guidelines on how to trim fat from cooking have emerged from the proliferation of literature and research.

Unless your doctor tells you otherwise, do not try to eliminate all the fat from your cooking. Fat contributes to flavor, texture, and overall satisfaction. If you don't feel satisfied, you might eat more. When you want a smear of cream cheese on a bagel or a dollop of mayonnaise on a tomato, go for the real thing if doctor's orders allow. Eat in moderation and make the food you eat enjoyable.

Ways to Reduce the Fat

- Use cooking spray in place of liquid cooking oil to grease pans.
- Use nonstick cookware.
- Steam, broil, grill, or bake food to avoid the fat used for sautéing and frying.
- Rely on chicken and beef stock, wine, and water to moisten and baste foods while they cook, instead of additional oil or butter.
- Use herbs and spices to flavor foods, instead of additional butter or cream.
- Learn about fat-cutting techniques such as replacing whole eggs with egg whites and using applesauce and puréed prunes in baked products in place of some of the butter.
- Skin poultry before or after cooking.
- Use water-packed tuna instead of the oil-packed version.
- Use ground turkey breast instead of ground beef.
- Trim meat and poultry of external fat before cooking.
- Substitute flavorful fat-free spreads such as jams, jellies, chutneys, or mustards for butter or margarine.

LYCHEE See LITCHI.

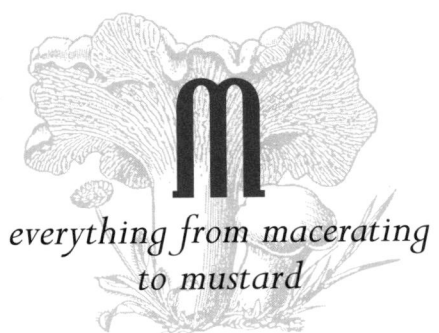

everything from macerating to mustard

m

MACADAMIA NUT See NUT.

MACE See SPICE.

MACERATING To soak fruit in juice, sugar, liqueur, or other flavoring and tenderizing mediums. Although similar to marinating, macerating applies specifically to fruit. To meld fruit flavors, let them soak together. On the other hand, to keep delicate flavors distinct, to prevent bleeding of bright colors, or to protect soft fruits from the crush of heavier, firmer fruits, soak each fruit separately. Always use a nonreactive bowl, as the acid in fruits can react with certain metals to create "off" flavors.

MÂCHE See GREENS, SALAD.

MADELEINE PAN See BAKEWARE.

MALT Malt is produced by first allowing soaked barley grains to germinate and then drying, roasting, and grinding them to a powder. When malt is mentioned, most of us think of ice cream and chocolate syrup blended with it into a frosty treat. But malt plays a quiet, yet important, role in foods from vinegar to beer to bagels.

Pure malt powder is used in the production of beer and whiskey and in bread making to boost yeast growth; improve flavor, structure, and crust color; and extend shelf life. Malted milk powder is a mixture of malt sugar and powdered milk. Malt syrup can replace honey or maple syrup, resulting in a subtler flavor and lighter color.

MANDARIN ORANGE Named after officials in the Chinese emperors' courts who wore orange robes and headpieces with distinctive buttons resembling the fruit. Mandarin oranges are less acidic and smaller than oranges, with a slightly flattened shape. They are distinguished by delicate strands of pith that lie beneath thin, loose skins. Their classification, *Citrus reticulata,* refers to this netlike filigree that encloses the sweet, juicy segments.

In the United States, mandarin oranges are commonly known as tangerines, although in the citrus trade this term actually designates specific varieties with a darker, red-orange peel. Mandarins grown in Florida, where they were first introduced from Tangier, Morocco, by way of Spain, generally carry the name *tangerine*. In Great Britain, *tangerine* identifies mandarin varieties from the Mediterranean region that are pale in color and mild in flavor.

Popular members of the whole mandarin group include the sweet Satsuma from Japan; the smooth, juicy Clementines from Algeria, Spain, and France; the ubiquitous red-orange Dancy tangerine from Florida; and the large, knobbly-skinned King mandarin from Southeast Asia. Tangors, such as the tart Temple orange, are a hybrid of mandarins and oranges. Tangelos result from a cross between a mandarin and a pomelo or grapefruit. The honey-flavored Minneola, with its distinctive stem-end neck, is perhaps the most recognized of the tangelos.

Easy to peel, mandarin oranges make appealing snacks for eating out of hand. While many do have seeds, the most common ones in markets tend to have few or no seeds. As festive in appearance as they are delicious, they are traditionally part of the celebrations at Christmas and Chinese New Year. See also ORANGE.

Selecting Choose fruits that are deep in color, heavy for their size, and free of dull or soft spots. Although some will have loose skins, avoid those that appear overly bumpy or puffy, for they are most probably old and overripe. Although the specific peak months vary according to variety and origin, mandarin oranges are generally at their best from November to March. They are also available in cans, their segments preserved in sugar syrup.

Storing Display colorful mandarin oranges at room temperature for up to 1 week. For longer storage of up to 1 month, keep them in a plastic bag in the refrigerator. Store canned segments in a cool, dry place for up to 2 years; once opened, they should be transferred to a nonreactive container and refrigerated for up to 1 week.

Preparing Although at their best simply eaten out of hand, mandarin oranges also are good in light sauces for poultry, fish, and pork, infusing them with subtle citrus flavor. They should be added at the end of cooking and just heated through to preserve their delicate flavor.

MANDOLINE A flat, rectangular tool ideal for cutting food quickly and easily. Mandolines usually come with an assortment of smooth and corrugated blades, so food can be sliced, julienned, or

waffle-cut. The advantages of using a mandoline are precision and regularity. It takes time to acquire the knife skills to transform a mountain of potatoes into the uniform pieces needed to make *frites* or into paper-thin slices for chips, or to trim a knobby celery root into perfect julienne strips, but once armed with a mandoline, even a novice cook can easily cut vegetables like a seasoned cooking professional.

Mandolines are available in a variety of designs. Some must be steadied by hand or placed over a bowl, while others have fold-away legs that permit you to stand them up at an ergonomic angle. You can choose a high-quality stainless-steel commercial model or a simpler plastic version. Look for one with a hand guard that keeps your fingers clear of the cutting edge as you move the ingredient across the extremely sharp mandoline blade.

MANGO This highly aromatic fruit was first cultivated in India. Now, mangoes are among the most commonly eaten fresh fruits in the world. Diced ripe mangoes are

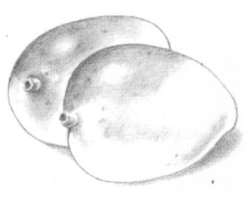

excellent in chutney to accompany pork, chicken, or fish. Mangoes complement coconut, pineapple, raspberries, and smoked chicken; puréed mango, strained and mixed with lime juice, makes a delectable dessert sauce for cakes, ice cream, or pastries. The brightly flavored mango chutneys of India depend on underripe green fruits, and the crisp, unripe fruit is shredded for popular salads in Southeast Asia.

Selecting The best mangoes are in the markets from May through September, but fresh fruits are available all year long, since different varieties are imported from around the world. When shopping for ripe mangoes, choose ones that emit a full aroma at their stem end, give slightly to gentle pressure, and have perfectly smooth skin. Mangoes will also ripen after purchase, although those picked too early will be particularly fibrous near the pit. Depending on the variety, they can range in color from all green to all red, with blushes of every shade of yellow and orange in between. Those with yellow in their skin tend to be the most flavorful, but do not buy any that are wrinkled or have soft spots. Most fruits sold in supermarkets weigh about ¾ pound each. For convenience, look for already peeled and cut mangoes packaged in jars or in plastic containers in the refrigerated section of the produce aisle.

Mango nectar, mango purée, and dried mango spears are available in health-food stores, supermarkets, and Indian markets.

Storing Keep not-quite-ripe mangoes at room temperature for a few days until ripened. You can place them inside a paper bag to speed up the ripening process. Like other tropical fruits, mangoes do not fare well when exposed to cold temperatures for long periods of time. After they are ripe, refrigerate them for no more than 2 or 3 days—or preferably not at all. Puréed mangoes can be frozen for up to

1 year. Keep unopened cans of mango nectar in a cool, dry place, but refrigerate them after opening. Store dried mango in an airtight container in the refrigerator for up to 6 months.

Preparing Always peel the fruit before serving. Slit the thick, sometimes leathery skin with a knife tip and pull it off in strips.

Caution!

Because the mango is a distant cousin of poison oak and poison ivy, some people will have allergic reactions to its skin. If you have any irritation or simply suspect that you are allergic, use gloves while peeling mangoes. Be sure to remove all of the skin before serving.

HOW TO *Eat a Mango*

In the tropics, where mangoes are as common as apples are in Washington, the locals have developed distinctive ways to eat the fruits. If you try either of the following methods, be prepared for a bit of a mess.

1. Score the skin so the fruit can be partially peeled, and then eat the mango similar to the manner in which one consumes a banana.
2. Roll an unpeeled ripe mango on a tabletop so the pulp almost liquefies, and then suck the pulp out of the stem end using a straw.

HOW TO *Cut a Mango*

The large, flat pit at the center of a mango can present a challenge when slicing and dicing the fruit.

1. Peel the mango.
2. Stand the mango up on one of its narrow edges, with the stem end pointing toward you.
3. With a large, sharp knife, cut down about 1 inch to one side of the stem, just grazing the side of the pit. You should have 1 large mango "half." Repeat with the other side of the fruit.
4. Place the mango halves cut side down on the cutting board and slice as desired.
5. Trim off the flesh left encircling the pit.

HOW TO *Make Quick Mango Cubes*

1. With the peel still on, cut the mango in halves as above.
2. Following a crisscross grid pattern, carefully score the cut side of the mango halves just down to the skin. Do not pierce the skin.

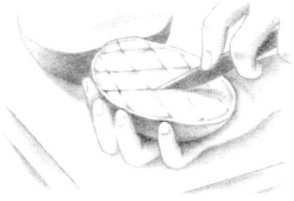

3. Using your thumbs to press against the skin side, turn the halves inside out. The cubes of mango will pop out.

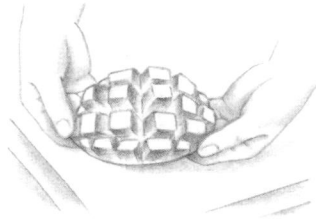

4. Cut across the bottom of the cubes, along the peel, to release the cubes. Trim off the flesh left encircling the pit.

Quick Bite

In India, where mangoes are revered for their sweetness, versatility, and abundance, giving a basket of the fruit is a gesture of friendship.

MAPLE SYRUP Pure maple syrup is made from the boiled sap of the sugar maple tree. The caramel-colored, maple-flavored corn syrup commonly drizzled on waffles and pancakes and called "pancake syrup" has no relation to the real thing. In early spring, throughout Canada and the northern United States, most notably in New York and New England, taps for collecting sap appear on the trunks of maple

⁓ Making the Grade ⁓

GRADE A Grade A Light or Fancy, sometimes called Grade AA, is clear gold and has a wonderfully subtle flavor. The most expensive of the maple syrups, its delicate character does not hold up in cooking. It is usually made into maple candies and is a favorite topping for pancakes, waffles, and ice cream. Grade A Medium is also used as a topping for the same familiar breakfast items and ice cream. Dedicated maple-syrup lovers will buy Grade A Dark, which is similar to Grade B.

GRADE B This maple syrup is produced only in Vermont. Preferred by some for its depth of flavor and pronounced caramel notes, others find it rather too strong and dark.

GRADE C Develops a robust, molasses-like flavor. Used primarily in making commercial table syrups.

trees. Sugaring season, as it is called, lasts for a month or so, as long as the nights are cold and the days are warm enough to get the sap rising. A long boiling reduces the clear, fresh sap to a rich, aromatic, amber syrup. Good-quality maple syrup will taste of vanilla and caramel. To make a single gallon of maple syrup, up to 40 gallons of fresh sap must be boiled down.

Selecting Blended maple syrups contain anywhere from 2 to 15 percent real maple syrup. Pure maple syrup is expensive, but it is so flavorful that less is needed. Maple syrup is graded according to its quality and color. In general, the lighter the color, the milder-tasting the syrup.

Storing Smaller amounts that can be used within 2 months can be kept in an airtight container in a cool, dry place. Store large

m

amounts of syrup in an airtight glass container in the refrigerator indefinitely.

Preparing Use maple syrup much as you would honey. Add it to barbecue sauces, muffins, quick breads, frostings, glazes, fresh fruit salads, and salad dressings. And, of course, drizzle it generously over pancakes and waffles.

MARGARINE This century-old substitute for butter is made from hydrogenated vegetable oil. Hydrogenation is the process by which food manufacturers transform liquid oil into solid fat. Margarine has less saturated fat than butter and no cholesterol, but because of the trans fatty acids it contains, it is not the healthful alternative to butter it once was believed to be.

Quick Bite

The hydrogenation of oils creates compounds known as trans fatty acids, now believed to be more harmful to your health in high amounts than regular saturated fats. The more an oil is hydrogenated, the stiffer it becomes and the more trans fats are created. This explains the increasing popularity of softer tub margarine, which has 50 to 80 percent less trans fat than the firmer stick form.

Because hydrogenated oils have a higher melting point than butter, they will scorch less readily when heated, which makes margarine useful for panfrying and browning or for greasing cake pans destined for hot ovens. For the same reason, margarine does not melt at body temperature, which is part of the reason it lacks butter's nutty flavor and "melt-in-your-mouth" richness. Manufacturers sometimes add vitamins, food coloring, and milk or cream to create a more butterlike product. Blending dairy butter or cream into margarine makes it more flavorful but also adds cholesterol.

Quick Tip

Because reduced-fat margarine contains a high proportion of water, do not use it in place of regular margarine in baking or frying. The results will be disappointing.

Selecting Margarine is widely available in the refrigerated dairy section of supermarkets, molded into firm sticks like butter, or packaged as a soft spread in plastic tubs. Reduced-fat and fat-free margarine also are available. Other forms of margarine, such as liquid squeezed from a plastic bottle and a powder that may be sprinkled on food at the table, help make it even more convenient.

Storing Keep margarine in the refrigerator for up to 2 months or in the freezer for up to 18 months. Store margarine to be frozen in a zippered plastic freezer bag or wrapped in freezer-weight plastic.

MARINATING A marinade is a highly flavored, acid-based liquid mixture in which meat, fish, or vegetables soak for a set amount of time. Marinating flavors the food and has some tenderizing effect on the surface of meat and fish. Research has shown that the flavoring and tenderizing effects are relatively slight, as the acid can penetrate only the surface of any food. Its effects are greatest on smaller, thin cuts.

Marinating meat.

Marinades usually contain three types of ingredients: oil to help keep meat moist, acid to tenderize protein, and flavorings such as spices and herbs. Marinades that do not have a significant liquid component are sometimes called dry marinades or, more often, rubs. The combinations are endless, but choosing an appropriate oil or acid will add depth to the mix. Some basic examples include sesame oil and rice vinegar for an Asian flair, citrus juice and a light oil for a refreshing, subtle flavor with seafood, or a robust red wine vinegar and olive oil for roasted meats.

Marinating Savvy

- Always use containers made of non-reactive material such as glass, stainless steel, or plastic. See NONREACTIVE.
- Place spices and aromatics in cheese-cloth or a mesh tea ball for easy removal from a marinade.
- If you plan to baste meat, fish, or poultry with some of its marinade during cooking, reserve a portion of the marinade at the beginning, before adding the food to it.

Caution!

Never use a meat's or poultry's marinade as a sauce for serving without first bringing it to a boil and letting it boil for 5 minutes, as it contains raw juices from the meat.

- Use heavy-duty zippered plastic bags to coat food evenly and neatly with wet marinades. Place the food in a bag and pour in the marinade. Fold down any excess plastic at the top, press out as much air as possible, and then seal.

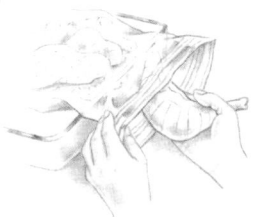

Placing poultry in a bag to marinate.

The thicker or bigger the food, the longer it will need to marinate. Thin slices of chicken may need only 15 minutes, while a large roast may require several days. Scoring a thick cut of meat will help a marinade to penetrate it. Use a small, sharp knife to make shallow cuts in the meat's surface.

Scoring poultry to help it marinate.

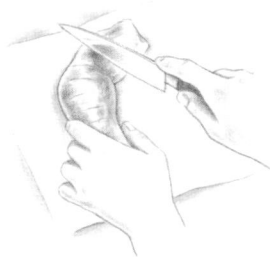

- Do not marinate meat or poultry at room temperature for more than 2 hours. For longer marinating, always refrigerate.
- Drain food and pat dry before cooking, especially if you want to sear and brown meat. Small pieces of onion, garlic, and fresh herbs from a marinade still clinging to meat will scorch over high heat.
- Take care when marinating delicate fish and shellfish. If left in acids too long, they will become firm and opaque. This is fine for seviche, but not for seafood that needs further cooking.

See also RUB.

MARIONBERRY See BERRY.

MARJORAM See HERB.

MASA HARINA See FLOUR; TORTILLA.

MASCARPONE See CHEESE.

MASHING Starchy vegetables such as potatoes, parsnips, squash, and beans can be cooked until soft, then mashed to a smooth

purée. Mash a small amount of cooked vegetable solids (potato, turnip, carrot) in a
soup or stew to thicken it. A masher, a special tool with a sturdy handle connected to
a wavy thick wire or a round cutout grid,
is an age-old tool for crushing food.

Potato mashers.

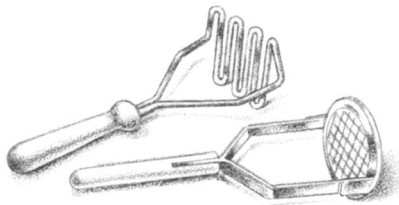

Potatoes can become unpleasantly gummy
if they are whipped rather than mashed, so
avoid using a food processor.

See also RICING.

MATZO Also spelled matzoh. A flat,
brittle bread baked without any leavening.
It is traditionally eaten during Passover, a
holiday commemorating the flight of the
Jews from Egypt, when, in their haste, they
did not have time to let their bread rise.
Matzo meal, ground from the bread, gives
bulk to matzo balls and replaces flour in
baked goods. Like bread crumbs, matzo
meal can also be used to bind, thicken, and
coat other foods. Matzo meal cake flour,
made from matzo ground to a fine powder,
is used primarily for cakes.

MAYONNAISE A creamy, cold sauce of
egg yolks, oil, and lemon juice or vinegar
blended into a thick emulsion. Whipping
together mayonnaise was once the test of a
dedicated cook, but now making it at home
is simple with a food processor, a blender,
or an electric mixer.

Recently, homemade mayonnaise has
raised concerns because of the slight possibility of salmonella bacteria in raw eggs. If
you wish to limit your potential exposure
to bacteria as much as possible for health
reasons, avoid making mayonnaise with raw
eggs. Store-bought mayonnaise, which is
made with pasteurized eggs, can be cus-
tomized with the addition of any number
of ingredients, from minced fresh herbs
to curry powder to mustard.

Selecting Prepared real mayonnaise and
its popular imitation version labeled
"mayonnaise-type salad dressing" are widely
available in jars. Mayonnaise is sold in low-
fat and low-cholesterol versions. Prepared
mayonnaises are good and inarguably convenient, but homemade mayonnaise will
have a superior flavor.

Storing Once opened, jars of prepared
mayonnaise should be kept in the refrigerator for no longer than 6 months. Refrigerate homemade mayonnaise as well, but
do not keep it for more than 3 days. Do
not leave salads that contain mayonnaise
unrefrigerated for more than 2 hours.

Preparing Be extremely careful not to
contaminate mayonnaise. Always use clean
utensils for scooping it out of the jar, and
never return leftover mayonnaise to the
original batch.

Quick Tip

Don't worry if your homemade mayonnaise
separates into a mess of curds as you are
making it. The rescue is easy. Simply beat another egg yolk in a clean bowl. Then, gradually
add the broken mayonnaise, whisking steadily
until it reforms. Balance the additional egg
with more oil and seasonings.

See also EGG; EMULSION.

MEASURING See opposite page.

MEASURING CUP AND SPOON
See COOKING TOOLS; MEASURING.

Measuring

Although experienced cooks have learned to add "a little of this" or "a lot of that" without bothering to measure, understanding the fundamentals of measuring helps prevent problems in baking or when trying new recipes. Certain ingredients require special attention to ensure accurate measurement.

Reading the Recipe Read the ingredient list of a recipe closely to check whether an item is measured *before* or *after* some form of preparation. For example, "1 cup walnuts, chopped" calls for measuring the walnuts *before* chopping, while "1 cup chopped walnuts" directs you to measure the nuts *after* chopping. Preparing an ingredient before or after measuring can make a big difference in the amount actually used. Using the same example, 1 cup chopped walnuts is actually more walnuts than 1 cup walnuts, chopped, because you can fit more chopped walnuts into a measuring cup than unchopped ones. Although the differences are sometimes not visible to the eye, they can seriously affect the outcome of recipes, especially when you are engaged in the exacting chemistry of baking.

Measuring Equipment Every kitchen should have both dry and wet measuring cups, which are not interchangeable. For accurate measuring, use the correct type of measuring cup.

Dry measuring cups are graduated cups in a standard set ranging from ¼ cup to 1 cup. Sometimes a ⅛-cup measure is also included. They are usually made of heavy-duty plastic or stainless steel. Each cup, when leveled at its brim, measures a specific amount. Look for a 2-cup dry measure; recipes frequently call for this amount.

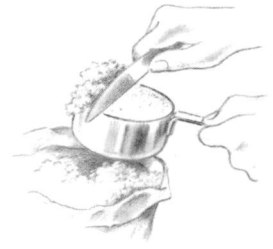
Measuring a dry ingredient.

Liquid measuring cups look like pitchers with rulers printed vertically on the side. They are clear glass or plastic, have pour spouts, extra room at the top for sloshing liquid, and continuous markings for fluid ounces and cups. The two most common sizes are 1 quart and 1 cup, and some manufacturers include metric markings as well. Although a 2-cup size is less common, seek one out, as it is convenient to have on hand. When measuring a liquid, place the cup on a flat surface, let the liquid settle, then read it at eye level.

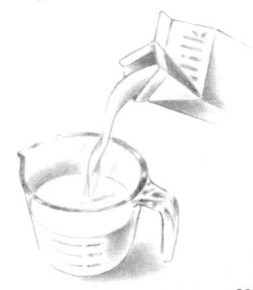
Measuring a liquid.

continued

Measuring, continued

Measuring spoons come in a set of ¼ teaspoon, ½ teaspoon, 1 teaspoon, and 1 tablespoon. The occasional set will include ½ tablespoon or ⅛ teaspoon. You can use them for both dry and liquid ingredients. As with the dry cups, after filling a measuring spoon, level off the dry ingredient with a flat edge.

PLASTIC, STAINLESS STEEL, OR GLASS? Plastic dry measures are light and can be strong, but plastic can also absorb oils and strong flavors. Metal ones are generally more durable, but avoid aluminum spoons, which will react with acidic ingredients such as lemon juice and vinegar to create an "off" flavor.

Plastic and glass liquid measures allow you to heat ingredients in the microwave, but Pyrex glass measures can even be used on gas stoves to scald liquids.

Whatever the material, look for measuring cups with comfortable handles securely attached, easy-to-read numbers that won't wear away, and the ability to nest for compact storage.

Quick Tip

If you don't have a ½ tablespoon measure, measure out 1½ teaspoons.

How to Measure If a measure includes no adjective, such as 1 tablespoon sugar or 1 cup sugar, then a level measure, that is, one that is even with the rim of the table-spoon or cup, is understood. A "heaping" measure, such as 1 heaping tablespoon sugar, is generously rounded above the rim. A "rounded" measure, such as 1 rounded tablespoon sugar, calls for a slightly

rounded dome above the rim, or slightly less than "heaping." Finally, 1 scant table-spoon sugar means slightly less than full. In other words, the ingredient is not level with the top of the measuring spoon but just below it.

BROWN SUGAR Pack moist brown sugar into the measuring cup firmly enough for it to retain its shape when it is tapped out of the cup.

CORN SYRUP Lightly coat the measuring cup with oil or butter before pouring in corn syrup, and it will slip out easily and cleanly. This also works for honey, molasses, and other sticky ingredients.

FLOUR Weighing flour is the most accurate way to measure it, but most American recipes are not written this way. There are two ways to use volume measures for flour. For the spoon-and-sweep method, lightly fill the measuring cup with a separate scoop or spoon. Level off the flour with the back of a knife, making it flush with the edge of the cup. Do not tamp down the flour. For the scoop-and-sweep method, fluff up the flour with a fork or whisk, dip the cup into the flour to scoop it up, and then sweep the top level. With the latter method you will end up with slightly more flour in the cup. Unless a recipe indicates which to use, pick a method and use it every time for consistent results in your baking.

Although all-purpose flour is commonly sold presifted, check the ingredient list of your recipe. If it specifically states sifted flour, sift it again for accurate measuring, since volume varies greatly between sifted and unsifted flour.

SHORTENING Fill a large measuring cup with cold water to the 1 cup level. Add shortening in large spoonfuls until the water registers the required amount plus 1 cup. Dump the water and you will have the exact amount of shortening needed. (Gently pat the shortening dry before using it in a mixture or for panfrying.)

Measurement Equivalents

3 teaspoons	= 1 tablespoon	= ½ fluid ounce				
	2 tablespoons	= 1 fluid ounce				
	4 tablespoons	= 2 fluid ounces	= ¼ cup			
	5 tablespoons plus 1 teaspoon		= ⅓ cup			
	16 tablespoons	= 8 fluid ounces	= 1 cup			
		16 fluid ounces	= 2 cups	= 1 pint		
		32 fluid ounces	= 4 cups	= 2 pints	= 1 quart	
		128 fluid ounces	= 16 cups	= 8 pints	= 4 quarts	= 1 gallon

Metric Conversions

VOLUME

U.S. to Metric	
1 teaspoon	5 milliliters
1 tablespoon	15 milliliters
¼ cup	59 milliliters
1 cup	236 milliliters
1 pint	473 milliliters
1 quart	946 milliliters
1 gallon	3.8 liters

Metric to U.S.	
10 milliliters	2 teaspoons
30 milliliters	1 fluid ounce
100 milliliters	½ cup minus 1 tablespoon
500 milliliters	2 cups plus 2 tablespoons
1 liter	4¼ cups, or 1 quart plus ¼ cup
2 liters	8½ cups, or ½ gallon plus ½ cup

WEIGHT-MASS

U.S. to Metric		
1 ounce	28.4 grams	
1 pound	454 grams	0.45 kilogram

Metric to U.S.	
100 grams	3.5 ounces
500 grams	1.1 pounds
1 kilogram	2.2 pounds

LINEAR

1 centimeter	0.4 inch
1 inch	2.5 centimeters
1 meter	39.4 inches

m

continued

Measuring, continued

Temperature Temperature is a key factor in good cooking. Every well-equipped cook should have three types of thermometer: a meat thermometer, a candy thermometer, and a deep-fat thermometer. Meat thermometers come in two varieties: one that remains in the meat throughout the cooking and the instant-read type, which is inserted at the presumed moment of doneness and gives an accurate reading within several seconds. The latter kind is also handy for testing water temperature for activating yeast and similar tasks. Thermometers that work equally well for both candy making and deep-frying are available (those designed solely for frying measure slightly higher temperatures). An oven thermometer is also handy, used to calibrate your oven so it can be set precisely to required cooking temperatures. See also COOKING TOOLS.

TO OBTAIN FAHRENHEIT:
Multiply the Celsius figure by 9, divide by 5, then add 32. After 65°F, Celsius figures are often rounded off.
$$F° = 9C°/5 + 32$$

TO OBTAIN CELSIUS:
Subtract 32 from the Fahrenheit figure, multiply by 5, then divide by 9.
$$C° = 5(F° − 32)/9$$

Key Temperatures in Cooking

FAHRENHEIT	CELSIUS	DESCRIPTION
0°	−17°	
32°	0°	Freezing (water)
100° to 110°	38° to 43°	Yeast activation
130°	54°	Scalding
160°	71°	Safe internal temperature for meat, poultry, and eggs
160° to 180°	71° to 82°	Poaching
185° to 205°	85° to 96°	Simmering
212°	100°	Boiling (at sea level)
234°	112°	Soft ball (sugar)
244°	117°	Firm ball
250°	121°	Hard ball
275°	135°	
300°	149°	
350°	177°	
400°	204°	
450°	232°	
500°	260°	

MELON Long enjoyed only by aristocrats, sweet and fragrant melons now tumble from piled-up pyramids at every neighborhood market. Thin wedges of cantaloupe are ubiquitous inclusions on brunch plates, icy melon sorbets are refreshing desserts, and many agree that the essence of summer is a big wedge of watermelon with plenty of seeds to spit. Many melon varieties exist, but they can be divided into two broad categories: muskmelons and watermelons. Winter melon and bitter melon are members of the squash family.

Muskmelons A single ripe muskmelon can fill an entire room with its fragrance. Depending on the variety, rinds range in color from cream to yellow to pale green, with various patterns and combinations of streaks. Inside, the flesh can be white, pale orange, or the lightest of greens. They have a hollow center where all their seeds are connected in a fibrous mass. Two general types of muskmelons exist, distinguished by the texture of their skin. Netted melons, such as cantaloupe, have fine, raised ridges and are generally at their peak from mid-summer to early fall. Smooth-skinned melons, such as honeydew, have less aroma, juicier flesh, more delicate flavor, and a longer storage life. Belonging to a category of muskmelons known as winter melons (not related to the winter melon squash mentioned above), they are at their best—full of flavor—during the cooler months of autumn.

CANTALOUPE Popular in the United States. Beige netted skin, with undertones of green. Flesh is orange, moist, and fragrant. Cantaloupes are best in July and August.

CASABA Golden yellow, slightly wrinkled and ridged rind and creamy, pale yellow flesh. Any green in the skin indicates an unripe specimen. Peak season is September and October.

CHARENTAIS One of the true cantaloupes of France. The flesh is orange, while the skin is smooth, gently ribbed, and very pale green with radiating streaks of darker green. Best in July and August.

CHRISTMAS Also know as Santa Claus melon. Elongated and resembling a small, dark green watermelon with bright yellow streaks. Creamy white flesh tinged with pale green is similar in taste to honeydew. Peaks in December.

CRENSHAW Large, smooth-skinned, and slightly pointed at the stem end. Bright yellow rind mottled with dark green spots. Very fragrant flesh, cream to salmon colored, with a rich, spicy flavor. Best in August and September.

HONEYDEW Smooth skin that ripens from pale green to creamy yellow. Its pale green flesh is sweet and juicy. A hybrid with pink flesh is sometimes available. Peak season is from June to October.

PERSIAN Fine, brownish netting over dark green skin. Firm, sweet flesh is orange with faint pink tones. At its best in August and September.

Selecting Ripe muskmelons have a strong, sweet fragrance and give slightly when pressed at both ends. Muskmelons allowed to ripen on the vine will break away cleanly, leaving only a shallow, symmetrical indentation. A melon picked while unripe, in order to facilitate shipping, will have a green stem, ragged fibers, or an irregular scar where the stem once was. For varieties with a netted skin, look for netting that is pronounced and evenly distributed. Smooth-skinned melons should be just that, smooth. A fully ripe melon may have tiny cracks at the stem end. Choose a melon heavy for its size and free of blemishes, shriveled peel, or soft, moldy areas.

Storing Although it will not obtain the flavor of a vine-ripened melon, an unripe melon will sweeten slightly if left in a paper bag at room temperature for a few days. An exception is the honeydew, which will stay only as sweet as it was when harvested. Once ripe, melons will keep for up to 5 days in the refrigerator or a dark, cool place. Seal whole and cut melons in plastic wrap or an airtight container, as they readily absorb the odors and flavors of other foods while they transfer their own.

Preparing Cut muskmelons in half and scoop out their seeds with a large spoon. To keep the melon moist, peel and cut off slices only as needed.

Quick Tip

Muskmelons will taste sweeter if served at room temperature or only slightly chilled. Remove from the refrigerator about 30 minutes before cutting and serving.

Watermelons The flesh of watermelon, true to its name, is almost 95 percent water. Native to West Africa, watermelons were and are crucial sources of water in arid areas and in countries with polluted waterways. Lovingly tended, they can grow to 100 pounds, but most come to market at a comfortable armful of 10 to

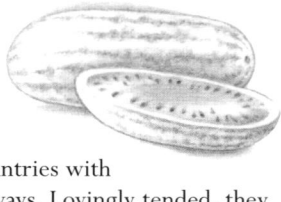

15 pounds. Unlike muskmelons, watermelons belong to a small, simple family. The choices are basically round or oblong, solid green or striped, with or without seeds. Watermelons have deep pink to bright red flesh that is crisp, juicy, and sweet. Yellow- and now orange-fleshed hybrids are sometimes available. Dark, shiny seeds are scattered throughout their flesh. Melons labeled seedless may still harbor a few soft, white, perfectly edible seeds. Watermelon seeds, roasted and dyed red, are served in Asia as a symbol of abundance during the Lunar New Year, and the rinds are made into pickles around the world.

Selecting Judging the ripeness of a whole watermelon is an inexact science, but a few indicators can point toward a sweet and juicy specimen. Look for a large, pale yellow (but not white, soft, or moldy) patch on one side, showing that it was left on the vine longer and may be sweeter than others. Shoppers knocking on watermelons in the produce section are listening for a particularly resonant thud that reveals the melon is juicy and full of water. Check cut watermelons for firm flesh with a deep red color and no white streaks. Watermelons are available year-round, but they are at their best during the summer months.

Storing Keep whole and cut watermelons in the refrigerator, because after they are picked from the vine, their flesh becomes increasingly dry and fibrous in warm temperatures. Although best eaten as soon as possible, a whole watermelon can stay in the refrigerator for up to 1 week. If it is too big, store it in a cold, dark place for no more than 3 days. Seal cut pieces in plastic wrap or an airtight container.

MELTING When certain solid ingredients must be incorporated into a mixture, melting them is often the best way to achieve uniform texture. Although solid at room temperature, foods such as butter, chocolate, gelatin, peanut butter, and sugar will become liquid if heated. Generally, melting calls for gentle heating in a double boiler or a microwave and frequent stirring.

MERINGUE One of the wonders of the kitchen is sweet, white, fluffy, delicate meringue, produced by beating a simple mixture of egg whites and sugar. Meringue can be either soft, glossy and smooth for spooning onto pies and other desserts, or hard, made with more sugar and baked until crisp, light, and dry. In Europe, hard meringues are important components in many classic desserts. Soft meringues are more popular in the United States.

Meringue Savvy A bowl and a whisk are all you need for whipping up meringue, but it helps to know a few secrets. Here are some tips that will keep your meringue up and your frustration down:

- While older egg whites will whip up more easily and to higher proportions, fresh egg whites have stronger proteins that hold air better and remain more stable once whipped.

- Separate eggs while they are still cold from the refrigerator, but set the whites aside for at least 30 minutes before whipping them. Room-temperature egg whites are easiest to whip.

- Make sure no egg yolk gets into the whites, which would prevent them from whipping up.

- Make sure your bowl and beaters are absolutely clean and free of fat.

- If possible, use a copper bowl. A harmless chemical reaction increases the beaten whites' volume and makes them more stable.

- If you do not have a copper bowl, add a small amount of cream of tartar or lemon juice before whipping the egg whites to increase their stability and volume.

Meringue Glossary

meringues are made in several styles, and each goes by a few different names. Following here are the classics.

DACQUOISE A Swiss meringue with finely chopped almonds or hazelnuts folded into it. Also known as a japonaise meringue, dacquoise is traditionally piped into spiraled rounds and then baked to form cake layers.

FRENCH MERINGUE Also called cold or simple meringue. After the egg whites are whipped to soft peaks with a small amount of sugar, the remaining sugar is folded in gently. French meringue is the lightest and most fragile of all meringues and must always be baked or incorporated into a batter and then cooked. Excellent for lightening batters and topping desserts.

ITALIAN MERINGUE A dense, stable meringue that is extremely smooth and shiny, created by slowly pouring hot sugar syrup into the egg whites during whipping. When baked, it has a more melting texture than the others. Since the meringue has been cooked by the hot sugar syrup, Italian meringue may be served with no further cooking. Ideal spread on filled pies and folded into puddings.

SWISS MERINGUE Also known as warm or cooked meringue, since the sugar (usually confectioners') and egg whites are beaten over hot water to dissolve the sugar completely and increase the height of the egg foam. It is a sturdy meringue and can be stored in the refrigerator for several days. Used in icings and decorations.

- Superfine sugar is ideal for making meringue, since it dissolves more quickly and completely than regular granulated sugar.
- Use the back of a spoon to swirl meringue peaks atop a pie.

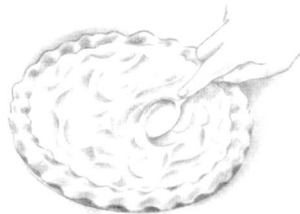

- Use or bake meringue immediately after preparing it.
- To avoid even the slightest discoloration, do not leave egg whites sitting in either aluminum or copper bowls.

Meringue Blues Got a problem with your meringue? Find the simple explanation here.

THERE ARE BEADS OF MOISTURE ON MY SOFT MERINGUE TOPPING. Meringue was overcooked. Use an oven thermometer to check your oven temperature, and don't cook your meringue topping on a cold filling, as the top can overcook before the meringue is cooked through.

MOISTURE IS OOZING FROM THE BOTTOM OF MY MERINGUE TOPPING. "Weeping" is caused by undercooking meringue. Cooking meringue topping on a cold filling can cause the bottom of the meringue to undercook.

Quick Tip

Serve meringue desserts soon after preparing. Soft meringue will begin weeping in warm, humid weather, and hard meringue will become soggy after it comes in contact with moist ingredients.

MESCLUN See GREENS, SALAD.

MEZZALUNA Meaning "half-moon" in Italian, the mezzaluna has a curved, crescent-shaped blade that chops herbs and small vegetables more quickly, safely, and easily than a chef's knife. With a wooden handle at each end, it is held with both hands and used with a rocking motion. Also known as a crescent cutter, it may be used on a cutting board or in a shallow wooden bowl designed for this purpose. See also KNIFE.

MICROWAVE OVEN Teenagers everywhere know microwave ovens are handy for making popcorn, and even the most traditional cook will admit there's no faster, easier way to melt butter or soften petrified brown sugar. Even better, many vegetables cooked in a microwave oven retain more nutrients and achieve perfect crisp-tenderness. Microwave ovens quickly defrost frozen meat or reheat leftovers.

Microwaves work by heating the moisture in a food. Anything that contains moisture can be cooked in a microwave; the less moist a food is, the longer it will take to cook. Lacking dry heat, microwave ovens do not brown meat, but for dishes that are normally steamed, simmered, or poached, they provide excellent moist cooking.

The appliance has been much maligned, yet nearly every kitchen boasts one and they do come in handy. Microwaves come in all shapes and sizes, some small enough to hang from a cupboard, others large and imposing. The technology has developed over the years so that today microwaves are easy, efficient, and safe. Most cooks think of them as another timesaving device or kitchen tool, rather than a replacement for conventional ovens and stove tops.

Microwave Savvy

- Microwaves of different wattage will produce varying results. The standard for most published microwave recipes is 700 watts. If yours has a different wattage (check your owner's manual), here is a general formula for converting cooking times in recipes: add or subtract 10 seconds for every 50 watts that your oven is below or above 700 watts, respectively. Experiment until you have a good sense of the power levels of your particular appliance.

- Since corners concentrate microwave energy, use round pans and plates to promote even cooking, and arrange appropriate foods in a circle.

- If your microwave does not have a turntable or a fan, be sure to rotate the dish and stir food frequently, especially thick liquids and chunky mixtures.

- Although microwaves do not heat up containers, they do heat up the food, which in turn makes the containers hot. Be sure to use pot holders when taking them from the microwave.

- Cut food into uniform-sized pieces for even cooking.

- Do not arrange whole foods or large pieces too snugly in the dishes. Allow a little space around each food so that the microwaves can reach it on all sides.

- It will take about twice as long to cook 2 potatoes as 1 potato, and nearly three times as long to cook 3 potatoes. For this reason, when cooking large amounts of food, it soon becomes just as efficient to use the conventional oven.

- If covering food with plastic wrap, turn back a corner or cut a small hole in the wrap to vent the dish. Don't let the plastic touch the food directly.

- Do not put metal in the microwave. (This includes foil wrappers and the shiny trim on dishes.) Use only plastic, glass, or ceramic containers that are specified microwave-safe.

- Pierce foods sealed in skins or membranes (egg yolks, sausages, tomatoes, potatoes) with a toothpick or fork to vent steam and prevent explosions.

- When melting chocolate, do not expect it to melt to a liquid pool. Remove it when it is soft and shiny and then stir the chocolate to liquefy fully.

- Food continues cooking after removal, so undercook dishes slightly in the microwave for perfect doneness.

See also OVEN.

MIE(N) See NOODLE.

MILK The milk of cows, goats, sheep, oxen, buffaloes, and yaks has been part of the human diet for thousands of years. Today, the term *milk* commonly refers to cow's milk. High in nutrients, milk and its products compose one of the fundamental food groups. Whether simply poured into a glass or transformed into béchamel sauce, cultured into nutritious yogurt or frozen into ice cream, milk is essential to the cuisines of many countries.

Quick Tip

Milk loses vitamins and flavor when exposed to sunlight or fluorescent light. If you buy your milk in glass bottles, keep it in the dark as much as possible or transfer it to a clean, airtight container that blocks out light.

The rich flavor of milk comes from its emulsified fats; its distinctive white color derives from casein protein; and its faintly sweet flavor reveals the presence of lactose, a type of sugar found only in milk. Most processed milk is fortified with vitamin D, which helps the body absorb calcium, and vitamin A.

Milk Glossary

The corner grocery store carries a wide range of cow's milk products—in cartons, in cans, in bottles, in boxes, on the shelf, in the refrigerated case. Here are the basic choices.

ACIDOPHILUS MILK Contains beneficial bacteria, *Lactobacillus acidophilus,* which aid in the digestion of milk.

BUTTERMILK Traditionally the liquid drained from churned butter. Today, milk is commercially cultured to develop the tangy flavor and creamy texture of buttermilk. For more details, see BUTTERMILK.

CONDENSED MILK Also known as sweetened condensed milk. Basically, condensed milk is evaporated milk with a high proportion of sugar (40 percent). It is also high in fat, at around 8 percent. Condensed milk has an ivory color, a syrupy consistency, and a glossy surface. It is sold in cans and used mainly in confections and desserts. After opening, transfer the milk to an airtight container and refrigerate for up to 2 weeks.

EVAPORATED MILK Has had about 60 percent of its water removed by heat. The process darkens the milk's color slightly to a pale ivory and gives it a faint caramelized flavor. Evaporated milk is sealed and sterilized in cans or cartons. Stable when heated, it is sometimes used in thick sauces and puddings that might otherwise curdle. It can be reconstituted with an equal amount of water, although it will taste a bit sweeter than fresh milk. Once you open a can, transfer the milk to an airtight glass or plastic container and keep it in the refrigerator for up to 1 week. Also available in low-fat and nonfat forms.

HALF-AND-HALF A mixture of milk and cream. It will not whip up but can be used in any recipe calling for a pouring cream. See also CREAM.

HOMOGENIZED MILK Forced through tiny holes to break its fat globules into small particles that will remain suspended evenly throughout the milk. Nonhomogenized milk will have cream that rises to the top. Almost all of the milk sold today is homogenized.

LACTOSE-REDUCED MILK Low-fat or nonfat milk with at least 70 percent of its lactose, or milk sugar, converted to more easily digested simple sugars. Over half of the world's population lacks the enzyme required to break down lactose, but adding the enzyme directly to milk reduces the amount of indigestible sugar. Breaking down the complex lactose sugar molecule into two simple sugars with higher sweetening power creates a milk that is sweeter in flavor as well as easier to digest.

LACTOSE-FREE MILK Low-fat or nonfat milk in which 99 percent of its lactose has been broken down. See Lactose-Reduced Milk, above.

LOW-FAT MILK Also known as partially skimmed milk, low-fat milk may contain either 1 or 2 percent fat. It has fewer calories and less fat than whole milk, but otherwise provides the same nutritional value.

NONFAT MILK Nonfat, or skim, milk must contain less than 0.2 percent fat.

PASTEURIZED MILK Heated briefly and then quickly cooled, a process that destroys most of the harmful bacteria in raw milk and extends its shelf life. Almost all milk sold in the United States has been pasteurized.

Milk Glossary, continued

POWDERED MILK Also called dry milk, this is pasteurized milk that has been dehydrated. It can be whole, low fat, or nonfat. To reconstitute, mix the powder with water. Although considered stable, the flavor of dry milk will deteriorate if the powder is exposed to light or air. Transfer dry milk powder to an airtight glass container, and keep it in the refrigerator for longer shelf life. Once reconstituted, the milk must be refrigerated; it will keep for up to 1 week. Powdered milk is used to boost the nutritional value of foods and to thicken sauces, and it is used in baking as well.

RAW MILK Has not been pasteurized. Many countries have banned raw milk, since bacteria can easily contaminate it. Stringently regulated (certified herds and hygienic premises), it is available in some health-food stores in the United States.

ULTRAPASTEURIZED MILK Heated to a higher temperature for a shorter period of time than pasteurized milk. It has a longer shelf life but also less flavor.

ULTRA HEAT PASTEURIZED (UHT) MILK Undergoes an extra-high heat treatment that effectively destroys all organisms present in the milk. Packed into aseptic containers, it can be stored unopened at room temperature for up to 3 months. Once opened, however, it should be stored in the refrigerator and should not be kept longer than 36 hours.

WHOLE MILK Contains around 3.5 percent fat. If not homogenized, it will have a layer of cream.

Selecting Choose cartons with the latest sell-by date for the freshest milk. The dates are conservative, so milk is usually still good for up to 5 days afterward, although it may have lost flavor by then.

Storing Unfortunately, bacteria also benefit from milk's abundant nutrients. To avoid contamination, keep milk in the refrigerator (no higher than 40°F) as much as possible. Buy milk at the end of your grocery shopping, avoid leaving the whole carton out on the table or counter for more than a few minutes, and do not pour milk that has been left at room temperature back into a carton of chilled milk. Since milk easily absorbs other odors and flavors, close cartons and bottles securely.

See also BUTTER; SCALDING; YOGURT.

Quick Tip

Milk curdles when mixed with acidic ingredients, such as lemon juice. To prevent curdling, mix a small amount of cornstarch into the acidic ingredient or the milk before combining them, then heat gently.

MILLET See GRAIN.

MINCING To chop food as finely as possible. Herbs and aromatics such as garlic are commonly minced to help release their flavor and meld them texturally into a mixture. The gently curved blade of a chef's knife allows for the two-handed rocking motion that makes quick work of mincing a pile of garlic or parsley. Be sure the knife is sharp, for a dull blade will crush and bruise ingredients instead of cleanly mincing them.

See also CHOPPING; GARLIC; HERB; KNIFE; MEZZALUNA; ONION.

MINT See HERB.

MIREPOIX See CELERY.

MIRLITON See CHAYOTE.

MISO See SOY FOODS.

MIXER Two basic types of motor-driven electric mixers are available, stand or standing and handheld or portable, and each has its place in the kitchen. Stand mixers are stationary machines good for large amounts and heavy batters.

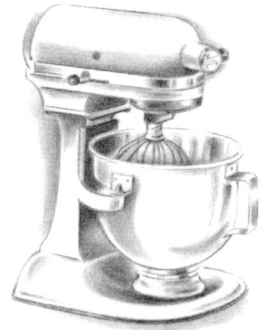

Stand mixer.

The basic set of attachments usually includes a wire whisk for beating egg whites or whipping cream, a paddle for creaming together butter and sugar and mixing batters, and a dough hook for kneading bread.

Attachments for stand mixer.

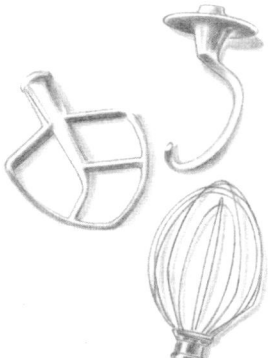

Handheld mixers are small, light portable machines. Lacking the power and special attachments of stand mixers, these appliances are adequate for most batters and soft doughs but they do not work well for stiff doughs. For long mixing tasks, such as making buttercream or beating large volumes of egg whites, handheld mixers can become tiring to hold. However, they can be used with nearly any bowl or pan, even those set over a pan of simmering water on the stove top.

Handheld mixer.

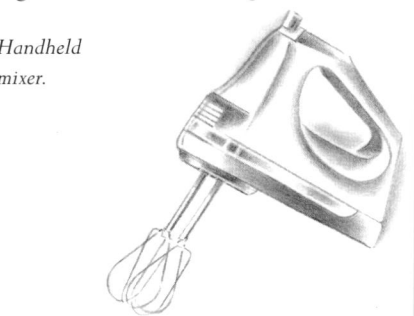

MIXING Mixing is the simple combining of two or more ingredients or mixtures. Some delicate batters require only a few turns of a spoon, leaving visible lumps but maintaining tenderness and airy height. Other recipes specify complete blending of ingredients until evenly distributed. A variety of equipment, from wooden spoons to whisks, mixers to blenders, allows a cook to obtain exactly the consistency needed. See also BEATING; BLENDING; MIXER; WHIPPING; WHISKING.

MIXING BOWL The well-equipped kitchen includes bowls in a range of materials, shapes, and sizes suitable for a variety of cooking and baking tasks. For example, whipping egg whites and creaming butter call for deep bowls. Some useful features include a turned rim or a beak for mess-free pouring, cup measurements marked

Materials for Mixing Bowls

CERAMIC Earthy and sturdy and standard in kitchens for centuries. Ceramic bowls change temperature slowly, keeping hot contents warm and cold ingredients cool. Be sure the glaze is food-safe.

COPPER For mixing egg whites. The moving whisk actually scrapes up minute amounts of copper ions that bond to the egg whites' unraveling proteins and stabilize them in the airy foam. Never mix acidic ingredients in copper; the food will react, taking on an unpleasant color and flavor. See NONREACTIVE.

GLASS Attractive for showing off colorful foods at the table, but not the most practical for mixing. Glass can be heavy and fragile, and its slippery surface can keep beaten egg whites from climbing and foaming up properly. Specially tempered heat- or flameproof Pyrex is available, fashioned either into bowls or into large measuring cups that can double as mixing bowls.

PLASTIC Light and convenient, and useful for storing or transporting foods when lidded. Avoid mixing delicately flavored ingredients or batters in them, however, since plastic can retain odors, flavors, and oils even after washing. In particular, residual oil can prevent egg whites from properly foaming.

STAINLESS STEEL There should be at least one stainless-steel bowl in every kitchen, if not a nesting set of various sizes. Stainless steel won't react with food, as copper or aluminum will, and is lighter and more durable than ceramic or glass.

on the side, airtight covers for storing prepared ingredients, rubber rings on the bottom for nonskid mixing, and the ability to nest, thus keeping storage space to a minimum. Knowing the advantages of certain materials, though, is the most important part of deciding which bowl to use.

MIZUNA See GREENS, SALAD.

MOLASSES A syrup used to sweeten baked goods, top breakfast dishes, and flavor sauces. Widely available in jars, molasses is a by-product of sugar refinement, a process that requires repeated boiling of cane syrup.

Selecting Each step in the molasses-making process produces a different type of molasses. Mixed with pure cane syrup, light molasses has the lightest flavor and color of any molasses and can be used as a topping for pancakes or waffles. Dark molasses is thicker, darker, stronger in flavor and less sweet than light molasses. It may be used interchangeably with light molasses and gives a distinctive flavor to baked beans, barbecue sauces, certain cookies, and gingerbread.

Quick Tip

Both light and dark molasses may be bleached with sulfur dioxide. Processed without sulfur, unsulfured molasses has a milder flavor.

Blackstrap molasses, also known as black treacle, is darker still than dark molasses and has a pronounced bitter flavor that some find overly strong. Considered healthier because it contains a high amount of minerals, it can sometimes be found in health-food stores. It should not be substituted for light or dark molasses in recipes.

Storing All styles of molasses can be kept in a cool, dark place for up to 1 year.

MOLDING Forming food into a specific shape, with special containers or simply by hand. Molded foods—fanciful terrines, rainbow gelatin salads, bright-colored ice-cream bombes, icy punch rings—recall a time when cooks regularly allowed hours for the preparation of meals.

Molds come in a wide range of sizes, shapes, and materials. Although today's more natural approach to food presentation has helped to banish large molds to decorative outposts on kitchen walls, many cooks still depend on ramekins, timbales, terrines, and rings to create dinner party fare. See also UNMOLDING.

MONTEREY JACK See CHEESE.

MOREL See MUSHROOM.

MORTAR & PESTLE Before electricity and food processors revolutionized the kitchen, a cook needed a mortar and pestle to grind, purée, and blend ingredients. Purists still eschew electrically powered machines for making a pesto, mole, or curry, insisting that such preparations require a mortar and pestle to crush the spices and herbs in a way that best releases their flavors and to give the cook better control over the end texture.

A bowl-shaped mortar holds the ingredients, while the club-shaped pestle crushes and grinds them. Mortars vary in magnitude and material, from palm-sized porcelain bowls etched with decorative ridges to substantial marble vessels to huge stone blocks that serve as permanent fixtures in many Indian homes. Although a pestle is often made of the same material as the mortar, it can also be carved from hardwood. Either the mortar or pestle must have an abrasive surface to work effectively.

Quick Bite

Molcajete y tejolote is the Mexican term for mortar and pestle. They are traditionally made of a rough-textured black volcanic rock called basalt.

MOUSSE A mousse is an airy, rich concoction of sweet or savory ingredients. It may be a suspension of fruit or chocolate in whipped cream served as an elegant dessert; or finely ground seafood lightened with cream and gelatin; or puréed chicken livers enriched with butter and seasonings. Some chilled mousses, also known as cold soufflés, contain beaten egg whites for extra height and lightness. A mousse that includes egg yolks, such as a classic chocolate mousse recipe, has a dense and creamy texture. Most mousses are served chilled, but both hot and frozen variations exist. Although closely related, molded Bavarian creams and chiffons, the fillings for ever-popular chiffon pies, have firmer textures that allow them to hold their shape.

MOZZARELLA See CHEESE.

MUENSTER Or Münster. See CHEESE.

MUFFIN Straddling the line between cake and bread, a muffin can be as healthful as bran studded with fresh or dried fruits or as decadent as a chocolate-chip variation topped with streusel and drizzled with a glaze. Although once a yeast bread, the modern muffin is usually leavened with baking powder or baking soda and is baked in distinctive pans with cup-shaped compartments. Muffin flavors range from apple and blueberry to banana-walnut and lemon-poppyseed. Muffins can be savory—such as cornmeal or oat muffins to accompany meals—as well as sweet.

Muffin Savvy

■ There are two kinds of muffin batter. Some batters are made by adding all the dry ingredients into the wet ones and mixing quickly; others are made like cakes, where butter and sugar are creamed together and dry and wet ingredients are alternately added. For the first style of batter, the ingredients should be mixed quickly with only a few turns of a spoon, just enough to bring the wet ingredients and dry ingredients together into a rough, lumpy mix. Any more stirring will create tough muffins.

■ Toss fruit and nuts with a little flour to coat them lightly before stirring them into the batter with the last few strokes of mixing. The thin layer of flour will help suspend them evenly throughout the muffins.

■ Fill any empty muffin cups halfway with water to ensure even cooking of the batter-filled cups and to prevent the pan from warping.

■ If you do not have a convection oven, turn the pan 180 degrees halfway through cooking for even browning.

■ Speed pan cleanup by using paper or foil muffin-cup liners.

HOW TO *Prepare Muffins in Advance*

1. Prepare pans and batter and fill pans, adding any nut or crunch toppings.
2. Place unbaked pans of muffin batter into the freezer. When firm, transfer the muffins to an airtight container or zippered freezer-weight plastic bag and freeze for 2 to 4 weeks.
3. To bake, preheat the oven and grease the same pan. Place the frozen batter back in the cups and bake without thawing, allowing about 15 minutes extra baking time.

Muffin Blues Got a problem with your muffins? Find the simple explanation here.

MUFFINS BROWN ON TOP BEFORE COOKING THROUGH. Oven heat was too high; pan was placed too close to top of oven.

MUFFINS DON'T RISE HIGH ENOUGH. Batter was allowed to sit for too long before baking; oven heat was too low.

MUFFINS HAVE CRATERS OR UNEVEN TOPS. Oven heat was too high.

MUFFINS HAVE HARD, SHINY TOPS AND LONG, VERTICAL INTERIOR TUNNELS. Batter was overmixed, developing the gluten and toughening the muffin.

MUFFINS STICK TO THE PAN. The pan was not greased sufficiently, or the muffins were left sitting too long in the pan after its removal from the oven.

MUFFINS TOPS HAVE A CENTER KNOB AND A SPREADING BASE. Too much batter was put into each muffin cup.

See also BAKEWARE.

MULBERRY See BERRY.

MULLING To sweeten and infuse a drink with spices and fruit. Mulled wine or cider, heated gently with such flavoring ingredients as sugar syrup, cinnamon sticks, cloves, allspice, and orange peel makes a comforting treat in the wintertime. Whole spices may be placed in a tea ball to save the trouble of straining the wine or cider. A mulled drink is often fortified with spirits.

MUNG BEAN See BEAN, DRIED.

MUNG BEAN NOODLE See NOODLE.

MÜNSTER Or Muenster. See CHEESE.

MUSHROOM See page 298.

MUSLIN See CHEESECLOTH.

Mushroom

Almost 40,000 varieties of mushroom exist in the world, but only a fraction of them make it to the table, where they are enjoyed for their rich, earthy flavor. For culinary purposes, mushrooms are divided into two categories: cultivated and wild.

Today, as demand for different varieties increases, mushroom growers are able to cultivate more and more types, and the line between cultivated and wild is blurring. The most flavorful—and most expensive—mushrooms, however, are still gathered by foragers in forests under trees or on old stumps. Highly prized mushrooms, such as the matsutake and the morel, have eluded all attempts at cultivation. Around the world, mushroom hunting after the rains of spring or during the cool mornings of autumn is still a thriving—and ultimately delicious—tradition.

Although mushrooms can be cooked by almost any method, they taste wonderful when simply sautéed in olive oil, with a little garlic, over high heat. Mushrooms are also good tossed with olive oil (be judicious; these little sponges can soak up a lot of oil) and seasonings, then roasted or grilled gill side up to retain their juices. To grill small mushrooms, thread them on skewers.

Caution!

Some wild mushrooms are fatally toxic, and they can closely resemble edible varieties. Do not pick or eat wild mushrooms unless a trained expert collector familiar with local varieties identifies them. Supermarket "wild" mushrooms generally are farmed and certainly not poisonous.

A Guide to Mushrooms

BUTTON MUSHROOM See White Mushroom, page 300.

CHANTERELLE Also known as girolle. Bright golden yellow and shaped like a trumpet, this distinctive mushroom is appreciated for its apricot-flavored 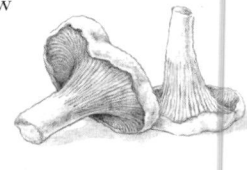 overtones. A less-common black variety, called black trumpet or trumpet of death, is close in flavor but has a more delicate texture. Chanterelles are not cultivated to date.

CHINESE BLACK MUSHROOM Always sold dried. The best are actually beige to brown with cream-colored cracks radiating over the caps. See also Shiitake, page 300.

CLOUD EAR MUSHROOM Ruffled, brown-black Chinese mushroom with almost no flavor. Its crunch stands up to heat, however, and it adds texture to soups, 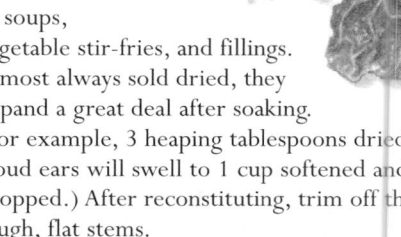 vegetable stir-fries, and fillings. Almost always sold dried, they expand a great deal after soaking. (For example, 3 heaping tablespoons dried cloud ears will swell to 1 cup softened and chopped.) After reconstituting, trim off the tough, flat stems.

CREMINO MUSHROOM The common brown mushroom. Cremini (the Italian plural) are closely related to common white mushrooms and can be used whenever white mushrooms are called for, but they have a light brown color, firmer texture, and fuller flavor. Cremini mature to become portobellos.

ENOKI Tiny, white Asian mushrooms with long, thin stems and caps shaped like pinheads, enoki are crisp and delicate in flavor. Available fresh during the winter or water-packed in cans or plastic tubs, they make beautiful garnishes for salads and clear soups.

MATSUTAKE A delicacy in Japan, the matsutake appears beneath pine trees for a brief period in midautumn. It has a slightly pointed, thick, dark brown cap and a meaty stem. Not cultivated and difficult to find, the matsutake appears in the northwest region of the United States, but the most flavorful ones come from Japan. Sauté them or wrap in foil and place on the grill.

MOREL Considered the king of mushrooms, the morel has an intense, musky flavor that makes it highly sought after. The uncultivated mushroom has a dark, elongated, spongelike cap and hollow stem. The crevices tend to fill with sand and insects, so you may want to treat them as an exception to the no-washing rule: immerse them briefly in a large bowl of water and agitate to dislodge all the sand. You can halve them lengthwise for easier cleaning.

Morels are especially delicious in cream sauces or scrambled eggs.

OYSTER MUSHROOM Cream to pale gray mushroom, with a fan shape and a subtle flavor of shellfish. They used to be wild only but are now cultivated. Look for smaller, younger oysters, since they become tough and bitter as they grow older. They weep a great amount of liquid, so are best grilled, roasted, or stir-fried. Cook oyster mushrooms just until heated through to preserve their silken texture.

PORCINO MUSHROOM Also known as cepe and bolete. Porcini (Italian for "little pigs")

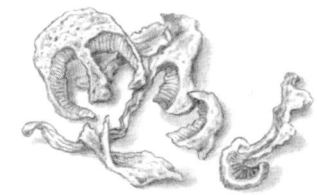

Dried porcini.

are indeed nicely plump, with a firm texture, sweet fragrance, and full, earthy flavor. An uncultivated variety, they have caps similar to cremini in shape and color, but their stems are thick and swollen. Although popular in Europe, the fresh mushrooms are difficult to find in the United States, where dried porcini are used instead. They are excellent in soups, pasta sauces, and risotto. Thinly slice young, fresh ones and dress with a simple vinaigrette.

PORTOBELLO MUSHROOM A cultivated mushroom, the portobello is in fact a mature cremino, allowed to grow until the cap is about 6 inches wide and dark brown. Portobellos have a rich,

continued

smoky flavor and meaty texture. Leave the caps whole for grilling or roasting, or slice and sauté them to top pasta or polenta. Food mixed or cooked with portobello mushrooms will take on some of their color, turning an unpleasant gray, so prepare the mushrooms separately and add just before serving. The thick, tough stems should be removed (and may be saved for stocks, soups, or sauces).

SHIITAKE The most popular mushroom in Japan and now widely cultivated. Buff to dark brown, they are available fresh and dried. Fresh shiitake should have smooth, plump caps, while better-quality dried ones will have pale cracks in the cap's surface. Dried shiitake and Chinese black mushrooms are interchangeable. Shiitake take well to grilling, roasting, stir-frying, and sautéing. Remove their thin, tough stems before using.

STRAW MUSHROOM Grown on straw left in rice paddies after harvest. These small, globe-shaped mushrooms have a distinct earthy flavor and a color ranging from beige to brown. Only available canned outside of Asia, they are a common addition to soups and stir-fries.

TREE OR WOOD EAR MUSHROOM Smaller, more delicate variety of the cloud ear, resembling crinkled black flakes. They are used much like cloud ears.

WHITE MUSHROOM The cultivated, all-purpose mushroom sold in grocery stores. Sometimes called button mushrooms, although the term refers specifically to young, tender ones with closed caps. For general cooking, use the medium-sized mushrooms with little or no gills showing. The large ones are excellent for stuffing.

Selecting Fresh mushrooms should be firm and have smooth, unblemished caps. Avoid any that are broken, limp, wrinkled, soggy, or moldy. Stems with gray, dried ends indicate that the mushrooms have been stored too long. Some mushrooms have closed caps, like the common button mushroom. For these varieties, if the caps are open so that the gills are exposed, the mushrooms are too old. For varieties where the gills are exposed, like portobellos, check that the gills are unbroken. As mushrooms age, they dry out, so the heaviest mushrooms should be the freshest. If you plan to cook mushrooms whole, select those with caps of the same size for even cooking. Check that packaged, pre-sliced mushrooms are not wrinkled or discolored. Mushrooms are also available whole or sliced in jars, preserved in a brine or marinated with oil and herbs.

Storing Refrigerate fresh mushrooms for no more than 3 or 4 days, keeping them in a paper bag to absorb excess moisture. Spread delicate varieties in a single layer on a tray and cover them with a damp cloth. If sealed in plastic, mushrooms will become slimy and mold quickly.

Preparing Mushrooms absorb water readily, becoming soggy and flavorless if left to soak. While some cooks insist that you should not wash mushrooms at all, a quick rinse and a thorough drying with paper towels immediately before cooking will not hurt them. If you have time or plan to cook only a few mushrooms, wipe them clean with a damp cloth or brush. Special mushroom brushes are available for gentle removal of dirt, or a toothbrush with soft bristles will work. Trim the dried end of tender stems; but if the stems are tough, remove them completely (and save them for soup or stock).

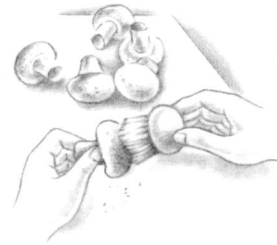

Brushing a mushroom.

When mushrooms are sautéed, they will at first give off a great deal of liquid when they hit the hot pan. Continue to cook them until they have reabsorbed all their flavorful juices and the pan is almost dry. Some mushrooms will shrink to less than half their original size.

HOW TO *Reconstitute Dried Mushrooms*

Reconstituted, or rehydrated, dried mushrooms may be substituted for fresh ones in most cooked dishes, although they may take longer to become tender. Cooks love dried mushrooms for their intense flavors and firmer textures.

1. Cover dried mushrooms with warm water or stock, letting sliced ones or pieces soak for 30 minutes and whole ones for 1 hour. Or for fuller flavor, reconstitute them in cold liquid overnight in the refrigerator.

2. Do not discard the flavorful soaking liquid. Strain it through cheesecloth or a coffee filter and use it in the same recipe as the mushrooms, or add it to other soups or sauces.

Quick Bite

Duxelles, a classic French mixture of finely chopped mushrooms and aromatics, is cooked until rich and flavorful. It is used primarily in sauces and fillings.

Mushroom Savvy

■ Toss raw white mushrooms, whole or sliced, with lemon juice to prevent discoloring.

■ To keep white mushrooms snowy white, rub them with a paper towel that has been dipped in acidulated water.

■ Cooking pale mushrooms in a pan of aluminum or cast iron will darken them, although it won't affect their flavor.

■ For the best flavor and texture in a finished dish, sauté mushrooms before adding them to a soup, sauce, or risotto.

■ For a more complex flavor, try replacing a small portion of the fresh mushrooms called for in a recipe with rehydrated dried ones.

■ To stretch wild mushrooms, mix them with less expensive cremini or white button mushrooms. Experiment with different combinations, but avoid mixing highly flavored ones with delicate varieties, or the flavors will not be balanced.

HOW TO *Make Duxelles*

1. Finely chop mushrooms—any variety will do—along with tender stems. (Because they will shrink significantly, use about twice the volume of fresh mushrooms as you will need cooked for the dish.) Wrap them in a kitchen towel, a handful at a time, and squeeze to remove as much moisture as possible.

2. In a skillet over medium-high heat, briskly sauté the mushrooms with finely chopped shallots or onion in unsalted butter, stirring occasionally, until the mushrooms and shallots or onion are lightly browned and the mushrooms begin to separate. The timing will depend on the type and quantity of mushroom used.

3. When the mushrooms are dry and tender, season with salt and freshly ground pepper. (Sometimes ground nutmeg is added as well.) Remove from the heat and use immediately or let cool, cover, and refrigerate.

See also TRUFFLE.

MUSSEL A saltwater mollusk with slightly pointed shells ranging in color from blue-green to yellowish brown to inky black. Mussels have cream to orange-colored meat 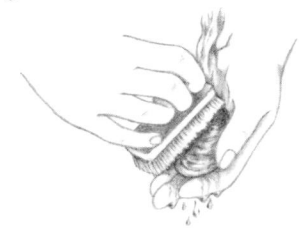 that is sweeter than that of oysters or clams. Mussels are an excellent buy, too, since they generally are less expensive than other shellfish.

The majority of the mussels available in the marketplace today are cultivated. Although there are dozens of different species, the two mostly widely available are the Atlantic blue or common mussel and the Pacific green-lipped or New Zealand mussel. The blue mussel, which is actually quite black, is 2 to 3 inches long. The green-lipped mussel is larger, 3 to 4 inches long, but its meat is also tougher.

Selecting Buy live mussels from a reputable fishmonger. They should have a fresh sea smell, with no trace of ammonia. Tap the mussels, and do not buy them if they stay open, indicating a dead or at least de-hydrated mussel. To cut preparation time, look for already-shucked and cooked mussels chilled in the seafood section or freezer case of your supermarket. Already-shucked mussels are also available frozen, and occasionally mussels can be found frozen on the half shell. Mussels are also available smoked and canned.

Storing Remove live mussels from their packaging, place them in a bowl, cover them completely with a moist kitchen towel, and refrigerate. Dampen the towel if it dries out during storage. Since they also need air, do not cover mussels with water or seal them in a plastic bag. Fresh mussels are best if used as soon as possible; keep them for no more than 1 day. To freeze, place live mussels in a zippered plastic freezer bag and store for no more

than 3 months. Defrost frozen mussels slowly in the refrigerator before cooking.

Preparing Scrub grit off the shells of fresh mussels with a stiff-bristled brush, then debeard each mussel, as needed.

Scrubbing a mussel.

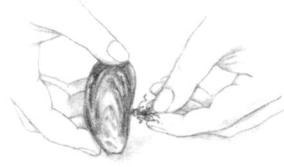

HOW TO *Debeard a Mussel*

1. Remove the beard, the little tuft of fibers the mussel uses to connect to rocks or pilings, by cutting and scraping it with a knife or scissors. You may also pull it sharply down toward the hinged point of the shells with your fingers, but this does tend to pull away a bit of the meat, so many cooks prefer to cut it.

Do not debeard mussels more than an hour before cooking, since doing so kills them. All mussels used to come with a very tough beard, but today farm-raised ones have hardly any beard, making cleaning them less of a chore.

While cleaning them, discard any mussels that are very light, as they are likely dead, or any that are heavy with sand. Remember that live mussels will close tightly, if a little slowly, when touched. If in doubt, try twisting the shells sideways in opposite directions, as if unscrewing a bottle cap. The shells of dead mussels will break apart easily. The mussels should open up again after cooking. Check cooked mussels and discard any that failed to open.

Caution!

Since mussels are susceptible to water contaminants and "red tides" of poisonous plankton, be sure to read posted signs and check with local health or game agencies before collecting your own mussels.

To shuck mussels, or remove the shells, steam them with 1 inch of liquid for 2 to 3 minutes, just until they loosen and open slightly. With a small knife—preferably one designed for shucking clams—pry open the shells and cut the meat away. Reserve the steaming liquid to use in the sauce.

Smaller mussels are best for steaming, while the larger ones lend themselves to stuffing, broiling, or grilling.

See also DEBEARDING; SHELLFISH.

MUSTARD, PREPARED At its simplest, prepared mustard is a mixture of ground mustard seed and water. But this basic paste has been refined around the world by the addition of everything from wine, beer, vinegar, fruit juice, and honey to a multitude of herbs and aromatics. Prepared mustards can be smooth or coarse-grained, depending on whether the seeds are finely ground or left mostly whole. They turn up on deli sandwiches and hot dogs and are stirred into vinaigrettes and glazes.

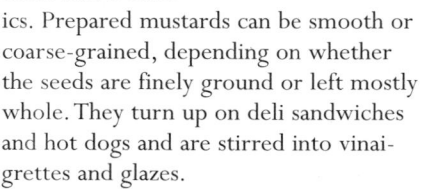

Selecting Finer mustards are available in glass jars, while the popular American style

Prepared-Mustard Glossary

AMERICAN MUSTARD The classic ballpark mustard. Made from yellow seeds, it is mild, yet with an edge of sharp pungency. Its bright yellow color comes from the addition of ground turmeric.

CHINESE MUSTARD Hot, pale yellow mustard served in Chinese restaurants, made by mixing powdered mustard with water.

DIJON MUSTARD Silky smooth and slightly tangy. Originating in Dijon, France, the mustard contains brown or black seeds, white wine, and herbs.

ENGLISH MUSTARD Very hot. Made from a combination of brown or black seeds and yellow seeds that have been ground very finely, along with wheat flour and turmeric. Usually mixed from powder.

GERMAN MUSTARD Mild or hot, hearty, and slightly sweet, to complement German sausages. It can be coarse or smooth. It has a dark color since the whole seed is used.

is found in convenient squeeze bottles. As with other condiments, experiment with different mustards, finding those you like.

Storing Since naturally occurring compounds effectively inhibit the growth of bacteria in prepared mustard, it will keep indefinitely in a tightly lidded glass or ceramic container in the refrigerator.

See also SPICE.

MUSTARD GREENS See GREENS, DARK.

MUSTARD SEED See SPICE.

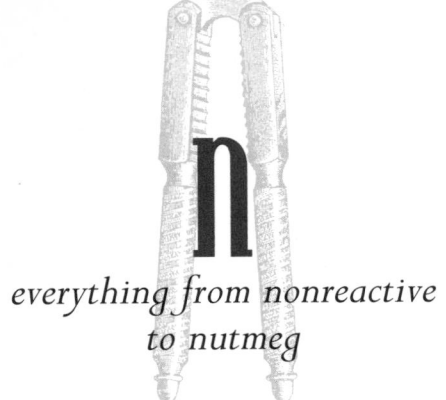

everything from nonreactive to nutmeg

NAVY BEAN See BEAN, DRIED.

NECTARINE See PEACH.

NONREACTIVE Every cook who regularly reads recipes has seen the following phrase, "combine the ingredients in a nonreactive bowl or pan." The meaning behind this instruction is quite simple: acidic ingredients such as tomatoes, citrus juice, vinegar, wine, and most vegetables will react with certain metals, resulting in a chemical reaction that creates an "off" flavor and unappealing (though harmless) dark color. A nonreactive pan or bowl is one made of or lined with a material—most commonly stainless steel, enamel, glass—that will not react with acidic ingredients. Reactive materials include nonanodized aluminum, unlined copper, or cast iron. Cast iron is the least problematic reactive material, however, and it can generally be used for preparing acidic food if the food is not left in the pan for an extended period of time.

NONSTICK See BAKEWARE; COOKWARE.

NOODLE See opposite page.

NOPAL CACTUS The nopal, also known as the prickly pear cactus, is grown both for its succulent, oval, flat pads, or paddles, and its sweet, egg-shaped fruits called prickly pears. The thorn-covered paddles, or *nopales* in Spanish, have a taste reminiscent of green beans, and the cleaned pads are cut up, cooked, and served as a vegetable, in salads, or in scrambled eggs. The fruits, also known as Indian figs and, in Spanish, *tunas,* appear in late summer on the mature joints of the plant. They range from pale yellow to magenta to red and are eaten out of hand or puréed and used as a dessert sauce or for making sorbet.

Selecting Look in Latin markets and well-stocked supermarkets for firm, slim paddles that are free of wrinkles and blemishes. They should have a fresh, bright green color. Fresh paddles are occasionally sold, both whole and cut up, with the spines removed, a real time-saver. Cactus pieces are also sold in cans or jars. Choose firm prickly pears that have a slight sheen.

Storing Refrigerate fresh paddles or fruits in plastic bags for up to 4 days. Once opened, canned cactus pieces should be refrigerated for no more than 1 week. If left on a countertop, underripe prickly pear fruits will soften within a few days.

Preparing To remove nopal spines, don heavy gloves or use a thick towel to hold the paddle, then pare away the bumps that conceal the tiny thorns and trim off the tough, fibrous base. Do not peel away all the green skin that sheaths the paddle. Cut as directed in individual recipes, then cook in boiling salted water until tender, 10 to 20 minutes, depending on the freshness and age of the cactus; drain, rinse well to rid the pieces of sliminess, and use as desired.

Prickly pears are usually sold with the spines removed (watch out for overlooked ones) but must be peeled and seeded before eating.

Noodle

Stemming perhaps from the perennial debate between those who believe the Chinese noodle predated spaghetti and those who insist Italians made pasta long before the time of Marco Polo, the terms *noodle* and *pasta* refer more to geographic distinctions than culinary classifications.

For details about the most popular and widespread Western-style noodles, see PASTA. Of course, pasta is not the only noodle story in the West. German, Dutch, and Eastern European noodle dishes like spaetzle and kugel are some of the world's most enduring comfort foods.

In Asia, where noodles symbolize long life, they are eaten throughout the day. A big bowl of noodle soup is a standard breakfast, stir-fried noodles from the corner vendor make a quick lunch, and seafood-crowned crisp fried noodles are served at formal dinners. Noodle uses vary, but most can be served with stir-fried meats, seafood, and vegetables. Try tossing your favorite stir-fry dish with cooked noodles in place of serving it over rice. They are also refreshing served cold, with simple sauces and thinly sliced vegetables.

Oodles of Noodles The flour, whether bean, rice, or wheat, used to make Asian noodles generally also categorizes them.

BUCKWHEAT NOODLES Popular in Japan, where they are known as soba, these grayish beige noodles have square-cut edges and a nutty, faintly sweet flavor. They are available fresh and dried, and are used in soups or chilled and accompanied with a dipping sauce during summer. Cook dried buckwheat noodles in boiling water until al dente.

CELLOPHANE NOODLES See Mung Bean Noodles, page 306.

DUMPLING WRAPPERS Rolled into thin sheets from the same dough as wheat noodles and then cut into squares or rounds, dumpling wrappers vary in size and thickness. Paper-thin squares are shaped into tender wontons for soup, slightly thicker rounds encase pot stickers, and larger sheets make crisp, golden brown egg rolls. Packaged in plastic, fresh wrappers keep for up to 1 week if sealed well and refrigerated. You'll find them in the refrigerator cases of Asian markets. When selecting them, thumb the stack of wrappers to check that their edges are firm and separate easily.

EGG NOODLES Much like Italian egg pasta, egg noodles are cut or extruded from a dough of wheat flour, eggs, and salt. The noodles can be narrow or wide, thin or thick, round or square, and are available dried or fresh, in tangled skeins or neat bundles. Check the packaging carefully; some noodles labeled "egg flavored" are artificially flavored. Asian egg noodles can be boiled and added to soups, braised with sauces, fried into a crisp cake, or stir-fried with meat and vegetables. Shrimp- and crab-flavored Asian egg noodles contain roe

continued

Noodle, continued

from the shellfish to complement seafood dishes. Boil fresh egg noodles for 2 to 3 minutes until al dente. See also PASTA.

MIE(N) See Wheat Noodles, below.

MUNG BEAN NOODLES Also called cellophane noodles, transparent noodles, glass noodles, or bean thread noodles, mung bean noodles are dried noodles made from ground mung bean flour and water. They resemble thin, white wires when dry but become soft and transparent after cooking. They are usually bundled in 1½-ounce skeins. Soften in warm water for 20 minutes before using in thin soups and stir-fried noodle dishes. If you wish to cut the noodles into shorter lengths, do so with scissors after soaking. Deep-fried without soaking, they expand into a nest of puffy, white crisps.

RICE NOODLES Made from rice flour and water, rice noodles vary in size from very thin dried rice sticks to wide, ribbonlike noodles. They appear in pad thai, spring rolls, and Vietnamese soups. Soak dried rice noodles in warm water for 20 minutes, cook them for 2 to 3 minutes just until al dente, and then rinse them in cold water. Soak but do not precook if you plan to stir-fry them; the sauce will soften and cook them just enough. Unlike mung bean noodles, dried rice noodles can overcook easily and turn to mush. Look for them in clear plastic packages, most often sold dried either as loose skeins or tightly tied into bricklike bundles. Fresh rice noodles, sold cut into ribbons usually about ¾ inch wide or in sheets to be cut as desired by the cook, are available in Asian markets. They are served hot or at room temperature. Wider versions generally are used in stir-fried dishes, while narrower ones are added to soups. Cook them for 1 to 2 minutes in boiling water to heat them through and make them pliable.

RICE VERMICELLI Often confused with rice noodles, dried rice vermicelli are more creamy in color, very straight, and packaged in small, ribbon-tied bundles. They cook extremely quickly, often needing only a soaking in hot water before being drained. They are delicate in texture and flavor and are used in both sweet and savory dishes, from Indonesian soups to Indian desserts. Like mung bean noodles, they expand to feathery, crisp threads when deep-fried.

SOBA NOODLES See Buckwheat Noodles, page 305.

SOMEN NOODLES See Wheat Noodles, below.

UDON NOODLES See Wheat Noodles, below.

WHEAT NOODLES Called *mie* or *mien,* a term derived from Chinese, in many Asian countries, wheat noodles are made from wheat flour, water, and salt and are sold fresh and dried. Without eggs, they tend to be lighter in color than egg noodles but come in the same variety of sizes and shapes. In Japan, thin wheat noodles are called *somen,* and thick, hearty wheat noodles are known as *udon.* After they have been boiled, wheat noodles may be fried into crisp pancakes, braised in a thick sauce, or added to soups.

WONTON WRAPPERS See Dumpling Wrappers, page 305.

Selecting Noodles are available dried, fresh, and frozen, with the last two primarily found in Asian markets. In general, fresh noodles are the best. Check packages for firm noodles that separate easily and avoid any that look soft, gray, or clumped. Dried noodles should not have pale spots or many broken pieces.

Storing Keep fresh noodles sealed in plastic in the refrigerator for up to 3 days. Fresh noodles freeze well, but defrost them completely before cooking. Store dried noodles in a cool, dark place for up to 6 months.

Preparing See specific noodle entries above for special instructions. Fresh and dried noodles are usually boiled before they are used. In general, cook noodles in a large pot of unsalted boiling water, stirring gently from time to time to separate the noodles while they cook. They should be cooked briefly, just until they are al dente. Once the water has returned to a boil and depending on size, fresh or thawed noodles require only 1 to 2 minutes, while dried noodles may need 2 to 3 minutes, or longer. Drain noodles in a colander and rinse them with cold water, tossing constantly, to stop the cooking and wash away excess starch that would cloud stocks and overthicken stir-fries and braises. Use as directed. (Not all cooks agree that noodles should be rinsed with cold water. Follow the recipe or use your own judgment.)

If coated with a tiny amount of oil and wrapped well, cooked noodles can be refrigerated for a day. Although not traditionally done in Asian cooking, some Westerners like to cook fresh egg noodles directly in soups without precooking, so that the extra starch coating the noodles will thicken the stock into more of a sauce consistency.

See also AL DENTE; PASTA.

NORI See SEAWEED.

NUT See page 308.

NUTMEG Although long prescribed as medicine and burnt as incense, nutmeg did not enter the kitchen until the 16th century. It is the seed of a tropical evergreen tree: brown, oblong, and closely wrapped in a brilliant red, lacy membrane. (The membrane, or aril, becomes the similarly flavored spice known as mace.) Whole nutmegs resemble unshelled pecans. The spice's warm sweetness complements creamy sauces, egg and cheese dishes, spiced cakes and cookies, fruit desserts, vegetables, and hot drinks. In France, a pinch of ground nutmeg is the secret ingredient in many spinach dishes.

Selecting Both whole and ground nutmeg are widely available, but nutmeg you grind or grate yourself from the whole spice far surpasses the packaged powdered spice.

Storing Keep ground and whole nutmeg in airtight containers away from light and heat. Whole nutmeg will keep for up to 2 years, but the flavor of ground nutmeg will dissipate after 6 months.

Preparing Grate whole nutmeg on specialized nutmeg graters, which have tiny rasps and usually a small compartment for storing a nutmeg or two. The finest rasps of a box grater may also be used. Nutmeg is powerful; even a tiny pinch will flavor an entire dish. Add it at the start of cooking to allow its flavor to mellow and meld with other ingredients.

See also GRATING; SPICE.

NUTRITION See FAT & OIL; FOOD GUIDE PYRAMID; LABEL TERMS; LOW-FAT COOKING.

Nut

Nuts find favor in kitchens the world over. Almonds thicken romesco sauce in Spain, cashews add crunch to curries in India, pecan halves generously fill pies in the American South, and rose-scented pistachios nestle among filo layers in Greece.

An essential ingredient in virtually every cuisine, nuts provide richness, flavor, body, crunch, and vital nutrients in dishes both sweet and savory. In their purest form, with their varied shapes and hues, unshelled nuts piled high in a festive bowl help mark the autumn season.

Most nuts have a hard shell, a protective coating developed by plants to shield their seeds from hungry animals. Inside each shell is usually one edible kernel. Once a staple in the diets of early hunter-gatherers, nuts are dense in nutrients, especially potassium, iron, vitamin E, and the B vitamins. But since they boast a high amount of fat and calories as well as proteins, nuts are best used in moderate amounts. Fortunately, even a light sprinkle of nuts will add noticeable flavor and texture to a variety of dishes such as pasta, salad, or ice cream.

A Guide to Nuts

ALMOND The meat found inside the pit of a dry fruit related to peaches, the almond is delicate and fragrant. It has a pointed, oval shape and a smooth texture that lends itself well to elegant presentations.

BRAZIL NUT Enclosed in a dark, hard, roughly textured shell shaped like a small orange segment, Brazil nuts taste somewhat like the meat of a coconut. They are the seeds of 250-foot-high trees that grow only in tropical regions of South America and require great labor to harvest. Best eaten as snacks or used in desserts.

CANDLENUT Looking like large macadamias, and sold packaged in Asian markets, these nuts of a native Malaysian bush are traditionally ground and mixed into the curries and spice pastes of the region to add body and richness. Macadamia or Brazil nuts or cashews may be substituted. The nut's name comes from the fact that Malaysian natives sometimes used the ground nuts as candles.

CASHEW A smooth, kidney-shaped nut from a tree native to Africa and India. They are always sold removed from their hard shell and caustic lining. Most commonly eaten whole as a snack, cashews also make excellent nut butter.

CHESTNUT Known as *marrons* in France, chestnuts are large and wrinkled and have a smooth, shiny, mahogany-colored shell shaped like a turban slightly flattened on one side. Unlike other nuts, they contain a high amount of starch and little oil. Often treated as a vegetable and almost always cooked, such as in a puréed soup or mixed with Brussels sprouts, sweet and rich chestnuts are also popular simply roasted whole and eaten while still hot.

You must cook chestnuts by briefly boiling or roasting them to loosen their tough outer shells and thin, bitter skins. Note that if you let the chestnuts cool after roasting or blanching them, they will again become difficult to peel. If they do cool, simply return them to a hot oven or hot water for 5 minutes to warm them up. For large amounts, roast or blanch and peel the nuts in batches, working steadily and without distractions.

HOW TO *Boil Chestnuts*

1. Using a small, sharp knife, score, or shallowly cut, an X in the flat side of the nut, being careful not to cut through the nutmeat.

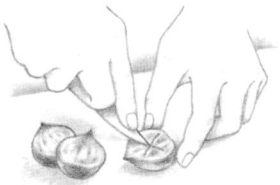

2. Put the nuts into a large pot of boiling water and boil for 12 to 15 minutes. (They take 30 to 45 minutes if you're going to eat them plain.)
3. Drain and return the nuts to the still-hot pot (turn off the heat below it). Cover the pot to keep the nuts warm.
4. Take the nuts 1 or 2 at time from the pot, using a kitchen towel or pot holder. Peel back the scored X using your fingers or the knife. Peel off the outer shell and the thin, beige inner skin. Discard both the outer and inner skins.

HOW TO *Roast Chestnuts*

1. Using a small, sharp knife, score, or shallowly cut, an X in the flat side of the nut. Be careful not to cut through the nutmeat.

2. Lay the nuts in a single layer on an ungreased baking sheet and roast in a 350°F oven until the nuts are fragrant and the scored portions begin to separate from the shells, 15 to 20 minutes. (If you're going to eat them plain, increase the heat to 400°F and bake until they give slightly when pressed with oven mitt—protected fingers.)

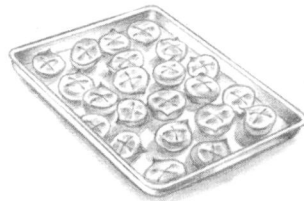

3. Transfer the nuts to a platter or heatproof surface and cover with a damp kitchen towel to keep them warm.
4. Using a kitchen towel or pot holder, pick up each nut and, using your fingers or the knife, peel back the scored X. Peel off the hard outer shell and the thin, beige, soft inner skin. Discard both outer shell and inner skin. Discard any nuts that, once peeled, look dried out.

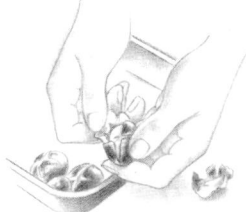

5. Eat the chestnuts immediately or use as directed in a recipe.

Quick Tip

Chestnuts have traditionally been roasted in fireplaces. They should be scored with an X first and nestled in the hot ashes of a dying fire. After 15 to 20 minutes, they will be fragrant and easy to shell.

continued

Nut, continued

COCONUT Like the almond, the coconut is the actual seed of a tree, a palm that grows in almost every tropical area. A dark brown, fibrous husk and a very hard shell enclose the rich, white flesh inside. See also COCONUT.

FILBERT See Hazelnut, below.

HAZELNUT Also known as filberts, grape-sized hazelnuts have hard shells that come to a point like an acorn, cream-colored flesh, and a sweet, rich, buttery flavor. Difficult to crack, they usually are sold already shelled.

MACADAMIA NUT Usually sold shelled, this rich nut originated in Australia but is now also grown widely in Hawaii. Smooth, off-white, and round, it resembles a large chickpea. Macadamias add crunch and sweet, buttery flavor to curries, salads, rice, cookies, candies, and ice cream.

PEANUT Actually not a nut but rather a type of legume that grows on underground stems, peanuts are seeds nestled inside waffle-veined pods that become thin and brittle once dried. The peanut has long been a nutritious staple throughout South America, Africa, and Asia, where it often flavors curries and garnishes salads. The peanut is also well known in North America in its puréed state as peanut butter; see also PEANUT BUTTER.

PECAN A native of North America, the pecan has two deeply crinkled lobes of nutmeat, much like its relative, the walnut. Hundreds of varieties exist, but they all have smooth, brown, oval shells that break easily. Their flavor is sweeter and more delicate than closely related walnuts.

PINE NUT The seed of pine trees, nestled in the scales of their cones. Pine nuts are small, rich nuts with an elongated, slightly tapered shape and a resinous, sweet flavor. Important in southern Europe and the Middle East, they appear in salads, stuffings, and sauces (most famously, pesto), as well as in baked goods and desserts.

PISTACHIO Used widely in Mediterranean, Middle Eastern, and Indian cuisines, the pistachio has a thin but hard shell that is creamy tan and rounded. Bright red nuts owe their color to vegetable dye. Pistachios are often used in desserts. As the nut ripens, its shell cracks to reveal a light green kernel inside.

WALNUT The furrowed, double-lobed nutmeat of the walnut has a rich, assertive flavor. The most common variety is the English walnut, also known as Persian walnut, which has a light brown shell that cracks easily. Black walnuts, native to North America, have dark shells that are extremely difficult to break. Almost always sold whole, black walnuts are a challenge to find and have a stronger, slightly astringent flavor desirable for desserts. The mild white walnut, or butternut, has a light tan shell.

Selecting Nuts in the shell remain fresh longer and are preferable if you have the time and inclination to shell them yourself. Look for whole nuts that are free of holes, cracks, and mold. Shake their shells; a rattling sound inside indicates old and dried nutmeats. Look for whole nuts sold in bulk at health-food stores or in specialty markets. Buying nuts in bulk is economical, but be sure that the store has a rapid turnover so you can purchase the nuts as fresh as possible. Nuts in the shell are best from autumn to early winter.

Shelled nuts should be plump and crisp. Avoid kernels that look withered or lack a snap when broken. Shelled nuts come whole, halved, chopped, and sometimes ground. Almonds can also be blanched (skinned), slivered, or sliced, and chestnuts are available dried, vacuum-packed, candied, or puréed. Supermarkets stock shelled nuts in plastic bags or vacuum-sealed jars and cans year-round.

Many nuts are available raw, roasted, or dry-roasted. Commercial roasted nuts tend to have more flavor, since they are actually fried in oil. On the other hand, no additional oil is used in the preparation of dry-roasted nuts. Nuts for snacking may be salted, smoked, or sweetened. Popular flavorings include garlic, jalapeño, and honey.

Occasionally, fresh green almonds or walnuts appear at farmers' markets during the late summer. Their tender, buttery flesh is a treat for snacking or grinding into a flavorful spread.

Storing Since they contain high amounts of oil, nuts will eventually turn rancid. Raw, unshelled nuts keep well for 6 months to 1 year if stored away from light, heat, and moisture. On the other hand, shelled nuts, especially chopped and unsalted ones, are convenient but have a shorter shelf life. Store shelled nuts in an airtight container for 1 to 2 months at room temperature, 3 to 6 months in the refrigerator, or 9 months to 1 year in the freezer in a zippered plastic freezer bag. (Exceptions: pistachios with partially opened shells will keep for only about half as long as other nuts; fresh chestnuts should be kept for no more than 1 week at room temperature, 1 month in the refrigerator, or 6 months in the freezer.) Be sure to check nuts for freshness before adding to recipes; rancid nuts will ruin the flavor of other foods.

Quick Tip

Generally, you will obtain about ½ pound nutmeats, or approximately 2 cups, from 1 pound unshelled nuts.

Although nut butters can remain at room temperature for several weeks, it is best to keep them in the refrigerator, where they will keep for up to 6 months. Since they are highly perishable, keep nut oils in the refrigerator for up to 4 months once they have been opened. Store nut flours in an airtight container or zippered plastic freezer bag in the freezer for 6 to 9 months.

Cracking Nuts Although you can shell some nuts, such as pistachios, with simply a press of your fingertips, others have hard shells that require more effort and additional equipment. Black walnuts and Brazil nuts call for a sturdy nutcracker, and macadamias demand a small hammer. There are two basic types of nutcrackers. The familiar stainless-steel lever with two grooved arms connected by a hinge usually comes with thin picks for removing the nutmeats. This effective and versatile cracker is also handy for opening lobster shells. Wooden screw-type nutcrackers have a small cup that holds a nut while you twist a knob that squeezes and eventually cracks the shell. Special nutcrackers are available for obtaining whole, intact nutmeats from pecans and walnuts.

continued

n

Nut, continued

For best results, soften the shells by covering them in boiling water and setting them aside to soak for about 15 minutes. Drain and dry well before cracking. Alternatively, bake the whole nuts in a 350°F oven for 15 to 20 minutes to make the shells more brittle. Let cool before cracking. Crack nuts lightly in several different places rather than in one big, crushing squeeze. Walnuts and pecans should be cracked along the seam in order to get an unbroken nut.

Quick Tip

If, after cracking nuts, you find a lot of shell bits mixed in with the kernels, pour the nutmeats into a large bowl of cold water. Slowly stir the nuts and let the pieces of shell float to the surface of the water. After skimming off the shells, drain and dry the nutmeats completely before using.

Skinning Nuts Some nuts have a thin, dark protective skin that can taste rather bitter. Blanching or toasting, depending on the type of nut, will loosen the skin for easy removal.

HOW TO *Skin Nuts by Blanching*

Works for almonds or pistachios.
1. Place the shelled nuts in a large bowl and pour boiling water over them.
2. Let sit for about 1 minute.
3. Drain in a colander and rinse with cold running water to cool.
4. Pinch each nut to slip the skin off.

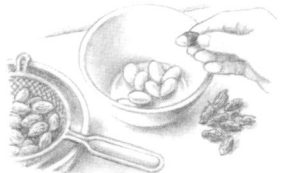

HOW TO *Skin Nuts by Toasting*

Works for hazelnuts, walnuts, and peanuts.
1. Toast the nuts in a dry skillet over medium heat for 10 to 15 minutes, or until fragrant and golden. Shake the pan or stir occasionally as the nuts toast. Alternatively, toast in the oven; see Toasting Nuts, below.

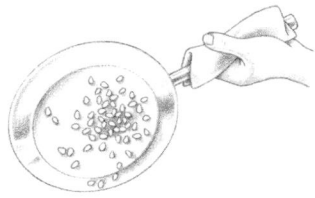

2. While they are still warm, wrap them completely in a coarse-textured kitchen towel and rub vigorously to remove the skins.
3. An easy (albeit messy) way to sift nuts from the loose skins: Transfer the nuts and skins to a shallow bowl or pan. Toss while you blow or fan them over a sink or outdoors. The papery skins will fly up, leaving behind the nuts.

Chopping Nuts For the best texture, chop nuts by hand with a large, sharp knife. A food processor can crush and extract too much oil from nuts, quickly reducing them to a paste. However, if you are in a hurry or have a lot of nuts to chop, the food processor is the easiest way to do it. Pay attention and do not overwork them. Pulse the machine instead of running it continuously, in order to control 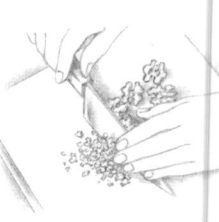 the texture better. If you plan to use chopped nuts in a baking recipe, add a little of the flour or sugar from the list of dry ingredients to absorb excess oil as you process the nuts. This will help keep the nuts dry and help them spread evenly throughout the batter or dough.

Grinding Nuts When nuts are ground, they release their natural oils. The cook must be vigilant when grinding nuts, for they can easily end up as nut butter. A 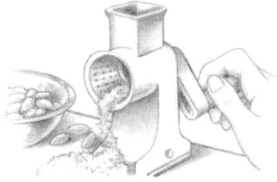 rotary nut mill, a simple contraption with a hamper for holding the nuts and a manually turned arm, assures the baker of perfectly dry ground nuts every time. For less precise grinds, a food processor can be used. For best results, combine the nuts with a little of the flour or sugar called for in the recipe you are preparing and process for no more than 5 to 10 seconds at a time. Be sure to watch the nuts carefully to prevent overprocessing.

Quick Tip

Full-flavored oils pressed from nuts, like hazelnuts and walnuts, add depth to dressings and sauces. Try substituting 1 to 2 tablespoons walnut oil or hazelnut oil for the same amount of butter or vegetable oil in recipes for pancake batters, cakes, or muffins. Nut oil does go rancid, so always check its flavor before adding it to a recipe.

Toasting Nuts Whether you plan to sprinkle almonds over a salad or fold walnuts into a batter, toasting nuts will intensify their flavor and give them a crisp texture and attractive golden color. Large amounts of nuts are best toasted in the oven. Spread them in a single layer on a baking sheet and bake them in a 325°F oven, stirring occasionally to prevent overbrowning at the edges of the pan, until the nuts are golden, fragrant, and coated in a thin layer of their own oil. Depending on the type of nut and the size of the pieces, this may take 10 to 20 minutes.

Quick Bite

Some desserts and sauces call for nut flours, or meals. Look in Italian markets for chestnut and almond flour and in Asian markets for peanut flour.

Toasting nuts in a microwave oven is quick and convenient. Although they will not turn golden, they will have much the same flavor as traditionally toasted nuts. Microwave them on a plate for 3 to 4 minutes, stirring them once about halfway through if the oven does not have a turntable. You can also toast small amounts of nuts in a dry skillet on the stove top. Cook the nuts over medium heat, stirring frequently, until they are golden. Keep a close eye on the nuts, especially pine nuts and sliced almonds, for they burn quickly.

Immediately transfer the nuts to a plate or paper towel and let them cool completely before using. Nuts will continue to toast, so cook them just a shade lighter than desired. They will become darker and crispier as they cool. Nuts easily develop acrid flavor if overbrowned, so just the exterior should be toasted, and the interior should remain lighter colored.

If needed, toast nuts in advance and store them in an airtight container at room temperature for up to 1 week.

See also BLANCHING; FAT & OIL; THICKENING.

Quick Tip

Most nuts contain 70 to 97 percent fat calories (except starchy chestnuts, which have only 8 percent). Fortunately, much of the fat is cholesterol-lowering monounsaturated and polyunsaturated fatty acids. Tropical nuts, especially the coconut, contain higher amounts of saturated fat.

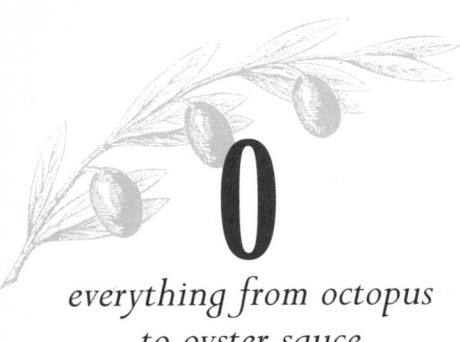

O

*everything from octopus
to oyster sauce*

OAT See GRAIN.

OCTOPUS Relatively unusual in mainstream American cuisine, octopus is well loved in Japan and in some of the Mediterranean countries. A diet of clams and scallops gives the octopus a rich flavor, but its meat can be quite tough and rubbery if not properly tenderized and cooked.

Like its relative the squid, octopus is best when cooked quickly over high heat or very slowly over low heat. It can be eaten raw, lightly pickled, sautéed, grilled, fried, boiled, or stewed. Its black ink colors and flavors sauces, stews, pastas, and risottos.

Selecting Look for fresh or frozen octopus in Japanese markets or specialty fish markets. If buying a whole octopus, ask the fishmonger to clean it for you, since it is an involved process. Usually, already-peeled and portioned tentacles are sold, and these can be found precooked.

Storing Keep octopus in the refrigerator, using it as soon as possible and keeping it for no more than 2 days. Defrost frozen octopus completely before cooking.

Preparing To tenderize octopus before cooking, pound well with a meat mallet, or plunge it several times into boiling water and then let it simmer for 5 to 6 minutes. Slice the tentacles crosswise or on a bias.

OFFAL See ORGAN MEATS.

OIL See FAT & OIL.

OKRA A slender, grayish green, ridged pod that contains numerous small, edible seeds, okra originated in Africa. Also called ladies' fingers, the tasty pods are now common fare throughout warmer climates, from India to the American South. Its mild flavor, similar to that of green beans, is often enlivened with spicy sauces, while its viscous quality thickens soups and stews such as gumbo. Okra is also delicious deep-fried.

Selecting Choose okra that is bright in color and free of bruises or soft spots. Its skin can be smooth or slightly fuzzy, depending on the variety. Okra pods grow up to 9 inches long, but they become increasingly tough and fibrous. Look for young, tender pods that are less than 4 inches in length. Although okra is available throughout the year in the South, it is most plentiful elsewhere in the country from May to October. Frozen okra (good for simmered dishes) and pickled okra are also marketed.

Storing The pods will keep for up to 3 days in the refrigerator, wrapped in a paper towel inside a perforated plastic bag. You also can blanch them briefly and freeze them for up to 8 months.

Preparing Small pods can be cooked whole, with only their tops sliced off. Larger pods are better if thickly sliced. If you don't like the sliminess typical of okra, however, cut off only the stem and do not cut the pod.

OLALLIEBERRY See BERRY.

OLIVE First cultivated in the Mediterranean basin thousands of years ago, the olive is one of the oldest and most important crops in the world. The fruit of a hardy, long-lived tree, fresh olives are too bitter to eat, even when completely ripe. After harvest, they are either pressed to make olive oil or coaxed by long curing into table olives.

The color of olives depends on when they are picked. Green olives are harvested before they ripen, while black olives have been left on the tree until completely ripe. Both are cured, and methods vary according to country and region, but the process basically involves months of sitting in oil, salt, water, brine, or in the sun. Alternatively, they can be processed in an alkaline solution for only a few days. With the American industrial method, half-ripe olives are bathed in lye and oxidized to develop a black color. These are called California or Mission olives and are the soft, mild ones available in cans.

Olives packed in brine stay plump, smooth, and relatively firm. Salt- or oil-cured olives become dry, wrinkled, and pleasantly bitter in flavor, and the best obtain a silky texture and rich flavor.

Selecting Olives are available pitted or unpitted. They may be packed in brine, dried in salt, marinated in oil with herbs and spices, or even stuffed with pimientos, anchovies, or almonds. Look for them in cans, jars, and plastic containers in the refrigerated section of the supermarket, and in bulk in the deli section. Choose evenly colored olives free of white spots.

Storing Covered completely with water, brine, or oil, olives will keep for 1 year in the refrigerator. Store salt-packed olives in an airtight, nonmetallic container for up to 6 months.

Olive Glossary

GAETA Brownish black and with a nutty flavor, the Gaeta, from Italy, is salt-cured but soft and smooth.

GREEK When "Greek olives" are called for in a recipe, most likely Kalamata olives are meant.

KALAMATA Most popular variety from Greece. Almond shaped, purplish black, rich, and meaty, the Kalamata is brine-cured and then packed in oil or vinegar.

MOROCCAN Can refer to either a large brine-cured, reddish green olive or a salt-cured, wrinkled, black one. Moroccan green olives are soft and salty-tart, while Moroccan black olives boast a glistening, silky texture and a meaty, slightly smoky, and pleasantly bitter flavor.

NIÇOISE A small, brownish black olive from Provence. Brine-cured, then packed in oil with lemon and herbs, the mellow and nutty olives appear in stews and authentic tapenade.

PICHOLINE Medium-sized, green, smooth, and very salty olives from France.

SICILIAN Large, green, tart, and meaty olives sometimes flavored with red pepper or fennel.

SPANISH Large, green, and dense, these olives are commonly pitted and stuffed with pimientos, almonds, or anchovies.

Preparing To remove the pits of smaller olives, use a cherry pitter or an olive pitter.

HOW TO *Pit Olives When You Don't Own a Pitter*

1. Spread the olives in a single layer on a cutting board.
2. Crush them gently with a rolling pin, the bottom of a pan, or the flat side of a chef's knife.
3. Most of the pits should roll out of the cracked olives. You can quickly pop out any stubborn pits with your fingers. Or carefully open the olive with a small sharp knife to remove the pit.

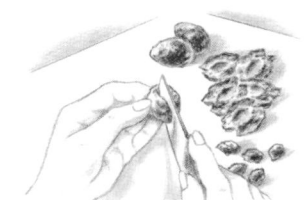

See also FAT & OIL.

OMELET An egg dish in which beaten eggs are cooked in a shallow pan, producing a firm exterior and soft interior. The omelet is usually folded over or rolled around a savory filling. Rolled omelets are called French omelets, and they might be filled with a simple scattering of fresh herbs or shredded cheese or more bountiful additions. There are also flat omelets, which resemble frittatas, and soufflé omelets, in which the egg whites are beaten to create a light and fluffy end result. Omelets can be made with whole eggs, egg whites alone, or a mixture of whole eggs and egg whites.

Any skillet may be used, but specialized omelet pans with rounded flared sides, often nonstick, make it easier to turn the omelet out of the pan, folding it in the process.

When beating eggs for omelets, try not to beat too much air into them. Foamy eggs interfere with an omelet's texture.

HOW TO *Make an Omelet*

1. Break the eggs called for in a recipe into a mixing bowl. Using a wire whisk or a fork, beat the eggs and a little water, just until the eggs are blended and only slightly frothy.

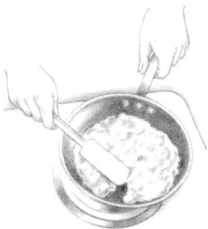

2. Heat an omelet pan or a skillet over medium heat. Add the butter and, once it melts and foams, the eggs. As the eggs begin to set along the edges and bottom, use a spatula or fork to push the edges toward the center, tilting the pan to let the liquid egg on top flow to the edges and run underneath.
3. When the eggs are almost set but still slightly moist on top, spoon the prepared filling, if using, over the half opposite from you. Shake the pan to loosen the omelet, then tilt the pan to let the filled half slide halfway up the side of the pan. Use the spatula or fork to fold the far edge over itself or the filling.

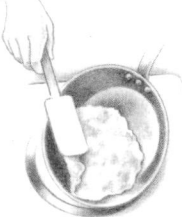

4. Gently roll the omelet onto the serving plate, folding it over itself (and any filling).

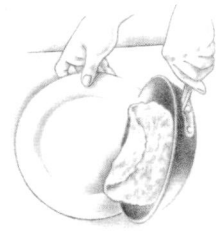
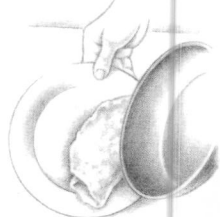

Onion

Belonging to the same family as garlic and leeks, this multi-layered bulb is a staple in nearly every kitchen. "Cook the onions until soft and golden" is the familiar first step in countless savory dishes, from tomato sauces to beef stews.

Onions are crisp and pungent when raw and become soft and sweet when cooked. Two types of onions are available, fresh or spring onions and dried or storage onions, the latter being the kind most of us think of when we consider the onion. Fresh onions include green onions and such sweet onions as Vidalia or Maui. Dried onions have been cured by drying, a process that causes their skins to tighten and protect against spoilage. The curing also concentrates their flavor, dries their skins, and brings out the colors that help shoppers identify the different types.

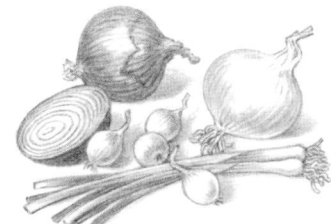

Assorted onions.

A Guide to Onions

GREEN ONION Also known as scallion or, sometimes, spring onion. Green onions are the immature shoots of the bulb onion, with a narrow white base that has not yet begun to swell and long, flat green leaves. Recipes often specify whether to use only the white base, the green tops, or both. Green onions have a mild flavor and can be enjoyed raw in salads, while their chopped or minced green tops are often used as a garnish. They are used extensively in Chinese cooking, especially in stir-fries. Whole green onions can also be grilled—in this form a popular addition to Mexican plates—or braised like leeks, and the white base of green onions may be used as a substitute for harder-to-find shallots.

Quick Tip

A spring onion, though often equated with the green onion, is actually an immature version of a white or red onion and has a slightly swollen white or red base. The tastes of the green onion and the spring onion are very similar, however, and the two varieties are interchangeable in recipes.

MAUI, VIDALIA, AND WALLA WALLA ONIONS Fresh onions that are mild, sweet, and juicy and named for their place of origin, since, due to soil and climate, they lose their characteristic sweetness if grown elsewhere. Maui and Vidalia onions, from Hawaii and Georgia, respectively, come into season during spring, and Walla Walla, from Washington, during late summer. Worth hunting down in well-stocked supermarkets and finer produce markets, they are best

continued

Onion, continued

eaten raw in sandwiches, in salads, or, enthusiasts insist, out of hand. Usually sold loose.

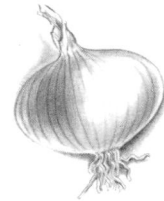

Vidalia onion.

PEARL AND BOILING ONIONS Pearl onions are small, dried onions no more than 1 inch in diameter. They are traditionally white, although red ones are now available. Boiling onions are also white and slightly larger. Both pearl and boiling onions have a mild flavor similar to that of green onions. They are often served as a garnish for stews, roasted meats, and marinated salads, or used for braised or creamed onions. Also available pickled or frozen.

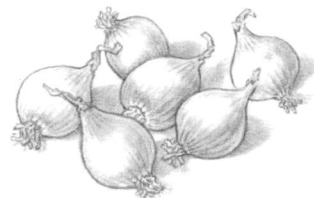

Pearl onions.

HOW TO *Peel Pearl and Boiling Onions*

Peeling a pile of pearl onions may seem daunting, but blanching them first will help the task pass more quickly and easily.

1. Bring a large pot of water to a full boil.
2. Put the onions in the boiling water. Cook for 1 minute, counting from when the water returns to a boil.
3. Drain the onions in a colander. Rinse them under cold running water, tossing continuously, until they are cool.
4. With a sharp paring knife, trim the root and stem ends of each onion.

5. Pinch the onions to remove their skins.

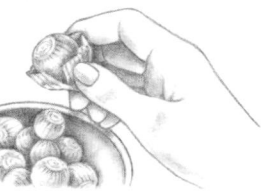

6. Many cooks score, or shallowly cut, an X in each pearl onion's root end to shorten cooking time, ensure even cooking, and help keep the layers from telescoping.

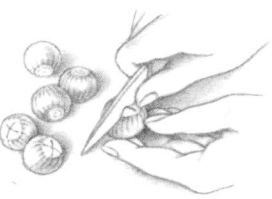

RED ONION Also called Italian onion and Bermuda onion. Mild and slightly sweet, this purplish red onion is delicious raw in salads, sandwiches, and relishes and briefly cooked in vegetable mixes. Extended cooking will dull the color to gray. Sweet elongated varieties, found in farmers' markets, are called torpedo onions.

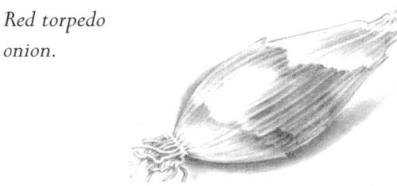

Red torpedo onion.

SHALLOT This small member of the onion family looks like a large clove of garlic covered with papery bronze or reddish skin. Shallots have white flesh lightly streaked with purple, a crisp texture, and a flavor that is subtler than that of an onion. They are often used for flavoring sauces and salad dressings that would be overpowered by the stronger taste of onion. The white part of a green onion may be substituted for a shallot.

SPANISH ONION Very large, round yellow onion. Similar to yellow onions and used in the same way.

WHITE ONION More pungent than the red onion, but milder and less sweet than the yellow, the white onion is a favorite of the Mexican cook. Large, slightly flattened, mild white onions are sometimes called white Spanish onions.

YELLOW ONION The yellow globe onion is the common, all-purpose onion sold in supermarkets. It can be globular, flattened, or slightly elongated and, since it is dried, has a parchmentlike golden brown skin. It usually is too harsh for serving raw but becomes rich and sweet when cooked, making it the ideal onion for caramelizing.

Selecting Choose fresh onions that look perky. For green onions, the shoots should be green with white bulb ends. For Vidalia and Maui, seek out fresh-looking, tubular green stems. For dried onions, choose firm specimens with smooth, dry skins. Avoid any with soft spots, particularly at the stem end; green shoots; moldy areas; or moist, wrinkled skins.

Storing Store green onions in a perforated plastic bag for up to 2 weeks in the refrigerator. Keep other onions in a cool, dark, well-ventilated place. Do not leave them in plastic bags, using instead a basket or crate to allow air circulation. Storing them alongside other vegetables (such as potatoes) that may give off gases or moisture will spoil the onions quickly. Discard

---

Quick Tip

To mellow an onion's bite, slice or cut the onion as desired. Soak the pieces in cold water for 30 to 60 minutes, changing the water several times. Drain and pat dry with a paper towel. Alternatively, raw chopped onion can be rinsed in a colander and then wrapped in a kitchen towel and squeezed to eliminate excess moisture. This method is especially useful when preparing raw onion to add to uncooked dishes like salsa.

---

onions that begin growing shoots, as they will taste bitter.

Preparing Nearly everyone wants the secret to preventing the tears that spring to your eyes when chopping a strong onion. Ideas range from the folksy (clamp a wooden spoon or kitchen match between your teeth) to the somewhat scientific (freeze the onions briefly to slow enzymes, or light candles to burn off irritating sulfur compounds) to the purely pragmatic (wear swimming goggles) to the foolish (keep your eyes closed). Since most of the tear-inducing sulfuric compounds are concentrated near the roots, trimming the stem end first, peeling downward, and cutting the root end last may help delay the onset of tears. The easiest preventives are to use your sharpest knife, avoid touching your face with oniony fingers, and work as quickly as you possibly can.

Onions can be chopped in a food processor, but the pieces will be irregular. More important, the processor's blade also

Quick Tip

Rub your hands with lemon juice or your equipment with a mixture of salt and vinegar to remove the smell of onions.

continued

Onion, continued

crushes the onion, releasing more juice and altering its flavor and texture.

When using green onions, you need only trim away the root end and any wilted or brown portions of the tops; both the green and white parts can be used, and recipes generally specify.

Cut all onions as close to cooking or serving time as possible. Their flavor deteriorates while their aroma intensifies over time.

HOW TO *Slice an Onion or a Shallot*

1. Peel the onion.
2. Slice a small piece from the onion's side to create a flat surface.

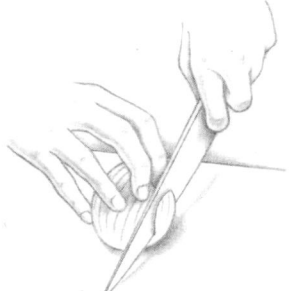

3. Place the onion flat side down on a cutting board. Now that the onion is stable, proceed to slice it, keeping fingertips safely clear of the blade.

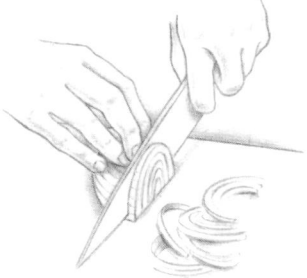

Note that this technique is useful for slicing nearly all round fruits and vegetables.

HOW TO *Chop an Onion or a Shallot*

1. Cut the onion in half lengthwise from stem to root end, then peel it.
2. Put an onion half flat side down on a cutting board, hold the stem end with your fingertips safely curled under and away from the blade, and, with the knife tip pointed toward the stem end, make a series of parallel vertical cuts through the onion half, at right angles to the cutting board. Do not cut all the way through the stem end.

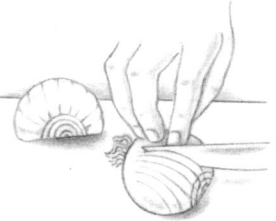

3. Turn your knife so that it is parallel with the cutting board and perpendicular to the first series of cuts, and make a series of horizontal cuts in the onion half, again not cutting through the stem end. The onion half should stay in one piece, more or less.

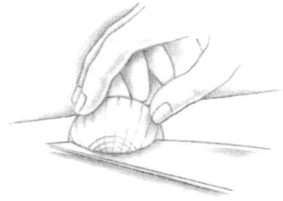

4. To chop the onion, simply slice the onion across the first cuts made in step 1.

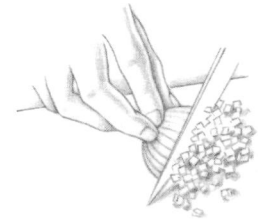

See also LEEK.

ORANGE The orange was first cultivated in China more than two thousand years ago and is now grown around the world. Long a symbol of abundance and prosperity, orange trees decorate royal palaces, their flowers grace bridal bouquets, and their juicy, sweet-tart fruit appears on tables fresh, juiced, and incorporated into countless savory and sweet dishes.

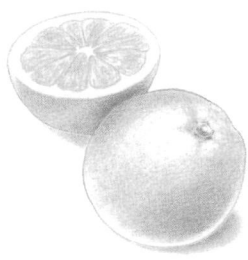

These international fruits fall into two broad categories: sweet and bitter. Sweet oranges are further divided into three groups: common, navel, and blood. The most popular common orange is the Valencia, considered the best for juicing because of its thin skin and juicy pulp. Navel oranges are sweet, easy to peel, and almost always seedless, making them ideal for eating out of hand. Blood oranges, originally from Sicily, have distinctive red flesh and juice and a flavor reminiscent of berries. As versatile as they are dramatic, blood oranges can be eaten out of hand or used in salads, sauces, desserts, and drinks.

Blood oranges.

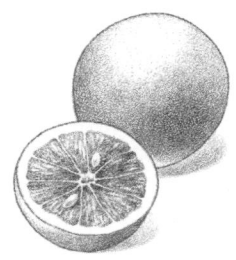

Bitter oranges have dry pulp, a thick rind, and an extremely bitter flavor. Hardly candidates for the fruit bowl, bitter oranges and their flavorful peels make excellent marmalades, candies, sauces, syrups, and liqueurs. Seville and Bergamot, oils from the latter being what gives Earl Grey tea its elusive flavor and aroma, are the two best-known varieties.

Selecting Choose oranges that are heavy for their size and have smooth skins. Don't look askance at an orange with brown surface patches. The imperfect peel may be hiding an extra dose of juice and sweetness. Color is not a good indicator of quality, since oranges are sometimes dyed and fully ripened oranges may regreen, particularly Valencias. Do avoid fruits with soft or moldy spots, however.

Oranges are available all year, but they have different peak seasons depending on variety. Valencias are at the height of their season from May through July, navels are best from January through March, and blood oranges peak from mid-December through March.

Storing Oranges can be left at room temperature for 1 week or kept in the refrigerator for up to 3 weeks.

Preparing For best flavor, serve oranges raw or cook them only briefly. Before peeling an orange, squeeze it between your palms or roll it on a countertop, pressing down. This will make the orange a little juicier and easier to peel. Special plastic orange peelers have a small cutting edge and a flat, curved blade that is slipped beneath the peel to separate it quickly and cleanly from the flesh. But, often the best way to serve oranges as a snack is to cut them, peel and all, into thick wedges.

Quick Tip

Don't overlook the pleasures of cooking with oranges. Add a little orange juice to the cooking water for rice to get a tangy pilaf to serve with chicken or lamb. Or toss orange segments with sliced fennel and endive for a refreshing appetizer salad.

HOW TO *Section an Orange*

1. Slice off the orange's top and bottom.
2. Stand the orange upright. Following the contour of the fruit, slice off the peel, pith, and membrane in thick strips.

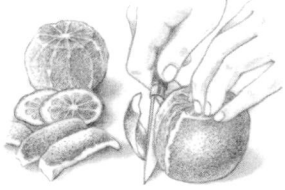

3. Holding the fruit over a bowl, cut along each side of the membrane between the sections, letting each freed section drop into the bowl.

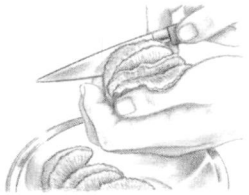

See also JUICING; ZESTING.

OREGANO See HERB.

ORGANIC With consumers ever more concerned about the quality and safety of the foods they eat, the term *organic* continues to rise in the public consciousness and appear on food labels in farmers' markets, health-food stores, and supermarkets alike. While government definitions may vary, the term generally refers to foods—whether plant or animal in origin—produced naturally, without the use of chemical-based pesticides, fungicides, or antibiotics. While the jury remains out on whether organic products are inherently safer or more nutritious, or whether those produced by conventional means are less so, organic products do offer one distinctive advantage: often, they are grown locally, ensuring that the products found in your market will be fresher, more flavorful, and possibly higher in nutrients.

ORGAN MEATS Sometimes also referred to by the term "offal," these types of animal proteins derive from internal organs. In general, when properly prepared and cooked, they combine very soft, tender texture with distinctive flavor. Most common types include liver, which may come from beef, veal, lamb, chicken, goose, or duck; kidneys, of which veal and lamb have the mildest flavor; sweetbreads, the tender and subtly sweet thymus glands of veal, lamb, or pork; and brains from lamb or veal, which are surprisingly delicate in both taste and texture.

OVEN Nowadays, ovens keep time, schedule dinner, clean themselves, and can even turn a roasting chicken for you. Despite all the available bells and whistles, ovens can be divided into three basic kinds. Each uses different types of energy and, more important, has different heating characteristics. Knowing what each one can and cannot do will help ensure that your roast is moist and flavorful, your casseroles creamy, and your cookies perfectly golden brown. Now available is a combination oven that offers all three functions.

Oven Options Three basic oven types are available for home kitchens.

THERMAL OVEN Uses radiant heat from gas flames or electric elements to cook foods with dry heat. Hot spots can occur, so be sure to check the food and turn it as needed for even cooking. Large pans or baking sheets can block heat and create noticeable variances in temperature between racks. Electric ovens tend to cook food more quickly and evenly than gas ovens. Most standard stoves are fitted with thermal ovens.

CONVECTION OVEN Has a fan that blows heated air throughout the oven. No matter how many pans or what their size, food cooks quickly and evenly in the moving air. A convection oven can cut cooking time by one-third, and most recipes will need to be adjusted accordingly. These ovens are excellent for smaller cuts of meat and for cookies, breads, cakes, and pies. Large roasts can dry out, however, and are best cooked more slowly in a conventional thermal oven. A convection oven is generally more expensive than a thermal model of comparable quality.

MICROWAVE OVEN Uses moist heat generated by the food itself, produced when its molecules are agitated by short, high-frequency microwaves. See also MICROWAVE OVEN.

OVEN MITT See COOKING TOOLS.

OYSTER This unassuming bivalve has enjoyed a long and varied history. Early Romans extolled the oyster's aphrodisiac qualities, while American colonists begrudgingly depended on 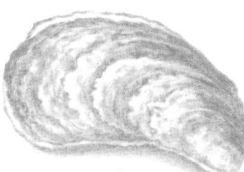 them to survive long, harsh winters. Few combinations are as simple and elegant as freshly shucked oysters and chilled Champagne. Lemon, lime, saffron, coconut milk, chiles, lemongrass, leeks, miso, and cream all complement oysters. Oysters also star in soups, stews, and fillings.

Selecting Always buy oysters from reputable merchants who can vouch that they come from safe, clean, unpolluted waters. Fresh live oysters in the shell have a mild, sweet smell. Their shells should be closed tightly and feel heavy with water. Do not buy any oysters that remain open when touched. A strong fishy or ammonium odor indicates the oysters are no longer fresh, so pass them by. Any oysters intended for eating raw should be bought fresh and shucked within a few hours of serving. Do not buy shucked oysters for eating raw unless you know that the fishmonger shucked them specially for your order.

When buying containers of shucked oysters, check that the shellfish are plump and their liquor is clear, without a trace of milkiness. Some grocery stores and fish markets sell frozen shucked oysters. Also available are canned smoked oysters.

While oysters are spawning during the summer months, their flesh becomes soft, milky, and less sweet. They are not toxic but simply taste unpleasant. In the United States and Europe, oysters are in season during the months that have the letter r in them—in other words, from September to April. Now, however, with sterile varieties cultivated, oysters are increasingly available all year long. A clear exception to the alphabet rule is the Kumamoto oyster, which spawns during the autumn months.

Storing Spread live oysters in a large container and cover them with a damp cloth. If needed, keep them in the refrigerator for 1 to 2 days, making sure the cloth stays moist. They will die if submerged in tap water, stored on ice, or sealed in an airtight container. Cover shucked oysters in their own liquor and refrigerate them in an airtight container for no more than 2 days. Store cans of smoked oysters in a cool, dry place for up to 2 years. Keep frozen oysters for up to 3 to 4 months.

Preparing Before opening oysters, be sure to scrub them with a stiff brush and rinse well. When opening, reserve their liquor and use it in place of other liquids when making soups and sauces. Add oysters toward the end of cooking, allowing just enough time to heat them through. Overcooking toughens them.

*Scrubbing
an oyster.*

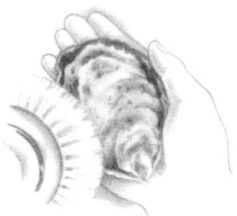

WHICH WAY IS UP? The top shells of
oysters tend to be flatter than the more
bowl-shaped bottom shells. For serving
on the half shell, open the oyster with its
top shell facing up, and leave the oyster
in its bottom shell.

Caution!

Since oysters are susceptible to water contaminants and "red tides" of poisonous plankton,
be sure to read posted signs and check with
local health or game agencies before collecting your own oysters.

HOW TO *Open Oysters*

Oyster knives have thick handles for easy
gripping and turning. Their wide, dull
blades are strong enough to lever open the
shell. (Although similar, oyster knives are
stubbier than clam knives.) Stainless-steel
oyster knives will not transfer any metallic
flavor to the oyster.

Oyster knife.

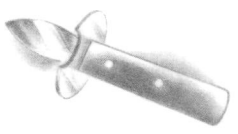

1. For protection and a better grip, use a folded
   cloth or an oven mitt to hold the oyster in one
   hand. (Right-handers should hold the shell with
   their left hand, and vice versa.) Position the
   shell so the rounded edge points out toward
   the space between your thumb and your
   fingers and the hinge end points toward you.

2. Holding the oyster knife in your other hand,
   insert its tip into the dark, rounded spot at the
   oyster's hinge. (The shell's ridges and dark rays
   emanate from the hinge.)

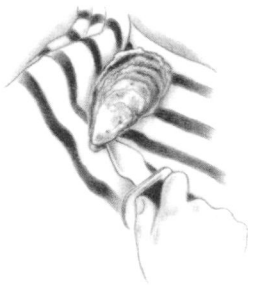

3. Twist the knife sharply to break the hinge.
4. Once the shell opens, slip the knife carefully up
   along the inside surface of the top shell, sever-
   ing the adductor muscle that grips it. Take care
   not to cut the oyster itself or to spill its liquor.

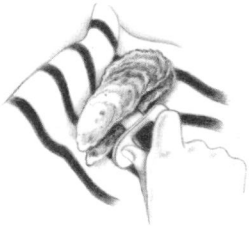

5. Lift the top shell away and discard.
6. Carefully cut the muscle under the oyster to
   loosen it from the bottom shell. Remove any
   small particles of shell.

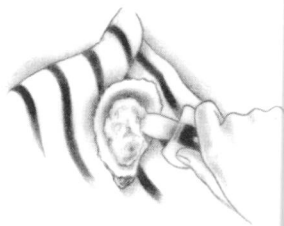

Speed Shucking There are a few ways
to open a large number of oysters quickly
for use in a recipe. Do not try to use these
methods for raw oysters on the half shell,

✒ Oyster Glossary ✒

Since water-filtering oysters readily take on the flavor of their environment, they traditionally are named after the area where they grow. In general, colder waters develop a firmer texture and sharper, saltier flavor, while warmer waters create a milder, softer oyster.

ATLANTIC OYSTER Tends to have a bumpy, elongated shell and a briny flavor with strong mineral notes. Varieties include Blue Point, Cape Cod, Chesapeake, Kent Island, Long Island, Malpeque, and Wellfleet. Atlantic oysters, also called Eastern oysters, account for most of the oysters sold at market.

PACIFIC OYSTER Also known as Japanese oysters, these specimens have more subtle, slightly fruity flavors and more distinctly fluted shells than their Atlantic cousins. Popular varieties are the Hama Hama, Hog Island, Quilcene, and Tomales Bay. The sweet, popular Kumamoto oyster is actually a separate species, but it is often grouped with the Pacific oysters.

OLYMPIA OYSTER A species indigenous to the American Northwest. Olympia oysters are tiny (about the size of a quarter), slow growing (taking 4 years to mature), and highly prized for their flavor. They are almost always served on the half shell.

FLAT OYSTER Native to European waters but now grown in both the Atlantic and Pacific. Varieties found in the waters off Maine and northern California have especially intense flavors. Small oysters inside large, round shells, they are commonly known by the name Belon, after a French region where they were once abundant.

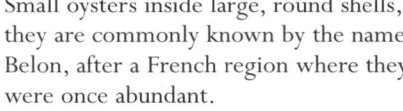

because they will be partially cooked and thus very unpleasant.

The first way is to steam them for about 1 minute. Use very little water, so the liquor that drains from the open oysters will not be overly diluted. Another trick is to spread the oysters in a large, shallow baking dish and heat the oysters in a 375°F oven just until they open, 1 to 2 minutes. Or, you can microwave them on High for about 1 minute.

See also SHELLFISH.

OYSTER SAUCE A thick, dark brown sauce made from oyster extracts and sea-sonings. With its distinctive smoky-sweet flavor, this all-purpose seasoning is used in Cantonese cuisine to give body, deep color, and rich flavor to the sauces in noodle, meat, vegetable, and seafood dishes. Stir-fried Chinese broccoli simply drizzled with oyster sauce is a popular dish.

Selecting The best brands, made only from dried oysters and salt, have a briny, slightly sweet flavor. Now, however, soy sauce, sugar, and cornstarch may replace some or all of the oysters.

Storing An unopened bottle will keep indefinitely. Once opened, it will keep for up to 2 years in the refrigerator.

O

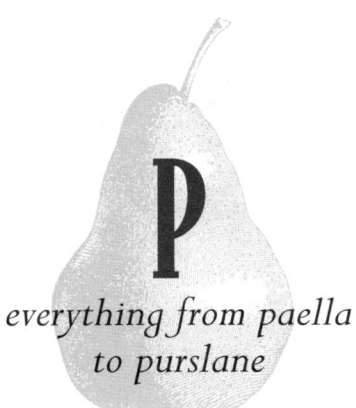

everything from paella to purslane

PAELLA Originating in the Valencia region of Spain, paella is a dish of saffron-infused rice cooked with various meats, seafood, and vegetables. It is prepared in a large, round, shallow pan called a *paellera* that usually ranges from 13 to 14 inches in diameter. At its most traditional, *paella valenciana* contains chicken, rabbit, snails, broad green beans, white beans, tomatoes, and saffron; but countless variations exist, from an elaborate all-seafood dish to a hearty recipe using chorizo sausage to a version that consists of only tomatoes and rice. Italian Arborio rice may be substituted for the Spanish medium-grain rice (the Spanish call it short-grain rice; the best comes from Calasparra and is called Bomba) used in paella; unlike risotto, however, paella should never be stirred once the other ingredients have been added.

Paellera.

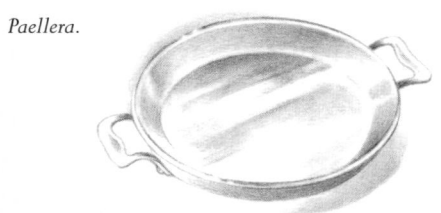

PAK-CHOI See BOK CHOY.

PALM See HEART OF PALM.

PAN BROILING See BROILING.

PANCAKE Variously known as griddle-cakes, flapjacks, hoecakes, and Indian cakes, these flat, round cakes are made from a thin batter poured onto the surface of a hot griddle or skillet and cooked on both sides. Pancakes are a staple of America's breakfast table. More famous incarnations include yeasted flannel cakes, modest silver dollar cakes, Dutch babies, and Rhode Island's cornmeal johnnycake. Most pancakes are slightly leavened, although some, like crepes and johnnycakes, are not. Commonly topped with butter, fresh fruit, and maple syrup, pancakes are now made in many colors and flavors, including whole wheat with banana and walnuts, lemon ricotta with blueberries, and jalapeño-cornmeal. Although once made with sourdough starter, most pancake recipes are now leavened with baking powder or baking soda.

Pancake Savvy When making pancakes, keep the following in mind:

- Using a whisk, stir the batter only a few times, stopping as soon as it begins to come together and all the ingredients are moistened. The batter should have small lumps. Too much stirring will develop the gluten in the flour and create tough pancakes.
- Use a griddle or heavy pan and heat it thoroughly before spooning or ladling in the batter.
- Turn a pancake only once, when bubbles appear on the surface and the bottom is golden brown.
- Serve pancakes as soon after cooking as possible. Ideally, flip them from the pan directly onto a plate set in front of a hungry eater.

■ If you must hold pancakes before serving, do not stack them more than 2 or 3 high, or they will steam and become soggy.
See also CREPE; WAFFLE.

PANCETTA This flavorful bacon, which derives its name from the Italian word for "belly," has a moist, silky texture. It is made by rubbing a slab of pork belly with a mix of spices that may include cinnamon, cloves, or juniper berries, then rolling the slab into a tight cylinder and curing it for at least 2 months. Since it is not smoked, pancetta is moister than American slab bacon. In Italy, chopped pancetta sautéed in olive oil is used to flavor soups, sauces, meats, and vegetables. 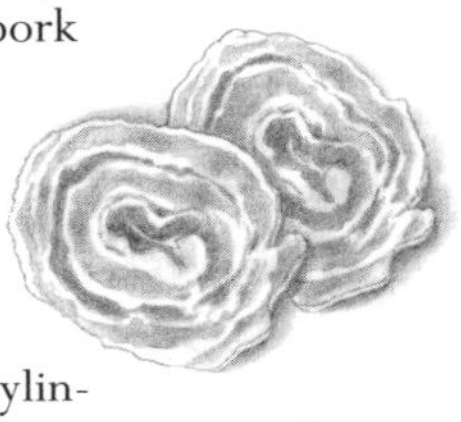
Selecting Pancetta may be purchased from a good butcher or Italian deli. Ask for it to be sliced thin or thick. When unfurled, the slices look like strips of bacon.
Storing Keep sliced pancetta wrapped in plastic in the refrigerator for up to 2 weeks.
Preparing Pancetta is generally chopped before use in a recipe.
See also BACON.

PANFRYING See FRYING.

PANKO See BREAD CRUMBS.

PAN ROASTING See ROASTING.

PAN SIZES Cookware and bakeware come in a wide range of sizes. A household's pots and pans, from pressure cookers to skillets to saucepans to roasting pans, are typically selected according to the needs of that household, both in terms of number and size. Some specialty pans, such as a fish poacher, are a fairly standard size,

Volume of Standard Baking Pans

PAN DIMENSIONS*	VOLUME
Square	
8 x 8 x 1½ inches	6 cups
8 x 8 x 2 inches	8 cups
9 x 9 x 2 inches	10 cups
10 x 10 x 2 inches	12 cups
12 x 12 x 2 inches	16 cups
Rectangular	
11 x 7 x 2 inches	8 cups
13 x 9 x 2 inches	12 cups
Jelly roll	
10½ x 15½ x 1 inch	10 cups
12½ x 17½ x 1 inch	12 cups
Loaf	
8 x 4 x 2½ inches	4 cups
8½ x 4½ x 2½ inches	6 cups
9 x 5 x 3 inches	8 cups
Round	
6 x 2 inches	3¾ cups
8 x 1½ inches	4 cups
8 x 2 inches	7 cups
9 x 1½ inches	6 cups
9 x 2 inches	8½ cups
10 x 2 inches	10¾ cups
12 x 2 inches	15½ cups
14 x 2 inches	21 cups
Springform	
9 x 2¾ inches	10 cups
9 x 3 inches	12 cups
10 x 2¾ inches	12 cups
Bundt	
9 x 3 inches	9 cups
10 x 3½ inches	12 cups
Tube	
9 x 3 inches	10 cups
10 x 4 inches	16 cups
8 x 2½-inch heart	8½ cups
9½ x 6½-inch oval	6 cups

*Measured on inside of pan.

while others, such as saucepans, come in several capacities. In general, however, if a cook substitutes, for example, a 3-quart saucepan for the $2\frac{1}{2}$-quart pan specified in a recipe, little adjustment is needed to the cooking process.

The sizes of bakeware, in contrast, are more critical. If you use a larger cake or bread pan than that called for in a recipe, for example, you will need to shorten the baking time. The batter or dough will be shallower and have more surface area, thus cooking more quickly. Likewise, the same batter or dough put into a smaller, deeper pan will require more time in the oven to cook them through and perhaps a slightly lower oven temperature to keep from over-browning with the increased cooking time. When purchasing bakeware, remember that the largest pan that will fit in most home ovens is about 17 by 14 inches. Also, when measuring the dimensions of insulated pans or other heavy baking dishes made of glass or ceramic, be sure to measure only the inside space and not include the thickness of the sides themselves.

You can determine a pan's volume by filling it with water, then pouring the water into a large liquid measure or marked pitcher. Use the chart on page 327 to compare the volumes of pan sizes when substituting one pan for another.

See also BAKEWARE; COOKWARE.

PAPAYA With its distinctive earthy aroma and flavor, papaya is the quintessential tropical fruit, although botanically speaking it is actually a berry. Native to Central America, it is now cultivated from Hawaii to South Africa to the Philippines. The papaya looks somewhat like a large pear, with thin, pale green skin that ripens to blotches of yellow and orange. Some people think it resembles a melon and call papayas "tree melons." Such

nomenclature may be a result of the fruit's hollow center, which holds a shiny mass of small, slick black seeds, which are edible and have a slightly peppery flavor. Some English speakers call the fruit papaw, a name that also refers, confusingly, to a sweet fruit with a custardlike flesh that is native to North America.

In Southeast Asia and Latin America, crunchy green papaya is treated like a vegetable and appears shredded in salads. Unripe papaya contains papain, a powerful digestive enzyme that rapidly breaks down proteins. Cooks throughout the world rub meat with green papaya or wrap meat in the tree's leaves to marinate and tenderize. Today, papain is the active ingredient in most powdered meat tenderizers.

Selecting Since they bruise easily, most papayas are transported while still hard, with shippers knowing they will ripen in storage. Try to buy a papaya that gives slightly when pressed. Look for skin that is smooth and has already started to turn yellow. Different varieties come in varying sizes, from palm-sized 6-ounce to giant 20-pound fruit, but most of the papayas in markets weigh about 1 pound. Since the tree simultaneously flowers and bears fruit and is cultivated around the world, papayas are available year-round. Look for the nectar in cans at Asian and Latin American markets. Dried papaya spears are available in bulk and packaged in plastic bags at well-stocked supermarkets and health-food stores.

Storing Leave papayas at room temperature to ripen. Once the fruit is ripe, you can peel, cut, and store it in an airtight container in the refrigerator for up to 2 days. The fruit quickly loses its flavor when chilled. Keep unopened cans of papaya nectar for up to 1 year in a cool, dry place; once opened, refrigerate for 2 or 3 days. Store dried papaya in an airtight container in the refrigerator for up to 6 months.

Preparing Small papayas can be halved and eaten with a spoon like custard. A squeeze of lime juice deepens the flavor. For larger fruit, remove the skin with a vegetable peeler, cut the papaya in half, and scoop out its seeds with a large spoon. The seeds can be rinsed and added to salads or other dishes to deliver a peppery bite.

Can't Wait for Your Papaya to Ripen?

Here's a shortcut to reduce the bitterness of a slightly underripe papaya:

1. Cut several shallow score lines through the skin along the length of the fruit. Expose the flesh but avoid cutting into it.
2. Prop the papaya, with its stem down, in a large glass or jar.
3. Leave it at room temperature overnight or, preferably, 1 day. The exposure to air deactivates the bitter papain enzyme. This will make the fruit taste sweeter. (This will not, however, make an already-ripe fruit sweeter.)

PAPRIKA See SPICE.

PARBOILING To cook food partially in boiling water, sometimes as a preparatory step before combining ingredients with different cooking times or finishing with another cooking method. Parboiling is closely related to blanching but usually implies longer cooking. Although parboiling traditionally referred to cooking food until nearly half done, modern cookbooks often use the term for brief cooking times as well, which can confuse longtime cooks.

PARCHMENT PAPER Treated to resist moisture and grease, parchment paper provides a nonstick surface for lining cake pans and baking sheets. Because parchment has undergone a process that strengthens it and makes the surface smooth and impermeable, the paper keeps the food from sticking and makes cleanup easier. Essential in a classic French kitchen, parchment paper folds into tidy packages for cooking food (called *en papillote*), covers floating fruit while it poaches, lines the bottom of cake pans, and folds quickly and neatly into pastry cones for decorating cakes (see also PIPING). Parchment can withstand high heat in the oven, but it must never be used in the broiler or directly on a burner. If touched by a flame or an electric burner, it will ignite. Parchment also maintains its strength when wet. Look for rolls of parchment paper in grocery stores and cookware shops. Large sheets and precut triangles are available at baking-supply stores. Waxed paper cannot replace parchment in cooking or baking; it will burn and smoke when heated.

PARING Another term for peeling; see PEELING.

PARMESAN An aged, firm cheese of medium butterfat content with a pale yellow to medium straw yellow color and a piquant, slightly salty flavor. Made from partially skimmed cow's milk, Parmesan is aged for 1 to 3 years in large wheels to achieve a granular texture and a rich, complex flavor that is at once mild, savory, 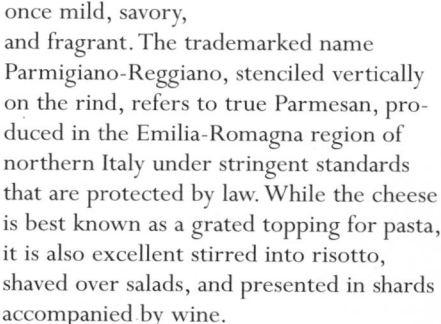 and fragrant. The trademarked name Parmigiano-Reggiano, stenciled vertically on the rind, refers to true Parmesan, produced in the Emilia-Romagna region of northern Italy under stringent standards that are protected by law. While the cheese is best known as a grated topping for pasta, it is also excellent stirred into risotto, shaved over salads, and presented in shards accompanied by wine.

P

Selecting For fuller flavor, buy Parmesan in wedges, never pregrated. The cheese dries out and begins to diminish in flavor soon after grating and should be kept whole for as long as possible.

Storing Keep wrapped tightly in plastic wrap or aluminum foil in the refrigerator for up to 2 weeks or wrapped airtight in the freezer for several months.

Quick Tip

If Parmesan begins drying out, wrap it first in a damp cloth and then loosely in aluminum foil. Refrigerate for 1 day. Remove the cheese from the cloth and seal it again tightly in plastic wrap or aluminum foil.

Preparing Grate or shave Parmesan only as needed just before using in a recipe or serving. If possible, during meals provide a small hand grater so diners may top their own pasta with cheese.

See also CHEESE.

PARMIGIANO-REGGIANO See PARMESAN.

PARSLEY See HERB.

PARSLEY, CHINESE Another name for cilantro; see HERB.

PARSNIP A relative of the carrot, this ivory-colored root closely resembles its brighter, more familiar cousin. Parsnips have a slightly sweet flavor and a tough, starchy texture that softens with cooking. Excellent roasted, steamed, boiled, or baked, parsnips can be prepared in almost any way that potatoes or carrots are. Because they become mushy more quickly than other root vegetables, add them toward the end of cooking to stews and soups. Very young, tender parsnips may be grated or thinly sliced and added raw to salads.

Selecting Although now available year-round, parsnips are at their peak during the winter months, when the frosty weather converts their starches to sugar. In fact, some devotees of the root find spring-dug parsnips the sweetest of all. (Today, cold storage helps do the same at other times of the year.) Look for small to medium parsnips that are firm and unblemished. Larger ones can be tough and stringy and have a woody core that must be removed.

Storing Wrapped in a perforated plastic bag, parsnips will keep in the refrigerator for up to 1 month.

Preparing Scratch parsnips with your fingernail to check for waxy coating. If the vegetables are waxed, be sure to peel them. Otherwise, they may be scrubbed with a vegetable brush or peeled, as you wish. Cut out and discard the tough, fibrous core found in large parsnips. Because they undergo discoloring when exposed to air, cook cut parsnips immediately or sprinkle them with lemon juice.

See also STEAMING.

PASSION FRUIT Though it is juicy, highly aromatic, and undeniably seductive, this tropical fruit was named not for any aphrodisiac qualities but by Spanish Jesuit missionaries in South America who thought the structure and patterns of its flower recalled the Crucifixion. Passion fruit may be enjoyed simply by slicing open the palm-sized, purplish sphere and spooning it straight from its skin. The yellow-orange pulp, at once sweet and tart, also adds exotic flavor and aroma to fruit salads, sauces, dressings, desserts, and beverages. Even the crunchy, spicy-tasting, glossy black seeds may be eaten, although they are often discarded. Commercially packaged passion fruit juice and nectar are also available.

Selecting The passion fruit is at its best when it looks its worst, the skin uniformly wrinkled and sometimes showing traces of mold. Eat such specimens within a day or so. Otherwise, buy smooth-skinned fruits, which will ripen within 3 to 5 days.

Storing Keep underripe passion fruits at room temperature until wrinkled. Refrigerate fully ripe fruits and use within 2 days. Freeze whole ripe fruits or their pulp for up to 6 months.

Preparing Use a sharp knife to halve a ripe passion fruit. To separate seeds from pulp, rub through a sieve.

PASTA See page 332.

PASTRY Another term for unleavened dough, as opposed to bread dough. Pie and tart dough is often referred to as pastry. See FILO; PIE & TART.

PASTRY BAG See BAKING TOOLS.

PASTRY BLENDER See BAKING TOOLS.

PASTRY BOARD See BAKING TOOLS.

PASTRY BRUSH See BAKING TOOLS.

PASTRY CLOTH See BAKING TOOLS.

PASTRY WEIGHTS Another term for pie weights; see BAKING TOOLS; BLIND BAKING.

PÂTÉ Taken from the French word for paste, a pâté is typically a rich, finely ground meat mixture. It can be made from almost any meat or combination of meats,

the most common being pork, veal, and rabbit, as well as chicken liver and foie gras. It may also be made from fish and shellfish. Some pâtés are blended to a silky smooth texture. Others are chunky and rustic. Still others are studded with ingredients, such as blanched asparagus, hard-boiled eggs, peppercorns, pistachios, diced mushrooms, strips of ham, or whole truffles. Pâtés can be served either hot or cold, with a crust or without. Purists will insist that any meat mixture cooked and served in a terrine dish should also be called a terrine, and that it is only a "pâté" if and when it is unmolded. Today, this distinction is rarely followed, so the two terms are often used interchangeably.

Selecting Look for prepared pâté in the deli section of food markets or specialty grocers. It is available packaged in miniature plastic terrine dishes or as individual slices wrapped in plastic.

Quick Tip

To test the flavor of a homemade pâté (or any meat mixture) before it is cooked, fry up a little patty in a small skillet. Taste and then adjust the seasoning of the mixture. The flavors will mellow as the pâté sits, so season with a bold hand. Also, food served at room temperature needs more seasoning because the lower temperature masks many flavors.

Storing Keep pâté in the refrigerator, sealed in plastic wrap or an airtight container. Serve it within 1 week. The flavor of homemade pâté improves if left to rest for 2 to 3 days in the refrigerator. Freezing pâté is not recommended, for its texture will suffer.

Preparing Before serving pâté, let it sit at room temperature for 30 minutes or so to take the chill off and bring out its flavor.

See also TERRINE.

Pasta

"Paste," as the Latin root of *pasta* unglamorously translates, doesn't begin to hint at the glorious dishes that result from combining flour and water (and sometimes eggs or flavorings) and forming the mixture into sheets, ribbons, or shapes. Pasta, for all its simplicity, is one of the world's most versatile foods.

Although popular legend has it that Marco Polo discovered noodles on his travels to China in the late 13th century and brought them home to his countrymen, more reputable sources suggest that Italians and Asians learned how to shape and boil pastes of ground wheat independently of each other. Although the term *pasta* used to refer only to wheat noodles found in Italian cooking, pasta long ago transcended Italy's borders to become a dish of universal appeal. Today, nearly every country in the world incorporates pasta into its cuisine, whether it is topped with a sauce, stuffed or layered and baked, added to soups, or dressed with a vinaigrette.

Another common Western-style noodle is the egg noodle. Both fresh and dried, these have a delicate character and silky finish. They are wonderful tossed with a sauce, of course, but also are a fine addition to soups (undercook them, then stir them in for the last few minutes of cooking); serve as a satisfying base for stews; and accompany main dishes, often tossed with butter and grated cheese.

Pick of the Pastas Hundreds of pasta shapes exist, many of them with descriptive or fanciful Italian names. More than 30 of the most commonly available types, both dried and fresh, are listed below. Choose the sizes and shapes of pasta that suit the sauce or other treatment you are using:

thin strands for light sauces; small shapes for broths or soups; broader strands, ribbons, or tubes, or larger shapes for more robust or chunky sauces; and wide ribbons or large, hollow tubes or shapes for layered or filled baked dishes.

ACINI DI PEPE Small "peppercorns." Spherical shapes for adding to soups.

AGNOLOTTI Crescent-shaped filled pasta.

BUCATINI Long, narrow tubes resembling hollow spaghetti; good for chunky, full-flavored sauces.

CANNELLONI Rolled tubes of fresh or dried pasta used for stuffing.

CAPELLINI/CAPELLI D'ANGELO "Little hairs" or "angel hair," resembling fine spaghetti strands. Best for simple, light, smooth sauces.

CONCHIGLIE "Shells" in various sizes. Used for soups or, in the case of larger shells, stuffing and baking.

DITALI Tubes resembling "thimbles," tossed with sauces or used in salads or soups. Ditalini are small ditali, used primarily in soups.

FARFALLE Bite-sized "butterflies." Also called bow ties. Farfalline are the smaller version.

FEDELINI Thin spaghetti strands; good served with medium- to full-bodied sauces.

FETTUCCINE Long, wide "ribbons," often fresh pasta. Good for hearty, rich, and chunky sauces.

FUSILLI "Fuses." Long, twisted strands or short, corkscrew-shaped tubes. Best with chunky, substantial sauces.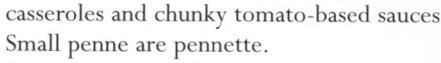

GEMELLI "Twins." Two short, intertwined strands, served with sauces or in salads or baked dishes.

LASAGNE Large, flat ribbons of dried pasta or ribbons or squares of fresh pasta, for layering. Sometimes made with ruffled edges.

LINGUINE "Little tongues." Flat, narrow ribbons of the same general length as spaghetti; best when served with light, smooth sauces or medium-bodied sauces.

LUMACHE "Snails." Large shells for stuffing.

MACARONI Small, short tubes curved like elbows; great for casseroles and salads.

MANICOTTI "Muffs." Hollow tubes for stuffing.

MOSTACCIOLI "Moustaches." Narrow tubes served with sauces or in salads or baked dishes.

ORECCHIETTE "Little ears." Small, indented circular shapes, good for chunky sauces.

ORZO "Barley." Slender, seedlike shapes that look not unlike large grains of rice. Good for soups.

PAPPARDELLE Wide ribbons of fresh pasta used with hearty sauces.

PENNE "Quills." Narrow tubes with angled ends resembling pen nibs. Traditionally used for casseroles and chunky tomato-based sauces. Small penne are pennette.

PERCIATELLI Another name for bucatini.

RADIATORI Bite-sized, ridged shapes resembling "radiators"; served with sauces or in salads or baked dishes.

RAVIOLI Classic stuffed pasta, usually square but often round.

RIGATONI Ridged bite-sized tubes. Hold up well under robust, chunky tomato sauces and in baked dishes.

ROTELLE Many-spoked wheels; served with sauces that catch in the spokes or in salads or baked dishes.

RUOTE More bite-sized wheels; served with sauces or in salads or baked dishes.

SEMI DI MELONE "Melon seeds." Similar to orzo.

SPAGHETTI Long, thin, cylindrical strands. From the word *spago,* "string." Spaghettini is a thinner version of spaghetti.

STELLINE "Little stars." Tiny shapes used typically in soups.

TAGLIARINI Long, flat, narrow ribbons, usually of fresh pasta. Also referred to as tagliolini.

TAGLIATELLE Ribbons similar to but slightly wider than fettuccine, usually of fresh pasta. Good with hearty, sturdy sauces.

TORTELLINI "Little pies." Small, circular stuffed pasta.

TUBETTI Short, stout "tubes" served in soups or with sauces. Tubettini are small tubetti.

VERMICELLI "Little worms." A slender form of spaghetti similar to spaghettini. Good for light, smooth sauces.

ZITI Hollow tubes in short and long forms, for hearty sauces.

continued

P

Pasta, continued

Selecting Pasta is sold in a wide variety of shapes and sizes (see Pick of the Pastas, page 332) and in both dried and fresh forms. Well-stocked food stores and Italian delicatessens offer the best selection of both dried and fresh pastas. The finest dried pasta begins with semolina flour ground from durum wheat, the hardest variety grown, which gives the resulting pasta shapes their desired firmness and elasticity. Fresh pasta is made from either all-purpose or semolina flour combined with eggs. Sometimes another ingredient, such as spinach, tomato, beet, saffron, or squid ink, is added to provide color and a subtle flavor. Despite a recent tendency in this country to consider fresh pasta better than dried, each has its place in a menu. Dried pasta goes best with tomato or oil-based sauces, while more tender fresh pasta is better suited to sauces featuring butter, cream, or cheese.

When buying dried egg noodles, check that eggs are, in fact, one of the ingredients listed; many are imitation egg noodles.

Storing Dried pasta keeps well in the manufacturer's packaging at room temperature for up to 2 months. Transferred to an airtight container away from moisture, heat, and light, it will keep for up to 1 year. Wrap homemade or store-bought fresh pasta in plastic and store in the refrigerator for no more than 3 days, or wrap in freezer-weight plastic and store in the freezer for up to 1 month.

About Cooking Pasta Both fresh and dried pastas should be cooked al dente, tender but still chewy. Use a two-handled pot large enough to let the pasta float freely during cooking, and plan on 5 quarts of water for each 1 pound of fresh pasta or 1 to 1¼ pounds of dried pasta. These amounts usually are sufficient for 8 first-course servings or 4 main-course servings.

Bring the water to a full rolling boil, salt it, and then add the pasta. (Unsalted water may result in bland pasta, and the finished dish may demand heavier seasoning.) As soon as the water returns to the boil, start timing. Cooking time will vary with the pasta's dryness, shape, and size. Fresh pasta usually cooks within 1 to 3 minutes, depending on thickness. Commercial dried pasta generally cooks in 3 to 15 minutes; check the manufacturer's packaging for suggested times. To test for doneness, at the earliest possible suggested time, remove a strand or piece with tongs, a long-handled fork, or a slotted spoon, let cool briefly, then bite into it.

Removing pasta for testing.

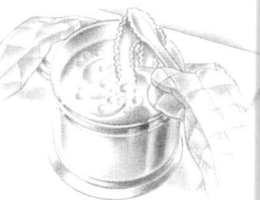

If the pasta seems too chewy, cook 1 minute more before testing again. As soon as it is ready, drain the pasta immediately, pouring it through a colander set in the kitchen sink.

The only exception to cooking pasta at a rolling boil is fresh filled pastas such as ravioli, which are more tender and should be simmered so they will not break apart.

HOW TO *Make Homemade Pasta*

1. On a work surface, heap the flour specified in a pasta recipe and make a well in its center. Break the eggs into the well.

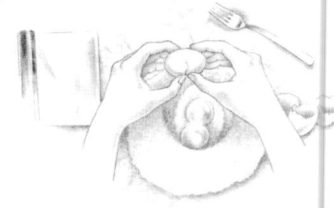

2. With a fork, lightly beat the eggs. Then, in a circular motion, gradually incorporate flour from the sides of the well until combined.

3. With the heel of your hand, knead the dough—pushing it down and away and turning it repeatedly, using a dough scraper if it sticks—until it is smooth and elastic, at least 5 minutes. If it sticks or seems a little soft, sprinkle it with flour. Gather the dough into a ball.

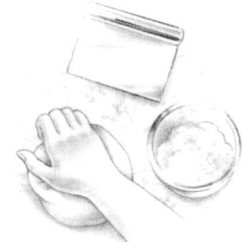

ROLLING AND CUTTING BY HAND

4. On a clean work surface dusted with flour, flatten the kneaded dough with your hand. With a flour-dusted rolling pin, roll it out to desired thickness as given in a recipe.

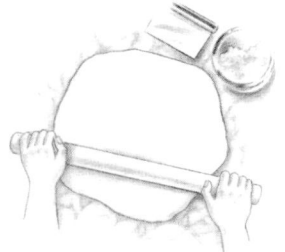

5. Loosely roll up the pasta around the rolling pin and unroll onto a flour-dusted kitchen towel, leaving it until dry to the touch but still flexible, about 10 minutes (less if the air is very dry).

6. On the work surface, roll the pasta into a cylinder. With a small, sharp knife, cut crosswise into ribbons of desired width.

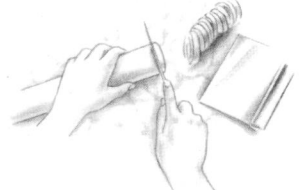

ROLLING AND CUTTING BY MACHINE

Start by following steps 1 to 3 above.

4. Adjust the rollers of a hand-cranked pasta machine to the widest setting. Cut the kneaded dough into manageable portions of 2 to 3 ounces each. Lightly dust a portion of dough and crank it through the rollers.

5. Lightly dust the sheet of dough with flour and fold it into thirds.

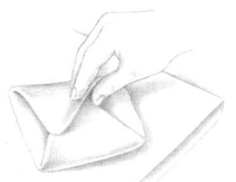

6. Reset the rollers one width narrower; roll the dough again. Repeat the process until the dough reaches desired thickness.

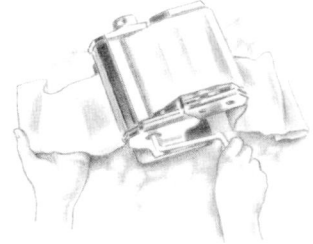

7. Secure a cutting attachment to the machine. Cut the pasta sheet into easily manageable lengths and crank each length through the cutter to make pasta strands.

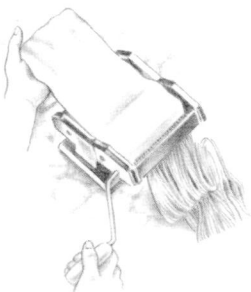

See also FLOUR; NOODLE.

P

PEA, FRESH The pea is one of the major groups within the vast legume family. Peas can be divided into three general categories: whole pea pods eaten young and fresh, shelled peas eaten fresh, and shelled peas that are dried.

Peas eaten fresh as whole pods include the broad, flat snow peas that star in Chinese stir-fries, as well as plumper, rounder, bright green sugar snap peas.

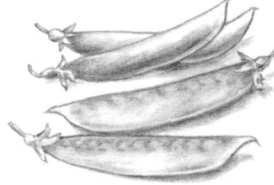

Sugar snap and snow peas.

The most common variety for shelling is the English, or garden, pea. Baby peas, or *petits pois,* refer to tiny, sweet English peas, while so-called early or June peas are larger and have more starch. The smaller ones need barely any cooking and are wonderful stirred into risotto at the last minute with a little grated Parmesan cheese. Most are harvested for freezing.

The final category of peas, those that are usually dried, include yellow and green split peas, chickpeas, and black-eyed peas. These are better grouped with beans and lentils because of their similar flavors and uses. See BEAN, DRIED.

Black-eyed peas are sometimes available fresh in the summer. If you buy them still in the pod, you'll need to shell them before using them.

Selecting Choose fresh peas with crisp, smooth, glossy, bright green pods. Avoid any that are wilted, dried, puffy, or blemished. Try to purchase them from a farmers' market for the sweetest flavor.

Canned peas bear so little resemblance to fresh peas that it is better to go without if they are the only option. Frozen shelled peas, on the other hand, are decent substitutes, especially if they will be cooked with other ingredients. Look for those labeled "baby" or "petite" for smaller, more delicate peas. Snow peas are available frozen as well, but frozen snow peas turn fairly soft and flavorless once cooked.

Storing Because their natural sugar begins converting to starch immediately after they are picked, peas should be prepared and eaten as soon as possible, preferably the day of purchase. Peas will stay crisp for 3 to 4 days if stored in a plastic bag in the refrigerator, but do not expect them to retain their characteristic sweetness after a day.

Preparing For whole pea pods, snap off the tips of the pods, pulling down the length of the pod to remove any tough strings as well. Although many modern hybrids have no strings or the peas are processed before reaching the store, it doesn't hurt to check. Whether pods or shelled, peas are best if steamed or blanched very briefly to retain their crisp texture and vibrant color.

Quick Tip

If raw snow peas wilt, let them stand in cold water for 10 to 15 minutes to recrisp them.

HOW TO *Shell English Peas*

Shell peas just before cooking to prevent them from drying out.

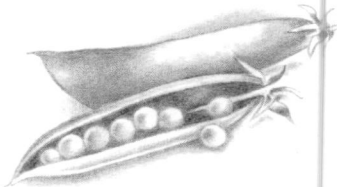

1. Work over a large bowl. After checking for and removing any strings as described above, squeeze the pod and press your thumb against the seam to split it open.

2. Continuing the same movement, sweep your thumb down along the inside of the pod to pop out the peas.

3. Discard the pod. (If making soup, save a few to sweeten the simmering stock.)

4. If needed, refrigerate the peas for up to 1 day. Cover with damp paper towels or cold water to keep them moist.

See also BEAN, FRESH; BLANCHING; BOILING; STEAMING.

PEACH A sweet and fragrant peach, ripe enough to drip juice down your chin, is one of the joys of summer. Native to China, where legends tell of this fruit's power to confer immortality, peaches now also grow in temperate regions of North America and Europe. Related to cherries, apricots, and plums, peaches are members of the stone fruit family, their flesh concealing a large, wrinkled pit. Peaches are often classified as clingstone or freestone, depending on how difficult or easy it is to separate the pit from the flesh. The flesh ranges from bright yellow to white, the latter being less common and more perishable but also generally sweeter and juicier. In more recent years, the fruit's downy skin has fallen into disfavor among consumers. Popular hybrids reduce the fuzz to a mere softness.

Peaches make excellent jams, pies, and sauces. Use them in salsas or marinades for pork or toss thin slices into a green salad. For dessert, enjoy peach halves prepared simply: poached in spiced white wine or broiled with a touch of butter and lime juice. Or bake peaches in a wide variety of homestyle classics, from peach pie to peach cobbler to peach variations of upside-down cakes.

Selecting Choose peaches that give slightly to gentle pressure, that emanate a flowery fragrance, and that are free of bruises and blemishes. The amount of red in a peach's skin depends on its variety and has little relation to its ripeness. Avoid any with tinges of green, however; they were picked too early and may never ripen properly. Once picked, a peach will eventually become softer and juicier but not significantly sweeter. Unfortunately, most peaches arrive at market stone hard. Handle even unripe peaches with care, for their flesh bruises easily. Peaches come to market from May to October, but most varieties peak in late June to early August.

Peach halves and slices are available canned in sugar syrup, water, or fruit juice. Other forms convenient for cooking include frozen slices and dried chunks.

Storing Keep peaches at room temperature in a smooth bowl until they are ripe. (The ridges of a basket can leave bruised indentations in ripening peaches.) Hasten the ripening process by placing them in a paper bag with an apple or a banana. Once they are soft, store peaches in the refrigerator in a plastic bag for 4 to 5 days.

Keep dried and canned peaches in a cool place away from light and moisture.

Preparing Wash peaches just before cooking or serving. If there's a good deal of fuzz, rub the peach briefly while washing. The fuzz will come right off. Like many fruits, fresh peaches will have a sweeter, fuller flavor if served at room temperature. Since the flesh of peaches discolors when exposed to air, toss cut pieces immediately with citrus juice, wine, or liqueur.

Quick Bite

Although the nectarine looks like a peach with smooth skin and is a member of the extended peach family, it is not, as some folks believe, a hybrid. Like the peach, however, it comes either freestone or cling, with yellow or white flesh, and it is sweet and juicy.

HOW TO *Halve a Peach*

1. Using a small, sharp knife, cut the peach in half lengthwise, cutting carefully around the round pit at the center.

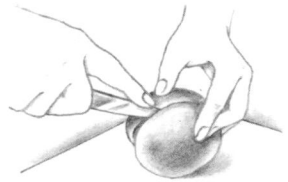

2. Rotate the halves in opposite directions to separate them.

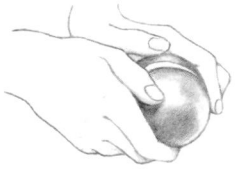

3. Scoop out the pit with the tip of a knife and discard.

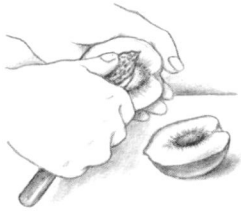

For peeling peaches, see BLANCHING.

PEANUT First grown in South America, peanuts quickly spread to Asia, Africa, and the American South aboard the ships of early Spanish and Portuguese explorers and slave traders. Known also as groundnuts, goobers (from the African word *nguba*), or goober peas, peanuts belong to the legume family, along with lentils, beans, and peas. The vinelike plant is unique in that its flower stalks, after fertilizing themselves, each grow a stem that bores into the soil. The seedpods then develop and mature underground. The primary types grown commercially are the jumbo Virginia, the oval Valencia, the smaller and rounder Spanish variety covered with a red skin, and the runner peanut with evenly sized kernels, which are ideal for producing peanut butter. The world's leading growers are India and China, where the plants flourish in the hot climates.

Peanuts are one of the most common ingredients in snacks and sweets, adding texture as well as flavor to cookies, candies—who isn't tempted by peanut brittle?—and countless snack mixes. With a high amount of protein and tremendous thickening power, peanuts appear in soups, stews, breads, and sauces around the

Quick Tip

If a recipe calls for 1 pound shelled peanuts, you will need to buy about 1½ pounds peanuts in the shell.

world, from West African chicken and peanut stew to Sichuan noodles tossed with a peanut-sesame-chile sauce to the rich, creamy sauce made from peanuts and coconut milk that accompanies saté, a specialty of Indonesia's many street vendors.

The colorless oil derived from pressed peanuts has a mild flavor and a particularly high smoking point, making it ideal for stir-frying and deep-frying. It is especially typical of Asian cuisines.

Selecting Peanuts are sold in a wide variety of ways. They are available with or without their shells, with or without their papery skins, roasted or unroasted, salted or unsalted, mixed with other nuts or alone. Although usually dried, they occasionally appear fresh at farmers' markets during the late-summer harvest. If buying them whole, shake the peanuts to check that they do not rattle in their shells, a sure sign that the nuts inside are old and dry. Once shelled, they are most commonly roasted and then vacuum-packed in cans or glass jars. Bags of unroasted (raw) skinned peanuts can be found in Asian and Latin American markets.

Storing Because of their oil content, peanuts go rancid fairly quickly if left at room temperature. Wrap unshelled peanuts in a plastic bag and keep them in the refrigerator for up to 6 months. Store unopened jars or cans of peanuts at room temperature for up to 1 year; once you open them, be sure to refrigerate them. They will stay fresh for 3 months in the refrigerator and for 2 years in the freezer. Store peanut oil for no longer than 2 months in an airtight container away from light and heat.

Preparing To shell peanuts, firmly and evenly press your thumb lengthwise along the shell. It will easily split and pull away.

See also FAT & OIL; NUT; PEANUT BUTTER.

PEANUT BUTTER This creamy or slightly crunchy peanut spread, made by grinding shelled dry-roasted peanuts to a paste, has come a long way from its humble beginnings. Commercially developed as an easily digested source of protein, peanut butter is now enjoyed by young and old alike in sandwiches, cookies, candies, and such unforgettable snacks as peanut butter fudge or "ants on a log," the classic combination of celery stalks, peanut butter, and raisins. It is also used in some savory dishes such as a spicy peanut soup.

Selecting Peanut butter is available smooth or chunky, that is, with chopped peanuts stirred in for texture. Many commercial peanut butters include additives to improve spreadability and flavor. Natural peanut butters have a slightly grainy texture and a layer of oil that must be stirred back

in before using. Variations include honey flavored, grape jelly or marshmallow swirled, and reduced fat.

Storing Some brands contain salt, sweeteners, stabilizers, and preservatives. These peanut butters can be kept for up to 1 year in a cool, dark place. The oils of "natural" or "old-fashioned" peanut butter will separate over time. Keep these peanut butters in the refrigerator for up to 6 months.

Preparing Use peanut butter as a convenient replacement for ground roasted peanuts in sauces or soups. The flavor of peanut butter pairs well with chocolate, banana, caramel, and marshmallow.

PEAR A perfectly ripe pear has soft, juicy flesh with delicately floral flavor. Sweet, fragrant pears are available year-round, but their peak season is during the cold months of winter, a time when their freshness is especially welcome. The many different varieties of pear are all generously curved in the fruit's well-known shape, but they range in color, contour, texture, and flavor. The French in particular have long admired and cultivated pears.

Selecting Pears are picked when mature but still hard, rather than when they are ripe. This prevents them from becoming too granular and soft. Look for smooth,

Bartlett and Comice pears.

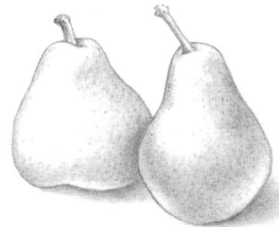

unblemished fruits with their stems still attached. They should be fragrant and just beginning to soften near the stem. They must be left at room temperature to soften and sweeten and are ready to eat when they

Pear Glossary

Although thousands of pear varieties have been developed since the fruit was first cultivated 4,000 years ago in Asia, today relatively few choices are available commercially.

ANJOU An almost egg-shaped pear with green skin, often with a yellow tinge even when ripe, although a rarer red variety blushes to reddish green. A ripe Anjou is juicy, yet keeps its shape when sliced for salads, cooked in desserts, or baked whole. In season from October to May.

BARTLETT Known as the Williams pear in Europe, with thin skin that ripens from dark green to light green and then yellow and an aromatic, slightly musky flesh that is very soft when ripe. This good eating and all-purpose cooking pear is available from August to November. The sturdier red Bartlett is not always as juicy.

BOSC A versatile pear with a long, tapered neck, green skin with distinct brown russeting, and sweet, creamy white flesh. Excellent for eating fresh and for baking or poaching. Eat Bosc pears when they yield only slightly to finger pressure. In season from September to May.

COMICE Widely available, Comice is the best pear for eating out of hand, with sweet, meltingly juicy, "buttery" flesh and a hint of spiciness. It is quite round, with hardly noticeable shoulders, and its greenish yellow skin blushes to a soft red. It also bakes well. The Comice is fragile and is not a good traveler. In season from October to January.

SECKEL Among the smallest of pears. Ideal for making preserves, it has smooth, dark green skin with reddish hues and firm, slightly granular flesh. In season from August to January.

WINTER NELLIS A short pear with almost no neck and with a brownish green peel with russeted dots. The slightly spicy flesh is enjoyed raw, holds its shape well when baked or poached, and is good for preserving. In season from November to May.

wrinkle a little at the stem end and are slightly soft at the blossom end. Pears are also available dried and canned in light sugar syrup or in fruit juice.

Storing Handle pears gently, for they bruise easily. Leave them at room temperature for a few days to ripen. Pears are notorious for having an extremely brief period of ripeness between being still too hard to eat and heading toward spoiling. They can be refrigerated in plastic bags for 3 to 5 days, depending on their degree of ripeness, but for the best flavor, be sure to bring them back to room temperature before eating. Because of their delicate texture, pears do not freeze well.

Keep canned pears for up to 2 years in a cool, dry place. Refrigerate dried pears

Quick Bite

The colorless French pear brandy known as *poire Williams* is made from Bartlett pears.

in an airtight container or zippered plastic bag for up to 6 months.

Preparing Pears can be left unpeeled for eating fresh, but be sure to peel pears before cooking. Although the peel is edible, some fruits may have tough skins with a slightly bitter flavor that is accentuated when cooked. When cutting pears for salads or hors d'oeuvres, halve them lengthwise, then scoop out the core with a small spoon or melon baller. Like cut apples, cut pears should be tossed with a little lemon juice to prevent discoloring.

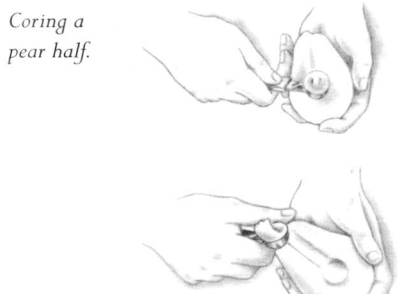

Coring a pear half.

To core a whole pear while leaving the stem end intact, use a small spoon, a grapefruit spoon, or the large end of a melon baller to scoop out the seeds and membrane from the pear's blossom end.

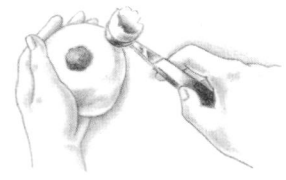

Coring a whole pear.

See also PEAR, ASIAN.

PEAR, ASIAN A relative newcomer in the American produce aisle, the Asian pear somehow manages to be both superbly crisp and extremely juicy. Belonging to a species completely different from regular pears, Asian pears resemble large, pale yellow-green apples. They are also known as Japanese pears, Chinese pears, and apple pears. Asian pears have a flowery fragrance, a mildly sweet flavor, and a slightly granular texture that bursts with juice from the first bite.

Asian pears are best enjoyed fresh as a snack or dessert. You can cut them into translucent, paper-thin slices for salads, cheese trays, and dessert garnishes. They can be cooked in many of the same ways as regular pears, but they require significantly longer cooking and remain relatively firm. The delicate flavor of Asian pears is lost if they are mixed with more strongly flavored fruits or ingredients. Stick to such subtle partners as citrus fruits, ginger, lemongrass, or almonds.

Selecting Varying in skin color from soft green to clear yellow depending on the variety, Asian pears often have a delicate scattering of russeted spots. They are sometimes sold wrapped in protective webbing to prevent bruising. Unlike regular pears, Asian pears are a little firm when ripe.

Storing Once ripened at room temperature, store Asian pears in a plastic bag in the refrigerator. They will keep well for up to 2 weeks, far longer than regular pears.

Preparing Asian pears can be left unpeeled for eating fresh but should be peeled before cooking.

PECAN See NUT.

PECORINO ROMANO See CHEESE.

PECTIN Pectin is a water-soluble carbohydrate, a flavorless, gelatinlike substance found naturally in fruits, valued for its ability to "set" or jell jams, jellies, and preserves. Concentrated in the seeds and skin of tart and underripe fruits, pectin diminishes as the fruit fully ripens. Pectin works effectively only when the correct balance of sugar and acid is present. The acid, which allows the release of the pectin, is often present in the fruit itself, and then cooking with sugar produces a soft set.

Some fruits naturally contain more pectin than others. For example, apples are naturally high in pectin, while peaches and strawberries contain low amounts. For making preserves from fruit with a low pectin content, you can buy liquid or powdered pectin to add as directed.

Selecting Liquid and powdered pectin are available in major supermarkets. Pectin sugar, which combines powdered pectin and sugar for use in preserving, may be found in specialty-food or baking-supply stores.

Storing Keep liquid and powdered pectin and pectin sugar in airtight containers away from light and moisture.

Preparing Different forms of pectin are not interchangeable and vary in how they are used. Follow instructions on the package and in specific recipes. With low-pectin fruits, additional pectin, a high-pectin fruit, or a greater amount of sugar must be added to set jams, jellies, and candies.

Pectin Content of Various Fruits

HIGH PECTIN

apple; cranberry; currants, red and black; lemon; orange; plum; quince

LOW PECTIN

banana; cherry; grapes; mango; peach; pineapple; strawberry

PEELING Removing the skin from fruits and vegetables is one of the first steps in preparing many dishes. Although peels frequently are edible and contain concentrated amounts of nutrients, they may add unwanted texture, color, or bitterness to a dish. Some fruits, vegetables, and nuts, such as peaches, tomatoes, and almonds, have thin skins that slip off more easily after blanching. Others, such as peppers and eggplant, have skins that will peel away quickly once they are roasted or charred.

A simple vegetable peeler or a sharp paring knife is used for peeling most foods. You can buy special peelers designed for specific foods. Unusual-shaped utensils for peeling asparagus, avocados, oranges, and pineapples are practical if you serve any of them frequently or in large amounts. See also BLANCHING.

PEPPER, BELL See BELL PEPPER.

PEPPER, HOT See CHILE.

PEPPERCORN See SPICE.

PERSIMMON In late autumn, bright orange persimmons hang from leaf-bare trees like small lanterns. Dramatic in color and demanding in temperament, these showy fruits reward the patient cook with a rich, sweet flavor that epitomizes the harvest season. Originally cultivated in China and later carried from Japan to the West by Commodore Perry, the persimmons most familiar to us today belong to the *kaki* species. Many countries still know the fruit by this name. A species native to the United States is now difficult to find, although the word *persimmon* derives, in fact, from an Algonquian word.

Two basic varieties are available, both derived from the *kaki* persimmon but each with different characteristics. The Hachiya is large, acorn shaped with a pointed end, and deep orange. It must be ripened until meltingly soft to rid it of its mouth-puckering astringency. Once ripe, the flesh

Hachiya and Fuyu persimmons.

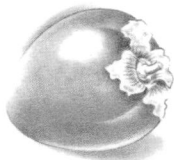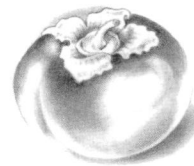

is creamy and rich, with a flavor hinting of honey and pumpkin. Puréed, it is wonderful added to muffin and quick-bread batters, custard, pudding, ice cream, or pie. It also makes flavorful jams, jellies, and confections. The Fuyu persimmon has a lighter color and a smaller, rounder shape, like a tomato. Popular for eating out of hand, it is still crisp when ripe and is also completely free of the bitter tannin present in the unripe Hachiya. Halved and broiled briefly, with butter and brown sugar, Fuyus can accompany roast pork or poultry.

Selecting Choose plump fruits heavy for their size and free of blemishes. Their skin should be smooth and shiny, with no hint of yellow. Look for intact stem caps that are green, not gray and brittle. Handle the Hachiya persimmons carefully, for any bruises will encourage rot as they ripen. For this reason, it's a good idea to buy them still a little firm (not rock hard) and let them ripen in peace on your countertop. Persimmons are in peak season from late October to late February.

Storing Arrange Hachiya persimmons stem down on a plate or in a large shallow bowl, and then leave them at room temperature for 1 to 2 weeks until ripe, when they will be very soft, and the flesh, encased in the now-wrinkled skin, will feel almost liquefied. To speed up ripening, place them inside a paper bag with a banana or an apple. Some claim that freezing persimmons will hasten the ripening, but this only softens them without developing their sweetness. Once ripe, persimmons should be eaten right away or refrigerated in a plastic bag for 2 days. Persimmon purée freezes well for up to 1 year.

Preparing Peel ripe Hachiya persimmons before eating. Fuyus can be eaten unpeeled.

PHYLLO See FILO.

PIE & TART See page 344.

PIE PLATE See BAKEWARE.

PIE WEIGHTS See BAKING TOOLS; BLIND BAKING.

PILAF See RICE.

PIMIENTO Also spelled pimento. From the Spanish for pepper, the pimiento is a sweet, scarlet pepper about 4 inches long. Essential to Hungarian cuisine, ground dried pimientos are better known as paprika. With wide shoulders tapering to a point, the fresh pepper has the shape of a heart. Its thick flesh is more flavorful than that of red bell peppers, and it ranges in heat from mild to hot.

Selecting Fresh pimientos can be found in specialty markets from late summer to early fall. Select firm, smooth peppers with no soft spots. Pimientos are available year-round whole, chopped, or sliced, preserved in brine or vinegar in cans or jars.

Storing Wrapped in a paper towel and then in a plastic bag, a fresh pimiento will keep refrigerated for about 1 week. Store unopened jars and cans for up to 1 year in a cool, dark place. Once opened, jarred pimientos begin to mold rather quickly.

Preparing See BELL PEPPER.

Pie & Tart

"Good apple pies," wrote Jane Austen, "are a considerable part of our domestic happiness." So, too, any lover of the pastry maker's art might add, are pumpkin pies, strawberry tarts, lemon meringue pies, chocolate cream pies, mincemeat tarts, Key lime pies, and other sweet—or occasionally savory—treats that combine a filling with one or two layers of crust.

Pies, which are usually baked in a pie pan with sloping sides, may feature two crusts or just a bottom crust. The crust is usually made from pastry dough that bakes up crisp and flaky. Some pies, however, may feature a more crumbly, tender pastry like those found in tarts. Still other pies use crusts made of crushed cookie or graham cracker crumbs, like those that form the crust for some cheesecakes.

Tarts almost always have only a bottom crust, which tends to be firmer, richer, and more crumbly than pie pastry. Rustic tarts, like a *pizza rustica,* may also be made with more chewy, breadlike, yeast-leavened dough. Tarts are usually baked in tart pans, which have straight or fluted vertical sides and sometimes removable bottoms that let you slip the rim away after baking and cooling. Some tarts, however, are free-form—shaped by hand on a baking sheet. Some of these may also be called *galettes.*

About Crusts "Flaky" and "tender" are the two basic styles of crust. Flaky crust is achieved by keeping the fat in discrete, cold bits within the dough. Once the dough reaches the oven, the bits of fat melt, giving off puffs of steam that lift the pastry into flakes and create air pockets. This airy, flaky texture defines a classic pie crust. A tender crust is flavorful and crumbly, like short-bread, and is created by blending fat and flour more thoroughly. The fat in the dough literally cuts the gluten strands in the flour, making them short and fragile. This is often desirable for tarts.

Such variety alone can lead to the impression that making pies and tarts is difficult work. In truth, however, it is fairly easy to master the basics.

Quick Tip

Crusts with sugar will brown more quickly than those without. A high-sugar crust may scorch if not watched carefully.

Some makers of pies and tarts swear by vegetable shortening for their pastry, while others prefer butter, margarine, lard, or suet. There are even old-fashioned pie crusts made with vegetable oil. Each type of fat contributes its own characteristics to the final results. For any particular recipe, choose a fat—or combination of fats—that gives you the effect you prefer and best complements the filling.

Which Fat Should I Use?

BUTTER Makes a rich-tasting, tender crust.

VEGETABLE SHORTENING Produces the flakiest results, without contributing distinctive flavor of its own.

BUTTER PLUS VEGETABLE SHORTENING
Combines flakiness with tenderness and
rich flavor, a combination that many bakers
swear by. Replace up to half the butter
called for in a recipe with shortening.
LARD Makes an extremely light, flaky, rich
but almost flavorless crust. Some bakers
think it complements a savory filling better
than a sweet one.
MARGARINE Makes a slightly oily dough
with good flavor. Use only solid stick
margarine, never whipped.
SUET Makes a rich-tasting, firm-textured
crust that is best for savory fillings.
Pie and Tart Crust Savvy When
making pie and tart crusts, keep the following tips in mind:

- For a flaky, airy pie crust, keep all ingredients and equipment cold and work
  quickly. For a tender, crumbly crust, use
  ingredients and equipment at room temperature and blend the fat and flour
  well. See CUTTING IN and RUBBING IN
  for more details.
- Measure pastry ingredients precisely.
  Even slightly wrong proportions of
  flour, fat, and liquid can produce less-
  than-ideal crusts.
- Bake pies and tarts using nonreflective
  cookware, so heat will transfer well to
  the crust and cook it properly.
- Bake pies and tarts on the bottom rack
  in the oven for crisper bottom crusts.

Quick Tip

When a fully baked tart shell is to be filled with
fresh fruit, its inside is sometimes sealed to
prevent the fruit's juices—or the pastry cream
base for the fruit—from making the pastry
soggy. The sealant often is little more than a
brushing of melted jam or jelly. Alternatively,
melted chocolate may be used, which hardens
to a thin, crisp coating that also complements
the flavor of the fruit.

HOW TO *Roll Out Pie or Tart*
Pastry Dough
Beginning bakers often like to roll out
dough between two sheets of waxed or
parchment paper or plastic wrap. This prevents the dough from sticking to the work
surface and also makes the dough easy to
transfer to the pan. With a little practice,
however, you will become able to roll out
easily any ordinary nonsticky dough.

1. Sprinkle flour lightly over both the work surface and the rolling pin. If using a pastry sleeve
   or pastry cloth, rub flour into it, too.
2. Using your hands, shape the dough into a flat,
   round disk. Place it on the work surface and
   tap it 3 times with the rolling pin, at the top,
   middle, and bottom of the disk, to flatten and
   spread it out a bit. Give the disk a quarter turn
   and tap it again 3 times to spread it out.
3. Starting with the pin in the center of the disk,
   roll the pin away from you toward the far edge.
   Stop rolling and lift the pin at a finger's width
   from the edge of the dough (so that the edge
   does not become too thin). Bring the pin back
   to the center of the disk and roll it toward you,
   again stopping just shy of the edge. Use firm
   and steady pressure as you roll the pin, and
   work quickly so that the fat in the dough does
   not have time to melt too much.
4. Give the dough a quarter turn and repeat
   step 3. Turning the dough after each couple of
   strokes prevents it from sticking to the work
   surface. A second safeguard against sticking:
   add sprinklings of flour beneath the dough and
   on the rolling pin. Repeat turning and rolling
   until the dough is rolled out about ⅛ inch thick,
   with about 1 inch to spare around the circumference of your pan for pies or ½ inch for tarts,
   or as directed in a recipe.
5. Place your pie or tart pan in the center of the
   dough circle and, with a small knife, trim the
   dough into a neat circle, including the extra
   ½ or 1 inch around the outside of the pan. Save
   any trimmings, if you like, to make decorations
   for a top crust.

continued

P

Pie & Tart, continued

HOW TO *Transfer Dough and Make a Pie or Tart Crust*

1. Roll the round of dough loosely around the rolling pin and unroll it over the pie or tart pan, draping it loosely over the top of the pan.

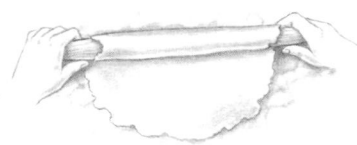

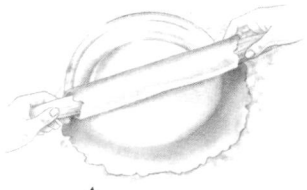

2. Lift up the edges of the dough circle as you gently ease it into the contours of the pan. Do not stretch the dough.

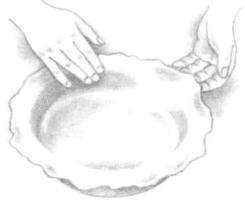

3. If not already done, use a knife or scissors to trim the overhanging dough to 1 inch for pies, ½ inch for tarts.

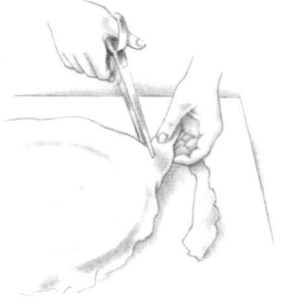

4. FOR PIES:

Tuck the overhang under itself to create a rim. This rim may be decoratively fluted or crimped (see page 348); for a double-crust pie, wait until the top crust is laid over the filling before crimping and sealing them (see opposite).

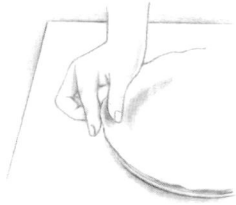

FOR TARTS:

Fold the overhang back into the pan and pat it into the sides of the pan, making the tart's sides a little thicker than the bottom.

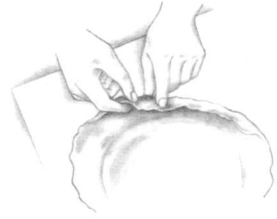

Press the dough well into the sides of the pan, raising the dough slightly above the rim of the pan. The crust will likely shrink slightly during baking.

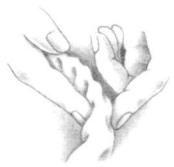

5. Before baking, place the crust in the freezer for 15 minutes to "relax the dough." The process of making dough and rolling it out develops a network of elastic gluten strands in the flour, and this cooling-down period will help avoid a chewy crust.

HOW TO *Make a Double-Crust Pie*

Follow these guidelines for forming a top crust on a pie.

1. After filling the pie and rolling out the top crust as directed in the specific recipe, brush the rim of the bottom crust with water.

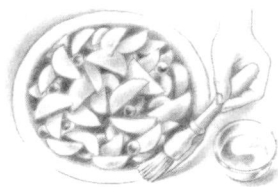

   Transfer the rolled-out top crust as described above, laying it over the pie.

2. Trim the pastry all around so you have about ½ inch of overhang.

3. Fold the overhang under the bottom crust.

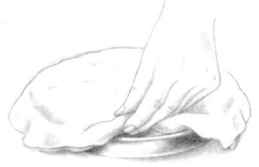

4. With the tines of a fork, crimp, or press firmly, around the rim to seal the crusts together.

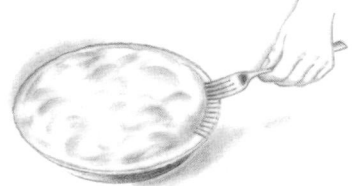

5. With a small knife, cut 4 or 5 vents, or slits, in the top crust so steam can escape from the filling during baking.

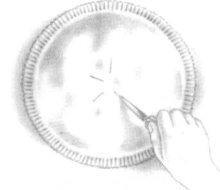

HOW TO *Make a Lattice Top*

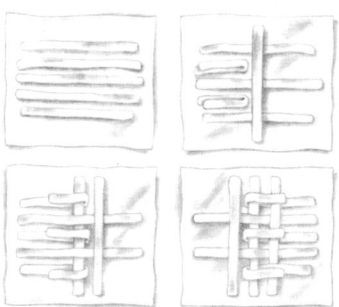

1. With a straight or fluted pastry wheel or a sharp knife, cut the rolled-out dough for the top crust into 12 strips of varying lengths, each about ½ inch wide.

2. Invert the pie pan on top of a sheet of waxed paper and run the tip of a table knife around its rim to make a visible indentation in the paper. Place the paper on top of a rimless baking sheet and spray lightly with nonstick spray.

3. Using the circle as a guide, lift up every other strip and place it on the paper, arranging the strips parallel and 1 inch apart, with the longest in the middle and the shortest at the sides.

4. Fold back every other strip halfway and lay the longest remaining strip perpendicular to the unfolded strips across their centers. Unfold the folded strips over the perpendicular one. Fold back the other strips and place another strip parallel to and 1 inch from the first perpendicular one. Continue to form one side of the lattice, then repeat to form the other side.

5. Glaze the lattice, if desired. Brush the rim of the filled bottom crust with water. Slide one edge of the lattice to the edge of the baking sheet. Line up the edge of the lattice with one side of the crust. While securely holding the waxed paper and baking sheet together, carefully slide them out from under the lattice, draping the lattice on top of the pie.

6. Press down on the edges of the lattice to secure them to the crust. Use kitchen scissors or the tip of a small, sharp knife to trim the edges of the lattice even with the rim.

continued

P

Pie & Tart, continued

Other Decorative Effects

Experiment with all sorts of simple techniques to make the tops of your pies look more attractive.

CRIMPING Pressing around the rim of a pie crust or pastry with the tines of a kitchen fork, the blunt side of a knife, or a special crimping tool. See also CRIMPING.

EGG GLAZE For a shiny top crust, beat together 1 egg yolk with 1 teaspoon milk or cream and brush over the crust before baking.

FLUTING Press your thumb at regular intervals all around the rim of a single-crust pie to give it a scalloped edge. Or, use the thumb of one hand and the thumb and forefinger of the other to pinch the pastry around the rim in V shapes. Double-crust pies are better crimped (above) to seal the crusts together. See also FLUTING.

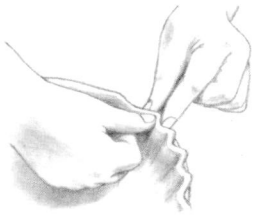

PASTRY CUTOUTS Reserve scraps of pastry dough left over from trimming the crusts for a double-crust pie. Roll them out and cut them into decorative shapes such as leaves or representations of the fruit being used in the pie. Moisten the undersides with water and place them in a pattern on the top crust.

SUGAR SPRINKLES Before baking, lightly brush the top crust with cold water and then sprinkle with granulated sugar or coarser sugar granules. The sugar will bake into sparkling jewel-like crystals.

VENTS Instead of cutting simple steam vents, use small cookie or candy cutters or the tip of a small, sharp knife to cut a pattern of decorative vents. It is easiest to do this before setting the top crust.

Pie and Tart Blues Got a problem with your pie or tart? Find the simple explanation here.

PASTRY CRACKS DURING ROLLING OUT. If small cracks cannot be repaired by pressing them together with your fingers, dough is too dry. Cover with a damp kitchen towel and refrigerate for 30 minutes. If problem persists, discard the dough and start over.

CRUST SHRINKS FROM SIDES OF PAN DURING BAKING. Dough was stretched too tightly while being put in pan. Always loosely drape and press dough into pan to avoid shrinkage, chill it briefly before baking, and weight it during blind baking.

CRUST EDGES BROWN TOO FAST. Your oven may be too hot or its heat not distributed evenly. Shield the crust edges during the final minutes of baking by covering with strips of aluminum foil, shiny side out.

CRUST ISN'T BROWNING QUICKLY ENOUGH. Oven is too cool, or there's not enough fat in the dough. Turn up the oven slightly, taking care not to overbake the pie. Even if the crust doesn't brown sufficiently, it should still be cooked through and tasty.

FILLING BUBBLES OVER AND DRIPS. Pie may be too full; pie dish may not be deep enough; or filling may be too moist. Next time, use a deeper dish or include a little more starch in the filling to thicken the juices. Meanwhile, place a sheet of aluminum foil on the rack below the pie (or place a foil-lined baking sheet directly underneath the pie) to catch drips.

TOP CRUST SAGS. The pie may not have enough filling, or dish may be too deep. To help support the crust in deep-dish pies, use a pie bird, an old-fashioned ceramic device—sometimes shaped like a bird—placed upright in the center of the filling.

See also BAKEWARE; BAKING TOOLS; BLIND BAKING; CRIMPING; FLUTING; ROLLING OUT; UNMOLDING.

PINCH This measuring term refers to the tiny amount of an ingredient that is picked up by pinching together thumb and forefinger. This informal measuring technique is used especially when adding a hint of strongly flavored ground spices such as cayenne or nutmeg and sometimes when seasoning with salt or pepper. A pinch is generally considered to be $\frac{1}{16}$ teaspoon.

PINEAPPLE Its oval shape and rugged, scalelike texture inspired the Spanish to name the pineapple after a *piña,* or "pinecone." Long cultivated in South America and the West Indies, the pineapple took Europe by storm after the explorers returned with samples of the fruit, odd and unwieldy on the outside but fragrant, sweet, and juicy inside. The pineapple now grows in hot regions from Hawaii to Malaysia and ranks as one of the world's most popular tropical fruits. It is also used as a symbol of hospitality.

Selecting Pineapples at the market usually weigh between 3 and 7 pounds. Look for a pineapple that gives slightly when pressed and sports deep green, fresh, healthy leaves. A center leaf usually pulls out easily from a ripe specimen. A ripe pineapple will smell fragrant, but an overly sweet, strong odor reveals that it has begun to ferment. As a pineapple ripens, it turns yellow from the bottom end up, but color is not an accurate indicator of the fruit's maturity. Avoid any pineapple with dried, wilted, or yellowed leaves. Check that the eyes on the skin are dry, pale, and free of mold. Dark, damp eyes reveal that it has been refrigerated too long. These fruits also tend to have browned flesh. This is more of a problem in winter, when pineapples imported from below the equator have to travel long distances to the market.

Look in the refrigerated section of the produce department for already peeled and cored pineapples; whole or sliced, they come in plastic containers or sealed in Cryovac. Pineapples are also available canned in juice or sugar syrup as slices, chunks, or crushed pulp. The fruit is also frozen, dried, and candied.

Storing Although a pineapple will not become any sweeter once picked, it will soften if left at room temperature for a few days. Once it is ready, use it as soon as possible. Otherwise, peel it, cut the flesh into pieces, and store it in an airtight container in the refrigerator for up to 4 days.

HOW TO *Peel a Pineapple*
1. Cut off the crown of leaves and the bottom end.
2. Set the pineapple straight up on one end and pare off the skin, cutting just below the surface in long, vertical strips and leaving the small brown eyes on the fruit. (If you cut deeper, much of the fruit will then be wasted.)

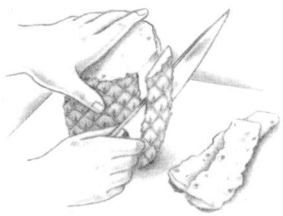

3. Place the pineapple on its side. Lining up the knife's blade with the diagonal rows of eyes, cut shallow furrows, following a spiral pattern to remove all the eyes.

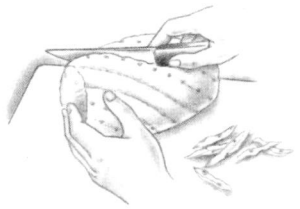

continued

4. Today's pineapple hybrids have softer, less fibrous cores that do not require trimming. Still, it's always a good idea to take a taste of the core and, if at all woody, remove it with a knife or small cookie cutter.

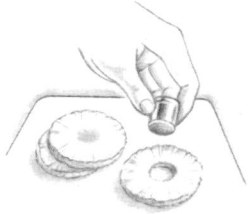

Quick Tip

Pineapple contains an enzyme, bromelin, which readily breaks down protein. Meat marinated in fresh pineapple juice will become mushy quickly, and any gelatin dish containing even a hint of pineapple will not set. But since heat completely destroys the enzyme, you can use cooked or canned pineapple in such cases.

PINE NUT See NUT.

PINK BEAN See BEAN, DRIED.

PINTO BEAN See BEAN, DRIED.

PIPING Frosting, whipped cream, or a similar mixture can be spooned into the wide end of a pastry bag and piped out of the narrow end through a tip to make a variety of decorative effects or to write messages on cakes. The same technique can also be used

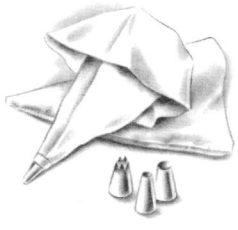

to form decorative rosettes or scrollwork of soft mashed potatoes, which may then be browned in the oven or beneath a broiler.

Bound with eggs and flour, the piped potato shapes may be fried as croquettes.

Many different tips can be inserted into the narrow end of a conical pastry bag for different piping styles. The bag is then filled and held with one hand guiding the tip and the other squeezing the mixture from the top of the bag out through the tip.

Disposable pastry bags are available. You also can fashion one from parchment paper, or cut a small corner off a plastic bag. Parchment cones are best for delicate work because their openings usually are very small. Plastic bags work for small, less precise jobs requiring narrow piping lines, such as decorating large cookies or applying stripes of melted chocolate to cupcakes.

HOW TO *Use a Pastry Bag*
To dress up a cake, decorate it with piped greetings, colorful flowers, or scalloped borders. Use frostings that are firm enough to hold their shape, yet soft enough to flow smoothly. Decorating bags with couplers and screw-on tips are most convenient because they allow you to switch tips quickly, but any 12- to 16-inch pastry bag will work fine.

1. Fold the edge of the bag down about 6 inches to create a cuff. If necessary, you can prop the bag upright inside a glass or tall container while you fill it. Fill the pastry bag no more than halfway, as overfilled bags are difficult to hold and tend to leak frosting out the top.

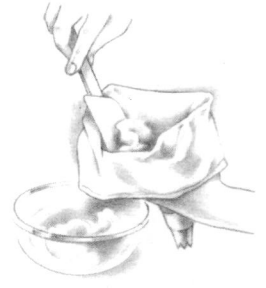

2. Unfold the cuff, press all the frosting down toward the tip, squeeze out as much air as possible, and then twist the bag several times to seal.

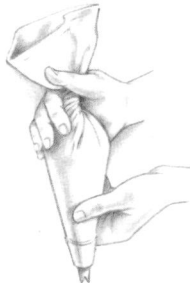

3. Grip the bag at the twisted part with your dominant hand; squeeze only with this hand. Lightly support the bottom of the bag, just behind its tip, with your other hand; this hand will guide your movements as you pipe. You may wish to practice on a sheet of waxed paper.

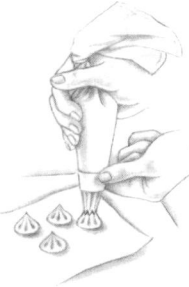

4. Hold the pastry bag at a 45-degree angle and maintain a small gap between the tip and the surface of the cake. Squeeze with steady pressure for an even line. More force will create larger shapes and less force smaller ones. Twist the bag regularly to keep it smooth and taut over the frosting.

Quick Tip

Before starting to pipe, practice on waxed paper. Then, as a guide, lightly trace designs and words in the frosting with a toothpick.

HOW TO *Make a Parchment Paper Cone for Piping*

1. Cut a triangle from parchment paper with two equal sides, each measuring about 15 inches long. The base of the triangle should measure about 17 inches.

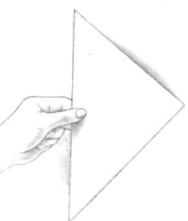

2. Curl one of the points of the base of the triangle over and position it at the top point of the triangle.

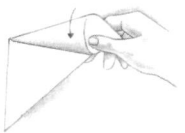

3. Wrap the third point under the other two points. Pull the paper as you work to make a tightly rolled cone.

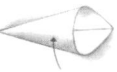

4. Fold the stacked points together. Tuck them securely inside the top. Fill the cone.

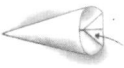

5. Using scissors, snip off the tip of the cone. Smaller openings produce more delicate lines.

See also BAKING TOOLS; FROSTING, ICING & GLAZE; PARCHMENT PAPER.

PISTACHIO See NUT.

PITA See BREAD.

PIZZA Italian visitors to America may sometimes be surprised by the thick, gooey concoctions we often call pizza. On the other hand, when faced with an authentic Italian pizza, thin and minimalist, some American tourists in Italy may dismiss it as a glorified cracker. Even in the States, three schools of pizza making vie for top honors: In the Northeast, tomato-smeared slices tend toward the thin and crispy. Chicago or Sicilian-style pizzas, appropriately nicknamed deep-dish, bake up thick, soft, and cheesy in special pans with high sides. An individual-sized crisp crust topped with ingredients from cuisines the world over and then baked in a wood-fired oven sets the California style.

Pizza and pizza wheel for cutting.

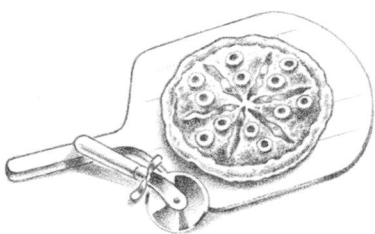

Although take-out, delivery, and frozen pizzas have become the ultimate noncook's convenience, making your own pizza at home is simple. Good-quality frozen and refrigerated pizza dough is available now in most supermarkets. In the time it takes to wait for the delivery of a pizza, you can shape, top, bake, and then eat a hot homemade one.

Quick Tip

Use a pizza wheel, a rotating circular blade, for cutting slices, starting at the center and rolling outward so you won't drag the toppings across the pizza.

HOW TO *Shape a Pizza Crust*

1. After punching down the pizza dough, use your hands to shape the ball into a flattened disk.

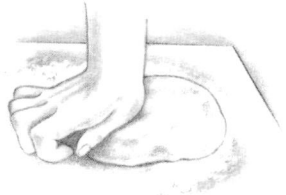

2. On a floured work surface, gently press, lift, and stretch the dough into the desired flat shape and thickness. For a soft crust, press it out to a thickness of ½ inch; for a crisp crust, press it out to a thickness of about ¼ inch.

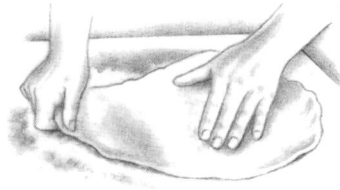

3. Press with your fingertips to form a slightly raised rim.

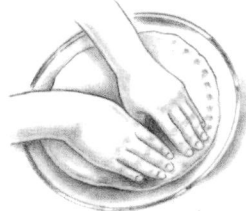

Topping Ideas An empty pizza shell is like a blank canvas. Some combinations, both classic and contemporary, to inspire the chef and artist in you:

- Chopped tomatoes, anchovies, and fresh or dried oregano
- Thinly sliced tomatoes, slivered garlic, and torn fresh basil leaves
- Roasted onions, zucchini, red bell pepper, and yellow squash
- Pancetta, spinach, and ricotta

- Caramelized onions, anchovies, and black olives
- Sautéed Swiss chard, plumped currants, and pine nuts
- Fontina, Gorgonzola, mozzarella, and goat cheeses
- Sliced mushrooms, onion, and spinach
- Asparagus tips, julienned ham, and shredded Gruyère cheese
- Artichoke hearts, red bell pepper, black olives, and pesto
- Crumbled Italian sausage and julienned red, yellow, and green bell pepper
- Sliced smoked chicken, arugula, and Asiago cheese
- Gorgonzola, caramelized onions, pine nuts, and fresh thyme
- Smoked salmon, dill, and capers
- Tuna, tapenade, and capers

Pizza Savvy Follow these insider's tips to help you achieve perfect pizzas at home:

- Preheat the oven fully. The best pizzas bake quickly in very hot ovens.
- Use a pizza stone or baking stone, or ceramic baker's tiles, placed on the lowest oven rack. These will absorb heat as your oven preheats, approximating the radiant heat of a traditional baker's oven. When the pizza is cooked directly on top, without a pan, the stone or tiles help absorb moisture from the dough, producing a crisp crust.
- Buy a baker's peel, a thin-edged metal or wooden paddle used for transferring pizzas or breads into or removing them from the oven. It slides easily under a pizza crust, making for smooth, mishap-free moving.
- Patch any tears in the crust before topping the pizza. This will keep sauce or toppings from bleeding through during baking, thus preventing the pizza from sticking to the pan, stone, or tiles.
- Don't add too much sauce. Excess sauce makes a pizza soggy.
- Don't add too many toppings. A heavy load of toppings makes pizza harder to cut and eat.

See also BAKING TOOLS; PREHEATING.

PIZZA PAN See BAKEWARE.

PLANTAIN Beloved of Caribbean, Latin American, African, and Indian cooks, this fruit, a close relative of the banana, tastes like a less sweet, blander version of its cousin but has a higher starch content that allows it to be cooked in many more ways. Unlike the banana, the plantain is eaten only when cooked, as all but the very ripest raw plantains are high in mouth-puckering tannin. Also unlike the banana, the sturdy plantain won't fall apart or become mushy when deep-fried, panfried, baked, or stewed, so it may be used like a vegetable in many dishes. Its bland flavor can be paired with a variety of sauces and combined with a large number of other ingredients. A popular way of serving plantains is to make *tostones:* cut plantains into thick slices, smash them to break their fibers, and fry them. Thinner slices are sometimes fried and eaten as a snack, like potato chips. Fried plantains are also wonderful mashed and served with roasted meats.

Selecting Plantains are available year-round. Look for them in major supermarkets or in Latin markets, where they may be labeled *platanos.* Choose fruits that are firm and have peels free of tears or breaks. Fully ripe plantains will have an almost completely black skin and be soft to the touch. Buy plantains at this stage of ripeness for dishes in which they are mashed or quickly cooked; they are much sweeter than in their less-ripe state. For sautéing, deep-frying, and stewing, use firm green plantains, with a yellow-green skin, or semiripe plantains, with black-spotted yellow skins.

P

Storing Leave plantains at room temperature for several days, or until they reach the desired ripeness. Afterward, refrigerate them for up to 1 week. They will not ripen any further once refrigerated, however. Like bananas, plantains freeze well. Simply wrap the peeled fruit tightly in plastic wrap and freeze for 2 to 3 weeks.

Preparing Plantains are harder to peel than bananas, as the peel tends to cling to the fruit. Because the skin contains a substance that can leave dark stains on your hands and fingernails, rub your hands with a very small amount of oil or with a lime half before you begin to peel.

HOW TO *Peel a Plantain*

1. Cut off the top and bottom of the plantain, then cut it in half crosswise.
2. Make a lengthwise cut through the skin down to the flesh on either side of each half and peel back the skin.

PLASTIC WRAP First introduced to consumers in the early 1950s as an improvement on waxed paper, plastic wrap has become an almost indispensable kitchen asset. Most often used for storage, the wrap is also used in microwave cooking to trap steam and aid in heat distribution.

Brands differ widely in quality. Some are easy to use and cling tightly to a variety of surfaces, while others don't trap moisture well and allow food to dry out. Some wraps have a frustrating tendency to cling to themselves, making them impossible to unravel. Experiment until you find a wrap that works well.

In recent years, consumers have voiced concern about the chemical plasticizers found in plastic wrap (and plastic containers used for food), as these substances are thought by some to be potential health hazards. When microwaving, you may wish to prevent the plastic wrap from touching food directly; or look for plastic wrap made from polyethylene.

When wrapping food for freezing, be sure to use freezer-weight plastic wrap or bags. Insufficient wrapping can lead to freezer burn, the drying out and discoloration that occurs when ice crystals from the food's surface evaporate into the drier air of the freezer. Freezer burn degrades the taste and texture of the food.

See also ALUMINUM FOIL; PARCHMENT PAPER; WAXED PAPER.

PLUCKING To pull the feathers from poultry and game birds. Modern processing practices have made plucking all but obsolete for most home cooks. Sometimes, however, a few feathers (usually tiny pinfeathers) remain on poultry, especially specialty game birds from small producers. Use your fingers, tweezers, or needlenosed pliers to remove these.

PLUM Thanks to crossbreeding, hundreds of varieties of this summer-ripening stone fruit exist. Take a trip to the farmers' market during plum season and you'll find plums in colors that range from yellow and green to many shades of pink, purple, and scarlet. Among the most common are Santa Rosa, Greengage, Red Ace, Damson, and prune plum, also called Italian plum. More unusual varieties include Queen Rosa, Black Amber, and Elephant Heart. Small beach plums, wild plums that grow near beaches or alongside country roads on the East Coast, are excellent for jams and jellies.

Quick Tip

One of the simplest of summer desserts is plums poached in a mixture of water, sugar, and lemon juice. Reduce the cooking liquid and spoon it over the warm plums.

In general, cooking plums are smaller and more acidic than the larger, juicier plum varieties. The latter are best used uncooked in tarts, shortcakes, and other desserts and for eating out of hand.

Selecting The first plums of the season ripen in mid-May, and fruits remain in the market through mid-September. To find a ripe plum, hold one in the palm of your hand. It should feel heavy and there should be some give, particularly at the blossom end. Tasting is the best indication of ripeness, so if you are shopping at a farmers' market, ask for a sample before you buy.

Storing To soften hard plums, put them in a paper bag and let sit at room temperature for a couple of days. Because their sugars must develop on the tree, plums won't sweeten appreciably once they've been picked. Perfectly ripe plums can be refrigerated for 3 to 5 days.

Quick Tip

Always taste plums before cooking. Tart varieties usually demand the addition of sugar, sometimes more than a recipe indicates. Balance the flavor of sweeter varieties with a squeeze of fresh lemon juice.

Preparing If you're using plum slices or halves in a pie or tart, leave the skins intact. They lend a pretty color to the finished dish. But if you're making a plum purée to flavor an ice cream or for jelly or jam, the skins will be unpleasantly acidic and should be removed. When plums are fully ripe, the skin should easily pull away, although it may need to be coaxed with a knife. If the plums are quite firm and the skin clings stubbornly to the fruit, slice a small X in the skin and blanch for 1 to 2 minutes in boiling water. The skins will then slip off easily.

See also PRUNE.

PLUMPING To rehydrate dried fruit, such as raisins, currants, prunes, and dried apricots, by soaking them in a liquid, most often warm water. Some recipes call for soaking the fruit in an unheated spirit, such as rum; the soaking liquid is then used in the recipe as well. Plumping softens dried fruits, making them more pleasant to eat and easier to incorporate into batters and sauces; it also restores flavor to dried fruits that have hardened during storage.

HOW TO *Plump Dried Fruits*
1. Cover the fruits with warm or hot water.
2. Cover and let stand for 10 to 20 minutes.
3. Drain, reserving the soaking liquid if called for in the recipe.

See also DRIED FRUIT; LIQUEUR.

PLUM SAUCE A mixture of plums, apricots, chiles, vinegar, and sugar, this thick, amber-colored, sweet-and-sour sauce is a frequently used condiment in Chinese restaurants. A popular accompaniment to roast duck, it's often called duck sauce and also is served with egg rolls, spareribs, and roast pork.

Selecting Look for jars of plum sauce in Asian markets or the Asian-foods section of supermarkets.

Storing Once opened, the jar of sauce should be placed in the refrigerator, where it will keep for up to 1 year.

PLUNGING After partial or complete cooking, foods are sometimes plunged, or immersed quickly, in cold water to stop the cooking, to brighten and set the color, or both. The French term for this technique translates to "refresh"; another term used is "shock." The water should be ice cold, especially for green vegetables, which need the dramatic temperature change to brighten them after blanching.

P

To plunge, have a large container of cold or ice water ready. Either remove the food from its cooking pan with a skimmer or slotted spoon, or simply pour the food and its cooking water into a sieve or colander set in the sink; then use the skimmer, spoon, sieve, or colander to transfer the food to the container of cold water. Use a large container, so the food won't warm up the water immediately. Remove the food as soon as it has cooled, 2 to 3 minutes, and don't leave it for more than 4 minutes. Soaking in water too long will leach out flavor and ruin texture, particularly in the case of green vegetables.

See also BLANCHING.

POACHING The technique of gently cooking foods in not-quite-simmering water or other seasoned liquid. The water should barely move, although a few small bubbles may break the surface. Although poaching and simmering are often used interchangeably, technically poaching is cooking food at a slightly lower temperature (160° to 180°F) than a simmer (185°F). Many recipes for poaching, however, specify cooking the food, especially larger pieces, at a low simmer.

Poaching is ideal for delicate foods that need careful treatment to avoid breaking apart or overcooking, such as eggs, fish, chicken, asparagus, and pears. It also is used for foods that need long cooking in order to tenderize them, such as beef or pork. (Two examples are classic French pot-au-feu and tough cuts of beef and pork to be shredded for Mexican dishes.) Usually, foods are poached either whole, as for whole chickens and fish, or in large pieces, as for chicken breasts and fish fillets. This helps to keep the food moist.

Either water or a flavored liquid is used to poach foods. In the latter case, the liquid will add flavor to the food being poached, and the liquid may then be used as the basis for a sauce for the cooked food. A common poaching liquid for savory foods is court-bouillon, a light, quickly made stock. Poaching chicken in chicken stock or fish in fish stock is also common. Pears and other fruits may be poached in wine or in simple syrup to which flavorings are added. Eggs and vegetables are usually poached in salted water that has already reached the almost-simmering stage. In the case of eggs, a small amount of vinegar sometimes is added to help the eggs hold their shape.

Poaching eggs.

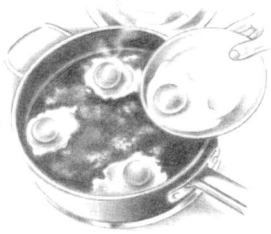

In poaching, the food to be cooked is partially or completely submerged in liquid, in a pan not much larger than the food, and the pan is usually covered to prevent excessive evaporation. Whole fish are classically cooked in a fish poacher, a long, covered narrow pan just large enough for a good-sized fish; many such pans include a perforated platform with handles for lifting the fish in and out. The fish may also be wrapped in a long length of cheesecloth that extends beyond its ends and sides; when the fish is cooked, the ends of the cloth are used to lift the fish out of the poacher or pot. Some recipes, especially French ones for delicate foods such as fillets of sole, call for the pan to be covered with a circle of buttered waxed paper or parchment paper, rather than a lid. This prevents the excessive heat and steam buildup caused by a tight lid. The dish is then poached in the oven.

Fish poacher.

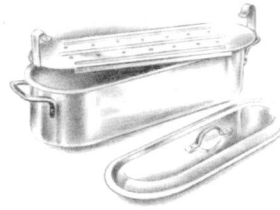

Quick-cooking foods like eggs or smaller cuts of meat and fish are added to the water once it has reached the almost-simmering stage, while larger foods, like whole chickens, are added to cold water that is brought just to a boil and then reduced to poaching temperature. This prevents overcooking of small foods and allows larger foods to heat gently and remain tender. The cooking time is clocked from the moment the liquid reaches the poaching stage. Smaller pieces of food are removed from the pan as soon as they are ready to avoid overcooking, while larger pieces, such as whole chickens or large pieces of meat, may be left to cool in the liquid.

Caution!

Note that poached eggs are not cooked to 160°F, the temperature needed to kill salmonella bacteria. For more information, see EGG.

See also COOKWARE.

POBLANO See CHILE.

POLENTA One of the glories of Italian cooking, polenta is cornmeal that is cooked in either water or stock until it thickens and the grains of the cornmeal become tender. In Italy, polenta may be either yellow or white, made from either coarsely ground or finely ground cornmeal, but the classic version is made from coarsely and evenly ground yellow corn. Traditionally, it was poured right onto the middle of a

wooden table or onto a wooden board as soon as it was ready and then cut with a string for serving after cooling.

Polenta can be spooned up straight from the pot when still soft. Just-cooked polenta is often enriched and softened with butter and Parmesan cheese and served as a base for a thick stew, absorbing savory meat juices and adding its own sweet taste of corn. It is a wonderful hot cereal as well, topped with butter, milk, and sugar or with poached eggs and grated cheese. Polenta in this stage is often referred to as "soft polenta," though true soft polenta, a southern Italian variation of polenta also known as *polentina,* is a thinner, porridgelike mixture that stays softer longer as it cools. The softness of polenta depends on the amount of liquid used. More liquid renders a softer polenta. Polenta that is to be cooled and cooked further is made with less liquid, so it is firmer and easier to cut.

Soft polenta can be poured into a flat pan and cooled until firm, then cut into shapes to be grilled, fried, sautéed, or baked. Thin slices can be layered with tomato sauce, cheese, and vegetables and baked like lasagne. Squares of firm polenta can be browned in butter or oil or brushed with oil and broiled or grilled, and then used in place of toast as the base for appetizers topped with sautéed greens, grilled peppers, or mushrooms.

Traditional Italian cooks make polenta in a special unlined copper polenta pot. They add the cornmeal to boiling water or stock in a slow, steady stream and stir with a wooden spoon, ideally in the same direction throughout cooking, until the polenta thickens to a golden mass and pulls away from the sides of the pan and the polenta grains are tender to the tongue. This usually takes 40 to 45 minutes. A serviceable polenta can be made after about 20 minutes of cooking, as it will have thickened and

P

cooked sufficiently by this time, but only the long-cooked kind will have a tender, silken texture. Some food writers are now recommending stirring-free oven-baked polenta.

Adding polenta to boiling liquid.

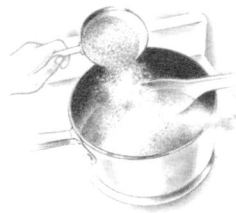

Stirring polenta.

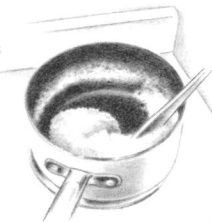

Selecting Choose an imported Italian polenta cornmeal or, if you prefer, stone-ground domestic cornmeal in a fine grind. Stone-ground cornmeal has more fiber and minerals than the more commonly available degerminated cornmeal, and some cooks find it has a richer corn flavor as well. Polenta is available in instant form, too, although for the best consistency, instant polenta should be cooked for about 15 minutes, which is longer than the instructions on most packages indicate. To purists, the flavor and texture of instant polenta suffer in comparison to regular polenta; it is best reserved for dishes in which polenta is one of several ingredients. Polenta is also available cooked, cooled, and shaped into plastic-wrapped cylinders, a great time-saver for making fried and grilled sliced polenta.

Storing Stone-ground cornmeal must be refrigerated. Degerminated cornmeal has a longer shelf life and can be stored at cool room temperature.

Quick Tip

The kind of pot you use for cooking polenta makes a difference. To keep the polenta from sticking and scorching, make sure the pot is heavy. Unless you have a copper polenta pot, enameled cast iron is the best choice.

See also CORNMEAL; GRAIN.

POMEGRANATE This deep red fruit has a thick, leathery skin, which when split open reveals an abundance of seeds—each surrounded by slightly translucent, ruby-red pulp—sectioned between tough white membranes. The pomegranate is an important food throughout the Middle East, where its fruity, sweet-sour juice is used in stews, sauces, marinades, glazes, salads, and drinks. Pomegranate seeds add sparkle and crunch to salads and make a pretty garnish for soup. Use them, too, in tarts and fruit desserts. Pomegranate juice is used to flavor syrups and drinks and to make sorbet and ice cream.

Quick Bite

Pomegranate molasses, or concentrated pomegranate juice, is an essential ingredient in many eastern Mediterranean cuisines. The thick, deep red, sweet-tart juice is used to flavor salad dressings and in sauces for grilled fish and chicken. Look for it in Middle Eastern groceries and in well-stocked supermarkets and specialty-food stores.

Selecting Pomegranates arrive in the market in the fall and early winter. Look for deeply colored, large fruits, which will have a greater proportion of the clear red, juicy, crisp pulp. Heavy fruits promise more juice. The tough skin should be thin and nearly bursting with seeds. Press the fruits gently; if they release a powdery cloud, return them to the bin; the pulp is dry as dust.

Storing Pomegranates have a much longer shelf life than most fresh fruits. They can be kept at room temperature for 3 to 5 days or refrigerated in a plastic bag for up to 3 weeks. The seeds and the whole fruit can be frozen for about 3 months.

HOW TO *Seed a Pomegranate*

1. Working over a bowl, cut off the peel from the blossom end of the fruit, removing it with some of the white pith, but taking care not to pierce the seeds.
2. Don't cut into the fruit with a knife. You'll break the seeds, releasing their juice and making a mess of your kitchen and clothing. Instead, lightly score, or shallowly cut, the peel into quarters, starting at the blossom end and working down to the stem end. Carefully break the fruit apart with your hands, pull back the skin, and use your fingertips to remove the seeds.

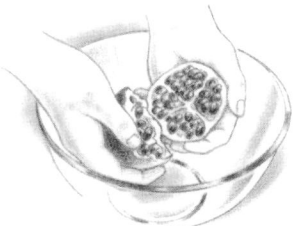

Quick Tip

Work over a bowl and wear an apron when seeding pomegranates. Their bright red juices leave stubborn stains on whatever they touch.

Quick Tip

For a refreshing drink, roll a pomegranate on a hard surface, pressing down firmly, to release the juice from the seeds. Cut a small hole in the peel, insert a straw, and sip.

POPOVER This classic quick bread is characterized by a crisp, brown exterior and moist, almost hollow center. Made from a thin batter of equal parts flour and milk enriched with butter and eggs, popovers have no added leavening. Operating on the same principles as the paste for cream puffs and the batters for Yorkshire pudding and Dutch babies, popover batter rises when the liquid in the batter turns to steam and the proteins in the eggs and flour coagulate to form an elastic shell that traps the steam inside. Although you can use standard muffin pans or individual custard cups, for best results use old-fashioned cast-iron popover pans, which have deep cups, or the newer black-steel popover pans, whose deep cups are attached only by metal strips. Many recipe writers call for the batter to be poured into preheated pans and put immediately into a hot oven, but others insist that popovers made in unheated pans and started in a cold oven will rise just as high. Try both ways yourself and decide.

Popover molds.

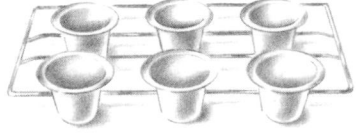

Popover Savvy When making popovers, keep the following in mind:
- Make sure that the popover batter is cold. It should be refrigerated for at least 1 hour or as long as overnight

P

before baking. If using black-steel popover pans, reduce the oven temperature
by 25°F.

- For the highest-rising popovers, use a
pan with smaller cups. The batter will
have nowhere to go but up. Fill cups of
any size no more than two-thirds full.
- Make sure the popover cups are well
buttered or sprayed with cooking spray
to prevent sticking.
- Place individual popover molds on a
baking sheet.
- While popovers are baking, do not open
the oven door for the first 30 minutes.
- After 30 minutes, pierce the side of
each popover with a small, sharp knife
to allow steam to escape and prevent
a soggy interior. Continue baking until
you reach the specific time.

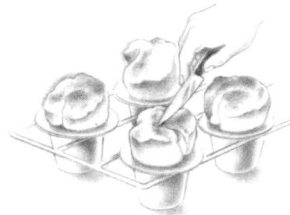

- After baking, pierce the popovers again,
unmold quickly, and serve at once.

POPPY SEED See SPICE.

PORCINO See MUSHROOM.

PORK A marvel of fertility and abundance, the pig, source of pork, has long
been one of the most valuable farm animals. Prolific, omnivorous, easy to raise,
and possessing an abundance of succulent
meat and fat, the pig is the primary source
of meat in many cultures. Almost every
part of the pig is eaten, from its feet to the
bits and pieces left over from hog butchering, which become scrapple and head-
cheese. The fresh meat is used in stews,

roasts, steaks, and chops. When cured, it
becomes ham, bacon, and sausages that can
be eaten on their own or used as flavoring
in other dishes. In fact, the keeping ability
of cured pork has always been one of the
greatest assets of this versatile meat.

Thanks to its sweet, mild taste, pork
pairs well with fruit, particularly dried
fruit such as prunes, which may be used in
a stuffing for a pork loin roast or made into
a sauce to accompany sliced pork or grilled
kabobs. Applesauce is a classic pork accompaniment, and quince also seems to go naturally with this meat. Or, try a mango or
papaya salsa with grilled pork. Such piquant
and spicy ethnic condiments as hoisin sauce
also complement this popular meat.

Pork may be divided into two distinct
categories: fresh and cured. Chances are
you will find a wider variety of cured pork
products available in your market than different cuts of fresh pork.

Selecting Fresh pork should have a clean
smell, white fat, and dark pink or rosy pink
flesh, depending on the cut. The premium
cuts, such as loin roasts and chops, are
available in any supermarket or specialty
butcher shop. Pork shoulder, fresh leg of
pork, picnic shoulder, fat back, fresh pigs'
feet, and fresh hocks may have to be ordered, but you will probably find them
readily available in ethnic markets such as
Chinese, German, or Mexican.

Storing Keep fresh pork in the cold bottom rear of the refrigerator for 2 to 3 days.
Pork wrapped in butcher paper should be
rewrapped in waxed paper or plastic and,
to catch any escaping juices, placed on a
plate. Carefully wrap pork to be frozen in
freezer-weight plastic wrap or zippered
plastic freezer bags; freeze large cuts for up
to 6 months, smaller cuts and ground pork
for up to 3 months.

Store all other cured pork products in
the refrigerator. Even though bacon, ham,

Pork Glossary

Pork cuts.

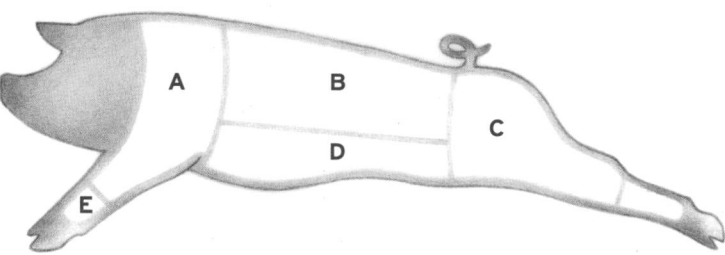

Like any food animal, a butchered pig is divided into primal cuts, the wholesale cuts from which smaller pieces of meat are carved for the market. The two primal cuts of pork most often sold in fresh form are the loin and the pork shoulder. Meat from three other primal cuts, the leg, the side and belly, and the picnic shoulder, is more often cured but occasionally sold fresh.

SHOULDER (A) The shoulder is divided into the upper and lower shoulder section. The upper shoulder, known as pork shoulder, pork butt, or Boston shoulder, is highly valued in many ethnic cuisines. Because it is marbled with fat, this cut is juicy and flavorful. It is ground, cut into kabobs, cut into cubes for stews, cooked as pot roasts, or cut into steaks. In Mexican cuisine, this is the meat used to make *carnitas;* in Chinese cuisine, it is cut into shreds and used in stir-fries or ground and used in spicy fillings; and in regional American cooking, it is used in soups and in stuffings for chicken and turkey and is ground for meat loaf and meatballs. Many of the recipes that today call for tenderloin, such as kabobs and stir-fries, have traditionally used the fattier pork shoulder. It may be boned for ease in cutting.

The foreleg and lower shoulder of the pig, known as the picnic shoulder, is usually smoked for picnic ham, but it is occasionally available fresh. This cut can be used in all the same ways as pork shoulder. The bottom portion of the picnic shoulder is cut off to make pork hocks, which can be added whole to flavor soups and stews and often are found smoked. The picnic shoulder may be boned.

LOIN (B) This upper back section is the most tender part of the pig. The front part of the loin, known as the blade and center loin, has rich, tender meat that is cut into large blade roasts or sliced into bone-in blade chops. Toward the center of the loin, the meat becomes juicier and more tender still.

Center-cut loin chop.

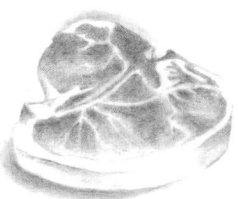

continued

P

Pork Glossary, continued

The loin may be cut into chops for grilling, broiling, or sautéing. A section with rib bones attached may be shaped and tied into the descriptively named crown roast. The tender back ribs from this section are excellent for barbecuing.

The sirloin, the back section of the loin, is the source of the tenderloin, a narrow cylinder about a foot long and 3 inches in diameter. The most tender of all pork cuts, it may be quickly roasted, grilled, or stir-fried; cut into medaillons; or flattened into scallops. The tenderloin is usually served with a sauce to complement its mild flavor and buttery texture. Loin chops also may be cut from this section for grilling, broiling, or sautéing.

The ribs from a boned pork loin are sold as baby back ribs.

LEG (C) A fresh leg of pork, which is one of the hind legs of the pig, usually becomes a smoked ham, but in the old days it was often roasted and served as a festive farmhouse dinner.

SIDE AND BELLY (D) Below the loin, or upper back, section of the pig are the sides and belly, the source of spareribs and fresh side pork, respectively. Pork spareribs are usually barbecued or grilled but, as with beef ribs, can also be braised. Fresh side pork is sometimes cooked, but usually it is smoked and turned into bacon, or salted and turned into salt pork.

Spareribs.

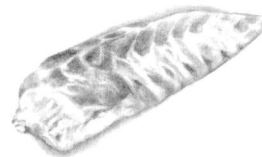

FEET (E) Also known as trotters. Fresh pigs' feet are usually found only in ethnic meat markets these days. They may be prepared in a variety of ways, including roasting, pickling, smoking, and braising in a flavorful sauce.

and some sausages are cured, they will lose flavor and begin to spoil in the refrigerator. It is best to use them within about 1 week.

Preparing The biggest challenge when cooking pork is to keep it from drying out. Over the years, pigs in the United States have been bred to have a lower fat content, and in some cuts there is little internal fat to insulate and lubricate the meat. Many cooks find that cooking pork gently to an internal temperature of 150° to 160°F ensures the best flavor, tenderness, and juiciness. However, an internal temperature of 160°F is needed to destroy any bacteria in pork (see also Pork Safety, below). Avoid cooking pork to temperatures above 160°F, with the exception of slow-cooked barbecue, which is cooked until the meat falls from the bone.

Even in its new lean incarnation, however, pork is still more succulent and tender than most beef cuts, and the various pork cuts can be cooked by either moist or dry heat. In other words, a cut of pork can be cooked almost any way you want to cook it: broiled, braised, roasted, panfried, poached, stir-fried, or grilled. Some cooks also help keep fresh pork moist nowadays by presoaking it in brine. For more information, see BRINE.

Quick Tip

Keep a piece of boned pork shoulder, well wrapped, in your freezer to use in stir-fries. Simply cut off thin slices of the meat with a chef's knife and stir-fry without defrosting to add to vegetable mixtures.

Pork Safety Though the internal doneness temperatures suggested in Preparing, above, yield what many cooks feel is the optimum taste and texture for pork, they are lower than those suggested by the U.S. Food Safety and Inspection Service guidelines. In order to destroy any lurking bacteria, cook pork to an internal temperature of 160°F. See also DONENESS.

Quick Bite

For many years, trichinosis was a major health concern in the consumption of pork, as this disease of microscopic parasites can be deadly in meat that is not thoroughly cooked. Thanks to advances in the sanitary conditions of pig husbandry, the incidence of trichinosis is rare today in the United States—but raw meats and poultry may harbor other harmful bacteria and should still be fully, diligently cooked.

Never taste pork before it is cooked. If you need to test the seasoning in a mixture containing uncooked pork, cook a small portion of the mixture until no trace of pink remains in the center, then taste it.

Thoroughly wash your hands, cutting board, knives, grinder, and any other utensils that have touched raw pork in hot, soapy water after use.

Don't use a marinade in which pork sat to baste the cooking meat or to serve with the cooked meat unless the marinade has first been brought to a boil and then boiled for about 5 minutes.

See also BACON; CANADIAN BACON; HAM; PANCETTA; PROSCIUTTO; ROASTING; SAUSAGE.

PORTOBELLO See MUSHROOM.

POTATO The Incas of Peru gave us this ancient vegetable. Not only did they cultivate more varieties than we now enjoy, but they also freeze-dried them at high altitudes for long keeping. This vegetable, a member of the nightshade family and once considered exotic by Europeans, is today a symbol of normality and comfort. Easy to grow and to store, the starchy, faintly earthy-tasting potato is compatible with many other foods and endlessly adaptable to various cooking methods.

Red, russet, and white potatoes.

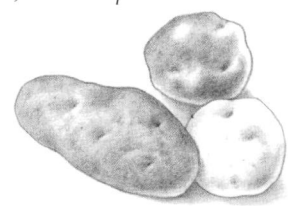

The reliable tuber may be boiled and puréed into mashed potatoes, baked and topped with sour cream, or thinly sliced and layered with cheese and cream to bake in a gratin. It is cut into long, thin sticks and deep-fried for French fries, cut into paper-thin slices and deep-fried for potato chips, or cut into wedges and roasted until crisp. It is simmered in stews and soups, made into a variety of potato salads, or grated and panfried as hash browns or potato pancakes. In addition, potato flour is used as a thickening agent, potato cooking water and puréed potatoes add moisture and flavor to yeast breads, and potatoes are used to make vodka. Even the skins of potatoes are fried or rebaked and eaten.

P

Potato Glossary

Thousands of potato varieties grow in the world, although we see only a handful in the markets. Increasingly, specialty potatoes are finding their way into produce bins.

RUSSET POTATO Also called baking potato, Idaho, or russet Burbank (named for Luther Burbank, a famed American horticulturalist, who developed the variety in Massachusetts in 1872). Large and oval, with a dry, reddish brown skin. Its starchy flesh is perfect for baking and mashing, and for making French fries and potato gnocchi. Specialty russets include the Lehmi, a large, brown potato with white flesh, similar to classic baking potatoes but more flavorful; and the Butterfinger, with brown russet skin and golden flesh.

RED OR WHITE POTATO Also known simply as the boiling or all-purpose potato. These round potatoes have a thin red or white skin and a waxy flesh that keeps its shape, making them perfect for grating for hash browns and potato pancakes; slicing for cottage fries; cutting into chunks for roasting; or boiling and then cubing or slicing for potato salads. Specialty red potatoes include Red Gold, flavorful tubers with yellow flesh and netted red skin; Red Dale, which are slightly flattened potatoes with white flesh and red skin; All Red, which have both rosy skin and flesh; and Rose Fir, which have pink skin and yellow flesh. Long white potatoes, which were developed in California and are also called white rose potatoes, are a specialty white potato that is oval and has a thin, cream-colored skin and relatively few, very small eyes.

YUKON GOLD Thin-skinned potatoes with a yellowish skin and golden, fine-grained, buttery-tasting flesh. These all-purpose potatoes hold their shape well when boiled, and so may be used in all the same ways as red, white, and new potatoes, but they also make colorful mashed potatoes. Yellow Finn is a similar variety.

NEW POTATO An immature potato, usually of the round red or round white variety, although you may also find new Yellow Finn and Rose Fir potatoes. Most often available in spring and early summer, new potatoes are low in starch and perfect for potato salad, for roasting and grilling, and to use in creamed dishes. Be aware that not all small red and white potatoes are new. A true new potato is freshly harvested, will have a thin skin, and will not keep long.

FINGERLING POTATOES Certain varieties of white potato are called fingerlings because of their narrow, knobby shape. Waxy fingerlings may be used in all the same ways as new potatoes and are good steamed or boiled and served with butter or olive oil.

BLUE OR PURPLE POTATOES With a dark blue or purple skin and flesh, these potatoes will catch your eye in the market. They can be mashed or boiled.

Selecting Most potato varieties are available year-round, although new potatoes may appear only in the spring and early summer and sporadically at other times. Choose firm specimens that are not blemished, wrinkled, tinged with green, or cracked. The buds, commonly called eyes, of the potatoes should not have sprouted.

Quick Tip

If you've oversalted a soup or stew, cut a boiling potato into slices and add it to the pot. Simmer the mixture for 5 to 10 minutes, and then remove the potato slices, which will have absorbed some of the salt.

Different potatoes are used in cooking in different ways. There are three basic types of potato: starchy or mealy, waxy, and all-purpose. Starchy or mealy potato varieties, such as russets, are best for baking and mashing because they cook up dry and fluffy but do not hold their shape well. Waxy potatoes, such as red or white potatoes, are low in starch. Use them for potato salads and other recipes where you want them to hold their shape and are not relying on their starch content to thicken a soup or sauce. All-purpose (that is, medium-starch-content) potatoes, such as Yukon Golds, are good for both uses.

Storing Store potatoes in a cool, dark place with good air circulation for up to 2 weeks; do not refrigerate and do not store in the same bin with onions. These vegetables together produce gases that cause rapid spoilage. New potatoes have a much shorter shelf life than other potatoes. To make the most of their fresh, sweet flavor and texture, use them within 2 or 3 days of purchase.

Preparing Potatoes are used both peeled and unpeeled. If you plan to eat the peels, try to use organic potatoes, as commer-

Quick Tip

If you must peel and cut potatoes ahead, put them in a bowl of cold water to keep them from discoloring, unless the recipe directs you not to do so. Some recipes, such as for latkes, rely on the surface starch of just-cut potatoes to bind the potato mixture during cooking. Other recipes, such as for French fries, will direct you to rinse potatoes in order to remove the starch that might otherwise cause the pieces to stick to one another or to the pan.

cially grown ones are subjected to a wide variety of pesticides that concentrate in the skin. Whether or not you peel the potatoes, scrub them well with a stiff brush under cold running water to remove any dirt. (When washing new potatoes, be aware that their thin skins will come off if scrubbed too hard.) If baking, prick the skins in a few places with a fork. If peeling, use a potato peeler, cutting out the eyes with a paring knife or the tip of the peeler if necessary. If the flesh is tinged with green spots, be sure to pare away all traces of them, for they will taste bitter.

Quick Tip

For the fluffiest, lump-free mashed potatoes, use a ricer or food mill. See RICING.

See also BOILING; MASHING; PURÉEING; STEAMING.

POT HOLDER See COOKING TOOLS.

POUNDING To tenderize or flatten food by pounding it with a heavy object. Thin, relatively tough cuts of meat, such as round steaks, are tenderized by pounding them with a meat mallet. This tool has blunt teeth on two of its sides that break down

P

the connective tissue of the meat. Swiss steak and country-fried or chicken-fried steak are tenderized in the same way.

Some recipes call for pounding or pressing food to ensure faster and more even cooking. Boned chicken and turkey breasts and beef, lamb, veal, or pork fillets may be pounded thin so that they will cook quickly or be thin enough to roll around a filling. To flatten a fillet evenly, place it between two sheets of waxed paper or plastic wrap and strike it with glancing blows, working from the center to the edge with the smooth side of a meat mallet or with a meat pounder (a smooth, heavy disk on a short handle), rolling pin, or the bottom of a heavy skillet. The idea is not to pound down directly on the food but to come at it from an angle as if to spread it out. Slices of veal tenderloin are pounded to make veal scallops (or scallopini), and pork tenderloin is pounded to make pork scallops.

See also SCALLOP.

POWDERED SUGAR See SUGAR.

PRAWN See SHRIMP.

PREBAKING See BLIND BAKING.

PREHEATING The process of bringing an oven, a grill, or a pan to the desired cooking temperature before adding food to be cooked. Without adequate preheating, the actual cooking time will not match the time given in a recipe, and food may cook unevenly, stick tenaciously, or fail to rise, brown, reduce, or otherwise transform itself as the recipe requires.

An oven should be preheated for 15 to 20 minutes before baking. Preheating is particularly important for baked goods, which need to be exposed to the correct temperature at the very beginning of baking in order for the leavening process to take place. When using a baking stone to bake pizzas or breads, the oven should be preheated for at least 45 minutes, to allow the stone to heat through completely. To make sure your oven is preheated to the correct temperature, use an oven thermometer. It is equally important to preheat skillets and sauté pans before pan broiling, sautéing, and stir-frying to prevent foods from sticking.

Quick Bite

Many recipes will tell you to preheat a broiler. This is needed for electric broilers, not gas ones, and electric broilers need only about 5 minutes of preheating.

PRESSURE COOKER This special cooking pot is equipped with an airtight locking lid that forces pressure to build up inside the pot as the liquid within it comes to a boil. The trapped steam causes the internal temperature to rise beyond what it would be capable of doing in a covered pot, decreasing cooking times by two-thirds or more. Dried beans can be cooked in 20 minutes or less, as compared to hours of normal cooking. The increased

Quick Tip

Buy a pressure cooker with a minimum 6-quart capacity. Since safety precautions demand that pressure cookers never be completely filled, anything smaller will be limiting.

pressure also softens the fibers in foods, which makes pressure cookers ideal for cooking tough cuts of meats.

While early models sometimes exploded under pressure and were considered dangerous by some cooks, current designs include safety features that make such problems impossible.

PRICKLY PEAR See NOPAL CACTUS.

PROOFING Yeast, a living organism that can weaken over time, may be tested or proofed to determine whether it is active and capable of leavening bread dough. The yeast is mixed with warm water and allowed to sit for a few minutes until creamy or foamy, which indicates that it is active. Today's commercial active dry yeast is quite reliable, and if used before the expiration date on the package, it should not require proofing. Proofing, however, also gives yeast a head start on multiplying before it is added to the other ingredients, thus giving it a boost in raising the dough. It is also recommended for compressed fresh yeast, which is more perishable than active dry yeast. See YEAST for more detail.

The second rise, or fermentation period, of a yeast dough, after it has been shaped, may also be referred to as proofing.

PROSCIUTTO This Italian ham is a seasoned, salt-cured, air-dried rear leg of pork. Prosciutto is not smoked or cooked, and it is treated with a minimum of salt, but it is cured enough to be eaten without cooking. The result is a meat with a distinctive fragrance and a subtle flavor that make prosciutto one of the world's favorite hams. Aged from 10 months to 2 years,

prosciutto from Parma in the Italian region of Emilia-Romagna is considered the best. The process for curing Parma prosciutto is dictated by law and is overseen by the Parma Ham Consortium.

Prosciutto's intense flavor goes a long way. It is best when served raw or only lightly cooked, since cooking can toughen the meat. Sweet melon wedges, fresh figs, and ripe pears are classic accompaniments that provide a sweet foil to the slightly salty flavor of the ham; together they make a fine first course. Prosciutto is also an excellent addition to an antipasto platter. Just a few paper-thin slices will make a luxurious sandwich on thick bread with butter and arugula. Prosciutto is often used in recipes as a flavoring agent as well. Add a bit of shredded prosciutto to pasta and egg dishes. Drape whole slices or scatter chopped bits on just-baked pizza.

Quick Tip

A blanched prosciutto rind makes a good seasoning for soup, such as minestrone. Ask the butcher to set one aside for you and blanch it before use. If your butcher carries bone-in prosciutto, ask him for the bone to use for making soups.

Selecting Under the rind, a whole prosciutto should be covered with a thick layer of creamy white fat that fades to rose where it touches the meat. The meat itself should be a soft, rosy pink. Before buying any prosciutto, ask for a taste. It should have a sweet, earthy flavor with a slight saltiness in the background. Don't buy any ham that tastes even slightly rancid, an indication that it has not been stored properly.

For prosciutto from Parma, check for the five-pointed Parma crown seared into the side of the intact ham. All consortium-approved hams bear this seal.

In general, prosciutto is sliced paper-thin, for otherwise it may be rather tough. This is best done by the butcher using a mechanical slicer. Once sliced, the delicate flavor of the ham begins to fade, so try to buy it the day you plan to serve it. Thin slices should not be stacked one directly on top of another, but separated by pieces of waxed paper or plastic; otherwise, you'll tear them as you try to pull them apart.

Storing Store sliced prosciutto well wrapped and sealed in the refrigerator. Bring to room temperature about an hour before serving. Never freeze prosciutto, or you'll ruin its creamy texture and diminish its flavor.

See also HAM; PORK.

PROVOLONE See CHEESE.

PRUNE Although this dried plum too seldom gets the respect it deserves, it is an absolutely delicious fruit. For centuries, prunes have been a specialty of the Agen district of Bordeaux in France. Today, most of the prunes eaten in the United States are produced in California, but the most common plum for drying is still the prune d'Agen, introduced to California by French settlers in the mid-1800s. Prune plums are freestone fruits whose pits separate easily from the flesh. They also have a high sugar content that allows them to dry without fermenting.

Many traditional recipes for prunes date back to medieval times and combine the fruits with meat and other savory ingredients. The sweet, rich flavor of the fruit marries well with pork, lamb, or duck. One classic French recipe combines prunes with eel, and another pairs them with tripe. As a special treat, stuff a slit prune with a bit of foie gras. Prunes also lend themselves to desserts. Poach them in wine or Armagnac, alone or with other dried or fresh fruits, to make a compote; or use them in cakes, tarts, and puddings.

Selecting Prunes are graded according to size, from small to jumbo. Bigger is usually better. They should be plumper and moister than other dried fruits, with an even blackish purple color. Some are sold with the pits still in them, others pitted.

Storing Store prunes in a tightly covered container in a cool, dry place for up to a month. You can store them for up to 6 months in the refrigerator. Dried foods readily absorb other flavors, so keep prunes away from strong-flavored foods.

Quick Tip

Because of the concentrated sugar content of prunes, crystals sometimes form on their surface. This does not affect their quality, but you can rid prunes of the crystals by dipping them briefly in boiling water and then drying them.

Preparing If the prunes are very dry, plump them in hot water for 15 to 20 minutes. If they are to be cooked, lengthy soaking is unnecessary, as they will continue to plump as they cook.

See also DRIED FRUIT; PLUM; PLUMPING.

PUDDING The term *pudding* is a source of confusion for some people, and with good reason. In Britain, it seems as if the name is pinned to nearly every dessert. For Americans, however, the definition narrows to a handful of distinct categories. First, and most familiar, are thick, creamy, cornstarch-thickened milk puddings, of which the most popular flavors are chocolate, vanilla, butterscotch, banana, and coconut. Next in popularity are probably rice puddings, which may be thickened custard style with eggs or simply by the starch in the rice itself. The same description applies to tapioca puddings, which feature the pearly granules of the cassava root.

More robust puddings are based on bread or on batters or doughs. Bread puddings start with firm-textured, sometimes stale bread, soaked and bound with milk and egg, sweetened with sugar, and flavored or embellished in a variety of ways. Most bread puddings are baked in the oven. Other starchy puddings may also be baked, such as the cornmeal-and-maple Indian pudding. Another cakelike variety traditional to the English kitchen is the steamed pudding, in which a rich and flavorful batter is cooked for several hours in an enclosed ceramic or metal mold in a large pot of simmering water. The results are incomparably moist and flavorful, the classic example being the Christmas pudding redolent of spices and dried fruit.

Pudding Savvy When making pudding, keep the following in mind:

- For cornstarch puddings, use a heavy-bottomed saucepan to prevent sticking and scorching, and stir and scrape constantly with a wooden spoon.
- For rice puddings, avoid using precooked "converted" rice, which will not thicken sufficiently.
- Avoid overcooking tapioca pudding, simmering only until the granules or pearls are translucent. The pudding will continue to thicken as it cools.
- When making bread puddings, feel free to experiment with a different type of bread than what is called for in the recipe and to substitute milk for cream.

- For a steamed pudding, set the mold atop a trivet in the pot, to keep the bottom of the pudding from overcooking. Be sure to replenish the pot with more boiling water, maintaining the level just over halfway up the mold's side.

PUFF PASTRY The high, flaky layers of a French napoleon or mille-feuille (literally, "thousand leaf"), the crisp, delicate folds of a fruit-filled turnover, and other ethereal baked goods depend for their rich taste and fine texture on this classic pastry dough. Puff pastry is made by rolling out a simple dough of flour, salt, water, and butter; layering it with more butter; folding it envelope fashion; refrigerating it to firm up the butter; and then rolling out the dough again and repeating the whole process. The end result is several hundred ultrathin layers of dough and butter that literally puff up in the oven. Making puff pastry dough from scratch takes more time and patience than skill. Fortunately, commercial puff pastry dough may be found packaged and frozen in well-stocked food stores.

Selecting Shop around for a good-quality brand of puff pastry dough that includes real butter. Check any sell-by or use-by dates on the packaging.

Storing Keep the carefully wrapped dough in the freezer until ready to use.

Preparing Following package instructions, defrost the dough in the refrigerator, keeping it cold until ready to roll it out.

PUMPKIN A popular cold-weather member of the gourd family. Pumpkins are round to oblong with a distinctive ridged shell, and range in color from pale ivory to a deep red-tinged orange. The biggest pumpkins found in the market usually tip the scale at 30 pounds or more, and some, grown by ambitious farmers or gardeners seeking to win agricultural prizes or to outdo their neighbors, can weigh more than 200 pounds. Others weigh just a few ounces and will fit in the palm of your hand. For cooking, seek out small, sweet varieties with a thick flesh and a fairly small seed cavity, such as the Sugar Pie, Baby Bear, or Cheese pumpkin. Field pumpkins have a fibrous flesh that is not good for cooking. Reserve them for jack-o'-lanterns.

When making savory pumpkin dishes, turn to seasonings such as garlic, onions, herbs, or curry to balance the pumpkin's natural sugars. Bakers of pies, custards, muffins, and quick breads can rely on maple syrup, molasses, brown sugar, and warm spices like nutmeg and cinnamon to emphasize pumpkin's sweet side.

There are many excellent brands of canned pumpkin purée, all of which offer considerable convenience to pumpkin-loving cooks. Some are unsweetened and plain, while others, labeled as pie filling, include sugar and spices.

Selecting Choose pumpkins that feel solid and heavy for their size. As they age, they dry out and become lighter. The skin should be hard, with no cracks, blemishes, or soft spots.

Storing Hard shells protect pumpkins from easy spoilage. Most will keep for a month or longer if stored in a cool, dry place. Once cut, pumpkins should be wrapped tightly in plastic, refrigerated, and used within 3 to 4 days.

Preparing The greatest challenge to cooking a pumpkin is cutting it open. Steady the pumpkin on a thick towel, very carefully insert a large, heavy knife near the stem, and cut down through the curved side. Always cut away from you. Turn the pumpkin 180 degrees and repeat on the other side. A more dramatic, messier

method is simply to drop the pumpkin onto newspapers spread on a hard floor. It will break into pieces. Once you've cracked into the pumpkin, use a large metal spoon to scrape out the seeds and any fibrous strings in the seed cavity. If you like, save the seeds for roasting (see below).

HOW TO *Make Pumpkin Purée*

1. Place a small whole pumpkin on a baking sheet and roast it in a preheated 350°F oven until it can be easily pierced with a knife, 1 to 1½ hours. For a shorter roasting time, slice the pumpkin in half and roast it cut side down in 1 inch of water in a baking dish for about 45 minutes, or until tender.
2. Let cool, then cut the pumpkin in half crosswise (if not already done) and scoop out and discard the seeds. Scoop out the flesh with a large spoon and purée the flesh in a blender or food processor or with a food mill.

HOW TO *Roast Pumpkin Seeds*

The seeds of the pumpkin can be cleaned off and toasted to serve as a snack or to use in recipes as an ingredient or a garnish. Toasting makes the hulls crisp and edible.

1. Wipe or pick off any pumpkin flesh or strands. Sauté pumpkin seeds in a little canola oil until lightly browned.
2. Transfer them to a baking sheet and sprinkle with salt.
3. Bake in a preheated 350°F oven until crisp, about 10 minutes.
4. Drain on paper towels, cool, and store in a covered container in the refrigerator for up to 1 month.

See also SQUASH; STEAMING.

PUNCHING DOWN

Once a yeast dough has gone through its first rise, it is punched down, or pressed, before a second rise. This step redistributes the yeast to give it a fresh food supply as it continues to

Quick Tip

If you have to leave your dough while it is rising, and you can't return until past the time it's due to double in bulk, punch the dough down and refrigerate it. This will slow the process and keep the dough from overrising in your absence—and may actually result in better bread, as each added rise will improve the texture and taste of the final loaf.

ferment and raise the dough, and it expels larger carbon dioxide bubbles that have already been created by the fermenting yeast, resulting in a more even crumb to the bread. Punching down also keeps the elastic gluten in the bread from becoming overstretched or broken by the gases trapped within the dough, which would result in a heavy and coarse baked bread.

To punch down, press down on the mass of dough with both hands. Bread dough that is removed from the bowl and shaped before the second rise—or that doesn't call for a second rise—doesn't need to be punched down, as the act of handling the dough achieves the same end.

Punching down.

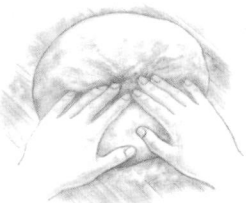

See also BREAD; RELAXING; RISING; YEAST.

PURÉEING Reducing solid food to a smooth, thick consistency by blending, mashing, or pushing it through some kind of sieving device. Puréed vegetables, such as mashed potatoes, make a comforting side dish. They are also used for soups, dips, and spreads and to add body to sauces. Fruit purées are used as fillings for cookies, cakes, and tarts.

There are many tools to help the cook prepare purées. Food can be mashed into a purée in a mortar using a pestle or pushed through a strainer with a wooden spoon. A chinois is a specialized conical strainer with a wooden pestle for just this purpose. Handheld immersion blenders do a fine job of puréeing without your having to transfer hot food from its pot. Food processors may be used to make coarser purées, while blenders are unsurpassed as a quick way of making very smooth purées. Many cooks prefer using a food mill for making purées, as many food mills have two or more plates with different-sized holes that allow the cook to control the degree of smoothness of the purée, from fine to coarse.

See also BLENDER; FOOD MILL; FOOD PROCESSOR; STRAINER.

PURSLANE Once gathered only in the wild but now also grown for market, this green resembles jumbo clover. The succulent, fleshy leaves have a pleasant tang. In the American Southwest, the green is known by the Spanish term *verdolages.*
Selecting Purslane is in season from late spring to early summer. Choose bright green, relatively small and tender leaves.
Storing Refrigerate, enclosed loosely in a plastic bag. Use within 3 or 4 days.
Preparing Add sprigs of fresh purslane to mixed green salads or chop them up as a garnish for sliced tomatoes. Purslane may also be cooked like spinach; used as an embellishment for pastas, mashed potatoes, and soups; or quickly sautéed on its own.

See also GREENS, DARK; GREENS, SALAD; HERB.

P

Q·R

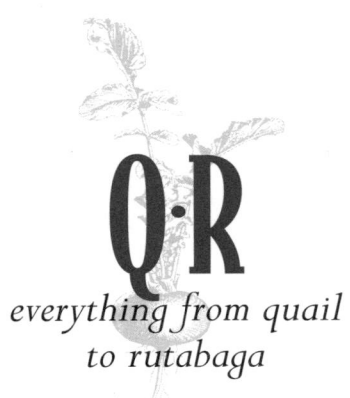

everything from quail
to rutabaga

q·r

QUAIL The American quail is a non-migratory, stay-at-home bird, prized for its light, lean flesh and sweet, nutty flavor. It is not related to European quail, although they resemble each other.

Quail are small and delicate birds, weighing about 6 ounces, with most of the meat in the breast. They are almost always served whole or halved. If a recipe calls for boned or butterflied quail, ask the butcher to do this for you, as it requires a fair amount of precision. (A boned quail is really only partially boned, with the legs and wings left intact.) Quail are generally roasted, fried, or grilled. Boned quail can be stuffed and roasted; butterflied quail is often marinated or rubbed with a spice mixture and then grilled.

Selecting The quail sold today are farm raised. Better butchers offer frozen quail (which are fine) or can special-order fresh. Asian markets are another good source for quail. When buying frozen birds, avoid torn packages or packages with pink-tinged ice (indicating thawing and refreezing). When buying fresh quail, look for plump birds with even color.

Storing Cook quail within 2 days of purchase. Refrigerate them as soon as you get home, in the original packaging. Thaw frozen quail in the refrigerator.

Preparing Allow at least 2 quail per person for a main course. Prepare as for any poultry: remove the innards, wash and pat dry, and pluck any remaining feathers with a sturdy pair of tweezers or needle-nosed pliers. It is often necessary to truss the birds or secure them with small metal skewers to help them maintain their shape during cooking.

QUATRE ÉPICES (KAH-tray-PEACE) Literally "four spices," a mixture of spices sold bottled in nearly every grocery in France. *Quatre épices* commonly appears in ingredient lists in French recipes, signaling Gallic cooks to use their own favorite mixture. *Quatre épices* usually combines white pepper, cinnamon or ginger, nutmeg, and clove, in proportions that vary. The blend seasons soups and stews as well as sausages, pâtés, and marinades for meats.

QUICHE A savory custard usually baked like a pie in a pastry crust and flavored with ingredients such as ham, cheese, mushrooms, and vegetables. The quiche originated in Lorraine in eastern France, where it is traditionally served as an hors d'oeuvre. Many different kinds are made in the area, as well as in neighboring Alsace, but the so-called quiche Lorraine, a common brunch dish in the United States, is the best known. To make this classic tart, bacon bits are layered atop a flaky pastry shell and then a mixture of eggs beaten with cream and seasoned with salt and pepper is poured into the crust. Sometimes Gruyère cheese, onion, or leeks may be included as well.

Quick Bread

There are yeast breads, and there are quick breads. Banana bread, muffins, biscuits, popovers, and corn bread are examples of quick breads. Yeast breads are leavened with yeast, while quick breads rapidly rise thanks to baking powder and/or baking soda, resulting in denser, moister textures.

They rarely require kneading (some doughs for biscuits and scones are kneaded briefly), and do not need to rise before baking, hence their name.

Quick-bread batters frequently contain fats and sweeteners, as well as flour and liquid. They also may be mixed with fresh or dried fruit, nuts, vegetables, cheese, herbs, spices, and other ingredients to create rich and flavorful breads and muffins.

To test a quick bread for doneness, open the oven at the earliest time specified in the recipe and insert a toothpick into the center of the loaf or muffin. It should come out clean or with only a few moist crumbs clinging to it. As they bake, the tops of some quick bread loaves may crack and split.

Quick Bread Savvy When making quick breads, keep the following in mind:

- Careful measuring of both liquid and dry ingredients is needed to achieve the correct texture in quick breads. (This is true of all baking, from breads to cakes to cookies.) See BAKING; MEASURING.
- Replace baking powder or baking soda that has been open in your pantry for more than 6 months, as its leavening power gradually dissipates.
- Coat baking containers thoroughly with fat such as butter, oil, or cooking spray to prevent sticking and promote browning. A light dusting of flour over the fat also helps (or use a baking spray that includes flour).
- Mixing batters with a light hand, just until combined but still slightly lumpy, keeps flour's gluten from overdeveloping and producing a tough texture.
- Bake quick breads as soon as possible after mixing. The leavening effect of the baking powder or baking soda gradually wears off if not exposed to heat. See BAKING POWDER & BAKING SODA for more details about how these chemical leaveners work.
- For convenience, you can mix the dry and wet ingredients separately and hold them apart until you are ready to combine them and bake the bread.
- When the minimum baking time called for in the recipe has elapsed, check for doneness by inserting a long wooden toothpick or thin wooden skewer into the center. (Old cookbooks often called for a clean broom straw.) If it comes out clean, the quick bread is done.
- Let quick-bread loaves or muffins cool in their pans for about 10 minutes, allowing them time to firm up. Then unmold and transfer to a wire rack to complete cooling, so their crusts won't grow damp from moisture trapped in the pan.

See also BISCUIT; CORN BREAD; FLOUR; MUFFIN; POPOVER.

q·r

QUINCE A relative of the rose, the quince has a heady aroma that can fill a room. These fruits, which look something like misshapen yellow apples, have hard, dry flesh, with an overwhelmingly astringent flavor; once cooked, however, it becomes a deep rose pink and increases in fragrance. Even cooked, however, quinces remain sour and need the addition of other ingredients to be palatable.

Quinces are old-fashioned fruits, predating their close cousins apples and pears. They were great favorites of the Romans, and the early American colonists eagerly planted quince trees in their orchards. The fruit has fallen from favor in more recent centuries, probably because it requires long cooking and cannot be eaten raw as a quick snack.

An extraordinary amount of pectin is packed into quinces, making them ideal for jellies and jams, especially those containing other fruits lower in pectin, such as pears. Quinces take well to all sorts of cooking methods, too. They can be poached, stewed, baked, or braised. They hold their shape even after long cooking and are traditionally combined with meats and used to flavor stews in the kitchens of Iran, Morocco, and Romania. Quinces are a wonderful addition to fruit compotes and make delicious pies and tarts. Quince paste, made by cooking the pulp with a high proportion of sugar, is served with soft cheese as a favorite European and Latin American dessert.

Selecting Quinces are available from October through December. Look for them in farmers' markets and specialty-food stores. They are harder to find in supermarkets. Large, smooth fruits are easiest to peel and are less wasteful than smaller ones. Blemishes and scars aren't an issue, since quinces are always cooked, but fruits that are too battered tend to spoil more quickly than others. Buy them before they ripen, when they are still quite firm and their skin is just beginning to turn from green to gold.

Storing Store unripe quinces at room temperature for up to 1 week or longer, where they will ripen from green to yellow and fill the room with their fragrance. Once they are ripe, refrigerate them in a plastic bag for up to 2 weeks. Ripe quinces bruise easily, so wherever you store them make sure that they won't be jostled and bumped.

Preparing Although edible, the peel of a quince can be somewhat bitter and is usually removed before cooking. The hard flesh will resist a knife. You may need a hefty cleaver and an extra bit of effort and care to cut the fruit open. Remove the core and the seeds unless you're planning to put the quince through a food mill or otherwise strain it.

QUINOA See GRAIN.

RAAB See BROCCOLI RABE.

RACLETTE See CHEESE.

RADICCHIO See CHICORY; GREENS, SALAD.

RADISH Although radishes come in a tremendous diversity of sizes, shapes, and colors, they all belong to a single subspecies of the mustard family. Aside from the familiar round red radishes, there are thin white ones, known as icicle radishes; Easter egg radishes that range in color from purple and white to lavender and red; and deep red, elongated French breakfast radishes, which fade to white at the root. Central Europeans serve grated black radishes as a first course. Although radishes are sometimes boiled, steamed, or sautéed, their flavor and texture are perhaps best appreciated when raw. They are sliced and used to add color and crunch to salads. Spring radishes, accompanied with sweet butter and bread, are a classic French hors d'oeuvre.

Red radish.

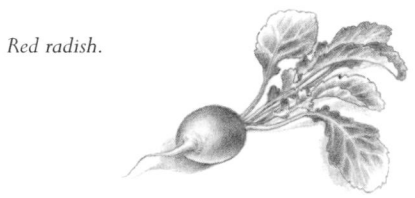

In addition, several different Asian radishes exist, which are cooked, pickled, or eaten raw. The most common is the daikon, a cylindrical vegetable that grows up to 20 inches long and about 2 inches in diameter. It is used extensively in Japanese cooking. Fried dishes are almost always accompanied by fresh daikon, as it is thought to aid the digestion of oily foods. It is grated and eaten in salads or pickled to eat with rice, and it turns up in long, thin threads on platters of sushi. The Chinese also use daikon, but they prefer to cook chunks of it in stews and other dishes.

Daikon.

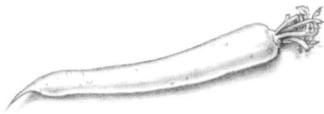

Selecting Look for smaller, round radishes in spring and elongated ones as summer arrives. Large Asian radishes are in season in autumn, and black radishes are in season in winter. Some more unusual varieties of radish are found in Asian gro-

ceries and farmers' markets. All radishes should be firm, with smooth skins and unwilted green leaves.

Storing If you are planning to serve the radishes whole as an hors d'oeuvre, don't remove the leaves; serve the radishes within a day or two of purchase. Otherwise, remove the leaves before storing small radishes in a perforated bag in the refrigerator for up to 1 week. Large radishes such as daikon can be refrigerated for up to 2 weeks. Use the greens in salads or cook them like other greens. See also GREENS, DARK; GREENS, SALAD.

Preparing Scrub the radishes and trim both ends, unless you are serving them as an hors d'oeuvre, in which case you may want to trim the root end but leave 1 inch of the leaves.

Quick Tip

If the radishes you buy are not as crisp as they should be, put them into a bowl of ice water and refrigerate them for a few hours.

RAISIN While you might think that a raisin is a raisin is a raisin, there are actually several different types of this popular dried fruit. All raisins are, of course, simply dried grapes, but the type of grape used determines the characteristics of the raisin. In addition to the common dark, seedless raisins made from sun-dried Thompson grapes that turn up in cereal boxes, dot oatmeal cookies, and are mixed with nuts and seeds in nearly every hiker's supply of trail mix, there are golden raisins, also called sultanas, which are Thompson grapes that have been treated with sulfur dioxide and dried in a dehydrator. During the winter holiday season, fat Muscat raisins are sometimes available. These large, plump raisins have an intense fruity flavor that is favored by many bakers. And tiny dried

q·r

currants are not really currants at all, but actually dried Zante grapes.

Rich in iron, raisins make a great snack for eating out of hand. Add them to cookies, cakes, and yeast breads. Raisins also go well with many savory dishes. Add them to salads or use them to flavor stews.
Selecting Look for plump, moist raisins. They are usually the freshest.
Storing Raisins can be stored in a covered container at room temperature for about a month, or refrigerated for up to 6 months.
Preparing If your raisins are dry and hard, soak them in hot water for about 20 minutes to plump them.

See also DRIED FRUIT.

RAMEKIN A small, round ceramic baking dish, usually 3 to 4 inches in diameter, used for making individual portions of sweet and savory dishes. Custard cups or individual soufflé dishes may be substituted. The term also refers to a small baked pastry filled with a creamy cheese filling.

RAPE See BROCCOLI RABE.

RAPINI See BROCCOLI RABE.

RASPBERRY See BERRY.

REACTIVE A metal that produces a chemical reaction when it comes in contact with an acidic food is said to be reactive. Copper, aluminum, and, to a lesser extent, cast iron are reactive metals. See also ACID; NONREACTIVE.

RECONSTITUTING To bring dehydrated foods back to their original consistency or strength, usually by adding liquid. This term is also used for the process of correcting a sauce that has separated.

See also REHYDRATING.

RED BEAN See BEAN, DRIED.

REDUCING Simmering or boiling a liquid in order to decrease its quantity through evaporation, while concentrating the flavor and thickening the consistency. Reducing is a handy sauce-making technique, typically used when food is being sautéed. Braising liquids, stocks, wine, cream, balsamic vinegar, and other liquids can all be reduced to make flavorful sauces. For a perfectly smooth texture, strain reduced sauces before serving. Meat and poultry stocks are particularly desirable for reduction sauces, since as they reduce their proteins give the sauce a silky, viscous texture unmatched by any starch-thickened sauce. Be careful when using commercial broths for reduction, as they may contain a good deal of salt, which will become concentrated. Opt for reduced-sodium broth when you're planning to make a reduced sauce, and salt to taste at the end.

HOW TO *Make a Simple Reduction Sauce*
For a quick sauce to accompany sautéed poultry or meat, deglaze the pan:
1. Add a small amount of wine, vermouth, or chicken or meat stock to the pan after removing the sautéed food.
2. Stir with a wooden spoon over medium-high heat, scraping up the browned particles from the bottom of the pan, until the liquid has reduced in volume slightly and has thickened.
3. Pour the reduction sauce over the sautéed food, through a strainer if desired, and serve.

Quick Tip

Season reduction sauces after they've reached the desired consistency. If you season them before reducing, you may find them too strong tasting and salty.

See also DEGLAZING.

REFRESHING See BLANCHING; PLUNGING.

REHYDRATING The process of restoring moisture to dried foods, also called plumping. Although drying is a wonderful way of preserving foods, often giving them a more intense and intriguing flavor than when fresh, it can leave foods with an unpalatable texture. By soaking dried foods in liquid, usually hot water, you can rehydrate them, essentially putting back some of the moisture that was lost during the drying process, making the food tender and pliable again. See also MUSHROOM; PLUMPING; SUN-DRIED TOMATO.

RELAXING Allowing dough to rest after punching down so that the elastic gluten strands in it can relax. For bread, relaxing the dough makes it easier to shape and helps to ensure a well-risen loaf.

The dough for flat breads, such as pizza and focaccia, will often resist being rolled out or pressed into pans, tightening up when you try to do so. When this happens, cover the dough with a kitchen towel and let it relax or rest for about 10 minutes, then finish rolling it out or pressing it into a pan. You will find the relaxed dough much easier to handle.
See also BREAD; RESTING; RISING.

RELISH A sweet or savory condiment, usually made of cooked or pickled fruits or vegetables. Relishes include the green pickle relish used for hot dogs, piccalilli, pickled vegetables, corn relish, spiced pears, and pickled watermelon rind. Pickles and chutneys are types of relishes, although relishes are generally considered more spicy than either.

RENDERING No matter how snowy white it appears, all animal fat in its natural state contains some amount of meat tissue, and the only way to separate the fat from the tissue is to melt it, a process known as rendering. As the fat melts, it separates from the bits of meat tissue, which sink to the bottom of the pan. The pure fat is then strained to remove these crisp bits, which are known as cracklings and are sometimes used, like crumbled bacon, as a garnish or as an ingredient. The fat of poultry, especially ducks and geese, is rendered when the birds are roasted. It is simply a matter of straining the pan drippings to capture the rendered fat. When bacon is cooked, it renders most or all of its fat, producing a favorite cooking medium in many kitchens.
Lard and schmaltz (rendered chicken fat), duck fat, and goose fat can all be purchased from specialty-food purveyors.

RESERVING Saving an ingredient or recipe component for use later in the recipe or for another dish.
See also SETTING ASIDE.

q·r

RESTING To allow food to sit undisturbed for a period of time during the course of preparing a dish. Resting is an important step in bread recipes, as it allows the gluten to relax, making the dough easier to shape and giving the final product a better texture. Pie dough is allowed to rest in the refrigerator, usually for a minimum of 30 minutes, to chill and firm the fat and to allow the moisture to distribute evenly throughout the dough. The cold slows down the development of gluten, which is desirable in bread dough but not in pastry. The batter for crepes should be allowed to rest in the refrigerator before using. The flour particles will then expand in the liquid, and the resulting crepes will be more tender.

Roasted meats should be allowed to rest after cooking and before carving or slicing. During cooking, the meat near the surface dries out due to evaporation and because some of its juices have been forced farther into the interior. Carving the meat right out of the oven results in dry edges and loss of juices from the center of the roast. A resting period allows the juices to redistribute themselves through the meat, making it uniformly juicier. Keep in mind that the internal temperature of meat and poultry will rise 5° to 10°F during resting, so account for this when judging roasting times.

See also RELAXING; ROASTING.

RHUBARB Although technically a vegetable, rhubarb is treated like a fruit in the kitchen. Its long, celery-like stalks range in color from cherry red to pale pink. Rhubarb usually is cooked with a good dose of sugar to balance its tartness. The delicious transformation after sweetening and cooking has earned rhubarb the nickname "pie plant."

Although hothouse-grown rhubarb is available all year in some areas, field-grown rhubarb is a spring crop, with the bulk appearing in April and May. Rhubarb is often paired with strawberries, which appear in the same season and whose sweetness provides a nice contrast. Oranges are another common flavor pairing. A favorite for pies and tarts, rhubarb also makes wonderful jams and preserves. Rhubarb chutneys and relishes are an excellent accompaniment to roast pork or duck.

Caution!

Rhubarb leaves are mildly toxic and should always be discarded.

Selecting Look for crisp, firm stalks without blemishes or cuts and with good color. Avoid rhubarb stalks that are turning from red or pink to green. Field-grown rhubarb has a bright red color and a more pronounced flavor than pale pink hothouse-grown stalks. Any leaves attached to the stalks should be fresh looking, not wilted, although the leaves should not be eaten.

Storing Whole stalks can be refrigerated for up to 3 days. Store them in the crisper in perforated plastic bags.

Quick Tip

To enjoy rhubarb long after its season has passed, cut the stalks into chunks, put into heavy-duty plastic freezer bags, and freeze for up to 8 months.

Preparing Trim away the leaves and stalk ends and peel any brown spots. If stalks are fibrous, remove the strings with a vegetable peeler. Stalks that are more than 1½ inches wide should be halved lengthwise.

Rice

From steaming bowls of plump, clingy rice served alongside Japanese sashimi to aromatic rice accompanying Middle Eastern kabobs to creamy Italian risotto, this seed of a species of grass is the most widely eaten of all the grains.

More than 40,000 distinct varieties of rice have been identified, explaining the diverse characteristics of rice dishes around the world. Nevertheless, far fewer types of rice lend themselves to commercial cultivation, and these may be readily classified into a handful of easily identifiable categories.

Rice Styles One or more of the following terms are likely to be found on the packaging of rice you encounter for sale. Some define a specific variety or type of rice, while others specify characteristics the rice has when cooked.

ARBORIO RICE Northern Italian variety of medium-grain rice with a high surface-starch content that dissolves when the rice is simmered and stirred, forming a creamy sauce that complements the chewy rice as in the classic Italian dish risotto. Two other, similar Italian varieties, Carnaroli and Vialone Nano, may be substituted. So, too, may other medium-grain rice varieties. See also Medium-Grain Rice, page 380.

AROMATIC RICE Varieties that give off pronounced aromas when cooked, such as Della, basmati, jasmine, and pecan rice.

BASMATI RICE Highly aromatic, long-grain variety, grown primarily in India, Iran, and the United States, with a sweet, nut-like taste and perfume. Both white and brown basmati rices are sold. Basmati is the best rice to use in pilafs. American-grown basmati rice is sometimes commercially labeled Texmati after its state of origin.

BLACK RICE Southeast Asian variety of unmilled sticky rice with a black hull that turns dark purple when cooked.

BROWN RICE Refers to any rice that has not been processed by milling or polishing, leaving its brown hull intact. Brown rice takes longer to cook than comparable white rice and has a chewier texture and a nutlike taste. Technically speaking, both black and red rice are brown rice.

CONVERTED RICE Refers to commercially sold white rice that was parboiled before the removal of its bran. This rice cooks quickly and is high in B vitamins.

DELLA RICE A hybrid rice of the American South similar to basmati. It has a taste and aroma that has been likened to popcorn.

GLUTINOUS RICE A short-grain rice that becomes soft, moist, sticky, and translucent when cooked. Also called sticky or sweet rice. Uncooked, it is opaque and almost as round as a pearl. It is also ground into flour. There is no substitute for glutinous rice in sticky rice desserts.

JASMINE RICE A long-grain rice variety from Thailand with a sweet floral scent.

LONG-GRAIN RICE Any rice variety with grains three to five times longer than they are wide. When cooked, the grains are generally fluffy and separate. Long-grain rice is traditionally used in such dishes as pilafs, which are cooked in stock and may include vegetables, poultry, meat, or seafood.

continued

Rice, continued

MEDIUM-GRAIN RICE Rice varieties with grains 2 to 3 times longer than they are wide. Note that the United States is the only country that uses "medium grain" as a category of rice. In other countries, all rice is divided into either "short grain" or "long grain." Therefore, the rice used in Spain for paella and in Italy for risotto is referred to as short grain, although both are more accurately described as medium grain.

PECAN RICE An aromatic long-grain white rice grown in Louisiana and enjoyed for a taste and scent reminiscent of pecans.

RED RICE Long-, medium-, or short-grain rice variety with red-colored bran, sold unmilled and enjoyed for its bright color.

RICE FLOUR See FLOUR.

SHORT-GRAIN RICE Most common in Asian and Caribbean kitchens, these almost-spherical grains yield very sticky, chewy results when cooked. Short-grain rice is used in many desserts. It is also ground into rice flour, to be used as a thickening agent.

SUSHI RICE Medium-grain white rice. What makes sushi rice so distinctive is the method of cooking that involves soaking and rinsing the grains as well as fanning them while they cool.

WHITE RICE Any rice that has been milled to remove its brown hull and bran.

WILD RICE Not actually a type of rice at all, but the seed of an aquatic grass. It is native to Minnesota, where it grows wild. It is also cultivated. The dark brown, un-polished kernels have a rich, nutlike flavor and texture. See also WILD RICE.

Selecting Most food stores today carry several different kinds of rice. For an even wider selection, seek out specific types in natural-food stores, ethnic markets, or specialty-food shops.

Storing Store rice in an airtight container away from moisture, heat, and light. White rice will keep for up to 2 years; brown rice, other unhulled rices, and wild rice will keep for up to 1 year, or longer if refrigerated.

Preparing Many cooks rinse rice before using it to remove excess starch that may create a gummy texture. Place the rice in a large pot and rinse it several times, gently swishing the rice with your fingers, until the water runs clear.

Rice may be boiled in a large quantity of liquid and then drained, like pasta; simmered in a covered pan with a carefully measured amount of liquid, which steams the grains; cooked in a microwave oven with a measured amount of liquid; or prepared in an Asian-style rice cooker, following the manufacturer's instructions. Substituting stock, coconut milk, or another savory or sweet liquid for its cooking water flavors rice as it cooks.

HOW TO *Steam Rice*

For plain rice follow these simple instructions and proportions, adding, if you wish, $\frac{1}{4}$ to $\frac{1}{2}$ teaspoon salt for each 1 cup rice.

1. Combine water (in the proportion listed below, depending on the type of rice) and rice in a small saucepan that has a tight-fitting lid.
2. Bring to a boil over high heat, stir, reduce the heat to low, cover, and cook until tender, according to the times suggested.
3. After cooking, let the rice sit undisturbed for 10 to 20 minutes to "steam" it before serving.

BROWN RICE Simmer, covered, in 2 parts water to 1 part rice until tender, 45 to 60 minutes.

LONG-GRAIN RICE Simmer, covered, in 1¾ parts water to 1 part rice for 15 to 20 minutes.

SHORT- OR MEDIUM-GRAIN RICE Simmer, covered, in 1½ parts water to 1 part rice for 15 to 20 minutes.

WILD RICE Simmer, covered, in 3 parts water to 1 part rice until tender but still chewy, about 1 hour; drain off any excess liquid.

See also NOODLE; PAELLA; RICE COOKER; RISOTTO.

RICE COOKER Also called a rice steamer, this electric appliance takes the guesswork and worry out of cooking rice. The cooker sits on the countertop. It is fitted with an insert for steaming rice. Some models have additional inserts for steaming other foods such as vegetables. Rice cookers typically cook from 2 to 24 cups of rice, depending on the size.

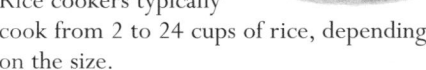

RICE PAPER Thin, dried translucent paper made from rice flour, water, and salt is known as rice paper, rice sheets, or spring roll wrappers. Indispensable to the Vietnamese kitchen, rice papers are distinguished by the cross-hatching that results from being dried on bamboo mats under a tropical sun.
Selecting Rice papers may be round or triangular, and they come in a range of sizes from small to large. Vietnamese spring rolls are usually made from 8-inch round rice papers, which come in 1-pound packages of about 50 papers.
Storing Rice papers will keep indefinitely in a tightly closed plastic bag stored on a cupboard shelf.
Preparing Brush or spray each paper with water on both sides, or simply dip it quickly in a bowl of cold water and shake to remove the excess water. Set the moistened rice paper on paper towels for 1 to 2 minutes to soften. Fill and roll. Spring rolls made with rice paper may be served without further cooking or deep-fried.

RICE VERMICELLI See NOODLE.

RICE VINEGAR See VINEGAR.

RICE WINE There are several variations of this sweet wine, which is made from glutinous rice. (See RICE.) Sake, the traditional Japanese beverage, is often served warm to pour into tiny cups or wooden boxes, though some sake is meant to be sipped chilled. Rice wine is also used in cooking, most often in sauces and marinades. Mirin, or sweet sake, a sweetened rice wine, is used exclusively for cooking and is an important ingredient in Japanese cuisine. Dry sherry may be substituted.

The best-known Chinese rice wine is Shaoxing. Like sake, it is often served warm. It is considered an essential ingredient in Chinese cooking, from stir-fries to braises. This is the spirit that is used in large quantities in "drunken" Chinese dishes, such as drunken shrimp. A dry sherry is the only substitute.
Selecting Look for rice wine in the ethnic-foods section of the supermarket or in Asian groceries.
Storing Rice wine will keep indefinitely in a cool, dark place.

Quick Bite

Although sake is called rice *wine*, it is actually made in a process that is more akin to that used to make beer.

RICING Ricing is a method of making a fluffy mash or purée. It is most commonly used for making extremely fine mashed potatoes. A ricer looks like a small pot with holes in the bottom and a plunger attached to the rim. Cooked potatoes are put in the "pot," which is positioned over a warmed bowl. The potatoes are then forced through the perforations with the plunger, which turns them into soft ricelike kernels. Finally, hot milk or cream and butter is gently stirred into the riced potatoes. The resulting texture is very refined and smooth.

You can also rice other sturdy vegetables, such as carrots, parsnips, or celery root.

Ricing potatoes.

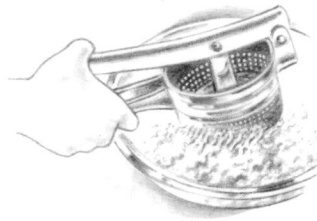

Quick Tip

If you use organic potatoes, you can cook and rice them without having to peel them. Scrub the potatoes well before cooking to remove dirt. After they are cooked, cut them into chunks if necessary and put them through the ricer, stopping periodically to scrape off the peels from the plunger.

See also COOKING TOOLS; POTATO.

RICOTTA See CHEESE.

RIND The tough, and usually thick, exterior coat of some foods, such as melons, citrus fruits, slab bacon, and ham. Citrus rinds consist of both the colored zest and the white pith. (See also ZESTING.) Like melon rinds, citrus rinds are generally inedible. But they may be cooked or packed in salt for an extended time to soften them, as for preserved lemons. Citrus rinds can also be candied. Melon rinds, or peels, particularly those of watermelons, are preserved by pickling. Ham and bacon rinds are often removed before cooking, but are sometimes reserved to use as a flavoring and thickening agent in soups and stews. Many aged cheeses have a rind, which varies in texture, thickness, and color, depending on the cheese. See also CHEESE.

RIPENING Fruits are best eaten at the point of ripeness, that is, when they have reached their peak of flavor and texture. Fruits play a key role in a plant's reproduction process: fruits are carried away and eaten by animals, dispersing their seeds far and wide. So it is to a plant's advantage that its fruit be as appealing to the animal senses as possible at the moment when its seeds become viable. There are four main sensory indicators of ripeness: a change in color, usually from green to a bright shade; a burst of scent; a softening of texture; and a decrease in acid content, highlighting the fruit's sugar content and sweet taste.

It's not always easy to come across fruits at their point of ripeness. Pears, for example, often are hard when you buy them and should sit at room temperature for a few days before eating out of hand. Some fruits are picked unripe for distribution to markets and so need to ripen after purchase. Bananas, plantains, peaches, and tomatoes are picked before they reach their peak and will benefit from sitting at room temperature. Avocados, in fact, do not ripen fully until *after* they have been picked.

To hasten the ripening process and to prevent fruit from spoiling before it ripens completely, put the fruit in a paper bag to trap the ethylene gas the fruit emits. Be sure to punch several holes in the bag to let the fruit breathe.

RISING The increase in volume of a mixed batter or dough is referred to as rising. A leavener causes these mixtures to increase in volume. Heat and steam alone are enough to induce some batters or light doughs to rise. Three other kinds of leaveners are eggs and butter (both aerating leaveners—beaten to incorporate air, which expands to raise the batter), yeast, and chemical leaveners such as baking soda and baking powder.

See also BAKING POWDER & BAKING SODA; EGG; LEAVENING; YEAST.

RISOTTO Like pasta and polenta, risotto is an example of the Italian talent of turning the simplest ingredients into a sublime dish. It is made from certain varieties of medium-grain rice that possess an outer layer of soft starch. During cooking, the rice is constantly stirred while hot liquid is gradually added, causing the starch to dissolve and form a creamy sauce that complements the chewy rice.

The varieties of Italian rice most commonly used are Arborio, Carnaroli, and Vialone Nano; Arborio is by far the best known and most widely available in the United States.

There are two styles of risotto made in Italy: the cohesive and slightly sticky dish from Lombardy and Emilia-Romagna is what we usually think of as risotto in the United States. The best-known example is probably *risotto alla milanese,* made with saffron and a sprinkling of Parmesan cheese. The second style, from the Veneto, is thinner and more like a porridge; the best-known example is the *risi e bisi* of Venice, which is rice with peas.

Risotto can be plain, with only Parmesan cheese added, or it can incorporate one or more of a wide variety of flavoring ingredients. Any risotto usually starts with finely chopped onion cooked in butter or, less frequently, olive oil. The rice is added and stirred just long enough to coat the grains. Next, about ½ cup of liquid is added at a time, and the rice is stirred constantly until almost all the liquid is absorbed. Often dry white wine is the first liquid addition, followed by a hot stock, typically chicken. This step is repeated, along with constant stirring, until the rice is creamy on the outside and al dente at the center: tender but firm to the bite. This process takes 20 to 30 minutes of closely monitored cooking and stirring.

Risotto may be served as a first course, side dish, or main course. It may also be molded before serving. In one classic dish, it is made from the stock of a poached chicken, and the bird is served in the center of a ring of the risotto. Risotto is the basis for *arancini* and *suppli,* deep-fried cheese-stuffed croquettes. It may also be formed into cakes, sautéed, and served as a side dish or as a bed for other foods.

Risotto Savvy When making risotto, keep the following in mind:

- The right pan is the secret to a good risotto. The pan must be large, of about 1-quart capacity for each serving made, and heavy enough to keep the rice from scorching or cooking too fast during the lengthy process of becoming risotto. An enameled cast-iron saucepan is ideal.
- Taste-test the rice after about 20 minutes, but plan for 25 to 35 minutes of total cooking time.
- If you run out of liquid before the rice is al dente, use hot water to finish the cooking process.
- Often the final step in making risotto is to stir in 1 or 2 tablespoons of butter or a good amount of grated Parmesan cheese, or both, depending on the other

ingredients. This process takes from 1 to 2 minutes and makes the final dish even creamier. Use a light hand: if you stir too vigorously, the rice will become gummy.

■ Although it will not be quite as creamy, you can partially cook the risotto ahead of time and finish it just before serving. To do so, cook the risotto until half of the hot liquid has been added, remove it from the pan, and spread it out on a rimmed baking sheet to arrest the cooking process. Return the rice to the heat and complete the risotto's preparation right before serving, adding a little more cheese or butter, or both, than called for in the recipe.

See also RICE.

ROASTING
This dry-heat method of oven-cooking foods in an uncovered pan should be reserved for tender meats with plenty of marbling or interior fat. Though marinating, coating with oil or butter, and basting will also help keep the surface of roasted meat moist, nothing will keep a roast's center moist if you overcook it. Paying attention to the internal temperature is the only final assurance of juicy, succulent meat. Leaner meats also can be roasted, but they should be well barded to supplement their moisture (see BARDING).

Quick Tip

Every kind of poultry, protected by its fatty skin, can be roasted whole or cut into pieces; brush the cut side of the pieces well with oil.

Cooks have developed various techniques for keeping the interior of roasted meats moist while developing a rich, brown exterior. Larger roasts are best cooked at a lower roasting temperature of 325° to 350°F, to help prevent the outer section of the roast from overcooking before the

center is done. If the roast isn't as brown as it should be by the end, the temperature can be raised to 400°F for the last minutes of cooking. Smaller roasts, including beef tenderloins, do better roasting quickly at higher temperatures. They need the higher heat to brown since they are not in the oven as long.

Quick Tip

Let roasted meats and poultry rest at room temperature for 15 to 25 minutes, depending on size, before carving and serving. In a cold kitchen, you can loosely cover the meat with aluminum foil to keep in heat, but some cooks find this softens a crisp, brown exterior.

Equipment A roasting pan has low sides in order to allow the oven heat to reach as much of the surface of the food as possible, while catching any juices from the roasting food. For roasts and poultry, choose a heavy roasting pan to keep the bottom of the food and the pan juices from burning. Although a pan with a nonstick surface makes cleanup easy, a regular surface allows more brown bits to stick to the pan during roasting, which means better gravy.

Roasting pan with rack.

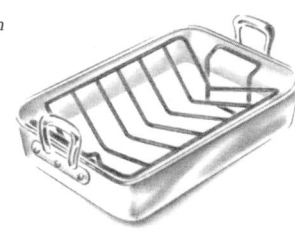

A metal rack keeps the bottom of the food from stewing in the pan drippings and sticking to the pan. It also produces clearer pan drippings, which means better-tasting gravy. You can use a wire cake rack in a pinch, but a V-shaped nonstick roasting rack is preferable, as it elevates the food

Roasting Times for Various Foods			
FOOD	OVEN TEMPERATURE	APPROXIMATE TIME	INTERNAL TEMPERATURE
BEEF			
Prime rib	550°F to preheat, 350°F to roast	18 to 20 minutes per pound	Medium-rare: 130° to 140°F*
Rolled roast	550°F to preheat, 350°F to roast	25 to 30 minutes per pound	Medium-rare: 130°F to 140°F*
Tenderloin (whole)	500°F to preheat, 400°F to roast	10 minutes per pound	Rare: 120° to 130°F;* Medium-rare: 130° to 140°F*
LAMB			
Boneless leg	450°F to preheat, 325°F to roast	20 to 25 minutes per pound	Medium-rare: 130°F*
Rack	400°F	25 minutes total	Medium-rare: 130°F*
PORK			
Boneless loin or shoulder	450°F to preheat, 325°F to roast	30 to 35 minutes per pound	Medium: 150° to 160°F*
Tenderloin	500°F	18 to 20 minutes total	Medium: 150° to 160°F*
VEAL, leg, shoulder, or loin (barded)	425°F to preheat, 325°F to roast	15 to 20 minutes per pound (turn once)	Medium: 145° to 155°F*
CHICKEN (whole)	450°F to preheat, 350°F to roast	20 to 25 minutes per pound	150° to 160°F* in breast; 165° to 175°F in thigh
TURKEY (whole)	450°F to preheat, 325°F to roast	15 to 20 minutes per pound (10- to 15-pound birds); 13 to 15 minutes per pound (birds over 16 pounds)	170°F in breast; 185°F in thigh
FISH	500°F	8 to 9 minutes per inch of thickness	135° to 137°F
VEGETABLES			
Asparagus	500°F	8 to 10 minutes total	
Beets (whole)	300°F	45 to 75 minutes total	
Winter squash (whole)	375°F	45 to 90 minutes total	

Although the internal temperatures for meats and poultry in this chart yield what many cooks feel are the optimum taste and texture for these foods, they are lower than those suggested by the U.S. Food Safety and Inspection Service guidelines; see DONENESS.

more and allows more of its surface to brown. You can also place the meat or poultry on a bed of aromatic vegetables, such as chopped carrots, onions, and celery. The vegetables serve the same function as a rack, with the added benefit that they may be puréed and combined with the degreased pan juices and the deglazing liquid to make a sauce for the roasted food.

About Vegetables Vegetables such as whole potatoes and sweet potatoes in their skin, sliced and oiled root vegetables, and softer vegetables such as tomatoes take well to roasting, as it concentrates their natural sugars and heightens their flavor. Beets roasted in their skins are a revelation, becoming almost as sweet as candy, and asparagus comes out crisp-tender and deep green. Except for baked potatoes, vegetables should be given a coating of olive oil before roasting: place them in a baking dish or roasting pan, sprinkle or spray with olive oil, and toss them to coat. Toss again with salt, pepper, and other seasonings.

Roasting Times Note in the chart on page 385 that the doneness temperatures are different for different meats and birds, and that cooking times are approximate. Keep in mind that the internal temperature of roasts and birds will continue to rise after they are out of the oven. In many cases, the oven is preheated to a high temperature, and the temperature is then reduced when the food is put in the oven to roast. The chart is based on unstuffed, room-temperature meats and poultry. For stuffed meats and smaller stuffed poultry, add a few minutes more per pound; the same rule also applies to stuffed turkeys over 12 pounds.

Pan Roasting Like pan broiling, this term refers (usually) to cooking in a dry skillet on the stove top. Pan roasting differs from pan broiling in that the heat is lower and the food is cooked more gently. In Mexican cooking, fresh chiles, tomatoes, onions, tomatillos, and garlic are all pan roasted on a *comal,* a flat carbon-steel griddle, until browned and tender. This concentrates the flavor in the vegetables as they cook by evaporating some of their moisture and giving them a slightly charred taste. You can use a griddle or a cast-iron skillet over medium heat for pan roasting these types of vegetables. You may want to line the griddle or pan with aluminum foil for easier cleanup. (They can also be cooked under a broiler.)

Another version of pan roasting is used for boneless chicken breasts and salmon, tuna, or swordfish fillets: the food is seared on one side—in a little oil heated over medium-high heat in a cast-iron or other heavy, ovenproof skillet—for a few minutes. The food is not turned, and the skillet is placed in a preheated 450°F oven for about 10 minutes, resulting in chicken or fish with a very crisp exterior and a tender, juicy interior.

See also BARDING; DEGLAZING; DONENESS; LARDING; MARINATING; RESTING; TEMPERATURE; individual types of poultry and meat.

ROCK CORNISH GAME HEN See CORNISH GAME HEN.

ROCKET See ARUGULA.

ROLLING OUT To flatten dough using a rolling pin. Pie dough and cookie dough are rolled out on a work surface, such as a countertop or pastry board, which is usually floured first to prevent sticking. Pastry sleeves (for the pins) and pastry cloths (for the surfaces) may be used to prevent sticking, too. A recipe usually specifies the final size and/or thickness of the dough and the shape. Bread doughs can be rolled out for pizza and various flat breads.

HOW TO *Roll Out Dough*

1. Sprinkle flour lightly over both the work surface and the rolling pin.
2. Using your hands, shape the dough into a flat, round disk. Place it on the work surface and tap it 3 times with the rolling pin, at the top, middle, and bottom of the disk, to flatten and spread it out a bit. Give the disk a quarter turn and tap it again 3 times to spread it out.
3. Starting with the pin in the center of the disk, firmly and steadily roll the pin away from you to within a finger's width of the far edge.
4. Give the dough a quarter turn and repeat the rolling. Continue in this manner, giving the dough a quarter turn and rolling away from you until the dough is the thickness indicated in the recipe. If the dough begins to stick, lift it and sprinkle flour beneath it.

Rolling Out Savvy for Pie, Tart, and Cookie Doughs

■ Some sticky doughs need to be placed between two sheets of waxed or parchment paper before rolling. Beginners may like to roll out all doughs this way, since it prevents any sticking to the work surface and makes the transfer to the pan easy. With practice, you will be able to roll out dough without paper.

Rolling out between waxed paper sheets.

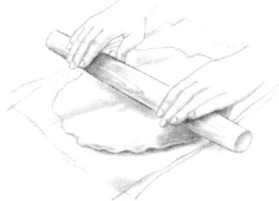

When you are ready to transfer the dough, remove the top layer of paper and gently flip the dough round over.

■ Although many recipes recommend chilling the dough disk before rolling it out, in order to relax it, this step can make the dough difficult to roll. Sometimes, it's better to chill dough just after you have cut the fat into the flour but before you have added water (if you find the fat is starting to melt) or after the dough has been rolled out and shaped.

■ Any time the dough begins to stick to the work surface or the rolling pin, lift up the dough and lightly flour the surface, the pin, and the top of the dough. You can also turn the dough over periodically, lightly flouring all the surfaces.

■ Periodically shape the dough into a circle with your cupped hands. If the edges begin to crack, press them together with your fingertips.

■ Make sure you roll the dough evenly, to avoid thin spots and holes. Patch any holes with a piece of dough brushed with a little water.

■ Do not push too hard on the dough with the rolling pin. Instead, flatten it with firm, quick, steady strokes.

■ Pie pastry is usually rolled out ⅛ inch thick. If the dough is too thick, it can be tough after baking; if too thin, it can fall apart or tear as you put it in the pie pan.

See also BAKEWARE; COOKIE; PIE & TART; RESTING.

ROLLING PIN See BAKING TOOLS.

ROMAN BEAN See BEAN, DRIED.

ROMANO BEAN See BEAN, FRESH.

ROSEMARY See HERB.

ROUNDED A "rounded" measure is one in which the ingredient forms a lightly rounded dome above the rim of the measuring spoon or measuring cup. See also MEASURING.

ROUX See SAUCE; THICKENING.

RUB Mixtures of spices and herbs, often in the form of powders and pastes, rubs are pressed or massaged onto the surface of meat or poultry. Many recipes call for allowing the foods to sit for several hours to absorb the flavors. The salt and spices draw the juices of the meat or poultry to the surface, so that eventually the food literally marinates in its own flavored juices. Rubs can also be applied directly before cooking. Either way, these concentrated dry mixtures are cousins to marinades, which are acid-based liquid concoctions that bathe the food, flavoring and tenderizing.

To help it adhere, a rub may contain a small amount of alcohol or juice to bind the dry ingredients, or the food may be lightly coated with oil.

Rub Savvy When using rubs, keep the following in mind:
- For better flavor, toast spices before combining in a rub.
- Before using a rub, let it stand overnight to meld and develop its flavors.

See also MARINATING.

RUBBING IN To break and flatten fat into small pea-sized pieces by rubbing it into flour with your fingertips. Used in the making of pie or biscuit dough, this technique is designed to create layers of fat and flour to ensure flaky or tender pastry. Many cooks prefer using fingers rather than cutting in the fat with two knives or a pastry cutter, as they believe the result is more thorough. When making flaky pastry, rubbing in must be done quickly and carefully to avoid melting the butter with the heat of your fingertips. The butter should remain in discrete pieces. For a crumbly, tender crust, the fat is worked into the flour more thoroughly, so this is not a concern. See also BISCUIT; CUTTING IN; PIE & TART.

RUM See SPIRITS.

RUTABAGA This member of the cabbage family looks something like an overgrown turnip, to which it is closely related. Sometimes known as swedes, Swedish turnips, and yellow turnips, rutabagas come in a variety of colors, from brown to yellow to white. Their firm, yellow flesh has a strong mustardlike taste that mellows and becomes sweeter when cooked. They can be substituted for turnips in most recipes, and cooking time will depend on age, with smaller young ones taking as little as 10 minutes and older, larger, and tougher roots taking up to an hour.

Rutabagas make wonderful purées, especially when enriched with butter or cream, or when combined with milder vegetables such as potatoes that offset their sometimes strong flavor. Braise them in chicken stock or use them in gratins. Cut into slices or chunks and brushed with oil, rutabagas are excellent roasted and stewed, either alone or mixed with other root vegetables.

Selecting Rutabagas are best during the cool-weather months of the late fall and early winter. Small ones are generally sweeter. Rutabagas should be firm and heavy for their size. Avoid those that look faded, have a strong smell, or feel at all soft. Some look shiny, which indicates they are coated with clear paraffin to hold in moisture. This is harmless and comes off with the peel.

Storing Keep rutabagas in a cool, dark place for up to 10 days, or store in a plastic bag in the refrigerator for up to 1 month.

Preparing Trim the ends and peel with a paring knife. Sprinkle cut pieces with lemon juice to prevent discoloring.

RYE See GRAIN.

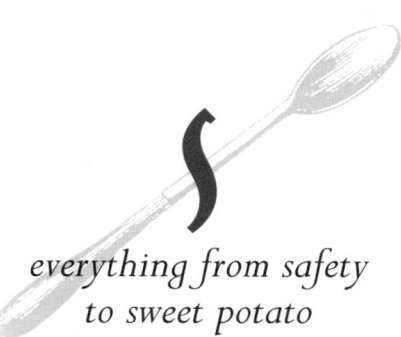

*everything from safety
to sweet potato*

SAFETY A few simple precautions and smart habits will help ensure safety in the kitchen. See also FOOD SAFETY.

Guarding against Accidents

- Keep knives sharpened and fingers clear of the blade during use. See also KNIFE.
- Always dry your hands thoroughly before handling any electrical appliances or their plugs or cords.
- Keep pan handles away from the edge of the stove and from adjacent hot burners or pilot lights.
- Do not leave metal spoons or other utensils inside pots during cooking, since they will heat up.
- To avoid splattering or scalding, never mix hot fats with water.
- Do not drop food into hot fat or boiling water; gently slip it in, using a slotted spoon or long-handled tongs. You may want to wear oven mitts to protect your hands.
- Always be especially cautious at every stage of frying and deep-frying, from heating fats or oils to adding food, regulating temperatures, and removing food and leaving oil to cool.
- When pouring hot liquids, pour away from yourself to avoid spills.

Guarding against Fire

- Keep your hands, sleeves, hair, pot holders, kitchen towels, cookbooks, and other flammable objects well clear of your stove's burners and pilot lights.
- Keep a fully charged, up-to-date fire extinguisher in your kitchen. Know where it is and how to use it.
- Whenever a fire breaks out, call for help immediately.
- For a fire contained in a small pan on the stove, turn off the heat and cover the pan with a tight-fitting lid to smother the flames; or, from a safe distance, toss handfuls of baking soda at the base of the flames to extinguish them. Do not try to move the pan. If the pan contains oil or fat, do not throw water on it. Water will spread a grease fire.
- Use the fire extinguisher to put out any small fires away from the stove. Do not attempt to fight large or quickly moving fires. Instead, yell "Fire!" and get everyone out of the house. Phone the fire department from a neighbor's house.

SAFFRON See SPICE.

SAGE See HERB.

SALAD Salads can consist of one ingredient or many; can be cooked or raw, hot or cold; and can be served as an appetizer, main course, or dessert. The one constant seems to be that they are usually dressed in a sauce that contains a tart element, such as vinegar or lemon juice. Most salads have at least one raw ingredient, and at least one that is either a vegetable or a fruit.

A salad should celebrate the freshness of its seasonal ingredients. Make sure that your vegetables, fruits, and salad greens are at their height of flavor and look their best.

See also DRESSING; GREENS, SALAD; VINAIGRETTE.

SALAD SAVOY See GREENS, SALAD.

SALMON A king among culinary fish, salmon has a beautiful, flavorful flesh rich in heart-beneficial omega-3 oils. Salmon is often included on lists of the most healthful foods, as it is also high in protein and A and B-complex vitamins, but it is favored by cooks and diners above all for its taste, appearance, and texture.

As a firm, meaty, oily fish, salmon is a good choice for poaching, baking, pan roasting, panfrying, steaming, broiling, and grilling. It is used fresh or canned as an ingredient in chowders and other stews, and in casseroles, gratins, and creamed dishes and to make salmon cakes. Fresh salmon's deep color and sweet, full flavor are complemented by assertive and colorful sauces and salsas such as tapenade, aioli, and pesto. Smoked salmon is always a delicacy, no matter what smoking method is used.

Salmon is native to both North American coasts. Atlantic Coast salmon stocks have declined greatly due to pollution in the United States, although Canada still provides Atlantic salmon. The majority of salmon comes from the Pacific Coast in Alaska. Salmon is now farmed in Norway, Chile, and the United States, but the farmed product has a blander flavor and softer texture.

Of the different species of salmon, the large Chinook, or king, salmon is the most prized for cooking. The silver, or coho, salmon is smaller, looks a lot like a trout, and has slightly leaner flesh. The sockeye, or red, salmon and the pink, or humpback, salmon are often used for canning. The chum, or dog, salmon is a lean fish with a pale color.

Selecting Farm-raised salmon are sold year-round. Wild Atlantic salmon is in season from summer to early winter, and wild Pacific salmon is available from spring through fall. The smallest Chinook salmon is around 6 pounds, and it is available whole or cut into chunks, steaks, or fillets. Like all fish, fresh salmon should smell sweet and clean and have clear eyes and firm flesh.

Storing Plan to cook fresh salmon the day it is purchased, or within 24 hours at the most. Wrap large fish in plastic wrap and place smaller fish in a zippered plastic bag, then refrigerate. Place the fish on a bed of ice cubes or crushed ice in the refrigerator if storing for more than a few hours.

Preparing Whole and chunk salmon are easily skinned and boned after cooking. Salmon fillets, however, must be checked carefully before cooking for pinbones, which are often buried vertically in the thickest part of the flesh. To find the bones, press the flesh gently with your fingers, then remove the bones using sturdy tweezers or needle-nosed pliers.

See also FISH.

SALT Since the dawn of civilization, salt has been a valuable commodity whose availability helped to found some cultures, while other cultures often created extensive trade routes to reach it. Salt is the most basic of seasonings. It is the one essential flavoring ingredient in almost all savory dishes, and a tiny amount helps to bring out the flavors in many sweet dishes. Salt substitutes such as ground seaweed and lemon juice will also heighten flavor, but they add a flavor of their own that can distract from food in a way that the proper amount of salt does not.

Aside from flavoring foods, salt performs a range of chemical actions that are important in cooking and preserving. It draws moisture away from bacteria and mold cells in food, for example, slowing their growth. In early history, when adequate food storage was crucial, salt was valued for its ability to preserve food as much as for its flavor. Many foods, such as bacon, ham, cured sausage, and pickles, originated because food had to be salted to keep it from spoiling.

Of the various kinds of salt available, the most common is table salt, which usually contains added iodine (a practice started in the 1920s as a public-health measure to help prevent hypothyroidism, or the formation of goiters) along with additives that prevent it from caking and keep it pouring easily. Table salt is granular and is made by evaporation in vacuum pans.

Sea salt, by contrast, has no additives, but it has more minerals than table salt. Naturally evaporated, sea salt is available in coarse or fine grains that are shaped like hollow, flaky pyramids. As a result, it adheres better to foods and dissolves more quickly than table salt. It also has more flavor than table salt, and sometimes a smaller amount is sufficient to season the same amount of food. Sea salt is also preferred for bread making, as its mineral content helps in the development of gluten. Most sea salt comes from France, England, or the United States. Salts from different areas carry a subtle difference in flavor. One of the most prized sea salts is the grayish-ivory Fleur du Sel from Brittany.

Kosher salt is another favorite of cooks because its large flakes are easy to handle. This coarse-grained salt, made by compressing granular salt, has no additives. It is used in the preparation of kosher meats, as its large surface and jagged shape help to draw more blood from meat, one of the aims of koshering. Since it is not as salty as table salt, it can be used more liberally. Besides, kosher salt has a superior flavor.

Rock salt is mined from salt deposits rather than being processed by evaporation. It has less taste than other salts and is pri-

marily used in making ice cream in hand-cranked ice cream makers (because salt lowers the freezing point of water, making the melting ice cold enough to freeze the ice cream) and as a bed for roasting oysters on the half shell and other foods (the bed of salt keeps the foods level).

Pickling salt is finely ground and has no additives. It is used in pickling and canning because it dissolves quickly and won't cloud liquids.

Salt Savvy When using salt, keep the following in mind:

- Add a spoonful of salt to the boiling water when you cook soft-boiled or hard-boiled eggs. It will help the egg white coagulate quickly to close any cracks in the eggs.
- Add salt to emulsions based on egg yolks to help thicken the yolks.
- Because salt absorbs moisture, drawing it out of foods, many recipes specify salting eggplant, cucumber, and zucchini to make them less watery.
- Add salt to boiling water for cooking vegetables and pasta to replace the salt leached from the food by boiling. Add salt to water after it comes to a boil, not before (Italians believe that adding salt to water before it boils makes the water taste bitter).
- A pinch of salt at the beginning of the cooking process will help to develop the flavor in almost any food (the exception is corn on the cob; salt toughens it), but wait until the end of cooking to season to taste with salt, or the dish may become too salty during cooking. This is especially true for any dish that cooks a long time, any reduced sauces or other liquids, and dishes containing such salty foods as cheese, ham, or anchovies.
- Although many cookbooks advise against salting dried beans until the very end of cooking, based on a belief that an excess

of salt will toughen the beans, tests have shown that a pinch of salt will not interfere with their cooking. Salt beans very lightly, however, as the liquid will reduce during the long cooking process, concentrating the saltiness.

■ To remove salt from an oversalted dish, add more unsalted liquid, vegetables, or starches such as potatoes, pasta, or rice. You can alleviate the saltiness of some sauces by diluting the sauce with unsalted liquid (you may then need to add thickener) or a tiny bit of brown sugar and/or vinegar.

■ Some people feel that salt draws off too much moisture when roasting or grilling meats, but the actual effect of salt on meat cooked by dry heat is minimal.

■ If you live in a coastal area, you probably ingest more than enough iodine from your drinking water (which absorbs iodine from the soil near seawater) and from eating seafood, so that you do not need iodized salt. If you live in the Midwest, particularly in one of the North Central states, you should use iodized salt to protect against hypothyroidism.

SAUCE The French brought the technique of saucing foods to its height, but every cuisine in the world has developed sauces that are as distinctive and varied as the cultures from which they come. Any liquid used to dress a food is technically a sauce, although the narrower definition of sauce usually refers to a liquid of some thickness. Thinner sauces are usually called dressings, vinaigrettes, or condiments. The basic French sauces may be classified by the method used to thicken them. Because each kind is the basis for a variety of other sauces, the French call these mother sauces. **WHITE SAUCES** White sauces are thickened with a roux, which is a mixture of butter and flour. The roux is cooked for 2 to 3 minutes to eliminate the raw taste of the flour, but it is not allowed to color. The two main white sauces are béchamel, which has milk added to the roux, and velouté, which uses a white stock as the liquid. Classic cream sauces are made by adding cream to either a béchamel or a velouté sauce. Béchamel is the sauce used to make creamed dishes of vegetables, chicken, eggs, and pastas, and it is also the basis for most savory soufflés. A velouté sauce is usually the basis for many dishes made with poultry, fish, or meat, as well as many creamed soups.

Quick Bite

Modern-day cream sauces are often made without a roux and gain thickness by simply reducing heavy cream with savory elements such as pan drippings or seasonings. See REDUCING for more details.

BROWN SAUCES Brown sauces are the most prestigious sauces in the entire system of classic French sauce making. Traditionally, brown sauces were based on rich, meaty beef and veal stock that was slowly reduced over a matter of days to concentrate its flavor. The resulting sauce is referred to as demi-glace and is used as the base of a legion of brown sauces. Demi-glace is deep and complex, with a thick, glossy texture derived from the gelatin naturally present in the stock. For economy's sake, many chefs now shortcut the process by using brown roux (cooked until the flour turns a nut brown) to thicken their reduced stock. Brown sauce is often flavored with wine, tomatoes, or herbs, and traditionally served with beef, lamb, duck, and other meats. **BUTTER SAUCES** Butter sauces are divided into two groups: those thickened with butter and egg yolks, and those thickened with butter only. The first group contains the celebrated hollandaise and béarnaise sauces. Like all butter sauces, they are delicate and will separate if overheated. The egg yolks must be whisked constantly over the correct level of heat as they thicken, and the melted or clarified butter must be beaten very gradually into the yolks. Finally, the sauce must be kept warm, if necessary, over tepid water. If these sauces separate they can often be saved. Hollandaise is best known as a topping for poached eggs, while béarnaise is served with steak and grilled fish.

Beurre blanc represents the second group. It is made by gradually beating small cubes of cold butter into a reduced mixture of shallots, vinegar, and white wine. It should be served as soon as it is made, but it may be kept a short time over tepid water. If this sauce separates, you can save it by beating 1 tablespoon of the sauce in a cold bowl, then gradually beating in the rest of the sauce by teaspoonfuls. Beurre blanc is traditionally served with fish.

MAYONNAISE Mayonnaise, thickened by gradually beating oil into beaten egg yolks, is the well-known sandwich spread and binder for dishes such as egg salad, chicken salad, and tuna salad. It is also used as a dressing for composed salads. You can vary mayonnaise by adding green herbs or flavored oils. Aioli, the famed garlic mayonnaise of Provence, may be served with meat, fish, chicken, or vegetables. Tartar sauce is another flavored mayonnaise, made by adding mustard, capers, chopped dill pickle, and herbs. If any of these mayonnaise-based sauces separates, beat a fresh egg yolk in a dry, warm bowl, then beat in the rest of the sauce by teaspoonfuls.

VINAIGRETTE Vinaigrettes are French sauces that are usually considered salad dressings in the United States, although many chefs also use them to top meats, fish, and chicken. See also VINAIGRETTE.

TOMATO SAUCE Tomato sauce is thickened by cooking tomatoes until they dissolve and their pulp reduces. Usually flavored with onion, garlic, and herbs, it is used in a myriad of dishes, including pizzas and a wide variety of pastas.

OTHER SAVORY SAUCES Other sauces include gravy and simple pan sauces made by using stock and/or wine to deglaze a pan used to sauté meat, chicken, or fish. Among many other sauces around the world are Philippine *adobos,* Mexican moles, fresh and cooked salsas, Spanish *romesco* sauce, Indian *raita,* chile sauce, barbecue sauce, and teriyaki sauce, as well as those often considered as condiments and flavorings, such as Worcestershire sauce and soy sauce.

SWEET SAUCES Sweet sauces, part of the realm of desserts, constitute another large category and are as varied as the ingredients they feature. Those based largely on sugar include caramel and butter-and-cream-enriched butterscotch sauces. Chocolate sauces range from fluid cream-enriched versions to thick hot fudge. Cream- and egg-based sauces have thick, velvety texture and rich flavor. They range from simple lightly whipped cream to the airy beaten egg sauce known as a sabayon to thick custard sauces such as the classic French crème anglaise. Puréed fruits give vibrant color and taste to other sweet sauces, such as light but flavorful raspberry *coulis* and thick, old-fashioned applesauce.

See also BARBECUE SAUCE; CURDLING; DEGLAZING; DRESSING; GRAVY; MAYONNAISE; REDUCING; STOCK; THICKENING.

SAUCEPAN See COOKWARE.

SAUERKRAUT A dish of salted, fermented green cabbage. Although known as a German specialty, sauerkraut likely originated in Asia or ancient Rome, where fermentation was widely used to preserve vegetables. Traditional recipes for sauerkraut call for layering shredded cabbage with pickling salt and sometimes other seasonings such as juniper berries or caraway seeds, and then allowing it to ferment. The strong, pungent flavor of raw sauerkraut mellows with long, slow cooking. There are many devotees who won't consider eating a hot dog without a generous topping of sauerkraut. It goes well, too, with other sausages and alongside roast pork. *Choucroute garnie,* braised sauerkraut served as a bed for bacon, ham, and sausages, is a classic Alsatian dish.

Selecting Purchase sauerkraut in bulk or in a clear plastic bag so that you can see what you're getting. It should be moist but not soupy.

Storing Like other fermented foods, sauerkraut has a long shelf life. Refrigerated in its own juices in a nonmetal container, it will last for 1 month or longer.

Preparing Sauerkraut can be served raw or braised with stock, hot or at room temperature. Rinse raw sauerkraut before serving. Always taste sauerkraut before cooking. If it is very salty, you may want to soak it in cold water for 15 minutes and then drain it before using.

SAUSAGE Most sausages are made from ground meat and fat mixed with salt and other seasonings and packed into casings, although country sausage is made by simply forming bulk sausage meat into patties or into rolls to be sliced and cooked. Originally concocted to use up every last scrap of meat after hog butchering, including the intestines, which serve as casings, sausages are often made of pork, although almost any meat, fish, poultry, shellfish, or game may be used. While sausages are traditionally high in fat, many lower-fat versions are now available, as are vegetarian sausages made from vegetables and/or bean curd. The three basic sausage categories are fresh, cooked, and semidry or dry.

Fresh Sausages Made with raw meat, fresh sausages must be cooked, whether or not they have been lightly smoked. The best-known fresh sausages include bockwurst, made of veal sometimes mixed with pork; chorizo, made with pork and available in the spicy Mexican version and the milder, usually smoked, Spanish version; and Italian sausage, which is also made with pork and may be either spicy or mild. In recent years, some sausage makers have introduced new varieties of fresh sausages, often made with chicken, turkey, or seafood mixed with ingredients such as apples, herbs, and sun-dried tomatoes. Like other fresh sausages, these varieties contain no preservatives.

Fresh sausages are excellent grilled or sautéed. They may be eaten whole, or sliced and sautéed further, then added to casseroles or sautés. Try sliced sautéed Italian sausages in tomato sauce over polenta or pasta, or sauté sliced chicken sausages in a skillet dish with vegetables.

HOW TO *Sauté Fresh Sausages*

1. Puncture the casing of each sausage twice on each of its four sides with the tines of a fork.
2. In a skillet, bring water to a depth of about ¼ inch to a simmer and add the sausages. Cook until the water evaporates.
3. Continue to cook, turning the sausages as necessary in the fat they have released, until they are browned on all sides, 5 to 10 minutes, adding a little olive oil if necessary for very lean sausages.
4. Cut open the sausages to make sure the sausages are cooked through if serving whole. If serving sliced, transfer the sausages to a cutting board and cut them into 1-inch-wide diagonal slices. Return the slices to the pan and sauté them until browned on both sides.

HOW TO *Grill Fresh Sausages*

1. Puncture the sausages as above.
2. Cook over medium-hot coals until browned on all sides.
3. Cover the grill and cook for several more minutes, turning the sausages once or twice. The total cooking time will be 10 to 12 minutes.

Mexican chorizos and Italian sausages are often removed from their casings and cooked as a recipe ingredient.

Cooked Sausages These sausages may also be smoked or unsmoked. They are fully cooked at purchase but most are usually re-heated to serve. Some of the most common are andouille, a smoked sausage made of tripe and often used in Cajun cooking or sliced and eaten cold; bratwurst, a pork or pork-and-veal sausage, which is also available fresh; and knockwurst, which is made from one of several meats and is usually eaten whole. Bologna and frankfurters are thoroughly Americanized sausages; the first is served sliced and eaten cold on sand-wiches, while frankfurters are the beloved grilled or boiled hot dog. Mortadella is a popular Italian cooked sausage and is eaten as a cold cut.

Andouille sausage.

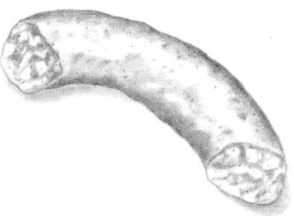

Bratwurst.

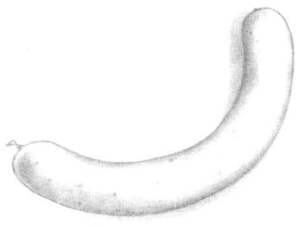

Mortadella sausage.

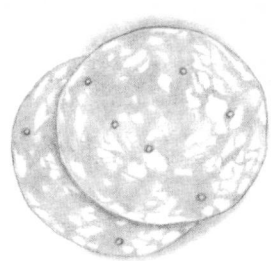

Semidry and Dry Sausages Both semidry and dry sausages may be eaten without cooking, as they have been cured, or preserved, by extensive smoking and/or drying. They may be eaten cold, reheated, or used in cooking. Semidry sausages, sometimes called summer sausages, are smoked to remove some of their moisture and preserve them during the heat of summer. Dry sausages are dried for 1 to 6 months and may or may not be smoked. They include kielbasa, a smoked garlic sausage of Polish origin usually made of pork. Most often cooked in casseroles, soups, and stews, or poached and served with sauerkraut or potatoes, it may also be eaten cold. Linguiça, a pork sausage native to Portugal, is flavored with garlic and red pepper. It is used, like chorizo, as an ingre-dient in other dishes, and it may also be grilled. Pepperoni and salami are dried sau-sages of Italian origin. Pepperoni, spicy with red and black pepper, is a favorite antipasto ingredient and pizza topping. Salami comes in many different styles and sizes and is usually sliced and eaten on sandwiches or as an hors d'oeuvre.

Storing Store uncooked fresh sausages in the refrigerator for up to 2 or 3 days or in the freezer for up to 2 months. Spanish chorizo and other smoked fresh sausages will keep, refrigerated, for 1 week. Store cooked sausage in the refrigerator for up to 1 week or freeze for up to 2 months. You can keep semidry sausages at room temperature for up to 3 days or refrigerate them for up to 3 weeks. Unsliced dry sausage may be kept at room temperature for up to 6 weeks. Once it has been sliced, refrigerate it for up to 2 weeks.

SAUTÉING One of the basic French cooking methods, sautéing takes its name from the verb *sauter,* meaning "to jump." In its classic form, this action is a skillful one that some home cooks envy: the pan is moved briskly back and forth, lifting slightly on the backward motion to make the contents jump. But the food can just as easily be stirred as tossed. Sautéed foods are cooked quickly, usually over medium or medium-high heat, in a small amount of fat. The food is tossed or stirred in the pan to cook its outside evenly without overcooking the inside.

Foods to be sautéed should be cut into small pieces or fairly thin slices, so they can cook quickly. Chicken, tender cuts of meat, tender vegetables, and tougher, starchy vegetables that have been blanched are all good choices for sautéing. Be sure to dry all foods to be sautéed on paper towels before adding them to the pan, to keep moisture from steaming the foods and, if you wish, to allow the foods to brown slightly. For the same reason, don't crowd the pan. Too much food can lower the temperature in the pan as well as trap moisture that will cause the food to steam instead of brown.

Use either a sauté pan (a wide pan with straight sides) or a skillet (a wide pan with slightly sloping sides). If you want the flavor of butter in your dish, use half butter and half oil, as butter alone will burn quickly over medium to high heat. Another alternative is to use clarified butter, which will not burn as quickly. (See BUTTER.) Pure olive oil, canola oil, and other vegetable oils may be used alone or with butter for sautéing.

HOW TO *Sauté*

1. Preheat the pan briefly over medium to medium-high heat and then add the oil and/or butter and heat for a few seconds until the oil is fragrant, the surface of the oil wavers, and small bubbles appear, or until the butter has foamed and begins to subside.
2. Add the food, in batches if necessary, and stir, toss, or turn it as it cooks, watching carefully to make sure it does not burn and adjusting the heat as necessary.
3. Sauté the food according to the recipe instructions. Foods may or may not be browned or cooked through, and some foods, such as onions, may be sautéed briefly just to bring out their flavor.

See also BUTTER; FAT & OIL; FRYING.

SAUTÉ PAN See COOKWARE.

SAVORY See HERB.

SCALDING Heating a liquid, usually milk, to almost simmering. Because milk scorches and boils over easily, recipes that require hot milk specify scalding as a safeguard against overcooking.

HOW TO *Scald Milk*

1. To keep milk from spilling over the pan edges as it simmers, select a saucepan large enough to allow for a few inches of rising.
2. Fill the pan with a little cold water, swirl, and then pour it out. The thin layer of water prevents milk from sticking to the pan.
3. Pour the milk into the pan and place it over medium heat. Stir occasionally to prevent scorching at the bottom and to dissolve the thin film that will form on the surface.
4. Heat just until small bubbles appear around the edge of the pan. Watch the milk carefully, for it can boil over quickly.

See also MILK.

SCALE See BAKING TOOLS.

SCALLION Also known as green onion; see ONION.

SCALLOP (MEAT) A slice of boneless meat or fish. Pork, veal, beef loin, turkey breasts, and other tender cuts may all be sliced into boneless cutlets, which are then pounded to an even thinness to tenderize them and so that they can be cooked quickly. (See also POUNDING.) Scallops may be breaded and are usually sautéed. Veal scallopini, Wiener schnitzel, and French *escalopes* are all meat scallop dishes.

SCALLOP (SHELLFISH) A popular mollusk, plump and flavorful. In the United States, the bivalves are shucked almost immediately after they are caught, while in Europe they are often sold in their pretty shells. The edible portion is actually the adductor muscle used to open and close the shell. Scallop roe and milt (eggs and male reproductive glands) are delicious but quite perishable and, with rare exceptions, are discarded when scallops are shucked. Scallops are often served creamed in scallop shells as coquilles Saint-Jacques. They may also be seared quickly and served with a sauce.

Scallops in their shells.

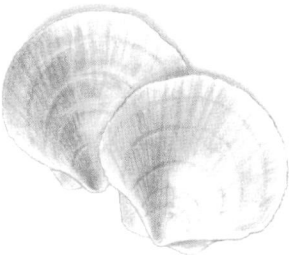

Selecting Choose sea scallops that are creamy white or slightly pink, rather than bright white, an indication that they have been soaked (see below). Bay scallops should be pale pink or light orange.

Although shucked scallops will always have some odor, choose those with the mildest scent. If you are lucky enough to find scallops still in their shells, snap them up. They cost more than shucked scallops, but their fresh taste is well worth the expense. The shells usually gape open a bit. They should close slightly when pinched and smell fresh. Don't turn up your nose if offered quick-frozen scallops. Because they are frozen as soon as they are shucked, these scallops often have a better flavor than those that have languished in a ship's hold for several days before they were delivered to the market.

Some wholesalers soak sea scallops in a tripolyphosphate solution to help preserve them. Although soaking may make the scallops last longer, the meat absorbs much of the water, which increases the weight (and thus the price) of the scallops and dilutes their flavor. Wholesalers are required to label their scallops "soaked" or "dry" (unsoaked), but retailers do not always pass this information on to their customers. Two indicators will help you to identify treated scallops. Unsoaked ones range in color from pale ivory to pale coral. If the scallops offered to you are shiny and bright white, you can be almost certain that they've been soaked. Another clue is that soaked scallops tend to clump together, while unsoaked ones remain separate.

Dried scallops are considered a delicacy by the Chinese. Called *conpoy* and sold by weight (large ones fetch exorbitant prices), they are used in steamed dishes and soups.

Storing Buy scallops the day you plan to serve them and keep them refrigerated until ready to cook. If still in the shell, put the scallops in a bowl and cover the bowl with a damp kitchen towel. Shuck them just before cooking.

Preparing Scallops in the shell are easier to shuck than oysters or clams.

Scallops take well to a wide range of recipes and cooking methods. The only caveat is to watch your cooking time carefully. Scallops need just a few minutes of heat to cook. If left for too long, they quickly turn rubbery and dry. If you like raw fish, you should know that scallops are one of the safest shellfish to eat raw. Like all shellfish, they filter large amounts of seawater for the nutrients they need to stay alive and accumulate some toxins in the process. But the scallop's filtration mechanism is discarded during shucking and what is eaten is likely to contain few toxins.

Scallop Glossary

BAY SCALLOP The most highly regarded of all scallops, these little morsels— about ½ inch in diameter—have a sweet, delicate flavor. Bay scallops are harvested from a small region of the Atlantic Ocean and are rarely found outside of East Coast fish markets during their short season, which begins in October and runs through March. Unscrupulous markets sometimes try to pass off less-expensive calico scallops or cut and trimmed sea scallops as bay scallops.

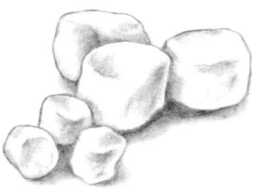

Bay scallops and sea scallops.

CALICO SCALLOP Tinier than bay scallops, calicos are found off the east coast of Florida and in the Gulf of Mexico. They are quite good and are often offered at a very reasonable price. The important thing to remember when preparing them is not to overcook them. Because shucking the small shells is too expensive for most processors, the shells are steamed open and the scallops arrive in the market already partially cooked, so they must be exposed to heat for no more than a few minutes during cooking.

SEA SCALLOP These are the most common scallops. At about 1½ inches in diameter, they are larger than bay scallops but not quite as tender. Because scallop boats fishing for sea scallops stay out on the ocean for weeks at a time, freshness is always an issue with sea scallops.

SINGING PINK SCALLOP Also known as swimming scallops, these are named for their translucent pink shell, about 3 inches in diameter, which propels them through the water by opening and closing. They are found in the Puget Sound of the Pacific Northwest.

HOW TO *Shuck Scallops*

1. Slide a knife sideways into the crack between the shells. Rotate the knife to open the shell.

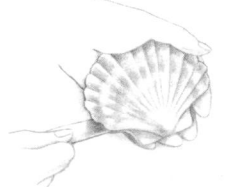

2. Run the knife around the scallop meat to free it and then remove it, along with any roe.
3. Peel the tough white tissue off the side of the scallop and discard it, along with the dark-colored innards.

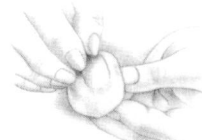

SCALLOPING To cook vegetables or seafood in milk or cream, usually topped with bread crumbs and sometimes cheese. Typical dishes include scalloped potatoes and scalloped oysters.

SCANT This term is used to describe measurements, such as "1 scant table-spoon," that are slightly less than full. See also MEASURING.

SCHMALTZ See FAT & OIL.

SCISSORS See COOKING TOOLS.

SCORING Making shallow cuts in food. Scoring is done for several reasons: It can help flatten a piece of meat, such as flank steak. It allows marinades or seasonings to flavor the interior of the meat. It can aid in the tenderizing of a piece of meat by cutting through some of the tough meat fibers. Whole fish are often scored in the thickest part to allow heat to penetrate to help the flesh cook evenly. Scoring the fat layer of whole hams encourages the fat to drain and creates a decorative appearance.

Breads are often scored, or slashed, before baking, both for decoration and to help them rise. Breads that are not scored can burst from the pressure that builds up inside the baking loaf or fail to rise at all if the crust sets before the bread has a chance to expand. Scoring the dough before it bakes provides an escape route for the gases. Similarly, pastry crusts are vented and pricked to allow steam to escape during baking. See also SLASHING.

SCRAPER A dough, or bench, scraper; see BAKING TOOLS.

SCRUBBING Many foods, such as potatoes and clams, carry dirt from the fields or impurities from the sea and should be scrubbed clean before eating. In fact, any vegetable that is cooked or eaten unpeeled, including citrus fruit that is to be zested, should be scrubbed. Special vegetable brushes made for this purpose are sold in supermarkets and cooking-supply shops, although you can use any brush with firm bristles. Scrub foods under cold running water, brushing or rubbing vigorously to remove all traces of dirt. If the brush scrubs off a vegetable's skin with the dirt, for example, if you are cleaning mushrooms, try a softer brush, or simply use your thumb to rub away the dirt.

SEAFOOD Although the dictionary definition of seafood is "edible *marine* fish and shellfish," the word is often used to mean all edible fish and shellfish, freshwater as well as seawater. See also FISH; SHELLFISH.

SEARING To brown a food—usually meat, poultry, or seafood—quickly over high heat, usually to prepare it for a second, moist cooking method such as braising or stewing. For years, cooks believed that searing sealed in juices and kept the meat from drying out, but food scientists have proven that it does just the opposite, drawing juices to the surface and releasing them into the pan or fire. But cooking meat over high heat with a small amount of fat sets off a series of reactions between the sugars and the proteins, essentially caramelizing the surface, which results in a more complex and richer flavor. The crisp, browned surface of a seared piece of meat is also more appetizing than the dull, gray look of meat that hasn't been properly browned before moist cooking.

Searing Savvy When getting ready to sear, keep the following in mind:

■ Be sure to pat meat dry with paper towels before searing, or the moisture will hinder proper browning.

searing

- Use a large, heavy pan such as a cast-iron frying pan or a dutch oven.
- Oil the food to be seared rather than the pan, for an oiled pan will soon start to smoke at the high temperatures needed for searing.
- Allow space between pieces of meat or one piece of meat and the sides of the

Seasoning Chart

KIND OF FOOD	SEASONING
Beans or peas, dried	Bay leaf, parsley, thyme
Beans, green	Basil, marjoram, savory, thyme
Beef	Allspice, bay leaf, black pepper, celery seed, chili powder, cumin, garlic, ginger, nutmeg, thyme
Beets	Basil, dill, ginger, mint, parsley
Carrots	Cinnamon, cloves, dill, lemon juice, mint, nutmeg, parsley, savory, tarragon, thyme
Cauliflower	Chives, curry powder, lemon juice, nutmeg, parsley
Chicken	Bay leaf, chives, cinnamon, cloves, cumin, curry powder, garlic, ginger, lemon, marjoram, mustard, rosemary, sage, tarragon, thyme
Corn	Basil, chives, chili powder, dill, lime juice, parsley
Duck	Orange, parsley, sage, thyme
Eggplant	Basil, cumin, garlic, parsley, thyme
Fish	Bay leaf, chervil, chives, cumin, curry, dill, marjoram, mint, mustard, oregano, paprika, parsley, saffron, savory, tarragon, thyme
Goose	Allspice, caraway, marjoram, thyme
Lamb	Cumin, curry powder, garlic, mint, oregano, rosemary
Peas	Basil, marjoram, mint, parsley, savory, tarragon
Pork	Allspice, bay leaf, cumin, fennel, garlic, ginger, marjoram, mustard, rosemary, sage, thyme
Potatoes	Chives, dill, garlic, parsley
Spinach	Curry powder, garlic, nutmeg
Squash, summer	Basil, chives, garlic, marjoram, oregano, parsley, savory
Squash, winter	Allspice, cinnamon, cloves, ginger, lemon, mace, nutmeg
Sweet potatoes	Cayenne, cinnamon, cloves, lime juice, mace, nutmeg
Tomatoes	Basil, chives, garlic, marjoram, oregano, parsley, savory, tarragon, thyme
Turkey	Bay leaf, rosemary, sage, savory
Veal	Basil, bay leaf, lemon, parsley, savory, tarragon, thyme

pan. Too much food crowding the pan will lower the temperature, trap moisture, and create steam, preventing the meat from browning properly.

■ Turn the meat frequently to brown it evenly on all sides.

■ Make the most of the pan drippings created by searing by deglazing the pan before continuing with the recipe.

See also BRAISING; BROWNING.

SEASONING The use of aromatic herbs and spices to enhance the flavors of ingredients in a dish is called seasoning. Some seasonings naturally seem to go well with some foods—rosemary with lamb, nutmeg with spinach—but seasoning is also a matter of taste. Much of the satisfaction of cooking comes from learning which flavors you like to bring together. Keep an assortment of spices and dried herbs, as well as fresh herbs, if you can, and experiment by replacing the seasonings called for in different dishes or changing the amounts. Start out with a small amount of seasoning, and learn as you go. To bring out the fullest flavors, season each component of a recipe and taste as you go along. (But take care not to taste meat, poultry, or seafood before it is done.) Never serve a dish without one last tasting to see if it needs a final seasoning.

See the chart at left for some tried-and-true combinations of ingredients and herbs and spices to use as a starting point when mixing and matching flavors.

The term *seasoning* also refers to the treating of cast-iron cookware to prevent it from rusting and foods from sticking. Pans are heated and coated with oil before the first use and whenever the coating starts to wear away and rust starts to appear.

HOW TO *Season a Cast-Iron Pan*
1. Heat the pan over high heat until a drop of water sizzles and evaporates immediately.

2. Coat the inside of the pan with vegetable oil, using paper towels to spread the oil and rub it well into the metal. Blot up any excess. If seasoning a new pan, repeat several times until the pan blackens.

See also ADJUSTING THE SEASONING; TASTING.

SEAWEED The ocean yields this foodstuff, rich in nutrients and tasting of the sea, which is widely used in Asian cooking. The Japanese use more kinds of seaweed than any other culture, beginning with the nori used in making sushi. Dried nori, like many other seaweeds, is available in Japanese markets, most natural-food stores, and some supermarkets. It comes in dark green, dark brown, or black thin sheets that are either toasted or untoasted. Dark brown to grayish black, kombu is kelp that is dried, cut, and folded. It is often mixed with dried bonito flakes as an ingredient in dashi, the typical Japanese stock. Wakame is a deep green or brown seaweed shaped like long strings and eaten in soups and salads. Agar-agar is sold in long strands or sticks. It may be soaked and eaten in soups like noodles, but its primary use throughout East Asia is as a gelatin-like thickener. In the West, agar-agar is prized by vegetarians as a replacement for animal-based gelatin.

HOW TO *Use Agar-Agar as a Gelatin*
1. To jell 4 cups of liquid, measure out about $2/3$ ounce strips or sticks, break into pieces, and soak in water to cover for about 20 minutes.
2. Wring the pieces dry. Put them in a saucepan with cold water to cover.
3. Bring to a boil over medium heat. Reduce the heat to a simmer and cook, stirring occasionally, until dissolved.
4. Add the ingredients to be jelled and bring just to a boil. Mold and chill them as required.

SEEDING For details on various techniques for removing seeds, see entries for individual foods.

SEIZING When melted chocolate comes into contact with any amount of moisture, the fine, dry particles of cocoa solids suspended in the cocoa butter can clump together, hardening the chocolate in a phenomenon known as seizing, or stiffening.

Paradoxically, a larger amount of liquid (at least 25 percent of the weight of the chocolate) will prevent seizing. This explains why some recipes can successfully instruct you to add liquid to chocolate as it melts. As long as you have at least 1 tablespoon of liquid for each 2 ounces of chocolate, the chocolate will not seize.

You can salvage seized chocolate by taking it off the heat and working in a bit of water, a tablespoon at a time. This restored chocolate will be smooth and shiny and fine for use in icings and fillings, but it will not work in recipes where the chocolate must set up, such as for candies. In these instances, you will need to discard the chocolate and start over.

When melting chocolate in a double boiler, always do so over barely simmering water, as briskly simmering or boiling water creates steam. Steam is moist and will cause chocolate to seize if the two come in contact. Melting chocolate in a microwave will also prevent seizing. Cool the chocolate uncovered to prevent contact with steam.

See also CHOCOLATE; TEMPERING.

SEMOLINA See GRAIN.

SEPARATING To separate the white of an egg from the egg yolk. This is more easily done when an egg is cold, and several different techniques may be used. For details, see EGG.

The word *separate* is also used to describe the curdling action of sauces; for more information, see CURDLING.

SERRANO See CHILE.

SESAME PASTE See TAHINI.

SESAME SEED Sesame seeds are widely used in Indian, Asian, African, Middle Eastern, and Latin American cuisines. In fact, these tiny, flat seeds have been used in cooking for at least 5,000 years. Brown, red, and black sesame seeds are available, but the most commonly available ones are a pale tan. They add a nutty flavor to any food and are often sprinkled over savory dishes as a garnish. Many breads and cookies are strewn with sesame seeds before baking. Ground sesame seeds are used to make halvah, a Middle Eastern candy, and tahini, a paste used in many Middle Eastern dishes. The seeds are crushed to make two kinds of highly polyunsaturated oil, one pale in color and often used in salad dressings and for deep-frying, and the other made with toasted sesame seeds and commonly called Asian sesame oil. This dark brown oil is highly flavorful and is used to season savory Asian dishes, but is seldom used for cooking.

Storing Because of their high oil content, sesame seeds can go rancid quickly and should be stored in the refrigerator.

See also FAT & OIL.

SETTING To firm up a food by letting it sit at room temperature or by chilling it. Some foods that need to set before serving are baked custards, lasagne, gelatin dishes, candies, chocolate decorations, and frostings and icings. The recipe method should either tell you how much time a dish will need in order to set or indicate this in some way other than time.

Some recipe components, such as custards incorporating eggs or mixtures including gelatin, need to thicken before they are added to other ingredients. This is done by refrigerating the mixture until thickened, usually for about 2 hours, or by placing a bowl containing the mixture in a larger bowl filled with ice cubes and stirring constantly until the mixture thickens.

SETTING ASIDE To put a component of a dish to one side while preparing other parts of the dish. When a recipe instructs you to set aside part of a dish and to keep it warm, you should cover it with a lid, a plate, or aluminum foil and keep it in a warm place, perhaps on the stove top. In some cases, a recipe will specify keeping a component or a finished dish warm in a low (180° to 200°F) oven, in a hot water bath, or over tepid or hot water. Other solutions, depending on the food, are candle warmers, electric heating trays, and the warming ovens found in some stoves.

Quick Tip

Some sauces, such as hollandaise, will separate if kept over water that is hotter than tepid. A solution to keeping such delicate sauces warm is to pour them into a thermos.

The term *reserve* is used when preparing an ingredient that yields two components, such as pears and their poaching liquid, or diced mushrooms and their soaking liquid. One component is used in the recipe sooner than the other, which is reserved for a later stage. Or, the second component may be reserved for use in another recipe altogether.

SHALLOT See ONION.

SHEARS See COOKING TOOLS.

SHELLFISH From raw oysters on the half shell to chilled cooked jumbo shrimp peeled and ready to dip in cocktail sauce to garlicky steamed mussels, shellfish offer a wide array of gastronomic delights.

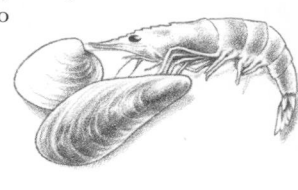

For all their variety, shellfish may be easily grouped into two broad categories: crustaceans and mollusks. Crustaceans are the more animated group, scurrying or swimming about with legs or fins, their bodies protected by a tough external skeleton. These include crabs, lobsters, crayfish, and shrimp. Mollusks include bivalves, shellfish that live within two hinged shell halves, such as oysters, clams, and mussels; cephalopods, whose shells are actually penlike bones within their bodies, such as squid and octopus; and finally univalves, or gastropods, which have one shell that protects their soft bodies, such as abalone, snails, and conch.

See also individual shellfish.

SHELLING Removing the hard outer covering of a food such as nuts or shellfish. Eggs and vegetables such as green peas and fava beans are also shelled.

See individual foods; SHUCKING.

SHERBET See SORBET.

SHIITAKE See MUSHROOM.

SHIRRING A way of baking eggs. Although eggs are essential to many baked goods, such as cakes and quick breads, they may also be baked themselves, in a ramekin or custard cup. When a bit of cream or butter is added before baking, the baked eggs become shirred eggs.

SHOCKING See BLANCHING; PLUNG-
ING.

SHORTENING Any solid fat can be
referred to as shortening, particularly in
baking and frying recipes, although this
is not the current usage of the word. When
modern recipes call for shortening, they
mean vegetable shortening. See FAT & OIL;
VEGETABLE SHORTENING.

SHREDDING To cut food into thin,
narrow strips. Medium-soft cheeses, such
as Cheddar and Monterey jack, and vegetables, such as carrots, usually are shredded
on the largest holes of a box grater. Grating, on the other hand, means to reduce
foods (such as Parmesan cheese) into tiny
particles using the fine rasps of a grater.
Cabbage and other stiff leaf vegetables are
shredded by cutting them with a large knife
into long pieces about ¼ inch wide. To
shred soft leaves such as spinach and basil,
roll individual leaves or stacks of leaves
into a tight roll and cut crosswise into thin
shreds with a large knife. (Very thin shreds
are called chiffonade.) Mandolines and
food processors fitted with a shredding disk
may also be used to shred.
    See also FOOD PROCESSOR; GRATING;
MANDOLINE.

SHRIMP There are thousands of shrimp
varieties in the world. The main ones eaten
in the United States are Gulf shrimp from
the Gulf of Mexico; tiger shrimp from
Asian waters,
easily identi-
fied by their
black stripes;
and Monterey
prawns, also
known as spot
prawns. Available in many different
colors, from pink to brown and white,

shrimp also vary in size, from "colossal" to
"miniature." The most common sizes are
jumbo (10 to 15 shrimp per pound); large
(16 to 20 shrimp per pound); medium
(25 to 30 shrimp per pound); and miniature (about 100 shrimp per pound). Jumbo
and large shrimp are also labeled U-15 or
U-12 to indicate there are fewer than 15 or
12 per pound. Miniature shrimp are also
known as bay shrimp and are almost always
purchased already cooked.

Quick Bite

Giant and jumbo shrimp are often called
prawns in the United States, although true
prawns are actually either a type of freshwater
shrimp or certain miniature members of the
lobster family.

Shrimp are a favorite food for appetizers, often served with cocktail sauce, and
for grilling, sautéing, and stir-frying. Boiled
with flavorings, they are eaten straight
from the shell, or they may be shelled and
cooked in soups such as shrimp bisque, or
in flavorful stews such as the Greek dish
of shrimp with feta and tomatoes or Cajun
shrimp jambalaya and gumbo.
    Dried shrimp are used to make shrimp
paste, a pungent fermented flavoring used
widely in Asia. It comes in two forms, as
a thick, moist paste and as a dried paste.
The former is usually labeled shrimp sauce
or shrimp paste and is easily found in
Chinese and Southeast Asian markets. The
latter is variously labeled *kapi* (Thailand),
trasi (Indonesia), and *blacan* (Malaysia).
Commonly found in Southeast Asian markets, it is sold in small bricks. Once opened,
the fresh paste must be refrigerated, while
the dried paste will keep for months in a
cool, dry cupboard. Either way, store the
pungent-smelling shrimp paste sealed in
an airtight jar or zippered plastic bag.

Bay shrimp.

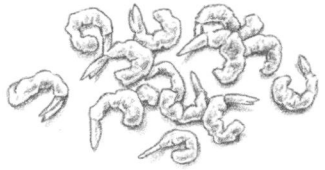

Selecting Choose firm, sweet-smelling fresh shrimp still in the shell when possible. All but the freshest shrimp will have had their heads already removed. Most shrimp sold has been previously frozen and thawed. You may do better buying still-frozen shrimp, since its quality is the same or better than thawed, and you'll be able to decide more freely when to use it. Previously frozen shrimp should not be refrozen. Bay shrimp are usually available only shelled and cooked.

Pass over shrimp with yellowing or black-spotted shells, an "off" odor, or a gritty feel. In general, avoid preshelled and deveined shrimp. Their texture and flavor will likely have suffered more during the freezing process than shrimp in the shell. Shrimp cooked without their shells are also less flavorful than those cooked in their shells.

Most Gulf shrimp, tiger shrimp, and Chinese white shrimp are available year-round, while Monterey prawns are in markets from spring through fall.

Storing Fresh raw shrimp should be used the day of purchase or within 24 hours at the longest. Keep them in a zippered plastic bag in the refrigerator on a bed of ice before using. Cooked shrimp may be refrigerated for up to 3 days. Frozen shrimp may be kept for up to 3 months. Once defrosted, shrimp should not be refrozen, or their texture will deteriorate.

Preparing Shrimp are often shelled and deveined before they are cooked. See instructions below.

To freshen frozen shrimp before cooking, soak in salted water for 10 to 15 minutes, then rinse well. Shrimp are very sensitive to heat and must be cooked quickly, or they will turn tough and chewy. When possible, cook shrimp in their shells; unshelled grilled shrimp are always juicier. The Chinese customarily stir-fry large shrimp in their shells for the same reason.

Rinse and drain canned shrimp before using them. Thaw frozen shrimp in the refrigerator.

HOW TO *Shell Shrimp*

1. If the shrimp still has its head, pull it off or lop it off with a knife.
2. Carefully pull off the legs on the inside curve of the shrimp.
3. Peel off the shell, beginning at the head end of the shrimp, pulling off the tail as well unless the recipe calls for it to be left attached.

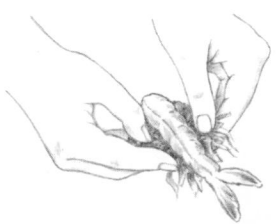

HOW TO *Devein Shrimp*

Shrimp may be deveined before or after cooking.

1. Shell the shrimp. See How to Shell Shrimp, page 405.
2. With a small knife, cut a shallow groove along the back of the shrimp.

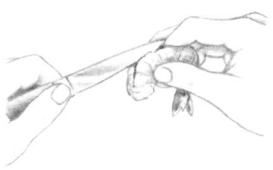

3. With the tip of the knife, gently lift and scrape away the dark vein, then rinse the shrimp under cold running water (if raw). Drain the shrimp on paper towels and proceed with the recipe.

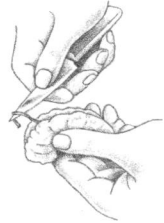

See also BUTTERFLYING.

SHUCKING To remove a bivalve, such as an oyster, a mussel, a scallop, or a clam, from its shell. Peas and beans are sometimes said to be shucked, rather than shelled, while to shuck corn means to remove its husk and silk. When shucking bivalves such as clams and oysters, make sure you have the right equipment. The correct knives make all the difference in safety and ease of shucking.

See also CLAM; CORN; MUSSEL; OYSTER; SCALLOP.

SIEVE See STRAINER.

SIFTING Passing an ingredient through a sifter or strainer to aerate it, give it a uniform consistency, and eliminate any large particles. Although most all-purpose flour is sold presifted, some baking recipes still specify sifted all-purpose flour. Because sifting significantly increases volume, you should not sift before measuring unless a recipe specifies this. (A good baking recipe is written so that you know by the order of the words if the flour is to be measured before sifting: "1 cup sifted flour" means that you are measuring sifted flour—in other words, you should sift before measuring—while "1 cup flour, sifted" means to measure the flour first, then sift it.) In recipes that do not specify sifted flour, the flour should be stirred or whisked to aerate it before measuring and sifted afterward if desired.

Flour sifters are metal or plastic canisters that force flour through a layer (or two or three) of wire mesh. A simple fine-mesh strainer may be used instead, its rim tapped to pass the flour through.

Sifter.

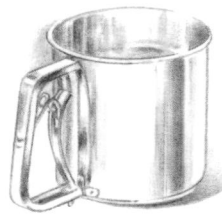

Sifting flour with other dry ingredients such as salt and baking soda is the best way to combine and aerate these ingredients so that they distribute evenly and readily into a batter, although you can also stir or whisk these ingredients together instead.

Soft pastry and cake flours clump easily and should always be sifted to remove any lumps. Trying to remove lumps later in the mixing process can result in overmixing and may toughen a dough.

Confectioners' sugar and cocoa powder regularly clump and often should be sifted before using. Use the back of a spoon to push these ingredients through a fine-mesh strainer, rather than sifting them in a flour sifter; they will be sifted more efficiently this way, and you won't have to clean the flour sifter before using it for flour.

See also STRAINER.

SIMMERING When liquid is maintained at a temperature just below a boil, about 185°F, it is called a simmer. Tiny bubbles barely breaking on the surface signal that a liquid has reached a gentle, or low, simmer. If the bubbles are larger and move a little more rapidly, the liquid is at a full simmer, or is "simmering rapidly" or "briskly." The temperature in this case will be closer to 200°F. Once the bubbles are quite large and numerous, filling much of the liquid and breaking when they reach the surface, the liquid is at a boil. Simmering is the ideal temperature for many soups and sauces, but only a gentle simmer or a slightly lower temperature should be used for braising or poaching meat and fish. See also BOILING; BRAISING; POACHING.

SIMPLE SYRUP See SUGAR.

SKEWERS See COOKING TOOLS.

SKILLET Also known as a frying pan; see COOKWARE.

SKIMMING To remove the top layer from the surface of a liquid. Many soups and stocks produce a white scum, or foam, during the cooking process that should be skimmed off and discarded. Use a large spoon or a skimmer to skim solids from liquids. A skimmer has a long handle and a slightly concave head

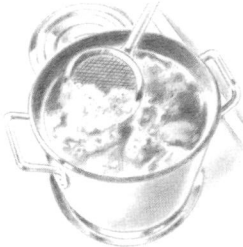

made of fine wire mesh or perforated metal. The fat that rises to the top of soups and stocks is often skimmed in a process called degreasing. Cream that rises to the surface of whole milk is also skimmed off to make heavy cream or to be churned into butter.

See also DEGREASING.

SKINNING Removing the thin outer membrane of a food. Poultry is often skinned to quicken the cooking process, to allow seasoning to penetrate the flesh more easily, or to lower the fat content of the final dish. Vegetables such as tomatoes and fava beans and foods such as hazelnuts and almonds also are often skinned, or peeled, for reasons of appearance, texture, or taste.

SLASHING Making shallow cuts with a sharp blade in the surface of a food, such as bread dough or whole fish, before cooking. See also SCORING.

Slashing bread dough.

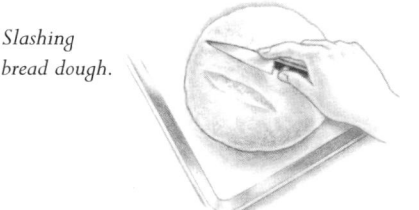

SLICING To cut a food into relatively flat pieces of varying possible thicknesses, as with bread or meat, or into wedges, as with cake or pie. Food is often sold by the slice in delicatessens. See also CHOPPING.

SLIVERING Cutting a small piece of food, such as a garlic clove or an almond, into thin pieces. Garlic is often slivered and inserted into pieces of meat to add flavor, and almonds are sold already slivered for use in desserts and other dishes. Thin wedges of pie or cake also may be referred to as slivers.

SLOW COOKER See CROCKPOT.

SMASHING Crushing a food, usually in order to release its flavor. See also BRUISING; CRUSHING.

SMOKE POINT The temperature at which a fat begins to break down and emit smoke. Some fats have a higher smoke point than others, and so are preferred for cooking techniques that employ a high heat, such as deep-frying. Also, keeping oil hot for any extended period of time will lower the smoke point. Each time you use a batch of oil for deep-frying, its smoke point is lowered.

Caution!

Beyond the smoke point, oils reach the flash point, at which stage they burst into flames.

Butter has one of the lowest smoke points of all fats, as the milk solids suspended in the butterfat begin to burn after only a few seconds over medium heat. Combining vegetable oil with butter will raise the smoke point, allowing you to add the taste of butter to sautéed food without burning the butter. Clarified butter, which has been separated from its milk solids, has a higher smoke point while retaining the flavor of butter. The smoke point of different types of oils varies, with safflower, peanut, canola, and corn oil having high smoke points and extra-virgin olive oil having a relatively low one.

Oil that has reached the smoke point gives off a noxious smell and may be chemically altered into saturated fat.

See FAT & OIL; FRYING.

SMOKING To preserve and flavor a food by either hot smoking or cold smoking. In most cases, particularly with cold smoking,

Quick Tip

To give a smoky flavor to foods cooked on an outdoor grill, buy aromatic wood chips such as apple or oak and soak them in water to cover for about 30 minutes. Drain the chips and sprinkle them over lighted coals, then cover the grill while cooking the food.

foods are partially cured in brine beforehand. Cold smoking, a slow-curing method, happens at low temperatures of 70° to 90°F, can take several weeks, and is done in traditional or makeshift smokehouses. Cold-smoked foods retain more moisture than hot-smoked foods and will have a more tender texture. Salmon is a frequent candidate for cold smoking. Hot smoking takes place at higher temperatures of 100° to 190°F for as long as it takes to cook the food partially or completely. It may be done in a commercial charcoal-water smoker, a tall, cylindrical device that concentrates the smoke from charcoal and smoking woods. These smokers are constructed in layers, with a fuel grate and water pan in the bottom, topped by one or more cooking racks; adjustable vents control the amount of smoke. Outdoor grills can be modified to smoke foods as well, by adding smoking woods to a charcoal fire and covering the grill during cooking. Stove-top smokers are also available.

See also GRILLING.

SNAIL As any gardener knows, the snail loves the tender leaves of salad greens and other vegetables. Snails also love grape leaves; when the ancient Romans brought grapevines to France, they also brought one of their favorite foods, the snail. Today, the large, black Burgundy, or vineyard, snail is considered to be the premium food snail, and an entire ritual has developed around their consumption in the French wine country of the same name, and wherever snails are available. The petit-gris snail, as its name indicates, is smaller and gray; it is found in the southern part of France.

Specially designed serving pieces known as snail plates, tongs, and forks make eating snails easier. A snail plate includes small indentations that hold snail shells securely in place. Snail tongs let the diner handily grip each usually butter-drenched snail shell while extracting its meat with a narrow two-pronged snail fork.

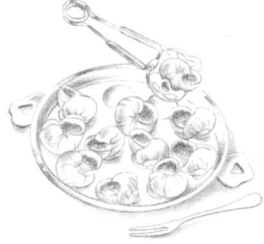

Snail serving plate.

Selecting Fresh farm-raised snails are available in some specialty markets; these have already been cleansed. You are much more likely to find canned snails, however, the best ones being imported from Burgundy. Snails are also available frozen. **Storing** If you should find fresh snails, eat them on the day they are bought. **Preparing** Fresh snails must be washed, soaked for 2 hours in a mixture of salt, vinegar, and a pinch of flour, then washed again and blanched. Then they are removed from their shells, and the black end of the tail is removed and discarded. Next, the snails are braised in a mixture of white wine and stock for 3 to 4 hours before they

are allowed to cool. If using the shells for serving, they must be boiled for 30 minutes in water with a pinch of baking soda, then drained, rinsed, and dried. Canned snails have already gone through all these steps; the shells are purchased separately to use and reuse for serving.

SNAP BEAN See BEAN, FRESH.

SOAKING To immerse a food in liquid. Some foods must be soaked to make them more tender or to remove salt or brine. Salt-packed anchovies and capers, and salt-dried fish such as cod, benefit from a cold-water soak to rinse away some of their salt. Without soaking, these foods would remain unpalatably salty and hard. See also BEAN, DRIED.

SORBET The name for this family of frozen desserts has a ring of elegance, and like many elegant things, much of its style derives from simplicity. Sorbets are made with merely fresh fruit (or sometimes chocolate, coffee, wine, or herbal infusions), sugar, usually water, and lemon juice, without the addition of milk, cream, or eggs. Sorbets were the rage in the late 19th and early 20th centuries, when they were often served as palate-cleansers between rich, heavy courses of formal meals. A *sorbetto,* the more intense Italian version, generally has more fruit and less water, resulting in a softer, less icy texture. Fruit ices, also known by the Italian name *granita* or the French *granité,* resemble sorbets but have more grainy textures, the result of being frozen in a simple freezer tray and repeatedly scraped and refrozen to form icy particles. A sherbet, similar to a sorbet, usually includes some milk or cream or, sometimes, egg whites, resulting in a flavor and consistency midway between those of sorbet and ice cream.

S

Sorbet Savvy When making sorbets and other related desserts, keep the following in mind:

- Use only fresh fruit for fruit-flavored sorbets. Those made with cooked or canned fruit will taste like cold jam.
- When making syrup for sorbets, use a hydrometer to measure its density and a candy thermometer to measure its temperature, following any specifications given in recipes. For sorbet to freeze properly, the syrup must have the correct density.
- For making granitas and other ices, use a stainless-steel pan, which will help the mixture freeze faster. As a layer of crystals forms, scrape it up occasionally with a metal spoon, until the desired consistency is reached.
- Alternatively, freeze mixtures for granitas in ice-cube trays until almost but not completely solid, then chop to the desired consistency in a food processor.
- If you enjoy serving sorbets, consider investing in a countertop electric machine that will stir and freeze the mixture.

See also ICE CREAM.

SORREL See GREENS, DARK; HERB.

SOUFFLÉ The soufflé is an airy concoction of beaten egg whites stabilized by a thicker base, often a béchamel sauce. Its name is based on the verb *souffler,* meaning "to blow" or "to puff up." The classic soufflé may be either savory, as in a cheese or vegetable soufflé, or sweet, as in a chocolate, lemon, or berry soufflé. In either case, it emerges hot and trembling from the oven and is eaten at once. But cold dessert soufflés, stabilized usually by gelatin and often by freezing, also exist, although they more properly should be called mousses. Soufflés may be cooked in one large soufflé dish or in individual ones; layered with other foods, such as poached eggs or fish fillets; baked in a shallow casserole or gratin dish; or baked in a water bath and served unmolded. Some soufflés are served with sauces, such as the whipped cream or berry coulis accompanying chocolate soufflés.

The French porcelain soufflé dish, with its high, straight sides, allows the soufflé to rise to its most dramatic heights. If you don't have a soufflé dish, use a charlotte mold, or fit a round casserole dish with a collar. The batter should come to within 1 inch of the rim. For savory recipes, the sides of the dish are buttered and sprinkled with bread crumbs or grated cheese to help the soufflé mixture climb upward as the beaten egg whites expand in the oven. In dessert soufflés, the buttered dish is sprinkled with sugar. Some recipes for savory soufflés forgo the bread crumbs or grated cheese and instead chill the buttered dish. The cold butter gives the soufflé mixture some traction on the dish's sides.

Soufflé dishes.

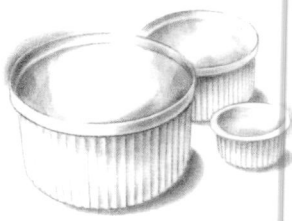

The French prefer their soufflés undercooked by American standards, that is, creamy in the center. This is a matter of taste, however, and you may prefer a drier, more fully cooked soufflé, especially if you are concerned about the possibility of salmonella from undercooked eggs. If so, bake your soufflé until a skewer inserted from the side into the center of the soufflé crown comes out clean. Some especially dense soufflés, such as those made of chocolate, will always remain a bit moist in the center.

HOW TO *Make a Soufflé Collar*

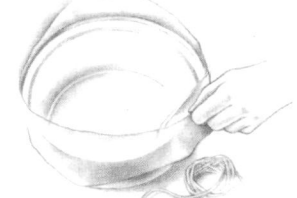

1. Measure the circumference of the mold and cut a strip of aluminum foil or heavy brown paper 1 or 2 inches longer than the circumference and 6 to 8 inches wide.
2. Fold the foil or paper in half lengthwise and tie it around the dish with kitchen string. It should rise no more than 2 to 3 inches above the rim.
3. Butter and sprinkle the exposed interior of the foil or paper when you prepare the interior of the dish.

SOUP Served for any course, including dessert, soup can be hot or cold, and it can be made from almost any ingredient. Among the various kinds are clear soups, which range from a simple stock to a clarified consommé and may have other ingredients, such as dumplings, added; cream soups, which have milk or cream added to a base of stock and are usually thickened with either puréed ingredients or a roux; and soups that blur the line between soups and stews, like chili, gumbo, and bouillabaisse. (In general, a stew has larger pieces of food cooked in a relatively smaller quantity of thicker, saucelike liquid.)

Storing Store soup, tightly covered, in the refrigerator for 2 to 3 days, depending on the soup. Some soups are better the day after they are made, as the flavors have had a chance to meld and deepen. Degrease meat soups after chilling, and reheat slowly over low heat. Most frozen soups will keep for 3 to 6 months. Do not freeze soups with potatoes, however, as they will turn into mush.

Soup Savvy When making soup, keep the following in mind:

■ When a soup recipe calls for stock or broth, start with the best quality. If you don't make and store your own, look for good frozen, vacuum-packed, or canned broth, choosing a brand that has a flavor you like and that is not too salty.

■ Many soups can be made vegetarian simply by substituting vegetable stock or broth for meat, chicken, or seafood stock or broth.

■ Conversely, vegetarian soups can gain more robust appeal for meat eaters by the use of meat or poultry stock or the addition of smoked ham or bacon.

■ In summer, consider serving a cold soup such as Spanish gazpacho, cream of avocado or cucumber, or iced melon soup.

■ To give puréed soups sufficient body, include starchy or full-bodied ingredients such as potatoes, carrots, tomatoes, bread crumbs, or cooked grains.

■ Because soups reduce in volume during cooking, concentrating their flavors, season them only at the end of cooking.

■ Don't forget to garnish your soups, adding flavor and texture while enhancing their appearance. Easy garnishes include puréed bell pepper, pesto, herbs, shredded cheese, or croutons.

See also STEW; STOCK.

SOUR CREAM Sour cream is cream that has been deliberately soured. By adding a bacterial culture to the cream, producers can control the souring process as the lactose in the cream converts to lactic acid. Sour cream comes in low-fat and nonfat versions. When sour cream is used in baking, its lactic acid makes for a more tender crumb, and the sour cream lends cakes and muffins a pleasingly tart taste. Sour cream is sometimes used in salad dressings, such as for carrot-and-raisin salad or coleslaw, and for topping baked potatoes. Many sauces are enriched with sour cream as well, although the cream should be added at the very end of cooking, as it will curdle if exposed to high heat.

Storing Check sour cream containers for sell-by dates before purchasing, then store in the refrigerator for up to 1 week.

SOYBEAN See BEAN, DRIED; SOY FOODS.

SOY FOODS
The humble soybean is mother to an entire family of soy foods that are high in protein and vitamins.

BEAN CURD Called *tofu* in Japanese and *dou-fu* in Chinese, bean curd comes in silken, soft, medium, firm, and extra-firm ivory-colored blocks and has a mild flavor. It comes packed in water and should be drained, rinsed, and drained again before use. If you are deep-frying bean curd or using it in some other preparation that would suffer from too much liquid, place it on a plate, top with a second plate and a weight, such as a 1-pound can, and let stand for about 1 hour, to release more moisture. Bean curd is also sold pressed, pickled, and dried in sheets and sticks.

TEMPEH Indonesian tempeh, a firm, slab form of fermented bean curd with a yeasty flavor, is a favorite meat substitute for vegetarians, as it is as high in protein as beef or chicken while containing no cholesterol. Often made with a mix of fermented grains to add flavor and texture, tempeh can be baked, broiled, grilled, stir-fried, or deep-fried and used like cooked meat in salads, sandwiches, soups, and casseroles.

SOY SAUCE The ubiquitous seasoning of Asia, soy sauce is made from fermented soybean meal and wheat. Look for soy sauce labeled as naturally brewed. Synthetic versions made with sweeteners and coloring agents are inferior. Tamari sauce, soy

sauce made without wheat, is thicker and more intense. Japanese soy sauce *(shoyu)* is a fairly light soy sauce that is less salty than Chinese soy. The two main types of Chinese soy sauce are dark and light (or thin). Dark soy sauce has had molasses added, and because it is rich and flavorful, it is often used with red meats and other robust foods.

MISO A staple food in Japan, this fermented soybean paste is made by crushing boiled soybeans; adding wheat, barley, or rice; inoculating the mix with a yeastlike culture; and then aging it. White miso, also called light or yellow miso, is aged from 2 to 6 months. It has a mild, sweet flavor and is used in soups, sauces, and salad dressings. Red, or dark, miso is aged from 3 months to 3 years. It has a strong, salty taste and is used in robust dishes.

SOY MILK Made by puréeing soybeans with water, and then straining, cooking, and filtering the purée, soy milk is sold plain or sweetened and flavored and is also used as the basis for soy-based cheeses.

Soybeans are also the basis for a number of other condiments and pastes, such as salted black beans, bean paste, hot bean sauce, hoisin sauce, and sweet bean sauce. All of these intense-tasting sauces may be added to stir-fries and other dishes to deepen the flavor. Look for soybean sprouts in Asian markets, or look for fresh soybeans in their pods in natural-food stores and some Asian markets for sprouting at home. The young, tender green soybeans in the pod are also a wonderful and nutritious snack. About 2 inches long, and called by their Japanese name, *edamame,* they are simply boiled in their shells in heavily salted water for 5 to 10 minutes, drained, cooled to room temperature, and popped from their pods and eaten.

SPATULA See BAKING TOOLS; COOKING TOOLS.

Spice

The average person's love for spices comes second only to his or her love for salt and sugar. These highly scented seeds, barks, roots, and fruits have been commodities since prehistory. They have been used since ancient times in sacred rituals, to anoint royalty, to mask the taste of spoiling foods, and to add aroma and flavor to prepared dishes.

For centuries, spices had to be brought overland by camel from Asia and India, and the spice trade was monopolized by the Arabs. By medieval times, spices were almost as valuable as gold, and Venice controlled their commerce, becoming a great power in the process. Christopher Columbus was only one of many European explorers who hoped to break the Venetian hold on the spice trade by finding a sea route westward to the spice lands. North America just happened to be in the way.

Coriander, star anise, and cumin.

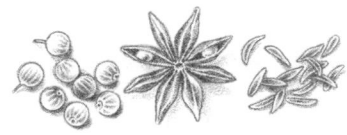

Spices are still valuable today, for only a small amount is needed to add a haunting or heady fragrance and taste to food. The cuisines of India and Indonesia, the two countries where most spices are still grown, use a wide range of them. Spain, Mexico, Ethiopia, and North Africa also depend on blends of spices to perfume their foods, reflecting their ancient connections with Arabic cuisine. Northern European countries continue to demonstrate their love of spices in a wide range of foods both sweet and savory, including gingerbread, sauerbraten, honey cake, mulled wine, and cardamom-scented butter cookies.

The Spice Pantry

ALLSPICE The berry of an evergreen tree, allspice tastes like a combination of cinnamon, nutmeg, and cloves. It is used ground or whole in many sweet and savory dishes, including some cakes, cookies, breads, braised meat dishes, tomato sauces, marinades, pickled foods, and stewed fruits.

ANISEED The seed of the anise plant, belonging to the parsley family, aniseed is used whole and ground and has a licorice taste. It is a popular addition to European baked goods, especially Italian breads and cookies. Aniseed is one of the flavorings used in the liqueurs pastis and anisette.

ANNATTO SEED Also called achiote, annatto seeds are the small, hard seeds of the annatto tree. The dark red seeds are ground and used in spice pastes or as part of a

continued

Spice, continued

dry-rub mixture for grilled and roasted meats, giving the food a musky, earthy taste and a reddish color. Annatto seeds are used in Indian, Spanish, and Mexican cooking, especially in seasoning pastes for meat and stews and to color rice.

CARAWAY SEED Caraway seed is a member of the parsley family. It has a strong, pungent taste that is closely identified with rye bread. Caraway seed is used in many other breads throughout northern and central Europe and is added to rich meat and poultry dishes and casseroles. It is almost always used whole.

CARDAMOM This intense spice is the dried fruit of a plant in the ginger family. Cardamom has an exotic, highly aromatic flavor and is used ground in curries, fruit dishes, and baked goods.

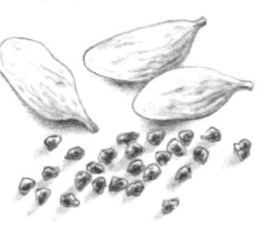

It may also be added whole to mulled wine, the spicy tea known as chai, and braised dishes. Cardamom is sold in small round pods or as whole or ground black seeds. The seeds are best removed from the pod and ground, although the whole pod also may be ground.

CAYENNE A very hot ground red pepper made from dried cayenne and other chiles, cayenne is used sparingly in a wide variety of preparations—hummus, salsas, chili, curries, chutneys—to add heat or to heighten flavor. Because different blends vary in heat, and because only a little is needed, always begin with a very small amount and add more to taste in small increments.

CELERY SEED This tiny dried seed of the wild celery plant has a strong celery flavor and is used whole in potato salad, coleslaw, and pickling mixtures. Use it sparingly.

CINNAMON While in American cooking cinnamon appears most often in sweets, such as apple pie and cinnamon rolls, the Greeks, Indians, and Moroccans use it in both sweet and savory dishes. The dried bark of a tree, cinnamon comes from two sources: the commonly available cassia cinnamon, which is a dark red-brown and has a strong, sweet taste; and pale tan, delicate-tasting Ceylon cinnamon, which is grown only in Sri Lanka and is considered by many to be true cinnamon. Buy cinnamon in stick form or already ground. To grind your own, first break or crush the stick into pieces.

CLOVE Shaped like a small nail with a round head, the almost-black clove is the dried bud of a tropical evergreen tree. It has a strong, sweet flavor with a peppery quality. Ground cloves are added to desserts such as spice cakes and to meat dishes such as sauerbraten, while whole cloves are used to stud hams and to flavor pickling mixtures.

Quick Bite

The word *clove* derives from the French word *clou*, which means "nail."

CORIANDER SEED The dried ripe fruit of fresh coriander, or cilantro. Coriander is a relative of parsley. Its tiny, round ridged "seeds" have an aroma said to be like a combination of lemon, sage, and caraway. The ground seeds add an exotic flavor to both savory and sweet foods, including stews and baked goods. Coriander is used in Indian, Scandinavian, and Middle Eastern cuisines, among others.

CUMIN The seed of another parsley family member, cumin has a sharp, strong flavor and is much used in Latin American, Indian, and Moroccan cooking. Mixed with ground chile, it is one of the ingredients in chili powder and is used in assertively flavored dishes like Mexican black beans and Texas chili. Cumin is available ground and whole. For superior flavor, buy whole seeds and toast them before grinding.

FENNEL SEED The seed of the common fennel has a licorice-like flavor and is used in savory dishes such as bouillabaisse, sausage, and pork stews and 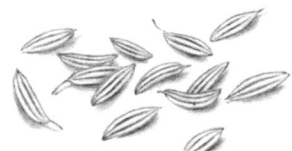 roasts. It is also used in some breads and desserts and to flavor liqueurs. Fennel seed may be used ground or whole.

FENUGREEK The characteristic bittersweet aroma of curry powder is due in part to the tiny yellow-brown seeds of the fenugreek plant. Highly aromatic, fenugreek seeds are actually legumes and are eaten as such in Ethiopia. They are also used to flavor Indian chutneys and Moroccan breads. The seeds are best purchased whole, as they quickly lose flavor after grinding. Fenugreek seeds should be toasted and soaked in water until soft before grinding.

GINGER Indispensable in Asian cooking, the warm, perfumy taste and spice of ginger is also a favorite flavoring of American and British cooks. See also GINGER.

JUNIPER BERRY This pea-sized berry from the evergreen juniper bush is blue-black and pungent. Juniper berries are used to flavor gin; in marinades for assertive-tasting meats such as lamb, venison, and 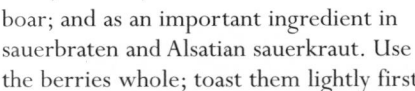 boar; and as an important ingredient in sauerbraten and Alsatian sauerkraut. Use the berries whole; toast them lightly first

and then crush them before adding to marinades or sauces.

MACE When the bright red, lacy membrane that covers the nutmeg seed is removed and dried, it turns orange-yellow and is sold as mace, usually in ground form. When sold whole, it is called blade mace. The flavor is a deeper and more pungent version of nutmeg. The spice is used in Indian, Moroccan, and Indonesian dishes and is also added to baked goods such as pound cake and to fruit dishes. Ground mace loses its flavor quickly, so buy it in small amounts and refrigerate it.

MUSTARD The seeds of the mustard plant come in three colors: white (also called yellow), brown, and black. Mustard seeds, which have a pungent, hot taste, are used whole as a primary ingredient in pickling mixtures and for flavoring marinades. Dry, or powdered, English mustard is used in sauces and dressings, and it may also be used to make prepared mustard at home. See also MUSTARD, PREPARED.

Quick Tip

Water triggers the chemical reaction in mustard seed that produces its distinctive hot flavor. If a recipe calls for dry mustard, mix it with a little tap water, let it stand for 10 minutes for the flavors to develop, and then add the paste to the other ingredients. One teaspoon of dry mustard is roughly equivalent to 1 tablespoon of prepared mustard.

NUTMEG The oval brown seed of a soft fruit, a nutmeg is about ¾ inch long, with a warm, sweet, spicy flavor. It has a hard shell that is in turn covered by the membrane that becomes mace. A beloved spice, nutmeg is used to dust

continued

Spice, continued

custards and eggnog and is one of the spices used to flavor sweet potato and winter squash dishes, pumpkin pie, spice cakes, breads, and cookies. The whole nutmeg keeps its flavor much longer than ground nutmeg. Specialized nutmeg graters, usually with small compartments for storing a nutmeg or two, are available for this purpose.

Quick Tip

If you do not have a nutmeg grater or other fine grater, very carefully shave a whole nutmeg seed crosswise with a sharp knife. The shavings will break apart into coarse powder. Mince them more finely with a knife, if needed.

See also NUTMEG.

PAPRIKA Made from ground dried red peppers and ranging from orange-red to red, paprika is used both as a garnish and as a flavoring. A dusting of paprika gives color to foods such as potato salad, macaroni salad, deviled eggs, fish, and creamed dishes. It is also used to give color and flavor to sausages and is an ingredient in spice mixes and rubs. Hungary and Spain make the finest paprika. Three basic types are available: sweet, half-sweet, and hot. Sweet paprika is often specified in recipes.

PEPPER Although small in size, peppercorns pack a wallop of piquancy that is essential to many dishes and is the natural flavor partner of salt. Both black and white peppercorns, which are the same spice picked at different stages of ripeness and processed differently, are used whole or ground to varying degrees of fineness.

Black peppercorns.

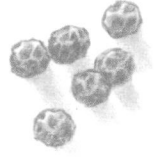
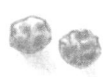

White peppercorns, which are actually tan, are slightly milder than their black kin and are used for aesthetic reasons in light-colored preparations such as cream sauce. Green peppercorns are harvested when still green and unripe, then packed in water or brine or dehydrated. They are less pungent than black and white peppercorns. So-called pink peppercorns are not true peppercorns but rather the brightly hued berries of a type of rose plant. All pepper is much more aromatic when freshly ground.

POPPY SEED Tiny in size and ranging from beige to blue-black in color, poppy seeds add crunch and a slight nutty flavor to foods. Black poppy seeds are used in central European cooking as a filling ingredient and as a garnish for baked goods such as strudel, cake, and cookies as well as for yeast breads and noodle dishes. Beige and brown poppy seeds are used in Indian and Middle Eastern cuisines. Because they are high in oil, poppy seeds should be stored in the refrigerator. Toasting the seeds brings out their flavor.

SAFFRON In flavor, saffron, the stigmas of a type of crocus, is pungent and earthy, with a slight bitterness. When soaked in liquid, it turns the liquid a dark yellow. Because it must be hand-picked, and because each crocus has only three stigmas, saffron is the world's most expensive spice. Only a tiny bit, however, is needed to tint and flavor rice (paella, risotto), chicken, breads, and many other dishes. It is available as "threads" (stigmas) or powdered. Thread saffron, although more expensive, is preferable, as powdered saffron is sometimes adulterated with other ingredients to extend it, and it loses flavor more rapidly.

Saffron is usually soaked in a small amount of hot water or other liquid before it is added to any dish. When possible, add saffron toward the end of the cooking process to preserve its highly aromatic flavor.

STAR ANISE Although it has an aniselike flavor, star anise is a seed-bearing pod from a Chinese evergreen tree related to the magnolia. The brown pods are indeed star shaped; each contains eight seeds. Slightly more bitter in flavor than aniseed, star anise is used in Asian cuisine to flavor teas and savory dishes. In the West, it is used in baked goods. Star anise is often used whole or snapped into points, and is also ground as one of the spices in Chinese five-spice powder.

TURMERIC Like saffron, turmeric is valued for both its taste and its bright color. The root of a plant belonging to the ginger family, turmeric is used fresh and dried. Fresh turmeric resembles fresh ginger in shape but is smaller and has orange-tinted skin. It is primarily used in Southeast Asian and South Asian cooking, in stews and curries. Dried and ground, the bright-orange flesh becomes yellow-orange. Ground turmeric is one of the primary ingredients in Indian curry powder and is also used to impart color to some prepared mustards.

VANILLA The favorite sweet flavoring of many Americans, vanilla is indigenous to the New World. In whole form, vanilla beans are the dried fruit of a tropical orchid; they are also used to make vanilla extract. See also VANILLA.

Selecting Ideally, spices should be bought whole and ground just before use. But in the interest of convenience, cooks stock many spices in two forms, whole and ground. Buy your spices, especially ground ones, in the smallest amounts you can, as they lose flavor over time. It's better to go to a natural-food store or a specialty-food shop that sells spices in bulk and buy only a little of each than to buy jars or cans of spices that will grow stale and have to be thrown out. Be sure your merchant stores spices in a cool, dark place.

Storing Keep spices in tightly closed containers in a cool, dark place such as a pantry, rather than beside the stove or elsewhere in a bright kitchen. Some cooks keep their spices in alphabetical order for ease of selection. If you buy your spices in bulk, purchase some empty glass spice jars for storing them. Whole spices kept this way will last for about 1 year; ground spices should be replaced after 6 months.

Preparing For grinding small quantities of spices, use a mortar and pestle or a pepper mill reserved for spices. Or buy a small electric coffee grinder and use it only for grinding spices. Grind just the amount you need. To add whole spices to stews and mulled wine, tie them in a cheesecloth square or place them in a tea ball for easy removal. If using an orange or onion and whole cloves, stud the orange or onion with the cloves. Whole peppercorns should be bruised or cracked before using.

Putting spices in a tea ball.

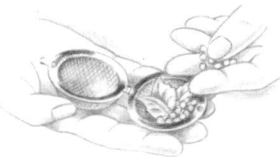

To intensify their flavor, toast spices in a dry skillet. It is best to toast whole spices before grinding, but ground spices may be toasted if you keep a close eye on them. Some recipes call for frying spices in oil. Take great care not to burn them.

HOW TO *Toast Spices*

1. Put the spices in a small, heavy skillet (cast iron is ideal) over medium heat.
2. Toast, stirring constantly, until fragrant. Immediately empty the spices into a bowl and stir them to stop the cooking.

Spirits

Alcoholic spirits can be distilled from almost any food that contains sugar and can be fermented. The list ranges from apples, corn, and potatoes to barley, watermelons, milk, cactus, grape skins, and wine itself.

The Arabs originated the art of distilling, in which a fermented solution is boiled in a pot still, a large, closed kettle with a long, very narrow spout. Alcohol, which has a lower boiling point than water, evaporates first, and the resulting steam condenses and is channeled off.

Spirits such as whiskey, rum, gin, and vodka are labeled with their proof, a number that indicates the alcohol content of the beverage and is always twice the actual percentage. For example, 80 proof bourbon is 40 percent alcohol. Distilled spirits, such as whiskey, are barreled at well over 100 proof and then diluted with water when bottled to reach the desired proof.

Quick Bite

The term *proof* derives from an old custom of testing the quality of liquor by mixing it into a little gunpowder and holding it over a flame. If it ignited, the spirit was said to be "proved," indicating that it contained at least 50 percent alcohol (100 proof). If it only fizzled, the spirit didn't prove and was labeled inferior.

The Liquor Cabinet Spirits are used as appetizers, as digestives, and in cooking. Some of the most common spirits follow.

AQUAVIT Distilled from grain or potatoes, this Scandinavian liquor is flavored with caraway. It is kept in the freezer and served as single shots before or after dinner.

BOURBON See Whiskey, below.

BRANDY Brandy, which has an ancient heritage, is distilled from wine or fermented fruit juice. Cognac is brandy that comes from six regions clustered around the town of Cognac in western France. Known as the best of all brandies, Cognac is distilled from wine made from Charente grapes and is aged in Limousin oak in a highly controlled process. It is usually sipped after dinner, but it is also used in desserts, sauces, and consommés. Cognac is added to French onion soup and used to flambé a variety of both sweet and savory foods. Armagnac is brandy made from wine in the Gascony area of France. It is aged in black oak and has a pungent aroma and a more robust flavor than Cognac. It is also taken after dinner and is occasionally used in cooking.

Fruit brandies, also known as eaux-de-vie, or "waters of life," are strong, colorless spirits distilled from fermented fruit juice. Most of these are made in eastern France, Germany, and Switzerland. They are drunk before or after dinner and are widely used in desserts, especially those made with fruit. Fruit brandies are made from pears (poire Williams), raspberries (framboise), cherries (kirsch), and other fruits, including prunes and apricots. Calvados, an apple brandy, comes from northern France, where apples are plentiful but grapes are not grown. A dry brandy aged in oak, Calvados is taken after dinner and, in

Normandy, even as a digestive between two courses of a long meal. It is also an important ingredient in the dishes of Norman cuisine.

Calvados.

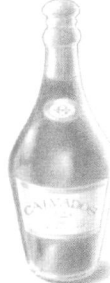

GIN This grain-based liquor gets its distinctive flavor from juniper berries and is often enjoyed as an ingredient in before-dinner mixed drinks. The most popular of these beverages is the dry martini, but dozens of gin mixed drinks exist, from gin and tonic to the Negroni (Campari, sweet vermouth, and gin) to the gimlet (lime juice and gin) to the salty dog (grapefruit juice, gin, and salt).

RUM Distilled from sugarcane juice or molasses, this Caribbean liquor comes in different colors, each stronger in flavor, from milk white or silver to golden, amber, dark, and Demerara, the darkest one. With its slightly sweet taste, rum is enjoyed straight, particularly in the Caribbean; in a Cuba libre and other highballs; and in a variety of cocktails, from a classic daiquiri to a martini in which the rum stands in for the gin. It is also widely used in Caribbean cooking, especially in fruit desserts, in ice cream, and in baked goods.

SCOTCH See Whiskey, below.

TEQUILA Made from fermented agave juice and named after its place of origin, Tequila, Mexico, this heady spirit ranges in color from white to golden and is the basis of the popular margarita. It is also drunk neat, with salt and a squeeze of lime, or sipped alternately with *sangrita,* a spicy mixture of tomato and lime juices.

VODKA Originally made from potatoes, today vodka is usually made from grain. Unaged and clear, vodka has little taste and so may be blended with a variety of other liquids. It is kept in the freezer to drink neat and also is sold in flavored form. A flavored, or infused, vodka is treated with one of a wide variety of ingredients, from lemon zest to chile. Vodka is occasionally used in cooking, as in a vodka-flavored cream sauce for pasta. It is also used as a base for homemade liqueurs.

WHISKEY Including bourbon, Canadian, Irish, rye, and Scotch, whiskeys are all made from grain. Scotch whisky, correctly spelled without an *e,* is also called simply Scotch. It is made throughout Scotland, and five kinds are produced: grain whisky, which is used in blended Scotch; and four distinctive malts, all made from malted barley in different areas of the country. Most Scottish malt whiskies are blended, except for the "single," or unblended, whiskies of the Highlands and other areas, which are considered the finest. Scotch is drunk on the rocks before dinner and is used in some mixed drinks. Bourbon takes its name from a county in Kentucky and is made from fermented grain, primarily corn. Indeed, so-called straight bourbon must be at least 51 percent corn. This slightly sweet whiskey is served before dinner over ice or in drinks such as eggnog. In cooking it may be added to barbecue sauce or baked beans, or used in bourbon balls or fruitcakes.

Quick Tip

Two common small bar tools that simplify measuring are the jigger (1½ ounces) and the pony (1 ounce), both small cups with flared sides. Sometimes they are available as a single double-ended measure. Most drinks call for 1½ ounces of alcohol; some call for 1 or 2 ounces.

See also LIQUEUR; WINE.

SPINACH See GREENS, DARK; GREENS, SALAD.

SPIRITS See page 418.

SPLIT PEA See BEAN, DRIED.

SPOON Stirring and spooning up food are simple tasks, but having a selection of different kinds of spoons to choose from makes them even easier. Wooden spoons are indispensable in the kitchen, as they are sturdy, do not scratch bowls or pans, or add a metallic taste to foods, and their handles do not get hot. Their only drawback is that they need to be washed by hand, not in a dishwasher, and if allowed to soak in water for extended periods, they will eventually warp, crack, and split. Metal spoons are nice for stirring large quantities of thick foods, such as stews, although their primary use is transferring food from one container to another. The slotted spoon is not used for stirring, but it is an essential tool for removing solid foods from liquid. The ladle is a necessary utensil for serving soups and sauces in the kitchen and at table. Scoops are used to remove dry foods from their containers. Ice-cream scoops come in several different sizes, and devoted cookie makers value them for scooping uniform balls of dough nearly as much as for scooping ice cream.

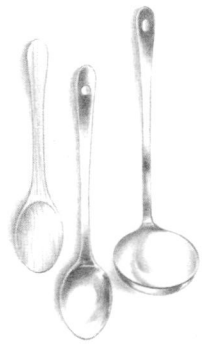

Wooden and metal spoons and ladle.

Measuring spoons help keep even the most intuitive cook on track. Choose metal ones that are linked, so you won't lose any. Precise measurements are critical in many recipes, especially those for baked goods.

See also BAKING TOOLS; COOKING TOOLS; MEASURING.

SPRINGFORM PAN See BAKEWARE; CAKE.

SPROUT Beans and seeds, germinated until they form a tender stalk and often their first leaves, are valued for their fresh, crisp taste and high nutritional content. Sprouts are rich in enzymes, which aid digestion, and are much higher in vitamins than are unsprouted seeds and beans.

Caution!

Raw sprouts have emerged as a possible source of food-borne illness. They may carry the pathogenic salmonella and _E. coli_ bacteria. Alfalfa and clover sprouts have been involved in outbreaks most often, but all raw sprouts may pose a risk. If you are pregnant or older, are cooking for young children or older people, have a compromised immune system, or want to limit your exposure to bacterial risk as much as possible, you should cook all sprouts before eating them.

Any live seed can be sprouted, but the most commonly available sprouts are mung bean, alfalfa, radish, sunflower, and red clover sprouts. Mung bean sprouts, often called simply bean sprouts, are used in stir-fries and salads. Radish sprouts, sunflower sprouts, and red clover sprouts are also good salad ingredients, and alfalfa sprouts are often used in sandwiches and in stuffed pita breads. Broccoli sprouts have recently become popular, as they have been shown to be higher in nutrition than full-grown broccoli. Lentil and wheat berry sprouts are also available in many natural-food stores. Soybean sprouts are available in both natural-food stores and Asian markets.

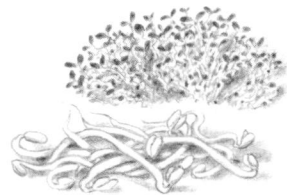

Alfalfa and soybean sprouts.

Selecting Sprouts should be as fresh as possible. Try to buy them in bulk, rather than packaged, so you can make sure they are not dry, wilted, discolored, or slimy. Recent studies have shown that sprouts that are past their prime may actually be detrimental to one's health. To be absolutely sure of freshness, try growing your own.

Storing Place sturdy sprouts, such as mung bean, sunflower, and radish sprouts, in an airtight plastic container and store in the refrigerator for up to 3 days. Store delicate sprouts, such as alfalfa, in a perforated plastic bag in the crisper of the refrigerator for no more than 2 days.

Preparing Rinse the sprouts lightly with cool water and shake dry. Pull them apart and, if you don't like the looks of the little tails on mung and soy sprouts, pull them off and discard them. They are, however, edible. Soy sprouts, which are a little larger and thicker than other sprouts, should always be cooked instead of eaten raw.

Toss sprouts into a stir-fry or into boiling water for only about a minute, so they will stay crunchy. Scatter raw sprouts over salads or use in sandwiches.

SQUAB A young farm-raised pigeon with a rich, succulent meat. Because the birds never fly (exercise that builds muscles and toughens meat), their flesh is also

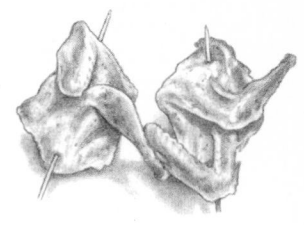

exceedingly tender. Usually weighing under 1 pound, they may be substituted for poussins and Cornish hens. Like duck, the meat of a squab is all somewhat dark and rich.

Selecting When shopping for squab, look for ones that are plump and firm. Fresh squab is available in some markets during the summer months. It may also be ordered from specialty-meat markets and from Asian meat markets. The rest of the year, rely on frozen birds.

Storing Store squab in the coldest part of the refrigerator, usually the rear bottom shelf or in a meat drawer. If not prepared within 48 hours, freeze until ready to use. Defrost frozen squab in their packaging in the refrigerator.

Preparing Like other birds, squab takes well to a wide range of cooking methods. It can be roasted, grilled, broiled, sautéed, or smoked but should never be cooked above medium-rare. The birds are done when the juices are still slightly pink. If overcooked, the meat takes on a gamy, liverlike flavor.

See also DONENESS.

SQUASH The large, sprawling squash clan, all members of the gourd family and native to the Americas, may be neatly divided into two branches: winter squash and summer squash. Winter squashes are allowed to mature until their flesh is thick and their shells are hard, and they have a long shelf life. They come in many shapes, colors (white to red to green to near-black), and sizes. Summer squashes are generally eaten while small and tender, and are best eaten young and fresh. The blossoms of winter and summer squashes are eaten as well.

Squash Blossoms Squash blossoms, particularly those of pumpkins and zucchini, can be sautéed and used in quesadillas, pastas, or soups. They can also be filled with a seasoned white cheese, then battered and deep-fried.

Zucchini with blossoms.

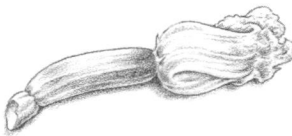

Summer Squash All summer squashes are similar in flavor. They may be shredded or cut into thin slices and eaten raw or cooked by sautéing, stir-frying, boiling, steaming, or broiling. Zucchini and crookneck yellow squash can be cut into lengthwise slices, coated with olive oil, and grilled, while pattypans or scallopini may be sliced crosswise and cooked the same way. Sliced summer squashes can be battered and panfried or deep-fried. All summer squashes can be halved, hollowed out, filled, and baked; or they may be made into soups and stews, perhaps most notably ratatouille. Enormously versatile, they can be steamed whole, or sliced and sautéed as a side dish or as a topping for pasta.

CROOKNECK SQUASH
This bright yellow squash is about the same size as zucchini, but with a curved neck.

PATTYPAN SQUASH
Also known as scallop squash, this pale green, yellow, or white squash is about 4 inches in diameter, with scalloped edges.
SCALLOPINI Shaped like the pattypan, the scallopini is larger, thicker, and speckled green, like zucchini.
ZUCCHINI These narrow green squashes, some of which grow to an enormous size and capture ribbons at county fairs, are

best eaten when small and young, before their tender flesh begins to toughen. Zucchini come in bright gold as well as the better-known green. A pale green round zucchini, known as Ronde de Nice, is sometimes available in farmers' markets and better produce stores. It is especially nice for panfrying. See also ZUCCHINI.

Selecting Summer Squash Look for small summer squash early in summer. Throughout the season, select firm, unblemished specimens.

Storing Summer Squash Put summer squashes in a perforated plastic bag and keep them in the crisper section of the refrigerator for up to 3 days. Use squash blossoms within 24 hours; place them in one layer on a baking sheet lined with paper towels and refrigerate them until using.

Preparing Summer Squash Trim the ends of summer squashes, then hollow them with a tablespoon if you plan to stuff them, or slice, chop, or shred them as called for in a recipe.

Acorn and pattypan squashes.

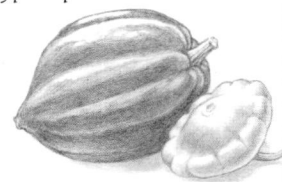

Winter Squash Compared to summer squashes, winter squashes have a strong taste and dense texture (with the exception of the long strands of the spaghetti squash). They may be baked whole or in halves, slices, or cubes; or they may be cubed or sliced, then steamed or simmered and puréed if you like. Small winter squashes such as acorns and golden nuggets are the perfect size for halving, stuffing, and baking. Large squashes such as butternuts may be sliced and baked, or cut into pieces, then cooked and puréed. Sliced or cubed squash is also good in soups and stews or glazed and baked.

ACORN SQUASH About 6 inches in diameter, this squash has a dark green, ribbed shell and orange flesh.

BANANA SQUASH A squash with peach-colored skin and orange flesh, shaped like its namesake, although it can grow several feet long. It is often sold cut into pieces.

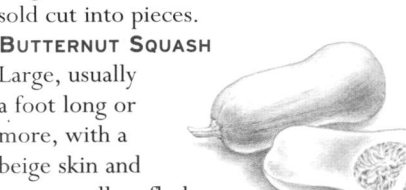

BUTTERNUT SQUASH Large, usually a foot long or more, with a beige skin and orange-yellow flesh, the butternut is identifiable by the round bulb at one end. It has a flavorful, dense flesh and is especially good for baking and puréeing.

DELICATA SQUASH A squash with green-striped yellow skin and yellow flesh that tastes a bit like a sweet potato. It is about 3 inches in diameter and 6 to 8 inches long.

GOLDEN NUGGET SQUASH Resembles a small pumpkin about 4 inches in diameter.

HUBBARD SQUASH Weighing 10 pounds or more, the Hubbard has yellow flesh and gray-green, blue, or dark green skin with small bumps. It makes an excellent purée that is a good substitute for pumpkin in pies.

KABOCHA SQUASH This squash, with its bright green skin marked with paler green stripes, has pale orange flesh. It usually weighs 2 to 3 pounds and may be substituted for acorn squash in recipes.

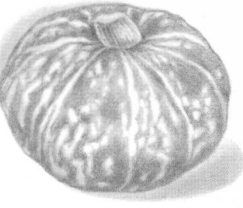

PUMPKIN Divided into field and cooking varieties; see PUMPKIN.

SPAGHETTI SQUASH Roughly the shape and size of a football, with bright yellow skin. Baked whole, the cooked flesh of the spaghetti squash forms long, thin strands when pulled from the shell with a fork, thus its name.

Spaghetti squashes should be baked whole, then halved and their strands pulled out; serve them like pasta.

SWEET DUMPLING SQUASH Actually an Asian gourd about 4 inches in diameter, the sweet dumpling has a very flavorful flesh and can be cooked and eaten like a winter squash. It is best when fully mature, its skin yellow with dark-orange stripes.

TABLE QUEEN Resembling an acorn squash in size and shape, this variety, also sometimes known as a golden acorn, has a bright orange shell and sweet, mild-tasting flesh.

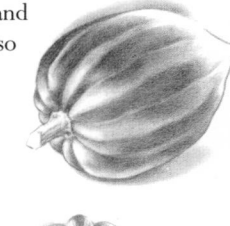

TURBAN SQUASH This exotic-looking specimen has a top-knot and a multihued skin in oranges, yellows, and greens. It comes in varied sizes and shapes.

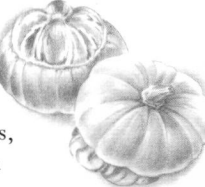

Selecting Winter Squash Some winter squash varieties are available year-round, but the widest selection is found during fall and winter. Squashes should be firm and unblemished and feel heavy for their size. To stuff and bake winter squash, choose a small squash, such as an acorn, that will yield two servings. For puréeing and cubing, choose a larger squash with more meat, such as the butternut.

Storing Winter Squash Cut winter squashes may be kept in the refrigerator for up to 1 week; whole winter squashes may be kept for months in a cool, dark place.

Preparing Winter Squash Using a chef's knife, cut winter squashes into halves or wedges. Using a large metal spoon, spoon out the seeds and strings, then peel the squash.

Scooping out the seeds.

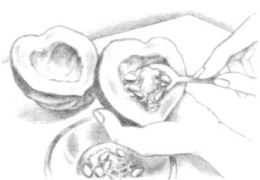

HOW TO *Roast (or Bake) a Winter Squash*

1. Using a large, sharp knife, carefully cut the squash in half lengthwise through its stem and flower ends. If the skin is very hard, use a kitchen mallet to tap the knife carefully once it is securely wedged in the squash.

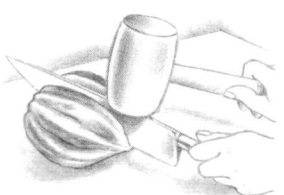

2. Place the squash halves cut side down in a baking dish and add water to a depth of 1 inch to the dish. Bake at 350°F until the squash is tender when pierced with a fork, 30 minutes to 1¼ hours, depending on variety. Add more water to the dish if it evaporates.

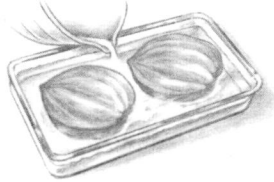

3. Once the squash is cooked and tender, scooping out the seeds and fibers is easy.

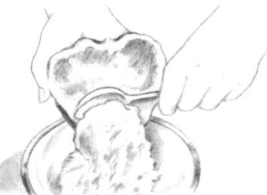

See also STEAMING.

SQUID One of the best values in the fish market, squid, sometimes called by its Italian name, calamari, is also one of the most delicious items you'll find there. This member of the cephalopod family (see SHELLFISH) has a sweet, mild flavor that takes well to a wide range of preparations. Many shops sell it already cleaned, cutting down dramatically on the cook's labor.

Whatever recipe or cooking method you choose, cook squid quickly, for 1 or 2 minutes, or slowly, for at least 1 hour. Otherwise, your squid will have the taste and texture of rubber bands.

Cuttlefish, which is similar in appearance to squid but much larger, is popular in Japan and some Mediterranean countries. Because its body walls are thicker than those of squid, it must be tenderized (see POUNDING) before cooking.

Selecting Fresh squid is shiny and firm, with a delicate ocean smell. The membrane that covers the squid should be gray. A purple or pink cast indicates that the squid may not be fresh.

Storing Squid is highly perishable and should be refrigerated on a bed of ice for no more than 2 days before cooking and serving. If you purchase frozen squid, don't defrost it more than a day before you plan to use it.

HOW TO *Clean Squid*

1. Pull the head and tentacles away from the body, or pouchlike part, of the squid. The innards, including the ink sac, should come away with the head.

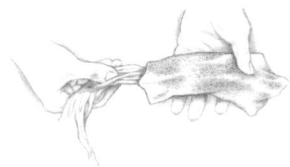

2. Reach into the pouch and remove the long, plasticlike quill and discard it.

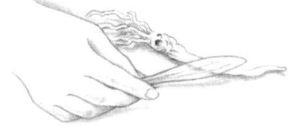

3. Cut off the tentacles from the rest of the head just below the eyes and discard the head and innards. Squeeze the cut end of the tentacles to remove the hard, round "beak" at the base and discard it.

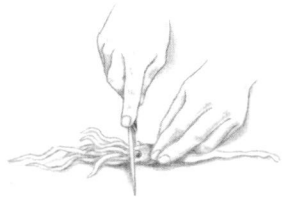

4. Rinse the squid body, inside and out, and the tentacles under cold running water and pull off the gray membrane that covers the pouch. You may want to use a paring knife to help scrape it off. If the 2 small fins on either side of the pouch come off, reserve them to cook with the squid. Once cleaned, the pouch, fins, and tentacles can be sliced or left whole.

STAR ANISE See SPICE.

STARFRUIT Also known as the star apple or carambola, this bright yellow, 4- to 6-inch-long subtropical fruit, a native of China and India, gets its name because of its deeply ribbed exterior, which forms a star when the fruit is cut crosswise. The juicy flesh has a taste reminiscent of pineapple, plum, and lemon. It may be enjoyed raw or cooked in sweet and savory dishes.

Selecting Choose shiny-skinned, firm specimens. It's okay if they have a touch of green to them, as they will ripen well in your kitchen.

Storing Keep at room temperature until uniformly golden, a sign of ripeness; then refrigerate and eat within several days.

Preparing The fruit may be eaten peel and all. Cut crosswise for the most attractive presentation.

STARTER See YEAST.

STEAMER BASKET See COOKING TOOLS.

STEAMING To cook food over boiling water in a covered pan. Also, to cook some foods, such as mussels and clams, in a small amount of simmering liquid in a covered pan. Steaming is an especially good cooking method for delicate foods such as fish and vegetables, as it cooks by a more gentle process than boiling, simmering, or even poaching, thereby retaining the food's shape, color, flavor, and texture. In addition, steamed foods will not take on excess water, which could dilute their inherent flavor. Steaming is the technique of choice for cauliflower and broccoli, as it keeps them from becoming waterlogged. Steaming is also the most healthful of all cooking techniques, because it uses no fat, and it allows more nutrients to remain intact.

Caution!

Take care when uncovering a steaming pot. Be sure to avert your face and lift the lid away from you as you uncover the pot, and wear oven mitts to protect your hands and arms from the hot steam. It can scald you just as boiling water can.

Steamers are large pots fitted with a perforated basket and a lid. Often pasta pots will include a steamer basket that can be used in place of the perforated pasta basket. Collapsible steamer baskets can turn almost any saucepan or stockpot into a steamer. They have feet that keep the basket above the level of the water, and a ring for lifting the basket out of the pan. In lieu of a steamer basket, a metal colander or strainer can be set inside a large saucepan or a stockpot. Chinese bamboo steamer baskets are designed to fit snugly against the sides of a wok above the water. They can be stacked three high, so you can steam a meal of meat, fish, and vegetables, all in separate baskets but in the same pot.

Steaming Times for Various Foods

Artichoke, medium	40 minutes
Asparagus	
Thin spears	3 to 4 minutes
Thick spears	5 to 6 minutes
Beets	30 to 35 minutes
Broccoli	
Florets	4 to 5 minutes
Spears	5 to 6 minutes
Brussels sprouts	7 to 11 minutes
Cabbage, cut into wedges	6 minutes
Carrots, ¼-inch-thick, 2-inch-long pieces	6 to 8 minutes
Cauliflower	
Head	12 to 15 minutes
Florets	4 to 6 minutes
Corn on the cob	5 minutes
Fennel	
Whole, trimmed	20 to 35 minutes
Quartered	7 to 10 minutes
Green beans	4 to 5 minutes
Kale	4 to 5 minutes
Parsnips, 1½-inch pieces	8 to 10 minutes
Peas	2 minutes
Potatoes	
New	12 minutes
2-inch chunks	15 minutes
Pumpkin & winter squashes	
Peeled 2-inch chunks	15 to 20 minutes
Spinach, 1 pound	4 to 5 minutes
Sweet potatoes	
Whole	40 to 50 minutes
1-inch chunks	12 to 15 minutes
Swiss chard	
Leaves	4 to 6 minutes
Ribs, in 2-inch pieces	10 to 12 minutes
Zucchini, ¼-inch slices	5 to 7 minutes

Foods may also be steamed in the microwave or by tightly sealing them in parchment paper or aluminum foil and cooking them in the oven.

Steaming Savvy When steaming foods, keep the following in mind:

- Fill the pot with several inches of water if using a steamer, or about ½ inch of water if using a collapsible steamer basket. Make sure the water will not touch the bottom of the basket or other container used to hold the food.
- Bring the water to a boil, then fill the steamer basket with food and add the basket to the pot. Cover and cook for the time specified in the recipe. Remove the basket as soon as the food is cooked.
- If the food must steam for a long time, and especially if you are using a small amount of water with a collapsible basket, check periodically to make sure the water has not boiled dry. Add more boiling water as needed.
- When steaming vegetables, especially strong-flavored ones like broccoli and cauliflower, try cooking by smell: when the vegetable begins to give off its fragrance, it is crisp-tender.

Vegetables are hands down the most popular food category to cook by steaming. Use the times suggested in the chart at left as guidelines only, relying more on taste and tenderness to help you determine when a vegetable is done to your liking.

STEEPING Extracting flavor from an ingredient by soaking it in a hot liquid. The point is to transfer the flavor from the solid ingredient to the liquid, which is then consumed or used as a flavoring. Steeping tea leaves in hot water makes tea. Ice creams are often flavored by steeping a flavoring such as coffee beans in the cream base and then straining out the beans after the base has taken on their flavor.

STEMMING To remove the stem from a fruit or vegetable. Many fruits and vegetables arrive in the market with their inedible stems still attached. Some stems, such as those on cherries, can simply be plucked off. Others foods, like artichokes, have thick stems that must be cut away with a knife. Greens and herbs such as spinach, watercress, basil, and parsley are usually stemmed before using, as the stems tend to be fibrous and somewhat bitter. See individual foods.

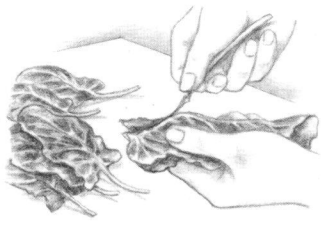

Stemming spinach.

STEW A stew is made by simmering pieces of meat, fish, and/or vegetables slowly in liquid. Usually thicker and more substantial than a soup, a stew is commonly served as a main course. It is similar to a braise, although stews generally use more liquid and the food for them is cut into smaller pieces.

Stews are among the basic dishes found in almost every cuisine, from the meat or seafood stews of France to the clay pots of Asia. A few famous French stews are the daube (which can also be a whole piece of braised beef), the ragout, and *boeuf bourguignonne*. The meat for stews is often browned to add flavor to the liquid, which gradually thickens as the meat cooks, although some dishes, such as fish stews and *blanquette de veau* (white veal stew) are made without browning.

Stews are economical, as they are usually made with foods that require long cooking for tenderness, such as root vegetables and tougher cuts of meat. They also have the advantage of usually tasting better the day after they are made. Refrigerating a stew overnight allows the flavors of the different ingredients to deepen.

Stew Savvy When making stew, keep the following in mind:

- When browning meat or vegetables for stews, follow the rules for searing: dry the food first on paper towels, add it to hot oil without crowding, and don't stir too often, to allow the meat to brown and to create browned bits on the bottom of the pan, which will flavor the sauce.

- An enameled cast-iron dutch oven or covered casserole is a perfect vessel for stewing, as it allows you to brown, cook, store, reheat, and serve the stew in the same container.

- The liquid in a stew should cover or almost cover the pieces of food.

- Stews and braises may be cooked on top of the stove, but medium-low oven heat allows for more even cooking and for a lower temperature, thus ensuring more tender results.

- Add quicker-cooking foods, such as potatoes and peas, when the meat is tender, and then cook them until tender, usually only 10 to 20 minutes. If you are making the stew a day ahead, add these foods the next day when reheating it.

- To make a stew 1 day ahead, let it cool to room temperature, then refrigerate. The next day, lift off any congealed fat from the surface, then slowly reheat the stew.

See also SOUP.

STIR-FRYING An Asian cooking technique of rapidly frying small pieces of foods in oil over high heat. The wok is the perfect implement for stir-frying, as it exposes the food to the maximum cooking surface while keeping it from flying out of the pan as you stir. A large, deep cast-iron skillet or heavy sauté pan is a good substitute, however. Almost any vegetable or meat can be stir-fried, as long it is cut into small pieces. Although Asian-flavored dishes are the most obvious choices for stir-fries, you can also fashion simple Italian-style stir-fries, using such ingredients as sun-dried tomatoes, basil, and fresh vegetables, to top pasta or to serve as side dishes.

HOW TO *Stir-fry*

For approximately 1 pound of vegetables and ½ pound meat or tofu.

1. All food to be stir-fried should be cut into bite-sized pieces about 1½ inches long or into ½-inch dice. Cut red meat into strips against the grain, cut chicken or fish into thin slices or strips or into dice, and cut tofu into dice. Shrimp should be left whole and may be shelled or not. Vegetables such as carrots and zucchini should be cut into matchsticks or very thin slices, while long, thin vegetables such as green beans and asparagus should be cut on the diagonal to help them cook more quickly.

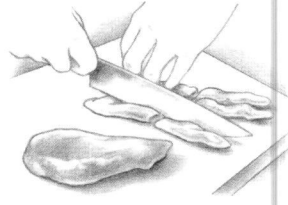

Cutting chicken into strips.

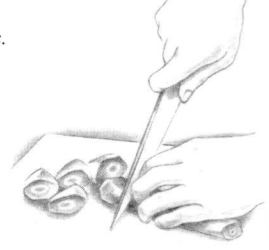

Cutting vegetables into small pieces.

2. Marinate meat, chicken, fish, shellfish, or tofu for about 15 minutes in a little soy sauce and vegetable oil, flavored with garlic, grated fresh ginger, and dry sherry or Shaoxing rice wine.

3. Preheat the wok over high heat until hot, then pour about 1½ tablespoons canola or peanut oil into the wok. Carefully tilt and rotate the pan in a circle so that the oil is distributed 6 inches up the sides of the pan. The oil should spread out in fragrant waves.

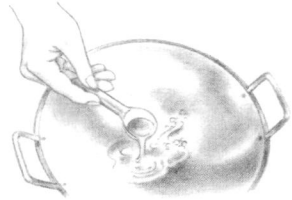

4. Add the meat or other foods; stir the food rapidly and push it up the sides of the wok until the meat, fish, chicken, or tofu is just beginning to brown, 2 to 3 minutes; shrimp should just have turned pink. Using a slotted spoon, transfer the meat to a bowl and set aside.

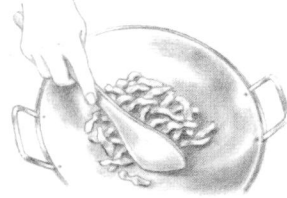

5. Add another tablespoon of oil to the pan, heat, and stir-fry the vegetables until their color turns bright, about 1 minute.

6. Add 2 to 3 tablespoons stock or water and cover the pan.

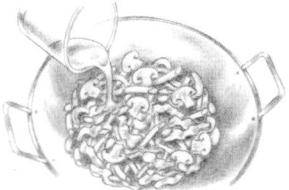

Reduce the heat to medium-high and cook for a few minutes, or just until the vegetables are crisp-tender. Vegetables such as broccoli, carrots, and cauliflower will take 3 to 4 minutes; bell peppers and zucchini will take 1 to 2 minutes; tender vegetables such as bean sprouts and snow peas need only 30 seconds or less.

7. Return the meat, chicken, fish, shellfish, or tofu to the pan along with the marinade and any other flavoring ingredients, such as black beans, soy sauce, chile oil, or Asian sesame oil. If you would like a thickened sauce, dissolve 2 teaspoons cornstarch in about ⅓ cup cold stock or water, add to the pan at the very end of cooking, and stir until the liquid is thickened. Serve at once.

See also COOKWARE.

STOCK The word *stock* is often used interchangeably with *broth* to describe the liquid made by cooking a food such as chicken, beef, fish, or vegetables in water for a few hours. More specifically, a stock is a homemade broth, a well-flavored liquid made by cooking meat and/or bones, fish parts and/or bones, the shells of shellfish, or vegetables with aromatic ingredients such as spices, herbs, onions, garlic, and other vegetables. Stock is used as the basis for countless soups, stews, and sauces and is used as a source of flavor and moisture in many other savory dishes.

Stock Savvy When making stock, keep the following in mind:

■ The more meat you use, the more flavorful your stock will be.

■ Ask your butcher for meaty soup bones or chicken parts for making stock (ask him or her to saw and/or chop them into 2- to 3-inch pieces for you). Or you can make your own stockpile by freezing leftover bones, meat scraps, chicken carcasses, bony chicken parts (backs, necks, and wings), and giblets (without the livers), both cooked and uncooked.

- Some strong-flavored vegetables, such as turnips and members of the cabbage family, will overpower the flavor of the stock, while starchy vegetables, like potatoes, will cloud and thicken the stock, and other vegetables, like beets, will color it.
- Don't let a stock being made with meat, fish, or chicken come to a boil, or it will become cloudy. Always cook the stock at a low simmer.
- Don't cover the pot completely while it is cooking, or the stock can sour. Cook with the lid askew so steam can escape, and let the stock cool uncovered.
- See SKIMMING and DEGREASING for tips on those processes.
- If you do not have homemade stock on hand, use a good-quality, low-salt commercial broth.

See also BROTH.

STOCKPOT See COOKWARE.

STRAINER A strainer, also called a sieve, is used to separate lumps or larger particles of food from smaller ones. It also is used to drain pieces of food of their liquid, and to purée soft foods, which are pushed through the strainer with the back of a large spoon.

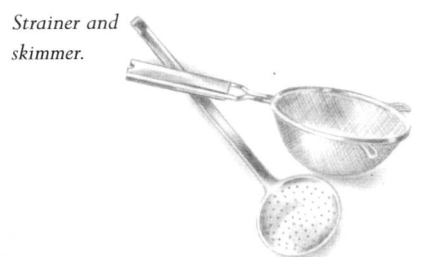

Strainer and skimmer.

Wire-mesh strainers come in a variety of sizes, from very small to large, with either fine or coarse mesh. Some strainers have a long handle, plus a metal hook that allows them to fit onto a bowl; others are freestanding. Strainers are used in blanching, to move food quickly from boiling water into an ice bath. Use fine-mesh strainers to strain delicate foods such as consommés and custard sauces; to make the strainer even more effective, line it with a double thickness of cheesecloth.

The chinois is a conical French-style strainer, named after its resemblance to a Chinese hat of the same shape. A fine-mesh chinois is used to clarify stocks, while others with coarser mesh are used in making jelly. A chinois of perforated metal instead of mesh is used to make very smooth purées. It employs a long, pointed wooden pestle that is used to force the food through the perforations. Lacking the pestle, you can use the back of a large spoon or the bottom of a ladle.

Chinois.

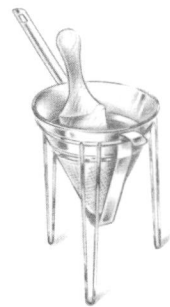

The colander is a freestanding strainer, with two handles and perforated holes; it is used to rinse foods and to drain foods such as pasta and vegetables.

Colander.

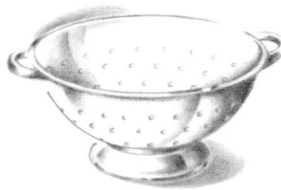

See also BLANCHING; COOKING TOOLS; PURÉEING.

STRAINING To pass a liquid or dry ingredient through a strainer in order to separate out unwanted particles. Straining is different from draining, in which food is rid of its liquid. The word *strain* also means to purée food by pressing it through a strainer or sieve with the back of a large spoon or another implement. See also PURÉEING; STRAINER.

STRAWBERRY See BERRY.

STRING BEAN See BEAN, FRESH.

STUDDING To decorate and/or flavor food by inserting seasonings such as garlic, spices, or nuts into the surface of the food. Whole cloves are commonly used to stud hams, while lamb and pork roasts are sometimes studded with garlic slivers or anchovy fillets. Breads containing raisins or other dried fruit are said to be studded with the fruit.

STUFFING Any mixture of food used to stuff another food and then cooked is called stuffing. Another word for stuffing is "dressing," a usage more common in the South and East. (In other parts of the country, dressing is cooked alongside the bird rather than stuffed into it.) Stuffed Thanksgiving turkey is the classic example, but any food with a natural or hollowed-out cavity, such as other kinds of poultry, squashes, vegetables, and fruits, may be filled with a stuffing. Other foods, such as meats, may be butterflied, stuffed, and tied closed or may have pockets cut into them for stuffing.

Although it was long believed that stuffing helped to flavor a bird, the stuffing is actually the main flavor beneficiary: the stuffing in a bird is always moister and more delicious than stuffing baked separately. Because a stuffed turkey takes longer to cook, however, and may become drier than a turkey without stuffing, many cooks prefer to bake the stuffing separately. If you do choose to stuff poultry, make sure that you stuff the bird loosely, giving the stuffing room to expand, and be sure to observe the safety rules given below.

One of the simplest stuffings for poultry and meats is a bread stuffing made from torn pieces, cubes, or crumbs of bread mixed with herbs, eggs, butter, chopped celery and onions, and stock. Torn pieces of bread seasoned with lemon, butter, and parsley is another, rather rustic stuffing. Foods such as nuts, vegetables, and oysters, may be added to bread stuffing. Other favorite poultry and meat stuffings have a base of corn bread, rice, or wild rice. Pork is often stuffed with a mixture of dried fruits; fresh fruits may be stuffed with sweet or savory mixtures.

Stuffing Safety

- Prepare stuffing just before roasting. This way, warm stuffing can be put into the bird and directly into the oven. A made-ahead and refrigerated stuffing will take longer to cook. If you do make it ahead, warm it before filling the bird.
- Never put stuffing into a bird the day before (or even several hours before) roasting. The warm stuffing can breed bacteria from the bird.
- Cook stuffing to 165°F on an instant-read thermometer. If it is not done and the bird is, transfer the stuffing to a baking dish and bake until it tests done.
- If adding meat to a stuffing, cook it thoroughly first. Stuffings made with raw meats may not cook through properly.

Quick Tip

Figure on ½ cup of stuffing for each pound of meat when stuffing poultry.

- To serve, spoon all the stuffing out of the bird at once. Do not let it sit more than 2 hours in the turkey or chicken.
- Store leftover stuffing separately from the bird in the refrigerator for no longer than 2 days.

SUBSTITUTIONS & EQUIVALENTS The following chart lists the equivalent weight or amount for specific measurements of certain foods, as well as acceptable substitutes for certain foods, when available.

Substitutions and Equivalents

FOOD	AMOUNT	EQUIVALENT/WEIGHT	SUBSTITUTE
Almonds, whole	1 cup	³⁄₄ cup ground	
Anchovy			Fresh sardines or anchovy paste
Apples	3 whole	2¹⁄₂ cups sliced	
Apricots, dried	1 cup	6 oz	
Arrowroot			Same amount of cornstarch; twice as much flour
Bacon	1 lb 1 slice, cooked	30 thin slices or 15 thick slices 1 tbsp, crumbled	
Baking powder	1 tsp		¹⁄₄ tsp baking soda plus ⁵⁄₈ tsp cream of tartar or ¹⁄₂ cup buttermilk or yogurt
Bananas	3 to 4 (1 lb)	1¹⁄₂ cups mashed, 2 cups sliced	
Barley	1 cup	3¹⁄₂ cups cooked	
Beans, dried	1 cup (7 oz)	2 to 2¹⁄₂ cups cooked	
Beans, green	1 lb	3 cups	
Beans, shelling	1 lb	1 cup shelled	
Bean sprouts	1 cup	4 oz	
Beets	1 lb, trimmed	2 cups cooked and sliced	
Bread crumbs, dried	¹⁄₄ cup	1 slice bread	
Bread crumbs, fresh	¹⁄₂ cup	1 slice bread	
Bread cubes, fresh	1 cup	1 slice bread	
Bulgur wheat	1 cup	3¹⁄₂ cups cooked	
Butter	¹⁄₂ stick 1 stick 2 sticks 4 sticks 4 tbsp	4 tbsp, ¹⁄₄ cup, 2 oz 8 tbsp, ¹⁄₂ cup, 4 oz 1 cup, 8 oz 2 cups, 16 oz (1 lb)	 ⁷⁄₈ cup vegetable oil or 1 cup lard 3 tbsp clarified butter

Substitutions and Equivalents, continued

Food	Amount	Equivalent/Weight	Substitute
Buttermilk	1 cup	8 oz	1 cup milk plus 1 tbsp fresh lemon juice, or 1 cup plain yogurt
Cabbage	1 head (1 lb)	4½ cups shredded or sliced	
Carrots	6 to 7 (1 lb)	3 cups shredded or sliced	
Cauliflower	2 lb	3 cups cut and cooked	
Celery	1 large rib	½ cup sliced or chopped	
Celery root	1 lb	3 cups grated or julienned	
Cheese	1 cup grated 1 cup crumbled feta 1 cup ricotta	4 oz 5 oz 8 oz	
Cherries	1 lb	2 to 2½ cups pitted	
Chestnuts	1½ lb	2½ cups peeled	
Chicken	1 whole (3½ lb)	3 cups cooked meat	
Chickpeas, dried	1 cup	2½ cups cooked	
Chocolate	1 square (1 oz)	4 tbsp grated	
Chocolate chips	6-oz pkg	1 cup morsels or bits	
Coconut, shredded	1 cup	4 oz	
Corn	2 ears	1 cup kernels	
Corn bread	8-in round or 9-in square	4 cups crumbs for stuffing	
Cornmeal	1 cup	4 cups cooked	
Cornstarch	1 tbsp		2 tbsp flour or 1 tbsp arrowroot
Couscous	1 cup	2½ cups cooked	
Crab	1 lb live	1 cup cooked meat	
Cracker and cookie crumbs	1 cup		28 soda crackers, 7 graham crackers, or 22 vanilla wafers
Cranberries	12-oz bag	3 cups	
Cream, heavy	1 cup	2 cups whipped	
Cream cheese	3-oz pkg	6 tbsp	
Cucumber	2 medium	3 cups sliced	

Substitutions and Equivalents, continued			
FOOD	**AMOUNT**	**EQUIVALENT/WEIGHT**	**SUBSTITUTE**
Currants, dried	1 cup	5 oz	
Dates	8 oz whole	1¼ cups chopped	
Eggs	1 large		¼ cup liquid egg substitute
	1 whole, large		2 yolks plus 1 tbsp water (for baking)
	1 white, large	2 tbsp	
	1 yolk, large	1 tbsp	
	5 whole, 7 whites, or 14 yolks, large	1 cup	
	3 large		2 jumbo, 3 extra-large, 3 medium, or 4 small
	4 large		3 jumbo, 4 extra-large, 5 medium, or 5 small
	6 large		5 jumbo, 5 extra-large, 7 medium, or 8 small
Figs, dried	1 lb	3 cups chopped	
Filo leaves	1-lb pkg	about 25 leaves	
Flour, all-purpose and whole wheat	1 lb 1 cup 1 cup	3½ cups unsifted	1 cup plus 2 tbsp cake flour 1 cup self-rising flour; omit any salt and baking powder listed in the recipe
Flour, cake	1 lb 1 cup	4½ cups sifted	1 cup less 2 tbsp all-purpose flour (with 2 tbsp cornstarch added if possible)
Flour, self-rising, unsifted	1 cup	5 oz	1 cup all-purpose flour plus 1½ tsp baking powder and ½ tsp salt
Garlic	2 medium cloves	1 tsp minced	
Gelatin	1 envelope	1 tbsp	4 sheets gelatin
Ginger, fresh	2-inch piece	2 tbsp grated or chopped	
Green onions, white part only	1 bunch (about 7)	½ cup chopped	
Hazelnuts, shelled	1 cup	5 oz	
Herbs	1 tbsp (3 tsp) fresh	1 tsp dried herbs	

substitutions & equivalents

Substitutions and Equivalents, continued

Food	Amount	Equivalent/Weight	Substitute
Horseradish, fresh	1 tbsp grated		2 tbsp prepared horseradish
Kasha (buckwheat groats)	1 cup	2½ to 3 cups cooked	
Leeks	2 lb trimmed	4 cups sliced or chopped	
Lemons	1 medium	1 to 3 tbsp juice, 1½ tsp zest	
Lentils, dried	1 cup	2½ cups cooked	
Lettuce, butter	1 head	4 cups torn leaves	
Lettuce, leaf and romaine	1 head (1 lb)	8 cups torn leaves	
Limes	1 medium	1½ to 2 tbsp juice	
Lobster	2 lb live	⅔ to 1 cup cooked meat	
Mangoes	1 lb	1½ cups chopped	
Milk, whole	1 cup		• ½ cup evaporated milk and ½ cup water; reduce the sugar in the recipe slightly • 1 cup skim milk plus 1 tbsp cream or melted butter
Mushrooms, fresh	4 oz	1 cup sliced, 1½ cups chopped	
Mustard, dry	1 tsp		1 tbsp prepared mustard
Nectarines	3 to 4 (1 lb)	2 cups sliced	
Nuts, whole	4 oz	¾ to 1 cup chopped, 1 cup ground	
Oats	1 cup	2 cups cooked	
Onions	1 medium	½ to ⅔ cup chopped	
Oranges	1 medium	⅓ cup juice, 2 to 3 tbsp zest	
Pasta	8 oz	3½ cups cooked	
Peaches	4 medium (1 lb)	2 cups peeled and sliced	
Pears	3 medium (1 lb)	2 cups peeled and sliced	
Peas	1 lb in shell 10-oz pkg	1 cup shelled 2 cups	
Pecans	1 cup	4 oz	
Peppers, bell	1 large	1 cup chopped	
Pineapple	1 medium	3 cups cubes	
Pistachios	1 lb in shell	2 cups shelled	
Plums	6 medium (1 lb)	2½ cups halved and pitted	

Substitutions and Equivalents, continued

FOOD	AMOUNT	EQUIVALENT/WEIGHT	SUBSTITUTE
Potatoes, white and sweet	1 lb	3 cups sliced, 2 cups mashed	
Prunes	1 lb	2 ½ cups pitted	
Pumpkin	3 to 4 lb	3 ½ cups puréed	
Purée	½ cup	About 1 cup berries, fruit, or cooked vegetables	
Raisins	1 cup	5 oz	
Rhubarb	1 lb	2 cups cooked	
Rice, brown	1 cup	3 to 4 cups cooked	
Rice, white and wild	1 cup	3 cups cooked	
Shallots	1 large	1 tbsp minced	
Shortening	1 lb	2 cups	2 cups butter (baking)
Shrimp	1 lb jumbo 1 lb large 1 lb medium	10 to 15 16 to 20 25 to 30	
Sour cream	1 cup	8 oz	1 cup plain yogurt
Spinach	1 lb bunched, or 10-oz bag	¾ cup chopped and cooked	
Split peas	2 cups	2 ½ cups cooked	
Squash, summer	1 lb	3 ½ cups sliced	
Squash, winter	3 lb	3 cups puréed	
Sugar, brown	1 lb 1 cup	2 ¼ cups packed	1 cup granulated sugar combined with 2 tbsp light or dark molasses
Sugar, confectioners'	1 lb	3 ½ to 4 cups	
Sugar, granulated	1 cup	8 oz	⅞ cup honey
Tapioca, instant	1 tbsp		1 tbsp flour
Tapioca flour	½ tbsp		1 tbsp flour
Tomatillos	5 to 6 whole		13-oz can, drained
Tomatoes	3 medium (1 lb)	1 ½ cups chopped	
Tomato sauce	2 cups		¾ cup tomato paste plus 1 cup water

Substitutions and Equivalents, continued

FOOD	AMOUNT	EQUIVALENT/WEIGHT	SUBSTITUTE
Vanilla	1 tsp extract		1-inch piece vanilla bean, halved and scraped
Yeast, active dry	1 pkg	2¼ tsp	1 cake (0.06 oz) compressed yeast
Yogurt, plain	1 cup	8 oz	

SUET See FAT & OIL.

SUGAR The Arabs introduced sugar to Europe and cultivated sugarcane in Sicily and Spain. Later it was shipped there from the sugarcane fields cultivated in the New World colonies. It was an expensive luxury until 1747, when a German physicist discovered that sugar could also be extracted from a type of beet. Only then did it become widely available in Europe. Today, it is sold in many different forms and has become an essential ingredient in cooking. Sugar sweetens, helps foods to caramelize and to stay fresh longer, encourages yeast to grow in bread dough, gives stability to egg whites, and preserves foods.

Granulated Sugar The most common sugar is granulated white sugar, which has been extracted from sugarcane or beets and refined by boiling, centrifuging, chemical treatment, and straining. For baking recipes, buy only sugar that is specifically labeled cane sugar; beet sugar will have an unpredictable effect on many recipes.

SUPERFINE When finely ground, granulated sugar becomes superfine sugar,

Quick Tip

To make your own superfine sugar, simply whirl granulated sugar in a blender or in a food processor fitted with the metal blade.

known as castor or caster sugar in England. Because it dissolves rapidly, it is preferred for cold recipes such as mixed drinks (it is also sold as bar sugar) and delicate mixtures such as beaten egg whites.

Confectioners' Sugar Crushed to a powder and mixed with a little cornstarch to prevent lumping, granulated sugar becomes confectioners' (or powdered) sugar, known as icing sugar in England. It is used for dusting foods and decorating plates and in icings and candies. Even though confectioners' sugar has been treated, it still forms little lumps in the package and should be sifted before using in most recipes.

Dusting a cake with confectioners' sugar.

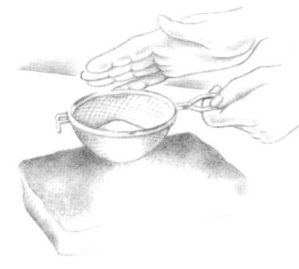

Brown Sugar Brown sugar is simply granulated sugar colored with molasses. It has a rich flavor and a soft, moist texture and is available as mild-flavored light brown sugar or the more strongly flavored dark brown sugar. Granulated brown sugar, also called Brownulated sugar, is good for sprinkling because it is dry and doesn't clump. It should not be used as a substitute for brown sugar in baking, however.

BROWN SUGAR SAVVY When using brown sugar, keep the following in mind:

- To soften hardened brown sugar, place a cut piece of apple in a container or plastic bag of brown sugar and close it tightly for a day or so. It can also be softened by sprinkling it with a little water and placing it in a 200°F oven for a few minutes.
- To sprinkle brown sugar evenly over dishes such as crème brûlée, push it through a small sieve with the back of a spoon.
- To keep brown sugar soft, refrigerate it in a tightly closed container.

Other Sugars

COARSE SUGAR Coarse sugar, also called sugar crystals or sanding sugar, comes in large granules and is used to decorate cookies, cakes, sweet breads, and candies. It is available in some cookware stores and in specialty-food stores.

COLORED SUGAR Colored sugar comes in different hues and in both coarse and fine grains. It is used for decorating cakes and cookies and is available in most well-stocked supermarkets.

DATE SUGAR Date sugar is made from ground dried dates. It does not dissolve well, but it may be used in cooking and some baking.

JAGGERY SUGAR Also called palm sugar, jaggery is made from palm tree sap or sugarcane. This unrefined sugar has dark, coarse grains and is used in Indian and Southeast Asian cooking. It is available as a soft spread and as a solid cake. Look for it in Indian markets. Dark brown sugar may be substituted for piloncillo and jaggery.

MAPLE SUGAR Maple sugar is made by boiling maple sap almost dry. It is twice as sweet as granulated white sugar and is often made into molded candies attractively packaged for gift giving.

PILONCILLO SUGAR Piloncillo is an unrefined Mexican sugar that is formed into blocks or dark brown tapered cones. It is available in Latin markets.

RAW SUGAR The sugars marketed as "raw" in the United States are actually partially refined. Turbinado, which has light brown coarse crystals, has been washed with steam. Demerara sugar and Barbados sugar are also raw sugars that have been purified. A sugar that retains much of the nutritive value of unrefined sugar is Sucanat, which is a dark brown granulated sugar made by dehydrating the juice of organically grown sugarcane. It has a nutty, molasses-like flavor. Organic sugar is also made from evaporated sugarcane juice, clarified to make a light tan granulated sugar that pours easily and has a warm, clean flavor.

ROCK SUGAR Amber-colored rock sugar, used in some Chinese dishes, comes in large crystals and is made by cooking sugar until it begins to caramelize. It is not as sweet as granulated white sugar.

HOW TO *Make Simple Syrup*

Make a jar of this syrup and keep it on hand in your refrigerator to use in making cocktails, ice cream and sorbet mixtures, frostings and candies, and for poaching fruit. For a heavy syrup, use equal parts sugar and water; for a medium syrup, use 2 parts water and 1 part sugar; and for a thin syrup, use 3 parts water and 1 part sugar. Plan on the following yield: 1 cup sugar will make about 1 cup heavy syrup, 2 cups medium syrup, or 3 cups thin syrup.

1. Combine equal parts granulated sugar and water in a heavy saucepan. Place over low heat and stir until the sugar has dissolved.
2. Bring to a boil and cook without stirring for 1 minute. Pour into a glass jar. Cover and refrigerate indefinitely.

See also CANDY MAKING; CORN SYRUP; HONEY; MAPLE SYRUP; MOLASSES.

SUGAR SYRUP See CANDY MAKING; SUGAR.

SUNCHOKE See JERUSALEM ARTICHOKE.

SUN-DRIED TOMATO Fresh tomatoes dried in the sun (or in special dehydrators or in a very low oven) take on a deep, intense tomato flavor and chewy, dense texture. Sun-dried tomatoes make a simple topping for a pizza or can be tucked inside a sandwich. Use them in salads or to season braises and stews.

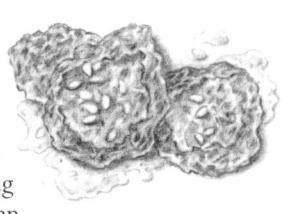

Selecting Sun-dried tomatoes are sold dry, often loose in plastic bags or in bulk, or packed in jars of olive oil. Those packed in oil tend to be sweeter and have more flavor than the dry-packed ones.

Storing Once opened, jars of oil-packed sun-dried tomatoes should be stored in the refrigerator. Dry-packed tomatoes should be stored airtight in a cool, dry place. They will last indefinitely.

Preparing Oil-packed sun-dried tomatoes can be used straight from the jar, after being drained. Dry-packed ones must be rehydrated before using.

HOW TO *Rehydrate Dry-Packed Sun-Dried Tomatoes*

1. In a bowl, cover the tomatoes with hot water and let stand for about 30 minutes.
2. Drain the tomatoes, reserving the soaking liquid. It can lend a good tomato flavor to soups, braises, and stews.

Quick Tip

A second, more flavorful, way to rehydrate dry-packed sun-dried tomatoes is to cover them with extra-virgin olive oil and let stand for 24 hours. Refrigerate the tomatoes in the oil and keep them for several months. Use the oil for salad dressing, drizzle it over toasted bread, or toss it with hot pasta.

The oil in which sun-dried tomatoes are packed has a rich tomato flavor and is often too good to be discarded. Taste it and use it for making salad dressings or brush it over pizzas still warm from the oven.

SWEATING A French technique of cooking food, usually vegetables, over low heat in a little fat in a covered pan. Sweating causes the food to release its juices and to cook without browning, thereby concentrating the flavor of the food. A variation of this technique is the preliminary step in many recipes that calls for sautéing onions, shallots, and/or garlic until translucent or just tender.

SWEETBREADS The thymus glands of calves or lambs. Each gland has two lobes, one elongated and the other round, both with the same subtle, rich flavor and delicate texture. Veal sweetbreads are widely considered better, while those of lamb are less common. Sweetbreads are blanched, then often breaded and fried and sauced.

Selecting Look for sweetbreads that are plump, compact, and surrounded by a shiny membrane. There should be no dark spots.

Storing Sweetbreads are highly perishable. Refrigerate them as soon as you get home, and serve the day of purchase.

Preparing Sweetbreads must be peeled and firmed before cooking. Long cooking will destroy their delicate texture; cook them quickly to preserve their tenderness. Sweetbreads can be poached whole or sliced and sautéed.

HOW TO *Peel and Firm Sweetbreads*

1. Cover the sweetbreads with water, bring to a gentle boil, reduce the heat to low, and simmer for about 5 minutes.
2. Drain and transfer to a bowl of cold water. Pull off the membrane that covers each sweetbread and remove any fat and tubes, working with the sweetbreads in the water.
3. Drain and put the sweetbreads on a tray and cover with plastic wrap. Top with a plate and weight it evenly with heavy cans or other items. Refrigerate until firm, about 3 hours.

SWEETENED CONDENSED MILK

See MILK.

SWEET PEPPER See BELL PEPPER.

SWEET POTATO Another of the New World's contributions to the world larder, the sweet potato has either yellow-brown skin and yellow flesh, or dark reddish or purplish skin and dark orange flesh. The latter is commonly known in the United States as a yam, although it is a different species from the true yam.

Sweet potato (below) vs. "yam" (above).

Both types of sweet potato may be cooked in a wide variety of ways. Baked whole, they are served with or without a sweet or savory topping. Cubed or sliced, they are baked with a sweet glaze. They also can be cooked and puréed and served alongside meat or poultry—often pork, ham, or turkey—or used to make a pie filling similar to pumpkin pie. A staple of Southern and tropical cooking, sweet potatoes are puréed and topped with marshmallows, then baked as a Thanksgiving side dish; added in chunks to stews and soups; and candied as a holiday treat in Mexico.

Selecting Sweet potatoes are available year-round, but their true seasons are fall and winter. Choose firm, unblemished sweet potatoes without any breaks in their thin skin.

Storing Sweet potatoes do not keep well. Store them in a cool, dark place, but plan to use them within a week or so.

Preparing To bake whole sweet potatoes, scrub them well first and prick their skins in a few places with a fork. Place them on a baking sheet to catch their juices, and bake in a preheated 400°F oven until they are tender when pierced with a knife, about 45 minutes. They may then be peeled and sliced or cut into chunks for glazing, or puréed. You can also peel uncooked sweet potatoes and cook them in salted boiling water until tender before glazing or puréeing.

See also STEAMING; YAM.

SWISS CHARD See GREENS, DARK; STEAMING.

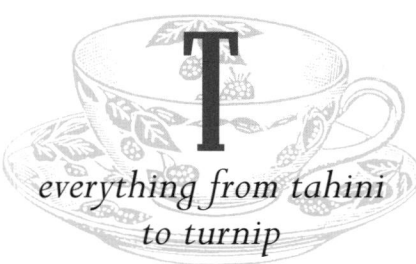

everything from tahini to turnip

TAHINI This paste, made from ground sesame seeds, has a rich, creamy flavor and a concentrated sesame taste. Tahini, also called sesame paste, is used in the popular chickpea spread known as hummus and in baba ghanoush, a Middle Eastern eggplant purée. It is also combined with lemon juice and seasonings to make *taratoor,* a thin Middle Eastern sauce used as a dip for vegetables and pita bread, as a dressing for salads, and as a sauce for fish, vegetables, and falafel. The oil often separates from the paste and should be stirred in before using.
Storing After opening, tahini can be refrigerated for up to 2 months.

Quick Tip

Turn a jar of tahini upside down occasionally and let it stand for a few days so that the oil redistributes itself throughout the paste.

TAMARIND Also known as Indian date, tamarind is the fruit of a tropical tree. The long, dark pods are filled with small seeds and a distinct sweet-and-sour pulp that is dried and used in Indian, Southeast Asian, and Middle Eastern kitchens in much the same way that cooks in the West use lemon

juice. Tamarind is available in several forms. In addition to whole pods, you may find blocks of tamarind paste and frozen pouches of pulp. There is also frozen nectar, sweetened tamarind syrup, and tamarind concentrate.

Tamarind pulp.

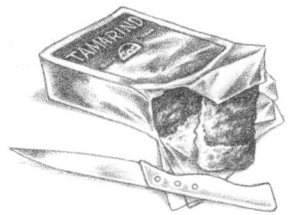

Tamarind pairs beautifully with aromatic seasonings such as ginger, garlic, chiles, and coconut milk, and Indian cooks have long used it in chutneys, relishes, curries, and preserves. In Mexico, tamarind is used to flavor one version of the refreshing fruit drinks known as *aguas frescas*. Western cooks have begun to experiment with the fruit, using it in sorbets and salad dressings. Tamarind's natural acidity helps to tenderize tougher cuts of meats, making it a popular ingredient for marinades in both Asian and Latin American kitchens.
Selecting Locating tamarind in pod form may take a bit of searching. It is increasingly available in large supermarkets, but you may need to search your local specialty-food stores and Asian, Latin, or Middle Eastern markets to find it. Fresh whole pods should bend easily in your hands. As an alternative, look for packaged blocks of paste or frozen pouches of pulp.
Storing Pods and unopened packages of tamarind paste will keep indefinitely when stored in a cool, dry place. Once opened, packages of paste can be refrigerated for about 3 months.
Preparing To use the whole dried pods: For 1 cup of tamarind pulp you will need about $4\frac{1}{2}$ ounces dried pods. Open the pods and remove the seeds. Combine the

t

pods with 1 cup of warm water and let soak for about 20 minutes. Pour through a fine-mesh sieve, pressing the pulp through the sieve with the back of a large wooden spoon. Stir to combine, then refrigerate in a tightly sealed glass jar for up to 1 week.

HOW TO *Use Packaged Tamarind Paste*
1. Use a knife to cut off about 2 ounces of the pulp. In a bowl, combine the pulp with about ½ cup warm water.
2. Soak for about 20 minutes before straining. Makes about ¾ cup.

TAMARI SAUCE See SOY FOODS.

TANGERINE See MANDARIN ORANGE.

TAPAS (TOP-uhs) Small, flavorful appetizers that appear in bars and restaurants all over Spain. Tapas may be hot or cold, as simple as a bowl of olives or a more involved dish such as Spanish tortilla, which is related to an omelet; fried squid; or grilled pork with romesco sauce.

TAPENADE Capers, anchovies, and garlic are some of the other ingredients that go into this classic Provençal olive spread. The ingredients are mashed into a paste, preferably with a mortar and pestle, and the paste is used as a spread for grilled bread, smeared on pizzas, or used as a dip for vegetables and crudités. It may also be used as an ingredient in sauces, such as for pasta, and marinades, especially for grilled foods. A little tapenade goes a long way, as its flavor is highly concentrated and salty. The ingredients (other than olives) and their proportions often vary, although the word *tapenade* comes from the Provençal word *tapeno,* meaning capers, and these tiny buds are usually considered an essential part of the dish. Some tapenades contain lemon juice or other seasonings and/or tuna fish. By contrast, *olivada* is an Italian spread made only of black olives, olive oil, and black pepper.

Both green and black tapenades, made from either green or black olives, are usually available in jars in specialty-food stores and many supermarkets in the United States. In their home in the south of France, a dazzling variety of tapenades, freshly made from a wide range of olives, are sold at weekly street markets.
Storing Once opened, tapenade should be kept in the refrigerator for up to 6 months.

See also ANCHOVY; CAPER; OLIVE.

TAPIOCA A starchy substance derived from the root of the cassava plant, tapioca can be used to thicken sauces and fruit fillings for pies, as well to make a dessert enjoyed by children everywhere. Tapioca comes in three basic forms, pearl (small dried balls of tapioca starch), granulated (coarsely broken-up pearl tapioca), or instant (very finely granulated pearl tapioca). Asian markets and some supermarkets carry tapioca flour, also called tapioca starch, which is used much like cornstarch.
Selecting For tapioca pudding, choose either pearl, granulated, or instant tapioca. To thicken sauces and fruit fillings, choose either instant tapioca or tapioca flour.
Storing All forms of tapioca will keep indefinitely in a cool, dark place.
Preparing Pearl tapioca should be soaked in cold water for an hour before using. Granulated and instant tapioca do not need soaking. As a thickener, 1 tablespoon instant tapioca or 1½ teaspoons tapioca flour can be substituted for 1 tablespoon flour.

TARRAGON See HERB.

TART See PIE & TART.

TARTAR SAUCE See SAUCE.

TART PAN See BAKEWARE.

TASTING The tasting of a dish during and after preparation is one of the keys to good cooking because the level of the seasoning needed can be affected by many factors. For example, some fruits need more or less sugar, depending on their natural sugars and degree of ripeness, while some vegetables and other foods not at their peak of flavor may need more seasoning. Temperature also affects the taste of foods. Flavors are strongest when heated, so chilled and frozen foods need relatively more seasoning. Ice cream, for example, must be made from a base that tastes very sweet at room temperature, as freezing will dull the sweetness. The good cook tastes a dish throughout the making of it. If a dish doesn't taste right at any stage of preparation, it won't taste right when it's done.

Recipes often specify salt and other ingredients "to taste" or give a range of amounts, as some people need to limit their salt intake and others prefer their dishes more or less spicy or piquant. When using salt or such assertive flavors as cayenne or rosemary, always use the smallest amount specified. You can always add more later to suit your taste—but you can't take it away.

"To taste" is not always meant literally, however. In foods that can't be tasted with pleasure, such as salted raw eggplant, or that could endanger your health, such as raw poultry or meat mixtures, this phrase means to use the seasoning lightly or moderately, as you prefer. (Some people are careful not to taste batters made with raw egg, because of concern for salmonella. A small portion of a raw meat mixture can be cooked until it has lost all pinkness throughout and then tasted for seasoning.)

Whether or not a recipe method says to "taste and adjust the seasoning," always taste a completed dish before you plan to serve it, and add more of any of the seasonings it seems to need. This is particularly true for highly or complexly seasoned dishes that depend for their success on the proper balance of seasonings.

See also ADJUSTING THE SEASONING.

TEA A cup of tea manages to be both calming and stimulating at the same time. Perhaps that's why tea always has gone hand in hand with meditation and reflection. The amount of theophylline, a close relative of caffeine, in black tea is just enough to keep you awake and aware, while the act of drinking the hot, fragrant brew seems to offer comfort and solace. Native to China, tea began to be cultivated there around 2000 B.C. Exported to Europe in the 17th century, it created a sensation, especially in England, where it is still favored over coffee, that other stimulating beverage.

There are three common types of tea leaves: black, green, and oolong. (A fourth kind, white tea, is very rare.) These three all come from the same species of plant, which produces different-tasting teas depending on where the plant was grown and how it was processed. The best teas grow at the highest altitudes and consist of the smallest new-growth leaves and the unopened leaf buds, picked by hand. Black tea leaves are fermented, then heated and dried. Green tea leaves, by contrast, are steamed and dried without fermenting, and oolong tea is made from leaves that are partially fermented. Black tea leaves produce a dark, full-flavored brew, while green tea

t

is a pale greenish yellow with a flowery flavor and astringent taste. Oolong tea is lighter than black tea and darker than green. The best known is Formosa oolong, which is appreciated for its bright and fruity flavor.

Quick Bite

Tea is sometimes used to dye white fabric a subtle shade of beige.

The names of black teas can be confusing. Many black tea blends, for example, were long ago given an arbitrary name, such as Earl Grey, English breakfast, or Prince of Wales, designed to intrigue the British consumer. Other teas—such as Assam and Ceylon—are instead named for their place of origin. Still other black teas are named for the size of their leaves, such as pekoe (medium leaves) and orange pekoe (small leaves), while the *souchong* in Lapsang Souchong signifies large leaves.

Green teas have a grassy, slightly bitter taste that seems to go perfectly with Asian food. Like black tea, green tea is high in vitamin C, while containing less theophylline, tea's natural stimulant. In addition, both black and green teas are beneficial to healthy teeth and gums.

A number of flavored teas exist, from Earl Grey (which is flavored with bergamot oil) and teas scented with flowers to newer teas flavored with fruits such as mango and peach. Herbal teas, known also as tisanes, are not technically teas but rather infusions of herbs and other flavorings. They are valued for their reputed health benefits, which vary from herb to herb.

In the United States, tea is often served cold, sweetened and iced, usually with lemon. Bottled iced teas are also popular. Instant iced tea and decaffeinated black tea may be found in supermarkets.

Tea is also used as a cooking ingredient, the best-known examples being tea-smoked duck and tea eggs. The latter are flavored and colored by steeping them in tea. Green tea is used to make a refreshing ice cream.

Selecting The world of tea is wide and varied. As with wine, there are so many different styles and flavors that you could spend years learning about this drink. Common commercial brands are made from blends of inferior bits of leaves. Look instead for high-quality teas sold in coffeehouses, tea shops, or specialty-food stores. Herbal teas are available in natural-food stores.

Storing Teas are available in loose form or in tea bags in foil- or plastic-lined packages. Store tea in its packaging in an airtight container in a cool, dark place for up to 1 year.

Preparing Although the tea bag is a marvel of convenience, it does not make the best tea, as the leaves are unable to circulate in the hot water and fully release their essence. The best solution is to spoon loose tea into the bottom of a pot. If you prefer not to deal with a few tea leaves in the bottom of your cup, use a strainer or a pot that comes with its own infuser, or buy the largest metal-mesh tea ball you can.

Tea ball.

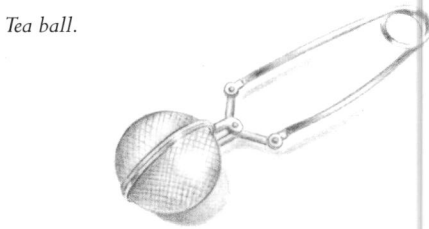

Quick Tip

Tea balls also come in handy for holding spices when mulling wine or cider or for holding herbs to make a bouquet garni.

HOW TO *Make a Pot of Tea*

1. Choose a ceramic teapot that is just the size of the amount of tea you are making. Bring a teapotful of water to a boil in a kettle.
2. Pour the boiling water into the teapot, cover the pot with its lid, and set it aside to warm. Fill the kettle with 1 cup fresh cold spring water or filtered water per cup of tea you are brewing and bring it just to a boil.
3. Turn off the kettle and let it sit for a minute. (Like coffee, tea is best when made with water that is slightly below boiling temperature.) Empty the teapot. Add 1 level teaspoon loose tea per cup to the teapot, to the teapot's infuser, or to a large metal-mesh tea ball. Add the infuser or tea ball, if using, to the pot and pour in the hot water. Cover the pot.
4. Let the tea steep for 1 to 3 minutes for green tea and 3 to 6 minutes for black tea. Oolong teas take from 6 to 8 minutes, while herbal teas need 8 to 12 minutes.
5. Stir the tea in the pot or in the infuser or swirl the tea ball around in the tea to extract more flavor from the leaves, then remove the infuser or ball from the pot. If necessary, pour the tea through a strainer into each cup.
6. If you have made more than 2 cups, use a tea cozy or wrap the teapot in a thick kitchen towel to help keep the tea hot.

HOW TO *Make Sun-Brewed Iced Tea*

1. Fill a clear glass or plastic container with cold water, keeping track of the amount of water as you fill the container.
2. Measure 3 tablespoons of leaves per quart of water. Place in a tea ball (you may need more than one).
3. Placing the container in direct sunlight, steep the tea in the water for 2 to 3 hours, or until it is strong enough for your taste.

TECHNIQUES Those folks fortunate enough to have grown up in a household with a good cook who shared his or her knowledge will find the ability to execute cooking techniques an almost natural occurrence when they are finally in their own kitchen. After years of watching while standing beside someone who is comfortable in the kitchen, these students will instinctively know how to seed a tomato, measure a cup of flour, or truss a chicken. When a recipe calls for reducing a sauce, blanching a green vegetable, clarifying a stock, barding a lean bird, or deglazing a pan, they will act almost without thinking.

Not everyone is so fortunate. But anyone can learn to become a good cook by trial and error, persistence, and openness to gleaning insights from any source he or she can find.

The complete mastery of cooking techniques begins with understanding how to perform the most basic kitchen tasks, such as chopping an onion, dredging a chicken breast, beating egg whites until stiff, or frosting a cake. Depending on the specific interests of a particular cook, it can extend to such exotic techniques as opening a sea urchin, assembling a *pâté en croûte,* hanging a game bird to age and season, or fashioning a marzipan blossom. Technique reaches all the way to presentation, whether the recipe calls for piping an attractive filling for stuffed eggs, hollowing out a pineapple to hold a fruit salad, or floating paper-thin vegetable slices atop a clear soup.

For complete information on basic cooking techniques, see individual technique listings throughout this book.

TEMPEH See SOY FOODS.

TEMPERATURE The definitions of some key temperatures vary, as you will see if you compare temperature charts among several different cookbooks. The chart on page 446 shows commonly accepted temperatures for different stages of cooking, oven heats, and other conditions.

Key Temperatures Chart

Freezer	0°F
Refrigerator	8° to 40°F
Cool room temperature	65°F
Warm room temperature	70° to 75°F
Lukewarm (tepid) liquid	95°F
Warm liquid	105° to 115°F
Hot liquid	120°F
Boiling water	212°F
Warm temperature for rising bread	80°F
Low/slow oven	180° to 200°F
Warm oven	300° to 325°F
Moderate oven	350° to 375°F
Hot oven	400° to 450°F
Very hot oven	475° to 500°F

See also DONENESS; HIGH-ALTITUDE COOKING; MEASURING; ROASTING; SAFETY.

TEMPERING Tempering means to melt and cool chocolate to very specific temperatures in order to create a shiny, smooth patina once it rehardens. Tempering also means to heat beaten eggs slightly before adding them to hot liquid, in order to keep them from curdling.

Tempered chocolate is preferred for candy coatings, molded candies, and decorations because it is silkier and more malleable and flavorful than untempered chocolate, and it breaks with a "snap" when bitten. Tempering chocolate also prevents "bloom," the white coating caused by excessive heat or humidity.

To temper bittersweet or semisweet chocolate, the melted chocolate is heated to 115° to 118°F, which breaks down the microscopic structure of the cocoa butter crystals. The chocolate is then cooled to 89° to 91°F, which causes the crystals to align perfectly. (The temperatures for tempering milk chocolate and white chocolate are slightly lower.)

HOW TO *Temper Bittersweet or Semisweet Chocolate*
This is one of the simplest ways to temper chocolate. It is sometimes known as the quick tempering method.

1. Chop the chocolate with a large chef's knife. Melt two-thirds of the chocolate in a double boiler over not-quite-simmering water until it reaches a temperature of 115° to 118°F on a candy thermometer. Make sure the bottom of the chocolate pan does not touch the water, and stir the chocolate occasionally as it melts.

2. Remove the upper portion of the double boiler from the bottom portion. Stir in the remaining one-third chopped chocolate until the mixture cools to 89° to 91°F, or until a little of the chocolate dabbed on your upper lip or inside wrist feels cool.

3. Place the pan in a larger pan of tepid water or on a heating pad to keep the chocolate at a constant 89° to 91°F while you work with it. If the temperature falls so much that the chocolate becomes hard to work with, you may reheat it to a maximum of 91°F. If you exceed this temperature, however, the chocolate will lose temper and you will have to repeat the entire process again.

Quick Tip

To test whether chocolate is in temper, spoon a little on a saucer and refrigerate it until hardened and set, 2 to 3 minutes. If it looks glossy, the chocolate is in temper.

To temper eggs, beat a little hot milk or cream into the beaten eggs, then gradually whisk the egg mixture into the hot liquid.

TEMPURA In its simplest description, Japanese tempura is batter-coated, deep-fried fish and vegetables. The basic method was introduced to the island nation by Portuguese missionaries in the 16th century (the word *tempura* reputedly comes from the Portuguese *tempora,* a day of abstinence from meat), but the Japanese developed it into an art, producing lacy, nongreasy, crisp morsels. The requisite dipping sauce is made from fish stock, soy sauce, and mirin (sweet cooking wine).

TENDERIZING See POUNDING.

TEQUILA See SPIRITS.

TERIYAKI A favorite Japanese dish among Americans, although its definition differs depending on whether you are in Japan or the United States. In the former, teriyaki is a sauce brushed onto chicken, fish, or meat during the final stages of grilling or panfrying, while in the latter the term refers to chicken, fish, or meat that has been marinated in the sauce before grilling, or sometimes simply coated with the sauce just before grilling. The bottled sweet sauce is widely available in supermarkets and can be used as a glaze on nearly any grilled food. You can make a simple home version by mixing equal parts sake, mirin (sweet cooking wine), or sherry and dark soy sauce with sugar to taste.

TERRINE A rectangular or oval heat-proof cooking and serving dish. Pâté mixtures are classically cooked in terrines. When served from the dish, the food is also called a terrine, or *pâté en terrine,* although it may also simply be called a pâté. The dishes are usually made of heavy 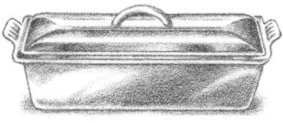 earthenware or enameled iron, but porcelain or Pyrex are also used.

See also PÂTÉ.

THAWING The process of restoring frozen food to room temperature is called thawing, or defrosting. Frozen poultry, meat, and fish should be thawed in the refrigerator to keep bacteria from multiplying. Large pieces of meat (over 4 pounds) will take 4 to 7 hours per pound to defrost this way; steaks and chops will take 8 to 14 hours or overnight. A whole chicken will take 12 to 16 hours, while a frozen turkey, depending on size, can take 2 to 5 days to thaw fully; figure on 3 to 4 hours per pound of poultry.

Thin pieces of meat, fish, or chicken may be thawed at room temperature in less than 2 hours. Or, put the food in a zippered plastic bag and immerse it in a large container or sink of cold water. This will generally cut the thawing time by about one-third. Food defrosted this way, however, will lose more of its juices and be drier when cooked.

Caution!

Thawing food in warm water is not safe. This encourages the growth of bacteria.

Meat, fish, or chicken may also be thawed in a microwave, although it will also lose some of its moisture and must be watched carefully. Wrap the food in waxed paper and microwave on Low in 5-minute increments; let the food stand for 5 minutes; and then check to see if it has thawed. Repeat as necessary until the food is barely thawed. Food thawed this way should be cooked immediately.

Vegetables may be safely thawed at room temperature or by cooking them in a small amount of boiling water.

See also FOOD SAFETY; FREEZING.

THERMOMETER See BAKING; COOK-
ING TOOLS; SAFETY; TEMPERATURE.

THICKENING Sauces depend on numerous ingredients and techniques for the
alchemy that turns a thin liquid into a
velvety substance to dress or accompany
food. Other dishes, from soups to desserts,
also use thickeners to give them body. Following is a list of thickening agents and
methods used in various cuisines and dishes.
Agar-agar A seaweed-based gelatin
used in Asia and preferred by vegetarians
to animal-derived gelatin. See SEAWEED.
Arrowroot Often used in place of cornstarch or flour in puddings and sauces, as
it doesn't have the chalky taste of undercooked cornstarch and it is more easily
digested than wheat. Use half as much
arrowroot as flour and the same amount
as cornstarch, and stir it into liquid before
adding it to a dish. Arrowroot will give a
sauce a lovely sheen. The thickening effect
will not hold up to reheating.
Butter A little butter (1 tablespoon per
¼ cup of sauce) stirred into sauce at the
end of cooking will "finish" or "mount" the
sauce, adding gloss and flavor and thickening it very slightly. Serve immediately.
Cornstarch Used in Asian cooking to
thicken stir-fry sauces and in American
cooking to thicken some pie fillings and
puddings, cornstarch will give a sauce a
glossy sheen. It should be dissolved in cold
liquid before being added to other ingredients: stir 1 tablespoon cornstarch into
2 tablespoons water in a small cup until
dissolved. This amount will thicken about
1 cup liquid. To substitute for flour, use
half as much cornstarch as flour. Cornstarch can have a chalky taste if it is undercooked, so when adding it to sauces, be
sure to stir for several minutes over heat.
Boiling can cause a cornstarch-thickened
sauce to separate. See also CORNSTARCH.

Cream Heavy cream added to a hot sauce
or soup will thicken it slightly. Add 2 tablespoons per ¼ cup of sauce. Beaten heavy
cream is used to thicken mousses and some
puddings and other desserts.
Egg Yolks When olive oil or melted
butter is beaten into egg yolks, the yolks
gradually absorb the liquid and emulsify,
thickening to make mayonnaise and butter
sauce, respectively. Egg yolks beaten with
wine and sugar over heat thicken to make
zabaglione, also called sabayon or sabayon
sauce, and when whisked over heat with
warm milk and sugar they thicken to
become crème anglaise, or custard sauce.
Heat gently to avoid curdling.
Flour Flour is a common thickener, but it
must be used correctly. When you add flour
directly into a liquid, it may clump. It will
also add the raw taste of flour to a mixture
unless the mixture is cooked for at least
several minutes after the flour is added.
Flour can be gradually whisked into a small
amount of milk, water, or stock until all
lumps disappear. The mixture, known as a
slurry, is then added to another liquid and
cooked to thicken it. Or, flour may be
mixed with fat, as when making a roux (see
below), and cooked for a few minutes to
remove the raw flour taste before it is incorporated into a liquid.

Quick Tip

The consistency of a gravy or sauce depends
on the amount of flour used: for thin, use
1 tablespoon flour for 1 cup of liquid; for
medium-thick, use 2 tablespoons flour for
1 cup of liquid; and for thick, use 3 tablespoons
of flour for 1 cup of liquid.

BEURRE MANIÉ A French technique for
thickening and enriching sauces and stews
at the end of cooking is to blend equal
parts flour and soft butter to make a paste,

beurre manié. The sauce is removed from the heat, the paste is whisked in, and the sauce is stirred over heat until thickened.

Roux Another mixture of flour and fat, roux is the basis of a béchamel sauce and is also used to thicken soups and other foods. It is made by heating fat and whisking in flour. After cooking out the raw taste of the flour, liquid is whisked in. A white roux is cooked for 2 to 3 minutes over medium heat. It is usually made with butter, although a mixture of butter and olive oil or all olive oil can be used. For some dishes, the roux is cooked to a pale tan. This blond roux has a toasted taste. Brown roux, cooked until dark and nutty in taste, is made with butter, drippings, or lard, and is one of the foundations of Cajun and Creole cuisine. The darker a roux, however, the less thickening power it has.

For a thin sauce or for soup, make a roux of 1 tablespoon butter mixed with 1 tablespoon flour per 1 cup liquid. For a thicker sauce, use 2 tablespoons butter and 2 tablespoons flour per 1 cup liquid.

Gelatin This animal protein–based substance is dissolved in liquid to add to mixtures that are then allowed to set and thicken. See GELATIN.

Reduction Boiling or simmering a liquid to reduce it in volume both thickens it and concentrates its flavor. See REDUCING.

Starch Pasta cooking water contains starch, so a bit of this water may be reserved and added to a pasta sauce. Potato cooking water is also a good source of starch for thickening sauces.

Tapioca Either tapioca flour or instant tapioca may be used to thicken fruit pie fillings (as long as they are not baked in a lattice-top pie), puddings, or sauces. Don't boil a mixture after tapioca flour has been added, or its consistency can turn gluey. To substitute for flour, use an equivalent amount. See TAPIOCA.

Tomato Paste Use tomato paste to thicken and intensify the taste of a tomato-based sauce. See also TOMATO.

Vegetable Purée Some cooks use puréed vegetables to thicken soups and sauces in place of butter, cream, flour, or egg yolks, both for the sake of lowering calories and fat content and for the clean, interesting tastes that vegetable purées provide. Many soups, such as corn, bean, and potato, are made by puréeing some of the contents for thickness and leaving the rest whole for texture.

THYME See HERB.

TIN FOIL See ALUMINUM FOIL.

TOASTING To heat foods until they are fragrant or lightly browned in order to bring out their flavor and/or to crisp them. Bread is toasted in a toaster, under a broiler, or on a grill to make such toasts as croutons and *crostini,* which are used plain or as a base for butter or other spreads or foods. Nuts, spices, and dried chiles may all be toasted to intensify their flavor before using them in recipes. The quickest way to toast these foods is in a dry pan over medium heat. The food should be stirred frequently and watched carefully to prevent it from burning. The minute it becomes fragrant and/or lightly browned, empty it onto a baking sheet or into a bowl. Even if taken off the heat, the food will continue to cook in the pan, and it might burn. Some cooks prefer to toast nuts in the oven; but watch them very carefully or they may burn. See CHILE; NUT; SPICE.

TOFU The Japanese word for bean curd, or soybean curd. See SOY FOODS.

TOMATILLO Although they look like small green tomatoes and are called *tomates*

t

verdes in Mexico, tomatillos are relatives of the Cape gooseberry, not the tomato. Strip away the papery husk that encloses them to get at one of the essential ingredients for *salsa verde,* the popular Mexican table sauce. Tomatillos have a lemony, herbal flavor that's sharply tart when raw and somewhat tempered by cooking. Some recipes, such as those for raw green salsas, use raw tomatillos, while most others specify poaching them until tender or roasting them on a griddle or in a skillet. Tomatillos are also used in pork stews and in green moles. Canned tomatillos, available in many Latino food stores, lack the spark of fresh but are an acceptable substitute.

Selecting Tomatillos are available off and on throughout the year; they are at their best from August through November. They are most commonly found in Latino markets but are increasingly available in supermarkets and specialty-produce stores. Choose firm, unblemished tomatillos with tightly clinging husks.

Storing Keep tomatillos in a perforated plastic bag in the refrigerator crisper for up to 2 weeks.

Preparing Tomatillos must be husked before use. Use your fingers to peel the brown papery husk under warm running water, and the husk and the sticky, resinous substance that lightly coats the fruit will rinse right off.

Once husked, fresh tomatillos may be added to sauces raw and chopped, to simmer with other ingredients. Some recipes call for them to be briefly boiled in water until their skins split, about 15 minutes. Still other recipes require that they be roasted, either on a dry griddle, in a dry cast-iron frying pan, or on the end of a long-handled fork over a low flame, turning the tomatillo until its surface is evenly golden brown and its flesh is slightly soft, 5 to 10 minutes. No further peeling is required.

TOMATO Once feared as poison, then considered a possible aphrodisiac, the "love apple" now adds its vivid color and delicious flesh to innumerable dishes. Like the potato, this fruit (which is generally treated as a vegetable) is a member of the nightshade family and is native to South America.

After finally gaining acceptance as food in Europe and the United States, tomatoes became an inextricable part of many cuisines, especially those of the Mediterranean. In Italy, they are used to make sauce for pasta, pizza, and many other dishes and are served sliced in salads. Slices of tomato, for example, are served with sliced fresh mozzarella and fresh basil leaves, and the trio is sprinkled with olive oil. Other dishes that depend on tomatoes for their character include minestrone, gazpacho, ratatouille, Greek salad, and tomato soup. And, of course, tomatoes are a staple of New World cuisine, from the American South's fried green tomatoes to Texas's chili con carne, from Latin America's *salsa cruda* to bacon, lettuce, and tomato sandwiches.

Today's health-conscious cooks know that, far from being poisonous, the tomato is high in vitamin C and cancer-fighting antioxidants. The tomato comes in a wide range of sizes, from tiny currant tomatoes no bigger than blueberries to fat beefsteaks up to 5 inches in diameter. The colors are varied, too, from white to purple-black to reddish black, with green-striped zebra tomatoes somewhere in between. Dedicated gardeners have traced and reintroduced a number of heirloom tomatoes, that is, old-fashioned varieties that don't work as well for modern commercial processing. (They may not keep as long, have thinner skins that won't stand up to jostling, or may just have a taste that, delicious though it may be, is less of a crowd-pleaser.) Look for heirloom tomatoes in a wide variety of colors and patterns, with evocative names like Elephant Heart, Lemon Boy, and Golden Jubilee. At the other end of the spectrum, hybridists have introduced many new varieties for the sake of variation in color, size, and other attributes, including thriving in a range of growing conditions.

Sun-dried tomatoes and tomato sauce, purée, and paste are commonly used to flavor a wide variety of dishes. Tomato sauce can be used straight from the can in sauces and casseroles. Tomato purée is a more concentrated version of the sauce, while tomato paste is the thickest and most intense mixture of all. Tomato purée and tomato paste are often used as flavoring agents in soups and sauces.

Selecting Although tomatoes are available year-round, they are at the top of the list of produce that is best when eaten at the height of its natural season. You can find hothouse or imported Mexican tomatoes during the off-season, but in general it is a good idea to wait until local vines are producing, usually June through September, to serve them sliced. If you must choose fresh tomatoes out of season, plum tomatoes and cherry tomatoes are the best bet, as they have more flavor and a better texture than hothouse slicing tomatoes. Otherwise, use canned (or packaged) imported plum tomatoes, usually called Italian tomatoes. They will have a much better flavor than will poor-quality fresh tomatoes.

For the best summer tomatoes, visit farm stands, farmers' markets, and natural-food stores for vine-ripened tomatoes, or grow your own. Most supermarket tomatoes are picked unripe and then ripened with ethylene gas, so they never develop a full flavor. Choose organic tomatoes, if possible, as they are likely to be more flavorful.

Storing Store ripe tomatoes at room temperature for up to 3 days. If they are slightly unripe, put them in a sunny place for several days and they will ripen further. Although whole fresh tomatoes should not be refrigerated, cut tomatoes should be wrapped in plastic or waxed paper and refrigerated. Put leftover canned tomatoes, sauce, purée, and paste in glass jars, cover, and refrigerate for several days.

Preparing Wash and dry tomatoes to be sliced. Cut out the stem end and leave the tomatoes whole or cut them into crosswise or lengthwise slices or into wedges, or chop, according to the recipe. Pull off the stems of cherry tomatoes.

Chopping a tomato.

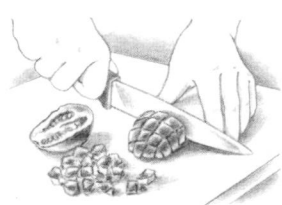

Some recipes call for peeled and/or seeded tomatoes, usually when the tomatoes are to be chopped for a sauce. For peeling tomatoes, see BLANCHING.

Tomato Glossary

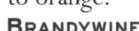

BEEFSTEAK Large, meaty, and delicious variety, bright red to orange.

BRANDYWINE A rich red heirloom tomato with a purple or green tinge.

CHERRY TOMATO Miniature, sweet tomatoes available in yellow, red, and orange. Look for red Sweet 100s or orange Sun Golds, both especially sweet and intensely flavored.

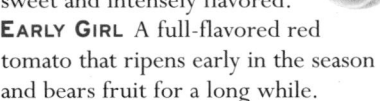

EARLY GIRL A full-flavored red tomato that ripens early in the season and bears fruit for a long while.

GREEN TOMATO Both a specific tomato variety and the unripe version of red tomatoes. The variety is eaten like any ripe tomato, while unripe green tomatoes are fried or made into conserves.

PEAR TOMATO Another category of cherry tomatoes is the tiny pear tomato, shaped like its namesake and available in yellow, red, and orange varieties.

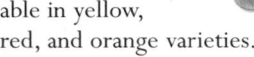

PLUM TOMATO Also known as Roma or egg tomatoes, these have a meaty, flavorful flesh that is particularly good for making sauce.

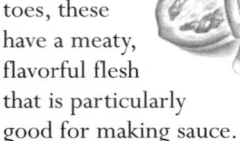

HOW TO *Seed Tomatoes*
1. Cut the tomatoes in half crosswise.
2. Holding each half in turn over a sink or bowl, lightly squeeze and shake it to dislodge the seeds. Use a finger if needed to help ease the seeds out of each half.

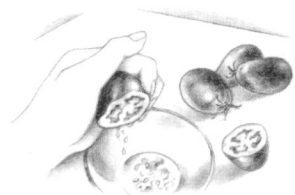

A Clever Way to Purée Tomatoes
1. Cut a tomato in half and seed it.
2. Using the small rasps, grate the cut side of the tomato half on a handheld grater.
3. Spread your fingers and press the tomato skin flat as its edges curl up, so that you grate only its pulp. You should end up with a flattened piece of tomato skin.
4. Discard the skin.

See also SUN-DRIED TOMATO.

TOMATO PASTE See TOMATO.

TOMATO PURÉE See TOMATO.

TONGS See COOKING TOOLS.

TOOLS Although only a few basic cooking tools are essential, the right tool can make a difference in the quality of the finished dish and can make cooking more enjoyable. For guidance in developing your own selection of culinary tools, see BAKING TOOLS; COOKING TOOLS.

TORTILLA When the Spanish conquistadores came to Mexico, they found the Indians preparing thin cakes of ground corn, as they had done for centuries. The

Spanish dubbed them *tortillas,* meaning "little round cakes." (In Spain, the word *tortilla* describes a round omelet. The best-known Spanish tortilla is the potato tortilla, popular as a tapa and as a lunch dish. See also FRITTATA; UNMOLDING.)

Corn tortillas were originally made completely by hand from fresh *masa,* a paste made from dried corn that has been softened in a solution of water and the mineral lime. Some are still made that way, but most tortillas today are factory produced. Some cooks use fresh *masa* but form the tortillas in a tortilla press rather than pat them out by hand. When fresh *masa* is unavailable, *masa harina,* a flour made from dried *masa,* is used. After wheat was introduced to Mexico, flour tortillas were developed in the northern part of the country.

Selecting Fresh hand-patted corn tortillas are sometimes available from restaurants or Latino markets. They are thicker and more uneven than tortillas made in a tortilla press, and they are especially good for serving as a bread alongside Mexican food. Look for the freshest corn tortillas you can find. Those purchased directly from a restaurant, market, or tortilla factory will be more pliable and tender than those that have sat in plastic in a supermarket for days. To make your own tortillas, try to get fresh *masa* from one of the same places, as it is easier to work with than dough made from *masa harina.*

Quick Tip

To heat corn or flour tortillas, wrap them in aluminum foil or put them in a clay tortilla warmer and heat in a low oven for about 20 minutes. To heat in a microwave, wrap the tortillas in plastic wrap and heat for 1 minute on one side and 30 seconds on the other.

Quick Tip

Don't throw away stale tortillas. Cut them into triangles and fry or bake them for tortilla chips, or cut them into shreds and fry or bake them for a salad or soup garnish. Mexicans cut stale tortillas into shreds or bits and use them in tortilla soup or bake them with chiles and cheese as casseroles called *chilaquiles.*

Storing Keep tortillas in an airtight plastic bag in the refrigerator. They will keep for several days but are best used sooner rather than later.

See also CORN.

TOSSING To mix ingredients lightly, or to coat them with a sauce or dressing by turning them over several times with two large spoons or your two hands. A somewhat riskier method is to pick up the container and jerk it so that the ingredients fly up in the air a few inches. Salads are customarily tossed to coat them with dressing. Other ingredients such as cooked vegetables that might be crushed or smashed by stirring are also tossed. Professional chefs often toss foods while sautéing or frying them in order to cook them quickly over high heat without burning. See also SALAD; SAUTÉING; STIR-FRYING.

TREE OR WOOD EAR MUSH-ROOM See MUSHROOM.

TRITICALE See GRAIN.

TRUFFLE No other food has developed quite the same mystique as this knobby, aromatic underground fungus. Until now it has been impossible to cultivate, so finding it has traditionally been a matter of having a good truffle dog or pig who could smell a truffle buried in the earth under oak trees

t

in Europe. The two most valuable kinds of truffle are the black truffle (sometimes called "black gold") of France, particularly from the Périgord and Quercy areas, and from Umbria in Italy, and the white truffle of the Piedmont in Italy. Truffles have a strong, earthy aroma and are used to flavor a variety of foods. The white truffle is even more powerfully scented than the black, although its flavor is somewhat milder. Black truffles may be cut into very thin slices or matchsticks and added to pâtés and terrines, and they are often used to flavor foie gras. Minced or shaved black truffles are used as a counterpoint to mild foods such as eggs and are added to sauces for meats and poultry for rich flavor. White truffles are used raw, grated or shaved, over cooked pasta, polenta, or risotto.

Black truffles.

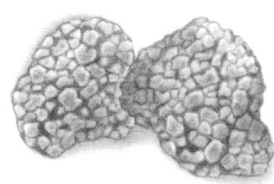

White truffle.

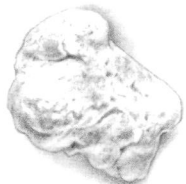

Selecting Truffle season begins in late autumn and lasts through the winter. Look for fresh truffles in specialty-food stores. A single truffle is usually packed on a bed of rice in a glass jar. The rice absorbs moisture and keeps the truffle from spoiling. (Be sure to cook the rice, which will have taken on the flavor of the truffle.) Whole, minced, or sliced truffles are available in jars or cans year-round, as is truffle paste in tubes and truffle oil in bottles. Truffle oil is an espe-

cially good way to add the truffle's haunting fragrance to pasta dishes, salads, and main courses. Sprinkle it on hot foods just before serving to preserve the truffle flavor.

Quick Tip

To scent eggs with a truffle, remove it from its jar and bury it in a bowl of eggs in their shells. Cover and refrigerate for 2 to 3 days.

Storing Keep a fresh truffle, in its jar of rice, in the refrigerator, but use within a few days of purchase, or the truffle will dry out and lose fragrance. Canned and jarred truffles, truffle paste, and truffle oil will keep indefinitely in a cool, dark place. Refrigerate them after opening.

Preparing For fresh truffles, brush the truffle clean with a soft mushroom brush or damp kitchen towel. Peel black truffles, saving the peel to flavor other dishes or to infuse olive oil, but use white truffles unpeeled. Grate truffles on a grater, or cut them into paper-thin slices, or shavings, with a vegetable peeler, a mandoline, or a tool called a truffle slicer. Slices of black truffles may be used whole or minced with a chef's knife.

Quick Bite

Chocolate truffles are so-called because their irregular spherical forms and cocoa dusting mimic the appearance of a black truffle with its coating of earth.

TRUSSING To tie a food, usually poultry or boned roasts, into a rounded, compact shape before cooking. Trussing gives a roast a plump, tidy form that holds even when the trussing string is removed. This technique should be reserved for birds that are presented whole at table, as poultry actually cooks more evenly untrussed.

HOW TO *Truss Poultry*

1. Have ready the bird, kitchen scissors, and kitchen string.

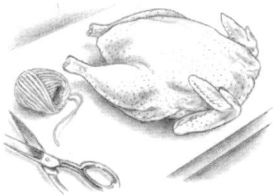

Tuck the first joint of each wing under the second joint.

2. Cut a long piece of kitchen string (4 to 5 times the length of the bird) and lay it across the board. Place the bird on its back on top of the string, so that the string is just under the tail. Cross the string over the legs, pulling them together and crossing the ends of the drumsticks; then loop the string under the end of the crossed drumsticks.

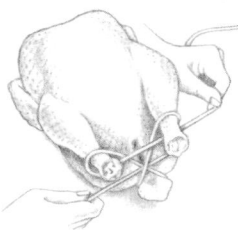

3. Fold the tail up into the cavity and pull on the string until it is tight. Pull each end of the string up toward the breast.

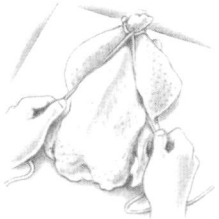

4. Turn the bird breast side down, bringing each string end over each wing and tucking the neck skin under the string. Cross the string ends and pull them tight. Tie securely in a knot and clip

the string ends. To remove string after the bird is cooked and has rested, cut it at the knot and pull it free.

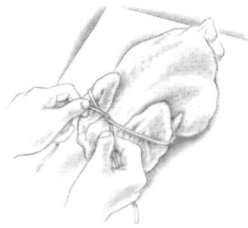

TUBE PAN See BAKEWARE; CAKE.

TUNA A prized food fish, the tuna comes from a family of large fish with rich, oily, firm flesh. Tuna is the most popular fish for canning and is widely available in cans in several different forms. The albacore, a small tuna (10 to 60 pounds) with the palest flesh of all the tunas, is mild in flavor and almost white in color when cooked. The bluefin is a very large fish—it can grow to more than 1,000 pounds—whose mature flesh is dark red and strongly flavored. Bonitos are small fish (up to 25 pounds) and have the most pronounced flavor among all the tunas. Skipjack tunas are usually quite small (6 to 8 pounds), with meat similar to that of the yellowfin. Yellowfin tuna, which can reach a weight of 300 pounds, is called ahi in Hawaiian. It has slightly more flavor than albacore.

Because its meat is oily and firm, tuna takes well to pan roasting or grilling. It is typically cooked until seared on the outside and rare on the inside. Fresh tuna is also used for Japanese sashimi and sushi. Canned tuna is served as part of an antipasto plate and is used to make salads, sandwiches, and casseroles.

Selecting Fresh albacore is usually available from spring through fall, while yellowfin is available year-round but is most plentiful in summer. The different kinds of fresh tuna are interchangeable for cooked dishes, although yellowfin steaks are often preferred for grilling and pan roasting. For sushi and sashimi, look for the freshest-possible fish, usually labeled "sushi-grade," "sashimi grade," "tuna loin," or "tuna belly."

When choosing canned tuna, imported Italian tuna packed in olive oil is considered the premium kind for antipasto, salads, and sandwiches, although you may prefer a lower-calorie tuna packed in spring water. Domestic tuna is also packed in vegetable oil. Solid albacore tuna is the most expensive domestic canned tuna, followed by chunk light tuna, and then flaked light tuna. Solid albacore can be somewhat dry, however, and some cooks prefer chunk light tuna. "Dolphin-safe" or "line-caught" tuna has been caught by methods that do not endanger dolphins.

Storing Pat fresh tuna dry with paper towels and put it in a heavy-duty zippered plastic bag. Place the bag on top of a bowl of ice cubes or cracked ice and refrigerate. Cook the fish the day you buy it. If you must wait, it should be kept no longer than 24 hours. Freezing degrades the texture and flavor of fish somewhat, but if you must freeze tuna, place it in a freezer-weight plastic bag and freeze for up to 1 month. Defrost in the refrigerator. Unopened canned tuna may be kept indefinitely.

Preparing Fresh tuna may be grilled, broiled, panfried, pan roasted, or poached. Canned tuna is usually drained before using in a recipe.

TURKEY Benjamin Franklin wanted to make the turkey the national bird of the United States, and it unofficially becomes just that every year at Thanksgiving, when Americans consume this bird in incredible numbers. Turkey is nearly as popular at Christmas and is also eaten throughout the year, often as a low-fat substitute for red meat. Ground turkey is made into turkey burgers and meat loaves, and sliced cooked turkey breast is a favorite meat for sandwiches. Turkey breast halves are roasted whole, sliced raw and sautéed, or boned, stuffed, rolled, and roasted.

Sooner or later, though, every cook is faced with roasting a whole turkey, and an entire culture of techniques, advice, and lore has grown up around this process. Turkeys are cooked in covered roasters or paper or plastic bags; roasted under a tent of aluminum foil; packed in a thick layer of salt and baked; grilled; roasted breast down; boned, rolled, and roasted; or soaked in brine, then roasted. Whole turkeys are even deep-fried. All of these methods have one aim in mind: to produce a bird with juicy meat throughout. And for most people, the juicy meat must be combined with crisp, well-browned skin. The great problem in cooking a turkey, of course, is that by the time the skin is crisp and the dark meat is done, the white meat is usually overcooked and dried out.

A simple way to combat this is to roast the turkey at a moderate temperature of 325°F and to cover the breast of the turkey with aluminum foil to keep it moist, and then remove the foil toward the end of roasting so the breast will brown.

Selecting For the best taste, pick a turkey over 10 pounds; if you want a small bird, a capon or a turkey breast half is a better choice. Figure on ¾ pound per person for serving, although you will probably want twice that (or more) for leftovers. If at all possible, choose a fresh bird (frozen turkeys have drier meat) that was raised free range and fed organic grain. Although they are more expensive, these turkeys have more flavor than those raised on factory farms. Order them from specialty butchers or natural-food stores.

Storing Store turkey in its original wrapping in the cold bottom back shelf of the refrigerator. Cook fresh or thawed turkey within 2 days. Pick up your whole turkey the day before it is to be roasted, unless it is frozen, in which case it will most likely take longer than a day to thaw (see THAWING). Fresh turkey may be frozen for up to 6 months, but previously frozen turkey should not be refrozen.

Preparing Two hours before roasting, remove the whole bird from the refrigerator, remove the packaging, and remove the package of giblets from the body and/or neck cavity. Remove the giblets from their packaging and rinse them. Use them now (with the exclusion of the liver) to make a stock to use in the turkey gravy, or place them in a bowl, cover it with plastic wrap, and refrigerate until ready to use. Rinse the turkey inside and out (both neck and body cavities) under cold water. Remove and discard any bloody bits. Pat the bird dry inside and out with paper towels. Pluck any leftover feathers, using tweezers or needle-nose pliers if necessary. Fold the wings under the bird. Let the bird sit at room temperature on a baking sheet until roasting.

If stuffing the bird, do so just before putting it into the oven, packing the stuffing loosely into the neck and body cavities to allow it room to expand. If not stuffing the bird, sprinkle the cavities with salt and pepper and put an onion half and a coarsely chopped carrot and celery rib inside the body cavity.

See also CARVING; DONENESS; GIBLETS; GRAVY; ROASTING; STUFFING; TRUSSING.

TURMERIC See SPICE.

TURNING OUT Removing a food, such as a baked pastry or a molded dessert, from its container; see UNMOLDING.

TURNIP Like so many other root vegetables, the turnip, which grows well in poor soil, has long been a staple of northern European cooking. It typically has crisp white flesh and a white skin with a purple cap, 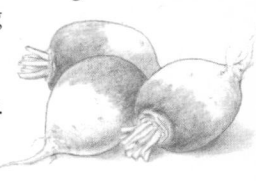 although some varieties have yellow flesh, and the cap might be green, red, white, or even black. Very young turnips are tender and have a mild, sweet flavor. The flavor grows stronger and the flesh woodier with age. Young turnips are delicious raw, eaten like radishes, or they may be cooked whole, along with their greens. Turnips are delightful in soups and stews, braised in butter, puréed with potatoes, glazed, roasted along with other root vegetables, or served in braises with duck and pork.

Selecting Although available year-round, turnips are at their best in winter. Baby turnips, with their greens attached, are 1 to 2 inches in diameter. Older turnips are usually 3 to 4 inches in diameter and are sold with their greens removed. Choose unblemished, firm, sweet-smelling turnips.

Storing Keep baby turnips, with their greens attached, in a perforated plastic bag in the refrigerator crisper for 1 to 2 weeks. Older turnips will keep for several weeks in a cool, dark place.

Preparing Peel and trim baby turnips, but leave them whole. Peel older turnips and slice them or cut them into chunks. If older turnips have a strong smell, blanch them for 3 to 5 minutes to remove some of the harshness.

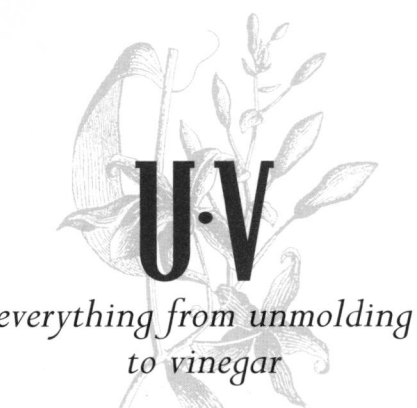

U·V

*everything from unmolding
to vinegar*

U·V

UNMOLDING To remove a food from the container in which it cooked or set, a step that can sometimes be the trickiest part of making the dish. Preparing the mold beforehand and cooking the dish properly are the keys to successful unmolding. Nonstick bakeware and cookware have been a boon to unmolding foods easily. A coating of cooking spray is added insurance against food's sticking to the pan and falling apart as it leaves the mold. Cast-iron skillets and other similar pans must be properly seasoned; many cooks wash them only in hot water (without soap) in order to preserve the seasoning.

To unmold such foods as frittatas and Spanish tortillas in order to cook them on the second side, make sure to use enough butter and/or oil at the beginning and to heat it well before adding the food to the pan. Make sure the mixture is browned on the bottom, and shake the pan to loosen it, or dislodge it with a thin spatula if necessary. You may invert a plate over the pan and then quickly invert both plate and pan if the pan is small and light enough; or you can slide the food out of the pan onto a plate, cooked side down, then top it with the upside-down pan and invert the two.

Jelled foods are easier to unmold if the mold has been oiled or sprayed with cooking spray before filling. To unmold, dip the base of the mold into a pan of very hot water for no more than 4 or 5 seconds. Remove the mold from the water and rock it slightly to see whether the food has loosened inside the mold. If not, dip it again in hot water. Rinse the serving plate with cold water, then place it upside down over the mold. Holding the mold and plate together tightly, invert the two quickly and place on the countertop. Tap the bottom of the mold to make sure the food drops onto the plate. If all else fails, loosen the edges of the food by slipping a thin knife along the inside edge of the mold, and then leave the mold upside down on the serving plate until the food falls out.

*Lowering mold
into hot water.*

*Setting plate
upside down
on mold.*

*Inverting mold
and plate
together.*

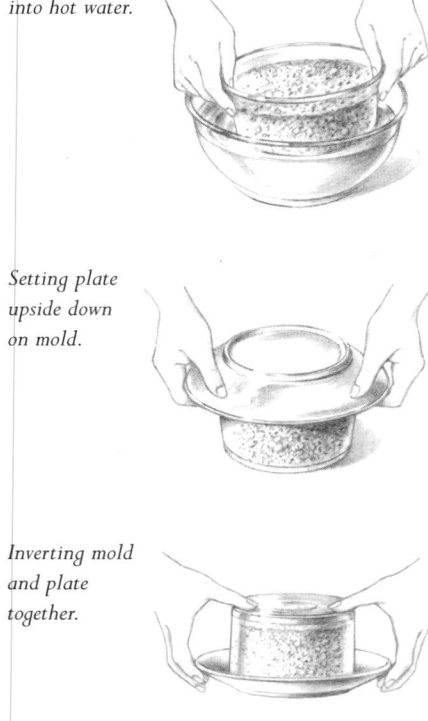

Most cakes, muffins, and loaf breads are cooked until they begin to pull away from the sides of the pan. Usually, they are allowed to cool for a few minutes in their pan on a wire rack, during which time they shrink slightly, making them easier to unmold. Run a thin knife around the inside edges of the pan before unmolding.

For ease in unmolding cakes, make sure to follow the recipe instructions for preparing the pans. Some cakes require a circle of parchment paper in the bottom and/or a coating of butter, and some need a sprinkle of flour or sugar over the butter. Many cakes are baked in springform pans in order to unmold them easily, while most tarts and tart shells are baked in a tart pan with a removable bottom. When using this type of pan, place it on a baking sheet for baking, and slide the tart pan onto a wire rack to cool. To unmold, push up on the false bottom of the pan so that the pan ring falls away. Cut and serve a filled tart while it is sitting on the pan's false bottom.

See also BAKING; MOLDING; PIE & TART; SEASONING.

VANILLA Lending perfume, depth, and nuance to a wide variety of dishes, including some savory ones, vanilla is one of the West's prime flavors for ice creams, cookies, cakes, custards, pastry cream, and puddings. It may be used either in its whole-bean form or as vanilla extract, a commercial product made by chopping the beans, soaking them in a mixture of alcohol and water, and then aging the solution. Because the beans are hand-pollinated and hand-picked, they are expensive, but they may be reused several times.

Vanilla beans.

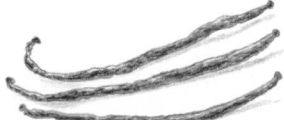

Selecting Whole beans, which are sold in bulk or packaged singly in plastic cylinders, are available in natural-food stores, specialty-food stores, and some supermarkets. They should be moist and pliable. The best-quality beans will develop a natural coating of vanillin, a white powder. Of the three most common kinds—Tahitian, Mexican, and Bourbon-Madagascar—the Mexican and Bourbon-Madagascar beans are more strongly scented, while Tahitian are more delicate. Mexican beans are in short supply, however, while Bourbon-Madagascar beans make up about three-fourths of the total supply.

The best vanilla extracts identify the type of bean used. Buy only pure vanilla extract, not imitation vanilla, which is made of artificial flavorings and has an inferior taste. Vanilla powder, the ground vanilla bean, is available by mail order and from some specialty-food stores. Some cooks prefer it because its flavor does not dissipate when it is heated.

Storing Vanilla beans sold in a plastic cylinder should be kept in the cylinder, and loose beans should be placed in an airtight jar. Keep in a cool, dark place for up to 6 months. The tightly capped extract keeps indefinitely stored in a cool, dark place.

Preparing Use the whole bean, or cut the bean in half lengthwise, scrape out the seeds, and add them, with the pod, to the liquid in the dish you are preparing. Some recipes will instruct you to steep the vanilla bean first. After use, rinse and dry whole beans, store as above, and reuse.

Scraping a vanilla bean.

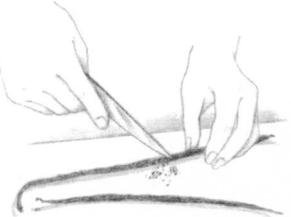

U·V

When adding vanilla extract to hot food, first let the food cool for a few minutes. When the extract is added to hot food, the alcohol evaporates, taking with it some of the vanilla flavor.

HOW TO *Make Vanilla Sugar*

Use vanilla sugar as a replacement for regular granulated sugar to add flavor in desserts, sauces, and drinks. One tablespoon vanilla sugar equals ¼ teaspoon vanilla extract in flavoring power.

1. Bury a vanilla bean—whole or halved—in 1 cup granulated or confectioners' sugar.
2. Cover tightly and let sit for at least 24 hours. Replace sugar as it is used and replace the bean after 1 year.

HOW TO *Make Homemade Vanilla Extract*

1. Cut a vanilla bean in half lengthwise and crosswise. Place the pieces in a clean glass jar.
2. Add ¾ cup vodka. Cover tightly and let steep for 6 months before using.

VEAL The meat of a calf up to the age of 3 months, or sometimes slightly older but still less than 6 months (when it becomes "baby beef"). The most tender and white veal is from a milk-fed calf that is no more than 3 months old. "Formula-fed" veal is raised on a diet of milk solids, milk fats, and other various nutrients and may be up to 4 months old. This kind of veal, sometimes referred to as "Dutch method" veal, is tender and pale but inferior in flavor to that of true milk-fed veal. The tenderness of the meat is also a result of restricting the calf's movement, which in recent years has raised concerns and protest. Most producers have responded by improving conditions; a good-quality butcher should be able to tell you about the practices of his or her suppliers.

When a calf is weaned from milk and fed on grass and grain, its flesh becomes redder due to the iron in the food, and some cooks prefer this "free-range" veal, as it has a meatier flavor.

Veal is a traditional European meat. The relative lack of pastureland in Europe has always made it practical to slaughter cattle at a younger age. Thus, France has developed such dishes as *blanquette de veau,* Germany has its traditional Wiener schnitzel, and Italy has its veal scallopini, among a host of other veal dishes.

Selecting For traditional dishes calling for veal scallopini or chops, look for milk-fed veal, distinguished by its creamy pink color and fine-grained texture. The redder meat of free-range veal is especially good in more hearty dishes such as stews.

Storing Ground veal may be refrigerated for up to 2 days, steaks or chops for 3 days, and roasts for 4 days. Freeze ground veal for up to 3 months; steaks, chops, and roasts may be frozen for up to 9 months.

Preparing Unlike beef, veal is low in fat and has little or no marbling. Thus all veal cuts, except the ones from the loin, leg, and rib, should be cooked by methods that involve moisture, such as stewing or braising, or else barded (see BARDING) to give them extra insulation during cooking.

Unlike beef and lamb, roasted veal should be cooked no less than medium (145° to 155°F). Braised and stewed cuts are cooked until tender.

VEGETABLE See individual vegetables; BLANCHING; BOILING; BRAISING; ROASTING; STEAMING.

VEGETABLE OIL See COOKING SPRAY; FAT & OIL.

VEGETABLE PEAR See CHAYOTE.

VEGETABLE PEELER See COOKING TOOLS.

U·V

Veal Glossary

Veal cuts.

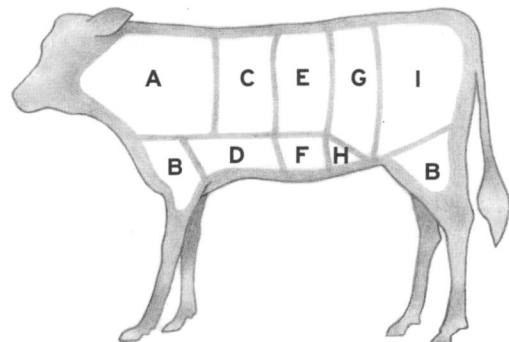

A C E G I
B D F H B

From the primal, or wholesale, cuts of veal come the smaller roasts, chops, and other cuts available from the butcher.

SHOULDER (A) Source of roasts for braising, stewing, or roasting. The shoulder may also be cut into steaks, which likewise should be braised. Ground veal is often shoulder meat.

SHANK (B) The shank is cut into slices and sold as veal shanks or osso buco. Many cooks feel hind shanks make better osso buco. This gelatinous meat is rich in flavor, and long braising turns the meat and its marrow meltingly tender. The same cut is a fine choice for making stock.

Veal shanks.

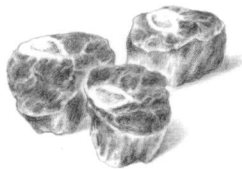

RIB (C) Veal rib, or rack of veal, may be roasted as a rack or a crown roast, or boned and roasted. Usually, however, it is cut into rib chops.

BREAST (D) The breast is a source of less expensive cuts that are traditionally stuffed and braised. The breast may be used for ground veal.

LOIN (E) The loin, the section beneath the ribs and above the leg, is the source of whole loin roast, either bone in or boned and stuffed, for roasting or braising. The loin is also cut into chops, which may be sautéed or grilled.

Veal loin chops.

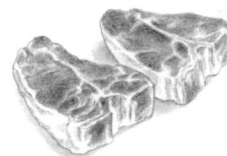

FLANK (F) Combined with trimmings from other cuts to make ground veal.

SIRLOIN (G) Cut into chops, which may be sautéed or grilled. The sirloin is also cut into roasts for grilling or broiling.

TIP (H) Sliced into cutlets, which are often pounded to become veal scallops.

Veal scallops.

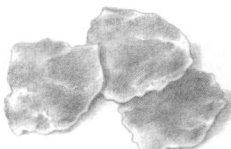

ROUND (I) Source of rump and round roasts for roasting, as well as round steaks for braising.

VEGETABLE SHORTENING A solid white fat made by hydrogenating a vegetable oil, such as cottonseed or soybean. (The hydrogenation process consists of pumping hydrogen atoms into the oil.)

Because about 10 percent of its volume is air, shortening requires less creaming than butter does. And shortening contains millions of tiny bubbles, which trap the air that's beaten in during the creaming process, making tender, light-textured cakes. Shortening remains solid even at warm room temperature, so there's no risk of its melting and absorbing flour the way that butter can. This ability to remain solid over a wide temperature range means that cookies made with shortening hold their shape and don't spread the way ones made with butter do. And unlike butter, which contains a small percentage of water, shortening is 100 percent fat. This lack of water means that shortening makes flakier pie crusts and crisper cookies than butter does. Shortening also is used for deep-frying because it has a high smoke point.

Recently, the use of vegetable shortening has caused health concerns because the hydrogenation of vegetable oil converts the oil into saturated fat and creates trans fatty acids. Some researchers believe that these saturated fats are more harmful to the body than regular saturated fats.

Because it's virtually flavorless, shortening is often combined with butter in baked goods, in order to get both the delicious flavor of butter and the flakiness created by using shortening.

Quick Tip

Butter may be substituted for shortening in most baking recipes.

Storing Once opened, store shortening in the refrigerator for up to 1 year.

VELOUTÉ See SAUCE.

VENISON See GAME.

VERMOUTH See WINE.

VINAIGRETTE The most basic of salad dressings, *sauce vinaigrette* is a simple mixture of oil and vinegar, plus seasonings. The proportions usually run 3 or 4 parts oil to 1 part vinegar. Vinaigrettes as simple as oil and vinegar plus seasonings shaken together in a glass jar offer a multitude of possibilities. By first whisking the vinegar with a spoonful of mustard and then drizzling in the oil as you whisk, you can create a creamier, better emulsified vinaigrette that will coat evenly. Experiment with different oils, vinegars, herbs, and spices.

Quick Tip

Before recycling a just-emptied mustard jar, add oil, vinegar, salt, and pepper and shake to make a mustard-flavored vinaigrette.

Vinaigrettes may also be used as marinades or as a sauce for meat, chicken, seafood, vegetables, and grains. See also EMULSION; SAUCE.

VINEGAR The first vinegar was probably a wine gone bad: *vin aigre,* French for "sour wine." A multiplicity of uses was soon found for this fortuitous discovery. Not only did it provide just the right tartness for dressing salad greens when mixed with oil, but it also preserved foods, cleaned surfaces, brightened hair, and was used as a medicine and a poultice. Before refrigeration, the keeping quality of vinegar was of major importance. It was used to pickle meats, fruits, and vegetables, preventing spoilage while altering taste and texture in ways resembling cooking. Several traditional dishes, such as pickled herring, dill pickles, piccalilli, sauerbraten, and adobo, remind us of this function. Today, vinegar is made from a variety of red or white wines, and you will even find varietal wine vinegars in some specialty-food stores. Sherry vinegar, which originated in Spain, has a nutty taste and is especially good on vegetables and in dressings.

In addition to wine vinegars, there are a number of vinegars based on fruit and grain, including cider vinegar and rice vinegar. Cider vinegar, a fruity vinegar made from apples and used in many traditional American recipes, was once more common in this country than wine vinegar. Distilled white vinegar, made from grain alcohol, is used in pickling and in other recipes where its clean taste is desired. Malt vinegar, a mild vinegar made from malted barley, is popular in England as a dressing for fish and chips. Rice vinegar, made from fermented rice, is widely used in Asian cuisines. It is used to add a slight acidity in cooked dishes and to make dressings for delicate greens. It is available either plain or sweetened; the latter is marketed as seasoned rice vinegar. The Chinese make white, red, and black rice vinegars, with the deeply flavored black type used in cooking and as a condiment and the milder red type used in much the same way. Many vinegars, whatever their source, are further seasoned by the addition of fresh herbs, fruit, garlic, or other ingredients.

Herb-flavored vinegar.

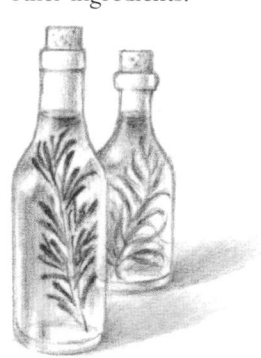

Balsamic Vinegar A specialty of the Italian region of Emilia-Romagna, primarily in the town of Modena, balsamic is an aged vinegar made from the pure wine must—unfermented grape juice, which may contain stems, skins, and seed—of white Trebbiano grapes. Authentic balsamic vinegar is designated by the word *tradizionale* or an Italian consortium seal on the label and is aged for as little as 1 year and on up to 25 years, 50 years, 75 years, and sometimes far longer, slowly evaporating and growing sweeter and mellower with time. It is aged in airy attics in a series of wooden casks of decreasing sizes, each a different wood that contributes to its flavor. Long-aged balsamic is an intense, expensive, syrupy vinegar that should be used sparingly; only a few drops are necessary. True balsamic that is aged for a shorter time is also available. Younger balsamic makes a superb salad dressing and is used, often reduced, in sauces for other foods, or is sprinkled over fruit.

What is often sold as balsamic vinegar is a relatively inexpensive duplication of the true product, made from grape must mixed with high-quality vinegar, but it makes a decent salad dressing.

Quick Tip

When making a vinaigrette with balsamic vinegar, use 3 parts olive oil or less to 1 part balsamic. Its flavor is less sharp than that of some other vinegars.

Storing All vinegar should be stored in glass bottles in cool, dark cupboards. It keeps indefinitely. Although vinegar may cloud with time, it is still usable and may simply need to be filtered through a heavy paper towel or coffee filter.

VODKA See SPIRITS.

U·V

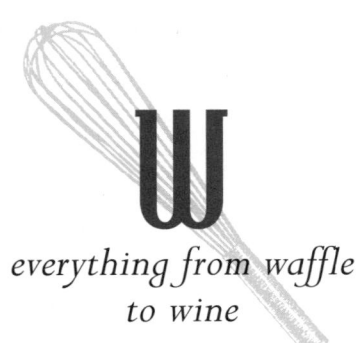

*everything from waffle
to wine*

WAFFLE Cunningly devised to combine the maximum amount of crisp-tender crust while trapping the maximum amount of syrup or sauce, a waffle can be sweet or savory. Waffles are usually leavened by baking powder and/or baking soda, but they may also be made from a yeast dough. Like pancakes, they may be lightened with foamy beaten egg whites or made more tender by incorporating buttermilk, sour cream, or yogurt. Standard waffles have a grid of small depressions, while Belgian waffles are thicker and have larger and deeper depressions, a crisp exterior, and an airy interior.

Waffle iron.

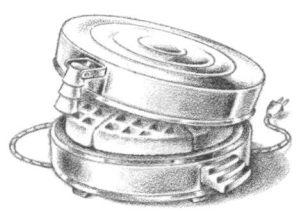

Waffles are a traditional breakfast or brunch dish, topped with maple syrup, yogurt, or a fruit sauce, but savory waffles may also be served as a quick, light lunch or supper, topped with creamed chicken, tuna, or vegetables.

Waffle irons come in a variety of shapes, including squares, circles, and hearts. They may be heated on the top of the stove, like European cookie irons, but are more commonly electric. Most of today's waffle irons are nonstick, but if you prefer one with a regular surface, make sure to season it according to the manufacturer's instructions. Seasoned or nonstick waffle irons do not need greasing. Make sure that the light on an electric iron indicates that the iron is ready to use, and wait until the top of the iron lifts easily away from the waffle to remove it from the iron. Do not immerse an electric waffle iron in water, and do not wash the grids after use. If crumbs have stuck to the surface, simply brush them out.

See also CREPE; PANCAKE.

WALNUT See NUT.

WATER BATH A water bath, sometimes called a bain-marie, is created by setting a baking dish or pan holding food inside a larger pan and then pouring either hot or nearly boiling water into the larger pan. The water, which should reach about halfway up the sides of the dish containing the food, insulates the food from the direct heat of the oven or stove, promoting gentle, moist, even cooking. Water baths provide a moist environment for baking delicate foods such as custards, mousses, cheesecakes, and puddings, or they can keep sauces, soups, or coffee warm on the stove top, acting as a sort of double boiler.

Water bath.

Although specialty water baths, or bain-marie pans, are available, it is easy to fashion a water bath from pans you already have on hand. The safest way to assemble a water bath intended for the oven is to line a large pan such as a roasting pan with a folded kitchen towel, and place the towel-lined pan on a pulled-out oven rack.

Quick Bite

Lining the water bath's outer pan with a folded towel keeps custard cups from rattling and shaking as they cook and also insulates them from the hot pan bottom.

Place the baking dish holding the food inside the larger pan, then pour the hot water into the larger pan. If using a springform pan, wrap it in aluminum foil before setting it in the water to prevent any leakage. Be sure the outer pan is large enough to hold a substantial amount of water, or the water will evaporate too quickly. Finally, slide the rack carefully into the oven. It's advisable to check the water level at regular intervals during cooking, pouring in more hot water as necessary.

Quick Bite

Bain-marie means "Marie's bath" in French, and some historians believe that the name for this mild cooking method alludes to the gentle nature of the Virgin Mary.

WATER CHESTNUT Cultivated in streams, ponds, and rivers throughout China and Southeast Asia, water chestnuts are the underwater stem tips of a type of water grass found in many parts of the world. In the past, the seeds of the water chestnut were sometimes used for making rosaries, inspiring a second name: Jesuit's nut. When it is fresh, the popular Asian vegetable looks something like a more spherical cousin of the tree-borne chestnut. It has a wonderfully crisp texture, welcome in stir-fries and salads, and a sweet, refreshing flavor all its own. Canned water chestnuts, whether whole or sliced, lack the sweetness of fresh ones and offer little more than a mild flavor and crunchy texture.

Selecting Look for fresh water chestnuts in Asian markets. Choose those that are rock hard with a slight sheen. Soft spots and a dull color are signs of mushy, soured fruit. Test various brands of canned water chestnuts until you find a good one.

Quick Tip

If using canned water chestnuts, cook them in boiling water for about 10 minutes, drain, and rinse with cold water. This will help rid them of any metallic flavors they may have absorbed from the can.

Storing Refrigerate fresh water chestnuts in a plastic bag for up to a week. Canned water chestnuts should be transferred to a plastic or glass container, covered with water, and refrigerated for up to 10 days.

Preparing If using fresh water chestnuts, rinse off any dirt. Cut off the flat top and bottom and peel the skin with a small knife or vegetable peeler. Cut out any yellow or brown bits of flesh. Keep peeled water chestnuts immersed in cold water until ready to use to prevent discoloration.

WATERCRESS Characterized by a refreshingly peppery flavor, watercress grows wild along streams and is cultivated in water. Like other members of the mustard

W

family, it has an agreeably assertive taste that makes it a classic filling for tea sandwiches; a dull green, lively tasting soup; a refreshing salad, either on its own or combined with other greens or with fruit; and an attractive garnish.

Selecting Watercress is available year-round, but it is at its peak in late spring and early summer. Look for brightly colored leaves. Pass over those that droop or are tinged with yellow.

Storing Place in a perforated plastic bag in the refrigerator for up to 2 days.

Preparing Wash and pick over the sprigs, discarding all but the freshest ones. Remove and discard the thick stems, then dry the watercress in a salad spinner. Or, line a baking sheet with paper towels and top with a layer of rinsed watercress sprigs. Repeat until all the watercress is washed, top with a final layer of paper towels, and gently roll up to dry.

See also GREENS, SALAD.

WATERMELON See MELON.

WAX BEAN See BEAN, FRESH.

WAXED PAPER Waxed paper is tissue-thin paper that has been coated on both sides with wax. This moisture-resistant, grease-resistant paper has largely been replaced in today's kitchens by aluminum foil, plastic bags and plastic wrap, and parchment paper, but it still has a place in the kitchen, especially since it is more ecologically friendly than plastic or foil. It does have some limitations, however. Waxed paper tears easily, and moisture or grease will eventually begin to soak through. Also, unlike parchment paper or foil, it cannot be directly exposed to heat in the oven, as its coating will melt. Nonetheless, it is often used to line cake pans to prevent sticking, as the batter protects the paper

from direct heat. Chocolate decorations and some candies such as divinity may also be spooned or piped onto waxed paper to set. Waxed-paper sandwich bags may be used for microwaving leftovers. Waxed paper is also useful for wrapping frozen food to be thawed in a microwave oven.

Quick Tip

Roll out pie dough and other sticky pastry between sheets of waxed paper. The dough won't adhere to its slick surface, allowing you to remove the paper easily.

WEIGHTS AND MEASURES See MEASURING.

WELL DONE When a food is cooked through completely, it is referred to as well done. In the case of meat, no trace of pink should remain. See also DONENESS; individual meats.

WET INGREDIENTS This term refers to the liquid ingredients in a baking recipe. Wet ingredients are usually water and/or milk, eggs, and liquid flavorings such as lemon juice, brandy, wine, or vanilla extract. Flour, sugar, salt, and other ingredients such as baking powder or baking soda are called dry ingredients. The wet ingredients are generally mixed together until blended, and dry ingredients are sifted or stirred together until blended. The wet and dry ingredients are then mixed together until blended or just combined. See also BAKING; DRY INGREDIENTS; MEASURING.

WHEAT See GRAIN.

WHIPPING Beating a food such as heavy cream or egg whites to increase its volume by incorporating air into it. Whipped ingredients are sometimes used to lighten the texture of heavier mixtures, such as adding whipped cream to custard to make it less dense, or folding whipped egg whites into a cake batter to facilitate rising.

Whipping can be accomplished using a wire whisk, an electric mixer, or a rotary beater. A balloon whisk will add the maximum amount of air to whipped cream or beaten egg whites.

Surprisingly, both egg whites and heavy cream are more quickly whipped by hand than with an electric mixer. Hand-beaten whites mound higher and are more stable than those beaten with an electric beater, while hand-beaten whipped cream is smoother and lighter.

Quick Tip

To whip egg whites or heavy cream, use a large bowl. The larger the bowl, the easier it is to incorporate air. A deep bowl also prevents the cream from splattering.

See also CREAM; EGG; WHISKING.

WHISKEY See SPIRITS.

WHISKING To beat, or whip, rapidly with a whisk, an implement with a head of thin looped metal wires and a metal or wooden handle.

Wire whisks.

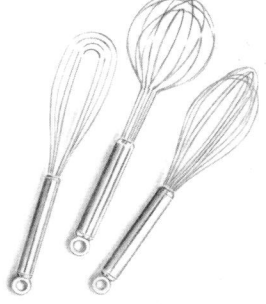

Also known as whips, whisks are made in various sizes and shapes and with differ-

ent thicknesses, flexibilities, and quantities of wire, depending on the kind of food for which they will be used. Sauce whisks are the basic model, used to mix ingredients thoroughly without adding excess air. Balloon whisks, which are more rounded, are used to incorporate air into egg whites and cream. Flat whisks are used for stirring gravies and sauces as they thicken, while also pressing out and smoothing lumps. Tiny whisks are made for whisking mixtures in cups or small pans.

See also BAKING TOOLS; COOKING TOOLS.

WHITE BEAN See BEAN, DRIED.

WHITE MUSTARD CABBAGE See BOK CHOY.

WILD RICE A different species of grain from true rice, this seed of a marsh grass is native to the northern Great Lakes of the United States, where it has long been harvested in boats by Native Americans. It now is also farmed elsewhere in the Midwest, in Canada, and in California. Wild rice is dark brown, almost black in color, and the long, narrow grains are pointed on both ends. With a pronounced nutty flavor, wild rice is pleasantly chewy and is a perfect accompaniment to game or wild mushrooms. It is especially good as an autumn pilaf or stuffing, mixed with nuts and raisins or currants. Wild rice may be substituted for white or brown rice in most recipes. Keep in mind, however, that its texture is firmer and it takes longer to cook. Combine it with white or brown rice to make a milder-tasting dish.

See also RICE.

WINE See page 468.

WOK See COOKWARE.

Wine

Certain connoisseurs have presented the convincing argument that wine is not so much a beverage as a food, citing its complex flavor, aroma, and body and the many ways in which those characteristics can interact with other elements of a meal.

Wine has indeed been an integral part of good dining for millennia, since humankind first discovered the happy results of fermentation in grape juice caused by airborne yeasts, followed by the subtle, yet profound, changes that can occur as wine ages in a cask or bottle. A thoughtfully chosen wine can greatly enhance the pleasure derived from the food it accompanies.

The Wine Cellar A significant factor in wine's compatibility with food lies in the fact that it can be made from many different grape varieties, each of which has unique characteristics of flavor, body, and color that are imparted to the finished wine. When a wine is made entirely or predominately from one grape variety, it is said to be a varietal wine. Today, most wines made in the Americas, Australia, and New Zealand are made and labeled as varietals. Most European wines, by contrast, are traditionally named after the regions in which they are produced. But each such region, as a rule, makes its wines from a predominant type of grape, and its wines will demonstrate that grape's signature varietal qualities as well as those of the land and climate in which the grapes were grown.

CABERNET SAUVIGNON (cab-er-NAY SO-vi-nyon) A robust red wine often described as fruity, spicy, or herbaceous, made from the same grape as the wines of Médoc and Graves in the Bordeaux region of France. Good with hearty red meat dishes, whether roasted, grilled, stewed, or braised.

CHAMPAGNE AND OTHER SPARKLING WINES Most often based on Chardonnay grapes, Champagne or sparkling wine describes a process rather than a grape. These wines delight with their fine bubbles of carbon dioxide, produced in the most authentic, highest-quality form by a secondary fermentation within the bottle. Dry Champagne or sparkling wine, which may be labeled "brut" or "extra sec," is appropriate nearly any time you would serve light white wine. It's excellent with foods such as caviar, fresh oysters, shrimp, salty cheeses, nuts, eggs, and smoked salmon.

Quick Bite

Though the term is used loosely in this country, *Champagne* specifically refers to sparkling wine made in the Champagne region of France, where the manufacturing process (called the *méthode champenoise*) and labeling are strictly controlled.

CHARDONNAY A rich and fruity white wine, which can range in taste from big and oaky to buttery and spicy to bracingly dry and flinty. The same grape yields the great white Burgundies of France—Chablis, Côte de Beaune, Mâcon, Meursault, and

Montrachet. Serve big, buttery Chardonnays with roast chicken, seafood, or creamy pastas, or even grilled veal or red meat; spicy Chardonnays with appetizers, light grilled meat or poultry, or pasta with tomato sauces; and flinty Chardonnays with raw or cooked shellfish or broiled whitefish.

GEWÜRZTRAMINER (guh-VURTZ-tra-meen-er) Popular in Germany, northeastern France, northern Italy, the United States, Australia, and New Zealand, this fruity, highly aromatic, spicy white wine is especially good with assertively spiced Asian dishes and with smoked fish and meats.

MERLOT (mer-LOW) Soft, rich, fruity, and full-bodied, this red wine comes from a grape also featured in the wines of Saint-Émilion and Pomerol in the Bordeaux region of France. Excellent with grilled or braised red meat, roast duck, or even grilled seafood.

PINOT NOIR (PEE-noh NWAHR) Many people consider this wine, with its silken body and a complex flavor and bouquet abounding in fruity, spicy, and floral characteristics, to be the greatest of the red wines. The same grape produces the renowned red wines of France's Burgundy region. Pinot noir may be served with a wide range of rich or complex-tasting dishes, from chicken braised in red wine to spicy Asian dishes.

RIESLING (REESE-ling) A crisp, floral white wine native to Germany, with a flavor that may variously bring to mind summer tree fruits, flint, or even a hint of smoke. Serve drier Rieslings on their own as a refreshing aperitif or with light appetizers or seafood; sweeter versions go well with blue cheeses or spicy food.

ROSÉ AND BLUSH WINES Made from red wine grapes of numerous varietals, these pink-tinged wines result from briefly leaving the skins in contact with the juice. Fresh and fruity, they go well with a wide range of casual foods, particularly well-seasoned Mediterranean dishes such as French seafood stews or Spanish paella.

SAUVIGNON BLANC (SO-vi-nyon BLAHNK) Crisp and acidic with herbaceous or grassy overtones, this white wine—made with a grape featured in France's great white Bordeaux—goes well with seafood of any kind or with dishes featuring (similarly acidic) tomato sauces. It is also known as Fumé Blanc.

ZINFANDEL Based on a popular California grape, Zinfandel is most often produced today as a hearty red wine with a flavor that brings to mind berries, cherries, and spices. It goes especially well with roasted or grilled red meats, robust stews, and game. Zinfandel is also produced in a lighter style similar to the Beaujolais Nouveau of France, ideal for drinking with casual meals of tomato-based pasta dishes or grilled poultry. So-called white Zinfandel is made by leaving the crushed grapes only briefly in contact with their skins, then straining the skins away. The result is a popular "blush" wine with a deep pink tint and a light, fruity flavor.

Selecting Wine Many food stores today carry a good range of reasonably priced wines. For the best selection, however, seek out a reputable wine store. A first-rate

Quick Bite

When applied to wine, the term *dry* refers to the amount of residual sugar in the wine. The less sugar, the drier the wine. Sweeter wines may be referred to as dessert wines or late-harvest wines.

continued

Wine, continued

merchant will be able to guide you to good bottles within your budget that will complement the foods you plan to serve. See The Wine Cellar, page 468, for a few pointers; for extra guidance on particular wine makers and on the best-quality vintages—that is, specific years in which wines are bottled—consult one of the many books or periodicals on the subject.

Storing Wine Bottles you plan to drink within a few days or weeks may be stored in your pantry, away from heat or light. For long-term storage of high-quality wines, keep the bottles undisturbed in an environment with a controlled constant temperature of 50° to 55°F, to slow their aging. They should rest on their sides in a wine rack to keep their corks moist and swollen, thus preventing outside air from coming into contact with the wine.

Serving Wine Red wines are best appreciated at cool room temperature, within the range of 55° to 65°F. More robust reds may be served at the warmer end of that range, and the lightest reds should be poured slightly cooler. The ideal serving temperature for white wines ranges from 40° to 50°F, with sparkling wines at the colder end of that range and big, full-bodied white wines at the warmer. Wines may be chilled in the refrigerator for up to 2 hours before serving time, or for about 20 minutes in an ice bucket filled with equal parts cold water and ice cubes. When using an ice bucket, fold a clean kitchen towel or napkin around the neck of the bottle to help catch drips when the bottle is removed for pouring.

Several styles of corkscrews are available; for details, see CORKSCREW. To open Champagne or sparkling wine, place a folded towel or napkin over the cork. With one hand, hold the bottle steady and pointing away from you and other people while you use your other hand to untwist and remove the wire cage that holds the cork in place. Then, grip the cork and gently twist the bottle to loosen the cork, letting the pressure within the bottle slowly force it out while you keep the cork in your grasp. Never cavalierly shoot the cork out of the bottle, which can lead to possible injury as well as loss of wine.

Loosening the cage.

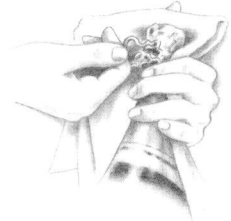

Twisting the bottle.

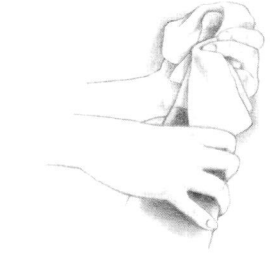

When pouring wine, fill glasses to only about two-thirds of their capacity, allowing

Quick Bite

Opening a bottle of wine ahead of time to allow it to "breathe" is not generally necessary. While exposure to air does change and bring out the flavors of wine, wine is well aerated as it is poured into a glass. A very young or tannic wine may be decanted and allowed to breathe and mellow for up to several hours before serving. This step is not recommended for older wines, as their bouquet fades rather quickly after pouring.

room at the top of the bowl for the wine's bouquet to develop upon exposure to air and for its aroma to be fully appreciated by those who drink it.

WINEGLASSES You will find wineglasses within a wide price range and in many different colors, patterns, sizes, and shapes. To best appreciate good wine, look for clear, unadorned glasses that do not interfere with the view of the wine's color and clarity. The rim of a wineglass should be narrower than the widest point of the bowl, to capture and hold the wine's bouquet. Generally, the bowls of glasses for red wine are more spherical, allowing more room for their bigger bouquets to develop. The bowls of white wineglasses, while still rounded, tend to be taller and narrower. All-purpose glasses for everyday use are also available. Champagne and sparkling wine are best appreciated in tall, slender glasses called flutes, which help to conserve their signature effervescence.

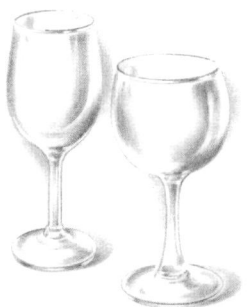

White and red wineglasses.

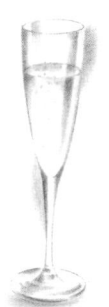

Champagne flute.

Wine connoisseurs always hold their wineglasses by the stem, not by the bowl, for two reasons. One is that touching the bowl with your fingers will subtly heat the wine, altering its flavor. While this might be a fine point for most wine drinkers, we can all appreciate the second concern: touching the bowl of the wineglass will leave unsightly fingerprints.

Matching Wine with Food "Red with meat, white with poultry and seafood"; so goes the old saw about matching wine and food. There is some wisdom in that advice, based on the logical assumption that a hearty red wine will better complement a hearty roast beef, while a more delicate white is a more sensible choice for, say, a delicate fish fillet. But pairing wine and food can become, depending on how you choose to look at it, far more complicated or even simpler.

Complexity is a factor when you consider the effects of sauces and seasonings not only on a given dish but also on the taste of the particular wine you pair with it. For instance, grilled fish with an aromatic rub of Indian spices might go very well with a light, fruity red Pinot Noir. Or the wine itself might dictate a departure from the rule, as when a particular white Chardonnay is big, buttery, and oaky enough to stand up to a chop.

While such examples illustrate how many fine considerations are possible in food and wine pairing, with a slight shift of perspective the same examples may also be seen as making a far more reassuring point. That is, if you enjoy drinking any particular type of wine, there is no good reason why you shouldn't feel free to try it as a companion to any food that you think it might complement.

Cooking with Wine While you would not want to pour a rare, expensive vintage wine into your stockpot, you should cook

continued

Wine, continued

with a wine that you'd actually want to drink. Avoid any products labeled "cooking wine," which tend to be needlessly seasoned, inferior products. Wines can add flavor to soups, such as a classic sherry-laced consommé; sauces, such as beurre blanc or a quick pan sauce made by deglazing with white wine; braises and stews, including such traditional French dishes as beef bourguignonne and coq au vin; and even desserts, such as pears poached in red wine.

Quick Bite

When cooking with wine, for the best pairing of wine and food at table, pour a wine made with the same grape variety to accompany the dish. Or, cook with the same wine you're serving.

Fortified Wines Some special types of wine are preserved through fortification, by the addition of brandy or a neutral spirit to raise the wine's total level of alcohol from the usual 7 to 14 percent to a range of 17 to 21 percent. Three of the most popular forms of fortified wine are Madeira, Port, and sherry.

MADEIRA From the Portuguese island of the same name, Madeira ranges in flavor from nutty and dry aperitifs to sweet after-dinner varieties.

PORT A classic, rich-tasting, and sweet fortified wine of Portugal, Port is excellent after dinner with nuts and cheeses. It comes in several styles, ranging from sweet, red ruby Port to drier tawny Port to complex, red vintage Port.

Port glass.

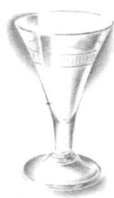

SHERRY A specialty of the Jerez region of Spain, sherry is now also made elsewhere. In its driest form, it may be served as an aperitif or with well-seasoned appetizers, while sweet sherries go well with mild to sharp cheeses after dinner. Fino sherries are characteristically very dry and tangy and drunk younger than oloroso sherries, which are aged to create a lovely brown color and rich, nutty bouquet.

Sherry glass.

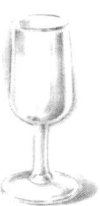

VERMOUTH This fortified white wine is flavored with various spices, herbs, and fruits. Dry vermouth, which contains just 2 to 4 percent sugar, can be served as an aperitif and is an essential ingredient in many cocktails, starting with the martini. Sweet vermouth, sometimes called Italian or red vermouth, has a minimum of 14 percent sugar, and is used for sweet cocktails such as Manhattans or is enjoyed alone over ice.

Quick Tip

Keep a bottle of dry vermouth on hand to use in recipes that call for white wine. Because it is fortified, once opened, it will last indefinitely stored in a cool cupboard. Use a little vermouth and stock to deglaze a pan that was used to sauté chicken or meat, thereby making a simple sauce.

See also ALCOHOL; CORKSCREW; DECANTING; DEGLAZING; LIQUEUR; REDUCING; SPIRITS.

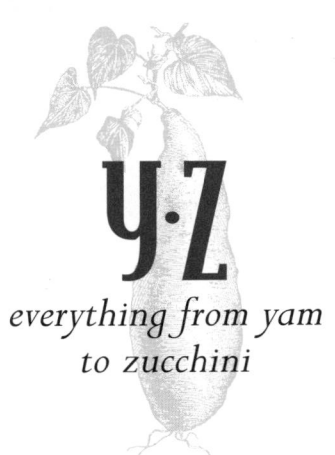

y·z

everything from yam to zucchini

YAM In the United States, orange-fleshed sweet potatoes are often referred to as yams. The true yam is a different species of plant, however, and is not widely available in this country.

Throughout Latin America, much of Asia, India, West Africa, the South Pacific, and the Caribbean, yams are one of the most important crops, with an annual production topping 25 million tons. There are over 600 varieties, which range in size from a few ounces to several hundred pounds. They may be brown, black, or tan, with white, pink, or yellow flesh. Shapes vary, too. Some yams resemble a giant animal foot or a misshapen hand, while others look like large potatoes. They have a slightly nutty flavor, with a texture that ranges from firm and chewy to moist and tender. Yams—boiled, stewed, fried, or baked—are often served as a foil to spicy sauces and to rich foods such as pork and ham. Grated and steamed yams are sometimes used to flavor breads and cakes.

Selecting Yams are available year-round in some Latin, Japanese, or African markets. Look for ones that are rock hard with no cracks or soft spots. Before you buy a yam, scrape it with your fingernail. It

should be slippery and juicy inside. If it's dry, leave it at the market. Yams and sweet potatoes are interchangeable in most recipes.

Storing Yams can be stored at room temperature for up to 1 week.

Preparing Yams can cause skin irritation, so it is a good idea to wear rubber gloves when handling them. Scrub yams well and use a paring knife to cut away the skin and underlayer. Cut the yams into chunks or slices as needed for specific recipes. Rinse and keep in a bowl of acidulated water (to prevent oxidation) until ready for use.

See also SWEET POTATO.

YEAST Yeast has been called the soul of bread, for it is the living substance that animates dough, eating its sugars and giving off carbon dioxide and ethyl alcohol to expand the gluten in the flour and raise the bread. Although many different strains of yeast exist, there are two main categories: brewer's yeast, also called nutritional yeast, and baker's yeast. Both are living single-cell organisms, but only baker's yeast is a leavener. Brewer's yeast is grown on hops and is used to make beer. Because it is high in B vitamins, it is also sold in natural-food stores as a nutritional supplement.

Baker's Yeast Baker's yeast is available as active dry and as compressed fresh yeast.

ACTIVE DRY YEAST Active dry yeast may be purchased in 4-ounce jars, in bulk in natural-food stores, or in small (¼-ounce) foil-lined envelopes. One envelope of dry yeast equals about 2¼ teaspoons. Check the expiration date on the package, then proof it if desired (see page 474). Store yeast in the freezer to prolong its shelf life.

Active dry yeast may be either regular or quick-rise, also known as rapid-rise yeast. This accelerated yeast will cut the rising time of a bread in half, but most bakers find that a shorter rising time makes for less flavor in the finished loaf. Quick-rise yeast does not need to be dissolved separately. It may be combined with the other dry ingredients, to which a warm liquid is added, thus activating the yeast.

A third kind of active dry yeast, instant dried yeast, is three times more powerful than regular dry yeast. Also called European yeast, it is a stronger, more stable yeast developed for commercial bakers. Some bakers feel that it has an objectionable taste, and it should not be used in sweet bread doughs or those that require long, slow risings.

COMPRESSED FRESH YEAST Compressed fresh yeast comes in small (0.06-ounce) foil-wrapped packages and is found in the refrigerated section of some markets. Since it has largely been replaced by active dry yeast, compressed yeast can be difficult to locate. It can be ordered in larger blocks from commercial bakers if you plan to do a lot of baking. Compressed yeast is much more perishable than dry yeast, however, and will keep under refrigeration for only about 10 days. Use it by the expiration date on the package. It may be frozen for up to 2 months and should be defrosted at room temperature and used at once. Proofing is recommended for fresh yeast; see A Word on Proofing, below. One cake of compressed yeast is equivalent to one package of active dry yeast.

A Word on Proofing Proofing yeast means to test the yeast to make sure it is still active, or alive. It is not really necessary for today's active dry yeast, but many bakers feel it doesn't hurt to check. It's a good idea to proof fresh yeast, as it is more perishable. Since all yeasts except quick-rise and instant dried are first dissolved in water before being mixed with dry ingredients, the dissolving process is essentially the same as proofing. Simply check to make sure that the mixture is bubbly or creamy after it sits for 5 to 10 minutes.

HOW TO *Proof Yeast*

1. Dissolve active dry yeast in a small bowl of warm (105° to 115°F) water (or another liquid, if called for in the recipe). Fresh yeast cake should be crumbled into lukewarm (90° to 100°F) liquid. If the water is too hot, it will kill the yeast; if the water is too cold, the yeast will not be activated.
2. If desired, add a pinch of sugar or another sweetener, such as honey, for the yeast to feed on (this is not necessary). Flour works well, too. Do not add salt; it inhibits the yeast.
3. Let the mixture stand for 5 to 10 minutes. If it becomes creamy, active dry yeast is indeed active and can be used for baking. Fresh yeast should bubble and foam. If it does, continue immediately with the recipe. If not, discard the yeast and purchase new yeast.

Yeast starters and sourdough starters are also used to leaven bread; they may be made at home or purchased. Yeast starter is a mixture of flour, water, sugar, and yeast that has been allowed to ferment. A portion of the starter is used as the leavener for yeast bread, and the remaining starter is kept alive indefinitely by replenishing it with equal parts flour and water. Sourdough starters are made without any (or with a very small amount of) baker's yeast. Instead, a mixture of flour and water, and sometimes a crushed vegetable or fruit, is allowed to sit at room temperature, where it will capture the wild yeasts always present in the atmosphere. Flour also contains some wild yeasts. A kitchen where yeast bread has been made from baker's yeast in the past is more likely to have an abundance of wild yeasts present in the air.

See also BAKING; BREAD.

YEAST BREAD See BREAD.

YOGURT Made from milk fermented with friendly bacterial cultures, yogurt is thick and tart with a custardlike texture. Like the milk it is made from, yogurt can be full fat, low fat, or nonfat. Available plain or sweetened and flavored, yogurt is made from cow's, goat's, or sheep's milk. Enjoy yogurt straight from the container, use it as a salad dressing or a topping for both savory and sweet dishes, or let it lend both body and flavor to sauces and soups.

The bacterial cultures in yogurt (*Lactobacillus bulgaricus* and *Streptococcus thermophilus;* a third kind, *Lactobacillus acidophilus,* is also sometimes added) are prized as an aid in digestion. They also give yogurt tenderizing properties that make it useful as a marinade for meats. Bakers like yogurt for the tender crumb it produces in quick breads and cakes. Frozen yogurt is refreshing, although freezing makes the friendly bacteria inactive. Likewise, heating yogurt over 120°F will kill the bacteria.

Yogurt may be drained in cheesecloth for several hours or overnight to make a thick substance known as yogurt cheese, which is used to make dips, desserts, and spreads for canapés and sandwiches. When making yogurt cheese and homemade yogurt, be sure to use a natural yogurt, made without gelatin or other stabilizers.

Selecting Check the sell-by date and make sure the yogurt you buy is fresh.

Storing Store in the refrigerator. Yogurt grows tarter with age, so enjoy it soon after purchase.

Yogurt Savvy When cooking with yogurt, keep the following in mind:

- Bring yogurt to room temperature before heating. When adding yogurt to hot food, make sure to do so toward the end of the cooking process, or it can curdle. For longer cooking, the yogurt should be stabilized (see below).
- To substitute yogurt for milk, cream, sour cream, or buttermilk in baking, add ½ teaspoon baking soda per cup of yogurt.

- For a lower-fat soft whipped cream, use half the amount of heavy cream. Beat it until stiff peaks form, then blend in an equal amount of plain nonfat yogurt.

HOW TO *Stabilize Yogurt for Cooking*

1. Stir 1 tablespoon all-purpose flour into 1 cup plain yogurt until blended. Use to replace cream in soups, casseroles, and sauces.

HOW TO *Make Yogurt at Home*

1. In a large, heavy saucepan, bring 1 quart whole, low-fat, or nonfat milk just to a boil, stirring to prevent a skin from forming. If a skin does form, skim it off with a spoon.
2. Remove from the heat and let cool to 112° to 115°F, or until a few drops sprinkled on your inner wrist are almost body temperature.
3. If using low-fat or nonfat milk, or for a high-protein yogurt made with whole milk, put ⅓ cup instant nonfat dried milk in a clean ceramic or glass bowl. Gradually whisk in about ½ cup of the warm milk until the mixture is smooth. Whisk in 2 tablespoons plain yogurt (made without gelatin or stabilizers) until well blended. Slowly whisk in the remaining warm milk until blended.
4. Cover tightly with plastic wrap. Set in a warm place (90° to 115°F) and let stand, without moving or otherwise disturbing the bowl, until thickened, 6 to 8 hours or overnight. (An oven with a gas pilot light is a good choice; if you have an electric oven, preheat it to 120°F, then turn it off. Or wrap the bowl in a heavy bath towel and place it on top of the refrigerator.) The longer the yogurt stands, the tarter and thicker the end product will be.
5. Use the yogurt at once, or refrigerate it. For the best flavor, use within 4 days.

ZESTING Citrus zest, the colored portion of the peel, is rich in flavorful oils that can perk up all sorts of foods. When used to flavor baked goods or salads, zest is

Y·Z

usually grated or minced. Large strips of zest should be removed from braises, stews, and sauces before serving.

When zesting fruit, be sure to scrub the fruit well to remove any wax or chemicals. Even better, buy organic citrus fruit if you need the peel. Use only the thin, colored layer of the rind, taking care not to include the bitter white pith. Zest may be removed with a tool known as a zester, which is designed to be pulled across the fruit's rind, removing the zest in thin strips. This is the best method for making attractive zest strips to use as a garnish or decoration.

y·z

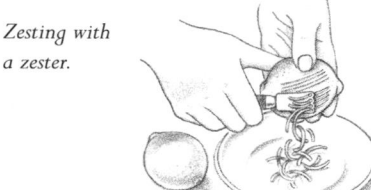

Zesting with a zester.

A vegetable peeler or a paring knife is a useful tool for removing zest in long strips, but these pieces may be larger and more irregular than needed, needing to be trimmed with a chef's knife. Zest strips may be chopped or minced, or zest may be removed with the fine rasps of a handheld grater, a technique that produces tiny bits of zest and eliminates any need for chopping it.

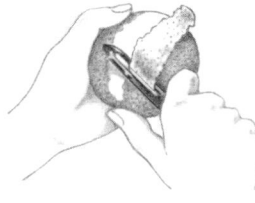

Zesting with a peeler.

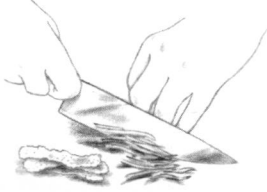

Slicing zest strips.

ZUCCHINI Nearly every backyard vegetable gardener has experienced a bumper crop of zucchini. Fortunately, this best-known member of the summer squash family is highly versatile. It can be cut into sticks and eaten raw; sliced and sautéed or fried; shredded or cooked and puréed in soups; cut into lengthwise slices, oiled, and grilled; and hollowed out, stuffed, and baked. It is a classic ingredient in ratatouille and other Provençal vegetable dishes, as well as in Middle Eastern stews. Shredded zucchini is also an ingredient in delicious quick breads and muffins.

Immature zucchini measuring no more than 3 to 5 inches long sometimes turn up at the market with their brilliant yellow flowers still attached. Marketed as baby zucchini, these tender, tiny squashes are favored for their delicate flavor and the fine texture of their flesh. The flowers are also edible and can be stuffed, battered, and fried or used as a filling for omelets.

Selecting Zucchini are available year-round, thanks to imports from Mexico. Local zucchini are at their best and most abundant in summer. Look for small zucchini for the most tender bite. The best have thin skins with a bright, even color and no blemishes or scars.

Storing Zucchini are at their best just after harvest. Serve them soon after you buy them, or store them for up to 3 days in a perforated plastic bag in the crisper of your refrigerator.

Preparing There's no need to peel zucchini; simply wash, trim the ends, and then slice, chop, or shred as desired. Some recipes call for salting zucchini to remove excess moisture.

See also SQUASH.

for further Reading

GENERAL FOOD REFERENCE

Chalmers, Irena. *The Great Food Almanac: A Feast of Facts from A to Z.* San Francisco: Collins Publishers, 1994.

Clingerman, Polly. *The Kitchen Companion.* Gaithersburg, Md.: The American Cooking Guild, 1994.

Davidson, Alan. *The Oxford Companion to Food.* New York: Oxford University Press, 1999.

Fortin, François, ed. *The Visual Food Encyclopedia.* New York: Macmillan, 1996.

Herbst, Sharon Tyler. *The Food Lover's Tiptionary.* New York: Hearst Books, 1994.

———. *The New Food Lover's Companion.* 2nd ed. Hauppauge, N.Y.: Barron's Educational Series, 1995.

Herbst, Sharon Tyler, and Ron Herbst. *Wine Lover's Companion.* Hauppauge, N.Y.: Barron's Educational Series, 1995.

Horn, Jane, ed. *Cooking A to Z: The Complete Culinary Reference Source.* New and rev. ed. Santa Rosa, Ca.: Cole Group, 1997.

Kamman, Madeleine. *The New Making of a Cook: The Art, Techniques, and Science of Good Cooking.* New York: William Morrow & Co., 1997.

Lang, Jenifer Harvey, ed. *Larousse Gastronomique: The New American Edition of the World's Greatest Culinary Encyclopedia.* New York: Crown Publishers, 1988.

Mariani, John F. *The Dictionary of American Food and Drink.* New York: Hearst Books, 1994.

Willan, Anne. *La Varenne Pratique: The Complete Illustrated Cooking Course.* New York: Crown Publishers, 1989.

FOOD HISTORY

Root, Waverly. *Food: An Authoritative and Visual History and Dictionary of the Foods of the World.* New York: Smithmark, 1980.

Sokolov, Raymond. *Why We Eat What We Eat: How the Encounter Between the New World and the Old Changed the Way Everyone on the Planet Eats.* New York: Summit Books, 1991.

Trager, James. *The Food Chronology: A Food Lover's Compendium of Events and Anecdotes, from Prehistory to the Present.* New York: Henry Holt & Co., 1995.

FOOD SAFETY

Bailey, Janet. *Keeping Food Fresh.* New York: Harper & Row, 1985.

Kilham, Christopher S. *The Bread & Circus Whole Food Bible: How to Select and Prepare Safe Healthful Foods without Pesticides or Chemical Additives.* Reading, Ma.: Addison-Wesley Publishing Co., 1991.

Mendelson, Cheryl. *Home Comforts: The Art and Science of Keeping House.* New York: Scribner, 1999.

FOOD SCIENCE

Corriher, Shirley O. *Cookwise: The Hows and Whys of Successful Cooking.* New York: William Morrow & Co., 1997.

Hillman, Howard. *Kitchen Science: A Guide to Knowing the Hows and Whys for Fun and Success in the Kitchen.* Rev. ed. Boston: Houghton Mifflin Co., 1989.

continued

McGee, Harold. *On Food and Cooking: The Science and Lore of the Kitchen.* New York: Scribner, 1984. Reprint, New York: Fireside, 1997.

COOKWARE AND TOOLS

Ettlinger, Steve. *The Kitchenware Book.* New York: Macmillan, 1992.

SPECIALTY

Alford, Jeffrey, and Naomi Duguid. *Seductions of Rice: A Cookbook.* New York: Artisan, 1998.

Bremness, Lesley, and Jill Norman. *The Complete Book of Herbs & Spices: The Ultimate Sourcebook to Herbs, Spices & Aromatic Seeds.* New York: Viking Studio Books, 1995.

Choate, Judith. *The Bean Cookbook.* New York: Simon & Schuster, 1992.

Clarke, Oz. *The Essential Wine Book: An Indispensable Guide to the World of Wines.* New York: Fireside, 1997.

Cost, Bruce. *Bruce Cost's Asian Ingredients: Buying and Cooking the Staple Foods of China, Japan, and Southeast Asia.* New York: William Morrow & Co., 1988.

Davidson, Alan. *Fruit: A Connoisseur's Guide and Cookbook.* New York: Simon & Schuster, 1991.

DeWitt, Dave, and Nancy Gerlach. *The Whole Chile Pepper Book.* Boston: Little, Brown & Co., 1990.

Ellis, Merle. *Cutting-up in the Kitchen: The Butcher's Guide to Saving Money on Meat & Poultry.* San Francisco: Chronicle Books, 1975.

Jenkins, Steven. *Cheese Primer.* New York: Workman Publishing Co., 1996.

Perry, Sara, et al. *The Complete Coffee Book: A Gourmet Guide to Buying, Brewing, and Cooking.* San Francisco: Chronicle Books, 1991.

Peterson, James. *Fish and Shellfish.* New York: William Morrow & Co., 1996.

Pratt, James Norwood. *The Tea Lover's Treasury.* San Francisco: 101 Productions, 1982.

Rosengarten, Frederic, Jr. *The Book of Spices.* Wynnewood, Pa.: Livingston Publishing Co., 1969.

Schneider, Elizabeth. *Uncommon Fruits & Vegetables: A Commonsense Guide.* New York: Harper & Row, 1986.

Wood, Rebecca. *The Splendid Grain.* New York: William Morrow & Co., 1997.

About the Contributors

ABOUT THE AUTHORS

MARY GOODBODY is a nationally known food writer and cookbook editor based in Connecticut. She has written or contributed to more than 45 books, including *The Basque Table; Sunday Dinner;* and *Spring Evenings, Summer Afternoons.* More recently, she collaborated on *Alfred Portale's 12 Seasons Cookbook, Prime Time: The Lobels' Guide to Great Grilled Meats,* and *No Need to Knead,* which was nominated for a 1999 James Beard Cookbook Award. Ms. Goodbody is also a senior contributing editor for *Chocolatier* and *Pastry Art & Design* magazines and is the editor for the *IACP (International Association of Culinary Professionals) Food Forum Quarterly.*

CAROLYN MILLER is a writer and book editor living in San Francisco. She is the author of *Savoring San Francisco: Recipes from the City's Neighborhood Restaurants* and *The Christmas Table: A Holiday Menu Cookbook.* Her writing has also been featured in many cookbooks, including *Chocolate: A Sweet Indulgence* and *Espresso: Culture and Cuisine.* In addition, she has edited innumerable other cookbooks for publishers nationwide.

THY TRAN is a San Francisco–based food and travel writer who specializes in the history and culture of cooking. A graduate of the California Culinary Academy, she has honed her craft working at numerous restaurants, catering, and testing recipes and writing for national food magazines. Ms. Tran is the owner of Wandering Spoon, a cooking school in San Francisco, where she teaches classes on traditional Asian ingredients and techniques.

ABOUT THE ILLUSTRATOR

ALICE HARTH, a San Francisco–based artist and graphic designer whose clients have included magazines, book publishers, and food producers, illustrated the multi-volume Williams-Sonoma *Kitchen Library* and *Lifestyles* series. Ms. Harth studied fine art and design at the University of California at Los Angeles. In addition to good food, travel, drawing, and painting are her passions.

We invite suggestions for future editions. Please send comments to kitchencompanion@weldonowen.com, or write to Kitchen Companion, Weldon Owen Inc., 814 Montgomery Street, San Francisco, CA 94133.

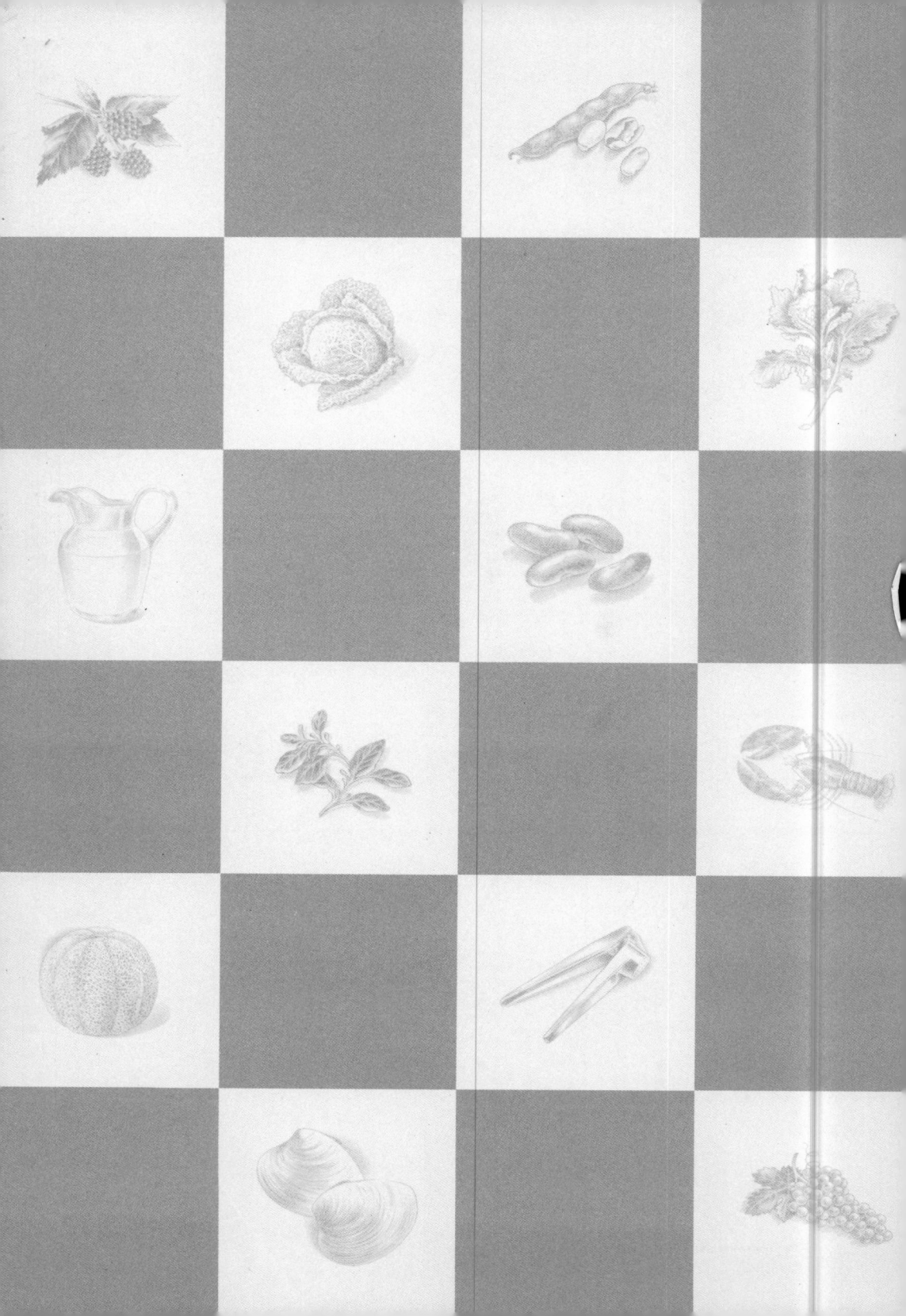